S0-CFU-756

FIRST EDITION

# PDR®
# Concise Drug Guide for Advanced Practice Clinicians

PAULA CHEVRIER, APRN

# PDR® Concise Drug Guide for Advanced Practice Clinicians

FIRST EDITION
*Senior Director, Editorial & Publishing:* Bette LaGow
*Manager, Professional Services:* Michael Deluca, PharmD, MBA
*Drug Information Specialists:* Anila Patel, PharmD; Nermin Shenouda, PharmD; Greg Tallis, RPh
*Contributing Editor:* Cathy Kim, PharmD
*Project Editors:* Kathleen Engel, Lori Murray
*Associate Editors:* Sabina Borza, Elise Philippi
*Senior Director, Client Sevices:* Stephanie Struble
*Project Manager:* Christina Klinger
*Manager, Production Purchasing:* Thomas Westburgh
*Manager, Art Department:* Livio Udina
*Electronic Publishing Designers:* Deana DiVizio, Carrie Faeth, Jaime Pinedo
*Production Associate:* Joan K. Akerlind
*Traffic Assistant:* Kim Condon

---

*Senior Director, Copy Sales:* Bill Gaffney
*Senior Product Manager:* Richard Buchwald

THOMSON PDR
*Executive Vice President, PDR:* Kevin D. Sanborn
*Vice President, Client Services & Publishing:* Christopher Young
*Vice President, Clinical Relations:* Mukesh Mehta, RPh
*Vice President, Operations:* Brian Holland
*Vice President, Strategic Marketing:* Valerie E. Berger
*Vice President, Pharmaceutical Sales:* Anthony Sorce



**Officers of Thomson Healthcare Inc.:** *President and Chief Executive Officer:* Robert Cullen; *Chief Medical Officer:* Alan Ying, MD; *Senior Vice President and Chief Technology Officer:* Frank Licata; *Chief Strategy Officer:* Courtney Morris; *Executive Vice President, Payer Decision Support:* Jon Newpol; *Executive Vice President, Provider Markets:* Terry Cameron; *Executive Vice President, Marketing and Innovation:* Doug Schneider; *Senior Vice President, Finance:* Phil Buckingham; *Vice President, Human Resources:* Pamela M. Bilash; *General Counsel:* Darren Pocsik

ISBN: 1-56363-677-8 Printed in Canada

# Contents

# Foreword

Advanced practice clinicians are assuming increased responsibility for clinical care, with many now having prescribing authority and practicing independently of their supervising physicians. With this increased autonomy of practice comes an increased need for accurate, easy-to-access information on evaluation and management of common problems. A trusted textbook has been the traditional source of such decision-support information–be it in print or online (such as the one I author and edit)–but equally important on a daily basis is accurate prescribing information. *Physicians' Desk Reference®* has been a standard resource of drug prescribing information for physicians for decades. This *PDR® Concise Drug Guide for Advanced Practice Clinicians* provides a subset of information from *PDR* organized and edited specifically for advanced practice clinicians working in busy practice settings.

The guide features terse all-you-need-to-know summaries of commonly used drugs prescribed in the ambulatory setting for treatment of problems likely to be encountered by advanced practice clinicians. Each drug entry contains must-have information: drug class, dosage, how supplied, warnings/precautions, adverse reactions, and use in pregnancy. Supplementing these entries are useful tables on such topics as drug management of common conditions, over-the-counter preparations, and recommendations for immunization.

The busy clinician will find this guide a trusted, constant companion, with its FDA-approved prescribing information. Generations of physicians have found *PDR* an essential tool in their daily practice, and this new guide should find an equally special place in the office of advanced practice clinicians.

**Allan H. Goroll, MD**
Professor of Medicine
Harvard Medical School
Editor, *Primary Care Medicine*, 6th edition

# How to Use This Book

The *PDR® Concise Drug Guide for Advanced Practice Clinicians* allows you to quickly locate important drug information so you can care for patients with confidence. With over 1,800 monographs providing current, organized information, this handy reference is the perfect companion for the busy medical professional or student.

This compact guide is divided into four discrete sections. The first section consists of concise drug monographs based on FDA-approved prescribing information. These monographs are organized alphabetically by brand name. When a brand is no longer available, the generic name is used. Monographs consist of:

- Brand name
- Generic name
- Manufacturer
- FDA/DEA schedule
- Black Box Warnings
- Therapeutic Class
- Indications
- Dosage (adults, pediatrics, special populations)
- How Supplied (dosage form/strength)
- Contraindications
- Warnings/Precautions
- Interactions
- Adverse Reactions
- Pregnancy category/Nursing considerations

The second section is comprised of an extensive collection of tables and key references to help clinicians with decisions about prescribing medications and drug therapy. Tables provided include drug information centers, poison control centers, immunization schedules, drug comparisons (both Rx and OTC), and much more. Within the drug comparison tables, drugs are organized alphabetically and by class for effortless access. These tables and references may include, but are not limited to:

- Brand/generic name
- How Supplied (dosage form/strength)
- Indications
- Initial and Max dosages
- Usual dosage range

The third section contains indices—all of the drugs are indexed by brand and generic name, as well as pharmacologic category, for quick location and investigation.

The final section of the *PDR® Concise Drug Guide for Advanced Practice Clinicians* contains a Visual Identification Guide featuring hundreds of product images, listed by brand name. This section helps you quickly verify the identity of a capsule, tablet, or other solid oral medication. Each product image contains both the generic and brand name, strength, and the name of its supplier. Other strengths and dosage forms may be available; please check FDA-approved prescribing information for a complete listing of all strengths and dosage forms.

**Important Information About Product Labeling**

Entries in the *PDR® Concise Drug Guide for Advanced Practice Clinicians* are drawn from FDA-approved product labeling as published in *Physicians' Desk Reference®* or supplied by the manufacturer. The entries are compiled and updated on a regular basis by a staff of experienced pharmacists. While diligent efforts have been made to ensure the accuracy of each entry, it is essential to bear in mind that the information presented here is merely a synopsis of key points in the official labeling, and that the complete labeling contains additional precautionary information that may be of significance in specific cases. Similarly, please remember that only common and dangerous adverse reactions and interactions are included here, and that numerous less-prevalent adverse effects may be reported in the complete labeling. If an entry leaves any question unanswered, be sure to consult *Physicians' Desk Reference* or the manufacturer for additional information.

The function of the publisher is the compilation, organization, and distribution of this information. In organizing and presenting the material in the *PDR Concise Drug Guide for Advanced Practice Clinicians*, the publisher does not warrant or guarantee any of the products described, or perform any independent analysis in connection with any of the product information contained herein.

The *PDR® Concise Drug Guide for Advanced Practice Clinicians* assumes no obligation to obtain and include any information in these entries other than that provided by the manufacturer. The publisher does not warrant, guarantee, or advocate the use of any product described herein. The publisher and editors do not assume, and expressly disclaim, any liability for error, omissions, or typographical errors in the information contained herein or for misuse of any of the products listed.

# DRUG MONOGRAPH KEY

**BRAND NAME** FDA/DEA Class*

Combined Generic (Manufacturer)

**Black Box Warning: A brief description of the black box warning(s) that appear in the beginning of the official FDA-approved labeling for the monograph.**

**OTHER BRAND NAMES:** Brand name drugs that have the same generic components as the monograph drug.

**THERAPEUTIC CLASS:** Based on the active ingredients and their mechanism of action.

**INDICATIONS:** Only includes FDA-approved indications.

**DOSAGE:** Dosages for adults and pediatrics as indicated in the official FDA-approved labeling.

**HOW SUPPLIED:** Product description including strength, formulation, [package size], and scored tablet information.

**CONTRAINDICATIONS:** Details harmful conditions related to the use of the drug and disease states or patient populations where the use of the monograph drug should be avoided.

**WARNINGS/PRECAUTIONS:** Details harmful conditions related to the use of the drug and disease states or patient populations where caution is dictated.

**ADVERSE REACTIONS:** Denotes side effects and adverse reactions listed in the official FDA-approved labeling as occurring with greater frequency (generally at a rate of ≥3%) or deemed significant based on the clinical judgment of the editors. Other side effects may be included if deemed serious or life-threatening. For complete prescribing information please refer to the official FDA-approved labeling.

**INTERACTIONS:** Includes the effects and implications of other drugs and food on the monograph drug based on official FDA-approved labeling.

**PREGNANCY:** Indicated pregnancy and nursing considerations and, when available, the FDA pregnancy rating system category.†

### *FDA/DEA CLASS

**OTC:** Available over-the-counter.
**RX:** Requires a prescription.
**CII:** Controlled substance; high potential for abuse.
**CIII:** Controlled substance; some potential for abuse.
**CIV:** Controlled substance; low potential for abuse.
**CV:** Controlled substance; subject to state and local regulation.

### †FDA USE-IN-PREGNANCY RATINGS

The FDA use-in-pregnancy rating system weighs the degree to which available information has ruled out risk to the fetus against the drug's potential benefit to the patient. The ratings, and the interpretation, are as follows:

| CATEGORY | INTERPRETATION |
|---|---|
| A | **CONTROLLED STUDIES SHOW NO RISK.** Adequate, well-controlled studies in pregnant women have failed to demonstrate a risk to the fetus in any trimester of pregnancy. |
| B | **NO EVIDENCE OF RISK IN HUMANS.** Adequate, well-controlled studies in pregnant women have not shown increased risk of fetal abnormalities despite adverse findings in animals, or, in the absence of fetal risk. The chance of fetal harm is remote, but remains a possibility. |
| C | **RISK CANNOT BE RULED OUT.** Adequate, well-controlled human studies are lacking, and animal studies have shown a risk to the fetus or are lacking as well. There is a chance of fetal harm if the drug is administered during pregnancy; but the potential benefits may outweigh the potential risk. |
| D | **POSITIVE EVIDENCE OF RISK.** Studies in humans, or investigational or post-marketing data, have demonstrated fetal risk. Nevertheless, potential benefits from the use of the drug may outweigh the potential risk. For example, the drug may be acceptable if needed in a life-threatening situation or serious disease for which safer drugs cannot be use or are ineffective. |
| X | **CONTRAINDICATED IN PREGNANCY.** Studies in animals or humans, or investigational or post-marketing reports, have demonstrated positive evidence of fetal abnormalities or risk which clearly outweighs any possible benefit to the patient. |

# Concise Drug Monographs

## 1-DAY

OTC

tioconazole (Personal Products Company)

**THERAPEUTIC CLASS:** Azole antifungal

**INDICATIONS:** Treatment of recurrent vaginal yeast infections.

**DOSAGE:** *Adults:* Insert contents of applicator intravaginally once hs. *Pediatrics:* >12 yrs: Insert contents of applicator intravaginally once hs.

**HOW SUPPLIED:** Oint: 6.5% [4.6g]

**WARNINGS/PRECAUTIONS:** Do not use if abdominal pain, fever (>100°F), chills, nausea, vomiting, diarrhea, or foul smelling discharge. Avoid tampons. Do not rely on condoms or diaphragm to prevent STDs or pregnancy until 3 days after last use.

**ADVERSE REACTIONS:** Vulvovaginal burning.

**PREGNANCY:** Safety in pregnancy and nursing not known.

## 8-MOP

RX

methoxsalen (Valeant)

**Risk of ocular damage, aging skin, and skin cancer. Do not interchange with Oxsoralen-Ultra® without re-titration.**

**THERAPEUTIC CLASS:** Psoralen

**INDICATIONS:** Photochemotherapy (methoxsalen with long wave UVA radiation) is for symptomatic control of severe, recalcitrant, disabling psoriasis (supported by a biopsy) unresponsive to other therapies and repigmentation of idiopathic vitiligo. Photopheresis (methoxsalen with long wave UVA radiation of WBC) for palliative treatment of skin manifestations of cutaneous T-cell lymphoma unresponsive to other therapies.

**DOSAGE:** *Adults:* Take with food or milk. Vitiligo: 20mg 2-4 hrs before UV exposure. Psoriasis: Initial: <30kg: 10mg. 30-50kg: 20mg. 51-65kg: 30mg. 66-80kg: 40mg. 81-90kg: 50mg. 91-115kg: 60mg. >115kg: 70mg. Take 2 hrs before UVA exposure. Titrate: May increase by 10mg after 15th treatment under certain conditions. Max: Do not treat more often than every other day.

**HOW SUPPLIED:** Cap: 10mg

**CONTRAINDICATIONS:** History of light sensitive diseases (eg, lupus erythematosus, porphyria cutanea tarda, erythropoietic protoporphyria, variegate porphyria, xeroderma pigmentosum, albinism), history/active melanoma, invasive squamous cell carcinoma, aphakia.

**WARNINGS/PRECAUTIONS:** May develop serious burns if exceed recommended dose or exposure. Increase risk of squamous cell carcinoma in fair skinned patients or with pre-PUVA exposure to prolonged tar/UVB treatment, ionizing radiation, or arsenic. Diligently observe and treat basal cell carcinomas. Patients should wear UVA-absorbing, wrap-around sunglasses for 24 hrs after methoxsalen ingestion to avoid cataractogenicity. Sunlight/UV radiation exposure may cause premature skin aging. Monitor for carcinomas with history of x-ray, genz ray, or arsenic therapy. Caution with hepatic impairment. Avoid vertical UVA chamber with cardiac disease. Ophthalmologic exam before therapy, then yearly. Obtain CBC, anti-nuclear antibody test, renal and LFTs before therapy, then 6-12 months after. Avoid sunbathing 24 hrs before or 48 hrs post treatment. Avoid sun exposure 8 hrs after ingestion. Protect eyes, abdominal skin, breasts, genitalia, and other sensitive areas during PUVA therapy.

**ADVERSE REACTIONS:** Nausea, nervousness, insomnia, depression, pruritus, erythema.

**INTERACTIONS:** Caution with photosensitizers such as anthralin, coal tar and its derivatives, griseofulvin, phenothiazines, nalidixic acid, halogenated salicylanilides, sulfonamides, tetracyclines, thiazides, and certain organic staining dyes (eg, methylene blue, toluidine blue, rose bengal, methyl orange).

**PREGNANCY:** Category C, caution in nursing.

## A/T/S RX
erythromycin (Taro)

**THERAPEUTIC CLASS:** Macrolide antibiotic

**INDICATIONS:** Acne vulgaris.

**DOSAGE:** *Adults:* (Gel) Clean and dry area. Apply qd-bid. Do not rub in. D/C if no improvement after 6-8 weeks. (Sol) Clean and dry area. Apply bid.

**HOW SUPPLIED:** Gel: 2% [30g]; Sol: 2% [60mL]

**WARNINGS/PRECAUTIONS:** Avoid eyes, nose, mouth, and other mucous membranes. D/C if overgrowth of antibiotic-resistant organisms occurs.

**ADVERSE REACTIONS:** Peeling, dryness, pruritus, erythema, oiliness, eye irritation, burning, desquamation.

**INTERACTIONS:** Caution with concomitant topical acne therapy, possible cumulative irritant effect.

**PREGNANCY:** (Gel) Category B, not for use in nursing; (Sol) Category C, caution in nursing.

## ABBOKINASE RX
urokinase (Abbott)

**THERAPEUTIC CLASS:** Thrombolytic agent

**INDICATIONS:** Lysis of acute massive pulmonary emboli (PE) and PE accompanied by unstable hemodynamics.

**DOSAGE:** *Adults:* LD: 4400 IU/kg IV at 90 mL/hr over 10 minutes. Maint: 4400 IU/kg/hr IV at 15mL/hr for 12 hrs. Flush line after each cycle.

**HOW SUPPLIED:** Inj: 250,000IU

**CONTRAINDICATIONS:** Active internal bleeding, intracranial neoplasm, arteriovenous malformation, aneurysm, bleeding diathesis, severe uncontrolled arterial HTN. Recent (within 2 months) CVA, intracranial or intraspinal surgery, trauma including resuscitation.

**WARNINGS/PRECAUTIONS:** Prior to use obtain Hct, platelet count, and aPTT. Increased risk of bleeding; fatalities due to hemorrhage, including intracranial and retroperitoneal, reported. Avoid IM injections, nonessential patient handling, frequent venipunctures. Use upper extremity vessels when performing arterial punctures. Increased risk of bleeding with recent (within 10 days) major surgery, obstetrical delivery, organ biopsy, previous puncture of noncompressible vessels, serious GI bleeding, high likelihood of left heart thrombus, subacute bacterial endocarditis, hemostatic defects including those secondary to severe hepatic or renal disease, pregnancy, cerebrovascular disease, diabetic hemorrhagic retinopathy, and any other condition in which bleeding may be a significant hazard or difficult to manage. May carry risk of transmitting infectious agents.

**ADVERSE REACTIONS:** Bleeding, fatal hemorrhage, anaphylaxis, allergic-type or infusion reactions.

**INTERACTIONS:** Increased risk of serious bleeding with other thrombolytic agents, anticoagulants, or agents inhibiting platelet function (eg, ASA, other NSAIDs, dipyridamole, GP IIb/IIIa inhibitors).

**PREGNANCY:** Category B, caution with nursing.

## ABBOKINASE OPEN-CATH RX
urokinase (Abbott)

**THERAPEUTIC CLASS:** Thrombolytic agent

**INDICATIONS:** Restoration of patency to IV catheters, obstructed by clotted blood or fibrin.

**DOSAGE:** *Adults:* Drug amount should equal the internal volume of the catheter, may repeat in resistant cases.

**HOW SUPPLIED:** Inj: 5000IU, 9000IU

**CONTRAINDICATIONS:** Active internal bleeding, history of CVA, recent (within 2 months) intracranial/intraspinal surgery or trauma including resuscitation, intracranial neoplasm, arteriovenous malformation, aneurysm, bleeding diathesis, severe uncontrolled arterial HTN.

**WARNINGS/PRECAUTIONS:** Manufactured from human source material; risk of infection transmission. Avoid excessive pressure during administration. Watch for drug precipitates in catheters. Do not use vigorous suction to determine catheter occlusion.

**ADVERSE REACTIONS:** Bleeding, fever, chills, bronchospasm, skin rash, nausea, vomiting, transient hypotension, HTN, dyspnea, tachycardia, cyanosis, back pain, hypoxemia, acidosis.

**PREGNANCY:** Category B, caution in nursing.

## ABELCET — RX

amphotericin B (lipid complex) (Enzon)

**THERAPEUTIC CLASS:** Polyene antifungal

**INDICATIONS:** Treatment of invasive fungal infections in patients refractory or intolerant to conventional amphotericin B therapy.

**DOSAGE:** *Adults:* 5mg/kg IV at 2.5mg/kg/h.
*Pediatrics:* 5mg/kg IV at 2.5mg/kg/h.

**HOW SUPPLIED:** Inj: 5mg/mL

**WARNINGS/PRECAUTIONS:** Anaphylaxis reported. D/C if respiratory distress occurs. Monitor SCr, LFTs, serum electrolytes, CBC during therapy.

**ADVERSE REACTIONS:** Chills, fever, increased SCr, multiple organ failure, nausea, hypotension, respiratory failure, vomiting, dyspnea, sepsis, diarrhea, headache, heart arrest, HTN, hypokalemia, infection, kidney failure, pain, thrombocytopenia.

**INTERACTIONS:** Antineoplastics may potentiate renal toxicity, bronchospasm, hypotension. Corticosteroids and corticotropin may potentiate hypokalemia predisposing patients to cardiac dysfunction. May potentiate digitalis toxicity. Increased risk of flucytosine toxicity. Acute pulmonary toxicity reported with leukocyte transfusions. Nephrotoxic drugs (eg, aminoglycosides, pentamidine) enhance potential for renal toxicity. Cyclosporine within several days of bone marrow ablation associated with nephrotoxicity. Hypokalemia effect may enhance curariform effect of skeletal muscle relaxants.

**PREGNANCY:** Category B, not for use in nursing.

## ABILIFY — RX

aripiprazole (Bristol-Myers Squibb/Otsuka America)

**Elderly patients with dementia-related psychosis treated with atypical antipsychotic drugs are at an increased risk of death; most appeared to be cardiovascular (eg, heart failure, sudden death) or infectious (eg, pneumonia) in nature. Aripiprazole is not approved for the treatment of patients with dementia-related psychosis.**

**OTHER BRAND NAMES:** Abilify Discmelt (Bristol-Myers Squibb/Otsuka America)

**THERAPEUTIC CLASS:** Partial $D_2/5HT_{1A}$ agonist/$5HT_{2A}$ antagonist

**INDICATIONS:** (PO) Treatment of schizophrenia. Treatment of acute manic and mixed episodes associated with bipolar disorder. (Inj) Treatment of agitation associated with schizophrenia or bipolar disorder, manic or mixed.

**DOSAGE:** *Adults:* (PO) Schizophrenia: Initial/Target: 10 to 15mg qd. Titrate: Should not increase before 2 weeks. Bipolar mania: Initial: 30mg qd. Titrate:

May decrease to 15mg qd based on assessment and tolerability. Oral solution can be given on a mg-per-mg basis up to 25mg. Patients receiving 30mg tablets should receive 25mg of the solution. (Inj) Agitation: 9.75 mg IM. Range: 5.25-15mg IM. Max: 30mg/day; Initiate PO therapy as soon as possible. Concomitant CYP3A4 Inhibitors (eg, ketoconazole): Reduce usual aripiprazole dose by 50%. Concomitant CYP2D6 Inhibitors (eg, quinidine, fluoxetine, paroxetine): Reduce usual aripiprazole dose by 50%. Concomitant CYP3A4 Inducers (eg, carbamazepine): Double aripiprazole dose (to 20mg or 30mg). Periodically reassess for maintenance therapy.

**HOW SUPPLIED:** ODT: (Discmelt) 10mg, 15mg; Tab: 2mg, 5mg, 10mg, 15mg, 20mg, 30mg; Sol: 1mg/mL [50mL, 150mL, 480mL]. Inj: 7.5mg/ml.

**WARNINGS/PRECAUTIONS:** May develop tardive dyskinesia, NMS. Monitor for hyperglycemia, worsening of glucose control with DM, FBG levels with diabetes risk. Increased incidence of cerebrovascular adverse events (stroke) in elderly dementia patients. Not approved for treatment of patients with dementia related psychosis. Orthostatic hypotension reported; caution with cardiovascular disease, conditions predisposed to hypotension (eg, dehydration, hypovolemia). May lower seizure threshold. Potential for cognitive and motor impairment. May disrupt body's temperature regulation. Possible esophageal dysmotility and aspiration; caution in patients at risk for aspiration pneumonia. Observe vigilance in treating psychosis associated with Alzheimer's.

**ADVERSE REACTIONS:** Headache, asthenia, rash, blurred vision, rhinitis, cough, tremor, anxiety, insomnia, nausea, vomiting, lightheadedness, somnolence, constipation, akathisia.

**INTERACTIONS:** May potentiate effect of antihypertensives. Caution with anticholinergic agents, other centrally acting drugs. Avoid alcohol. CYP3A4 inducers (eg, carbamazepine) may lower blood levels. CYP3A4 inhibitors (eg, ketoconazole, itraconazole) or 2D6 inhibitors (eg, quinidine, fluoxetine, paroxetine) can increase blood levels.

**PREGNANCY:** Category C, not for use in nursing.

## ABRAXANE RX

paclitaxel protein-bound particles (Abraxis Oncology)

**Do not administer to patients with metastatic breast cancer who have baseline neutrophil counts of less than 1,500 cells/mm³. Perform peripheral blood cell counts on all patients to monitor occurence of bone marrow suppression, primarily neutropenia. Should only be administered under the supervision of a physician experienced in the use of cancer chemotherapeutic agents. Do not substitute for or with other paclitaxel formulations.**

**THERAPEUTIC CLASS:** Antimicrotubule agent

**INDICATIONS:** Treatment of breast cancer after failure of combination chemotherapy for metastatic disease or relapse within 6 months of adjuvant chemotherapy. Prior therapy should have included an anthracyline unless clinically contraindicated.

**DOSAGE:** *Adults:* 260mg/m² IV over 30 minutes every 3 weeks. Severe neutropenia (neutrophil <500 cells/mm³ for a week or longer) or severe sensory neuropathy (Grade 3 or 4): Hold dose to neutrophil >1500 cells/mm³ or sensory neuropathy resolves to Grade 1 or 2. Reduce subsequent courses to 220mg/m², if recurrence reduce subsequent courses to 180mg/m².

**HOW SUPPLIED:** Inj: 100mg

**CONTRAINDICATIONS:** Patients with baseline neutrophil counts of < 1,500 cells/mm³.

**WARNINGS/PRECAUTIONS:** Perform frequent blood counts to monitor for bone marrow suppresion. Men should be advised to not father a child while receiving treatment. Remote risk for transmission of viral diseases; theoretical risk for transmission of Creutzfeldt-Jacob disease. Sensory neuropathy occurs frequently. Reports of injection site reactions.

**ADVERSE REACTIONS:** Neutropenia, infectious episodes, anemia, hypotension, ECG abnormalities, dyspnea, cough, sensory neuropathy, ocular/visual disturbances, arthralgia, myalgia, nausea, vomiting, asthenia, abnormal liver function test.

**PREGNANCY:** Category D, not for use in nursing.

## ABREVA OTC
docosanol (GlaxoSmithKline Consumer)

**THERAPEUTIC CLASS:** Antiviral

**INDICATIONS:** To treat cold sore/fever blisters on the face or lips.

**DOSAGE:** *Adults:* Apply to affected area on face or lips at 1st sign of cold sore/fever blister (tingle). Use 5x/day until healed.
*Pediatrics:* >12 yrs: Apply to affected area on face or lips at 1st sign of cold sore/fever blister (tingle). Use 5x/day until healed.

**HOW SUPPLIED:** Cre: 10% [2g]

**WARNINGS/PRECAUTIONS:** Avoid in or near eyes, and inside mouth. Discontinue if sore worsens or does not heal in 10 days.

**PREGNANCY:** Safety in pregnancy and nursing is not know.

## ACCOLATE RX
zafirlukast (AstraZeneca LP)

**THERAPEUTIC CLASS:** Leukotriene receptor antagonist

**INDICATIONS:** Prophylaxis and chronic treatment of asthma.

**DOSAGE:** *Adults:* 20mg bid. Administer 1 hr ac or 2 hrs pc.
*Pediatrics:* >12 yrs: 20mg bid. 5-11 yrs: 10mg bid. Administer 1 hr ac or 2 hrs pc.

**HOW SUPPLIED:** Tab: 10mg, 20mg

**WARNINGS/PRECAUTIONS:** Not for treatment of acute asthma attacks. Bioavailability decreases with food. Hepatic dysfunction and systemic eosinophilia reported.

**ADVERSE REACTIONS:** Headache, infection, nausea, diarrhea, hypersensitivity reactions including angioedema.

**INTERACTIONS:** Potentiates warfarin. Caution with drugs metabolized by CYP2C9 (eg, tolbutamide, phenytoin, carbamazepine) or CYP3A4 (eg, dihydropyridine calcium-channel blockers, cyclosporine, cisapride, astemizole). Increased levels with ASA. Decreased levels by erythromycin, theophylline. May increase theophylline levels.

**PREGNANCY:** Category B, not for use in nursing.

## ACCUNEB RX
albuterol sulfate (Dey)

**THERAPEUTIC CLASS:** $Beta_2$ agonist

**INDICATIONS:** Relief of bronchospasm with asthma.

**DOSAGE:** *Pediatrics:* 2-12 yrs: Initial: 0.63mg or 1.25mg tid-qid via nebulizer. 6-12 yrs with severe asthma, >40kg or 11-12 yrs: Initial: 1.25mg tid-qid.

**HOW SUPPLIED:** Sol: 1.25mg/3mL, 0.63mg/3mL [3mL, $25^s$]

**WARNINGS/PRECAUTIONS:** Hypersensitivity reactions reported. Fatalities reported with excessive use. Caution with cardiovascular disorders, especially coronary insufficiency, arrhythmias and HTN. May need concomitant anti-inflammatory agents. Can produce paradoxical bronchospasm. Caution with DM. May cause hypokalemia.

**ADVERSE REACTIONS:** Asthma exacerbation, otitis media, allergic reaction, gastroenteritis, cold symptoms.

**INTERACTIONS:** Avoid other short-acting sympathomimetic bronchodilators and epinephrine. Extreme caution within 2 weeks of MAOI or TCA use. Monitor digoxin. ECG changes and/or hypokalemia with non-$K^+$-sparing diuretics may worsen. May be antagonized by β-blockers.

**PREGNANCY:** Category C, not for use in nursing.

## ACCUPRIL — RX

quinapril HCl (Parke-Davis)

**ACE inhibitors can cause death/injury to developing fetus during 2nd and 3rd trimesters. Stop therapy if pregnancy detected.**

**THERAPEUTIC CLASS:** ACE inhibitor

**INDICATIONS:** Treatment of hypertension. Adjunct therapy in heart failure with diuretics and/or digitalis.

**DOSAGE:** *Adults:* HTN: If possible, d/c diuretic 2-3 days prior to therapy. Initial: 10-20mg qd; 5mg qd with concomitant diuretic. Titrate at intervals of at least 2 weeks. Usual: 20-80mg/day given qd-bid. CrCl >60mL/min: Initial: 10mg/day. CrCl 30-60mL/min: Initial: 5mg/day. CrCl 10-30mL/min: Initial: 2.5mg/day. Heart Failure: Initial: 5mg bid. Titrate at weekly intervals. Usual: 10-20mg bid. CrCl >30mL/min: Initial: 5mg/day. CrCl 10-30mL/min: Initial: 2.5mg/day.

**HOW SUPPLIED:** Tab: 5mg*, 10mg, 20mg, 40mg *scored

**CONTRAINDICATIONS:** History of ACE inhibitor associated angioedema.

**WARNINGS/PRECAUTIONS:** D/C if angioedema, jaundice, or if marked LFT elevation occurs. Risk of hyperkalemia with DM, renal dysfunction. Persistent nonproductive cough reported. Monitor WBCs in renal or collagen vascular disease. Anaphylactoid reactions reported. Fetal/neonatal morbidity and death reported. Monitor for hypotension in high risk patients (heart failure, surgery/anesthesia, hyponatremia, high dose diuretic therapy, recent intensive diuresis, dialysis, or severe volume and/or salt depletion,etc.). Caution with CHF, renal dysfunction, and renal artery stenosis. Less effective on BP in blacks and more reports of angioedema than nonblacks.

**ADVERSE REACTIONS:** Fatigue, headache, dizziness, cough, nausea, vomiting, hypotension, chest pain.

**INTERACTIONS:** Decreases tetracycline absorption (possibly due to magnesium content in quinapril); consider interaction with drugs that interact with magnesium. May increase lithium levels. Hypotension risk with diuretics. Increase risk of hyperkalemia with $K^+$-sparing diuretics, $K^+$ supplements, or $K^+$-containing salt substitutes.

**PREGNANCY:** Category C (1st trimester) and D (2nd and 3rd trimesters), not for use in nursing.

## ACCURETIC — RX

hydrochlorothiazide - quinapril HCl (Parke-Davis)

**ACE inhibitors can cause death/injury to developing fetus during 2nd and 3rd trimesters. Stop therapy if pregnancy detected.**

**THERAPEUTIC CLASS:** ACE inhibitor/thiazide diuretic

**INDICATIONS:** Treatment of hypertension. Not for initial therapy.

**DOSAGE:** *Adults:* Initial (if not controlled on quinapril monotherapy): 10mg-12.5mg or 20mg-12.5mg tab qd. Titrate: May increase after 2-3 weeks. Initial (if controlled on HCTZ 25mg/day but significant $K^+$ loss): 10mg-12.5mg or 20mg-12.5mg tab qd. If previously treated with 20mg quinapril and 25mg HCTZ, may switch to 20mg-25mg tab qd.

**HOW SUPPLIED:** Tab: (Quinapril-HCTZ) 10mg-12.5mg*, 20mg-12.5mg*, 20mg-25mg* *scored

**CONTRAINDICATIONS:** History of ACE inhibitor associated angioedema, anuria, sulfonamide hypersensitivity.

**WARNINGS/PRECAUTIONS:** D/C if angioedema, jaundice, or marked LFT elevation occurs. Risk of hyperkalemia with DM, renal dysfunction. Persistent nonproductive cough reported. Monitor WBCs in renal or collagen vascular disease. Anaphylactoid reactions reported. Fetal/neonatal morbidity and death reported. Monitor for hypotension in high risk patients (heart failure, surgery/anesthesia, hyponatremia, severe volume/salt depletion, etc.). Caution with CHF, renal or hepatic dysfunction, and renal artery stenosis. Less effective on BP in blacks and more reports of angioedema than nonblacks. May exacerbate or activate SLE. Monitor serum electrolytes. Avoid if CrCl <30mL/min/1.73m$^2$. May increase cholesterol, TG, and uric acid levels and decrease glucose tolerance.

**ADVERSE REACTIONS:** Dizziness, headache, cough, myalgia.

**INTERACTIONS:** Decreases tetracycline absorption (possibly due to magnesium content in quinapril); consider interaction with drugs that interact with magnesium. Increase risk of hyperkalemia with $K^+$-sparing diuretics, $K^+$-supplements, or $K^+$-containing salt substitutes. Potentiates orthostatic hypotension with alcohol, barbiturates, and narcotics. Adjust insulin and antidiabetic drugs. Impaired absorption with cholestyramine, colestipol. Corticosteroids and ACTH deplete electrolytes. May decrease response to pressor amines. Potentiates other antihypertensives. May increase responsiveness to skeletal muscle relaxants. Risk of lithium toxicity. NSAIDs decrease diuretic effects.

**PREGNANCY:** Category C (1st trimester) and D (2nd and 3rd trimesters), not for use in nursing.

## ACCUTANE

isotretinoin (Roche Labs)

RX

**Not for use by females who are or may become pregnant, or if breast feeding. Birth defects have been documented. Approved for marketing only under special restricted distribution program called iPLEDGE™. Must have 2 (-) pregnancy tests. Repeat pregnancy test monthly. Use 2 forms of contraception at least 1 month prior, during, and 1 month following discontinuation. Must fill written prescriptions within 7 days; refills require new prescriptions. May dispense maximum of 1 month supply. Prescriber and patient must be registered with iPLEDGE.**

**OTHER BRAND NAMES:** Claravis (Barr) - Sotret (Ranbaxy) - Amnesteem (Genpharm)

**THERAPEUTIC CLASS:** Retinoid

**INDICATIONS:** Severe recalcitrant nodular acne unresponsive to conventional therapy, including systemic antibiotics.

**DOSAGE:** *Adults:* Initial/Usual: 0.5-1mg/kg/day given bid for 15-20 weeks. Max: 2mg/kg/day (for very serious cases). Adjust for side effects and disease response. May discontinue if nodule count reduced by >70% prior to completion. Repeat only if necessary after 2 months off drug. Take with food. *Pediatrics:* >12 yrs: Initial/Usual: 0.5-1mg/kg/day given bid for 15-20 weeks. Max: 2mg/kg/day (for very serious cases). Adjust for side effects and disease response. May discontinue if nodule count reduced by >70% prior to completion. Repeat only if necessary after 2 months off drug. Take with food.

**HOW SUPPLIED:** Cap: 10mg, 20mg, 40mg

**CONTRAINDICATIONS:** Pregnancy, paraben sensitivity (preservative in gelatin cap).

**WARNINGS/PRECAUTIONS:** Acute pancreatitis, impaired hearing, anaphylactic reactions, inflammatory bowel disease, elevated TG and LFTs, hepatotoxicity, premature epiphyseal closure, and hyperostosis reported. May cause depression, psychosis, aggressive and/or violent behaviors, rarely suicidal ideation/attempts and suicide; may need further evaluation after discontinuation. May cause decreased night vision, and corneal opacities. Associated with pseudotumor cerebri. Check lipids before therapy, and then at intervals until response established (within 4 weeks). D/C if significant decrease in WBC, hearing or visual impairment, abdominal pain, rectal bleeding, or severe diarrhea occurs. Monitor LFTs before therapy, weekly or biweekly until response established. May develop musculoskeletal symptoms. Avoid prolonged UV rays or sunlight, and donating blood up to 1 month after discontinuing therapy. Caution with genetic predisposition for age-related osteoporosis, history of childhood osteoporosis, osteomalacia, other bone metabolism disorders (eg, anorexia nervosa). Spontaneous osteoporosis, osteopenia, bone fractures, and delayed fracture healing reported; caution in sports with repetitive impact.

**ADVERSE REACTIONS:** Cheilitis, dry skin and mucous membranes, conjunctivitis, blood dyscrasias, epistaxis, decreased HDL, elevated cholesterol and TG, elevated blood sugar, arthralgias, back pain, hearing/vision impairment, rash, photosensitivity reactions, psychiatric disorders.

**INTERACTIONS:** Avoid Vitamin A. Limit alcohol consumption. Tetracyclines increase incidence of pseudotumor cerebri. Pregnancy reported with oral and injectable/implantable contraceptives. Avoid St. John's Wort; may cause breakthrough bleeding with oral contraceptives. Caution with drugs that cause drug-induced osteoporosis/osteomalacia and affect vitamin D metabolism (eg, corticosteroids, phenytoin).

**PREGNANCY:** Category X, not for use in nursing.

## ACCUZYME — RX

urea - papain (Healthpoint)

**THERAPEUTIC CLASS:** Proteolytic enzyme (debriding agent)

**INDICATIONS:** Debridement of necrotic tissue and liquefaction of slough in acute and chronic lesions such as pressure ulcers, varicose and diabetic ulcers, burns, postoperative wounds, pilonidal cyst wounds, carbuncles and other traumatic or infected wounds.

**DOSAGE:** *Adults:* (Oint, Spray) Clean wound, then apply qd-bid. Cover with dressing. Irrigate wound at each re-dressing.

**HOW SUPPLIED:** (Papain-Urea) Oint: 830000 U/g-10% [6g, 30g]; Spray: 830000 U/g-10% [33mL]

**WARNINGS/PRECAUTIONS:** Avoid eyes.

**ADVERSE REACTIONS:** Transient burning, skin irritation.

**INTERACTIONS:** May be inactivated by hydrogen peroxide, and salts of heavy metals (eg, lead, silver, mercury).

**PREGNANCY:** Safety in pregnancy and nursing is not known.

## ACEON — RX

perindopril erbumine (Solvay)

> **ACE inhibitors can cause death/injury to developing fetus during 2nd and 3rd trimesters. Stop therapy if pregnancy detected.**

**THERAPEUTIC CLASS:** ACE inhibitor

**INDICATIONS:** Treatment of hypertension (HTN). Risk reduction of cardiovascular mortality or nonfatal myocardial infarction in patients with stable coronary artery disease (CAD).

**DOSAGE:** *Adults:* HTN: If possible, discontinue diuretic 2-3 days prior to therapy. Initial: 4mg qd; 2-4mg/day given qd-bid with concomitant diuretic. Maint: 4-8mg/day given qd-bid. Resume diuretic if BP not controlled. Max: 16mg/day. Elderly (>65 yrs): Initial: 4mg/day given qd-bid. Max (usual):

8mg/day. Renal Impairment: CrCl >30mL/min: Initial: 2mg/day. Max: 8mg/day. CAD: Initial: 4mg qd for 2 weeks. Maint: 8mg qd. Elderly (>70 yrs): Initial: 2mg qd for 1 week. Titrate: 4mg qd for week 2. Maint: 8mg qd.

**HOW SUPPLIED:** Tab: 2mg*, 4mg*, 8mg* *scored

**CONTRAINDICATIONS:** History of ACE inhibitor associated angioedema.

**WARNINGS/PRECAUTIONS:** Discontinue if angioedema, jaundice, or if marked LFT elevation occurs. Risk of hyperkalemia with DM, renal dysfunction. Persistent nonproductive cough reported. Monitor WBCs in renal and collagen vascular disease. Anaphylactoid reactions reported. Fetal/neonatal morbidity and death reported. Monitor for hypotension in high risk patients (heart failure, surgery/anesthesia, hyponatremia, prolonged diuretic therapy, or volume and/or salt depletion). Caution with CHF, renal dysfunction, and renal artery stenosis. Less effective on BP in blacks and more reports of angioedema than nonblacks. Avoid if CrCl <30mL/min.

**ADVERSE REACTIONS:** Cough, headache, asthenia, dizziness, diarrhea, edema, respiratory infection, lower extremity pain.

**INTERACTIONS:** May increase lithium levels. Hypotension risk with diuretics. Increase risk of hyperkalemia with $K^+$-sparing diuretics, drugs that increase serum $K^+$, or $K^+$ supplements. Caution with gentamicin.

**PREGNANCY:** Category C (1st trimester) and D (2nd and 3rd trimesters), caution in nursing.

## ACETADOTE RX

acetylcysteine (Cumberland)

**THERAPEUTIC CLASS:** Acetaminophen antidote

**INDICATIONS:** Prevent or lessen hepatic injury within 8-10 hrs of potentially hepatotoxic dose of acetaminophen.

**DOSAGE:** *Adults:* LD: Infuse 150mg/kg IV over 15 minutes. Maint: 50mg/kg over 4 hrs followed by 100mg/kg over 16 hrs.

**HOW SUPPLIED:** Inj: 200mg/ml [30ml]

**WARNINGS/PRECAUTIONS:** Caution in patients with asthma or history of brochospasm; can cause serious anaphylactoid reactions. Acute flushing and erythema of skin may occur. Caution in patients <40kg; avoid fluid overload; adjust D5W volume.

**ADVERSE REACTIONS:** Rash, urticaria, pruritus, nausea, vomiting, bronchospasm, angioedema.

**PREGNANCY:** Category B, caution in nursing.

## ACID JELLY RX

acetic acid - ricinoleic acid - oxyquinoline sulfate (Hope)

**THERAPEUTIC CLASS:** Topical acidic medium

**INDICATIONS:** Adjunct therapy to restore and maintain vaginal acidity.

**DOSAGE:** *Adults:* 1 applicatorful intravaginally every am and pm. Duration depends on response.

**HOW SUPPLIED:** Gel: (Acetic Acid-Oxyquinoline-Ricinoleic Acid) 0.92%-0.025%-0.7%

**WARNINGS/PRECAUTIONS:** Monitor vaginal pH (normal range pH 4-5).

**ADVERSE REACTIONS:** Local stinging, burning.

**PREGNANCY:** Category C, caution in nursing.

## ACIPHEX RX

rabeprazole sodium (Eisai/PriCara)

**THERAPEUTIC CLASS:** Proton pump inhibitor

**INDICATIONS:** Healing and maintenance treatment of erosive or ulcerative gastroesophageal reflux disease (GERD). Healing of duodenal ulcers (DU). Treatment of symptomatic GERD and pathological hypersecretory conditions (eg, Zollinger-Ellison syndrome). In combination with amoxicillin and clarithromycin, to reduce the risk of duodenal ulcer recurrence with *H.pylori* infection.

**DOSAGE:** *Adults:* Erosive/Ulcerative GERD: Healing: 20mg qd for 4-8 weeks. May repeat for 8 weeks if needed. Maint: 20mg qd. Symptomatic GERD: 20mg qd for 4 weeks. May repeat for 4 weeks if needed. DU: 20mg qd after morning meal for up to 4 weeks. May need additional therapy. *H.pylori* Triple Therapy: 20mg + clarithromycin 500mg + amoxicillin 1g, all bid (qam and qpm) with food for 7 days. Zollinger-Ellison Syndrome: Initial: 60mg qd. Titrate: Adjust according to need. Maint: Up to 100mg qd or 60mg bid. May treat up to 1 year. Swallow tabs whole; do not chew, crush, or split.

**HOW SUPPLIED:** Tab, Delayed Release: 20mg

**WARNINGS/PRECAUTIONS:** Symptomatic response does not preclude the presence of gastric malignancy. Caution with severe hepatic impairment.

**ADVERSE REACTIONS:** Headache. Diarrhea and taste perversion with triple therapy.

**INTERACTIONS:** May alter absorption of pH-dependent drugs (eg, ketoconazole, digoxin). May increase digoxin plasma levels and decrease ketoconazole levels. Monitor PT/INR with warfarin. Increased rabeprazole and clarithromycin levels with triple therapy.

**PREGNANCY:** Category B, not for use in nursing.

## ACLOVATE RX

alclometasone dipropionate (GlaxoSmithKline)

**THERAPEUTIC CLASS:** Corticosteroid

**INDICATIONS:** Corticosteroid responsive dermatoses.

**DOSAGE:** *Adults:* Apply bid-tid. Reassess if no improvement after 2 weeks. *Pediatrics:* >1 yr: Apply bid-tid. Reassess if no improvement after 2 weeks.

**HOW SUPPLIED:** Cre, Oint: 0.05% [15g, 45g, 60g]

**WARNINGS/PRECAUTIONS:** May produce reversible HPA axis suppression, manifestations of Cushing's syndrome, hyperglycemia, and glucosuria. Use appropriate antifungal or antibacterial agent with dermatological infections. Peds may be more susceptible to systemic toxicity. Avoid occlusive dressings. Avoid diaper area. Not for use in diaper dermatitis. D/C if irritation occurs. Caution in peds.

**ADVERSE REACTIONS:** Itching, burning, erythema, dryness, irritation, papular rash.

**PREGNANCY:** Category C, caution in nursing.

## ACTHIB RX

haemophilus B conjugate (Sanofi Pasteur)

**THERAPEUTIC CLASS:** Vaccine

**INDICATIONS:** Solo or combined with DTP (Aventis Pasteur) for active immunization of children 2-18 months for prevention of invasive disease caused by *H.influenzae* type B and/or diphtheria, tetanus, and pertussis. Combined with Tripedia® (TriHIBit®) for active immunization of children 15-18 months for prevention of invasive disease caused by *H.influenzae* type B and diphtheria, tetanus, and pertussis.

**DOSAGE:** *Pediatrics:* Reconstituted with DTP or Saline: 0.5mL IM in deltoid or thigh at 2, 4, and 6 months old; 4th dose at 15-18 months; 5th dose at 4-6 yrs. Reconstituted with Tripedia® (as 4th dose in series): 0.5mL IM in deltoid or thigh given at 15-18 months; 5th dose at 4-6 yrs. Previously Unvaccinated: 7-11 months old: 2 doses at 8 week intervals with a booster at 15-18 months. 12-14 months: 1 dose followed by a booster 2 months later.

**HOW SUPPLIED:** Inj: 10mcg

**WARNINGS/PRECAUTIONS:** Immunosuppressed patients may not obtain expected antibody response. Have epinephrine injection (1:1000) available.

**ADVERSE REACTIONS:** Local: tenderness, erythema, induration. Systemic: fever, irritability, drowsiness, anorexia, nausea, diarrhea, vomiting.

**INTERACTIONS:** Immunosuppressive therapies may reduce effectiveness.

**PREGNANCY:** Category C, safety in nursing not known.

## ACTHREL

corticorelin ovine triflutate (Ferring) RX

**THERAPEUTIC CLASS:** CRH (human) peptide analogue

**INDICATIONS:** For use in differentiating pituitary and ectopic production of ACTH in patients with ACTH-dependent Cushing's syndrome.

**DOSAGE:** *Adults:* 1mcg/kg IV single dose. If repeated evaluation is needed, repeat test at the same time of day as the original test. Administer over 30 seconds and not as a bolus injection to decrease side effects. Doses >1mcg/kg are not recommended.

**HOW SUPPLIED:** Inj: 0.1mg

**WARNINGS/PRECAUTIONS:** Transient tachycardia, decreased BP, loss of consciousness, and asystole reported at higher than recommended doses.

**ADVERSE REACTIONS:** Flushing of the face, neck, and upper chest, the urge to take a deep breath.

**INTERACTIONS:** Pretreatment with dexamethasone inhibits or blunts plasma ACTH response. Major hypotensive reaction reported with heparin.

**PREGNANCY:** Category C, caution in nursing.

## ACTICIN

permethrin (Mylan Bertek) RX

**THERAPEUTIC CLASS:** Pyrethroid scabicidal agent

**INDICATIONS:** Treatment of scabies.

**DOSAGE:** *Adults:* Massage into skin from head to soles of feet. Wash off after 8-14 hrs. One treatment should be adequate. Retreat if living mites present after 14 days.
*Pediatrics:* >2 months: Massage into skin from head (scalp, temples and forehead) to soles of feet. Wash off after 8-14 hrs. One treatment should be adequate. Retreat if living mites present after 14 days.

**HOW SUPPLIED:** Cre: 5% [60g]

**CONTRAINDICATIONS:** Allergy to synthetic pyrethroid or pyrethrin.

**WARNINGS/PRECAUTIONS:** May temporarily exacerbate infection (eg pruritus, edema, erythema). Avoid eyes. D/C if hypersensitivity occurs.

**ADVERSE REACTIONS:** Burning, stinging, pruritus, erythema, numbness, tingling, rash.

**PREGNANCY:** Category B, not for use in nursing.

## ACTIGALL

RX

ursodiol (Watson)

**THERAPEUTIC CLASS:** Bile acid

**INDICATIONS:** Treatment of radiolucent, noncalcified gallbladder stones <20mm in diameter in patients unable to undergo cholecystecomy. Prevention of gallstone formation in obese patients experiencing rapid weight loss.

**DOSAGE:** *Adults:* Treatment: 8-10mg/kg/day given bid-tid. Obtain ultrasound at 6 month intervals for 1 year. Continue therapy after stones have dissolved and confirm with repeat ultrasound within 1-3 months. Prevention: 300mg bid.

**HOW SUPPLIED:** Cap: 300mg

**CONTRAINDICATIONS:** Calcified cholesterol stones, radiopaque stones, radiolucent bile pigment stones, unremitting acute cholecystitis, cholangitis, biliary obstruction, gallstone pancreatitis, biliary-gastrointestinal fistula, bile acid hypersensitivity.

**WARNINGS/PRECAUTIONS:** Therapy is not associated with liver damage. Monitor LFTs at the initiation of therapy and periodically thereafter. Caution in elderly.

**ADVERSE REACTIONS:** Abdominal pain, constipation, diarrhea, dyspepsia, flatulence, nausea, arthralgia, coughing, viral infection, vomiting, bronchitis, pharyngitis, back pain, myalgia, headache, sinusitis, upper respiratory tract infection.

**INTERACTIONS:** Decreased absorption with bile acid sequestrants and aluminum based antacids. Estrogens, oral contraceptives, and clofibrate encourage gallstone formation.

**PREGNANCY:** Category B, caution in nursing.

## ACTIQ

CII

fentanyl citrate (Cephalon)

**May cause life-threatening hypoventilation in opioid non-tolerant patients. Only for cancer pain in opioid tolerant patients with malignancies. Keep out of reach of children and discard properly. Concomitant use with moderate and strong CYP3A4 inhibitors may cause fatal respiratory depression.**

**THERAPEUTIC CLASS:** Narcotic agonist analgesic

**INDICATIONS:** Management of breakthrough cancer pain in patients with malignancies who are already receiving and are tolerant to opioid therapy.

**DOSAGE:** *Adults:* Initial: 0.2mg (consume over 15 minutes). Titrate: Redose 15 minutes after previous dose is completed. No more than 2 units per breakthrough pain episode. May increase to next higher available strength if several breakthrough episodes (1-2 days) require more than 1 unit per pain episode. Repeat titration for each new dose. Max: 4 units/day. Prescribe 6 units with each new titration. The lozenge should be sucked, not chewed, and consumed over 15 minutes.
*Pediatrics:* ≥16 yrs: Initial: 0.2mg (consume over 15 minutes). Titrate: Redose 15 minutes after previous dose is completed. No more than 2 units per breakthrough pain episode. May increase to next higher available strength if several breakthrough episodes (1-2 days) require more than 1 unit per pain episode. Repeat titration for each new dose. Max: 4 units/day. Prescribe 6 units with each new titration. The lozenge should be sucked, not chewed, and consumed over 15 minutes.

**HOW SUPPLIED:** Loz: 0.2mg, 0.4mg, 0.6mg, 0.8mg, 1.2mg, 1.6mg

**CONTRAINDICATIONS:** Opioid non-tolerant patients and management of acute or postoperative pain.

**WARNINGS/PRECAUTIONS:** Caution with COPD, hepatic or renal dysfunction. Risk of clinically significant hypoventilation. Extreme caution with evidence of increased intracranial pressure or impaired consciousness. Can produce morphine-like dependence. Increased risk of dental decay; ensure proper oral hygiene. Caution with bradyarrhythmias, liver or kidney dysfunction. Patients on concomitant CNS depressants must be monitored for a change in opioid effects. May impair mental and/or physical status.

**ADVERSE REACTIONS:** Respiratory depression, circulatory depression, headache, hypotension, shock, nausea, vomiting, constipation, dizziness, dyspnea, anxiety, somnolence.

**INTERACTIONS:** Concomitant use with other CNS depressants, including opioids, sedatives, hypnotics, general anesthetics, phenothiazines, tranquilizers, skeletal muscle relaxants, sedating antihistamines, potent inhibitors of CYP3A4 (eg, erythromycin, ketoconazole, itraconazole, ritonavir, troleandomycin, clarithromycin, nelfinavir and nefazodone) or moderate inhibitors (eg amprenavir, aprepitant, diltiazem, erythromycin, fluconazole, fosamprenavir, and verapamil) and alcohol may result in increased plasma concentrations. Avoid grapefruit juice. Avoid within 14 days of MAOIs.

**PREGNANCY:** Category C, not for use in nursing.

## ACTIVASE — RX

alteplase (Genentech)

**THERAPEUTIC CLASS:** Thrombolytic agent

**INDICATIONS:** To improve ventricular function, reduce incidence of congestive heart failure, and reduce mortality with AMI. Management of acute ischemic stroke and acute massive PE.

**DOSAGE:** *Adults:* AMI: Accelerated Infusion: >67kg: 15mg IV bolus, then 50mg over next 30 minutes, and then 35mg over next 60 minutes. <67kg: 15mg IV bolus, then 0.75mg/kg (max 50mg) over next 30 minutes, then 0.5mg/kg (max 35mg) over next 60 minutes. Max: 100mg total dose. 3-Hr Infusion: >65kg: 60mg in 1st hr (give 6-10mg as IV bolus), then 20mg over 2nd hr, then 20mg over 3rd hr. Less than 65kg: 1.25mg/kg over 3 hrs as described above. Stroke: 0.9mg/kg IV over 1 hr (max 90mg total dose). Administer 10% of total dose as IV bolus over 1 minute. PE: 100mg IV over 2 hrs. Start heparin at end or immediately after infusion when PTT or PT <2x normal.

**HOW SUPPLIED:** Inj: 50mg, 100mg

**CONTRAINDICATIONS:** (AMI, PE) Active internal bleeding, history of CVA, recent intracranial/intraspinal surgery or trauma, intracranial neoplasm, arteriovenous (AV) malformation, aneurysm, bleeding diathesis, severe uncontrolled HTN. (Stroke) Active internal bleeding, AV malformation, intracranial neoplasm or hemorrhage, aneurysm, bleeding diathesis, uncontrolled HTN, SAH, seizure at on stroke onset. Recent intracranial or intraspinal surgery, serious head trauma, previous stroke.

**WARNINGS/PRECAUTIONS:** Weigh benefits/risks with recent major surgery, cerebrovascular disease, recent GI or GU bleeding, recent trauma, HTN, left heart thrombus, acute pericarditis, subacute bacterial endocarditis, hemostatic defects, severe hepatic dysfunction, pregnancy, diabetic hemorrhagic retinopathy or other hemorrhagic ophthalmic conditions, septic thrombophlebitis or occluded AV cannula at a seriously infected site, elderly, any other bleeding condition that is difficult to manage. For stroke, also weigh benefits/risks with severe neurological deficit or major early infarct signs on CT. Cholesterol embolism and internal/superficial bleeding reported. Arrhythmias may occur with reperfusion. Avoid IM injection, noncompressible arterial puncture, and internal jugular or subclavian venous puncture. Caution with readministration.

**ADVERSE REACTIONS:** Bleeding.

**INTERACTIONS:** Increased risk of bleeding with heparin, vitamin K antagonists, drugs altering platelets (eg, ASA, dipyridamole, abciximab) given before, during, or after alteplase therapy.

**PREGNANCY:** Category C, caution in nursing.

## ACTIVELLA RX

estradiol - norethindrone (Novo Nordisk)

**Estrogens and progestins, should not be used for the prevention of cardiovascular disease or dementia. Increased risks of MI, stroke, invasive breast cancer, PE, and DVT in postmenopausal women (50-79 yrs of age) reported. Increased risk of developing probable dementia in postmenopausal women ≥65 yrs of age reported.**

**THERAPEUTIC CLASS:** Estrogen/progestogen combination

**INDICATIONS:** For women with intact uterus, treatment of moderate to severe vasomotor symptoms associated with menopause, vulvar/vaginal atrophy and prevention of postmenopausal osteoporosis

**DOSAGE:** *Adults:* 1 tab qd.

**HOW SUPPLIED:** Tab: (Estradiol-Norethindrone) 1mg-0.5mg

**CONTRAINDICATIONS:** Pregnancy, breast cancer, abnormal genital bleeding, estrogen-dependent neoplasia, DVT, thromboembolic disorders, stroke, liver dysfunction or disease.

**WARNINGS/PRECAUTIONS:** Risk of gallbladder disease, endometrial and breast cancer, fetal congenital reproductive tract disorder, elevated BP, and hypercalcemia with breast cancer or bone metastases. Possible risk of cardiovascular disease. Increased risk of DVT, stroke, and PE; increased risk of endometrial, breast, and ovarian cancer with prolonged use. Risk of probable dementia-unknown risk in postmenopausal women under 65 years of age. Monitor for fluid retention with asthma, epilepsy, migraine, and cardiac/renal dysfunction. Avoid in post-menopausal women without a uterus. D/C if vision disturbances or thrombotic disorders occur. Caution with depression, DM. Acceleration of PT, PTT. Hypercoagulability effects. Impaired glucose tolerance. Increased triglycerides, fibrin/fibrinogen, and plasmin/plasminogen activity.

**ADVERSE REACTIONS:** Back pain, headache, nasopharyngitis, sinusitis, insomnia, upper respiratory tract infection, breast pain, postmenopausal bleeding/vaginal hemorrhage, endometrial thickening, uterine fibroid, pain in extremities, nausea, and diarrhea.

**PREGNANCY:** Category X, caution in nursing.

## ACTONEL RX

risedronate sodium (Procter & Gamble)

**THERAPEUTIC CLASS:** Bisphosphonate

**INDICATIONS:** Prevention and treatment of osteoporosis in postmenopausal women, glucocorticoid-induced osteoporosis in men and women. Increase bone mass in men with osteoporosis. Treatment of Paget's disease in men and women.

**DOSAGE:** *Adults:* Paget's Disease: 30mg qd for 2 months. May retreat after 2 months. Postmenopausal Osteoporosis: 5mg qd or 35mg once weekly or 75mg on 2 consecutive days each month. Glucocorticoid-Induced Osteoporosis: 5mg qd. Increase Bone Mass in Men with Osteoporosis: 35mg once weekly. Take at least 30 min before the first food or drink of the day other than water. Swallow tab in upright position with 6-8 oz of plain water. Do not lie down for 30 min after dose.

**HOW SUPPLIED:** Tab: 5mg, 30mg, 35mg, 75mg

**CONTRAINDICATIONS:** Hypocalcemia; inability to stand or sit upright for at least 30 min.

**WARNINGS/PRECAUTIONS:** May cause upper GI disorders (eg, dysphagia, esophagitis, esophageal or gastric ulcer). Treat hypocalcemia and other disturbances of bone and mineral metabolism before therapy. Give supplemental calcium and vitamin D if dietary intake is inadequate. Avoid with severe renal impairment (CrCl <30mL/min). Osteonecrosis, primarily in the jaw, has been reported. Postmarketing severe and occasionally incapacitating bone, joint, and/or muscle pain, has been reported.

**ADVERSE REACTIONS:** Asthenia, diarrhea, abdominal pain, nausea, constipation, peripheral edema, arthralgia, leg cramps, headache, dizziness, sinusitis, rash, tinnitus.

**INTERACTIONS:** Calcium supplements and calcium-, aluminum-, and magnesium-containing agents may interfere with absorption; space doses.

**PREGNANCY:** Category C, not for use in nursing.

## ACTONEL WITH CALCIUM RX

calcium carbonate - risedronate sodium (Procter & Gamble)

**THERAPEUTIC CLASS:** Bisphosphonate

**INDICATIONS:** Treatment and prevention of postmenopausal osteoporosis.

**DOSAGE:** *Adults:* Risedronate: 35mg once weekly (Day 1 of the 7-day treatment cycle). Take at least 30 minutes before 1st food or drink of the day other than water. Swallow tab in upright position with 6-8 oz of plain water. Do not lie down for 30 minutes after dose. Calcium: 1250mg qd with food on each of the remaining 6 days (Days 2-7 of the 7-day treatment cycle).

**HOW SUPPLIED:** Tab: (Risedronate Sodium) 35mg; Tab: (Calcium Carbonate) 1250mg

**CONTRAINDICATIONS:** Risedronate: Hypocalcemia; inability to stand or sit upright for at least 30 minutes. Calcium: Hypercalcemia from any cause (eg, hyperparathyroidism, hypercalcemia of malignancy, or sarcoidosis).

**WARNINGS/PRECAUTIONS:** Risedronate: May cause upper GI disorders (eg, dysphagia, esophagitis, esophageal or gastric ulcer). Treat hypocalcemia and other disturbances of bone and mineral metabolism before therapy. May cause osteonecrosis, primarily in the jaw. Avoid with severe renal impairment (CrCl <30mL/min). Calcium: Should not be used to treat hypocalcemia. Daily intake above 2000mg has been associated with increased risk of adverse effects, including hypercalcemia and kidney stones. Patients with achlorhydria may have decreased absorption of calcium. Severe and occasionally incapacitating bone, joint, and/or muscle pain in patient taking bisphosphonates, have been reported.

**ADVERSE REACTIONS:** Risedronate: Infection, pain, flu syndrome, abdominal pain, headache, asthenia, HTN, constipation, dyspepsia, nausea, arthralgia, nausea, diarrhea, dizziness, myalgia. Calcium: Constipation, flatulence, nausea, abdominal pain, and bloating.

**INTERACTIONS:** Risedronate: Calcium supplements, and calcium-, aluminum-, and magnesium-containing agents may interfere with absorption; space doses. Calcium: May reduce absorption of levothyroxine, fluoroquinolones, tetracycline. Calcium absorption reduced when taken with systemic glucocorticoids. Reduced urinary excretion of calcium with use of thiazide diuretics. Absorption of calcium increased with use of Vitamin D and analogues. May interfere with absorption of iron. Take iron and calcium at different times of the day.

**PREGNANCY:** Category C, not for use in nursing.

## ACTOPLUS MET RX

metformin HCl - pioglitazone HCl (Takeda)

**Lactic acidosis is a rare, but serious, metabolic complication. Symptoms at onset is nonspecific and include malaise, myalgia and increasing somnolence. Lactic acidosis is a medical emergency and must be treated in a hospital. Drug should be discontinued immediately if a patient with lactic acidosis is taking metformin.**

**THERAPEUTIC CLASS:** Thiazolidinedione/biguanide

**INDICATIONS:** Adjunct to diet and exercise, to improve glycemic control in type 2 diabetes mellitus in patients already treated with a combination of pioglitazone and metformin or whose diabetes is not adequately controlled with metformin alone, or for those patients who have initially responded to pioglitazone alone and require additional glycemic control.

**DOSAGE:** *Adults:* Individualize dose. Prior Pioglitazone/Metformin: Base on current regimen. Prior Metformin Monotherapy or Pioglitazone Monotherapy: Initial: 15mg-500mg or 15mg-850mg qd-bid. Titrate: Gradually increase after assessing adequacy of therapeutic response. Max: (Pioglitazone) 45mg, (Metformin) 2550mg. Elderly/Debilitated/Malnourished: Conservative dosing; do not titrate to max dose.

**HOW SUPPLIED:** Tab: (Pioglitazone-Metformin) 15mg-500mg, 15mg-850mg

**CONTRAINDICATIONS:** Renal disease or renal failure (eg, serum creatinine levels ≥1.5mg/dL [males], ≥1.4mg/dL [females], or abnormal creatinine clearance) and acute or chronic metabolic acidosis, including diabetic ketoacidosis, with or without coma. Tempoarily discontinue in patients undergoing radiologic studies involving intravascular administration of iodinated contrast materials.

**WARNINGS/PRECAUTIONS:** (Metformin) Lactic acidosis reported (rare); increased risk with renal dysfunction, increased age, DM, CHF, and other conditions with risk of hypoperfusion and hypoxemia. Avoid in patients ≥80 yrs unless reanl function is normal. Monitor renal function and for ketoacidosis and metabolic acidosis. Avoid in renal/hepatic impairment. Discontinue in hypoxic states (eg, CHF, shock, acute MI), loss of blood glucose control due to stress (give insulin), acidosis, dehydration, sepsis. Temporarily discontiue prior to surgery (due to restricted food intake) and procedures requiring intravascular iodinated contrast materials. May decrease serum $B_{12}$ levels. Increased risk of hypoglycemia in elderly, debilitated/malnourished, adrenal or pituitary insufficiency, or alcohol intoxication. Monitor renal function. Alcohol is known to potentiate the effect of metformin on lactate metabolism. (Pioglitazone) May cause fluid retention and exacerbation/initiation of heart failure; discontinue if cardiac status deteriorates. Avoid if NYHA Class III of IV cardiac status. Use lowest approved dose if systolic heart failure (NYHA Class II). Not for use in type 1 diabetes or for diabetic ketoacidosis treatment. Caution with edema. Dose related weight gain reported. Ovulation in premenopausal anovulatory patients may occur; risk of pregnancy with inadequate contraception. May decrease Hgb and Hct. Avoid with active liver disease, if ALT levels >2.5X ULN. Discontinue if jaundice occurs or ALT >3X ULN on therapy. Macular edema reported.

**ADVERSE REACTIONS:** Upper respiratory tract infection, diarrhea, nausea, edema, headache, UTI, sinusitis, dizziness, weight increase, new onset or worsening diabetic macular edema.

**INTERACTIONS:** (Pioglitazone) Possible loss of contraception with ethinyl estradiol and norethindrone; caution when co-administering. Ketoconazole may inhibit pioglitazone metabolism; evaluate glycemic control more frequently. Risk for hypoglycemia with insulin or oral hypoglycemic agents. May cause reduction of midazolam levels. (Metformin) Furosemide, nifedipine, cimetidine, cationic drugs (eg, digoxin, amiloride, procainamide, quinidine, quinine, ranitidine, trimethoprim, vancomycin, triamterene, morphine) may increase metformin levels. Thiazides, other diuretics, corticosteroids, phenothiazines, thyroid products, estrogens, oral contraceptives, phenytoin, nicotinic acid, sympathomimetics, calcium channel blockers, isoniazid may cause hyperglycemia. Risk of hypoglycemia with alcohol. Excess alcohol may increase potential for lactic acidosis. May decrease furosemide levels. An enzyme inhibitor of CYP2C8 (such as gemfibrozil) may significantly increase the AUC of pioglitazone and an enzyme inducer of CYP2C8 (such as rifampin) may significantly decrease the AUC of pioglitazone.

**PREGNANCY:** Category C, not for use in nursing.

## ACTOS
pioglitazone HCl (Takeda)

RX

**THERAPEUTIC CLASS:** Thiazolidinedione

**INDICATIONS:** Adjunct to diet and exercise, to improve glycemic control in type 2 diabetes mellitus. May use in combination with a sulfonylurea, metformin, or insulin.

**DOSAGE:** *Adults:* Monotherapy: Initial: 15-30mg qd. Max: 45mg/day. Combination Therapy: Initial: 15-30mg qd. Max: 30mg/day. Decrease insulin dose by 10-25% if hypoglycemia occurs or if plasma glucose is <100mg/dL. Decrease sulfonylurea dose with hypoglycemia also.

**HOW SUPPLIED:** Tab: 15mg, 30mg, 45mg

**WARNINGS/PRECAUTIONS:** May cause fluid retention and exacerbation/initiation of heart failure; discontinue if cardiac status deteriorates. Avoid if NYHA Class III or IV cardiac status. Use lowest approved dose if systolic heart failure (NYHA Class II). Not for use in type 1 diabetes or for diabetic ketoacidosis treatment. Caution with edema. Dose related weight gain reported. Ovulation in premenopausal anovulatory patients may occur; risk of pregnancy with inadequate contraception. May decrease Hgb and Hct. Avoid with active liver disease, if ALT levels >2.5X ULN, or if jaundice occurred with troglitazone. Check LFTs before therapy, every 2 months for 1 year, and periodically thereafter, or if hepatic dysfunction symptoms occur. Discontinue if jaundice occurs or ALT >3X ULN on therapy. Macular edema reported.

**ADVERSE REACTIONS:** Upper respiratory tract infection, myalgia, tooth disorder, headache, sinusitis, pharyngitis, transient CPK level elevations, CHF, weight gain, aggravated DM, edema, dyspnea, new onset or worsening of diabetic macular edema.

**INTERACTIONS:** Possible loss of contraception with ethinyl estradiol and norethindrone; caution when co-administering. Ketoconazole may inhibit pioglitazone metabolism; evaluate glycemic control more frequently. Risk for hypoglycemia with insulin or oral hypoglycemic agents. May cause reduction of midazolam levels. An enzyme inhibitor of CYP2C8 (such as gemfibrozil) may significantly increase the AUCof pioglitazone and an enzyme inducer of CYP2C8 (such as rifampin) may significantlydecrease the AUC of pioglitazone.

**PREGNANCY:** Category C, not for use in nursing.

## ACULAR
ketorolac tromethamine (Allergan)

RX

**THERAPEUTIC CLASS:** NSAID

**INDICATIONS:** Ocular itching due to seasonal allergic conjunctivitis. Postoperative inflammation in cataract extraction.

**DOSAGE:** *Adults:* 1 drop qid. Post-op Inflammation: Begin 24 hrs post-op and continue for 2 weeks.
*Pediatrics:* >3 yrs: 1 drop qid. Post-op Inflammation: Begin 24 hrs post-op and continue for 2 weeks.

**HOW SUPPLIED:** Sol: 0.5% [3mL, 5mL, 10mL]

**WARNINGS/PRECAUTIONS:** May increase ocular tissue bleeding in conjunction with ocular surgery. Avoid use with contact lenses. D/C if corneal epithelium breakdown occurs. Caution in known bleeding tendencies, complicated ocular surgeries, corneal denervation, corneal epithelial defects, DM, ocular surface diseases (eg, dry eye syndrome), rheumatoid arthritis, or repeat ocular surgeries within a short period of time. Caution if used >24 hrs prior to surgery and use beyond 14 days post-surgery.

**ADVERSE REACTIONS:** Transient stinging/burning, superficial keratitis or infections, allergic reactions, ocular inflammation, corneal edema, iritis.

**INTERACTIONS:** Potential for cross-sensitivity to acetylsalicylic acid, phenylacetic acid derivatives, and other NSAIDs. Caution with agents that may prolong bleeding time. Increased potential for healing problems with topical steroids.

**PREGNANCY:** Category C, caution in nursing.

## ADACEL RX

tetanus toxoid - diphtheria toxoid, reduced - pertussis vaccine acellular, adsorbed (Sanofi Pasteur)

**THERAPEUTIC CLASS:** Vaccine

**INDICATIONS:** Active booster immunization against tetanus, diphtheria, and pertussis in persons 11-64 years of age.

**DOSAGE:** *Adults:* ≤64 yrs: 0.5mL IM (deltoid).
*Pediatrics:* ≥11 yrs: 0.5mL IM (deltoid).

**HOW SUPPLIED:** Inj: (Tetanus-Diphtheria-Pertussis) 5 LF- 2 LF-2.5mcg/0.5mL

**CONTRAINDICATIONS:** Encephalopathy not attributable to another identifiable cause within 7 days from initial vaccination. Progressive neurological disorder, uncontrolled epilepsy, or progressive encephalopathy.

**WARNINGS/PRECAUTIONS:** Evaluate risks/benefits of subsequent doses if temperature ≥105ºF within 48 hrs not due to another identifiable cause; if collapse/shock occurs; persistent crying for ≥3 hrs within 48 hrs; and convulsions with or without fever within 3 days of vaccine. Continue with Td vaccine if pertussis must be withheld. Have epinephrine (1:1000) available. May not achieve expected immune response in immunosuppressed patients. Avoid injection into blood vessel. Should not be administered into the buttocks nor by the intradermal route.

**ADVERSE REACTIONS:** Injection site reactions, fever, headache, body aches, tiredness, chills, sore joints, nausea, lymph node swelling, diarrhea, and vomiting.

**INTERACTIONS:** Immunosuppressives (eg, irradiation, antimetabolites, alkylating agents, cytotoxic drugs, and corticosteroids) may reduce the immune response to vaccines.

**PREGNANCY:** Category C, caution in nursing

## ADALAT CC RX

nifedipine (Schering)

**OTHER BRAND NAMES:** Afeditab CR (Watson)

**THERAPEUTIC CLASS:** Calcium channel blocker (dihydropyridine)

**INDICATIONS:** Treatment of hypertension.

**DOSAGE:** *Adults:* Initial: 30mg qd. Titrate over 7-14 days. Usual: 30-60mg qd. Max: 90mg/day. Take on empty stomach. Swallow tab whole.

**HOW SUPPLIED:** Tab, Extended Release: (Adalat CC, Afeditab CR) 30mg, 60mg, (Adalat CC) 90mg

**WARNINGS/PRECAUTIONS:** May cause hypotension; monitor BP initially or with titration. May exacerbate angina from β-blocker withdrawal. CHF risk, especially with aortic stenosis or β-blockers. Peripheral edema reported. May increase angina or MI with severe obstructive CAD. Caution in elderly.

**ADVERSE REACTIONS:** Headache, flushing, heat sensation, dizziness, peripheral edema, fatigue, asthenia.

**INTERACTIONS:** β-blockers may increase risk of CHF, severe hypotension, or angina exacerbation. Possible hypotension with fentanyl. Monitor digoxin, quinidine, and coumarin levels. CYP3A4 inhibitors (eg, ketoconazole, erythromycin, protease inhibitors) may increase levels. Avoid grapefruit juice. Cimetidine may increase levels. CYP3A4 inducers (eg, phenytoin, St. John's wort) may decrease levels.

**PREGNANCY:** Category C, not for use in nursing.

# ADDERALL

**CII**

amphetamine salt combo (Shire US)

**High potential for abuse; avoid prolonged use. Misuse of amphetamine may cause sudden death and serious cardiovascular adverse events.**

**THERAPEUTIC CLASS:** Sympathomimetic amine

**INDICATIONS:** Treatment of attention deficit disorder with hyperactivity (ADHD) and narcolepsy.

**DOSAGE:** *Adults:* Narcolepsy: Initial: 10mg/day. Titrate: May increase by 10mg/day every week. Usual: 5-60mg/day. Give 1st dose upon awakening, and additional doses q4-6h.
*Pediatrics:* ADHD: 3-5 yrs: Initial: 2.5mg qd. Titrate: May increase by 2.5mg weekly. ≥6 yrs: 5mg qd-bid. May increase by 5mg weekly. Max (usual): 40mg/day. Narcolepsy: 6-12 yrs: Initial: 5mg/day. May increase by 5mg weekly. ≥12 yrs: Initial: 10mg/day. Titrate: May increase by 10mg/day every week. Usual: 5-60mg/day. Give 1st dose upon awakening, and additional doses q4-6h.

**HOW SUPPLIED:** Tab: 5mg*, 7.5mg*, 10mg*, 12.5mg*, 15mg*, 20mg*, 30mg*
*scored

**CONTRAINDICATIONS:** Advanced arteriosclerosis, symptomatic cardiovascular disease, moderate to severe HTN, hyperthyroidism, glaucoma, agitated states, history of drug abuse, during or within 14 days of MAOI use.

**WARNINGS/PRECAUTIONS:** May exacerbate symptoms of behavior disturbance and thought disorder in psychotic patients. Caution when using stimulants to treat patients with comorbid bipolar disorder because of concern for possible induction of mixed/manic episode in such patients. Stimulants at usual doses can cause treatment emergent psychotic or manic symptoms (eg, hallucinations, delusional thinking, mania) in children and adolescents without prior history of psychotic illness. Aggressive behavior or hostility reported in clinical trials and the postmarketing experience of some medications indicated for the treatment of ADHD. Monitor growth in children. May lower convulsive threshold; d/c in presence of seizures. Visual disturbances reported with stimulant treatment. May exacerbate Tourette's syndrome and phonic or motor tics. Caution with HTN and monitor BP. Interrupt occasionally to determine if patient requires continued therapy. Sudden death reported in children with structural cardiac abnormalities; avoid use in children or adults with structural cardiac abnormalities.

**ADVERSE REACTIONS:** HTN, tachycardia, palpitations, CNS overstimulation, dry mouth, GI disorders, anorexia, impotence, urticaria, rash, angioedema, anaphylaxis, Stevens Johnson Syndrome.

**INTERACTIONS:** GI acidifying agents (guanethidine, reserpine, glutamic acid, etc) and urinary acidifying agents (ammonium chloride, etc) decrease efficacy. MAOIs may cause hypertensive crisis. Potentiated by GI and urinary alkalinizers, propoxyphene overdose. Potentiated effects of both agents with TCAs. May delay absorption of phenytoin, ethosuximide, phenobarbital. Potentiates meperidine, norepinephrine, phenobarbital, phenytoin. Antagonized by haloperidol, chlorpromazine, lithium. Antagonizes adrenergic blockers, antihistamines, antihypertensives, veratrum alkaloids (antihypertensive). Avoid co-administration with alkalinizing agents (eg, antacids).

**PREGNANCY:** Category C, not for use in nursing.

# ADDERALL XR

amphetamine salt combo (Shire US)

**High potential for abuse; avoid prolonged use. Misuse of amphetamine may cause sudden death and serious cardiovascular adverse events.**

**THERAPEUTIC CLASS:** Sympathomimetic amine

**INDICATIONS:** Treatment of attention deficit hyperactivity disorder (ADHD).

**DOSAGE:** *Adults:* Initial: 20mg qam. Currently Using Adderall: Switch to Adderall XR at the same total daily dose, taken once daily. Titrate at weekly intervals as needed. Swallow cap whole or open cap and sprinkle contents on applesauce; do not chew beads.
*Pediatrics:* ≥6 yrs: Initial: 10mg qam. Titrate: May increase weekly by 5-10mg/day. Max: 30mg/day. 13 to 17 yrs: Initial: 10mg/day. Titrate: May increase to 20mg/day after one week. Currently Using Adderall: Switch to Adderall XR at the same total daily dose, taken once daily. Titrate at weekly intervals as needed. Swallow cap whole or open cap and sprinkle contents on applesauce; do not chew beads.

**HOW SUPPLIED:** Cap, Extended-Release: 5mg, 10mg, 15mg, 20mg, 25mg, 30mg

**CONTRAINDICATIONS:** Advanced arteriosclerosis, symptomatic cardiovascular disease, moderate to severe HTN, hyperthyroidism, glaucoma, agitated states, history of drug abuse, during or within 14 days of MAOI use.

**WARNINGS/PRECAUTIONS:** May exacerbate symptoms of behavior disturbance and thought disorder in psychotic patients. Caution when using stimulants to treat patients with comorbid bipolar disorder because of concern for possible induction of mixed/manic episode in such patients. Stimulants at usual doses can cause treatment emergent psychotic or manic symptoms (eg, hallucinations, delusional thinking, mania) in children and adolescents without prior history of psychotic illness. Aggressive behavior or hostility reported in clinical trials and postmarketing experience of some medications indicated for the treatment of ADHD. Monitor growth in children. May lower convulsive threshold; d/c in presence of seizures. Visual disturbances reported with stimulant treatment. May exacerbate Tourette's syndrome and phonic or motor tics. Caution with HTN and monitor BP. Interrupt occasionally to determine if patient requires continued therapy. Sudden death reported in children with structural cardiac abnormalities; avoid use in children or adults with structural cardiac abnormalities. May decrease appetite.

**ADVERSE REACTIONS:** Abdominal pain, asthenia, fever, infection, viral infection, loss of appetite, diarrhea, nausea, vomiting, emotional lability, insomnia, nervousness, weight loss, dry mouth, headache, urticaria, anaphylaxis.

**INTERACTIONS:** GI acidifying agents (guanethidine, reserpine, glutamic acid, etc) and urinary acidifying agents (ammonium chloride, etc) decrease efficacy. MAOIs may cause hypertensive crisis. Potentiated by GI and urinary alkalinizers, propoxyphene overdose. Potentiated effects of both agents with TCAs. May delay absorption of phenytoin, ethosuximide, phenobarbital. Potentiates meperidine, norepinephrine, phenobarbital, phenytoin. Antagonized by haloperidol, chlorpromazine, lithium. Antagonizes adrenergic blockers, antihistamines, antihypertensives, veratrum alkaloids (antihypertensive). Avoid co-administration of alkalinizing agents (eg, antacid).

**PREGNANCY:** Category C, not for use in nursing.

## ADENOCARD

RX

adenosine (Astellas)

**THERAPEUTIC CLASS:** Endogenous nucleoside

**INDICATIONS:** Conversion of paroxysmal supraventricular tachycardia (including Wolff-Parkinson-White syndrome) to sinus rhythm (SR).

**DOSAGE:** *Adults:* 6mg rapid IV bolus infusion over 1-2 seconds. If not converted to SR within 1-2 minutes, give 12mg rapid IV bolus; may give 2nd 12mg dose if needed. Max: 12mg/dose.
*Pediatrics:* <50kg: 0.05-0.1mg/kg rapid IV bolus. If not converted to SR within 1-2 minutes, give additional bolus doses incrementally increasing amount by 0.05-0.1mg/kg. Follow each bolus with a saline flush. Continue process until SR or a maximum single dose of 0.3mg/kg is used. >50kg: 6mg rapid IV bolus infusion over 1-2 seconds. If not converted to SR within 1-2 minutes, give 12mg rapid IV bolus; may give 2nd 12mg dose if needed. Max: 12mg/dose.

**HOW SUPPLIED:** Inj: 3mg/mL [2mL, 4mL]

**CONTRAINDICATIONS:** 2nd- or 3rd-degree AV block (except with pacemaker), sinus node disease such as sick sinus syndrome or symptomatic bradycardia (except with pacemaker).

**WARNINGS/PRECAUTIONS:** May produce short-lasting heart block. Transient or prolonged asystole, respiratory alkalosis, ventricular fibrillation reported. Caution with obstructive lung disease (eg, emphysema, bronchitis). Avoid with bronchoconstriction/bronchospasm (eg, asthma). D/C if severe respiratory difficulties develop. New arrhythmias may appear on ECG at time of conversion. Caution in elderly.

**ADVERSE REACTIONS:** Facial flushing, dyspnea/shortness of breath, chest pressure, nausea.

**INTERACTIONS:** Antagonized by methylxanthines (eg, theophylline, caffeine); may need larger adenosine dose. Potentiated by dipyridamole; use lower adenosine dose. Caution with digoxin, verapamil; ventricular fibrillation reported and potential for additive/synergistic depressant effects on the SA and AV nodes. Possible higher degrees of heart block with carbamazepine.

**PREGNANCY:** Category C, safety in nursing not known.

## ADENOSCAN

RX

adenosine (Astellas)

**THERAPEUTIC CLASS:** Vasodilator

**INDICATIONS:** Adjunct to thalium-201 myocardial perfusion scintigraphy in patients unable to exercise adequately.

**DOSAGE:** *Adults:* 140mcg/kg/min IV for 6 minutes (total dose 0.84mg/kg). Inject thallium-201 at midpoint of infusion.

**HOW SUPPLIED:** Inj: 3mg/mL

**CONTRAINDICATIONS:** 2nd-or 3rd-degree AV block (except with a pacemaker), sinus node disease, bronchosconstrictive or bronchospastic lung disease.

**WARNINGS/PRECAUTIONS:** Fatal cardiac arrest, sustained ventricular tachycardia, MI reported. Exerts depressant effect on SA and AV nodes and may cause 1st-, 2nd-, 3rd-degree AV block or sinus bradycardia. May precipitate significant hypotension. Caution with autonomic dysfunction, stenotic valvular heart disease, pericarditis, stenotic carotid artery disease with CVA, uncorrected hypovolemia. Increase in BP reported. May cause bronchoconstriction in asthmatics.

**ADVERSE REACTIONS:** Flushing, chest discomfort, dyspnea, headache, throat, neck or jaw discomfort, GI disturbances, dizziness, ST segment depression, 1st and 2nd degree AV block, paresthesia, hypotension, nervousness, arrhythmia.

**INTERACTIONS:** Potential synergistic effects with other cardioactive drugs (eg, β-blockers, cardiac glycosides, and calcium channel blockers). Diminished effects with adenosine receptor antagonists (eg, theophylline, caffeine). Withold drugs that may inhibit or augment effects for at least 5 half-lives.

**PREGNANCY:** Category C, safety in nursing not known.

## ADIPEX-P — CIV

phentermine HCl (Gate)

**THERAPEUTIC CLASS:** Anorectic sympathomimetic amine

**INDICATIONS:** Short term adjunct for exogenous obesity if initial BMI >30 kg/m² or >27 kg/m² with other risk factors (eg, hypertension, diabetes hyperlipidemia).

**DOSAGE:** *Adults:* Usual: 37.5mg before breakfast or 1-2 hrs after breakfast. Alternate Schedule: 18.75mg qd-bid. Avoid late evening dosing.
*Pediatrics:* >16 yrs: Usual: 37.5mg before breakfast or 1-2 hrs after breakfast. Alternate Schedule: 18.75mg qd-bid. Avoid late evening dosing.

**HOW SUPPLIED:** Cap: 37.5mg; Tab: 37.5mg* *scored

**CONTRAINDICATIONS:** Advanced arteriosclerosis, cardiovascular disease, moderate to severe HTN, hyperthyroidism, glaucoma, agitated states, history of drug abuse, within 14 days of MAOI use.

**WARNINGS/PRECAUTIONS:** Only for short-term therapy. Primary pulmonary HTN and valvular heart disease reported. Abuse potential. Caution with mild HTN. Tolerance may develop.

**ADVERSE REACTIONS:** Primary pulmonary hypertension, regurgitant valvular heart disease, palpitation, tachycardia, BP elevation, CNS overstimulation, dry mouth, impotence, urticaria.

**INTERACTIONS:** May alter insulin requirements. Avoid alcohol and other weight loss products including SSRIs. Valvular heart disease and primary pulmonary hypertension reported with fenfluramine and dexfenfluramine. May decrease effects of guanethidine.

**PREGNANCY:** Category C, not for use in nursing.

## ADRIAMYCIN — RX

doxorubicin HCl (Bedford)

**Severe local tissue necrosis will occur if extravasation occurs. Do not give IM/SC route. Myocardial toxicity may occur during or after therapy. Increased risk of CHF with high cumulative doses, previous anthracycline/anthracenedione therapy, pre-existing heart disease, radiotherapy to mediastinal/pericardial area, concomitant cardiotoxic drugs. Increased risk of delayed cardiotoxicity in pediatrics. Secondary acute myelogenous leukemia reported. Reduce dose in hepatic impairment. Severe myelosuppression may occur.**

**THERAPEUTIC CLASS:** Anthracycline

**INDICATIONS:** To produce regression in disseminated neoplastic conditions such as acute lymphoblastic and myeloblastic leukemias, Wilms' tumor, neuroblastoma, soft tissue/bone sarcomas, carcinomas of the breast, ovary, bladder and thyroid, gastric and bronchogenic carcinomas, Hodgkin's disease, malignant lymphoma in which the small cell histologic type is the most responsive compared to other cell types.

**DOSAGE:** *Adults:* Monotherapy: 60-75mg/m² IV every 21 days. Use the lower dose with inadequate bone marrow reserves due to old age, prior therapy, or neoplastic marrow infiltration. Concomitant Chemotherapy: 40-60mg/m² IV every 21-28 days. Hyperbilirubinemia: Reduce dose by 50% if 1.2-3mg/dL; reduce dose by 75% if 3.1-5mg/dL.
*Pediatrics:* Monotherapy: 60-75mg/m² IV every 21 days. Use the lower dose with inadequate bone marrow reserves due to old age, prior therapy, or neoplastic marrow infiltration. Concomitant Chemotherapy: 40-60mg/m² IV

every 21-28 days. Hyperbilirubinemia: Reduce dose by 50% if 1.2-3mg/dL; reduce dose by 75% if 3.1-5mg/dL.

**HOW SUPPLIED:** Inj: 2mg/mL, 10mg, 20mg, 50mg

**CONTRAINDICATIONS:** Marked myelosuppression induced by previous treatment with other antitumor agents or radiotherapy. Previous therapy with complete cumulative doses of doxorubicin, daunorubicin, idarubicin, or other anthracyclines and anthracenes.

**WARNINGS/PRECAUTIONS:** Irreversible myocardial toxicity may occur. Bone marrow depression and arrhythmias reported. Enhanced toxicity with hepatic impairment; evaluate hepatic function before dosing. Imparts a red coloration to urine for 1-2 days after administration. May induce"tumor lysis syndrome" and hyperuricemia with rapidly growing tumors. Periodically monitor CBC, hepatic function, and radionuclide left ventricular ejection fraction. May cause prepubertal growth failure and gonadal impairment.

**ADVERSE REACTIONS:** Myelosuppression, cardiotoxicity, alopecia, nausea, vomiting, mucositis, ulceration and necrosis of colon, fever, chills, urticaria, phlebosclerosis, facial flushing.

**INTERACTIONS:** May potentiate toxicity of other anticancer therapies. May exacerbate cyclophosphamide-induced hemorrhagic cystitis. May enhance hepatotoxicity of 6-mercaptopurine. May increase radiation induced toxicity of the myocardium, mucosae, skin, and liver. Acute"recall" pneumonitis in pediatrics with actinomycin-D. Paclitaxel infused before doxorubicin may decrease clearance of doxorubicin and increase neutropenia and stomatitis episodes, than the reverse sequence of administration. Enhanced neutropenia and thrombocytopenia reported with IV progesterone. Cyclosporine may prolong and exacerbate hematologic toxicity. Phenobarbital increases elimination. May decrease phenytoin levels. Streptozocin may inhibit hepatic metabolism. Live vaccines may be hazardous in those undergoing cytotoxic chemotherapy. Necrotizing colitis reported with cytarabine. Seizures and coma reported with cyclosporine, cisplatin or vincristine. Possible increased risk of cardiotoxicity with calcium channel blockers. Increased risk of CHF with radiotherapy to mediastinal/pericardial area or cardiotoxic drugs.

**PREGNANCY:** Category D, not for use in nursing.

## ADRUCIL

fluorouracil (Sicor) RX

**Hospitalize patient during initial therapy due to possible severe toxic reactions.**

**THERAPEUTIC CLASS:** Antimetabolite

**INDICATIONS:** Palliative management of colon, rectum, breast, stomach, and pancreatic carcinomas.

**DOSAGE:** *Adults:* 12mg/kg IV qd for 4 days. Max: 800mg/day. If no toxicity, give 6mg/kg IV on 6th, 8th, 10th, and 12th days. Skip days 5, 7, 9, and 11. Inadequate Nutritional State: 6mg/kg IV for 3 days. If no toxicity, give 3mg/kg IV on 5th, 7th, and 9th days. Max: 400mg/day. Skip days 4, 6, and 8. Maint (Use Schedule 1 or Schedule 2): Schedule 1: If no toxicity, repeat 1st course every 30 days after last day of previous course. Schedule 2: When toxic signs from initial course subside, give 10-15mg/kg/week IV single dose; do not exceed 1g/week.

**HOW SUPPLIED:** Inj: 50mg/mL

**CONTRAINDICATIONS:** Poor nutritional state, depressed bone marrow function, potentially serious infection.

**WARNINGS/PRECAUTIONS:** Extreme caution in poor risk patients with history of high-dose irradiation, previous use of alkylating agents, hepatic/renal dysfunction, widespread bone marrow involvement by metastatic tumors. Dipyrimidine dehydrogenase deficiency prolongs 5-fluorouracil clearance; can cause severe toxicity. May cause fetal harm in pregnancy. Other therapy interfering with nutrition or depressing bone marrow function increases toxicity. Discontinue with stomatitis, esophagopharyngitis, leukopenia, intractable vomiting, diarrhea, GI ulceration or bleeding, thrombocytopenia, or hemorrhage from any site. Palmar-plantar erythrodysesthesia syndrome (hand-foot syndrome) reported. Perform WBC with differential before each dose. Narrow margin of safety; monitor patients very closely.

**ADVERSE REACTIONS:** Stomatitis, esophagopharyngitis, diarrhea, anorexia, nausea, emesis, leukopenia, alopecia, dermatitis.

**INTERACTIONS:** Leucovorin calcium may enhance toxicity.

**PREGNANCY:** Category D, not for use in nursing.

## ADVAIR

RX

salmeterol xinafoate - fluticasone propionate (GlaxoSmithKline)

> **Long-acting $\beta_2$-adrenergic agonists, such as salmeterol, may increase the risk of asthma-related deaths.**

**THERAPEUTIC CLASS:** Corticosteroid/beta$_2$ agonist

**INDICATIONS:** For long-term, maintenance treatment of asthma. (250/50mcg only): Treatment of COPD with chronic bronchitis.

**DOSAGE:** *Adults:* Asthma: 1 inh q12h. Without Prior Inhaled Corticosteroid (CS): Initial: 100/50 bid. Max: 500/50 bid. Current Inhaled CS: Beclomethasone: ≤160mcg/day use 100/50 bid, 320mcg/day use 250/50Bid, 640mcg/day use 500/50 bid. Budesonide: ≤400mcg/day use 100/50 bid, 800-1200mcg/day use 250/50 bid, 1600mcg/day use 500/50 bid. Flunisolide: ≤1000mcg/day use 100/50 bid, 1250-2000mcg/day use 250/50 bid. Flunisolide HFA: ≤320mcg/day use 100/50 bid, 640mcg/day use 250/50 bid. Fluticasone HFA: ≤176mcg/day use 100/50 bid, 440mcg/day use 250/50 bid, 660-880mcg/day use 500/50 bid. Fluticasone Powder: ≤200mcg/day use 100/50 bid, 500mcg/day use 250/50 bid, 1000mcg/day use 500/50 bid. Mometasone: 220mcg/day use 100/50 bid, 440mcg/day use 250/50 bid, 880mcg/day use 500/50 bid. Triamcinolone: ≤1000mcg/day use 100/50 bid, 1100-1600mcg/day use 250/50 bid. If no response within 2 weeks, increase to higher strength. COPD: (250/50 only): 1 inh q12h. Rinse mouth after use. *Pediatrics:* ≥12 yrs: 1 inh q12h. Without Prior Inhaled CS: Initial: 100/50 bid. Max: 500/50 bid. Current Inhaled CS: Beclomethasone: ≤160mcg/day use 100/50 bid, 320mcg/day use 250/50 Bid, 640mcg/day use 500/50 bid. Budesonide: ≤400mcg/day use 100/50 bid, 800-1200mcg/day use 250/50 bid, 1600mcg/day use 500/50 bid. Flunisolide: ≤1000mcg/day use 100/50 bid, 1250-2000mcg/day use 250/50 bid. Flunisolide HFA: ≤320mcg/day use 100/50 bid, 640mcg/day use 250/50 bid. Fluticasone HFA: ≤176mcg/day use 100/50 bid, 440mcg/day use 250/50 bid, 660-880mcg/day use 500/50 bid. Fluticasone Powder: ≤200mcg/day use 100/50 bid, 500mcg/day use 250/50 bid, 1000mcg/day use 500/50 bid. Mometasone: 220mcg/day use 100/50 bid, 440mcg/day use 250/50 bid, 880mcg/day use 500/50 bid. Triamcinolone: ≤1000mcg/day use 100/50 bid, 1100-1600mcg/day use 250/50 bid. If no response within 2 weeks, increase to higher strength. 4-11 yrs: (100/50mcg only): Symptomatic on Inhaled CS: 1 inh q12h. Rinse mouth after use.

**HOW SUPPLIED:** Disk (Inhalation): (Fluticasone-Salmeterol) (100/50) 0.1mg-0.05mg/inh, (250/50) 0.25mg-0.05mg/inh, (500/50) 0.5mg-0.05mg/inh [60 blisters]

**CONTRAINDICATIONS:** Status asthmaticus or other acute asthma or COPD episodes.

**WARNINGS/PRECAUTIONS:** See Contraindications. Deaths due to adrenal insufficiency have occurred with transfer from systemic corticosteroids to inhaled corticosteroids. Resume oral corticosteroids during stress or severe asthma attack. Observe for adrenal insufficiency, systemic corticosteroid withdrawal effects, hypercorticism, reduction in growth velocity (pediatrics). More susceptible to infection. Not for acute bronchospasm. Discontinue if bronchospasm occurs after dosing. Caution with TB; untreated systemic fungal, bacterial, viral or parasitic infections; or ocular herpes simplex. *Candida* infection of mouth and pharynx, glaucoma, hypersensitivity reactions, increased IOP, cataracts reported. Monitor for increasing use of $\beta_2$ agonists. QTc interval prolongation reported with large doses. Discontinue if paradoxical bronchospasm occurs. Caution with cardiovascular disorders.

**ADVERSE REACTIONS:** Upper respiratory tract inflammation, pharyngitis, sinusitis, cough, hoarseness, headaches, GI effects, musculoskeletal pain, palpitations.

**INTERACTIONS:** Extreme caution with TCAs or MAOIs during or within 14 days of use. Antagonized by β-blockers. Caution with non-potassium sparing diuretics; ECG changes, hypokalemia may develop. Potentiated by ketoconazole, other CYP3A4 inhibitors.

**PREGNANCY:** Category C, caution in nursing.

## ADVAIR HFA

RX

salmeterol xinafoate - fluticasone propionate (GlaxoSmithKline)

**Long-acting $\beta_2$-adrenergic agonists, such as salmeterol, may increase the risk of asthma-related deaths.**

**THERAPEUTIC CLASS:** Corticosteroid/beta$_2$ agonist

**INDICATIONS:** For long-term, maintenance treatment of asthma.

**DOSAGE:** *Adults:* Asthma: 2 inh q12h. Without Prior Inhaled Corticosteroid (CS): Initial: 2 inh of 45/21 bid or 1 inh of 115/21 bid. Max: 2 inh of 230/21 bid. Current Inhaled CS: Beclomethasone: ≤160mcg/day use 2 inh of 45/21 bid, 320mcg/day use 2 inh of 115/21 bid, 640mcg/day use 2 inh of 230/21 bid. Budesonide: ≤400mcg/day use 2 inh of 45/21 bid, 800-1200mcg/day use 2 inh of 115/21 bid, 1600mcg/day use 2 inh of 230/21 bid. Flunisolide: ≤1000mcg/day use 2 inh of 45/21 bid, 1250-2000mcg/day use 2 inh of 115/21 bid. Flunisolide HFA: ≤320mcg/day use 2 inh of 45/21 bid, 640mcg/day use 2 inh of 115/21 bid. Fluticasone Aerosol: ≤176mcg/day use 2 inh of 45/21 bid, 440mcg/day use 2 inh of 115/21 bid, 660-880mcg/day use 2 inh of 230/21 bid. Fluticasone Powder: ≤200mcg/day use 2 inh of 45/21 bid, 500mcg/day use 2 inh of 115/21 bid, 1000mcg/day use 2 inh of 230/21 bid. Mometasone Powder: 220mcg/day use 2 inh of 45/21 bid, 440mcg/day use 2 inh of 115/21 bid, 880mcg/day use 2 inh of 230/21 bid. Triamcinolone: ≤1000mcg/day use 2 inh of 45/21 bid, 1100-1600mcg/day use 2 inh of 115/21 bid. If no response within 2 weeks, increase to higher strength.
*Pediatrics:* ≥12 yrs: Asthma: 2 inh q12h. Without Prior Inhaled Corticosteroid (CS): Initial: 2 inh of 45/21 bid or 1 inh of 115/21 bid. Max: 2 inh of 230-21 bid. Current Inhaled CS: Beclomethasone: ≤160mcg/day use 2 inh of 45/21 bid, 320mcg/day use 2 inh of 115/21 bid, 640mcg/day use 2 inh of 230/21 bid. Budesonide: ≤400mcg/day use 2 inh of 45/21 bid, 800-1200mcg/day use 2 inh of 115/21 bid, 1600mcg/day use 2 inh of 230/21 bid. Flunisolide: ≤1000mcg/day use 2 inh of 45/21 bid, 1250-2000mcg/day use 2 inh of 115/21 bid. Flunisolide HFA: ≤320mcg/day use 2 inh of 45/21 bid, 640mcg/day use 2 inh of 115/21 bid. Fluticasone Aerosol: ≤176mcg/day use 2 inh of 45/21 bid, 440mcg/day use 2 inh of 115/21 bid, 660-880mcg/day use 2 inh of 230/21 bid. Fluticasone Powder: ≤200mcg/day use 2 inh of 45/21 bid, 500mcg/day use 2 inh of 115/21 bid, 1000mcg/day use 2 inh of 230/21 bid. Mometasone powder: 220mcg/day use 2 inh of 45/21 bid, 440mcg/day use 2 inh of 115/21 bid, 880mcg/day use 2 inh of 230/21 bid. Triamcinolone: ≤1000mcg/day use 2 inh of 45/21 bid, 1100-1600mcg/day use 2 inh of 115/21 bid. If no response within 2 weeks, increase to higher strength.

**HOW SUPPLIED:** MDI: (Fluticasone-Salmeterol) (45/21) 0.045mg-0.021mg/inh, (115/21) 0.115mg-0.021mg/inh, (230/21) 0.230mg-0.021mg/inh [120 inhalations]

**CONTRAINDICATIONS:** Status asthmaticus or other acute asthma.

**WARNINGS/PRECAUTIONS:** See Contraindications. Deaths due to adrenal insufficiency have occurred with transfer from systemic corticosteroids to inhaled corticosteroids. Resume oral corticosteroids during stress or severe asthma attack. Observe for adrenal insufficiency, systemic corticosteroid withdrawal effects, hypercorticism, reduction in growth velocity (pediatrics). More susceptible to infection. Not for acute bronchospasm. Discontinue if bronchospasm occurs after dosing. Caution with TB; untreated systemic fungal, bacterial, viral or parasitic infections; or ocular herpes simplex. Candida infection of mouth and pharynx, glaucoma, hypersensitivity reactions, increased IOP, cataracts reported. Monitor for increasing use of $\beta_2$ agonists. QTc interval prolongation reported with large doses. Discontinue if paradoxical bronchospasm occurs. Caution with cardiovascular disorders.

**ADVERSE REACTIONS:** Upper respiratory tract infection, throat irritation, upper respiratory tract inflammation, headaches, nausea, vomiting, musculoskeletal pain, menstruation symptoms.

**INTERACTIONS:** Extreme caution with TCAs or MAOIs during or within 14 days of use. Antagonized by β-blockers. Caution with non-potassium sparing diuretics; ECG changes, hypokalemia may develop. Potentiated by ketoconazole, other CYP3A4 inhibitors.

**PREGNANCY:** Category C, caution in nursing.

## ADVICOR — RX

niacin - lovastatin (Kos)

**THERAPEUTIC CLASS:** B-complex vitamin/HMG-CoA reductase inhibitor

**INDICATIONS:** Treatment of primary hypercholesterolemia and mixed dyslipidemia (Types IIa, IIb) in patients on lovastatin therapy requiring further TG lowering or HDL raising who may benefit from addition of niacin; or in patients on niacin therapy requiring further LDL lowering who may benefit from addition of lovastatin. Not for initial therapy.

**DOSAGE:** *Adults:* >18 yrs: Initial: 500mg-20mg qhs. Titrate: Increase by no more than 500mg of niacin every 4 weeks. Max: 2000mg-40mg. Concomitant Cyclosporine/Fibrates: Max: 1000mg-20mg. Swallow tab whole. Take with low-fat snack.

**HOW SUPPLIED:** Tab: (Niacin Extended Release-Lovastatin) 500mg-20mg, 750mg-20mg, 1000mg-20mg

**CONTRAINDICATIONS:** Active liver disease, unexplained persistent elevations in serum transaminases, active PUD, arterial bleeding, pregnancy, nursing mothers.

**WARNINGS/PRECAUTIONS:** Do not substitute for equivalent dose of immediate-release niacin. Myopathy, rhabdomyolysis, severe hepatotoxicity reported. Caution with history of liver disease or jaundice, heavy alcohol use, hepatobilliary disease, peptic ulcer, diabetes, unstable angina, acute phase of MI, gout, renal dysfunction. Monitor LFTs prior to therapy, every 6-12 weeks for 1st 6 months, and periodically thereafter. May elevate PT, uric acid levels. Discontinue if AST or ALT >3X ULN persist, if myopathy diagnosed or suspected, and a few days before surgery. May reduce phosphorous levels.

**ADVERSE REACTIONS:** Flushing, asthenia, flu syndrome, headache, infection, pain, GI effects, hyperglycemia, pruritus, rash.

**INTERACTIONS:** May potentiate ganglionic blockers, vasoactive drugs. Decreased niacin clearance with ASA. Separate bile acid sequestrants by 4-6 hrs. Avoid concomitant alcohol and hot drinks; may increase flushing and pruritus. Antidiabetic agents may need adjustment. Caution with niacin-containing nutritional supplements. Increased risk of skeletal muscle disorders with CYP3A4 inhibitors (eg, cyclosporine, itraconazole, ketoconazole, erythromycin, clarithromycin, protease inhibitors, nefazodone, >1 quart/day of grapefruit juice), verapamil, fibrates (eg, gemfibrozil). Monitor warfarin. Caution with drugs that diminish levels or activity of steroid hormones (eg, ketoconazole, spironolactone, cimetidine). Caution with acute MI and nitrates, calcium channel blockers, and adrenergic blockers.

**PREGNANCY:** Category X, not for use in nursing.

## ADVIL MIGRAINE

OTC

ibuprofen (Wyeth Consumer)

**THERAPEUTIC CLASS:** NSAID

**INDICATIONS:** Treatment of migraine headache.

**DOSAGE:** *Adults:* 2 caps with water. Max: 2 caps/24hrs.

**HOW SUPPLIED:** Cap: 200mg

**WARNINGS/PRECAUTIONS:** May cause severe allergic reaction (eg, hives, facial swelling, asthma, shock).

**INTERACTIONS:** Risk of stomach bleeding with alcohol.

**PREGNANCY:** Safety in pregnancy and nursing not known.

## AEROBID

RX

flunisolide (Forest)

**OTHER BRAND NAMES:** Aerobid-M (with menthol) (Forest)

**THERAPEUTIC CLASS:** Corticosteroid

**INDICATIONS:** Maintenance treatment of asthma as prophylactic therapy in patients ≥6 years and to reduce or eliminate the need for oral systemic corticosteroidal therapy.

**DOSAGE:** *Adults:* Initial: 2 inh bid. Max: 4 inh bid. Rinse mouth after use. *Pediatrics:* 6-15 yrs: 2 inh bid. Rinse mouth after use.

**HOW SUPPLIED:** MDI: 0.25mg/inh [7g]

**CONTRAINDICATIONS:** Primary treatment of status asthmaticus or other acute asthma attacks.

**WARNINGS/PRECAUTIONS:** Deaths due to adrenal insufficiency have occurred with transfer from systemic corticosteroids to inhaled corticosteroids. Resume oral corticosteroids during stress or severe asthma attack. Observe for adrenal insufficiency, systemic corticosteroid withdrawal effects, and growth suppression (children). More susceptible to infections. Not for acute bronchospasm. D/C if bronchospasm occurs after dosing. Caution with tuberculosis of the respiratory tract; untreated systemic fungal, bacterial, viral or parasitic infections; or ocular herpes simplex. *Candida* infection of the mouth and pharynx reported.

**ADVERSE REACTIONS:** Upper respiratory infection, diarrhea, stomach upset, cold symptoms, nasal congestion, headache, nausea, vomiting, sore throat, unpleasant taste.

**PREGNANCY:** Category C, caution with nursing.

## AGENERASE

RX

amprenavir (GlaxoSmithKline)

**Oral solution contains propylene glycol; risk of toxicity in pediatrics <4 yrs, pregnant women, hepatic or renal failure, and concomitant disulfiram or metronidazole.**

**THERAPEUTIC CLASS:** Protease inhibitor

**INDICATIONS:** Treatment of HIV infection in combination with other antiretrovirals.

**DOSAGE:** *Adults:* (Cap) 1200mg bid. Hepatic Impairment (Child-Pugh score 5-8): 450mg bid. (Child-Pugh score 9-12) 300mg bid. Avoid high-fat meals.

(Sol): 1400mg bid
*Pediatrics:* (Cap) 13-16 yrs: 1200mg bid. 13-16 yrs and <50kg or 4-12yrs: 20mg/kg bid or 15mg/kg tid. Max: 2400mg/day. Hepatic Impairment (Child-Pugh score 5-8): 450mg bid. (Child-Pugh score 9-12) 300mg bid. Avoid high-fat meals. (Sol) >16 yrs or 13-16 yrs and >50kg: 1400mg bid. 4-12 yrs or 13-16 yrs and <50kg: 22.5mg/kg bid or 17mg/kg tid. Max: 2800mg/day.

**HOW SUPPLIED:** Cap: 50mg; Sol: 15mg/mL [240mL]

**CONTRAINDICATIONS:** (Cap, Sol) Drugs highly dependent on CYP450 3A4 for clearance (eg, dihydroergotamine, ergonovine, ergotamine, methylergonovine, cisapride, pimozide, midazolam, triazolam). (Sol) <4 yrs, pregnancy, hepatic or renal failure, concomitant disulfiram or metronidazole. (Cap) Flecanide and propafenone if coadministered with ritonavir.

**WARNINGS/PRECAUTIONS:** Caution with sulfonamide allergy. Spontaneous bleeding may occur with hemophilia A and B. Possible redistribution or accumulation of body fat. Caps and solution are not interchangeable on mg-mg basis. Severe life-threatening reactions including Stevens-Johnson syndrome reported. New onset and exacerbation of diabetes and hyperglycemia reported. May elevate LFTs; caution with hepatic impairment. May increase cholesterol and triglycerides; monitor before therapy and periodically thereafter.

**ADVERSE REACTIONS:** Severe skin reactions, rash, paresthesias, depression, nausea, vomiting, diarrhea, abdominal pain, hyperlipidemia.

**INTERACTIONS:** Serious/life-threatening interactions may occur with amiodarone, lidocaine (systemic), TCAs, and quinidine. Monitor INR with warfarin. Avoid supplemental vitamin E. Avoid astemizole, terfenadine, pimozide, ergonovine, methylergonovine, midazolam, triazolam, dihydroergotamine, ergotamine, and cisapride. Possible loss of virologic response and resistance with rifampin and St. John's wort. Give 50% of rifabutin dose. Increased risk of rhabdomyolysis with lovastatin, simvastatin. Increased sildenafil levels. Take 1 hr before or after antacids and didanosine. Increased levels of ketoconazole, itraconazole, alprazolam, clorazepate, diazepam, flurazepam, and calcium channel blockers. Oral contraceptives (ethinyl estradiol/norethindrone) may decrease efficacy and lead to resistance; use alternative non-hormonal contraception. Decreases methodone levels. Phenobarbital, phenytoin, and carbamazepine decrease levels. Increased bepridil levels; life-threatening reaction can occur. Decreased levels with dexamethasone. Monitor levels of cyclosporine, tacrolimus, rapamycin, and TCAs. Avoid solution administration with ritonavir solution. Reduce dose with ritonavir caps. Elevated LFTs, cholesterol, and TG with low-dose ritonavir. Use lowest possible dose of atorvastatin or consider other HMG-CoA reductase inhibitor.

**PREGNANCY:** (Cap) Category C, (Sol) Contraindicated in pregnancy; not for use in nursing.

## AGGRASTAT RX

tirofiban HCl (Medicure)

**THERAPEUTIC CLASS:** Glycoprotein IIb/IIIa inhibitor

**INDICATIONS:** In combination with heparin, for treatment of acute coronary syndrome, in patients being medically managed or undergoing PTCA or atherectomy.

**DOSAGE:** *Adults:* Initial: 0.4mcg/kg/min IV for 30 minutes. Maint: 0.1mcg/kg/min IV. Continue through angiography and for 12-24 hrs after angioplasty or atherectomy. CrCl <30mL/min: Administer half of the usual rate of infusion.

**HOW SUPPLIED:** Inj: 0.05mg/mL, 0.25mg/mL

**CONTRAINDICATIONS:** Active internal bleeding, acute pericarditis, severe HTN, concomitant parenteral GP IIb/IIIa inhibitor, hemorrhagic stroke, aortic dissection, thrombocytopenia with prior exposure. Bleeding diathesis, stroke, major surgical procedure, or severe physical trauma within past 30 days. History of intracranial hemorrhage or neoplasm, arteriovenous malformation, aneurysm.

**WARNINGS/PRECAUTIONS:** Bleeding reported. Monitor platelets, Hgb, Hct before treatment, within 6 hrs after loading infusion, and daily during therapy. Monitor platelets earlier if previous GP IIb/IIIa inhibitor use. Determine APTT before and during therapy with heparin. Caution with platelets <150,000/mm$^3$, hemorrhagic retinopathy, chronic hemodialysis patients, femoral access site in percutaneous coronary intervention. Minimize vascular and other trauma. D/C if thrombocytopenia confirmed or if bleeding cannot be controlled by pressure.

**ADVERSE REACTIONS:** Bleeding, nausea, fever, headache, edema, anaphylaxis.

**INTERACTIONS:** Avoid other parenteral GP IIb/IIIa inhibitors. Increased bleeding with heparin and ASA. Caution with other drugs that affect hemostasis (eg, warfarin). Increased clearance with levothyroxine, omeprazole.

**PREGNANCY:** Category B, not for use in nursing.

## AGGRENOX — RX

aspirin - dipyridamole (Boehringer Ingelheim)

**THERAPEUTIC CLASS:** Platelet aggregation inhibitor

**INDICATIONS:** Reduce the risk of stroke in patients with transient brain ischemia or complete ischemic stroke due to thrombosis.

**DOSAGE:** *Adults:* 1 cap bid (am and pm).

**HOW SUPPLIED:** Cap: (Dipyridamole Extended Release-ASA) 200mg-25mg

**CONTRAINDICATIONS:** NSAID allergy, children or teenagers with viral infections, syndrome of asthma, rhinitis, nasal polyps.

**WARNINGS/PRECAUTIONS:** Increased risk of bleeding with chronic, heavy alcohol use. Caution with inherited or acquired bleeding disorders, severe CAD, and hypotension. Monitor for signs of GI ulcers and bleeding. Avoid with history of peptic ulcer disease, severe renal failure (CrCl <10mL/min). Risk of hepatic dysfunction. Not interchangeable with individual components of aspirin and Persantine® Tablets. Avoid in 3rd trimester of pregnancy.

**ADVERSE REACTIONS:** Headache, dyspepsia, abdominal pain, nausea, diarrhea, vomiting, fatigue, arthralgia, pain, hemorrhage.

**INTERACTIONS:** May decrease effects of ACE inhibitors, cholinesterase inhibitors, phenytoin, β-blockers. Potentiates adenosine, acetazolamide, methotrexate, oral hypoglycemics, valproic acid. Anticoagulants increase risk of bleeding. Decreased effects of diuretics in renal or cardiovascular disease. NSAIDs may increase risk of bleeding and decrease renal function. May antagonize uricosuric agents.

**PREGNANCY:** Category B (dipyridamole), Category D (aspirin), caution in nursing.

## AGRYLIN — RX

anagrelide HCl (Shire US)

**THERAPEUTIC CLASS:** Platelet-reducing agent

**INDICATIONS:** Treatment of thrombocythemia secondary to myeloproliferative disorders.

**DOSAGE:** *Adults:* Initial: 0.5mg qid or 1mg bid for at least 1 week. Moderate Hepatic Impairment: Initial: 0.5mg qd for at least 1 week. Titrate: Increase by no more than 0.5mg/day per week. Max: 10mg/day or 2.5mg/dose. Adjust lowest effective dose to reduce and maintain platelets <600,000/mcL. Monitor platelets every 2 days during first week, then weekly thereafter until reach

maintenance dose.
*Pediatrics:* Initial: 0.5mg qd. Titrate: Increase by no more than 0.5mg/day per week. Max: 10mg/day or 2.5mg/dose. Adjust to lowest effective dose to reduce and maintain platelets <600,000/mcL. Monitor platelets every 2 days during first week, then weekly thereafter until reach maintenance dose.

**HOW SUPPLIED:** Cap: 0.5mg, 1mg

**CONTRAINDICATIONS:** Severe hepatic impairment.

**WARNINGS/PRECAUTIONS:** Caution with heart disease, renal or hepatic dysfunction. Perform pre-treatment cardiovascular exam and monitor during treatment; may cause cardiovascular effects (eg, vasodilation, tachycardia, palpitations, CHF). Monitor closely for renal toxicity if creatinine >2mg/dL or hepatic toxicity if bilirubin, SGOT, or LFTs >1.5X ULN). Monitor blood counts, renal and hepatic function while platelets are lowered. Increase in platelets after therapy interruption. Reduce dose in moderate hepatic impairment.

**ADVERSE REACTIONS:** Headache, palpitations, asthenia, edema, GI effects, dizziness, pain, dyspnea, fever, chest pain, rash, tachycardia, malaise, pharyngitis, cough, paresthesia.

**INTERACTIONS:** Sucralfate may interfere with absorption. Exacerbated effects of products that inhibit cyclic AMP PDE III (inotropes: milrinone, enoximone, amrinone, olparinone, cilostazol).

**PREGNANCY:** Category C, not for use in nursing.

## AK-FLUOR RX

fluorescein sodium (Akorn)

**THERAPEUTIC CLASS:** Diagnostic dye

**INDICATIONS:** Indicated in diagnostic fluorescein angiography or angioscopy of the fundus and iris vasculature.

**DOSAGE:** *Adults:* Perform intradermal skin test before IV use if suspect potential allergy. Inject contents of ampule rapidly into antecubital vein. A syringe with fluorescein is attached to transparent tubing and a 25 gauge scalp vein needle for injection. Insert needle and draw patient's blood to hub of syringe so small air bubble separates patient's blood in tubing from fluorescein. With room lights on, inject blood back into vein while watching skin over needle tip. If needle extravasated, patient's blood will bulge skin; stop injection before injecting fluorescein. When certain there is no extravasation, turn room light off and complete fluorescein injection. Luminescence appears in retina and choroidal vessels in 9-14 seconds.
*Pediatrics:* Perform intradermal skin test before IV use if suspect potential allergy. Dose is 35mg/10lbs. Inject contents of ampule/vial rapidly into antecubital vein. A syringe with fluorescein is attached to transparent tubing and a 25 gauge scalp vein needle for injection. Insert needle and draw patient's blood to hub of syringe so small air bubble separates patient's blood in tubing from fluorescein. With room lights on, inject blood back into vein while watching skin over needle tip. If needle extravasated, patient's blood will bulge skin; stop injection before injecting fluorescein. When certain there is no extravasation, turn room light off and complete fluorescein injection. Luminescence appears in retina and choroidal vessels in 9-14 seconds.

**HOW SUPPLIED:** Inj: 10% [5mL], 25% [2mL]

**WARNINGS/PRECAUTIONS:** Avoid extravasation; severe local tissue damage can occur. Caution with history of allergy or bronchial asthma. Have emergency tray (eg, 0.1% epinephrine IV/IM, antihistamine, soluble steroid, IV aminophylline) and oxygen available. Avoid angiography in pregnancy, especially 1st trimester. Skin attains temporary yellowish discoloration and urine attains bright yellow color.

**ADVERSE REACTIONS:** Nausea, vomiting, headache, GI distress, syncope, hypotension, cardiac arrest, basilar artery ischemia, severe shock, convulsions, thrombophlebitis.

**PREGNANCY:** Safety in pregnancy not known, caution in nursing.

## ALACOL DM RX

phenylephrine HCl - dextromethorphan hbr - brompheniramine maleate (Ballay)

**THERAPEUTIC CLASS:** Antihistamine/antitussive/sympathomimetic

**INDICATIONS:** Relief of cough and upper respiratory symptoms including nasal congestion, associated with allergy or the common cold.

**DOSAGE:** *Adults:* 10mL q4h. Max: 6 doses/24 hrs.
*Pediatrics:* >12 yrs: 10mL q4h. 6-12 yrs: 5mL q4h. 2-6 yrs: 2.5mL q4h. Max: 6 doses/24 hrs.

**HOW SUPPLIED:** Syrup: (Brompheniramine-Dextromethorphan-Phenylephrine) 2mg-10mg-5mg/5mL

**CONTRAINDICATIONS:** Newborns, premature infants, nursing, severe HTN or CAD, with MAOIs, lower respiratory tract conditions including asthma.

**WARNINGS/PRECAUTIONS:** Caution with persistent or chronic cough (eg, associated with asthma, emphysema, smoking, excessive phlegm). Persistent cough may be a sign of a serious condition. May diminish mental alertness. May produce excitation in children. Caution with asthma, narrow-angle glaucoma, GI obstruction, urinary bladder neck obstruction, DM, HTN, heart and thyroid disease.

**ADVERSE REACTIONS:** Sedation, thickening of bronchial secretions, dizziness, dryness of mouth, nose, and throat.

**INTERACTIONS:** Additive effects with alcohol, CNS depressants (eg, hypnotics, sedatives, tranquilizers, anxiolytics). MAOIs may prolong/intensify anticholinergic effects of antihistamines and phenylephrine. May reduce effects of antihypertensives.

**PREGNANCY:** Category C, contraindicated in nursing.

## ALAMAST RX

pemirolast potassium (Vistakon)

**THERAPEUTIC CLASS:** Mast cell stabilizer

**INDICATIONS:** Prevention of ocular itching due to allergic conjunctivitis.

**DOSAGE:** *Adults:* 1-2 drops in affected eye qid.
*Pediatrics:* >3 yrs: 1-2 drops in affected eye qid.

**HOW SUPPLIED:** Sol: 0.1% [10mL]

**WARNINGS/PRECAUTIONS:** May reinsert soft contact lens after 10 minutes, if eyes are not red. Contains lauralkonium chloride; may be absorbed by soft contact lens.

**ADVERSE REACTIONS:** Headache, rhinitis, cold/flu symptoms, ocular burning/discomfort, dry eye, foreign body sensation.

**PREGNANCY:** Category C, caution in nursing.

## ALBALON RX

naphazoline HCl (Allergan)

**THERAPEUTIC CLASS:** Decongestant

**INDICATIONS:** Topical ocular vasoconstrictor.

**DOSAGE:** *Adults:* 1-2 drops q3-4h prn.

**HOW SUPPLIED:** Sol: 0.1% [15mL]

**CONTRAINDICATIONS:** Anatomically narrow angle or narrow angle glaucoma.

**WARNINGS/PRECAUTIONS:** CNS depression leading to coma may occur in children and infants. Caution with HTN, cardiovascular abnormalities, DM, hyperthyroidism, infection, or injury.

**ADVERSE REACTIONS:** Mydriasis, increased redness, irritation, discomfort, blurring, punctate keratitis, lacrimation, increased IOP, dizziness, headache, nausea, sweating, nervousness, drowsiness, weakness, HTN, cardiac irregularities, hyperglycemia.

**INTERACTIONS:** Maprotiline, TCAs may potentiate pressor effects of naphazoline. Hypertensive crisis may occur with MAOIs.

**PREGNANCY:** Category C, caution in nursing.

## ALBENZA RX

albendazole (GlaxoSmithKline)

**THERAPEUTIC CLASS:** Broad-spectrum anthelmintic

**INDICATIONS:** Treatment of parenchymal neurocysticercosis and cystic hydatid disease of the liver, lung, and peritoneum.

**DOSAGE:** *Adults:* Hydatid Disease: >60kg: 400mg bid. <60kg: 7.5mg/kg bid up to 800mg/day. Take with meals for 28 days, then 14 days drug-free, repeat for a total of 3 cycles. Neurocysticercosis: Same dose as Hydatid disease. Treat for 8-30 days.
*Pediatrics:* >6 yrs: Hydatid Disease: >60kg: 400mg bid. <60kg: 7.5mg/kg bid up to 800mg/day. Take with meals for 28 days, then 14 days drug-free, repeat for a total of 3 cycles. Neurocysticercosis: Same dose as Hydatid disease. Treat for 8-30 days.

**HOW SUPPLIED:** Tab: 200mg

**WARNINGS/PRECAUTIONS:** Monitor blood counts at the beginning of each 28-day cycle, and every 2 weeks during therapy. May continue if total WBC and absolute neutrophil count decrease are modest and do not progress. Not for use in pregnancy unless no other therapy is appropriate. Avoid pregnancy at least 1 month after discontinuing therapy. Discontinue immediately if become pregnant. Treatment for neurocysticercosis should include anticonvulsants and steroids. Examine for retinal lesions before therapy. Elevated LFTs reported.

**ADVERSE REACTIONS:** Abnormal LFTs, abdominal pain, nausea, vomiting, headache.

**INTERACTIONS:** Monitor theophylline levels after therapy. Increased levels with dexamethasone, praziquantel, and cimetidine.

**PREGNANCY:** Category C, caution in nursing.

## ALBUMINAR RX

albumin (ZLB Behring)

**OTHER BRAND NAMES:** Albuminar-5 (ZLB Behring) - Albuminar-25 (ZLB Behring)

**THERAPEUTIC CLASS:** Human albumin

**INDICATIONS:** (5%, 25%) Emergency treatment of shock and burns and in other similar conditions where the restoration of blood volume is urgent. (5%) Acute hypoproteinemia where sodium restriction is not a problem. (25%) Hypoproteinemia with or without edema.

**DOSAGE:** *Adults:* Shock: Initial: (5%) 500mL given as rapidly as tolerated. May repeat 30 minutes later if needed. Guide therapy by clinical response, BP, an assessment of relative anemia. (25%) Dose dependent on BP, degree of pulmonary congestion, Hct. May repeat 15-30 minutes later if needed. Severe Burns: (5%) Large volumes of crystalloid with lesser amount of albumin 5%. May increase ratio of albumin to crystalloid after 24 hrs to maintain plasma albumin level 2.5g/100mL or total serum protein level 5.2g/100mL.

Burns: (25%) Large volumes of crystalloid during 1st 24 hrs. More albumin than crystalloid after 24 hrs is required. Hypoproteinemia: (5%) Use to replace protein lost. (25%) 200-300mL to reduce edema and normalize serum protein.

**HOW SUPPLIED:** Inj: 5%, 25%

**CONTRAINDICATIONS:** Severe anemia, cardiac failure, history of human albumin allergy.

**WARNINGS/PRECAUTIONS:** Avoid if turbid or sediment in bottle. Do not begin administration >4 hrs after container has been entered. Made from human plasma; risk of viral disease transmission. Supplement with RBCs or whole blood when administer large quantities. Slower administration with HTN. Observe for bleeding points due to quick response of BP. Caution with low cardiac reserve or with no albumin deficiency.

**ADVERSE REACTIONS:** Anaphylaxis, nausea, vomiting, increased salivation, chills, febrile reactions, urticaria, pruritus, edema, erythema, hypotension, bronchospasm, rash.

**PREGNANCY:** Category C, safety in nursing not known.

## ALBUTEROL RX

albuterol sulfate (Various)

**OTHER BRAND NAMES:** Proventil (Schering)

**THERAPEUTIC CLASS:** Beta$_2$ agonist

**INDICATIONS:** (Aerosol) Prevention and treatment of bronchospasm with reversible obstructive airway disease. Prevention of Exercise-Induced Bronchospasm (EIB). (Sol) Relief of bronchospasm with reversible obstructive airway disease and acute attacks of bronchospasm in patients ≥12 yrs. (Tab, Tab, Extended Release) Relief of bronchospasm with reversible obstructive airway disease in patients ≥6 yrs. (Syrup) Relief of bronchospasm in patients ≥2 yrs with reversible obstructive airway disease.

**DOSAGE:** *Adults:* Bronchospasm: (Aerosol) 2 inh q4-6h or 1 inh q4h. (Repetabs) Initial: 4-8mg q12h. Max: 32mg/day. (Sol) 2.5mg tid-qid by nebulizer. (Syrup, Tabs) 2-4mg tid-qid. Max: 32mg/day (8mg qid). Elderly/Beta-Adrenergic Sensitivity: (Syrup, Tabs) Initial: 2mg tid-qid. Max: (Tabs) 8mg tid-qid. EIB: (Aerosol) 2 inh 15 minutes before activity. *Pediatrics:* Bronchospasm: >14 yrs: (Syrup) Initial: 2-4mg tid-qid. Max: 8mg qid. >12 yrs: (Aerosol) 2 inh q4-6h or 1 inh q4h. (Sol) 2.5mg tid-qid by nebulizer. (Tabs) Initial: 2-4mg tid-qid. Max: 8mg qid. >12 yrs: (Repetabs) Initial: 4-8mg q12h. Max: 32mg/day. 6-14 yrs: (Syrup) Initial: 2mg tid-qid. Max: 24mg/day. 6-12 yrs: (Repetabs) Initial: 4mg q12h. Max: 24mg/day. (Tabs) Initial: 2mg tid-qid. Max: 24mg/day. 2-5 yrs: (Syrup) Initial: 0.1mg/kg tid (not to exceed 2mg tid). Titrate: May increase to 0.2mg/kg/day. Max: 4mg tid. EIB: >12 yrs: (Aerosol) 2 inh 15 minutes before activity.

**HOW SUPPLIED:** Aerosol: 0.09mg/inh [17g]; Sol (neb): 0.083% [3mL, 25$^s$], 0.5% [20mL]; Syrup: 2mg/5mL; Tab: 2mg*, 4mg*; Tab, Extended Release (Repetabs): 4mg *scored

**WARNINGS/PRECAUTIONS:** Hypersensitivity reactions reported. Monitor for worsening asthma. Fatalities reported with excessive use. Caution with cardiovascular disorders, especially coronary insufficiency, arrhythmias and HTN. May need concomitant corticosteroids. Can produce paradoxical bronchospasm. Caution with DM, hyperthyroidism, seizures. May cause transient hypokalemia.

**ADVERSE REACTIONS:** Tachycardia, increased BP, tremor, nervousness, dizziness, nausea/vomiting, palpitations, paradoxical bronchospasm, heartburn, rhinitis, respiratory tract infection.

**INTERACTIONS:** Avoid other sympathomimetic agents. Extreme caution with MAOIs and TCAs. Monitor digoxin. May worsen ECG changes and/or hypokalemia with nonpotassium-sparing diuretics. Antagonized by β-blockers.

**PREGNANCY:** Category C, not for use in nursing.

## ALCORTIN RX

iodoquinol - hydrocortisone (Primus)

**THERAPEUTIC CLASS:** Corticosteroid/Anti-infective

**INDICATIONS:** "Possibly" Effective: Contact or atopic dermatitis, impetiginized eczema, nummular eczema, endogenous chronic infectious dermatitis, stasis dermatitis, pyoderma, nuchal eczema and chronic eczematoid otitis externa, acne urticata, localized or disseminated neurodermatitis, lichen simplex chronicus, anogenital pruritus (vulvae, scroti, ani), folliculitis, bacterial dermatoses, mycotic dermatoses such as tinea (capitis, cruris, corporis, pedis), monliasis, intertrigo.

**DOSAGE:** *Adults:* Apply to affected area(s) tid-qid.
*Pediatrics:* >12 yrs: Apply to affected area(s) tid-qid.

**HOW SUPPLIED:** Gel: (Hydrocortisone-Iodoquinol) 2%-1% [2g]

**WARNINGS/PRECAUTIONS:** For external use only. Avoid eyes. Discontinue if irritation develops. May stain skin, hair, or fabrics. Risk of systemic absorption with treatment of extensive areas or use of occlusive dressings. Increased risk of systemic absorption in children. Iodoquinol may interfere with thyroid tests. False-positive phenylketonuria test reported.

**ADVERSE REACTIONS:** Burning, itching, irritation, dryness, folliculitis, hypertrichosis, acneiform eruptions, hypopigmentation, perioral dermatitis, allergic dermatitis, skin maceration, secondary infection, skin atrophy, striae, miliaria.

**PREGNANCY:** Category C, caution in nursing.

## ALDACTAZIDE RX

spironolactone - hydrochlorothiazide (Pharmacia & Upjohn)

**Tumorigenic in chronic toxicity animal studies; avoid unnecessary use. Not for initial therapy.**

**THERAPEUTIC CLASS:** $K^+$-sparing diuretic/thiazide diuretic

**INDICATIONS:** Management of edematous conditions (CHF, hepatic cirrhosis with edema/ascites, nephrotic syndrome) and hypertension.

**DOSAGE:** *Adults:* Edema: 100mg/day per component qd or in divided doses. Maint: 25-200mg/day per component. HTN: 50-100mg/day per component qd or in divided doses.

**HOW SUPPLIED:** Tab: (Spironolactone-HCTZ) 25mg-25mg, 50mg-50mg*
*scored

**CONTRAINDICATIONS:** Acute renal impairment, significantly impaired renal excretory function, hyperkalemia, acute or severe hepatic dysfunction, anuria, sulfonamide hypersensitivity.

**WARNINGS/PRECAUTIONS:** Monitor for fluid/electrolyte imbalance. Caution with renal and hepatic dysfunction. Hyperchloremic metabolic acidosis reported with decompensated hepatic cirrhosis. Mild acidosis, gynecomastia, transient BUN elevation, hypercalcemia, hyperglycemia, hyperuricemia, hypomagnesemia, and sensitivity reactions may occur. Discontinue if hyperkalemia occurs. Risk of dilutional hyponatremia. Enhanced effects in post-sympathetectomy patient. May increase cholesterol and TG levels. May manifest latent DM.

**ADVERSE REACTIONS:** Gastric bleeding, ulceration, gynecomastia, impotence, agranulocytosis, fever, urticaria, confusion, ataxia, renal dysfunction, blood dyscrasias, electrolyte disturbances, weakness.

**INTERACTIONS:** Risk of hyperkalemia with $K^+$-sparing diuretics, $K^+$-supplements, NSAIDs, ACE inhibitors. Alcohol, barbiturates, or narcotics potentiate orthostatic hypotension. Corticosteroids, ACTH may intensify electrolyte depletion. Reduced vascular response to norepinephrine. Increased response to nondepolarizing skeletal muscle relaxants. Risk of digoxin, lithium toxicity. NSAIDs may reduce effects. Antidiabetic agents may need adjustment.

**PREGNANCY:** Category C, not for use in nursing.

## ALDACTONE

RX

spironolactone (Pharmacia & Upjohn)

**Tumorigenic in chronic toxicity animal studies; avoid unnecessary use.**

**THERAPEUTIC CLASS:** $K^+$-sparing diuretic

**INDICATIONS:** Management of primary hyperaldosteronism (diagnosis, short-term preoperative and long-term maintenance treatment); edematous conditions (CHF, hepatic cirrhosis with edema/ascites, nephrotic syndrome); hypertension. Treatment and prophylaxis of hypokalemia.

**DOSAGE:** *Adults:* Hyperaldosteronism: (Diagnostic) 400mg/day for 3-4 weeks or 400mg/day for 4 days. (Preoperative) 100-400mg/day. Maint: Lowest effective dose. Edema: Initial: 100mg/day given qd or in divided doses for at least 5 days. Maint: 25-200mg/day given qd-bid. HTN: Initial: 50-100mg/day given qd or in divided doses. Titrate: Adjust at 2 week intervals. Hypokalemia: 25-100mg/day.

**HOW SUPPLIED:** Tab: 25mg, 50mg*, 100mg* *scored

**CONTRAINDICATIONS:** Anuria, acute renal insufficiency, significantly impaired renal excretory function, hyperkalemia.

**WARNINGS/PRECAUTIONS:** Monitor for fluid/electrolyte imbalance. Caution with renal and hepatic dysfunction. Hyperchloremic metabolic acidosis reported with decompensated hepatic cirrhosis. Mild acidosis, gynecomastia, transient BUN elevation may occur. Discontinue and monitor ECG if hyperkalemia occurs. Risk of dilutional hyponatremia.

**ADVERSE REACTIONS:** Gastric bleeding, ulceration, gynecomastia, impotence, agranulocytosis, fever, urticaria, confusion, ataxia, renal dysfunction.

**INTERACTIONS:** Risk of hyperkalemia with $K^+$-sparing diuretics, $K^+$ supplements, NSAIDs, ACE inhibitors. Alcohol, barbiturates, or narcotics potentiate orthostatic hypotension. Corticosteroids, ACTH may intensify electrolyte depletion. Reduced vascular response to norepinephrine. Increased response to nondepolarizing skeletal muscle relaxants. Risk of digoxin, lithium toxicity. NSAIDs may reduce effects.

**PREGNANCY:** Category C, not for use in nursing.

## ALDARA

RX

imiquimod (Graceway)

**THERAPEUTIC CLASS:** Immune response modifier

**INDICATIONS:** Actinic keratoses on face or scalp in immunocompetent adults. External genital and perianal warts/condyloma acuminata. Biopsy-confirmed, primary superficial basal cell carcinoma (sBCC) in immunocompetent adults, with a maximum tumor diameter of 2cm, located on the trunk (excluding anogenital skin), neck, or extremities (excluding hands and feet), only when surgical methods are medically less appropriate and patient follow-up can be assured.

**DOSAGE:** *Adults:* Use before bedtime. Actinic Keratosis: Usual: Apply 2x/week to defined area on face or scalp (but not both concurrently). Wash off after 8 hrs with soap and water. Max: 16 weeks. External Genital and Perianal Warts/Condyloma: Usual: Apply 3x/week. Wash off after 6-10 hrs with soap and water. Use until warts are clear. Max: 16 weeks. May suspend use for several days to manage local reactions. Do not occlude treatment area. sBCC: Apply 5x/week for 6 weeks. If tumor diameter is 0.5 to <1cm, use 4mm (10mg)

of cream. If tumor is ≥1 to <1.5cm, use 5mm (25mg) of cream. If tumor is ≥1.5 to 2cm, use 7mm (40mg) of cream. Max diameter of tumor: ≤2cm. Treatment area should include a 1cm margin of skin around the tumor. Wash off after 8 hrs with soap and water.
*Pediatrics:* >12 yrs: External Genital and Perianal Warts/Condyloma: Usual: Apply 3x/week before bedtime. Wash off after 6-10 hrs with soap and water. Use until warts are clear. Max: 16 weeks. May suspend use for several days to manage local reactions. Do not occlude treatment area.

**HOW SUPPLIED:** Cre: 5% [12 pkt]

**WARNINGS/PRECAUTIONS:** Not for urethral, intra-vaginal, cervical, rectal, or intra-anal human papilloma viral disease. Avoid sexual contact while cream is on skin. May weaken condoms and diaphragms; avoid concurrent use. Avoid or minimize exposure to sunlight. May exacerbate inflammatory skin conditions. Avoid contact with eyes, lips, nostrils. Avoid after surgery or with sunburn until tissue is healed.

**ADVERSE REACTIONS:** Wart (erythema, erosion, flaking, edema) and application site reactions (bleeding, burning, itching, pain) , flu-like symptoms, headache.

**INTERACTIONS:** Avoid topical drugs immediately after treatment of warts.

**PREGNANCY:** Category C, safety in nursing not known.

## ALESSE

RX

levonorgestrel - ethinyl estradiol (Wyeth)

**OTHER BRAND NAMES:** Lessina (Barr) - Aviane (Duramed)

**THERAPEUTIC CLASS:** Estrogen/progestogen combination

**INDICATIONS:** Prevention of pregnancy.

**DOSAGE:** *Adults:* Start 1st Sunday after menses begin or the 1st day of menses. *21-day:* 1 tab qd for 21 days, stop 7 days, then repeat. *28-day:* 1 tab qd for 28 days, then repeat.

**HOW SUPPLIED:** Tab: (Ethinyl Estradiol-Levonorgestrel) 0.02mg-0.1mg

**CONTRAINDICATIONS:** Thrombophlebitis, DVT or thromboembolic disorders, pregnancy, cerebrovascular or coronary artery disease, undiagnosed abnormal genital bleeding, cholestatic jaundice of pregnancy or jaundice with prior pill use, hepatic adenomas or carcinomas, active liver disease (as long as liver function has not returned to normal), breast cancer or other estrogen-dependent neoplasia, thrombogenic valvulopathies, thrombogenic rhythm disorders, diabetes with vascular involvement, uncontrolled hypertension.

**WARNINGS/PRECAUTIONS:** Cigarette smoking increases risk of serious cardiovascular side effects. This risk increases with age (especially >35 yrs) and heavy smoking. Increased risk of MI, vascular disease, thromboembolism, stroke and gallbladder disease. Retinal thrombosis, hepatic neoplasia, carcinoma of breast and reproductive organs reported. May cause glucose intolerance. May increase BP, elevate LDL levels or cause other lipid changes, fluid retention, breakthrough bleeding, and spotting. May cause or exacerbate migraine. May develop visual changes with contact lens. Diarrhea and/or vomiting may reduce absorption. Increased risk of MI with HTN, hyperlipidemia, obesity, and diabetes. Discontinue if develop jaundice, significant depression or ophthalmic irregularities. Perform annual physical exam. Use before menarche is not indicated. May affect certain endocrine, LFTs and blood components.

**ADVERSE REACTIONS:** Nausea, vomiting, breakthrough bleeding, spotting, amenorrhea, migraine, depression, vaginal candidiasis, edema, weight changes.

**INTERACTIONS:** Reduced effects, increased breakthrough bleeding, and menstrual irregularities with rifampin, barbiturates, phenylbutazone, phenytoin, griseofulvin, topiramate, some protease inhibitors, modafinil, ampicillin, tetracyclines, and possibly with St. John's wort. Troleandomycin may increase risk of intrahepatic cholestasis. Ascorbic acid, APAP, CYP3A4 inhibitors (eg, indinavir, fluconazole, troleandomycin), atorvastatin may increase plasma levels. Increased plasma levels of cyclosporine, theophylline, and corticosteroids.

**PREGNANCY:** Category X, not for use in nursing.

## ALEVE

OTC

naproxen sodium (Bayer Healthcare)

**THERAPEUTIC CLASS:** NSAID

**INDICATIONS:** Relief of minor aches and pains. Reduction of fever.

**DOSAGE:** *Adults:* Initial: 1 to 2 tabs, then 1 tab q8-12h. Max: 660mg/24hrs or 440mg/12hrs. Elderly: >65 yrs: 1 tab q12h.
*Pediatrics:* >12 yrs: Initial: 1 to 2 tabs, then 1 tab q8-12h. Max: 660mg/24hrs or 440mg/12hrs.

**HOW SUPPLIED:** Tab: 220mg

**WARNINGS/PRECAUTIONS:** Avoid during last trimester of pregnancy. Do not use >10 days for pain or >3 days for fever.

**INTERACTIONS:** Increased risk of GI bleeding with alcohol.

**PREGNANCY:** Safety in pregnancy or nursing not known.

## ALFENTANIL

CII

alfentanil HCl (Various)

**OTHER BRAND NAMES:** Alfenta (Akorn)

**THERAPEUTIC CLASS:** Opioid analgesic

**INDICATIONS:** As an analgesic adjunct given in incremental doses in the maintenance of anesthesia with barbiturate/nitrous oxide/oxygen. As an analgesic administered by continuous infusion with nitrous oxide/oxygen in the maintenance of general anesthesia. As a primary anesthetic agent for the induction of anesthesia in patients undergoing general surgery in which endotracheal intubation and mechanical ventilation are required. As the analgesic component for monitored anesthesia care (MAC).

**DOSAGE:** *Adults:* Individualize dose. Spontaneous Breathing/Assisted Ventilation: Induction: 8-20mcg/kg. Maint: 3-5mcg/kg q 5-20 minutes or 0.5-1mcg/kg/min. Total: 8-40mcg/kg. Assisted or Controlled Ventilation: Incremental Injection: Induction: 20-50mcg/kg. Maint: 5-15mcg/kg q 5-20 minutes. Total: Up to 75mcg/kg. Continuous Infusion: Induction: 50-75mcg/kg. Maint: 0.5-3mcg/kg/min (average rate 1-1.5mcg/kg/min). Total: Dependent on duration of procedure. Anesthetic Induction: Induction: 130-245 mcg/kg. Maint: 0.5-1.5mcg/kg/min or general anesthetic. Total: dependent on duration of procedure. Monitored Anesthesia Care (MAC): Induction: 3-8mcg/kg. Maint: 3-5 mcg/kg q 5-20 minutes or 0.25-1mcg/kg/min. Total: 3-40mcg/kg.

**HOW SUPPLIED:** Inj: 500mcg/mL

**WARNINGS/PRECAUTIONS:** May cause delayed respiratory depression, respiratory arrest, bradycardia, asystole, arrhythmias, and hypotension; an opioid antagonist, resuscitative and intubation equipment and oxygen should be readily available. Use in caution with patients with head injury, increased intracranial pressure, pulmonary disease, and liver or kidney dysfunction. Initial dose of alfentanil should be appropriately reduced in elderly and debilitated patients.

**ADVERSE REACTIONS:** Respiratory depression, skeletal muscle rigidity, nausea, vomiting, HTN, hypotension, bradycardia, tachycardia, dizziness, skeletal muscle movements, apnea, chest wall rigidity.

**INTERACTIONS:** Coadministration with CNS depressants such as barbiturates, tranquilizers, opioids, or inhalation general anesthetics may enhance CNS effects and postoperative respiratory depression. Erythromycin may significantly inhibit alfentanil clearance and increase the risk of prolonged or delayed respiratory depression.Cimetidine reduces clearance of alfentanil and may extend duration of action.

**PREGNANCY:** Category C, caution in nursing

## ALIMTA RX
pemetrexed (Lilly)

**THERAPEUTIC CLASS:** Antifolate

**INDICATIONS:** In combination with cisplatin for the treatment of patients with unresectable malignant pleural mesothelioma who are not candidates for curative surgery. Monotherapy for the treatment of patients with locally advanced or metastatic non-small cell lung cancer (NSCLC) after prior chemotherapy

**DOSAGE:** *Adults:* Premedication: Dexamethasone: 4mg bid day before, day of, and day after pemetrexed. Folic Acid: At least 5 daily doses (350-1000mcg) during 7 days prior to pemetrexed. Continue for 21 days after last pemetrexed dose. Vitamin $B_{12}$: 1000mcg IM once during week preceding first pemetrexed dose and every 3 cycles thereafter. Treatment: Mesothelioma: 500mg/m$^2$ IV over 10 minutes on Day 1 of each 21 day cycle with cisplatin 75mg/m$^2$ infused over 2 hours beginning 30 minutes after pemetrexed. NSCLC: 500mg/m$^2$ IV over 10 minutes on Day 1 of each 21 day cycle. Hematologic Toxicity: Nadir ANC <500mm$^3$/Nadir Platelets ≥50,000/mm$^3$: 75% of previous dose (both drugs). Nadir Platelets <50,000/mm$^3$: 50% of previous dose (both drugs). Nonhematologic Toxicity: Grade 3/4 (except Grade 3 transaminase elevation or mucositis)/Diarrhea Requiring Hospitalization: 75% of previous dose (both drugs). Grade 3/4 Mucositis: 50% of previous pemetrexed dose. Neurotoxicity: CTC Grade 2: 50% of previous cisplatin dose. Discontinue with Grade 3/4 neurotoxicity; Grade 3/4 hematologic or nonhematologic toxicities after 2 dose reductions (except Grade 3 transaminase elevations). Avoid with CrCl <45mL/min.

**HOW SUPPLIED:** Inj: 500mg

**WARNINGS/PRECAUTIONS:** May suppress bone marrow function. With pleural effusions, ascites, consider draining prior to therapy. Monitor CBCs, for nadir and recovery before each dose and on days 8 and 15 of each cycle. Do not begin new cycle unless ANC ≥1500 cells/mm$^3$, platelets ≥100,000 cells/mm$^3$, CrCl ≥45mL/min.

**ADVERSE REACTIONS:** Nausea, fatigue, dyspnea, vomiting, hematologic effects, constipation, chest pain, anorexia, fever, infection, stomatitis, pharyngitis, rash/desquamation.

**INTERACTIONS:** Delayed clearance with nephrotoxic or tubularly secreted drugs (eg, probenecid). Reduced clearance with ibuprofen; caution with CrCl <80mL/min. In mild-moderate renal insufficiency, avoid NSAIDs with short elimination half-lives from 2 days prior to 2 days following therapy. Interrupt NSAID dosing with longer half-lives from at least 5 days before to 2 days following therapy.

**PREGNANCY:** Category D, not for use in nursing.

## ALINIA RX
nitazoxanide (Romark)

**THERAPEUTIC CLASS:** Antiprotozoal agent

**INDICATIONS:** Treatment of diarrhea caused by *Cryptosporidium parvum* and *Giardia lamblia.*

**DOSAGE:** *Adults:* ≥12 yrs: *G.lamblia* Diarhhea: 500mg q12h for 3 days. Take with food.

*Pediatrics: C.parvum/G.lamblia* Diarrhea: 1-3 yrs: 100mg (5mL) q12h for 3 days. 4-11yrs: 200mg (10mL) q12h for 3 days. *G.lamblia* Diarrhea: ≥12 yrs: 500mg (1 tab or 25mL) q12h for 3 days. Take with food.

**HOW SUPPLIED:** Sus: 100mg/5mL [60mL]; Tab: 500mg [60$^s$, 3-Day Therapy Packs, 6$^s$]

**WARNINGS/PRECAUTIONS:** Caution with hepatic and biliary disease, renal disease. Contains 1.48g sucrose/5mL. Safety and effectiveness have not been established in HIV positive or immunodeficient patients.

**ADVERSE REACTIONS:** Abdominal pain, diarrhea, headache, nausea.

**INTERACTIONS:** Highly protein bound; caution with other highly plasma protein-bound drugs with narrow therapeutic indices.

**PREGNANCY:** Category B; caution in nursing.

## ALKERAN

melphalan HCl (Celgene) RX

**Severe bone marrow suppression resulting in bleeding or infection may occur. Potentially mutagenic and leukemogenic.**

**THERAPEUTIC CLASS:** Nitrogen mustard alkylating agent

**INDICATIONS:** (Inj) Palliative treatment of multiple myeloma where oral therapy is not appropriate. (Tab) Palliative treatment of multiple myeloma and palliation of nonresectable epithelial carcinoma of the ovary.

**DOSAGE:** *Adults:* (Inj) Usual: 16mg/m$^2$ IV at 2-week intervals for 4 doses. After recover from toxicity, resume at 4-week intervals. Renal Impairment (BUN >30mg/dL): Reduce dose up to 50%. (Tab) Multiple Myeloma: 6mg qd. Adjust weekly based on blood counts. After 2-3 weeks, d/c for up to 4 weeks and monitor blood counts. Maint: 2mg qd. Epithelial Ovarian Cancer: 0.2mg/kg qd for 5 days. Repeat every 4-5 weeks depending on hematologic tolerance.

**HOW SUPPLIED:** Inj: 50mg; Tab: 2mg

**CONTRAINDICATIONS:** Prior resistance to agent.

**WARNINGS/PRECAUTIONS:** Marked bone marrow suppression with excessive doses. Monitor platelets, Hgb, WBCs, and differential before therapy and each dose. Use blood counts for dosing to avoid toxicity. Do not readminister if hypersensitivity occurs. Secondary malignancies reported. Ovary function suppression (eg, amenorrhea) may occur in premenopausal women. Reversible and irreversible testicular suppression reported. Extreme caution with compromised bone marrow reserve or if marrow function recovering from previous cytotoxic therapy. Caution in renal dysfunction; reduce IV dose. (Tab) If leukocytes <3000 cells/mcL or platelets <100,000 cells/mcL; d/c until peripheral blood counts recover. Avoid live vaccines in the immunocompromised.

**ADVERSE REACTIONS:** Bone marrow suppression, alopecia, hemolytic anemia, pulmonary fibrosis, interstitial pneumonitis. (Inj) Hypersensitivity reactions (eg, urticaria, pruritus, edema, tachycardia). (Tab) Hepatic disorders (eg, abnormal LFTs, hepatitis, jaundice)

**INTERACTIONS:** (Inj) Severe renal failure reported with oral cyclosporine. Cisplatin may alter melphalan clearance from inducing renal dysfunction. May reduce the threshold for BCNU lung toxicity. Nalidixic acid may increase incidence of severe hemorrhagic necrotic enterocolitis in peds.

**PREGNANCY:** Category D, not for use in nursing.

## ALL CLEAR OTC

polyethylene glycol 300 - naphazoline HCl (Bausch & Lomb)

**THERAPEUTIC CLASS:** Decongestant/lubricant

**INDICATIONS:** To relieve eye redness due to minor eye irritations. Temporary relief of burning and irritation due to dryness of the eye and as a protectant against further irritation.

**DOSAGE:** *Adults:* 1-2 drops in affected eye up to qid.
*Pediatrics:* >6 yrs: 1-2 drops in affected eye up to qid.

**HOW SUPPLIED:** Sol: (Naphazoline-Polyethylene Glycol 300) 0.012%-0.2% [15mL]

**WARNINGS/PRECAUTIONS:** Overuse may cause more redness. Remove contact lenses before use. Do not touch container tip to any surface to avoid contamination. D/C if eye pain or vision changes occur, if redness or irritation continues, or if condition worsens or persists >72 hrs. Supervision required in patients with glaucoma.

**PREGNANCY:** Safety in pregnancy or nursing not known.

## ALL CLEAR AR OTC

hydroxypropyl methylcellulose - naphazoline HCl (Bausch & Lomb)

**THERAPEUTIC CLASS:** Decongestant/lubricant

**INDICATIONS:** Temporary relief of discomfort due to minor irritations of the eye or to exposure to wind or sun. To prevent further irritation or to relieve eye dryness. To relieve eye redness due to minor eye irritations.

**DOSAGE:** *Adults:* 1-2 drops in affected eye up to qid.
*Pediatrics:* >8 yrs: 1-2 drops in affected eye up to qid.

**HOW SUPPLIED:** Sol: (Naphazoline-Hydroxypropyl Methylcellulose) 0.03%-0.5% [15mL]

**WARNINGS/PRECAUTIONS:** Overuse may cause more redness. Remove contact lenses before use. Do not touch container tip to any surface to avoid contamination. D/C if eye pain or vision changes occur, if redness or irritation continues, or if condition worsens or persists >72 hrs. Supervision required in patients with glaucoma.

**PREGNANCY:** Safety in pregnancy or nursing not known.

## ALLEGRA RX

fexofenadine HCl (Sanofi-Aventis)

**THERAPEUTIC CLASS:** $H_1$ antagonist

**INDICATIONS:** (Sus) Relief of symptoms associated with seasonal allergic rhinitis in children 2-11 yrs. Treatment of uncomplicated skin manifestations of chronic idiopathic urticaria in children 6 months to 11 yrs. (Tab) Relief of symptoms associated with seasonal allergic rhinitis and treatment of uncomplicated skin manifestations of chronic idiopathic urticaria in adults and children ≥6 yrs.

**DOSAGE:** *Adults:* Tab: Rhinitis/Urticaria: 60mg bid or 180mg qd. Renal Dysfunction: Initial: 60mg qd.
*Pediatrics:* Tab: >12 yrs: Rhinitis/Urticaria: 60mg bid or 180mg qd. Renal Dysfunction: Initial: 60mg qd. 6-11 yrs: Rhinitis/Urticaria: 30mg bid. Renal Dysfunction: Initial: 30mg qd. Sus: Rhinitis: 2-11 yrs: 30mg (5mL) bid. Renal Dysfunction: 30mg (5mL) qd. Urticaria: 2-11 yrs: 30mg (5mL) bid. Renal Dysfunction: 30mg (5mL) qd. 6 months to <2 yrs: 15mg (2.5mL) bid. Renal Dysfunction: 15mg (2.5mL) qd.

**HOW SUPPLIED:** Tab: 30mg, 60mg, 180mg; Sus: 30mg/5mL

**ADVERSE REACTIONS:** Headache, cough, upper respiratory tract infection, back pain, fever, pain, otitis media, chronic idiopathic urticaria.

**INTERACTIONS:** Increased plasma levels with erythromycin or ketoconazole. Avoid concomitant aluminum- and magnesium-containing antacids. Fruit juices (eg, grapefruit, orange and apple) may decrease levels.

**PREGNANCY:** Category C, caution in nursing.

## ALLEGRA-D RX

fexofenadine HCl - pseudoephedrine HCl (Sanofi-Aventis)

**THERAPEUTIC CLASS:** $H_1$ antagonist/sympathomimetic amine

**INDICATIONS:** Relief of symptoms of seasonal allergic rhinitis.

**DOSAGE:** *Adults:* 60-120mg tab bid or 180-240mg qd without food. Renal Dysfunction: Initial: 60-120mg tab qd; avoid 180-240mg tab. Do not crush or chew.
*Pediatrics:* >12 yrs: 60-120mg tab bid or 180-240mg qd without food. Renal Dysfunction: Initial: 60-120mg tab qd; avoid 180-240mg tab. Do not crush or chew.

**HOW SUPPLIED:** Tab, Extended Release: (Fexofenadine-Pseudoephedrine) (12 Hour) 60-120mg, (24 Hour) 180-240mg

**CONTRAINDICATIONS:** Narrow-angle glaucoma, urinary retention, severe HTN, severe CAD, within 14 days of MAOI therapy.

**WARNINGS/PRECAUTIONS:** Caution with HTN, DM, ischemic heart disease, increased IOP, hyperthyroidism, renal impairment, or prostatic hypertrophy. May produce CNS stimulation with convulsions or cardiovascular collapse with hypotension.

**ADVERSE REACTIONS:** Headache, insomnia, nausea, dry mouth, dyspepsia, throat irritation.

**INTERACTIONS:** Increased plasma levels with erythromycin or ketoconazole. Avoid MAOIs. Increased ectopic pacemaker activity can occur with digitalis. Caution with other sympathomimetic amines. Reduced effects of antihypertensive drugs which interfere with sympathetic activity (eg, methyldopa, mecamylamine, reserpine).

**PREGNANCY:** Category C, caution with nursing.

## ALLERX RX

pseudoephedrine HCl - methscopolamine nitrate - chlorpheniramine maleate (Adams)

**THERAPEUTIC CLASS:** Antihistamine/anticholinergic/decongestant

**INDICATIONS:** Temporary relief of symptoms associated with allergic rhinitis, vasomotor rhinitis, sinusitis, and the common cold.

**DOSAGE:** *Adults:* 1 AM Dose tab in morning and 1 PM Dose tab in evening.
*Pediatrics:* >12 yrs: 1 AM Dose tab in morning and 1 PM Dose tab in evening.

**HOW SUPPLIED:** Tab, Extended Release: (AM Dose) (Methscopolamine-Pseudoephedrine) 2.5mg-120mg; (PM Dose) (Chlorpheniramine-Methscopolamine) 8mg-2.5mg

**CONTRAINDICATIONS:** Severe HTN or CAD, MAOI use or within 14 days of discontinuation, nursing mothers taking MAOIs, narrow-angle glaucoma, urinary retention, peptic ulcer, during asthma attack.

**WARNINGS/PRECAUTIONS:** Caution with elderly, HTN, DM, ischemic heart disease, hyperthyroidism, prostatic hypertrophy, cardiovascular disease, increased IOP. May produce CNS stimulation with convulsions or cardiovascular collapse with hypotension. Excitability reported especially in children.

**ADVERSE REACTIONS:** Drowsiness, lassitude, nausea, giddiness, dry mouth, blurred vision, cardiac palpitations, flushing, increased irritability.

**INTERACTIONS:** May enhance effects of TCAs, barbiturates, alcohol, other CNS depressants. May diminish antihypertensive effects of reserpine, veratrum alkaloids, methyldopa, mecamylamine. Increased sympathomimetic effect with β-blockers and MAOIs. Contraindicated with or within 14 days of discontinuing MAOIs. Hypotension potentiated with sildenafil or other organic nitrates; avoid concomitant use. Caution with hyperactivity to sympathomimetics.

**PREGNANCY:** Category C, not for use in nursing.

## ALOCRIL RX
nedocromil sodium (Allergan)

**THERAPEUTIC CLASS:** Mast cell stabilizer

**INDICATIONS:** Treatment of itching associated with allergic conjunctivitis.

**DOSAGE:** *Adults:* 1-2 drops bid. Continue throughout period of exposure.
*Pediatrics:* >3 yrs: 1-2 drops bid. Continue throughout period of exposure.

**HOW SUPPLIED:** Sol: 2% [5mL]

**WARNINGS/PRECAUTIONS:** Avoid wearing contacts while symptoms of allergic conjunctivitis persist.

**ADVERSE REACTIONS:** Headache, ocular burning, irritation, stinging, unpleasant taste, nasal congestion, asthma, conjunctivitis, eye redness, photophobia, rhinitis.

**PREGNANCY:** Category B, caution in nursing.

## ALOMIDE RX
lodoxamide tromethamine (Alcon)

**THERAPEUTIC CLASS:** Mast cell stabilizer

**INDICATIONS:** Ocular disorders including vernal keratoconjunctivitis, vernal conjunctivitis, and vernal keratitis.

**DOSAGE:** *Adults:* 1-2 drops qid for up to 3 months.
*Pediatrics:* >2 yrs: 1-2 drops qid for up to 3 months.

**HOW SUPPLIED:** Sol: 0.1% [10mL]

**WARNINGS/PRECAUTIONS:** Do not wear soft contacts during treatment. Transient burning and stinging upon instillation.

**ADVERSE REACTIONS:** Ocular pruritus, blurred vision, dry eye, tearing, discharge, hyperemia, crystalline deposits, foreign body sensation.

**PREGNANCY:** Category B, caution in nursing.

## ALOPRIM RX
allopurinol sodium (Nabi)

**THERAPEUTIC CLASS:** Xanthine oxidase inhibitor

**INDICATIONS:** Management of elevated serum and urinary uric acid levels in patients with leukemia, lymphoma, and solid tumor malignancies receiving cancer therapy when oral therapy is not tolerated.

**DOSAGE:** *Adults:* Initial: 200-400mg/m²/day IV as qd or in divided doses every 6, 8, or 12 hrs. Max: 600mg/day. CrCl 10-20mL/min: 200mg/day. CrCl 3-10mL/min: 100mg/day. CrCl <3mL/min: 100mg/day at extended intervals.
*Pediatrics:* Initial: 200mg/m²/day IV as qd or in divided doses every 6, 8, or 12 hrs.

**HOW SUPPLIED:** Inj: 500mg

**CONTRAINDICATIONS:** Previous severe reaction to therapy.

**WARNINGS/PRECAUTIONS:** D/C at first appearance of hypersensitivity; increased risk in decreased renal function. Monitor LFTs during early stages of therapy in liver disease. Monitor renal function and uric acid levels; adjust dose if needed. Maintain sufficient fluid intake to yield a daily urinary output >2 L. Drowsiness, hepatotoxicity, bone marrow suppression reported.

**ADVERSE REACTIONS:** Skin rash, eosinophilia, local injection site reaction, nausea, vomiting, diarrhea, renal failure/insufficiency.

**INTERACTIONS:** Decrease mercaptopurine and azathioprine dose to 1/3 to 1/4 of usual dose. Increased risk of skin rash with ampicillin, amoxicillin. Increased toxicity and risk of hypersensitivity with thiazide diuretics; monitor renal function. Caution with anticoagulants. Hypoglycemia reported with chlorpropamide. Enhanced myelosuppressive effects of cyclophosphamide, other cytotoxic agents. Increased cyclosporine levels. Increased urinary excretion of uric acid with uricosuric agents. Monitor PT with dicumarol.

**PREGNANCY:** Category C, caution with nursing.

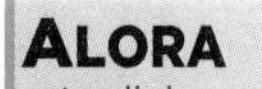

## ALORA — RX

estradiol (Watson)

> **Estrogens increase risk of endometrial cancer. Estrogens, with or without progestins, should not be used for the prevention of cardiovascular disease or dementia. Increased risks of MI, stroke, invasive breast cancer, PE, and DVT in postmenopausal women (50-79 yrs of age) reported. Increased risk of developing probable dementia in postmenopausal women ≥65 yrs of age reported.**

**THERAPEUTIC CLASS:** Estrogen

**INDICATIONS:** Treatment of moderate to severe vasomotor symptoms associated with menopause. Treatment of vulvar/vaginal atrophy. Treatment of hypoestrogenism due to hypogonadism, castration, or primary ovarian failure. Prevention of postmenopausal osteoporosis.

**DOSAGE:** *Adults:* Apply to lower abdomen, upper quadrant of the buttocks or the hip; avoid breasts and waistline. Rotate application sites. Vasomotor Symptoms/Vulvar/Vaginal Atrophy/Hypoestrogenism: Initial: Apply 0.05mg/day twice weekly. Titrate: Adjust dose to control symptoms. Use continuously without an intact uterus. Use cyclic schedule (3 weeks on, 1 week off) with an intact uterus without a progestin. Discontinue or taper at 3-6 month intervals. In women who are taking oral estrogens, initiate therapy 1 week after withdrawal of oral estrogens or sooner if menopausal symptoms reappear in less than 1 week. Osteoporosis Prevention: Apply 0.025mg/day twice weekly. Titrate: May increase depending on bone mineral density and adverse events.

**HOW SUPPLIED:** Patch: 0.025mg/24 hrs, 0.05mg/24 hrs [$8^{s}$ $24^{s}$], 0.075mg/24 hrs, 0.1mg/24 hrs [$8^{s}$]

**CONTRAINDICATIONS:** Pregnancy, undiagnosed abnormal genital bleeding, breast cancer unless being treated for metastatic disease, estrogen-dependent neoplasia, DVT/PE, active or recent (eg, within past year) arterial thromboembolic disease (eg, stroke, MI), liver dysfunction or disease.

**WARNINGS/PRECAUTIONS:** May increase risk of cardiovascular events (eg, MI, stroke), venous thrombosis, and PE; d/c immediately if any of these events occur or are suspected. May increase risk of breast/endometrial cancer, and gallbladder disease. May lead to severe hypercalcemia with breast cancer and bone metastases; monitor and d/c if hypercalcemia occurs. Retinal vascular thrombosis reported; monitor and d/c if papilledema or retinal vascular lesions occur. Consider addition of a progestin if no hysterectomy. May elevate BP; monitor at regular intervals. May cause elevations of plasma triglycerides with pre-existing hypertriglyceridemia. Caution with history of cholestatic jaundice associated with past estrogen use or with pregnancy; d/c with recurrence. May lead to increased thyroid-binding globulin levels; monitor thyroid function. May cause fluid retention; caution with cardiac/renal dysfunction. Caution with severe hypocalcemia. May increase risk of ovarian cancer. May exacerbate endometriosis, asthma, DM, epilepsy, migraine, porphyria; use with caution.

**ADVERSE REACTIONS:** Redness/irritation at application site, altered uterine/vaginal bleeding, vaginal candidiasis, breast tenderness/enlargement, GI effects, melasma, CNS effects, weight changes, edema, altered libido.

**INTERACTIONS:** CYP3A4 inducers (eg, St. John's wort, phenobarbital, carbamazepine, rifampin) may decrease levels which may decrease therapeutic effects and/or change uterine bleeding profile. CYP3A4 inhibitors (eg, erythromycin, clarithromycin, ketoconazole, itraconazole, ritonavir, grapefruit juice) may increase levels which may result in side effects.

**PREGNANCY:** Category X, caution in nursing.

## ALOXI RX

palonosetron HCl (MGI Pharma)

**THERAPEUTIC CLASS:** 5-$HT_3$ antagonist

**INDICATIONS:** Prevention of acute nausea and vomiting associated with initial and repeat courses of moderately and highly emetogenic cancer chemotherapy. Prevention of delayed nausea and vomiting associated with initial and repeat courses of moderately emetogenic cancer chemotherapy.

**DOSAGE:** *Adults:* 0.25mg IV single dose 30 minutes before start of chemotherapy. Repeated dosing within a 7 day interval is not recommended.

**HOW SUPPLIED:** Inj: 0.25mg/5mL

**WARNINGS/PRECAUTIONS:** Caution with, or at risk of developing, prolongation of cardiac conduction intervals, particulary QTc (eg, hypokalemia, hypomagnesemia, congenital QT syndrome). Caution with diuretics which induce electrolyte abnormalities, drugs which cause QT prolongation (eg, antiarrhythmics), and cumulative high-dose anthracycline therapy.

**ADVERSE REACTIONS:** Headache, constipation, diarrhea, dizziness.

**PREGNANCY:** Category B, not for use in nursing.

## ALPHAGAN P RX

brimonidine tartrate (Allergan)

**THERAPEUTIC CLASS:** Selective $alpha_2$ agonist

**INDICATIONS:** Treatment of open-angle glaucoma and ocular hypertension.

**DOSAGE:** *Adults:* 1 drop tid, give q8h. Space dosing of other topical products that lower IOP by 5 minutes.
*Pediatrics:* >2 yrs: 1 drop tid, give q8h. Space dosing of other topical products that lower IOP by 5 minutes.

**HOW SUPPLIED:** Sol: 0.1% [5mL, 10mL, 15mL], 0.15% [5mL, 10mL, 15mL] (contains Purite®)

**CONTRAINDICATIONS:** Concomitant MAOI therapy.

**WARNINGS/PRECAUTIONS:** Caution with severe cardiovascular disease, hepatic or renal dysfunction, depression, cerebral or coronary insufficiency, Raynaud's phenomenon, orthostatic hypotension, thromboangiitis obliterans. Wait 15 minutes before reinserting contacts with 0.2% solution. Monitor IOP.

**ADVERSE REACTIONS:** Oral dryness, ocular hyperemia, ocular pruritus, burning, stinging, ocular allergic reaction, blurred vision, foreign body sensation, fatigue, drowsiness, headache, conjunctival follicles.

**INTERACTIONS:** May potentiate CNS depressants. May reduce BP; caution with β-blockers, antihypertensives, cardiac glycosides. Caution with TCAs. May be given with other topical products to lower IOP.

**PREGNANCY:** Category B, not for use in nursing.

## ALREX
RX

loteprednol etabonate (Bausch & Lomb)

**THERAPEUTIC CLASS:** Corticosteroid

**INDICATIONS:** Relief of signs and symptoms of seasonal allergic conjunctivitis.

**DOSAGE:** *Adults:* 1 drop qid.

**HOW SUPPLIED:** Sus: 0.2% [5mL, 10mL]

**CONTRAINDICATIONS:** Viral diseases of the cornea and conjunctiva including epithelial herpes simplex keratitis, vaccinia, and varicella. Mycobacterial infection and fungal diseases of the eye.

**WARNINGS/PRECAUTIONS:** Caution with glaucoma, herpes simplex, diseases causing thinning of cornea/sclera and other ocular viral infections. Prolonged use can cause glaucoma or secondary ocular infections (eg, fungal). Monitor IOP beyond 10 days of therapy. Wait 10 minutes after instillation before inserting soft contact lenses. Re-evaluate if no response after 2 days.

**ADVERSE REACTIONS:** Elevated IOP, foreign body sensation, itching, chemosis, epiphora, blurred vision, burning on instillation, discharge, dry eyes, photophobia.

**PREGNANCY:** Category C, caution in nursing.

## ALTABAX
RX

retapamulin (GlaxoSmithKline))

**THERAPEUTIC CLASS:** Pleuromutilin antibacterial

**INDICATIONS:** Topical treatment of impetigo caused by susceptible strains of microorganisms, in patients ≥9 months.

**DOSAGE:** *Adults*: Apply thin layer (up to 100 $cm^2$ in total area) bid for 5 days. May cover with sterile bandage or gauze.
*Pediatrics:* ≥9 months: Apply thin layer (up to 2% total BSA) bid for 5 days. May cover with sterile bandage or gauze.

**HOW SUPPLIED:** Oint: 1% [5g, 10g, 15g]

**WARNINGS/PRECAUTIONS:** D/C if sensitization or irritation occurs. Not intended for oral, intranasal, ophthalmic or intravaginal use. May cause superinfection during therapy.

**ADVERSE REACTIONS:** Application site reactions.

**INTERACTIONS:** Co-administration with ketoconazole may increase levels.

**PREGNANCY:** Category B, caution in nursing.

## ALTACE
RX

ramipril (King)

**ACE inhibitors can cause death/injury to developing fetus during 2nd and 3rd trimesters. Stop therapy if pregnancy detected.**

**THERAPEUTIC CLASS:** ACE inhibitor

**INDICATIONS:** Hypertension, alone or with thiazide diuretics. To decrease hospitalization and mortality in stable post-MI patients that show signs of congestive heart failure. To reduce risk of MI, stroke, and cardiovascular (CV) death in patients >55 yrs who are at risk due to history of coronary artery disease, stroke, peripheral vascular disease, or diabetes with at least 1 other CV risk factor.

**DOSAGE:** *Adults:* HTN: Initial: 2.5mg qd. Maint: 2.5-20mg/day given qd or bid. Add diuretic if BP not controlled. CrCl <40mL/min: Initial: 1.25mg qd. Titrate/Max: 5mg/day. CHF Post-MI: Initial: 2.5mg bid, 1.25mg bid if hypotensive. Titrate: Increase to 5mg bid. CrCl <40mL/min: Initial: 1.25mg qd.

Titrate: May increase to 1.25mg bid. Max: 2.5mg bid. Reduction in risk of MI, stroke, death (>55 yrs): Initial: 2.5mg qd for 1 week. Increase to 5mg qd for the next 3 weeks. Maint: 10mg qd. Reduce/discontinue diuretic if possible. With Volume Depletion/Renal Artery Stenosis: Initial: 1.25mg qd.

**HOW SUPPLIED:** Cap: 1.25mg, 2.5mg, 5mg, 10mg

**CONTRAINDICATIONS:** History of ACE inhibitor associated angioedema.

**WARNINGS/PRECAUTIONS:** D/C if angioedema, jaundice, or if marked LFT elevation occurs. Risk of hyperkalemia with DM, renal dysfunction. Persistent nonproductive cough and anaphylactoid reactions reported. Monitor WBCs in renal and collagen vascular disease. Fetal/neonatal morbidity and death reported. Monitor for hypotension in high risk patients (heart failure, surgery/anesthesia, hyponatremia, high dose diuretic therapy, recent intensive diuresis, dialysis, or severe volume and/or salt depletion, etc). Caution with CHF, renal dysfunction, severe liver cirrhosis and/or ascites, and renal artery stenosis. Less effective on BP in blacks and more reports of angioedema than nonblacks. May reduce RBC, Hgb, WBC or platelets. May cause agranulocytosis, pancytopenia, and bone marrow depression.

**ADVERSE REACTIONS:** Hypotension, cough, dizziness, fatigue, angina, impotence, Stevens-Johnson syndrome.

**INTERACTIONS:** May increase lithium levels. Hypotension risk with diuretics. Increase risk of hyperkalemia with $K^+$-sparing diuretics, $K^+$ supplements, or $K^+$-containing salt substitutes. NSAIDs may worsen renal failure and increase serum potassium.

**PREGNANCY:** Category C (1st trimester) and D (2nd and 3rd trimesters), not for use in nursing.

## ALTOPREV

RX

lovastatin (Sciele)

**THERAPEUTIC CLASS:** HMG-CoA reductase inhibitor

**INDICATIONS:** Adjunct to diet, to slow progression of coronary atherosclerosis in coronary heart disease. Adjunct to diet, for reduction of elevated total cholesterol (total-C), LDL-C, Apo B, and TG, and to increase HDL-C in patients with primary hypercholesterolemia (heterozygous familial and non-familial) and mixed dyslipidemia (Fredrickson types IIa and IIb). To reduce risk of MI, unstable angina and coronary revascularization procedures associated with asymptomatic cardiovascular disease with average to moderately elevated Total-C and LDL-C, and below average HDL-C.

**DOSAGE:** *Adults:* Initial: 20, 40, or 60mg qhs. Consider immediate release lovastatin in patients requiring smaller reductions. May adjust at intervals of ≥4 weeks. Concomitant Fibrates/Niacin (≥1g/day): Try to avoid. Max: 20mg/day. Concomitant Amiodarone/Verapamil: Max: 20mg/day. CrCl <30mL/min: Consider dose increase of >20mg/day carefully and implement cautiously. Swallow whole; do not chew or crush.

**HOW SUPPLIED:** Tab: Extended Release: 20mg, 40mg, 60mg

**CONTRAINDICATIONS:** Active liver disease, unexplained persistent elevations of serum transaminases, pregnancy, nursing mothers.

**WARNINGS/PRECAUTIONS:** May increase serum transaminases and CPK levels; consider in differential diagnosis of chest pain. D/C if AST or ALT >3x ULN persist, if myopathy diagnosed or suspected, and a few days before major surgery. Monitor LFTs prior to therapy, at 6 weeks, 12 weeks, then periodically or with dose elevation. Caution with heavy alcohol use and/or history of hepatic disease. Caution with dose escalation in renal insufficiency. Lovastatin immediate-release found to be less effective with homozygous familial hypercholesterolemia. Rhabdomyolysis (rare), myopathy reported.

**ADVERSE REACTIONS:** Nausea, abdominal pain, insomnia, dyspepsia, headache, asthenia, myalgia.

**INTERACTIONS:** Due to increased risk of myopathy: suspend lovastatin if itraconazole, ketoconazole, erythromycin or clarithromycin must be used;

avoid other CYP3A4 inhibitors (protease inhibitors, nefazodone, >1 quart/day of grapefruit juice); avoid gemfibrozil (reduce max lovastatin dose if must be used); reduce max lovastatin dose with amiodarone, verapamil, if must be used; caution with other fibrates, >1g/day of niacin. Avoid use with cyclosporine. Monitor warfarin. May blunt adrenal and/or gonadal steroid production; caution with steroid hormone suppressive drugs (eg, ketoconazole, spironolactone, cimetidine).

**PREGNANCY:** Category X, not for use in nursing.

## AMARYL

glimepiride (Sanofi-Aventis) RX

**THERAPEUTIC CLASS:** Sulfonylurea (2nd generation)

**INDICATIONS:** Adjunct to diet and exercise, to improve glycemic control in type 2 diabetes mellitus. May use in combination with metformin or insulin.

**DOSAGE:** *Adults:* Initial: 1-2mg qd with breakfast or 1st main meal. Titrate: After 2mg, may increase by up to 2mg every 1-2 weeks. Maint: 1-4mg qd. Max: 8mg qd. Amaryl/Metformin: Add Metformin to 8mg qd for better glucose control. Amaryl/Insulin Therapy: If FBG >150mg/dL on 8mg qd, add low dose insulin; increase insulin weekly as needed. Renal Insufficiency: Initial: 1mg qd. Elderly/Debilitated/Malnourished/Hepatic Insufficiency: Dose conservatively to avoid hypoglycemia.

**HOW SUPPLIED:** Tab: 1mg*, 2mg*, 4mg* *scored

**CONTRAINDICATIONS:** Diabetic ketoacidosis.

**WARNINGS/PRECAUTIONS:** Increased cardiovascular mortality. Hypoglycemia risk if debilitated, malnourished, or with adrenal, pituitary, renal or hepatic insufficiency. Hypoglycemia may be masked in elderly. May lose blood glucose control with stress. Secondary failure may occur. D/C if skin reactions persist or worsen.

**ADVERSE REACTIONS:** Dizziness, nausea, asthenia, headache, hypoglycemia.

**INTERACTIONS:** Potentiated hypoglycemia with alcohol, NSAIDs, highly protein bound drugs, such as salicylates, sulfonamides, chloramphenicol, coumarins, probenecid, MAOIs, miconazole, and β-blockers. Risk of hyperglycemia with diuretics, corticosteroids, phenothiazines, thyroid products, estrogens, oral contraceptives, phenytoin, nicotinic acid, sympathomimetics, and isoniazid. Monitor for hypoglycemia when switching from long-acting sulfonylurea, and with combination therapy with insulin and metformin. Hypoglycemia may be masked with β-blockers/sympatholytic agents.

**PREGNANCY:** Category C, not for use in nursing.

## AMBIEN

zolpidem tartrate (Sanofi-Aventis) **CIV**

**THERAPEUTIC CLASS:** Imidazopyridine hypnotic

**INDICATIONS:** Short-term treatment of insomnia.

**DOSAGE:** *Adults:* Tab: Usual: 10mg qhs. Elderly/Debilitated/Hepatic Insufficiency: Initial: 5mg. Decrease dose with other CNS-depressants. Max: 10mg qd. Use should be limited to 7-10 days. Re-evaluate if patient needs to take for more than 2-3 weeks.

**HOW SUPPLIED:** Tab: 5mg, 10mg

**WARNINGS/PRECAUTIONS:** Monitor elderly and debilitated patients for impaired motor performance. Caution with depression and conditions that could affect metabolism or hemodynamic responses.

**ADVERSE REACTIONS:** Drowsiness, dizziness, headache, nausea, drugged feeling, dyspepsia, myalgia, confusion, dependence.

**INTERACTIONS:** Increased effect with alcohol and other CNS depressants. Rifampin may decrease effects. Flumazenil may reverse effect.

**PREGNANCY:** Category B, not for use in nursing.

## AMBIEN CR

CIV

zolpidem tartrate (Sanofi-Aventis)

**THERAPEUTIC CLASS:** Imidazopyridine hypnotic

**INDICATIONS:** Treatment of insomnia, characterized by difficulties with sleep onset and/or sleep maintenance.

**DOSAGE:** *Adults:* 12.5mg qhs. Elderly/Debilitated/Hepatic Insufficiency: 6.25mg qhs. Swallow whole; do not divide, crush, or chew.

**HOW SUPPLIED:** Tab, Extended-Release: 6.25mg, 12.5mg

**WARNINGS/PRECAUTIONS:** Use smallest possible effective dose, especially in the elderly. Abnormal thinking and behavior changes have been reported with the use of sedative/hypnotics. Caution with depression and conditions that could affect metabolism or hemodynamic responses. Signs and symptoms of withdrawal reported with abrupt discontinuation of sedative/hypnotics. Monitor elderly and debilitated patients for impaired motor and/or cognitive performance.

**ADVERSE REACTIONS:** Headache, somnolence, dizziness, nausea, hallucinations, back pain, myalgia, fatigue.

**INTERACTIONS:** Increased effect with alcohol and other CNS depressants. Rifampin may decrease effects. Flumazenil reverses effect.

**PREGNANCY:** Category C, not for use in nursing.

## AMBISOME

RX

amphotericin B (Astellas)

**THERAPEUTIC CLASS:** Polyene antifungal

**INDICATIONS:** Empiric therapy for presumed fungal infection in febrile, neutropenic patients. Treatment of *Aspergillus, Candida* or *Cryptococcus* infections refractory to amphotericin B deoxycholate or where renal impairment or unacceptable toxicity precludes its use. Treatment of visceral leishmaniasis and cryptococcal meningitis in HIV infected patients.

**DOSAGE:** *Adults:* Empiric Therapy: 3mg/kg/day IV. Systemic Infections (*Aspergillus, Candida, Cryptococcus*): 3-5mg/kg/day IV. Cryptococcal Meningitis in HIV: 6mg/kg/day IV. Visceral Leishmaniasis: Immunocompetent: 3mg/kg/day IV on days 1-5, 14, 21. May repeat course if needed. Immunocompromised: 4mg/kg/day IV on days 1-5, 10, 17, 24, 31, 38. *Pediatrics:* 1 month-16 yrs: Empirical Therapy: 3mg/kg/day IV. Systemic Infections (*Aspergillus, Candida, Cryptococcus*): 3-5mg/kg/day IV. Cryptococcal Meningitis in HIV: 6mg/kg/day IV.Visceral Leishmaniasis: Immunocompetent: 3mg/kg/day IV on days 1-5, 14, 21. May repeat course if needed. Immunocompromised: 4mg/kg/day IV on days 1-5, 10, 17, 24, 31, 38.

**HOW SUPPLIED:** Inj: 50mg

**WARNINGS/PRECAUTIONS:** If anaphylaxis occurs, d/c all further infusions. Significantly less toxic than amphotericin B deoxycholate. Monitor renal, hepatic, hematopoietic function and electrolytes (especially $K^+$, $Mg^+$).

**ADVERSE REACTIONS:** Chills, asthenia, back pain, pain, infection, chest pain, HTN, hypotension, tachycardia, GI hemorrhage, diarrhea, nausea, vomiting, hyperglycemia, hypokalemia, dyspnea.

**INTERACTIONS:** Antineoplastic agents may potentiate renal toxicity, bronchospasm, hypotension. Corticosteroids and corticotropin may potentiate hypokalemia. May potentiate digitalis toxicity. May increase flucytosine toxicity. Acute pulmonary toxicity with leukocyte transfusions reported. Caution with imidazoles (eg, ketoconazole, clotrimazole, miconazole, fluconazole). Nephrotoxic drugs enhance potential for renal toxicity. May enhance curariform effect of skeletal muscle relaxants due to hypokalemia. Imidazoles (eg, ketocoazole, miconazole) may induce fungal resistance; caution with combination therapy in immunocompromised patients.

**PREGNANCY:** Category B, not for use in nursing.

## AMERGE RX

naratriptan HCl (GlaxoSmithKline)

**THERAPEUTIC CLASS:** 5-$HT_{1D,1B}$ agonist

**INDICATIONS:** Acute treatment of migraine with or without aura.

**DOSAGE:** *Adults:* >18 yrs: 1mg or 2.5mg taken with fluids; may repeat dose once after 4 hrs. Max: 5mg/24 hrs. Mild-Moderate Renal/Hepatic Impairment. Initial: Lower dose. Max: 2.5mg/24 hrs. Safety of treating >4 headaches/30 days not known.

**HOW SUPPLIED:** Tab: 1mg, 2.5mg

**CONTRAINDICATIONS:** Uncontrolled HTN, ischemic cardiac, cerebrovascular or peripheral vascular syndromes, other significant CVD, severe renal or hepatic impairment and basilar or hemiplegic migraine. Within 24 hrs of another 5-$HT_1$ agonist, ergotamine-containing or ergot containing drug (dihydroergotamine or methysergide).

**WARNINGS/PRECAUTIONS:** Confirm diagnosis. Supervise 1st dose and monitor cardiac function in those at risk of CAD (eg, HTN, hypercholesterolemia, smoker, obesity, diabetes, CAD family history, postmenopausal women, males >40 yrs). Monitor cardiovascular function with long term intermittent use. May cause vasospastic reactions or cerebrovascular events. Caution with renal or hepatic dysfunction. Avoid in elderly.

**ADVERSE REACTIONS:** Paresthesias, dizziness, drowsiness, malaise/fatigue, throat and neck symptoms (eg, pain/pressure sensation).

**INTERACTIONS:** Ergotamine-containing and ergot-type (dihydroergotamine or methysergide) drugs may cause prolonged vasospastic reactions. Avoid other 5-$HT_1$ agonist drugs within 24 hr period due to additive effects. SSRIs may cause weakness, hyperreflexia, and incoordination.

**PREGNANCY:** Category C, caution in nursing.

## AMEVIVE RX

alefacept (Biogen Idec)

**THERAPEUTIC CLASS:** Immunosuppressive agent

**INDICATIONS:** Treatment of moderate to severe chronic plaque psoriasis for candidates of systemic therapy or phototherapy.

**DOSAGE:** *Adults:* 7.5mg IV bolus or 15mg IM once weekly for 12 weeks. May initiate retreatment with an additional 12-week course if CD4+ T lymphocyte counts are within normal range and a 12-week minimum interval has passed since the previous course of treatment. CD4+ T Lymphocyte Counts <250 cells/microliter: Withhold dose. Discontinue if counts remain below 250 cells/microliter for 1 month.

**HOW SUPPLIED:** Inj: (IV) 7.5mg, (IM) 15mg

**CONTRAINDICATIONS:** HIV.

**WARNINGS/PRECAUTIONS:** Do not initiate with CD4+ T-lymphocyte counts below normal; monitor weekly. Caution with history or risk of malignancy; discontinue if malignancy develops. May increase risk of infection or reactivate latent, chronic infections; avoid with clinically important infections, caution with chronic or history of recurrent infections; discontinue if serious infection develops. Discontinue if serious hypersensitivity reactions occur. Caution in elderly. Avoid concurrent phototherapy.

**ADVERSE REACTIONS:** Pharyngitis, dizziness, increased cough, nausea, pruritus, myalgia, chills, injection site pain/inflammation, lymphopenia, malignancies, serious infections, hypersensitivity reactions.

**INTERACTIONS:** Avoid with other immunosuppressive agents.

**PREGNANCY:** Category B, not for use in nursing.

## AMICAR RX
aminocaproic acid (Xanodyne)

**THERAPEUTIC CLASS:** Monoamino carboxylic acid anti-fibrinolytic

**INDICATIONS:** To enhance hemostasis when fibrinolysis contributes to bleeding.

**DOSAGE:** *Adults:* IV: 16-20mL (4-5g) in 250mL diluent during 1st hr, then 4mL/hr (1g) in 50mL of diluent. PO: 5g during 1st hr, then 5mL (syr) or 1g (tabs) per hr. Continue therapy for 8 hrs or until bleeding is controlled.

**HOW SUPPLIED:** Inj: 250mg/mL; Syrup: 1.25g/5mL; Tab: 500mg*, 1000mg* *scored

**CONTRAINDICATIONS:** Active intravascular clotting process, disseminated intravascular coagulation without concomitant heparin.

**WARNINGS/PRECAUTIONS:** Avoid in hematuria of upper urinary tract origin due to risk of intrarenal obstruction from glomerular capillary thrombosis or clots in renal pelvis and ureters. Skeletal muscle weakness with necrosis of muscle fibers reported after prolonged therapy. Consider cardiac muscle damage with skeletal myopathy. Avoid rapid IV infusion. Thrombophlebitis may occur. Contains benzyl alcohol; do not administer to neonates due to risk of fatal"gasping syndrome". Do not administer without a definite diagnosis of hyperfibrinolysis.

**ADVERSE REACTIONS:** Edema, headache, anaphylactoid reactions, injection site reactions, pain, bradycardia, hypotension, abdominal pain, diarrhea, nausea, vomiting, agranulocytosis, increased CPK, confusion, dyspnea, pruritus, tinnitus.

**INTERACTIONS:** Increase risk of thrombosis with Factor IX Complex concentrates, Anti-Inhibitor Coagulant concentrates.

**PREGNANCY:** Category C, caution in nursing.

## AMIDATE RX
etomidate (Hospira)

**THERAPEUTIC CLASS:** General anesthetic

**INDICATIONS:** For induction of general anesthesia. For supplementation of subpotent anesthetic agents, such as nitrous oxide in oxygen, during maintenance of anesthesia for short operative procedures.

**DOSAGE:** *Adults:* 0.2-0.6mg/kg IV. Usual: 0.3mg/kg IV, over 30 to 60 seconds. *Pediatrics:* >10 yrs: 0.2-0.6mg/kg IV. Usual: 0.3mg/kg IV, over 30 to 60 seconds.

**HOW SUPPLIED:** Inj: 2mg/mL

**WARNINGS/PRECAUTIONS:** Not for prolonged infusion. Reduction of plasma cortisol and aldosterone concentrations have occurred; consider exogenous replacement during severely stressful conditions.

**ADVERSE REACTIONS:** Transient venous pain, transient skeletal muscle movements, including myoclonus, hyper/hypoventilation, apnea of short duration, hyper/hypotension, tachycardia, bradycardia.

**PREGNANCY:** Category C, caution in nursing.

## AMIKIN

RX

amikacin sulfate (Sandoz)

**Potential for ototoxicity and nephrotoxicity. Neuromuscular blockade, respiratory blockade reported. Avoid potent diuretics, and other neurotoxic, nephrotoxic, and ototoxic drugs.**

**OTHER BRAND NAMES:** Amikin Pediatric (Sandoz)

**THERAPEUTIC CLASS:** Aminoglycoside

**INDICATIONS:** Short-term treatment of serious infections caused by gram-negative bacteria such as septicemia, and respiratory tract, bone/joint, CNS (including meningitis), skin and soft tissue, and intra-abdominal infections; burns and postoperative infections; complicated and recurrent urinary tract infections (UTI); and staphylococcal disease.

**DOSAGE:** *Adults:* (IM/IV)15mg/kg/day given q8h or q12h. Max: 15mg/kg/day. Heavier Weight Patients: Max: 1.5g/day. Recurrent Uncomplicated UTI: 250mg bid. Duration: 7-10 days. Stop therapy if no response after 3-5 days. Reduce dose if suspect renal dysfunction. Discontinue if azotemia increases or if a progressive decrease in urinary output occurs.
*Pediatrics:* 15mg/kg/day given bid-tid. Newborns: LD: 10mg/kg. MD: 7.5mg/kg q12h. Duration: 7-10 days.

**HOW SUPPLIED:** Inj: 50mg/mL, 250mg/mL

**CONTRAINDICATIONS:** History of serious toxic reactions to aminoglycosides.

**WARNINGS/PRECAUTIONS:** May aggravate muscle weakness; caution with muscular disorders (eg, myasthenia gravis, parkinsonism). May cause fetal harm in pregnancy. Contains sodium bisulfite, allergic reactions may occur especially in asthmatics. Maintain adequate hydration. Assess kidney function before therapy then daily.

**ADVERSE REACTIONS:** Ototoxicity, neuromuscular blockage, nephrotoxicity, skin rash, drug fever, headache, paresthesia, tremor, nausea, arthralgia, anemia, hypotension.

**INTERACTIONS:** Increased nephrotoxicity with cephalosporins. Significant mutual inactivation may occur with β-lactams (eg, penicillin, cephalosporins). Cross-allergenicity between aminoglycosides. Avoid diuretics, potent diuretics (eg, ethacrynic acid, furosemide), bacitracin, cisplatin, amphotericin B, paromomycin, polymyxin B, colistin, vancomycin, other aminoglycosides, and other neurotoxic, nephrotoxic and ototoxic drugs. Increased risk of neuromuscular blockade and respiratory paralysis with anesthetics, neuromuscular blockers, or massive transfusions of citrate-anticoagulated blood.

**PREGNANCY:** Category D, not for use in nursing.

## AMILORIDE/HCTZ

RX

hydrochlorothiazide - amiloride HCl (Various)

**THERAPEUTIC CLASS:** $K^+$-sparing diuretic/thiazide diuretic

**INDICATIONS:** Treatment of hypertension or congestive heart failure if hypokalemia occurs on thiazides or kaliuretic diuretics alone, or if maintenance of normal serum $K^+$ levels is clinically important.

**DOSAGE:** *Adults:* Initial: 1 tab qd. Titrate: May increase to 2 tabs qd or in divided doses. Max: 2 tabs/day. May give intermittently once diuresis is achieved. Take with food.

**HOW SUPPLIED:** Tab: (Amiloride-HCTZ) 5mg-50mg* *scored

**CONTRAINDICATIONS:** Hyperkalemia, anuria, sulfonamide hypersensitivity, acute or chronic renal insufficiency, diabetic neuropathy. Concomitant $K^+$-sparing agents (eg, spironolactone, triamterene), $K^+$ supplements, salt substitutes, $K^+$- rich diet (except with severe hypokalemia).

**WARNINGS/PRECAUTIONS:** Risk of hyperkalemia (>5.5mEq/L) especially with renal impairment or DM; d/c if hyperkalemia occurs. Monitor for fluid/electrolyte imbalance. Caution in severely ill (risk of respiratory or metabolic acidosis). Increases BUN, cholesterol, and TG levels. D/C at least 3 days before glucose tolerance test. May precipitate gout or exacerbate SLE.

**ADVERSE REACTIONS:** Nausea, anorexia, rash, headache, weakness, hyperkalemia, dizziness.

**INTERACTIONS:** May potentiate other antihypertensives. Risk of lithium toxicity. Increased risk of hyperkalemia with ACE inhibitors, angiotensin II receptor antagonists, indomethacin, cyclosporine, tacrolimus. May increase responsiveness to nondepolarizing muscle relaxants. May decrease response to norepinephrine. Antidiabetic agents may need adjustment. Alcohol, barbiturates, or narcotics may potentiate orthostatic hypotension. NSAIDs may decrease effects. Cholestyramine, colestipol impair absorption. ACTH, corticosteroids intensify electrolyte depletion. Increased response to nondepolarizing muscle relaxants.

**PREGNANCY:** Category B, not for use in nursing.

## AMINO-CERV RX

urea - cystine - inositol - methionine - sodium propionate (Milex)

**THERAPEUTIC CLASS:** Healing agent

**INDICATIONS:** Treatment of mild cervicitis, postpartum cervicitis, postpartum cervical tears, and post-surgical cervical procedures.

**DOSAGE:** *Adults:* Postpartum: When bleeding subsides, 1 applicatorful intravaginally qhs for 4 weeks. Mild Cervicitis: 1 applicatorful intravaginally qhs for 2 weeks. Following Surgical Cervical Procedure: Apply a small amount immediately after, then qhs for 2-4 weeks. Cold Coning: 1 applicatorful intravaginally qhs for 4 weeks; start 24 hrs post surgery.

**HOW SUPPLIED:** Cre: (Cystine-Inositol-Methionine-Sodium Propionate-Urea) 0.35%-0.83%-0.83%-0.5%-8.34% [82.5g]

**PREGNANCY:** Safety in pregnancy and nursing not known.

## AMITIZA RX

lubiprostone (Sucampo/Takeda)

**THERAPEUTIC CLASS:** Chloride channel activator

**INDICATIONS:** Treatment of chronic idiopathic constipation in adults.

**DOSAGE:** *Adults:* 24mcg bid with food.

**HOW SUPPLIED:** Cap: 24mcg

**CONTRAINDICATIONS:** History of mechanical gastrointestinal obstruction.

**WARNINGS/PRECAUTIONS:** Potential to cause fetal loss; women who could become pregnant should have a negative pregnancy test prior to initiation of therapy and comply with effective contraceptive measures.

**ADVERSE REACTIONS:** Nausea, diarrhea, abdominal distention/pain/discomfort, flatulence, vomiting, loose stools, sinusitis, urinary/upper respiratory tract infections, headache, dizziness, peripheral edema, arthralgia.

**PREGNANCY:** Category C, not for use in nursing.

## AMITRIPTYLINE

RX

amitriptyline HCl (Various)

**Antidepressants increased the risk of suicidal thinking and behavior (suicidality) in short-term studies in children and adolescents with Major Depressive Disorder (MDD) and other psychiatric disorders.**

**THERAPEUTIC CLASS:** Tricyclic antidepressant

**INDICATIONS:** Treatment of depression, especially endogenous depression.

**DOSAGE:** *Adults:* PO: Initial: (Outpatient) 75mg/day in divided doses or 50-100mg qhs. (Inpatient) 100mg/day. Titrate: (Outpatient) Increase by 25-50mg qhs. (Inpatient) Increase to 200mg/day. Maint: 50-100mg qhs. Max: (Outpatient) 150mg/day. (Inpatient) 300mg/day. IM: Initial: 20-30mg qid. Elderly: 10mg tid or 20mg qhs.

**HOW SUPPLIED:** Inj: 10mg/mL; Tab: 10mg, 25mg, 50mg, 75mg, 100mg, 150mg

**CONTRAINDICATIONS:** MAOI use or within 14 days, acute recovery period following MI.

**WARNINGS/PRECAUTIONS:** Caution with history of seizures, urinary retention, angle-closure glaucoma, increased IOP, hyperthyroidism, cardiovascular disorders, liver dysfunction. Increases symptoms with schizophrenia and manic-depression. D/C several weeks before elective surgery. May alter blood glucose levels.

**ADVERSE REACTIONS:** MI, stroke, seizure, paralytic ileus, urinary retention, constipation, blurred vision, dry mouth, hyperpyrexia, rash, bone marrow depression, testicular swelling, gynecomastia (male), breast enlargement (female), alopecia, edema.

**INTERACTIONS:** See Contraindications. May block antihypertensive effects of guanethidine. Potentiates other CNS depressants, alcohol, barbiturates. Increased levels with CYP2D6 inhibitors (eg, quinidine, cimetidine, SSRIs) and enzyme substrates (eg, phenothiazines, propafenone, flecainide). Avoid within 5 weeks of fluoxetine use. Caution with thyroid drugs. Delirium reported with disulfiram and ethchlorvynol. Paralytic ileus and hyperpyrexia with anticholinergics. Monitor with sympathomimetics and neuroleptics.

**PREGNANCY:** Category C, not for use in nursing.

## AMOXAPINE

RX

amoxapine (Watson)

**Antidepressants increased the risk of suicidal thinking and behavior (suicidality) in short-term studies in children and adolescents with Major Depressive Disorder (MDD) and other psychiatric disorders.**

**THERAPEUTIC CLASS:** Tricyclic antidepressant

**INDICATIONS:** Treatment of neurotic or reactive depressive disorders, endogenous and psychotic depression, and depression accompanied by anxiety or agitation.

**DOSAGE:** *Adults:* Initial: 50mg bid-tid. Titrate: May increase to 100mg bid-tid by end of first week. Usual: 200-300mg/day. Max: Outpatients: 400mg/day; Inpatients: 600mg/day. Elderly: Initial: 25mg bid-tid. Titrate: May increase to 50mg bid-tid by end of first week. Max: 300mg/day. Doses ≤300mg/day may be given as single dose at bedtime.

**HOW SUPPLIED:** Tab: 25mg*, 50mg*, 100mg*, 150mg* *scored

**CONTRAINDICATIONS:** During or within 14 days of MAOIs, recent MI.

**WARNINGS/PRECAUTIONS:** Discontinue if NMS, TD, rash and/or drug fever occur. Caution with history of urinary retention, angle-closure glaucoma, or increased IOP, suicidal tendencies. May induce sinus tachycardia, changes in conduction time, arrhythmias. MI, stroke reported. Extreme caution with history of seizure disorders. Activation of mania, increased psychosis reported. May impair mental/physical abilities.

**ADVERSE REACTIONS:** Drowsiness, dry mouth, constipation, blurred vision.

**INTERACTIONS:** Avoid MAOIs (during or within 14 days of therapy). Additive effects with alcohol, barbiturates, other CNS depressants. Increased levels in poor metabolizers of CYP2D6, quinidine, cimetidine, other antidepressants, phenothiazines, propafenone, flecainide. Caution with SSRIs.

**PREGNANCY:** Category C, caution in nursing.

## AMOXIL RX

amoxicillin (GlaxoSmithKline)

**THERAPEUTIC CLASS:** Semisynthetic ampicillin derivative

**INDICATIONS:** Infections of the ear, nose, throat, genitourinary tract, skin and skin structure, lower respiratory tract due to susceptible (beta lactamase negative) organisms; gonorrhea (acute uncomplicated). *H. pylori* eradication to reduce the risk of duodenal ulcer recurrence.

**DOSAGE:** *Adults:* Ear/Nose/Throat/SSSI/GU: (Mild/Moderate) 500mg q12h or 250mg q8h. (Severe) 875mg q12h or 500mg q8h. LRTI: 875mg q12h or 500mg q8h. Gonorrhea 3g as single dose. H.pylori: (Dual Therapy) 1g + 30mg lansoprazole, both tid X 14 days. (Triple Therapy) 1g + 30mg lansoprazole + 500mg clarithromycin, all q12h X 14 days. CrCl 10-30mL/min: 250-500mg q12h. <10mL/min: 250-500mg q24h. Hemodialysis: 250-500mg or 250mg q24h, additional dose during and at the end.
*Pediatrics:* Neonates: ≤12 weeks: Max: 30mg/kg/day divided q12h. >3 months: Ear/Nose/Throat/SSSI/GU: (Mild/Moderate): 25mg/kg/day given q12h or 20mg/kg/day given q8h. (Severe): 45mg/kg/day given q12h or 40 mg/kg/day given q8h. LRTI: 45mg/kg/day given q12h or 40mg/kg/day given q8h. Gonorrhea: (Prepubertal) 50mg/kg with 25mg/kg probenecid as single dose. (Not for < 2yrs). >40kg: Dose as adult.

**HOW SUPPLIED:** Cap: 250mg, 500mg; Sus: 50mg/mL [15mL, 30mL], 125mg/5mL [80mL, 100mL, 150mL], 200mg/5mL [5mL, 50mL, 75mL, 100mL], 250mg/5mL [80mL, 100mL, 150mL], 400mg/5mL [5mL, 50mL, 75mL, 100mL]; Tab: 500mg, 875mg; Tab, Chewable: 200mg, 400mg

**WARNINGS/PRECAUTIONS:** Monitor renal, hepatic, and blood with prolonged use. 200mg, 400mg chewable tabs contain phenylalanine.

**ADVERSE REACTIONS:** Nausea, vomiting, diarrhea, pseudomembranous colitis, hypersensitivity reactions, blood dyscrasias, superinfection (prolonged use).

**INTERACTIONS:** Increased levels with probenecid. Chloramphenicol, macrolides, sulfonamides, tetracyclines may interfere with bactericidal effects. False (+) for urine glucose with Clinitest®, Benedict's or Fehling's solution.

**PREGNANCY:** Category B, caution in nursing.

## AMPHOCIN RX

amphotericin B (Pharmacia & Upjohn)

**Treatment primarily for progressive and potentially life-threatening fungal infections. Not for noninvasive fungal infections (eg, oral thrush, vaginal and esophageal candidiasis) in patients with normal neutrophil counts. Extreme caution to prevent overdose; verify product name and dose if dose >1.5mg/kg.**

**THERAPEUTIC CLASS:** Polyene antifungal

**INDICATIONS:** Treatment of life-threatening fungal infections including aspergillosis, cryptococcosis, North American blastomycosis, systemic candidiasis, coccidioidomycosis, histoplasmosis, zygomycosis, sporotrichosis, and infections due to Conidiobolus and Basidiobolus species. May be useful for treatment of American mucocutaneous leishmaniasis.

**DOSAGE:** *Adults:* Administer by slow IV infusion. Test dose: 1mg in 20mL of D5W over 20-30 minutes. Treatment: Initial: 0.25mg/kg. Severe Infection: Initial: 0.3mg/kg. Give smaller initial dose if impaired cardio/renal function or severe reaction to test dose. Titrate: Increase by 5-10mg/day, depending on cardio-renal status, up to 0.5-0.7mg/kg/day. Max: 1.5mg/kg/day. If interrupt therapy >7 days, resume with lowest dose.

**HOW SUPPLIED:** Inj: 50mg

**WARNINGS/PRECAUTIONS:** Acute reactions (eg, fever, shaking chills, hypotension, anorexia, nausea, vomiting, tachypnea) 1-3 hrs after start infusion. Avoid rapid infusion. Caution with renal impairment. Decreased risk of nephrotoxicity with hydration and sodium repletion. Acute pulmonary reactions reported with leukocyte infusions; separate infusions and monitor pulmonary function. Leukoencephalopathy reported. Monitor renal function, LFTs, electrolytes, blood counts, Hgb.

**ADVERSE REACTIONS:** Fever, malaise, weight loss, hypotension, tachypnea, anorexia, nausea, vomiting, diarrhea, dyspepsia, normochromic normocytic anemia, injection site pain, renal dysfunction.

**INTERACTIONS:** Antineoplastics may potentiate renal toxicity, bronchospasm, hypotension. Corticosteroids and corticotropin may potentiate hypokalemia. May increase flucytosine toxicity. Caution with imidazoles (eg, ketoconazole, clotrimazole, miconazole, fluconazole). Increased risk of renal toxicity with nephrotoxic drugs (eg, aminoglycosides, cyclosporine, pentamidine). May enhance curariform effect of skeletal muscle relaxants (eg, tubocurarine) or digitalis toxicity with hypokalemia.

**PREGNANCY:** Category B, not for use in nursing.

## AMPHOJEL — OTC

aluminum hydroxide (Wyeth)

**THERAPEUTIC CLASS:** Antacid

**INDICATIONS:** For temporary relief of heartburn, upset stomach, sour stomach, and/or acid indigestion.

**DOSAGE:** *Adults:* 10mL 5-6 times daily, between meals and qhs. Max: 60mL/24hrs.

**HOW SUPPLIED:** Sus: 320mg/5mL

**WARNINGS/PRECAUTIONS:** Extreme caution with renal failure, dialysis. Prolonged use of aluminum-containing antacids with renal failure may result in or worsen dialysis osteomalacia. Elevated tissue aluminum levels contribute to development of dialysis encephalopathy and osteomalacia syndromes.

**ADVERSE REACTIONS:** Constipation.

**INTERACTIONS:** May interact with prescription drugs. Avoid with tetracycline.

**PREGNANCY:** Safety in pregnancy and nursing not known.

## AMPHOTEC — RX

amphotericin B cholesteryl sulfate (InterMune)

**THERAPEUTIC CLASS:** Polyene antifungal

**INDICATIONS:** Treatment of invasive aspergillosis in patients with renal impairment, unacceptable toxicity, or previous failure to amphotericin deoxycholate.

**DOSAGE:** *Adults:* Test Dose: Infuse small amount over 15-30 minutes. Treatment: 3-4mg/kg/day IV at 1mg/kg/hr.
*Pediatrics:* Test Dose: Infuse small amount over 15-30 minutes. Treatment: 3-4mg/kg/day IV at 1mg/kg/hr.

**HOW SUPPLIED:** Inj: 50mg, 100mg

**WARNINGS/PRECAUTIONS:** Anaphylaxis may occur. Discontinue if severe respiratory distress occurs. Acute reactions (eg, fever, shaking chills, hypotension, nausea, tachypnea) 1-3 hrs after start infusion. Monitor renal/hepatic function, electrolytes, CBC, PT during therapy.

**ADVERSE REACTIONS:** Chills, fever, headache, hypotension, tachycardia, HTN, nausea, vomiting, thrombocytopenia, increased creatinine, hypokalemia, dyspnea, hypoxia.

**INTERACTIONS:** Antineoplastics may potentiate renal toxicity, bronchospasm, hypotension. Corticosteroids and corticotropin may potentiate hypokalemia. May increase flucytosine toxicity. Caution with imidazoles (eg, ketoconazole, clotrimazole, miconazole, fluconazole). Increased risk of renal toxicity with nephrotoxic drugs (eg, aminoglycosides, cyclosporine, pentamidine). May enhance curariform effect of skeletal muscle relaxants (eg, tubocurarine) or digitalis toxicity with hypokalemia.

**PREGNANCY:** Category B, not for use in nursing.

## AMPICILLIN RX

ampicillin (Various)

**THERAPEUTIC CLASS:** Semi-synthetic penicillin derivative

**INDICATIONS:** Genitourinary tract (GU) infections, including gonorrhea, respiratory and GI tract infections, and meningitis.

**DOSAGE:** *Adults:* GI/GU: 500mg qid. Use larger doses in chronic or severe infections. Gonorrhea: 3.5g single dose with 1g probenecid. Respiratory: 250mg qid. Treat minimum 48-72 hrs after eradication. Treat minimum 10 days for hemolytic strains of strep.
*Pediatrics:* >20kg: GI/GU: 500mg qid. Respiratory: 250mg qid. <20kg: GI/GU: 25mg/kg qid. Respiratory: 50mg/kg/day given tid-qid. Do not exceed adult doses. Use larger doses in chronic or severe infections. Treat minimum 48-72 hrs after eradication. Treat minimum 10 days for hemolytic strains of strep.

**HOW SUPPLIED:** Cap: 250mg, 500mg; Sus: 125mg/5mL, 250mg/5mL [100mL, 200mL]

**CONTRAINDICATIONS:** Infections caused by penicillinase-producing organisms.

**WARNINGS/PRECAUTIONS:** Possible cross-sensitivity with cephalosporins. Pseudomembranous colitis and anaphylatic reactions may occur.

**ADVERSE REACTIONS:** Stomatitis, nausea, vomiting, diarrhea, rash, SGOT elevation, blood dyscrasias, eosinophilia, thrombocytopenic purpura, hypersensitivity reactions, superinfection (prolonged use).

**INTERACTIONS:** Increased risk of rash with allopurinol. Bacteriostatic antibiotics (eg, chloramphenicol, erythromycins, sulfonamides or tetracyclines) may interfere with bactericidal activity. May decrease the effectiveness of oral contraceptives. Increased blood levels with probenecid.

**PREGNANCY:** Category B, not for use in nursing.

## AMPICILLIN INJECTION RX

ampicillin sodium (Apothecon)

**THERAPEUTIC CLASS:** Synthetic penicillin

**INDICATIONS:** Treatment of respiratory tract, urinary tract, and GI infections, bacterial meningitis, septicemia, endocarditis.

**DOSAGE:** *Adults:* IM/IV: Respiratory Tract: >40kg: 250-500mg q8h. <40kg: 25-50mg/kg/day given q6-8h. GI/GU caused by N.gonorrhea females: >40kg: 500mg q6h. <40kg: 50mg/kg/day given q6-8h. Urethritis caused by N.gonorrhea (males): 500mg q8-12h for 2 doses; may retreat if needed. Bacterial Meningitis: 150-200mg/kg/day given q3-4h. Septicemia: 150-200mg/kg/day IV for 3 days, continue with IM q3-4h. Treat for minimum of 10

days and 48-72hrs after being asymptomatic.
*Pediatrics:* Bacterial Meningitis: 150-200mg/kg/day given q3-4h. Septicemia: 150-200mg/kg/day IV given q3-4h for 3 days, continue with IM q3-4h. Treat for minimum of 10 days and 48-72hrs after being asymptomatic.

**HOW SUPPLIED:** Inj: 125mg, 250mg, 500mg, 1g, 2g, 10g

**WARNINGS/PRECAUTIONS:** Caution with renal impairment. Cross-sensitivity with other β-lactams. May cause skin rash, especially in mononucleosis; avoid use. Pseudomembranous colitis reported. May result in overgrowth of nonsusceptible organisms.

**ADVERSE REACTIONS:** Headache, nausea, vomiting, oral and vaginal candidiasis, diarrhea, urticaria, allergic reactions, anaphylaxis, serum sickness-like reactions, exfoliative dermatitis.

**INTERACTIONS:** Potentiated by probenecid. Decreases effects of oral contraceptives. Allopurinol increases incidence of skin rash.

**PREGNANCY:** Category B, caution in nursing.

## AMRIX RX

cyclobenzaprine HCl (ECR)

**THERAPEUTIC CLASS:** Skeletal muscle relaxant (central-acting)

**INDICATIONS:** Adjunct to rest and physical therapy to relieve muscle spasm associated with acute, painful musculoskeletal conditions. Use for only short periods of time (up to 2-3 weeks).

**DOSAGE:** *Adults:* Usual: 15mg qd. Titrate: May increase to 30mg qd if needed. Use for longer than 2-3 weeks not recommended.

**HOW SUPPLIED:** Cap, Extended-Release: 15mg, 30mg

**CONTRAINDICATIONS:** MAOI use during or within 14 days. Hyperpyretic crisis seizures and deaths associated with concomitant use of cyclobenzaprine (or stucturally similar to TCAs) and MAOIs reported. Acute recovery phase of MI, arrhythmias, heart block conduction disturbances, CHF, hyperthyroidism.

**WARNINGS/PRECAUTIONS:** Avoid in hepatic impairment and elderly patients. Caution with history of urinary retention, angle-closure glaucoma, increased IOP, and use of anticholinergic medication. May impair mental and/or physical performance.

**ADVERSE REACTIONS:** Drowsiness, dry mouth, dizziness.

**INTERACTIONS:** Contraindicated with MAOIs. Enhances effects of alcohol, barbiturates and other CNS depressants. TCAs may block antihypertensive action of guanethidine and similar compounds and may enhance seizure risk with tramadol.

**PREGNANCY:** Category B, caution in nursing.

## AMVISC PLUS RX

sodium hyaluronate (Bausch & Lomb)

**THERAPEUTIC CLASS:** Surgical aid

**INDICATIONS:** Surgical aid in ophthalmic anterior and posterior segment procedures (eg, cataract extraction, intraocular lens (IOL) implantation, corneal transplant surgery, glaucoma filtering surgery, surgical procedures to reattach retina).

**DOSAGE:** *Adults:* Cataract Surgery/IOL Implant: Infuse required amount slowly through needle/cannula into anterior chamber. Perform prior to cataract extraction and IOL insertion. May apply to IOL prior to insertion. May inject prn during procedure. Corneal Transplant: Remove corneal button and fill anterior chamber until level with cornea surface. Place donor graft on top and suture into place. May use prn during procedures. Glaucoma Filtration: Inject through corneal paracentesis to restore and maintain anterior chamber volume during trabeculectomy. May use prn during procedures. Intraocular Injection With Scleral Buckling Procedures For Retina Reattachment: After release subretinal fluid and develop buckling by tying mattress sutures, inject air into vitreous cavity and exchange with sodium hyaluronate (2-4mL) injected with 22-30 gauge needle passed via pars plana epithelium.

**HOW SUPPLIED:** Sol: 16mg/mL [0.5mL, 0.8mL]

**WARNINGS/PRECAUTIONS:** Do not use excessive quantity. Remove from anterior chamber at end of surgery. Administer appropriate therapy if post-op IOP above expected levels. Avoid reuse of cannula. Diffuse particulates and haziness reported after injection.

**ADVERSE REACTIONS:** Transient post-op inflammation and increased IOP.

**PREGNANCY:** Safety in pregnancy or nursing not known.

## ANAFRANIL

RX

clomipramine HCl (Mallinckrodt)

**Antidepressants increased the risk of suicidal thinking and behavior (suicidality) in short-term studies in children and adolescents with Major Depressive Disorder (MDD) and other psychiatric disorders. Clomipramine is not approved for use in pediatric patients except for patients with obsessive compulsive disorder.**

**THERAPEUTIC CLASS:** Tricyclic antidepressant

**INDICATIONS:** Treatment of obsessive-compulsive disorder.

**DOSAGE:** *Adults:* Initial: 25mg/day with meals. Titrate: Increase within 2 weeks to 100mg/day. Increase further over several weeks. Max: 250mg/day. Maint: May give total daily dose at bedtime.
*Pediatrics:* >10 yrs: Initial: 25mg/day with meals. Titrate: Increase within 2 weeks to 3mg/kg or 100mg/day, whichever is smaller. Increase further over several weeks. Max: 3mg/kg/day or 200mg/day. Maint: May give total daily dose at bedtime.

**HOW SUPPLIED:** Cap: 25mg, 50mg, 75mg

**CONTRAINDICATIONS:** MAOI use within 14 days, acute recovery period following MI.

**WARNINGS/PRECAUTIONS:** Increased risks with electroconvulsive therapy. Discontinue prior to elective surgery. Avoid abrupt withdrawal. Caution with seizure disorder, conditions predisposing to seizures (eg, brain damage, alcoholism), urinary retention, narrow-angle glaucoma, adrenal medulla tumors, increased IOP, hyperthyroidism, cardiovascular disorders, liver dysfunction, significant renal dysfunction. Monitor hepatic enzymes with liver dysfunction. Weight changes, sexual dysfunction, blood dyscrasias, elevated liver enzymes reported. Hypomania/mania reported with affective disorder. Psychosis reported with schizophrenia.

**ADVERSE REACTIONS:** Dry mouth, constipation, nausea, dyspepsia, anorexia, weight gain, increased sweating, increased appetite, myoclonus, nervousness, libido change, dizziness, tremor, somnolence, impotence, visual changes.

**INTERACTIONS:** See Contraindications. Caution with anticholinergics, sympathomimetics, thyroid and CNS drugs. Blocks effects of clonidine, guanethidine. Increased levels with haloperidol, methyphenidate, highly protein bound drugs, CYP2D6 inhibitors (eg, quinidine, cimetidine, SSRIs) and enzyme substrates (eg, phenothiazines, propafenone, flecainide). At least 5 weeks must elapse before starting TCA therapy after fluoxetine discontinuation. Decreased levels with enzyme inducers (eg, barbiturates, phenytoin). Additive effects with CNS depressants, barbiturates, alcohol. NMS reported with neuroleptics. Increases phenobarbital and highly protein bound drugs (eg, warfarin, digoxin) plasma levels.

**PREGNANCY:** Category C, not for use in nursing.

## ANALPRAM-HC

RX

pramoxine HCl - hydrocortisone acetate (Ferndale)

**THERAPEUTIC CLASS:** Corticosteroid/anesthetic

**INDICATIONS:** Corticosteroid responsive dermatoses of the anal region.

**DOSAGE:** *Adults:* Apply tid-qid. May use occlusive dressings in psoriasis or recalcitrant conditions. For cleansing anogenital area, spread lotion on cotton or tissue and wipe affected area.
*Pediatrics:* Apply tid-qid. May use occlusive dressings in psoriasis or recalcitrant conditions. For cleansing anogenital area, spread lotion on cotton or tissue and wipe affected area.

**HOW SUPPLIED:** Cre: (Hydrocortisone-Pramoxine) 1%-1%, 2.5%-1% [30g]; Lot: 2.5%-1% [60mL]

**WARNINGS/PRECAUTIONS:** May produce reversible HPA axis suppression, manifestations of Cushing's syndrome, hyperglycemia, and glucosuria. D/C use if irritation occurs. Avoid eyes. Peds may be more susceptible to systemic toxicity. Use appropriate therapy with infections.

**ADVERSE REACTIONS:** Burning, itching, irritation, dryness, folliculitis, hypertrichosis, acneiform eruptions, hypopigmentation, perioral dermatitis, allergic contact dermatitis, secondary infection, skin maceration, skin atrophy, striae, miliaria.

**PREGNANCY:** Category C, caution in nursing.

## ANAMANTLE HC

RX

lidocaine HCl - hydrocortisone acetate (Kenwood Therapeutics)

**THERAPEUTIC CLASS:** Corticosteroid/local anesthetic

**INDICATIONS:** Relief of itching, pain, soreness, discomfort due to hemorrhoids, anal fissures, pruritus ani.

**DOSAGE:** *Adults:* Apply rectally bid.

**HOW SUPPLIED:** Cre: (Hydrocortisone-Lidocaine): 0.5%-3% [7g]

**CONTRAINDICATIONS:** Tuberculosis, fungal lesions, skin vaccinia, varicella, acute herpes simplex.

**WARNINGS/PRECAUTIONS:** Caution with impaired liver function, debilitated, elderly. Discontinue if irritation occurs. Not for prolonged use. May cause adrenal suppression with systemic absorption.

**ADVERSE REACTIONS:** Transient stinging or burning, transient blanching, erythema.

**INTERACTIONS:** Additive adverse effects with Class I antiarrhythmics.

**PREGNANCY:** Category B, caution in nursing.

## ANAPROX DS

RX

naproxen sodium (Roche Labs)

**NSAIDs may cause an increased risk of serious cardiovascular thrombotic events, MI, stroke and serious GI adverse events including bleeding, ulceration, and perforation of the stomach or intestines. Contraindicated for the treatment of peri-operative pain in the setting of coronary artery bypass graft (CABG) surgery.**

**OTHER BRAND NAMES:** Anaprox (Roche Labs)

**THERAPEUTIC CLASS:** NSAID

**INDICATIONS:** Relief of signs and symptoms of rheumatoid arthritis (RA), osteoarthritis (OA), ankylosing spondylitis, juvenile arthritis (JA), tendinitis, bursitis, and acute gout. Management of pain and primary dysmenorrhea.

**DOSAGE:** *Adults:* RA/OA/AS: 275mg bid or 550mg bid. Max: 1650mg/day. Acute Gout: 825mg followed by 275mg q8h. Pain/Dysmenorrhea/Tendinitis/Bursitis: 550mg followed by 550mg q12h or 275mg q6-8h prn. Max: 1375mg day 1, then 1100mg/day.

**HOW SUPPLIED:** (Anaprox) Tab: 275mg; (Anaprox DS) Tab: 550mg* *scored

**CONTRAINDICATIONS:** History of ASA or NSAID allergy that cause symptoms of asthma, rhinitis, nasal polyps, and hypotension. Treatment of peri-operative pain in the setting of CABG surgery.

**WARNINGS/PRECAUTIONS:** May lead to onset of new HTN or worsening of pre-existing HTN; monitor BP closely. Fluid retention, edema, and peripheral edema reported; caution with fluid retention, HTN, or heart failure. Renal papillary necrosis and other renal injury reported after long-term use. Not recommended for use with advanced renal disease; if therapy must be initiated, monitor renal function. Anaphylactoid reactions may occur. May cause serious skin adverse events (eg, exfoliative dermatitis, Stevens-Johnson syndrome, and toxic epidermal necrolysis). Avoid in late pregnancy; may cause premature closure of ductus arteriosis. Monitor Hgb levels with long-term therapy if initial Hgb ≤10g. Monitor for visual changes or disturbances. May cause elevations of LFTs; d/c if liver disease develops or systemic manifestations occur. Caution with high doses in chronic alcoholic liver disease and elderly. Anemia may occur; with long-term use, monitor Hgb/Hct if signs or symptoms of anemia develop. May inhibit platelet aggregation and prolong bleeding time; monitor with coagulation disorders. Caution with asthma and avoid with aspirin-sensitive asthma.

**ADVERSE REACTIONS:** Edema, drowsiness, dizziness, constipation, heartburn, abdominal pain, nausea, headache, tinnitus, dyspnea, pruritus, skin eruptions, ecchymoses.

**INTERACTIONS:** Avoid other products containing naproxen. Decreased plasma levels with ASA. May reduce tubular secretion of methotrexate; monitor for toxicity. May diminish antihypertensive effect and potentiate renal disease with ACE inhibitors. May reduce natriuretic effect of furosemide and thiazides. May increase lithium levels; monitor for toxicity. Synergistic effects on GI bleeding with warfarin. Observe for dose adjustment with hydantoins, sulfonamides, or sulfonylureas. May reduce antihypertensive effects of propranolol and other β-blockers. Probenecid may increase half-life.

**PREGNANCY:** Category C, not for use in nursing.

## ANCEF

RX

cefazolin (GlaxoSmithKline)

**THERAPEUTIC CLASS:** Cephalosporin (1st generation)

**INDICATIONS:** Treatment of serious respiratory tract, urinary tract (UTI), skin and skin structure, biliary tract, bone and joint, and genital infections, septicemia, endocarditis, and perioperative surgical prophylaxis.

**DOSAGE:** *Adults:* Moderate-Severe Infection: 500mg-1g q6-8h. Mild Gram-Positive Cocci Infection: 250-500mg q8h. Uncomplicated UTI: 1g q12h. Pneumococcal Pneumonia: 500mg q12h. Severe Life Threatening Infection (eg, Endocarditis, Septicemia): 1-1.5g q6h; Max: 12g/day (rare). Perioperative Surgical Prophylaxis: 1g IM/IV 0.5-1 hr before surgery. For Procedures ≥2 hrs: 500mg-1g IM/IV during surgery. Maint: 500mg-1g IM/IV q6-8h for 24 hrs post-op. Continue for 3-5 days for devastating procedures (eg, open-heart surgery and prosthetic arthroplasty). CrCl 35-54mL/min: Full dose q8h. CrCl 11-34mL/min: Half usual dose q12h. CrCl <10mL/min: Half usual dose q18-24h. Apply reduced dosage recommendations after initial LD is given.
*Pediatrics:* Mild-Moderately Severe Infection: 25-50mg/kg/day in 3-4 equal doses. Severe Infection: 100mg/kg/day in divided doses. CrCl 40-70mL/min: 60% of normal daily dose in equally divided doses q12h. CrCl 20-40mL/min: 25% of normal daily dose in equally divided doses q12h. CrCl 5-20mL/min: 10% of normal daily dose q24h. Apply reduced dosage recommendations after initial LD is given.

**HOW SUPPLIED:** Inj: 1g

**WARNINGS/PRECAUTIONS:** Prolonged use may result in overgrowth of nonsusceptible organisms. Possible cross-sensitivity between penicillins, cephalosporins, and other β-lactam antibiotics. Pseudomembranous colitis reported. Elevated levels with renal insufficiency can lead to seizures. Caution with colitis and other GI diseases. Safety in premature infants and neonates not established.

**ADVERSE REACTIONS:** Diarrhea, oral candidiasis, vomiting, nausea, stomach cramps, anorexia, allergic reactions, blood dyscrasias, renal failure, transient rise in SGOT/SGPT/BUN/SCr/alkaline phosphatase, local reactions.

**INTERACTIONS:** Decreased renal tubular secretion with probenecid.

**PREGNANCY:** Category B, caution in nursing.

## ANCOBON

flucytosine (Valeant)

RX

**Extreme caution with renal dysfunction. Monitor hematologic, renal, and hepatic status closely.**

**THERAPEUTIC CLASS:** 5-fluorocytosine antifungal

**INDICATIONS:** Treatment of septicemia, endocarditis, and urinary tract infections caused by *Candida*. Treatment of meningitis and pulmonary infection caused by *Crytococcus*.

**DOSAGE:** *Adults:* 50-150mg/kg/day given q6h. Renal Impairment: Reduce initial dose. Take a few caps over 15 minutes to reduce nausea/vomiting.

**HOW SUPPLIED:** Cap: 250mg, 500mg

**WARNINGS/PRECAUTIONS:** Caution with renal dysfunction and bone marrow depression. Bone marrow depression can be irreversible and fatal.

**ADVERSE REACTIONS:** Myocardial toxicity, chest pain, dyspnea, rash, pruritus, urticaria, photosensitivity, nausea, vomiting, jaundice, renal failure, pyrexia, crystalluria, anemia, leukopenia, eosinophilia, thrombocytopenia, ataxia, hearing loss, neuropathy.

**INTERACTIONS:** Antagonized by cytosine. Drugs that impair glomerular filtration may prolong half-life. Antifungal synergism with polyene antibiotics (eg, amphotericin B).

**PREGNANCY:** Category C, not for use in nursing.

## ANDRODERM

testosterone (Watson)

CIII

**THERAPEUTIC CLASS:** Androgen

**INDICATIONS:** Testosterone replacement therapy in males due to primary or secondary hypogonadism.

**DOSAGE:** *Adults:* Initial: 5mg/day. Maint: 2.5mg-7.5mg/day. Apply patch nightly to intact skin of the back, abdomen, upper arm or thigh. Rotate sites; avoid same site for 7 days. Do not apply to scrotum or oily, damaged, irritated areas. May apply 2 patches at same time.
*Pediatrics:* >15 yrs: Initial: 5mg/day. Maint: 2.5mg-7.5mg/day. Apply patch nightly to intact skin of the back, abdomen, upper arm or thigh. Rotate sites; avoid same site for 7 days. Do not apply to scrotum or oily, damaged, irritated areas. May apply 2 patches at same time.

**HOW SUPPLIED:** Patch: 2.5mg/24 hrs [60s], 5mg/24 hrs [30s]

**CONTRAINDICATIONS:** Breast or prostate cancer in men. Women.

**WARNINGS/PRECAUTIONS:** Prolonged use is associated with serious hepatic effects. Increased risk for prostatic hyperplasia/carcinoma in elderly. Risk of edema with pre-existing cardiac, renal, or hepatic disease; discontinue if edema occurs. Risk of virilization of female sex partner. Monitor LFTs, Hgb, Hct, PSA, cholesterol, lipids.

**ADVERSE REACTIONS:** Gynecomastia, pruritus/erythema/vesicles/blister at application site, prostate abnormalities, headache, depression.

**INTERACTIONS:** May potentiate effects of anticoagulants, oxyphenbutazone. May decrease blood glucose and insulin requirements in diabetics. Pretreatment with ointments may reduce testosterone absorption.

**PREGNANCY:** Category X, not for use in nursing.

## ANDROGEL

testosterone (Unimed)

CIII

**THERAPEUTIC CLASS:** Androgen

**INDICATIONS:** Testosterone replacement in males with primary hypogonadism or hypogonadotrophic hypogonadism.

**DOSAGE:** *Adults:* Apply 5g qd to clean, dry, intact skin of shoulders and upper arms and/or abdomen. Allow to dry prior to dressing. Titrate: May increase to 7.5g qd, then 10g qd if response not achieved. Do not apply to scrotum/genitals.

**HOW SUPPLIED:** Gel: 1% [2.5g, 5g packets, 75g pump]

**CONTRAINDICATIONS:** Breast or prostate carcinoma in men. Women. Pregnant women should avoid skin contact with application sites in men.

**WARNINGS/PRECAUTIONS:** Prolonged use is associated with serious hepatic effects. Increased risk for prostatic hyperplasia/carcinoma in elderly. Risk of edema with pre-existing cardiac, renal, or hepatic disease; discontinue if edema occurs. Risk of virilization of female sex partner. Monitor LFTs, Hgb, Hct, PSA, cholesterol, lipids. May potentiate sleep apnea. Transfer of testosterone can occur with skin to skin contact. Gels are flammable; avoid fire, flame, or smoking during use.

**ADVERSE REACTIONS:** Acne, alopecia, application site reaction, asthenia, emotional lability, gynecomastia, HTN, prostate disorder.

**INTERACTIONS:** May elevate oxyphenbutazone levels. May decrease blood glucose and insulin requirements. Increased clearance of propranolol. Corticosteroids may enhance edema.

**PREGNANCY:** Category X, not for use in nursing.

## ANECTINE

succinylcholine chloride (Sandoz)

RX

**Rare reports of acute rhabdomyolysis with hyperkalemia followed by ventricular dysrhythmias, cardiac arrest, and death in children with undiagnosed skeletal muscle myopathy. Reserve in children for emergency intubation where securing airway is necessary.**

**THERAPEUTIC CLASS:** Skeletal muscle relaxant (depolarizing)

**INDICATIONS:** Adjunct to general anesthesia to facilitate tracheal intubation and to provide skeletal muscle relaxation during surgery or mechanical ventilation.

**DOSAGE:** *Adults:* Short Surgical Procedure: Average Dose: 0.6mg/kg IV. Range: 0.3-1.1mg/kg IV. Blockade develops in 1 minute, may persist up to 2 minutes. Long Surgical Procedure: 2.5-4.3mg/min IV; or 0.3-1.1mg/kg initial IV injection, then 0.04-0.07mg/kg IV at appropriate intervals. IM (if vein not accessible): Up to 3-4mg/kg IM. Max: 150mg/total dose. Effect observed in 2-3 minutes.
*Pediatrics:* Procedure to Secure Airway: Infants/Small Children: 2mg/kg IV. Older Children/Adolescents: 1mg/kg IV. IM (if vein not accessible): Infants/Older Children: Up to 3-4mg/kg IM. Max: 150mg/total dose. Effect observed in 2-3 minutes.

**HOW SUPPLIED:** Inj: 20mg/mL

**CONTRAINDICATIONS:** Personal or familial history of malignant hyperthermia, skeletal muscle myopathies. Acute phase of injury following major burns, multiple trauma, extensive skeletal muscle denervation, upper motor neuron injury.

**WARNINGS/PRECAUTIONS:** Avoid administration before unconsciousness has been induced. May induce arrhythmias or cardiac arrest in electrolyte abnormalities or massive digitalis toxicity. Caution with chronic abdominal infection, subarachnoid hemorrhage, conditions causing degeneration of central and peripheral nervous system, fractures, muscle spasms, reduced plasma cholinesterase activity, and acute phase of injury following major burns, multiple trauma, extensive skeletal muscle denervation, upper motor neuron injury. Malignant hyperthermia reported. Higher incidence of bradycardia progressing to asystole with 2nd dose. May increase IOP, intracranial or intragastric pressure. With prolonged therapy, Phase I block will progress to Phase II block associated with prolonged respiratory paralysis and weakness. Confirm Phase II block before therapy. Hypokalemia or hypocalcemia prolong neuromuscular blockade.

**ADVERSE REACTIONS:** Respiratory depression, cardiac arrest, malignant hyperthermia, arrhythmia, bradycardia, tachycardia, HTN, hypotension, hyperkalemia, increased IOP, muscle fasciculation, jaw rigidity, post-op muscle pains.

**INTERACTIONS:** Enhanced effects with promazine, oxytocin, certain non-penicillin antibiotics, β-blockers, procainamide, lidocaine, trimethaphan, lithium carbonate, magnesium salts, quinine, aprotinin, chloroquine, diethylether, isoflurane, desflurane, metoclopramide, terbutaline, and drugs that reduce plasma cholinesterase activity (eg, chronically administered oral contraceptives, glucocorticoids, certain MAOIs) or inhibit plasma cholinesterase. Increased risk of malignant hyperthermia with volatile anesthetics.

**PREGNANCY:** Category C, caution in nursing.

## ANEXSIA **CIII**

acetaminophen - hydrocodone bitartrate (Mallinckrodt)

**THERAPEUTIC CLASS:** Opioid analgesic

**INDICATIONS:** Relief of moderate to moderately severe pain.

**DOSAGE:** *Adults:* (5-500mg) Usual: 1-2 tabs q4-6h prn. Max: 8 tabs/day. (7.5-650mg) Usual: 1 tab q4-6h prn. Max: 6 tabs/day.

**HOW SUPPLIED:** Tab: (Hydrocodone-APAP) 5mg-325mg, 7.5mg-325mg, 5mg-500mg, 7.5mg-650mg

**WARNINGS/PRECAUTIONS:** Caution in elderly, debilitated, severe hepatic or renal dysfunction, hypothyroidism, Addison's disease, prostatic hypertrophy, urethral stricture, pulmonary disease, and postoperative use. Impairs mental/physical abilities. May obscure diagnosis or clinical course of acute abdominal conditions or head injuries. May produce dose-related respiratory depression. Monitor for tolerance. Suppresses cough reflex.

**ADVERSE REACTIONS:** Lightheadedness, dizziness, sedation, nausea, vomiting, constipation, rash, respiratory depression.

**INTERACTIONS:** Additive CNS depression with other narcotic analgesics, antihistamines, antipsychotics, antianxiety agents, alcohol and other CNS depressants. Increased effect of antidepressant or hydrocodone with MAOIs or TCAs.

**PREGNANCY:** Category C, not for use in nursing.

## ANGELIQ

RX

estradiol - drospirenone (Berlex)

**Estrogens and progestins should not be used for prevention of cardiovascular disease or dementia. Increased risk of MI, stroke, invasive breast cancer, PE, and DVT in postmenopausal women (50-79 yrs of age) reported. Increased risk of developing probable dementia in postmenopausal women ≥65 yrs of age reported.**

**THERAPEUTIC CLASS:** Estrogen/progestogen combination

**INDICATIONS:** Treatment of moderate to severe vasomotor symptoms and/or vulvar/vaginal atrophy associated with menopause.

**DOSAGE:** *Adults:* 1 tab qd. Re-evaluate after 3-6 months.

**HOW SUPPLIED:** Tab: (Drospirenone-Estradiol) 0.5mg-1mg

**CONTRAINDICATIONS:** Pregnancy, undiagnosed abnormal genital bleeding, breast cancer, estrogen-dependent neoplasia, DVT/PE, active or recent (eg, within past year) arterial thromboembolic disease (eg, stroke, MI), liver dysfunction or disease, renal insufficiency, adrenal insufficiency.

**WARNINGS/PRECAUTIONS:** Not for use in renal insufficiency, hepatic dysfunction, and adrenal insufficiency due to increased risk of hyperkalemia. May increase risk of cardiovascular events (eg, MI, stroke), venous thrombosis, and PE; d/c immediately if any of these events occur or are suspected. May increase risk of breast/endometrial cancer, and gallbladder disease. May lead to severe hypercalcemia with breast cancer and bone metastases; monitor and d/c if hypercalcemia occurs. Retinal vascular thrombosis reported; monitor and d/c if papilledema or retinal vascular lesions occur. May elevate BP; monitor at regular intervals. May cause elevations of plasma triglycerides with pre-existing hypertriglyceridemia. Caution with history of cholestatic jaundice associated with past estrogen use or with pregnancy; d/c with recurrence. May lead to increased thyroid-binding globulin levels; monitor thyroid function. May cause fluid retention; caution with cardiac/renal dysfunction. Caution with severe hypocalcemia. May increase risk of ovarian cancer. May exacerbate endometriosis, asthma, DM, epilepsy, migraine, porphyria, SLE, and hepatic hemangiomas; use with caution.

**ADVERSE REACTIONS:** Abdominal pain, pain in extremity, back pain, flu syndrome, enlarged abdomen, headache, upper respiratory infection, sinusitis, breast pain, vaginal hemorrhage.

**INTERACTIONS:** CYP3A4 inducers (eg, St. John's wort, phenobarbital, carbamazepine, rifampin) may decrease levels which may decrease therapeutic effects and/or change uterine bleeding profile. CYP3A4 inhibitors (eg, erythromycin, clarithromycin, ketoconazole, itraconazole, ritonavir, grapefruit juice) may increase levels which may result in side effects. Increased risk of hyperkalemia with ACE inhibitors, angiotensin receptor blockers, NSAIDs, potassium-sparing diuretics, potassium supplements, and heparin.

**PREGNANCY:** Contraindicated in pregnancy, caution in nursing.

## ANGIOMAX

RX

bivalirudin (The Medicines Company)

**THERAPEUTIC CLASS:** Thrombin inhibitor

**INDICATIONS:** Adjunct to aspirin for anticoagulation in patients with unstable angina undergoing percutaneous transluminal coronary angioplasty (PTCA) or percutaneous coronary intervention (PCI). Patients with, or at risk of, HIT/HITTS undergoing PCI.

**DOSAGE:** *Adults:* Initial: 0.75mg/kg IV bolus, then 1.75mg/kg/hr for duration of PCI procedure. Additional bolus of 0.3mg/kg can be given if needed based on ACT. Continuation of infusion for up to 4 hrs post-procedure is optional. After 4 hrs, if needed, an additional 0.2mg/kg/hr IV for up to 20 hrs may be initiated. Renal Impairment: CrCl <30mL/min: 1mg/kg/hr infusion. Hemodialysis:

0.25mg/kg/hr infusion. Reduction in bolus dose not necessary; monitor anticoagulation.

**HOW SUPPLIED:** Inj: 250mg

**CONTRAINDICATIONS:** Active major bleeding.

**WARNINGS/PRECAUTIONS:** Not for IM administration. Hemorrhage can occur at any site. Discontinue with unexplained symptom, fall in BP or Hct. There is no known antidote to treatment, but can be hemodialyzable.

**ADVERSE REACTIONS:** Bleeding, back pain, pain, nausea, vomiting, headache, hypotension, HTN, bradycardia, dyspepsia, urinary retention, insomnia, anxiety, abdominal pain, fever, nervousness.

**INTERACTIONS:** Increased risk of major bleed with heparin, warfarin, thrombolytics.

**PREGNANCY:** Category B, caution in nursing.

## ANIMI-3 RX

folic acid - vitamin B6 - vitamin B12 - omega-3 acids

(PBM Pharmaceuticals)

**THERAPEUTIC CLASS:** Prenatal Vitamin

**INDICATIONS:** Improving nutritional status before, during and after pregnancy and in conditions requiring essential fatty acid, Vitamin $B_{12}$, $B_6$ and folic acid supplementation.

**DOSAGE:** *Adults:* 1 cap qd or bid.

**HOW SUPPLIED:** Cap: Folic Acid 1mg-Vitamin $B_6$ 12.5mg-Vitamin $B_{12}$ 500µg-Omega-3 Acids 500mg

**WARNINGS/PRECAUTIONS:** Folic acid doses >0.1mg/day may obscure pernicious anemia. in that hematological remission can occur while neurological manifestations remain progressive.

**ADVERSE REACTIONS:** Allergic sensitization.

## ANSAID RX

flurbiprofen (Pharmacia & Upjohn)

**NSAIDs may cause an increased risk of serious cardiovascular thrombotic events, MI, stroke and serious GI adverse events including bleeding, ulceration, and perforation of the stomach or intestines. Contraindicated for the treatment of peri-operative pain in the setting of coronary artery bypass graft (CABG) surgery.**

**THERAPEUTIC CLASS:** NSAID

**INDICATIONS:** Relief of the signs and symptoms of rheumatoid arthritis or osteoarthritis.

**DOSAGE:** *Adults:* Initial: 200-300mg/day given bid, tid or qid. Max: 300mg/day or 100mg/dose.

**HOW SUPPLIED:** Tab: 50mg, 100mg

**CONTRAINDICATIONS:** ASA, with ASA triad, or other NSAID allergy that precipitates acute asthmatic attack, urticaria, or rhinitis. Treatment of peri-operative pain in the setting of CABG surgery.

**WARNINGS/PRECAUTIONS:** May lead to onset of new HTN or worsening of pre-existing HTN; monitor BP closely. Fluid retention and edema reported; caution with fluid retention or heart failure. Renal papillary necrosis and other renal injury reported after long-term use. Not recommended for use with advanced renal disease; if therapy must be initiated, monitor renal function. Anaphylactoid reactions may occur. Avoid in late pregnancy; may cause premature closure of ductus arteriosis. May cause elevations of LFTs; d/c if liver disease develops or systemic manifestations occur. Caution in elderly. Anemia may occur; monitor Hgb/Hct with long-term use. May inhibit platelet aggregation and prolong bleeding time; monitor with coagulation disorders. Caution with asthma and avoid with aspirin-sensitive asthma. Monitor for visual changes or disturbances.

**ADVERSE REACTIONS:** Dyspepsia, diarrhea, abdominal pain, constipation, headache, nausea, edema.

**INTERACTIONS:** Caution with anticoagulants; serious bleeding reported. ASA is not recommended. May decrease hypotensive effects of β-blockers. May decrease diuretic effects.

**PREGNANCY:** Category C, not for use in nursing.

## ANTABUSE

disulfiram (Odyssey)

RX

**Do not give if in a state of alcohol intoxication, or without full knowledge. Instruct relatives accordingly.**

**THERAPEUTIC CLASS:** Alcohol oxidation inhibitor

**INDICATIONS:** Aid in the management of selected chronic alcoholics who want to remain sober for supportive and psychotherapeutic treatment.

**DOSAGE:** *Adults:* Initial: Up to 500mg/day as a single dose for 1-2 weeks. Maint: 125-500mg/day. Max: 500mg/day. Abstain from alcohol at least 12 hours prior to therapy.

**HOW SUPPLIED:** Tab: 250mg

**CONTRAINDICATIONS:** Severe myocardial disease, coronary occlusion, psychoses, hypersensitivity to thiuram derivatives in pesticides and rubber vulcanization, and if receiving or recently received metronidazole, paraldehyde, alcohol, or alcohol-containing preparations (eg, cough syrups).

**WARNINGS/PRECAUTIONS:** Avoid in alcohol intoxication or without patients full knowledge. Antabuse-alcohol reaction; can cause respiratory and cardiovascular problems. Avoid alcohol containing products (eg, sauces, vinegars, cough mixtures, after shave lotions, back rubs) and ethylene dibromide or its vapors. Reactions with alcohol up to 14 days after ingestion. Evaluate for hypersensitivity if history of rubber contact dermatitis. Hepatic toxicity/failure has been reported. Perform baseline and follow-up LFTs (10-14 days) and monitor CBC and SMA-12. Caution with diabetes mellitus, hypothyroidism, epilepsy, cerebral damage, chronic and acute nephritis, hepatic cirrhosis or insufficiency.

**ADVERSE REACTIONS:** Optic neuritis, peripheral neuritis, polyneuritis peripheral neuropathy, hepatitis, skin eruptions, drowsiness, fatigability, impotence, headache, acneform eruptions, allergic dermatitis, metallic or garlic-like aftertaste.

**INTERACTIONS:** Increases phenytoin level; monitor for toxicity. May prolong PT; adjust oral anticoagulants. Stop therapy if unsteady gait or marked changes in mental status with isoniazid.

**PREGNANCY:** Safety not known in pregnancy, not for use in nursing.

## ANTARA

fenofibrate (Reliant)

RX

**THERAPEUTIC CLASS:** Fibric acid derivative

**INDICATIONS:** Adjunct to diet, for treatment of hypertriglyceridemia (Types IV and V) and to reduce elevated LDL-C, Total-C, TG, Apo B, and to increase HDL-C in primary hypercholesterolemia or mixed dyslipidemia (Types IIa and IIb).

**DOSAGE:** *Adults:* Hypercholesterolemia/Mixed Dyslipidemia: Initial: 130mg qd. Hypertriglyceridemia: Initial: 43-130mg/day. Titrate: Adjust if needed after repeat lipid levels at 4-8 week intervals. Max: 130mg/day. Renal Dysfunction/Elderly: Initial: 43mg/day. Take with meals.

**HOW SUPPLIED:** Cap: 43mg, 130mg

**CONTRAINDICATIONS:** Hepatic or severe renal dysfunction (including primary cirrhosis), unexplained persistent hepatic function abnormality, pre-existing gallbladder disease.

**WARNINGS/PRECAUTIONS:** Monitor LFTs regularly; discontinue if >3X ULN. May cause cholelithiasis; discontinue if gallstones found. Discontinue if myopathy or marked CPK elevation occurs. Decreased Hgb, Hct, WBCs, thrombocytopenia, and agranulocytosis reported; monitor CBCs during first 12 months of therapy. Acute hypersensitivity reactions (rare) and pancreatitis reported. Rare cases of rhabdomyolysis. Evaluate for myopathy. Monitor lipids periodically initially, discontinue if inadequate response after 2 months on 130mg/day. Minimize dose in severe renal impairment. Caution in elderly.

**ADVERSE REACTIONS:** Abdominal pain, back pain, headache, abnormal LFTs, respiratory disorder, increased creatinine phosphokinase, increased SGPT/SGOT.

**INTERACTIONS:** May potentiate coumarin anticoagulants; reduce anticoagulant dose and monitor PT/INR. Avoid HMG-CoA reductase inhibitors unless benefits outweigh risks. Bile acid sequestrants may impede absorption; take at least 1 hr before or 4-6 hrs after the resin. Evaluate benefits/risks with immunosuppressants (eg, cyclosporine) and other nephrotoxic agents.

**PREGNANCY:** Category C, not for use in nursing.

## ANTIVERT — RX

meclizine HCl (Pfizer)

**THERAPEUTIC CLASS:** Antihistamine

**INDICATIONS:** Management of nausea, vomiting and dizziness associated with motion sickness. Management of vertigo associated with diseases affecting the vestibular system.

**DOSAGE:** *Adults:* Motion Sickness: 25-50mg 1 hr prior to trip/departure, repeat q24h prn. Vertigo: 25-100mg/day in divided doses.
*Pediatrics:* >12 yrs: Motion Sickness: 25-50mg 1 hr prior to trip/departure, repeat q24h prn. Vertigo: 25-100mg/day in divided doses.

**HOW SUPPLIED:** Tab: 12.5mg, 25mg, 50mg* *scored

**WARNINGS/PRECAUTIONS:** Caution with asthma, glaucoma, prostatic hypertrophy.

**ADVERSE REACTIONS:** Drowsiness, dry mouth, blurred vision (rare).

**INTERACTIONS:** Avoid alcoholic beverages.

**PREGNANCY:** Category B, safety in nursing is not known.

## ANTIZOL — RX

fomepizole (Orphan Medical)

**THERAPEUTIC CLASS:** Alcohol dehydrogenase inhibitor

**INDICATIONS:** Antidote for ethylene glycol or methanol poisoning either alone or with hemodialysis (HD).

**DOSAGE:** *Adults:* IV: LD: 15mg/kg. Maint: 10mg/kg q12h for 4 doses, then 15mg/kg q12h until levels are undetectable or <20mg/dL. Dose at Beginning of HD: If >6 hrs since last dose, give next scheduled dose. Dose During HD: Give q4h. Dose at time when HD is Complete: Give 50% of dose if 1-3 hrs between the last dose and the end of HD. If >3 hrs between last dose and end of HD, give next dose.

**HOW SUPPLIED:** Sol: 1g/mL

**CONTRAINDICATIONS:** Pyrazole hypersensitivity.

**WARNINGS/PRECAUTIONS:** Do not give undiluted or as a bolus injection. Monitor for allergic reactions (eg, mild rash, eosinophilia). Monitor LFTs, WBC during therapy.

**ADVERSE REACTIONS:** Headache, nausea, dizziness, increased drowsiness, bad/metallic taste.

**INTERACTIONS:** Reduced elimination of ethanol and fomepizole (PO).

**PREGNANCY:** Category C, caution in nursing.

## ANUSOL-HC CREAM RX

hydrocortisone (Salix)

**OTHER BRAND NAMES:** Proctosol HC (NuCare) - Proctozone-HC (Rising) - Proctocream HC (Schwarz Pharma)

**THERAPEUTIC CLASS:** Corticosteroid

**INDICATIONS:** Corticosteroid responsive dermatoses.

**DOSAGE:** *Adults:* Apply bid-qid. May use occlusive dressings for psoriasis or recalcitrant conditions; d/c dressings if infection develops.
*Pediatrics:* Apply bid-qid. May use occlusive dressings for psoriasis or recalcitrant conditions; d/c dressings if infection develops.

**HOW SUPPLIED:** Cre: 2.5% [30g]

**WARNINGS/PRECAUTIONS:** May cause reversible adrenal suppression, manifestations of Cushing's syndrome, hyperglycemia, glucosuria. Caution when applied to large surface areas or under occlusive dressings. Use appropriate therapy with infections. Pediatrics may be more susceptible to systemic toxicity. D/C if irritation occurs. Avoid eyes.

**ADVERSE REACTIONS:** Burning, itching, irritation, dryness, folliculitis, hypertrichosis, acneiform eruptions, hypopigmentation, perioral dermatitis, allergic contact dermatitis, maceration skin, secondary infection, skin atrophy, striae, miliaria.

**PREGNANCY:** Category C, caution in nursing.

## ANUSOL-HC SUPPOSITORY RX

hydrocortisone acetate (Salix)

**OTHER BRAND NAMES:** Anucort HC (G & W Labs) - Hemorrhoidal HC (Alpharma)

**THERAPEUTIC CLASS:** Corticosteroid

**INDICATIONS:** For use in inflamed hemorrhoids and post irradiation (factitial) proctitis. Adjunct for chronic ulcerative colitis, cryptitis, other anorectum inflammation and pruritus ani.

**DOSAGE:** *Adults:* Nonspecific Proctitis: 1 sup rectally bid for 2 weeks. More Severe Cases: 1 sup rectally tid or 2 sup rectally bid. Factitial Proctitis: Use up to 6-8 weeks.

**HOW SUPPLIED:** Sup: (Anusol-HC) 25mg [12ˢ 24ˢ]

**WARNINGS/PRECAUTIONS:** D/C if irritation develops. D/C if infection develops that does not respond to appropriate therapy. May stain fabric. Only use after adequate proctologic exam.

**ADVERSE REACTIONS:** Burning, itching, irritation, dryness, folliculitis, hypopigmentation, allergic contact dermatitis, secondary infection.

**PREGNANCY:** Category C, not for use in nursing.

## ANZEMET RX

dolasetron mesylate (Sanofi-Aventis)

**THERAPEUTIC CLASS:** 5-$HT_3$ antagonist

**INDICATIONS:** (Inj) Prevention of nausea/vomiting associated with emetogenic cancer chemotherapy including high dose cisplatin. Prevention and treatment of post-op nausea/vomiting. (Tab) Prevention of nausea/vomiting associated with moderately emetogenic cancer chemotherapy and prevention of post-op nausea/vomiting.

**DOSAGE:** *Adults:* (Inj) Prevention of Chemotherapy Nausea/Vomiting: 1.8mg/kg IV single dose or 100mg IV 30 minutes before chemotherapy. Prevention/Treatment of Post-op Nausea/Vomiting: 12.5mg IV single dose 15 minutes before cessation of anesthesia or as soon as nausea/vomiting presents. (Tab) Prevention of Chemotherapy Induced Nausea/Vomiting: 100mg PO within 1 hr before chemotherapy. Prevention of Postoperative Nausea/Vomiting: 100mg PO within 2 hrs before surgery.
*Pediatrics:* 2-16 yrs: (Inj) Prevention of Chemotherapy Nausea/Vomiting: 1.8mg/kg IV single dose 30 minutes before chemotherapy. Max: 100mg. May mix Inj in apple or grape juice and take orally within 1 hr before chemotherapy. Prevention/Treatment of Post-op Nausea/Vomiting: 0.35mg/kg IV single dose 15 minutes before cessation of anesthesia or as soon as nausea/vomiting presents. Max: 12.5mg single dose. May mix 1.2mg/kg Inj in apple or grape juice and take orally within 2 hrs before surgery. Max: 100mg/dose. (Tab) Prevention of Chemotherapy Induced Nausea/Vomiting: 1.8mg/kg PO within 1 hr before chemotherapy. Max: 100mg. Prevention of Postoperative Nausea/Vomiting: 1.2mg/kg PO within 2 hrs before surgery. Max: 100mg.

**HOW SUPPLIED:** Inj: 20mg/mL; Tab: 50mg, 100mg

**WARNINGS/PRECAUTIONS:** Caution in patients with or may develop cardiac conduction interval prolongation, especially those with congenital QT syndrome, hypokalemia and hypomagnesemia. Cross sensitivity may occur with other 5-$HT_3$ antagonists. Can cause ECG interval changes.

**ADVERSE REACTIONS:** Headache, diarrhea, fever, fatigue, dizziness, abnormal hepatic function, chills/shivering, urinary retention, abdominal pain, HTN.

**INTERACTIONS:** Increased risk of prolongation of cardiac conduction intervals with diuretics, antiarrhythmics, drugs that prolong $QT_c$ interval and cumulative high dose anthracycline therapy. Increased levels with cimetidine. Decreased levels with rifampin. Decreased clearance with IV atenolol.

**PREGNANCY:** Category B, caution in nursing.

## APHTHASOL OTC

amlexanox (GlaxoSmithKline Consumer)

**THERAPEUTIC CLASS:** Inflammatory mediator inhibitor

**INDICATIONS:** Treatment of aphthous ulcers in people with normal immune systems.

**DOSAGE:** *Adults:* Begin at 1st sign of aphthous ulcer. Apply 1/4 inch qid, pc and qhs, following oral hygiene. Use until ulcer heals. Re-evaluate if healing or pain reduction has not occurred after 10 days of use.

**HOW SUPPLIED:** Paste: 5% [5g]

**WARNINGS/PRECAUTIONS:** Wash hands immediately after applying paste. D/C if rash or contact mucositis occurs. Avoid eyes.

**ADVERSE REACTIONS:** Transient pain, stinging, burning.

**PREGNANCY:** Category B, caution in nursing.

## APIDRA RX

insulin glulisine, rdna (Sanofi-Aventis)

**THERAPEUTIC CLASS:** Insulin

**INDICATIONS:** To control hyperglycemia in diabetes.

**DOSAGE:** *Adults:* Individualize dose. Inject SQ within 15 min before a meal or within 20 min after starting a meal.

**HOW SUPPLIED:** Inj: 100 U/mL [3mL, 10mL]

**CONTRAINDICATIONS:** Episodes of hypoglycemia.

**WARNINGS/PRECAUTIONS:** Monitor glucose. Rapid onset and short duration of action; follow dosage directions. Longer-acting insulin or insulin infusion pump may be required to maintain glucose control. When used in an external pump for SQ infusion, do not dilute or mix with any other insulin. Caution when changing insulin strength, manufacturer, type, or species. Concomitant antidiabetic therapy may need adjustment. As with other insulin therapy hypoglycemic reactions and local/systemic allergic reactions may occur.

**ADVERSE REACTIONS:** Allergic reactions, injection site reactions, lipodystrophy, pruritus, rash, hypoglycemia.

**INTERACTIONS:** Decreased effect with corticosteroids, danazol, diazoxide, diuretics, sympathomimetic agents (eg, epinephrine, albuterol, terbutaline), glucagon, isoniazid, phenothiazine derivatives, somatropin, thyroid hormones, estrogens, progestogens (eg, in oral contraceptives), protease inhibitors, and atypical antipsychotic medications (eg, olanzepine and clozapine). Increased effect with ACEIs, MAOIs, oral antidiabetics, disopyramide, fibrates, fluoxetine, pentoxifylline, propoxyphene, salicylates, sulflonomide antibiotics. Decreased or increased effect with β-blockers, clonidine, lithium salts, and alcohol. Pentamidine may cause hypoglycemia followed by hyperglycemia.

**PREGNANCY:** Category C, caution in nursing.

## APOKYN RX

apomorphine HCl (Mylan Bertek)

**THERAPEUTIC CLASS:** Non-ergoline dopamine agonist

**INDICATIONS:** Acute, intermittent treatment of hypomobility,"off" episodes ("end-of-dose wearing off" and unpredictable"on/off" episodes) associated with advanced Parkinson's disease.

**DOSAGE:** *Adults:* Initial: Test Dose: 2mg SC; closely monitor BP. Titrate: Increase by 1mg every few days; assess efficacy/tolerability. Max: 6mg/day. Renal Impairment: Initial: 1mg SC.

**HOW SUPPLIED:** Inj: 10mg/mL [2mL, 3mL]

**CONTRAINDICATIONS:** Concomitant use with $5HT_3$ antagonists (eg, ondansetron, granisetron, dolasetron, palonosetron, alosetron).

**WARNINGS/PRECAUTIONS:** Avoid IV administration; serious adverse events reported (thrombus formation and PE). Nausea, vomiting, syncope, symptomatic hypotension, falls, hallucinations, falling asleep during activities of daily living, coronary events (eg, angina, MI, cardiac arrest, suddden death) reported. May prolong QT interval; potential proarrhythmic effects; caution with drugs that prolong QT/QTc interval. Caution with sulfite sensitivity. May cause or worsen dyskinesias. Withdrawal-emergent hyperpyrexia and confusion reported with rapid dose reduction/withdrawal/changes in therapy. Fibrotic complications (eg, retroperitoneal fibrosis, pulmonary infiltrates, pleural effusion/thickening, cardiac valvulopathy) reported. May cause priapism. Caution with hepatic/renal impairment.

**ADVERSE REACTIONS:** Yawning, somnolence, dizziness, rhinorrhea, edema, chest pain, increased sweating, flushing, pallor.

**INTERACTIONS:** See Contraindications. Antihypertensives and vasodilators may increase risk of hypotension, MI, serious pneumonia/falls, bone and joint injuries. Dopamine antagonists (eg, phenothiazines, butyrophenones, thioxanthenes, metoclopramide) may diminish effectiveness.

**PREGNANCY:** Category C, not for use in nursing.

## APTIVUS

RX

tipranavir (Boehringer Ingelheim)

**Tipranavir co-administered with 200mg ritonavir has been associated with reports of both fatal and non-fatal intracranial hemorrhage as well as clinical hepatitis And hepatic decompensation including some fatalities. Extra vigilance is warranted in patients with chronic hepatitis B or hepatitis C co-infection, as these patients have an increased risk of hepatotoxicity.**

**THERAPEUTIC CLASS:** Protease inhibitor

**INDICATIONS:** Co-administered with 200mg of ritonavir for treatment of HIV-1 infected patients with evidence of viral replication, who are highly treatment-experienced or have HIV-1 strains resistant to multiple protease inhibitors.

**DOSAGE:** *Adults:* 500mg with 200mg ritonavir bid with food.

**HOW SUPPLIED:** Cap: 250mg

**CONTRAINDICATIONS:** Moderate to severe (Child-Pugh Class B and C) hepatic insufficiency. Concomitant administration with amiodarone, bepridil, flecainide, propafenone, quinidine, astemizole, terfenadine, dihydroergotamine, ergonovine, ergotamine, methylergonovine, cisapride, pimozide, midazolam, triazolam.

**WARNINGS/PRECAUTIONS:** Must be co-administered with ritonavir. Caution with hepatic impairment; monitor LFTs during therapy. Caution in patients at risk of increased bleeding from trauma, surgery or other medical conditions, or who are receiving medications known to increase risk of bleeding (eg, antiplatelet agents, anticoagulants). Reports of new-onset DM, exacerbation of pre-existing DM, hyperglycemia; rash and rash accompanied with joint pain/stiffness, throat tightness, generalized pruritus; increased bleeding with hemophilia Types A and B; and increased total cholesterol and triglycerides. Caution with known sulfonamide allergy. D/C with severe rash. Possible redistribution/accumulation of body fat. Immune reconstitution syndrome reported with combination therapy.

**ADVERSE REACTIONS:** Diarrhea, nausea, vomiting, abdominal pain, pyrexia, fatigue, asthenia, bronchitis, headache, depression, insomnia, cough, rash.

**INTERACTIONS:** See Contraindications. Do not use with rifampin, St. John's wort, lovastatin, simvastatin, meperidine, methadone. Decreased levels of abacavir, didanosine, zidovudine, amprenavir, lopinavir, saquinavir. Increased levels of fluoxetine, paroxetine, sertraline; adjust dose. Caution with itraconazole, ketoconazole, voriconazole, diltiazem, felodipine, nicardipine, nisoldipine, verapamil, disulfiram/metronidazole, atorvastatin, cyclosporine, sirolimus, tacrolimus. Starting dose of sildenafil should not exceed 25mg within 48 hours, tadalfil 10mg every 72 hours, and vardenafil 2.5mg every 72 hours. Decreased levels of ethinyl estradiol; use alternative forms of birth control. Dosage reduction needed for clarithromycin by 50% if CrCl 30-60mL/min and 75% if <30mL/min; rifabutin by 75%; despiramine. Increased levels with fluconazole. Monitor glucose with glimepiride, glipizide, glyburide, pioglitazone, repaglinide, tolbutamine. Monitor INR with warfarin.

**PREGNANCY:** Category C, not for use in nursing.

## ARALEN

RX

chloroquine (Sanofi-Aventis)

**THERAPEUTIC CLASS:** Aminoquinolone

**INDICATIONS:** Treatment of extraintestinal amebiasis and acute attacks of malaria. Suppression of malaria.

**DOSAGE:** *Adults:* Malaria: Initial: 1g, then 500mg 6-8 hrs later, then 500mg qd for 2 consecutive days (total of 2.5g in 3 days). Suppression: 500mg on the same day each week. Start 2 weeks before exposure (double initial dose if <2 weeks before exposure) and continue for 8 weeks after return. Extraintestinal Amebiasis: 1g qd for 2 days, then 500mg qd for at least 2-3 weeks. Treatment usually combined with intestinal amebicide.
*Pediatrics:* Malaria: Total dose of 25mg base/kg taken over 3 day, as follows: 1st Dose: 10mg base/kg (max 600mg base single dose). 2nd Dose: 5mg base/kg (300mg base single dose) 6 hrs after 1st dose. 3rd Dose: 5mg base/kg 18 hrs after 2nd dose. 4th Dose: 5mg base/kg 24 hrs after 3rd dose. Suppression: 5mg base/kg/week. Max: 300mg base/dose. Start 2 weeks before exposure (double initial dose if <2 weeks before exposure) and continue for 8 weeks after return.

**HOW SUPPLIED:** Tab: (Phosphate) 500mg (500mg tab=300mg base)

**CONTRAINDICATIONS:** Retinal or visual field changes.

**WARNINGS/PRECAUTIONS:** Caution with G6PD deficiency, pre-existing auditory damage, hepatic impairment, alcoholism, porphyria, psoriasis, elderly, and history of seizures. Monitor CBCs, vision, reflexes with prolonged use. D/C if visual or hematological disturbances, muscle weakness, hearing defects develop.

**ADVERSE REACTIONS:** Headache, pruritus, psychic stimulation, visual disturbances, pleomorphic skin eruptions, GI effects, convulsions.

**INTERACTIONS:** Caution with hepatotoxic drugs. Space dosing of antacids/kaolin by 4 hours. Increased levels with cimetidine; avoid concomitant use. Space dosing of ampicillin by at least 2 hours. May increase cyclosporine levels; monitor closely.

**PREGNANCY:** Avoid in pregnancy except for treatment of malaria if benefits outweigh risks. Not for use in nursing.

## ARAMINE RX

metaraminol bitartrate (Merck)

**THERAPEUTIC CLASS:** Sympathomimetic amine

**INDICATIONS:** Prevention and treatment of the acute hypotensive state occurring with spinal anesthesia. Adjunct treatment of hypotension due to hemorrhage, reactions to medications, surgical complications, and shock associated with brain damage due to trauma or tumor.

**DOSAGE:** *Adults:* Hypotension Prevention: 2-10mg IM/SC. Hypotension Adjunct Treatment: Adjust 15-100mg IV infusion to maintain desired BP. Severe Shock: 0.5-5mg direct IV injection, followed by 15-100mg IV infusion.

**HOW SUPPLIED:** Inj: 10mg/mL

**CONTRAINDICATIONS:** Cyclopropane or halothane anesthesia.

**WARNINGS/PRECAUTIONS:** Contains sodium bisulfate; may cause allergic reaction especially in asthmatics. Avoid excessive BP response. Possible prolonged BP elevation after discontinuation. Caution with cirrhosis, heart or thyroid disease, HTN, or diabetes. If used for long periods, the resulting vasoconstriction may prevent adequate expansion of circulating volume and cause perpetuation of shock. May provoke relapse in patients with history of malaria.

**ADVERSE REACTIONS:** Tachycardia, arrhythmia, abscess formation/tissue necrosis/sloughing at injection site.

**INTERACTIONS:** See Contraindications. Caution in digitalized patients; digitalis with sympathomimetic amines may cause ectopic arrhythmias. MAOIs or TCAs may potentiate pressor effect; lower initial dose of metaraminol.

**PREGNANCY:** Category C, caution in nursing.

## ARANESP

darbepoetin alfa (Amgen)

RX

**Erythropoiesis-stimulating agents (ESAs) may increase risk for death and/or serious cardiovascular events when administered to a target Hgb >12g/dL. Use lowest dose that will gradually increase Hgb concentration to lowest level sufficient to avoid need for RBC transfusion. When ESAs are used preoperatively for reduction of allogenic RBC transfusions, a higher incidence of DVT was reported in patients not receiving prophylactic anticoagulation; darbepoetin alfa is not approved for this indication.**

**THERAPEUTIC CLASS:** Erythropoiesis stimulator

**INDICATIONS:** Treatment of anemia associated with chronic renal failure (CRF), and anemia in patients with non-myeloid malignancies due to chemotherapy.

**DOSAGE:** *Adults:* CRF: Initial: 0.45mcg/kg IV/SQ weekly. Conversion from Epoetin Alfa: Base dose on weekly epoetin dose. Give once weekly if receiving epoetin 2-3x/week. Give every 2 weeks if receiving epoetin once weekly. (See labeling for more information). Titrate: Adjust to target Hgb <12g/dL. If Hgb increases >1g/dL in a 2-week period or is approaching 12g/dL, decrease dose by 25%. If Hgb continues to increase, hold dose until Hgb begins to decrease, and reinitiate at 25% below previous dose. Do not increase more than once monthly. Malignancy: Initial: 2.25mcg/kg SQ weekly. Titrate: Increase to 4.5mcg/kg if Hgb increases <1g/dL after 6 weeks of therapy. If Hgb increases by >1g/dL in a 2-week period or if Hgb >12g/dL, decrease dose by 25%. If Hgb >13g/dL, hold dose until Hgb falls to 12g/dL and reinitiate at 25% below previous dose.

**HOW SUPPLIED:** Inj: Syringe: 0.025mg/0.42mL, 0.04mg/0.4mL, 0.06mg/0.3mL, 0.1mg/0.5mL, 0.15mg/0.3mL, 0.2mg/0.4mL, 0.3mg/0.6mL, 0.5mg/mL; SDV: 0.025mg/mL, 0.04mg/mL, 0.06mg/mL, 0.1mg/mL, 0.15mg/0.75mL, 0.2mg/mL, 0.3mg/mL

**CONTRAINDICATIONS:** Uncontrolled HTN.

**WARNINGS/PRECAUTIONS:** Pure red cell aplasia and severe anemia (with or without other cytopenias) may occur. Due to increased Hgb, increased risk of cardiovascular events including death may occur. Control BP before therapy. Seizures reported. Increased risk of thrombotic events. Pure red cell aplasia reported; discontinue if this occurs. Evaluate etiology if lack/loss of response occurs. Permanently discontinue if serious allergic reaction occurs. Monitor renal function, fluid, and electrolytes. Albumin solution carries risk of transmission of viral diseases. May need interval of 2-6 weeks between dose adjustment and response. Monitor Hgb weekly until stabilized and maintenance dose is established, and for at least 4 weeks after dosage change. Monitor iron status before and during therapy. Increases RBCs and decreases plasma volume.

**ADVERSE REACTIONS:** Thrombic events, infection, myalgia, HTN, hypotension, headache, diarrhea, fatigue, edema, nausea, vomiting, fever, dyspnea.

**PREGNANCY:** Category C, caution in nursing.

## ARAVA

leflunomide (Sanofi-Aventis)

RX

**Avoid pregnancy during treatment or before completion of drug elimination procedure after treatment.**

**THERAPEUTIC CLASS:** Pyrimidine synthesis inhibitor

**INDICATIONS:** Treatment of active rheumatoid arthritis to reduce signs/symptoms, inhibit structural damage, or improve physical function.

**DOSAGE:** *Adults:* LD: 100mg qd for 3 days. Maint: 20mg qd. If not tolerated and/or ALT elevations >2 but ≤3X ULN: Reduce to 10mg qd. If elevations persist or >3X ULN, d/c and give cholestyramine or charcoal. Max: 20mg/day.

**HOW SUPPLIED:** Tab: 10mg, 20mg

**CONTRAINDICATIONS:** Pregnancy.

**WARNINGS/PRECAUTIONS:** May cause immunosuppression. Avoid with severe immunodeficiency, bone marrow dysplasia, severe, uncontrolled infections, significant hepatic impairment, or evidence of hepatitis B or C. Rare reports of pancytopenia, agranulocytosis, thrombocytopenia, Stevens-Johnson syndrome, toxic epidermal necrolysis, and potentially fatal severe liver injury. Monitor WBCs, platelets, Hgb, Hct, LFTs (esp ALT) at baseline then monthly for 6 months, and every 6-8 weeks thereafter; monitor monthly with concomitant MTX and/or other immunosuppressive agents. D/C with evidence of bone marrow suppression. Women of childbearing potential must have negative pregnancy test. Caution with renal impairment.

**ADVERSE REACTIONS:** Diarrhea, respiratory infections, HTN, alopecia, rash, nausea, bronchitis, abdominal/back pain, abnormal liver enzymes, urinary tract infections, dyspepsia.

**INTERACTIONS:** Decreased levels with cholestyramine or activated charcoal. Increased side effects with hepatotoxic substances. Increased levels with rifampin; caution with concomitant use. May increase levels of diclofenac, ibuprofen, or tolbutamide. Avoid vaccination with live vaccines.

**PREGNANCY:** Category X, not for use in nursing.

## AREDIA RX

pamidronate disodium (Novartis)

**THERAPEUTIC CLASS:** Bone resorption inhibitor

**INDICATIONS:** Treatment of moderate to severe hypercalcemia of malignancy, Paget's disease. Adjunct to standard anti-neoplastic therapy for treatment of osteolytic bone metastases of breast cancer and osteolytic lesions of multiple myeloma.

**DOSAGE:** *Adults:* Moderate Hypercalcemia: 60-90mg IV single dose over 2-24 hrs. Severe Hypercalcemia: 90mg IV single dose over 2-24 hrs. Retreatment: May repeat after 7 days. Paget's Disease: 30mg IV over 4 hrs for 3 consecutive days. Osteolytic Bone Lesions of Multiple Myeloma: 90mg IV over 4 hrs once a month. Osteolytic Bone Metastases of Breast Cancer: 90mg IV over 2 hrs every 3-4 weeks. Max: 90mg/single dose for all indications. Renal Dysfunction With Bone Metastases: Withhold dose if SrCr increases by 0.5mg/dL (normal baseline) or by 1mg/dL (abnormal baseline). Resume when SrCr returns to within 10% of baseline.

**HOW SUPPLIED:** Inj: 30mg, 90mg

**WARNINGS/PRECAUTIONS:** Associated with renal toxicity; monitor serum creatinine prior to each treatment. Monitor serum calcium, electrolytes, phosphate, magnesium, CBC with differential, Hct/Hgb closely. Monitor for 2 weeks post-treatment if pre-existing anemia, leukopenia, thrombocytopenia. Increased risk of renal adverse reactions with renal impairment; monitor renal function. Avoid treatment of bone metastases in severe renal impairment. Reports of osteonecrosis of jaw in cancer patients treated with bisphosphonates; avoid invasive dental procedures.

**ADVERSE REACTIONS:** Malaise, fever, convulsions, hypomagnesemia, hypocalcemia, hypokalemia, fluid overload, hypophosphatemia, nausea, diarrhea, constipation, anorexia, abnormal hepatic function, bone pain, dyspnea.

**PREGNANCY:** Category D, caution in nursing.

## ARGATROBAN

argatroban (GlaxoSmithKline)

RX

**THERAPEUTIC CLASS:** Direct thrombin inhibitor

**INDICATIONS:** Prophylaxis or treatment of thrombosis in heparin-induced thrombocytopenia (HIT). As an anticoagulant in patients with or at risk for HIT undergoing percutaneous coronary intervention (PCI).

**DOSAGE:** *Adults:* Thrombosis: Discontinue heparin and obtain baseline aPTT. Initial: 2mcg/kg/min IV. Check aPTT after 2 hrs. Titrate: Increase dose until aPTT is 1.5-3x the initial baseline. Max: 10mcg/kg/min. Moderate Hepatic Impairment: Initial: 0.5mcg/kg/min. PCI: Initial: 350mcg/kg bolus with 25mcg/kg/min IV. Check activated clotting time (ACT) 5-10 minutes after bolus. Proceed with PCI if ACT >300 seconds. If ACT <300 seconds, give additional 150mcg/kg bolus and increase infusion to 30mcg/kg/min. Check ACT 5-10 minutes later. If ACT >450 seconds, decrease to 15mcg/kg/min and check ACT 5-10 minutes later. Continue infusion dose at therapeutic ACT (300-450 seconds) during procedure. May give additional 150mcg/kg bolus and increase infusion to 40mcg/kg/min if dissection, impending abrupt closure, thrombus formation, or inability to achieve/maintain ACT >300 seconds. After PCI, may use lower infusion rate if anticoagulation is needed.

**HOW SUPPLIED:** Inj: 100mg/mL

**CONTRAINDICATIONS:** Overt major bleeding.

**WARNINGS/PRECAUTIONS:** Discontinue all parenteral anticoagulants before administering. Extreme caution in conditions associated with an increased danger of hemorrhage (eg, severe HTN, immediately following lumbar puncture, bleeding disorder, GI lesions, spinal anesthesia, major surgery, etc). Caution in hepatic impairment. Avoid high doses in PCI patients with significant hepatic disease or AST/ALT >3X ULN. Monitor aPTT. For PCI, obtain ACT before dose, 5-10 minutes after bolus and infusion rate change, at the end of PCI, and every 20-30 minutes during prolonged procedures.

**ADVERSE REACTIONS:** GI bleed, GU bleed, Hct/Hgb decrease, hypotension, fever, diarrhea, sepsis, cardiac arrest, nausea, ventricular tachycardia, vomiting, allergic reactions, chest pain (in PCI).

**INTERACTIONS:** Initiate after cessation of heparin therapy; allow time for heparin's effect on the aPTT to decrease. Prolongation of PT and INR with warfarin. Antiplatelets, thrombolytics, and other anticoagulants may increase risk of bleeding. Discontinue all anticoagulants before argatroban administration.

**PREGNANCY:** Category B, not for use in nursing.

## ARICEPT

donepezil HCl (Eisai/Pfizer)

RX

**OTHER BRAND NAMES:** Aricept ODT (Eisai/Pfizer)

**THERAPEUTIC CLASS:** Acetylcholinesterase inhibitor

**INDICATIONS:** Treatment of dementia of the Alzheimer's type.

**DOSAGE:** *Adults:* Mild to Moderate Alzheimer's Disease: Initial: 5mg qhs. Titrate: May increase to 10mg after 4-6 weeks. Severe Alzheimer's Disease: 10mg qhs. Start with 5mg qhs and increase to 10mg after 4-6 weeks.

**HOW SUPPLIED:** Tab: 5mg, 10mg; Tab, Disintegrating: 5mg, 10mg

**CONTRAINDICATIONS:** Hypersensitivity to piperidine derivatives.

**WARNINGS/PRECAUTIONS:** May exaggerate succinylcholine-type muscle relaxation during anesthesia. May have vagotonic effects on sinoatrial and atrioventricular node; may cause bradycardia or heart block. May increase gastric acid secretion; monitor for GI bleeding. May cause bladder outflow obstruction or seizures. Caution with asthma or COPD.

**ADVERSE REACTIONS:** Nausea, diarrhea, insomnia, vomiting, muscle cramps, fatigue, anorexia, dizziness, depression, somnolence, weight decrease, infection, hypertension, back pain.

**INTERACTIONS:** Synergistic effect with neuromuscular blocking agents (eg, succinylcholine) and cholinergic agonists (eg, bethanechol). May interfere with anticholinergic medications. CYP2D6 and CYP3A4 inducers (eg, phenytoin, carbamazepine, dexamethasone, rifampin, phenobarbital) may increase elimination rate.

**PREGNANCY:** Category C, not for use in nursing.

## ARIMIDEX

RX

anastrozole (AstraZeneca LP)

**THERAPEUTIC CLASS:** Aromatase inhibitor (non-steroidal)

**INDICATIONS:** Treatment of advanced breast cancer in postmenopausal women with disease progression following tamoxifen therapy. First-line treatment of postmenopausal women with hormone receptor positive or hormone receptor unknown locally advanced or metastatic breast cancer. Adjuvant treatment of postmenopausal women with hormone-receptor positive early breast cancer. (Patients with ER-negative disease and who did not respond to previous tamoxifen therapy rarely respond.)

**DOSAGE:** *Adults:* Adjuvant/Advanced/Metastatic Breast Cancer: 1mg qd. Continue until tumor progression for advanced breast cancer.

**HOW SUPPLIED:** Tab: 1mg

**WARNINGS/PRECAUTIONS:** May cause fetal harm during pregnancy. Avoid in premenopausal women. May cause reduction in bone mineral density. May elevate serum cholesterol.

**ADVERSE REACTIONS:** Joint disorders, mood disturbances, pharyngitis, depression, hypertension, osteoporosis, peripheral edema, bone fractures, asthenia, headache, hot flushes, dyspnea, nausea, vomiting, cough, pain, edema.

**INTERACTIONS:** Avoid tamoxifen, estrogen-containing therapies.

**PREGNANCY:** Category D, caution in nursing.

## ARIXTRA

RX

fondaparinux sodium (GlaxoSmithKline)

**Risk of paralysis by spinal/epidural hematoma with neuraxial anesthesia or spinal puncture. Increased risk with indwelling epidural catheters for analgesia, drugs affecting hemostasis (eg, NSAIDs, platelet inhibitors, anticoagulants), and traumatic or repeated epidural or spinal puncture.**

**THERAPEUTIC CLASS:** Specific factor Xa inhibitor

**INDICATIONS:** Prophylaxis of DVT in patients undergoing hip fracture surgery, including extended prophylaxis; hip replacement surgery; knee replacement surgery; abdominal surgery who are at risk of thromboembolic complications. With concomitant warfarin, treatment of acute PE when initial therapy is administered in hospital and acute DVT.

**DOSAGE:** *Adults:* DVT Prophylaxis: 2.5mg SQ qd, starting 6-8 hrs post-op for 5-9 days (up to 11 days). Hip Fracture Surgery: Extended prophylaxis up to 24 additional days is recommended. DVT/PE Treatment: <50kg: 5mg SQ qd. 50-100kg: 7.5mg SQ qd. >100kg: 10mg SQ qd. Add concomitant warfarin ASAP (usually within 72 hrs) and continue for 5-9 days (up to 26 days) until INR=2-3.

**HOW SUPPLIED:** Inj: (Syringe) 2.5mg/0.5mL, 5mg/0.4mL, 7.5mg/0.6mL, 10mg/0.8mL

**CONTRAINDICATIONS:** Severe renal impairment (CrCl <30mL/min), body weight <50kg undergoing hip fracture, hip/knee replacement or abdominal surgery, bacterial endocarditis, active major bleeding, thrombocytopenia with a positive *in vitro* test for anti-platelet antibody.

**WARNINGS/PRECAUTIONS:** Not for IM injection. Cannot use interchangeably unit for unit with heparin or other low molecular weight heparins. Risk of hemorrhage increases with renal impairment. Caution with moderate renal dysfunction, elderly, history of HIT, bleeding diathesis, uncontrolled arterial HTN, recent GI ulceration, diabetic retinopathy, hemorrhage. Monitor renal function periodically. Extreme caution in conditions with an increased risk of hemorrhage (eg, bleeding disorders, hemorrhagic stroke, etc). Perform routine CBC, SCr, stool occult blood tests. Discontinue if platelets <100,000/mm³. Thrombocytopenia reported. Major bleeding with abdominal surgery reported.

**ADVERSE REACTIONS:** Hemorrhage, thrombocytopenia, local reactions (eg, rash, pruritus), AST/ALT elevations, anemia, fever, nausea, edema, constipation, vomiting.

**INTERACTIONS:** Discontinue agents that may enhance risk of hemorrhage (eg, platelet inhibitors); monitor closely if co-administered.

**PREGNANCY:** Category B, caution in nursing.

## ARMOUR THYROID

RX

thyroid (Forest)

**THERAPEUTIC CLASS:** Thyroid replacement hormone

**INDICATIONS:** Treatment of hypothyroidism. As a pituitary TSH suppressant in the treatment or prevention of various types of euthyroid goiters. Diagnostic agent in suppression tests to differentiate suspected mild hyperthyroidism or thyroid gland autonomy. Management of thyroid cancer.

**DOSAGE:** *Adults:* Hypothyroidism: Initial: 30mg qd. Titrate: Increase by 15mg q2-3 weeks. Myxedema with Cardiovascular Disorder: 15mg qd. Maint: 60-120mg/day. Thyroid Cancer: Higher doses then replacement therapy is required. Myxedema Coma: Levothyroxine Sodium: Initial: 400mcg IV then 100-200mcg/day IV. Continue with oral therapy when stabilized. Thyroid Suppression: 1.56mg/kg/day for 7-10 days. Elderly: Initial: Use lower dose (eg, 15-30mg qd).
*Pediatrics:* Hypothyroidism: 0-6months: 4.8-6mg/kg/day; 6-12 months: 3.6-4.8mg/kg/day; 1-5 yrs: 3-3.6mg/kg/day; 6-12 yrs: 2.4-3mg/kg/day; >12 yrs: 1.2-1.8mg/kg/day.

**HOW SUPPLIED:** Tab: 15mg, 30mg, 60mg, 90mg, 120mg, 180mg, 240mg, 300mg

**CONTRAINDICATIONS:** Untreated thyrotoxicosis; uncorrected adrenal cortical insufficiency.

**WARNINGS/PRECAUTIONS:** Do not use in the treatment of obesity; larger doses in euthyroid patients can cause serious or even life threatening toxicity. Caution with cardiovascular disease, DM, diabetes insipidus, elderly, and adrenal cortical insufficiency.

**INTERACTIONS:** May increase insulin or oral hypoglycemic requirements. Reduced absorption with cholestyramine and colestipol; space dosing by 4-5 hours. Altered effect of oral anticoagulants; monitor PT/INR. Estrogens increase thyroxine-binding globulin; increase in thyroid dose may be needed. Serious or life-threatening side effects can occur with sympathomimetic amines. Androgens, corticosteroids, estrogens, iodine-containing preparations, and salicylates may interfere with thyroid lab tests.

**PREGNANCY:** Category A, caution in nursing.

## AROMASIN

exemestane (Pharmacia)

RX

**THERAPEUTIC CLASS:** Aromatase inactivator

**INDICATIONS:** In postmenopausal women, treatment of advanced breast cancer that has progressed after tamoxifen therapy. Adjuvant treatment of postmenopausal women with estrogen-receptor positive early breast cancer who have received 2-3 years of tamoxifen and are switched to exemestane for a total completion of 5 consecutive years to adjuvant hormonal therapy.

**DOSAGE:** *Adults:* Early/Advanced: 25mg qd after a meal. Continue in the absence of recurrence of contralateral breast cancer until completion of 5 years of adjuvant endocrine therapy in postmenopausal women with early breast cancer treated with 2-3 years of tamoxifen. Continue until tumor progression is evident. Concomitant Potent CYP3A4 Inducers (eg, rifampicin, phenytoin): 50mg qd after a meal.

**HOW SUPPLIED:** Tab: 25mg

**WARNINGS/PRECAUTIONS:** Fetal harm in pregnancy. Avoid in premenopausal women.

**ADVERSE REACTIONS:** Fatigue, nausea, hot flashes, pain, depression, insomnia, anxiety, dyspnea, dizziness, headache, vomiting, increased sweating, edema, HTN, anorexia.

**INTERACTIONS:** Avoid coadministration with estrogen-containing agents. Potent CYP3A4 inducers (eg, rifampin, phenytoin, carbamazepine, phenobarbital, St. John's wort) may decrease plasma levels.

**PREGNANCY:** Category D, caution in nursing.

## ARRANON

nelarabine (GlaxoSmithKline)

RX

**Severe neurologic events reported; close monitoring is strongly recommended. Discontinue for neurologic events of NCI Common Toxicity Criteria ≥ grade 2.**

**THERAPEUTIC CLASS:** Deoxyguanosine analogue

**INDICATIONS:** Treatment of T-cell acute lymphoblastic leukemia and T-cell lymphoblastic lymphoma in patients whose disease has not responded to or has relapsed following treatment with at least two chemotherapy regimens.

**DOSAGE:** *Adults:* 1500mg/m$^2$ IV over 2 hrs on days 1, 3, and 5 repeated every 21 days. CrCl <50ml/min: Insufficient data to support dose recommendation. *Pediatrics:* 650mg/m$^2$/day IV over 1 hr daily for 5 consecutive days. Repeat every 21 days. CrCl <50ml/min: Insufficient data to support dose recommendation.

**HOW SUPPLIED:** Inj: 5mg/mL

**WARNINGS/PRECAUTIONS:** Leukopenia, thrombocytopenia, anemia, neutropenia/febrile neutropenia reported; regularly monitor CBC including platelets. Intravenous hydration recommended for management of hyperuricemia with risk of tumor lysis syndrome; may also consider allopurinol. Avoid administration of live vaccines. Closely monitor toxicities with severe renal impairment (eg, CrCl <30mL/min) and/or severe hepatic impairment (eg, bilirubin >3mg/dL); increased risk of adverse reactions.

**ADVERSE REACTIONS:** See Black Box Warning, Warnings/Precautions. Pediatrics: headache, increased transaminases, decreased blood potassium, decreased/increased blood albumin, vomiting. Adults: fatigue, nausea, diarrhea, vomiting, constipation, cough, dyspnea, dizziness, pyrexia, blurred vision.

**PREGNANCY:** Category D, not for use in nursing.

## ARTHROTEC

RX

misoprostol - diclofenac sodium (Searle)

**Contraindicated in pregnancy. Must have (-) pregnancy test 2 weeks before therapy. Provide oral and written hazards of misoprostol. Begin on 2nd or 3rd day of the next normal menstrual period. Use reliable contraception. NSAIDs may cause an increased risk of serious cardiovascular thrombotic events, MI, stroke and serious GI adverse events including bleeding, ulceration, and perforation of the stomach or intestines. Contraindicated for the treatment of peri-operative pain in the setting of coronary artery bypass graft (CABG) surgery.**

**THERAPEUTIC CLASS:** NSAID/prostaglandin $E_1$ analogue

**INDICATIONS:** Treatment of the signs and symptoms of osteoarthritis (OA) or rheumatoid arthritis (RA) in patients at high risk of developing NSAID-induced gastric and duodenal ulcers.

**DOSAGE:** *Adults:* OA: 50mg tid. RA: 50mg tid-qid. OA/RA: If not tolerable, give 50-75mg bid (less effective in preventing ulcers). Do not crush, chew, or divide.

**HOW SUPPLIED:** Tab: (Diclofenac-Misoprostol) 50mg-0.2mg, 75mg-0.2mg

**CONTRAINDICATIONS:** Pregnancy. ASA or other NSAID allergy that precipitates asthma, urticaria or other allergic reactions. Treatment of peri-operative pain in the setting of CABG surgery.

**WARNINGS/PRECAUTIONS:** May lead to onset of new HTN or worsening of pre-existing HTN; monitor BP closely. Fluid retention and edema reported; caution with fluid retention or heart failure. Renal papillary necrosis and other renal injury reported after long-term use. Not recommended for use with advanced renal disease; if therapy must be initiated, monitor renal function. May cause elevations of LFTs; discontinue if abnormal LFTs persist/worsen, liver disease develops or systemic manifestations occur. Anaphylactoid reactions may occur. May cause serious skin adverse events (eg, exfoliative dermatitis, Stevens-Johnson syndrome, and toxic epidermal necrolysis). Avoid in late pregnancy; may cause premature closure of ductus arteriosis. Caution in elderly. Anemia may occur; with long-term use, monitor Hgb/Hct if signs or symptoms of anemia. May inhibit platelet aggregation and prolong bleeding time; monitor with coagulation disorders. Caution with asthma and avoid with aspirin-sensitive asthma. Aseptic meningitis with fever and coma reported. Avoid with hepatic porphyria.

**ADVERSE REACTIONS:** Abdominal pain, diarrhea, dyspepsia, nausea, flatulence, GI disorders.

**INTERACTIONS:** Avoid magnesium-containing antacids, salicylates, ASA, other NSAIDs. Caution with anticoagulants; may have synergistic GI bleeding effects with warfarin. May decrease effects of antihypertensives, diuretics. Increased serum potassium with $K^+$-sparing diuretics. May alter response to insulin or oral hypoglycemics. Monitor for digoxin, methotrexate, cyclosporine, phenobarbital, and lithium toxicities.

**PREGNANCY:** Category X, not for use in nursing.

## ASACOL

RX

mesalamine (Procter & Gamble)

**THERAPEUTIC CLASS:** Anti-inflammatory agent

**INDICATIONS:** Treatment of mild to moderately active ulcerative colitis and maintenance of remission of ulcerative colitis.

**DOSAGE:** *Adults:* Mild-Moderate Active Ulcerative Colitis: Usual: 800mg tid for 6 weeks. Maintenance of Remission: 1.6g/day in divided doses.

**HOW SUPPLIED:** Tab, Delayed Release: 400mg

**CONTRAINDICATIONS:** Hypersensitivity to salicylates.

**WARNINGS/PRECAUTIONS:** Exacerbation of colitis reported upon initiation of therapy; symptoms abate with discontinuation. Caution with sulfasalazine hypersensitivity. Caution with renal dysfunction or history of renal disease. Monitor renal function prior to therapy and periodically after. Pyloric stenosis could delay mesalamine release in the colon.

**ADVERSE REACTIONS:** Diarrhea, headache, nausea, pharyngitis, abdominal pain, pain, eructation, dizziness, asthenia, fever, dysmenorrhea, arthralgia, dyspepsia, vomiting.

**PREGNANCY:** Category B, caution in nursing.

## ASMANEX RX

mometasone furoate (Schering)

**THERAPEUTIC CLASS:** Corticosteroid

**INDICATIONS:** Maintenance treatment of asthma as prophylactic therapy in patients ≥12 years; to reduce or eliminate the need for oral corticosteroidal therapy.

**DOSAGE:** *Adults:* Previous Therapy with Bronchodilators Alone or Inhaled Corticosteroids: Initial: 220mcg qpm. Max: 440mcg qpm or 220mcg bid. Previous Therapy with Oral Corticosteroids: Initial: 440mcg bid. Max: 880mcg/day. Titrate to lowest effective dose once asthma stability is achieved.
*Pediatrics:* ≥12 yrs: Previous Therapy with Bronchodilators Alone or Inhaled Corticosteroids: Initial: 220mcg qpm. Max: 440mcg qpm or 220mcg bid. Previous Therapy with Oral Corticosteroids: Initial: 440mcg bid. Max: 880mcg/day. Titrate to lowest effective dose once asthma stability is achieved.

**HOW SUPPLIED:** Twisthaler: 220mcg/inh

**CONTRAINDICATIONS:** Primary treatment of status asthmaticus or other acute episodes of asthma where intensive measures are required.

**WARNINGS/PRECAUTIONS:** Deaths due to adrenal insufficiency have occurred with transfer from systemic corticosteroids to inhaled corticosteroids. Wean slowly from systemic corticosteroid therapy. Resume oral corticosteroids during stress or severe asthma attack. May unmask allergic conditions previously suppressed by systemic corticosteroid therapy. May increase susceptibility to infections. Not for rapid relief of bronchospasm or other acute episodes of asthma. Discontinue if bronchospasm occurs after dosing. Observe for systemic corticosteroid withdrawal effects, hypercorticism, reduced bone mineral density, and adrenal suppression; reduce dose slowly if needed. Decreased growth velocity may occur in pediatric patients. *Candida* infections in the mouth and pharynx reported. Caution with active or quiescent TB infection of the respiratory tract; untreated systemic fungal, bacterial, viral, or parasitic infections; or ocular herpes simplex. Glaucoma, increased IOP, and cataracts reported.

**ADVERSE REACTIONS:** Headache, allergic rhinitis, pharyngitis, upper respiratory tract infection, sinusitis, oral candidiasis, dysmenorrhea, musculoskeletal pain, back pain, dyspepsia, myalgia, abdominal pain, nausea.

**INTERACTIONS:** Ketoconazole may increase plasma levels.

**PREGNANCY:** Category C, caution in nursing.

## ASPIRIN WITH CODEINE CIII

aspirin - codeine (Various)

**THERAPEUTIC CLASS:** Opioid analgesic

**INDICATIONS:** For relief of mild, moderate, and moderate to severe pain.

**DOSAGE:** *Adults:* 1-2 tabs of 325mg-30mg q4h prn. 1 tab of 325mg-60mg q4h prn.

**HOW SUPPLIED:** Tab: (ASA-Codeine) 325mg-30mg, 325mg-60mg

**CONTRAINDICATIONS:** Severe bleeding, disorders of coagulation or primary hemostasis (eg, hemophilia, hypoprothrombinemia, von Willebrand's disease, thrombocytopenia, thromboasthenia), ill defined hereditary platelet dysfunction, severe vitamin K deficiency, severe hepatic damage, anticoagulant therapy, peptic ulcer, serious GI lesions.

**WARNINGS/PRECAUTIONS:** May cause anaphylactic shock, severe allergic reactions. Serious bleeding can occur with peptic ulcer, GI lesions, and bleeding disorders. May prolong bleeding time if given preoperatively. Enhanced respiratory depression and cerebrospinal fluid pressure with head injury or intracranial lesion. May obscure signs of acute abdominal conditions or head injury. Caution in children and teenagers with chickenpox or flu. Caution in elderly, debilitated, severe renal/hepatic impairment, gallbladder disease or gallstones, respiratory impairment, arrhythmias, inflammatory GI tract disorders, hypothyroidism, Addison's disease, prostatic hypertrophy, urethral stricture, coagulation disorders, head injuries, or acute abdominal conditions.

**ADVERSE REACTIONS:** Lightheadedness, dizziness, drowsiness, nausea, vomiting, constipation, hearing impairment, tinnitus, diminished vision, headache, respiratory depression, sweating.

**INTERACTIONS:** May enhance effects of MAOIs, oral anticoagulants, oral antidiabetic agents, insulin, 6-MP, methotrexate, penicillins, sulfonamides, NSAIDs, narcotic analgesics, alcohol, general anesthetics, tranquilizers, corticosteroids. May diminish effects of uricosurics. Accumulation to toxic levels can occur with para-aminosalicylic acid, furosemide, and vitamin C.

**PREGNANCY:** Category C, not for use in nursing.

## ASTELIN — RX

azelastine HCl (MedPointe)

**THERAPEUTIC CLASS:** Antihistamine

**INDICATIONS:** Treatemnt of the symptoms of seasonal allergic rhinitis and vasomotor rhinitis.

**DOSAGE:** *Adults:* 2 sprays per nostril bid.
*Pediatrics:* Seasonal Allergic/Vasomotor Rhinitis: >12 yrs: 2 sprays per nostril bid. Seasonal Allergic Rhinitis: 5-11 yrs: 1 spray per nostril bid.

**HOW SUPPLIED:** Spray: 137mcg/spray [30mg]

**ADVERSE REACTIONS:** Bitter taste, somnolence, weight increase, headache, nasal burning, pharyngitis, paroxysmal sneezing, dry mouth, nausea.

**INTERACTIONS:** Avoid alcohol or other CNS depressants; additive CNS impairment may occur. Increased azelastine levels with cimetidine.

**PREGNANCY:** Category C, caution in nursing.

## ASTRAMORPH PF — CII

morphine sulfate (Abraxis)

**THERAPEUTIC CLASS:** Opioid analgesic

**INDICATIONS:** Management of pain unresponsive to non-narcotic analgesics.

**DOSAGE:** *Adults:* IV: Initial: 2-10mg/70kg. Epidural Injection: Initial: 5mg in lumbar region. Titrate: If inadequate pain relief within 1 hr, increase by 1-2mg. Max: 10mg/24hrs. Continuous Epidural: Initial: 2-4mg/24hrs. Give additional 1-2mg if needed. Intrathecal: 0.2-1mg single dose, do not repeat; may follow with 0.6mg/hr naloxone infusion to reduce incidence of side effects. Elderly/Debilitated: Epidural: <5mg/24hrs. Intrathecal: Lower dose.

**HOW SUPPLIED:** Inj: 0.5mg/mL, 1mg/mL

**CONTRAINDICATIONS:** Allergy to opiates, acute bronchial asthma, upper airway obstruction. Epidural/intrathecal routes with injection site infection, anticoagulants, bleeding diathesis, within 2 weeks of IV corticosteroids.

**WARNINGS/PRECAUTIONS:** Have resuscitation equipment, trained personnel and narcotic antagonists available; severe respiratory depression may occur. Avoid rapid administration. May be habit-forming. Caution with head injury, increased intracranial/intraocular pressure, decreased respiratory reserve, hepatic/renal dysfunction, elderly, debilitated. High doses may cause seizures. Smooth muscle hypertonicity may cause biliary colic, urinary difficulty or retention. Orthostatic hypotension may occur with hypovolemia or myocardial dysfunction. Acute respiratory failure reported with COPD or acute asthmatic attack. Limit epidural/intrathecal route to lumbar area.

**ADVERSE REACTIONS:** Respiratory depression, hypotension, pruritus, urinary retention, nausea, vomiting, constipation, anxiety, cough reflex depression, oliguria.

**INTERACTIONS:** CNS depressants (eg, alcohol, sedatives, antihistamines) and psychotropics (eg, MAOIs, phenothiazines, TCAs) potentiate CNS depression. Neuroleptics may increase respiratory depression.

**PREGNANCY:** Category C, safety in nursing not known.

## ATACAND — RX

candesartan cilexetil (AstraZeneca LP)

**Can cause death/injury to developing fetus during 2nd and 3rd trimesters. Stop therapy if pregnancy detected.**

**THERAPEUTIC CLASS:** Angiotensin II receptor antagonist

**INDICATIONS:** Treatment of hypertension, alone or with other antihypertensives. Treatment of heart failure (NYHA class II-IV, ejection fraction ≤40%) to reduce risk of death and hospitalizations.

**DOSAGE:** *Adults:* HTN: Monotherapy without Volume Depletion: Initial: 16mg qd. Usual: 8-32mg/day given qd-bid. May add diuretic if BP not controlled. Intravascular Volume Depletion/Moderate Hepatic Impairment: Lower initial dose. Heart Failure: Initial: 4mg qd. Usual: 32mg qd. Titrate: Double dose q 2 weeks as tolerated.

**HOW SUPPLIED:** Tab: 4mg, 8mg, 16mg, 32mg

**WARNINGS/PRECAUTIONS:** Can cause fetal injury/death. Correct volume or salt depletion before therapy or monitor closely. Changes in renal function may occur; caution with renal artery stenosis, CHF. Risk of hypotension; caution in major surgery and anesthesia, or when initiating therapy in heart failure.

**ADVERSE REACTIONS:** Back pain, dizziness, upper respiratory infection.

**INTERACTIONS:** Increases lithium levels.

**PREGNANCY:** Category C (1st trimester) and D (2nd and 3rd trimesters), not for use in nursing.

## ATACAND HCT — RX

hydrochlorothiazide - candesartan cilexetil (AstraZeneca LP)

**Can cause death/injury to developing fetus during 2nd and 3rd trimesters. Stop therapy if pregnancy detected.**

**THERAPEUTIC CLASS:** Angiotensin II receptor antagonist/thiazide diuretic

**INDICATIONS:** Treatment of hypertension. Not for initial therapy.

**DOSAGE:** *Adults:* Initial: If BP not controlled on HCTZ 25mg/day or controlled but serum $K^+$ decreased: 16mg-12.5mg tab qd. If BP not controlled on 32mg candesartan/day, give 32mg-12.5mg qd; may increase to 32mg-25mg qd.

**HOW SUPPLIED:** Tab: (Candesartan-HCTZ) 16mg-12.5mg, 32mg-12.5mg

**CONTRAINDICATIONS:** Anuria, sulfonamide hypersensitivity.

**WARNINGS/PRECAUTIONS:** Can cause fetal injury/death. Correct volume or salt depletion before therapy. Caution with hepatic or renal dysfunction, renal artery stenosis, severe CHF, history of allergies, and asthma. May exacerbate or activate SLE. Monitor serum electrolytes. Avoid if CrCl <30mL/min. Hyperuricemia, hyperglycemia, hypokalemia, hypomagnesemia, hypercalcemia may occur. Enhanced effects in post-sympathectomy patient. May increase cholesterol and triglyceride levels. Risk of hypotension; caution in major surgery or anesthesia.

**ADVERSE REACTIONS:** Upper respiratory infection, back pain, influenza-like symptoms, dizziness, headache.

**INTERACTIONS:** Potentiates orthostatic hypotension with alcohol, barbiturates, and narcotics. Adjust insulin and antidiabetic drugs. Impaired absorption with cholestyramine, colestipol. Corticosteroids and ACTH deplete electrolytes. May decrease response to pressor amines. Potentiates other antihypertensives. May increase responsiveness to skeletal muscle relaxants. Risk of lithium toxicity. NSAIDs decrease diuretic effects.

**PREGNANCY:** Category C (1st trimester) and D (2nd and 3rd trimesters), not for use in nursing.

## ATGAM

RX

lymphocyte immune globulin, anti-thymocyte globulin (equine)

(Pharmacia & Upjohn)

**Administer in facility equipped and staffed with adequate lab and supportive medical resources.**

**THERAPEUTIC CLASS:** Lymphocyte-selective immunosuppressant

**INDICATIONS:** Management of allograft rejection in renal transplantation. Treatment of moderate to severe aplastic anemia unsuitable for bone marrow transplantation.

**DOSAGE:** *Adults:* Renal Transplant: Delaying Rejection Onset: 15mg/kg/day for 14 days, then every other day for 14 days for total of 21 doses in 28 days. Give 1st dose 24 hrs before or after transplant. Rejection Treatment: 10-15mg/kg/day for 14 days. May give additional alternate day therapy up to a total of 21 doses. May delay 1st dose until diagnosis of 1st rejection episode. Aplastic Anemia: 10-20mg/kg/day for 8-14 days. May give additional alternate day therapy up to a total of 21 doses.
*Pediatrics:* Renal Transplant: Delaying Rejection Onset: 15mg/kg/day for 14 days, then every other day for 14 days for total of 21 doses in 28 days. Give 1st dose 24 hrs before or after transplant. Rejection Treatment: 10-15mg/kg/day for 14 days. May give additional alternate day therapy up to a total of 21 doses. May delay 1st dose until diagnosis of 1st rejection episode. Aplastic Anemia: 10-20mg/kg/day for 8-14 days. May give additional alternate day therapy up to a total of 21 doses.

**HOW SUPPLIED:** Inj: 50mg/mL

**CONTRAINDICATIONS:** History of severe systemic reaction to this product or other equine gamma globulin agents.

**WARNINGS/PRECAUTIONS:** Potency of agent may vary from lot to lot. Discontinue if anaphylaxis (eg, respiratory distress, hypotension) occurs, or if severe and unremitting thrombocytopenia or leukopenia occur in renal transplant patients. Risk of infectious transmission due to equine and human blood components. Monitor for leukopenia, thrombocytopenia, or infection (eg, CMV). Decide whether or not to continue therapy based on clinical circumstances (eg, infection).

**ADVERSE REACTIONS:** Fever, chills, leukopenia, thrombocytopenia, rash, pruritus, urticaria, wheal, flare, arthralgia, headache, phlebitis, chest/back pain, diarrhea, vomiting, nausea, dyspnea, hypotension, night sweats, stomatitis.

**INTERACTIONS:** Previously masked reactions may appear with corticosteroid or immunosuppressant dose reduction. Do not dilute with dextrose or use highly acidic infusions.

**PREGNANCY:** Category C, caution in nursing.

## ATIVAN CIV

lorazepam (Biovail)

**THERAPEUTIC CLASS:** Benzodiazepine

**INDICATIONS:** Management of anxiety.

**DOSAGE:** *Adults:* Initial: 2-3mg/day given bid-tid. Usual: 2-6mg/day in divided doses. Insomnia: 2-4mg qhs. Elderly/Debilitated: 1-2mg/day in divided doses. *Pediatrics:* >12 yrs: Initial: 2-3mg/day given bid-tid. Usual: 2-6mg/day in divided doses. Insomnia: 2-4mg qhs.

**HOW SUPPLIED:** Tab: 0.5mg, 1mg*, 2mg* *scored

**CONTRAINDICATIONS:** Acute narrow-angle glaucoma.

**WARNINGS/PRECAUTIONS:** Avoid with primary depression or psychosis. Withdrawal symptoms with abrupt discontinuation. Careful supervision if addiction-prone. Caution with elderly, and renal or hepatic dysfunction. Monitor for GI disease with prolonged therapy. Periodic blood counts and LFTs with long-term therapy.

**ADVERSE REACTIONS:** Sedation, dizziness, weakness, unsteadiness, transient amnesia, memory impairment.

**INTERACTIONS:** CNS-depressant effects with barbiturates, alcohol. Diminished tolerance to alcohol and other CNS depressants.

**PREGNANCY:** Not for use in pregnancy or nursing.

## ATIVAN INJECTION CIV

lorazepam (Baxter)

**THERAPEUTIC CLASS:** Benzodiazepine

**INDICATIONS:** Treatment of status epilepticus and preanesthetic medication in adults.

**DOSAGE:** *Adults:* >18 yrs: Status Epilepticus: 4mg IV (given slowly at 2mg/min); may repeat 1 dose after 10-15 minutes if seizures recur or fail to cease. Preanesthetic Sedation: Usual: 0.05mg/kg IM; 2mg or 0.044mg/kg IV (whichever is smaller). Max: 4mg IM/IV.

**HOW SUPPLIED:** Inj: 2mg/mL, 4mg/mL

**CONTRAINDICATIONS:** Acute narrow-angle glaucoma, sleep apnea syndrome, severe respiratory insufficiency. Not for intra-arterial injection.

**WARNINGS/PRECAUTIONS:** Monitor all parameters to maintain vital function. Risk of respiratory depression or airway obstruction in heavily sedated patients. May cause fetal damage during pregnancy. Increased risk of CNS and respiratory depression in elderly. Avoid with hepatic/renal failure. Caution with mild to moderate hepatic/renal disease. Avoid outpatient endoscopic procedures. Possible propylene glycol toxicity in renal impairment. Extreme caution when administering injections to elderly, very ill, or to patients with limited pulmonary reserve, hypoventilation and/or hypoxic cardiac arrest may occur. Gasping syndrome, characterized by central nervous system depression, metabolic acidosis, gasping respirations, and high levels of benzyl alcohol, may occur.

**ADVERSE REACTIONS:** Respiratory depression/failure, hypotension, somnolence, headache, hypoventilation.

**INTERACTIONS:** Additive CNS depression with other CNS depressants (eg, ethyl alcohol, phenothiazines, barbiturates, MAOIs). Increased sedation, hallucinations and irrational behavior with scopolamine. Decreased clearance with valproate, probenecid. Increased clearance with oral contraceptives. Severe adverse effects with clozapine and haloperidol reported.

**PREGNANCY:** Category D, not for use in nursing.

# ATRIPLA

RX

efavirenz - emtricitabine - tenofovir disoproxil fumarate

(Bristol-Myers Squibb/Gilead Sciences)

**Lactic acidosis and severe hepatomegaly with steatosis, including fatal cases, have been reported with the use of nucleoside analogs alone or in combination with other antiretrovirals. Not indicated for the treatment of chronic hepatitis B virus (HBV) infection and the safety and efficacy have not been established in patients co-infected with HBV and HIV. Severe acute exacerbations of hepatitis B have been reported in patients who have discontinued Emtriva or Viread. Hepatic function should be monitored closely with both clinical and laboratory follow-up for at least several months in patients who discontinue Atripla and are coinfected with HIV and HBV. If appropriate, initiation of anti-hepatitis B therapy may be warranted.**

**THERAPEUTIC CLASS:** Non-nucleoside reverse transcriptase inhibitor/nucleoside analog combination

**INDICATIONS:** For use alone as a complete regimen or in combination with other antiretroviral agents for the treatment of HIV-1 infection in adults.

**DOSAGE:** *Adults:* ≥18 yrs: 1 tab qd on empty stomach. Bedtime dosing may improve tolerability of nervous system effects.

**HOW SUPPLIED:** Tab: (Efavirenz-Emtricitabine-Tenofovir DF) 600mg-200mg-300mg

**CONTRAINDICATIONS:** Concomitant astemizole, cisapride, midazolam, triazolam, ergot derivatives, voriconazole, bepridil, pimozide.

**WARNINGS/PRECAUTIONS:** Obesity and prolonged nucleoside exposure may be risk factors for lactic acidosis and severe hepatomegaly with steatosis. Suspend treatment if clinical or laboratory findings suggestive of lactic acidosis or pronounced hepatotoxicity. Test for presence of HBV prior to initiation; post-treatment exacerbations reported. Monitor hepatic function for several months with discontinuation and with co-infection with HIV and HBV. Serious psychiatric adverse experiences reported. CNS symptoms reported. May cause renal impairment. Monitor SrCr and phosphorous with risk or with a history of renal dysfunction and with concomitant nephrotoxic agents. Avoid in pregnancy; use barrier contraception with other contraception methods and obtain (-) pregnancy test before therapy. Severe skin rash reported. Monitoring of liver enzymes recommended with known or suspected history of hepatitis B or C infection and with other medications associated with liver toxicity. Bone monitoring should be considered for HIV infected patients with a history of pathologic bone fracture or are at risk for osteopenia. Caution with history of seizures. Possible redistribution/accumulation of body fat. Immune reconstitution syndrome reported.

**ADVERSE REACTIONS:** Diarrhea, nausea, fatigue, sinusitis, upper respiratory tract infections, drowsiness, headache, dizziness, depression, insomnia, abnormal dreams, rash, laboratory abnormalities.

**INTERACTIONS:** Efavirenz is a CYP3A4 inducer *in vivo*, increasing the biotransformation of some drugs metabolized by CYP3A4. Co-administration of efavirenz with drugs primarily metabolized by 2C9, 2C19, and 3A4 isozymes may result in altered plasma concentrations of the co-administered drug. Drugs which induce CYP3A4 activity (eg, phenobarbital, rifampin, rifabutin) may increase clearance of efavirenz resulting in lowered plasma concentrations. Levels of efavirenz may be decreased by lopinavir/ritonavir, nelfinavir, saquinavir (SGC), rifabutin, rifampin, carbamazepine. St. John's wort to suboptimal levels, leading to loss of virologic response and possible resistance. Levels of efavirenz are increased by ritonavir, clarithromycin, sertraline, voriconazole, diltiazem. Efavirenz decreased levels of atazanavir, indinavir, lopinavir/ritonavir, saquinavir (SGC), clarithromycin, rifabutin, carbamazepine, methadone, sertraline and significantly reduced levels of voriconazole, itraconazole, atorvastatin, pravastatin, simvastatin, diltiazem. Efavirenz increased levels of nelfinavir, ritonavir, ethinyl estradiol. Co-administration of emtricitabine and tenofovir DF with drugs that are eliminated by active tubular secretion may increase concentrations of emtricitabine, tenofovir, and/or the co-administered drug. Drugs that decrease renal function may increase concentrations of emtricitabine and/or tenofovir. Levels of tenofovir increased by atazanavir, lopinavir/ritonavir may potentiate tenofovir-associated adverse events, including renal disorders. Tenofovir decreased levels of atazanavir, atazanavir/ritonavir. Co-administration of tenofovir DF with didanosine buffered tablets or EC capsules significantly increases the $C_{max}$ and AUC of didanosine; patients receiving this combination should be monitored closely for didanosine-associated adverse events. Related drugs not for co-administration include Emtriva, Viread, Truvada, and Sustiva. Should no

**PREGNANCY:** Category D, not for use in nursing.

## ATROPINE SULFATE

RX

atropine sulfate (Various)

**THERAPEUTIC CLASS:** Anticholinergic

**INDICATIONS:** Antisialagogue for preanesthetic medication to prevent or reduce secretions of the respiratory tract. To restore cardiac rate and arterial pressure during anesthesia when vagal stimulation produced by intra-abdominal surgical traction causes a sudden decrease in pulse rate and cardiac action. To lessen degree of AV heart block when increased vagal tone is a major factor in the conduction defect (possibly due to digitalis). To overcome severe bradycardia and syncope due to hyperactive carotid sinus reflex, as an antidote (with external cardiac massage) for cardiovascular collapse from the injudicious use of choline ester (cholinergic) drug. In the treatment of anticholinesterase poisoning from organophosphorus insecticides, and as an antidote for the"rapid" type of mushroom poisoning due to presence of the alkaloid muscarine, in certain species of fungus such as *Amanita muscaria*.

**DOSAGE:** *Adults:* Usual: 0.5mg IM/IV/SC. Range: 0.4-0.6mg. If used as an antisialagogue, inject IM prior to anesthesia induction. Bradyarrhythmias: 0.4-1mg every 1-2 hrs prn. Max: 2mg/dose. May be used as an antidote for cardiovascular collapse resulting from injudicious administration of choline ester. When cardiac arrest has occurred, external cardiac massage or other method of resuscitation is required to distribute the drug after IV injection. Anticholinesterase Poisoning From Insecticide Poisoning: 2-3mg IV. Repeat until signs of atropine intoxication appear. Mushroom Poisoning: Administer sufficient doses to control parasympathomimetic signs before coma and cardiovascular collapse supervene.
*Pediatrics:* Range:0.1mg (newborn) to 0.6mg (>12 yrs). Inject SC 30 minutes before surgery. Bradyarrhythmias: Range: 0.01-0.03mg/kg IV.

**HOW SUPPLIED:** Inj: 0.05mg/mL, 0.1mg/mL, 0.4mg/mL, 0.5mg/mL, 1mg/mL

**CONTRAINDICATIONS:** Glaucoma, pyloric stenosis, or prostatic hypertrophy except in doses used for preanesthetic medication.

**WARNINGS/PRECAUTIONS:** Avoid overdose in IV administration. Increased susceptibility to toxic effects in children. Caution in patients >40 yrs. Conventional doses may precipitate glaucoma in susceptible patients, convert partial organic pyloric stenosis into complete obstruction, lead to complete urinary retention in patients with prostatic hypertrophy or cause inspissation of bronchial secretions and formation of dangerous viscid plugs in patients with chronic lung disease.

**ADVERSE REACTIONS:** Dryness of the mouth, blurred vision, photophobia, tachycardia, anhidrosis.

**PREGNANCY:** Category C, safety in nursing not known.

## ATROVENT RX
ipratropium bromide (Boehringer Ingelheim)

**OTHER BRAND NAMES:** Atrovent HFA (Boehringer Ingelheim)

**THERAPEUTIC CLASS:** Anticholinergic bronchodilator

**INDICATIONS:** Maintenance treatment of bronchospasm associated with COPD, including chronic bronchitis and emphysema.

**DOSAGE:** *Adults:* (MDI, HFA MDI) Initial: 2 inh qid. Max: 12 inh/24hrs. (Sol) 1 vial (500mcg/2.5mL) nebulized tid-qid; separate doses by 6-8 hrs.
*Pediatrics:* >12 yrs: (MDI) Initial: 2 inh qid. Max: 12 inh/24hrs. (Sol) 1 vial (500mcg/2.5mL) nebulized tid-qid; separate doses by 6-8 hrs.

**HOW SUPPLIED:** MDI: 0.018mg/inh [14g], (HFA) 0.017mg/inh [12.9g]; Sol (neb): 0.02% [2.5mL, 25$^s$]

**CONTRAINDICATIONS:** Hypersensitivity to atropine or its derivatives. (MDI) History of hypersensitivity to soya lecithin or related food products (eg, soybeans, peanuts).

**WARNINGS/PRECAUTIONS:** Not for acute episodes. Immediate hypersensitivity reaction reported. Caution with narrow-angle glaucoma, prostatic hypertrophy or bladder-neck obstruction.

**ADVERSE REACTIONS:** Nervousness, bronchitis, dyspnea, dizziness, headache, nausea, blurred vision, dry mouth, exacerbation of symptoms.

**INTERACTIONS:** Caution with anticholinergic-containing drugs.

**PREGNANCY:** Category B, caution in nursing.

## ATROVENT NASAL RX
ipratropium bromide (Boehringer Ingelheim)

**THERAPEUTIC CLASS:** Anticholinergic agent

**INDICATIONS:** (0.03%) Relief of rhinorrhea associated with allergic and nonallergic perennial rhinitis. (0.06%) Relief of rhinorrhea associated with the common cold.

**DOSAGE:** *Adults:* (0.03%) 2 sprays per nostril bid-tid. (0.06%) 2 sprays per nostril tid-qid. Do not use >4 days with common cold.
*Pediatrics:* (0.03%) >6 yrs: 2 sprays per nostril bid-tid. (0.06%) >12 yrs: 2 sprays per nostril tid-qid. 5-11 yrs: 2 sprays per nostril tid. Do not use >4 days with common cold.

**HOW SUPPLIED:** Spray: (0.03%) 21mcg/spray [31g], (0.06%) 42mcg/spray [16.6g]

**CONTRAINDICATIONS:** Hypersensitivity to atropine or its derivatives.

**WARNINGS/PRECAUTIONS:** Immediate hypersensitivity reaction reported. Caution with narrow-angle glaucoma, prostatic hypertrophy or bladder-neck obstruction.

**ADVERSE REACTIONS:** Epistaxis, nasal dryness, dry mouth, dry throat, headache, upper respiratory infection, pharyngitis.

**INTERACTIONS:** May produce additive effects with other anticholinergic agents.

**PREGNANCY:** Category B, caution in nursing.

## AUGMENTIN RX
amoxicillin - clavulanate potassium (GlaxoSmithKline)

**THERAPEUTIC CLASS:** Aminopenicillin/beta lactamase inhibitor

**INDICATIONS:** Treatment of lower respiratory tract (LRTI), skin and skin structure (SSSI), and urinary tract infections (UTI), otitis media (OM), sinusitis.

**DOSAGE:** *Adults:* (Dose based on amoxicillin) 500mg q12h or 250mg q8h. Severe Infections/RTI: 875mg q12h or 500mg q8h. May use 125mg/5mL or 250mg/5mL sus in place of 500mg tab and 200mg/5mL sus or 400mg/5mL sus in place of 875mg tab. CrCl <30mL/min: Do not give 875mg tab. CrCl 10-30mL/min: 250-500mg q12h. CrCl <10mL/min: 250-500mg q24h. Hemodialysis: 250-500mg q24h, give additional dose during and at the end of dialysis.
*Pediatrics:* (Dose based on amoxicillin) >40kg: Use adult dose. >12 weeks: Sinusitis/OM/LRTI/Severe Infections: (Sus/Tab, Chewable) 45mg/kg/day given q12h or 40mg/kg/day given q8h. Less Severe Infections: 25mg/kg/day given q12h or 20mg/kg/day given q8h. <12 weeks:15mg/kg q12h (use 125mg/5mL sus).

**HOW SUPPLIED:** (Amoxicillin-Clavulanate) Sus: 125-31.25mg/5mL [75mL, 100mL, 150mL] 200-28.5mg/5mL [50mL, 75mL, 100mL], 250-62.5mg/5mL [75mL, 100mL, 150mL], 400-57mg/5mL [50mL, 75mL, 100mL]; Tab: 250-125mg, 500-125mg, 875-125mg*; Tab, Chewable: 200-28.5mg, 250-62.5mg, 400-57mg *scored

**CONTRAINDICATIONS:** History of penicillin allergy or amoxicillin-clavulanate associated cholestatic jaundice/hepatic dysfunction.

**WARNINGS/PRECAUTIONS:** Pseudomembranous colitis reported. Possibility of superinfection. Caution with hepatic dysfunction. Monitor renal, hepatic, and hematopoietic functions with prolonged use. Avoid with mononucleosis. Fatal hypersensitivity reactions reported. Take with food to reduce GI upset. Chewable tabs and suspension contain phenylalanine. The 250mg tab and chewable tab are not interchangeable due to unequal clavulanic acid amounts. Only use 250mg tab in pediatrics >40kg. False (+) for urine glucose with Clinitest® and Benedict's or Fehling's solution.

**ADVERSE REACTIONS:** Diarrhea/loose stools, nausea, skin rashes, urticaria, vomiting, vaginitis.

**INTERACTIONS:** Increased and prolonged plasma levels with probenecid. May reduce effects of oral contraceptives. Allopurinol may increase incidence of rash. May increase PT with anticoagulant therapy.

**PREGNANCY:** Category B, caution in nursing.

## AUGMENTIN ES-600 RX

amoxicillin - clavulanate potassium (GlaxoSmithKline)

**THERAPEUTIC CLASS:** Aminopenicillin/beta lactamase inhibitor

**INDICATIONS:** Treatment of recurrent or persistent acute otitis media.

**DOSAGE:** *Pediatrics:* (Dose based on amoxicillin) 3 months-12 yrs: <40kg: 45mg/kg q12h for 10 days.

**HOW SUPPLIED:** Sus: (Amoxicillin-Clavulanate) 600mg-42.9mg/5mL [50mL, 75mL, 100mL, 150mL]

**CONTRAINDICATIONS:** History of penicillin allergy or amoxicillin-clavulanate associated cholestatic jaundice/hepatic dysfunction.

**WARNINGS/PRECAUTIONS:** Pseudomembranous colitis reported. Possibility of superinfection. Caution with hepatic dysfunction. Monitor renal, hepatic, and hematopoietic functions with prolonged use. Avoid with mononucleosis. Fatal hypersensitivity reactions reported. Contains phenylalanine. False (+) for urine glucose with Clinitest® and Benedict's or Fehling's solution.

**ADVERSE REACTIONS:** Diaper rash, diarrhea, vomiting, moniliasis, rash.

**INTERACTIONS:** Increased and prolonged plasma levels with probenecid. May reduce effects of oral contraceptives. Allopurinol may increase incidence of rash. May increase PT with anticoagulant therapy.

**PREGNANCY:** Category B, caution in nursing.

## AUGMENTIN XR

RX

amoxicillin - clavulanate potassium (GlaxoSmithKline)

**THERAPEUTIC CLASS:** Aminopenicillin/beta lactamase inhibitor

**INDICATIONS:** Treatment of community acquired pneumonia (CAP) or acute bacterial sinusitis due to confirmed or suspected β-lactamase producing pathogens.

**DOSAGE:** *Adults:* Sinusitis: 2 tabs q12h for 10 days. CAP: 2 tabs q12h for 7-10 days. Take at the start of a meal.
*Pediatrics:* >16 yrs: Sinusitis: 2 tabs q12h for 10 days. CAP: 2 tabs q12h for 7-10 days. Take at the start of a meal.

**HOW SUPPLIED:** Tab, Extended Release: (Amoxicillin-Clavulanate) 1000mg-62.5mg

**CONTRAINDICATIONS:** History of penicillin allergy or amoxicillin-clavulanate associated cholestatic jaundice/hepatic dysfunction, severe renal impairment (CrCl <30mL/min), hemodialysis.

**WARNINGS/PRECAUTIONS:** Pseudomembranous colitis reported. Possibility of superinfection. Caution with hepatic dysfunction. Monitor renal, hepatic, and hematopoietic functions with prolonged use. Avoid with mononucleosis. Fatal hypersensitivity reactions reported. Not interchangeable with other Augmentin products due to unequal clavulanic acid amounts. False (+) for urine glucose with Clinitest® and Benedict's or Fehling's solution.

**ADVERSE REACTIONS:** Diarrhea, nausea, genital moniliasis, abdominal pain, vaginal mycosis.

**INTERACTIONS:** Increased and prolonged plasma levels with probenecid. May reduce effects of oral contraceptives. Allopurinol may increase incidence of rash. May increase PT with anticoagulant therapy.

**PREGNANCY:** Category B, caution in nursing.

## AUROTO

RX

glycerin - antipyrine - benzocaine (Alpharma)

**OTHER BRAND NAMES:** Benzotic (Alba) - A/B Otic (Qualitest)

**THERAPEUTIC CLASS:** Analgesic/hygroscopic agent

**INDICATIONS:** To reduce pain in acute otitis media. For cerumen removal.

**DOSAGE:** *Adults:* Otitis Media: Fill ear canal and insert moistened cotton plug. Repeat q1-2h, until pain and congestion resolve. Cerumen Removal: Fill ear canal tid for 2-3 days before cerumen removal; insert moistened cotton plug. Use after removal to dry out canal and relieve discomfort.

**HOW SUPPLIED:** Sol: (Antipyrine-Benzocaine) 54mg-14mg/mL (Auralgan) [10mL], (Auroto) [15mL]

**CONTRAINDICATIONS:** Perforated tympanic membrane.

**WARNINGS/PRECAUTIONS:** Discontinue if irritation occurs.

**PREGNANCY:** Category C, caution in nursing.

## AVAGE

RX

tazarotene (Allergan)

**THERAPEUTIC CLASS:** Retinoic acid derivative

**INDICATIONS:** Adjunct to a comprehensive skin care and sunlight avoidance program, in the mitigation (palliation) of facial fine wrinkling, facial mottled hyper- and hypopigmentation, and benign facial lentigines.

**DOSAGE:** *Adults:* >17 yrs: Cleanse and dry skin. Apply a pea-sized (1/4 inch or 5mm diameter) amount to face (including eyelids, if desired) qhs.

**HOW SUPPLIED:** Cre: 0.1% [30g]

**CONTRAINDICATIONS:** Women who are or may become pregnant.

**WARNINGS/PRECAUTIONS:** Use adequate birth control measures. Obtain negative pregnancy test within 2 weeks before therapy. Begin therapy during normal menstrual period. Avoid mouth, eyes, sunlight exposure (including sunlamps), or sunburned or eczematous skin. Stop therapy or reduce dosing interval with pruritus, burning, skin redness, or peeling. Weather extremes (eg, wind, cold) may be irritating. Sunscreen (minimum SPF 15) and protective clothing should be used.

**ADVERSE REACTIONS:** Desquamation, erythema, burning sensation, dry skin, skin irritation, pruritus, irritant contact dermatitis.

**INTERACTIONS:** Avoid topical agents that have a strong drying effect. Caution with photosensitizers (eg, thiazides, tetracyclines, fluoroquinolones, phenothiazines, sulfonamides).

**PREGNANCY:** Category X; caution in nursing.

## AVALIDE RX

irbesartan - hydrochlorothiazide (Bristol-Myers Squibb/Sanofi-Aventis)

**Can cause death/injury to developing fetus during 2nd and 3rd trimesters. Stop therapy if pregnancy detected.**

**THERAPEUTIC CLASS:** Angiotensin II receptor antagonist/thiazide diuretic

**INDICATIONS:** Treatment of hypertension. Not for initial therapy.

**DOSAGE:** *Adults:* Initial: 150mg irbesartan qd. Titrate: May increase to 300mg irbesartan qd. Elderly: Start at low end of dosing range. Intravascular Volume Depletion: Initial: 75mg irbesartan qd. Avoid with CrCl ≤30mL/min.

**HOW SUPPLIED:** Tab: (Irbesartan-HCTZ) 150mg-12.5mg, 300mg-12.5mg, 300mg-25mg

**CONTRAINDICATIONS:** Anuria, sulfonamide hypersensitivity.

**WARNINGS/PRECAUTIONS:** Can cause fetal injury/death. Correct volume or salt depletion before therapy. Caution with hepatic or renal dysfunction, renal artery stenosis, severe CHF, history of allergies, elderly, and asthma. May exacerbate or activate SLE. Monitor serum electrolytes. Avoid if CrCl ≤30mL/min. Hyperuricemia, hyperglycemia, hypokalemia, hypomagnesemia, hypercalcemia may occur. Enhanced effects in post-sympathectomy patient. May increase cholesterol and triglyceride levels. Caution in elderly.

**ADVERSE REACTIONS:** Dizziness, fatigue, musculoskeletal pain, influenza, edema, nausea, vomiting.

**INTERACTIONS:** Potentiation of orthostatic hypotension may occur with alcohol, barbiturates, and narcotics. Dosage adjustment of insulin or oral hypoglycemic agents may be required. Impaired absorption with cholestyramine, colestipol. Corticosteroids and ACTH deplete electrolytes. May decrease response to pressor amines. Potentiates other antihypertensives. May increase responsiveness to skeletal muscle relaxants. Increased risk of lithium toxicity. NSAIDs may reduce diuretic effects.

**PREGNANCY:** Category C (1st trimester) and D (2nd and 3rd trimesters), not for use in nursing.

## AVANDAMET RX

metformin HCl - rosiglitazone maleate (GlaxoSmithKline)

**THERAPEUTIC CLASS:** Thiazolidinedione/biguanide

**INDICATIONS:** Adjunct to diet and exercise, to improve glycemic control in type 2 diabetes mellitus when treatment with dual rosiglitazone and metformin therapy is appropriate.

**DOSAGE:** *Adults:* Prior Metformin Therapy of 1g/day: Initial: 2mg-500mg tab bid. Prior Metformin Therapy of 2g/day: Initial: 2mg-1g tab bid. Prior Rosiglitazone Therapy of 4mg/day: Initial: 2mg-500mg tab bid. Prior Rosiglitazone Therapy of 8mg/day: 4mg-500mg tab bid. Titrate: May increase by increments of 4mg rosiglitazone and/or 500mg metformin. Max: 8mg-2g/day. Elderly/Debilitated/Malnourished: Conservative dosing; do not titrate to max dose. Take with meals.

**HOW SUPPLIED:** Tab: (Rosiglitazone-Metformin) 1mg-500mg, 2mg-500mg, 4mg-500mg, 2mg-1g, 4mg-1g

**CONTRAINDICATIONS:** Renal disease/dysfunction (SrCr >1.5mg/dL [males], >1.4mg/dL [females], abnormal CrCl), metabolic acidosis, diabetic ketoacidosis. Discontinue temporarily (48 hrs) for radiologic studies with intravascular iodinated contrast materials.

**WARNINGS/PRECAUTIONS:** Lactic acidosis reported (rare); increased risk with renal dysfunction, increased age, DM, CHF, and other conditions with risk of hypoperfusion and hypoxemia. Avoid use in patients >80 yrs unless renal function is normal. Monitor renal function and for ketoacidosis and metabolic acidosis. Discontinue in hypoxic states (eg, CHF, shock, acute MI), loss of blood glucose control due to stress, acidosis and prior to surgical procedures (due to restricted food intake). May decrease serum vitamin $B_{12}$ levels. Increased risk of hypoglycemia with concomitant use with other hypoglycemic agents, elderly, debilitated/malnourished, adrenal or pituitary insufficiency, or alcohol intoxication. May cause fluid retention and exacerbation/initiation of heart failure; discontinue if cardiac status deteriorates. Avoid with NYHA Class III or IV cardiac status. Not for use in type 1 diabetes or for diabetic ketoacidosis treatment. Caution with edema. Dose related weight gain reported. Ovulation in premenopausal anovulatory patients may occur; risk of pregnancy with inadequate contraception. May decrease Hgb and Hct. Avoid with active liver disease, if ALT levels >2.5X ULN, or if jaundice occurred with troglitazone. Check LFTs before therapy, every 2 months for 1 year, and periodically thereafter, or if hepatic dysfunction symptoms occur. Discontinue if ALT >3X ULN on therapy. Not for use with insulin.

**ADVERSE REACTIONS:** Upper respiratory tract infection, headache, back pain, hyperglycemia, fatigue, sinusitis, diarrhea, viral infection, arthralgia, anemia.

**INTERACTIONS:** Furosemide, nifedipine, cimetidine and cationic drugs (eg, digoxin, amiloride, procainamide, quinidine, quinine, ranitidine, trimethoprim, vancomycin, triamterene, morphine) may increase metformin levels. Thiazides and other diuretics, corticosteroids, phenothiazines, thyroid products, estrogens, oral contraceptives, phenytoin, nicotinic acid, sympathomimetics, calcium channel blockers, and isoniazid may cause hyperglycemia. Risk of hypoglycemia with alcohol. Excess alcohol may increase potential for lactic acidosis. May decrease furosemide levels. Inhibitors of CYP2C8 (eg, gemfibrozil) may increase rosiglitazone AUC. Inducers of CYP2C8 (eg, rifampin) may decrease rosiglitazone AUC.

**PREGNANCY:** Category C, not for use in nursing.

## AVANDARYL RX

glimepiride - rosiglitazone maleate (GlaxoSmithKline)

**THERAPEUTIC CLASS:** Thiazolidinedione/sulfonylurea

**INDICATIONS:** Adjunct to diet and exercise to improve glycemic control in type 2 diabetes already being treated with combination of rosiglitazone and sulfonylurea, or with inadequate control on sulfonylurea alone, or with initial response to rosiglitazone alone requiring additional glycemic control.

**DOSAGE:** *Adults:* Give with first meal of day. Prior Sulfonylurea Monotherapy or Inital Response To Rosiglitazone Alone Requiring Additional Control: 4mg-1mg or 4mg-2mg qd. Switching From Prior Combination Therapy: Same dose of each component already being taken. Prior Thiazolidinedione Monotherapy:

Titrate dose. After 1-2 weeks with inadequate control, increase glimepiride component to in more than 2mg increments at 1-2 week intervals. Max: 8mg-4mg daily. Prior Sulfonylurea Monotherapy: May take 2-3 months for full effect of rosiglitazone; do not exceed 8mg of rosiglitazone daily. Titrate: May increase glimepiride component. Elderly/Debilitated/Malnourished/Renal, Hepatic or Adrenal Insufficiency: Initial: 4mg-1mg qd. Titrate carefully.

**HOW SUPPLIED:** Tab: (Rosiglitazone-Glimepiride) 4mg-1mg, 4mg-2mg, 4mg-4mg

**CONTRAINDICATIONS:** Diabetic ketoacidosis, with or without coma.

**WARNINGS/PRECAUTIONS:** (Glimepiride): Increased cardiovascular mortality. Hypoglycemia risk if debilitated, malnourished, or with adrenal, pituitary, renal or hepatic insufficiency. Hypoglycemia may be masked in elderly. May lose blood glucose control with stress. Secondary failure may occur. Discontinue if skin reactions persist or worsen. (Rosiglitazone): May cause fluid retention and exacerbation/initiation of heart failure; discontinue if cardiac status deteriorates. Avoid if NYHA Class III or IV cardiac status. Not for use in type 1 DM or diabetic ketoacidosis treatment. Caution with edema. May cause macular edema. Dose-related weight gain reported. Ovulation in premenopausal anovulatory patient may occur; risk of pregnancy with inadequate contraception. May decrease Hgb and Hct. Avoid with active liver disease, if ALT levels >2.5x ULN, or if jaundice occurred with rosiglitazone. Check LFTs before therapy, every 2 months for 1 yr, and periodically thereafter, or if hepatic dysfunction symptoms occur. Discontinue if ALT >3x ULN on therapy.

**ADVERSE REACTIONS:** Upper respiratory tract infection, injury, headache, hypoglycemia, anemia, edema.

**INTERACTIONS:** (Rosiglitazone): CYP2C8 inhibitors (eg, gemfibrozil) may increase the AUC. CYP2C8 inducers (eg, rifampin) may decrease the AUC. (Glimepiride): Risk of hyperglycemia with thiazides, corticosteroids, phenothiazines, thyroid products, estrogens, oral contraceptives, phenytoin, nicotinic acid, sympathomimetics, and isoniazid. Risk of severe hypoglycemia with oral miconazole.

**PREGNANCY:** Category C, not for use in nursing.

## AVANDIA

RX

rosiglitazone maleate (GlaxoSmithKline)

**THERAPEUTIC CLASS:** Thiazolidinedione

**INDICATIONS:** Adjunct to diet and exercise, to improve glycemic control in type 2 diabetes mellitus. May use in combination with metformin, insulin, or a sulfonylurea.

**DOSAGE:** *Adults:* >18 yrs: Initial: 2mg bid or 4mg qd. Titrate: May increase after 8-12 weeks to 4mg bid or 8mg qd. Max: 8mg/day as monotherapy or with metformin; 4mg/day in combination with sulfonylureas or insulin. Decrease insulin by 10-25% if hypoglycemic or FPG <100mg/dL; individualize further adjustments based on glucose lowering response.

**HOW SUPPLIED:** Tab: 2mg, 4mg, 8mg

**CONTRAINDICATIONS:** Combination use with metformin with renal impairment.

**WARNINGS/PRECAUTIONS:** May cause fluid retention and exacerbation/initiation of heart failure; discontinue if cardiac status deteriorates. Increased risk of CV events with NYHA Class 1 or 2 cardiac status; avoid with NYHA Class 3 or 4 cardiac status. Not for use in type 1 diabetes or for diabetic ketoacidosis treatment. Caution with edema. Macular edema reported. Dose related weight gain reported. Ovulation in premenopausal anovulatory patients may occur; risk of pregnancy with inadequate contraception. May decrease Hgb and Hct. Avoid with active liver disease, if ALT levels >2.5X ULN, or if jaundice occurred with troglitazone. Check LFTs before therapy, every 2 months for 1 year, and periodically thereafter, or if hepatic dysfunction symptoms occur. Discontinue if ALT >3X ULN on therapy.

**ADVERSE REACTIONS:** Upper respiratory tract infection, injury, headache, back pain, hyperglycemia, fatigue, sinusitis, anemia, edema.

**INTERACTIONS:** Risk of hypoglycemia when used in combination with other hypoglycemic agents.

**PREGNANCY:** Category C, not for use in nursing.

## AVAPRO

RX

irbesartan (Bristol-Myers Squibb/Sanofi-Aventis)

**Can cause death/injury to developing fetus during 2nd and 3rd trimesters. Stop therapy if pregnancy detected.**

**THERAPEUTIC CLASS:** Angiotensin II receptor antagonist

**INDICATIONS:** Hypertension, alone or with other antihypertensives. Diabetic nephropathy with an elevated serum creatinine and proteinuria (>300mg/day) in patients with type 2 diabetes and hypertension.

**DOSAGE:** *Adults:* HTN: Initial: 150mg qd. Titrate: May increase to 300mg qd. Intravascular Volume/Salt Depletion: Initial: 75mg qd. Nephropathy: Maint: 300mg qd.
*Pediatrics:* HTN: ≥17 yrs: Initial: 150mg qd. Titrate: May increase to 300mg qd. Intravascular Volume/Salt Depletion: Initial: 75mg qd.

**HOW SUPPLIED:** Tab: 75mg, 150mg, 300mg

**WARNINGS/PRECAUTIONS:** Can cause fetal injury/death. Correct volume or salt depletion before therapy. Changes in renal function may occur; caution with renal artery stenosis, severe CHF. Angioedema reported.

**ADVERSE REACTIONS:** Diarrhea, dyspepsia/heartburn, musculoskeletal trauma, fatigue, upper respiratory infection.

**PREGNANCY:** Category C (1st trimester) and D (2nd and 3rd trimesters), not for use in nursing.

## AVASTIN

RX

bevacizumab (Genentech)

**Fatal pulmonary hemorrhage has occurred in patients with non-small cell lung cancer treated with chemotherapy and bevacizumab; avoid with recent hemoptysis. Avoid if GI perforation or wound dehiscence develops; may be fatal.**

**THERAPEUTIC CLASS:** Vascular endothelial growth factor (VEGF) inhibitor

**INDICATIONS:** First- or second-line treatment of metastatic carcinoma of the colon or rectum in combination with 5-fluorouracil-based chemotherapy. First-line treatment of unresectable, locally advanced, recurrent or metastatic non-squamous, non-small cell lung cancer in combination with carboplatin and paclitaxel.

**DOSAGE:** *Adults:* Colon/Rectum Metastatic Carcinoma: 5mg/kg (in combination with bolus IFL) or 10 mg/kg (in combination with FOLFOX4) given once every 14 days . Lung Cancer: 15mg/kg q3wks. IV infusion over 90 minutes, 1st infusion is well tolerated, give 2nd infusion over 60 minutes and subsequent doses over 30 minutes.

**HOW SUPPLIED:** Inj: 25mg/mL [4mL, 16mL]

**WARNINGS/PRECAUTIONS:** Discontinue with GI perforation, wound dehiscence, nephrotic syndrome or serious hemorrhage. Increased risk of HTN; permanently discontinue if hypertensive crisis occurs. Monitor BP every 2-3 weeks during treatment. Increased incidence/severity of proteinuria. Potential for immunogenicity. CHF reported. Avoid initiation of therapy for at least 28 days following major surgery; surgical incision must be fully healed prior to start of therapy. Suspend treatment prior to elective surgery. Reversible posterior leukoencephalopathy syndrome reported; discontinue and treat HTN if present.

**ADVERSE REACTIONS:** Asthenia, pain, abdominal pain, headache, HTN, diarrhea, nausea, vomiting, anorexia, stomatitis, constipation, upper respiratory infection, epistaxis, dyspnea, exfoliative dermatitis, proteinuria.

**INTERACTIONS:** Increased risk of thromboembolic events when coadministered with chemotherapy; discontinue if severe arterial thromboembolic event occurs.

**PREGNANCY:** Category C, not for use in nursing.

## AVC
sulfanilamide (Novavax) RX

**THERAPEUTIC CLASS:** Antifungal agent

**INDICATIONS:** Treatment of vulvovaginitis caused by *Candida albicans*.

**DOSAGE:** *Adults:* 1 applicatorful intravaginally qd-bid. Continue for 30 days.

**HOW SUPPLIED:** Cre: 15% [120g]

**CONTRAINDICATIONS:** Sulfonamide sensitivity.

**WARNINGS/PRECAUTIONS:** Observe for skin rash or evidence of systemic toxicity. Goiter, diuresis, hypoglycemia, and deaths from hypersensitivity reactions, agranulocytosis, aplastic anemia, and blood dyscrasias reported with oral sulfonamides. Caution after 7th month of pregnancy.

**ADVERSE REACTIONS:** Local sensitivity reaction (eg, discomfort, burning).

**PREGNANCY:** Category C, not for use in nursing.

## AVELOX
moxifloxacin HCl (Schering) RX

**THERAPEUTIC CLASS:** Fluoroquinolone

**INDICATIONS:** Acute bacterial sinusitis, acute bacterial exacerbation of chronic bronchitis (ABECB), uncomplicated skin and skin structure infections (SSSI), complicated skin and skin structure infections (cSSSI), complicated intra-abdominal infections (cIAI), and community acquired pneumonia (CAP), including multi-drug resistant *S. pneumoniae*.

**DOSAGE:** *Adults:* ≥18 yrs: Sinusitis: 400mg PO/IV q24h for 10 days. ABECB: 400mg PO/IV q24h for 5 days. SSSI: 400mg PO/IV q24h for 7 days. cSSSI: 400mg PO/IV q24h for 7-21 days. cIAI: 400mg IV q24h for 5-14 days. CAP: 400mg PO/IV q24h for 7-14 days.

**HOW SUPPLIED:** Inj: 400mg/250mL; Tab: 400mg [ABC Pack, 5 tabs]

**WARNINGS/PRECAUTIONS:** Avoid in pregnancy, nursing, and patients <18 yrs. QT prolongation may be dose or infusion rate dependent; do not exceed recommended dose. Avoid with known QT interval prolongation, uncorrected hypokalemia. Caution with ongoing proarrhythmic conditions (eg, significant bradycardia, acute MI). Pseudomembranous colitis reported. Caution with CNS disorders (eg, severe cerebral arteriosclerosis, epilepsy). D/C if convulsions, CNS effects, hypersensitivity reaction, or tendon rupture occurs.

**ADVERSE REACTIONS:** Nausea, diarrhea, dizziness.

**INTERACTIONS:** Take oral formulation at least 4 hrs before or 8 hrs after aluminum-, magnesium-, or calcium-containing antacids, sucralfate, multivitamins with iron or zinc, and didanosine chewable/buffered tablets or oral solution. Avoid Class IA (eg, quinidine, procainamide) or Class III (eg, amiodarone, sotalol) antiarrhythmics. Caution with drugs that prolong the QT interval (eg, cisapride, erythromycin, antipsychotics, TCAs). NSAIDs may increase risk of CNS stimulation and convulsions. Monitor PT with warfarin. Corticosteroids in elderly may increase risk of tendon rupture. Do not add other substances, additives or medications to injection or infuse simultaneously through same IV line.

**PREGNANCY:** Category C, not for use in nursing.

## AVINZA

**CII**

morphine sulfate (Ligand)

> **Swallow capsules whole or sprinkle contents on applesauce. Do not crush, chew, or dissolve capsule beads. Avoid alcohol and alcohol-containing medications; consumption of alcohol may result in the rapid release and absorption of potentially fatal dose of morphine.**

**THERAPEUTIC CLASS:** Opioid analgesic

**INDICATIONS:** Relief of moderate to severe pain requiring continuous opioid therapy for an extended period of time.

**DOSAGE:** *Adults:* >18 yrs: Conversion from Other Oral Morphine Products: Give total daily morphine dose as a single dose q24h. Conversion from Parenteral Morphine: Initial: Give about 3x the previous daily parenteral morphine requirement. Conversion from Other Parenteral or Oral Non-Morphine Opioids: Initial: Give 1/2 of estimated daily morphine requirement q24h. Supplement with immediate-release morphine or short-acting analgesics if needed. Titrate: Adjust dose as frequently as every other day. Non-Opioid Tolerant: 30mg q24h. Titrate: Increase by increments <30mg every 4 days. The 60, 90, and 120mg caps are for opioid-tolerant patients. Max: 1600mg/day. Doses >1600mg/day contain a quantity of fumaric acid, which may cause renal toxicity.

**HOW SUPPLIED:** Cap, Extended Release: 30mg, 60mg, 90mg, 120mg

**CONTRAINDICATIONS:** Respiratory depression in the absence of resuscitative equipment, acute or severe bronchial asthma, paralytic ileus.

**WARNINGS/PRECAUTIONS:** Abuse potential. Extreme caution with COPD, cor pulmonale, decreased respiratory reserve (eg, severe kyphoscoliosis), hypoxia, hypercapnia, pre-existing respiratory depression, increased intracranial pressure, head injury. May cause orthostatic hypotension, syncope, severe hypotension with depleted blood volume. Caution with circulatory shock, biliary tract disease, severe renal/hepatic insufficiency, Addison's disease, hypothyroidism, prostatic hypertrophy, urethral stricture, elderly or debilitated, CNS depression, toxic psychosis, acute alcoholism, delirium tremens, seizure disorders. Avoid with GI obstruction. Withdrawal symptoms with abrupt discontinuation. Tolerance and physical dependence may develop. Potential for severe constipation; use laxatives, stool softeners at onset of therapy.

**ADVERSE REACTIONS:** Constipation, nausea, somnolence, vomiting, dehydration, headache, peripheral edema, diarrhea, abdominal pain, infection, UTI, flu syndrome, back pain, rash, sweating, fever, insomnia, depression, paresthesia, anorexia, dry mouth, asthenia, dyspnea.

**INTERACTIONS:** See Black Box Warning. Additive effects with alcohol, other opioids, illicit drugs that cause CNS depression. Reduce dose with other CNS depressants (eg, sedatives, hypnotics, general anesthetics, antiemetics, phenothiazines, tranquilizers, alcohol). May enhance neuromuscular blocking action of skeletal muscle relaxants. Avoid with mixed agonist/antagonists (eg, pentazocine, nalbuphine, butorphanol) and within 14 days of MAOI use. Monitor for increased respiratory and CNS depression with cimetidine.

**PREGNANCY:** Category C, not for use in nursing.

## AVITA

RX

tretinoin (Mylan Bertek)

**THERAPEUTIC CLASS:** Retinoic acid derivative

**INDICATIONS:** Acne vulgaris.

**DOSAGE:** *Adults:* Apply qpm to cleansed skin. May reduce dosing frequency if irritation occurs.

**HOW SUPPLIED:** Cre: 0.025% [20g, 45g]; Gel: 0.025% [20g, 45g]

**WARNINGS/PRECAUTIONS:** Avoid eyes, lips, paranasal creases, mucous membranes, and sunburned skin. May exacerbate acne during 1st weeks of therapy. Severe irritation with eczematous skin. Extreme weather may increase skin irritatation. Gel is flammable.

**ADVERSE REACTIONS:** Local skin reactions (red, edematous, blistered, crusted), photosensitivity, temporary skin pigmentation changes.

**INTERACTIONS:** Caution with other topicals with strong drying effects, high concentration of alcohol, astringents, spices, or lime. Caution with sulfur, resorcinol, or salicylic acid, allow effects of these agents to subside before application of tretinoin.

**PREGNANCY:** Category C, caution in nursing.

## AVODART

RX

dutasteride (GlaxoSmithKline)

**THERAPEUTIC CLASS:** Type I and II 5 alpha-reductase inhibitor (2nd generation)

**INDICATIONS:** Benign prostatic hyperplasia (BPH). To reduce risk of acute urinary retention, and need for BPH-related surgery.

**DOSAGE:** *Adults:* 0.5mg qd. Swallow caps whole.

**HOW SUPPLIED:** Cap: 0.5mg

**CONTRAINDICATIONS:** Women and children.

**WARNINGS/PRECAUTIONS:** Risk to male fetus; should not be handled by pregnant women. Monitor for obstructive uropathy with large residual urinary volume and/or severely diminished urinary flow. Avoid donating blood until 6 months after last dose. Caution with liver disease. Decreases serum PSA levels by about 40%-50%; adjust (double) PSA results after 6 months or more of therapy to compare with normal values.

**ADVERSE REACTIONS:** Impotence, decreased libido.

**INTERACTIONS:** CYP3A4 inhibitors (eg, ritonavir, ketoconazole, verapamil, diltiazem, cimetidine, ciprofloxacin) may increase blood levels.

**PREGNANCY:** Category X, not for use in nursing.

## AVONEX

RX

interferon beta-1a (Biogen Idec)

**THERAPEUTIC CLASS:** Biological response modifier

**INDICATIONS:** Treatment of relapsing forms of multiple sclerosis (MS) including patients who experienced a first clinical episode and have MRI features consistent with MS.

**DOSAGE:** *Adults:* 30mcg IM once a week.

**HOW SUPPLIED:** Kit: 33mcg

**CONTRAINDICATIONS:** Hypersensitivity to human albumin.

**WARNINGS/PRECAUTIONS:** Caution with depression, mood disorders, pre-existing seizure disorders. Depression, suicidal ideation, and development of new or worsening pre-existing other psychiatric disorders reported. Anaphylaxis (rare), suicidal ideation, psychosis, decreased peripheral blood counts, autoimmune disorders (eg, thrombocytopenia, hyper- and hypothyroidism), hepatic injury including hepatitis reported. Rare reports of severe hepatic injury, including cases of hepatic failure; monitor for signs of hepatic injury. Monitor closely with cardiac disease (eg, angina, CHF, arrhythmia). Risk of transmission of viral diseases. Abortifacient potential. Perform TFTs, LFTs, CBCs, differential WBCs, and platelets during therapy.

**ADVERSE REACTIONS:** Flu-like symptoms, myalgia, depression, fever, chills, asthenia, headache, pain, dizziness, nausea, sinusitis, upper respiratory tract infection, UTI.

**INTERACTIONS:** Caution with other drugs associated with hepatic injury.

**PREGNANCY:** Category C, not for use in nursing.

## AXERT RX

almotriptan malate (Ortho-McNeil)

**THERAPEUTIC CLASS:** 5-$HT_{1D,1B}$ agonist

**INDICATIONS:** Acute treatment of migraine with or without aura.

**DOSAGE:** *Adults:* >18 yrs: Initial: 6.25-12.5mg at onset of headache. May repeat after 2 hrs. Max: 2 doses/24 hrs. Hepatic/Renal Impairment: 6.25mg at onset of headache. Max: 12.5mg/24 hrs. Safety of treating >4 headaches/30 days not known.

**HOW SUPPLIED:** Tab: 6.25mg, 12.5mg

**CONTRAINDICATIONS:** Ischemic heart disease, coronary artery vasospasm, other significant CVD, uncontrolled HTN, within 24 hrs of another 5-$HT_1$ agonist or ergot type agent, hemiplegic or basilar migraine.

**WARNINGS/PRECAUTIONS:** Confirm diagnosis. Supervise first dose and monitor cardiac function in those at risk of CAD (eg, HTN, hypercholesterolemia, smoker, obesity, diabetes, CAD family history, postmenopausal women, males >40 yrs). Monitor cardiovascular function with long term intermittent use. May cause vasospastic reactions or cerebrovascular events. Caution with renal or hepatic dysfunction. Avoid in elderly.

**ADVERSE REACTIONS:** Nausea, somnolence, headache, paresthesia, dry mouth, coronary artery vasospasm, MI, ventricular tachycardia, fibrillation.

**INTERACTIONS:** Additive vasospastic reactions with ergotamines. SSRIs may cause weakness, hyperreflexia, and incoordination. Avoid other 5-$HT_1$ agonist drugs within 24 hr period. Clearance may be decreased by MAOIs. Increased levels possible with CYP3A4 inhibitors (eg, ketoconazole).

**PREGNANCY:** Category C, caution in nursing.

## AXID RX

nizatidine (Reliant)

**OTHER BRAND NAMES:** Axid Oral Solution (Braintree)

**THERAPEUTIC CLASS:** $H_2$ blocker

**INDICATIONS:** Short term treatment of active duodenal ulcer (DU) and benign gastric ulcer (GU). Maintenance therapy for duodenal ulcers. Treatment of endoscopically diagnosed esophagitis, including erosive and ulcerative esophagitis, and heartburn due to GERD.

**DOSAGE:** *Adults:* Active DU/Active Benign GU: Usual: 300mg qhs or 150mg bid up to 8 weeks. Healed DU: Maint: 150mg qhs, up to 1 year. GERD: 150mg bid up to 12 weeks. Renal Impairment: Treatment: CrCl 20-50mL/min: 150mg/day. CrCl <20mL/min: 150mg every other day. Maint: CrCl 20-50mL/min: 150mg every other day. CrCl <20mL/min: 150mg every 3 days.
*Pediatrics:* ≥12 yrs: (Sol) Erosive Esophagitis/GERD: 150mg bid up to 8 weeks. Max: 300mg/day. Renal Impairment: Treatment: CrCl 20-50mL/min: 150mg/day. CrCl <20mL/min: 150mg every other day. Maint: CrCl 20-50mL/min: 150mg every other day. CrCl <20mL/min: 150mg every 3 days.

**HOW SUPPLIED:** Cap: 150mg, 300mg; Sol: 15mg/mL

**WARNINGS/PRECAUTIONS:** Caution with renal dysfunction; reduce dose. Symptomatic response does not preclude the presence of gastric malignancy. False positive tests for urobilinogen with Multistix®.

**ADVERSE REACTIONS:** Headache, abdominal pain, pain, asthenia, diarrhea, nausea, flatulence, vomiting, dyspepsia, rhinitis, pharyngitis, dizziness, headache.

**INTERACTIONS:** May elevate serum salicylate levels with high dose ASA.

**PREGNANCY:** Category B, not for use in nursing.

## AYGESTIN RX

norethindrone acetate (Duramed)

**THERAPEUTIC CLASS:** Progestogen

**INDICATIONS:** Treatment of secondary amenorrhea, endometriosis, and abnormal uterine bleeding due to hormonal imbalance in the absence of organic pathology.

**DOSAGE:** *Adults:* Assume interval between menses is 28 days. Secondary Amenorrhea/Abnormal Uterine Bleeding: 2.5-10mg qd for 5-10 days during second half of menstrual cycle. Endometriosis: Initial: 5mg qd for 2 weeks. Titrate: Increase by 2.5mg qd every 2 weeks until 15mg/day. Continue for 6-9 months or until breakthrough bleeding demands temporary termination.

**HOW SUPPLIED:** Tab: 5mg* *scored

**CONTRAINDICATIONS:** Pregnancy, thrombophlebitis, thromboembolic disorders, cerebral apoplexy, liver impairment, breast carcinoma, undiagnosed vaginal bleeding, missed abortion, use as a pregnancy diagnostic test.

**WARNINGS/PRECAUTIONS:** D/C with migraine, vision loss, proptosis, diplopia, papilledema, or retinal vascular lesions. May cause thrombophlebitis, pulmonary embolism, and fluid retention. Caution with epilepsy, migraine, psychic depression, asthma, cardiac or renal dysfunction, depression, DM, and hyperlipidemia. May mask onset of climacteric. Not for use during the first trimester of pregnancy; risk to the fetus.

**ADVERSE REACTIONS:** Breakthrough bleeding, spotting, change in menstrual flow, amenorrhea, edema, weight changes, cervical changes, cholestatic jaundice, rash, melasma, chloasma, depression.

**PREGNANCY:** Category X, safety in nursing is not known.

## AZACTAM RX

aztreonam (Elan)

**THERAPEUTIC CLASS:** Monobactam

**INDICATIONS:** Treatment of septicemia and lower respiratory tract (eg, pneumonia, bronchitis), skin and skin-structure, urinary tract (UTI), gynecologic (eg, endometritis), and intra-abdominal (eg, peritonitis) infections. Adjunct therapy to surgery for management of infections.

**DOSAGE:** *Adults:* UTI: 500mg-1g IM/IV q8-12h. Moderately Severe Systemic Infections: 1-2g IM/IV q8-12h. Severe Systemic/Life-Threatening Infections/*Pseudomonas aeruginosa*: 2g IV q6-8h. Max: 8g/day. CrCl 10-30mL/min: Initial: LD: 1 or 2g. Maint: 50% of usual dose. CrCl <10mL/min: Initial: LD: 500mg, 1g or 2g. Maint: 25% of initial dose at usual intervals. Serious/Life-Threatening Infections: In addition to maintenance dose, give 1/8 initial dose after each hemodialysis session. IV route is recommended for single dose >1g or for bacterial septicemia, localized parenchymal abscess (eg, intra-abdominal abscess), peritonitis, or other severe systemic or life-threatening infections. Continue for at least 48 hrs after patient is asymptomatic or bacterial eradication.

*Pediatrics:* 9 months-16 yrs: Mild-Moderate Infections: 30mg/kg IV q8h. Moderate-Severe Infections: 30mg/kg IV q6-8h. Max: 120mg/kg/day. IV route is recommended for single dose >1g or for bacterial septicemia, localized parenchymal abscess (eg, intra-abdominal abscess), peritonitis, or other severe systemic or life-threatening infections. Continue for at least 48 hrs after patient is asymptomatic or evidence of bacterial eradication.

**HOW SUPPLIED:** Inj: 500mg, 1g, 2g, 1g/50mL, 2g/50mL

**WARNINGS/PRECAUTIONS:** Caution with hypersensitivity to other beta-lactams or allergens. Pseudomembranous colitis reported. May promote overgrowth of nonsusceptible organisms. Monitor with renal or hepatic impairment. Toxic epidermal necrolysis reported (rarely) in bone marrow transplant with multiple risk factors including sepsis.

**ADVERSE REACTIONS:** Diarrhea, nausea, vomiting, rash, abdominal cramps, vaginal candidiasis, discomfort/swelling at injection site, hypersensitivity reaction.

**INTERACTIONS:** Monitor renal function with aminoglycosides; increased risk of nephrotoxicity, ototoxicity. Toxic epidermal necrolysis reported (rarely) in bone marrow transplant with radiation therapy and other drugs associated with toxic epidermal necrolysis.

**PREGNANCY:** Category B, not for use in nursing.

## AZASAN RX

azathioprine (aaiPharma)

**Increased risk of neoplasia with chronic therapy. Mutagenic potential and possible hematological toxicities.**

**THERAPEUTIC CLASS:** Purine antagonist antimetabolite

**INDICATIONS:** Adjunct therapy for prevention of rejection in renal homotransplantation. Management of severe, active rheumatoid arthritis (RA) unresponsive to rest, aspirin, NSAIDs, or gold.

**DOSAGE:** *Adults:* Renal Homotransplantation: Initial: 3-5mg/kg/day, start at time of transplant. Maint: 1-3mg/kg/day. Rheumatoid Arthritis: Initial: 1mg/kg/day given qd-bid. Titrate: Increase by 0.5mg/kg/day after 6-8 weeks, then at 4 week intervals. Max: 2.5mg/kg/day. Maint: Lowest effective dose. Decrease by 0.5mg/kg/day or 25mg/day every 4 weeks. If no response by week 12, then considered refractory. Renal Dysfunction: Lower dose

**HOW SUPPLIED:** Tab: 25mg*, 50mg*, 75mg*, 100mg* *scored

**CONTRAINDICATIONS:** Pregnancy in RA treatment. Previous treatment of RA with alkylating agents (eg, cyclophosphamide,chlorambucil, melphalan) may increase risk of neoplasia.

**WARNINGS/PRECAUTIONS:** Dose-related leukopenia, thrombocytopenia, macrocytic anemia, and severe bone marrow suppression may occur. Monitor CBCs, including platelets, weekly during the 1st month, twice monthly for the 2nd and 3rd months, then monthly or more frequently if dose/therapy changes. Monitor for infections.

**ADVERSE REACTIONS:** Leukopenia, thrombocytopenia, infections, nausea, vomiting, hepatotoxicity.

**INTERACTIONS:** Reduce dose by 1/3-1/4 with allopurinol. Drugs affecting leukocyte production (eg, co-trimazole) may exaggerate leukopenia. ACE inhibitors may induce severe leukopenia.

**PREGNANCY:** Category D, not for use in nursing.

## AZASITE RX

azithromycin (Inspire)

**THERAPEUTIC CLASS:** Macrolide

**INDICATIONS:** Treatment of bacterial conjunctivitis caused by susceptible strains of microorganisms.

**DOSAGE:** *Adults:* Initial: 1 drop bid, 8 to 12 hrs apart, for first 2 days. Maint: 1 drop qd for next 5 days.
*Pediatric:* ≥1 yr: Initial: 1 drop bid, 8 to 12 hrs apart, for first 2 days. Maint: 1 drop qd for next 5 days.

**HOW SUPPLIED:** Sol: 1% [2.5mL]

**WARNINGS/PRECAUTIONS:** Not for injection; do not give systemically, inject subconjunctivally or into chamber of eye. Caution may cause hypersensitivity reactions. Growth of resistant organisms including fungi may occur with prolonged use. Avoid contact lens use.

**ADVERSE REACTIONS:** Eye irritation, burning, stinging and irritation upon instillation, contact dermatitis, corneal erosion, dry eye, dysgeusia, nasal congestion, ocular discharge, punctate keratitis, sinusitis.

**PREGNANCY:** Category B, caution in nursing.

## AZELEX RX

azelaic acid (Allergan)

**THERAPEUTIC CLASS:** Dicarboxylic acid antimicrobial

**INDICATIONS:** Mild-to-moderate inflammatory acne vulgaris.

**DOSAGE:** *Adults:* Wash and dry skin. Massage gently into affected area bid (am and pm).
*Pediatrics:* >12 yrs: Wash and dry skin. Massage gently into affected area bid (am and pm).

**HOW SUPPLIED:** Cre: 20% [30g, 50g]

**WARNINGS/PRECAUTIONS:** Avoid mouth, eyes, mucous membranes, and occlusive dressings.

**ADVERSE REACTIONS:** Pruritus, burning, stinging, tingling, hypopigmentation.

**PREGNANCY:** Category B, caution in nursing.

## AZILECT RX

rasagiline mesylate (Teva)

**THERAPEUTIC CLASS:** Monoamine oxidase inhibitor (Type B)

**INDICATIONS:** Treatment of signs and symptoms of idiopathic Parkinson's disease as initial monotherapy and adjunct therapy to levodopa.

**DOSAGE:** *Adults:* Monotherapy: 1mg qd. Adjunctive Therapy: Initial: 0.5mg qd. Titrate: May increase to 1mg qd. Adjust dose of levodopa with concomitant use. Concomitant Ciprofloxacin or Other CYP1A2 Inhibitors/Hepatic Impairment: 0.5mg qd.

**HOW SUPPLIED:** Tab: 0.5mg, 1mg

**CONTRAINDICATIONS:** Pheochromocytoma. Concomitant use with meperidine, tramadol, methadone, propoxyphene, dextromethorphan, St. John's wort, mirtazapine, cyclobenzaprine, sympathomimetic amines (eg, amphetamines, cold products containing pseudoephedrine, phenylephrine, phenylpropanolamine, and ephedrine), other MAOIs, cocaine, general anesthesia, local anesthesia containing vasoconstrictors.

**WARNINGS/PRECAUTIONS:** May increase incidence of melanoma. Concomitant use with levodopa may potentiate dopaminergic side effects and exacerbate pre-existing dyskinesia. Postural hypotension reported. Patients should be warned to restrict dietary tyramines and avoid amine-containing medications for 2 weeks after discontinuation.

**ADVERSE REACTIONS:** Headache, arthralgia, depression, fall, flu syndrome, dyskinesia, accidental injury, nausea, weight loss, constipation, postural hypotension, vomiting, dry mouth, rash, somnolence.

**INTERACTIONS:** See Contraindications. Concomitant use with SSRIs, SNRIs, tricyclic and tetracyclic antidepressants is not recommended due to severe CNS toxicity. Increased plasma concentrations up to 2-fold with concomitant ciprofloxacin and other CYP1A2. Severe hypertensive reactions reported with concomitant use of sympathomimetics.

**PREGNANCY:** Category C, caution in nursing.

## AZMACORT — RX

triamcinolone acetonide (Kos)

**THERAPEUTIC CLASS:** Corticosteroid

**INDICATIONS:** Maintenance treatment of asthma as prophylactic therapy in patients ≥6 yrs; to reduce or eliminate the need for oral corticosteroidal therapy.

**DOSAGE:** *Adults:* 2 inh tid-qid or 4 inh bid. Severe Asthma: Initial: 12-16 inh/day. Max: 16 inh/day. Rinse mouth after use.
*Pediatrics:* >12 yrs: 2 inh tid-qid or 4 inh bid. Severe Asthma: Initial: 12-16 inh/day. Max: 16 inh/day. 6-12 yrs: 1-2 inh tid-qid or 2-4 inh bid. Max: 12 inh/day. Rinse mouth after use.

**HOW SUPPLIED:** MDI: 100mcg/inh [20g]

**CONTRAINDICATIONS:** Primary treatment of status asthmaticus or other acute asthma attacks.

**WARNINGS/PRECAUTIONS:** Deaths due to adrenal insufficiency have occurred with transfer from systemic corticosteroids to inhaled corticosteroids. Resume oral corticosteroids during stress or severe asthma attack. Observe for adrenal insufficiency, systemic corticosteroid withdrawal effects, hypercorticism and growth suppression (children). More susceptible to infections. Not for acute bronchospasm. D/C if bronchospasm occurs after dosing. Caution with TB of respiratory tract; untreated systemic fungal, bacterial, viral or parasitic infections; or ocular herpes simplex. *Candida* infection of mouth and pharynx reported.

**ADVERSE REACTIONS:** Pharyngitis, sinusitis, headache, flu syndrome.

**INTERACTIONS:** Caution with prednisone.

**PREGNANCY:** Category C, caution in nursing.

## AZOPT — RX

brinzolamide (Alcon)

**THERAPEUTIC CLASS:** Carbonic anhydrase inhibitor

**INDICATIONS:** Open-angle glaucoma. Ocular hypertension.

**DOSAGE:** *Adults:* 1 drop tid. Space dosing other ophthalmic drugs by 10 minutes.

**HOW SUPPLIED:** Sus: 1% [5mL, 10mL, 15mL]

**WARNINGS/PRECAUTIONS:** Systemically absorbed. Avoid with sulfonamide allergy or severe renal impairment. Caution with hepatic impairment. Not studied in acute angle-closure glaucoma.

**ADVERSE REACTIONS:** Blurred vision, taste disturbances, blepharitis, dermatitis, dry eye, foreign body sensation, headache, hyperemia, ocular discharge, ocular discomfort, ocular keratitis, ocular pain, ocular pruritus, rhinitis.

**INTERACTIONS:** Caution with high-dose salicylates. Acid-base disturbances with oral carbonic anhydrase inhibitors. Avoid oral carbonic anhydrase inhibitors due to additive effects. Wait 10 minutes before using another ophthalmic drug.

**PREGNANCY:** Category C, not for use in nursing.

## AZULFIDINE RX

sulfasalazine (Pharmacia & Upjohn)

**THERAPEUTIC CLASS:** 5-Aminosalicylic acid derivative/sulfapyridine

**INDICATIONS:** Treatment of mild to moderate ulcerative colitis. Adjunct therapy in severe ulcerative colitis. To prolong remission period between acute attacks of ulcerative colitis.

**DOSAGE:** *Adults:* Initial: 3-4g/day in divided doses. May initiate at 1-2g/day to reduce GI intolerance. Maint: 2g/day.
*Pediatrics:* >2 yrs: 40-60mg/kg/day divided into 3-6 doses. Maint: 7.5mg/kg qid.

**HOW SUPPLIED:** Tab: 500mg* *scored

**CONTRAINDICATIONS:** <2 yrs, intestinal or urinary obstruction, porphyria, hypersensitivity to sulfonamides, salicylates.

**WARNINGS/PRECAUTIONS:** Caution with hepatic/renal impairment, blood dyscrasias, severe allergy, bronchial asthma, G6PD deficiency. Monitor CBC, WBC, LFTs, at baseline, every 2nd week for 1st 3 months, monthly for next 3 months, and every 3 months thereafter. Monitor renal function periodically. Maintain adequate fluid intake to prevent crystalluria and stone formation. D/C if hypersensitivity or toxic reaction occurs.

**ADVERSE REACTIONS:** Anorexia, headache, nausea, vomiting, gastric distress, reversible oligospermia.

**INTERACTIONS:** Reduces absorption of folic acid, digoxin.

**PREGNANCY:** Category B, caution in nursing.

## AZULFIDINE EN RX

sulfasalazine (Pharmacia & Upjohn)

**THERAPEUTIC CLASS:** 5-Aminosalicylic acid derivative/sulfapyridine

**INDICATIONS:** Mild to moderate ulcerative colitis, as an adjunct treatment of severe ulcerative colitis, and for the prolongation of the remission period between acute attacks of ulcerative colitis. Rheumatoid arthritis and polyarticular-course juvenile rheumatoid arthritis that has responded inadequately to salicylates or other NSAIDs.

**DOSAGE:** *Adults:* Ulcerative Colitis: Initial: 1-4g/day in divided doses at intervals not exceeding 8 hrs. Maint: 2g/day. Rheumatoid Arthritis: Initial: 0.5-1g/day. Maint: 2g/day given bid. Swallow tabs whole after meals.
*Pediatrics:* >2 yrs: Ulcerative Colitis: Initial: 40-60mg/kg/24hrs in 3-6 divided doses. Maint: 7.5mg/kg qid. Juvenile Rheumatoid Arthritis: 30-50mg/kg/day given bid. To reduce GI effects give 1/4 to 1/3 initial dose; increase weekly for 1 month. Max: 2g/day. Swallow tabs whole after meals.

**HOW SUPPLIED:** Tab, Delayed Release: 500mg

**CONTRAINDICATIONS:** Intestinal or urinary obstruction, porphyria, hypersensitivity to sulfonamides or salicylates.

**WARNINGS/PRECAUTIONS:** Caution with hepatic or renal impairment, blood dyscrasias, severe allergy, bronchial asthma or G6PD deficiency. Monitor CBC,

WBC, and LFTs prior to therapy and every other week for the 1st 3 months, once monthly for next 3 months, then every 3 months. Monitor renal function periodically. Maintain adequate fluid intake. Fatal hypersensitivity reactions reported. D/C if tabs pass undisintegrated or if hypersensitivity reactions occur.

**ADVERSE REACTIONS:** Anorexia, headache, nausea, vomiting, gastric distress, oligospermia, rash, pruritus, urticaria, fever, orange-yellow urine or skin.

**INTERACTIONS:** Reduces absorption of folic acid and digoxin. Increased incidence of GI adverse events with combination of sulfasalazine (2g/day) and MTX (7.5mg/week).

**PREGNANCY:** Category B, caution in nursing.

## BACITRACIN INJECTION RX

bacitracin (Pharmacia & Upjohn)

**May cause renal failure due to tubular and glomerular necrosis. Monitor renal function prior to, and daily during therapy. Fluid intake and urinary output should be maintained at proper levels to avoid kidney toxicity. Discontinue if renal toxicity occurs. Avoid other nephrotoxic drugs.**

**THERAPEUTIC CLASS:** Antibiotic

**INDICATIONS:** Treatment of pneumonia and empyema caused by staphylococci.

**DOSAGE:** Pediatrics: <2500g: 900U/kg/24h IM. >2500g: 1000U/kg/24h IM. Administer in 2-3 divided doses. Inject in upper outer quadrant of buttocks.

**HOW SUPPLIED:** Inj: 50,000U

**WARNINGS/PRECAUTIONS:** Use appropriate therapy if superinfection occurs.

**ADVERSE REACTIONS:** Albuminuria, cylindruria, azotemia, nausea, vomiting, pain at injection site, skin rashes, rising blood levels without increase in dosage.

**INTERACTIONS:** Avoid with other nephrotoxic drugs (eg, streptomycin, kanamycin, polymyxin B, polymyxin E, neomycin).

**PREGNANCY:** Safety in pregnancy or nursing not known.

## BACLOFEN RX

baclofen (Various)

**OTHER BRAND NAMES:** Kemstro (Schwarz)

**THERAPEUTIC CLASS:** GABA analog

**INDICATIONS:** Treatment of spasticity associated with multiple sclerosis. May be effective in spinal cord injuries and other spinal cord diseases.

**DOSAGE:** *Adults:* Initial: 5mg tid for 3 days. Titrate: May increase dose by 5mg tid every 3 days. Usual: 40-80mg/day. Max: 80 mg/day (20mg qid). Renal Impairment: Reduce dose.
*Pediatrics:* >12 yrs: Initial: 5mg tid for 3 days. Titrate: May increase dose by 5mg tid every 3 days. Usual: 40-80mg/day. Max: 80 mg/day (20mg qid). Renal Impairment: Reduce dose.

**HOW SUPPLIED:** Tab: (Generic) 10mg, 20mg; Tab, Disintegrating (ODT): (Kemstro) 10mg, 20mg

**WARNINGS/PRECAUTIONS:** Caution with psychosis, schizophrenia, confusional states; may exacerbate conditions. Caution with bladder sphincter hypertonia, peptic ulceration, seizures, elderly, cerebrovascular disorder, respiratory failure, hepatic or renal failure. Abnormal AST, alkaline phosphatase and blood glucose reported. Caution when used to maintain locomotion or to obtain increased function. Decreased alertness with operating machinery. Has not significantly benefited stroke patients. Avoid abrupt discontinuation; reduce dose slowly over 1-2 weeks.

**ADVERSE REACTIONS:** Drowsiness, dizziness, weakness, fatigue, confusion, daytime sedation, headache, insomnia, hypotension, nausea, constipation, urinary frequency.

**INTERACTIONS:** May potentiate antihypertensives. May increase CNS depressant effects with MAO inhibitors. Potentiated by TCAs. Mental confusion, hallucinations and agitation with levodopa plus carbidopa therapy. May increase blood glucose and require dosage adjustment of antidiabetic agents. Synergistic effects with magnesium sulfate and other neuromuscular blockers. Additive CNS effects with alcohol and other CNS depressants.

**PREGNANCY:** Category C, caution in nursing.

## BACTRIM RX

trimethoprim - sulfamethoxazole (AR Scientific)

**OTHER BRAND NAMES:** Bactrim DS (AR Scientific)

**THERAPEUTIC CLASS:** Sulfonamide/tetrahydrofolic acid inhibitor

**INDICATIONS:** Treatment of urinary tract infection (UTI), acute otitis media, acute exacerbation of chronic bronchitis (AECB), travelers' diarrhea, Shigellosis, and pneumocystitis carinii pneumonia (PCP).

**DOSAGE:** *Adults:* UTI: 800mg SMX-160mg TMP q12h for 10-14 days. Shigellosis: 800mg SMX-160mg TMP q12h for 5 days. AECB: 800mg SMX-160mg TMP q12h for 14 days. PCP Treatment: 15-20mg/kg TMP and 75-100mg/kg SMX per 24 hrs given q6h for 14-21 days. PCP Prophylaxis: 800mg SMX-160mg TMP qd. Traveler's Diarrhea: 800mg SMX-160mg TMP q12h for 5 days. CrCl: 15-30mL/min: 50% usual dose. CrCl: <15mL/min: Not recommended. *Pediatrics:* >2 months: UTI/Otitis Media: 4mg/kg TMP and 20mg/kg SMX q12h for 10 days. Shigellosis: 8mg/kg TMP and 40mg/kg SMX per 24 hrs given q12h for 5 days. PCP Treatment: 15-20mg/kg TMP and 75-100mg/kg SMX per 24 hrs given q6h for 14-21 days. PCP Prophylaxis: 150mg/m²/day TMP with 750mg/m²/day SMX given bid, on 3 consecutive days/week. Max: 320mg TMP/1600mg SMX/day. CrCl: 15-30mL/min: 50% usual dose. CrCl: <15mL/min: Not recommended.

**HOW SUPPLIED:** (Sulfamethoxazole [SMX]-Trimethoprim [TMP]) Tab: 400mg-80mg*; Tab, DS: 800mg-160mg* *scored

**CONTRAINDICATIONS:** Megaloblastic anemia due to folate deficiency, pregnancy, nursing, infants <2 months, marked hepatic damage, severe renal insufficiency if cannot monitor renal status.

**WARNINGS/PRECAUTIONS:** Fatal hypersensitivity reactions (eg, Stevens-Johnson syndrome, toxic epidermal necrolysis, fulminant hepatic necrosis, agranulocytosis, aplastic anemia) may occur. Pseudomembranous colitis, cough, SOB, and pulmonary infiltrates reported. Avoid with group A β-hemolytic streptococcal infections. Caution with hepatic/renal impairment, elderly, folate deficiency (eg, chronic alcoholics, anticonvulsants, malabsorption, malnutrition), bronchial asthma, and other allergies. In G6PD deficiency, hemolysis may occur. Increased incidence of adverse events with AIDS. Ensure adequate fluid intake and urinary output. Caution with porphyria, thyroid dysfunction.

**ADVERSE REACTIONS:** Nausea, vomiting, anorexia, rash, urticaria.

**INTERACTIONS:** Diuretics (especially thiazides) may increase risk of thrombocytopenia with purpura in elderly patients. Caution with warfarin, may prolong PT. Increased effects of phenytoin, oral hypoglycemics. Increased plasma levels of methotrexate, digoxin (especially in elderly). Marked but reversible nephrotoxicity reported with cyclosporine. May develop megaloblastic anemia with pyrimethamine >25mg/week. Increased levels with indomethacin. May decrease effects of TCAs. Single case of toxic delirium with amantadine.

**PREGNANCY:** Category C, contraindicated in nursing.

## BACTROBAN

RX

mupirocin (GlaxoSmithKline)

B

**THERAPEUTIC CLASS:** Bacterial protein synthesis inhibitor

**INDICATIONS:** (Oint) Topical treatment of impetigo due to *S.aureus* and *S.pyogenes*. (Cre) Treatment of secondarily infected traumatic skin lesions (up to 10 cm in length or 100 $cm^2$) due to *S.aureus* and *S.pyogenes*.

**DOSAGE:** *Adults:* (Oint) Apply tid. (Cre) Apply tid for 10 days. May cover with gauze. Re-evaluate if no response within 3-5 days.
*Pediatrics:* (Oint) 2-16 yrs: Apply tid. (Cre) 3 months-16 yrs: Apply tid for 10 days. May cover with gauze. Re-evaluate if no response within 3-5 days.

**HOW SUPPLIED:** Cre: 2% [15g, 30g]; Oint: 2% [22g]

**WARNINGS/PRECAUTIONS:** Avoid eyes. Discontinue if sensitization or irritation occurs. May cause superinfection with prolonged use. Caution with ointment in renal dysfunction. Avoid mucosal surfaces. Avoid open wounds or damaged skin with ointment.

**ADVERSE REACTIONS:** Burning, pain, pruritus, headache, rash, nausea.

**PREGNANCY:** Category B, caution in nursing.

## BALAMINE DM

RX

pseudoephedrine HCl - dextromethorphan hbr - carbinoxamine maleate (Ballay)

**THERAPEUTIC CLASS:** Antihistamine/cough suppressant/decongestant

**INDICATIONS:** Relief of cough and upper respiratory symptoms, including nasal congestion associated with allergy or the common cold.

**DOSAGE:** *Adults:* (Syrup) 5mL qid.
*Pediatrics:* (Syrup) >6 yrs: 5mL qid. 18 months-6yrs: 2.5mL qid. (Drops) 9-18 months: 1mL qid. 6-9 months: 0.75mL qid. 3-6 months: 0.5mL qid. 1-3 months: 0.25mL qid.

**HOW SUPPLIED:** Drops: (Carbinoxamine-Dextromethorphan-Pseudoephedrine) 2mg-3.5mg-25mg/mL [30mL]; Syrup: (Carbinoxamine-Dextromethorphan-Pseudoephedrine) 4mg-12.5mg-60mg/5mL

**CONTRAINDICATIONS:** Severe HTN or CAD, MAOI use or within 14 days of discontinuation, narrow-angle glaucoma, urinary retention, peptic ulcer, during asthma attack.

**WARNINGS/PRECAUTIONS:** Caution with elderly, atopic children, sedated/debilitated, patients confined to supine positions, HTN, DM, ischemic heart disease, hyperthyroidism, prostatic hypertrophy, asthma, and increased IOP. May produce CNS stimulation with convulsions or cardiovascular collapse with hypotension. Excitability reported especially in children. Caution while operating machinery.

**ADVERSE REACTIONS:** Sedation, dizziness, diplopia, vomiting, diarrhea, dry mouth, headache, arrhythmias, increased heart rate and BP, tremors, nervousness, insomnia.

**INTERACTIONS:** May enhance effects of TCAs, barbiturates, alcohol, other CNS depressants. May diminish antihypertensive effects of reserpine, veratrum alkaloids, methyldopa, mecamylamine. Increased sympathomimetic effect with beta-blockers and MAOIs. Additive cough-suppressant effect with narcotic antitussives. Contraindicated with or within 14 days of discontinuing MAOIs.

**PREGNANCY:** Category C, not for use in nursing.

## BARACLUDE RX

entecavir (Bristol-Myers Squibb)

**Lactic acidosis and severe, possibly fatal, hepatomegaly with steatosis reported. Reports of severe acute exacerbations of hepatitis B upon discontinuation of therapy. Follow-up liver function monitoring required.**

**THERAPEUTIC CLASS:** Guanosine nucleoside analogue

**INDICATIONS:** Treatment of chronic hepatitis B virus (HBV) infection with active viral replication and persistent elevations in serum aminotransferases (ALT or AST) or histologically active disease.

**DOSAGE:** *Adults:* Nucleoside-Treatment-Naive: 0.5mg qd. CrCl 30 to <50mL/min: 0.25mg qd. CrCl 10 to <30mL/min: 0.15mg qd. CrCl <10mL/min: 0.05mg qd. Receiving Lamivudine or Known Lamivudine Resistance Mutation: 1mg qd. CrCl 30 to <50mL/min: 0.5mg qd. CrCl 10 to <30mL/min: 0.3mg qd. CrCl <10mL/min: 0.1mg qd. Take on empty stomach.
*Pediatrics:* ≥16 yrs: Nucleoside-Treatment-Naive: 0.5mg qd. CrCl 30 to <50mL/min: 0.25mg qd. CrCl 10 to <30mL/min: 0.15mg qd. CrCl <10mL/min: 0.05mg qd. Receiving Lamivudine or Known Lamivudine Resistance Mutation: 1mg qd. CrCl 30 to <50mL/min: 0.5mg qd. CrCl 10 to <30mL/min: 0.3mg qd. CrCl <10mL/min: 0.1mg qd. Take on empty stomach.

**HOW SUPPLIED:** Sol: 0.05mg/mL; Tab: 0.5mg, 1mg

**WARNINGS/PRECAUTIONS:** Reduce dose in renal dysfunction (CrCl <50mL/min) including patients on hemodialysis or CAPD (continuous ambulatory peritoneal dialysis).Exacerbations of hepatitis After discontinuation of treatment

**ADVERSE REACTIONS:** Headache, fatigue, dizziness, nausea, hyperglycemia, lipase > or equal to 2.1 X ULN, glycosuria, hematuria and increase in total bilirubin.

**INTERACTIONS:** May increase serum concentrations of entecavir or coadministered drug with drugs that reduce renal function or compete for active tubular secretion.

**PREGNANCY:** Category C, not for use in nursing.

## BAYER ASPIRIN OTC

aspirin (Bayer Healthcare LLC)

**OTHER BRAND NAMES:** Bayer Extra Strength (Bayer Healthcare LLC) - Bayer Aspirin Regimen (Bayer Healthcare LLC) - Genuine Bayer Aspirin (Bayer Healthcare LLC) - Bayer Aspirin Children's (Bayer Healthcare LLC) - Bayer Aspirin Regimen with Calcium (Bayer Healthcare LLC)

**THERAPEUTIC CLASS:** Salicylate

**INDICATIONS:** To reduce the risk of death and nonfatal stroke with previous ischemic stroke or transient ischemia of the brain. To reduce risk of vascular mortality with suspected acute MI. To reduce risk of death and nonfatal MI with previous MI or unstable angina. To reduce risk of MI and sudden death in chronic stable angina pectoris. For patients who have undergone revascularization procedures with a pre-existing condition for which ASA is indicated. Relief of signs of rheumatoid arthritis (RA), juvenile rheumatoid arthritis (JRA), osteoarthritis (OA), spondyloarthropathies, arthritis, and pleurisy associated with SLE. For minor aches and pains.

**DOSAGE:** *Adults:* Ischemic Stroke/TIA: 50-325mg qd. Suspected Acute MI: Initial: 160-162.5mg qd as soon as suspect MI. Maint: 160-162.5mg qd for 30 days post-infarction, consider further therapy for prevention/recurrent MI. Prevention or Recurrent MI/Unstable Angina/Chronic Stable Angina: 75-325mg qd. CABG: 325mg qd, start 6 hrs post-surgery. Continue for 1 year. PTCA: Initial: 325mg, 2 hrs pre-surgery. Maint: 160-325mg qd. Carotid Endarterectomy: 80mg qd to 650mg bid, start pre-surgery. RA: Initial: 3g qd in

divided doses. Increase for anti-inflammatory efficacy to 150-300mcg/mL plasma salicylate level. Spondyloarthropathies: Up to 4g/day in divided doses. OA: Up to 3g/day in divided doses. Arthritis/SLE Pleurisy: Initial: 3g/day in divided doses. Increase for anti-inflammatory efficacy to 150-300mcg/mL plasma salicylate level. Pain: 325-650mg q4-6h. Max: 4g/day.
*Pediatrics:* JRA: Initial: 90-130mg/kg/day in divided doses. Increase for anti-inflammatory efficacy to 150-300mcg/mL plasma salicylate level. Pain: >12 yrs: 325-650mg q4-6h. Max: 4g/day.

**HOW SUPPLIED:** Tab: (Genuine Bayer Aspirin) 325mg; Tab: (Bayer Extra Strength) 500mg; Tab: (Bayer Aspirin Regimen with Calcium) 81mg; Tab, Chewable: (Bayer Aspirin Children's) 81mg; Tab, Delayed Release: (Bayer Aspirin Regimen) 81mg, 325mg

**CONTRAINDICATIONS:** NSAID allergy, viral infections in children or teenagers, syndrome of asthma, rhinitis, and nasal polyps.

**WARNINGS/PRECAUTIONS:** Increased risk of bleeding with heavy alcohol use (>3 drinks/day). May inhibit platelet function; can adversely affect inherited (hemophilia) or acquired (hepatic disease, vitamin K deficiency) bleeding disorders. Monitor for bleeding and ulceration. Avoid in history of active peptic ulcer, severe renal failure, severe hepatic insufficiency, and sodium restricted diets. Associated with elevated LFTs, BUN, and serum creatinine; hyperkalemia; proteinuria; and prolonged bleeding time. Avoid 1 week before and during labor.

**ADVERSE REACTIONS:** Fever, hypothermia, dysrhythmias, hypotension, agitation, cerebral edema, dehydration, hyperkalemia, dyspepsia, GI bleed, hearing loss, tinnitus, problems in pregnancy.

**INTERACTIONS:** Diminished hypotensive and hyponatremic effects of ACE inhibitors. May increase levels of acetazolamide, valproic acid. Increased bleeding risk with heparin, warfarin. Decreased levels of phenytoin. Decreased hypotensive effects of β-blockers. Decreased diuretic effects with renal or cardiovascular disease. Decreased methotrexate clearance; increased risk of bone marrow toxicity. Avoid NSAIDs. Increased effects of hypoglycemic agents. Antagonizes uricosuric agents.

**PREGNANCY:** Avoid in 3rd trimester of pregnancy and nursing.

## BAYER ASPIRIN EXTRA STRENGTH — OTC

aspirin (Bayer Healthcare LLC)

**THERAPEUTIC CLASS:** Salicylate

**INDICATIONS:** For the temporary relief of headache, pain and fever of colds, muscle aches and pains, menstrual pain, toothache pain, minor aches and arthritis pain.

**DOSAGE:** *Adults:* 500-1000mg q4-6h prn. Max: 4g/24hrs.
*Pediatrics:* >12 yrs: 500-1000mg q4-6h prn. Max: 4g/24hrs.

**HOW SUPPLIED:** Tab: 500mg

**WARNINGS/PRECAUTIONS:** Avoid in children or teenagers for chickenpox or flu symptoms; Reye's syndrome may occur. Do not take >10 days for pain or >3 days for fever. Avoid in asthma, stomach problems that persist or recur, gastric ulcers, or bleeding problems. Stop therapy if ringing in the ears or loss of hearing occurs.

**INTERACTIONS:** Avoid with drugs for anticoagulation, diabetes, gout, or arthritis. Increased risk of stomach bleeding with alcohol use (>3 drinks/day).

**PREGNANCY:** Avoid in 3rd trimester of pregnancy; safety in nursing not known.

B

## BAYRHO-D FULL DOSE RX

immune globulin (Bayer Biological)

**THERAPEUTIC CLASS:** Rh response inhibitor

**INDICATIONS:** To prevent isoimmunization of Rh-negative women (not sensitized to Rh-factor) exposed to Rh-positive blood following delivery of Rh-positive infant, ruptured tubal pregnancy, transfusion, abortion, amniocentesis or abdominal trauma. Prevention of Rh hemolytic disease of the newborn by administration to Rh-negative mother after subsequent birth of Rh-positive infant.

**DOSAGE:** *Adults:* 300mcg for <15mL fetal RBCs; if >15mL fetal RBCs, or if the dose calculation results in a fraction, administer the next higher whole number of vials/syringes. Postpartum Prophylaxis: 300mcg IM within 72 hrs of delivery. Antenatal Prophylaxis: 300mcg IM at about 28 weeks gestation, followed by 300mcg IM within 72 hrs of delivery if infant is Rh-positive. Following Threatened Abortion (any gestational stage)/Miscarriage/Abortion/Termination of Ectopic Pregnancy (at or beyond 13 weeks gestation)/Amniocentesis (at either 15-18 weeks gestation or during the 3rd trimester)/Abdominal Trauma (2nd or 3rd trimester): 300mcg IM. If abdominal trauma, amniocentesis, or other adverse event requires administration at 13-18 weeks gestation, another 300mcg IM should be given at 26-28 weeks.

**HOW SUPPLIED:** Inj: 300mcg (approx.)

**WARNINGS/PRECAUTIONS:** For IM administration only. Do not administer to neonates. Risk of transmitting infectious agents (eg, viruses). Increased potential for anaphylactic reactions with isolated IgA deficiency. Caution with thrombocytopenia or other bleeding disorders. Have epinephrine available. If father is Rh-negative, BayRho is not needed.

**ADVERSE REACTIONS:** Injection site reactions, slight temperature elevation, elevated bilirubin levels, sensitization/anaphylactic reactions (rare).

**INTERACTIONS:** May interfere with response to live vaccines; avoid within 3 months of BayRho.

**PREGNANCY:** Category C, safety in nursing not known.

## BAYRHO-D MINI-DOSE RX

immune globulin (Bayer Biological)

**THERAPEUTIC CLASS:** Rh response inhibitor

**INDICATIONS:** To prevent isoimmunization of Rh-negative women at time of spontaneous or induced abortion of up to 12 weeks gestation provided mother is Rh-negative and not already sensitized to the Rh antigen, or father is not known to be Rh-negative.

**DOSAGE:** *Adults:* 50mcg IM to prevent Rh sensitization to 2.5mL RBCs. Give within 3 hrs or as soon as possible within 72 hrs following termination of pregnancy.

**HOW SUPPLIED:** Inj: 50mcg (approx.)

**WARNINGS/PRECAUTIONS:** For IM administration only. Do not administer to neonates. Risk of transmitting infectious agents (eg, viruses). Increased potential for anaphylactic reactions with isolated IgA deficiency. Caution with thrombocytopenia or other bleeding disorders. Have epinephrine available.

**ADVERSE REACTIONS:** Injection site reactions, slight temperature elevation, sensitization/anaphylactic reactions (rare).

**INTERACTIONS:** May interfere with response to live vaccines; avoid within 3 months of BayRho.

**PREGNANCY:** Category C, safety in nursing not known.

## BECONASE AQ RX
beclomethasone dipropionate (GlaxoSmithKline)

**OTHER BRAND NAMES:** Beconase (Various)

**THERAPEUTIC CLASS:** Corticosteroid

**INDICATIONS:** Relief of symptoms of seasonal or perennial allergic and nonallergic rhinitis. Prevention of nasal polyp recurrence following surgical removal.

**DOSAGE:** *Adults:* (Beconase): 1 spray per nostril bid-qid. (Beconase AQ) 1-2 sprays per nostril bid. Max: 2 sprays per nostril bid.
*Pediatrics:* (Beconase) >12 yrs: 1 spray per nostril bid-qid. 6-12 yrs: 1 spray per nostril tid. (Beconase AQ) ≥6 yrs: 1-2 sprays per nostril bid. Max: 2 sprays per nostril bid.

**HOW SUPPLIED:** Aerosol: (Beconase) 42mcg/spray [6.7g, 16.8g]; Spray: (Beconase AQ) 42mcg/spray [25g]

**WARNINGS/PRECAUTIONS:** Risk of adrenal insufficiency and withdrawal symptoms when replacing systemic corticosteroids with a topical corticosteroids. Caution with active or quiescent TB, ocular herpes simplex, or untreated bacterial, fungal and systemic viral infections. Avoid with recent nasal trauma, surgery or septum ulcers. Risk for more severe/fatal course of infections (eg, chickenpox, measles) and for Candida infection of the nose and pharynx. Potential for growth velocity reduction in pediatrics.

**ADVERSE REACTIONS:** Nasopharyngeal irritation, sneezing, headache, nausea, lightheadedness, irritated/dry nose and throat, unpleasant taste/smell.

**INTERACTIONS:** Concomitant systemic corticosteroids increases risk of hypercorticism and/or HPA axis suppression.

**PREGNANCY:** Category C, caution in nursing.

## BELLAMINE-S RX
phenobarbital - belladonna alkaloids - ergotamine tartrate (Amide)

**THERAPEUTIC CLASS:** Anticholinergic/ergot derivative/barbiturate

**INDICATIONS:** Management of nervous tension and exaggerated autonomic response associated with menopausal (hot flushes, sweats, restlessness, insomnia), cardiovascular (palpitations, tachycardia, vasomotor disturbances), and GI disorders (hypermotility, hypersecretion,"nervous stomach". Interval treatment for recurrent, throbbing headache.

**DOSAGE:** *Adults:* 1 tab bid. Max: 16 tabs/week.

**HOW SUPPLIED:** Tab: (Belladonna Alkaloids-Ergotamine Tartrate-Phenobarbital) 0.2mg-0.6mg-40mg

**CONTRAINDICATIONS:** Peripheral vascular or coronary heart disease, HTN, impaired hepatic/renal function, sepsis, glaucoma, latent porphyria, pregnancy, nursing mothers, paradoxical reactions to phenobarbital, concomitant dopamine therapy.

**WARNINGS/PRECAUTIONS:** May be habit forming. Caution in asthma, obstructive uropathy. Possible vascular complications with ergot sensitivity.

**ADVERSE REACTIONS:** Paresthesias, blurred vision, palpitations, dry mouth, decreased GI motility, decreased sweating, urinary retention, tachycardia, drowsiness, flushing.

**INTERACTIONS:** Avoid dopamine. May decrease anticoagulant effect. Additive CNS depression with other CNS depressants, alcohol. Monitor for excessive vasoconstriction with beta blockers. Increases metabolism of griseofulvin, quinidine, doxycycline, estrogen. Monitor phenytoin levels. Sodium valproate, valproic acid decrease barbiturate levels. Additive anticholinergic effects with TCAs.

**PREGNANCY:** Category X, not for use in nursing.

B

## BENADRYL ALLERGY OTC

diphenhydramine HCl (McNeil)

**THERAPEUTIC CLASS:** Antihistamine

**INDICATIONS:** Relief of hay fever or upper respiratory allergies, and rhinorrhea/sneezing due to the common cold.

**DOSAGE:** *Adults:* 25-50mg q4-6h. Max: 300mg/24hrs.
*Pediatrics:* >12 yrs: 25-50mg q4-6h. Max: 300mg/24 hrs. 6-11 yrs: 12.5-25mg q4-6h. Max: 150mg/24hrs.

**HOW SUPPLIED:** Cap: 25mg; Sol: 12.5mg/5mL; Tab: 25mg; Tab, Chewable: 12.5mg

**WARNINGS/PRECAUTIONS:** Caution with emphysema, chronic bronchitis, glaucoma, or difficulty in urination due to prostate gland enlargement. May impair mental/physical abilities.

**ADVERSE REACTIONS:** Drowsiness, excitability (especially in children).

**INTERACTIONS:** Increased drowsiness with alcohol, sedatives, tranquilizers.

**PREGNANCY:** Safety in pregnancy and nursing not known.

## BENICAR RX

olmesartan medoxomil (Sankyo)

**Can cause death/injury to developing fetus during 2nd and 3rd trimesters. Stop therapy if pregnancy detected.**

**THERAPEUTIC CLASS:** Angiotensin II receptor antagonist

**INDICATIONS:** Hypertension, alone or with other antihypertensives.

**DOSAGE:** *Adults:* Monotherapy Without Volume Depletion: Initial: 20mg qd. Titrate: May increase to 40mg qd after 2 weeks if needed. May add diuretic if BP not controlled. Intravascular Volume Depletion (eg, with diuretics, impaired renal function): Lower initial dose; monitor closely.

**HOW SUPPLIED:** Tab: 5mg, 20mg, 40mg

**WARNINGS/PRECAUTIONS:** Can cause fetal injury/death. Symptomatic hypotension may occur in volume- and/or salt-depleted patients; monitor closely. Changes in renal function may occur; caution with severe CHF. Increases in serum creatinine or BUN reported with renal artery stenosis.

**ADVERSE REACTIONS:** Dizziness, transient hypotension.

**INTERACTIONS:** Risk of hypotension with high-dose diuretics.

**PREGNANCY:** Category C (1st trimester) and D (2nd and 3rd trimesters), not for use in nursing.

## BENICAR HCT RX

hydrochlorothiazide - olmesartan medoxomil (Sankyo)

**Can cause death/injury to developing fetus during 2nd and 3rd trimesters. Stop therapy if pregnancy detected.**

**THERAPEUTIC CLASS:** Angiotensin II receptor antagonist/thiazide diuretic

**INDICATIONS:** Hypertension. Not for initial therapy.

**DOSAGE:** *Adults:* If BP not controlled with olmesartan alone: Add HCTZ 12.5mg qd. May titrate to 25mg qd if BP uncontrolled after 2-4 weeks. If BP not controlled with HCTZ alone: Add olmesartan 20mg qd. May titrate to 40mg qd if BP uncontrolled after 2-4 weeks. Intravascular Volume Depletion (eg, with diuretics, impaired renal function): Lower initial dose; monitor closely. Elderly: Start at lower end of dosing range.

**HOW SUPPLIED:** Tab: (Olmesartan-HCTZ) 20mg-12.5mg, 40mg-12.5mg, 40mg-25mg

**CONTRAINDICATIONS:** Sulfonamide hypersensitivity.

**WARNINGS/PRECAUTIONS:** Can cause fetal injury/death. Correct volume or salt depletion before therapy or monitor closely. Caution with hepatic or severe renal dysfunction, progressive liver disease, history of allergies or asthma, renal artery stenosis, severe CHF. Avoid if CrCl <30mL/min. May exacerbate or activate SLE. Monitor serum electrolytes. Hyperuricemia, hyperglycemia, hypercalcemia, hypomagnesemia may occur. May increase cholesterol and triglyceride levels.

**ADVERSE REACTIONS:** Dizziness, upper respiratory tract infection, hyperuricemia, nausea.

**INTERACTIONS:** Potentiates orthostatic hypotension with alcohol, barbiturates, or narcotics. May need to adjust antidiabetics. Potentiates other antihypertensives. Impaired absorption with cholestyramine, colestipol. Corticosteroids, ACTH deplete electrolytes. May decrease response to pressor amines. May potentiate non-depolarizing skeletal muscle relaxants. Risk of lithium toxicity. NSAIDs decrease diuretic effects.

**PREGNANCY:** Category C (1st trimester) and D (2nd and 3rd trimesters), not for use in nursing.

## BENTYL

RX

dicyclomine HCl (Axcan Scandipharm)

**THERAPEUTIC CLASS:** Anticholinergic

**INDICATIONS:** Treatment of functional bowel/irritable bowel syndrome.

**DOSAGE:** *Adults:* (Tab/Syrup) Initial: 20mg qid. Usual: 40mg qid if tolerated. Discontinue if no improvement after 2 weeks or if doses >80mg/day are not tolerated. (Inj) 20mg IM qid for 1-2 days, followed by oral dicyclomine. Not for IV use.

**HOW SUPPLIED:** Cap: 10mg; Inj: 10mg/mL; Syrup: 10mg/5mL; Tab: 20mg

**CONTRAINDICATIONS:** GI tract obstruction, obstructive uropathy, severe ulcerative colitis, reflux esophagitis, glaucoma, myasthenia gravis, unstable cardiovascular status and in acute hemorrhage, nursing mothers, infants <6 months of age.

**WARNINGS/PRECAUTIONS:** Caution in autonomic neuropathy, hepatic/renal impairment, ulcerative colitis, hyperthyroidism, HTN, CHF, cardiac tachyarrhythmia, coronary heart disease, hiatal hernia, and prostatic hypertrophy. Heat prostration may occur in high environmental temperature. Monitor for diarrhea, may be the early symptom of intestinal obstruction. Psychosis reported. Serious respiratory symptoms, seizures, syncope and death reported in infants.

**ADVERSE REACTIONS:** Dry mouth, nausea, vomiting, blurred vision, dizziness, drowsiness, nervousness, mental confusion/excitement (especially in the elderly), mydriasis, increased ocular tension, urinary retention, dyspnea, apnea, tachycardia, decreased sweating, lactation suppression, impotence.

**INTERACTIONS:** Potentiated by amantadine, Class I antiarrhythmics (eg, quinidine), antihistamines, antipsychotics (eg, phenothiazines), benzodiazepines, MAOIs, narcotic analgesics (eg, meperidine), nitrates/nitrites, sympathomimetics, TCAs. Antagonizes the effects of antiglaucoma agents; do not give with corticosteroid eye drops. Antagonizes the effect of metoclopramide. May effect the GI absorption of delayed release digoxin. Decreased absorption with antacids. Antagonized by drugs treating achlorhydria and those used to test gastric secretion.

**PREGNANCY:** Category B, contraindicated in nursing.

## BENZAC AC

RX

benzoyl peroxide (Galderma)

**THERAPEUTIC CLASS:** Antibacterial/keratolytic

**INDICATIONS:** Topical treatment of acne vulgaris.

**DOSAGE:** *Adults:* (Sol) Wash area qd-bid. Rinse and dry area. (Gel) Apply qd-bid to clean affected area.

**HOW SUPPLIED:** Gel: 5%, 10% [60g]; Sol (Wash): 5%, 10% [240mL]

**WARNINGS/PRECAUTIONS:** External use only. Avoid contact with eyes, lips, mucous membranes. D/C if severe irritation occurs.

**ADVERSE REACTIONS:** Allergic contact dermatitis, dryness.

**PREGNANCY:** Category C, caution in nursing.

## BENZACLIN

RX

clindamycin - benzoyl peroxide (Dermik)

**THERAPEUTIC CLASS:** Antibacterial/keratolytic

**INDICATIONS:** Topical treatment of acne vulgaris.

**DOSAGE:** *Adults:* Wash face and pat dry. Apply bid (am and pm).
*Pediatrics:* >12 yrs: Wash face and pat dry. Apply bid (am and pm).

**HOW SUPPLIED:** Gel: (Clindamycin-Benzoyl Peroxide) 1%-5% [25g, 50g]

**CONTRAINDICATIONS:** Hypersensitivity to lincomycin. History of regional enteritis, ulcerative colitis, and antibiotic-associated colitis.

**WARNINGS/PRECAUTIONS:** Severe colitis reported with oral and parenteral clindamycin. Discontinue if severe diarrhea occurs. Avoid contact with eyes and mucous membranes.

**ADVERSE REACTIONS:** Dry skin, pruritus, peeling, erythema, sunburn.

**INTERACTIONS:** Cumulative irritancy possible with other topical acne agents. Avoid erythromycin agents.

**PREGNANCY:** Category C, not for use in nursing.

## BENZAGEL

RX

benzoyl peroxide (Dermik)

**OTHER BRAND NAMES:** Benzagel Wash (Dermik)

**THERAPEUTIC CLASS:** Antibacterial/keratolytic

**INDICATIONS:** Treatment of mild to moderate acne, used alone or as an adjunct.

**DOSAGE:** *Adults:* (Wash) Wash area qd-bid. Rinse and dry area. (Gel) Apply qd or more often to clean affected area. Very fair patients should start with single application qhs.
*Pediatrics:* >12 yrs: (Wash) Wash area qd-bid. Rinse and dry area. (Gel) Apply qd or more often to clean affected area. Very fair patients should start with single application qhs.

**HOW SUPPLIED:** Gel: 5%, 10% [42.5g], (Wash) 10% [60g]

**WARNINGS/PRECAUTIONS:** Discontinue if itching, redness, burning, swelling, or undue dryness occurs. Avoid contact with eyes and mucous membranes. May bleach colored fabrics or hair.

**ADVERSE REACTIONS:** Irritation, contact dermatitis.

**PREGNANCY:** Category C, caution in nursing.

## BENZAMYCIN

RX

erythromycin - benzoyl peroxide (Dermik)

**THERAPEUTIC CLASS:** Antibacterial/keratolytic

**INDICATIONS:** Topical treatment of acne vulgaris.

**DOSAGE:** *Adults:* Wash skin and dry. Apply bid (am and pm).
Pediatrics: >12 yrs: Wash skin and dry. Apply bid (am and pm).

**HOW SUPPLIED:** Gel: (Benzoyl Peroxide-Erythromycin) 5%-3% [46.6g, 60[s]]

**WARNINGS/PRECAUTIONS:** D/C if severe irritation occurs. Avoid eyes, mouth, and mucous membranes. Keep refrigerated after reconstitution and discard after 3 months.

**ADVERSE REACTIONS:** Dryness, urticaria, skin irritation, skin discoloration, oiliness, tenderness.

**INTERACTIONS:** Additive irritation with peeling, desquamating, or abrasive agents.

**PREGNANCY:** Category C, caution in nursing.

## BENZTROPINE

RX

benztropine mesylate (Various)

**OTHER BRAND NAMES:** Cogentin (Merck)

**THERAPEUTIC CLASS:** Anticholinergic agent

**INDICATIONS:** Adjunct in all forms of parkinsonism. Control of drug-induced extrapyramidal disorders.

**DOSAGE:** *Adults:* Parkinsonism: Initial: 0.5-1mg PO/IV/IM qhs. Titrate: May increase every 5-6 days by 0.5mg. Usual: 1-2mg PO/IV/IM qhs. Max: 6mg/day. Extrapyramidal Disorders: 1-4mg PO/IV/IM qd-bid. Acute Dystonic Reactions: 1-2mg IM/IV, then 1-2mg PO bid.

**HOW SUPPLIED:** Inj: 1mg/mL; Tab: 0.5mg, 1mg, 2mg

**CONTRAINDICATIONS:** Patients <3 yrs.

**WARNINGS/PRECAUTIONS:** May produce anhidrosis, caution in hot weather. Muscle weakness and dysuria may occur. Caution in pediatrics >3 years of age. Not recommended for tardive dyskinesia. Avoid with angle-closure glaucoma. Caution with CNS disease, mental disorders, tachycardia, prostatic hypertrophy, alcoholics, chronically ill, those exposed to hot environments.

**ADVERSE REACTIONS:** Tachycardia, paralytic ileus, constipation, vomiting, nausea, dry mouth, confusion, blurred vision, urinary retention, heat stroke, hyperthermia, fever.

**INTERACTIONS:** Paralytic ileus, hyperthermia and heat stroke reported with phenothiazines and TCAs. Caution with other atropine-like agents.

**PREGNANCY:** Safety in pregnancy and nursing not known.

## BETAGAN

RX

levobunolol HCl (Allergan)

**OTHER BRAND NAMES:** Betagan C Cap (Allergan)

**THERAPEUTIC CLASS:** Nonselective beta-blocker

**INDICATIONS:** Treatment of elevated intraocular pressure in chronic open-angle glaucoma and ocular hypertension.

**DOSAGE:** *Adults:* (0.5%) 1-2 drops qd; bid for more severe or uncontrolled glaucoma. (0.25%): 1-2 drops bid.

**HOW SUPPLIED:** Sol: (Betagan) 0.5% [2mL]; (Betagan, C Cap) 0.25% [5mL, 10mL], 0.5% [5mL, 10mL, 15mL]

**CONTRAINDICATIONS:** Bronchial asthma, COPD, overt cardiac failure, sinus bradycardia, 2nd- and 3rd-degree AV block, cardiogenic shock.

**WARNINGS/PRECAUTIONS:** Caution with cardiac failure, DM, COPD, cerebral insufficiency, pulmonary disease, bronchospastic disease, surgery and hepatic impairment. May mask symptoms of hypoglycemia and thyrotoxicosis. Contains sodium metabisulfite. Follow with a miotic in angle-closure glaucoma. Potentiates muscle weakness (eg, diplopia, ptosis).

**ADVERSE REACTIONS:** Ocular burning, ocular stinging, decreased heart rate, decreased blood pressure.

**INTERACTIONS:** Mydriasis with epinephrine. Additive effects with catecholamine-depleting drugs (eg, reserpine) and systemic β-blockers. AV conduction disturbance with calcium antagonists and digitalis. Left ventricular failure and hypotension with calcium antagonists also. Additive hypotensive effects with phenothiazine-related drugs. Risk of hypoglycemia with insulin and oral hypoglycemic agents.

**PREGNANCY:** Category C, caution in nursing.

## BETAMETHASONE DIPROPIONATE — RX

betamethasone dipropionate (Various)

**THERAPEUTIC CLASS:** Corticosteroid

**INDICATIONS:** Corticosteroid responsive dermatoses.

**DOSAGE:** *Adults:* (Cre, Oint) Apply qd-bid. (Lot) Apply a few drops bid, am and pm.
*Pediatrics:* (Cre, Oint) Apply qd-bid. (Lot) Apply a few drops bid, am and pm.

**HOW SUPPLIED:** Cre, Oint: 0.05% [15g, 45g]; Lot: 0.05% [20mL, 60mL]

**WARNINGS/PRECAUTIONS:** May produce reversible HPA axis suppression, manifestations of Cushing's syndrome, hyperglycemia, and glucosuria. Avoid occlusive dressings. Pediatrics are more prone to systemic toxicity. Discontinue if irritation occurs. Avoid eyes.

**ADVERSE REACTIONS:** Burning, itching, irritation, dryness, folliculitis, hypertrichosis, acneiform eruptions, hypopigmentation, perioral dermatitis, allergic contact dermatitis, skin maceration, secondary infection, skin atrophy, striae, miliaria.

**PREGNANCY:** Category C, caution in nursing.

## BETAPACE — RX

sotalol HCl (Berlex)

**To minimize risk of arrhythmia, place patients initiated or reinitiated on therapy for minimum of 3 days in a facility that can provide ECG monitoring and cardiac resuscitation. Perform CrCl before therapy. Do not substitute Betapace® for Betapace AF®.**

**THERAPEUTIC CLASS:** Beta-blocker (group II/III antiarrhythmic)

**INDICATIONS:** Treatment of documented life-threatening ventricular arrhythmias.

**DOSAGE:** *Adults:* Initial: 80mg bid. Titrate: Increase to 120-160mg bid if needed. Allow 3 days between dose increments. Usual: 160-320mg/day given bid-tid. Refractory Patients: 480-640mg/day. CrCl 30-59mL/min: Dose q24h. CrCl 10-29mL/min: Dose q36-48h. CrCl <10mL/min: Individualize dose. May increase dose with renal impairment after at least 5-6 doses.
*Pediatrics:* >2 yrs: Initial: 30mg/m² tid. Titrate: Wait at least 36 hrs between dose increases. Guide dose by response, heart rate and QTc. Max: 60mg/m². <2 yrs: See dosing chart in labeling. Reduce dose or discontinue if QTc >550msec. Renal Impairment: Reduce dose or increase interval. Preparation of 5mg/mL Oral Solution: Add five 120mg tabs to 120mL simple syrup in a 6oz plastic, amber bottle. Shake bottle to wet all tabs. Allow tabs to hydrate for 2

hrs then shake bottle intermittently over 2 hrs until tabs are completely disintegrated. Shake before administration. Store at room temp for 3 months.

**HOW SUPPLIED:** Tab: 80mg*, 120mg*, 160mg*, 240mg* *scored

**CONTRAINDICATIONS:** Bronchial asthma, sinus bradycardia, 2nd- and 3rd-degree AV block (unless a functioning pacemaker is present), long QT syndromes, cardiogenic shock, uncontrolled CHF.

**WARNINGS/PRECAUTIONS:** Caution with heart failure controlled by digitalis and/or diuretics, DM, left ventricular dysfunction, non-allergic bronchospasm, sick sinus syndrome, renal impairment, 2-weeks post-MI. Avoid with hypokalemia, hypomagnesemia, excessive QT interval prolongation (>550msec). Correct electrolyte imbalances before therapy. May provoke new or worsen ventricular arrhythmias. Avoid abrupt withdrawal. Use in surgery is controversial. May mask hypoglycemia, hyperthyroidism symptoms. Proarrhythmic events reported.

**ADVERSE REACTIONS:** Dyspnea, fatigue, dizziness, bradycardia, chest pain, palpitation, asthenia, abnormal ECG, hypotension, headache, lightheadedness, edema.

**INTERACTIONS:** May block epinephrine effects. Caution with drugs that prolong the QT interval (eg, Class I and III antiarrhythmics, phenothiazines, TCAs, bepridil, certain quinolones and oral macrolides, astemizole). Avoid within 2 hrs of aluminum- or magnesium-containing antacids. Potentiates rebound HTN with clonidine withdrawal. May potentiate bradycardia or hypotension with catecholamine-depleting drugs (eg, reserpine). Antidiabetic agents may need adjustment. Avoid Class 1A and Class III antiarrhythmics; potential to prolong refractoriness. $\beta_2$-agonists (eg, terbutaline) may need dose increase. Additive Class II effects with β-blockers. Additive conduction abnormalities with digoxin and calcium channel blockers. Caution with diuretics.

**PREGNANCY:** Category B, not for use in nursing.

## BETAPACE AF — RX

sotalol HCl (Berlex)

**To minimize risk of arrhythmia, place patients initiated or reinitiated on therapy for minimum of 3 days in a facility that can provide CrCl, ECG monitoring, and cardiac resuscitation. Do not substitute Betapace® for Betapace AF®.**

**THERAPEUTIC CLASS:** Beta-blocker (group II/III antiarrhythmic)

**INDICATIONS:** Maintenance of normal sinus rhythm with symptomatic atrial fibrillation/atrial flutter (AFIB/AFL) in patients who are currently in sinus rhythm.

**DOSAGE:** *Adults:* Initiate with continuous ECG monitoring. Give dose qd for CrCl 40-60mL/min and bid for CrCl >60mL/min. Initial: 80mg. Monitor QT 2-4hrs after each dose. Discontinue if QT >500msec. If QT <500msec after 3 days (after 5th or 6th dose if receiving qd dosing) discharge on current treatment. Alternately, may increase dose to 120mg during hospitalization, and follow for 3 days with bid dose and for 5 or 6 doses if receiving qd dose. Max: 160mg qd or bid depending on CrCl.
*Pediatrics:* >2 yrs: Initial: 30mg/m² tid. Titrate: Wait at least 36 hrs between dose increases. Guide dose by response, heart rate and QTc. Max: 60mg/m². <2 yrs: See dosing chart in labeling. Reduce dose or discontinue if QTc >550msec. Renal Impairment: Reduce dose or increase interval. Preparation of 5mg/mL Oral Solution: Add five 120mg tabs to 120mL simple syrup in a 6oz plastic, amber bottle. Shake bottle to wet all tabs. Allow tabs to hydrate for 2 hrs then shake bottle intermittently over 2 hrs until tabs are completely disintegrated. Shake before administration. Store at room temp for 3 months.

**HOW SUPPLIED:** Tab: 80mg*, 120mg*, 160mg* *scored

**CONTRAINDICATIONS:** Sinus bradycardia (<50bpm during waking hrs), sick sinus syndrome or 2nd- or 3rd-degree AV block (unless a functioning pacemaker is present), long QT syndromes, baseline QT interval >450msec, cardiogenic shock, uncontrolled heart failure, hypokalemia (<4meq/L), CrCl <40mL/min, bronchial asthma.

**WARNINGS/PRECAUTIONS:** Can cause serious ventricular arrhythmias. Avoid with hypokalemia, hypomagnesemia. Correct electrolyte imbalances before therapy. Bradycardia reported. Caution with heart failure controlled by digitalis and/or diuretics, non-allergic bronchospasm, sick sinus syndrome, left ventricular dysfunction, DM, renal dysfunction, post-MI. Avoid abrupt withdrawal. Use in surgery is controversial. May mask hypoglycemia, hyperthyroidism symptoms.

**ADVERSE REACTIONS:** Bradycardia, dyspnea, fatigue, dose-related QT interval prolongation, abnormal ECG, chest pain, diarrhea, nausea, vomiting, hyperhidrosis, dizziness.

**INTERACTIONS:** May block epinephrine effects. Avoid drugs that prolong the QT interval (eg, antiarrhythmics, phenothiazines, TCAs, bepridil, certain oral macrolides). Avoid within 2 hrs of aluminum- or magnesium-containing antacids. Potentiates rebound HTN with clonidine withdrawal. May potentiate bradycardia or hypotension with catecholamine-depleting drugs (eg, reserpine). Antidiabetic agents may need adjustment. $\beta_2$-agonists (eg, terbutaline) may need dose increase. Additive conduction abnormalities with digoxin and calcium channel blockers. Caution with diuretics.

**PREGNANCY:** Category B, not for use in nursing.

## BETASERON — RX

interferon beta-1b (Berlex)

**THERAPEUTIC CLASS:** Biological response modifier

**INDICATIONS:** Treatment in patients who have experienced a first clinical episode and have MRI features consistent with Multiple Sclerosis (MS). To reduce frequency of clinical exacerbations in patients with relapsing-remitting MS.

**DOSAGE:** *Adults:* Initial: 0.0625mg SQ every other day. Titrate: Increase over 6 wks to 0.25mg SQ every other day.

**HOW SUPPLIED:** Inj: 0.3mg

**CONTRAINDICATIONS:** Hypersensitivity to human albumin.

**WARNINGS/PRECAUTIONS:** Caution with depression. Injection site necrosis reported; d/c if multiple lesions occur. Perform Hgb, LFTs, CBC, differential WBC and platelet count before therapy and periodically thereafter.

**ADVERSE REACTIONS:** Injection site reactions/necrosis, flu-like symptoms, headache, lymphopenia, liver enzyme elevations, pain, fever, chills, diarrhea, abdominal pain, vomiting, constipation, nausea, myalgia, asthenia, malaise, hypertonia, sinusitis, sweating, dizziness, menstrual disorders.

**INTERACTIONS:** May inhibit antipyrine elimination.

**PREGNANCY:** Category C, not for use in nursing.

## BETAXOLOL HCL — RX

betaxolol HCl (Various)

**THERAPEUTIC CLASS:** Selective $beta_1$-blocker

**INDICATIONS:** Management of hypertension.

**DOSAGE:** *Adults:* Initial: 10mg qd. Titrate: May increase to 20mg qd after 7-14 days. Max (usual): 20mg/day. Severe Renal Impairment/Dialysis: Initial: 5mg qd. Titrate: May increase by 5mg/day every 2 weeks. Max: 20mg/day. Elderly: Initial: 5mg qd.

**HOW SUPPLIED:** Tab: 10mg, 20mg

**CONTRAINDICATIONS:** Sinus bradycardia, >1st-degree heart block, cardiogenic shock, overt cardiac failure.

**WARNINGS/PRECAUTIONS:** Caution in CHF controlled by digitalis and diuretics, bronchospastic disease, renal or hepatic dysfunction. Can cause cardiac failure. Avoid abrupt withdrawal. Withdrawal before surgery is controversial. May mask hypoglycemia and hyperthyroidism symptoms. May decrease IOP and interfere with glaucoma-screening test. Bradycardia may occur more often in elderly. May develop antinuclear antibodies (ANA).

**ADVERSE REACTIONS:** Bradycardia, fatigue, dyspnea, lethargy, impotence, dyspepsia, arthralgia, headache, dizziness, insomnia.

**INTERACTIONS:** May block epinephrine effects. Possible additive effects with catecholamine-depleting drugs (eg, reserpine). Discontinue gradually before clonidine withdrawal. Avoid oral calcium channel blockers with cardiac dysfunction; may increase cardiac adverse effects.

**PREGNANCY:** Category C, caution in nursing.

## BETIMOL RX

timolol (Vistakon)

**THERAPEUTIC CLASS:** Nonselective beta-blocker

**INDICATIONS:** Treatment of elevated intraocular pressure in patients with open-angle glaucoma or ocular hypertension.

**DOSAGE:** *Adults:* Initial: 1 drop 0.25% bid. May increase to a max of 1 drop 0.5% bid. Maint: If adequate control, may attempt 1 drop 0.25-0.5% qd.

**HOW SUPPLIED:** Sol: 0.25%, 0.5% [5mL, 10mL, 15mL]

**CONTRAINDICATIONS:** Bronchial asthma, history of bronchial asthma, severe COPD, sinus bradycardia, 2nd- or 3rd-degree AV block, overt cardiac failure, cardiogenic shock.

**WARNINGS/PRECAUTIONS:** Caution with cardiac failure, DM, cerebrovascular insufficiency. Severe cardiac and respiratory reactions reported. May mask symptoms of hypoglycemia and hyperthyroidism. Bacterial keratitis reported with contaminated containers. May reinsert contacts 5 minutes after applying drops. Avoid with COPD, bronchospastic disease. Not for use alone in angle-closure glaucoma. May potentiate muscle weakness. D/C if cardiac failure develops. Withdrawal before surgery is controversial.

**ADVERSE REACTIONS:** Burning/stinging on instillation, dry eyes, itching, foreign body sensation, eye discomfort, eyelid erythema, conjunctival injection, headache.

**INTERACTIONS:** May potentiate systemic β-blockers and catecholamine-depleting drugs (eg, reserpine). Oral/IV calcium antagonists can cause AV conduction disturbances, left ventricular failure, or hypotension. Digitalis can cause additive effects in prolonging AV conduction time. May antagonize epinephrine.

**PREGNANCY:** Category C, not for use in nursing.

## BETOPTIC S RX

betaxolol HCl (Alcon)

**THERAPEUTIC CLASS:** Selective beta$_1$-blocker

**INDICATIONS:** Chronic open-angle glaucoma. Ocular hypertension.

**DOSAGE:** *Adults:* 1-2 drops bid.

**HOW SUPPLIED:** Sus: 0.25% [2.5mL, 5mL, 10mL, 15mL]

**CONTRAINDICATIONS:** Sinus bradycardia, greater than 1st-degree AV block, cardiogenic shock or overt cardiac failure.

**WARNINGS/PRECAUTIONS:** Caution with cardiac failure, heart block, DM, asthma. May mask hypoglycemic symptoms and signs of hyperthyroidism.

May potentiate muscle weakness. D/C before general anesthesia. Avoid abrupt withdrawal.

**ADVERSE REACTIONS:** Transient ocular discomfort, blurred vision, corneal punctate keratitis, foreign body sensation, tearing, photophobia, tearing, itching, dryness of eye, erythema, inflammation, discharge, ocular pain, decreased visual acuity, crusty lashes.

**INTERACTIONS:** May potentiate systemic β-blockers and catecholamine-depleting drugs (eg, reserpine). May be potentiated by systemic β-blockers. May antagonize adrenergic psychotropics. May increase risk of hypoglycemia with insulin or oral hypoglycemic drugs.

**PREGNANCY:** Category C, caution with nursing.

## BEXXAR RX

tositumomab - iodine I 131 tositumomab (GlaxoSmithKline)

**Hypersensitivity reactions, including anaphylaxis, and prolonged and severe cytopenias reported. Can cause fetal harm if given during pregnancy. Contains radioactive component.**

**THERAPEUTIC CLASS:** Monoclonal antibody/CD20-blocker

**INDICATIONS:** Treatment of CD20 positive, follicular, non-Hodgkin's lymphoma (NHL), with and without transformation, in patients refractory to rituximab and who have relapsed following chemotherapy.

**DOSAGE:** *Adults:* Premedication: Day 1: Begin thyro-protective regimen of either SSKI (4 drops po tid), Lugol's solution (20 drops po tid), or potassium iodide (130mg po qd). Continue until 14 days post-therapeutic dose. Day 0: APAP 650mg and diphenhydramine 50mg. Dosimetric Step: IV: 450mg tositumomab over 60 minutes followed by 5mCi Iodine I 131 tositumomab (35mg) over 20 minutes. Day 0 + Day 2, 3, or 4 + Day 6 or 7: Whole body dosimetry and biodistribution. Day 6 or 7: Calculation of patient-specific activity of iodine I 131 tositumomab to deliver 75cGy total body irradiation or 65cGy if platelets ≥100,000 but <150,000 platelets/mm$^3$. Day 7 (up to Day 14): Premedicate with APAP and diphenhydramine. Therapeutic Step: IV: Do not administer if biodistribution is altered. 450mg tositumomab over 60 minutes followed by prescribed therapeutic dose of iodine I 131 tositumomab (35mg) over 20 minutes.

**HOW SUPPLIED:** Inj: For Dosimetric Dosing: Tositumomab: 225mg [2 single-use vials], 35mg [1 single-use vial]; Iodine I 131 Tositumomab: 1 single-use vial. For Therapeutic Dosing: Tositumomab: 225mg [2 single-use vials], 35mg [1 single-use vial]; Iodine I 131 Tositumomab: 1 or 2 single-use vials.

**CONTRAINDICATIONS:** Pregnant women.

**WARNINGS/PRECAUTIONS:** Obtain CBCs weekly for 10-12 weeks. Safety not established with >25% lymphoma marrow involvement, platelet <100,000 cells/mm$^3$, or neutrophil count <1500 cells/mm$^3$. Secondary malignancies reported. May cause hypothyroidism; monitor TSH prior to initiation and then annually. Thyroid blocking agents must be used; initiate at least 24 hrs before dosimetric dose and continue until 14 days after therapeutic dose. Caution with impaired renal function. Effective contraceptive methods should be used during, and for 12 months following treatment. Increased risk of serious allergic reactions if positive for human anti-murine antibodies (HAMA).

**ADVERSE REACTIONS:** Neutropenia, thrombocytopenia, anemia, asthenia, fever, infection, cough, pain, chills, headache, GI effects, myalgia, arthralgia, pharyngitis, dyspnea, rash.

**INTERACTIONS:** Weigh risks vs benefits of concomitant agents that interfere with platelet function and/or anticoagulation.

**PREGNANCY:** Category X, not for use in nursing.

## BIAXIN
clarithromycin (Abbott)

RX

**THERAPEUTIC CLASS:** Macrolide antibiotic

**INDICATIONS:** Adults: Pharyngitis/tonsillitis, acute maxillary sinusitis, acute bacterial exacerbation of chronic bronchitis (ABECB), community aquired pneumonia (CAP), uncomplicated skin and skin structure infections (SSSI), disseminated mycobacterial infections, combination therapy for *H.pylori* infection with duodenal ulcers. MAC prophylaxis in advanced HIV. *Pediatrics:* Pharyngitis/tonsillitis, CAP, acute maxillary sinusitis, acute otitis media, uncomplicated SSSI, disseminated mycobacterial infections. MAC prophylaxis in advanced HIV.

**DOSAGE:** *Adults:* Pharyngitis/Tonsillitis: 250mg q12h for 10 days. Sinusitis: 500mg q12h for 14 days. ABECB: 250-500mg q12h for 7-14 days. SSSI/CAP: 250mg q12h for 7-14 days. MAC Prophylaxis/Treatment: 500mg bid. *H.pylori:* Triple Therapy: 500mg + amoxicillin 1g + omeprazole 20mg, all q12h for 10 days; or 500mg + amoxicillin 1g + lansoprazole 30mg, all q12h for 10-14 days. Give additional omeprazole 20mg qd for 18 days with active ulcer. Dual Therapy: 500mg q8h + omeprazole 40mg qd for 14 days (give additional omeprazole 20mg qd for 14 days with active ulcer); or 500mg q8h or q12h + ranitidine bismuth citrate 400mg q12h for 14 days (give additional ranitidine bismuth citrate 400mg bid for 14 days with active ulcer). Avoid Biaxin and ranitidine bismuth citrate combination with CrCl<25mL/min.
*Pediatrics:* >6 months: Usual: 7.5mg/kg q12h for 10 days. MAC Prophylaxis/Treatment: >20 months: 7.5mg/kg bid, up to 500mg bid. CrCl <30mL/min: Give 50% dose or double interval.

**HOW SUPPLIED:** Sus: 125mg/5mL, 250mg/5mL [50mL, 100mL]; Tab: 250mg, 500mg

**CONTRAINDICATIONS:** Concomitant cisapride, pimozide, terfenadine, or other macrolide antibiotics.

**WARNINGS/PRECAUTIONS:** Avoid in pregnancy. Pseudomembranous colitis reported. Adjust dose with severe renal impairment. Colchicine toxicity reported, avoid concomitant use especially in elderly.

**ADVERSE REACTIONS:** Diarrhea, nausea, abnormal taste, dyspepsia, abdominal pain, headache, vomiting, rash.

**INTERACTIONS:** Increases serum levels of theophylline, digoxin, HMG-CoA reductase inhibitors, omeprazole, carbamazepine, drugs metabolized by CYP450. Decreases zidovudine plasma levels. Potentiates oral anticoagulant effects. Acute ergot toxicity with ergotamine or dihydroergotamine reported. Decreased clearance of triazolam. Avoid astemizole. Avoid ranitidine, bismuth citrate if CrCl <25mL/min or history of porphyria. Reduce dose with ritonavir if CrCl <60mL/min. Increased levels with fluconazole. Caution with concomitant colchicine use.

**PREGNANCY:** Category C, caution in nursing.

## BIAXIN XL
clarithromycin (Abbott)

RX

**THERAPEUTIC CLASS:** Macrolide antibiotic

**INDICATIONS:** Treatment of acute maxillary sinusitis, community acquired pneumonia (CAP), and acute bacterial exacerbation of chronic bronchitis (ABECB).

**DOSAGE:** *Adults:* Sinusitis: 1000mg qd for 14 days. ABECB/CAP: 1000mg qd for 7 days. CrCl <30mL/min: Give 50% dose or double interval. Take with food.

**HOW SUPPLIED:** Tab, Extended Release: 500mg [PAC 14 tabs]

**CONTRAINDICATIONS:** Concomitant cisapride, pimozide, terfenadine, or other macrolide antibiotics.

**WARNINGS/PRECAUTIONS:** Avoid in pregnancy. Pseudomembranous colitis reported. Adjust dose with severe renal impairment. Colchicine toxicity reported, avoid concomitant use especially in the elderly.

**ADVERSE REACTIONS:** Diarrhea, nausea, abnormal taste, dyspepsia, abdominal pain, headache, vomiting, rash.

**INTERACTIONS:** Increases serum levels of theophylline, digoxin, HMG-CoA reductase inhibitors, omeprazole, carbamazepine and drugs metabolized by CYP450. Decreases zidovudine plasma levels. Potentiates oral anticoagulant effects. Acute ergot toxicity with ergotamine or dihydroergotamine reported. Decreased clearance of triazolam. Avoid astemizole. Avoid ranitidine bismuth citrate if CrCl <25mL/min or history of porphyria. Reduce dose with ritonavir if CrCl <60mL/min. Increased levels with fluconazole. Caution with concomitant colchicine use.

**PREGNANCY:** Category C, caution in nursing.

## BICILLIN C-R — RX

penicillin G procaine - penicillin G benzathine (King)

**THERAPEUTIC CLASS:** Penicillin

**INDICATIONS:** Treatment of moderately severe to severe upper-respiratory tract (URTI) and skin and soft-tissue infections (SSTI), scarlet fever and erysipelas due to streptococci. Treatment of moderately severe pneumonia and otitis media due to pneumococci.

**DOSAGE:** *Adults:* Group A Strep: URTI/SSTI/Scarlet Fever/Erysipelas: 2.4MU IM. Treat at a single session using multiple IM sites, or use an alternative schedule and give 1/2 of the total dose on Day 1 and 1/2 on Day 3. Pneumococcal Infections (Except Meningitis): 1.2MU IM, repeat every 2-3 days until temperature is normal for 48 hrs. Administer IM into upper, outer quadrant of buttock.

*Pediatrics:* Group A Strep: URTI/SSTI/Scarlet Fever/Erysipelas: >60 lbs: 2.4MU IM. 30-60 lbs: 900,000U-1.2MU IM. <30 lbs: 600,000U IM. Treat at a single session using multiple IM sites, or use an alternative schedule and give 1/2 of the total dose on Day 1 and 1/2 on Day 3. Pneumococcal Infections (Except Meningitis): 600,000U IM, repeat every 2-3 days until temperature is normal for 48 hrs. Administer IM into upper, outer quadrant of buttock. Use the midlateral aspect of thigh in neonates, infants, and small children.

**HOW SUPPLIED:** Inj: (Penicillin G Benzathine-Penicillin G Procaine) 300,000-300,000U/mL

**CONTRAINDICATIONS:** Do not inject into or near an artery or nerve.

**WARNINGS/PRECAUTIONS:** Serious, fatal anaphylactic reactions reported; increased risk with hypersensitivity to penicillin, cephalosporins, and other allergens. Pseudomembranous colitis reported. Avoid IV, intra-arterial administration, or injection into/near major peripheral nerves or blood vessels may cause severe neurovascular and neurological damage. IM administration into anterolateral thigh may cause quadriceps femoris fibrosis and atrophy. Caution with asthma. Avoid with procaine sensitivity. May result in overgrowth of nonsusceptible organisms. Monitor culture after therapy completion to determine eradication. Monitor renal and hematopoietic systems periodically with prolonged and high-dose therapy.

**ADVERSE REACTIONS:** Maculopapular/exfoliative dermatitis, urticaria, laryngeal edema, fever, pseudomembranous colitis, hemolytic anemia, leukopenia, thrombocytopenia, neuropathy, nephropathy.

**INTERACTIONS:** Increased and prolonged levels with probenecid. Tetracycline may antagonize bacterial effect; avoid concomitant use.

**PREGNANCY:** Category B, caution in nursing.

## BICILLIN C-R 900/300

RX

penicillin G procaine - penicillin G benzathine (King)



**THERAPEUTIC CLASS:** Penicillin

**INDICATIONS:** Treatment of moderately severe to severe upper-respiratory tract (URTI) and skin and soft-tissue infections (SSTI), scarlet fever and erysipelas due to streptococci. Treatment of moderately severe pneumonia and otitis media due to pneumococci.

**DOSAGE:** *Pediatrics:* Group A Strep: URTI/SSTI/Scarlet Fever/Erysipelas: 1.2MU IM single dose. Pneumococcal Infections (Except Meningitis): 1.2MU IM every 2-3 days until temperature is normal for 48 hrs. Administer IM into upper, outer quadrant of buttock. Use midlateral aspect of thigh in neonates, infants, and small children.

**HOW SUPPLIED:** Inj: (Penicillin G Benzathine-Penicillin G Procaine) 900,000-300,000U/2mL

**CONTRAINDICATIONS:** Do not inject into or near an artery or nerve.

**WARNINGS/PRECAUTIONS:** Serious, fatal anaphylactic reactions reported; increased risk with hypersensitivity to penicillin, cephalosporins, and other allergens. Pseudomembranous colitis reported. Avoid IV, intra-arterial administration, or injection into/near major peripheral nerves or blood vessels may cause severe neurovascular and neurological damage. IM administration into anterolateral thigh may cause quadriceps femoris fibrosis and atrophy. Caution with asthma. Avoid with procaine sensitivity. May result in overgrowth of nonsusceptible organisms. Monitor culture after therapy completion to determine eradication. Monitor renal and hematopoietic systems periodically with prolonged and high-dose therapy.

**ADVERSE REACTIONS:** Maculopapular/exfoliative dermatitis, urticaria, laryngeal edema, fever, pseudomembranous colitis, hemolytic anemia, leukopenia, thrombocytopenia, neuropathy, nephropathy.

**INTERACTIONS:** Increased and prolonged levels with probenecid. Tetracycline may antagonize bactericidal effect.

**PREGNANCY:** Category B, caution in nursing.

## BICILLIN L-A

RX

penicillin G benzathine (King)

**THERAPEUTIC CLASS:** Penicillin

**INDICATIONS:** Treatment of mild to moderate upper respiratory tract infections (URTI) due to streptococci and venereal infections (eg, syphilis, yaws, bejel, pinta). Prophylaxis to prevent recurrence of rheumatic fever or chorea.

**DOSAGE:** *Adults:* Group A Strep: URTI: 1.2MU IM single dose. Primary/Secondary/Latent Syphilis: 2.4MU IM single dose. Late Syphilis (Tertiary/Neurosyphilis): 2.4MU IM every 7 days for 3 doses. Yaws/Bejel/Pinta: 1.2MU IM single dose. Rheumatic Fever/Glomerulonephritis Prophylaxis: 1.2MU IM once a month or 600,000U IM every 2 weeks. Administer IM into upper, outer quadrant of buttock.
*Pediatrics:* Group A Strep: URTI: Older Pediatrics: 900,000U IM single dose. <60 lbs: 300,000-600,000U IM single dose. Congenital Syphilis: 2-12 yrs: Adjust dose based on adult schedule. <2 yrs: 50,000U/kg IM single dose. Rheumatic Fever/Glomerulonephritis Prophylaxis: 1.2MU IM once a month or 600,000U every 2 weeks. Administer IM into upper, outer quadrant of buttock. Use the midlateral aspect of thigh in neonates, infants, and small children.

**HOW SUPPLIED:** Inj: 600,000U/mL

**CONTRAINDICATIONS:** Do not inject into or near an artery or nerve.

**WARNINGS/PRECAUTIONS:** Serious, fatal anaphylactic reactions reported; increased risk with hypersensitivity to penicillin, cephalosporins, and other allergens. Pseudomembranous colitis reported. Avoid IV, intra-arterial administration, or injection into/near major peripheral nerves or blood vessels may cause severe neurovascular and neurological damage. IM administration into anterolateral thigh may cause quadriceps femoris fibrosis and atrophy. Caution with asthma. May result in overgrowth of nonsusceptible organisms. Monitor culture after therapy completion to determine eradication.

**ADVERSE REACTIONS:** Maculopapular/exfoliative dermatitis, urticaria, laryngeal edema, fever, pseudomembranous colitis, hemolytic anemia, leukopenia, thrombocytopenia, neuropathy, nephropathy.

**INTERACTIONS:** Increased and prolonged levels with probenecid. Tetracycline may antagonize bactericidal effect.

**PREGNANCY:** Category B, caution in nursing.

## BiCNU

RX

carmustine (Bristol-Myers Squibb)

**Bone marrow suppression, thrombocytopenia, leukopenia reported. Monitor blood counts weekly for at least 6 weeks after dose. Base dose adjustments on nadir blood counts from prior dose. Pulmonary toxicity may be dose related ( >1400 mg/m$^2$ at greater risk) and can occur years after treatment.**

**THERAPEUTIC CLASS:** Nitrosourea alkylating agent

**INDICATIONS:** Palliative therapy as single or adjunct agent for treatment of brain tumors, multiple myeloma, Hodgkin's disease, and non-Hodgkin's lymphomas.

**DOSAGE:** *Adults:* Single Agent in Untreated Patients: 150-200mg/m$^2$ IV every 6 weeks, as a single dose or divide into daily injections (75-100mg/m$^2$ for 2 days). Adjust subsequent doses according to hematologic response. If leukocytes 2000-2999 and platelets 25,000-74,999, give 70% of dose. If leukocytes <2000 and platelets <25,000, then give 50% of dose.

**HOW SUPPLIED:** Inj: 100mg

**WARNINGS/PRECAUTIONS:** Long-term use may be associated with secondary malignancies. Monitor hepatic/renal function. Conduct baseline and periodic pulmonary function tests during treatment. Caution in elderly; monitor renal function.

**ADVERSE REACTIONS:** Delayed myelosuppression, pulmonary infiltrates/fibrosis, nausea, vomiting, hepatic toxicity, azotemia, renal failure, neuroretinitis, chest pain, headache, allergic reaction, hypotension, tachycardia.

**PREGNANCY:** Category D, not for use in nursing.

## BiDil

RX

hydralazine HCl - isosorbide dinitrate (NitroMed)

**THERAPEUTIC CLASS:** Vasodilator combination

**INDICATIONS:** Treatment of heart failure as an adjunct to standard therapy in self-identified black patients to improve survival, prolong time to hospitalization for heart failure, and improve patient-reported functional status.

**DOSAGE:** *Adults:* Initial: 1 tab tid. Max: 2 tabs tid.

**HOW SUPPLIED:** Tab: (Hydralazine-Isosorbide) 37.5mg-20mg

**CONTRAINDICATIONS:** Allergies to organic nitrates.

**WARNINGS/PRECAUTIONS:** May produce a clinical picture simulating systemic lupus erythematosus including glomerulonephritis. May cause symptomatic hypotension, tachycardia, peripheral neuritis. Caution in patients with acute MI, hemodynamic and clinical monitoring recommended. May aggravate angina associated with hypertrophic cardiomyopathy.

**ADVERSE REACTIONS:** Headache, dizziness, chest pain, asthenia, nausea, bronchitis, hypotension, sinusitis, ventricular tachycardia, palpitations, hyperglycemia, rhinitis, paresthesia, vomiting, amblyopia, hyperlipidemia.

**INTERACTIONS:** Increased vasodilatory effects with phosphodiesterase inhibitors (sildenafil, vardenafil, tadalafil). Increased risk of hypotension with potent parenteral antihypertensive agents. Caution with MAOIs.

**PREGNANCY:** Category C, caution in nursing.

## BILTRICIDE

praziquantel (Schering) RX

**THERAPEUTIC CLASS:** Trematodicide

**INDICATIONS:** Treatment of infections due to all species of schistosoma and due to liver flukes.

**DOSAGE:** *Adults:* Schistosomiasis: 3x 20mg/kg for 1 day. Clonorchiasis/Opisthorchiasis: 3x 25mg/kg for 1 day. Take with fluids during meals; do not chew. Dosage interval should not be <4 hrs or >6 hrs. *Pediatrics:* >4 yrs: Schistosomiasis: 3 X 20mg/kg for 1 day. Clonorchiasis/Opisthorchiasis: 3 X 25mg/kg for 1 day. Take with fluids during meals; do not chew. Dosage interval should not be <4 hrs or >6 hrs.

**HOW SUPPLIED:** Tab: 600mg [6$^{s}$]

**CONTRAINDICATIONS:** Ocular cysticercosis.

**WARNINGS/PRECAUTIONS:** Avoid driving or operating machinery until one day after treatment. Minimal increases in liver enzymes reported. Hospitalize if schistosomiasis or fluke infection is associated with cerebral cysticercosis.

**ADVERSE REACTIONS:** Malaise, headache, dizziness, abdominal discomfort, nausea.

**PREGNANCY:** Category B, not for use in nursing.

## BIOLON

sodium hyaluronate (Akorn) RX

**THERAPEUTIC CLASS:** Surgical aid

**INDICATIONS:** Surgical aid to protect corneal endothelium during cataract extraction (extra-capsular) procedures, intraocular lens (IOL) implantation, and anterior segment surgery.

**DOSAGE:** *Adults:* Cataract Surgery/IOL Implantation: Introduce 0.2-0.5mL slowly into anterior chamber by using cannula. Inject before or after delivery of the lens. May use to coat lens and surgical instruments prior to lens insertion. Can inject during surgery to replace any of the drug lost during surgery.

**HOW SUPPLIED:** Inj: 1% [0.5mL, 1mL]

**WARNINGS/PRECAUTIONS:** Precipitate will form with quaternary ammonium salts (eg, benzalkonium chloride). Use only with single-use cannula provided in package. Do not use excessive quantity. Remove all solution by irrigation or aspiration at end of surgery. Administer appropriate therapy if post-op IOP significantly rises. Cannulas are for single patient use only. Remove any cloudy or precipitated material by irrigation or aspiration. Injection of biological substances carry immunological, allergic, and other potential risks. Avoid trapping eye bubbles behind the agent.

**ADVERSE REACTIONS:** Increased IOP, superficial/conjunctival punctate keratitis, cystoid macular edema, posterior capsule opacity.

**INTERACTIONS:** Do not irrigate with solution containing quaternary ammonium salts (eg, benzalkonium chloride); precipitate will form.

**PREGNANCY:** Safety in pregnancy or nursing not known.

B

## BION TEARS OTC
dextran 70 - hydroxypropyl methylcellulose (Alcon)

**THERAPEUTIC CLASS:** Lubricant

**INDICATIONS:** Use as a protectant against further irritation or to relieve dryness of the eye.

**DOSAGE:** *Adults:* 1-2 drops in affected eye prn.

**HOW SUPPLIED:** Sol: (Dextran 70-Hydroxypropyl Methylcellulose) 0.1%-0.3% [0.45mL 28$^{s}$, 12mL]

**WARNINGS/PRECAUTIONS:** Do not touch container tip to any surface to avoid contamination. D/C if eye pain or vision changes occur, if redness or irritation continues, or if condition worsens or persists >72 hrs. Do not reuse once opened; discard.

**PREGNANCY:** Safety in pregnancy or nursing not known.

## BIOTHRAX RX
anthrax vaccine adsorbed (Bioport)

**THERAPEUTIC CLASS:** Vaccine

**INDICATIONS:** Active immunization against Bacillus anthracis in individuals who come in contact with animal products (eg, hides, hairs, bones) that come from anthrax endemic areas and that may be contaminated with spores. Also for individuals at high risk of exposure to these spores (eg, veterinarians, laboratory workers).

**DOSAGE:** *Adults:* 18-65 yrs: 0.5mL SQ for 3 doses given 2 weeks apart, followed by 3 additional doses of 0.5mL given at 6, 12, 18 months. Booster injections of 0.5mL recommended at 1-year intervals.

**HOW SUPPLIED:** Inj: 5mL

**WARNINGS/PRECAUTIONS:** May cause birth defects if given during pregnancy. Review history for vaccine sensitivities. Avoid with history of Guillain-Barre syndrome. Increased risk of local adverse reaction with history of anthrax disease. Possible inadequate immunization with impaired immune responsiveness (eg, congenital/acquired immunodeficiency). Postpone vaccination with moderate to severe illness. Caution with latex sensitivity.

**ADVERSE REACTIONS:** (Local) tenderness, erythema, SQ nodule, induration, warmth, pruritus, arm motion limitation. (Systemic) headache, respiratory difficulty, fever, malaise, myalgia, fever, anorexia, nausea, vomiting.

**INTERACTIONS:** Possible inadequate immunization with immunosuppressives. Chemotherapy, high-dose corticosteroid therapy >2 week duration, or radiation therapy may cause suboptimal vaccine response; defer vaccination until 3 months after completion of therapy.

**PREGNANCY:** Category D, safety in nursing not known.

## BLENOXANE RX
bleomycin sulfate (Bristol-Myers Squibb)

**Pulmonary fibrosis is the most severe toxicity reported (usually presents as pneumonitis occasionally progressing to pulmonary fibrosis); higher occurrence in elderly and if receiving >400 units total dose. A severe idiosyncratic reaction including hypotension, mental confusion, fever, chills, and wheezing reported in lymphoma patients.**

**THERAPEUTIC CLASS:** Cytotoxic glycopeptide antibiotic

**INDICATIONS:** Palliative treatment of squamous cell carcinoma (eg, head and neck, penis, cervix, vulva), Hodgkin's Disease, non-Hodgkin's lymphoma, testicular carcinoma (embryonal cell, choriocarcinoma, teratocarcinoma). As a sclerosing agent for treatment of malignant pleural effusion and prevention of recurrent pleural effusions.

**DOSAGE:** *Adults:* Squamous Cell Carcinoma/Non-Hodgkin's Lymphoma/Testicular Carcinoma: 0.25-0.5U/kg IV/IM/SQ weekly or twice weekly. For lymphoma patients, give <2U for the 1st two doses; continue with regular dosage schedule if no acute reaction occurs. Hodgkin's Disease: 0.25-0.5U/kg IV/IM/SQ weekly or twice weekly. Maint: After 50% response, give 1U/day or 5U weekly IV/IM. Malignant Pleural Effusion: 60U as a single dose bolus intrapleural injection.

**HOW SUPPLIED:** Inj: 15U, 30U

**WARNINGS/PRECAUTIONS:** Extreme caution with significant renal impairment or compromised pulmonary function. Pulmonary toxicity (dose and age related) may occur; frequent roentgenograms are recommended. Monitor for severe idiosyncratic reactions, especially after 1st and 2nd doses. Renal and hepatic toxicity reported. Can cause fetal harm during pregnancy. Risk of pulmonary toxicity with total dose >400U. Caution with dose selection in elderly.

**ADVERSE REACTIONS:** Pneumonitis, erythema, rash, striae, vesiculation, hyperpigmentation, skin tenderness, hyperkeratosis, nail changes, alopecia, pruritus, stomatitis, pulmonary toxicity.

**INTERACTIONS:** In combination with other antineoplastics, pulmonary toxicities may occur at lower doses.

**PREGNANCY:** Category D, not for use in nursing.

## BLEPH-10

sulfacetamide sodium (Allergan) RX

**OTHER BRAND NAMES:** AK-Sulf (Akorn)

**THERAPEUTIC CLASS:** Sulfonamide

**INDICATIONS:** (Oint, Sol) Treatment of conjunctivitis and other superficial ocular infections. (Sol) Adjunct to systemic sulfonamide therapy of trachoma.

**DOSAGE:** *Adults:* Conjunctivitis/Superficial Infections: (Sol) 1-2 drops q2-3h initially. (Oint) Apply 1/2 inch q3-4h and hs. Taper dose by decreasing frequency with improvement. Treat for 7-10 days. Trachoma: (Sol) 2 drops q2h with systemic therapy.
*Pediatrics:* >2 months: Conjunctivitis/Superficial Infections: (Sol) 1-2 drops q2-3h initially. (Oint) Apply 1/2 inch q3-4h and hs. Taper dose by decreasing frequency with improvement. Treat for 7-10 days. Trachoma: (Sol) 2 drops q2h with systemic therapy.

**HOW SUPPLIED:** Oint: (AK-Sulf) 10% [3.5g]; Sol: (Bleph-10) 10% [5mL, 15mL]

**WARNINGS/PRECAUTIONS:** Fatalities reported from severe reactions to sulfonamides. D/C if develop sign of hypersensitivity. Ointments may retard corneal wound healing.

**ADVERSE REACTIONS:** Local irritation, stinging, burning.

**INTERACTIONS:** Incompatible with silver preparations.

**PREGNANCY:** Category C, not for use in nursing.

## BLEPHAMIDE

prednisolone acetate - sulfacetamide sodium (Allergan) RX

**OTHER BRAND NAMES:** Blephamide S.O.P. (Allergan)

**THERAPEUTIC CLASS:** Sulfonamide/corticosteroid

**INDICATIONS:** For steroid-responsive inflammatory ocular conditions associated with bacterial infection or risks of bacterial infection (eg, corneal injury).

**DOSAGE:** *Adults:* (Sus) 2 drops into conjunctival sac q4h and qhs. (Oint) Apply 1/2 inch into conjunctival sac tid-qid and qd-bid at night. Re-evaluate if no improvement after 2 days. Decrease dose as condition improves. Max: 20mL or 8g prescribed initially.
*Pediatrics:* >6 yrs: (Sus) 2 drops into conjunctival sac q4h and qhs. (Oint) Apply 1/2 inch into conjunctival sac tid-qid and qd-bid at night. Re-evaluate if no improvement after 2 days. Decrease dose as condition improves. Max: 20mL or 8g prescribed initially.

**HOW SUPPLIED:** (Sulfacetamide-Prednisolone) Oint: 10%-0.2% [3.5g]; Sus: 10%-0.2% [5mL, 10mL]

**CONTRAINDICATIONS:** Most viral diseases of the cornea and conjunctiva (eg, epithelial herpes simplex keratitis, vaccinia, and varicella), mycobacterial infection of the eye, fungal diseases of ocular structures.

**WARNINGS/PRECAUTIONS:** Not for injection. Ocular HTN, glaucoma, secondary infections may occur with prolonged use. Acute anterior uveitis may occur. May mask or enhance infection with acute purulent conditions. Caution with glaucoma, treatment of herpes simplex. Monitor IOP. Staphylococcal isolates may be resistant to sulfonamides. Not effective in mustard gas keratitis and Sjogren's keratoconjunctivitis. Sensitization may recur with sulfonamides. May delay healing after cataract surgery. Fatalities reported due to adverse effects.

**ADVERSE REACTIONS:** Local irritation, intraocular pressure elevation, acute anterior uveitis, mydriasis, allergic sensitization (Stevens-Johnson syndrome, toxic epidermal necrolysis, fulminant hepatic necrosis, etc.).

**INTERACTIONS:** Incompatible with silver preparations. Local anesthetics related to p-amino benzoic acid may antagonize sulfonamides.

**PREGNANCY:** Category C, not for use in nursing.

## BONIVA RX

ibandronate sodium (Roche)

**THERAPEUTIC CLASS:** Bisphosphonate

**INDICATIONS:** Treatment and prevention of postmenopausal osteoporosis.

**DOSAGE:** *Adults:* 2.5mg qd or 150mg once monthly. Swallow whole with 6-8 oz. of water. Do not lie down for 60 minutes after dose. Take at least 60 minutes before first food, drink (other than water), medication, or supplementation.

**HOW SUPPLIED:** Tab: 2.5mg, 150mg

**CONTRAINDICATIONS:** Hypocalcemia; inability to stand or sit upright for at least 60 minutes.

**WARNINGS/PRECAUTIONS:** May cause upper GI disorders (eg, dysphagia, esophagitis, esophageal or gastric ulcer). Not recommended in severe renal impairment (CrCl <30mL/min). Reports of osteonecrosis, primarily in the jaw, and severe, incapacitating bone, joint, and/or muscle pain

**ADVERSE REACTIONS:** HTN, dyspepsia, nausea, back pain, arthalgia, abdominal pain, diarrhea, constipation, influenza, nasopharyngitis, headache, bronchitis.

**INTERACTIONS:** Calcium and other multivalent cations may interfere with absorption.

**PREGNANCY:** Category C, caution in nursing.

## BONTRIL SLOW-RELEASE CIII

phendimetrazine tartrate (Valeant)

**OTHER BRAND NAMES:** Bontril PDM (Valeant)

**THERAPEUTIC CLASS:** Anorectic sympathomimetic amine

**INDICATIONS:** Short term adjunct treatment of exogenous obesity.

**DOSAGE:** *Adults:* (Slow-Release) 105mg qam, 30-60 minutes before breakfast. (PDM) 35mg bid-tid, 1 hr before meals; may reduce to 17.5mg/dose. Max: 70mg tid.

*Pediatrics:* >12 yrs: (Slow-Release) 105mg qam, 30-60 minutes before breakfast. (PDM) 35mg bid-tid, 1 hr before meals; may reduce to 17.5mg/dose. Max: 70mg tabs tid.

**HOW SUPPLIED:** Cap, Extended Release: (Slow-Release) 105mg; Tab: (PDM) 35mg* *scored

**CONTRAINDICATIONS:** Advanced arteriosclerosis, symptomatic cardiovascular disease, moderate and severe HTN, hyperthyroidism, glaucoma, agitated states, history of drug abuse, concomitant CNS stimulants including MAOIs.

**WARNINGS/PRECAUTIONS:** Tolerance to anorectic effect develops within a few weeks, d/c if this occurs. Fatigue and depression with abrupt withdrawal after prolonged high dose therapy. Caution with mild HTN.

**ADVERSE REACTIONS:** Palpitation, tachycardia, BP elevation, overstimulation, restlessness, dizziness, dry mouth, diarrhea, constipation, nausea, libido changes, dysuria, insomnia.

**INTERACTIONS:** Hypertensive crisis if used within 14 days of MAOIs. May decrease hypotensive effects of guanethidine. May alter insulin requirements.

**PREGNANCY:** Not for use in pregnancy, safety in nursing not known.

## BOOSTRIX RX

tetanus toxoid - diphtheria toxoid - pertussis vaccine, acellular (GlaxoSmithKline)

**THERAPEUTIC CLASS:** Vaccine/toxoid combination

**INDICATIONS:** Active booster immunization against tetanus, diphtheria, and pertussis as a single dose in individuals 10-18 yrs of age.

**DOSAGE:** *Pediatrics:* 10-18 yrs: 0.5mL IM into the deltoid muscle.

**HOW SUPPLIED:** Inj: (Tetanus-Diphtheria-Pertussis) 5LF-2.5LF-8mcg/0.5mL.

**CONTRAINDICATIONS:** Hypersensitivity to any component; serious allergic reaction (eg, anaphylaxis) associated with previous dose. Encephalopathy not due to an identifiable cause within 7 days prior to pertussis immunization and progressive neurologic disorder, uncontrolled epilepsy, or progressive encephalopathy.

**WARNINGS/PRECAUTIONS:** May cause allergic reactions in latex sensitive patients. Caution if within 48 hrs of fever ≥105°F not due to another identifiable cause; collapse or shock-like state; persistent, inconsolable crying lasting ≥3 hrs. Caution if within 3 days of seizure with or without fever. Do not administer in patients with bleeding disorders such as hemophilia or thrombocytopenia, or patients on anticoagulant therapy unless potential benefit outweighs risk. Caution if Guillian Barre syndrome within 6 weeks of tetanus toxoid vaccine. Do not give Td, Tdap, or emergency dose of Td more frequently then every 10 yrs if patient has experienced Arthus-type reaction. Hypersensitivity reaction possible; epinephrine injection (1:1000) should be readily available.

**ADVERSE REACTIONS:** Local: pain, redness, swelling. Systemic: headache, fatigue, fever, nausea, vomiting, diarrhea, abdominal pain.

**INTERACTIONS:** Immunosuppressive therapies, including irradiation, antimetabolites, alkylating agents, cytotoxic drugs, and corticosteroids may reduce the immune response to vaccines.

**PREGNANCY:** Category C, caution in nursing.

## BOTOX RX

botulinum toxin type A (Allergan)

**THERAPEUTIC CLASS:** Purified neurotoxin complex

**INDICATIONS:** Treatment of strabismus and blepharospasm associated with dystonia, including benign essential blepharospasm or VII nerve disorders. Treatment of cervical dystonia to decrease severity of abnormal head position and neck pain. Treatment of severe primary axillary hyperhidrosis that is inadequately managed with topical agents

**DOSAGE:** *Adults:* Cervical Dystonia: Average Dose: 236U divided among affected muscles. Adjust to individual response. Max: 100U total dose in sternocleidomastoid muscles. Strabismus: Initial: Vertical Muscle and Horizontal Strabismus <20 Prism Diopters: 1.25-2.5U in any muscle. Horizontal Strabismus of 20-50 Prism Diopters: 2.5-5U in any one muscle. Persistent VI Nerve Palsy >1 Month: 1.25-2.5U into medial rectus muscle. Increase dose by 2-fold if previous dose results in incomplete paralysis. Max: 25U/muscle. Reassess 7-14 after each injection. Blepharospasm: Initial: 1.25-2.5U into medial and lateral pre-tarsal orbicularis oculi of the upper lid and into lateral pre-tarsal orbicularis oculi of the lower lid. Max: 200U/30 day. Primary Axillary Hyperhidrosis: 50 units per axilla.
*Pediatrics:* >16 yrs: Cervical Dystonia: 236U divided among affected muscles. Adjust dose to individual response. Max: 100U in sternocleidomastoid muscles. >12 yrs: Strabismus: Initial: Vertical Muscle and Horizontal Strabismus <20 Prism Diopters: 1.25-2.5U in any muscle. Horizontal Strabismus of 20-50 Prism Diopters: 2.5-5U in any one muscle. Persistent VI Nerve Palsy >1 Month: 1.25-2.5U into medial rectus muscle. Increase dose by 2-fold if previous dose results in incomplete paralysis. Max: 25U/muscle. Reassess 7-14 after each injection. Blepharospasm: Initial: 1.25-2.5U into medial and lateral pre-tarsal orbicularis oculi of the upper lid and into lateral pre-tarsal orbicularis oculi of the lower lid. Max: 200U/30 day.

**HOW SUPPLIED:** Inj: 100U

**WARNINGS/PRECAUTIONS:** Do not exceed dosing recommendations. Caution with peripheral motor neuropathic diseases (eg, amyotrophic lateral sclerosis, motor neuropathy), neuromuscular junctional disorders (eg, myasthenia gravis, Lambert-Eaton syndrome); increased risk of dysphagia and respiratory compromise. Contains albumin. Have epinephrine available if anaphylactic reaction occurs. Caution with inflammation at injection sites, excessive weakness or atrophy in target muscles. Injection of orbicularis muscle may reduce blinking. Caution to resume activities gradually. Retrobulbular hemorrhages compromising retinal circulation reported; have instruments to decompress orbit accessible. Increased risk of dysphagia in patients with smaller neck muscle mass and those with bilateral injections into sternocleidomastoid muscle; limit dose. Caution in elderly.

**ADVERSE REACTIONS:** (Cervical Dystonia) dysphagia, upper respiratory infection, neck pain, headache, (Blepharospasm) ptosis, keratitis, eye dryness, (Strabismus) ptosis, vertical deviation.

**INTERACTIONS:** May be potentiated with aminoglycosides, agents interfering with neuromuscular transmission (eg, curare-like compounds). Excessive neuromuscular weakness may be exacerbated if administer another botulinum toxin before effects resolve from the previous botulinum toxin injection.

**PREGNANCY:** Category C, caution in nursing.

## BOTOX COSMETIC

botulinum toxin type A (Allergan) RX

**THERAPEUTIC CLASS:** Purified neurotoxin complex

**INDICATIONS:** For temporary improvement in appearance of moderate to severe glabellar lines associated with corrugator or procerus muscle activity.

**DOSAGE:** *Adults:* <65 yrs: 0.1mL IM into each of 5 sites, 2 in each corrugator muscle and 1 in the procerus muscle for a total dose of 20 U. Intervals should be no more than every three months. Reconstitute with 2.5mL of 0.9% saline; store in refrigerator and use within 4 hrs.

**HOW SUPPLIED:** Inj: 100 U

**CONTRAINDICATIONS:** Infection at proposed injection sites.

**WARNINGS/PRECAUTIONS:** Do not exceed dosing recommendations. Caution with peripheral motor neuropathic diseases (eg, amyotrophic lateral sclerosis, motor neuropathy), neuromuscular junctional disorders (eg, myasthenia gravis, Lambert-Eaton syndrome); increased risk of dysphagia and respiratory compromise. Contains albumin. Have epinephrine available if anaphylactic reaction occurs. Caution with inflammation at injection sites, excessive weakness or atrophy in target muscles. Injection of orbicularis muscle may reduce blinking. Carefully test corneal sensation in eyes previously operated upon, avoid injection into lower lid area to avoid ectropion, and vigorously treat any epithelial defect. Inducing paralysis in extraocular muscles may produce spatial disorientation, double vision or past pointing; covering affected eye may alleviate symptoms. Caution with marked facial asymmetry, ptosis, excessive dermatochalasis, deep dermal scarring, thick sebaceous skin, or inability to substantially lessen glabellar lines by physically spreading them apart.

**ADVERSE REACTIONS:** Headache, respiratory infection, flu-syndrome, blepharoptosis, nausea.

**INTERACTIONS:** May be potentiated with aminoglycosides, agents interfering with neuromuscular transmission (eg, curare-like nondepolarizing blockers, lincosamides, polymyxins, quinidine, magnesium sulfate, anticholinesterases, succinylcholine chloride). Excessive neuromuscular weakness may be exacerbated if administer another botulinum toxin before effects resolve from the previous botulinum toxin injection.

**PREGNANCY:** Category C, caution in nursing.

## BRAVELLE

urofollitropin (Ferring) RX

**THERAPEUTIC CLASS:** Follicle stimulating hormone

**INDICATIONS:** With hCG, to induce ovulation in patients who previously received pituitary suppression. With hCG, for multiple follicular development (controlled ovarian stimulation) during assisted reproductive technologies (ART) cycles in patients who previously received pituitary suppression.

**DOSAGE:** *Adults:* Ovulation Induction: Initial: 150 IU SQ/IM qd for 1st 5 days. Adjust subsequent dose to individual response at intervals no less than every 2 days and not exceeding 75-150 IU/adjustment. Max: 450 IU/day. Dosing >12 days is not recommended. If adequate response, give 5000-10,000 U hCG 1 day following last dose. May repeat course if inadequate follicle development or ovulation without pregnancy occurs. ART: 225 IU SQ qd for 1st 5 days. Adjust subsequent dose to individual response at intervals no less than every 2 days and not exceeding 75-150 IU/adjustment. Max: 450 IU/day. Dosing >12 days is not recommended. If adequate follicular development, give 5000-10,000 U hCG to induce final follicular maturation in preparation for oocyte retrieval.

**HOW SUPPLIED:** Inj: 75 IU

B

**CONTRAINDICATIONS:** High FSH levels indicating primary ovarian failure, uncontrolled thyroid or adrenal dysfunction, organic intracranial lesions (eg, pituitary tumor), any cause of infertility other than anovulation, abnormal bleeding of undetermined origin, ovarian cysts or enlargement not due to polycystic ovary syndrome, pregnancy.

**WARNINGS/PRECAUTIONS:** Exclude primary ovarian failure. Ovarian enlargement may occur; monitor ovarian response. Ovarian hyperstimulation syndrome (OHSS), multiple births, hypersensitivity/anaphylactic reactions, serious pulmonary and vascular complications reported. Avoid hCG if ovaries are abnormally enlarged on last day of therapy. Monitor follicle growth and maturation with estradiol levels and ultrasonography.

**ADVERSE REACTIONS:** OHSS, vaginal hemorrhage, pelvic pain, nausea, headache, pain, UTI, respiratory disorder, hot flashes, abdominal enlargement or pain.

**PREGNANCY:** Category X, not for use in nursing.

## BREVIBLOC RX

esmolol HCl (Baxter)

**THERAPEUTIC CLASS:** Selective $beta_1$-blocker

**INDICATIONS:** For rapid control of ventricular rate in atrial fibrillation or atrial flutter in perioperative, postoperative, or other emergent circumstances. For noncompensatory sinus tachycardia. Treatment of tachycardia and hypertension that occur during induction and tracheal intubation, during surgery, on emergence from anesthesia, and in the postoperative period.

**DOSAGE:** *Adults:* Supraventricular Tachycardia: Titrate dose based on ventricular rate. Load: 0.5mg/kg over 1 min. Maint: 0.05mg/kg/min for next 4 min. May increase by 0.05mg/kg/min at intervals of 4 min or more up to 0.2mg/kg/min. Rapid slowing of ventricular response: Repeat 0.5mg/kg load over 1 min, then 0.1mg/kg/min for 4 min. If needed, another (final) load of 0.5mg/kg over 1 min, then 0.15mg/kg/min for 4 min up to 0.2mg/kg/min. May continue infusions for 24-48hrs. Intraoperative/Postoperative Tachycardia and/or HTN: Immediate Control: Initial: 80mg bolus over 30 sec. Maint: 0.15mg/kg/min. May titrate up to 0.3mg/kg/min. Gradual Control: Initial: 0.5mg/kg over 1 min. Maint: 0.05mg/kg/min for 4 min. Then, if needed, may repeat load and increase to 0.1mg/kg/min.

**HOW SUPPLIED:** Inj: 10mg/mL [10mL, 250mL], 20mg/mL [5mL, 100mL], 250mg/mL [10mL]

**CONTRAINDICATIONS:** Sinus bradycardia, heart block greater than first degree, cardiogenic shock or overt heart failure.

**WARNINGS/PRECAUTIONS:** Hypotension may occur; monitor BP and reduce dose or d/c if needed. May cause cardiac failure; withdraw at 1st sign of impending cardiac failure. Caution with supraventricular arrhythmias when patient is compromised hemodynamically or is taking other drugs that decrease peripheral resistance, myocardial filling/contractility, and/or electrical impulse propagation in the myocardium. Not for HTN associated with hypothermia. Caution in bronchospastic diseases; titrate to lowest possible effective dose and terminate immediately in the event of bronchospasm. Caution in diabetics; may mask tachycardia occurring with hypoglycemia. Caution in impaired renal function. Avoid concentrations >10mg/mL and infusions into small veins or through butterfly catheters. Sloughing of skin and necrosis reported with infiltration and extravasation. Use caution when discontinuing infusion in CAD patients.

**ADVERSE REACTIONS:** Hypotension, dizziness, diaphoresis, somnolence, confusion, headache, agitation, bronchospasm, nausea, infusion site reactions.

**INTERACTIONS:** Additive effects with catecholamine-depleting agents (eg, reserpine); monitor for hypotension or bradycardia. Levels increased by warfarin or morphine; titrate with caution. May increase digoxin levels; titrate with caution. May prolong effects of succinylcholine; titrate with caution.

Caution when using with verapamil in depressed myocardial function; fatal cardiac arrest may occur. Do not use to control supraventricular tachycardia with vasoconstrictive and inotropic agents (eg, dopamine, epinephrine, norepinephrine) because of the danger of blocking cardiac contractility when systemic vascular resistance is high. Patients with a history of severe anaphylactic reaction may be more reactive to repeated challenge and unresponsive to the usual doses of epinephrine used to treat allergic reaction.

**PREGNANCY:** Category C, caution in nursing.

## BREVITAL
methohexital sodium (King)

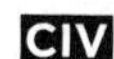

**Should be used only in hospital or ambulatory care settings that provide for continuous monitoring of respiratory and cardiac function. Immediate availability of resuscitative drugs and age- and size-appropriate equipment for bag/valve/mask ventilation and intubation and personnel trained in their use and skilled in airway management should be assured. For deeply sedated patients, a designated individual other than the practitioner performing the procedure should be present to continuously monitor the patient.**

**THERAPEUTIC CLASS:** Barbiturate anesthetic

**INDICATIONS:** IV induction of anesthesia prior to the use of other general anesthetic agents. IV induction of anesthesia and as an adjunct to subpotent inhalational anesthetic agents (such as nitrous oxide in oxygen) for short surgical procedures. For use along with other parenteral agents, usually narcotic analgesics, to supplement subpotent inhalational anesthetic agents (such as nitrous oxide in oxygen) for longer surgical procedures. IV anesthesia for short surgical, diagnostic, or therapeutic procedures associated with minimal painful stimuli. Agent for inducing a hypnotic state. Pediatrics (older than 1 month): Rectal or intramuscular induction of anesthesia prior to the use of other general anesthetic agents; rectal or intramuscular induction of anesthesia and as an adjunct to subpotent inhalational anesthetic agents for surgical procedures; rectal or intramuscular anesthesia for short surgical, diagnostic, or therapeutic procedures associated with minimal painful stimuli.

**DOSAGE:** *Adults:* Individualize dose.Induction: 1% solution administered at a rate of 1mL/5 seconds. Range: 50-120mg or more (average: 70mg). Usual dose: 1-1.5mg/kg. Maint: Intermittent: 20-40mg (2 to 4mL of a 1% solution) q 4-7 minutes. Continuous drip: Average rate of administration is 3mL of a 0.2% solution/minute (1 drop/second).
*Pediatrics:* ≥1 month:Individualize dose:Induction: IM: 6.6 to 10mg/kg IM of the 5% concentration. Rectal: 25mg/kg rectally of the 1% solution.

**HOW SUPPLIED:** Inj: 500mg, 2.5g

**CONTRAINDICATIONS:** Patients with latent or manifest porphyria.

**WARNINGS/PRECAUTIONS:** Seizures may be elicited in patients with previous history of convulsive activity. Caution in severe hepatic dysfunction, severe cardiovascular instability, shock-like condition, asthma, COPD, severe HTN or hypotension, MI, CHF, severe anemia, status asthmaticus, extreme obesity, debilitated patients or those with impaired function of respiratory, circulatory, renal, hepatic, or endocrine system. Unintended intra-arterial injection may produce platelet aggregates and thrombosis at the site of injection.

**ADVERSE REACTIONS:** Circulatory depression, thrombophlebitis, hypotension, tachycardia, respiratory depression, skeletal muscle hypersensitivity (twitching), emergence delirium.

**INTERACTIONS:** May influence the metabolism of other concomitantly used drugs, such as phenytoin, halothane, anticoagulants, corticosteroids, ethyl alcohol, and propylene-glycol-containing solutions. Prior chronic administration of barbiturates or phenytoin may reduce the effectiveness of methohexital. Additive CNS effects with other CNS depressants, including ethyl alcohol and propylene alcohol.

**PREGNANCY:** Category B, caution in nursing.

B

## BREVOXYL RX
benzoyl peroxide (Stiefel)

**THERAPEUTIC CLASS:** Antibacterial/keratolytic

**INDICATIONS:** Topical treatment of mild to moderate acne vulgaris.

**DOSAGE:** *Adults:* (Gel) Apply qd-bid to clean affected area. (Lotion) Shake well. Wet affected area and wash qd for 1st week, then bid thereafter if tolerated.
*Pediatrics:* >12 yrs: (Gel) Apply qd-bid to clean affected area. (Lotion) Shake well. Wet affected area and wash qd for 1st week, then bid thereafter if tolerated.

**HOW SUPPLIED:** Gel: 4%, 8% [42.5g, 90g]; Lot: (Cleanser) 4%, 8% [297g]; Lot: (Creamy Wash) 4%, 8% [170g]

**WARNINGS/PRECAUTIONS:** Avoid contact with hair, eyes, mucous membranes, carpeting, and fabrics.

**ADVERSE REACTIONS:** Erythema, peeling.

**PREGNANCY:** Category C, caution in nursing.

## BROMFED RX
pseudoephedrine HCl - brompheniramine maleate (Muro)

**OTHER BRAND NAMES:** Bromfed-PD (Muro) - Bromfenex (Ethex) - Bromfenex-PD (Ethex)

**THERAPEUTIC CLASS:** Antihistamine/decongestant

**INDICATIONS:** Treatment of symptoms of seasonal and perennial allergic rhinitis, and vasomotor rhinitis, including nasal congestion.

**DOSAGE:** *Adults:* (12mg-120mg) 1 cap q12h. (6mg-60mg) 1-2 caps q12h.
*Pediatrics:* >12 yrs: (12mg-120mg) 1 cap q12h. (6mg-60mg) 1-2 caps q12h. 6-11 yrs: (6mg-60mg) 1 cap q12h.

**HOW SUPPLIED:** (Brompheniramine-Pseudoephedrine) Cap, Extended Release: (PD) 6mg- 60mg, (Bromfed, Bromfenex) 12mg-120mg

**CONTRAINDICATIONS:** Severe HTN, CAD, narrow-angle glaucoma, MAOI therapy, urinary retention, peptic ulcer, during an asthmatic attack.

**WARNINGS/PRECAUTIONS:** Caution with HTN, DM, ischemic heart disease, hyperthyroidism, increased IOP, prostatic hypertrophy, and elderly. Caution while operating machinery.

**ADVERSE REACTIONS:** Drowsiness, lassitude, nausea, giddiness, dryness of the mouth, blurred vision, palpitations, flushing, increased irritability or excitement.

**INTERACTIONS:** Potentiated by MAOIs and β-blockers. Reduced antihypertensive effects of methyldopa, mecamylamine, reserpine, and veratrum alkaloids. Additive effects with alcohol and other CNS depressants.

**PREGNANCY:** Safety in pregnancy and nursing not known.

## BROVANA RX
arformoterol tartrate (Sepracor)

**Long-acting beta$_2$-adrenergic agonists may increase the risk of asthma-related death.**

**THERAPEUTIC CLASS:** Beta$_2$ agonist

**INDICATIONS:** Long term maintenance treatment of bronchoconstriction in patients with COPD, including chronic bronchitis and emphysema.

**DOSAGE:** *Adults:* Usual: 15mcg bid (am and pm). Max: 30mcg/day. Administer via nebulizer.

**HOW SUPPLIED:** Sol (neb): 15mcg/2mL [30$^{s}$, 60$^{s}$]

**CONTRAINDICATIONS:** Hypersensitivity to racemic formoterol

**WARNINGS/PRECAUTIONS:** Not indicated for the treatment of acute episodes of bronchospasm. Should not be initiated or used in children, patients with acutely deteriorating COPD. Fatalities reported with excessive use of inhaled sympathomimetics, avoid use with other long-acting beta$_2$-agonists. Discontinue regular use of short acting beta$_2$-agonists (e.g. four times a day) before initiating therapy. May produced life threatening paradoxical bronchospasm. Caution in patients with convulsive disorders, thyrotoxicosis, cardiovascular disorders especially coronary insufficiency, cardiac arrhythmias, and hypertension. Immediate hypersensitivity reactions may occur.

**ADVERSE REACTIONS:** Pain, chest pain, back pain , diarrhea, sinusitis, leg cramps, dyspnea, rash, flu syndrome, peripheral edema.

**INTERACTIONS:** Sympathetic effects may be poentiated with concomitant use of additional adrenergic agoinsts. Concomitant use with methylxanthines, steriods, or diuretics may potentiate hypokalemia. Caution with co-administration with non-potassium sparing diuretics may cause ECG changes.Use extreme caution in patients being treated with MAOIs, TCAs, or any drugs known to prolong the $QT_c$ interval. Caution wtih beta blockers.

**PREGNANCY:** Category C, caution in nursing.

## BUMETANIDE

bumetanide (Various) RX

**Can lead to profound water and electrolyte depletion with excessive use.**

**OTHER BRAND NAMES:** Bumex (Roche Labs)

**THERAPEUTIC CLASS:** Loop diuretic

**INDICATIONS:** Treatment of edema associated with CHF, hepatic disease, and renal disease including nephrotic syndrome.

**DOSAGE:** *Adults:* >18 yrs: PO: Usual: 0.5-2mg qd. Maint: May give every other day or every 3-4 days. Max: 10mg/day. IV/IM: Initial: 0.5-1mg over 1-2 minutes, may repeat every 2-3 hrs for 2-3 doses. Max: 10mg/day. Elderly: Start at low end of dosing range.

**HOW SUPPLIED:** Inj: 0.25mg/mL; Tab: 0.5mg*, 1mg*, 2mg* *scored

**CONTRAINDICATIONS:** Anuria, hepatic coma, severe electrolyte depletion.

**WARNINGS/PRECAUTIONS:** Monitor for volume/electrolyte depletion, hypokalemia, blood dyscrasias, hepatic damage. Elderly are prone to volume/electrolyte depletion. Caution in elderly, hepatic cirrhosis and ascites. Associated with ototoxicity, hypocalcemia, thrombocytopenia, hypomagnesemia, hypokalemia, and hyperuricemia. Hypersensitivity with sulfonamide allergy. Discontinue if marked increase in BUN or creatinine or if develop oliguria with progressive renal disease.

**ADVERSE REACTIONS:** Muscle cramps, dizziness, hypotension, headache, nausea, hyperuricemia, hypokalemia, hyponatremia, hyperglycemia, azotemia, increase serum creatinine.

**INTERACTIONS:** Avoid aminoglycosides, ototoxic and nephrotoxic drugs, indomethacin. Lithium toxicity. Probenecid reduces effects. Potentiates antihypertensives.

**PREGNANCY:** Category C, not for use in nursing.

## BUPRENEX

buprenorphine HCl (Reckitt Benckiser) CV

**THERAPEUTIC CLASS:** Opioid analgesic

**INDICATIONS:** Relief of moderate to severe pain.

B

**DOSAGE:** *Adults:* 0.3mg IM/IV q6h prn. Repeat if needed, 30-60 minutes after initial dose and then prn. High Risk Patients/Concomitant CNS depressants: Reduce dose by approximately 50%. May use single doses <0.6mg IM if not at high-risk.
*Pediatrics:* >13 yrs: 0.3mg IM/IV q6h prn. Repeat if needed, 30-60 minutes after initial dose and then prn. High Risk Patients/Concomitant CNS depressants: Reduce dose by approximately 50%. May use single doses <0.6mg IM if not at high-risk. 2-12 yrs: 2-6mcg/kg IM/IV q4-6h.

**HOW SUPPLIED:** Inj: 0.3mg/mL

**WARNINGS/PRECAUTIONS:** Significant respiratory depression reported; caution with compromised respiratory function. May increase CSF pressure; caution with head injury, intracranial lesions. Caution with debilitated, BPH, biliary tract dysfunction, myxedema, hypothyroidism, urethral stricture, acute alcoholism, Addison's disease, CNS disease, coma, toxic psychoses, delirium tremens, elderly, pediatrics, kyphoscoliosis or hepatic/renal/pulmonary impairment. May impair mental or physical abilities. May precipitate withdrawal in narcotic-dependence. May lead to psychological dependence.

**ADVERSE REACTIONS:** Nausea, dizziness, sweating, hypotension, vomiting, headache, miosis, hypoventilation.

**INTERACTIONS:** Caution with MAOIs, CNS and respiratory depressants. Respiratory and cardiovascular collapse reported with diazepam. Increased CNS depression with other narcotic analgesics, general anesthetics, antihistamines, benzodiazepines, phenothiazines, other tranquilizers, sedative-hypnotics. Decreased clearance with CYP3A4 inhibitors (eg, macrolides, azole antifungals, protease inhibitors). Increased clearance with CYP3A4 inducers (eg, rifampin, carbamazepine, phenytoin).

**PREGNANCY:** Category C, not for use in nursing.

## BuSpar RX

buspirone HCl (Bristol-Myers Squibb)

**THERAPEUTIC CLASS:** Atypical anxiolytic

**INDICATIONS:** Management of anxiety disorders, short-term relief of anxiety symptoms.

**DOSAGE:** *Adults:* Usual: 7.5mg bid. Titrate: May increase by 5mg/day every 2-3 days. Usual: 20-30mg/day. Max: 60mg/day. Use low dose with potent CYP450 3A4 inhibitors (eg, 2.5mg qd with nefazodone). Take consistently with or without food; bioavailabilty increased with food.

**HOW SUPPLIED:** Tab: 5mg*, 10mg*, 15mg*, 30mg* *scored

**WARNINGS/PRECAUTIONS:** Avoid with hepatic or renal impairment.

**ADVERSE REACTIONS:** Dizziness, nausea, headache, nervousness, lightheadedness, excitement.

**INTERACTIONS:** Avoid MAOIs and alcohol. Withdraw other CNS depressants gradually before therapy. Caution with psychotropics. Elevated liver transaminases reported with trazodone. Increases haloperidol levels. Verapamil, diltiazem, grapefruit juice, nefazodone, itraconazole, cimetidine, erythromycin increase plasma levels. May increase levels of both drugs with nefazodone; decrease dose of buspirone. Decreased plasma levels and effects with rifampin; may need to adjust buspirone dose. CYP3A4 inhibitors may increase plasma levels and CYP3A4 inducers may increase metabolism of buspirone; may need dose adjustment. Presystemic clearance may be decreased with food. May displace digoxin.

**PREGNANCY:** Category B, not for use in nursing.

## BYETTA RX
exenatide (Amylin/Lilly)

**THERAPEUTIC CLASS:** Incretin mimetic

**INDICATIONS:** Adjunctive therapy to improve glycemic control in patients with type 2 DM who are taking metformin, a sulfonylurea, a thiazolidinedione, a combination of metformin/sulfonylurea or metformin/thiazolidinedione, but have not achieved adequate glycemic control.

**DOSAGE:** *Adults:* 5mcg SQ bid, 60 minutes before am & pm meals. Titrate: May increase to 10mcg bid after 1 month. Reduction of sulfonylurea dose may be considered to reduce risk of hypoglycemia.

**HOW SUPPLIED:** Inj: 5mcg/dose, 10mcg/dose [60-dose Prefilled Pen]

**WARNINGS/PRECAUTIONS:** Not a substitute for insulin. Do not use with type 1 DM, for treatment of diabetic ketoacidosis, end-stage renal disease, severe renal impairment (CrCl <30mL/min), or severe GI disease. Increased incidence of hypoglycemia with sulfonylurea. Observe for signs and symptoms for hypersensitivity reactions; patients with abdominal pain should be investigated. When used with thiazolidinediones possible chest pain and/or chronic hypersensitivity pneumonitis.

**ADVERSE REACTIONS:** Nausea, vomiting, diarrhea, feeling jittery, dizziness, headache, dyspepsia, injection-site reactions; dysgeusia, somnolence, generalized pruritus and/or urticaria, macular or papular rash, angioedema, rare reports of anaphylactic reaction, abdominal pain, hypoglycemia.

**INTERACTIONS:** Caution with drugs that require rapid gastrointestinal absorption. Drugs that are dependent on threshold concentrations for efficacy (eg, contraceptives, antibiotics) should be taken 1 hour before. Caution with concomitant use of warfarin; could lead to increased INR and possibly bleeding.

**PREGNANCY:** Category C, caution in nursing.

## CADUET RX
amlodipine besylate - atorvastatin calcium (Pfizer)

**THERAPEUTIC CLASS:** Calcium channel blocker/HMG-CoA reductase inhibitor

**INDICATIONS:** When treatment with both amlodipine and atorvastatin is appropriate. (Amlodipine) Treatment of hypertension, chronic stable or vasospastic angina (Prinzmetal's or Variant Angina). (Atorvastatin) Adjunct to diet to reduce total cholesterol (total-C), LDL-C, TG, and Apo B levels, and to increase HDL-C in primary hypercholesterolemia (heterozygous familial and nonfamilial) and mixed dyslipidemia (Types IIa and IIb). Adjunct to diet for elevated serum TG levels (Type IV). Treatment of primary dysbetalipoproteinemia (Type III) inadequately responding to diet. Adjunct to other lipid-lowering treatments or if treatments are unavailable, to reduce total-C and LDL-C in homozygous familial hypercholesterolemia. Adjunct to diet to lower total-C, LDL-C and Apo B in boys and postmenarchal girls with heterozygous familial hypercholesterolemia.

**DOSAGE:** *Adults:* Dosing should be individualized and based on the appropriate combination of recommendations for the monotherapies. (Amlodipine): HTN: Initial: 5mg qd. Titrate over 7-14 days. Max: 10mg qd. Small, Fragile, or Elderly/Hepatic Dysfunction/Concomitant Antihypertensive: Initial: 2.5mg qd. Angina: 5-10mg qd. Elderly/Hepatic Dysfunction: 5mg qd. (Atorvastatin): Hypercholesterolemia/Mixed Dyslipidemia: Initial: 10-20mg qd (or 40mg qd for LDL-C reduction >45%). Titrate: Adjust dose if needed at 2-4 week intervals. Usual: 10-80mg qd. Homozygous Familial Hypercholesterolemia: 10-80mg qd.
*Pediatrics:* ≥10 yrs (postmenarchal): (Amlodipine): HTN: 2.5-5mg qd. 10-17 yrs (postmenarchal): (Atorvastatin): Heterozygous Familial Hypercholesterolemia: Initial: 10mg/day. Titrate: Adjust dose if needed at intervals of ≥4 weeks. Max: 20mg/day.

**HOW SUPPLIED:** Tab: (Amlodipine-Atorvastatin) 2.5mg-10mg, 2.5mg-20mg, 2.5mg-40mg, 5mg-10mg, 5mg-20mg, 5mg-40mg, 5mg-80mg, 10mg-10mg, 10mg-20mg, 10mg-40mg, 10mg-80mg

**CONTRAINDICATIONS:** Active liver disease, unexplained persistent elevations of serum transaminases, pregnancy, nursing mothers.

**WARNINGS/PRECAUTIONS:** May, rarely, increase angina or MI with severe obstructive CAD. Monitor LFTs prior to therapy, at 12 weeks after initiation, with dose elevation, and periodically thereafter. Reduce dose or withdraw if AST or ALT >3x ULN persist. Caution with heavy alcohol use and/or history of hepatic disease, severe aortic stenosis, CHF. D/C if markedly elevated CPK levels occur, if myopathy is diagnosed or suspected, or if predisposition to renal failure secondary to rhabdomyolysis.

**ADVERSE REACTIONS:** Headache, edema, palpitation, dizziness, fatigue, constipation, flatulence, dyspepsia, abdominal pain.

**INTERACTIONS:** Increases levels with erythromycin. Increases levels of oral contraceptives (norethindrone, ethinyl estradiol), digoxin. Cyclosporine, fibric acid derivatives, niacin, erythromycin, azole antifungals may increase risk of myopathy. Caution with drugs that decrease levels or activity of endogenous steroid hormones (eg, ketoconazole, spironolactone, cimetidine). Decreased levels with Maalox® TC, but LDL-C reduction not altered. Colestipol decreases levels when coadministered, but greater LDL-C reduction with coadministration than when each given alone. Avoid fibrates.

**PREGNANCY:** Category X, not for use in nursing

## CAFCIT — RX

caffeine citrate (Mead Johnson)

**THERAPEUTIC CLASS:** Methylxanthine

**INDICATIONS:** Short-term treatment of apnea of prematurity in infants.

**DOSAGE:** *Pediatrics:* 28-<33 weeks: LD: 1mL/kg IV. Maint: 0.25mL/kg IV/PO q24h beginning 24 hrs after LD.

**HOW SUPPLIED:** Inj: 20mg/mL [3mL]; Sol: 20mg/mL [3mL]

**WARNINGS/PRECAUTIONS:** Necrotizing enterocolitis, seizures reported. Rule out other possible causes of apnea before initiating therapy. Caution with cardiovascular disease, seizure disorder, renal/hepatic impairment. Monitor baseline caffeine levels if previously exposed to theophylline.

**ADVERSE REACTIONS:** Feeding intolerance, sepsis, hemorrhage, gastritis, GI hemorrhage, DIC, abnormal healing, dyspnea, cerebral hemorrhage, lung edema, dry skin, retinopathy of prematurity.

**INTERACTIONS:** Potential for interaction with CYP450 1A2 substrates, inducers, inhibitors. May need lower dose with cimetidine, ketoconazole. May need dose increase with phenobarbital, phenytoin.

**PREGNANCY:** Category C, safety in nursing not known.

## CAFERGOT TABLETS — RX

caffeine - ergotamine tartrate (Sandoz)

**THERAPEUTIC CLASS:** Ergot alkaloid

**INDICATIONS:** To abort or prevent vascular headaches.

**DOSAGE:** *Adults:* 2 tabs at start of attack. Repeat 1 tab every 1/2 hr prn. Max: 6 tabs/attack, 10 tabs/week. May give at bedtime as short-term preventive measure.

**HOW SUPPLIED:** Tab: (Ergotamine-Caffeine) 1mg-100mg

**CONTRAINDICATIONS:** Pregnancy, peripheral vascular disease, CHD, HTN, hepatic or renal dysfunction, sepsis.

**WARNINGS/PRECAUTIONS:** Do not exceed recommended dosage.

**ADVERSE REACTIONS:** Precordial distress, transient tachycardia or bradycardia, nausea, vomiting, localized edema, itching, numbness/tingling of fingers/toes, muscle pains, leg weakness.

**PREGNANCY:** Safety in pregnancy and nursing not known.



## CALAN

verapamil HCl (Pharmacia & Upjohn)

RX

**THERAPEUTIC CLASS:** Calcium channel blocker (nondihydropyridine)

**INDICATIONS:** Treatment of hypertension and vasospastic, unstable and chronic stable angina. With digitalis, for control of ventricular rate at rest and during stress in patients with chronic atrial flutter and/or atrial fibrillation. Prophylaxis of repetitive paroxysmal supraventricular tachycardia.

**DOSAGE:** *Adults:* HTN: Initial: 80mg tid. Usual: 360-480mg/day. Elderly/Small Stature: Initial: 40mg tid. Angina: Usual: 80-120mg tid. Elderly/Small Stature: Initial: 40mg tid. Titrate: Increase daily or weekly. A-Fib (Digitalized): Usual: 240-320mg/day given tid-qid. PSVT Prophylaxis (Non-Digitalized): 240-480mg/day given tid-qid. Max: 480mg/day. Severe Hepatic Dysfunction: Give 30% of normal dose.

**HOW SUPPLIED:** Tab: 40mg, 80mg*, 120mg* *scored

**CONTRAINDICATIONS:** Severe ventricular dysfunction, hypotension, cardiogenic shock, sick sinus syndrome or 2nd- or 3rd-degree AV block (except with functioning ventricular pacemaker), A-Fib/Flutter with an accessory bypass tract.

**WARNINGS/PRECAUTIONS:** Avoid with moderate to severe cardiac failure, and ventricular dysfunction if taking a β-blocker. May cause hypotension, AV block, transient bradycardia, PR interval prolongation. Monitor LFTs periodically; hepatocellular injury reported. Caution with hypertrophic cardiomyopathy, renal or hepatic dysfunction. Decrease dose with decreased neuromuscular transmission.

**ADVERSE REACTIONS:** Constipation, dizziness, nausea, hypotension, headache, edema, CHF, fatigue, elevated liver enzymes, dyspnea, bradycardia, AV block, rash, flushing.

**INTERACTIONS:** Additive effects on HR, AV conduction, and contractility with β-blockers. Potentiates other antihypertensives. May increase digoxin, carbamazepine, theophylline, cyclosporine and alcohol levels. Avoid disopyramide within 48 hrs before or 24 hrs after verapamil. Additive negative inotropic effects and AV conduction prolongation with flecainide. Avoid quinidine with hypertrophic cardiomyopathy. Monitor lithium. Increased clearance with phenobarbital. Rifampin may reduce oral bioavailability. May potentiate neuromuscular blockers; both agents may need dose reduction.

**PREGNANCY:** Category C, not for use in nursing.

## CALAN SR

verapamil HCl (Pharmacia & Upjohn)

RX

**THERAPEUTIC CLASS:** Calcium channel blocker (nondihydropyridine)

**INDICATIONS:** Treatment of hypertension.

**DOSAGE:** *Adults:* >18 yrs: Initial: 180mg qam. Titrate: If inadequate response, increase to 240mg qam, then 180mg bid; or 240mg qam plus 120mg qpm, then 240mg q12h. Elderly/Small Stature: Initial: 120mg qam. Take with food.

**HOW SUPPLIED:** Tab, Extended Release: 120mg, 180mg*, 240mg* *scored

**CONTRAINDICATIONS:** Severe ventricular dysfunction, hypotension, cardiogenic shock, sick sinus syndrome or 2nd- or 3rd-degree AV block (except with functioning ventricular pacemaker), A-Fib/Flutter with an accessory bypass tract.

**WARNINGS/PRECAUTIONS:** Avoid with moderate to severe cardiac failure, and ventricular dysfunction if taking a β-blocker. May cause hypotension, AV block, transient bradycardia, PR interval prolongation. Monitor LFTs periodically; hepatocellular injury reported. Caution with hypertrophic cardiomyopathy, renal or hepatic dysfunction. Decrease dose with decreased neuromuscular transmission.



**ADVERSE REACTIONS:** Constipation, dizziness, nausea, hypotension, headache, edema, CHF, fatigue, elevated liver enzymes, dyspnea, bradycardia, AV block, rash, flushing.

**INTERACTIONS:** Additive effects on HR, AV conduction, and contractility with β-blockers. Potentiates other antihypertensives. May increase digoxin, carbamazepine, theophylline, cyclosporine, and alcohol levels. Avoid disopyramide within 48 hrs before or 24 hrs after verapamil. Additive negative inotropic effects and AV conduction prolongation with flecainide. Avoid quinidine with hypertrophic cardiomyopathy. Monitor lithium. Increased clearance with phenobarbital. Rifampin may reduce oral bioavailability. May potentiate neuromuscular blockers; both agents may need dose reduction.

**PREGNANCY:** Category C, not for use in nursing.

## CAMPATH
alemtuzumab (Berlex)

RX

**Hematologic toxicity reported; avoid single doses >30mg or cumulative doses >90mg/week. Gradually escalate dose to avoid infusion reactions. Opportunistic infections reported.**

**THERAPEUTIC CLASS:** Monoclonal antibody/CD52-blocker

**INDICATIONS:** Treatment of B-cell chronic lymphocytic leukemia in patients treated with alkylating agents and failed fludarabine therapy.

**DOSAGE:** *Adults:* Initial: 3mg IV qd until tolerated, then increase to 10mg IV qd. Continue until tolerated, then increase to maint dose of 30mg (escalation to 30mg usually takes 3-7 days). Maint: 30mg IV 3x/week up to 12 weeks. Max: 30mg single dose or 90mg/week.

**HOW SUPPLIED:** Inj: 30mg/mL

**CONTRAINDICATIONS:** Active systemic infection, underlying immunodeficiency.

**WARNINGS/PRECAUTIONS:** Premedicate with oral antihistamine, acetaminophen to avoid infusion reactions. Monitor BP, hypotensive symptoms in ischemic heart disease, with antihypertensives. Discontinue if serious infection occurs. Monitor CBC, platelets weekly.

**ADVERSE REACTIONS:** Infusion reactions (eg, rigors, fever, nausea, vomiting, hypotension), infections, hematologic toxicity (eg, neutropenia, anemia, pancytopenia), fatigue, skeletal pain, anorexia, asthenia, peripheral edema, back pain, chest pain, HTN, tachycardia, headache, diarrhea, stomatitis, myalgias, dyspnea, cough.

**INTERACTIONS:** Avoid live viral vaccines.

**PREGNANCY:** Category C, not for use in nursing.

## CAMPRAL
acamprosate calcium (Forest)

RX

**THERAPEUTIC CLASS:** GABA analogue

**INDICATIONS:** Maintenance of abstinence from alcohol in patients with alcohol dependence who are abstinent at treatment initiation.

**DOSAGE:** *Adults:* 2 tabs tid. CrCl 30-50mL/min: 1 tab tid.

**HOW SUPPLIED:** Tab: 333mg

**CONTRAINDICATIONS:** Severe renal impairment (CrCl ≤30mL/min).

**WARNINGS/PRECAUTIONS:** Use does not eliminate or diminish withdrawal symptoms. Dose reduction required with renal impairment (CrCl ≤30-50mL/min). Suicidal events reported.

**ADVERSE REACTIONS:** Accidental injury, asthenia, pain, anorexia, diarrhea, flatulence, nausea, anxiety, depression, dizziness, dry mouth, insomnia, paresthesia, pruritus, sweating.

**INTERACTIONS:** Naltrexone may increase levels. Weight gain/weight loss may occur with antidepressants.

**PREGNANCY:** Category C, caution in nursing.

C

## CAMPTOSAR

irinotecan HCl (Pharmacia & Upjohn) RX

**Early and/or late forms of diarrhea, severe myelosuppression may occur. Interrupt and reduce subsequent doses if severe diarrhea occurs. Carefully monitor with diarrhea; give fluid/electrolyte replacement if dehydrated or give antibiotics if ileus, fever, or severe neutropenia develops.**

**THERAPEUTIC CLASS:** Topoisomerase I inhibitor

**INDICATIONS:** First-line therapy in combination with 5-fluorouracil (5-FU) and leucovorin (LV) for metastatic colon or rectal carcinomas, and for disease that has progressed or recurred following initial 5-FU therapy.

**DOSAGE:** *Adults:* Combination Therapy (5-FU/LV see labeling for dosage): 125mg/m$^2$ IV over 90 minutes on days 1, 8, 15, 22 for 6 weeks; or 180mg/m$^2$ IV over 90 minutes on days 1, 15, and 29 for 6 weeks. Both regimens: Begin next cycle on day 43. Single Therapy: 125mg/m$^2$ IV over 90 minutes on days 1, 8, 15, 22 followed by a 2 week rest; or 350mg/m$^2$ IV over 90 minutes once every 3 weeks. Premedicate with antiemetics at least 30 minutes prior to therapy. Dose modifications for reduced UGT1A1 activity, neutropenia, diarrhea, and other toxicities: See labeling. All dose modifications should be based on worst preceding toxicity.

**HOW SUPPLIED:** Inj: 20mg/mL

**CONTRAINDICATIONS:** Concomitant ketoconazole or St. John's wort.

**WARNINGS/PRECAUTIONS:** Due to increased toxicity, avoid use of irinotecan with the"Mayo Clinic" regimen of 5-FU/LV (given 4-5 days every 4 weeks). Treat/prevent early diarrhea with atropine IV/SQ and late diarrhea (occurring >24 hrs after dose) with loperamide PO. If late diarrhea occurs, delay therapy until return of pretreatment bowel function for at least 24 hrs without antidiarrheals; decrease subsequent doses if late diarrhea is grade 2, 3 or 4. Deaths due to sepsis reported following severe neutropenia. Temporarily hold therapy if neutropenic fever occurs or if neutrophils <1000/mm$^3$. Increased risk for neutropenia in patients homozygous for the UGT1A1 28 allele. Consider reduced initial dose. Heterozygous patients may also have increased risk. Hypersensitivity reactions, colitis, ileus, and renal impairment/failure, thromboembolic events reported. May cause fetal harm during pregnancy. Monitor for extravasation at infusion site. Consider atropine for cholinergic symptoms. Caution with modestly elevated baseline bilirubin levels (eg, 1-2mg/dL), abnormal glucuronidation of bilirubin, hepatic insufficiency, elderly with comorbidities, previous pelvic/abdominal irradiation. Careful monitoring of WBC with differential, Hgb, and platelets is recommended before each dose. Avoid in severe bone marrow failure, and fructose intolerant patients.

**ADVERSE REACTIONS:** Nausea, vomiting, diarrhea, abdominal pain, blood dyscrasias, asthenia, muscositis, anorexia, alopecia, fever, pain, constipation, infection, dyspnea, increased bilirubin.

**INTERACTIONS:** Exacerbated myelosuppression and diarrhea with antineoplastic agents having similar adverse effects. Avoid concurrent irradiation therapy. Possible hyperglycemia and lymphocytopenia with dexamethasone. Akathisia reported with prochlorperazine. Laxatives may worsen diarrhea. Consider withholding diuretics with irinotecan therapy. Decreased levels with CYP3A4 inducing anticonvulsants and St. John's wort.

Consider substituting non-enzyme inducing anticonvulsants 2 weeks prior to and during treatment. Increased levels with ketoconazole. Discontinue ketoconazole at least 1 week prior to and during therapy.

**PREGNANCY:** Category D, not for use in nursing.



## CANASA RX

mesalamine (Axcan Scandipharm)

**THERAPEUTIC CLASS:** Anti-inflammatory Agent

**INDICATIONS:** Treatment of active ulcerative proctitis.

**DOSAGE:** *Adults:* 1000mg rectally qhs. Retain suppository for at least 1-3 hrs.

**HOW SUPPLIED:** Sup: 1000mg

**CONTRAINDICATIONS:** Hypersensitivity to suppository vehicle (eg, saturated vegetable fatty acid esters) or salicylates.

**WARNINGS/PRECAUTIONS:** Discontinue if acute intolerance syndrome develops (eg, cramping, bloody diarrhea, abdominal pain, headache); consider sulfasalazine hypersensitivity. If rechallenge is considered, perform under careful observation. Caution with sulfasalazine hypersensitivity. Carefully monitor with renal dysfunction. Pancolitis, pericarditis (rare) reported.

**ADVERSE REACTIONS:** Dizziness, rectal pain, fever, acne, colitis, rash, hair loss.

**PREGNANCY:** Category B, caution in nursing.

## CANCIDAS RX

caspofungin acetate (Merck)

**THERAPEUTIC CLASS:** Glucan synthesis inhibitor

**INDICATIONS:** Treatment of esophageal candidiasis, invasive aspergillosis in patients refractory to or intolerant to other therapies, and candidemia and the following *Candida* infections: intra-abdominal abscesses, peritonitis, and pleural space infections. Empirical therapy for presumed fungal infections in febrile, neutropenic patients.

**DOSAGE:** *Adults:* Invasive Aspergillosis: LD: 70mg IV on Day 1. Maint: 50mg IV qd. Empirical Therapy: LD: 70mg IV on Day 1. Maint: 50mg IV qd. If 50mg is well tolerated but does not provide adequate clinical response, daily dose can be increased to 70mg. Fungal infections should be treated for a minimum of 14 days. Continue treatment 7 days after neutropenia and clinical symptoms are resolved. Esophageal Candidiasis: 50mg IV qd. Consider suppressive therapy in HIV patients. Candidemia/*Candida* Infections: LD: 70mg IV on Day 1. Maint: 50mg IV qd. Moderate Hepatic Insufficiency: LD: 70mg IV on Day 1. Maint: 35mg IV qd. Concomitant Rifampin: 70mg IV qd. Concomitant Nevirapine/Efavirenz/Carbamazepine/Dexamethasone/Phenytoin: May need to increase dose to 70mg IV qd. Base duration of treatment on severity of disease, clinical response, microbiological response, and recovery from immunosuppression.

**HOW SUPPLIED:** Inj: 50mg, 70mg

**ADVERSE REACTIONS:** Fever, infused vein complications, nausea, vomiting, flushing, rash, facial edema.

**INTERACTIONS:** Reduces blood levels of tacrolimus. Efavirenz, nevirapine, phenytoin, rifampin, dexamethasone, carbamazepine may decrease levels. Increased levels with cyclosporine; avoid concomitant use. Do not mix or co-infuse with other medications. Do not use with diluents containing dextrose.

**PREGNANCY:** Category C, caution in nursing.

## CAPEX
RX

fluocinolone acetonide (Galderma)



**THERAPEUTIC CLASS:** Corticosteroid

**INDICATIONS:** Treatment of seborrheic dermatitis of the scalp.

**DOSAGE:** *Adults:* Apply up to 1oz to scalp qd. Work into lather, rinse after 5 minutes.

**HOW SUPPLIED:** Shampoo: 0.01% [120mL]

**WARNINGS/PRECAUTIONS:** May produce reversible HPA axis suppression, manifestations of Cushing's syndrome, hyperglycemia, and glucosuria. Evaluate periodically for HPA axis suppression if applied to large surface area or with occlusive dressings. Discontinue if irritation occurs. Pediatrics may be more susceptible to systemic toxicity. Use appropriate therapy with infections.

**ADVERSE REACTIONS:** Allergic contact dermatitis, secondary infection, skin atrophy, striae, miliaria, burning, itching, irritation, hypopigmentation, perioral dermatitis, dryness, folliculitis, acneiform eruptions.

**PREGNANCY:** Category C, caution in nursing.

## CAPOZIDE
RX

captopril - hydrochlorothiazide (Par)

> **ACE inhibitors can cause death/injury to developing fetus during 2nd and 3rd trimesters. Stop therapy if pregnancy detected.**

**THERAPEUTIC CLASS:** ACE inhibitor/thiazide diuretic

**INDICATIONS:** Treatment of hypertension.

**DOSAGE:** *Adults:* Initial: 25mg-15mg tab qd. Titrate: Adjust dose at 6-week intervals. Max: 150mg captopril/50mg HCTZ per day. Replacement Therapy: Substitute combination for titrated components. Renal Impairment: Decrease dose or increase interval. Take 1 hr before meals.

**HOW SUPPLIED:** Tab: (Captopril-HCTZ) 25mg-15mg*, 25mg-25mg*, 50mg-15mg*, 50mg-25mg* *scored

**CONTRAINDICATIONS:** History of ACE inhibitor associated angioedema, anuria, sulfonamide hypersensitivity.

**WARNINGS/PRECAUTIONS:** Discontinue if angioedema, jaundice, or if marked LFT elevation occurs. Risk of hyperkalemia with DM, renal dysfunction. Monitor WBCs in renal and collagen vascular disease. Fetal/neonatal morbidity and death reported. Monitor for hypotension in high risk patients (eg, surgery/anesthesia, volume/salt depletion). Caution with renal or hepatic dysfunction. More reports of angioedema in blacks than nonblacks. May exacerbate or activate SLE. Monitor electrolytes. Hypercalcemia, hypomagnesemia, hyperuricemia may occur. With renal impairment, monitor WBCs and differential before therapy, every 2 weeks for 3 months, then periodically. Neutropenia with myeloid hypoplasia, persistent nonproductive cough, anaphylactoid reactions, proteinuria reported.

**ADVERSE REACTIONS:** Cough, hypotension, rash, pruritus, fever, arthralgia, eosinophilia, dysgeusia, neutropenia/thrombocytopenia.

**INTERACTIONS:** Increase risk of hyperkalemia with $K^+$-sparing diuretics, $K^+$ supplements, or $K^+$-containing salt substitutes. Potentiates orthostatic hypotension with alcohol, barbiturates, and narcotics. Adjust other antihypertensives, anticoagulants, antidiabetic or antigout drugs. Reduced absorption with cholestyramine, colestipol. Amphotericin B, corticosteroids, ACTH deplete electrolytes. May decrease methenamine effects. May decrease response to pressor amines. May potentiate non-depolarizing skeletal muscle relaxants, anesthetics. Risk of lithium toxicity. NSAIDs (eg, indomethacin) reduce effects. Enhanced hypotensive effects with MAOIs. Probenecid, sulfinpyrazone may need dose increase. Diazoxide enhances hyperglycemic, hyperuricemic and antihypertensive effects. Monitor serum calcium levels with calcium salts. Monitor potassium levels with cardiac glycosides. Caution with agents affecting sympathetic activity. Discontinue vasodilators before therapy. Caution and decrease vasodilator dose if resumed during therapy.



**PREGNANCY:** Category C (1st trimester) and D (2nd and 3rd trimesters), not for use in nursing.

## CAPTOPRIL — RX

captopril (Various)

> **ACE inhibitors can cause death/injury to developing fetus during 2nd and 3rd trimesters. Stop therapy if pregnancy detected.**

**OTHER BRAND NAMES:** Capoten (Par)

**THERAPEUTIC CLASS:** ACE inhibitor

**INDICATIONS:** Hypertension. CHF. To decrease hospitalization and mortality in stable post-MI patients with left ventricular dysfunction. Diabetic nephropathy (proteinuria >500mg/day) and slows progression of renal insufficiency in type I diabetes.

**DOSAGE:** *Adults:* Take 1 hour before meals. HTN: If possible, d/c recent antihypertensive drug for 1 week prior to therapy. Initial: 25mg bid-tid. Titrate: May increase to 50mg bid-tid after 1-2 weeks. Usual: 25-150mg bid-tid. Max: 450mg/day. CHF: Initial: 25mg tid; 6.25-12.5mg tid with risk of hypotension or salt/volume depletion. Usual: 50-100mg tid. Max: 450mg/day. Left Ventricular Dysfunction Post-MI: Initial: 6.25mg single dose, then 12.5mg tid. Titrate: Increase to 25mg tid over next several days, then to 50mg tid over next several weeks. Usual: 50mg tid. Diabetic Nephropathy: 25mg tid. Significant Renal Dysfunction: Decrease initial dose and titrate slowly.

**HOW SUPPLIED:** Tab: 12.5mg*, 25mg*, 50mg*, 100mg* *scored

**CONTRAINDICATIONS:** History of ACE inhibitor associated angioedema.

**WARNINGS/PRECAUTIONS:** D/C if jaundice or marked LFT elevation occurs. Risk of hyperkalemia with DM, renal dysfunction. Persistent nonproductive cough, anaphylactoid reactions, neutropenia with myeloid hypoplasia reported. Fetal/neonatal morbidity and death reported. Monitor for hypotension in high risk patients (surgery/anesthesia, dialysis, heart failure, volume/salt depletion, etc). Caution with CHF, renal dysfunction, renal artery stenosis, collagen vascular disease (especially with renal dysfunction). Monitor WBC before therapy, then every 2 weeks for 3 months, then periodically. Less effective on BP in blacks and more reports of angioedema than nonblacks.

**ADVERSE REACTIONS:** Proteinuria, rash, hypotension, dysgeusia, cough, MI, CHF.

**INTERACTIONS:** May increase lithium levels. NSAIDs may decrease antihypertensive effects. Hypotension risk with diuretics. Increased risk of hyperkalemia with $K^+$-sparing diuretics, $K^+$-containing salt substitutes, or $K^+$ supplements. Caution with vasodilators or agents affecting sympathetic activity. Augmented effect by antihypertensives that cause renin release (eg, thiazides).

**PREGNANCY:** Category C (1st trimester) and D (2nd and 3rd trimesters), not for use in nursing.

## CARAC — RX

fluorouracil (Dermik)

**THERAPEUTIC CLASS:** Antimetabolite

**INDICATIONS:** Topical treatment of multiple actinic or solar keratosis of the face and anterior scalp.

**DOSAGE:** *Adults:* >18 yrs: Apply thin film qd to lesions for up to 4 weeks. Apply 10 minutes after washing and drying area.

**HOW SUPPLIED:** Cre: 0.5% [30g]

**CONTRAINDICATIONS:** Pregnancy, dihydropyrimidine dehydrogenase (DPD) enzyme deficiency.

**WARNINGS/PRECAUTIONS:** Discontinue if symptoms of DPD enzyme deficiency develop. Avoid contact with eyes, eyelids, nostrils, mouth, and sun/UV light. Increased absorption with ulcerated or inflamed skin. Wash hands after application

**ADVERSE REACTIONS:** Application site reaction (eg, erythema, dryness, burning, erosion, pain, edema), eye irritation.

**PREGNANCY:** Category X, not for use in nursing.

## CARAFATE

RX

sucralfate (Axcan Scandipharm)

**THERAPEUTIC CLASS:** Duodenal ulcer adherent complex

**INDICATIONS:** (Sus/Tab) Short-term treatment of active duodenal ulcer. (Tab) Maintenance therapy of healed duodenal ulcers.

**DOSAGE:** *Adults:* Active Ulcer: (Sus/Tab) 1g qid for 4-8 weeks. Maint: (Tab) 1g bid. Take on empty stomach.

**HOW SUPPLIED:** Sus: 1g/10mL [414mL]; Tab: 1g* *scored

**WARNINGS/PRECAUTIONS:** Caution with chronic renal failure and dialysis.

**ADVERSE REACTIONS:** Constipation, diarrhea, nausea, vomiting, pruritus, rash, dizziness, insomnia, back pain, headache.

**INTERACTIONS:** Reduced absorption of cimetidine, digoxin, fluoroquinolones, ketoconazole, levothyroxine, phenytoin, quinidine, ranitidine, tetracycline, and theophylline; dose concomitant drugs 2 hrs before sucralfate. Monitor warfarin. Additive aluminum absorption with aluminum-containing products. Antacids should not be taken within 1/2 hr before or after sucralfate.

**PREGNANCY:** Category B, caution with nursing.

## CARBATROL

RX

carbamazepine (Shire US)

**Aplastic anemia and agranulocytosis reported. Obtain complete pretreatment hematological testing as a baseline. Discontinue if develop evidence of bone marrow depression.**

**THERAPEUTIC CLASS:** Carboxamide anticonvulsant

**INDICATIONS:** Treatment of partial seizures with complex symptomatology, generalized tonic-clonic seizures, and mixed seizure patterns of these or other partial or generalized seizures. Treatment of trigeminal neuralgia pain.

**DOSAGE:** *Adults:* Epilepsy: Initial: 200mg bid. Titrate: May increase weekly by 200mg/day. Maint: 800-1200mg/day. Max: 1200mg/day. Trigeminal Neuralgia: Initial (Day 1): 200mg qd. Titrate: May increase by 200mg/day q12h. Maint: 400-800mg/day. Max: 1200mg/day. Re-evaluate every 3 months. *Pediatrics:* Epilepsy: >12 yrs: Initial: 200mg bid. Titrate: May increase weekly by 200mg/day. Max: 12-15 yrs: 1000mg/day. >15 yrs: 1200mg/day. 6 months-12 yrs: May convert immediate-release dose >400mg/day to equal daily dose using bid regimen. Usual/Max: <35mg/kg/day.

**HOW SUPPLIED:** Cap, Extended Release: 200mg, 300mg

**CONTRAINDICATIONS:** History of bone marrow depression, MAOI use within 14 days, sensitivity to TCAs.

**WARNINGS/PRECAUTIONS:** Lyell's syndrome and Stevens-Johnson syndrome, multi-organ hypersensitivity reactions reported. Caution with history of adverse hematologic reaction to any drug, increased IOP, the elderly, mixed seizure with atypical absence seizure. Fetal harm with pregnancy. May activate latent psychosis. Caution with cardiac, hepatic, or renal damage. Perform eye exam and monitor LFTs and renal function at baseline and periodically.



**ADVERSE REACTIONS:** Dizziness, drowsiness, unsteadiness, nausea, vomiting, bone marrow depression, rash, urticaria, hypersensitivity reactions, photosensitivity reactions, CHF, edema, HTN, hypotension.

**INTERACTIONS:** See Contraindications. Metabolism is inhibited by CYP3A4 inhibitors (eg, cimetidine, macrolides, etc.) and induced by CYP3A4 inducers (eg, rifampin, phenytoin, trazodone, etc.). Decreases oral contraceptive effectiveness. Increases plasma levels of clomipramine, phenytoin, and primidone. Decreases levels of APAP, alprazolam, clonazepam, clozapine, dicumarol, doxycycline, ethosuximide, haloperidol, methsuximide, phensuximide, phenytoin, theophylline, valproate, warfarin. Increased risk of neurotoxic side effects with lithium.

**PREGNANCY:** Category D, not for use in nursing.

## CARBOPLATIN

carboplatin (Various) RX

**Bone marrow suppression, resulting in infection or bleeding reported. Anemia and anaphylactic-like reactions reported.**

**THERAPEUTIC CLASS:** Platinum coordination compound

**INDICATIONS:** Initial treatment of advanced ovarian carcinoma. Palliative treatment of advanced ovarian carcinoma recurrent after prior chemotherapy.

**DOSAGE:** *Adults:* Monotherapy: 360mg/m² IV on day 1 every 4 weeks. Concomitant Cyclophosphamide: 300mg/m² IV on day 1 every 4 weeks for 6 cycles, with cyclophosphamide 600mg/m² IV on day 1 every 4 weeks for 6 cycles. If platelets >100,000 or neutrophils >2000: Give 125% of dose. If platelets <50,000 or neutrophils <500: Give 75% of dose. Renal Impairment: Initial: CrCl 41-59mL/min: 250mg/m². CrCl 16-40mL/min: 200mg/m². Subsequent dose adjustments based on the degree of bone marrow suppression.

**HOW SUPPLIED:** Inj: 10mg/mL

**CONTRAINDICATIONS:** Severe bone marrow depression, significant bleeding. History of severe allergic reactions to cisplatin, platinum-containing compounds, or mannitol.

**WARNINGS/PRECAUTIONS:** Bone marrow suppression is dose-dependent and is the dose-limiting toxicity. May need transfusion for anemia. Bone marrow suppression increased in patients who recieved prior therapy. Neurotoxicity increased if >65 yrs and previous cisplatin treatment. LFT abnormalities and temporary loss of vision with high doses. Emesis reported.

**ADVERSE REACTIONS:** Blood dyscrasias, infection, bleeding, nausea, vomiting, peripheral neuropathies, ototoxicity, central neurotoxicity, elevated LFTs/bilirubin/serum creatinine, electrolyte loss, allergic reactions, alopecia, mucositis.

**INTERACTIONS:** Nephrotoxic compounds may potentiate renal adverse effects. Aminoglycosides may increase ototoxic or nephrotoxic effects.

**PREGNANCY:** Category D, not for use in nursing.

## CARDENE

nicardipine HCl (PDL) RX

**THERAPEUTIC CLASS:** Calcium channel blocker (dihydropyridine)

**INDICATIONS:** Treatment of hypertension. Management of chronic stable angina.

**DOSAGE:** *Adults:* >18 yrs: Initial: 20mg tid. Titrate: Increase dose every 3 days if needed. Usual: 20-40mg tid. Hepatic Dysfunction: Initial: 20mg bid.

**HOW SUPPLIED:** Cap: 20mg, 30mg

**CONTRAINDICATIONS:** Advanced aortic stenosis.

**WARNINGS/PRECAUTIONS:** Increased angina reported in patients with angina. Caution with CHF when titrating dose. Caution in hepatic/renal impairment, or reduced hepatic blood flow. May cause symptomatic hypotension. Measure BP 1-2 hrs and 8 hrs after dosing.

**ADVERSE REACTIONS:** Headache, pedal edema, vasodilation, palpitations, nausea, dizziness, asthenia, flushing, increased angina.

**INTERACTIONS:** Increased levels with cimetidine. Elevates cyclosporine levels. With β-blocker withdrawal, gradually reduce over 8-10 days. Monitor digoxin levels. Caution with fentanyl anesthesia.

**PREGNANCY:** Category C, not for use in nursing.

## CARDENE SR

nicardipine HCl (PDL)

RX

**THERAPEUTIC CLASS:** Calcium channel blocker (dihydropyridine)

**INDICATIONS:** Treatment of hypertension.

**DOSAGE:** *Adults:* Initial: 30mg bid. Usual: 30-60mg bid.

**HOW SUPPLIED:** Cap, Extended Release: 30mg, 45mg, 60mg

**CONTRAINDICATIONS:** Advanced aortic stenosis.

**WARNINGS/PRECAUTIONS:** Increased angina reported in patients with angina. Caution with CHF when titrating dose. Caution in hepatic/renal impairment, or reduced hepatic blood flow. May cause symptomatic hypotension. Measure BP 2-4 hrs after 1st dose or dose increase.

**ADVERSE REACTIONS:** Headache, pedal edema, vasodilation, palpitations, nausea, dizziness, asthenia, flushing, increased angina.

**INTERACTIONS:** Increased levels with cimetidine. Elevates cyclosporine levels. With β-blocker withdrawal, gradually reduce over 8-10 days. Monitor digoxin levels. Caution with fentanyl anesthesia.

**PREGNANCY:** Category C, not for use in nursing.

## CARDIZEM

diltiazem HCl (Biovail)

RX

**THERAPEUTIC CLASS:** Calcium channel blocker (nondihydropyridine)

**INDICATIONS:** Management of chronic stable angina or angina due to coronary artery spasm.

**DOSAGE:** *Adults:* Initial: 30mg qid (before meals and qhs). Adjust at 1-2 day intervals. Usual: 180-360mg/day.

**HOW SUPPLIED:** Tab: 30mg, 60mg*, 90mg*, 120mg* *scored

**CONTRAINDICATIONS:** Sick sinus syndrome and 2nd- or 3rd-degree AV block (except with functioning pacemaker), hypotension (<90mmHg systolic), acute MI, pulmonary congestion.

**WARNINGS/PRECAUTIONS:** Caution in renal, hepatic, or ventricular dysfunction. Monitor LFTs and renal function with prolonged use. Discontinue if persistent rash occurs. Symptomatic hypotension may occur. Acute hepatic injury reported.

**ADVERSE REACTIONS:** Headache, dizziness, asthenia, flushing, 1st-degree AV block, edema, nausea, bradycardia, rash.

**INTERACTIONS:** Increased levels of propranolol, digoxin, carbamazepine, cyclosporine; monitor closely. Increased levels of diltiazem with cimetidine. Potentiates the depression of cardiac contractility, conductivity, automaticity and vascular dilation with anesthetics. Additive cardiac conduction effects with digitalis or β-blockers. Potential additive effects with agents known to affect cardiac contractility and/or conduction. May increase levels of midazolam/triazolam. Avoid with CYP3A4 inducers.



**PREGNANCY:** Category C, not for use in nursing.

## CARDIZEM CD

RX

diltiazem HCl (Biovail)

**OTHER BRAND NAMES:** Cardizem LA (Kos) - Cartia XT (Andrx)

**THERAPEUTIC CLASS:** Calcium channel blocker (nondihydropyridine)

**INDICATIONS:** Treatment of hypertension. Management of chronic stable angina (LA) or angina due to coronary artery spasm.

**DOSAGE:** *Adults:* HTN: (CD, Cartia XT) Initial (monotherapy): 180-240mg qd. Titrate: Adjust at 2 week intervals. Usual: 240-360mg qd. Max: 480mg qd. (LA) Initial: 180-240mg qd. Adjust at 2 week intervals. Max: 540mg qd. Angina: (CD, Cartia XT) Initial: 120-180mg qd. Adjust at 1-2 week intervals. Max: 480mg/day. (LA) Initial: 180mg qd. Adjust at 1-2 week intervals.

**HOW SUPPLIED:** Cap, Extended Release: (Cardizem CD, Cartia XT) 120mg, 180mg, 240mg, 300mg, (Cardizem CD) 360mg; Tab, Extended Release: (Cardizem LA) 120mg, 180mg, 240mg, 300mg, 360mg, 420mg

**CONTRAINDICATIONS:** Sick sinus syndrome and 2nd- or 3rd-degree AV block (except with functioning pacemaker), hypotension (<90mmHg systolic), acute MI, pulmonary congestion.

**WARNINGS/PRECAUTIONS:** Caution in renal, hepatic, or ventricular dysfunction. Monitor LFTs and renal function with prolonged use. D/C if persistent rash occurs. Symptomatic hypotension may occur. Acute hepatic injury reported.

**ADVERSE REACTIONS:** Headache, dizziness, asthenia, flushing, 1st-degree AV block, edema, nausea, bradycardia, rash.

**INTERACTIONS:** May require dosage adjustment with concomitant CYP3A4 substrates. Increased levels of propranolol, digoxin, carbamazepine, lovastatin. Increased levels of diltiazem with cimetidine. May increase effects of benzodiazepines. Monitor digoxin, cyclosporine. Potentiates the depression of cardiac contractility, conductivity, automaticity and vascular dilation with anesthetics. Avoid concurrent use with CYP3A4 inducers (eg, rifampin). Additive cardiac conduction effects with digitalis or β-blockers. Potential additive effects with agents known to affect cardiac contractility and/or conduction.

**PREGNANCY:** Category C, not for use in nursing.

## CARDIZEM INJECTION

RX

diltiazem HCl (Biovail)

**OTHER BRAND NAMES:** Cardizem Lyo-Ject (Biovail) - Cardizem Monovial (Biovail)

**THERAPEUTIC CLASS:** Calcium channel blocker (nondihydropyridine)

**INDICATIONS:** Temporary control of rapid ventricular rate in atrial fibrillation/flutter (A-Fib/Flutter). Rapid conversion of paroxysmal supraventricular tachycardia (PSVT) to sinus rhythm.

**DOSAGE:** *Adults:* Bolus: (Injection/Lyo-Ject) 0.25mg/kg IV over 2 minutes. If no response after 15 minutes, may give 2nd dose of 0.35mg/kg over 2 minutes. Continuous Infusion: (Injection/Lyo-Ject/Monovial) 0.25-0.35mg/kg IV bolus, then 10mg/hr. Titrate: Increase by 5mg/hr. Max: 15mg/hr and duration up to 24 hrs.

**HOW SUPPLIED:** Inj: 5mg/mL, (Lyo-Ject) 25mg, (Monovial) 100mg

**CONTRAINDICATIONS:** Sick sinus syndrome and 2nd- or 3rd-degree AV block (except with functioning pacemaker), severe hypotension, cardiogenic shock, concomitant IV β-blockers or within a few hrs of use, A-Fib/Flutter associated with accessory bypass tract (eg, Wolff-Parkinson-White syndrome, short PR syndrome), ventricular tachycardia, (Lyo-Ject) neonates due to benzyl alcohol.

**WARNINGS/PRECAUTIONS:** Initiate in setting with resuscitation capabilities. Caution if hemodynamically compromised, and renal, hepatic, or ventricular dysfunction. Monitor ECG continuously and BP frequently. Symptomatic hypotension, acute hepatic injury reported. D/C if high-degree AV block occurs in sinus rhythm or if persistent rash occurs. Ventricular premature beats may be present on conversion of PSVT to sinus rhythm.

**ADVERSE REACTIONS:** Hypotension, injection site reactions (eg, itching, burning), vasodilation (flushing), arrhythmias.

**INTERACTIONS:** Caution with drugs that decrease peripheral resistance, intravascular volume, myocardial contractility or conduction. Increased AUC of midazolam, triazolam, buspirone, quinidine, and lovastatin; which may require a dose adjustment due to increased clinical effects or increased adverse events. Elevates carbamazepine levels, which may result in toxicity. Cyclosporine may need dose adjustment. Potentiates the depression of cardiac contractility, conductivity, automaticity and vascular dilation with anesthetics. Possible bradycardia, AV block, and contractility depression with oral β-blockers. Possible competitive inhibition of metabolism with drugs metabolized by CYP450. Avoid IV β-blockers and rifampin. Monitor for excessive slowing of HR and/or AV block with digoxin. Cimetidine increases peak diltiazem plasma levels and AUC.

**PREGNANCY:** Category C, not for use in nursing.

## CARDURA

RX

doxazosin mesylate (Pfizer)

**THERAPEUTIC CLASS:** $Alpha_1$-blocker (quinazoline)

**INDICATIONS:** Hypertension. Benign prostatic hyperplasia.

**DOSAGE:** *Adults:* HTN: Initial: 1mg qd (am or pm). Monitor BP 2-6 hrs and 24 hrs after 1st dose. Titrate: Increase to 2mg qd then upwards as needed. Max: 16mg/day. BPH: Initial: 1mg qd (am or pm). Titrate: May double the dose every 1-2 weeks. Max: 8mg/day.

**HOW SUPPLIED:** Tab: 1mg*, 2mg*, 4mg*, 8mg* *scored

**WARNINGS/PRECAUTIONS:** Monitor for orthostatic hypotension and syncope with 1st dose and dose increase. Caution with hepatic dysfunction. Rule out prostate cancer. Priapism (rare), leukopenia/neutropenia reported.

**ADVERSE REACTIONS:** Fatigue/malaise, hypotension, edema, dizziness, dyspnea, weight gain.

**PREGNANCY:** Category C, caution with nursing.

## CARDURA XL

RX

doxazosin mesylate (Pfizer)

**THERAPEUTIC CLASS:** $Alpha_1$-blocker (quinazoline)

**INDICATIONS:** Treatment of the signs and symptoms of benign prostatic hyperplasia.

**DOSAGE:** *Adults:* Initial: 4mg qd with breakfast. Titrate: May increase to 8mg after 3-4 weeks. Max: 8mg. Swallow whole; do not chew, divide, cut, or crush.

**HOW SUPPLIED:** Tab, Extended-Release: 4mg, 8mg

**WARNINGS/PRECAUTIONS:** Postural hypotension with or without symptoms (eg, dizziness) may develop; caution with symptomatic hypotension or hypotensive response to other medications. Rule out prostate cancer. Intraoperative Floppy Iris Syndrome has been observed during cataract surgery in some patients on or previously treated with $alpha_1$ blockers. Caution with preexisting severe GI narrowing (pathologic or iatrogenic). Caution with mild or moderate hepatic dysfunction; avoid with severe hepatic dysfunction. Discontinue with worsening of or new-onset angina pectoris symptoms.

**ADVERSE REACTIONS:** Dizziness, dyspnea, asthenia, headache, hypotension, postural hypotension, somnolence, respiratory tract infection, backache.

**INTERACTIONS:** Caution with potent CYP3A4 inhibitors (eg, atanazavir, clarithromycin, indinavir, itraconazole, ketoconazole, nefazodone, nelfinavir, ritonavir, saquinavir, telithromycin, voriconazole).

**PREGNANCY:** Category C, not for use in nursing.

## CARMOL 40

RX

urea (Doak)

**THERAPEUTIC CLASS:** Debriding/Healing Agent

**INDICATIONS:** Debridement and promotion of normal healing of hyperkeratotic surface lesions, particularly where healing is retarded by local infection, necrotic tissue, fibrinous or prurient debris or eschar. Treatment of hyperkeratotic conditions such as dry, rough skin, dermatitis, psoriasis, xerosis, ichthyosis, eczema, keratosis, corns and calluses, damaged ingrown and devitalized nails.

**DOSAGE:** *Adults:* Apply bid. Rub until absorbed.

**HOW SUPPLIED:** Cre: 40% [28.35g, 85g, 198.6g]; Gel: 40% [15mL]; Lot: 40% [236.6 mL]

**WARNINGS/PRECAUTIONS:** Avoid contact with eyes, lips, or mucous membranes.

**ADVERSE REACTIONS:** Transient stinging, burning, itching, or irritation

**PREGNANCY:** Category C, caution in nursing.

## CARTEOLOL

RX

carteolol HCl (Bausch & Lomb)

**THERAPEUTIC CLASS:** Nonselective beta-blocker

**INDICATIONS:** Reduction of IOP in chronic open-angle glaucoma and intraocular hypertension.

**DOSAGE:** *Adults:* 1 drop bid.

**HOW SUPPLIED:** Sol: 1% [5mL, 10mL, 15mL]

**CONTRAINDICATIONS:** Bronchial asthma, severe COPD, sinus bradycardia, 2nd- and 3rd-degree AV block, overt cardiac failure, cardiogenic shock.

**WARNINGS/PRECAUTIONS:** May be absorbed systemically. Caution with cardiac failure, bronchospasm, diminished pulmonary function, and DM. May mask symptoms of hypoglycemia and hyperthyroidism. Not for use alone in angle-closure glaucoma. May potentiate muscle weakness. Discontinue if develop cardiac failure. Withdrawal before surgery is controversial.

**ADVERSE REACTIONS:** Eye irritation, burning, tearing, conjunctival hyperemia, conjunctival edema, photophobia, decreased night vision, ptosis.

**INTERACTIONS:** May potentiate systemic effects with oral β-blockers. Possible hypotension and bradycardia with catecholamine-depleting drugs (eg, reserpine). May antagonize epinephrine.

**PREGNANCY:** Category C, caution in nursing.

## CASODEX

bicalutamide (AstraZeneca LP) RX

**THERAPEUTIC CLASS:** Non-steroidal antiandrogen

**INDICATIONS:** Treatment of stage $D_2$ metastatic carcinoma of the prostate in combination with a luteinizing hormone-releasing hormone (LHRH) analogue.

**DOSAGE:** *Adults:* 50mg qd at the same time each day. Initiate with LHRH analogue therapy.

**HOW SUPPLIED:** Tab: 50mg

**CONTRAINDICATIONS:** Women, pregnancy.

**WARNINGS/PRECAUTIONS:** Rare cases of death or hospitalization due to severe liver injury have been reported. Hepatitis and marked increases in liver enzymes leading to drug discontinuation have occured. Caution with moderate-severe hepatic impairment; serum transamine levels should be measured prior to starting treatment, at regular intervals for first four months, then periodically. Monitor PSA regularly to assess therapy. For patients who have objective progression of disease together with an elevated PSA, a treatment-free period of anti-androgen, while continuing LHRH analogue, may be considered. Gynecomastia, breast pain reported with single agent.

**ADVERSE REACTIONS:** Hot flashes, pain, back pain, asthenia, constipation, pelvic pain, infection, nausea, dyspnea, peripheral edema, diarrhea, hematuria, nocturia.

**INTERACTIONS:** Can displace coumarin anticoagulants, such as warfarin, from their protein-binding sites; monitor PT.

**PREGNANCY:** Category X, caution in nursing.

## CATAFLAM

diclofenac potassium (Novartis) RX

**NSAIDs may cause an increased risk of serious cardiovascular thrombotic events, MI, stroke and serious GI adverse events including bleeding, ulceration, and perforation of the stomach or intestines. Contraindicated for the treatment of peri-operative pain in the setting of coronary artery bypass graft (CABG) surgery.**

**THERAPEUTIC CLASS:** NSAID (benzeneacetic acid derivative)

**INDICATIONS:** Relief of signs and symptoms of osteoarthritis (OA) and rheumatoid arthritis (RA). Treatment of primary dysmenorrhea and relief of mild to moderate pain.

**DOSAGE:** *Adults:* OA: 50mg bid-tid. Max: 150mg/day. RA: 50mg tid-qid. Max: 200mg/day. Pain/Primary Dysmenorrhea: Initial: 50mg tid or 100mg on 1st dose, then 50mg on subsequent doses.

**HOW SUPPLIED:** Tab: 50mg

**CONTRAINDICATIONS:** ASA or other NSAID allergy that precipitates asthma, urticaria or allergic reactions. Treatment of peri-operative pain in the setting of CABG surgery.

**WARNINGS/PRECAUTIONS:** May lead to onset of new HTN or worsening of pre-existing HTN; monitor BP closely. Fluid retention and edema reported; caution with fluid retention or heart failure. Renal papillary necrosis and other renal injury reported after long-term use. Not recommended for use with advanced renal disease; if therapy must be initiated, monitor renal function. Anaphylactoid reactions may occur. May cause serious skin adverse events (eg, exfoliative dermatitis, Stevens-Johnson syndrome, and toxic epidermal necrolysis). Avoid in late pregnancy; may cause premature closure of ductus arteriosis. May cause elevations of LFTs; discontinue if liver disease develops or systemic manifestations occur. Caution in elderly. Anemia may occur; with long-term use, monitor Hgb/Hct if signs or symptoms of anemia develop. May inhibit platelet aggregation and prolong bleeding time; monitor with coagulation disorders. Caution with asthma and avoid with aspirin-sensitive asthma.

**ADVERSE REACTIONS:** Fluid retention, dizziness, rash, nausea, abdominal cramps, LFT abnormalities, constipation, diarrhea, heartburn, tinnitus, GI ulceration, HTN, insomnia, stomatitis, pruritus.



**INTERACTIONS:** Avoid with other diclofenac products. Increased adverse effects with ASA; avoid use. May enhance methotrexate toxicity; caution when co-administering. May increase nephrotoxicity of cyclosporine; caution when co-administering. May diminish antihypertensive effect of ACE-inhibitors. May reduce natriuretic effect of furosemide and thiazides; monitor for renal failure. May increase lithium levels; monitor for toxicity. Synergistic effects on GI bleeding with warfarin.

**PREGNANCY:** Category C, not for use in nursing.

## CATAPRES

RX

clonidine (Boehringer Ingelheim)

**OTHER BRAND NAMES:** Catapres-TTS (Boehringer Ingelheim)

**THERAPEUTIC CLASS:** Central alpha-adrenergic agonist

**INDICATIONS:** Treatment of hypertension.

**DOSAGE:** *Adults:* (Patch) Apply to hairless, intact area of upper arm or chest weekly. Taper withdrawal of previous antihypertensive. Initial: 0.1mg/24hr patch weekly. Titrate: May increase after 1-2 weeks. Max: 0.6mg/24hr. (Tab) Initial: 0.1mg bid. Titrate: May increase by 0.1mg weekly. Usual: 0.2-0.6mg/day in divided doses. Max: 2.4mg/day. (Patch, Tab) Renal Impairment: Adjust according to degree of impairment.

**HOW SUPPLIED:** Patch, Extended Release (TTS): 0.1mg/24hr [12[s]], 0.2mg/24hr [12[s]], 0.3mg/24hr [4[s]]; Tab: 0.1mg*, 0.2mg*, 0.3mg* *scored

**WARNINGS/PRECAUTIONS:** Avoid abrupt discontinuation. Tabs may cause rash if have allergic reaction to patch. Continue tabs to within 4 hrs of surgery resume and as soon as possible thereafter. Do not remove patch for surgery. Caution with severe coronary insufficiency, conduction disturbances, recent MI, cerebrovascular disease or chronic renal failure. Remove patch before defibrillation or cardioversion due to the potential risk of altered electrical conductivity or MRI due to the ocurrence of burns.

**ADVERSE REACTIONS:** Dry mouth, drowsiness, dizziness, constipation, sedation, impotence/sexual dysfunction, nausea, vomiting, alopecia, weakness, orthostatic symptoms, nervousness, localized skin reactions (patch).

**INTERACTIONS:** May potentiate CNS depression with alcohol, barbiturates, or other sedatives. Additive bradycardia and AV block with agents that affect sinus node function or AV nodal conduction (eg, digitalis, calcium channel blockers, and β-blockers). Hypotensive effect reduced by TCAs.

**PREGNANCY:** Category C, caution in nursing.

## CATHFLO ACTIVASE

RX

alteplase (Genentech)

**THERAPEUTIC CLASS:** Thrombolytic agent

**INDICATIONS:** To restore function to central venous access devices as assessed by ability to withdraw blood.

**DOSAGE:** *Adults:* >30kg: 2mg in 2mL. <30kg: 110% of catheter internal lumen volume, not to exceed 2mg in 2mL. If function not restored after 120 minutes, may instill 2nd dose. Max: 2mg/dose. Reconstitute to final concentration of 1mg/mL.
*Pediatrics:* >2 yrs: >30kg: 2mg in 2mL. 10 to <30kg: 110% of catheter internal lumen volume, not to exceed 2mg in 2mL. If function not restored after 120

minutes, may instill 2nd dose. Max: 2mg/dose. Reconstitute to final concentration of 1mg/mL.

**HOW SUPPLIED:** Inj: 2mg

**WARNINGS/PRECAUTIONS:** Before therapy, consider catheter dysfunction due to causes other than thrombus formation. Avoid excessive pressure when instilling alteplase into catheter. Discontinue and withdraw drug from catheter if serious bleeding in critical location occurs. Caution if active internal bleeding, infection in the catheter, any bleeding condition that is difficult to manage, thrombocytopenia, hemostatic defects, or if high risk for emobolic complications. Caution if any of the following occurred within 48 hrs: sugery, OB delivery, percutaneous biopsy of viscera or deep tissues, or puncture of non-compressible vessels.

**ADVERSE REACTIONS:** Sepsis, GI bleeding, venous thrombosis.

**PREGNANCY:** Category C, caution in nursing.

## CAVERJECT

RX

alprostadil (Pharmacia & Upjohn)

**OTHER BRAND NAMES:** Caverject Impulse (Pharmacia & Upjohn)

**THERAPEUTIC CLASS:** Prostaglandin $E_1$

**INDICATIONS:** Treatment of erectile dysfunction (ED) due to neurogenic, vasculogenic, psychogenic, or mixed etiology. Adjunct for diagnosis of ED.

**DOSAGE:** *Adults:* Intracavernosal Injection. Avoid visible veins; alternate site and side. Determine dose in office. If no initial response, may give next higher dose within 1 hr. If partial response, give next higher dose after 24 hrs. Vasculogenic/Psychogenic/Mixed Etiology: Initial: 2.5mcg. Partial Response: Increase by 2.5mcg, then by 5-10mcg until desired response. No Response: Increase by 5mcg, then by 5-10mcg until desired response. Neurogenic Etiology (Spinal Cord Injury): Initial: 1.25mcg. Partial/No Response: May give 2nd dose of 2.5mcg, 3rd dose of 5mcg, then may increase by 5mcg until desired response. Max: 60mcg/dose. Reduce dose if erection >1 hour. Give no more than 3 times weekly; allow 24 hrs between doses.

**HOW SUPPLIED:** Inj: 0.02mg/mL, (Impulse) 10mcg, 20mcg, (Powder) 5mcg, 10mcg, 20mcg, 40mcg

**CONTRAINDICATIONS:** Predisposition to priapism (eg, sickle cell anemia, multiple myeloma, leukemia), penis anatomical deformation (eg, angulation, cavernosal fibrosis, Peyronie's disease), penile implants, those in whom sexual activities are contraindicated, women, children or newborns.

**WARNINGS/PRECAUTIONS:** Impluse device is for single use only. Treat erections lasting >4 hrs immediately. Penile fibrosis, including Peyronie's disease reported. Follow-up with patient to detect penile fibrosis. If possible, treat underlying cause of ED before therapy. Blood at injection site increases risk of blood-borne disease transmission.

**ADVERSE REACTIONS:** Penile pain, priapism/prolonged erection, penile fibrosis, hematoma/bleeding at injection site.

**INTERACTIONS:** Increased injection site bleeding with anticoagulants (eg, warfarin, heparin). Avoid other vasoactive agents.

**PREGNANCY:** Not for use in women.

## CEDAX

RX

ceftibuten (Shionogi)

**THERAPEUTIC CLASS:** Cephalosporin (3rd generation)

**INDICATIONS:** Acute bacterial exacerbations of chronic bronchitis (ABECB), acute bacterial otitis media, pharyngitis and tonsillitis.

**DOSAGE:** *Adults:* ABECB/Otitis Media/Pharyngitis/Tonsillitis: 400mg qd for 10 days. Max: 400mg/day. CrCl 30-49mL/min: 4.5mg/kg or 200mg qd. CrCl 5-29mL/min: 2.25mg/kg or 100mg qd. Take 2 hrs before or at least 1 hr after a meal.
*Pediatrics:* >6 months: Pharyngitis/Tonsillitis/Otitis Media: 9mg/kg qd for 10 days. Max: 400mg. ABECB/Otitis Media/Pharyngitis/Tonsillitis: >12 yrs: 400mg qd for 10 days. Max: 400mg/day. CrCl 30-49mL/min: 4.5mg/kg or 200mg qd. CrCl 5-29mL/min: 2.25mg/kg or 100mg qd. Take 2 hrs before or at least 1 hr after a meal.

**HOW SUPPLIED:** Cap: 400mg; Sus: 90mg/5mL [30mL, 60mL, 90mL, 120mL]

**WARNINGS/PRECAUTIONS:** Pseudomembranous colitis reported. Caution with history of GI disease. Cross-sensitivity with cephalosporins and penicillins.

**ADVERSE REACTIONS:** Diarrhea, vomiting, abdominal pain, anorexia, dizziness, dyspepsia, dry mouth, dyspnea, dysuria, fatigue, flatulence, loose stooles, headache, pruritus, rash, rigors, urticaria, superinfection (prolonged use).

**PREGNANCY:** Category B, caution in nursing.

## CEENU

lomustine (Bristol-Myers Squibb) RX

**Bone marrow suppression (eg, thrombocytopenia, leukopenia) may contribute to bleeding and infections in compromised patients. Monitor blood counts weekly for 6 weeks after each dose. Adjust dose based on nadir blood counts from prior dose.**

**THERAPEUTIC CLASS:** Nitrosourea alkylating agent

**INDICATIONS:** Single or adjunct treatment in primary/metastatic brain tumors in patients who already received surgical and/or radiation therapy. Secondary combination therapy of Hodgkin's disease in patients who relapse/fail primary therapy.

**DOSAGE:** *Adults:* Single Regimen/Previously Untreated: 130mg/m$^2$ PO single dose every 6 weeks. Compromised Bone Marrow: 100mg/m$^2$ PO single dose every 6 weeks. Subsequent Doses: Adjust according to hematologic response. Leukocytes 2000-2999, platelets 25,000-74,999: Give 70% of dose. Leukocytes <2000, platelets <25,000: Give 50% of dose.
*Pediatrics:* Single Regimen/Previously Untreated: 130mg/m$^2$ PO single dose every 6 weeks. Compromised Bone Marrow: 100mg/m$^2$ PO single dose every 6 weeks. Subsequent Doses: Adjust according to hematologic response. Leukocytes 2000-2999, platelets 25,000-74,999: Give 70% of dose. Leukocytes <2000, platelets <25,000: Give 50% of dose.

**HOW SUPPLIED:** Cap: 10mg, 40mg, 100mg

**WARNINGS/PRECAUTIONS:** Pulmonary toxicity is dose-related. May develop secondary malignancies with long-term use. Monitor hepatic and renal function. Caution in elderly.

**ADVERSE REACTIONS:** Delayed myleosuppression, pulmonary infiltrates/fibrosis, nausea, vomiting, hepatotoxicity, azotemia, renal failure, stomatitis, alopecia, optic atrophy, visual disturbances, lethargy, ataxia.

**PREGNANCY:** Category D, not for use in nursing.

## CEFACLOR

cefaclor (Various) RX

**THERAPEUTIC CLASS:** Cephalosporin (2nd generation)

**INDICATIONS:** Treatment of otitis media, pharyngitis, tonsillitis, lower respiratory tract, urinary tract, and skin and skin structure infections caused by susceptible strains of microorganisms.

**DOSAGE:** *Adults:* Usual: 250mg q8h. Severe Infections/Pneumonia: 500mg q8h. Treat β-hemolytic strep for 10 days.
*Pediatrics:* >1 month: Usual: 20mg/kg/day given q8h. Otitis Media/Serious Infections: 40mg/kg/day. Max: 1g/day. May administer q12h for otitis media and pharyngitis. Treat β-hemolytic strep for 10 days.

**HOW SUPPLIED:** Cap: 250mg, 500mg; Sus: 125mg/5mL [75mL, 150mL], 187mg/5mL [50mL, 100mL], 250mg/5mL [75mL, 150mL], 375mg/5mL [50mL, 100mL]

**WARNINGS/PRECAUTIONS:** Cross sensitivity to penicillins and other cephalosporins may occur. Pseudomembranous colitis reported. Positive direct Coombs' tests reported. Caution with markedly impaired renal function, history of GI disease. False (+) for urine glucose with Benedict's, Fehling's solution, and Clinitest tablets.

**ADVERSE REACTIONS:** Hypersensitivity reactions, diarrhea, eosinophilia, genital pruritus and vaginitis, serum-sickness-like reactions, superinfection.

**INTERACTIONS:** Renal excretion inhibited by probenecid. May potentiate warfarin and other anticoagulants; monitor PT/INR.

**PREGNANCY:** Category B, caution in nursing.

## CEFACLOR ER — RX

cefaclor (Various)

**THERAPEUTIC CLASS:** Cephalosporin (2nd generation)

**INDICATIONS:** Acute bacterial exacerbation of chronic bronchitis (ABECB), secondary bacterial infections of acute bronchitis, pharyngitis, tonsillitis, and uncomplicated skin and skin structure infections (SSSI) caused by susceptible strains of microorganisms.

**DOSAGE:** *Adults:* ABECB/Acute Bronchitis: 500mg q12h for 7 days. Pharyngitis/Tonsillitis: 375mg q12h for 10 days. SSSI: 375mg q12h for 7-10 days. Take with meals. Do not crush, cut or chew tab.
*Pediatrics:* >16 yrs: ABECB/Acute Bronchitis: 500mg q12h for 7 days. Pharyngitis/Tonsillitis: 375mg q12h for 10 days. SSSI: 375mg q12h for 7-10 days. Take with meals. Do not crush, cut or chew tab.

**HOW SUPPLIED:** Tab, Extended Release: 375mg, 500mg

**WARNINGS/PRECAUTIONS:** Cross sensitivity to penicillins and other cephalosporins may occur. Pseudomembranous colitis reported. False (+) direct Coombs' tests reported. Caution with markedly impaired renal function, history of GI disease. False (+) for urine glucose with Benedict's, Fehling's solution, and Clinitest® tablets.

**ADVERSE REACTIONS:** Headache, rhinitis, diarrhea, nausea, vomiting, vaginitis, abdominal pain, pharyngitis, increased cough, pruritus, back pain, serum-sickness-like reactions, superinfection (prolonged use).

**INTERACTIONS:** Decreased absorption with antacids containing aluminum or magnesium hydroxide; space dose by 1 hr. Potentiated by probenecid. May potentiate warfarin, and other anticoagulants; monitor PT/INR.

**PREGNANCY:** Category B, caution in nursing.

## CEFIZOX — RX

ceftizoxime (Astellas)

**THERAPEUTIC CLASS:** Cephalosporin (3rd generation)

**INDICATIONS:** Treatment of lower respiratory tract, skin and skin structure, intra-abdominal, bone and joint, and urinary tract infections (UTI), gonorrhea, pelvic inflammatory disease (PID), meningitis, and septicemia.

**DOSAGE:** *Adults:* Uncomplicated UTI: 500mg q12h IM/IV. Other Sites: 1g q8-12h IM/IV. Severe/Refractory Infections: 1-2g IM/IV q8-12h. PID: 2g IV q8h. Life

Threatening Infections: 3-4g IV q8h. Uncomplicated Gonorrhea: 1g IM as single dose. Renal Impairment: LD: 500mg-1g IM/IV. Less Severe Infection: Maint: CrCl 50-79mL/min: 500mg q8h. CrCl 5-49mL/min: 250-500mg q12h. CrCl 0-4mL/min (Dialysis): 500mg q48h or 250mg q24h. Life Threatening Infection: Maint: CrCl 50-79mL/min: 0.75-1.5g q8h. CrCl 5-49mL/min: 0.5-1g q12h. CrCl 0-4mL/min (Dialysis): 0.5-1g q48h or 0.5g q24h.
*Pediatrics:* >6 months: 50mg/kg IM/IV q6-8h, up to 200mg/kg/day. Max: 6g/day for serious infections.

**HOW SUPPLIED:** Inj: 1g, 2g, 10g

**WARNINGS/PRECAUTIONS:** Pseudomembranous colitis reported. Caution with history of GI disease. Cross-sensitivity with cephalosporins and penicillins. Prolonged use may result in overgrowth of superinfection, positive Coombs test.

**ADVERSE REACTIONS:** Rash, pruritus, fever, BUN elevation, injection site reactions (eg, burning, cellulitis, phlebitis, pain, induration, tenderness), eosinophilia, thrombocytosis, elevated liver enzymes, GI effects.

**INTERACTIONS:** Risk of nephrotoxicity with aminoglycosides.

**PREGNANCY:** Category B, caution in nursing.

## CEFOL RX

multiple vitamin (Abbott)

**THERAPEUTIC CLASS:** Vitamin supplement

**INDICATIONS:** Vitamin C deficiency associated with deficient intake or increased need for Vitamin B-Complex, Folic Acid, and Vitamin E in non-pregnant patients.

**DOSAGE:** *Adults:* 1 tab qd.

**HOW SUPPLIED:** Tab: Calcium Pantothenate 20mg-Folic Acid 0.5mg-Niacinamide 100mg-Vitamin $B_1$ 15mg-Vitamin $B_2$ 10mg-Vitamin $B_6$ 5mg-Vitamin $B_{12}$ 6mcg-Vitamin C 750mg-Vitamin E 30 IU

**WARNINGS/PRECAUTIONS:** Folic acid alone is improper treatment of pernicious anemia and other megaloblastic anemias with Vitamin $B_{12}$-deficiency. Folic acid >0.1mg/day may obscure pernicious anemia.

**ADVERSE REACTIONS:** Allergic sensitization.

**PREGNANCY:** Safety in pregnancy and nursing not known.

## CEFOXITIN RX

cefoxitin sodium (Various)

**OTHER BRAND NAMES:** Mefoxin (Merck)

**THERAPEUTIC CLASS:** Cephalosporin (2nd generation)

**INDICATIONS:** Treatment of lower respiratory tract, urinary tract, intra-abdominal, gynecological, skin and skin structure, and bone and joint infections, and septicemia. For surgical prophylaxis.

**DOSAGE:** *Adults:* Usual: 1-2g IV q6-8h. Uncomplicated Infections: 1g IV q6-8h. Moderate-Severe: 1g IV q4h or 2g IV q6-8h. Gas Gangrene/Other Infections Requiring Higher Dose: 2g IV q4h or 3g IV q6h. Renal Insufficiency: LD: 1-2g IV. Maint: CrCl 30-50mL/min: 1-2g IV q8-12h. CrCl 10-29mL/min: 1-2g IV q12-24h. CrCl 5-9mL/min: 0.5-1g IV q12-24h. CrCl <5mL/min: 0.5-1g IV q24-48h. Hemodialysis: LD: 1-2g IV after dialysis. Maint: See renal insufficiency doses above. Prophylaxis: Uncontaminated GI Surgery/Hysterectomy: 2g IV 0.5-1 hr prior to surgery, then 2g IV q6h after first dose up to 24 hrs. C-Section: 2g IV single dose after umbilical cord is clamped, or 2g IV after umbilical cord is clamped followed by 2g IV 4 and 8 hrs after initial dose.
*Pediatrics:* >3 months: 80-160mg/kg/day divided into 4-6 equal doses. Max: 12g/day. Prophylaxis: Uncontaminated GI Surgery/Hysterectomy: 30-

40mg/kg IV 0.5-1 hr prior to surgery, then 30-40mg/kg IV q6h after first dose up to 24 hrs.

**HOW SUPPLIED:** Inj: 1g, 1g/50mL, 2g, 2g/50mL, 10g

**WARNINGS/PRECAUTIONS:** Possible cross-sensitivity between penicillins and cephalosporins. Pseudomembranous colitis reported. Caution with allergies, GI disease, particularly colitis. Prolonged use may result in overgrowth of nonsusceptible organisms. Monitor renal, hepatic, hematopoietic functions, especially with prolonged therapy. False positive for urine glucose with Clinitest tablets.

**ADVERSE REACTIONS:** Thrombophlebitis, rash, pseudomembranous colitis, pruritus, fever, dyspnesa hypotension, diarrhea, blood dyscrasias, elevated LFTs, changes in renal function tests, exacerbation of myasthenia gravis.

**INTERACTIONS:** Increased nephrotoxicity with concomitant aminoglycosides.

**PREGNANCY:** Category B, caution use in nursing.

## CEFTIN

RX

cefuroxime axetil (GlaxoSmithKline)

**THERAPEUTIC CLASS:** Cephalosporin (2nd generation)

**INDICATIONS:** (Sus/Tab) Pharyngitis/tonsillitis, acute otitis media, and impetigo. (Tab) Uncomplicated skin and skin structure (SSSI), and urinary tract infection (UTI), gonorrhea, early lyme disease, acute bacterial maxillary sinusitis, acute bacterial exacerbations of chronic bronchitis (ABECB) and secondary bacterial infections of acute bronchitis.

**DOSAGE:** *Adults:* (Tab) Pharyngitis/Tonsillitis/Sinusitis: 250mg bid for 10 days. ABECB/SSSI: 250-500mg bid for 10 days. Acute Bronchitis: 250-500mg bid for 5-10 days. UTI: 125-250mg bid for 7-10 days. Gonorrhea: 1000mg single dose. Lyme Disease: 500mg bid for 20 days.
*Pediatrics:* >13 yrs: (Tab) Pharyngitis/Tonsillitis/Sinusitis: 250mg bid for 10 days. ABECB/SSSI: 250-500mg bid for 10 days. Acute Bronchitis: 250-500mg bid for 5-10 days. UTI: 125-250mg bid for 7-10 days. Gonorrhea: 1000mg single dose. Lyme Disease: 500mg bid for 20 days. 3 months-12 yrs: (Sus) Pharyngitis/Tonsillitis: 10mg/kg bid for 10 days. Max: 500mg/day. Otitis Media/Sinusitis/Impetigo: 15mg/kg bid for 10 days. Max: 1000mg/day. (Tab-if can swallow whole) Pharyngitis/Tonsillitis: 125mg bid for 10 days. Otitis Media/Sinusitis: 250mg bid for 10 days.

**HOW SUPPLIED:** Sus: 125mg/5mL [100mL], 250mg/5mL [50mL, 100mL]; Tab: 125mg, 250mg, 500mg

**WARNINGS/PRECAUTIONS:** Tablets are not bioequivalent to suspension. Caution with colitis, renal impairment. Cross-sensitivity with cephalosporins and penicillins. Pseudomembranous colitis reported. False (+) for urine glucose with Benedict's, Fehling's solution, and Clinitest® tablets. May cause fall in PT; risk in patients stable on anticoagulants, if receiving protracted course of antibiotics, renal/hepatic impairment, or a poor nutritional state; give vitamin K as needed.

**ADVERSE REACTIONS:** Diarrhea, nausea, vomiting, vaginitis, (suspension in peds) taste dislike, superinfection (prolonged use).

**INTERACTIONS:** Probenecid increases plasma levels. Lower bioavailability with drugs that lower gastric acidity. Caution with agents causing adverse effects on renal function (diuretics).

**PREGNANCY:** Category B, not for use in nursing.

## CEFZIL

RX

cefprozil (Bristol-Myers Squibb)

C

**THERAPEUTIC CLASS:** Cephalosporin (2nd generation)

**INDICATIONS:** Mild to moderate pharyngitis/tonsillitis, otitis media, acute sinusitis, secondary bacterial infection of acute bronchitis, acute bacterial exacerbation of chronic bronchitis (ABECB), and uncomplicated skin and skin structure infections (SSSI).

**DOSAGE:** *Adults:* >13 yrs: Pharyngitis/Tonsillitis: 500mg q24h for 10 days. Acute Sinusitis: 250-500mg q12h for 10 days. ABECB/Acute Bronchitis: 500mg q12h for 10 days. SSSI: 250-500mg q12h or 500mg q24h. CrCl <30mL/min: 50% of standard dose.
*Pediatrics:* 2-12 yrs: Pharyngitis/Tonsillitis: 7.5mg/kg q12h for 10 days. SSSI: 20mg/kg q24h for 10 days. 6 months-12 yrs: Otitis Media: 15mg/kg q12h for 10 days. Acute Sinusitis: 7.5-15mg/kg q12h for 10 days. Do not exceed adult dose. CrCl <30mL/min: 50% of standard dose.

**HOW SUPPLIED:** Sus: 125mg/5mL, 250mg/5mL [50mL, 75mL, 100mL]; Tab: 250mg, 500mg

**WARNINGS/PRECAUTIONS:** Cross-sensitivity with cephalosporins and penicillins. False (+) direct Coombs' tests reported. Pseudomembranous colitis reported. Caution with GI disease, renal impairment, elderly. False (+) for urine glucose with Benedict's, Fehling's solution, and Clinitest® tablets. Suspension contains phenylalanine.

**ADVERSE REACTIONS:** Diarrhea, nausea, hepatic enzyme elevations, eosinophilia, genital pruritus, genital vaginitis, superinfection (prolonged use).

**INTERACTIONS:** Nephrotoxicity with aminoglycosides reported. Probenecid may increase plasma levels. Caution with agents causing adverse effects on renal function (diuretics).

**PREGNANCY:** Category B, caution in nursing.

## CELEBREX

RX

celecoxib (Searle)

**NSAIDs may cause an increased risk of serious cardiovascular thrombotic events, MI, stroke and serious GI adverse events including bleeding, ulceration, and perforation of the stomach or intestines. Contraindicated for the treatment of peri-operative pain in the setting of coronary artery bypass graft (CABG) surgery.**

**THERAPEUTIC CLASS:** COX-2 inhibitor

**INDICATIONS:** Relief of signs and symtoms of rheumatoid arthritis (RA) in adults, osteoarthritis (OA), and ankylosing spondylitis (AS). Management of acute pain in adults. Treatment of primary dysmenorrhea. To reduce the number of adematous colorectal polyps in familial adenomatous polyposis (FAP). Relief of signs and symptoms of juvenile rheumatoid arthritis (JRA) in patients ≥2 yrs.

**DOSAGE:** *Adults:* >18 yrs: OA: 200mg qd or 100mg bid. RA: 100-200mg bid. AS: 200mg qd or 100mg bid. Titrate: May increase to 400mg/day after 6 weeks. FAP: 400mg bid with food. Acute Pain/Primary Dysmenorrhea: Day 1: 400mg, then 200mg if needed. Maint: 200mg bid prn. Moderate Hepatic Insufficiency: Reduce daily dose by 50%.
*Pediatrics:* JRA: ≥2 yrs: 10-25 kg: 50mg bid. >25 kg: 100mg bid.

**HOW SUPPLIED:** Cap: 50mg, 100mg, 200mg, 400mg

**CONTRAINDICATIONS:** Sulfonamide hypersensitivity. Asthma, urticaria, or allergic type reactions after ASA or NSAID use. Treatment of peri-operative pain in the setting of CABG surgery.

**WARNINGS/PRECAUTIONS:** May lead to onset of new HTN or worsening of pre-existing HTN; monitor BP closely. Fluid retention and edema reported; caution with fluid retention or heart failure. Renal papillary necrosis and other renal injury reported after long-term use. Not recommended for use with advanced renal disease; if therapy must be initiated, monitor renal function. Anaphylactoid reactions may occur. May cause serious skin adverse events (eg, exfoliative dermatitis, Stevens-Johnson syndrome, and toxic epidermal necrolysis). Avoid in late pregnancy; may cause premature closure of ductus arteriosis. May cause elevations of LFTs; d/c if liver disease develops or systemic manifestations occur. Caution in elderly. Anemia may occur; with long-term use, monitor Hgb/Hct if signs or symptoms of anemia or blood loss develop. May inhibit platelet aggregation and prolong bleeding time (prolonged APTT); monitor with coagulation disorders. Caution with asthma and avoid with aspirin-sensitive asthma. Caution in pediatric patients with systemic onset JRA due to increased possibly of DIC.

**ADVERSE REACTIONS:** Dyspepsia, diarrhea, abdominal pain, nausea, dizziness, headache, sinusitis, upper respiratory infection, rash, fever, cough, arthralgia.

**INTERACTIONS:** Monitor oral anticoagulants; reports of serious bleeding, some fatal, with warfarin. Decrease effects of ACEIs, furosemide, and thiazides. Increased levels with fluconazole. Monitor lithium. Caution with CYP2C9 inhibitors and drugs metabolized by CYP2D6. Celecoxib is not a substitute for ASA for cardiovascular prophylaxis; may use with low-dose ASA but may increase GI complications.

**PREGNANCY:** Category C, not for use in nursing.

## CELESTONE — RX

betamethasone (Schering)

**THERAPEUTIC CLASS:** Glucocorticoid

**INDICATIONS:** Steroid responsive disorders.

**DOSAGE:** *Adults:* Initial: 0.6-7.2mg/day depending on disease. Maintain until sufficient response. Maint: Decrease dose by small amounts to lowest effective dose. Discontinue gradually.
*Pediatrics:* Initial: 0.6-7.2mg/day depending on disease. Maintain until sufficient response. Maint: Decrease dose by small amounts to lowest effective dose. Discontinue gradually.

**HOW SUPPLIED:** Syrup: 0.6mg/5mL [118mL]

**CONTRAINDICATIONS:** Systemic fungal infections.

**WARNINGS/PRECAUTIONS:** May need to increase dose before, during, and after stressful situations. May mask signs of infection or cause new infections. Prolonged use may produce posterior subcapsular cataracts, glaucoma, optic nerve damage, secondary ocular infections. Increases BP, salt/water retention, potassium and calcium excretion. More severe/fatal course of infections reported with chickenpox, measles. Caution with threadworm infestation, latent TB, hypothyroidism, cirrhosis, ocular herpes simplex, HTN, diverticulitis, fresh intestinal anastomosis, ulcerative colitis, osteoporosis, myasthenia gravis, renal insufficiency, peptic ulcer disease. Growth and development of children on prolonged therapy should be monitored. Monitor for psychic disturbances. Avoid abrupt withdrawal.

**ADVERSE REACTIONS:** Sodium retention, fluid retention, potassium loss, muscle weakness, myopathy, peptic ulcer, impaired wound healing, thin fragile skin, convulsions, menstrual irregularities, cataracts.

**INTERACTIONS:** Caution with ASA in hypoprothrombinemia. Increased susceptibility to infections with immunosuppressives. Avoid smallpox vaccines and other immunization procedures at high doses. Increased requirements of insulin or oral hypoglycemic agents.

**PREGNANCY:** Safety in pregnancy and nursing not known.

## CELESTONE SOLUSPAN RX

betamethasone acetate - betamethasone sodium phosphate (Schering)



**THERAPEUTIC CLASS:** Glucocorticoid

**INDICATIONS:** When oral therapy is not feasible, use IM route for steroid responsive treatment of endocrine, rheumatic, collagen, dermatologic, respiratory, ophthalmic, neoplastic, hematologic, and GI disorders, allergic and edematous states and Tuberculous meningitis with subarachnoid block and trichinosis with neurologic/myocardial involvement. Intra-articular or soft tissue administration for short-term adjunct treatment of synovitis, osteoarthritis (OA), rheumatoid arthritis (RA), bursitis, acute gouty arthritis, epicondylitis, acute nonspecific tenosynovitis. Intralesional injection for keloids, discoid lupus erythematosus, necrobiosis lipoidica diabeticorum, alopecia areata, lesions of: lichen planus, psoriatic plaques, granuloma, annulare, lichen simplex chronicus.

**DOSAGE:** *Adults:* Initial: 0.5-9mg/day IM. Parenteral dose is usually 1/2-1/3 the oral dose given q12h. Maintain until sufficient response occurs. Maint: Decrease in small increments at appropriate time intervals until lowest effective dose. Discontinue gradually. Bursitis/Tenosynovitis/Peritendinitis: 1mL intrabursal injection. Tenosynovitis/Tendinitis: Give 3-4 injections every 1-2 weeks. Chronic Bursitis: Reduce initial dose. Ganglion Cysts: 0.5mL into cyst. RA/OA: 0.5-2mL intra-articularly. Dermatologic Conditions: 0.2mL/sq cm intradermally. Max: 1mL/week.
*Pediatrics:* Initial: 0.5-9mg/day IM. Parenteral dose is usually 1/2-1/3 the oral dose given q12h. Maintain until sufficient response. Maint: Decrease in small increments at appropriate time intervals until reach lowest dose that sustains response. Discontinue gradually.

**HOW SUPPLIED:** Inj: (Betamethasone Acetate-Betamethasone Sodium Phosphate) 3mg-3mg/mL

**CONTRAINDICATIONS:** Systemic fungal infections.

**WARNINGS/PRECAUTIONS:** May need to increase dose before, during, and after stressful situations. May mask signs of infection or cause new infections. Prolonged use may produce posterior subcapsular cataracts, glaucoma, optic nerve damage, secondary ocular infections. Increases BP, salt/water retention, potassium and calcium excretion. More severe/fatal course of infections reported with chickenpox, measles. Caution with threadworm infestation, latent TB, hypothyroidism, cirrhosis, ocular herpes simplex, HTN, diverticulitis, fresh intestinal anastomosis, ulcerative colitis, osteoporosis, myasthenia gravis, renal insufficiency, peptic ulcer disease. Growth and development of children on prolonged therapy should be monitored. Monitor for psychic disturbances. Avoid abrupt withdrawal. (Intra-articular) Examine joint fluid to rule out a septic process. Avoid injection into previously infected joint.

**ADVERSE REACTIONS:** Sodium retention, fluid retention, potassium loss, muscle weakness, myopathy, peptic ulcer, impaired wound healing, thin fragile skin, convulsions, menstrual irregularities, cataracts.

**INTERACTIONS:** Caution with ASA in hypoprothrombinemia. Increased susceptibility to infections with immunosuppressives. Avoid smallpox vaccines and other immunization procedures at high doses. Increased requirements of insulin or oral hypoglycemic agents. Avoid diluents containing methylparaben, phenol, propylparaben; may cause flocculation of steroid.

**PREGNANCY:** Safety in pregnancy and nursing not known.

## CELEXA RX

citalopram hydrobromide (Forest)

**Antidepressants increased the risk of suicidal thinking and behavior (suicidality) in short-term studies in children and adolescents with Major Depressive Disorder (MDD) and other psychiatric disorders. Citalopram is not approved for use in pediatric patients.**

**THERAPEUTIC CLASS:** Selective serotonin reuptake inhibitor

**INDICATIONS:** Treatment of depression.

**DOSAGE:** *Adults:* Initial: 20mg qd, in the am or pm. Titrate: Increase by 20mg at intervals of no less than 1 week. Max: 40mg/day (non-responders may require 60mg/day). Elderly/Hepatic Impairment: 20mg/day; titrate to 40mg/day in nonresponders.

**HOW SUPPLIED:** Sol: 10mg/5mL [240mL]; Tab: 10mg, 20mg*, 40mg* *scored

**CONTRAINDICATIONS:** Concomitant MAOI or pimozide therapy.

**WARNINGS/PRECAUTIONS:** Activation of mania/hypomania, SIADH, hyponatremia reported. Close supervision with high risk suicide patients. Caution with history of mania or seizures, hepatic impairment, severe renal impairment, conditions that alter metabolism or hemodynamic responses. May impair judgment, thinking, or motor skills.

**ADVERSE REACTIONS:** Nausea, dyspepsia, vomiting, diarrhea, dry mouth, somnolence, insomnia, increased sweating, ejaculation disorder, rhinitis, anxiety, anorexia, skeletal pain, agitation.

**INTERACTIONS:** See Contraindications. Avoid alcohol. Caution with other CNS drugs, TCAs, lithium, carbamazepine, cimetidine. Increased risk of bleeding with warfarin, aspirin, NSAIDs. Rare reports of weakness, hyperreflexia, incoordination with SSRI's and sumatriptan. Clearance may be decreased with potent CYP3A4 (eg, ketoconazole, itraconazole, fluconazole, erythromycin) and CYP2C19 (eg, omeprazole) inhibitors. May increase metoprolol levels which leads to decreased cardioselectivity.

**PREGNANCY:** Category C, not for use in nursing.

## CELONTIN — RX
methsuximide (Parke-Davis)

**THERAPEUTIC CLASS:** Succinimide

**INDICATIONS:** Management of absence (petit mal) seizures refractory to other drugs.

**DOSAGE:** *Adults:* Initial: 300mg qd for 7 days. Titrate: Increase weekly by 300mg/day for 3 weeks if needed. Max: 1.2g/day.
*Pediatrics:* Initial: 300mg qd for 7 days. Titrate: Increase weekly by 300mg/day 3 weeks if needed. Max: 1.2g/day. Use 150mg caps in small children.

**HOW SUPPLIED:** Cap: 150mg, 300mg

**WARNINGS/PRECAUTIONS:** Fatal blood dyscrasias reported; monitor blood counts periodically or if signs of infection. SLE reported. Withdraw slowly if altered behavior appears. May increase frequency of grand mal seizures if given alone in mixed type of seizures. Avoid abrupt withdrawal. Caution with renal/hepatic disease.

**ADVERSE REACTIONS:** GI effects, blood dyscrasias, dermatologic manifestations, drowsiness, ataxia, dizziness, hyperemia, proteinuria, periorbital edema.

**INTERACTIONS:** May interact with other anticonvulsants; monitor serum levels periodically.

**PREGNANCY:** Safety in pregnancy and nursing not known.

## CENESTIN — RX
conjugated estrogens (Duramed)

**Estrogens increase risk of endometrial cancer. Estrogens, with or without progestins, should not be used for the prevention of cardiovascular disease. Increased risks of MI, stroke, invasive breast cancer, PE, and DVT in postmenopausal women reported.**

**THERAPEUTIC CLASS:** Estrogen

**INDICATIONS:** (0.45mg, 0.625mg, 0.9mg, 1.25mg) Treatment of moderate to severe vasomotor symptoms associated with menopause. (0.3mg) Treatment of vulvar and vaginal atrophy.

**DOSAGE:** *Adults:* Vasomotor Symptoms: Initial: 0.45mg/day. Adjust dose based on response. Discontinue or taper at 3-6 month intervals. Vulvar/Vaginal Atrophy: 0.3mg qd.

**HOW SUPPLIED:** Tab: 0.3mg, 0.45mg, 0.625mg, 0.9mg, 1.25mg

**CONTRAINDICATIONS:** Pregnancy, undiagnosed abnormal genital bleeding, breast cancer, estrogen-dependent neoplasia, DVT/PE, active or recent (eg, within past year) arterial thromboembolic disease (eg, stroke, MI), liver dysfunction or disease.

**WARNINGS/PRECAUTIONS:** May increase risk of cardiovascular events (eg, MI, stroke), venous thrombosis, and PE; d/c immediately if any of these events occur or are suspected. May increase risk of breast/endometrial cancer, and gallbladder disease. May lead to severe hypercalcemia with breast cancer and bone metastases; monitor and d/c if hypercalcemia occurs. Retinal vascular thrombosis reported; monitor and d/c if papilledema or retinal vascular lesions occur. Consider addition of a progestin if no hysterectomy. May elevate BP; monitor at regular intervals. May cause elevations of plasma triglycerides with pre-existing hypertriglyceridemia. Caution with history of cholestatic jaundice associated with past estrogen use or with pregnancy; d/c with recurrence. May lead to increased thyroid-binding globulin levels; monitor thyroid function. May cause fluid retention; caution with cardiac/renal dysfunction. Caution with severe hypocalcemia. May increase risk of ovarian cancer. May exacerbate endometriosis, asthma, DM, epilepsy, migraine, porphyria, SLE, and hepatic hemangiomas; use with caution.

**ADVERSE REACTIONS:** Abdominal pain, back pain, pain, headache, infection, vomiting, leg cramps, paresthesia, breast pain, metrorrhagia, endometrial thickening, vaginitis.

**INTERACTIONS:** CYP3A4 inducers (eg, St. John's wort, phenobarbital, carbamazepine, rifampin) may decrease levels which may decrease therapeutic effects and/or change uterine bleeding profile. CYP3A4 inhibitors (eg, erythromycin, clarithromycin, ketoconazole, itraconazole, ritonavir, grapefruit juice) may increase levels which may result in side effects.

**PREGNANCY:** Contraindicated in pregnancy; caution in nursing.

## CENOGEN ULTRA — RX

minerals - folic acid - multiple vitamin (US Pharmaceutical)

**THERAPEUTIC CLASS:** Prenatal vitamin

**INDICATIONS:** Vitamin and mineral supplementation for before, during, and after pregnancy.

**DOSAGE:** *Adults:* 1 cap qd between meals.

**HOW SUPPLIED:** Cap: Copper 0.8mg-Ferrous Fumarate 324mg-Folic Acid 1mg-Manganese 1.3mg-Niacinamide 30mg-Pantothenic Acid 10mg-Vitamin $B_1$ 10mg-Vitamin $B_2$ 6mg-Vitamin $B_6$ 5mg-Vitamin $B_{12}$ 0.015mg-Vitamin C 200mg

**CONTRAINDICATIONS:** Hemochromatosis, hemosiderosis, hemolytic or pernicious anemias.

**WARNINGS/PRECAUTIONS:** Accidental overdose of iron-containing products is a leading cause of fatal poisoning in children <6 yrs. Not for the treatment of pernicious anemia and other megaloblastic anemias where vitamin $B_{12}$ is deficient. Folic acid >0.1mg-0.4mg/day may obscure pernicious anemia.

**ADVERSE REACTIONS:** GI disturbances.

## CEPTAZ
RX

ceftazidime (GlaxoSmithKline)



**THERAPEUTIC CLASS:** Cephalosporin (3rd generation)

**INDICATIONS:** Treatment of lower respiratory tract (eg, pneumonia), skin and skin structure (SSSI), bone and joint, gynecologic, CNS (eg, meningitis), intra-abdominal, and urinary tract infections (UTI), and septicemia. For use in sepsis.

**DOSAGE:** *Adults:* Usual: 1g IM/IV q8-12h. Uncomplicated UTI: 250mg IM/IV q12h. Complicated UTI: 500mg IM/IV q8-12h. Bone and Joint Infection: 2g IV q12h. Uncomplicated Pneumonia/SSSI: 500mg-1g IM/IV q8h. Gynecological/Intra-Abdominal/Meningitis/Severe Life-Threatening Infection: 2g IV q8h. Lung Infection caused by Pseudomonas spp. in Cystic Fibrosis (normal renal function): 30-50mg/kg IV q8h. Max: 6g/day. CrCl 31-50mL/min: 1g q12h. CrCl 16-30mL/min: 1g q24h. CrCl 6-15mL/min: 500mg q24h. CrCl <5mL/min: 500mg q48h. For severe infections (6g/day), increase renal impairment dose by 50% or increase dosing interval. Apply reduced dosage recommendations after initial 1g LD is given. Hemodialysis: Give 1g before then 1g after each hemodialysis. Intra-Peritoneal Dialysis/Continuous Ambulatory Peritoneal Dialysis: Give 1g followed by 500mg q24h.
*Pediatrics:* >12 yrs: Usual: 1g IM/IV q8-12h. Uncomplicated UTI: 250mg IM/IV q12h. Complicated UTI: 500mg IM/IV q8-12h. Bone and Joint Infection: 2g IV q12h. Uncomplicated Pneumonia/SSSI: 500mg-1g IM/IV q8h. Gynecological/Intra-Abdominal/Meningitis/Severe Life-Threatening Infection: 2g IV q8h. Lung Infection caused by Pseudomonas spp. in Cystic Fibrosis (normal renal function): 30-50mg/kg IV q8h. Max: 6g/day. CrCl 31-50mL/min: 1g q12h. CrCl 16-30mL/min: 1g q24h. CrCl 6-15mL/min: 500mg q24h. CrCl <5mL/min: 500mg q48h. For severe infections (6g/day), increase renal impairment dose by 50% or increase dosing interval. Apply reduced dosage recommendations after initial 1g LD is given. Hemodialysis: Give 1g before then 1g after each hemodialysis. Intra-Peritoneal Dialysis/Continuous Ambulatory Peritoneal Dialysis: Give 1g followed by 500mg q24h.

**HOW SUPPLIED:** Inj: 10g

**WARNINGS/PRECAUTIONS:** Monitor renal function; potential for nephrotoxicity. Prolonged use may result in overgrowth of nonsusceptible organisms. Possible cross-sensitivity between penicillins, cephalosporins, and other beta-lactam antibiotics. Pseudomembranous colitis reported. Elevated levels with renal insufficiency can lead to seizures, encephalopathy, asterixis, coma, and neuromuscular excitability. Possible decrease in PT; caution with renal or hepatic impairment, poor nutritional state; monitor PT and give vitamin K if needed. Caution with colitis and other GI diseases. Distal necrosis can occur after inadvertent intra-arterial administration. Continue therapy for 2 days after the signs and symptoms of infection have disappeared, but in complicated infections longer therapy may be required. False positive for urine glucose with Benedict's, Fehling's solution, and Clinitest® tablets.

**ADVERSE REACTIONS:** Phlebitis and inflammation at injection site, pruritus, rash, fever, diarrhea.

**INTERACTIONS:** Nephrotoxicity reported with aminoglycosides or potent diuretics (eg, furosemide). Avoid with chloramphenicol; may decrease effect of beta-lactam antibiotics.

**PREGNANCY:** Category B, not for use in nursing.

## CEREBYX
RX

fosphenytoin sodium (Parke-Davis)

**THERAPEUTIC CLASS:** Hydantoin

**INDICATIONS:** Short term (up to 5 days) parenteral administration when other means of phenytoin administration are unavailable, inappropriate, or less advantageous, including to control general convulsive status epilepticus, prevent or treat seizures during neurosurgery, as a short term substitute for oral phenytoin.

**DOSAGE:** *Adults:* Doses, concentration in dosing solutions, and infusion rates are expressed as phenytoin sodium equivalents (PE). Status Epilepticus: LD: 15-20 PE/kg IV at 100-150mg PE/min then switch to maintenance dose. Non-Emergent Cases: LD: 10-20mg PE/kg IV (max 150mg PE/min) or IM. Maint: Initial: 4-6mg PE/kg/day. May substitute for oral phenytoin sodium at the same total daily dose.

**HOW SUPPLIED:** Inj: 50mg PE/mL (2mL, 10mL)

**CONTRAINDICATIONS:** Sinus bradycardia, sino-atrial block, 2nd- and 3rd-degree AV block, Adams-Stokes syndrome.

**WARNINGS/PRECAUTIONS:** Avoid abrupt discontinuation. Not for use in absence seizures. Hypotension and severe cardiovascular reactions and fatalities reported; continuously monitor ECG, BP, and respiration during and for at least 20 minutes after IV infusion and monitor phenytoin levels at least 2 hours after IV infusion or 4 hours after IM injection. Caution with severe myocardial insufficiency, porphyria, hepatic/renal dysfunction, hypoalbuminemia, elderly, and diabetes. Acute hepatotoxicity, lymphadenopathy, hemopoietic complications, hyperglycemia reported. D/C if rash or acute hepatotoxicity occurs. Neonatal postpartum bleeding disorder, congenital malformations and increased seizure frequency reported with use during pregnancy. Avoid use with seizures due to hypoglycemia or other metabolic causes. Caution with phosphate restriction because of phosphate load (0.0037 mmol phosphate/mg PE). May lower folate levels.

**ADVERSE REACTIONS:** Cardiovascular collapse and/or CNS depression, nystagmus, dizziness, pruritus, paresthesia, headache, somnolence, ataxia, tinnitus, stupor, nausea, hypotension, vasodilation, tremor, incoordination.

**INTERACTIONS:** Increased levels with acute alcohol intake, amiodarone, chloramphenicol, chlordiazepoxide, cimetidine, diazepam, dicumarol, disulfiram, estrogens, ethosuximide, fluoxetine, $H_2$-antagonists, halothane, isoniazid, methylphenidate, phenothiazines, phenylbutazone, salicylates, succinimides, sulfonamides, tolbutamide, trazodone. Decreased levels with carbamazepine, chronic alcohol abuse, reserpine. Decreases efficacy of anticoagulants, corticosteroids, coumarin, digitoxin, doxycycline, estrogens, furosemide, oral contraceptives, rifampin, quinidine, theophylline, vitamin D. Variable effects (increase or decrease levels) with phenobarbital, valproic acid and sodium valproate. Caution with drugs highly bound to serum albumin. TCAs may precipitate seizures.

**PREGNANCY:** Category D, not for use in nursing.

## CEREZYME — RX

imiglucerase (Genzyme)

**THERAPEUTIC CLASS:** Beta-glucocerebrosidase

**INDICATIONS:** Long-term enzyme replacement therapy in Type 1 Gaucher disease.

**DOSAGE:** *Adults:* Initial: 2.5U/kg TIW to 60U/kg once every 2 weeks IV infusion over 1-2 hours. Adjust dose based on therapeutic goals. *Pediatrics:* ≥2 yrs: Initial: 2.5U/kg TIW to 60U/kg once every 2 weeks IV infusion over 1-2 hours. Adjust dose based on therapeutic goals.

**HOW SUPPLIED:** Inj: 200U, 400U

**WARNINGS/PRECAUTIONS:** Monitor for IgG antibody formation during the 1st year of therapy. Reduce rate of infusion and pretreat with antihistamines and/or corticosteroids if anaphylactoid reactions occur. Caution in patients who developed antibodies or hypersensitivity reactions to alglucerase.

**ADVERSE REACTIONS:** Injection site reactions, pruritus, flushing, urticaria, angioedema, chest discomfort, dyspnea, coughing, cyanosis, hypotension, nausea, vomiting, rash, headache, fever.

**PREGNANCY:** Category C, caution in nursing.

## CERUBIDINE

RX

daunorubicin HCl (Bedford)

**Avoid IM/SQ route. Severe local tissue necrosis with extravasation. Myocardial toxicity may occur during or after terminate therapy; increased risk if cumulative dose >400-550mg/m$^2$ in adults, >300mg/m$^2$ in pediatrics >2 yrs, or >10mg/m$^2$ in pediatrics <2 yrs. Severe myelosuppression may occur. Reduce dose with impaired hepatic or renal function.**

**THERAPEUTIC CLASS:** Anthracycline

**INDICATIONS:** In combination with other anticancer drugs, for remission induction in acute nonlymphocytic leukemia (ANLL) in adults, and for remission induction in acute lymphocytic leukemia (ALL) in children and adults.

**DOSAGE:** *Adults:* ANLL: Combination Therapy: <60 yrs: 45mg/m$^2$/day IV on days 1, 2, 3 of 1st course and on days 1, 2 of subsequent courses. >60 yrs: 30mg/m$^2$/day IV on days 1, 2, 3 of 1st course and on days 1, 2 of subsequent courses. ALL: Combination Therapy: 45mg/m$^2$/day IV on days 1, 2, 3. Renal Impairment: If SCr >3mg%, reduce dose by 50%. Hepatic Impairment: If serum bilirubin 1.2-3mg%, reduce dose by 25%. If >3mg%, reduce dose by 50%. *Pediatrics:* ALL: Combination Therapy: 25mg/m$^2$ IV on day 1 every week. If complete remission not obtained after 4 courses, may give additional 1-2 courses. If <2 yrs or <0.5m$^2$ BSA, calculate dose based on weight (1mg/kg) instead of BSA.

**HOW SUPPLIED:** Inj: 20mg

**WARNINGS/PRECAUTIONS:** Avoid if pre-existing drug-induced bone marrow suppression occurs unless benefit warrants the risk. May cause fetal harm during pregnancy. May impart red color to urine. Monitor blood uric acid levels. Determine CBC frequently. Evaluate cardiac, renal, and hepatic function before each course.

**ADVERSE REACTIONS:** Cardiotoxicity, myelosuppression, alopecia, nausea, vomiting, diarrhea, abdominal pain, hyperuricemia, mucositis (3-7 days after therapy).

**INTERACTIONS:** Possible secondary leukemias with other antineoplastics or radiation therapy. Increased risk of cardiotoxicity with previous doxorubicin therapy or with concomitant cyclophosphamide. May need dose reduction with other myelosuppressants. Hepatotoxic agents (eg, high dose MTX) may increase risk of toxicity.

**PREGNANCY:** Category D, not for use in nursing.

## CERUMENEX

RX

triethanolamine polypeptide oleate (Purdue Frederick)

**THERAPEUTIC CLASS:** Ceruminolytic

**INDICATIONS:** Removal of impacted cerumen.

**DOSAGE:** *Adults:* Fill ear canal and insert cotton plug for 15-30 minutes. Flush with warm water. Repeat if needed.

**HOW SUPPLIED:** Sol: 10% [6mL, 12mL]

**CONTRAINDICATIONS:** Perforated tympanic membrane, otitis media.

**WARNINGS/PRECAUTIONS:** D/C if sensitization or irritation occurs. Extreme caution with allergies. Limit exposure of ear canal to 15-30 minutes. Avoid undue exposure of skin outside ear. Caution with external otitis.

**ADVERSE REACTIONS:** Mild erythema, pruritus of external ear, contact dermatitis, skin ulcerations, burning/pain at application site, skin rash.

**PREGNANCY:** Category C, caution in nursing.

## CERVIDIL

RX

dinoprostone (Forest)

C

**THERAPEUTIC CLASS:** Oxytocic agent

**INDICATIONS:** For cervical ripening initiation and/or continuation in patients at or near term with a medical or obstetrical need for labor induction.

**DOSAGE:** *Adults:* 10mg to release 0.3mg/hr over 12 hrs. Place one unit transversely in posterior fornix of the vagina immediately after removal from its foil package. Remove at onset of active labor or 12 hrs after insertion.

**HOW SUPPLIED:** Insert: 0.3mg/hr

**CONTRAINDICATIONS:** Fetal distress where delivery is not imminent, marked cephalopelvic disproportion, unexplained vaginal bleeding during this pregnancy, when oxytocic drugs are contraindicated, when prolonged uterus contraction may be detrimental to fetal safety or uterine integrity, concomitant IV oxytocic drugs, multipara with 6 or more previous term pregnancies.

**WARNINGS/PRECAUTIONS:** Avoid with history of cesarean section or uterine surgery. Caution with ruptured membranes, history of uterine hypertony, glaucoma, childhood asthma (even if no attacks in adulthood). Monitor uterine activity, fetal status, progression of cervical dilation and effacement. Remove if hyperstimulation occurs and before amniotomy.

**ADVERSE REACTIONS:** Uterine hyperstimulation, fetal distress.

**INTERACTIONS:** May augment activity of other oxytocic drugs; avoid concomitant use. Wait 30 minutes after removal of dinoprostone before useing oxytocin.

**PREGNANCY:** Category C, safety in nursing not known.

## CESAMET

CII

nabilone (Valeant)

**THERAPEUTIC CLASS:** Cannabinoid

**INDICATIONS:** Treatment of the nausea and vomiting associated with chemotherapy when conventional treatment has failed.

**DOSAGE:** *Adults:* Initial: 1 or 2mg bid; given 1-3 hrs before chemotherapy. A dose of 1 or 2mg the night before may be useful. Max: 6mg/day given in divided doses tid.

**HOW SUPPLIED:** Cap: 1mg

**WARNINGS/PRECAUTIONS:** Patients should remain under the supervision of a responsible adult during nabilone treatment, especially during initial use and dose adjustments. Caution when initiating therepy in patients with hypertension, heart disease, current or previous psychiatric disorders and in patients with a history of substance abuse. Avoid driving, operating heavy machinary, or engaging in any hazardous activity during treatment. May cause dizziness, euphoria, ataxia, anxiety, disorientation, depression, hallucinations, and psychosis. Adverse psychiatric reactions can persist for 48-72 hrs following cessation of treatment. Avoid with alcohol, sedatives, hypnotics, or other psychoactive substances. May cause tachycardia and orthostatic hypotension.

**ADVERSE REACTIONS:** Drowsiness, vertigo, dry mouth, euphoria, ataxia, headache, concentration difficulties, nausea, dysphoria, sleep/visual disturbance, asthenia, anorexia.

**INTERACTIONS:** Highly protein bound drugs may require dosage changes. Additive effects with alcohol, sedatives, hypnotics, or other psychactive drugs. Additive HTN, tachycardia, and possible cardiotoxicity with amphetamines, cocaine, and sympathomimetics. Increased tachycardia and drowsiness with anticholinergic agents. Potentiates effects of TCAs and CNS depressants.

Decreases clearance of antipyrine and barbiturates. Increased metabolism of theophylline.

**PREGNANCY:** Category C, not for use in nursing.

## CETROTIDE RX

cetrorelix acetate (Serono)

**THERAPEUTIC CLASS:** GnRH antagonist

**INDICATIONS:** For inhibition of premature LH surges in women undergoing controlled ovarian stimulation.

**DOSAGE:** *Adults:* Multiple-Dose Regimen: 0.25mg SQ qd; start on day 5 (AM or PM) or day 6 (AM). Continue until HCG administration. Single-Dose Regimen: 3mg SQ single dose when estradiol level indicates appropriate stimulation response, usually on Day 7. If HCG not given within 4 days, then give 0.25mg SQ qd until day of HCG administration.

**HOW SUPPLIED:** Inj: 0.25mg, 3mg

**CONTRAINDICATIONS:** Pregnancy, nursing, hypersensitivity to extrinsic peptide hormones or mannitol, severe renal impairment.

**WARNINGS/PRECAUTIONS:** Exclude pregnancy before initiating therapy.

**ADVERSE REACTIONS:** Ovarian hyperstimulation syndrome, nausea, headache.

**PREGNANCY:** Category X, not for use in nursing.

## CHANTIX RX

varenicline tartrate (Pfizer)

**THERAPEUTIC CLASS:** Nicotinic Acetylcholine Receptor Agonist

**INDICATIONS:** Aid to smoking cessation treatment.

**DOSAGE:** *Adults:* ≥18 yrs: Days 1-3: 0.5mg daily. Days 4-7: 0.5mg bid. Day 8-End of Treatment: 1mg bid. Severe Renal Impairment: Initial: 0.5mg daily. Titrate: Max: 0.5mg bid. End-Stage Renal Disease: Max: 0.5mg daily.

**HOW SUPPLIED:** Tab: 0.5mg, 1mg

**WARNINGS/PRECAUTIONS:** Physiological changes resulting from smoking cessation may alter pharmacokinetics or pharmacodynamics of some drugs.

**ADVERSE REACTIONS:** Nausea, insomnia, abnormal dreams, abdominal pain, constipation, headache, dysgeusia, upper respiratory tract disorder.

**INTERACTIONS:** Reduced renal clearance with cimetidine.

**PREGNANCY:** Category C, not for use in nursing.

## CHERACOL W/CODEINE CV

guaifenesin - codeine phosphate (Lee Pharmaceuticals)

**OTHER BRAND NAMES:** Guaituss AC (Alpharma) - Halotussin AC (Watson) - Cheratussin AC (Vintage) - Mytussin AC (Morton Grove)

**THERAPEUTIC CLASS:** Cough suppressant/expectorant

**INDICATIONS:** Relief of cough due to minor throat and bronchial irritation from a cold or inhaled irritants. Loosens phlegm and thins bronchial secretions to make coughs more productive.

**DOSAGE:** *Adults:* 10mL q4h. Max: 60mL/24 hrs.
*Pediatrics:* >12 yrs: 10mL q4h. Max: 60mL/24 hrs. 6 to <12 yrs: 5mL q4h. Max: 30mL/24 hrs.

**HOW SUPPLIED:** Syrup: (Codeine-Guaifenesin) 10-100mg/5mL [120mL]

**WARNINGS/PRECAUTIONS:** Use caution with persistant/chronic cough, cough with excessive phlegm, chronic pulmonary disease, or shortness of breath. May cause or aggravate constipation.

**ADVERSE REACTIONS:** Constipation, sedation.



**INTERACTIONS:** Increased sedation with sedatives, tranquilizers and antidepressants, especially MAOIs.

**PREGNANCY:** Safety in pregnancy and nursing not known.

## CHILDREN'S MYLANTA — OTC

calcium carbonate (J&J – Merck)

**THERAPEUTIC CLASS:** Antacid

**INDICATIONS:** For the relief of acid indigestion, sour stomach, and upset stomach due to these symptoms or overindulgence in food and drink.

**DOSAGE:** *Pediatrics:* 24-47 lbs or 2-5 yrs: 1 tab; 48-95 lbs or 6-11 yrs: 2 tabs. Max: 2-5 yrs: 3 tabs/24hrs; 6-11 yrs: 6 tabs/24hrs. Repeat as needed. Do not use for >2 weeks unless under supervision of a doctor.

**HOW SUPPLIED:** Tab, Chewable: 400mg

**INTERACTIONS:** Antacids may interact with other prescription drugs.

## CHLORAL HYDRATE — CIV

chloral hydrate (Pharmaceutical Associations)

**THERAPEUTIC CLASS:** Trichloroacetaldehyde monohydrate

**INDICATIONS:** Short-term sedative/hypnotic (<2 weeks). To allay anxiety or induce sedation preoperatively or prior to EEG evaluations. Alone or with paraldehyde to prevent or suppress alcohol withdrawal syndrome. To reduce anxiety associated with withdrawal of other drugs such as narcotics or barbiturates.

**DOSAGE:** *Adults:* Dilute in half glass of water, fruit juice, or ginger ale. Hypnotic: Usual: 500mg-1g 15-30 min before bedtime. Sedative: Usual: 250mg tid pc. Alcohol Withdrawal: Usual: 500mg-1g q6h prn. Max: 2g/day. *Pediatrics:* Hypnotic: 50mg/kg. Max: 1g/dose. Sedative: 8mg/kg tid. Max: 500mg tid. Prior to EEG: 20-25mg/kg.

**HOW SUPPLIED:** Syr: 500mg/5mL

**CONTRAINDICATIONS:** Marked hepatic or renal impairment.

**WARNINGS/PRECAUTIONS:** May be habit forming. Caution with depression, suicidal tendencies, history of drug abuse. Avoid with esophagitis, gastritis or gastric or duodenal ulcers, large doses with severe cardiac disease. May impair mental/physical abilities. Risk of gastritis, skin eruptions, parenchymatous renal damage with prolonged use. Withdraw gradually with chronic use.

**ADVERSE REACTIONS:** Nausea, vomiting, diarrhea, ataxia, dizziness.

**INTERACTIONS:** Reduces effectiveness of coumarin anticoagulants. May result in transient potentiation of warfarin-induced hypoprothrombinemia. Additive CNS effects with other CNS depressants (eg, paraldehyde, barbiturates, alcohol). Use with IV furosemide may cause diaphoresis, flushes, variable BP; use alternative hypnotic.

**PREGNANCY:** Category C, caution in nursing.

## CHLORPROMAZINE — RX

chlorpromazine (Various)

**THERAPEUTIC CLASS:** Phenothiazine

**INDICATIONS:** Treatment of schizophrenia. Control of nausea and vomiting. Relief of restlessness and apprehension before surgery. Treatment of acute intermittent porphyria. Adjunct treatment of tetanus. To control the manic type of manic-depressive illness. Relief of intractable hiccups. Treatment of severe behavioral problems in children. Short-term treatment of hyperactivity in children.



**DOSAGE:** *Adults:* Severe Behavioral Problems: Inpatient: Acute Schizophrenic/Manic State: 25mg IM, then 25-50mg IM in 1 hr if needed. Titrate: Increase over several days up to 400mg q4-6h until controlled then switch to PO. Usual: 500mg/day PO. Max: 1000mg/day PO. Less Acutely Disturbed: 25mg PO tid. Titrate: Increase gradually to 400mg/day. Outpatient: 10mg PO tid-qid or 25mg PO bid-tid. More Severe: 25mg PO tid. Titrate: After 1-2 days, increase by 20-50mg twice weekly until calm. Prompt Control of Severe Symptoms: 25mg IM, may repeat in 1 hr then 25-50mg PO tid. Nausea/Vomiting: Usual: 10-25mg PO q4-6h prn; 25mg IM then, if no hypotension, 25-50mg q3-4h prn until vomiting stops then switch to PO; 100mg rectally q6-8h prn. Nausea/Vomiting in Surgery: 12.5mg IM, may repeat in 1/2 hr; 2mg IV per fractional injection at 2 minute intervals. Max: 25mg. Presurgical Apprehension: 25-50mg PO 2-3 hrs pre-op; 12.5-25mg IM 1-2 hrs pre-op. Intractable Hiccups: 25-50mg PO tid-qid; if symptoms persist after 2-3 days, give 25-50mg IM; if symptoms still persist, give 25-50mg slow IV. Porphyria: 25-50mg PO tid-qid; 25mg IM tid-qid until PO therapy. Tetanus: 25-50mg IM tid-qid; 25-50mg IV. Elderly: Use lower doses, increase dose more gradually, monitor closely.
*Pediatrics:* 6 months-12 yrs: Severe Behavioral Problems: Outpatient: 0.25mg/lb PO q4-6h prn; 0.5mg/lb sup rectally q6-8h prn; 0.25mg/lb IM q6-8h prn. Inpatient: Start low and increase gradually to 50-100mg/day; ≥200mg/day in older children. Max: 500mg/day. <5 yrs (<50lbs): Max: ≤40mg/day IM; 5-12 yrs (50-100lbs): Max: ≤75mg/day IM. Nausea/Vomiting: 0.25mg/lb PO q4-6h; 0.5mg/lb sup rectally q6-8 prn. 0.25mg/lb IM q6-8h prn. Max: 6 months-5 yrs (or 50 lbs): <40mg/day. 5-12 yrs (or 50-100lbs): <75mg/day except in severe cases. During Surgery: 0.125mg/lb IM repeat in 1/2 hr if needed; 1mg IV per fractional injection at 2-minute intervals and not exceeding recommended IM dosage. Presurgical Apprehension: 0.25mg/lb PO 2-3 hrs (or IM 1-2 hrs) before operation. Tetanus: 0.25mg/lb IM/IV q6-8h. <50lbs: Max: ≤40mg/day; 50-100lbs: Max: ≤75mg/day.

**HOW SUPPLIED:** Cap, Extended Release: 30mg, 75mg, 150mg; Inj: 25mg/mL; Sup: 25mg, 100mg; Syrup: 10mg/5mL [120mL]; Tab: 10mg, 25mg, 50mg, 100mg, 200mg

**CONTRAINDICATIONS:** Comatose states, or with large amounts of CNS depressants. Hypersensitivity to phenothiazines.

**WARNINGS/PRECAUTIONS:** Tardive dyskinesia, NMS may occur. Caution with chronic respiratory disorders, acute respiratory infections (especially in children), glaucoma, cardiovascular, hepatic, or renal disease, history of hepatic encephalopathy due to cirrhosis. Suppresses cough reflex; aspiration of vomitus possible. Caution if exposed to extreme heat or organophosphates. Avoid in children/adolescents with signs of Reye's syndrome. Lowers seizure threshold. Reduce dose gradually to prevent side effects. May mask signs of overdoses to other drugs and obscure diagnosis of other conditions (eg, intestinal obstruction, brain tumor, Reye's syndrome). May produce false-positive PKU test. May elevate prolactin levels. Injection contains sulfites.

**ADVERSE REACTIONS:** Drowsiness, jaundice, agranulocytosis, hypotensive effects, EKG changes, dystonias, motor restlessness, pseudo-parkinsonism, tardive dyskinesia, anticholinergic effects, NMS, ocular changes.

**INTERACTIONS:** See Contraindications. May decrease effects of oral anticoagulants, guanethidine. Propranolol increases plasma levels of both agents. Thiazide diuretics may potentiate orthostatic hypotension. Potentiates effects of CNS depressants (eg, anesthetic, barbiturates, narcotics); reduce doses of these drugs by 1/4 to 1/2. Anticonvulsants may need adjustment; phenytoin toxicity reported. Do not use with Amipaque®; discontinue at least 48 hrs before myelography and resume at least 24 hrs after. Can cause alpha-adrenergic blockade. Caution with atropine or related drugs. Encephalopathic syndrome reported with lithium.

**PREGNANCY:** Safety in pregnancy not known. Not for use in nursing.

## CHLOR-TRIMETON OTC
chlorpheniramine maleate (Schering)



**THERAPEUTIC CLASS:** Antihistamine

**INDICATIONS:** Allergic rhinitis and conjunctivitis.

**DOSAGE:** *Adults:* (Tab/Syrup) 4mg q4-6h. (Tab, ER) 8mg q8-12h or 12mg q12h. Max: 24mg/day.
*Pediatrics:* >12 yrs: (Tab/Syrup) 4mg q4-6h. Tab, ER: 8mg q8-12h or 12mg q12h. Max: 24mg/day. 6-12 yrs: (Tab/Syrup) 2mg q4-6h. Max: 12mg/24hrs.

**HOW SUPPLIED:** Syrup: 2mg/5mL; Tab: 4mg; Tab, Extended Release: 8mg, 12mg

**WARNINGS/PRECAUTIONS:** Avoid with emphysema, chronic bronchitis, glaucoma, and difficulty in urination due to prostate gland enlargement.

**ADVERSE REACTIONS:** Drowsiness, excitability.

**INTERACTIONS:** Alcohol, sedatives, hypnotics potentiate CNS depression.

**PREGNANCY:** Safety in pregnancy or nursing not known.

## CHROMAGEN RX
vitamin C - vitamin B12 - dessicated stomach substance - ferrous fumarate (Savage)

**OTHER BRAND NAMES:** Anemagen (Ethex)

**THERAPEUTIC CLASS:** Iron/vitamin

**INDICATIONS:** Treatment of all anemias responsive to oral iron therapy.

**DOSAGE:** *Adults:* 1 cap qd.

**HOW SUPPLIED:** Cap: Dessicated Stomach Substance 100mg-Ferrous Fumarate 200mg-Vitamin $B_{12}$ 0.01mg-Vitamin C 250mg

**CONTRAINDICATIONS:** Hemochromatosis, hemosiderosis.

**ADVERSE REACTIONS:** Nausea, rash, vomiting, diarrhea, precordial pain, flushing.

**PREGNANCY:** Safety in pregnancy and nursing not known.

## CHROMAGEN FA RX
vitamin C - folic acid - vitamin B12 - ferrous fumarate (Savage)

**THERAPEUTIC CLASS:** Iron/vitamin

**INDICATIONS:** Treatment of all anemias responsive to oral iron therapy.

**DOSAGE:** *Adults:* 1 cap qd.

**HOW SUPPLIED:** (Ferrous Fumarate-Folic Acid-Vitamin $B_{12}$-Vitamin C) Cap: 200mg-1mg-0.01mg-250mg

**CONTRAINDICATIONS:** Hemochromatosis, hemosiderosis. Folic acid is contraindicated in pernicious anemia.

**WARNINGS/PRECAUTIONS:** Accidental overdose of iron-containing products is a leading cause of fatal poisoning in children <6 yrs. Avoid folic acid unless the diagnosis of pernicious anemia has been excluded.

**ADVERSE REACTIONS:** Nausea, rash, vomiting, diarrhea, precordial pain, flushing.

**PREGNANCY:** Safety in pregnancy and nursing is not known.

## CHROMAGEN FORTE

RX

vitamin C - folic acid - vitamin B12 - ferrous fumarate (Savage)

**THERAPEUTIC CLASS:** Iron/vitamin

**INDICATIONS:** Treatment of all anemias responsive to oral iron therapy.

**DOSAGE:** *Adults:* 1-2 caps qd.

**HOW SUPPLIED:** Cap: Ferrous Fumarate 460mg-Folic Acid 1mg-Vitamin $B_{12}$ 0.01mg-Vitamin C 60mg

**CONTRAINDICATIONS:** Hemochromatosis, hemosiderosis, pernicious anemia.

**WARNINGS/PRECAUTIONS:** Accidental overdose of iron-containing products is a leading cause of fatal poisoning in children <6 yrs. Avoid folic acid unless the diagnosis of pernicious anemia has been excluded.

**ADVERSE REACTIONS:** Nausea, rash, vomiting, diarrhea, precordial pain, flushing.

**PREGNANCY:** Safety in pregnancy and nursing not known.

## CHROMAGEN OB

RX

minerals - folic acid - multiple vitamin (Savage)

**THERAPEUTIC CLASS:** Prenatal vitamin

**INDICATIONS:** Vitamin and mineral supplementation for before, during, and after pregnancy.

**DOSAGE:** *Adults:* 1 cap qd with food.

**HOW SUPPLIED:** Cap: Calcium 200mg-Copper 2mg-Docusate Calcium 25mg-Folic Acid 1mg-Iron 28mg-Manganese 2mg-Niacinamide 5mg-Vitamin $B_1$ 1.6mg-Vitamin $B_2$ 1.8mg-Vitamin $B_6$ 20mg-Vitamin $B_{12}$ 0.012mg-Vitamin C 60mg-Vitamin D 400 IU-Vitamin E 30 IU-Zinc 25mg

**CONTRAINDICATIONS:** Hemochromatosis, hemosiderosis, Wilson's disease.

**WARNINGS/PRECAUTIONS:** Accidental overdose of iron-containing products is a leading cause of fatal poisoning in children <6 yrs. Folic acid alone is improper treatment of pernicious anemia and other megaloblastic anemias with vitamin $B_{12}$-deficiency. Folic acid >0.1mg/day may obscure pernicious anemia.

**ADVERSE REACTIONS:** Constipation, diarrhea, nausea, vomiting, dark stools, abdominal pain, nausea, rash, vomiting, diarrhea, precordial pain, flushing.

## CIALIS

RX

tadalafil (Lilly ICOS)

**THERAPEUTIC CLASS:** Phosphodiesterase type 5 inhibitor

**INDICATIONS:** Treatment of erectile dysfunction.

**DOSAGE:** *Adults:* Take once daily prior to sexual activity. Initial: 10mg. Range: 5-20mg. Renal Impairment: CrCl 31-50mL/min: Initial: 5mg. Max: 10mg/48 hrs. CrCl <30mL/min/Hemodialysis: Max: 5mg. Hepatic Impairment: Mild/Moderate: Max: 10mg. With Potent CYP3A4 Inhibitors (eg, ketoconazole, itraconazole, ritonavir): Max: 10mg/72 hrs.

**HOW SUPPLIED:** Tab: 5mg, 10mg, 20mg

**CONTRAINDICATIONS:** Concomitant nitrates.

**WARNINGS/PRECAUTIONS:** Avoid in men for whom sexual activity is inadvisable due to underlying CV status. Increased sensitivity to vasodilatory effect with left ventricular outflow obstruction. Avoid with MI (within last 90 days), unstable angina or angina occurring during sexual intercourse, NYHA Class 2 or greater heart failure (in the last 6 months), uncontrolled arrhythmias, hypotension (<90/50mmHg), or uncontrolled HTN (>170/100mmHg), stroke within the last 6 months, severe hepatic impairment (Childs-Pugh Class C), degenerative retinal disorders, including retinitis pigmentosa. Caution with predisposition to priapism (eg, sickle cell anemia, multiple myeloma, leukemia), anatomical deformation of the penis, bleeding disorders or active peptic ulceration. May cause transient decrease in BP. Caution with coadministration of PDE5 inhibitors and alpha-blockers. May cause additive hypotensive effect. Initiate at lowest dose once patient is stable on either therapy. Rare reports of non-arteritic anterior ischemic optic neuropathy (NAION) with PDE5 inhibitors.



**ADVERSE REACTIONS:** Headache, dyspepsia, back pain, myalgia, nasal congestion, flushing, limb pain, urticaria, Stevens-Johnson syndrome, exoliative dermatitis, migraine, visual field defect, retinal vein occlusion, retinal artery occlusion.

**INTERACTIONS:** See Contraindications. Increased levels with CYP3A4 inhibitors (eg, ketoconazole, HIV protease inhibitors, erythromycin, itraconazole, grapefruit juice). Decreased levels with CYP3A4 inducers (eg, rifampin, carbamazepine, phenytoin, phenobarbital). Additive hypotensive effects with alcohol, alpha blockers (eg, tamsulosin, doxazosin, alfuzosin), antihypertensives (eg, amlodipine, metoprolol, bendrofluazide, enalapril, angiotensin-II receptor blockers).

**PREGNANCY:** Category B, not for use in nursing.

## CILOXAN — RX

ciprofloxacin HCl (Alcon)

**THERAPEUTIC CLASS:** Fluoroquinolone

**INDICATIONS:** Bacterial conjunctivitis and corneal ulcers.

**DOSAGE:** *Adults:* Bacterial Conjunctivitis: Sol: 1-2 drops q2h while awake for 2 days, then 1-2 drops every 4 hrs while awake for 5 days. Oint: 1/2 inch tid for 2 days, then bid for 5 days. Corneal Ulcer: Sol: 2 drops every 15 minutes for the first 6 hrs, then 2 drops every 30 minutes for the rest of day 1, then 2 drops every hr on day 2, then 2 drops every 4 hrs on days 3-14. May continue if re-epithelialization has not occurred.
*Pediatrics:* Bacterial Conjunctivitis: >1 yr: Sol: 1-2 drops q2h while awake for 2 days, then 1-2 drops every 4 hrs while awake for 5 days. >2 yr: Oint: 1/2 inch tid for 2 days, then bid for 5 days. Corneal Ulcer: Sol: >1 yr: 2 drops every 15 minutes for the first 6 hrs, then 2 drops every 30 minutes for the rest of day 1, then 2 drops every hr on day 2, then 2 drops every 4 hrs on days 3-14. May continue if re-epithelialization has not occurred.

**HOW SUPPLIED:** Oint: 0.3% [3.5g]; Sol: 0.3% [2.5mL, 5mL, 10mL]

**WARNINGS/PRECAUTIONS:** Not for injection into eye. Superinfection may result with prolonged use. Fatal hypersensitivity reactions reported after 1st dose of systemic quinolone therapy. Avoid allowing tip of container to contact eye or surrounding structures. Avoid contact lenses with conjunctivitis. Risk of crystalline precipitate in cornea. Ointment may slow corneal healing and cause visual blurring.

**ADVERSE REACTIONS:** Local burning, white crystalline precipitants, lid margin crusting, crystals/scales, foreign body sensation, itching, conjunctival hyperemia, bad taste.

**INTERACTIONS:** Systemic quinolone therapy may increase theophylline levels, interfere with caffeine metabolism, enhance warfarin effects, and elevate serum creatinine with cyclosporine.

**PREGNANCY:** Category C, caution in nursing.

## CIMETIDINE
cimetidine (Various)

RX

C

**OTHER BRAND NAMES:** Tagamet (GlaxoSmithKline)

**THERAPEUTIC CLASS:** $H_2$ blocker

**INDICATIONS:** Short-term treatment of active duodenal ulcer (DU), active benign gastric ulcer (GU). Maintenance of healed duodenal ulcer. Treatment of GERD and/or pathological hypersecretory conditions (eg, Zollinger-Ellison syndrome). Prevention of upper GI bleeding in critically ill patients.

**DOSAGE:** *Adults:* (PO) Active DU: 800mg qhs or 300mg qid or 400mg bid for 4-8 weeks. Maint: 400mg qhs. Active Benign GU: 800mg qhs or 300mg qid for 6 weeks. GERD: 800mg bid or 400mg qid for 12 weeks. Hypersecretory Conditions: 300mg qid. Max: 2400mg/day. (Inj) 300mg IM/IV q6-8h. Max: 2400mg/day. Rapid Gastric pH Elevation: LD: 150mg IV, then 37.5mg/hr IV. Upper GI Bleed Prevention: Continuous IV infusion of 50mg/hr for 7 days. CrCl <30mL/min: Give half the recommended dose.
*Pediatrics:* >16 yrs: (PO) Active DU: 800mg qhs or 300mg qid or 400mg bid for 4-8 weeks. Maint: 400mg qhs. Active Benign GU: 800mg qhs or 300mg qid for 6 weeks. GERD: 800mg bid or 400mg qid for 12 weeks. Hypersecretory Conditions: 300mg qid. Max: 2400mg/day. (Inj) 300mg IM/IV q6-8h. Max: 2400mg/day. Rapid Gastric pH Elevation: LD: 150mg IV, then 37.5mg/hr IV. Upper GI Bleed Prevention: Continuous IV infusion of 50mg/hr for 7 days. CrCl <30mL/min: Give half the recommended dose.

**HOW SUPPLIED:** Inj: (HCl) 150mg/mL, 300mg/50mL; Sol: (HCl) 300mg/5mL; Tab: 300mg, 400mg*, 800mg* *scored

**WARNINGS/PRECAUTIONS:** Cardiac arrhythmias and hypotension reported following rapid IV administration (rare). Symptomatic response does not preclude the presence of gastric malignancy. Reversible confusional states reported, especially in severely ill patients. Elderly, renal and/or hepatic impairment are risk factors for confusional states. Risk of hyperinfection of strongyloidiasis in immunocompromised patients.

**ADVERSE REACTIONS:** Diarrhea, headache, dizziness, somnolence, reversible confusional states, impotence, increased serum transaminases, rash, gynecomastia, blood dyscrasias.

**INTERACTIONS:** Reduces metabolism of warfarin-type anticoagulants, phenytoin, propranolol, nifedipine, chlordiazepoxide, diazepam, certain TCAs, lidocaine, theophylline and metronidazole. Monitor PT/INR. Adverse effects reported with phenytoin, lidocaine and theophylline; monitor levels. May affect absorption of drugs (eg, ketoconazole) affected by gastric pH; give 2 hrs before cimetidine. Antacids may interfer with absorption of cimetidine; space the dosing.

**PREGNANCY:** Category B, not for use in nursing.

## CIPRO HC
hydrocortisone - ciprofloxacin HCl (Alcon)

RX

**THERAPEUTIC CLASS:** Antibacterial/corticosteroid combination

**INDICATIONS:** Acute otitis externa in adults and pediatric patients >1 year.

**DOSAGE:** *Adults:* 3 drops into affected ear bid for 7 days. Warm bottle in hand for 1-2 minutes to avoid dizziness. Shake well before use.
*Pediatrics:* >1 yr: 3 drops into affected ear bid for 7 days. Warm bottle in hand for 1-2 minutes to avoid dizziness. Shake well before use.

**HOW SUPPLIED:** Sus: (Ciprofloxacin-Hydrocortisone) 0.2%-1% [10mL]

**CONTRAINDICATIONS:** Perforated tympanic membrane, viral infections of external ear canal (eg, varicella and herpes simplex infections).

**WARNINGS/PRECAUTIONS:** D/C if hypersensitivity reaction occurs. Re-evaluate if no improvement after one week.

**ADVERSE REACTIONS:** Headache, pruritus.

**PREGNANCY:** Category C, not for use in nursing.



## CIPRO IV RX

ciprofloxacin (Schering)

**THERAPEUTIC CLASS:** Fluoroquinolone

**INDICATIONS:** Treatment of skin and skin structure (SSSI), bone and joint, complicated intra-abdominal infections, lower respiratory (LRTI), and urinary tract infections (UTI), nosocomial pneumonia, acute sinusitis, chronic bacterial prostatitis, post-exposure inhalational anthrax, empirical therapy for febrile neutropenia, complicated UTI and pyelonephritis in pediatrics.

**DOSAGE:** *Adults:* >18 yrs: IV: UTI: Mild-Moderate: 200mg q12h for 7-14 days. Complicated/Severe: 400mg q12h for 7-14 days. LRTI/SSSI: Mild-Moderate: 400mg q12h for 7-14 days. Complicated/Severe: 400mg q8h for 7-14 days. Bone and Joint: Mild-Moderate: 400mg q12h for >4-6 weeks. Complicated/Severe: 400mg q8h for >4-6 weeks. Nosocomial Pneumonia: 400mg q8h for 10-14 days. Complicated Intra-Abdominal: 400mg q12h (w/metronidazole) for 7-14 days. Acute Sinusitis: 400mg q12h for 10 days. Chronic Bacterial Prostatitis: 400mg q12h for 28 days. Febrile Neutropenia: 400mg q8h (w/piperacillin 50mg/kg q4h) for 7-14 days. Max: 24g/day. Inhalational Anthrax: 400mg q12h for 60 days. Administer over 60 minutes. CrCl 5-29mL/min: 200-400mg q18-24h.
*Pediatrics:* <18 yrs: Inhalational Anthrax: 10mg/kg q12h for 60 days. Max: 400mg/dose; 800mg/day. 1-17 yrs: Complicated UTI/Pyleonephritis: 6-10mg/kg q8h for 10-21 days. Max: 400mg/dose.

**HOW SUPPLIED:** Inj: 10mg/mL, 200mg/100mL, 400mg/200mL

**CONTRAINDICATIONS:** Concomitant administration with tizanidine.

**WARNINGS/PRECAUTIONS:** Convulsions, increased intracranial pressure, and toxic psychosis reported. Caution with CNS disorders or if predisposed to seizures. Severe, fatal hypersensitivity reactions may occur. Pseudomembranous colitis, achilles and other tendon ruptures reported. D/C at first sign of rash/hypersensitivity or if pain, inflammation, or ruptured tendon occur. May permit overgrowth of clostridia. Maintain hydration; avoid alkaline urine. Avoid excessive sunlight and UV light. Do not give via feeding tube. Monitor renal, hepatic and hematopoietic function with prolonged use. Adust dose with renal dysfunction.

**ADVERSE REACTIONS:** Nausea, diarrhea, CNS disturbances, local IV site reactions, hepatic enzyme abnormalities, eosinophilia, headache, restlessness rash.

**INTERACTIONS:** See Contraindications. Increases theophylline and caffeine levels and prolongs effects. Altered serum levels of phenytoin. Severe hypoglycemia with glyburide (rare). Potentiated by probenecid. Transient serum creatinine elevations with cyclosporine. Enhances oral anticoagulant effects. Caution with drugs that lower seizure threshold.

**PREGNANCY:** Category C, not for use in nursing.

## CIPRO ORAL RX

ciprofloxacin HCl (Schering)

**THERAPEUTIC CLASS:** Fluoroquinolone

**INDICATIONS:** Treatment of lower respiratory tract (LRTI), complicated intra-abdominal, skin and skin structure (SSSI), bone and joint, and urinary tract infections (UTI), acute exacerbations of chronic bronchitis, acute sinusitis, acute uncomplicated cystitis in females, chronic bacterial prostatitis, infectious diarrhea, typhoid fever, post-exposure inhalational anthrax, uncomplicated cervical and urethral gonorrhea, complicated UTI and pyelonephritis in pediatrics.

**DOSAGE:** *Adults:* >18 yrs: Acute Sinusitis/Typhoid Fever: 500mg q12h for 10 days. LRTI/SSSI: Mild-Moderate: 500mg q12h for 7-14 days. Severe/Complicated: 750mg q12h for 7-14 days. Cystitis/Acute Uncompilcated UTI: 250mg q12h for 3 days. Mild-Moderate UTI: 250mg q12h for 7-14 days. Severe/Complicated UTI: 500mg q12h for 7-14 days. Chronic Bacterial Prostatitis: 500mg q12h for 28 days. Intra-Abdominal: 500mg q12h (w/ metronidazole) for 7-14 days. Bone and Joint: Mild-Moderate: 500mg q12h for >4-6 weeks. Severe/Complicated: 750mg q12h for >4-6 weeks. Infectious Diarrhea: 500mg q12h for 5-7 days. Uncomplicated Urethral/Cervical Gonococcal: 250mg single dose. Inhalational Anthrax: 500mg q12h for 60 days. CrCl 30-50mL/min: 250-500mg q12h. CrCl 5-29mL/min: 250-500mg q18h. Hemodialysis/Peritoneal Dialysis: 250-500mg q24h (after dialysis). Administer at least 2 hrs before or 6 hrs after magnesium or aluminum containing antacids, sucralfate, Videx (didanosine) chewable/buffered tablets or pediatric powder, or other products containing calcium, iron or zinc. *Pediatrics:* <18 yrs: Inhalational Anthrax: 15mg/kg q12h for 60 days. Max: 500mg/dose. 1-17 yrs: Complicated UTI/Pyelonephritis: 10-20mg/kg q12h for 10-21 days. Max: 750mg/dose.

**HOW SUPPLIED:** Sus: 250mg/5mL, 500mg/5mL [100mL]; Tab: 250mg, 500mg, 750mg

**CONTRAINDICATIONS:** Concomitant administration with tizanidine.

**WARNINGS/PRECAUTIONS:** Convulsions, increased intracranial pressure, and toxic psychosis reported. Caution with CNS disorders or if predisposed to seizures. Severe, fatal hypersensitivity reactions may occur. Pseudomembranous colitis, achilles and other tendon ruptures reported. D/C at first sign of rash or if pain, inflammation, or ruptured tendon occurs. Maintain hydration; avoid alkaline urine. Avoid excessive sunlight and UV light. Do not give via feeding tube. Monitor renal, hepatic, and hematopoietic function with prolonged use. Adjust dose with renal dysfunction.

**ADVERSE REACTIONS:** Nausea, dizziness, headache, CNS disturbances, vomiting, diarrhea, rash, abdominal pain/discomfort.

**INTERACTIONS:** See Contraindications. Increases theophylline and caffeine levels and prolongs effects. Fatal reactions have occurred with theophylline. Magnesium or aluminum containing antacids, sucralfate, Videx (didanosine) chewable/buffered tablets or pediatric powder, and products containing calcium, iron, or zinc decrease serum and urine levels; space doses at least 2 hrs before or 6 hrs after administration. Altered serum levels of phenytoin. Severe hypoglycemia with glyburide (rare). Potentiated by probenecid. Transient serum creatinine elevations with cyclosporine. Enhances oral anticoagulant effects. Monitor PT. Caution with drugs that lower seizure threshold.

**PREGNANCY:** Category C, not for use in nursing.

## CIPRO XR

ciprofloxacin (Schering)

RX

**THERAPEUTIC CLASS:** Fluoroquinolone

**INDICATIONS:** Uncomplicated (acute cystitis) and complicated urinary tract infections (UTI), and acute uncomplicated pyelonephritis due to *E.coli*.

**DOSAGE:** *Adults:* ≥18 yrs: Uncomplicated UTI: 500mg qd for 3 days. Complicated UTI: 1000mg qd for 7-14 days. CrCl <30mL/min: 500 mg qd. Acute Uncomplicated Pyelonephritis: 1000mg qd for 7-14 days. CrCl <30mL/min: 500mg qd. Take with fluids. Administer at least 2 hrs before or 6 hrs after magnesium or aluminum containing antacids, sucralfate, Videx (didanosine) chewable/buffered tablets or pediatric powder, metal cations (eg, iron), multivitamins with zinc. Avoid concomitant administration with dairy products alone, or with calcium-fortified products. Space concomitant calcium intake (>800mg) by at least 2 hrs. Do not split, crush, or chew. Swallow tab whole. Dialysis: Give after procedure is completed.

**HOW SUPPLIED:** Tab, Extended Release: 500mg, 1000mg



**CONTRAINDICATIONS:** Concomitant administration with tizanidine.

**WARNINGS/PRECAUTIONS:** Convulsions, increased intracranial pressure and toxic psychosis reported. Caution with CNS disorders or if predisposed to seizures. Severe, fatal hypersensitivity reactions may occur. Pseudomembranous colitis, achilles, and other tendon ruptures reported. Discontinue at first sign of rash or if pain, inflammation, or ruptured tendon occurs. Maintain hydration; avoid alkaline urine. Avoid excessive sunlight and UV light. Not interchangeable with immediate-release tablets.

**ADVERSE REACTIONS:** Nausea, headache.

**INTERACTIONS:** See Contraindications. Increases theophylline and caffeine levels and prolongs effects. Serious/fatal reactions have occurred with theophylline. Magnesium or aluminum containing antacids, sucralfate, Videx (didanosine) chewable/buffered tablets or pediatric powder, and products containing calcium, iron, or zinc decrease serum and urine levels; space doses at least 2 hrs before or 6 hrs after administration. Altered serum levels of phenytoin. Severe hypoglycemia with glyburide (rare). Potentiated by probenecid. Transient serum creatinine elevations with cyclosporine. Enhances oral anticoagulant effects. Caution with drugs that lower seizure threshold.

**PREGNANCY:** Category C, not for use in nursing.

## CIPRODEX — RX

ciprofloxacin - dexamethasone (Alcon)

**THERAPEUTIC CLASS:** Antibacterial/corticosteroid combination

**INDICATIONS:** Acute otitis media in pediatric patients with tympanostomy tubes. Acute otitis externa.

**DOSAGE:** *Adults:* Acute Otitis Externa: 4 drops in affected ear(s) bid for 7 days. Warm bottle in hand for 1-2 minutes to avoid dizziness. Shake well before use.
*Pediatrics:* ≥6 months: 4 drops in affected ear(s) bid for 7 days. Warm bottle in hand for 1-2 minutes to avoid dizziness. Shake well before use.

**HOW SUPPLIED:** Sus: (Ciprofloxacin-Dexamethasone) 0.3%-0.1% [5mL, 7.5mL]

**CONTRAINDICATIONS:** Viral infections of external ear canal including herpes simplex infections.

**WARNINGS/PRECAUTIONS:** Discontinue if hypersensitivity reaction occurs. Reevaluate if no improvement after one week.

**ADVERSE REACTIONS:** Ear pain/discomfort/pruritus.

**PREGNANCY:** Category C, not for use in nursing.

## CLAFORAN — RX

cefotaxime sodium (Sanofi-Aventis)

**THERAPEUTIC CLASS:** Cephalosporin (3rd generation)

**INDICATIONS:** Treatment of lower respiratory tract, genitourinary, gynecologic, intra-abdominal, skin and skin structure, bone and joint, and CNS infections (eg, meningitis), bacteremia, and septicemia. For surgical prophylaxis.

**DOSAGE:** *Adults:* Gonococcal Urethritis/Cervicitis (males/females): 500mg single dose IM. Rectal Gonorrhea: 0.5g (females) or 1g (males) single dose IM. Uncomplicated Infections: 1g IM/IV q12h. Moderate-Severe Infections: 1-2g IM/IV q8h. Septicemia: 2g IV q6-8h. Life-Threatening Infections: 2g IV q4h. Max: 12g/day. Surgical Prophylaxis: 1g IM/IV 30-90 minutes before surgery.

Cesarean Section: 1g IV when umbilical cord is clamped, then 1g IV at 6 and 12 hrs after 1st dose. CrCl <20mL/min/1.73 $m^2$: Give 1/2 of usual dose.
*Pediatrics:* >50kg: Use adult dose. Max: 12g/day. 1month-12 yrs and <50kg: 50-180mg/kg/day IM/IV divided in 4-6 doses. 1-4 weeks: 50mg/kg IV q8h. 0-1 week: 50mg/kg IV q12h. CrCl <20mL/min/1.73 $m^2$: Give 1/2 of usual dose.

**HOW SUPPLIED:** Inj: 500mg, 1g, 2g, 10g

**WARNINGS/PRECAUTIONS:** Cross sensitivity to penicillins and other cephalosporins may occur. Pseudomembranous colitis reported. May result in overgrowth of nonsusceptible organisms. Caution with history of GI disease. Reduce dose with renal dysfunction. Granulocytopenia may occur with long-term use. Monitor blood counts if therapy >10 days. Monitor injection site for tissue inflammation. False positive direct Coombs' tests reported.

**ADVERSE REACTIONS:** Injection site reactions, rash, pruritus, fever, eosinophilia, colitis, diarrhea.

**INTERACTIONS:** Increased nephrotoxicity with aminoglycosides.

**PREGNANCY:** Category B, caution in nursing.

## CLARINEX

desloratadine (Schering)

RX

**OTHER BRAND NAMES:** Clarinex Syrup (Schering) - Clarinex RediTabs (Schering)

**THERAPEUTIC CLASS:** $H_1$ antagonist

**INDICATIONS:** Relief of perennial allergic rhinitis and chronic idiopathic urticaria in patients ≥6 months of age. Relief of seasonal allergic rhinitis in patients ≥2 yrs of age.

**DOSAGE:** *Adults:* 5mg qd. Hepatic/Renal Impairment: 5mg every other day. Dissolve RediTabs on tongue with or without water.
*Pediatrics:* Tabs: ≥12 yrs: 5mg qd. 6-11 yrs: 2.5mg qd. Syrup: ≥12 yrs: 10mL (5mg) qd. 6-11 yrs: 5mL (2.5mg) qd. 12 months-5 yrs: 2.5mL (1.25mg) qd. 6-11 months: 2mL (1mg) qd. Dissolve RediTabs on tongue with or without water.

**HOW SUPPLIED:** Tab: 5mg; Tab, Disintegrating: (RediTabs) 2.5mg, 5mg; Syrup: 0.5mg/mL

**WARNINGS/PRECAUTIONS:** Adjust dose with renal or hepatic impairment. Caution in elderly.

**ADVERSE REACTIONS:** Pharyngitis, dry mouth, headache, fever, diarrhea, cough, upper respiratory tract infection, cough, irritability, somnolence, bronchitis, otitis media, vomiting, nausea, fatigue.

**INTERACTIONS:** Erythromycin, ketoconazole increase plasma levels.

**PREGNANCY:** Category C, not for use in nursing.

## CLARINEX-D 24 HOUR

desloratadine - pseudoephedrine sulfate (Schering)

RX

**THERAPEUTIC CLASS:** $H_1$ antagonist/sympathomimetic amine

**INDICATIONS:** Relief of nasal and non-nasal symptoms of seasonal allergic rhinitis including nasal congestion.

**DOSAGE:** *Adults:* 1 tab qd. Renal Impairment: 1 tab qod.
*Pediatrics:* ≥12 yrs: 1 tab qd. Renal Impairment: 1 tab qod.

**HOW SUPPLIED:** Tab, Extended Release: (Desloratadine-Pseudoephedrine) 5mg-240mg

**CONTRAINDICATIONS:** Narrow-angle glaucoma, urinary retention, MAOI therapy or within 14 days of discontinuation, severe HTN, severe CAD, hypersensitivity or idiosyncrasy to adrenergic agents, or to other drugs of similar chemical structures.

**WARNINGS/PRECAUTIONS:** Caution with HTN, DM, ischemic heart disease, increased intraocular pressure, hyperthyroidism, renal impairment, or prostatic hypertrophy. CNS stimulation with convulsions or cardiovascular collapse with accompanying hypotension may be produced by sympathomimetic amines. Avoid with hepatic insufficiency.



**ADVERSE REACTIONS:** Dry mouth, headache, insomnia, fatigue, pharyngitis, somnolence

**INTERACTIONS:** Do not use with MAOIs or within 14 days of discontinuation. Antihypertensive effects of β-adrenergic blocking agents, methyldopa, mecamylamine, reserpine, and veratrum alkaloids may be reduced by sympathomimetics (eg, pseudoephedrine). Increased ectopic pacemaker activity with digitalis.

**PREGNANCY:** Category C, not for use in nursing.

## CLARIPEL RX

hydroquinone (Stiefel)

**THERAPEUTIC CLASS:** Depigmenting agent

**INDICATIONS:** Gradual treatment of ultraviolet induced dyschromia and discoloration resulting from use of oral contraceptives, pregnancy, hormone replacement therapy, or skin trauma.

**DOSAGE:** *Adults:* Apply bid.
*Pediatrics:* >12 yrs: Apply bid.

**HOW SUPPLIED:** Cre: 4% [28g, 45g]

**WARNINGS/PRECAUTIONS:** Avoid sun exposure on bleached skin. Claripel contains sunscreen. May produce unwanted cosmetic effects if not used as directed. Test for skin sensitivity. Discontinue if no lightening effect after 2 months of therapy, if blue-black skin discoloration occurs, or if itching, vesicle formation, or excessive inflammatory reactions occur. Contains sodium metabisulfite; may cause serious allergic type reactions. Avoid contact with eyes.

**ADVERSE REACTIONS:** Cutaneous hypersensitivity (contact dermatitis).

**PREGNANCY:** Category C, caution in nursing.

## CLARITIN OTC OTC

loratadine (Schering)

**OTHER BRAND NAMES:** Claritin Reditab OTC (Schering)

**THERAPEUTIC CLASS:** $H_1$ antagonist

**INDICATIONS:** Relief of symptoms due to hay fever or other upper respiratory allergies.

**DOSAGE:** *Adults:* (Reditab, Syrup, Tab) 10mg qd. Max: 10mg/d. Dissolve Reditab on tongue. Hepatic/Renal Impairment: May need to adjust dose.
*Pediatrics:* ≥6 yrs: (Reditab, Syr, Tab) 10mg qd. Max: 10mg/d. 2-5 yrs: (Syr) 5mg qd. Max: 5mg/d. Dissolve Reditab on tongue. Hepatic/Renal Impairment: May need to adjust dose.

**HOW SUPPLIED:** Syrup: 1mg/mL; Tab, Extended Release: (24 hr) 10mg; Tab, Disintegrating: (Reditab) 10mg

**WARNINGS/PRECAUTIONS:** Caution with hepatic or renal impairment.

**PREGNANCY:** Safety in pregnancy and nursing is not known.

## CLARITIN-D OTC

OTC

loratadine - pseudoephedrine sulfate (Schering)

**THERAPEUTIC CLASS:** $H_1$ antagonist/sympathomimetic amine

**INDICATIONS:** Relief of symptoms due to hay fever or other upper respiratory allergies. Reduces swelling of nasal passages. Relief of sinus congestion and pressure.

**DOSAGE:** *Adults:* 5-120mg tab q12h or 10-240mg tab qd (with full glass of water). Max: 10-240mg/24 hrs. Hepatic/Renal Impairment: May need to adjust dose. Do not divide, crush, chew or dissolve tabs.
*Pediatrics:* >12 yrs: 5-120mg tab q12h, or 10-240mg tab qd (with full glass of water). Max: 10-240mg/24 hrs. Hepatic/Renal Impairment: May need to adjust dose. Do not divide, crush, chew or dissolve tabs.

**HOW SUPPLIED:** Tab, Extended Release: (Loratadine-Pseudoephedrine) (12 Hour) 5-120mg, (24 Hour) 10-240mg

**WARNINGS/PRECAUTIONS:** Caution with hepatic or renal impairment, heart disease, thyroid disease, high BP, diabetes, enlarged prostate.

**ADVERSE REACTIONS:** Dizziness, insomnia, nervousness.

**INTERACTIONS:** Avoid during or within 14 days MAOIs.

**PREGNANCY:** Safety in pregnancy and nursing is not known.

## CLEAR EYES

OTC

glycerin - naphazoline HCl (Ross)

**THERAPEUTIC CLASS:** Decongestant/lubricant

**INDICATIONS:** Temporary relief of redness due to minor eye irritation. For protection against further irritation or dryness of the eye.

**DOSAGE:** *Adults:* 1-2 drops in affected eye up to qid.

**HOW SUPPLIED:** Sol: (Naphazoline-Glycerin) 0.012%-0.2% [15mL, 30mL]

**WARNINGS/PRECAUTIONS:** May temporarily enlarge pupils. Overuse may cause more redness. Do not touch container tip to any surface to avoid contamination. D/C if eye pain or vision changes occur, if redness or irritation continues, or if condition worsens or persists >72 hrs. Supervision required in patients with narrow angle glaucoma.

**PREGNANCY:** Safety in pregnancy or nursing not known.

## CLEAR EYES ACR

OTC

glycerin - zinc sulfate - naphazoline HCl (Ross)

**THERAPEUTIC CLASS:** Decongestant/lubricant/astringent

**INDICATIONS:** Temporary relief of redness and discomfort due to minor eye irritation. For protection against further eye irritation. Temporary relief of burning and irritation due to dryness of the eye.

**DOSAGE:** *Adults:* 1-2 drops in affected eye up to qid.

**HOW SUPPLIED:** Sol: (Naphazoline-Glycerin-Zinc) 0.012%-0.2%-0.25% [15mL, 30mL]

**WARNINGS/PRECAUTIONS:** May temporarily enlarge pupils. Overuse may cause more redness. Do not touch container tip to any surface to avoid contamination. D/C if eye pain or vision changes occur, if redness or irritation continues, or if condition worsens or persists >72 hrs. Supervision required in patients with narrow angle glaucoma.

**PREGNANCY:** Safety in pregnancy or nursing not known.

C

## CLEAR EYES CLR OTC

glycerin - hydroxypropyl methylcellulose (Ross)

**THERAPEUTIC CLASS:** Lubricant

**INDICATIONS:** To moisten daily wear soft lenses while on the eyes during the day. To moisten extended wear soft lenses upon awakening, prior to retiring at night, and as needed during the day.

**DOSAGE:** *Adults:* May use prn throughout the day. Minor Irritation, Discomfort, Blurring With Lenses: Instill 1-2 drops on eye and blink 2-3 times. Remove lenses if discomfort continues.

**HOW SUPPLIED:** Sol: [15mL, 30mL]

**WARNINGS/PRECAUTIONS:** Eye problems including corneal ulcers can occur; remove contacts if eye discomfort, excessive tearing, vision changes, or eye redness occur. Do not touch container tip to any surface to avoid contamination. Eye irritation, unusual eye secretions, reduced visual acuity, blurred vision, photophobia, and dry eyes may occur with contact lenses; remove lenses if any of these occur.

**ADVERSE REACTIONS:** Transient contact urticaria.

**PREGNANCY:** Safety in pregnancy and nursing not known.

## CLENIA RX

sulfur - sulfacetamide sodium (Upsher-Smith)

**THERAPEUTIC CLASS:** Sulfonamide/sulfur combination

**INDICATIONS:** Topical treatment of acne vulgaris, acne rosacea, and seborrheic dermatitis.

**DOSAGE:** *Adults:* (Cleanser) Wash qd-bid. Massage into skin for 10-20 seconds, then rinse and dry. (Cream) Initial: Apply qd. Titrate: Increase up to bid-tid prn.
*Pediatrics:* >12 yrs: (Cleanser) Wash qd-bid. Massage into skin for 10-20 seconds, then rinse and dry. (Cream) Initial: Apply qd. Titrate: Increase up to bid-tid prn.

**HOW SUPPLIED:** Cleanser: (Sulfacetamide-Sulfur) 10%-5% [170g, 340g]; Cre: 10%-5% [28g]

**CONTRAINDICATIONS:** Kidney disease.

**WARNINGS/PRECAUTIONS:** Discontinue if excessive irritation occurs. Avoid contact with eyes, eyelid, lips, or mucous membranes. Caution with denuded or abraded skin. Can cause reddening and scaling of epidermis.

**ADVERSE REACTIONS:** Dryness, erythema, itching, edema.

**PREGNANCY:** Category C, caution in nursing.

## CLEOCIN RX

clindamycin HCl (Pharmacia & Upjohn)

**Pseudomembranous colitis reported; may range in severity from mild to life threatening.**

**THERAPEUTIC CLASS:** Lincomycin derivative

**INDICATIONS:** Serious infections caused by anaerobes, streptococci, pneumococci and staphylococci.

**DOSAGE:** *Adults:* Serious Infection: 150-300mg PO q6h or 600-1200mg/day IM/IV given bid-qid. More Severe Infection: 300-450mg PO q6h or 1200-2700mg/day IM/IV given bid-qid. Life-threatening Infections: Up to 4800mg/day IV. Max: 600mg per IM injection. Take oral form with full glass of water. Treat β-hemolytic strep for at least 10 days.

*Pediatrics:* Birth-16 yrs: Serious Infection: 8-16mg/kg/day PO. More Severe Infection: 16-20mg/kg/day PO. 1 month-16 yrs: 20-40mg/kg/day IM/IV given tid-qid; use higher dose for more severe infection. <1 month: 15-20mg/kg/day IM/IV given tid-qid. Take oral form with full glass of water. Treat β-hemolytic strep for at least 10 days.

**HOW SUPPLIED:** Cap: (HCl) 75mg, 150mg, 300mg; Inj: (Phosphate) 150mg/mL, 300mg/50mL, 600mg/50mL, 900mg/50mL; Sus: (HCl) 75mg/5mL [100g]

**WARNINGS/PRECAUTIONS:** D/C if diarrhea occurs. May permit overgrowth of clostridia. Not for treatment of meningitis. Caution with atopic patients, GI disease (eg, colitis), hepatic disease and the elderly. Monitor blood, hepatic and renal function with long-term use. Do not give injection undiluted as a bolus. The 75mg and 100mg caps contain tartrazine.

**ADVERSE REACTIONS:** Abdominal pain, pseudomembranous colitis, esophagitis, nausea, vomiting, diarrhea, hypersensitivity reactions, metallic taste (Inj), jaundice, blood dyscrasias, pruritus, vaginitis, superinfection (prolonged use).

**INTERACTIONS:** Antagonism may occur with erythromycin. May potentiate neuromuscular blockers.

**PREGNANCY:** Category B, not for use in nursing.

## CLEOCIN T

RX

clindamycin phosphate (Pharmacia & Upjohn)

**THERAPEUTIC CLASS:** Lincomycin derivative

**INDICATIONS:** Acne vulgaris.

**DOSAGE:** *Adults:* Apply thin film bid.
*Pediatrics:* >12 yrs: Apply thin film bid. May use more than 1 pledget.

**HOW SUPPLIED:** Gel: 1% [30g, 60g]; Lot: 1% [60mL]; Sol: 1% [30mL, 60mL]; Swab (Pledgets): 1% [60$^{s}$]

**CONTRAINDICATIONS:** Hypersensitivity to lincomycin. History of regional enteritis, ulcerative colitis, or antibiotic-associated colitis.

**WARNINGS/PRECAUTIONS:** Avoid eyes, abraded skin, mucous membranes, and mouth. Caution in atopic patients. D/C if significant diarrhea occurs.

**ADVERSE REACTIONS:** Dryness, oily skin, erythema, peeling, burning, itching, pseudomembranous colitis (rare).

**INTERACTIONS:** May potentiate neuromuscular blockers.

**PREGNANCY:** Category B, not for use in nursing.

## CLEOCIN VAGINAL

RX

clindamycin phosphate (Pharmacia & Upjohn)

**OTHER BRAND NAMES:** Clindamax Vaginal (PharmaDerm) - Cleocin Vaginal Ovules (Pharmacia & Upjohn)

**THERAPEUTIC CLASS:** Lincomycin derivative

**INDICATIONS:** (Cream) Treatment of bacterial vaginosis in non-pregnant women and pregnant women during the 2nd and 3rd trimester. (Sup) Treatment of bacterial vaginosis in non-pregnant women.

**DOSAGE:** *Adults:* (Cream) 1 applicatorful intravaginally qhs. Treat non-pregnant females for 3 or 7 days. Treat pregnant females (2nd and 3rd trimester) for 7 days. (Sup) 1 suppository intravaginally qhs for 3 days.
*Pediatrics:* Post-Menarchal: (Sup) 1 suppository intravaginally qhs for 3 days.

**HOW SUPPLIED:** Cre: 2% [40g]; Sup, Vaginal: (Ovules) 100mg [3$^{s}$]

**CONTRAINDICATIONS:** Hypersensitivity to lincomycin. History of regional enteritis, ulcerative colitis, or antibiotic-associated colitis.

C

**WARNINGS/PRECAUTIONS:** Do not use condoms or contraceptive diaphragms within 72 hrs following treatment. Monitor for pseudomembranous colitis. Avoid eye contact. Do not engage in vaginal intercourse or use other vaginal products (such as tampons or douches) during treatment. Monitor for pseudomembranous colitis.

**ADVERSE REACTIONS:** Vaginitis, vulvovaginal disorder, candidiasis, moniliasis, pruritus, abnormal labor.

**INTERACTIONS:** May potentiate neuromuscular blockers.

**PREGNANCY:** Category B, not for use in nursing.

## CLIMARA

RX

estradiol (Berlex)

**Estrogens increase risk of endometrial cancer. Estrogens, with or without progestins, should not be used for the prevention of cardiovascular disease or dementia. Increased risks of MI, stroke, invasive breast cancer, PE, and DVT in postmenopausal women (50-79 yrs of age) reported. Increased risk of developing probable dementia in postmenopausal women ≥65 yrs of age reported.**

**THERAPEUTIC CLASS:** Estrogen

**INDICATIONS:** Treatment of moderate to severe vasomotor symptoms and/or vulvar/vaginal atrophy associated with menopause. Treatment of hypoestrogenism due to hypogonadism, castration, or primary ovarian failure. Prevention of postmenopausal osteoporosis.

**DOSAGE:** *Adults:* Apply 1 patch weekly to lower abdomen or upper area of buttocks (avoid breasts and waistline). Rotate application sites. Vasomotor Symptoms: Initial: 0.025mg/day patch once weekly. Titrate: Adjust dose as needed. Wait 1 week after withdrawal of oral therapy before initiating patch. Discontinue or taper at 3-6 month intervals. Osteoporosis Prevention: Minimum Effective Dose: 0.025mg/day once weekly.

**HOW SUPPLIED:** Patch: 0.025mg/day, 0.0375mg/day, 0.05mg/day, 0.06mg/day, 0.075mg/day, 0.1mg/day [4s]

**CONTRAINDICATIONS:** Pregnancy, undiagnosed abnormal genital bleeding, breast cancer, estrogen-dependent neoplasia, DVT/PE, active or recent (eg, within 1 year) thromboembolic disease (eg, stroke, MI), liver dysfunction or disease.

**WARNINGS/PRECAUTIONS:** May increase risk of cardiovascular events (eg, MI, stroke), venous thrombosis, and PE; d/c immediately if any of these events occur or are suspected. May increase risk of breast/endometrial cancer, and gallbladder disease. Retinal vascular thrombosis reported; monitor and d/c if papilledema or retinal vascular lesions occur. Consider addition of a progestin if no hysterectomy. May elevate BP; monitor at regular intervals. May cause elevations of plasma triglycerides with pre-existing hypertriglyceridemia. Caution with history of cholestatic jaundice associated with past estrogen use or with pregnancy; d/c with recurrence. May lead to increased thyroid-binding globulin levels; monitor thyroid function. May cause fluid retention; caution with cardiac/renal dysfunction. Caution with severe hypocalcemia. May increase risk of ovarian cancer. May exacerbate endometriosis, asthma, DM, epilepsy, migraine, porphyria; use with caution.

**ADVERSE REACTIONS:** Skin irritation, headache, arthralgia, depression, breast pain, leukorrhea, upper respiratory tract infection, sinusitis.

**INTERACTIONS:** CYP3A4 inducers (eg, St. John's wort, phenobarbital, carbamazepine, rifampin) may decrease levels which may decrease therapeutic effects and/or change uterine bleeding profile. CYP3A4 inhibitors (eg, erythromycin, clarithromycin, ketoconazole, itraconazole, ritonavir, grapefruit juice) may increase levels which may result in side effects.

**PREGNANCY:** Contraindicated in pregnancy, caution in nursing.

## CLIMARA PRO
estradiol - levonorgestrel (Berlex)

RX

**Estrogens and progestins should not be used for the prevention of cardiovascular disease or dementia. Increased risks of MI, stroke, invasive breast cancer, PE, and DVT in postmenopausal women (50-79 yrs of age) reported. Increased risk of developing probable dementia in postmenopausal women ≥65 yrs of age reported.**

**THERAPEUTIC CLASS:** Estrogen/progestogen combination

**INDICATIONS:** Treatment of moderate to severe vasomotor symptoms associated with menopause. Prevention of postmenopausal osteoporosis.

**DOSAGE:** *Adults:* Apply 1 patch weekly to lower abdomen (avoid breasts and waistline). Rotate application site; allow 1 week between same site. Re-evaluate periodically (3-6 month intervals).

**HOW SUPPLIED:** Patch: (Estradiol-Levonorgestrel): 0.045mg-0.015mg/day [4[s]]

**CONTRAINDICATIONS:** Pregnancy, undiagnosed abnormal genital bleeding, breast cancer, estrogen-dependent neoplasia, DVT/PE, active or recent (eg, within 1 year) thromboembolic disease (eg, stroke, MI), liver dysfunction or disease.

**WARNINGS/PRECAUTIONS:** May increase risk of cardiovascular events (eg, MI, stroke), venous thrombosis, and PE; d/c immediately if any of these events occur or are suspected. May increase risk of breast/endometrial cancer, and gallbladder disease. Retinal vascular thrombosis reported; monitor and d/c if papilledema or retinal vascular lesions occur. Consider addition of a progestin if no hysterectomy. May elevate BP; monitor at regular intervals. May cause elevations of plasma triglycerides with pre-existing hypertriglyceridemia. Caution with history of cholestatic jaundice associated with past estrogen use or with pregnancy; d/c with recurrence. May lead to increased thyroid-binding globulin levels; monitor thyroid function. May cause fluid retention; caution with cardiac/renal dysfunction. Caution with severe hypocalcemia. May increase risk of ovarian cancer. May exacerbate endometriosis, asthma, DM, epilepsy, migraine, porphyria; use with caution.

**ADVERSE REACTIONS:** Application site reaction, vaginal bleeding, breast pain, upper respiratory infection, back pain, headache, depression, arthralgia, flu syndrome, abdominal pain.

**INTERACTIONS:** CYP3A4 inducers (eg, St. John's wort, phenobarbital, carbamazepine, rifampin) may decrease levels which may decrease therapeutic effects and/or change uterine bleeding profile. CYP3A4 inhibitors (eg, erythromycin, clarithromycin, ketoconazole, itraconazole, ritonavir, grapefruit juice) may increase levels which may result in side effects.

**PREGNANCY:** Contraindicated in pregnancy, caution in nursing.

## CLINDAGEL
clindamycin phosphate (Galderma)

RX

**THERAPEUTIC CLASS:** Lincomycin derivative

**INDICATIONS:** Acne vulgaris.

**DOSAGE:** *Adults:* Apply thin film once daily.
*Pediatrics:* ≥12 yrs: Apply thin film once daily.

**HOW SUPPLIED:** Gel: 1% [40mL, 75mL]

**CONTRAINDICATIONS:** Hypersensitivity to lincomycin. History of regional enteritis, ulcerative colitis, or antibiotic-associated colitis.

**WARNINGS/PRECAUTIONS:** Discontinue if significant diarrhea occurs. Caution in atopic individuals.

**ADVERSE REACTIONS:** Peeling, pruritus, pseudomembranous colitis (rare).

**INTERACTIONS:** May potentiate neuromuscular blockers.

**PREGNANCY:** Category B, not for use in nursing.

## CLINDESSE RX
clindamycin phosphate (Ther-Rx)

**THERAPEUTIC CLASS:** Lincomycin derivative

**INDICATIONS:** Treatment of bacterial vaginosis in non-pregnant women.

**DOSAGE:** *Adults:* 1 applicatorful administered intravaginally any time of day.

**HOW SUPPLIED:** Cre: 2% [5g]

**CONTRAINDICATIONS:** Hypersensitivity to lincomycin. History of regional enteritis, ulcerative colitis, or antibiotic-associated colitis.

**WARNINGS/PRECAUTIONS:** Do not use condoms or contraceptive diaphragms within 5 days following treatment. Monitor for pseudomembranous colitis. Avoid eye contact. Do not engage in vaginal intercourse or use other vaginal products (such as tampons or douches) during treatment.

**ADVERSE REACTIONS:** Fungal vaginosis, vulvuvaginal pruritus.

**INTERACTIONS:** May potentiate neuromuscular blockers.

**PREGNANCY:** Category B, not for use in nursing

## CLOBEVATE RX
clobetasol propionate (Stiefel)

**THERAPEUTIC CLASS:** Corticosteroid

**INDICATIONS:** Inflammatory and pruritic manifestations of corticosteroid-responsive dermatoses.

**DOSAGE:** *Adults:* Apply thin layer bid. Limit treatment to 2 consecutive weeks. Max: 50g/week. Avoid with occlusive dressings.
*Pediatrics:* ≥12 yrs: Apply thin layer bid. Limit treatment to 2 consecutive weeks. Max: 50g/week. Avoid with occlusive dressings.

**HOW SUPPLIED:** Gel: 0.05% [45g]

**WARNINGS/PRECAUTIONS:** May produce reversible HPA axis suppression, Cushing's syndrome, hyperglycemia, and glucosuria. Pediatrics may be more susceptible to systemic toxicity. Discontinue if irritation occurs. Use appropriate antifungal or antibacterial with concomitant skin infections; discontinue if infection does not clear. Should not be used to treat rosacea or perioral dermatitis. Avoid use on face, groin, or axillae.

**ADVERSE REACTIONS:** Burning, stinging, irritation, pruritus, erythema, folliculitis, cracking and fissuring of the skin, numbness of fingers, skin atrophy, telangiectasia.

**PREGNANCY:** Category C, caution in nursing.

## CLOBEX RX
clobetasol propionate (Galderma)

**THERAPEUTIC CLASS:** Corticosteroid

**INDICATIONS:** (Lot) Relief of corticosteroid responsive dermatoses. Treatment of moderate to severe plaque psoriasis (<10% BSA). (Shampoo) Treatment of moderate to severe scalp psoriasis. (Spray) Treatment of moderate to severe plaque psoriasis affecting up to 20% BSA.

**DOSAGE:** *Adults:* ≥18 yrs: (Lot) Apply bid for up to 2 consecutive weeks. Psoriasis: Reassess after 2 weeks; may repeat for additional 2 weeks. Max: 50g/week or 50mL/week. (Shampoo) Apply thin film daily to dry scalp for up to 4 consecutive weeks. Leave in place for 15 mins before lathering and rinsing.

(Spray) Spray on affected area(s) bid. Rub in gently and completely. Reassess after 2 weeks; may repeat for additional 2 weeks. Limit treatment to 4 weeks. Max: 50g/week.

**HOW SUPPLIED:** Lot: 0.05% [30mL, 59mL]; Shampoo: 0.05% [118mL]; Spray: 0.05% [2oz]



**WARNINGS/PRECAUTIONS:** Not for use on the face, groin, axillae, eyes, lips, or for the treatment of rosacea or perioral dermatitis. May produce reversible HPA axis suppression, manifestations of Cushing's syndrome, hyperglycemia, and glucosuria. Discontinue if irritation occurs. Use appropriate antifungal or antibacterial agent with dermatological infections.

**ADVERSE REACTIONS:** Burning/stinging, pruritus, folliculitis, skin dryness, skin atrophy, telangiectasia.

**PREGNANCY:** Category C, caution in nursing.

## CLODERM

clocortolone pivalate (Healthpoint) RX

**THERAPEUTIC CLASS:** Topical corticosteroid

**INDICATIONS:** Corticosteroid-responsive dermatoses.

**DOSAGE:** *Adults:* Apply tid. Use with occlusive dressing for management of psoriasis or recalcitrant conditions.
*Pediatrics:* Apply TID. Use with occlusive dressing for management of psoriasis or recalcitrant conditions.

**HOW SUPPLIED:** Cre: 0.1% [15g, 45g, 90g]

**WARNINGS/PRECAUTIONS:** May produce reversible HPA axis suppression, manifestations of Cushing's syndrome, hyperglycemia, glucosuria. Caution when applied to large surface areas or under occlusive dressings. Use appropriate antifungal or antibacterial agent with dermatological infections. D/C if infection is not adequately controlled or if irritation develops.

**ADVERSE REACTIONS:** Burning, itching, irritation, dryness, folliculitis, hypertrichosis, acneform eruptions, hypopigmentation, perioral/allergic contact dermatitis, secondary infection, skin atrophy.

**PREGNANCY:** Category C, caution in nursing.

## CLOLAR

clofarabine (Genzyme) RX

**THERAPEUTIC CLASS:** Antimetabolite

**INDICATIONS:** Treatment of pediatric patients 1-21 years old with relapsed or refractory acute lymphoblastic leukemia after at least two prior regimens.

**DOSAGE:** *Pediatrics:* 1-21 yrs: 52mg/m$^2$ IV over 2 hours daily for 5 consecutive days. Treatment cycles are repeated following recovery or return to baseline organ function, approximately 2-6 weeks. Continuous IV fluids throughout 5 days of clofarabine therapy is recommended. The use of prophylactic steroids (eg, 100mg/m$^2$ hydrocortisone on Days 1-3) may be of benefit in preventing signs and symptoms of systemic inflammatory response syndrome (SIRS) or capillary leak. If patient develops signs and symptoms of SIRS or capillary leak, clofarabine therapy should be discontinued and appropriate supportive measures should be provided. Close monitoring of renal and hepatic function is required. If substantial increases in creatine or bilirubin occur, clofarabine therapy should be discontinued.

**HOW SUPPLIED:** Inj: 1mg/mL

**WARNINGS/PRECAUTIONS:** Suppression of bone marrow function should be anticipated. Increased risk of infection, including severe sepsis is possible. Monitor for signs and symptoms of tumor lysis syndrome, as well as cytokine release that could develop into SIRS/capillary leak syndrome and organ dysfunction. D/C immediately if SIRS or capillary leak syndrome develop. Severe bone marrow suppression, including neutropenia, anemia and thrombocytopenia have been observed. Dehydration may occur due to vomiting and diarrhea. Clofarabine should be discontinued if patient develops hypotension for any reason during the 5 days of administration. Since clofarabine is excreted primarily by the kidneys, drugs with known renal toxicity should be avoided during the 5 days of administration. Since the liver is a known target of clofarabine, concomitant use of medications known to induce hepatic toxicity should also be avoided. Patients taking medications known to affect BP or cardiac function should be closely monitored during administration.



**ADVERSE REACTIONS:** Vomiting, nausea, diarrhea, anemia, leukopenia, thrombocytopenia, neutropenia, febrile neutropenia, and infection.

**PREGNANCY:** Category D, not for use in nursing.

## CLOMID — RX
clomiphene citrate (Sanofi-Aventis)

**THERAPEUTIC CLASS:** Ovulatory stimulant

**INDICATIONS:** Treatment of ovulatory dysfunction in women desiring pregnancy.

**DOSAGE:** *Adults:* Initial: 50mg/day for 5 days. Start any time if no recent uterine bleeding. If progestin-induced bleeding is intended, or if spontaneous uterine bleeding occurs, start on the 5th day of the cycle. If ovulation does not occur, increase to 100mg qd for 5 days, 30 days after the 1st course. Max: 100mg qd for 5 days and 3 courses of therapy.

**HOW SUPPLIED:** Tab: 50mg* *scored

**CONTRAINDICATIONS:** Pregnancy, liver disease or history of liver dysfunction, abnormal uterine bleeding of undetermined origin, ovarian cysts or enlargement not due to polycystic ovarian syndrome, uncontrolled thyroid or adrenal dysfunction, organic intracranial lesion (eg, pituitary tumor).

**WARNINGS/PRECAUTIONS:** Increased incidence of visual symptoms with increasing total dose or therapy duration; d/c treatment and perform complete ophthalmological evaluation. Ovarian hyperstimulation syndrome reported; monitor for abdominal pain, nausea, vomiting, diarrhea, weight gain. Increased chance of multiple pregnancy. Perform pelvic exam before initiating therapy and before each course. Prolonged use may increase risk of borderline/invasive ovarian tumor.

**ADVERSE REACTIONS:** Ovarian enlargement, vasomotor flushes, nausea, vomiting, breast discomfort, abdominal-pelvic discomfort/distention/bloating, visual symptoms, headache, abnormal uterine bleeding.

**PREGNANCY:** Category X, caution in nursing.

## CLORPRES — RX
chlorthalidone - clonidine HCl (Mylan Bertek)

**THERAPEUTIC CLASS:** Central alpha-agonist/monosulfamyl diuretic

**INDICATIONS:** Treatment of hypertension. Not for initial therapy.

**DOSAGE:** *Adults:* Determine dose by individual titration. 0.1mg clonidine-15mg chlorthalidone tab qd-bid. Max: 0.6mg clonidine-30mg chlorthalidone/day.

**HOW SUPPLIED:** Tab: (Clonidine-Chlorthalidone) 0.1mg-15mg*, 0.2mg-15mg*, 0.3mg-15mg* *scored

**CONTRAINDICATIONS:** Anuria, sulfonamide hypersensitivity.

**WARNINGS/PRECAUTIONS:** Caution with severe renal disease, hepatic dysfunction, asthma, severe coronary insufficiency, recent MI, cerebrovascular disease. May develop allergic reaction to oral clonidine if sensitive to clonidine patch. Avoid abrupt withdrawal. Continue therapy to within 4 hrs of surgery and resume after. Monitor for fluid/electrolyte imbalance. Hyperuricemia, hypokalemia, and hyperglycemia may occur.

**ADVERSE REACTIONS:** Drowsiness, dizziness, constipation, sedation, nausea, vomiting, blood dyscrasias, hypersensitivity reactions, orthostatic symptoms, impotence.

**INTERACTIONS:** Potentiates other antihypertensives. May increase response to tubocurarine. May decrease arterial response to norepinephrine. Antidiabetic agents may need adjustment. Risk of lithium toxicity. TCAs may reduce effects of clonidine. Amitriptyline may enhance ocular toxicity. Enhanced CNS-depressive effects of alcohol, barbiturates or other sedatives. Orthostatic hypotension aggravated by alcohol, barbiturates, narcotics.

**PREGNANCY:** (Clonidine) Category C, caution in nursing. (Chlorthalidone) Category B, not for use in nursing.

## CLOZAPINE

clozapine (Various)

RX

**Risk of agranulocytosis, seizures, myocarditis, and other cardiovascular and respiratory effects. Conduct baseline WBC and differential before therapy, then regularly, and 4 weeks after discontinuation. Elderly patients with dementia-related psychosis treated with atypical antipsychotic drugs are at an increased risk of death; most appeared to be cardiovascular (eg, heart failure, sudden death) or infectious (eg, pneumonia) in nature. Clozapine is not approved for the treatment of patients with dementia-related psychosis.**

**OTHER BRAND NAMES:** Clozaril (Novartis)

**THERAPEUTIC CLASS:** Dibenzapine derivative

**INDICATIONS:** Management of severe schizophrenia when response to standard schizophrenia treatment fails. To reduce the risk of recurrent suicidal behavior with schizophrenia or schizoaffective disorder.

**DOSAGE:** *Adults:* Initial: 12.5mg qd-bid. Titrate: Increase by 25-50mg/day, up to 300-450mg/day by end of 2nd week, then increase weekly or bi-weekly by up to 100mg. Usual: 100-900mg/day given tid. Max: 900mg/day. If at risk of suicidal behavior then treat for at least 2 yrs then assess; reassess thereafter at regular intervals. To d/c, gradually reduce dose over 1-2 weeks. Monitor for psychotic symptoms if abrupt discontinuation warranted (eg, leukopenia).

**HOW SUPPLIED:** Tab: (Clozapine) 12.5mg, 25mg, 100mg; (Clozaril) 25mg*, 100mg* *scored

**CONTRAINDICATIONS:** Myeloproliferative disorders, uncontrolled epilepsy, paralytic ileus, history of clozapine induced agranulocytosis or severe granulocytopenia, severe CNS depression, coma, with agents with potential to cause agranulocytosis or suppress bone marrow function.

**WARNINGS/PRECAUTIONS:** Reserve treatment for severely ill patients unresponsive to other schizophrenia therapies. Monitor for hyperglycemia, worsening of glucose control with DM, FBG levels with diabetes risk. Significant risk of orthostatic hypotension, and tachycardia. May impair alertness with initial doses. May cause high fever, hyperglycemia, or pulmonary embolism. Cardiomyopathy reported; d/c unless benefit outweighs risk. Caution with prostatic enlargement, narrow angle glaucoma, and renal, hepatic, or cardiac/pulmonary disease. NMS and tardive dyskinesia reported. Acquire WBC and ANC at baseline, then weekly for 1st 6 months of therapy, then every 2 weeks for 6 months, and then every 4 weeks thereafter if WBCs and ANC are acceptable. Avoid initiation of treatment if WBCs <3500/mm$^3$, ANC <2000/mm$^3$, history of myeloproliferative disorder, previous clozapine-induced agranulocytosis or granulocytopenia. D/C treatment if WBCs <3000/mm$^3$, ANC <1500/mm$^3$, eosinophils >4000/mm$^3$, or if myocarditis develops. D/C over 1-2 weeks. Varying degrees of intestinal peristalsis impairment (eg, constipation, intestinal obstruction, paralytic ileus), ECG changes reported.

**ADVERSE REACTIONS:** Drowsiness, vertigo, headache, tremor, salivation, sweating, dry mouth, visual disturbances, tachycardia, hypotension, syncope, constipation, nausea, blood dyscrasias, fever.



**INTERACTIONS:** See Contraindications. Avoid with bone marrow suppressants, epinephrine, and carbamazepine. Caution with CNS-active drugs, anesthesia, alcohol, paroxetine, sertraline, fluvoxamine, benzodiazepines, other psychotropics, inhibitors/inducers of CYP1A2, 2D6, 3A4. Potentiates hypotensive effects of antihypertensives and anticholinergic effects of atropine-type drugs. Decrease dose with drugs metabolized by CYP2D6. Caution with general anesthesia. CYP450 inducers (eg, phenytoin, nicotine, rifampin) decrease plasma levels. CYP450 inhibitors (eg, cimetidine, caffeine, erythromycin, citalopram) increase plasma levels.

**PREGNANCY:** Category B, not for use in nursing.

## COGNEX — RX

tacrine HCl (Sciele)

**THERAPEUTIC CLASS:** Reversible cholinesterase inhibitor

**INDICATIONS:** Treatment of mild to moderate dementia of the Alzheimer's type.

**DOSAGE:** *Adults:* Initial: 10mg qid. Titrate: Increase to 20mg qid after 4 weeks, then increase at 4-week intervals to 30mg qid then to 40mg qid. ALT/SGPT: >3 to <5x ULN: Reduce dose by 40mg/day and resume dose titration when levels are normal. >5x ULN: Stop therapy and monitor; may rechallenge when ALT/SGPT levels are normal. D/C and do not rechallenge if jaundice and/or signs of hypersensitivity. Rechallenge: 10mg qid, may titrate if normal ALT/SGPT after 6 weeks. Monitor weekly for 16 weeks, then monthly for 2 months, and every 3 months thereafter. Take between meals.

**HOW SUPPLIED:** Cap: 10mg, 20mg, 30mg, 40mg

**CONTRAINDICATIONS:** Hypersensitivity to acridine derivatives, history of tacrine-associated jaundice (bilirubin >3mg/dL) or signs of hypersensitivity associated with ALT/SGPT elevations.

**WARNINGS/PRECAUTIONS:** Vagotonic effects; caution with conduction abnormalities, bradyarrhythmia, sick sinus syndrome. May increase risk of developing ulcers. Monitor LFTs every other week from weeks 4-16 from start of therapy, then every 3 months. Modify LFT monitoring based on LFTs (see dosage). Higher incidence of LFTs elevation in females. May cause seizures, bladder outflow obstruction, neutrophil abnormalities. May worsen cognitive function with abrupt withdrawal. Caution with liver disease, ulcers, asthma. D/C with clinical jaundice or hypersensitivity with ALT/SGPT elevations.

**ADVERSE REACTIONS:** Elevated LFTs, nausea, vomiting, diarrhea, dyspepsia, myalgia, anorexia, ataxia.

**INTERACTIONS:** May potentiate succinylcholine, cholinesterase inhibitors, cholinergic agonists, and theophylline. May interact with drugs metabolized by CYP450. Fluvoxamine increases levels. May antagonize anticholinergics. Monitor for GI disease with NSAIDs. Increased levels with cimetidine.

**PREGNANCY:** Category C, caution in nursing.

## COLACE — OTC

docusate sodium (Purdue Products)

**THERAPEUTIC CLASS:** Stool softener

**INDICATIONS:** (PO) Stool softener for constipation, painful anorectal conditions and in cardiac conditions.

**DOSAGE:** *Adults:* 50-200mg/day. (Retention or Flushing Enema) Add 5-10mL of liquid to enema fluid. Mix Liq/Syr into 6-8 oz of milk or juice. *Pediatrics:* >12 yrs: 50-200mg/day. 6-12 yrs: 40-120mg/day Liq. 3-6 yrs: 2mL

Liq tid. Mix Liq/Syr into 6-8 oz of milk, juice or formula. (Retention/Flushing Enema) Add 5-10mL of liquid to enema fluid.

**HOW SUPPLIED:** Cap: 50mg, 100mg; Liq: 10mg/mL; Syrup: 20mg/5mL

**WARNINGS/PRECAUTIONS:** Avoid with abdominal pain, nausea, or vomiting. D/C enema if rectal bleeding occurs or fail to have a bowel movement.



**ADVERSE REACTIONS:** Bitter taste, throat irritation, nausea, rash.

**PREGNANCY:** Safety in pregnancy and nursing not known.

## COLAZAL

balsalazide disodium (Salix)

RX

**THERAPEUTIC CLASS:** Anti-inflammatory Agent

**INDICATIONS:** Treatment of mild-to-moderate active ulcerative colitis in patients ≥5 yrs.

**DOSAGE:** *Adults:* 3 caps tid for up to 8 weeks (or 12 weeks if needed). May open capsule and sprinkle on applesauce.
*Pediatrics:* 5-17 yrs: 1 or 3 caps tid for 8 weeks. May open capsule and sprinkle on applesauce.

**HOW SUPPLIED:** Cap: 750mg

**CONTRAINDICATIONS:** Hypersensitivity to salicylates.

**WARNINGS/PRECAUTIONS:** May exacerbate symptoms of colitis. Prolonged gastric retention with pyloris stenosis. Caution with renal dysfunction or history of renal disease.

**ADVERSE REACTIONS:** Headache, abdominal pain, diarrhea, nausea, vomiting, respiratory problems, arthralgia, rhinitis, insomnia, fatigue, rectal bleeding, flatulence, fever, dyspepsia.

**INTERACTIONS:** Oral antibiotics may interfere with the release of mesalamine in the colon.

**PREGNANCY:** Category B, caution in nursing.

## COLCHICINE

colchicine (Various)

RX

**THERAPEUTIC CLASS:** Miscellaneous gout agent

**INDICATIONS:** Treatment and prophylaxis of acute gouty arthritis.

**DOSAGE:** *Adults:* Acute Treatment: Initial: 1-1.2mg, followed by 0.5-0.6mg q1h, or 1-1.2mg q2h or 0.5-0.6mg q2-3h until pain relief, GI discomfort or diarrhea ensues. Usual: 4-8mg/attack. Wait 3 days before retreatment. Prophylaxis: <1 attack/yr: 0.5-0.6mg/day given 3-4x/week. >1 attack/yr: 0.5-0.6mg qd. Severe Cases: 2-3 tabs of 0.5mg or 0.6mg daily. Surgical Gout Prophylaxis: 0.5-0.6mg tid 3 days before and 3 days after surgery.

**HOW SUPPLIED:** Tab: 0.5mg, 0.6mg

**CONTRAINDICATIONS:** Serious GI, renal, hepatic or cardiac disorders and blood dyscrasias.

**WARNINGS/PRECAUTIONS:** Caution in elderly and debilitated, or those with GI, renal, hepatic, cardiac and hematologic disorders. Discontinue if nausea, vomiting or diarrhea occurs. Monitor blood counts periodically with long-term therapy. May adversely affect spermatogenesis. Elevates SGOT and alkaline phosphatase. May cause false (+) for urine RBC and Hgb.

**ADVERSE REACTIONS:** Bone marrow depression, peripheral neuritis, purpura, myopathy, alopecia, dermatoses, reversible azoospermia, nausea, vomiting, diarrhea.

**INTERACTIONS:** Inhibited by acidifying agents. Potentiated by alkalinizing agents. Potentiates sympathomimetics and CNS depressants.

**PREGNANCY:** Category C, caution in nursing.

## COLCHICINE/PROBENECID

RX

colchicine - probenecid (Various)

C

**THERAPEUTIC CLASS:** Uricosuric

**INDICATIONS:** Chronic gouty arthritis complicated by frequent, recurrent acute gout attacks.

**DOSAGE:** *Adults:* Initial: 1 tab qd for 1 week, then 1 tab bid. Titrate: May increase by 1 tab/day every 4 weeks. Max: 4 tabs/day. May reduce dose by 1 tab every 6 months if acute attacks have been absent >6 months. Decrease dose with gastric intolerance. Renal Impairment: May need to increase dose. May not be effective if CrCl <30mL/min.

**HOW SUPPLIED:** Tab: (Colchicine-Probenecid) 0.5mg-500mg

**CONTRAINDICATIONS:** Blood dyscrasias, uric acid kidney stones, children <2 yrs and pregnancy. Do not use in acute gout attack.

**WARNINGS/PRECAUTIONS:** Exacerbation of gout may occur. Use APAP if analgesic needed. Severe allergic reaction and anaphylaxis reported (rare). D/C if hypersensitivity occurs. Caution with peptic ulcer. Monitor for glycosuria. Determine benefit/risk ratio with long-term therapy. Maintain liberal fluid intake and alkalization of urine.

**ADVERSE REACTIONS:** Headache, dizziness, hepatic necrosis, vomiting, nausea, anorexia, sore gums, uric acid stones, renal colic, anaphylaxis, fever, pruritus, blood dyscrasias, peripheral neuritis, muscular weakness, abdominal pain, diarrhea, alopecia, dermatitis.

**INTERACTIONS:** Probenecid increases plasma levels of penicillin and other beta-lactams; psychic disturbances reported. Salicylates and pyrazinamide antagonize uricosuric effects. Increased plasma levels of methotrexate, sulfonamides, sulfonylureas, thiopental or ketamine-induced anesthesia, some NSAIDs (eg, indomethacin, naproxen), lorazepam, APAP, and rifampin. Possible false high plasma levels of theophylline.

**PREGNANCY:** Contraindicated in pregnancy; safety in nursing not known.

## COLESTID

RX

colestipol HCl (Pharmacia & Upjohn)

**THERAPEUTIC CLASS:** Bile acid sequestrant

**INDICATIONS:** Adjunct to diet, to reduce elevated serum total and LDL-C in primary hypercholesterolemia.

**DOSAGE:** *Adults:* Initial: 2g, 1 packet or 1 scoopful qd-bid. Titrate: Increase by 2g qd or bid at 1-2 month intervals. Usual: 2-16g/day (tab) or 1-6 packets or scoopfuls qd or in divided doses. Always mix granules with liquid. Swallow tabs whole with plenty of liquid.

**HOW SUPPLIED:** Granules: 5g/packet [30ˢ 90ˢ], 5g/scoopful [300g, 500g]; Tab: 1g

**WARNINGS/PRECAUTIONS:** Exclude secondary causes of hypercholesterolemia and perform a lipid profile. May produce hyperchloremic acidosis with prolonged use. Monitor cholesterol and TG based on NCEP guidelines. May cause hypothyroidism. May interfere with normal fat absorption. Chronic use may produce or worsen constipation. Avoid constipation with symptomatic CAD. May increase bleeding tendency due to vitamin K deficiency.

**ADVERSE REACTIONS:** Constipation, musculoskeletal pain, headache, migraine headache, sinus headache.

**INTERACTIONS:** May interfere with absorption of folic acid, fat soluble vitamins (eg, A, D, K), oral phosphate supplements, hydrocortisone. May delay or reduce absorption of concomitant oral medication; take other drugs 1 hr before or 4 hrs after colestipol. Reduces absorption of chlorothiazide, tetracycline, furosemide, penicillin G, hydrochlorothiazide, and gemfibrozil. Caution with digitalis agents, propranolol.

**PREGNANCY:** Safety in pregnancy not known, caution in nursing.



## COLLAGENASE SANTYL RX
collagenase (Smith & Nephew)

**THERAPEUTIC CLASS:** Debriding agent

**INDICATIONS:** For debriding chronic dermal ulcers and severely burned areas.

**DOSAGE:** *Adults:* Clean and debride wound. Apply ointment qd; use more frequently if dressings becomes soiled. If needed, apply topical antibiotic agent before ointment.

**HOW SUPPLIED:** Oint: 250 U/g [15g, 30g]

**WARNINGS/PRECAUTIONS:** Use on skin with optimal pH (6-8); lower or higher pH may diminish efficacy. Monitor debilitated patients for systemic bacterial infections; may increase risk of bacteremia. Apply carefully within area of wound.

**INTERACTIONS:** Avoid soaks containing metal ions or acidic solutions due to the metal ion and low pH. Diminished effects with certain detergents/antiseptics containing heavy metal ions (eg, mercury, silver).

**PREGNANCY:** Safety in pregnancy and nursing not known.

## COLLYRIUM OTC
boric acid - sodium borate - sodium chloride (Bausch & Lomb)

**THERAPEUTIC CLASS:** Eye wash

**INDICATIONS:** To cleanse the eye to help relieve irritation by removing loose foreign material, air pollutants or chlorinated water.

**DOSAGE:** *Adults:* Fill eye cup with sol and apply cup to affected eye. Press tightly to prevent escape of liquid and tilt head backwards. Open eyelids wide and rotate eyeball to ensure thorough bathing with the wash. If not using cup, flush affected eye prn, controlling rate of solution flow by pressure on bottle.

**HOW SUPPLIED:** Sol: [120mL]

**WARNINGS/PRECAUTIONS:** Do not touch container tip to any surface to avoid contamination. D/C if eye pain or vision changes occur, if redness or irritation continues, or if condition worsens or persists.

**PREGNANCY:** Safety in pregnancy or nursing not known.

## COLOCORT RX
hydrocortisone (Paddock)

**THERAPEUTIC CLASS:** Corticosteroid

**INDICATIONS:** Adjunct treatment of ulcerative colitis, ulcerative proctitis, and ulcerative proctosigmoiditis.

**DOSAGE:** *Adults:* 1 enema qhs for 21 days or until remission. After 21 days, decrease to every other night for 2-3 weeks. Discontinue if no clinical improvement after 2-3 weeks. Difficult cases may require 2-3 months of therapy. Retain for 1 hr minimum, preferably all night.

**HOW SUPPLIED:** Enema: 100mg/60mL

**CONTRAINDICATIONS:** Systemic fungal infections, ileocolostomy during the immediate or early postoperative.

**WARNINGS/PRECAUTIONS:** Rectal wall damage with improper insertion. May mask signs of infection and cause new infections; avoid exposure to chickenpox and measles. Prolonged use may cause adrenocortical insufficiency, cataracts, glaucoma, optic nerve damage, and may enhance secondary ocular infections. May cause elevated BP, salt and water retention, increased potassium and calcium excretion and reactivation of TB. Caution with perforation, abscess, obstruction, fistulas, sinus tracts, peptic ulcer, diverticulitis, renal impairment, HTN, osteoporosis, ocular herpes simplex, and myasthenia gravis. Enhanced effects in hypothyroidism and cirrhosis. May need increased dose in stressful situation. Do not vaccinate against smallpox or perform other immunization procedure; risk of neurological complications and lack of antibody response. Observe growth in pediatrics. Psychic derangement may appear; caution with emotional instability or psychotic tendencies.



**ADVERSE REACTIONS:** Local pain/burning/bleeding, fluid retention, HTN, muscle weakness, osteoporosis, peptic ulcer, abdominal distention, impaired wound healing, ecchymosis, facial erythema, sweating, menstrual disorders, Cushingoid state, decreased glucose tolerance.

**INTERACTIONS:** Caution with ASA in hypoprothrombinemia. Avoid vaccinations.

**PREGNANCY:** Safety in pregnancy and nursing is not known.

## COLY-MYCIN M — RX

colistimethate sodium (King)

**THERAPEUTIC CLASS:** Polypeptide antibiotic

**INDICATIONS:** Treatment of acute or chronic infections due to certain gram-negative bacilli (eg, *Pseudomonas aeruginosa*, *Enterobacter aerogenes*, *E. coli*, *Klebsiella pneumoniae*).

**DOSAGE:** *Adults:* Usual: 2.5-5mg/kg/day IV/IM in 2-4 divided doses. Max: 5mg/kg/day. SCr 1.3-1.5mg/dL: 2.5-3.8mg/kg/day IV/IM in 2 divided doses. SCr 1.6-2.5mg/dL: 2.5mg/kg/day IV/IM in 1-2 divided doses. SCr 2.6-4mg/dL: 1.5mg/kg/day IV/IM q36h. Obesity: Base dose on IBW.
*Pediatrics:* Usual: 2.5-5mg/kg/day IV/IM in 2-4 divided doses. Max: 5mg/kg/day. SCr 1.3-1.5mg/dL: 2.5-3.8mg/kg/day IV/IM in 2 divided doses. SCr 1.6-2.5mg/dL: 2.5mg/kg/day IV/IM in 1-2 divided doses. SCr 2.6-4mg/dL: 1.5mg/kg/day IV/IM q36h. Obesity: Base dose on IBW.

**HOW SUPPLIED:** Inj: 150mg

**WARNINGS/PRECAUTIONS:** Transient neurological disturbances may occur; dose reduction may alleviate symptoms. Respiratory arrest reported after IM administration. Increased risk of apnea and neuromuscular blockade with renal impairment. Reversible dose-dependent nephrotoxicity reported. Pseudomembranous colitis reported. May permit overgrowth of clostridia. Use extreme caution with renal impairment; d/c with further impairment.

**ADVERSE REACTIONS:** GI upset, tingling of extremities and tongue, slurred speech, dizziness, vertigo, paresthesia, itching, urticaria, rash, fever, increased BUN and creatinine, decreased creatinine clearance, respiratory distress, apnea, nephrotoxicity, decreased urine output.

**INTERACTIONS:** Avoid certain antibiotics (eg, aminoglycosides, polymyxin); may interfere with nerve transmission at neuromuscular junction. Extreme caution with curariform muscle relaxants (eg, tubocurarine), succinylcholine, gallamine, decamethonium and sodium citrate; may potentiate neuromuscular blocking effect. Avoid sodium cephalothin; may enhance nephrotoxicity.

**PREGNANCY:** Category C, caution in nursing.

## Colyte

RX

sodium sulfate - sodium chloride - potassium chloride - sodium bicarbonate - polyethylene glycol 3350 (Schwarz)

**OTHER BRAND NAMES:** Colyte-Flavored (Schwarz) - Colyte w/ Flavor Packs (Schwarz)

**THERAPEUTIC CLASS:** Bowel cleanser

**INDICATIONS:** Bowel cleansing prior to colonoscopy or barium enema X-ray.

**DOSAGE:** *Adults:* Oral: 240mL every 10 minutes until fecal discharge is clear. Nasogastric Tube: 20-30mL/minute (1.2-1.8L/hr). Patient should fast at least 3 hrs before administration, except for clear liquids.

**HOW SUPPLIED:** Sol: (Polyethylene Glycol-Potassium Chloride-Sodium Bicarbonate-Sodium Chloride-Sodium Sulfate) 60g-0.745g-1.68g-1.46g-5.68g/L [3754mL, 4000mL]

**CONTRAINDICATIONS:** Ileus, gastric retention, GI obstruction, bowel perforation, toxic colitis, toxic megacolon.

**WARNINGS/PRECAUTIONS:** Caution with severe ulcerative colitis. Monitor therapy with impaired gag reflex, semi- or unconsciousness, and risk of regurgitation or aspiration especially with NG tube.

**ADVERSE REACTIONS:** Nausea, abdominal fullness/cramps, bloating, anal irritation, vomiting.

**INTERACTIONS:** Medications taken within 1 hr of start of administration may not be absorbed.

**PREGNANCY:** Category C, safety in nursing is unkown.

## CombiPatch

RX

estradiol - norethindrone acetate (Novartis)

**Estrogens and progestins should not be used for prevention of cardiovascular disease or dementia. Increased risks of MI, stroke, invasive breast cancer, PE, and DVT in postmenopausal women (50-79 yrs of age) reported. Increased risk of developing probable dementia in postmenopausal women ≥65 yrs of age reported.**

**THERAPEUTIC CLASS:** Estrogen/progestogen combination

**INDICATIONS:** In women with an intact uterus, for the treatment of moderate to severe vasomotor symptoms associated with menopause, vulvar/vaginal atrophy. Treatment of hypoestrogenism due to hypogonadism, castration, or primary ovarian failure.

**DOSAGE:** *Adults:* Continuous Combined Regimen: Apply 0.05mg/0.14mg patch on lower abdomen (avoid breasts and waistline). Apply twice weekly during 28-day cycle. Continuous Sequential Regimen: Wear estradiol-only patch for 1st 14 days of 28-day cycle, replace twice weekly. Apply 0.05mg/0.14mg patch for remaining 14 days, replace twice weekly. For both regimens, use 0.05mg/0.25mg patch if additional progestin required. Re-evaluate at 3-6 month intervals. Rotate sites; allow 1 week between same site.

**HOW SUPPLIED:** Patch: (Estradiol-Norethindrone) 0.05-0.14mg/day, 0.05-0.25mg/day [8$^{s}$, 24$^{s}$]

**CONTRAINDICATIONS:** Undiagnosed abnormal genital bleeding, breast cancer, estrogen-dependent neoplasia, DVT, PE, arterial thromboembolic disorder (eg, stroke, MI), liver dysfunction or disease.

**WARNINGS/PRECAUTIONS:** May increase risk of cardiovascular events (eg, MI, stroke), venous thrombosis, and PE; d/c immediately if any of these events occur or are suspected. May increase risk of breast/endometrial cancer, and gallbladder disease. May lead to severe hypercalcemia with breast cancer and bone metastases; monitor and d/c if hypercalcemia occurs. Retinal vascular thrombosis reported; monitor and d/c if papilledema or retinal vascular lesions occur. May elevate BP; monitor at regular intervals. May cause elevations of

C

plasma triglycerides with pre-existing hypertriglyceridemia. Caution with history of cholestatic jaundice associated with past estrogen use or with pregnancy; d/c with recurrence. May lead to increased thyroid-binding globulin levels; monitor thyroid function. May cause fluid retention; caution with cardiac/renal dysfunction. Caution with severe hypocalcemia. May increase risk of ovarian cancer. May exacerbate endometriosis, asthma, DM, epilepsy, migraine, porphyria, SLE, and hepatic hemangiomas; use with caution.

**ADVERSE REACTIONS:** Abdominal pain, back pain, asthenia, flu syndrome, application site reaction, nausea, nervousness, pharyngitis, respiratory disorder, breast pain, dysmenorrhea, menstrual disorder, vaginitis.

**INTERACTIONS:** CYP3A4 inducers (eg, St. John's wort, phenobarbital, carbamazepine, rifampin) may decrease levels which may decrease therapeutic effects and/or change uterine bleeding profile. CYP3A4 inhibitors (eg, erythromycin, clarithromycin, ketoconazole, itraconazole, ritonavir, grapefruit juice) may increase levels which may result in side effects.

**PREGNANCY:** Contraindicated in pregnancy, caution in nursing.

## COMBIVENT RX

albuterol sulfate - ipratropium bromide (Boehringer Ingelheim)

**THERAPEUTIC CLASS:** $Beta_2$ agonist/anticholinergic

**INDICATIONS:** Adjunct therapy for bronchospasm in COPD if currently on a regular aerosol bronchodilator and require a second bronchodilator.

**DOSAGE:** *Adults:* 2 inh qid. Max: 12 inh/24 hrs.

**HOW SUPPLIED:** MDI: (Albuterol-Ipratropium) 0.09mg-0.018mg/inh [14.7g]

**CONTRAINDICATIONS:** History of hypersensitivity to soya lecithin or related food products (eg, soybeans, peanuts).

**WARNINGS/PRECAUTIONS:** Paradoxical bronchospasm reported. Hypersensitivity reactions reported. Caution with coronary insufficiency, arrhythmias, narrow-angle glaucoma, prostatic hypertrophy, bladder-neck obstruction, HTN, DM, hyperthyroidism, seizures, renal or hepatic dysfunction, and in those unusually responsive to sympathomimetic amines. May produce transient hypokalemia. Fatalities reported with excessive use.

**ADVERSE REACTIONS:** Headache, cough, respiratory disorders, pain, dyspnea, bronchitis.

**INTERACTIONS:** Potential additive interactions with other anticholinergic drugs. Increased risk of cardiovascular effects with other sympathomimetics. β-blockers and albuterol inhibit effects of each other. ECG changes and/or hypokalemia may occur with non-$K^+$ sparing diuretics. Avoid MAOI's and TCA's.

**PREGNANCY:** Category C, not for use in nursing.

## COMBIVIR RX

lamivudine - zidovudine (GlaxoSmithKline)

**Zidovudine has been associated with hematologic toxicity (eg, granulocytopenia, severe anemia), especially with advanced HIV disease, and symptomatic myopathy reported with prolonged use. Lactic acidosis and severe, fatal hepatomegaly reported with nucleoside analogues.**

**THERAPEUTIC CLASS:** Nucleoside analogue

**INDICATIONS:** Treatment of HIV infection in combination with other antiretrovirals.

**DOSAGE:** *Adults:* 1 tab bid. Do not give if CrCl <50mL/min or with dose-limiting adverse events.
*Pediatrics:* >12 yrs: 1 tab bid. Do not give if CrCl <50mL/min or with dose-limiting adverse events.

**HOW SUPPLIED:** Tab: (Lamivudine-Zidovudine) 150mg-300mg

**WARNINGS/PRECAUTIONS:** Caution with granulocyte count <1000cells/$mm^3$ or Hgb <9.5g/dL; monitor blood counts frequently with advanced HIV and periodically with asymptomatic or early HIV. Hepatic decompensation occured when used with interferon alfa w/ or w/o ribavirin. Avoid with CrCl <50mL/min, and hepatic impairment. Myopathy, myositis may occur. Posttreatment exacerbation of hepatitis reported. Lamivudine-resistant hepatitis B virus reported. Caution in elderly. Possible redistribution or accumulation of body fat. Immune reconstitution syndrome reported.

**ADVERSE REACTIONS:** Headache, malaise, fatigue, fever, chills, nausea, diarrhea, anorexia, abdominal pain/cramps, neuropathy, insomnia, dizziness, neutropenia, musculoskeletal pain, myalgia, rash, cough, aplastic anemia, gynecomastia, oral mucosal pigmentation.

**INTERACTIONS:** Ganciclovir, interferon-alpha, other bone marrow suppressives and cytotoxic agents may increase the hematologic toxicity of zidovudine. Increased lamivudine exposure with trimethoprim 160mg/sulfamethoxazole 800mg. Avoid with zalcitabine, stavudine, doxorubicin, ribavirin, zidovudine, lamivudine, and fixed-dose combinations of abacavir, lamivudine, and zidovudine.

**PREGNANCY:** Category C, not for use in nursing.

## COMBUNOX

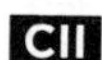

ibuprofen - oxycodone HCl (Forest)

**NSAIDs may cause an increased risk of serious cardiovascular thrombotic events, MI, stroke and serious GI adverse events including bleeding, ulceration, and perforation of the stomach or intestines. Contraindicated for the treatment of peri-operative pain in the setting of coronary artery bypass graft surgery.**

**THERAPEUTIC CLASS:** Opioid analgesic

**INDICATIONS:** Short term (<7 days) management of acute, moderate to severe pain.

**DOSAGE:** *Adults:* 1 tab/dose. Do not exceed 4 tabs/day and 7 days.

**HOW SUPPLIED:** Tab: (Oxycodone-Ibuprofen) 5mg-400mg

**CONTRAINDICATIONS:** Significant respiratory depression, acute or severe bronchial asthma, hypercarbia, paralytic ileus, or in patients who have experienced asthma, urticaria, allergic-type reactions after taking aspirin or NSAIDs.

**WARNINGS/PRECAUTIONS:** See Black Box Warning. May cause drug dependence and tolerance; potential for abuse. Risk of dose-related respiratory depression. May cause severe hypotension. Can lead to hypertension or worsening of pre-existing hypertension. Fluid retention and edema have been observed. Capacity to elevate CSF pressure may be exaggerated with head injury, other intracranial lesions or pre-existing increase in intracranial pressure. May obscure the diagnosis or clinical course with head injuries or acute abdominal conditions. Risk of GI ulceration, bleeding and perforation. Risk of anaphylactoid reactions. NSAIDs can cause exfoliative dermatitis, Stevens-Johnson syndrome, and toxic epidermal necrolysis (TEN). Caution with severe hepatic impairment, pulmonary or renal dysfunction, hypothyroidism, Addison's disease, acute alcoholism, convulsive disorders, CNS depression or coma, delirium tremens, kyphoscoliosis associated with respiratory depression, toxic psychosis, prostatic hypertrophy, urethral stricture, biliary tract disease, anemia, pre-existing asthma, elderly or debilitated, aseptic meningitis.

**ADVERSE REACTIONS:** Nausea, vomiting, flatulence, somnolence, dizziness, diaphoresis, asthenia, fever, headache, vasodilation, constipation, diarrhea, dyspepsia.

**INTERACTIONS:** (Oxycodone) Respiratory depression, hypotension and profound sedation with other CNS depressants (eg, narcotics, tranquilizers, sedatives, anesthetics, phenothiazines, alcohol). Concurrent use with anticholinergics may produce paralytic ileus. Mixed agonist/antagonist analgesics may reduce the analgesic effect and/or cause withdrawal. Do not use with, or within 14 days of discontinuing, MAOIs. May enhance skeletal muscle relaxant effects and increase respiratory depression. (Ibuprofen) May diminish antihypertensive effect of ACEIs. Use caution with anticoagulants, such as warfarin. May enhance methotrexate toxicity. May decrease natriuretic effect of furosemide and thiazides. Avoid use with aspirin. Decreases lithium clearance; monitor for toxicity.

**PREGNANCY:** Category C, caution in nursing.

## COMMIT — OTC
nicotine polacrilex (GlaxoSmithKline Consumer)

**THERAPEUTIC CLASS:** Nicotine

**INDICATIONS:** To reduce withdrawal symptoms associated with smoking cessation.

**DOSAGE:** *Adults:* Stop smoking completely before use. Use 4mg loz if time to 1st cigarette is within 30 minutes of waking. Use 2mg loz if your time to 1st cigarette is >30 minutes after waking. Weeks 1-6: 1 loz q1-2h. Weeks 7-9: 1 loz q2-4h. Weeks 10-12: 1 loz q4-8h. Use at least 9 loz/day for first 6 weeks. Max: 5 loz/6 hrs or 20 loz/day. Dissolve loz in mouth for 20-30 minutes (minimize swallowing) moving it from one side of your mouth to the other; do not chew or swallow whole. Do not eat/drink for 15 minutes before or during use.

**HOW SUPPLIED:** Loz: 2mg, 4mg

**WARNINGS/PRECAUTIONS:** Do not use if continue to smoke, chew tobacco, use snuff, use a nicotine patch, or other nicotine products. Caution with heart disease, recent MI, irregular heartbeat, HTN, stomach ulcers or diabetes. May increase BP and HR. D/C with mouth problems, persistent indigestion, severe sore throat, palpitations, irregular heartbeat, or with symptoms of nicotine overdose (nausea, vomiting, dizziness, weakness, palpitations). Contains phenylalanine. Use 1 loz at a time. Do not continuously use one after another. Use under medical supervision if <18 yrs of age.

**INTERACTIONS:** Antidepressants and antiasthmatic agents may need adjustment.

**PREGNANCY:** Safety in pregnancy and nursing is not known.

## COMPUTER EYE DROPS — OTC
glycerin (Bausch & Lomb)

**THERAPEUTIC CLASS:** Lubricant

**INDICATIONS:** To prevent further irritation or to relieve dryness of the eye.

**DOSAGE:** *Adults:* 1-2 drops in affected eye prn.

**HOW SUPPLIED:** Sol: 1% [15mL]

**WARNINGS/PRECAUTIONS:** Remove contact lenses before use. Do not touch container tip to any surface to avoid contamination. D/C if eye pain or vision changes occur, if redness or irritation continues, or if condition worsens or continues >72 hrs.

**PREGNANCY:** Safety in pregnancy or nursing not known.

## COMTAN — RX
entacapone (Novartis)

**THERAPEUTIC CLASS:** COMT inhibitor

**INDICATIONS:** Adjunct to levodopa/carbidopa for treatment of idiopathic Parkinson's disease if experience signs of end-of-dose "wearing-off."

**DOSAGE:** *Adults:* 200mg with each levodopa/carbidopa dose. Max: 1600mg/day. Withdraw slowly for discontinuation.

**HOW SUPPLIED:** Tab: 200mg

**WARNINGS/PRECAUTIONS:** Hypotension/syncope, diarrhea, hallucinations, dyskinesia, rhabdomyolysis, hyperpyrexia, confusion, and fibrotic complications may occur due to increased dopaminergic activity. Caution with hepatic impairment, biliary obstruction. Avoid rapid withdrawal or abrupt dose reduction. May impair mental and/or motor performance.



**ADVERSE REACTIONS:** Sweating, back pain, dyskinesia, hyperkinesia, hypokinesia, nausea, diarrhea, abdominal pain, urine discoloration.

**INTERACTIONS:** Avoid non-selective MAOIs (eg, phenelzine, tranylcypromine). Caution with drugs metabolized by COMT (eg, isoproterenol, epinephrine, norepinephrine, dopamine, dobutamine, alpha-methyldopa, apomorphine, isoetherine, bitolterol); increased heart rate, arrhythmias, and BP changes may occur. Additive sedative effects with CNS depressants. Probenecid, cholestyramine, and some antibiotics (eg, erythromycin, rifampicin, ampicillin, chloramphenicol) may interfere with biliary excretion.

**PREGNANCY:** Category C, caution with nursing.

## CONCERTA — CII

methylphenidate HCl (McNeil Consumer)

**THERAPEUTIC CLASS:** Sympathomimetic amine

**INDICATIONS:** Treatment of attention deficit hyperactivity disorder (ADHD) in patients ≥6 years old.

**DOSAGE:** *Adults:* Methylphenidate-Naive or Receiving Other Stimulant: Initial: 18mg qam. Titrate: Adjust dose at weekly intervals. Previous Methylphenidate Use: Initial: 18mg qam if previous dose 10-15mg/day; 36mg qam if previous dose 20-30mg/day; 54mg qam if previous dose 30-45mg/day. Initial conversion should not exceed 54mg/day. Titrate: Adjust dose at weekly intervals. Max: 72mg/day. Reduce dose or discontinue if paradoxical aggravation of symptoms occurs. Discontinue if no improvement after appropriate dosage adjustments over 1 month. Swallow whole with liquids. Do not crush, chew, or divide.
*Pediatrics:* >6 yrs: Methylphenidate-Naive or Receiving Other Stimulant: Initial: 18mg qam. Titrate: Adjust dose at weekly intervals. Max: 6-12 yrs: 54mg/day; 13-17 yrs: 72mg/day not to exceed 2mg/kg/day. Previous Methylphenidate Use: Initial: 18mg qam if previous dose 10-15mg/day; 36mg qam if previous dose 20-30mg/day; 54mg qam if previous dose 30-45mg/day. Initial conversion should not exceed 54mg/day. Titrate: Adjust dose at weekly intervals. Max: 72mg/day. Reduce dose or discontinue if paradoxical aggravation of symptoms occurs. Discontinue if no improvement after appropriate dosage adjustments over 1 month. Swallow whole with liquids. Do not crush, chew, or divide.

**HOW SUPPLIED:** Tab, Extended-Release: 18mg, 27mg, 36mg, 54mg

**CONTRAINDICATIONS:** Marked anxiety, tension, and agitation; glaucoma; motor tics or family history or diagnosis of Tourette's syndrome, during or within 14 days of MAOI use.

**WARNINGS/PRECAUTIONS:** Monitor growth during treatment in children. Not for severe depression or fatigue. May exacerbate symptoms of behavior disturbance and thought disorder in psychotic patients. Avoid with severe GI narrowing (eg, esophageal motility disorders, small bowel inflammatory disease, short-gut syndrome). May lower seizure threshold, especially in known EEG abnormalities. Caution with HTN, conditions affected by BP or HR elevation, history of drug abuse or alcoholism. Monitor during withdrawal from abusive use. Visual disturbances may occur (rare). Monitor CBC, differential, and platelets with prolonged use. Caution when using stimulants to treat patients with comorbid bipolar disorder because of concern for possible induction of mixed/manic episode in such patients. Stimulants at usual does can cause treatment emergent psychotic or manic symptoms (eg, hallucinations, delusional thinking, mania) in children and adolescents without prior history of psychotic illness. Aggressive behavior or hostility reported in clinical trials and postmarketing experience of some medications indicated for the treatment of ADHD. Avoid with known structural cardiac abnormalities or other serious cardiac problems.



**ADVERSE REACTIONS:** Headache, abdominal pain, anorexia, insomnia, upper respiratory tract infection.

**INTERACTIONS:** Avoid MAOIs. Potentiates anticoagulants, anticonvulsants (eg, phenobarbital, phenytoin, primidone), TCAs, and SSRIs. Caution with $\alpha_2$-agonists (eg, clonidine) and pressor agents.

**PREGNANCY:** Category C, caution in nursing.

## CONDYLOX RX

podofilox (Oclassen)

**THERAPEUTIC CLASS:** Antimitotic

**INDICATIONS:** (Gel) Topical treatment of external genital warts and perianal warts. (Sol) Topical treatment of external genital warts.

**DOSAGE:** *Adults:* Apply q12h for 3 days then discontinue for 4 days. May repeat for up to 4 treatment cycles. Max: 0.5g/day or 0.5mL/day and <10cm$^2$ of wart tissue.

**HOW SUPPLIED:** Gel: 0.5% [3.5g]; Sol: 0.5% [3.5mL]

**WARNINGS/PRECAUTIONS:** Confirm diagnosis before therapy. Avoid eyes. For cutaneous use only. Avoid use on the mucous membranes of genital area (eg, urethra, rectum, vagina).

**ADVERSE REACTIONS:** Inflammation, burning, erosion, pain, itching, bleeding.

**PREGNANCY:** Category C, not for use in nursing.

## COPEGUS RX

ribavirin (Roche Labs)

**Not for monotherapy treatment of chronic hepatitis C. Primary toxicity is hemolytic anemia. Avoid with significant or unstable cardiac disease. Contraindicated in pregnancy and male partners of pregnant women. Use 2 forms of contraception during therapy and for 6 months after discontinuation.**

**THERAPEUTIC CLASS:** Nucleoside analogue

**INDICATIONS:** Treatment of chronic hepatitis C, in combination with Pegasys, in adults with compensated liver disease not previously treated with interferon alpha. Patients in whom efficacy was demonstrated included patients with compensated liver disease and histological evidence of cirrhosis (Child-Pugh class A) and patients with HIV disease that is clinically stable.

**DOSAGE:** *Adults:* HCV: Give bid in divided doses. Treat for 24-48 weeks with Pegasys® 180mcg. Genotypes 1 and 4: <75kg: 1000mg/day for 48 weeks. >75kg: 1200mg/day for 48 weeks. Genotypes 2 and 3: 800mg/day for 24 weeks. HCV/HIV: 800mg qd. Treat for 48 weeks with Pegasys® 180mcg. Dose Modifications: Reduce to 600mg/day if Hgb <10g/dL with no cardiac history, or if Hgb decreases by >2g/dL during a 4 week-period with stable cardiac disease. Discontinue if Hgb <8.5g/L with no cardiac history or if Hgb <12g/dL after 4 weeks of dose reduction with stable cardiac disease. After dose modification, may restart at 600mg/day, then may increase to 800mg/day. CrCl <50mL/min: Avoid use.

**HOW SUPPLIED:** Tab: 200mg

**CONTRAINDICATIONS:** Pregnancy, male partners of pregnant women, hemoglobinopathies (eg, thalassemia major, sickle cell anemia). Autoimmune hepatitis, and hepatic decompensation (Child-Pugh score greater than 6, Class B and C) in chirrotic CHC patients when used in combination with Pegasys®.

**WARNINGS/PRECAUTIONS:** Discontinue with hepatic decompensation, confirmed pancreatitis, and hypersensitivity reaction. Severe depression, suicidal ideation, hemolytic anemia, bone marrow suppression, autoimmune and infectious disorders, pancreatitis, and diabetes reported. Pulmonary symptoms reported; monitor closely with evidence of pulmonary infiltrates or pulmonary function impairment and discontinue if appropriate. Assess for underlying cardiac disease (obtain EKG); fatal and nonfatal MI reported with anemia. Caution with cardiac disease, discontinue if cardiovascular status deteriorates. Hemolytic anemia reported; monitor Hgb or Hct initially then at week 2 and 4 (or more if needed) of therapy. Suspend therapy if symptoms of pancreatitis arise. Avoid if CrCl <50mL/min. Obtain negative pregnancy test prior to initiation then monthly, and for 6 months post-therapy.

**ADVERSE REACTIONS:** Injection site reaction, fatigue/asthenia, pyrexia, rigors, nausea/vomiting, neutropenia, anorexia, myalgia, headache, irritability/anxiety/nervousness, insomnia, alopecia.

**INTERACTIONS:** Avoid concomitant use with didanosine, stavudine and zidovudine. Hepatic decompensation can occur with concomitant use of NRTIs and Pegasys®/Copegus®.

**PREGNANCY:** Category X, not for use in nursing.

## CORDARONE

RX

amiodarone HCl (Wyeth)

**THERAPEUTIC CLASS:** Class III antiarrhythmic

**INDICATIONS:** Treatment of documented, life-threatening recurrent ventricular fibrillation and recurrent hemodynamically unstable ventricular tachycardia.

**DOSAGE:** *Adults:* Give LD in hospital. LD: 800-1600mg/day in divided doses for 1-3 weeks. After control is achieved, then 600-800mg/day for 1 month. Maint: 400mg/day; up to 600mg/day if needed. Use lowest effective dose. Take with meals. Elderly: Start at low end of dosing range.

**HOW SUPPLIED:** Tab: 200mg* *scored

**CONTRAINDICATIONS:** Severe sinus-node dysfunction causing marked sinus bradycardia; 2nd- and 3rd-degree AV block; when episodes of bradycardia have caused syncope (except when used with a pacemaker); cardiogenic shock. Hypersensitivity to iodine.

**WARNINGS/PRECAUTIONS:** Only for life-threatening arrhythmias due to its substantial toxicity (eg, pulmonary toxicity including pulmonary alveolar hemorrhage, hepatic injury, arrhythmia exacerbation). Hospitalize when giving LD. May cause a clinical syndrome of cough and progressive dyspnea. Discontinue if LFTs are 3X ULN or if the elevated baseline doubles; monitor LFTs regularly. Optic neuropathy, optic neuritis reported. Fetal harm in pregnancy. May develop reversible corneal micro deposits (eg, visual halos, blurred vision), photosensitivity, peripheral neuropathy (rare). May decrease $T_3$ levels, increase thyroxine levels, increase inactive reverse $T_3$ levels and can cause hypo- or hyperthyroidism. Hyperthyroidism may result in thyrotoxicosis and/or the possibility of arrhythmia breakthrough or aggravation. Adult Respiratory Distress syndrome reported with surgery. Correct $K^+$ or magnesium deficiency before therapy. Caution in elderly.

**ADVERSE REACTIONS:** Pulmonary toxicity (inflammation, fibrosis), arrhythmia exacerbation, hepatic injury, malaise, fatigue, tremor, poor coordination, paresthesis, nausea, vomiting, constipation, anorexia, ophthalmic abnormalities, photosensitivity.

**INTERACTIONS:** Risk of interactions after discontinuation due to its long half-life. May increase sensitivity to myocardial depressant and conduction effects of halogenated inhalation anesthetics. Elevates cyclosporine plasma levels.

Discontinue or reduce digoxin dose by 50%. Discontinue or decrease warfarin dose by 1/3-1/2. Avoid grapefruit juice. Caution with β-blockers, calcium channel blockers, lidocaine, methotrexate. May increase levels of quinidine, procainamide, phenytoin, flecainide. Initiate added antiarrhythmic drug at lower than usual dose. Discontinue or decrease quinidine dose by 1/3-1/2. Discontinue or decrease procainamide dose by 1/3. Caution with loratadine, trazadone, disopyramide, fluoroquinolones, macrolides, azoles; QT prolongation reported. Decreased levels with cholestyramine, rifampin, phenytoin, St. John's wort. Rhabdomyolysis/myopathy reported with simvastatin. Ineffective inhibition of platelet aggregation with clopidogrel. Fentanyl may cause hypotension, bradycardia, and decreased cardiac output. Increased levels with protease inhibitors; monitor for toxicity. Increased levels of CYP1A2, CYP2C9, CYP2D6, CYP3A4 substrates reported. Interactions reported with CYP3A4 inducers. CYP2C8 and CYP3A4 inhibitors may increase amiodarone levels.

**PREGNANCY:** Category D, not for use in nursing.

## CORDARONE IV

RX

amiodarone HCl (Wyeth)

**THERAPEUTIC CLASS:** Class III antiarrhythmic

**INDICATIONS:** Initiation of treatment and prophylaxis of frequently recurring ventricular fibrillation and hemodynamically unstable ventricular tachycardia refractory to other therapies.

**DOSAGE:** *Adults:* LD: 150mg over 1st 10 minutes (15mg/min), then 360mg over next 6 hrs (1mg/min), then 540mg over remaining 18 hrs (0.5mg/min). Maint: 0.5mg/minute for 2-3 weeks. Breakthrough Ventricular Tachycardia/Ventricular Fibrillation: 150mg supplement IV over 10 minutes. Increase rate to achieve suppression. Elderly: Start at low end of dosing range. Administer infusions >2hrs in a glass or polyolefin bottle containing $D_5W$. Amiodarone leaches out plasticizers (eg, DEHP from IV tubing) especially at higher infusion concentrations, and lower flow rates.

**HOW SUPPLIED:** Inj: 50mg/mL

**CONTRAINDICATIONS:** Cardiogenic shock, marked sinus bradycardia, 2nd- or 3rd-degree AV block (unless a functioning pacemaker is available). Hypersensitivity to iodine.

**WARNINGS/PRECAUTIONS:** Hypotension reported; do not exceed initial rate of infusion. Correct hypokalemia or hypomagnesemia before therapy to prevent exaggeration of $QT_c$ prolongation. Congenital goiter/hypothyroidism, hyperthyroidism, postoperative ARDS reported with oral therapy. Hyperthyroidism may result in thyrotoxicosis and/or the possibility of arrhythmia breakthrough or aggravation. Elevations of hepatic enzymes reported. May worsen or precipitate a new arrhythmia; monitor for $QT_c$ prolongation. Contains benzyl alcohol. Caution in elderly.

**ADVERSE REACTIONS:** Hypotension, fever, bradycardia, CHF, heart arrest, ventricular tachycardia, abnormal LFT's, nausea.

**INTERACTIONS:** Risk of interactions may persist after discontinuation due to long half-life. May increase PT with warfarin. May elevate plasma levels of cyclosporine, digoxin, quinidine, procainamide. May increase QT prolongation with disopyramide. Reduce flecainide dose to maintain therapeutic plasma levels. Cholestyramine may decrease levels and half-life. Increased levels with cimetidine. Decreased levels with phenytoin. Risk of bradycardia, hypotension with beta-blockers, fentanyl. Increases risk of AV block with verapamil or diltiazem and hypotension with calcium channel blockers. May increase sensitivity to myocardial depressant and conduction defects of halogenated inhalational anesthetics.

**PREGNANCY:** Category D, not for use in nursing.

## CORDRAN
flurandrenolide (Watson)

RX



**OTHER BRAND NAMES:** Cordran SP (Watson)

**THERAPEUTIC CLASS:** Corticosteroid

**INDICATIONS:** Treatment of corticosteroid responsive dermatoses.

**DOSAGE:** *Adults:* (Cre, Lot) Apply qd-qid depending on severity. For moist lesions, apply cream bid-tid. Apply lotion bid-tid. (Tape) Clean and dry skin. Shave or clip hair. Apply tape q12-24h.
*Pediatrics:* (Cre, Lot) Apply qd-qid depending on severity. For moist lesions, apply cream bid-tid. Apply lotion bid-tid. (Tape) Clean and dry skin. Shave or clip hair. Apply tape q12-24h.

**HOW SUPPLIED:** Cre (SP): 0.05% [15g, 30g, 60g]; Lot: 0.05% [15mL, 60mL]; Tape: 4mcg/$cm^2$

**CONTRAINDICATIONS:** (Tape) Not for lesions exuding serum or in intertriginous areas.

**WARNINGS/PRECAUTIONS:** Systemic absorption may produce reversible HPA axis suppression, manifestations of Cushing's syndrome, hyperglycemia, and glucosuria. Application of more potent steroids, use on large surfaces, prolonged use, or occlusive dressings may augment systemic absorption. Evaluate periodically for HPA suppression if large dose applied to large area or with occlusive dressings. Pediatrics are more susceptible to toxicity. D/C if irritation develops. May use occlusive dressing for psoriasis or recalcitrant conditions.

**ADVERSE REACTIONS:** Burning, itching, irritation, dryness, folliculitis, hypertrichosis, acneform eruptions, hypopigmentation, dermatitis. Occlusive dressing may cause skin maceration, secondary infection, skin atrophy, miliaria.

**PREGNANCY:** Category C, caution in nursing.

## COREG CR
carvedilol (GlaxoSmithKline)

RX

**OTHER BRAND NAMES:** Coreg (GlaxoSmithKline)

**THERAPEUTIC CLASS:** $Alpha_1$/Beta-blocker

**INDICATIONS:** Treatment of mild to severe heart failure of ischemic or cardiomypathic origin; left ventricular dysfunction (LVD) following MI; essential hypertension.

**DOSAGE:** *Adults:* Individualize dose. Take with food. Monitor dose increases. Take extended-release capsules in am and swallow whole. CHF: Tab: Initial: 3.125mg bid for 2 weeks. Titrate: May double dose every 2 weeks as tolerated. Max: 50mg bid if >85kg. Reduce dose if HR <55 beats/min. Cap, Extended-Release: Initial: 10mg qd for 2 weeks. Titrate: May double dose every 2 weeks as tolerated. Max: 80mg/day. Reduce dose if HR <55 beats/min. HTN: Tab: Initial: 6.25mg bid for 7-14 days. Titrate: May double dose at 7-14 day intervals. Max: 50mg/day. Cap, Extended-Release: Initial: 20mg qd for 7-14 days. Titrate: May double dose every 7-14 days as tolerated. Max: 80mg/day. LVD Post-MI: Tab: Initial: 6.25mg bid for 3-10 days. Titrate: May double dose every 3-10 days to target of 25mg bid. May begin with 3.125mg bid and slow up-titration rate if clinically indicated. Cap, Extended-Release: Initial: 20mg qd for 3-10 days. Titrate: May double dose every 3-10 days to target of 80mg qd.

**HOW SUPPLIED:** Tab: 3.125mg, 6.25mg, 12.5mg, 25mg; Cap, Extended-Release: 10mg, 20mg, 40mg, 80mg

**CONTRAINDICATIONS:** Bronchial asthma or related bronchospastic conditions, 2nd- or 3rd-degree AV block, sick sinus syndrome, severe bradycardia (without permanent pacemaker), cardiogenic shock, decompensated heart failure requiring IV inotropic therapy, severe hepatic impairment.

**WARNINGS/PRECAUTIONS:** Avoid abrupt discontinuation; taper over 1-2 weeks. Hepatic injury reported; discontinue and do not restart if develop hepatic injury. Hypotension reported with up-titration; avoid driving. May mask hypoglycemia and hyperthyroidism. May potentiate insulin-induced hypoglycemia and delay recovery of serum glucose levels. Decrease dose if pulse <55 beats/min. Monitor renal function during uptitration with low BP (SBP <100mmHg), ischemic heart disease, diffuse vascular disease and/or renal insufficiency. Worsening heart failure or fluid retention may occur with uptitration. Caution in pheochromocytoma, peripheral vascular disease, major surgery with anesthesia, Prinzmetal's variant angina, and bronchospastic disease.

**ADVERSE REACTIONS:** Bradycardia, fatigue, edema, hypotension, dizziness, headache, diarrhea, nausea, vomiting, hyperglycemia, weight increase, dyspnea, anemia, increased cough, arthralgia.

**INTERACTIONS:** CYP2D6 inhibitors (eg, quinidine, fluoxetine, paroxetine, and propafenone) may increase levels. Monitor for hypotension and bradycardia with catecholamine-depleting agents (eg, reserpine, MAOIs). Clonidine may potentiate BP and heart rate lowering effects. Rifampin may reduce plasma levels. Cimetidine may increase AUC. Monitor ECG and BP with calcium channel blockers (eg, verapamil, diltiazem). Monitor with insulin, oral hypoglycemics, cyclosporin, and digoxin. Caution with anesthetic agents which may depress myocardial function (eg, cyclopropane, trichloroethylene). Alcohol may affect release properties of the extended release caps; separate administration by ≥2 hrs.

**PREGNANCY:** Category C, not for use in nursing.

## CORGARD RX

nadolol (King)

**THERAPEUTIC CLASS:** Nonselective beta-blocker

**INDICATIONS:** Long-term management of angina pectoris. Treatment of hypertension.

**DOSAGE:** *Adults:* Angina Pectoris: Initial: 40mg qd. Titrate: Increase by 40-80mg every 3-7 days. Usual: 40-80mg qd. Max: 240mg/day. HTN: Initial: 40mg qd. Titrate: Increase by 40-80mg. Max: 320mg/day. CrCl 31-50mL/min: Dose q24-36h. CrCl 10-30mL/min: Dose q24-48h. CrCl <10mL/min: Dose q40-60h.

**HOW SUPPLIED:** Tab: 20mg*, 40mg*, 80mg*, 120mg*, 160mg* *scored

**CONTRAINDICATIONS:** Bronchial asthma, sinus bradycardia and >1st-degree conduction block, cardiogenic shock, overt cardiac failure.

**WARNINGS/PRECAUTIONS:** Caution in well-compensated cardiac failure, nonallergic bronchospasm, renal dysfunction. Exacerbation of ischemic heart disease with abrupt withdrawal. Withdrawal before surgery is controversial. May mask hyperthyroidism or hypoglycemia symptoms. Can cause cardiac failure.

**ADVERSE REACTIONS:** Bradycardia, peripheral vascular insufficiency, dizziness, fatigue.

**INTERACTIONS:** Additive hypotension and/or bradycardia with catecholamine-depleting drugs. Antidiabetic agents may need adjustment. General anesthetics may exaggerate hypotension. May block epinephrine effects.

**PREGNANCY:** Category C, not for use in nursing.

C

## CORLOPAM
fenoldopam mesylate (Abbott)

RX

**THERAPEUTIC CLASS:** Dopamine $D_1$-like receptor agonist

**INDICATIONS:** For short-term (up to 48 hrs), in-hospital management of severe hypertension when rapid, but quickly reversible, emergency reduction of blood pressure is clinically indicated, including malignant hypertension with deteriorating end-organ function.

**DOSAGE:** *Adults:* Range: Initial: 0.01-0.8 mcg/kg/min IV. Titrate: Increase/decrease by 0.05-0.1mcg/kg/min no more frequently than every 15 minutes. May use for up to 48 hrs. Refer to prescribing information for detailed dosing information.

**HOW SUPPLIED:** Inj: 10mg/mL

**WARNINGS/PRECAUTIONS:** Contains sodium metabisulfite; may cause allergic-type reactions especially in asthmatics. Caution in glaucoma or intraocular HTN. Dose-related tachycardia reported. Symptomatic hypotension may occur; monitor BP. Avoid hypotension with acute cerebral infarction or hemorrhage. Hypokalemia reported; monitor serum electrolytes.

**ADVERSE REACTIONS:** Headache, nausea, flushing, extrasystoles, palpitations, bradycardia, heart failure, elevated BUN/glucose/transaminase, chest pain, leukocytosis, bleeding, dyspnea.

**INTERACTIONS:** Avoid beta-blockers; unexpected hypotension may occur.

**PREGNANCY:** Category B, caution in nursing.

## CORMAX
clobetasol propionate (Watson)

RX

**OTHER BRAND NAMES:** Cormax Scalp (Watson)

**THERAPEUTIC CLASS:** Corticosteroid

**INDICATIONS:** Corticosteroid responsive dermatoses.

**DOSAGE:** *Adults:* Apply bid. Limit treatment to 2 consecutive weeks. Max: 50g/week or 50mL/week.
*Pediatrics:* >12 yrs: (Cre, Sol) Apply bid. Limit treatment to 2 consecutive weeks. Max: 50g/week or 50mL/week.

**HOW SUPPLIED:** Cre: 0.05% [15g, 30g, 45g]; Sol (Scalp): 0.05% [25mL, 50mL]

**CONTRAINDICATIONS:** Primary infections of the scalp with solution.

**WARNINGS/PRECAUTIONS:** Not for treatment of rosacea or perioral dermatitis. May produce reversible HPA axis suppression, manifestations of Cushing's syndrome, hyperglycemia, and glucosuria. Reassess diagnosis if no improvement after 2 weeks. D/C if irritation occurs. Pediatrics may be more susceptible to systemic toxicity. Use appropriate antifungal or antibacterial agent with dermatological infections. Avoid occlusive dressings.

**ADVERSE REACTIONS:** Burning, stinging, pruritus, skin atrophy, cracking/fissuring of skin, irritation, (sol) tingling, (sol) folliculitis.

**PREGNANCY:** Category C, caution in nursing.

## CORTANE-B
chloroxylenol - hydrocortisone - pramoxine HCl (Blansett)

RX

**OTHER BRAND NAMES:** Zoto HC (Sciele)

**THERAPEUTIC CLASS:** Antimicrobial/Corticosteroid/Topical anesthetic

**INDICATIONS:** Treatment of superficial infections of the external ear and to control inflammation and itching.

**DOSAGE:** *Adults:* Instill 4-5 drops tid-qid. A gauze or wick may be inserted into ear canal after first administration. Add additional drops to saturate wick q4h. Remove wick after 24 hrs and continue to instill. Do not treat for >10 days.
*Pediatrics:* Instill 3 drops tid-qid. A gauze or wick may be inserted into ear canal after first administration. Add additional drops to saturate wick q4h. Remove wick after 24 hrs and continue to instill. Do not treat for >10 days.



**HOW SUPPLIED:** Sol: (Chloroxylenol-Hydrocortisone-Pramoxine) 1mg-10mg-10mg/mL [10mL]

**CONTRAINDICATIONS:** Varicella, vaccinia, perforated ear drum or when medication can reach the middle ear.

**WARNINGS/PRECAUTIONS:** Caution in long-standing otitis media. If local irritation or sensitization occurs, discontinue. Systemic absorption has produced HPA axis, manifestations of Cushing's syndrome, hyperglycemia, and glucosuria.

**ADVERSE REACTIONS:** Itching, burning, irritation, dryness, folliculitis, hypertrichosis, acneform eruptions, hypopigmentations.

**PREGNANCY:** Category C, caution in nursing.

## CORTEF RX

hydrocortisone (Pharmacia & Upjohn)

**THERAPEUTIC CLASS:** Corticosteroid

**INDICATIONS:** Steroid responsive disorders.

**DOSAGE:** *Adults:* Initial: 20-240mg/day depending on disease. Adjust until a satisfactory response. Maint: Decrease in small amounts to lowest effective dose. Acute Exacerbations of Multiple Sclerosis: Initial: (Tab) 200mg/day of prednisolone for 1 week, then 80mg every other day for 1 month (20mg hydrocortisone=5mg prednisolone).
*Pediatrics:* Initial: 20-240mg/day depending on disease. Adjust until a satisfactory response. Maint: After favorable response, decrease in small amounts to lowest effective dose. Acute Exacerbations of Multiple Sclerosis: Initial: (Tab) 200mg/day of prednisolone for 1 week, then 80mg every other day for 1 month (20mg hydrocortisone=5mg prednisolone).

**HOW SUPPLIED:** Sus: (Hydrocortisone Cypionate) 10mg/5mL [120mL]; Tab: (Hydrocortisone) 5mg, 10mg, 20mg

**CONTRAINDICATIONS:** Systemic fungal infections.

**WARNINGS/PRECAUTIONS:** May need to increase dose before, during, and after stressful situations. May mask signs of infections. Avoid abrupt withdrawal. Prolonged use may produce glaucoma, optic nerve damage, secondary ocular infections. Increases BP, salt/water retention, potassium excretion. More severe/fatal course of infections reported with chickenpox, measles. Caution with TB, hypothyroidism, cirrhosis, ocular herpes simplex, HTN, diverticulitis, fresh intestinal anastomosis, ulcerative colitis, osteoporosis, myasthenia gravis, renal insufficiency, peptic ulcer disease. Growth and development of children on prolonged therapy should be monitored. Monitor for psychic disturbances. Kaposi's sarcoma reported.

**ADVERSE REACTIONS:** Fluid and electrolyte disturbances, HTN, osteoporosis, muscle weakness, cushingoid state, menstrual irregularities, nervousness, insomnia, impaired wound healing, DM, ulcerative esophagitis, excessive sweating, increases intracranial pressure, carbohydrate intolerance, glaucoma, cataracts.

**INTERACTIONS:** Reduced efficacy and increased clearance with hepatic enzyme inducers (eg, phenobarbital, phenytoin, and rifampin). Decreased clearance with ketoconazole and troleandomycin. Increases clearance of chronic high dose ASA; caution with hypoprothrombinemia. Effects on oral anticoagulants are variable; monitor PT. Increased insulin and oral hypoglycemic requirements in DM. Avoid live vaccines with immunosuppressive doses. Possible decreased vaccine response with killed or inactivated vaccines with immunosuppressive doses.

**PREGNANCY:** Safety in pregnancy and nursing not known.

## CORTIFOAM

RX

hydrocortisone acetate (Schwarz)

**THERAPEUTIC CLASS:** Corticosteroid

**INDICATIONS:** Adjunct therapy in ulcerative proctitis of the distal part of the rectum for patients who cannot retain corticosteroid enemas.

**DOSAGE:** *Adults:* 1 applicatorful rectally qd-bid for 2-3 weeks, and every 2nd day thereafter. Maint: Decrease in small amounts to lowest effective dose. Discontinue if no improvement within 2-3 weeks.

**HOW SUPPLIED:** Foam: 10% [15g]

**CONTRAINDICATIONS:** Obstruction, abscess, perforation, peritonitis, fresh intestinal anastomoses, extensive fistulas and sinus tracts.

**WARNINGS/PRECAUTIONS:** Absorption may be greater than from other corticosteroid enemas. May elevate BP, cause salt and water retention, IOP, or increase potassium and calcium excretion. Caution with recent MI, hypo- or hyperthyroidism, Strongyloides infestation, TB, CHF, HTN, renal insufficiency, peptic ulcers, diverticulitis, nonspecific ulcerative colitis, cirrhosis, risk of osteoporosis. May produce reversible HPA axis suppression, posterior subcapsular cataracts, glaucoma with possible optic nerve damage. May mask signs of infection or cause new infections. Kaposi's sarcoma reported with chronic use. Avoid with cerebral malaria, systemic fungal infections, active ocular herpes simplex, postoperative ileorectostomy. Rule out latent or active amebiasis. Avoid exposure to chickenpox and/or measles. Observe growth in pediatrics. Withdraw gradually. Acute myopathy observed with high steroid doses. May aggravate existing emotional instability or psychosis. Discontinue if severe reaction occurs.

**ADVERSE REACTIONS:** Bradycardia, acne, abdominal distention, convulsions, depression, abnormal fat deposits, fluid/electrolyte disturbances, muscle weakness, osteoporosis, peptic ulcer, pancreatitis, impaired wound healing, headache, psychic disturbances, suppression of growth in children, glaucoma, hyperglycemia, weight gain, thromboembolism, malaise, hypersensitivity reactions.

**INTERACTIONS:** Avoid live vaccines with immunosuppressive doses. Risk of hypokalemia with amphotericin B injection, potassium depleting agents, digitalis glycosides. Caution with aminoglutethimide or neuromuscular blockers. Decreased clearance or metabolism with macrolide antibiotics, estrogens, ketoconazole. Increased metabolism with hepatic enzyme inducers (eg, barbiturates, phenytoin, carbamazepine, rifampin). Withdraw anticholinesterase agents 24 hrs prior to initiation. Inhibits response to warfarin; monitor PT/INR. May increase blood glucose levels; may need to adjust antidiabetic agents. May decrease isoniazid and salicylate levels. Caution with ASA in hypoprothrombinemia. Cyclosporine may increase activity of both drugs; convulsions reported with concomitant use. Increased clearance with cholestyramine. Increased risk for gastrointestinal side effects with ASA and other NSAIDs.

**PREGNANCY:** Category C, caution in nursing.

## CORTISPORIN

RX

bacitracin zinc - neomycin sulfate - polymyxin B sulfate - hydrocortisone acetate (King)

**THERAPEUTIC CLASS:** Antibacterial/corticosteroid

**INDICATIONS:** Corticosteroid responsive dermatoses with secondary infection.

**DOSAGE:** *Adults:* Apply bid-qid for maximum of 7 days.

**HOW SUPPLIED:** Cre: (Neomycin-Polymyxin-Hydrocortisone) 0.35%-10,000 U/g-0.5% [7.5g]; Oint: (Bacitracin-Neomycin-Polymyxin-Hydrocortisone) 400 U-0.35%-5,000 U/g-1% [15g]

**CONTRAINDICATIONS:** Use in eyes or external ear canal if eardrum is perforated. Tuberculous, fungal, or viral skin lesions.

**WARNINGS/PRECAUTIONS:** Avoid prolonged use or use over a large area. Prolonged use may result in secondary infection. May encourage spread of infection. Occlusive dressings will increase systemic absorption. Percutaneous absorption may cause growth cessation in pediatrics. D/C if redness, irritation, swelling, or pain persists.

**ADVERSE REACTIONS:** Allergic sensitization, burning, itching, irritation, dryness, folliculitis, hypertrichosis, acneiform eruptions, secondary infection, skin maceration, striae.

**PREGNANCY:** Category C, caution with nursing.

## CORTISPORIN OPHTHALMIC — RX

hydrocortisone - bacitracin zinc - neomycin sulfate - polymyxin B sulfate (King)

**THERAPEUTIC CLASS:** Antibacterial/corticosteroid

**INDICATIONS:** Ocular inflammation associated with infection or risk of infection.

**DOSAGE:** *Adults:* (Sus) 1-2 drops q3-4h depending on severity. (Oint) Apply q3-4h depending on severity. Max: 8g or 20mL for initial prescription.

**HOW SUPPLIED:** Oint: (Neomycin-Bacitracin-Polymyxin-Hydrocortisone) 3.5mg-400U-10,000U-1%/g [3.5g]; Sus: (Neomycin-Polymyxin-Hydrocortisone) 3.5mg-10,000U-1%/mL [7.5mL]

**CONTRAINDICATIONS:** Viral diseases of the cornea and conjunctiva including epithelial herpes simplex keratitis, vaccinia, and varicella. Mycobacterial infection and fungal diseases of the eye.

**WARNINGS/PRECAUTIONS:** Caution with glaucoma, herpes simplex, diseases causing thinning of cornea/sclera and other ocular viral infections. Prolonged use can cause glaucoma or secondary ocular infections (eg, fungal). Monitor IOP after 10 days of therapy. Re-evaluate if no response after 2 days. May delay healing and increase incidence of bleb formation after cataract surgery.

**ADVERSE REACTIONS:** Allergic sensitization reactions (itching, swelling, conjunctival erythema), elevation of IOP, infrequent optic nerve damage, secondary infection.

**PREGNANCY:** Category C, not for use in nursing.

## CORTISPORIN OTIC — RX

neomycin - hydrocortisone - polymyxin B sulfate (King)

**THERAPEUTIC CLASS:** Antibacterial/corticosteroid combination

**INDICATIONS:** (Sol/Sus) Treatment of superficial bacterial infections of the external auditory canal. (Sus) Treatment of infections of mastoidectomy and fenestration cavities.

**DOSAGE:** *Adults:* Clean and dry ear canal. Dropper: 4 drops tid-qid for up to 10 days. Alternate Regimen: Insert cotton wick into ear canal, then saturate cotton. Repeat q4h to keep cotton moist. Replace wick q24h.
*Pediatrics:* Clean and dry ear canal. Dropper: 3 drops tid-qid for up to 10 days. Alternate Regimen: Insert cotton wick into ear canal, then saturate cotton. Repeat q4h to keep cotton moist. Replace wick q24h.

**HOW SUPPLIED:** Sol, Sus: (Neomycin-Hydrocortisone-Polymyxin B) 0.35%-1%-10,000 U/mL [10mL]

**CONTRAINDICATIONS:** Herpes simplex, vaccinia, and varicella infections.

**WARNINGS/PRECAUTIONS:** Caution with perforated eardrum, chronic otitis media. Prolonged use may result in secondary infection. Re-evaluate if no improvement after 1 week. D/C after 10 days. Solution contains sulfites. May cause cutaneous sensitization.

**ADVERSE REACTIONS:** Skin sensitization, burning, itching, irritation, dryness, folliculitis, hypertrichosis, acneiform eruptions, secondary infection.

**PREGNANCY:** Category C, caution in nursing.



## CORTISPORIN-TC OTIC RX

colistin sulfate - neomycin sulfate - thonzonium bromide - hydrocortisone acetate (King)

**THERAPEUTIC CLASS:** Antibacterial/corticosteroid combination

**INDICATIONS:** Treatment of infections of the external auditory canal, mastoidectomy and fenestration cavities.

**DOSAGE:** *Adults:* Clean and dry ear canal. Dropper: 5 drops (calibrated dropper) or 4 drops (dropper bottle) tid-qid. Alternate Regimen: Insert cotton wick into ear canal, then saturate cotton. Repeat q4h to keep cotton moist. Replace wick q24h.

*Pediatrics:* Clean and dry ear canal. Dropper: 4 drops (calibrated dropper) or 3 drops (dropper bottle) tid-qid. Alternate Regimen: Insert cotton wick into ear canal, then saturate cotton. Repeat q4h to keep cotton moist. Replace wick q24h.

**HOW SUPPLIED:** (Colistin-Hydrocortisone-Neomycin-Thonzonium) Sus: 3mg-10mg-3.3mg-0.5mg/mL [10mL]

**CONTRAINDICATIONS:** Herpes simplex, vaccinia, and varicella infections.

**WARNINGS/PRECAUTIONS:** Caution with perforated eardrum, chronic otitis media. Prolonged use may result in secondary infection. Re-evaluate if no improvement after 1 week. D/C after 10 days.

**ADVERSE REACTIONS:** Cutaneous sensitization.

**PREGNANCY:** Safety in pregnancy and nursing not known.

## CORTROSYN RX

cosyntropin (Amphastar)

**THERAPEUTIC CLASS:** Synthetic ACTH

**INDICATIONS:** Diagnostic agent used to screen for adrenocortical insufficiency.

**DOSAGE:** *Adults:* 0.25-0.75mg IM/IV injection or 0.25-0.75mg IV over 4-8 hrs. (See labeling for method details).

*Pediatrics:* >2 yrs: 0.25-0.75mg IM/IV injection or 0.25-0.75mg IV over 4-8 hrs. <2 yrs: 0.125mg IM/IV injection or IV over 4-8 hrs. (See labeling for method details).

**HOW SUPPLIED:** Inj: 0.25mg

**WARNINGS/PRECAUTIONS:** Exhibits slight immunologic activity. Patients known to be sensitized to natural ACTH with markedly positive skin tests will, with few exceptions, react negatively when tested intradermally. Falsely high fluorescence measurements with high plasma bilirubin or if plasma contains free Hgb.

**ADVERSE REACTIONS:** Hypersensitivity/anaphylactic reactions (rare), bradycardia, tachycardia, HTN, peripheral edema, rash.

**INTERACTIONS:** May potentiate electrolyte loss associated with diuretics.

**PREGNANCY:** Category C, caution in nursing.

## CORVERT
RX

ibutilide fumarate (Pharmacia & Upjohn)

C

**THERAPEUTIC CLASS:** Class III antiarrhythmic

**INDICATIONS:** For rapid conversion of atrial fibrillation or flutter (A-Fib/Flutter) of recent onset to sinus rhythm.

**DOSAGE:** *Adults:* >60kg: 1mg over 10 minutes. <60kg: 0.01mg/kg over 10 minutes. If arrhythmia still present within 10 minutes after the end of the initial infusion, repeat infusion 10 minutes after completion of 1st infusion.

**HOW SUPPLIED:** Inj: 0.1mg/mL

**WARNINGS/PRECAUTIONS:** Proarrhythmic; can cause potentially fatal arrhythmias. Administer in setting with continuous ECG monitoring and person able to treat acute ventricular arrhythmia. Adequately anticoagulate if A-Fib >2-3 days. Correct hypokalemia and hypomagnesemia before therapy. Caution in elderly.

**ADVERSE REACTIONS:** Sustained and nonsustained polymorphic ventricular tachycardia, sustained and nonsustained monomorphic ventricular tachycardia, bundle branch and AV block, ventricular and supraventricular extrasystoles, hypotension, bradycardia.

**INTERACTIONS:** Avoid Class IA (eg, disopyramide, quinidine, procainamide) and other Class III (eg, amiodarone, sotalol) antiarrhythmics with or within 4 hrs postinfusion of ibutilide. Increase proarrhythmia potential with drugs that prolong the QT interval (eg, phenothiazines, TCAs). Supraventricular arrhythmias may mask cardiotoxicity associated with excessive digoxin levels.

**PREGNANCY:** Category C, not for use in nursing.

## CORZIDE
RX

nadolol - bendroflumethiazide (King)

**THERAPEUTIC CLASS:** Nonselective beta-blocker/thiazide diuretic

**INDICATIONS:** Management of hypertension. Not for initial therapy.

**DOSAGE:** *Adults:* Initial: 40mg-5mg tab qd. Max: 80mg-5mg tab qd. CrCl >50mL/min: Dose q24h. CrCl 31-50mL/min: Dose q24-36h. CrCl 10-30mL/min: Dose q24-48h. CrCl <10mL/min: Dose q40-60h.

**HOW SUPPLIED:** Tab: (Nadolol-Bendroflumethiazide) 40mg-5mg*, 80mg-5mg* *scored

**CONTRAINDICATIONS:** Bronchial asthma, sinus bradycardia and >1st-degree conduction block, cardiogenic shock, overt cardiac failure, anuria, sulfonamide hypersensitivity.

**WARNINGS/PRECAUTIONS:** Caution in well-compensated cardiac failure, nonallergic bronchospasm, progressive hepatic disease, and renal or hepatic dysfunction. Exacerbation of ischemic heart disease with abrupt withdrawal. Withdrawal before surgery is controversial. May mask hyperthyroidism or hypoglycemia symptoms. Can cause cardiac failure, sensitivity reactions, hypokalemia, hyperuricemia, hypomagnesemia, hypophosphatemia. May activate or exacerbate SLE. Monitor for fluid/electrolyte imbalance. Enhanced effects in postsympathectomy patient. May manifest latent DM. May decrease PBI levels.

**ADVERSE REACTIONS:** Bradycardia, peripheral vascular insufficiency, dizziness, fatigue, nausea, vomiting, blood dyscrasias, hypersensitivity reactions.

**INTERACTIONS:** Additive hypotension and/or bradycardia with catecholamine-depleting drugs. Antidiabetic agents, anticoagulants, other antihypertensives, antigout agents may need adjustment. General anesthetics may exaggerate hypotension. May block epinephrine effects. Lithium toxicity. Alcohol, barbiturates, narcotics potentiate orthostatic hypotension. Amphotericin B, ACTH, corticosteroids intensify electrolyte imbalance.

Monitor calcium levels with calcium salts. Monitor digoxin. Cholestyramine and colestipol may delay or decrease absorption. Enhanced hyperglycemic, hyperuricemic, and antihypertensive effects with diazoxide. Enhanced hypotensive effects with MAOIs. Possible decreased effectiveness with methenamine. Decreased arterial responsiveness with pressor amines. Probenecid, sulfinpyrazone may need dose increase. May potentiate nondepolarizing muscle relaxants, preanesthetics, and anesthetics. NSAIDs may decrease effects.



**PREGNANCY:** Category C, not for use in nursing.

## COSMEGEN

dactinomycin (Ovation) RX

**Drug is highly toxic; handle and administer with care. Avoid inhalation or contact with skin and mucous membranes. Extremely corrosive to soft tissue. Severe damage to soft tissue will occur with extravasation during IV use.**

**THERAPEUTIC CLASS:** Actinomycin antibiotic

**INDICATIONS:** Concomitant treatment of Wilms' tumor, childhood rhabdomyosarcoma, Ewing's sarcoma, and metastatic nonseminomatous testicular carcinoma. Monotherapy for gestational trophoblastic neoplasia, and as palliative and/or adjunctive treatment of solid malignancies.

**DOSAGE:** *Adults:* Wilms' Tumor/Childhood Rhabdomyosarcoma/Ewing's Sarcoma: 15mcg/kg IV daily for 5 days. Testicular Cancer: 1000mcg/m$^2$ IV on day 1 of combination therapy. Gestational Trophoblastic Neoplasia: Monotherapy: 12mcg/kg IV daily for 5 days. Combination Therapy: 500mcg/m$^2$ IV on days 1 and 2. Solid Malignancies: 50mcg/kg IV for lower extremity or pelvis. 35mcg/kg IV for upper extremity. May need lower dose with obese patients, or with previous chemotherapy or radiation use. Dose intensity per 2-week cycle should not exceed 15mcg/kg/day or 400-600mcg/m$^2$ daily for 5 days. Calculate dose for obese or edematous patients based on BSA. Elderly: Start at low end of dosing range.
*Pediatrics:* >6-12 months: Wilms' Tumor, Childhood Rhabdomyosarcoma/Ewing's Sarcoma: 15mcg/kg IV daily for 5 days. Testicular Carcinoma: 1000mcg/m$^2$ IV on day 1 of combination therapy. Gestational Trophoblastic Neoplasia: Monotherapy: 12mcg/kg IV daily for 5 days. Combination Therapy: 500mcg/m$^2$ IV on days 1 and 2. Solid Malignancies: 50mcg/kg IV for lower extremity or pelvis. 35mcg/kg IV for upper extremity. May need lower dose with obese patients, or with previous chemotherapy or radiation use. Dose intensity per 2-week cycle should not exceed 15mcg/kg/day or 400-600mcg/m$^2$ daily for 5 days. Calculate dose for obese or edematous patients based on BSA.

**HOW SUPPLIED:** Inj: 0.5mg

**CONTRAINDICATIONS:** At or about the time of infection with chickenpox or herpes zoster.

**WARNINGS/PRECAUTIONS:** Monitor renal, hepatic, and bone marrow functions frequently. Can cause fetal harm during pregnancy. Possible anaphylactoid reactions. If stomatitis, diarrhea, or severe hematopoietic depression occurs; d/c until recovery. Caution in elderly; increased risk of myelosuppression. Veno-occlusive disease (primarily hepatic) reported.

**ADVERSE REACTIONS:** Nausea, vomiting, fatigue, lethargy, fever, cheilitis, esophagitis, abdominal pain, liver toxicity, anemia, blood dyscrasias, skin eruptions, acne, alopecia.

**INTERACTIONS:** Increased GI toxicity, marrow suppression, and incidence of secondary tumors with radiation. May reactivate erythema from previous radiation therapy. Caution if used within 2 months of irradiation for treatment of right-sided Wilms' tumor; hepatomegaly and elevated AST levels reported. Only use with radiotherapy for Wilms' tumor if benefit outweighs risks.

**PREGNANCY:** Category D, not for use in nursing.

## COSOPT RX
dorzolamide HCl - timolol maleate (Merck)

C

**THERAPEUTIC CLASS:** Carbonic anhydrase inhibitor/nonselective beta-blocker

**INDICATIONS:** Treatment of ocular hypertension and open-angle glaucoma insufficiently responsive to β-blockers.

**DOSAGE:** *Adults:* 1 drop bid. Space dosing of other ophthalmic drugs by 10 minutes.
*Pediatrics:* ≥2 yrs: 1 drop bid. Space dosing of other ophthalmic drugs by 10 minutes.

**HOW SUPPLIED:** Sol: (Dorzolamide-Timolol) 2%-0.5% [5mL, 10mL]

**CONTRAINDICATIONS:** Bronchial asthma, history of bronchial asthma, severe COPD, sinus bradycardia, 2nd- or 3rd-degree AV block, overt cardiac failure, cardiogenic shock.

**WARNINGS/PRECAUTIONS:** Caution with sulfonamide allergy, cardiac failure, DM, COPD, bronchospastic disease, surgery and hepatic impairment. May mask symptoms of hypoglycemia and thyrotoxicosis. Bacterial keratitis reported with contaminated containers. Avoid in severe renal impairment. D/C if hypersensitivity or ocular reaction occur. Reinsert contact lenses 15 minutes after applying drops.

**ADVERSE REACTIONS:** Taste perversion, ocular burning, conjunctival hyperemia, blurred vision, superficial punctate keratitis, eye itching.

**INTERACTIONS:** Avoid oral carbonic anhydrase inhibitors, oral β-blockers, or topical β-blockers due to potential additive effects. Oral/IV calcium antagonists can cause AV-conduction disturbances, left ventricular failure or hypotension. Potentiated systemic β-blockade with concomitant CYP2D6 inhibitors. Reserpine can cause additive effects, hypotension and/or bradycardia. AV conduction time prolonged with digitalis. Quinidine may potentiate β-blockade. Increased risk of hypoglycemia with insulin or oral hypoglycemic agents. Wait 10 minutes before using another ophthalmic drug.

**PREGNANCY:** Category C, not for use in nursing.

## COUMADIN RX
warfarin sodium (Bristol-Myers Squibb)

**May cause major or fatal bleeding.**

**OTHER BRAND NAMES:** Jantoven (USL Pharma)

**THERAPEUTIC CLASS:** Vitamin K-dependent coagulation factor inhibitor

**INDICATIONS:** Prophylaxis and treatment of venous thrombosis, PE, and thromboembolic disorders associated with atrial fibrillation and/or cardiac valve replacement. To reduce risk of death, recurrent MI, and thromboembolic events after MI.

**DOSAGE:** *Adults:* >18 yrs: Adjust dose based on PT/INR. Give IV as alternate to PO. Initial: 2-5mg qd. Usual: 2-10mg qd. Venous Thromboembolism (including pulmonary embolism): INR 2-3. Atrial Fibrillation: INR 2-3. Post-MI: Initiate 2-4 weeks post-infarct and maintain INR 2.5-3.5. Mechanical/Bioprosthetic Heart Valve: INR 2-3 for 12 weeks after valve insertion, then INR 2.5-3.5 long term.

**HOW SUPPLIED:** Inj: (Coumadin) 5mg; Tab: (Coumadin, Jantoven) 1mg*, 2mg*, 2.5mg*, 3mg*, 4mg*, 5mg*, 6mg*, 7.5mg*, 10mg* *scored

**CONTRAINDICATIONS:** Hemorrhagic tendencies, blood dyscrasias, CNS surgery, ophthalmic or traumatic surgery, inadequate lab facility, threatened abortion, eclampsia, preeclampsia, major regional lumbar block anesthesia, malignant HTN, pregnancy and unsupervised senile, alcoholic or psychotic patients. Bleeding of GI, GU or respiratory tract, aneurysms, pericarditis and pericardial effusion, bacterial endocarditis, cerebrovascular hemorrhage, spinal puncture, procedures with potential for uncontrollable bleeding.

**WARNINGS/PRECAUTIONS:** Monitor PT/INR; many endogenous and exogenous factors may affect PT/INR. Weigh benefits/risks with severe-moderate hepatic or renal insufficiency, infectious disease, intestinal flora disturbance, lactation, surgery, trauma, severe-moderate HTN, protein C deficiency, polycythemia vera, vasculitis, severe DM, indwelling catheters. D/C if tissue necrosis, systemic cholesterol microembolization ("purple toe syndrome") occurs. Caution with HIT, DVT, elderly. Warfarin resistance, allergic reactions reported.

**ADVERSE REACTIONS:** Tissue or organ hemorrhage/necrosis, paresthesia, vasculitis, fever, rash, abdominal pain, hepatic disorders, fatigue, headache, alopecia.

**INTERACTIONS:** Interacts with protein bound drugs, hepatic enzyme inducers and inhibitors. Avoid streptokinase and urokinase. Caution with drugs that may cause hemorrhage (eg, NSAIDs, ASA). Potentiates hypoglycemic and anticonvulsant drugs. See product labeling for extensive list.

**PREGNANCY:** Category X, weigh benefits/risks with nursing.

## COVERA-HS

verapamil HCl (Searle) RX

**THERAPEUTIC CLASS:** Calcium channel blocker (nondihydropyridine)

**INDICATIONS:** Management of hypertension and angina.

**DOSAGE:** *Adults:* Initial: 180mg qhs. Titrate: May increase to 240mg qhs, then 360mg qhs, then 480mg qhs, if needed. Swallow tab whole. Elderly: Start at the low end of the dosing range.

**HOW SUPPLIED:** Tab, Extended Release: 180mg, 240mg

**CONTRAINDICATIONS:** Severe ventricular dysfunction, hypotension, cardiogenic shock, sick sinus syndrome or 2nd- or 3rd-degree AV block (except with functioning ventricular pacemaker), A-Fib/Flutter with an accessory bypass tract.

**WARNINGS/PRECAUTIONS:** Avoid with moderate to severe cardiac failure, and ventricular dysfunction if taking a β-blocker. May cause hypotension, AV block, transient bradycardia, PR interval prolongation. Monitor LFTs periodically; hepatocellular injury reported. Give 30% of normal dose with severe hepatic dysfunction. Caution with hypertrophic cardiomyopathy, renal or hepatic dysfunction. Decrease dose with decreased neuromuscular transmission.

**ADVERSE REACTIONS:** Constipation, dizziness, nausea, hypotension, headache, edema, CHF, pulmonary edema, fatigue, dyspnea, bradycardia, AV block, rash, flushing.

**INTERACTIONS:** Additive effects on HR, AV conduction, and contractility with β-blockers. Potentiates other antihypertensives. May increase digoxin, carbamazepine, theophylline, cyclosporine, and alcohol levels. Avoid disopyramide within 48 hrs before or 24 hrs after verapamil. Additive negative inotropic effects and AV conduction prolongation with flecainide. Avoid quinidine with hypertrophic cardiomyopathy. Monitor lithium. CYP3A4 inhibitors (eg, erythromycin, ritonavir) and grapefruit juice may increase levels. CYP3A4 inducers (eg, rifampin, phenobarbital) may decrease levels. Increased bleeding time with ASA. May potentiate neuromuscular blockers; both agents may need dose reduction. Caution with inhalation anesthetics.

**PREGNANCY:** Category C, not for use in nursing.

## COZAAR
RX

losartan potassium (Merck)



**Can cause death/injury to developing fetus during 2nd and 3rd trimesters. Stop therapy if pregnancy detected.**

**THERAPEUTIC CLASS:** Angiotensin II receptor antagonist

**INDICATIONS:** Hypertension (HTN), alone or with other antihypertensives. To reduce the risk of stroke in patients with HTN and left ventricular hypertrophy (LVH), but evidence shows this does not apply to black patients. Diabetic nephropathy with an elevated serum creatinine and proteinuria (urinary albumin to creatinine ratio >300mg/g) in patients with type 2 diabetes and hypertension.

**DOSAGE:** *Adults:* HTN: Initial: 50mg qd. Usual: 25-100mg/day given qd-bid. Intravascular Volume Depletion/Hepatic Impairment: Initial: 25mg qd. HTN with LVH: Initial: 50mg qd. Add hydrochlorothiazide (HCTZ) 12.5mg qd and/or increase losartan to 100mg qd, followed by an increase in HCTZ to 25mg qd based on BP response. Nephropathy: Initial: 50 mg qd. Titrate: Increase to 100mg qd based on BP response.

**HOW SUPPLIED:** Tab: 25mg, 50mg, 100mg

**WARNINGS/PRECAUTIONS:** Can cause fetal injury/death. Correct volume or salt depletion before therapy. Changes in renal function may occur; caution with renal artery stenosis, severe CHF. Angioedema reported. Consider dose adjustment with hepatic dysfunction.

**ADVERSE REACTIONS:** Dizziness, cough, upper respiratory infection, diarrhea.

**INTERACTIONS:** $K^+$-sparing diuretics (eg, spironolactone, triamterene, amiloride), $K^+$ supplements, or $K^+$-containing salt substitutes may increase serum $K^+$. May reduce excreation of lithium; monitor lithium levels. Combination with NSAIDs, including COX-2 inhibitors, may lead to further deterioration of renal function.

**PREGNANCY:** Category C (1st trimester) and D (2nd and 3rd trimesters), not for use in nursing.

## CRESTOR
RX

rosuvastatin calcium (AstraZeneca LP)

**THERAPEUTIC CLASS:** HMG-CoA reductase inhibitor

**INDICATIONS:** Adjunct to diet in primary hypercholesterolemia (heterozygous familial and non familial) and mixed dyslipidemia (Types IIa and IIb) to reduce elevated total-C, LDL-C, Apo B, non HDL-C, and triglyceride (TG) levels and to increase HDL-C. Adjunct to diet for elevated serum TG levels (Type IV). Adjunct to other lipid-lowering agents or if these are unavailable, to reduce LDL-C, total-C, and Apo B in homozygous familial hypercholesterolemia.

**DOSAGE:** *Adults:* Hypercholesterolemia/Mixed Dyslipidemia: Initial: 10mg qd (or 5mg qd for less aggressive LDL-C reductions; 20mg qd with LDL-C >190mg/dL). Titrate: Adjust dose if needed at 2-4 week intervals. Range: 5-40mg qd. Homozygous Familial Hypercholesterolemia: 20mg qd. Max: 40mg qd. Concomitant Cyclosporine: Max: 5mg qd. Concomitant Gemfibrozil: Max: 10mg qd. Severe Renal Impairment: CrCl <30mL/min (not on hemodialysis): Initial: 5mg qd. Max: 10mg qd.

**HOW SUPPLIED:** Tab: 5mg, 10mg, 20mg, 40mg

**CONTRAINDICATIONS:** Active liver disease, unexplained persistent elevations of serum transaminases, pregnancy, nursing mothers.

**WARNINGS/PRECAUTIONS:** Rare cases of rhabdomyolysis with acute renal failure secondary to myoglobinuria have been reported. Monitor LFTs prior to therapy, at 12 weeks or with dose elevation, and periodically thereafter. Reduce dose or withdraw if AST or ALT >3X ULN persist. Caution with heavy alcohol use, history of hepatic disease, renal impairment, hypothyroidism, elderly. Discontinue if markedly elevated CPK levels occur, if myopathy is diagnosed or suspected, or if predisposition to renal failure secondary to rhabdomyolysis. Approximately 2-fold elevation in median exposure in Asian subjects.



**ADVERSE REACTIONS:** Pharyngitis, headache, diarrhea, dyspepsia, nausea.

**INTERACTIONS:** Increased levels and risk of myopathy with cyclosporine, fibrates, niacin. Avoid gemfibrozil. Caution with drugs that decrease levels or activity of endogenous steroid hormones (eg, ketoconazole, spironolactone, cimetidine). Increases levels of oral contraceptives (norgestrel, ethinyl estradiol). Increases INR with warfarin. Space antacid dosing by 2 hours.

**PREGNANCY:** Category X, not for use in nursing.

## CRINONE

progesterone (Serono)

RX

**OTHER BRAND NAMES:** Prochieve (Columbia Labs)

**THERAPEUTIC CLASS:** Progestogen

**INDICATIONS:** (4%) Treatment of secondary amenorrhea. (8%) Progesterone replacement or supplementation in Assisted Reproductive Technology (ART) and treatment of secondary amenorrhea after failure to respond to 4%.

**DOSAGE:** *Adults:* ART: 90mg of 8% intravaginally qd if require progesterone supplementation. 90mg of 8% intravaginally bid with partial or complete ovarian failure requiring progesterone replacement. If pregnancy occurs, continue until placental autonomy is achieved, up to 10-12 weeks. Secondary Amenorrhea: 4% intravaginally every other day up to 6 doses. If fails, 8% intravaginally every other day up to 6 doses.

**HOW SUPPLIED:** Gel: (Crinone, Prochieve) 4% [45mg, $6^s$], (Crinone, Prochieve) 8% [90mg, $6^s$ $18^s$]

**CONTRAINDICATIONS:** Undiagnosed vaginal bleeding, liver dysfunction, malignancy of breast or genital organs, missed abortion, thrombophlebitis, thromboembolic disorders, history of hormone-associated thrombophlebitis or thromboembolic disorders.

**WARNINGS/PRECAUTIONS:** D/C if signs of thrombotic disorders develop. Include pap smear in pretreatment exam. Caution with depression, DM, epilepsy, migraine, asthma, cardiac or renal dysfunction.

**ADVERSE REACTIONS:** Bloating, abdominal pain/cramps, depression, headache, nausea, vaginal discharge, fatigue, genital pruritus.

**PREGNANCY:** Safety in pregnancy or nursing not known.

## CRIXIVAN

indinavir sulfate (Merck)

RX

**THERAPEUTIC CLASS:** Protease inhibitor

**INDICATIONS:** Treatment of HIV infection in combination with other antiretrovirals.

**DOSAGE:** *Adults:* 800mg q8h on empty stomach. Hepatic Insufficiency or Concomitant Delavirdine, Itraconazole, Ketoconazole: 600mg every 8 hrs. Concomitant Efavirenz or Rifabutin: 1g every 8 hrs (reduce rifabutin dose by 1/2). Maintain adequate hydration (1.5L fluid/24 hrs).

**HOW SUPPLIED:** Cap: 100mg, 200mg, 333mg, 400mg

**CONTRAINDICATIONS:** Concomitant terfenadine, cisapride, astemizole, triazolam, midazolam, alprazolam, ergot derivatives.

**WARNINGS/PRECAUTIONS:** D/C or suspend during acute nephrolithiasis/urolithiasis. Tubulointerstitial nephritis seen with asymptomatic severe leukocyturia; monitor frequently with urinalyses.

Consider discontinuation with severe leukocyturia. Immune reconstitution syndrome, hemolytic anemia, hyperglycemia, hyperbilirubinemia, hepatitis And liver failure reported. Spontaneous bleeding may occur with hemophilia A and B. Monitor hepatic function. Maintain adequate hydration. Possible redistribution or accumulation of body fat. Caution in elderly.



**ADVERSE REACTIONS:** Nephrolithiasis, GI discomfort, headache, fatigue, insomnia, hyperbilirubinemia, hyperglycemia, hemolytic anemia, renal failure, hematuria, nausea.

**INTERACTIONS:** See Contraindications. Increased risk of myopathy with HMG-CoA reductase inhibitors metabolized by CYP3A4. Increased levels with delavirdine, itraconazole, ketoconazole; reduce dose. Decreased levels with efavirenz, rifabutin, St. John's wort, rifampin. Avoid coadministration with atazanavir. Increases rifabutin and calcium channel blocker levels. Administer didanosine 1 hr apart on empty stomach. Caution with phenobarbital, phenytoin, carbamazepine, and dexamethasone. Substantially increases sildenafil plasma levels; increased risk of sildenafil adverse events (eg, hypotension, visual changes, priapism). Decreases metabolism of alprazolam; increased risk of alprazolam adverse effects (eg, sedation, respiratory depression)

**PREGNANCY:** Category C, not for use in nursing.

## CROFAB — RX

crotalidae polyvalent immune fab (ovine) (Savage)

**THERAPEUTIC CLASS:** Venom specific immunoglobulin Fab fragment

**INDICATIONS:** Management of minimal to moderate North American crotalid envenomation. Use within 6 hrs to prevent clinical deterioration and systemic coagulation abnormalities.

**DOSAGE:** *Adults:* Initial: 4-6 vials IV over 60 minutes. Observe patient for 1 hr following dose to determine if envenomation is controlled. If needed, administer additional 4-6 vials until envenomation controlled. Once control is achieved, give 2 vials q6h for up to 18 hrs (3 doses). Additional 2-vial doses may be given based on clinical course.
*Pediatrics:* Initial: 4-6 vials IV over 60 minutes. Observe patient for 1 hr following dose to determine if envenomation is controlled. If needed, administer additional 4-6 vials until envenomation controlled. Once control is achieved, give 2 vials q6h for up to 18 hrs (3 doses). Additional 2-vial doses may be given based on clinical course.

**HOW SUPPLIED:** Inj: 1g/vial

**CONTRAINDICATIONS:** Hypersensitivity to papaya or papain.

**WARNINGS/PRECAUTIONS:** Recurrent coagulopathy may persist for 1-2 weeks; monitor for symptoms. Risk of anaphylactic reaction. Sensitization may occur; caution with a repeat course of treatment for subsequent envenomation episode. Contains ethyl mercury; use with caution in children. Use caution with conditions that cause coagulation defects (eg, cancer, collagen disease, CHF, diarrhea, elevated temperature, hepatic disorders, hyperthyroidism, poor nutritional state, steatorrhea, vitamin K deficiency.

**ADVERSE REACTIONS:** Urticaria, rash.

**PREGNANCY:** Category C, caution in nursing.

## CUBICIN — RX

daptomycin (Cubist)

**THERAPEUTIC CLASS:** Cyclic lipopeptide

**INDICATIONS:** Susceptible complicated skin and skin structure infections (cSSSI). *Staphylococcus aureus* bloodstream infections (bacteremia).

**DOSAGE:** *Adults:* ≥18 yrs: Administer as IV infusion over 30 minutes. cSSSI: 4mg/kg once every 24 hrs for 7-14 days. *S. aureus* Bacteremia: 6mg/kg once every 24 hrs for minimum 2-6 weeks. Renal impairment: CrCl <30mL/min, Hemodialysis or CAPD: (cSSSI) 4mg/kg or (*S. aureus* Bacteremia) 6mg/kg once every 48 hrs.

**HOW SUPPLIED:** Inj: 500mg

**WARNINGS/PRECAUTIONS:** Pseudomembranous colitis and neuropathy reported. Monitor CPK levels weekly; discontinue with unexplained signs & symptoms of myopathy and CPK elevation >1000 U/L (~5X ULN), or with CPK levels ≥10X ULN. Persisting or relapsing S. aureus infection or poor clinical response should have repeat blood cultures.

**ADVERSE REACTIONS:** Constipation, nausea, injection site reactions, headache, diarrhea, insomnia, rash, vomiting, abnormal LFTs, superinfection, pharyngolaryngeal pain, pain in extremity and pulmonary eosinophilia.

**INTERACTIONS:** Caution with tobramycin; may affect levels. Monitor PT/INR for first several days with warfarin. Consider temporarily suspending statins. HMG-CoA reductase inhibitors may cause myopathy; consider suspending these agents with concomitant therapy.

**PREGNANCY:** Category B, caution in nursing.

## CUPRIMINE

RX

penicillamine (Aton)

**Supervise closely due to toxicity, special dosage considerations, and therapeutic benefits.**

**OTHER BRAND NAMES:** Depen (Wallace)

**THERAPEUTIC CLASS:** Copper chelating agent

**INDICATIONS:** Treatment of Wilson's disease, cystinuria, and severe, active rheumatoid arthritis (RA) when conventional therapy has failed.

**DOSAGE:** *Adults:* Wilson's Disease: Determine dosage by 24-hr urinary copper excretion. Maint: 0.75-1.5g/day for 3 months. Max: Up to 2g/day, based on serum free copper. Cystinuria: Initial: 250mg qd. Usual: 250mg-1g qid. RA: Initial: 125-250mg/day. Titrate: May increase by 125-250mg/day every 1-3 months. If needed after 2-3 months, increase by 250mg/day every 2-3 months. D/C if no improvement after 3-4 months at dose of 1-1.5g/day. Maint: 500-750mg/day. Max: 1.5g/day. Give on empty stomach, 1 hr before or 2 hrs after meals, and 1 hr apart from any other drug, food or milk. Supplemental pyridoxine 25mg/day recommended.
*Pediatrics:* Cystinuria: 30mg/kg/day given qid.

**HOW SUPPLIED:** Cap: (Cuprimine): 250mg; Tab: (Depen) 250mg* *scored

**CONTRAINDICATIONS:** Pregnancy (except for treatment of Wilson's disease or certain cases of cystinuria), nursing, RA patients with renal insufficiency, history of penicillamine-related aplastic anemia or agranulocytosis.

**WARNINGS/PRECAUTIONS:** Aplastic anemia, agranulocytosis, drug fever, thrombocytopenia, Goodpasture's syndrome, myasthenia gravis, pemphigus foliaceus/vulgaris, obliterative bronchiolitis, proteinuria and hematuria reported. Routine urinalysis, CBC with differentials, Hgb and platelet count every 2 weeks for 6 months, then monthly.

**ADVERSE REACTIONS:** Rash, urticaria, anorexia, epigastric pain, nausea, vomiting, diarrhea, leukopenia, thrombocytopenia, proteinuria.

**INTERACTIONS:** Hematologic and renal adverse reactions increase with gold therapy, antimalarial or cytotoxic drugs, oxyphenbutazone and phenylbutazone. Systemic levels lowered by iron; separate doses by 2 hrs. Mineral supplements may block response to therapy.

**PREGNANCY:** Category D, not for use in nursing.

## CUTIVATE

RX

fluticasone propionate (GlaxoSmithKline)

C

**THERAPEUTIC CLASS:** Corticosteroid

**INDICATIONS:** Corticosteroid responsive dermatoses.

**DOSAGE:** *Adults:* (Cre) Atopic Dermatitis: Apply qd-bid. Other Dermatoses: Apply bid. Re-evaluate if no improvement after 2 weeks. (Oint) Apply bid. Avoid occlusive dressings.
*Pediatrics:* >3 months: (Cre) Atopic Dermatitis: Apply qd-bid. Other Dermatoses: Apply bid. Reassess if no improvement after 2 weeks. Avoid in diaper area. Oint not approved in peds. Avoid occlusive dressings.

**HOW SUPPLIED:** Cre: 0.05% [15g, 30g, 60g]; Oint: 0.005% [15g, 30g, 60g]

**WARNINGS/PRECAUTIONS:** Caution with cre in peds. May produce reversible HPA axis suppression, manifestations of Cushing's syndrome, hyperglycemia, and glucosuria. D/C if irritation occurs. Use appropriate antifungal or antibacterial agent with dermatological infections. Peds may be more susceptible to systemic toxicity. Caution when applied to large surface areas. Avoid with pre-existing skin atrophy. Not for use in rosacea or perioral dermatitis.

**ADVERSE REACTIONS:** Stinging, burning, dryness, pruritus, erythema, irritation, hypertrichosis.

**PREGNANCY:** Category C, caution in nursing.

## CYANIDE ANTIDOTE PACKAGE

RX

amyl nitrite - sodium nitrite - sodium thiosulfate (Akorn)

**THERAPEUTIC CLASS:** Antidote

**INDICATIONS:** Treatment of cyanide poisoning.

**DOSAGE:** *Adults:* Apply1 ampule of Amyl Nitrite to a handkerchief and hold in front of patient's mouth for 15 seconds followed by a rest for 15 seconds. Then reapply until Sodium Nitrite can be administered. Discontinue Amyl Nitrite and give Sodium Nitrite IV 300mg at the rate of 2.5-5mL/minute. Immediately after, inject 12.5g of Sodium Thiosulfate. If the poison was taken by mouth, gastric lavage should be performed as soon as possible. If signs of poisoning reappear, repeat Sodium Nitrite and Sodium Thiosulfate at one-half the original dose.
*Pediatrics:* Apply 1 ampule of Amyl Nitrite to a handkerchief and hold in front of patient's mouth for 15 seconds followed by a rest for 15 seconds. Then reapply until Sodium Nitrite can be administered. Discontinue Amyl Nitrite and give 6-8mL/$m^2$ of Sodium Nitrite IV; max: 10mL. Immediately after, inject 7g/$m^2$ of Sodium Thiosulfate; max: 12.5g. If the poison was taken by mouth, gastric lavage should be performed as soon as possible. If signs of poisoning reappear, repeat Sodium Nitrite and Sodium Thiosulfate at one-half the original dose.

**HOW SUPPLIED:** Sodium Nitrite: 300mg/10mL [2 ampules]; Sodium Thiosulfate: 12.5mg/50mL [2 vials]; Amyl Nitrite Inhalant: 0.3mL [12 ampules]

**WARNINGS/PRECAUTIONS:** Sodium Nitrite and Amyl Nitrite in high doses induce methemoglobinemia and can cause death.

**PREGNANCY:** Safety in pregnancy and nursing is not known.

## CYCLESSA

RX

desogestrel - ethinyl estradiol (Organon)

**OTHER BRAND NAMES:** Velivet (Duramed Pharms Barr)

**THERAPEUTIC CLASS:** Estrogen/progestogen combination

**INDICATIONS:** Prevention of pregnancy.

**DOSAGE:** *Adults:* Start 1st Sunday after menses begins or the 1st day of menses. 1 tab qd for 28 days, then repeat.

**HOW SUPPLIED:** Tab: (Ethinyl Estradiol-Desogesterol) 0.025mg-0.1mg, 0.025mg-0.125mg, 0.025mg-0.15mg

**CONTRAINDICATIONS:** Thrombophlebitis, DVT or thromboembolic disorders, pregnancy, cerebrovascular or coronary artery disease, undiagnosed abnormal genital bleeding, cholestatic jaundice of pregnancy or jaundice with prior pill use, hepatic adenomas or carcinomas, breast cancer or other estrogen-dependent neoplasia, hepatic tumors, active liver disease, and heavy smoking (≥15 cigarettes/day) and over age 35.

**WARNINGS/PRECAUTIONS:** Cigarette smoking increases risk of serious cardiovascular side effects. This risk increases with age (especially >35 yrs) and heavy smoking. Increased risk of MI, vascular disease, thromboembolism, stroke and gallbladder disease. Retinal thrombosis, hepatic neoplasia, carcinoma of breast and reproductive organs reported. May cause glucose intolerance. May increase BP, elevate LDL levels or cause other lipid changes, fluid retention, breakthrough bleeding, and spotting. May cause or exacerbate migraine. May develop visual changes with contact lens. Increased risk of MI with HTN, hyperlipidemia, obesity, and diabetes. Increased risk of stroke with thrombophilias, hyperlipidemias, obesity, and migraine (especially with aura). Discontinue if develop jaundice, significant depression or ophthalmic irregularities. Perform annual physical exam. Use before menarche is not indicated. May affect certain endocrine, LFTs and blood components. Should not be used if pregnant. Does not protect against STD's. Caution in nursing mothers and those who have lipid disorders.

**ADVERSE REACTIONS:** Nausea, vomiting, breakthrough bleeding, spotting, amenorrhea, migraine headache, mood changes including depression, vaginal candidiasis, edema, weight or appetite changes, and fluid retention.

**INTERACTIONS:** Reduced effects, increased breakthrough bleeding, and menstrual irregularities with some antibiotics, antifungals, anticonvulsants. Anti-HIV protease inhibitors may affect safety and efficacy. St. John's wort may induce hepatic enzymes and reduce effectiveness as well as resulting in breakthrough bleeding. Increased plasma concentrations of cyclosporine, prednisolone, and theophylline.

**PREGNANCY:** Category X, not for use in nursing.

## CYCLOCORT RX

amcinonide (Astellas)

**THERAPEUTIC CLASS:** Corticosteroid

**INDICATIONS:** Corticosteroid responsive dermatoses.

**DOSAGE:** *Adults:* Apply bid-tid depending on severity.
*Pediatrics:* Apply bid-tid depending on severity.

**HOW SUPPLIED:** Cre, Oint: 0.1% [15g, 30g, 60g]; Lot: 0.1% [20mL, 60mL]

**WARNINGS/PRECAUTIONS:** Systemic absorption may produce reversible HPA axis suppression, manifestations of Cushing's syndrome, hyperglycemia, and glucosuria. Discontinue if irritation occurs. Use appropriate antifungal or antibacterial agent with dermatological infections. Pediatrics may be more susceptible to systemic toxicity. Caution when applied to large surface areas or with occlusive dressings.

**ADVERSE REACTIONS:** Itching, stinging, soreness, burning, irritation, folliculitis, hypertrichosis, hypopigmentation, perioral dermatitis, skin maceration, striae, miliaria, skin atrophy, secondary infection, contact dermatitis.

**PREGNANCY:** Category C, not for use in nursing.

## CYMBALTA
RX

duloxetine HCl (Lilly)



**Antidepressants increased the risk of suicidal thinking and behavior (suicidality) in short-term studies in children and adolescents with major depressive disorder (MDD) and other psychiatric disorders. Duloxetine is not approved for use in pediatric patients.**

**THERAPEUTIC CLASS:** Serotonin and norepinephrine reuptake inhibitor

**INDICATIONS:** Treatment of MDD, diabetic peripheral neuropathic pain, generalized anxiety disorder (GAD).

**DOSAGE:** *Adults:* MDD: Initial: 40mg/day (given as 20mg bid) to 60mg/day (given qd or as 30mg bid). Re-evaluate periodically. Diabetic Peripheral Neuropathic Pain: 60mg/day given qd. May lower starting dose if tolerability is a concern. Renal Impairment: Consider lower starting dose with gradual increase. GAD: Initial: 60mg qd or 30mg qd for one week to adjust before increasing to 60mg qd. Titrate: increase by increments of 30mg qd. Max: 120 mg qd. Do not chew or crush.

**HOW SUPPLIED:** Cap, Delayed-Release: 20mg, 30mg, 60mg

**CONTRAINDICATIONS:** During or within 14 days of MAOI therapy, uncontrolled narrow-angle glaucoma.

**WARNINGS/PRECAUTIONS:** Monitor for clinical worsening and/or suicidality. May increase risk of serum transaminase elevations. May cause hepatotoxicity. Avoid with chronic liver disease. May increase BP; obtain baseline and monitor periodically. Orthostatic hypotension and syncope have been reported. Avoid abrupt cessation and in patients with severe renal impairment/ESRD or hepatic insufficiency. Caution with conditions that may slow gastric emptying, history of mania or seizures. May increase risk of mydriasis; caution in patients with controlled narrow-angle glaucoma. Serotonin syndrome may occur; caution with concomitant use of serotonergic drugs. Hyponatremia reported.

**ADVERSE REACTIONS:** Nausea, dry mouth, constipation, diarrhea, vomiting, decreased appetite, fatigue, dizziness, somnolence, increased sweating, blurred vision, insomnia, erectile dysfunction.

**INTERACTIONS:** See Contraindications. Avoid within 14 days of MAOI therapy. Upon discontinuation, wait at least 5 days before starting MAOI therapy. Avoid thioridazine, CYP1A2 inhibitors (eg, fluvoxamine, some quinolone antibiotics), substantial alcohol use. Increased levels with potent CYP2D6 inhibitors (eg, paroxetine, fluoxetine, quinidine). Caution with drugs metabolized by CYP2D6 having a narrow therapeutic index (eg, TCAs, phenothiazines, Type 1C antiarrhythmics), and CNS-active drugs. May increase free concentration levels of highly protein-bound drugs. Potential for interaction with drugs that affect gastric acidity. Caution with serotonergic drugs (including triptans, tramadol, SNRIs).

**PREGNANCY:** Category C, not for use in nursing.

## CYPROHEPTADINE
RX

cyproheptadine HCl (Various)

**THERAPEUTIC CLASS:** Serotonin/histamine antagonist

**INDICATIONS:** Perennial and seasonal rhinitis, vasomotor rhinitis, allergic conjunctivitis, uncomplicated allergic skin manifestations, blood or plasma allergic reactions, cold urticaria, and dermatographism. Adjunct to anaphylaxis.

**DOSAGE:** *Adults:* Initial: 4mg tid. Usual: 4-20mg/day. Max: 0.5mg/kg/day. *Pediatrics:* 7-14 yrs: Usual: 4mg bid-tid. Max: 16mg/day. 2-6 yrs: Usual: 2mg bid-tid or 0.25mg/kg/day. Max: 12mg/day.

**HOW SUPPLIED:** Syrup: 2mg/5mL; Tab: 4mg* *scored

**CONTRAINDICATIONS:** Newborn or premature infants, nursing mothers, concomitant MAOIs, angle-closure glaucoma, stenosing peptic ulcer, symptomatic prostatic hypertrophy, bladder neck obstruction, pyloroduodenal obstruction, elderly, debilitated.

**WARNINGS/PRECAUTIONS:** Caution with bronchial asthma, increased IOP, hyperthyroidism, CVD, HTN, and elderly. May impair mental/physical abilities.



**ADVERSE REACTIONS:** Drowsiness, somnolence, sedation, dizziness, confusion, restlessness, excitation, nervousness, insomnia, blurred vision, hypotension, palpitation, dry mouth, urinary frequency and retention.

**INTERACTIONS:** Avoid MAOIs. Additive effects with alcohol and other CNS depressants.

**PREGNANCY:** Category B, not for use in nursing.

## CYSTOSPAZ RX

hyoscyamine sulfate (Amerifit)

**THERAPEUTIC CLASS:** Anticholinergic

**INDICATIONS:** Management of hypermotility disorders of the lower urinary tract. Adjunct therapy of PUD, IBS, acute enterocolitis, and other GI disorders. To control gastric secretion, visceral spasm, and hypermotility in cystitis, pylorospasm and associated abdominal cramps. To reduce symptoms of mild dysenteries, diverticulitis, and biliary/renal colic.

**DOSAGE:** *Adults:* 0.15-0.3mg up to qid prn.

**HOW SUPPLIED:** Tab: 0.15mg

**CONTRAINDICATIONS:** Glaucoma, obstructive uropathy, GI obstructive disease, paralytic ileus, intestinal atony in elderly or debilitated, unstable cardiovascular status in acute hemorrhage, severe ulcerative colitis, toxic megacolon, myasthenia gravis.

**WARNINGS/PRECAUTIONS:** Heat prostration can occur with high environmental temperature. Diarrhea may indicate incomplete intestinal obstruction. Caution with autonomic neuropathy, hyperthyroidism, coronary heart disease, CHF, arrhythmia, HTN, and hiatal hernia associated with reflux esophagitis. Avoid with tachycardia. May cause drowsiness, blurred vision.

**ADVERSE REACTIONS:** Dry mouth, urinary hesitancy/retention, blurred vision, palpitations, mydriasis, cycloplegia, increased ocular tension, headache, nervousness, drowsiness, urticaria, decreased sweating.

**INTERACTIONS:** Additive adverse effects with other antimuscarinics, amantadine, haloperidol, phenothiazines, MAOIs, TCAs, and some antihistamines. Antacids may interfere with absorption.

**PREGNANCY:** Category C, caution in nursing.

## CYTADREN RX

aminoglutethimide (Novartis)

**THERAPEUTIC CLASS:** Adrenocortical steroid synthesis inhibitor

**INDICATIONS:** Suppression of adrenal function in selected patients with Cushing's syndrome.

**DOSAGE:** *Adults:* Initial: 250mg PO q6h. Titrate: May increase by 250mg/day q1-2 wks. Max: 2000mg. Discontinue if skin rash persists for >5-8 days or becomes severe. If glucocorticoid replacement therapy is needed, give 20-30mg of hydrocortisone PO in the morning.

**HOW SUPPLIED:** Tab: 250mg* *scored

**WARNINGS/PRECAUTIONS:** May cause adrenocortical hypofunction, especially under conditions of stress; monitor closely. May suppress aldosterone production by the adrenal cortex and may cause orthostatic or persistent hypotension; monitor BP. May cause fetal harm. Therapy should be initiated in a hospital. May impair mental/physical abilities.

**ADVERSE REACTIONS:** Drowsiness, morbilliform skin rash, nausea, anorexia, dizziness.

**INTERACTIONS:** Alcohol may potentiate effects. May accelerate metabolism of dexamethasone; if glucocorticoid replacement is needed, hydrocortisone should be prescribed. May diminish the effects of coumarin and warfarin.

**PREGNANCY:** Category D, not for use in nursing.



## CYTOGAM RX

cytomegalovirus immune globulin (human) (MedImmune)

**THERAPEUTIC CLASS:** Immunoglobulin

**INDICATIONS:** Prophylaxis of cytomegalovirus (CMV) disease associated with kidney, lung, liver, pancreas and heart transplantation.

**DOSAGE:** *Adults:* Initial: 150mg/kg 72 hrs post-transplant. Maint: Kidney Transplant: Weeks 2,4,6, and 8: 100mg/kg IV. Week 12 and Week 16: 50mg/kg IV. Liver/Pancreas/Lung/Heart Transplant: Week 2, 4, 6, and 8: 150mg/kg IV. Week 12 and Week 16: 100mg/kg IV. Administration: Initial: 15mg/kg/hr IV; may increase to 30mg/kg/hr if no adverse reactions after 30 minutes (after 15 minutes for subsequent doses), then increased to 60mg/kg/hr. Max: 150mg/kg/dose.

**HOW SUPPLIED:** Inj: 50mg/mL

**CONTRAINDICATIONS:** Selective immunoglobulin A deficiency.

**WARNINGS/PRECAUTIONS:** Consider use with ganciclovir for transplantation other than kidney from CMV seropositive donors into seronegative recipients. Risk of transmission of blood-borne viral agents. Renal dysfunction, acute renal failure, osmotic nephrosis and death reported; caution in pre-existing renal impairment, DM, >65 yrs, volume depletion, sepsis, or paraproteinemia. Confirm patient is not volume depleted prior to therapy. Monitor vital signs continuously. Monitor renal function before and during therapy, and urine output. D/C if renal function deteriorates, anaphylaxis occurs, or aseptic meningitis syndrome.

**ADVERSE REACTIONS:** Flushing, chills, muscle cramps, back pain, fever, nausea, vomiting, arthralgia, wheezing, increased BUN and serum creatinine, angioneurotic edema.

**INTERACTIONS:** Defer live virus vaccines (eg, measles, mumps, rubella) for 3 months; may interfere with immune response. Caution with nephrotoxic drugs.

**PREGNANCY:** Category C, safety in nursing not known.

## CYTOMEL RX

liothyronine sodium (King)

**THERAPEUTIC CLASS:** Thyroid replacement hormone

**INDICATIONS:** Hypothyroidism. As a pituitary TSH suppressant in the treatment and prevention of euthyroid goiters, including thyroid nodules, and Hashimoto's and multinodular goiter. Diagnostic agent in suppression tests to differentiate mild hyperthyroidism or thyroid gland autonomy.

**DOSAGE:** *Adults:* Mild Hypothyroidism: Initial: 25mcg qd. Titrate: May increase by up to 25mcg qd every 1-2 weeks. Maint: 25-75mcg qd. Myxedema: Initial: 5mcg qd. Titrate: May increase by 5-10mcg qd every 1-2 weeks up to 25mcg qd, then increase by 5-25mcg qd every 1-2 weeks. Maint: 50-100mcg/day. Goiter: Initial: 5mcg/day. Titrate: May increase by 5-10mcg qd every 1-2 weeks up to 25mcg qd, then by 12.5-25mcg qd every 1-2 weeks. Maint: 75mcg qd. Elderly/Coronary Artery Disease: Initial: 5mcg qd. Titrate: Increase by no more than 5mcg qd every 2 weeks. Thyroid Suppression Therapy: 75-100mcg qd for 7 days. Radioactive iodine uptake is determined before and after administration of hormone.
*Pediatrics:* Congenital Hypothyroidism: Initial: 5mcg qd. Titrate: Increase by

5mcg qd every 3-4 days until desired response. Maint: <1 yr: 20mcg qd. 1-3yrs: 50mcg qd. >3 yrs: 25-75mcg/day.

**HOW SUPPLIED:** Tab: 5mcg, 25mcg*, 50mcg* *scored

**CONTRAINDICATIONS:** Uncorrected adrenal cortical insufficiency and untreated thyrotoxicosis.



**WARNINGS/PRECAUTIONS:** Do not use in the treatment of obesity; larger doses in euthyroid patients can cause serious or even life threatening toxicity. Caution with angina pectoris and elderly; use lower doses. Rule out hypogonadism and nephrosis prior to therapy. With prolonged and severe hypothyroidism supplement with adrenocortical steroids. May aggravate diabetes mellitus or insipidus and adrenal cortical insufficiency. Add glucocorticoid with myxedema coma. Excessive doses may cause craniosynostosis in infants.

**ADVERSE REACTIONS:** Allergic skin reactions (rare).

**INTERACTIONS:** Hypothyroidism decreases and hyperthyroidism increases sensitivity to oral anticoagulants; monitor PT/INR. Monitor insulin and oral hypoglycemic requirements. Decreased absorption with cholestyramine; space dosing by 4-5 hrs. Large dose may cause life-threatening toxicities with sympathomimetic amines. Estrogens increase thyroxine-binding globulin; increase in thyroid dose may be needed. Additive effects of both agents with TCAs. HTN and tachycardia with ketamine. May potentiate digitalis toxicity. Increased adrenergic effects of catecholamines; caution with CAD.

**PREGNANCY:** Category A, caution in nursing.

## CYTOSAR-U

RX

cytarabine (Pharmacia & Upjohn)

**Associated with bone marrow suppression, nausea, vomiting, oral ulceration, hepatic dysfunction, diarrhea, and abdominal pain. For induction therapy, treat in a facility able to monitor drug tolerance and toxicity.**

**THERAPEUTIC CLASS:** Antimetabolite

**INDICATIONS:** Adjunct therapy for remission induction in acute non-lymphocytic leukemia (ANLL). Found useful in the treatment of acute lymphocytic leukemia (ALL) and blast phase of chronic myelocytic leukemia (CML). Prophylaxis and treatment of meningeal lymphoma.

**DOSAGE:** *Adults:* ANLL: Induction: 100mg/m²/day continuous infusion or 100mg/m² IV q12h for days 1-7. Meningeal Leukemia: Give intrathecally. Range: 5-75mg/m² given qd to every 4 days. Usual: 30mg/m² every 4 days until CSF normal, followed by 1 additional treatment.
*Pediatrics:* ANLL: Induction: 100mg/m²/day continuous infusion or 100mg/m² IV q12h for days 1-7. Meningeal Leukemia: Give intrathecally. Range: 5-75mg/m² given qd to every 4 days. Usual: 30mg/m² every 4 days until CSF normal, followed by 1 additional treatment.

**HOW SUPPLIED:** Inj: 100mg, 500mg, 1g, 2g

**WARNINGS/PRECAUTIONS:** Caution with pre-existing drug-induced bone marrow suppression, hepatic or renal dysfunction. Perform leukocyte and platelet counts daily during induction therapy. Monitor bone marrow, hepatic and renal functions, platelets, and leukocytes frequently. Sudden respiratory distress, cardiomyopathy, alopecia reported with high dose therapy. Severe and fatal CNS, GI, and pulmonary toxicity reported. Contains benzyl alcohol; fatal"Gasping Syndrome" in premature infants reported. Acute pancreatitis, hyperuricemia reported.

**ADVERSE REACTIONS:** Anorexia, nausea, vomiting, diarrhea, oral/anal inflammation or ulceration, hepatic dysfunction, fever, rash, thrombophlebitis, bleeding (all sites).

**INTERACTIONS:** Antagonizes susceptibility of gentamicin for K.pneumoniae. May inhibit efficacy of flucytosine. Monitor digoxin. Acute pancreatitis reported in patients receiving prior L-asparaginase treatment.

Cardiomyopathy and death reported during high dose therapy with cyclophosphamide.

**PREGNANCY:** Category D, not for use in nursing.



## CYTOTEC RX
misoprostol (Searle)

**Can cause abortion, premature birth, or birth defects. Uterine rupture reported when used to induce labor or induce abortion beyond 8th week of pregnancy. Not for use by pregnant women to reduce risk of NSAID-induced ulcers. Only use in women of childbearing age if at high risk of GI ulcers or complications with NSAID therapy; patient must then have negative serum pregnancy test within 2 weeks before therapy, maintain contraceptive measures, and begin therapy on 2nd or 3rd day of menstrual period.**

**THERAPEUTIC CLASS:** Prostaglandin $E_1$ analogue

**INDICATIONS:** Prevention of NSAID-induced gastric ulcers in patients at high risk of developing gastric ulcers.

**DOSAGE:** *Adults:* 200mcg qid, or if not tolerated, 100mcg qid. Take for the duration of NSAID therapy. Take with meals; last dose at bedtime.

**HOW SUPPLIED:** Tab: 100mcg, 200mcg* *scored

**CONTRAINDICATIONS:** Pregnant women to reduce risk of NSAID-induced ulcers, prostaglandin allergy.

**ADVERSE REACTIONS:** Diarrhea, abdominal pain, nausea, flatulence, headache, dyspepsia.

**INTERACTIONS:** Avoid with magnesium-containing antacids to decrease incidence of diarrhea.

**PREGNANCY:** Category X, not for use in nursing.

## CYTOXAN RX
cyclophosphamide (Bristol-Myers Squibb)

**THERAPEUTIC CLASS:** Nitrogen mustard alkylating agent

**INDICATIONS:** Treatment of malignant lymphomas, Hodgkin's disease, lymphocytic lymphoma, mixed-cell type or histiocytic lymphoma, Burkitt's lymphoma, multiple myeloma, chronic lymphocytic leukemia, chronic granulocytic leukemia, acute myelogenous and monocytic leukemia, acute lymphoblastic leukemia in children, mycosis fungoides, neuroblastoma, ovary adenocarcinoma, retinoblastoma, breast carcinoma. Treatment of biopsy proven"minimal change" nephrotic syndrome in children, but not as primary therapy.

**DOSAGE:** *Adults:* Malignant Diseases (Without Hematologic Deficiency): Monotherapy: Initial: 40-50mg/kg IV in divided doses over 2-5 days, or 10-15mg/kg IV given every 7-10 days, or 3-5mg/kg twice weekly. Oral Dosing: Initial/Maint: 1-5mg/kg/day PO. Adjust dose according to antitumor activity and/or leukopenia. May need to reduce dose when combined with other cytotoxic drugs.
*Pediatrics:* Malignant Diseases (Without Hematologic Deficiency): Monotherapy: Initial: 40-50mg/kg IV in divided doses over 2-5 days, or 10-15mg/kg IV given every 7-10 days, or 3-5mg/kg twice weekly. Oral Dosing: Initial/Maint: 1-5mg/kg/day PO. Adjust dose according to antitumor activity and/or leukopenia. May need to reduce dose when combined with other cytotoxic drugs. Nephrotic Syndrome: 2.5-3mg/kg/day PO for 60-90 days.

**HOW SUPPLIED:** Inj (Lyophilized): 500mg, 1g, 2g; Tab: 25mg, 50mg

**CONTRAINDICATIONS:** Severely depressed bone marrow function.

**WARNINGS/PRECAUTIONS:** Second malignancies, cardiac dysfunction, and hemorrhagic cystitis reported. May cause fetal harm in pregnancy. Serious, fatal infections may develop if severely immunosuppressed. Monitor for toxicity with leukopenia, thrombocytopenia, tumor cell infiltration of bone marrow, previous X-ray therapy or cytotoxic therapy, and impaired hepatic and/or renal function. Monitor hematologic profile for hematopoietic suppression. Examine urine for red blood cells. Anaphylactic reactions reported. Possible cross-sensitivity with other alkylating agents. May cause sterility. May interfere with normal wound healing. Consider dose adjustment with adrenalectomy.

**ADVERSE REACTIONS:** Impairment of fertility, amenorrhea, nausea, vomiting, anorexia, abdominal discomfort, diarrhea, alopecia, leukopenia, thrombocytopenia, hemorrhagic ureteritis, interstitial pneumonitis, malaise, asthenia, renal tubular necrosis.

**INTERACTIONS:** Chronic, high doses of phenobarbital increase metabolism and leukopenic activity. Potentiates succinylcholine chloride effects and doxorubicin-induced cardiotoxicity. Alert anesthesiologist if treated within 10 days of general anesthesia.

**PREGNANCY:** Category D, not for use in nursing.



## D.H.E. 45 RX

dihydroergotamine mesylate (Valeant)

**Serious and life-threatening peripheral ischemia reported with potent CYP450 3A4 inhibitors (eg, protease inhibitors, macrolides). Elevated levels of dihydroergotamine increases risk of vasospasm leading to cerebral ischemia or ischemia of the extremities. Concomitant use with CYP450 3A4 inhibitors is contraindicated.**

**THERAPEUTIC CLASS:** Alpha adrenergic antagonist/vasoconstrictor

**INDICATIONS:** Acute treatment of migraine with or without aura. Acute treatment of cluster headache episodes.

**DOSAGE:** *Adults:* 1mL IV/IM/SQ. May repeat at 1 hr intervals. Max: 3mL/24hrs IM/SC or 2mL/24hrs IV and 6mL/week.

**HOW SUPPLIED:** Inj: 1mg/mL

**CONTRAINDICATIONS:** Ergot alkaloids hypersensitivity, ischemic heart disease, coronary artery vasospasm (eg, Prinzmetal's variant angina), uncontrolled HTN, hemiplegic or basilar migraine, peripheral artery disease, sepsis, following vascular surgery, severe renal/hepatic dysfunction, pregnancy, nursing, with potent CYP3A4 inhibitors (eg, ritonavir, nelfinavir, indinavir, erythromycin, clarithromycin, troleandomycin, ketoconazole, itraconazole), concomitant peripheral and central vasoconstrictors, and within 24 hrs after taking 5-$HT_1$ agonists, methysergide, ergotamine-containing, or ergot-type agents.

**WARNINGS/PRECAUTIONS:** Confirm migraine diagnosis. Risk of adverse cardiac, cerebrovascular, and vasospastic events and fatalities. Avoid with cardiac risk factors (eg, HTN, hypercholesterolemia, smoker, obesity, DM, strong family history of CAD, females who are surgically/physiologically postmenopausal, or males >40 yrs) unless cardiovascular evaluation is done. Perform cardiovascular monitoring with long-term use. Significant BP elevations reported.

**ADVERSE REACTIONS:** Vasospasm, angina, paraesthesia, HTN, dizziness, anxiety, dyspnea, headache, flushing, diarrhea, rash, increased sweating.

**INTERACTIONS:** Potentiated BP elevation with peripheral and central vasoconstrictors. Additive coronary vasospastic effect with sumatriptan; avoid within 24 hrs of each other. Propranolol and nicotine may potentiate the vasoconstrictive action. Increased plasma levels and peripheral vasoconstriction with macrolides. Contraindicated with CYP3A4 inhibitors (eg, macrolides, protease inhibitors). Caution with less potent CYP3A4 inhibitors (eg, saquinavir, nefazodone, fluconazole, grapefruit juice, fluoxetine, fluvoxamine, zileuton, clotrimazole).

**PREGNANCY:** Category X, contraindicated in nursing.

## DACOGEN

RX

decitabine (MGI Pharma)

**THERAPEUTIC CLASS:** DNA methyltransferase inhibitor

**INDICATIONS:** Treatment of myelodysplastic syndromes.

**DOSAGE:** *Adults*:Initial: 15mg/m² IV over 3 hrs q8h for 3 days. Repeat cycle every 6 weeks. Treat for ≥4 cycles. Adjust dose based on hematology lab values, renal function, and serum electrolytes.

**HOW SUPPLIED:** Inj: 50mg

**WARNINGS/PRECAUTIONS:** May cause fetal harm. Avoid pregnancy in women of childbearing potential. Men should be advised not to father a child while receiving treatment and for 2 months afterwards. Neutropenia and thrombocytopenia may occur; monitor CBC and platelets periodically (at minimum, before each cycle). Caution with renal and hepatic dysfunction. Avoid with serum creatinine >2mg/dL, transaminase >2 times normal, or serum bilirubin >1.5mg/dL.

**ADVERSE REACTIONS:** Neutropenia, thrombocytopenia, anemia, fatigue, pyrexia, nausea, cough, petechiae, constipation, diarrhea, hyperglycemia, febrile neutropenia, leukopenia, headache, insomnia.

**PREGNANCY:** Category D, not for use in nursing.

## DALLERGY

RX

phenylephrine HCl - methscopolamine nitrate - chlorpheniramine maleate (Laser)

**THERAPEUTIC CLASS:** Antihistamine/anticholinergic/ sympathomimetic

**INDICATIONS:** Relief of upper respiratory symptoms associated with allergies and the common cold.

**DOSAGE:** *Adults:* 1 tab or 10mL q4-6h. Max: 4 doses/24hrs.
*Pediatrics:* >12 yrs: 1 tab or 10mL q4-6h. 6-12 yrs: 1/2 tab or 5mL q4-6h. Max: 4 doses/24hrs.

**HOW SUPPLIED:** (Chlorpheniramine-Methscopolamine-Phenylephrine) Syrup: 2mg-0.625mg-10mg/5mL; Tab: 4mg-1.25mg-10mg*; Tab, Extended Release: 12mg-2.5mg-20mg *scored

**CONTRAINDICATIONS:** Severe HTN, severe CAD, MAOI therapy, narrow angle glaucoma, urinary retention, PUD, during asthma attack.

**WARNINGS/PRECAUTIONS:** Caution in HTN, DM, ischemic heart disease, hyperthyroidism, increased IOP, prostatic hypertrophy. Adverse events are more common in elderly. May cause excitability in children.

**ADVERSE REACTIONS:** Drowsiness, lassitude, nausea, giddiness, dry mouth, blurred vision, cardiac palpitations, flushing, increased irritability or excitement.

**INTERACTIONS:** Increased effect of sympathomimetic amines with MAOIs and β-blockers. May reduce antihypertensive effect of methyldopa, mecamylamine, reserpine, and veratrum alkaloids. Additive effect with alcohol, other CNS depressants.

**PREGNANCY:** Category C, caution in nursing.

## DALLERGY JR

RX

phenylephrine HCl - chlorpheniramine maleate (Laser)

**THERAPEUTIC CLASS:** Antihistamine/sympathomimetic amine

**INDICATIONS:** Relief of upper respiratory symptoms associated with allergies and the common cold.

**DOSAGE:** *Adults:* 2 caps q12h. Max: 2 doses/24h.
*Pediatrics:* >12 yrs: 2 caps q12h. 6-12 yrs: 1 cap q12h. Max: 2 doses/24h.

**HOW SUPPLIED:** Cap: (Chlorpheniramine-Phenylephrine) 4mg-20mg

**CONTRAINDICATIONS:** Severe HTN, severe CAD, MAOI therapy, narrow angle glaucoma, urinary retention, PUD, during asthma attack.

**WARNINGS/PRECAUTIONS:** Caution with HTN, DM, ischemic heart disease, hyperthyroidism, increased IOP, prostatic hypertrophy, the elderly. May cause excitability especially in children.

**ADVERSE REACTIONS:** Drowsiness, lassitude, nausea, giddiness, dry mouth, blurred vision, cardiac palpitations, flushing, increased irritability or excitement.

**INTERACTIONS:** Increased sympathomimetic effect with MAOIs and β-blockers. May reduce antihypertensive effect of methyldopa, mecamylamine, reserpine, and veratum alkaloids. Additive effect with alcohol and other CNS depressants.

**PREGNANCY:** Category C, caution in nursing.

## DALMANE CIV

flurazepam HCl (Valeant)

**THERAPEUTIC CLASS:** Benzodiazepine

**INDICATIONS:** Treatment of insomnia.

**DOSAGE:** *Adults:* Usual: 15-30mg at bedtime. Elderly/Debilitated: Initial: 15mg at bedtime.
*Pediatrics:* >15 yrs: Usual: 15-30mg at bedtime.

**HOW SUPPLIED:** Cap: 15mg, 30mg

**CONTRAINDICATIONS:** Pregnancy.

**WARNINGS/PRECAUTIONS:** Caution in elderly, debilitated, severely depressed, those with suicidal tendencies, hepatic/renal impairment, respiratory disease. Ataxia and falls reported in elderly and debilitated.Withdrawal symptoms after discontinuation; avoid abrupt discontinuation.

**ADVERSE REACTIONS:** Confusion, dizziness, drowsiness, lightheadedness, ataxia.

**INTERACTIONS:** Additive effects with alcohol and other CNS depressants.

**PREGNANCY:** Not for use in pregnancy or nursing.

## DANTRIUM RX

dantrolene sodium (Procter & Gamble Pharmaceuticals)

**Associated with hepatotoxicity; monitor hepatic function. Discontinue if no benefit after 45 days.**

**THERAPEUTIC CLASS:** Direct acting skeletal muscle relaxant

**INDICATIONS:** To control manifestations of clinical spasticity from upper motor neuron disorders (eg, spinal cord injury, stroke, cerebral palsy, multiple sclerosis). Preoperatively to prevent or attenuate development of malignant hyperthermia, and after a malignant hyperthermia crisis.

**DOSAGE:** *Adults:* Chronic Spasticity: Initial: 25mg qd for 7 days. Titrate: Increase to 25mg tid for 7 days, then 50mg tid for 7 days, then 100mg tid. Max: 100mg qid. If no further benefit at next higher dose, decrease to previous lower dose. Malignant Hyperthermia: Pre-Op: 4-8mg/kg/day given tid-qid for 1-2 days before surgery, with last dose given 3-4 hrs before surgery. Post-Op Following Malignant Hyperthermia Crisis: 4-8mg/kg/day given qid for 1-3 days.
*Pediatrics:* >5 yrs: Chronic Spasticity: Initial: 0.5mg/kg qd for 7 days. Titrate: Increase to 0.5mg/kg tid for 7 days, then 1mg/kg tid for 7 days, then 2mg/kg

tid. Max: 100mg qid. If no further benefit at next higher dose, decrease to previous lower dose.

**HOW SUPPLIED:** Cap: 25mg, 50mg, 100mg

**CONTRAINDICATIONS:** Active hepatic disease, where spasticity is utilized to sustain upright posture and balance in locomotion, when spasticity is utilized to obtain or maintain increased function.



**WARNINGS/PRECAUTIONS:** Monitor LFTs at baseline, then periodically. Increased risk of hepatocellular disease in females and patients >35 yrs. Caution with pulmonary, cardiac, and liver dysfunction. Photosensitivity reaction may occur; limit sunlight exposure.

**ADVERSE REACTIONS:** Drowsiness, dizziness, weakness, malaise, fatigue, diarrhea, hepatitis, tachycardia, aplastic anemia, thrombocytopenia, depression, seizure.

**INTERACTIONS:** Increased drowsiness with CNS depressants. Caution with estrogens; risk of hepatotoxicity. Avoid with calcium channel blockers; risk of cardiovascular collapse. May potentiate vecuronium-induced neuromuscular block.

**PREGNANCY:** Safety in nursing not known. Not for use in nursing.

## DANTRIUM IV

RX

dantrolene sodium (Procter & Gamble Pharmaceuticals)

**THERAPEUTIC CLASS:** Direct acting skeletal muscle relaxant

**INDICATIONS:** Adjunct management of fulminant hypermetabolism of skeletal muscle characteristic of malignant hyperthermia crises. For pre- and post-operative use to prevent or attenuate development of malignant hyperthermia.

**DOSAGE:** *Adults:* Malignant Hyperthermia: Initial: Minimum 1mg/kg IV push. Continue until symptoms subside or max cumulative dose 10mg/kg. Pre-Op Malignant Hyperthermia Prophylaxis: 2.5mg/kg 1.25 hrs before anesthesia and infuse over 1 hr. May need additional therapy during anesthesia/surgery if symptoms arise. Post-Op Prophylaxis: Initial: 1mg/kg or more as clinical situation dictates.
*Pediatrics:* Malignant Hyperthermia: Initial: Minimum 1mg/kg IV push. Continue until symptoms subside or max cumulative dose 10mg/kg.

**HOW SUPPLIED:** Inj: 20mg

**WARNINGS/PRECAUTIONS:** Use with supportive therapies to treat malignant hyperthermia. Take steps to prevent extravasation. Fatal and non-fatal hepatic disorders reported. Do not operate automobile or engage hazardous activity for 48 hrs after therapy. Caution at meals on day of administration because difficulty in swallowing/choking reported. Monitor vital signs if receive pre-operatively.

**ADVERSE REACTIONS:** Loss of grip strength, weakness in legs, drowsiness, dizziness, pulmonary edema, thrombophlebitis, urticaria, erythema.

**INTERACTIONS:** Plasma protein binding reduced by warfarin and clofibrate, and increased by tolbutamide. Avoid with calcium channel blockers; possible risk of cardiovascular collapse. Caution with tranquilizers. Possible increased metabolism by drugs known to induce hepatic microsomal enzymes. May potentiate vecuronium-induced neuromuscular block.

**PREGNANCY:** Category C, safety in nursing not known.

## DAPSONE

RX

dapsone (Jacobus)

**THERAPEUTIC CLASS:** Leprostatic agent

**INDICATIONS:** Treatment of dermatitis herpetiformis and leprosy.

**DOSAGE:** *Adults:* Dermatitis Herpetiformis: Initial: 50mg/day. Usual: 50-300mg/day, may increase dose if needed. Reduce to minimum maintenance dose. Leprosy: Give with 1 or more anti-leprosy drugs. Maint: 100mg/day. *Pediatrics:* Same schedule as adults but with correspondingly smaller doses.

**HOW SUPPLIED:** Tab: 25mg*, 100mg* *scored

**WARNINGS/PRECAUTIONS:** Agranulocytosis, aplastic anemia and other blood dyscrasias reported. CBC weekly for the 1st month, monthly for 6 months and semi-annually thereafter. D/C if significant reduction in leukocytes, platelets or hemopoiesis occurs. Treat severe anemia prior to therapy. D/C if sensitivity occurs. Caution in those with G6PD deficiency, methemoglobin reductase deficiency, or hemoglobin M. Toxic hepatitis And cholestatic jaundice reported. Monitor LFT's.

**ADVERSE REACTIONS:** Hemolysis, peripheral neuropathy, nausea, vomiting, abdominal pain, pancreatitis, vertigo, blurred vision, tinnitus, insomnia, fever, headache, psychosis, phototoxicity, pulmonary eosinophilia, tachycardia, albuminuria, renal papillary necrosis, male infertility.

**INTERACTIONS:** Rifampin lowers plasma levels. Folic acid antagonists (eg, pyrimethamine) may increase hematologic reactions. Dapsone and trimethoprim each raise the level of the other.

**PREGNANCY:** Category C, not for use in nursing.

## DAPTACEL RX

tetanus toxoid - diphtheria toxoid - pertussis vaccine acellular, adsorbed (Aventis)

**THERAPEUTIC CLASS:** Vaccine

**INDICATIONS:** Active immunization against diphtheria, tetanus, and pertussis.

**DOSAGE:** *Pediatrics:* 6 weeks-up to 7 yrs: 0.5mL IM at intervals of 6-8 weeks, and at 17-20 months old. The interval between 3rd and 4th dose should be at least 6 months. May use to complete series in infants who received >1 dose of whole-cell pertussis (DTP). Usual age for 1st dose is 2 months old.

**HOW SUPPLIED:** Inj: (Diphtheria-Pertussis-Tetanus-) 15Lf U-23mcg-5Lf U/0.5mL

**CONTRAINDICATIONS:** Adults and pediatrics >7 yrs. Administration after immediate anaphylactic reaction, or encephalopathy not attributable to another identifiable cause within 7 days from initial vaccination. Moderate or serious illness. Outbreak of poliomyelitis.

**WARNINGS/PRECAUTIONS:** Stopper contains dry natural latex rubber. Evaluate risks/benefits of subsequent doses if temperature >105°F, or if collapse/shock occurs, or persistent crying for >3 hrs within 48 hrs, and convulsions with or without fever within 3 days of vaccine. Continue with DT vaccine if pertussis must be withheld. Avoid in coagulation disorder. Increased risk of neurological events with family history of convulsions; administer antipyretic at time of and for 24 hrs after immunization. Enhanced risk of manifestation of underlying neurological within 2-3 days following vaccine. May not achieve expected immune response in immunosuppressed patients. Avoid injection into blood vessel.

**ADVERSE REACTIONS:** Local tenderness, fever, fretfulness, anorexia, drowsiness, vomiting.

**INTERACTIONS:** Caution with anticoagulants. Immunosuppressives (eg, irradiation, antimetabolites, alkylating agents, cytotoxic drugs, corticosteroids) may reduce immune response to vaccine. Adequate immune response may not occur after recent immune globulin injection.

**PREGNANCY:** Category C, safety in nursing not known.

## DARAPRIM RX

pyrimethamine (GlaxoSmithKline)

D

**THERAPEUTIC CLASS:** Folic acid antagonist

**INDICATIONS:** Adjunct treatment of toxoplasmosis and acute malaria. Prophylaxis of malaria.

**DOSAGE:** *Adults:* Toxoplasmosis: Initial: 50-75mg qd with 1-4g/day of sulfonamide. After 1-3 weeks, reduce dose of each drug to 1/2 of previous dose for additional 4-5 weeks. Acute Malaria: 25mg qd for 2 days with sulfonamide. As monotherapy in semi-immune persons, 50mg for 2 days. Follow with prophylaxis dose through periods of early recrudescence and late relapse. Malaria Prophylaxis: 25mg once weekly.
*Pediatrics:* Toxoplasmosis: 0.5mg/kg bid. After 2-4 days, reduce to 0.25mg/kg bid for 1 month. Use with usual pediatric sulfonamide dose. Acute Malaria: 4-10 yrs: As monotherapy in semi-immune persons, 25mg for 2 days. Follow with prophylaxis dose through periods of early recrudescence and late relapse. Malaria Prophylaxis: >10 yrs: 25mg once weekly. 4-10 yrs: 12.5 once weekly. <4 yrs: 6.25mg once weekly.

**HOW SUPPLIED:** Tab: 25mg* *scored

**CONTRAINDICATIONS:** Megaloblastic anemia due to folate deficiency.

**WARNINGS/PRECAUTIONS:** Dose for toxoplasmosis approaches toxic levels; reduce dose or d/c if develop folate deficiency. Administer leucovorin 5-15mg qd (po, IV, or IM) until normal hematopoiesis. May be carcinogenic. Pediatric deaths reported with accidental ingestion. Use small initial dose with convulsive disorders to avoid nervous system toxicity. Caution with renal or hepatic dysfunction or if possible folate deficiency (eg, pregnancy, malabsorption syndrome, alcoholism). Perform semiweekly blood counts, including platelets with high doses.

**ADVERSE REACTIONS:** Hypersensitivity reactions (eg, Stevens-Johnson syndrome, toxic epidermal necrolysis) hyperphenylalinemia (with sulfonamides), anorexia, vomiting, blood dyscrasias, cardiac rhythm disorders.

**INTERACTIONS:** Concurrent phenytoin may affect folate levels. Increased risk of bone marrow suppression with antifolic drugs (eg, sulfonamides or trimethoprim-sulfamethoxazole). Mild hepatotoxicity reported with lorazepam.

**PREGNANCY:** Category C, not for use in nursing.

## DARVOCET A500 CIV

acetaminophen - propoxyphene napsylate (aaiPharma)

**THERAPEUTIC CLASS:** Opioid analgesic

**INDICATIONS:** Relief of mild-to-moderate pain.

**DOSAGE:** *Adults:* Usual: 1 tab q4h prn for pain. Max: 6 tabs/24 hrs. Elderly: Increase dosing interval. Hepatic/Renal Impairment: Reduce daily dose.

**HOW SUPPLIED:** Tab: (Propoxyphene-APAP) 100mg-500mg

**WARNINGS/PRECAUTIONS:** Drug dependence potential. Not for suicidal or addiction-prone patients. Caution with hepatic or renal impairment, elderly.

**ADVERSE REACTIONS:** Dizziness, sedation, nausea, vomiting, liver dysfunction.

**INTERACTIONS:** Additive CNS-depressant effects with alcohol, sedatives, tranquilizers, muscle relaxants, antidepressants. Increases plasma levels of antidepressants, anticonvulsants, coumarins. Severe neurologic signs, including coma reported with carbamazepine.

**PREGNANCY:** Not for use in pregnancy, safety not known in nursing.

## DARVOCET-N

CIV

acetaminophen - propoxyphene napsylate (aaiPharma)

**THERAPEUTIC CLASS:** Opioid analgesic

**INDICATIONS:** Relief of mild-to-moderate pain.

**DOSAGE:** *Adults:* Usual: 100mg propoxyphene napsylate and 650mg APAP q4h prn for pain. Max: 600mg propoxyphene napsylate/day. Elderly: Increase dosing interval. Hepatic/Renal Impairment: Reduce daily dose.

**HOW SUPPLIED:** Tab: (Propoxyphene-APAP) 50mg-325mg, 100mg-650mg

**WARNINGS/PRECAUTIONS:** Drug dependence potential. Not for suicidal or addiction-prone patients. Caution with hepatic/renal impairment, elderly.

**ADVERSE REACTIONS:** Dizziness, sedation, nausea, vomiting, liver dysfunction.

**INTERACTIONS:** Additive CNS-depressant effects with alcohol, sedatives, tranquilizers, muscle relaxants, antidepressants. Increases plasma levels of antidepressants, anticonvulsants, coumarins. Severe neurologic signs, including coma reported with carbamazepine.

**PREGNANCY:** Not for use in pregnancy, safety not known in nursing.

## DARVON

CIV

propoxyphene HCl (aaiPharma)

**THERAPEUTIC CLASS:** Opioid analgesic

**INDICATIONS:** Relief of mild-to-moderate pain.

**DOSAGE:** *Adults:* Usual: 65mg q4h as needed for pain. Max: 390mg/day. Elderly: Increase dose interval. Hepatic/Renal Impairment: Reduce daily dose.

**HOW SUPPLIED:** Cap: 65mg

**WARNINGS/PRECAUTIONS:** Drug dependence potential. May impair mental/physical ability for operating machinery. Caution with hepatic or renal impairment and the elderly. Not for suicidal or addiction-prone patients. Do not exceed recommended dose.

**ADVERSE REACTIONS:** Dizziness, sedation, nausea, vomiting, liver dysfunction.

**INTERACTIONS:** Additive CNS-depressant effect with other CNS depressants, including alcohol. Increases plasma levels of antidepressants, anticonvulsants, and coumarins. Severe neurologic signs, including coma reported with carbamazepine. Caution with tranquilizers, antidepressants and with excess alcohol use.

**PREGNANCY:** Not for use in pregnancy, unknown use in nursing.

## DARVON COMPOUND 65

CIV

aspirin - caffeine - propoxyphene HCl (aaiPharma)

**THERAPEUTIC CLASS:** Opioid analgesic

**INDICATIONS:** Relief of mild-to-moderate pain.

**DOSAGE:** *Adults:* Usual: 1 cap q4h as needed for pain. Max: 390mg propoxyphene/day. Elderly: Increase dose interval. Hepatic/Renal Impairment: Reduce daily dose.

**HOW SUPPLIED:** Cap: (Propoxyphene-ASA-Caffeine) 65mg-389mg-32.4mg

**CONTRAINDICATIONS:** Suicidal or addiction-prone patients.

**WARNINGS/PRECAUTIONS:** Drug dependence potential. May impair mental/physical ability for operating machinery. Caution use in peptic ulcer disease, coagulation disorders, hepatic/renal impairment and the elderly. ASA may increase risk of Reye syndrome. Not for suicidal or addiction-prone patients. Do not exceed recommended dose.

**ADVERSE REACTIONS:** Dizziness, sedation, nausea, vomiting, liver dysfunction.

**INTERACTIONS:** Enhances anticoagulant effects. Inhibits effect of uricosuric agents. Additive CNS-depressant effect with other CNS depressants, including alcohol. Increases plasma levels of antidepressants, anticonvulsants and coumarins. Severe neurologic signs, including coma reported with carbamazepine. Caution with tranquilizers, antidepressants and with excess alcohol use.



**PREGNANCY:** Not for use in pregnancy, unknown use in nursing.

## DARVON-N CIV

propoxyphene napsylate (aaiPharma)

**THERAPEUTIC CLASS:** Opioid analgesic

**INDICATIONS:** Relief of mild-to-moderate pain.

**DOSAGE:** *Adults:* Usual: 100mg q4h prn pain. Max: 600mg/day. Elderly: Increase dose interval. Hepatic/Renal Impairment: Reduce daily dose.

**HOW SUPPLIED:** Tab: 100mg

**WARNINGS/PRECAUTIONS:** Avoid in suicidal or addiction-prone patients. May produce drug dependence in higher than recommended doses. May impair mental/physical ability. Caution with hepatic or renal impairment. Do not exceed recommended dose and limit alcohol intake.

**ADVERSE REACTIONS:** Dizziness, sedation, nausea, vomiting, constipation, abdominal pain, skin rashes, lightheadedness, headache, weakness, euphoria, dysphoria, hallucination.

**INTERACTIONS:** Additive CNS-depressant effect with other CNS depressants, including alcohol. Increases plasma levels of antidepressants, anticonvulsants and warfarin-like drugs. Severe neurologic signs, including coma reported with carbamazepine. Caution with tranquilizers, antidepressants and excess alcohol use.

**PREGNANCY:** Safety in pregnancy and nursing not known.

## DAUNOXOME RX

daunorubicin citrate liposome (Gilead)

**Monitor for cardiac toxicity. Severe myelosuppression may occur. Reduce dose with hepatic dysfunction. A triad of back pain, flushing, and chest tightness reported during 1st 5 minutes of infusion; resume infusion at slower rate.**

**THERAPEUTIC CLASS:** Anthracycline

**INDICATIONS:** First line cytotoxic therapy for advanced HIV-associated Kaposi's sarcoma.

**DOSAGE:** *Adults:* 40mg/m$^2$ IV infusion; repeat every 2 weeks until evidence of progressive disease or until other complications of HIV preclude continuation.

**HOW SUPPLIED:** Inj: 2mg/mL

**WARNINGS/PRECAUTIONS:** Primary toxicity is myelosuppression; careful hematologic monitoring (prior to each dose) required. Evaluate cardiac function before each course and determine left ventricular ejection fraction (LVEF) at total cumulative dose of 320mg/m$^2$, and every 160mg/m$^2$ thereafter. Monitor LVEF at cumulative doses prior to therapy and every 160mg/m$^2$ in those with prior anthracycline therapy, pre-existing cardiac disease, or previous radiotherapy. Avoid extravasation. Can cause fetal harm during pregnancy.

**ADVERSE REACTIONS:** Myelosuppression, alopecia, cardiomyopathy with CHF, nausea, vomiting, fatigue, fever, diarrhea, cough, dyspnea, abdominal pain, anorexia, rigors, back pain, increased sweating, rhinitis, neuropathy.

**PREGNANCY:** Category D, safety in nursing not known.



## DAYPRO

RX

oxaprozin (Pharmacia & Upjohn)

**NSAIDs may cause an increased risk of serious cardiovascular thrombotic events, MI, stroke and serious GI adverse events including bleeding, ulceration, and perforation of the stomach or intestines. Contraindicated for the treatment of peri-operative pain in the setting of coronary artery bypass graft (CABG) surgery.**

**THERAPEUTIC CLASS:** NSAID (propionic acid derivative)

**INDICATIONS:** Relief of signs and symptoms of osteoarthritis (OA), rheumatoid arthritis (RA), and juvenile rheumatoid arthritis (JRA).

**DOSAGE:** *Adults:* RA: 1200mg qd. Max: 1800mg/day in divided doses (not to exceed 26mg/kg/day). OA: 1200mg qd, give 600mg qd for low weight or milder disease. Max: 1800mg/day in divided doses (not to exceed 26mg/kg/day). Renal Dysfunction/Hemodialysis: Initial: 600mg qd. *Pediatrics:* 6-16yrs: JRA: >55kg: 1200mg qd. 32-54kg: 900mg qd. 22-31kg: 600mg qd.

**HOW SUPPLIED:** Tab: 600mg* *scored

**CONTRAINDICATIONS:** Complete or partial syndrome of nasal polyps, angioedema and bronchospastic reactivity to ASA or other NSAIDs. Treatment of peri-operative pain in the setting of CABG surgery.

**WARNINGS/PRECAUTIONS:** May lead to onset of new HTN or worsening of pre-existing HTN; monitor BP closely. Fluid retention and edema reported; caution with fluid retention or heart failure. Renal papillary necrosis and other renal injury reported after long-term use. Not recommended for use with advanced renal disease; if therapy must be initiated, monitor renal function. Anaphylactoid reactions may occur. May cause serious skin adverse events (eg, exfoliative dermatitis, Stevens-Johnson syndrome, and toxic epidermal necrolysis). Avoid in late pregnancy; may cause premature closure of ductus arteriosis. May cause elevations of LFTs; d/c if liver disease develops or systemic manifestations occur. Caution in elderly. Anemia may occur; with long-term use, monitor Hgb/Hct if signs or symptoms of anemia develop. May inhibit platelet aggregation and prolong bleeding time; monitor with coagulation disorders. Caution with asthma and avoid with aspirin-sensitive asthma. Rash and/or mild photosensitivity reactions reported.

**ADVERSE REACTIONS:** Constipation, diarrhea, dyspepsia, flatulence, nausea, rash.

**INTERACTIONS:** Avoid with ASA. Caution with oral anticoagulants. Monitor BP with β-blockers.

**PREGNANCY:** Category C, not for use in nursing.

## DAYTRANA

CII

methylphenidate (Shire)

**THERAPEUTIC CLASS:** Sympathomimetic amine

**INDICATIONS:** Treatment of attention deficit hyperactivity disorder (ADHD).

**DOSAGE:** *Adults:* Individualize dose. Apply to hip area 2 hrs before effect is needed and remove 9 hrs after application. Recommended Titration Schedule: Week 1: 10mg/9 hrs. Week 2: 15mg/9 hrs. Week 3: 20mg/9 hrs. Week 4: 30mg/9 hrs.
*Pediatrics:* ≥6 yrs: Individualize dose. Apply to hip area 2 hrs before effect is needed and remove 9 hrs after application. Recommended Titration Schedule:

Week 1: 10mg/9 hrs. Week 2: 15mg/9 hrs. Week 3: 20mg/9 hrs. Week 4: 30mg/9 hrs.

**HOW SUPPLIED:** Patch: 10mg/9 hrs, 15mg/9 hrs, 20mg/9 hrs, 30mg/9 hrs [10$^s$, 30$^s$]

**CONTRAINDICATIONS:** Marked anxiety, tension, and agitation; glaucoma; motor tics or family history or diagnosis of Tourette's syndrome; treatment with MAOIs and within minimum of 14 days following discontinuation.

D

**WARNINGS/PRECAUTIONS:** Avoid use with known structural cardiac abnormalities; sudden death reported. D/C if contact sensitization is suspected. Monitor growth during treatment. May exacerbate symptoms of behavior disturbance and thought disorder in psychotic patients. Caution when using stimulants to treat patients with comorbid bipolar disorder because of concern for possible induction of mixed/manic episode in such patients. Stimulants at usual doses can cause treatment emergent psychotic or manic symptoms (eg, hallucinations, delusional thinking, mania) in children and adolescents without prior history of psychotic illness. Aggressive behavior or hostility reported in clinical trials and postmarketing experience of some medications indicated for the treatment of ADHD. May lower convulsive threshold; d/c in the presence of seizures. Caution with HTN; monitor BP. Caution when underlying medical conditions might be compromised by increases in BP or HR (eg, pre-existing HTN, heart failure, recent MI, or hyperthyroidism). Visual disturbances reported. Caution with history of drug dependence or alcoholism. Avoid exposing application site to external heat sources (eg, heating pads, electric blankets, heated water beds, etc). Monitor CBC, differential, and platelet counts during prolonged therapy.

**ADVERSE REACTIONS:** Nausea, vomiting, nasopharyngitis, weight decrease, anorexia, decreased appetite, affect lability, insomnia, tic, nasal congestion.

**INTERACTIONS:** See Contraindications. Caution with pressor agents. May decrease effectiveness of antihypertensive agents. May inhibit metabolism of coumarin anticoagulants, anticonvulsants (eg, phenobarbital, phenytoin, primidone), some tricyclic drugs (eg, imipramine, clomipramine, desipramine), and SSRIs. Monitor drug levels (or coagulation times with coumarin) and consider dose adjustments with concomitant use. Serious adverse events reported with concomitant clonidine use.

**PREGNANCY:** Category C, caution in nursing.

## DDAVP

RX

desmopressin acetate (Sanofi-Aventis)

**OTHER BRAND NAMES:** DDAVP Nasal Spray (Sanofi-Aventis) - DDAVP Rhinal Tube (Sanofi-Aventis)

**THERAPEUTIC CLASS:** Synthetic vasopressin analog

**INDICATIONS:** (Spray/Tube/Tab) Primary nocturnal enuresis. (Inj/Spray/Tube/Tab) Central (cranial) diabetes insipidus. Temporary polyuria and polydipsia after head trauma or surgery in the pituitary region. (Inj) Hemophilia A and von Willebrand's disease (Type I).

**DOSAGE:** *Adults:* Nocturnal Enuresis: (Tab) Initial: 0.2mg PO qhs. Titrate: May increase up to 0.6mg. (Spray/Tube) Initial: 20mcg intranasally qhs. Titrate: Decrease to 10mcg or increase up to 40mcg if needed. Max: 4-8 weeks. Administer 1/2 dose in each nostril. Diabetes Insipidus: (Tab) Initial: 0.05mg bid. Titrate: Increase/decrease by 0.1-1.2mg/day given bid-tid. Maint: 0.1-0.8mg/day in divided doses. (Spray/Tube) Usual: 0.1-0.4mL/day given qd-tid. (Inj) 1-2mcg IV/SQ bid. Hemophilia A and von Willebrand's Disease: 0.3mcg/kg IV. Add 50mL diluent. Give 30 minutes preoperatively.
*Pediatrics:* Nocturnal Enuresis: >6 yrs: (Tab) Initial: 0.2mg PO hs. Titrate: May increase up to 0.6mg. (Spray/Tube) Initial: 20mcg intranasally qhs. Titrate: Decrease to 10mcg or increase up to 40mcg if needed. Max: 4-8 weeks. Administer 1/2 dose per nostril. Diabetes Insipidus: (Tab) >4 yrs: Initial: 0.05mg bid. Titrate: Increase/decrease by 0.1-1.2mg/day given bid-tid. Maint: 0.1-

0.8mg/day in divided doses. (Spray/Tube) 3 months-12 yrs: Usual: 0.05-3mL/day given qd-bid. (Inj) >12 yrs: 1-2mcg IV/SQ bid. Hemophilia A and von Willebrand's Disease: >3 months: (Inj) 0.3mcg/kg IV. Add 50mL diluent if >10kg; add 10mL diluent if <10kg. Give 30 minutes preoperatively.

**HOW SUPPLIED:** Inj: 4mcg/mL; Nasal Spray: 10mcg/inh [5mL]; Tab: 0.1mg*, 0.2mg*; Rhinal Tube: 0.01% [2.5mL] *scored



**WARNINGS/PRECAUTIONS:** Mucosal changes with nasal forms may occur; d/c until resolved. Decrease fluid intake in pediatrics and elderly to decrease risk of water intoxication and hyponatremia; monitor osmolality. Caution with coronary artery insufficiency, hypertensive cardiovascular disease, fluid and electrolyte imbalance (eg, cystic fibrosis). Anaphylaxis reported with IV use. Caution with IV use if history of thrombus formation. For diabetes insipidus, dosage must be adjusted according to diurnal pattern of response; estimate response by adequate duration of sleep and adequate, not excessive, water turnover.

**ADVERSE REACTIONS:** Inj: Headache, nausea, abdominal cramps, vulval pain, injection site reactions, facial flushing, BP changes. Spray: Headache, dizziness, rhinitis, nausea, nasal congestion, sore throat, cough, respiratory infection, epistaxis. Tab: Nausea, flushing, abdominal cramps, headache, increased SGOT, water intoxication, hyponatremia.

**INTERACTIONS:** Caution with other pressor agents.

**PREGNANCY:** Category B, caution in nursing.

## DECADRON OPHTHALMIC RX

dexamethasone sodium phosphate (Merck)

**THERAPEUTIC CLASS:** Corticosteroid

**INDICATIONS:** (Oint, Sol) Treatment of inflammation of the palpebral and bulbar conjunctiva, cornea, and anterior segment of the globe. (Sol) Treatment of inflammation of the external auditory canal.

**DOSAGE:** *Adults:* Eye: (Oint) Apply tid-qid. Decrease to bid, then to qd with improvement. (Sol) Initial: 1-2 drops every hr during day and q2h during the night. Decrease to 1 drop q4h, then 1 drop tid-qid with improvement. Ear: (Sol) Clean and dry ear canal. Instill 3-4 drops into ear canal bid-tid, gradually reduce dose with favorable response.

**HOW SUPPLIED:** Oint: 0.05% [3.5g]; Sol: 0.1% [5mL]

**CONTRAINDICATIONS:** (Oint, Sol) Viral diseases of the cornea and conjunctiva including epithelial herpes simplex keratitis, vaccinia, and varicella. Mycobacterial infection and fungal diseases of the eye. (Sol) Eardrum membrane perforation, sulfite hypersensitivity.

**WARNINGS/PRECAUTIONS:** (Oint, Sol) Prolonged use may cause ocular HTN, glaucoma, optic nerve damage, cataracts, increased secondary infections, fungal infections. Monitor IOP after 10 days of therapy. May mask or enhance existing infection in acute, purulent conditions. Perforations may occur in diseases causing thinning of the cornea or sclera. Periodic slit-lamp microscopy if use in herpes simplex infections. Solution contains sulfites.

**ADVERSE REACTIONS:** Glaucoma, optic nerve damage, visual acuity and field defects, cataracts, secondary ocular infections, corneal globe perforation.

**PREGNANCY:** Category C, not for use in nursing.

## DECLOMYCIN RX

demeclocycline HCl (Wyeth)

**THERAPEUTIC CLASS:** Tetracycline derivative

**INDICATIONS:** Treatment of infections due to rickettsiae, *Mycoplasma pneumoniae*, *B.recurrentis*, agents of psittacosis, ornithosis, lymphomagranuloma venereum or granuloma inguinale. Treatment of gram-negative infections (eg, respiratory, urinary tract ), gram-positive infections (eg, respiratory tract, skin and soft tissue), trachoma, inclusion conjunctivitis. When PCN is contraindicated, treatment of gonorrhea, syphilis, listeriosis, anthrax, *Clostridium* species, and others. Adjunct therapy for amebicides.



**DOSAGE:** *Adults:* Usual: 150mg qid or 300mg bid. Gonorrhea: Initial: 600mg, then 300mg q12h for 4 days. Gonorrhea: 600mg followed by 300mg q12h for 4 days to a total of 3g. Renal/Hepatic Impairment: Reduce dose and/or extend dose intervals. Continue therapy for at least 24-48 hrs after symptoms subside. Treat strep infections for at least 10 days. Take at least 1 hr before or 2 hrs after meals with plenty of fluids.
*Pediatrics:* >8 yrs: Usual: 3-6mg/lb/day given bid-qid. Gonorrhea: 600mg followed by 300mg q12h for 4 days to a total of 3g. Renal/Hepatic Impairment: Reduce dose and/or extend dose intervals. Continue therapy for at least 24-48 hrs after symptoms subside. Treat strep infections for at least 10 days. Take at least 1 hr before or 2 hrs after meals with plenty of fluids.

**HOW SUPPLIED:** Tab: 150mg, 300mg

**CONTRAINDICATIONS:** Hypersensitivity to any of the tetracyclines.

**WARNINGS/PRECAUTIONS:** May cause fetal harm during pregnancy. Use during tooth development (last half of pregnancy, infancy, <8 yrs), or long-term use, or repeated short-term use may cause permanent discoloration of the teeth. Pseudotumor cerebri (adults), bulging fontanels (infants) reported. Caution with renal or hepatic impairment. Long-term use may cause reversible, nephrogenic diabetes insipidus syndrome. May result in overgrowth of nonsusceptible organisms; d/c if superinfection develops. CNS symptoms may occur; caution when operating machinery. May decrease bone growth in premature infants. Monitor hematopoietic, renal, and hepatic function with long-term use. D/C at first evidence of skin erythema after sun/UV light exposure.

**ADVERSE REACTIONS:** GI problems, rash, esophageal ulceration, hypersensitivity reactions, dizziness, headache, tinnitus, blood dyscrasias, photosensitivity reactions, enamel hypoplasia, elevated BUN.

**INTERACTIONS:** Decreases PT; may need to decrease dose of anticoagulants. May interfere with bactericidal action of penicillin; avoid concomitant use. May decrease efficacy of oral contraceptives; use alternate method. Decreased absorption with antacids and iron-containing products. Fatal renal toxicity with methoxyflurane reported. Foods/dairy products interfere with absorption.

**PREGNANCY:** Category D, not for use in nursing.

## DECONAMINE RX

pseudoephedrine HCl - chlorpheniramine maleate (Kenwood Therapeutics)

**OTHER BRAND NAMES:** Kronofed-A (Ferndale) - De-Congestine TR (Qualitest) - Deconamine SR (Kenwood Therapeutics)

**THERAPEUTIC CLASS:** Antihistamine/decongestant

**INDICATIONS:** Temporary relief of symptoms associated with rhinorrhea, sneezing, and nasal congestion.

**DOSAGE:** *Adults:* (Cap, SR) 1 cap q12h, (Tab) 1 tab tid-qid. (Syrup) 5-10mL tid-qid.
*Pediatrics:* >12 yrs: (Cap, SR) 1 cap q12h, (Tab) 1 tab tid-qid. (Syrup) 5-10mL tid-qid. 2-6 yrs: (Syrup) 2.5mL tid-qid. Max: 10mL/24hrs. 6-12 yrs: 2.5-5mL tid-qid. Max: 20mL/24hrs.

**HOW SUPPLIED:** (Chlorpheniramine-Pseudoephedrine) Cap, Sustained Release: 8mg-120mg; Syrup: 2mg-30mg/5mL; Tab: 4mg-60mg

**CONTRAINDICATIONS:** Severe HTN, severe CAD, concomitant MAOIs.

**WARNINGS/PRECAUTIONS:** Extreme caution in narrow angle glaucoma, stenosing peptic ulcer, pyloroduodenal obstruction, symptomatic prostatic hypertrophy, bladder neck obstruction. Caution in bronchial asthma, emphysema, chronic pulmonary disease, HTN, ischemic heart disease, DM, increased IOP, hyperthyroidism. May cause excitability in children. May produce CNS stimulation with convulsions or cardiovascular collapse with hypotension.

**ADVERSE REACTIONS:** Drowsiness, urticaria, drug rash, hypotension, hemolytic anemia, sedation, epigastric distress, urinary frequency, nervousness, dizziness.



**INTERACTIONS:** Hypertensive crisis may occur with MAOIs. May reduce antihypertensive effect of methyldopa, reserpine, veratrum alkaloids, mecamylamine. Sedative effects potentiated by alcohol, other CNS depressants.

**PREGNANCY:** Category C, not for use in nursing.

## DELATESTRYL CIII

testosterone enanthate (Savient)

**THERAPEUTIC CLASS:** Androgen

**INDICATIONS:** Testosterone replacement in males with primary hypogonadism and hypogonadotropic hypogonadism. To stimulate puberty in males with delayed puberty. May also be used secondarily in females with advancing inoperable metastatic (skeletal) mammary cancer who are 1-5 years postmenopausal.

**DOSAGE:** *Adults:* Dose based on age, sex, and diagnosis. Adjust dose according to response and adverse reactions. Male Hypogonadism: 50-400mg IM every 2-4 weeks. Delayed Puberty: 50-200mg every 2-4 weeks for a limited duration (eg, 4-6 months). Breast Cancer: 200-400mg every 2-4 weeks. *Pediatrics:* Dose based on age, sex, and diagnosis. Adjust dose according to response and adverse reactions. Male Hypogonadism: 50-400mg IM every 2-4 weeks. Delayed Puberty: 50-200mg every 2-4 weeks for a limited duration (eg, 4-6 months). Caution in children.

**HOW SUPPLIED:** Inj: 200mg/mL

**CONTRAINDICATIONS:** Breast or prostate carcinoma in men. Pregnancy.

**WARNINGS/PRECAUTIONS:** D/C if hypercalcemia occurs in breast cancer or immobilized patients; monitor calcium levels. Risk of hepatic adenomas, hepatocellular carcinoma, and peliosis hepatitis with prolonged high doses. D/C if jaundice, cholestatic hepatitis, or abnormal LFTs occur. Avoid use in elderly who has age related hypogonadism. D/C if edema occurs in patients with pre-existing cardiac, renal, or hepatic disease; restart at lower dose. Risk of compromised stature in children; monitor bone growth every 6 months. Monitor for virilization in females. Caution with a history of MI or CAD due to altered serum cholesterol levels. Monitor cholesterol, LFTs, Hct, Hgb periodically.

**ADVERSE REACTIONS:** Amenorrhea, virilization, menstrual irregularities, gynecomastia, excessive frequency/duration of penile erections, male pattern baldness, increased/decreased libido, oligospermia, hirsutism, acne, fluid and electrolyte disturbances, nausea, hypercholesterolemia, clotting factor suppression, polycythemia, altered LFTs, oligospermia, anxiety, depression.

**INTERACTIONS:** Potentiates oral anticoagulants and oxyphenbutazone. May decrease blood glucose and insulin requirements. ACTH and corticosteroids may enhance edema.

**PREGNANCY:** Category X, not for use in nursing.

## DELESTROGEN

RX

estradiol valerate (King)

**Estrogens increase the risk of endometrial cancer. Estrogens and progestins should not be used for the prevention of cardiovascular disease. Increased risks of MI, stroke, invasive breast cancer, PE, and DVT in postmenopausal women (50-79 yrs of age) reported. Increased risk of developing probable dementia in postmenopausal women ≥65 yrs of age reported.**



**THERAPEUTIC CLASS:** Estrogen

**INDICATIONS:** Treatment of moderate to severe vasomotor symptoms and vulvar/vaginal atrophy associated with menopause. Treatment of hypoestrogenism due to hypogonadism, castration, or primary ovarian failure. Palliative treatment of advanced androgen-dependent prostate carcinoma.

**DOSAGE:** *Adults:* Vasomotor Symptoms/Vaginal/Vulval Atrophy: 10-20mg IM every 4 weeks. Discontinue or taper at 3-6 month intervals. Hypoestrogenism: 10-20mg IM every 4 weeks. Prostate Carcinoma: 30mg or more every 1 or 2 weeks.

**HOW SUPPLIED:** Inj: 10mg/mL, 20mg/mL, 40mg/mL

**CONTRAINDICATIONS:** Pregnancy, undiagnosed abnormal genital bleeding, breast cancer, estrogen-dependent neoplasia, thrombophlebitis, thromboembolic disorders.

**WARNINGS/PRECAUTIONS:** May increase risk of cardiovascular events (eg, MI, stroke), venous thrombosis, and PE; d/c immediately if any of these events occur or are suspected. May increase risk of breast/endometrial cancer, and gallbladder disease. May lead to severe hypercalcemia with breast cancer and bone metastases; monitor and d/c if hypercalcemia occurs. Retinal vascular thrombosis reported; monitor and d/c if papilledema or retinal vascular lesions occur. Consider addition of a progestin if no hysterectomy. May elevate BP; monitor at regular intervals. May cause elevations of plasma triglycerides with pre-existing hypertriglyceridemia. Caution with history of cholestatic jaundice associated with past estrogen use or with pregnancy; d/c with recurrence. May lead to increased thyroid-binding globulin levels; monitor thyroid function. May cause fluid retention; caution with cardiac/renal dysfunction. Caution with severe hypocalcemia. May increase risk of ovarian cancer. May exacerbate endometriosis, asthma, DM, epilepsy, migraine, porphyria, SLE, and hepatic hemangiomas; use with caution. May cause hypercoagulability. May develop uterine bleeding and mastodynia.

**ADVERSE REACTIONS:** Altered vaginal bleeding, vaginal candidiasis, breast tenderness/enlargement, GI effects, CNS effects, chloasma, melasma, weight changes, edema, altered libido.

**PREGNANCY:** Contraindicated in pregnancy, caution in nursing.

## DEMADEX

RX

torsemide (Roche Labs)

**THERAPEUTIC CLASS:** Loop diuretic

**INDICATIONS:** Treatment of edema associated with CHF, renal disease, chronic renal failure or hepatic disease. Treatment of hypertension.

**DOSAGE:** *Adults:* PO/IV (bolus over 2 minutes or continuous): CHF: Initial: 10-20mg qd. Max: 200mg single dose. Chronic Renal Failure: Initial: 20mg qd. Max: 200mg single dose. Hepatic Cirrhosis: Initial: 5-10mg qd with aldosterone antagonist or $K^+$-sparing diuretic. Titrate: Double dose. Max: 40mg single dose. HTN: Initial: 5mg qd. Titrate: May increase to 10mg qd in 4-6 weeks, then may add additional antihypertensive agent.

**HOW SUPPLIED:** Inj: 10mg/mL; Tab: 5mg*, 10mg*, 20mg*, 100mg* *scored

**CONTRAINDICATIONS:** Anuria, sulfonamide hypersensitivity.

**WARNINGS/PRECAUTIONS:** Caution with cirrhosis and ascites in hepatic disease. Tinnitus and hearing loss (usually reversible) reported. Avoid excessive diuresis, especially in elderly. Caution with brisk diuresis, inadequate oral intake of electrolytes, and cardiovascular disease, especially with digitalis glycosides. Monitor for electrolyte/volume depletion. Hyperglycemia, hypokalemia, hypermagnesemia, hypercalcemia, gout reported. May increase cholesterol and TG.

**ADVERSE REACTIONS:** Headache, excessive urination, dizziness, cough, ECG abnormality, asthenia, rhinitis, diarrhea.

**INTERACTIONS:** Caution with high dose salicylates, aminoglycosides. Lithium toxicity. Indomethacin partially inhibits natriuretic effect. Avoid simultaneous cholestyramine administration. Probenecid decreases effects. Reduces spironolactone clearance. Risk of hypokalemia with ACTH, corticosteroids. Possible renal dysfunction with NSAIDs.

**PREGNANCY:** Category B, caution in nursing.



## DEMEROL INJECTION — CII

meperidine HCl (Hospira)

**THERAPEUTIC CLASS:** Opioid analgesic

**INDICATIONS:** For relief of moderate to severe pain. For preoperative medication, anesthesia support, and obstetrical analgesia.

**DOSAGE:** *Adults:* Pain: Usual: 50-150mg IM/SQ q3-4h prn. Preoperative: Usual: 50-100mg IM/SQ 30-90 minutes before anesthesia. Anesthesia Support: Use repeated slow IV injections of fractional doses (eg, 10mg/mL) or continuous IV infusion of a more dilute solution (eg, 1mg/mL). Titrate as needed. Obstetrical Analgesia: Usual: 50-100mg IM/SQ when pain is regular, may repeat at 1- to 3-hr intervals. Elderly: Start at lower end of dosage range and observe. With Phenothiazines/Other Tranquilizers: Reduce dose by 25 to 50%). IM method preferred with repeated use. For IV injection: Reduce dose and administer slowly, preferably using diluted solution.
*Pediatrics:* Pain: Usual: 0.5-0.8mg/lb IM/SQ, up to 50-150mg, q3-4h prn. Preoperative: Usual: 0.5-1mg/lb IM/SQ, up to 50-100mg, 30-90 minutes before anesthesia. With Phenothiazines/Other Tranquilizers: Reduce dose by 25 to 50%). IM method preferred with repeated use. For IV injection: Reduce dose and administer slowly, using diluted solution.

**HOW SUPPLIED:** Inj: 25mg/mL, 50mg/mL, 75mg/mL, 100mg/mL

**CONTRAINDICATIONS:** MAOI during or within 14 days of use.

**WARNINGS/PRECAUTIONS:** May develop tolerance and dependence; abuse potential. Extreme caution with head injury, increased intracranial pressure, intracranial lesions, acute asthmatic attack, chronic COPD or cor pulmonale, decreased respiratory reserve, respiratory depression, hypoxia, and hypercapnia. Rapid IV infusion may result in increased adverse reactions. Caution with acute abdominal conditions, atrial flutter, supraventricular tachycardias. May aggravate convulsive disorders. Caution and reduce initial dose with elderly or debilitated, renal/hepatic impairment, hypothyroidism, Addison's disease, prostatic hypertrophy or urethral stricture. Severe hypotension may occur post-op or if depleted blood volume. Orthostatic hypotension may occur. May impair mental/physical abilities. Not for use in pregnancy prior to labor. May produce depression of respiration and psychophysiologic functions in the newborn when used as an obstetrical analgesic.

**ADVERSE REACTIONS:** Lightheadedness, dizziness, sedation, nausea, vomiting, sweating, respiratory/circulatory depression.

**INTERACTIONS:** See Contraindications. Caution and reduce dose with other CNS depressants (eg, narcotics, anesthetics, phenothiazines, tranquilizers, sedative-hypnotics, TCAs, alcohol).

**PREGNANCY:** Safety in pregnancy and nursing not known.

## DEMEROL ORAL CII
meperidine HCl (Sanofi-Aventis)

**THERAPEUTIC CLASS:** Opioid analgesic

**INDICATIONS:** Moderate to severe pain.

D

**DOSAGE:** *Adults:* Usual: 50-150mg q3-4h prn. Concomitant Phenothiazines/Other Tranquilizers: Reduce dose by 25-50%. Dilute syrup in 1/2 glass of water.
*Pediatrics:* Usual: 1.1-1.8mg/kg up to 50-150mg q3-4h prn. Concomitant Phenothiazines/Other Tranquilizers: Reduce dose by 25-50%. Dilute syrup in 1/2 glass of water.

**HOW SUPPLIED:** Syrup: 50mg/5mL; Tab: 50mg*, 100mg *scored

**CONTRAINDICATIONS:** MAOI during or within 14 days of use.

**WARNINGS/PRECAUTIONS:** May develop tolerance and dependence; abuse potential. Extreme caution with head injury, increased intracranial pressure, intracranial lesions, acute asthma attack, chronic COPD, cor pulmonale, decreased respiratory reserve, respiratory depression, hypoxia, and hypercapnia. Caution with sickle cell anemia, pheochromocytoma, acute alcoholism, Addison's disease, CNS depression or coma, delirium tremens, elderly or debilitated, kyphoscoliosis associated with respiratory depression, myxedema, hypothyroidism, acute abdominal conditions, epilepsy, atrial flutter, other supraventricular tachycardias, renal or hepatic impairment, prostatic hypertrophy, urethral stricture, drug dependencies, neonates, and young infants. Severe hypotension may occur post-op or if depleted blood volume. Orthostatic hypotension may occur. Not for use in pregnancy prior to labor.

**ADVERSE REACTIONS:** Lightheadedness, dizziness, sedation, nausea, vomiting, sweating, respiratory depression.

**INTERACTIONS:** See Contraindications. Reduce dose with other CNS depressants (eg, narcotics, anesthetics, phenothiazines, tranquilizers, sedative-hypnotics, TCAs, alcohol). Mixed agonist/antagonist analgesics (eg, pentazocine, nalbuphine, butorphanol, buprenorphine) may reduce analgesic effects and/or precipitate withdrawal symptoms. Caution with acyclovir, cimetidine. Phenytoin may enhance hepatic metabolism. May enhance neuroblocking action of skeletal muscle relaxants. Increased levels with ritonavir; avoid concurrent administration.

**PREGNANCY:** Category C, not for use in nursing.

## DEMSER RX
metyrosine (Aton)

**THERAPEUTIC CLASS:** Tyrosine hydroxylase inhibitor

**INDICATIONS:** Treatment of pheochromocytoma for preoperative preparation and when surgery is contraindicated. Chronic treatment with malignant pheochromocytoma.

**DOSAGE:** *Adults:* Initial: 250mg qid. Titrate: May increase by 250-500mg/day. Max: 4g/day. Titrate based on clinical symptoms and catecholamine excretion. Usual: 2-3g/day. Preoperative Preparation: Take 5-7 days before surgery.
*Pediatrics:* >12 yrs: Initial: 250mg qid. Titrate: May increase by 250-500mg/day. Max: 4g/day. Titrate based on clinical symptoms and catecholamine excretion. Usual: 2-3g/day. Preoperative Preparation: Take 5-7 days before surgery.

**HOW SUPPLIED:** Cap: 250mg

**WARNINGS/PRECAUTIONS:** When used preoperatively or with alpha-adrenergic blockers, maintain intravascular volume intra- and postoperatively to avoid hypotension and decreased perfusion. Maintain adequate water intake to achieve urine volume of >2000mL to prevent crystalluria. Risk of hypertensive crisis or arrhythmias during tumor manipulation. Monitor BP and ECG continuously during surgery.

**ADVERSE REACTIONS:** Sedation, EPS, anxiety, depression, hallucinations, disorientation, confusion, diarrhea.

**INTERACTIONS:** Additive sedative effects with alcohol and other CNS depressants (eg, hypnotics, sedatives, tranquilizers). May potentiate EPS with phenothiazines and haloperidol.

**PREGNANCY:** Category C, caution in nursing.



## DEMULEN

RX

ethinyl estradiol - ethynodiol diacetate (Pharmacia & Upjohn)

**OTHER BRAND NAMES:** Zovia (Watson)

**THERAPEUTIC CLASS:** Estrogen/progestogen combination

**INDICATIONS:** Prevention of pregnancy.

**DOSAGE:** *Adults:* Start 1st Sunday after menses begins or the 1st day of menses. *21-day:* 1 tab qd for 21 days, stop 7 days, then repeat. *28-day:* 1 tab qd for 28 days, then repeat.

**HOW SUPPLIED:** (Ethinyl Estradiol-Ethynodiol Diacetate) Tab: (1/35) 0.035mg-1mg; (1/50) 0.05mg-1mg

**CONTRAINDICATIONS:** Thrombophlebitis, DVT or thromboembolic disorders, pregnancy, cerebrovascular or coronary artery disease, undiagnosed abnormal genital bleeding, cholestatic jaundice of pregnancy or jaundice with prior pill use, hepatic adenomas or carcinomas, breast cancer or other estrogen-dependent neoplasia.

**WARNINGS/PRECAUTIONS:** Cigarette smoking increases risk of serious cardiovascular side effects. This risk increases with age (especially >35 yrs) and heavy smoking. Increased risk of MI, vascular disease, thromboembolism, stroke and gallbladder disease. Retinal thrombosis, hepatic neoplasia, carcinoma of breast and reproductive organs reported. May cause glucose intolerance. May increase BP, elevate LDL levels or cause other lipid changes, fluid retention, breakthrough bleeding, and spotting. May cause or exacerbate migraine. May develop visual changes with contact lens. Increased risk of MI with HTN, hyperlipidemia, obesity, and diabetes. Discontinue if develop jaundice, significant depression or ophthalmic irregularities. Perform annual physical exam. Use before menarche is not indicated. May affect certain endocrine, LFTs and blood components.

**ADVERSE REACTIONS:** Nausea, vomiting, breakthrough bleeding, spotting, amenorrhea, migraine, depression, vaginal candidiasis, edema, weight changes.

**INTERACTIONS:** Reduced effects, increased breakthrough bleeding, and menstrual irregularities with rifampin, barbiturates, phenylbutazone, phenytoin, and possibly with griseofulvin, ampicillin, and tetracyclines. Troglitazone reduces plasma levels of hormones.

**PREGNANCY:** Category X, not for use in nursing.

## DENAVIR

RX

penciclovir (Novartis)

**THERAPEUTIC CLASS:** Nucleoside analogue antiviral

**INDICATIONS:** Treatment of recurrent herpes labialis (cold sores) in adults and children ≥12 yrs.

**DOSAGE:** *Adults:* Apply q2h while awake for 4 days. Start with earliest sign or symptom.

**HOW SUPPLIED:** Cre: 1% [1.5g]

**WARNINGS/PRECAUTIONS:** Only use on herpes labialis on the lips and face. Avoid mucous membranes or near the eyes. Effectiveness not established in immunocompromised patients.

**ADVERSE REACTIONS:** Headache, application site reaction.

**PREGNANCY:** Category B, not for use in nursing.



## DEPACON

RX

valproate sodium (Abbott)

**Fatal hepatic failure (<2 yrs at considerable risk), teratogenic effects (eg, neural tube defects), and life-threatening pancreatitis reported.**

**THERAPEUTIC CLASS:** Carboxylic acid derivative

**INDICATIONS:** Monotherapy and adjunctive therapy for treatment of simple and complex absence seizures, and complex partial seizures. Adjunct therapy for multiple seizure types.

**DOSAGE:** *Adults:* Simplex/Complex Absence Seizure: Initial: 15mg/kg/day. Titrate: Increase weekly by 5-10mg/kg/day until optimal response. Max: 60mg/kg/day. Complex Partial Seizure: Initial: 10-15mg/kg/day. Titrate: Increase weekly by 5-10mg/kg/day until optimal response. Max: 60mg/kg/day. Elderly: Reduce initial dose and titrate slowly. If dose >250mg/day, give in divided doses. Administer as 60 minute IV infusion, not >20mg/min. Not for use >14 days; switch to oral route as soon as clinically feasible. Decrease dose or discontinue if decreased food or fluid intake or if excessive somnolence occurs.
*Pediatrics:* >2 yrs: Simplex/Complex Absence Seizure: Initial: 15mg/kg/day. Titrate: Increase weekly by 5-10mg/kg/day until optimal response. Max: 60mg/kg/day. >10 yrs: Complex Partial Seizure: Initial: 10-15mg/kg/day. Titrate: Increase weekly by 5-10mg/kg/day until optimal response. Max: 60mg/kg/day. If dose >250mg/day, give in divided doses. Administer as 60 minute IV infusion, not >20mg/min. Not for use >14 days; switch to oral route as soon as clinically feasible. Decrease dose or discontinue with decreased food or fluid intake and if excessive somnolence.

**HOW SUPPLIED:** Inj: 100mg/mL

**CONTRAINDICATIONS:** Hepatic disease, significant hepatic dysfunction, known urea cycle disorders (UCD).

**WARNINGS/PRECAUTIONS:** Hyperammonemic encephalopathy in UCD patients; d/c if this occurs. Prior to therapy, evaluate for UCD in high risk patients (eg, history of unexplained encephalopathy, coma, etc). Measure ammonia levels if develop unexplained lethargy, vomiting, or mental status changes. Caution in elderly; monitor for fluid/nutritional intake, dehydration, somnolence. Monitor LFTs before therapy and during 1st 6 months. D/C if develop hepatic dysfunction, pancreatitis. Increased risk of hepatotoxicity with multiple anticonvulsants, congenital metabolic disorders, severe seizure disorder with mental retardation, organic brain disease, children <2 yrs. Avoid abrupt withdrawal. Monitor platelets and coagulation tests before therapy and periodically thereafter. Elevated liver enzymes and thrombocytopenia may be dose-related. Not for prophylaxis of post-traumatic seizures in acute head trauma. May interfere with urine ketone and thyroid function tests.

**ADVERSE REACTIONS:** Dizziness, headache, nausea, local reactions.

**INTERACTIONS:** Clonazepam may induce absence status in patients with absence seizures. Potentiates amitriptyline, nortriptyline, carbamazepine, diazepam, ethosuximide, lamotrigine, phenobarbital, primidone, phenytoin, tolbutamide, warfarin, zidovudine. Potentiated by ASA and felbamate. Antagonized by rifampin, carbamazepine, phenobarbital, phenytoin. Additive CNS depression with other CNS depressants (eg, alcohol).

**PREGNANCY:** Category D, not for use in nursing.

## DEPAKENE
valproic acid (Abbott) RX

**Fatal hepatic failure (<2 yrs at considerable risk), teratogenic effects (eg, neural tube defects), and life-threatening pancreatitis reported.**



**THERAPEUTIC CLASS:** Carboxylic acid derivative

**INDICATIONS:** Monotherapy and adjunctive therapy for treatment of simple and complex absence seizures, and complex partial seizures. Adjunct therapy for multiple seizure types.

**DOSAGE:** *Adults:* Simplex/Complex Absence Seizure: Initial: 15mg/kg/day. Titrate: Increase weekly by 5-10mg/kg/day until optimal response. Max: 60mg/kg/day. Complex Partial Seizure: Initial: 10-15mg/kg/day. Titrate: Increase weekly by 5-10mg/kg/day until optimal response. Max: 60mg/kg/day. If dose >250mg/day, give in divided doses. Elderly: Reduce initial dose. Swallow caps whole, do not chew.
*Pediatrics:* >10 yrs: Complex Partial Seizure: Initial: 10-15mg/kg/day. Titrate: Increase weekly by 5-10mg/kg/day until optimal response. Max: 60mg/kg/day. If dose >250mg/day, give in divided doses. Swallow caps whole, do not chew.

**HOW SUPPLIED:** Cap: 250mg; Syrup: 250mg/5mL

**CONTRAINDICATIONS:** Hepatic disease, significant hepatic dysfunction, known urea cycle disorders (UCD).

**WARNINGS/PRECAUTIONS:** Hyperammonemic encephalopathy in UCD patients; d/c if this occurs. Prior to therapy, evaluate for UCD in high risk patients (eg, history of unexplained encephalopathy, coma, etc). Measure ammonia levels if develop unexplained lethargy, vomiting, or mental status changes. Caution in elderly; monitor for fluid/nutritional intake, dehydration, somnolence. Monitor LFTs before therapy and during 1st 6 months. D/C if develop hepatic dysfunction, pancreatitis. Increased risk of hepatotoxicity with multiple anticonvulsants, congenital metabolic disorders, severe seizure disorder with mental retardation, organic brain disease, children <2 yrs. Avoid abrupt withdrawal. Hyperammonemia reported. Monitor platelets and coagulation tests before therapy and periodically thereafter. Elevated liver enzymes and thrombocytopenia may be dose-related. May interfere with urine ketone and thyroid function tests.

**ADVERSE REACTIONS:** Headache, asthenia, nausea, vomiting, diarrhea, abdominal pain, somnolence, tremor, dizziness, thrombocytopenia, ecchymosis, nystagmus, alopecia.

**INTERACTIONS:** Clonazepam may induce absence status in patients with absence seizures. Potentiates amitriptyline, nortriptyline, carbamazepine, diazepam, ethosuximide, lamotrigine, phenobarbital, primidone, phenytoin, tolbutamide, warfarin, zidovudine. Potentiated by ASA and felbamate. Antagonized by rifampin, carbamazepine, phenobarbital, phenytoin. Additive CNS depression with other CNS depressants (eg, alcohol).

**PREGNANCY:** Category D, not for use in nursing.

## DEPAKOTE
divalproex sodium (Abbott) RX

**Fatal hepatic failure (<2 yrs at considerable risk), teratogenic effects (eg, neural tube defects), and life-threatening pancreatitis reported.**

**THERAPEUTIC CLASS:** Valproate compound

**INDICATIONS:** (Tab, Cap) Management of simple and complex absence seizures; complex partial seizures; and adjunctively with multiple seizure types including absence seizures. (Tab) Treatment of mania associated with bipolar disorder and migraine prophylaxis.

**DOSAGE:** *Adults:* (Cap/Tab) Complex Partial Seizures: Initial: 10-15mg/kg/day. Titrate: Increase by 5-10mg/kg/week. Max: 60mg/kg/day. Absence Seizures: Initial: 15mg/kg/day. Titrate: Increase weekly by 5-10mg/kg/day. Max: 60mg/kg/day. Give in divided doses if >250mg/day. (Tab) Migraine: Initial: >16 yrs: 250mg bid. Max: 1000mg/day. Mania: 750mg daily in divided doses. Titrate: Increase dose rapidly to clinical effect. Max: 60mg/kg/day. Elderly: Reduce initial dose and titrate slowly. Decrease dose or d/c if decreased food or fluid intake or if excessive somnolence occurs.



*Pediatrics:* >10 yrs: (Cap/Tab) Complex Partial Seizures: Initial: 10-15mg/kg/day. Titrate: Increase by 5-10mg/kg/week. Max: 60mg/kg/day. Absence Seizures: Initial: 15mg/kg/day. Titrate: Increase weekly by 5-10mg/kg/day. Max: 60mg/kg/day. Give in divided doses if >250mg/day.

**HOW SUPPLIED:** Cap, Delayed Release: (Sprinkle) 125mg; Tab, Delayed Release: 125mg, 250mg, 500mg

**CONTRAINDICATIONS:** Hepatic disease, significant hepatic dysfunction, known urea cycle disorders (UCD).

**WARNINGS/PRECAUTIONS:** Hyperammonemic encephalopathy in UCD patients; d/c if this occurs. Prior to therapy, evaluate for UCD in high risk patients (eg, history of unexplained encephalopathy, coma, etc). Measure ammonia levels if develop unexplained lethargy, vomiting, or mental status changes. Caution with hepatic disease. Check LFTs prior to therapy, then frequently during first 6 months. Dose-related thrombocytopenia and elevated liver enzymes reported. Monitor platelet and coagulation tests prior to therapy, then periodically. Altered thyroid function tests and urine ketone test. May stimulate replication of HIV and CMV viruses. Avoid abrupt discontinuation.

**ADVERSE REACTIONS:** Nausea, vomiting, diarrhea, somnolence, dyspepsia, thrombocytopenia, asthenia, abdominal pain, tremor, headache, anorexia, diplopia, blurred vision, weight gain, ataxia, nystagmus.

**INTERACTIONS:** Potentiates carbamazepine, amitriptyline, nortriptyline, diazepam, ethosuximide, primidone, lamotrigine, phenobarbital, phenytoin, tolbutamide, zidovudine, lorazepam. Efficacy potentiated by ASA, felbamate. Efficacy reduced by rifampin, carbamazepine, phenobarbital, phenytoin, primidone. Clonazepam may induce absence status in patients with absence type seizures. CNS depression with alcohol and other CNS depressants. Monitor PT/INR with warfarin.

**PREGNANCY:** Category D, not for use in nursing.

## DEPAKOTE ER

RX

divalproex sodium (Abbott)

> **Fatal hepatic failure (<2 yrs at considerable risk), teratogenic effects (eg, neural tube defects), and life-threatening pancreatitis reported.**

**THERAPEUTIC CLASS:** Valproate compound

**INDICATIONS:** Migraine prophylaxis. Monotherapy and adjunct therapy for treatment of complex partial seizures, and simple and complex absence seizures. Adjunct for multiple seizure types that include absence seizures. Acute manic or mixed episodes associated with bipolar disorder.

**DOSAGE:** *Adults:* For qd dosing. Migraine: Initial: 500mg qd for 1 week. Titrate: Increase to 1000mg qd. Max: 1000mg/day. Complex Partial Seizures: Monotherapy/Adjunct Therapy: Initial: 10-15mg/kg/day. Titrate: Increase by 5-10mg/kg/week to optimal response. Usual: Less than 60mg/kg/day (accepted therapeutic range 50-100mcg/mL). When converting to monotherapy, reduce concomitant antiepilepsy drug by 25% every 2 weeks starting at initiation or delay 1-2 weeks after start of therapy. Simple and Complex Absence Seizures: Initial: 15mg/kg/day. Titrate: Increase weekly by 5-10mg/kg/day to optimal response. Max: 60mg/kg/day. Mania: Initial: 25mg/kg/day given once daily. Titrate: Increase dose rapidly to clinical effect. Max: 60mg/kg/day. Conversion from Depakote: Administer Depakote ER qd using a dose 8-20% higher than the total daily dose of Depakote. If cannot directly convert to Depakote ER, consider increasing to next higher Depakote total daily dose before converting to appropriate total daily Depakote ER dose. Elderly: Give lower initial dose and titrate slowly. Decrease dose or d/c if decreased food or fluid intake or if excessive somnolence occurs. Swallow whole; do not crush or chew. *Pediatrics:* ≥10yrs: For qd dosing. Complex Partial Seizures: Monotherapy/Adjunct Therapy: Initial: 10-15mg/kg/day. Titrate: Increase by 5-10mg/kg/week to optimal response. Usual: Less than 60mg/kg/day (accepted therapeutic range 50-100mcg/mL). When converting to monotherapy, reduce concomitant antiepilepsy drug by 25% every 2 weeks starting at initiation or delay 1-2 weeks after start of therapy. Simple and Complex Absence Seizures: Initial: 15mg/kg/day. Titrate: Increase weekly by 5-10mg/kg/day to optimal response. Max: 60mg/kg/day. Conversion from Depakote: Administer Depakote ER qd using a dose 8-20% higher than the total daily dose of Depakote. If cannot directly convert to Depakote ER, consider increasing to next higher Depakote total daily dose before converting to appropriate total daily Depakote ER dose. Swallow whole; do not crush or chew.

**HOW SUPPLIED:** Tab, Extended Release: 250mg, 500mg

**CONTRAINDICATIONS:** Hepatic disease, significant hepatic dysfunction, known urea cycle disorders (UCD).

**WARNINGS/PRECAUTIONS:** Hyperammonemic encephalopathy in UCD patients; d/c if this occurs. Prior to therapy, evaluate for UCD in high risk patients (eg, history of unexplained encephalopathy, coma, etc). If unexplained lethargy, vomiting, or mental status changes occur measure ammonia levels. Caution with hepatic disease and elderly. Check LFTs prior to therapy, then frequently during 1st 6 months. Dose-related thrombocytopenia and elevated liver enzymes reported. Thrombocytopenia significantly increases with plasma trough levels >110mcg/mL in females and >135mcg/mL in males. Monitor platelet and coagulation tests prior to therapy, then periodically. Altered thyroid function tests and urine ketone test. May stimulate replication of HIV and CMV viruses. Avoid abrupt discontinuation.

**ADVERSE REACTIONS:** Nausea, dyspepsia, diarrhea, vomiting, abdominal pain, increased appetite, asthenia, somnolence, infection, dizziness, tremor, weight gain, back pain, alopecia.

**INTERACTIONS:** Potentiates carbamazepine, amitriptyline, nortriptyline, diazepam, ethosuximide, primidone, lamotrigine, phenobarbital, phenytoin, tolbutamide, zidovudine, lorazepam. Efficacy potentiated by ASA, felbamate. Efficacy reduced by rifampin, carbamazepine, phenobarbital, phenytoin, primidone. Clonazepam may induce absence status in patients with history of absence type seizures. CNS depression with alcohol and other CNS depressants. Monitor PT/INR with warfarin.

**PREGNANCY:** Category D, not for use in nursing.

## DEPOCYT RX

cytarabine liposome (Enzon)

**Chemical arachnoiditis (eg, nausea, vomiting, headache, fever), a common adverse event, can be fatal if untreated. Treat concurrently with dexamethasone to reduce incidence and severity.**

**THERAPEUTIC CLASS:** Antimetabolite

**INDICATIONS:** Intrathecal treatment of lymphomatous meningitis.

**DOSAGE:** *Adults:* Induction: 50mg intrathecally every 14 days for 2 doses (weeks 1 and 3). Consolidation: 50mg intrathecally every 14 days for 3 doses (weeks 5, 7, and 9) followed by 1 additional dose at week 13. Maint: 50mg intrathecally every 28 days for 4 doses (weeks 17, 21, 25, and 29). Reduce to 25mg if drug-related neurotoxicity develops. Discontinue if toxicity persists.

**HOW SUPPLIED:** Inj: 10mg/mL

**CONTRAINDICATIONS:** Active meningeal infection.

**WARNINGS/PRECAUTIONS:** Intrathecal use of free cytarabine may cause myelopathy and other neurotoxicity. CSF blockage may increase free cytarabine levels and increase risk of neurotoxicity. Can cause fetal harm during pregnancy. Monitor for neurotoxicity. Anaphylactic reactions with IV free cytarabine. Transient elevations of CSF protein and WBC reported. Monitor hematopoietic system carefully.



**ADVERSE REACTIONS:** Chemical arachnoiditis (headache, fever, back pain, nausea, vomiting), confusion, somnolence, abnormal gait, peripheral edema, neutropenia, thrombocytopenia, urinary incontinence.

**INTERACTIONS:** Intrathecal cytarabine in combination with other chemotherapeutic agents or with cranial/spinal irradiation may increase risk of neurotoxicity and other adverse events.

**PREGNANCY:** Category D, not for use in nursing.

## DEPO-ESTRADIOL RX

estradiol cypionate (Pharmacia & Upjohn)

**Estrogens increase the risk of endometrial cancer. Estrogens, with or without progestins, should not be used for the prevention of cardiovascular disease or dementia. Increased risks of MI, stroke, invasive breast cancer, PE, and DVT in postmenopausal women (50-79 yrs of age) reported. Increased risk of developing probable dementia in postmenopausal women ≥65 yrs of age reported.**

**THERAPEUTIC CLASS:** Estrogen

**INDICATIONS:** Treatment of moderate to severe vasomotor symptoms associated with menopause and hypoestrogenism due to hypogonadism.

**DOSAGE:** *Adults:* Vasomotor Symptoms/Vaginal/Vulval Atrophy: 1-5mg IM every 3-4 weeks cyclically. Discontinue or taper at 3-6 month intervals. Hypoestrogenism: 1.5-2mg IM every month.

**HOW SUPPLIED:** Inj: 5mg/mL

**CONTRAINDICATIONS:** Pregnancy, undiagnosed abnormal genital bleeding, breast cancer, estrogen-dependent neoplasia, DVT/PE, active or recent (eg, within past year) arterial thromboembolic disease (eg, stroke, MI), liver dysfunction or disease.

**WARNINGS/PRECAUTIONS:** May increase risk of cardiovascular events (eg, MI, stroke), venous thrombosis, and PE; d/c immediately if any of these events occur or are suspected. May increase risk of breast/endometrial cancer, and gallbladder disease. May lead to severe hypercalcemia with breast cancer and bone metastases; monitor and d/c if hypercalcemia occurs. Retinal vascular thrombosis reported; monitor and d/c if papilledema or retinal vascular lesions occur. Consider addition of a progestin if no hysterectomy. May elevate BP; monitor at regular intervals. May cause elevations of plasma triglycerides with pre-existing hypertriglyceridemia. Caution with history of cholestatic jaundice associated with past estrogen use or with pregnancy; d/c with recurrence. May lead to increased thyroid-binding globulin levels; monitor thyroid function. May cause fluid retention; caution with cardiac/renal dysfunction. Caution with severe hypocalcemia. May increase risk of ovarian cancer. May exacerbate endometriosis, asthma, DM, epilepsy, migraine, porphyria, SLE, and hepatic hemangiomas; use with caution.

**ADVERSE REACTIONS:** Changes in vaginal bleeding pattern, breakthrough bleeding, vaginal candidiasis, breast tenderness/enlargement, nausea, vomiting, abdominal cramps, headache, migraine, dizziness, increase/decrease in weight.

**INTERACTIONS:** CYP3A4 inducers (eg, St. John's wort, phenobarbital, carbamazepine, rifampin) may decrease levels which may decrease therapeutic effects and/or change uterine bleeding profile. CYP3A4 inhibitors (eg, erythromycin, clarithromycin, ketoconazole, itraconazole, ritonavir, grapefruit juice) may increase levels which may result in side effects.

**PREGNANCY:** Contraindicated in pregnancy, caution in nursing.

# DEPO-MEDROL RX

methylprednisolone acetate (Pharmacia & Upjohn)



**THERAPEUTIC CLASS:** Glucocorticoid

**INDICATIONS:** Steroid responsive disorders.

**DOSAGE:** *Adults:* Local Effect: Rheumatoid/Osteoarthritis: Large Joint: 20-80mg. Medium Joint: 10-40mg. Small Joint: 4-10mg. Administer intra-articularly into synovial space every 1-5 weeks or more depending on relief. Ganglion/Tendinitis/Epicondylitis: 4-30mg into cyst/area of greatest tenderness. May repeat if necessary. Dermatologic Conditions: Inject 20-60mg into lesion. Distribute 20-40mg doses by repeated injections into large lesions. Usual: 1-4 injections. Systemic Effect: Substitute for Oral Therapy: IM dose should equal total daily PO methylprednisolone dose q24h. Prolonged Therapy: Administer weekly PO dose as single IM injection. Androgenital Syndrome: 40mg IM every 2 weeks. Rheumatoid Arthritis: 40-120mg IM weekly. Dermatologic Lesions: 40-120mg IM weekly for 1-4 weeks. Acute Severe Dermatitis (Poison Ivy): 80-120mg IM single dose. Chronic Contact Dermatitis: May repeat injections every 5-10 days. Seborrheic Dermatitis: 80mg IM weekly. Multiple Sclerosis: 200mg/day prednisolone for 1 week, then 80mg every other day for 1 month (4mg methylprednisolone=5mg prednisolone). Asthma/Allergic Rhinitis: 80-120mg IM.
*Pediatrics:* Use lower adult doses. Determine dose by severity of condition and response.

**HOW SUPPLIED:** Inj: 20mg/mL, 40mg/mL, 80mg/mL

**CONTRAINDICATIONS:** Intrathecal administration, systemic fungal infections.

**WARNINGS/PRECAUTIONS:** Dermal and subdermal atrophy reported; do not exceed recommended doses. May need to increase dose before, during, and after stressful situations. May mask signs of infection or cause new infections. Prolonged use may produce cataracts, glaucoma, secondary ocular infections. Increases BP, salt/water retention, potassium and calcium excretion. More severe/fatal course of infections reported with chickenpox, measles. Caution with Strongyloides, latent TB, hypothyroidism, cirrhosis, ocular herpes simplex, HTN, diverticulitis, fresh intestinal anastomoses, ulcerative colitis, osteoporosis, myasthenia gravis, renal insufficiency, peptic ulcer disease. Kaposi's sarcoma reported. Growth and development of children on prolonged therapy should be monitored. Monitor for psychic disturbances. Avoid abrupt withdrawal. Do not use intra-articularly, intrabursally, or for intratendinous administration in acute infection. Avoid injection into unstable and previously infected joints. Monitor urinalysis, blood sugar, BP, weight, chest x-ray, and upper GI x-ray (if ulcer history) regularly during prolonged therapy.

**ADVERSE REACTIONS:** Fluid and electrolyte disturbances, HTN, osteoporosis, muscle weakness, cushingoid state, menstrual irregularities, impaired wound healing, DM, ulcerative esophagitis, excessive sweating, increases intracranial pressure, carbohydrate intolerance, glaucoma, cataracts, urticaria, subcutaneous/cutaneous atrophy.

**INTERACTIONS:** Reduced efficacy with hepatic enzyme inducers (eg, phenobarbital, phenytoin, and rifampin). Increases clearance of chronic high dose ASA. Caution with ASA in hypoprothrombinemia. Effects on oral anticoagulants are variable; monitor PT. Increased insulin and oral hypoglycemic requirements in DM. Avoid live vaccines with immunosuppressive doses. Possible decreased vaccine response with killed or inactivated vaccines with immunosuppressive doses. Mutual inhibition of metabolism with cyclosporine; convulsions reported. Potentiated by ketoconazole and troleandomycin. Do not dilute or mix with other solutions.

**PREGNANCY:** Safety in pregnancy and nursing not known.

## DEPO-PROVERA RX

medroxyprogesterone acetate (Pharmacia & Upjohn)

**THERAPEUTIC CLASS:** Progestogen

**INDICATIONS:** Adjunct and palliative treatment of inoperable, recurrent, and metastatic endometrial or renal carcinoma.

**DOSAGE:** *Adults:* Initial: 400-1000mg IM weekly. Maint: 400mg/month if disease stabilizes and/or improves within a few weeks or months.

**HOW SUPPLIED:** Inj: 400mg/mL

**CONTRAINDICATIONS:** Pregnancy, undiagnosed vaginal bleeding, breast malignancy, thrombophlebitis, thromboembolic disorders, cerebral vascular disease, liver dysfunction.

**WARNINGS/PRECAUTIONS:** Avoid during 1st 4 months of pregnancy. May cause thromboembolic disorders, ocular disorders, fluid retention. Caution with depression, family history of breast cancer or patients with breast nodules. May mask the onset of climacteric.

**ADVERSE REACTIONS:** Menstrual irregularities, nervousness, dizziness, edema, weight changes, cervical changes, cholestatic jaundice, breast tenderness, galactorrhea, rash, acne, alopecia, hirsutism, depression, pyrexia, fatigue, insomnia, nausea.

**INTERACTIONS:** Aminoglutethimide may decrease serum levels. Caution with estrogen.

**PREGNANCY:** Safety in pregnancy and nursing not known.

## DEPO-PROVERA CONTRACEPTIVE RX

medroxyprogesterone acetate (Pharmacia & Upjohn)

**May cause significant loss of bone mineral density (BMD); greater with increasing duration of use and may not be completely reversible. Should be used as long-term birth control (>2yrs) only if other birth control methods are inadequate. Unknown if use during adolescence or early adulthood will reduce peak bone mass and increase risk of osteoporotic fractures in later life.**

**THERAPEUTIC CLASS:** Progestogen

**INDICATIONS:** Prevention of pregnancy.

**DOSAGE:** *Adults:* 150mg IM every 3 months (13 weeks) in gluteal or deltoid muscle. Give 1st injection during 1st 5 days of menses; within 1st 5 days postpartum if not nursing; or 6 weeks postpartum if nursing.

**HOW SUPPLIED:** Inj: 150mg/mL

**CONTRAINDICATIONS:** Pregnancy, undiagnosed vaginal bleeding, breast malignancy, thrombophlebitis, thromboembolic disorders, cerebral vascular disease, liver dysfunction.

**WARNINGS/PRECAUTIONS:** Loss of BMD, may cause bleeding irregularities, cancer risk, thromboembolic disorders, ocular disorders, unexpected pregnancies, ectopic pregnancy, anaphylaxis and anaphylactoid reaction, fluid retention, return of fertility, decrease in glucose metabolism. Caution with CNS or convulsive disorders. D/C if jaundice develops.

**ADVERSE REACTIONS:** Menstrual irregularities, weight changes, abdominal pain, dizziness, headache, asthenia, nervousness, decreased libido, depression, nausea, insomnia, leukorrhea, acne, vaginitis, pelvic pain.

**INTERACTIONS:** Aminoglutethimide may decrease serum levels.

**PREGNANCY:** Category X, safety in nursing not known.

## DEPO-SUBQ PROVERA 104

RX

medroxyprogesterone acetate (Pharmacia & Upjohn)

**May cause significant loss of bone mineral density (BMD); greater with increasing duration of use and may not be completely reversible. Should be used as long-term birth control (>2yrs) only if other birth control methods are inadequate. Unknown if use during adolescence or early adulthood will reduce peak bone mass and increase risk of osteoporotic fractures in later life.**



**THERAPEUTIC CLASS:** Progestogen

**INDICATIONS:** Prevention of pregnancy. Management of endometriosis-associated pain.

**DOSAGE:** *Adults:* 104mg SQ once every 3 months in the anterior thigh or abdomen. Give 1st injection during 1st 5 days of menses or 6 weeks postpartum if nursing.

**HOW SUPPLIED:** Inj: 104mg/0.65mL

**CONTRAINDICATIONS:** Pregnancy, undiagnosed vaginal bleeding, breast malignancy, thrombophlebitis, thromboembolic disorders, cerebral vascular disease, liver dysfunction.

**WARNINGS/PRECAUTIONS:** Loss of BMD, may cause bleeding irregularities, cancer risk, thromboembolic disorders, ocular disorders, unexpected pregnancies, ectopic pregnancy, anaphylaxis and anaphylactoid reaction, fluid retention, return of fertility, decrease in glucose metabolism. Caution with CNS or convulsive disorders. D/C if jaundice develops.

**ADVERSE REACTIONS:** Uterine bleeding irregularities, increased weight, decreased libido, acne, injection site reactions, headache, amenorrhea.

**INTERACTIONS:** Amioglutethimide may decrease serum levels.

**PREGNANCY:** Not for use in pregnancy, safety in nursing not known.

## DEPO-TESTOSTERONE

CIII

testosterone cypionate (Pharmacia & Upjohn)

**THERAPEUTIC CLASS:** Androgen

**INDICATIONS:** Testosterone replacement in males with primary hypogonadism and hypogonadotropic hypogonadism.

**DOSAGE:** *Adults:* Male Hypogonadism: 50-400mg IM every 2-4 weeks. Dose based on age, sex, and diagnosis. Adjust dose according to response and adverse reactions.
*Pediatrics:* >12 yrs: Male Hypogonadism: 50-400mg IM every 2-4 weeks. Dose based on age, sex, and diagnosis. Adjust dose according to response and adverse reactions.

**HOW SUPPLIED:** Inj: 100mg/mL, 200mg/mL

**CONTRAINDICATIONS:** Severe renal, hepatic and cardiac disease. Males with carcinoma of the breast or prostate gland. Pregnancy.

**WARNINGS/PRECAUTIONS:** May accelerate bone maturation without linear growth; monitor bone growth every 6 months. Risk of hepatic damage with long-term use. Discontinue if hypercalcemia occurs in immobilized patients. Discontinue with acute urethral obstruction, priapism, excessive sexual stimulation, or oligospermia; restart at lower doses. Risk of edema; caution with pre-existing cardiac, renal or hepatic disease. Caution in the elderly; increased risk of prostatic hypertrophy and prostatic carcinoma. Caution with BPH. Should not be used for enhancement of athletic performance. Do not administer IV. Monitor Hct, Hgb, cholesterol periodically.

**ADVERSE REACTIONS:** Gynecomastia, excessive frequency/duration of penile erections, male pattern baldness, increased/decreased libido, oligospermia, hirsutism, acne, fluid and electrolyte disturbances, nausea, hypercholesterolemia, clotting factor suppression, polycythemia, altered LFTs, priapism, anxiety, depression.

**INTERACTIONS:** Potentiates oral anticoagulants (eg, warfarin) and oxyphenbutazone. May decrease blood glucose and insulin requirements in diabetics.

**PREGNANCY:** Category X, not for use in nursing.



## Derma-Smoothe/FS RX

fluocinolone acetonide (Hill Dermaceuticals)

**THERAPEUTIC CLASS:** Corticosteroid

**INDICATIONS:** Treatment of atopic dermatitis and scalp psoriasis.

**DOSAGE:** *Adults:* Atopic Dermatitis: Apply tid. Scalp Psoriasis: Wet/dampen hair and scalp thoroughly. Massage into scalp and cover with shower cap. Wash hair with regular shampoo after minimum of 4 hrs and rinse thoroughly.
*Pediatrics:* Atopic Dermatitis: >2 yrs: Moisten skin and apply bid up to 4 weeks.

**HOW SUPPLIED:** Oil: 0.01% [120mL]

**WARNINGS/PRECAUTIONS:** May produce reversible HPA axis suppression, manifestations of Cushing's syndrome, hyperglycemia, and glucosuria. Pediatrics may be more susceptible to systemic toxicity. Use appropriate antifungal or antibacterial agent with dermatological infections. Contains refined peanut oil NF. Discontinue if develop hypersensitivity. Avoid face, diaper area, and intertriginous areas with pediatrics.

**ADVERSE REACTIONS:** Dryness, folliculitis, acneiform eruptions, perioral dermatitis, allergic contact dermatitis, secondary infections, skin atrophy, striae, miliaria, burning, itching, irritation, hypopigmentation.

**PREGNANCY:** Category C, caution in nursing.

## Dermatop RX

prednicarbate (Dermik)

**THERAPEUTIC CLASS:** Corticosteroid (medium-potency)

**INDICATIONS:** Corticosteroid responsive dermatoses.

**DOSAGE:** *Adults:* (Cre, Oint) Apply bid.
*Pediatrics:* >1 yr: (Cre) Apply bid. Max: 3 weeks of therapy. >10 yrs: (Oint) Apply bid.

**HOW SUPPLIED:** Cre, Oint: 0.1% [15g, 60g]

**WARNINGS/PRECAUTIONS:** May produce reversible HPA axis suppression, manifestations of Cushing's syndrome, hyperglycemia, and glucosuria. D/C if irritation occurs. Use appropriate antifungal or antibacterial agent with dermatological infections. Pediatrics may be more susceptible to systemic toxicity. Re-evaluate if no improvement after 2 weeks. Avoid eyes, occlusive dressings. Not for treatment of diaper dermatitis.

**ADVERSE REACTIONS:** Stinging, burning, dry skin, pruritus, urticaria, allergic contact dermatitis, edema, paresthesia, rash, skin atrophy.

**PREGNANCY:** Category C, caution in nursing.

## Desferal RX

deferoxamine mesylate (Novartis)

**THERAPEUTIC CLASS:** Iron-chelating agent

**INDICATIONS:** Treatment of acute iron intoxication and of chronic iron overload due to transfusion-dependent anemias.

**DOSAGE:** *Adults:* See labeling for solution preparation. Iron Intoxication: IM preferred for all patients not in shock. Only use IV slow infusion with cardiovascular collapse, and do not exceed 15mg/kg/hr for the 1st 1g. Subsequent IV dosing should not exceed 125mg/hr. IM: Initial: 1g, then 500mg q4h for 2 doses. Give subsequent 500mg doses q4-12h depending upon clinical response. Max: 6g/24 hrs. IV: 1g, then 500mg over 4 hrs for 2 doses. Give subsequent 500mg doses over 4-12 hrs depending upon clinical response. Max: 6g/24 hrs. Iron Overload: IM: 500mg-1g/day IM. In addition, 2g IV per unit of blood transfused; not to exceed 15mg/kg/hr. Max: 1g without transfusion or 6g even with >3 units of blood or PRBC. SQ: 1-2g (20-40mg/kg/day) SQ over 8-24 hrs using small pump for continuous infusion. Individualize duration.



*Pediatrics:* >3 yrs: See labeling for solution preparation. Iron Intoxication: IM preferred for all patients not in shock. Only use IV slow infusion with cardiovascular collapse, and do not exceed 15mg/kg/hr for the 1st 1g. Subsequent IV dosing should not exceed 125mg/hr. IM: Initial: 1g, then 500mg q4h for 2 doses. Give subsequent 500mg doses q4-12h depending upon clinical response. Max: 6g/24 hrs. IV: 1g, then 500mg over 4 hrs for 2 doses. Give subsequent 500mg doses over 4-12 hrs depending upon clinical response. Max: 6g/24 hrs. Iron Overload: IM: 500mg-1g/day IM. In addition, 2g IV per unit of blood transfused; not to exceed 15mg/kg/hr. Max: 1g without transfusion or 6g even with >3 units of blood or PRBC. SQ: 1-2g (20-40mg/kg/day) SQ over 8-24 hrs using small pump for continuous infusion. Individualize duration.

**HOW SUPPLIED:** Inj: 500mg, 2g

**CONTRAINDICATIONS:** Severe renal disease, anuria.

**WARNINGS/PRECAUTIONS:** Ocular and auditory disturbances reported with prolonged use, high doses, or low ferritin levels. Periodic visual acuity tests, slit-lamp exams, funduscopy, and audiometry with prolonged treatment. High doses with low ferritin levels associated with growth retardation. Adult respiratory distress syndrome, also in children, reported after high IV doses in acute iron intoxication or thalassemia. Give IM, slow SQ, or IV infusion; skin flushing, urticaria, hypotension, and shock reported with rapid IV injection. High dose may exacerbate neurological dysfunction in aluminum-related encephalopathy. May precipitate onset of dialysis dementia. Aluminum overload with deferoxamine may decrease serum calcium and aggravate hyperparathyroidism. D/C with mucormycosis, *Yersinia enterocolitica* or *Yersinia pseudotuberculosis* infections. Monitor pediatrics body weight and growth every 3 months. Caution in elderly patients.

**ADVERSE REACTIONS:** Injection site reactions, hypersensitivity reactions, tachycardia, hypotension, shock, abdominal discomfort, diarrhea, nausea, vomiting, blood dyscrasia, leg cramps, growth retardation, bone changes, reddish urine.

**INTERACTIONS:** Cardiac dysfunction reported with high dose vitamin C (>500mg/day in adults) in patients with severe chronic iron overload; avoid vitamin C supplements in cardiac failure patients. Only give vitamin C after 1 month of deferoxamine therapy and monitor cardiac function. Do not exceed vitamin C 200mg/day in adults; 50mg/day for pediatrics <10 yrs and 100mg/day for older children usually suffices. Concurrent prochlorperazine may lead to temporary impairment of consciousness. May distort imaging results with gallium-67; discontinue deferoxamine 48 hrs before scintigraphy.

**PREGNANCY:** Category C, caution in nursing.

## DESMOPRESSIN ACETATE — RX

desmopressin acetate (Ferring)

**THERAPEUTIC CLASS:** Synthetic vasopressin analog

**INDICATIONS:** Management of primary nocturnal enuresis, central cranial diabetes insipidus and temporary polyuria and polydipsia following head trauma or surgery.

**DOSAGE:** *Adults:* Central Cranial Diabetes Insipidus: 0.1-0.4mL/day as single dose or divided into 2-3 doses.
*Pediatrics:* Primary Nocturnal Enuresis: ≥6 yrs: 20mcg intranasally hs.

Administer 1/2 the dose into each nostril. Max: 40mcg/day. Central Cranial Diabetes Insipidus: >12 yrs: 0.1-0.4mL/day as single dose or divided into 2-3 doses. 3 months-12 yrs: 0.05-0.3mL/day as single dose or divided into 2-3 doses.

**HOW SUPPLIED:** Sol: 0.01% [5mL]

**WARNINGS/PRECAUTIONS:** For intranasal use only. Adjust fluid intake downward in order to decrease the potential for water intoxication and hyponatremia. May increase BP, caution in coronary insufficiency and cardiovascular disease. Caution in fluid and electrolyte imbalance. Anaphylaxis reported. Changes in the nasal mucosa may cause erratic absorption, use IV administration in these cases.

**ADVERSE REACTIONS:** Transient headache, nausea, nasal congestion, rhinitis, flushing, abdominal cramps, nosebleed, sore throat, cough, upper respiratory tract infection, water intoxication, hyponatremia, asthenia, dizziness, epistaxis, GI disorder, conjunctivitis, edema lachrymation disorder.

**INTERACTIONS:** Caution with pressor agents.

**PREGNANCY:** Category B, caution in nursing.

## DESOGEN RX

desogestrel - ethinyl estradiol (Organon)

**OTHER BRAND NAMES:** Apri (Duramed)

**THERAPEUTIC CLASS:** Estrogen/progestogen combination

**INDICATIONS:** Prevention of pregnancy.

**DOSAGE:** *Adults:* Start 1st Sunday after onset of menstruation or 1st day of menstruation. 1 tab qd for 28 days continuously, then repeat.

**HOW SUPPLIED:** Tab: (Ethinyl Estradiol-Desogestrel) 0.03mg-0.15mg

**CONTRAINDICATIONS:** Thrombophlebitis, DVT or thromboembolic disorders, pregnancy, cerebrovascular or coronary artery disease, undiagnosed abnormal genital bleeding, cholestatic jaundice of pregnancy or jaundice with prior pill use, hepatic adenomas or carcinomas, breast cancer or other estrogen-dependent neoplasia.

**WARNINGS/PRECAUTIONS:** Cigarette smoking increases risk of serious cardiovascular side effects. This risk increases with age (especially >35 yrs) and heavy smoking. Increased risk of MI, vascular disease, thromboembolism, stroke and gallbladder disease. Retinal thrombosis, hepatic neoplasia, carcinoma of breast and reproductive organs reported. May cause glucose intolerance. May increase BP, elevate LDL levels or cause other lipid changes, fluid retention, breakthrough bleeding, and spotting. May cause or exacerbate migraine. May develop visual changes with contact lens. Increased risk of MI with HTN, hyperlipidemia, obesity, and diabetes. D/C if jaundice, significant depression or ophthalmic irregularities develop. Perform annual physical exam. Use before menarche is not indicated. May affect certain endocrine, LFTs and blood components.

**ADVERSE REACTIONS:** Nausea, vomiting, breakthrough bleeding, spotting, amenorrhea, migraine, depression, vaginal candidiasis, edema, weight changes.

**INTERACTIONS:** Reduced effects, increased breakthrough bleeding, and menstrual irregularities with rifampin, barbiturates, phenylbutazone, phenytoin, and possibly with griseofulvin, ampicillin, and tetracyclines.

**PREGNANCY:** Category X, not for use in nursing.

## DESONATE RX

desonide (SkinMedica)

**THERAPEUTIC CLASS:** Corticosteroid

**INDICATIONS:** Mild to moderate atopic dermatitis.

**DOSAGE:** *Adults*: Apply thin layer bid to affected area and rub in gently. Not recommended beyond 4 consecutive weeks.
*Pediatrics*: ≥3 months: Apply a thin layer bid to the affected area and rub in gently. Not recommended beyond 4 consecutive weeks.

**HOW SUPPLIED:** Gel: 0.05% [15g, 30g, 60g]

**WARNINGS/PRECAUTIONS:** May produce reversible HPA axis suppression, manifestations of Cushing's syndrome, hyperglycemia, and glucosuria. Discontinue if irritation occurs. Pediatrics may be more susceptible to systemic toxicity. Caution when applied to large surface areas. Avoid occlusive dressings. Avoid use beyond 4 wks.

**ADVERSE REACTIONS:** Burning, rash, application site pruritus.

**PREGNANCY:** Category C, caution in nursing.



## DESOWEN

desonide (Galderma) RX

**THERAPEUTIC CLASS:** Corticosteroid

**INDICATIONS:** Corticosteroid responsive dermatoses.

**DOSAGE:** *Adults:* Apply bid-tid, depending on severity. Reassess if no improvement after 2 weeks.

**HOW SUPPLIED:** Cre, Oint: 0.05% [15g, 60g]; Lot: 0.05% [60mL, 120mL]

**WARNINGS/PRECAUTIONS:** May produce reversible HPA axis suppression, manifestations of Cushing's syndrome, hyperglycemia, and glucosuria. D/C if irritation occurs. Use appropriate antifungal or antibacterial agent with dermatological infections. Peds may be more susceptible to systemic toxicity. Caution when applied to large surface areas. Avoid occlusive dressings.

**ADVERSE REACTIONS:** Stinging, burning, irritation, erythema, contact dermatitis, worsening condition, skin peeling, dryness/scaliness.

**PREGNANCY:** Category C, caution in nursing.

## DESOXYN

methamphetamine HCl (Ovation) CII

**High potential for abuse. Avoid prolonged therapy in obesity.**

**THERAPEUTIC CLASS:** Sympathomimetic amine

**INDICATIONS:** Attention deficit disorder with hyperactivity. Short term adjunct to treat exogenous obesity.

**DOSAGE:** *Adults:* Obesity: 5mg, 1/2 hr before each meal. Do not exceed a few weeks of treatment.
*Pediatrics:* ADHD: >6 yrs: Initial: 5mg qd-bid. Titrate: Increase weekly by 5mg/day until optimum response. Usual: 20-25mg/day given bid. Obesity: >12 yrs: 5mg, 1/2 hr before each meal. Do not exceed a few weeks of treatment.

**HOW SUPPLIED:** Tab: 5mg

**CONTRAINDICATIONS:** Advanced arteriosclerosis, symptomatic cardiovascular disease, moderate to severe HTN, hyperthyroidism, glaucoma, agitated states, history of drug abuse, during or within 14 days of MAOI use.

**WARNINGS/PRECAUTIONS:** Tolerance to anorectic effect develops within a few weeks, do not exceed recommended dose to increase effect. Monitor growth in children. Caution with HTN. Do not use to combat fatigue or replace rest. Exacerbation of motor and phonic tics and Tourette's syndrome. May exacerbate behavior disturbance and thought disorder in psychotic pediatrics. Interrupt occasionally to determine if patient requires continued therapy.

**ADVERSE REACTIONS:** BP elevation, tachycardia, palpitation, dizziness, insomnia, tremor, diarrhea, constipation, dry mouth, urticaria, impotence, changes in libido.

**INTERACTIONS:** May alter insulin requirements. May decrease hypotensive effect of guanethidine. Avoid MAOIs. Caution with TCAs and indirect acting sympathomimetic amines. Antagonized by phenothiazines.

**PREGNANCY:** Category C, not for use in nursing.



## DETROL LA RX

tolterodine tartrate (Pharmacia & Upjohn)

**OTHER BRAND NAMES:** Detrol (Pharmacia & Upjohn)

**THERAPEUTIC CLASS:** Muscarinic antagonist

**INDICATIONS:** Treatment of overactive bladder with symptoms of urinary frequency, urgency or urge incontinence.

**DOSAGE:** *Adults:* (LA Cap) Usual: 4mg qd, may lower to 2mg. (Tab) Initial: 2mg bid, may lower to 1mg bid. (LA Cap, Tab) Significant Hepatic/Renal Dysfunction/Concomitant CYP3A4 Inhibitors: 1mg bid or 2mg LA cap qd.

**HOW SUPPLIED:** Cap, Extended-Release: 2mg, 4mg; Tab: 1mg, 2mg

**CONTRAINDICATIONS:** Urinary retention, gastric retention, uncontrolled narrow-angle glaucoma.

**WARNINGS/PRECAUTIONS:** Risk of urinary retention with significant bladder outflow obstruction and risk of gastric retention with GI obstructive disorders. Caution with renal impairment and narrow-angle glaucoma. Reduce dose with significant hepatic or renal dysfunction. May cause blurred vision, drowsiness, or dizziness.

**ADVERSE REACTIONS:** Dry mouth, dizziness, headache, abdominal pain, constipation, diarrhea, dyspepsia, fatigue, somnolence, aggravation of symptoms of dementia reproted.

**INTERACTIONS:** Reduce dose with concomitant CYP3A4 inhibitors (eg, erythromycin, clarithromycin, ketoconazole, itraconazole, and miconazole).

**PREGNANCY:** Category C, not for use in nursing.

## DEXAMETHASONE RX

dexamethasone (Various)

**OTHER BRAND NAMES:** Decadron (Merck)

**THERAPEUTIC CLASS:** Glucocorticoid

**INDICATIONS:** Treatment of steroid responsive disorders.

**DOSAGE:** *Adults:* Individualize for disease and patient response. Withdraw gradually. (Tab) Initial: 0.75-9mg/day PO. Maint: Decrease in small amounts to lowest effective dose. Cushing's Syndrome Test: 1mg PO at 11pm; draw blood at 8am next morning. Or, 0.5mg PO q6h for 48 hrs; or 2mg (to distinguish if excess pituitary ACTH or other causes) PO q6h for 48 hrs; obtain 24 hr urine collections. (Inj) Initial: 0.5-9mg/day IV/IM. Cerebral Edema: Initial: 10mg IV, then 4mg IM q6h until edema subsides. Reduce dose after 2-4 days and gradually discontinue over 5-7 days. Palliative Management of Recurrent/Inoperable Brain Tumors: Maint: 2mg IV/PO bid-tid. Acute Allergic Disorders: 4-8mg IM on 1st day, then 1.5mg PO bid for 2 days, then 0.75mg PO bid for 1 day, then 0.75mg PO qd for 2 days. (Inj) Usual: 0.2-9mg. Maint: Decrease in small amounts to lowest effective dose. Intra-Articular/Intralesional/Soft Tissue Injection: Usual: 0.2-6mg once every 3-5 days to once every 2-3 weeks. See labeling for Shock Treatment. Take with meals and antacids to prevent peptic ulcer.
*Pediatrics:* Individualize for disease and patient response. Withdraw gradually. (Tab) Initial: 0.75-9mg/day PO. Maint: Decrease in small amounts to lowest effective dose. Cushing's Syndrome Test: 1mg PO at 11pm; draw blood at 8am next morning. Or, 0.5mg PO q6h for 48 hrs; or 2mg (to distinguish if excess pituitary ATCH or other causes) PO q6h for 48 hrs; obtain 24 hr urine collections. (Inj) Initial: 0.5-9mg/day IV/IM. Cerebral Edema: Initial: 10mg IV,

then 4mg IM q6h until edema subsides. Reduce dose after 2-4 days and gradually discontinue over 5-7 days. Palliative Management of Recurrent/Inoperable Brain Tumors: Maint: 2mg IV/PO bid-tid. Acute Allergic Disorders: 4-8mg IM on 1st day, then 1.5mg PO bid for 2 days, then 0.75mg PO bid for 1 day, then 0.75mg PO qd for 2 days. (Inj) Usual: 0.2-9mg. Maint: Decrease in small amounts to lowest effective dose. Intra-Articular/Intralesional/Soft Tissue Injection: Usual: 0.2-6mg once every 3-5 days to once every 2-3 weeks. See labeling for shock treatment. Take with meals and antacids to prevent peptic ulcer.

**HOW SUPPLIED:** Inj: (Dexamethasone Sodium Phosphate) 4mg/mL, 10mg/mL; Sol: (Dexamethasone) 0.5mg/5mL, 1mg/mL; Tab: (Dexamethasone) 0.5mg*, 0.75mg*, 1mg*, 1.5mg*, 2mg*, 4mg*, 6mg* *scored

**CONTRAINDICATIONS:** Systemic fungal infections.

**WARNINGS/PRECAUTIONS:** Increase dose before, during, and after stressful situations. Avoid abrupt withdrawal. May mask signs of infection, activate latent amebiasis, elevate BP, cause salt/water retention, increase excretion of potassium and calcium. Prolonged use may produce cataracts, glaucoma, secondary ocular infections. Caution with recent MI, ocular herpes simplex, emotional instability, nonspecific ulcerative colitis, diverticulitis, peptic ulcer, renal insufficiency, HTN, osteoporosis, myasthenia gravis, threadworm infection, active tuberculosis. Enhanced effect with hypothyroidism, cirrhosis. Consider prophylactic therapy if exposed to measles or chickenpox. Risk of glaucoma, cataracts and eye infections. False negative dexamethasone suppression test with indomethacin.

**ADVERSE REACTIONS:** Fluid/electrolyte disturbances, muscle weakness, osteoporosis, peptic ulcer, pancreatitis, ulcerative esophagitis, impaired wound healing, headache, psychic disturbances, growth suppression (children), glaucoma, hyperglycemia, weight gain, nausea, malaise.

**INTERACTIONS:** Caution with ASA. Inducers of CYP3A4 (eg, phenytoin, phenobarbital, carbamazepine, rifampin) and ephedrine enhance clearance; increase steroid dose. Inhibitors of CYP3A4 (ketoconazole, macrolides) may increase plasma levels. Drugs that affect metabolism may interfere with dexamethasone suppression tests. Increased clearance of drugs metabolized by CYP3A4 (eg, indinavir, erythromycin). May increase or decrease phenytoin levels. Ketoconazole may inhibit adrenal corticosteroid synthesis and cause adrenal insufficiency during corticosteroid withdrawal. Antagonizes or potentiates coumarins. Hypokalemia with potassium-depleting diuretics. Live virus vaccines are contraindicated with immunosuppressive doses.

**PREGNANCY:** Safety in pregnancy not known, not for use in nursing.

## DEXEDRINE **CII**

dextroamphetamine sulfate (GlaxoSmithKline)

**High potential for abuse. Avoid prolonged use. Misuse may cause sudden death and serious CV adverse events.**

**OTHER BRAND NAMES:** Dexedrine Spansules (GlaxoSmithKline)

**THERAPEUTIC CLASS:** Sympathomimetic amine

**INDICATIONS:** Treatment of attention deficit disorder with hyperactivity (ADHD) and narcolepsy.

**DOSAGE:** *Adults:* Narcolepsy: Initial: 10mg/day. Titrate: May increase by 10mg/day every week. Usual: 5-60mg/day. For tabs, give 1st dose upon awakening and additional every 4-6 hrs. May give caps once daily. *Pediatrics:* Narcolepsy: 6-12 yrs: Initial: 5mg qd. Titrate: Increase weekly by 5mg/day. >12 yrs: Initial: 10mg qd. Titrate: Increase weekly by 10mg/day. Usual: 5-60mg/day in divided doses. ADHD: Initial: 3-5 yrs: 2.5mg qd. Titrate: Increase weekly by 2.5mg/day. >6 yrs: 5mg qd-bid. Titrate: Increase weekly by 5mg/day. Max: 40mg/day. For tabs, give 1st dose upon awakening and additional every 4-6 hrs. May give caps once daily.

D

**HOW SUPPLIED:** Cap, Extended-Release: (Spansules) 5mg, 10mg, 15mg; Tab: 5mg* *scored

**CONTRAINDICATIONS:** Advanced arteriosclerosis, symptomatic cardiovascular disease, moderate to severe HTN, hyperthyroidism, glaucoma, agitated states, history of drug abuse, during or within 14 days of MAOI use.

**WARNINGS/PRECAUTIONS:** May exacerbate symptoms of behavior disturbance and thought disorder in psychotic patients. Caution when using stimulants to treat patients with comorbid bipolar disorder because of concern for possible induction of mixed/manic episode in such patients. Stimulants at usual doses can cause treatment emergent psychotic or manic symptoms (eg, hallucinations, delusional thinking, mania) in children and adolescents without prior history of psychotic illness. Aggressive behavior or hostility reported in clinical trials and the postmarketing experience of some medications indicated for the treatment of ADHD. Caution with HTN. Tablets contain tartrazine; may cause allergy reactions. Exacerbation of motor and phonic tics and Tourette's syndrome. Monitor growth in children. Avoid with serious structural cardiac abnormalities, cardiomyopathy, serious heart rhythm abnormalities, CAD, or other serious cardiac problems. Avoid use in the presence of seizure. Visual disturbances reported with stimulant treatment.

**ADVERSE REACTIONS:** Palpitations, tachycardia, BP elevation, CNS overstimulation, restlessness, insomnia, dry mouth, GI disturbances, anorexia, urticaria, impotence.

**INTERACTIONS:** GI acidifying agents (guanethidine, reserpine, glutamic acid, etc.) and urinary acidifying agents (ammonium chloride, etc) decrease efficacy. MAOIs may cause hypertensive crisis. Potentiated by GI and urinary alkalinizers, propoxyphene overdose. Potentiated effects of both agents with TCAs. May delay absorption of phenytoin, ethosuximide, phenobarbital. Potentiates meperidine, norepinephrine, phenobarbital, phenytoin. Antagonized by haloperidol, chlorpromazine, lithium. Antagonizes adrenergic blockers, antihistamines, antihypertensives, veratrum alkaloids (antihypertensive).

**PREGNANCY:** Category C, not for use in nursing.

## DEXTROSTAT CII

dextroamphetamine sulfate (Shire US)

**High potential for abuse. Avoid prolonged use.**

**THERAPEUTIC CLASS:** Sympathomimetic amine

**INDICATIONS:** Treatment of narcolepsy and attention deficit disorder with hyperactivity (ADHD).

**DOSAGE:** *Adults:* Narcolepsy: Initial: 10mg/day. Titrate: May increase by 10mg/day every week. Usual: 5-60mg/day. Give 1st dose upon awakening, and additional doses every 4-6 hrs.
*Pediatrics:* Narcolepsy: 6-12 yrs: Initial: 5mg/day. Titrate: Increase weekly by 5mg/day. >12 yrs: Initial: 10mg/day. Titrate: Increase weekly by 10mg/day. Usual: 5-60mg/day in divided doses. ADHD: 3-5 yrs: Initial: 2.5mg/day. Titrate: Increase weekly by 2.5mg/day until optimum response. 6-16 yrs: Initial 5mg qd-bid. Titrate: Increase weekly by 5mg/day optimum response. Give 1st dose upon awakening, and additional doses q4-6h.

**HOW SUPPLIED:** Tab: 5mg*, 10mg* *scored

**CONTRAINDICATIONS:** Advanced arteriosclerosis, symptomatic cardiovascular disease, moderate to severe HTN, hyperthyroidism, glaucoma, agitated states, history of drug abuse, during or within 14 days of MAOI use.

**WARNINGS/PRECAUTIONS:** Caution in HTN. Contains tartrazine, may cause allergic reactions. Exacerbation of motor and phonic tics and Tourette's syndrome. May exacerbate behavior disturbance and thought disorder in psychotic pediatrics. Interrupt occasionally to determine if patient requires continued therapy. Monitor growth in children.

**ADVERSE REACTIONS:** BP elevation, tachycardia, palpitation, dizziness, insomnia, tremor, diarrhea, constipation, dry mouth, urticaria, impotence, changes in libido.

**INTERACTIONS:** GI acidifying agents (guanethidine, reserpine, glutamic acid, etc.) and urinary acidifying agents (ammonium chloride, etc.) decrease efficacy. MAOIs may cause hypertensive crisis. Potentiated by GI and urinary alkalinizers, propoxyphene overdose. Potentiated effects of both agents with TCAs. May delay absorption of phenytoin, ethosuximide, phenobarbital. Potentiates meperidine, norepinephrine, phenobarbital, phenytoin. Antagonized by haloperidol, chlorpromazine, lithium. Antagonizes adrenergic blockers, antihistamines, antihypertensives, veratrum alkaloids (antihypertensive).

**PREGNANCY:** Category C, not for use in nursing.



## DHT

dihydrotachysterol (Roxane) RX

**THERAPEUTIC CLASS:** Vitamin D analog

**INDICATIONS:** Treatment of acute, chronic, and latent forms of postoperative tetany, idiopathic tetany, and hypoparathyroidism.

**DOSAGE:** *Adults:* Initial: 0.8-2.4mg qd for several days. Maint: 0.2-1mg qd (average 0.6mg qd). Individualize dose and evaluate periodically.

**HOW SUPPLIED:** Tab: 0.125mg, 0.2mg, 0.4mg; Sol (Intensol): 0.2mg/mL [30mL]

**CONTRAINDICATIONS:** Hypercalcemia, abnormal sensitivity to the effects of Vitamin D, and hypervitaminosis D.

**WARNINGS/PRECAUTIONS:** Maintain normal serum phosphorous with renal osteodystrophy accompanied by hyperphosphatemia by using dietary phosphate restrictions and/or administration of phosphate binders. Caution in pregnancy or with renal stones. Monitor serum calcium regularly. Effects can persist for up to 1 month after discontinuation.

**INTERACTIONS:** Thiazide diuretics may cause hypercalcemia.

**PREGNANCY:** Category C, caution in nursing.

## DiaBeta

glyburide (Sanofi-Aventis) RX

**THERAPEUTIC CLASS:** Sulfonylurea (2nd generation)

**INDICATIONS:** Adjunct to diet and exercise, to improve glycemic control in type 2 diabetes mellitus.

**DOSAGE:** *Adults:* Initial: 2.5-5mg qd with breakfast or first main meal; give 1.25mg if sensitive to hypoglycemia. Titrate: Increase by no more than 2.5mg/day at weekly intervals. Maint: 1.25-20mg given qd or in divided doses. Max: 20mg/day. May give bid with >10mg/day. Renal/Hepatic Disease, Elderly, Debilitated, Malnourished, Adrenal or Pituitary Insufficiency: Initial: 1.25mg qd. Transfer From Other Oral Antidiabetic Agents: Initial: 2.5-5mg/day. Switch From Insulin: If >40U/day, decrease dose by 50% and give 5mg qd. Titrate: Progressive withdrawal of insulin and increase by 1.25-2.5mg/day every 2-10 days.

**HOW SUPPLIED:** Tab: 1.25mg*, 2.5mg*, 5mg* *scored

**CONTRAINDICATIONS:** Diabetic ketoacidosis.

**WARNINGS/PRECAUTIONS:** Increased risk of cardiovascular mortality. Risk of hypoglycemia, especially with renal and hepatic disease, elderly, debilitated or malnourished patients, and those with adrenal or pituitary insufficiency. May need to d/c and give insulin with stress (eg, fever, trauma). Secondary failure may occur. D/C if jaundice, hepatitis, or persistent skin reaction occur. Hematologic reactions and hyponatremia reported.

**ADVERSE REACTIONS:** Hypoglycemia, nausea, epigastric fullness, heartburn, allergic skin reactions, disulfiram-like reactions (rarely), hyponatremia, liver function abnormalities, photosensitivity reactions.



**INTERACTIONS:** Potentiated hypoglycemia with alcohol, NSAIDs, miconazole, fluoroquinolones, highly protein bound drugs, salicylates, sulfonamides, chloramphenicol, probenecid, coumarins, MAOIs, and β-blockers. Risk of hyperglycemia with diuretics, corticosteroids, phenothiazines, thyroid products, estrogens, oral contraceptives, phenytoin, nicotinic acid, sympathomimetics, calcium channel blockers, and INH. β-blockers may mask hypoglycemia. Increased or decreased coumarin effects. Disulfiram-like reactions (rarely) with alcohol.

**PREGNANCY:** Category C, not for use in nursing.

## DIABINESE RX

chlorpropamide (Pfizer)

**THERAPEUTIC CLASS:** Sulfonylurea (1st generation)

**INDICATIONS:** Adjunct to diet and exercise, to improve glycemic control in type 2 diabetes mellitus.

**DOSAGE:** *Adults:* Initial: 250mg qd. Titrate: After 5-7 days, adjust by 50-125mg/day every 3-5 days for control. Maint: 100-500 qd. Max: 750mg qd. Elderly/Debilitated/Malnourished/Renal or Hepatic Dysfunction: Initial: 100-125mg qd. Maint: Conservative dosing. Take with breakfast. Divide dose with GI intolerance. If <40U/day insulin, discontinue therapy. If >40U/day insulin, decrease dose by 50% and start chlorpropamide therapy. Adjust insulin dose depending on response.

**HOW SUPPLIED:** Tab: 100mg*, 250mg* *scored

**CONTRAINDICATIONS:** Diabetic ketoacidosis.

**WARNINGS/PRECAUTIONS:** Increased risk of cardiovascular mortality. Hypoglycemia risk especially with renal/hepatic insufficiency, elderly, debilitated, malnourished, and adrenal/pituitary insufficiency. Loss of blood glucose control when exposed to stress (fever, trauma, infection or surgery); d/c therapy and start insulin. Secondary failure can occur over a period of time.

**ADVERSE REACTIONS:** Hypoglycemia, cholestatic jaundice, diarrhea, nausea, vomiting, anorexia, pruritus, photosensitivity reactions, skin eruptions, blood dyscrasias, hepatic porphyria, disulfiram-like reactions.

**INTERACTIONS:** Potentiated hypoglycemia with NSAIDs, highly protein bound drugs, salicylates, sulfonamides, chloramphenicol, probenecid, coumarins, MAOIs, and β-blockers. Risk of hyperglycemia with diuretics, corticosteroids, phenothiazines, thyroid products, estrogens, oral contraceptives, phenytoin, nicotinic acid, sympathomimetics, calcium channel blockers, and isoniazid. Alcohol may produce disulfiram-like reaction. β-blockers may mask signs of hypoglycemia. Caution with barbiturates and miconazole.

**PREGNANCY:** Category C, not for use in nursing.

## DIAMOX SEQUELS RX

acetazolamide (Duramed)

**THERAPEUTIC CLASS:** Carbonic anhydrase inhibitor

**INDICATIONS:** Adjunct therapy for chronic open-angle glaucoma, secondary glaucoma and preoperatively in acute angle-closure glaucoma to lower IOP. Prophylaxis and amelioration of symptoms in acute mountain sickness.

**DOSAGE:** *Adults:* Glaucoma: 500mg bid. Acute Mountain Sickness: 500mg-1g/day in divided doses; 1g for rapid ascent. Initiate 24-48 hrs before ascent and continue for 48 hrs while at high altitude or longer as needed.

**HOW SUPPLIED:** Cap, Extended Release: 500mg

**CONTRAINDICATIONS:** In sodium or potassium depleted patients, marked hepatic or kidney impairment, cirrhosis, suprarenal gland failure, hyperchloremic acidosis, (with long-term therapy) chronic noncongestive angle-closure glaucoma.



**WARNINGS/PRECAUTIONS:** Rare reports of fatal sulfonamide hypersensitivity reactions (eg, Stevens-Johnson syndrome, toxic epidermal necrolysis, fulminant hepatic necrosis, anaphylaxis, agranulocytosis, aplastic anemia, other blood dyscrasias) have occurred. D/C drug if this occurs. Sensitizations may recur despite route of administration. Dose increase does not increase diuresis and may result in decreased diuresis and increased drowsiness. Use with caution if patient predisposed to acid/base imbalances (elderly with renal impairment), DM, or impaired alveolar ventilation. Monitor serum electrolytes. Obtain CBC and platelet count before therapy and at regular intervals during therapy.

**ADVERSE REACTIONS:** Paresthesia, hearing dysfunction, tinnitus, loss of appetite, taste alteration, GI disturbances, polyuria, drowsiness, confusion, metabolic acidosis, electrolyte imbalance, transient myopia.

**INTERACTIONS:** Caution with high-dose aspirin. Increased phenytoin levels; may increase occurrence of osteomalacia. Decreased levels of primidone, lithium. Increased effects of other carbonic anhydrase inhibitors, folic acid antagonists, quinidine, amphetamine. May prevent urinary antiseptic effect of methenamine. Increased risk of renal calculus formation with sodium bicarbonate. Increased levels of cyclosporine.

**PREGNANCY:** Category C, not for use in nursing.

## DIASTAT **CIV**

diazepam (Valeant)

**THERAPEUTIC CLASS:** Benzodiazepine

**INDICATIONS:** Management of refractory patients with epilepsy, on stable regimens of anti-epileptic drugs, who require intermittent use to control bouts of increased seizure activity.

**DOSAGE:** *Adults:* 0.2mg/kg rectally. Calculate amount and round upwards to next available dose. May give 2nd dose 4-12 hrs later. Max: 5 episodes/month or 1 episode every 5 days.
*Pediatrics:* >12 yrs: 0.2mg/kg. 6-11yrs: 0.3mg/kg. 2-5 yrs: 0.5mg/kg. Calculate amount and round upwards to next available dose. May give 2nd dose 4-12 hrs later. For rectal administration. Max: 5 episodes/month and 1 episode every 5 days.

**HOW SUPPLIED:** Kit: 2.5mg, 5mg, 10mg, 15mg, 20mg

**CONTRAINDICATIONS:** Acute narrow angle glaucoma, untreated open angle glaucoma.

**WARNINGS/PRECAUTIONS:** Produces CNS depression. Avoid abrupt withdrawal. Caution with elderly, hepatic/renal dysfunction, compromised respiratory function, neurologic damage. Not for daily chronic use. Withdrawal symptoms reported with discontinuation.

**ADVERSE REACTIONS:** Somnolence, dizziness, headache, pain, abdominal pain, nervousness, vasodilation, diarrhea, ataxia, euphoria, incoordination, asthma, rhinitis, rash.

**INTERACTIONS:** Potentiated by phenothiazines, narcotics, barbiturates, valproate, MAOIs, and other antidepressants. Potential inhibitors of CYP450 2C19 (eg, cimetidine, quinidine, tranylcypromine) and CYP450 3A4 (eg, ketoconazole, troleandomycin, clotrimazole) may decrease elimination. CYP450 2C19 (eg, rifampin) and CYP450 3A4 (eg, carbamazepine, phenytoin, dexamethasone, phenobarbital) inducers could increase elimination. May interfere with metabolism of substrates for CYP450 2C19 (eg, omeprazole, propranolol, imipramine) and CYP450 3A4 (eg, cyclosporine, paclitaxel, terfenadine, theophylline, warfarin).

**PREGNANCY:** Category D, not for use in nursing.



## DIAZEPAM INJECTION CIV

diazepam (Various)

**THERAPEUTIC CLASS:** Benzodiazepine

**INDICATIONS:** Management of anxiety disorders and short-term relief of anxiety symptoms. Symptomatic relief of acute alcohol withdrawal. Adjunct prior to endoscopic procedures, surgical procedures and cardioversion. Adjunct therapy in skeletal muscle spasm (eg, tetanus, etc), status epilepticus and severe recurrent convulsive disorders.

**DOSAGE:** *Adults:* Anxiety (moderate): 2-5mg IM/IV, may repeat in 3-4 hrs. Anxiety (severe): 5-10mg IM/IV, may repeat in 3-4 hrs. Alcohol Withdrawal (acute): 10mg IM/IV, then 5-10mg in 3-4 hrs if needed. Endoscopic Procedures: Usual: ≤10mg IV (up to 20mg) or 5-10mg IM 30 minutes prior to procedure. Muscle Spasm: 5-10mg IM/IV, then 5-10mg in 3-4 hrs if needed. Status Epilepticus/Severe Seizures: Initial: 5-10mg IV. Maint: May repeat at 10-15 minute intervals. Max: 30mg. Preoperative: 10mg IM. Cardioversion: 5-15mg IV, 5-10 minutes prior to procedure. Elderly/Debilitated: Usual: 2-5mg. *Pediatrics:* Tetanus: 30 days-5 yrs: 1-2mg IM/IV (slowly), may repeat every 3-4 hrs prn. ≥5 yrs: 5-10mg IM/IV, may repeat every 3-4 hrs. Status Epilepticus/Severe Seizures: 30 days-5 yrs: 0.2-0.5mg IV (slowly) every 2-5 minutes up to 5mg. ≥5 yrs: 1mg IV (slowly) every 2-5 minutes up to 10mg, may repeat in 2-4 hrs.

**HOW SUPPLIED:** Inj: 5mg/mL

**CONTRAINDICATIONS:** Acute narrow angle glaucoma, untreated open angle glaucoma.

**WARNINGS/PRECAUTIONS:** Inject slowly and avoid small veins with IV. Do not mix or dilute with other products in syringe or infusion flask. Extreme caution in elderly, severely ill and those with limited pulmonary reserve. Avoid if in shock, coma or acute alcohol intoxication with depressed vital signs. May impair mental/physical abilities. Increase in grand mal seizures reported. Caution with kidney or hepatic dysfunction. Not for obstetrical use. Withdrawal symptoms may occur. Hypotension and muscular weakness reported. Monitor blood counts and LFT's. Not for maintenance of seizures once controlled.

**ADVERSE REACTIONS:** Drowsiness, fatigue, ataxia, venous thrombosis and phlebitis (injection site).

**INTERACTIONS:** Phenothiazines, narcotics, barbiturates, MAOIs, and other antidepressants may potentiate effects. Delayed clearance with cimetidine. Reduce narcotic dose by at least one-third. Risk of apnea with concomitant barbiturates, alcohol, or other CNS depressants.

**PREGNANCY:** Not for use during pregnancy, safety in nursing unknown.

## DIBENZYLINE RX

phenoxybenzamine HCl (WellSpring)

**THERAPEUTIC CLASS:** Alpha blocker

**INDICATIONS:** To control episodes of hypertension and sweating associated with pheochromocytoma.

**DOSAGE:** *Adults:* Initial: 10mg bid. Titrate: Increase every other day to 20-40mg bid-tid, until BP is controlled.

**HOW SUPPLIED:** Cap: 10mg

**CONTRAINDICATIONS:** Conditions where fall in BP may be undesirable.

**WARNINGS/PRECAUTIONS:** Caution with marked cerebral or coronary arteriosclerosis, or renal damage. May aggravate symptoms of respiratory infections.

**ADVERSE REACTIONS:** Postural hypotension, tachycardia, ejaculation inhibition, nasal congestion, miosis, GI irritation, drowsiness, fatigue.

**INTERACTIONS:** Exaggerated hypotensive response and tachycardia with agents that stimulate both α and β-adrenergic receptors (eg, epinephrine). Blocks hyperthermia production by levarterenol, and blocks hypothermia production by reserpine.

**PREGNANCY:** Category C, not for use in nursing.



## DICLOXACILLIN
dicloxacillin sodium (Various)

RX

**THERAPEUTIC CLASS:** Penicillin (penicillinase-resistant)

**INDICATIONS:** Infections caused by penicillinase-producing staphylococci.

**DOSAGE:** *Adults:* Mild-Moderate Infection: 125mg q6h. Severe Infection: 250mg q6h for at least 14 days.
*Pediatrics:* <40kg: Mild-Moderate Infection: 12.5mg/kg/day in divided doses q6h. Severe Infection: 25mg/kg/day in divided doses q6h for at least 14 days.

**HOW SUPPLIED:** Cap: 250mg, 500mg; Sus: 62.5mg/5mL [100mL]

**WARNINGS/PRECAUTIONS:** Serious, fatal hypersensitivity reactions reported. Caution with history of allergy and/or asthma. Monitor renal, hepatic, and hematopoietic function with prolonged use. Not for use as initial therapy with serious, life-threatening infections, or with nausea, vomiting, gastric dilation, cardiospasm, or intestinal hypermotility.

**ADVERSE REACTIONS:** Allergic reactions, nausea, vomiting, diarrhea, stomatitis, black or hairy tongue, superinfection (prolonged use).

**INTERACTIONS:** Tetracycline may antagonize the bactericidal effects. Potentiated by probenecid.

**PREGNANCY:** Category B, caution in nursing.

## DIDREX
benzphetamine HCl (Pharmacia & Upjohn)

CIII

**THERAPEUTIC CLASS:** Anorectic sympathomimetic amine

**INDICATIONS:** Short term adjunct treatment of exogenous obesity.

**DOSAGE:** *Adults:* Initial: 25-50mg qd. Usual: 25-50mg qd-tid.
*Pediatrics:* >12 yrs: Initial: 25-50mg qd. Usual: 25-50mg qd-tid.

**HOW SUPPLIED:** Tab: 50mg* *scored

**CONTRAINDICATIONS:** Advanced arteriosclerosis, symptomatic cardiovascular disease, moderate to severe HTN, agitated states, hyperthyroidism, glaucoma, history of drug abuse, concomitant CNS stimulants, MAOI use within 14 days, pregnancy.

**WARNINGS/PRECAUTIONS:** Caution with mild HTN. Discontinue if tolerance develops. Psychological disturbances reported when used with restrictive dietary regimen.

**ADVERSE REACTIONS:** Palpitations, tachycardia, BP elevation, restlessness, dizziness, insomnia, headache, tremor, sweating, dry mouth, nausea, diarrhea, unpleasant tastes, urticaria, altered libido.

**INTERACTIONS:** Hypertensive crisis risk if used within 14 days of MAOIs. Potentiates TCAs. Avoid with other CNS stimulants. Decreases effects of antihypertensives. Potentiated by urinary alkalinizing agents and reduced effect with urinary acidifying agents. May alter insulin requirements.

**PREGNANCY:** Category X, not for use in nursing.

## DIDRONEL

RX

etidronate disodium (Procter & Gamble)

**THERAPEUTIC CLASS:** Bone metabolism regulator

**INDICATIONS:** Treatment of Paget's disease. Treatment and prevention of heterotopic ossification following total hip replacement or due to spinal cord injury.

**DOSAGE:** *Adults:* Give as single dose (preferred) or in divided doses. Paget's disease: Initial: 5-10mg/kg/day up to 6 months or 11-20mg/kg/day up to 3 months. May retreat after drug free period of 90 days only if evidence of active disease process. Heterotopic Ossification: Hip Replacement: 20mg/kg/day 1 month before and 3 months after surgery. Spinal Cord: 20mg/kg/day for 2 weeks, followed by 10mg/kg/day for 10 weeks.

**HOW SUPPLIED:** Tab: 200mg, 400mg* *scored

**CONTRAINDICATIONS:** Overt osteomalacia.

**WARNINGS/PRECAUTIONS:** Therapy response in Paget's Disease may be of slow onset and continue for months after stopping. Maintain adequate dietary intake of calcium and vitamin D. Diarrhea reported with enterocolitis. Monitor with renal impairment. Reduce dose with decreased GFR. Max dose (20mg/day) or long-term therapy (>6 months) may increase fracture risk. Rachitic syndrome reported in children at doses of 10mg/kg/day for prolonged periods (approaching or exceeding 1 year).

**ADVERSE REACTIONS:** Diarrhea, nausea, increased bone pain in Paget's, alopecia, arthropathy, esophagitis, hypersensitivity reactions, osteomalacia, amnesia, confusion.

**INTERACTIONS:** Vitamins with mineral supplements or antacids that contain calcium, iron, aluminum, or magnesium reduce absorption (separate dosing by 2 hours). Monitor PT with warfarin.

**PREGNANCY:** Category C, caution with nursing.

## DIFFERIN

RX

adapalene (Galderma)

**THERAPEUTIC CLASS:** Naphthoic acid derivative (retinoid-like)

**INDICATIONS:** Topical treatment of acne vulgaris.

**DOSAGE:** *Adults:* Apply qhs after washing.
*Pediatrics:* >12 yrs: Apply qhs after washing.

**HOW SUPPLIED:** Cre: 0.1% [45g]; Gel: 0.1%, 0.3% [45g]

**WARNINGS/PRECAUTIONS:** Avoid contact with eyes, lips, paranasal creases, mucous membranes, cuts, abrasions, eczematous or sunburned skin. Minimize sun exposure. Extreme weather may increase skin irritation.

**ADVERSE REACTIONS:** Erythema, scaling, dryness, pruritus, burning, sunburn, acne flares.

**INTERACTIONS:** Caution with other topicals with strong drying effects, high concentration of alcohol, astringents, spices, or lime. Allow effects of sulfur, resorcinol, or salicylic acid to subside before use.

**PREGNANCY:** Category C, caution in nursing.

## DIFLUCAN
fluconazole (Pfizer)

RX

**THERAPEUTIC CLASS:** Triazole antifungal

**INDICATIONS:** Treatment of vaginal, oropharyngeal, esophageal, and systemic candidiasis. Treatment of peritonitis and UTI caused by *Candida*. Treatment of cryptococcal meningitis. Prophylaxis in patients undergoing BMT.



**DOSAGE:** *Adults:* Vaginal Candidiasis: 150mg PO single dose. IV/PO: Oropharyngeal Candidiasis: 200mg 1st day then 100mg qd for minimum 2 weeks. Esophageal Candidiasis: 200mg 1st day then 100mg qd for minimum 3 weeks then treat 2 weeks following resolution of symptoms. Max: 400mg/day. Systemic Infections: 400mg/day. UTI/Peritonitis: 50-200mg/day. Cryptococcal Meningitis: 400mg 1st day then 200mg qd for 10-12 weeks after negative CSF culture. Suppression of relapse in AIDS: 200mg/day. Prophylaxis in BMT: 400mg/day. CrCl <50mL/min: Initial: LD 50-400mg. Maint: Give 50% of recommended dose.
*Pediatrics:* IV/PO: Oropharyngeal Candidiasis: 6mg/kg 1st day then 3mg/kg/day for minimum of 2 weeks. Esophageal Candidiasis: 6mg/kg 1st day then 3mg/kg/day for minimum 3 weeks and 2 weeks following resolution of symptoms. Max: 12mg/kg/day. Systemic Infections: 6-12mg/kg/day. Cryptococcal Meningitis: 12mg/kg 1st day then 6mg/kg/day for 10-12 weeks after negative CSF culture. Suppression of relapse in AIDS: 6mg/kg/day. CrCl <50mL/min: Initial: 50-400mg. Maint: Give 50% of recommended dose.

**HOW SUPPLIED:** Inj: 200mg/100mL, 400mg/200mL; Sus: 50mg/5mL, 200mg/5mL [35mL]; Tab: 50mg, 100mg, 150mg, 200mg

**CONTRAINDICATIONS:** Coadministration with cisapride or terfenadine (with multiple diflucan doses of >400mg). Caution if hypersensitive to other azoles.

**WARNINGS/PRECAUTIONS:** Monitor LFTs. D/C if hepatic dysfunction develops or exfoliative skin disorder progresses. Anaphylaxis reported.

**ADVERSE REACTIONS:** Headache, nausea, abdominal pain, diarrhea, skin rash, vomiting.

**INTERACTIONS:** Severe hypoglycemia with oral hypoglycemics. May increase PT with coumarin-type drugs. Increases levels of phenytoin, cyclosporine, cisapride, astemizole, zidovudine and theophylline. Rifampin enhances metabolism of fluconazole. Cimetidine may decrease levels. HCTZ may increase levels. Contraindicated with terfenadine and cisapride due to prolongation of QTc interval. Cardiac events (torsade de pointes) reported with cisapride. Uveitis reported with rifabutin. Nephrotoxicity reported with tacrolimus. May increase or decrease levels of ethinyl estradiol- and levonorgestrel-containing oral contraceptives.

**PREGNANCY:** Category C, not for use in nursing.

## DIGIBIND
digoxin immune fab (ovine) (GlaxoSmithKline)

RX

**THERAPEUTIC CLASS:** Antidote, digoxin toxicity

**INDICATIONS:** Treatment of life-threatening digoxin intoxication.

**DOSAGE:** *Adults:* Acute Ingestion of Unknown Amount: Usual: Administer 10 vials, observe response, then additional 10 vials if clinically indicated. Calculation: # vials = total digitalis body load (mg)/0.5mg of digitalis bound per vial. 1 vial will bind approximately 0.5mg of digoxin (or digitoxin). Digoxin Concentrations At Steady State: # of vials = (serum dig conc in ng/mL) x (wt in kg)/100. Digitoxin Concentrations At Steady State: # of vials = (serum digitoxin conc in ng/mL) x (wt in kg)/1000. If toxicity not adequately reversed after several hrs or appears to recur, may need readministration. See labeling for details.
*Pediatrics:* Acute Ingestion of Unknown Amount: Usual: Administer 10 vials, observe response, then additional 10 vials if clinically indicated. Calculation: #

vials = total digitalis body load (mg)/0.5mg of digitalis bound per vial. 1 vial will bind approximately 0.5mg of digoxin (or digitoxin). Digoxin Concentrations At Steady State: Dose (mg) = (# vials) (38mg/vial). Digitoxin Concentrations At Steady State: # of vials = (serum digitoxin conc in ng/mL) x (wt in kg)/1000. If toxicity not adequately reversed after several hrs or appears to recur, may need readministration. See labeling for details.



**HOW SUPPLIED:** Inj: 38mg

**WARNINGS/PRECAUTIONS:** Obtain digoxin level before initiation. Do not overlook possibility of multiple drug overdose. Risk of hypersensitivity is greater with allergies to papain, chymopapain, or other papaya extracts; skin testing may be appropriate for high risk individuals. $K^+$ levels may drop rapidly after administration; monitor closely. Digitalis toxicity may recur with renal dysfunction. Caution with cardiac dysfunction, further deterioration may occur from digoxin withdrawal. Can provide additional support with inotropes or vasodilators. Monitor for volume overload in children.

**ADVERSE REACTIONS:** Allergic reactions, exacerbation of low cardiac output, CHF.

**PREGNANCY:** Category C, caution in nursing.

## DILACOR XR

RX

diltiazem HCl (Watson)

**OTHER BRAND NAMES:** Diltia XT (Andrx)

**THERAPEUTIC CLASS:** Calcium channel blocker (nondihydropyridine)

**INDICATIONS:** Treatment of hypertension and management of chronic stable angina.

**DOSAGE:** *Adults:* HTN: Initial: 180-240mg qd. Usual: 180-480mg qd. Max: 540mg qd. >60 yrs: Initial: 120mg qd. Angina: Initial: 120mg qd. Titrate: Adjust at 1-2 week intervals. Max: 480mg/day. Swallow whole on an empty stomach in the am.

**HOW SUPPLIED:** Cap, Extended Release: 120mg, 180mg, 240mg

**CONTRAINDICATIONS:** Sick sinus syndrome, 2nd- or 3rd-degree AV block (except with functioning pacemaker), hypotension (<90mmHg systolic), acute MI, pulmonary congestion.

**WARNINGS/PRECAUTIONS:** Caution in renal, hepatic, or ventricular dysfunction. Monitor LFTs and renal function with prolonged use. Discontinue if persistent rash occurs. Symptomatic hypotension may occur. Acute hepatic injury reported.

**ADVERSE REACTIONS:** Rhinitis, pharyngitis, cough, flu syndrome, peripheral edema, myalgia, vomiting, sinusitis, asthenia, nausea, vasodilation, headache, constipation, diarrhea.

**INTERACTIONS:** Increased levels of propranolol. Increased levels of diltiazem with cimetidine. Monitor digoxin, cyclosporine. Potentiates cardiac contractility, conductivity, and automaticity; and vascular dilation with anesthetics. Additive cardiac conduction effects with digitalis or β-blockers. Potential additive effects with agents known to affect cardiac contractility and/or conduction.

**PREGNANCY:** Category C, not for use in nursing.

## DILANTIN

RX

phenytoin (Parke-Davis)

**THERAPEUTIC CLASS:** Hydantoin

**INDICATIONS:** (CER, CTB) Control of generalized tonic-clonic (grand mal) and complex partial (psychomotor, temporal lobe) seizures. Prevention and treatment of neurosurgically induced seizures. (Sus) Control of tonic-clonic (grand mal) and psychomotor (temporal lobe) seizures.

**DOSAGE:** *Adults:* (CER) Initial: 100mg tid. Titrate: May increase at 7-10 day intervals. Max: 200mg tid. May give once daily with extended release if controlled on 300mg daily. LD (clinic/hospital): 1g in 3 divided doses (400mg, 300mg, 300mg) given 2 hrs apart. Start maintenance 24 hrs later. (CTB) Initial: 100mg tid. Titrate: May increase at 7-10 day intervals. Usual: 300-400mg/day. Max: 600mg/day. May chew or swallow tab whole. Not for once daily dosing. (Sus) Initial: 125mg tid. Titrate: May increase at 7-10 day intervals. Max: 625mg/day.
*Pediatrics:* (CER, CTB, Sus) Initial: 5mg/kg/day given bid-tid. Titrate: May increase at 7-10 day intervals. Maint: 4-8mg/kg/day. Max: 300mg/day. >6 yrs: May require the minimum adult dose (300mg/day).

D

**HOW SUPPLIED:** Cap, Extended Release (CER): 30mg, 100mg; Sus: 125mg/5mL [237mL]; Tab, Chewable (CTB): 50mg* *scored

**WARNINGS/PRECAUTIONS:** Avoid abrupt discontinuation. Caution with porphyria, hepatic dysfunction, elderly, diabetes, debilitated. D/C if rash occurs. Lymphadenopathy reported. Serum sickness may occur with lymph node involvement. Gingival hyperplasia reported; maintain proper dental hygiene. Hyperglycemia, birth defects and osteomalacia reported. Monitor levels. Confusional states reported with increased levels. Increased seizure frequency during pregnancy. Neonatal coagulation defects reported within first 24 hrs of birth. Give Vitamin K to mother before delivery and to neonate after birth. Avoid use with seizures due to hypoglycemia or other metabolic causes.

**ADVERSE REACTIONS:** Nystagmus, ataxia, slurred speech, decreased coordination, confusion, dizziness, insomnia, transient nervousness, motor twitchings, headaches, nausea, vomiting, constipation, rash, hypersensitivity reactions.

**INTERACTIONS:** Increased levels with acute alcohol intake, amiodarone, chloramphenicol, chlordiazepoxide, diazepam, dicumarol, disulfiram, estrogens, $H_2$-antagonists, halothane, isoniazid, methylphenidate, phenothiazines, phenylbutazone, salicylates, succinamides, sulfonamides, tolbutamide, trazodone. Decreased levels with chronic alcohol abuse, carbamazepine, reserpine, sucralfate. Decreases effects of corticosteroids, coumarin anticoagulants, digitoxin, doxycycline, estrogens, furosemide, oral contraceptives, quinidine, rifampin, theophylline, vitamin D. Phenobarbital, sodium valproate, valproic acid may increase or decrease levels. May increase or decrease levels of phenobarbital, sodium valproate, valproic acid. Calcium antacids decrease absorption; space dosing. Moban® contains calcium ions which interfere with absorption. TCAs may precipitate seizures.Increased risk of phenytoin hypersensitivity with barbiturates, succinamides, oxazolidinediones.

**PREGNANCY:** Possibly teratogenic, weigh benefits versus risk; not for use in nursing.

## DILATRATE-SR — RX

isosorbide dinitrate (Schwarz)

**THERAPEUTIC CLASS:** Nitrate vasodilator

**INDICATIONS:** Prevention of angina pectoris.

**DOSAGE:** *Adults:* 40mg bid (Separate doses by 6 hrs). Max: 160mg/day. Should have >18 hr nitrate-free interval.

**HOW SUPPLIED:** Cap, Extended Release: 40mg

**WARNINGS/PRECAUTIONS:** Severe hypotension may occur; caution with volume depletion and hypotension. Hypotension may cause paradoxical bradycardia and increased angina pectoris. May aggravate angina caused by hypertrophic cardiomyopathy. Monitor for tolerance. Caution with CHF and acute MI.

**ADVERSE REACTIONS:** Headache, lightheadedness, hypotension, syncope, rebound HTN.

**INTERACTIONS:** Potentiates effects of other vasodilators such as alcohol. Severe hypotension with sildenafil.

**PREGNANCY:** Category C, caution in nursing.



## DILAUDID

hydromorphone HCl (Abbott)

CII

**Contains hydromorphone, a potent Schedule II opioid agonist which has the highest potential for abuse and risk of producing respiratory depression. HP formulation is a highly concentrated solution of hydromorphone; do not confuse with standard parenteral formulations of hydromorphone or other opioids as overdose and death could result.**

**OTHER BRAND NAMES:** Dilaudid-HP (Abbott)

**THERAPEUTIC CLASS:** Opioid analgesic

**INDICATIONS:** Management of pain. (HP) Relief of moderate-to-severe pain in opioid-tolerant patients who require larger than usual doses of opioids to provide adequate pain relief.

**DOSAGE:** *Adults:* Individualize dose. Initial: 1-2mg SQ/IM/IV q4-6h prn. (HP) Range: 1-14mg IM/SQ; adjust dose based on response. (Sol) 2.5-10mg PO q3-6h prn. (Tab) 2-4mg PO q4-6h prn. (Sup) Insert 1 PR q6-8h prn. Titrate: Increase dose as needed. Elderly: Start at lower end of dosing range.

**HOW SUPPLIED:** Inj: 1mg/mL, 2mg/mL, 4mg/mL, (HP) 10mg/mL, 250mg; Sol: 1mg/mL; Sup: 3mg; Tab: 2mg, 4mg, 8mg* *scored

**CONTRAINDICATIONS:** Intracranial lesions associated with increased intracranial pressure, COPD, cor pulmonale, emphysema, kyphoscoliosis, and in status asthmaticus. (HP-Inj) Obstetrical analgesia.

**WARNINGS/PRECAUTIONS:** See BlackBox Warnings. Increased respiratory depression with head injury and/or increased intracranial pressure. May mask acute abdominal conditions. Caution with elderly/debilitated, seizures, biliary tract surgery, renal/hepatic impairment, hypothyroidism, Addison's disease, BPH, and urethral stricture; initial dose should be reduced in these patients. May suppress cough reflex. Potential for physical/psychological tolerance or dependence, especially in patients with alcoholism and drug dependencies; monitor closely. Seizures reported in compromised patients receiving high doses. Dilaudid-HP should only be used in patients already receiving large doses of narcotics. 8mg tab and sol contains sulfites.

**ADVERSE REACTIONS:** Excessive sedation, lethargy, mental clouding, anxiety, dysphoria, nausea, vomiting, constipation, urinary retention, respiratory depression. Orthostatic hypotension and fainting reported with injection.

**INTERACTIONS:** Additive CNS depression with other narcotic analgesics, neuromuscular blocking agents, general anesthetics, phenothiazines, tranquilizers, sedative hypnotics, TCAs, alcohol, or other CNS depressants. Mixed agonist/antagonist analgesics may reduce the analgesic effect of hydromorphone and/or may precipitate withdrawal symptoms.

**PREGNANCY:** Category C, not for use in nursing.

## DIOVAN

valsartan (Novartis)

RX

**Can cause death/injury to developing fetus during 2nd and 3rd trimesters. Stop therapy if pregnancy detected.**

**THERAPEUTIC CLASS:** Angiotensin II receptor antagonist

**INDICATIONS:** Treatment of hypertension, alone or with other antihypertensives. Treatment of heart failure (NYHA Class II-IV) in patients intolerant of ACE inhibitors. Reduction of cardiovascular mortality in clinically stable patients with left ventricular failure or dysfunction following MI.

**DOSAGE:** *Adults:* HTN: Monotherapy Without Volume Depletion: Initial: 80mg or 160mg qd. Titrate: Increase to 320mg qd or add diuretic (greater effect than increasing dose >80mg). Hepatic/Renal Dysfunction: Caution with dosing. Heart Failure: Initial: 40mg bid. Titrate: Increase to 80mg or 160mg bid (use highest dose tolerated). Max: 320mg/day in divided doses. Post-MI: Initial: 20mg bid. Titrate: Increase to 40mg bid within 7 days, with subsequent titrations up to 160mg bid. Renal Dysfunction: Caution and possible dose reduction and/or discontinuation.



**HOW SUPPLIED:** Tab: 40mg, 80mg, 160mg, 320mg

**WARNINGS/PRECAUTIONS:** Can cause fetal injury/death. Changes in renal function may occur; caution with renal artery stenosis, severe CHF. Caution with hepatic dysfunction, renal dysfunction, and obstructive biliary disorder. Risk of hypotension; caution when initiating therapy in heart failure or post-MI. Correct volume or salt depletion before therapy.

**ADVERSE REACTIONS:** (HTN) Viral infection, fatigue, abdominal pain; (Heart Failure) dizziness, hypotension, diarrhea, arthralgia, fatigue, back pain.

**INTERACTIONS:** Avoid with concomitant ACE inhibitors and beta blockers with heart failure. Potassium-sparing diuretics, potassium supplements, or salt substitutes containing potassium may increase serum potassium levels, and in heart failure patients increase serum creatinine.

**PREGNANCY:** Category C (1st trimester) and D (2nd and 3rd trimesters), not for use in nursing.

## DIOVAN HCT

RX

valsartan - hydrochlorothiazide (Novartis)

**Can cause death/injury to developing fetus during 2nd and 3rd trimesters. Stop therapy if pregnancy detected.**

**THERAPEUTIC CLASS:** Angiotensin II receptor antagonist/thiazide diuretic

**INDICATIONS:** Treatment of hypertension. Not for initial therapy.

**DOSAGE:** *Adults:* Initial: Uncontrolled on Valsartan Monotherapy: Switch to 80mg-12.5mg, 160mg-12.5mg, or 320mg-12.5mg qd. Increase dose if uncontrolled after 3-4 weeks. Max: 320mg-25mg/day. Uncontrolled on 25mg HCTZ/day or Controlled on 25mg HCTZ/day with Hypokalemia: Switch to 80mg-12.5mg or 160mg-12.5mg tab qd. Titrate if uncontrolled after 3-4 weeks. Max: 320mg-25mg/day.

**HOW SUPPLIED:** Tab: (Valsartan-HCTZ) 80mg-12.5mg, 160mg-12.5mg, 160mg-25mg, 320mg-12.5mg, 320mg-25mg

**CONTRAINDICATIONS:** Anuria, sulfonamide hypersensitivity.

**WARNINGS/PRECAUTIONS:** Can cause fetal injury/death. Correct volume or salt depletion before therapy. Caution with hepatic or renal dysfunction, biliary obstructive disorders, renal artery stenosis, severe CHF, history of allergies, and asthma. May exacerbate or activate SLE. Monitor serum electrolytes. Avoid if CrCl <30mL/min. Hyperuricemia, hyperglycemia, hypokalemia, hypomagnesemia, hypercalcemia may occur. Enhanced effects in post-sympathectomy patient. May increase cholesterol and triglyceride levels.

**ADVERSE REACTIONS:** Cough, headache, dizziness, fatigue, viral infection, pharyngitis, diarrhea.

**INTERACTIONS:** Potentiates orthostatic hypotension with alcohol, barbiturates, and narcotics. Adjust insulin and antidiabetic drugs. Impaired absorption with cholestyramine, colestipol. Corticosteroids and ACTH deplete electrolytes. May decrease response to pressor amines. Potentiates other antihypertensives. May increase responsiveness to skeletal muscle relaxants. Risk of lithium toxicity. NSAIDs decrease diuretic effects.

**PREGNANCY:** Category C (1st trimester) and D (2nd and 3rd trimesters), not for use in nursing.

D

## DIPHENHYDRAMINE HCL INJECTION RX

diphenhydramine HCl (Various)

**THERAPEUTIC CLASS:** Antihistamine

**INDICATIONS:** Amelioration of allergic reactions to blood or plasma. Adjunct to epinephrine in anaphylaxis. For other uncomplicated immediate type allergic conditions when oral therapy is contraindicated. Treatment of motion sickness. For parkinsonism when oral therapy is not possible or contraindicated.

**DOSAGE:** *Adults:* Usual: 10-50mg IV or up to 100mg IM if needed. Max: 400mg/day.
*Pediatrics:* Usual: 5mg/kg/24hrs or 150mg/m²/24hrs IV/IM in 4 divided doses. Max: 300mg/day.

**HOW SUPPLIED:** Inj: 50mg/mL

**CONTRAINDICATIONS:** Neonates, premature infants, nursing, as a local anesthetic.

**WARNINGS/PRECAUTIONS:** Caution with narrow-angle glaucoma, stenosing peptic ulcer, pyloroduodenal obstruction, symptomatic prostatic hypertrophy, or bladder-neck obstruction. May cause excitation in pediatrics. Increased risk of dizziness, sedation, and hypotension in elderly. Caution with lower respiratory diseases, bronchial asthma, increased IOP, hyperthyroidism, cardiovascular disease, or HTN. Local necrosis with SQ or intradermal use.

**ADVERSE REACTIONS:** Sedation, drowsiness, dizziness, disturbed coordination, epigastric distress, thickening of bronchial secretions.

**INTERACTIONS:** Additive effects with alcohol, CNS depressants. MAOIs prolong and intensify anticholinergic effects.

**PREGNANCY:** Category B, contraindicated in nursing.

## DIPRIVAN RX

propofol (Abraxis)

**THERAPEUTIC CLASS:** General anesthetic

**INDICATIONS:** Sedative-hypnotic agent used for both induction and maintenance of anesthesia. For initiation and maintenance of monitored anesthesia care (MAC) sedation during diagnostic procedures and in conjunction with local/regional anesthesia in patients undergoing surgical procedures. To provide continuous sedation and control of stress responses in intubated, mechanically ventilated adult patients in ICU.

**DOSAGE:** *Adults:* General Anesthesia: <55 yrs: 40mg IV every 10 seconds until induction onset. Maint: 100-200mcg/kg/min IV or 20-50mg intermittently byIV bolus prn. Elderly/Debilitated/ASA III & IV: 20mg IV every 10 seconds until induction onset. Maint: 50-100mcg/kg/min IV. Cardiac Anesthesia: 20mg IV every 10 seconds until induction onset. Maint: 100-150mcg/kg/min IV with secondary opioid or 50-100mcg/kg/min IV with primary opioid. Neurosurgical Patients: 20mg IV every 10 seconds until induction onset. Maint: 100-200mcg/kg/min IV. MAC Sedation: 100-150mcg/kg/min IV infusion or 0.5mg/kg slow IV injection over 3-5 min followed immediately by maintenance infusion. Maint: 25-75mcg/kg/min IV infusion or 10-20mg incremental IV boluses. Elderly/Debilitated/ASA III & IV: Use doses similar to healthy adults. Avoid rapid boluses. Maint: 80% of the usual adult dose. ICU Sedation: Initial: 5mcg/kg/min IV infusion for 5 min. Increase 5-10mcg/kg/min IV over 5-10 min. Maint: 5-50mcg/kg/min IV or higher may be required.
Pediatrics: 3-16 yrs: General Anesthesia: 2.5-3.5mg/kg IV over 20-30 seconds. Maint: 2 months-16 yrs: 125-300mcg/kg/min IV.

**HOW SUPPLIED:** Inj: 10mg/mL

**WARNINGS/PRECAUTIONS:** Avoid rapid bolus administration in elderly, debilitated or ASA III/IV patients. Monitor oxygen saturation and for signs of significant hypotension, bradycardia, cardiovascular depression, apnea or airway obstruction. Caution with hyperlipoproteinemia, diabetic hyperlipemia, pancreatitis, epilepsy. Rare reports of anaphylaxis reactions, pulmonary edema, perioperative myoclonia, postoperative pancreatitis, bradycardia, asystole, cardiac arrest, rhabdomyolysis. Minimize transient local pain by using larger veins of forearm or antecubital fossa and/or prior lidocaine injection. May elevate serum TG. Do not infuse for >5 days without drug holiday to replace zinc losses; consider supplemental zinc with chronic use in those predisposed to zinc deficiency. In renal impairment, perform baseline urinalysis/urinary sediment then monitor on alternate days during sedation. (Neurosurgical Anesthesia) Use infusion or slow bolus to avoid significant hypotension and decreases in cerebral perfusion pressure. (Cardiac Anesthesia) Use slower rates of administration in premedicated and geriatric patients, patients with recent fluid shifts or those hemodynamically unstable. Correct fluid deficits prior to use.

**ADVERSE REACTIONS:** Bradycardia, arrhythmia, hypotension, HTN, tachycardia nodal, decreased cardiac output, CNS movement, injection site burning/stinging/pain, hyperlipemia, apnea, rash, pruritus, respiratory acidosis during weaning.

**INTERACTIONS:** Increased effects with narcotics (eg, morphine, meperidine, fentanyl), combinations of opioids and sedatives (eg, benzodiazepines, barbiturates, chloral hydrate, droperidol) and potent inhalational agents (eg, isoflurane, enflurane, halothane). Concomitant fentanyl may cause bradycardia in pediatrics.

**PREGNANCY:** Category B, not for use in nursing.

## DIPROLENE — RX

betamethasone (augmented) dipropionate (Schering)

**OTHER BRAND NAMES:** Diprolene AF (Schering)

**THERAPEUTIC CLASS:** Corticosteroid

**INDICATIONS:** Relief of inflammatory and pruritic manifestations of corticosteroid responsive dermatoses.

**DOSAGE:** *Adults:* (Gel, Lot) Apply qd-bid for no more than 2 weeks. Limit to (Gel) 50g/week, (Lot) 50mL/week. (Cre, Oint) Apply qd-bid, up to 45g/week. *Pediatrics:* >13 yrs: (Cre) Apply qd-bid for no more than 2 weeks. Limit to 45g/week. >12 yrs: (Gel, Lot) Apply qd-bid for no more than 2 weeks. Limit to (Gel) 50g/week, (Lot) 50mL/week. (Oint) Apply qd-bid, up to 45g/week.

**HOW SUPPLIED:** Cre (AF), Gel, Oint: 0.05% [15g, 50g]; Lot: 0.05% [30mL, 60mL]

**WARNINGS/PRECAUTIONS:** May produce reversible HPA axis suppression, manifestations of Cushing's syndrome, hyperglycemia and glucosuria. Discontinue if irritation occurs. Use appropriate antifungal or antibacterial agent with dermatological infections. Pediatrics may be more susceptible to systemic toxicity. Caution when applied to large surface areas. Not for use with occlusive dressings. Gel is not for use in rosacea or perioral dermatitis or on the face, groin, or in the axillae.

**ADVERSE REACTIONS:** Stinging, burning, dry skin, pruritus, folliculitis, acneiform papules, irritation, hypopigmentation, skin maceration, secondary infection, skin atrophy, striae, miliaria.

**PREGNANCY:** Category C, (Cre, Lot) not for use in nursing; (Gel, Oint) caution in nursing.

## DISPERMOX
amoxicillin (Ranbaxy)

RX

**THERAPEUTIC CLASS:** Semisynthetic ampicillin derivative



**INDICATIONS:** Infections of the ear, nose, throat, genitourinary tract, skin and skin structure, lower respiratory tract due to susceptible (beta lactamase negative) organisms; gonorrhea (acute uncomplicated).

**DOSAGE:** *Adults:* ENT/SSSI/GU: (Mild/Moderate): 500mg q12h or 250mg q8h. (Severe): 875mg q12h or 500mg q8h. LRTI: 875mg q12h or 500mg q8h. Gonorrhea: 3g as single oral dose. Do not chew or swallow dispersible tabs.
*Pediatrics:* Neonates: ≥12 weeks: Max: 30mg/kg/day divided q12h. >3 months: ENT/SSSI/GU: (Mild/Moderate): 25mg/kg/day given q12h or 20mg/kg/day given q8h. (Severe): 45mg/kg/day given q12h or 40 mg/kg/day given q8h. LRTI: 45mg/kg/day given q12h or 40mg/kg/day given q8h. Gonorrhea: (Prepubertal) 50mg/kg with 25mg/kg probenecid as single dose (regimen not for use if <2 yrs). >40kg: Dose as adult. Do not chew or swallow dispersible tabs.

**HOW SUPPLIED:** Tab, Dispersible: 200mg, 400mg, 600mg

**WARNINGS/PRECAUTIONS:** Monitor renal, hepatic, and blood with prolonged use. Dispersible tabs contain phenylalanine.

**ADVERSE REACTIONS:** Nausea, vomiting, diarrhea, pseudomembranous colitis, hypersensitivity reactions, blood dyscrasias, superinfection (prolonged use).

**INTERACTIONS:** Increased levels with probenecid. Chloramphenicol, macrolides, sulfonamides, tetracyclines may interfere with bactericidal effects. False (+) for urine glucose with Clinitest, Benedict's or Fehling's solution.

**PREGNANCY:** Category B, caution in nursing.

## DITROPAN XL
oxybutynin chloride (Ortho-McNeil)

RX

**OTHER BRAND NAMES:** Ditropan (Ortho-McNeil)

**THERAPEUTIC CLASS:** Anticholinergic agent

**INDICATIONS:** (All) Overactive bladder/bladder instability with symptoms of urge urinary incontinence, urgency, and frequency. (Tab, Extended Release) Detrusor overactivity associated with a neurological condition in pediatrics ≥6 years old.

**DOSAGE:** *Adults:* (Tab, Syrup) Usual: 5mg bid-tid. Max: 5mg qid. (Tab, Extended Release) Initial: 5 or 10mg qd. Titrate: May increase by 5mg weekly. Max: 30mg/day. Swallow XL whole with liquid; do not chew, divide or crush tab.
*Pediatrics:* >5 yrs: (Tab, Syrup) Usual: 5mg bid. Max: 5mg tid. ≥6 yrs: (Tab, Extended Release) Initial: 5mg qd. Titrate: May increase by 5mg weekly. Max: 20mg/day. Swallow XL whole with liquid; do not chew, divide, or crush tab.

**HOW SUPPLIED:** Syrup: 5mg/5mL; Tab: 5mg*; Tab, Extended Release: 5mg, 10mg, 15mg *scored

**CONTRAINDICATIONS:** (Tab/Syrup) Untreated angle closure glaucoma and narrow anterior chamber angles, GI tract obstruction, paralytic ileus, intestinal atony, megacolon, toxic megacolon complicating ulcerative colitis, severe colitis, myasthenia gravis, obstructive uropathy, unstable cardiovascular status in acute hemorrhage. (Tab, Extended-Release) Urinary retention, gastric retention, uncontrolled narrow-angle glaucoma, and in patients at risk for these conditions.

**WARNINGS/PRECAUTIONS:** Caution with hepatic or renal impairment, bladder outflow obstruction, GI obstruction/narrowing, ulcerative colitis, intestinal atony, myasthenia gravis, autonomic neuropathy, hyperthyroidism, CHD, CHF, arrhythmias, HTN, tachycardia, prostatic hypertrophy, and GERD.

Heat prostration can occur with high environmental temperatures. D/C if diarrhea develops. Tab, Extended-Release shell may be excreted in the stool.

**ADVERSE REACTIONS:** Dry mouth, constipation, somnolence, headache, diarrhea, nausea, blurred vision, dyspepsia, asthenia, pain, dizziness, rhinitis, dry eyes, UTI.

**INTERACTIONS:** Increased adverse effects with other anticholinergics. Increased drowsiness with alcohol or other sedatives. May alter GI absorption of other drugs due to GI motility effects. Increased levels with ketoconazole; caution with CYP3A4 inhibitors (eg, antimycotics, macrolides). Caution with bisphosphonates or other drugs that may exacerbate esophagitis.

**PREGNANCY:** Category B, caution in nursing.



## DIURIL

chlorothiazide (Salix) RX

**THERAPEUTIC CLASS:** Thiazide diuretic

**INDICATIONS:** (PO/IV) Adjunct therapy in edema associated with CHF, hepatic cirrhosis, corticosteroid and estrogen therapy, renal dysfunction. (PO) Management of hypertension.

**DOSAGE:** *Adults:* (PO/IV) Edema: 0.5-1g qd-bid. May give every other day or 3-5 days/week. Substitute IV for oral using same dosage. (PO) HTN: 0.5-1g qd or in divided doses. Max: 2g/day.
*Pediatrics:* (PO) Diuresis/HTN: Usual: 10-20mg/kg/day given qd-bid. Max: Infants up to 2 yrs: 375mg/day. 2-12 yrs: 1g/day. <6 months: Up to 15mg/kg bid may be required.

**HOW SUPPLIED:** Inj: 0.5g; Sus: 250mg/5mL [237mL]; Tab: 250mg*, 500mg* *scored

**CONTRAINDICATIONS:** Anuria, sulfonamide hypersensitivity.

**WARNINGS/PRECAUTIONS:** Caution in severe renal disease, liver dysfunction, electrolyte/fluid imbalance. Monitor electrolytes. Hyperuricemia, hyperglycemia, hypokalemia, hyponatremia, hypomagnesemia, hypercalcemia may occur. Increases in cholesterol and triglyceride levels reported. May exacerbate SLE. Sensitivity reactions reported. D/C prior to parathyroid test. Enhanced effects in post-sympathectomy patient. IV use not recommended in infants or children.

**ADVERSE REACTIONS:** Weakness, hypotension, pancreatitis, jaundice, diarrhea, vomiting, blood dyscrasias, rash, photosensitivity, electrolyte imbalance, impotence.

**INTERACTIONS:** May potentiate orthostatic hypotension with alcohol, barbiturates, narcotics. Adjust antidiabetic drugs. Possible decreased response to pressor amines. Corticosteroids, ACTH increase electrolyte depletion. May potentiate nondepolarizing skeletal muscle relaxants, antihypertensives. Lithium toxicity. NSAIDs decrease effects. Decreased PO absorption with cholestyramine, colestipol.

**PREGNANCY:** Category C, not for use in nursing.

## DOBUTAMINE

dobutamine (Various) RX

**THERAPEUTIC CLASS:** Inotropic agent

**INDICATIONS:** Short-term treatment of cardiac decompensation due to depressed contractility resulting from organic heart disease or from cardiac surgical procedures.

**DOSAGE:** *Adults:* Usual: 2.5-15mcg/kg/min, up to 40mcg/kg/min (rare). Adjust rate and duration based on BP, urine flow, ectopic activity, HR, and when possible on cardiac output, central venous or pulmonary wedge pressure.

**HOW SUPPLIED:** Inj: 12.5mg/mL [20mL, 40mL]

**CONTRAINDICATIONS:** Idiopathic hypertrophic subaortic stenosis.

**WARNINGS/PRECAUTIONS:** May increase HR or BP, especially systolic pressure; caution with atrial fibrillation and HTN. May precipitate or exacerbate ventricular ectopic activity. Hypersensitivity reactions (eg, skin rash, fever, eosinophilia, bronchospasm) reported. Contains sulfites. Monitor EKG, BP, pulmonary wedge pressure, and cardiac output. Correct hypovolemia prior to infusion. Caution in elderly. May decrease serum $K^+$ levels. Improvement may not be observed with marked mechanical obstruction (eg, severe valvular aortic stenosis). Safety following acute MI has not been established.

**ADVERSE REACTIONS:** Increased HR, BP and ventricular ectopic activity, hypotension, infusion site reactions, nausea, headache, anginal pain, palpitations, shortness of breath, decreased $K^+$ levels.

**INTERACTIONS:** Recent administration of β-blockers may reduce effectiveness and increase peripheral vascular resistance. Increased cardiac output and lower pulmonary wedge pressure with nitroprusside.

**PREGNANCY:** Category B, not for use in nursing.

## DOLOBID — RX

diflunisal (Merck)

**NSAIDs may cause an increased risk of serious cardiovascular thrombotic events, MI, stroke and serious GI adverse events including bleeding, ulceration, and perforation of the stomach or intestines. Contraindicated for the treatment of peri-operative pain in the setting of coronary artery bypass graft (CABG) surgery.**

**THERAPEUTIC CLASS:** NSAID

**INDICATIONS:** Acute or long-term symptomatic treatment of mild to moderate pain, osteoarthritis (OA), rheumatoid arthritis (RA).

**DOSAGE:** *Adults:* Pain: Initial: 1g, then 500mg q8-12h. OA/RA: 250-500mg bid. Max: 1500mg/day.
*Pediatrics:* >12 yrs: Pain: Initial: 1g, then 500mg q12h or 500mg q8h. OA/RA: 250-500mg bid. Max: 1500mg/day.

**HOW SUPPLIED:** Tab: 250mg, 500mg

**CONTRAINDICATIONS:** ASA or other NSAID allergy that precipitates acute asthmatic attack, urticaria, or rhinitis. Treatment of peri-operative pain in the setting of CABG surgery.

**WARNINGS/PRECAUTIONS:** May lead to onset of new HTN or worsening of pre-existing HTN; monitor BP closely. Fluid retention and edema reported; caution with fluid retention or heart failure. Renal papillary necrosis and other renal injury reported after long-term use. Not recommended for use with advanced renal disease; if therapy must be initiated, monitor renal function. Anaphylactoid reactions may occur. May cause serious skin adverse events (eg, exfoliative dermatitis, Stevens-Johnson syndrome, and toxic epidermal necrolysis). Avoid in late pregnancy; may cause premature closure of ductus arteriosis. May cause elevations of LFTs; d/c if liver disease develops or systemic manifestations occur. Caution in elderly. Anemia may occur; with long-term use, monitor Hgb/Hct if signs or symptoms of anemia develop. May inhibit platelet aggregation and prolong bleeding time; monitor with coagulation disorders. Caution with asthma and avoid with aspirin-sensitive asthma. Adverse eye findings reported. Hypersensitivity syndrome reported; d/c if hypersensitivity occurs. Reye's syndrome may develop.

**ADVERSE REACTIONS:** Nausea, dyspepsia, GI pain, diarrhea, rash, headache, insomnia, dizziness, tinnitus, fatigue.

**INTERACTIONS:** May prolong PT with oral anticoagulants. Decreases hyperuricemic effect of HCTZ, furosemide. Antacids may reduce plasma levels. Avoid other NSAIDs. May potentiate methotrexate, cyclosporine toxicities. Increased plasma levels of APAP. Decreased plasma levels with ASA. Caution with nephrotoxic or hepatotoxic drugs.

**PREGNANCY:** Category C, not for use in nursing.

## DOLOPHINE CII

methadone HCl (Roxane)

D

**Only approved hospitals and pharmacies can dispense oral methadone for the treatment of narcotic addiction. Methadone can be dispensed in any licensed pharmacy when used as an analgesic. Deaths, cardiac and respiratory, have been reported during initiation and conversion of painpatients to methadone treatment from treatment with other opioid agonists. Respiratory depression is the main hazard associated with methadone administration. QT interval prolongation and serious arrhythmias have been observed during treatment with methadone.**

**OTHER BRAND NAMES:** Methadone (Various)

**THERAPEUTIC CLASS:** Opioid analgesic

**INDICATIONS:** Detoxification and temporary maintenance treatment of narcotic addiction (heroin or other morphine-like drugs). Relief of severe pain.

**DOSAGE:** *Adults:* Detoxification: Initial: 15-20mg/day (up to 40mg/day may be required). Stabilize for 2-3 days, then may decrease every 1-2 days depending on patient symptoms. Max: 21 days. May not repeat earlier than 4 weeks after completing previous course. Pain: Usual: 2.5-10mg q3-4h PO/IM/SQ prn.

**HOW SUPPLIED:** Tab: 5mg, 10mg

**CONTRAINDICATIONS:** Methadone is contraindicated in any patient suspected or having a paralytic ileus, acute bronchial asthma or hypercarbia and respiratory depression.

**WARNINGS/PRECAUTIONS:** Do not inject agent. Extreme caution if use narcotic antagonists in patients physically dependent on narcotics. Can cause respiratory depression and elevate CSF pressure. Caution with head injuries, acute asthma attacks, COPD, cor pulmonale, decreased respiratory reserve, pre-existing respiratory depression, hypoxia, or hypercapnia. Reduce initial dose in elderly, debilitated, severe hepatic or renal impairment, hypothyroidism, Addison's disease, prostatic hypertrophy, or urethral stricture. Risk of tolerance, dependence, and abuse may occur. Impairs physical and mental abilities. Ineffective in relieving anxiety. May mask symptoms of acute abdominal conditions. May produce hypotension. May cause incomplete cross-tolerance and iatrogenic overdose, interactions with other CNS depressants, alcohol and other drugs of abuse. May cause cardiac conduction effects like prolonged QT interval and seroius arrhythmias.

**ADVERSE REACTIONS:** Lightheadedness, dizziness, sedation, sweating, nausea, vomiting, asthenia, cardiomyopathy, ECG abnormalities, abdominal pain, agitation, siezures, confusion, hallucinations, respiratory depression.

**INTERACTIONS:** May increase desipramine levels. Pentazocine may precipitate withdrawal. Decreased serum levels with rifampin. Caution and reduce dose with CNS depressants (eg, tranquilizers, sedative-hypnotics, phenothiazines, TCAs, alcohol). MAOIs may cause severe reactions. Use caution with concomitant administration of inducers/inhibitors of CYP450 (eg, azole antifungals, phenytoin).

**PREGNANCY:** Safety in pregnancy and nursing not known.

## DOMEBORO OTIC RX

acetic acid - aluminum acetate (Bayer)

**THERAPEUTIC CLASS:** Antibacterial/antifungal

**INDICATIONS:** Treatment of superficial infections of the external auditory canal.

**DOSAGE:** *Adults:* Rest head to the side with affected ear up. Instill 4-6 drops into external ear canal and maintain position for 5 minutes. Repeat q2-3h.

**HOW SUPPLIED:** Sol: (Acetic Acid-Aluminum Acetate) 2%-0.79% [60mL]

**CONTRAINDICATIONS:** Perforated tympanic membrane.

**WARNINGS/PRECAUTIONS:** Not for ophthalmic use. D/C if sensitization or irritation occurs. Assure that solution stays in contact with affected area for sufficient time.

**ADVERSE REACTIONS:** Local irritation.

**PREGNANCY:** Safety in pregnancy and nursing is not known.



## DONNATAL RX

phenobarbital - atropine sulfate - hyoscyamine sulfate - scopolamine hydrobromide (PBM Pharmaceuticals)

**OTHER BRAND NAMES:** Donnatal Extentabs (PBM Pharmaceuticals)

**THERAPEUTIC CLASS:** Anticholinergic/barbiturate

**INDICATIONS:** Adjunct therapy for irritable bowel syndrome, acute enterocolitis, duodenal ulcers.

**DOSAGE:** *Adults:* (Elixir/Tab) 1-2 tabs or 5-10mL tid-qid. (Extentabs) 1 tab q8-12h. Hepatic Disease: Use lower doses.
*Pediatrics:* (Elixir) 4.5kg: 0.5mL q4h or 0.75mL q6h. 9.1kg: 1mL q4h or 1.5mL q6h. 13.6kg: 1.5mL q4h or 2mL q6h. 22.7kg: 2.5mL q4h or 3.75mL q6h. 34kg: 3.75mL q4h or 5mL q6h. 45.4kg: 5mL q4h or 7.5mL q6h. Hepatic Disease: Use lower doses.

**HOW SUPPLIED:** (Atropine-Hyoscyamine-Phenobarbital-Scopolamine) Elixir: 0.0194mg-0.1037mg-16.2mg-0.0065mg/5mL; Tab: 0.0194mg-0.1037mg-16.2mg-0.0065mg; Tab, Extended Release: (Extentabs) 0.0582mg-0.3111mg-48.6mg-0.0195mg

**CONTRAINDICATIONS:** Glaucoma, obstructive uropathy, obstructive GI disease, paralytic ileus, intestinal atony in elderly or debilitated, unstable cardiovascular status in acute hemorrhage, severe ulcerative colitis, myasthenia gravis, hiatal hernia with reflux esophagitis, intermittent porphyria, and for patients in whom phenobarbital produces restlessness and/or excitement.

**WARNINGS/PRECAUTIONS:** Inconclusive whether anticholinergic/antispasmodic drugs aid in duodenal ulcer healing, decrease recurrence rate, or prevent complications. Heat prostration can occur with high environmental temperatures. Avoid with intestinal obstruction. May be habit forming; caution with history of physical and/or psychological drug dependence. Caution with hepatic disease, renal disease, autonomic neuropathy, hyperthyroidism, coronary heart disease, CHF, arrhythmias, tachycardia, HTN. May delay gastric emptying. Diarrhea may be an early symptom of incomplete intestinal obstruction, especially with ileostomy or colostomy; treatment would be inappropriate.

**ADVERSE REACTIONS:** Xerostomia, urinary hesitancy/retention, blurred vision, tachycardia/palpitation, mydriasis, cycloplegia, increased ocular tension, loss of taste, headache, nervousness, drowsiness, weakness, dizziness, insomnia, nausea, vomiting, impotence, suppression of lactation, constipation, bloated feeling, musculoskeletal pain, allergic reaction/drug idiosyncrasies, decreased sweating.

**INTERACTIONS:** Phenobarbital may decrease anticoagulant effects; adjust dose.

**PREGNANCY:** Category C, caution in nursing.

## DOPAMINE HCL
dopamine HCl (Various)

RX

**THERAPEUTIC CLASS:** Inotropic agent

**INDICATIONS:** For correction of hemodynamic imbalances present in shock due to MI, trauma, endotoxic septicemia, open-heart surgery, renal failure, and chronic cardiac decompensation.

**DOSAGE:** *Adults:* Initial: 2-5mcg/kg/min. Use 5mcg/kg/min in seriously ill. Increase in 5-10mcg/kg/min increments, up to 20-50mcg/kg/min.

**HOW SUPPLIED:** Inj: 40mg/mL, 80mg/mL, 160mg/mL

**CONTRAINDICATIONS:** Pheochromocytoma, uncorrected tachyarrhythmias or ventricular fibrillation.

**WARNINGS/PRECAUTIONS:** Contains sulfites. Monitor BP, urine flow, cardiac output and pulmonary wedge pressure. Correct hypovolemia, hypoxia, hypercapnia, and acidosis prior to use. Reduce infusion rate with increase in diastolic BP/marked decrease in pulse pressure; increase rate if hypotension occurs. Discontinue if hypotension persists. Reduce dose if increased ectopic beats occurs. Caution with history of occlusive vascular disease (eg, atherosclerosis, arterial embolism, Raynaud's disease, cold injury, diabetic endarteritis, and Buerger's disease); monitor for changes in skin color or temperature. Administer phentolamine if extravasation is noted. Avoid abrupt withdrawal.

**ADVERSE REACTIONS:** Tachycardia, palpitation, ventricular arrhythmia (high doses), dyspnea, nausea, vomiting, headache, anxiety, bradycardia, hypotension, HTN, vasoconstriction.

**INTERACTIONS:** Reduce dose to 1/10th of usual dose within 2 to 3 weeks of MAOI use. Potential additive effects on urine flow with diuretics. TCAs may potentiate pressor response. Antagonized by beta- and alpha-blockers, haloperidol. Extreme caution with cyclopropane or halogenated hydrocarbon anesthetics. Possible severe HTN with some oxytocic drugs. Hypotension and bradycardia reported with phenytoin.

**PREGNANCY:** Category C, caution in nursing.

## DORYX
doxycycline hyclate (Warner Chilcott)

RX

**THERAPEUTIC CLASS:** Tetracycline derivative

**INDICATIONS:** Treatment of susceptible infections including respiratory, urinary, skin and skin structure, lymphogranuloma, psittacosis, trachoma, uncomplicated urethral/endocervical/rectal, nongonococcal urethritis, rickettsiae, chancroid, plague, cholera, brucellosis, anthrax. When penicillin is contraindicated, treatment of syphilis, listeriosis, *Clostridium* species, and others. Adjunct therapy for amebiasis and severe acne.

**DOSAGE:** *Adults:* Usual: 100mg q12h on 1st day, followed by 100mg qd. Severe Infections/Chronic UTI: 100mg q12h. Uncomplicated Gonococcal Infections (Men, except anorectal infections): 100mg bid for 7 days, or 300mg followed in 1 hr by another 300mg dose. Acute Epididymo-Orchitis: 100mg bid for at least 10 days. Primary/Secondary Syphilis: 300mg/day in divided doses for at least 10 days. Nongonococcal Urethritis, Uncomplicated Urethral/Endocervical/Rectal Infection: 100mg bid for at least 7 days. Inhalational Anthrax (post-exposure): 100mg bid for 60 days. Treat Strep infections for 10 days.
*Pediatrics:* >8 yrs: >100lbs: 100mg q12h on 1st day, followed by 100mg qd. Severe Infections/Chronic UTI: 100mg q12h. <100lbs: 2mg/lb given bid on day 1, followed by 1mg/lb given qd-bid thereafter. Severe Infections: Up to 2mg/lb. Inhalational Anthrax (post-exposure): <100lbs: 1mg/lb bid for 60 days. >100lbs: 100mg bid for 60 days.

**HOW SUPPLIED:** Cap: 75mg, 100mg

**WARNINGS/PRECAUTIONS:** May cause fetal harm during pregnancy. Use during tooth development (last half of pregnancy, infancy, <8 yrs) may cause permanent discoloration of the teeth or enamel hypoplasia. Photosensitivity, increased BUN, superinfection may occur. Monitor hematopoietic, renal and hepatic values periodically with long term therapy. Bulging fontanels in infants and benign intracranial HTN in adults reported. May decrease bone growth in premature infants.



**ADVERSE REACTIONS:** Anorexia, nausea, vomiting, diarrhea, dysphagia, enterocolitis, rash, exfoliative dermatitis, renal toxicity, hypersensitivity reactions, blood dyscrasias.

**INTERACTIONS:** May require downward adjustments of anticoagulant dosage. May interfere with bactericidal action of penicillin; avoid concurrent use when possible. Avoid antacids containing aluminum, calcium, or magnesium, sodium bicarbonate, and iron-containing preparations.

**PREGNANCY:** Category D, not for use in nursing.

## DOSTINEX RX

cabergoline (Pharmacia & Upjohn)

**THERAPEUTIC CLASS:** Pituitary hormone

**INDICATIONS:** Treatment of hyperprolactinemic disorders, either idiopathic or due to pituitary adenomas.

**DOSAGE:** *Adults:* Initial: 0.25mg twice weekly. Titrate: May increase by 0.25mg twice weekly at 4 week intervals. Max: 1mg twice weekly. Discontinue after maintaining a normal serum prolactin level for 6 months. Efficacy >24 months not established.

**HOW SUPPLIED:** Tab: 0.5mg* *scored

**CONTRAINDICATIONS:** Uncontrolled HTN, hypersensitivity to ergot derivatives.

**WARNINGS/PRECAUTIONS:** Initial doses >1mg may produce orthostatic hypotension. Caution with hepatic impairment. Avoid with pregnancy-induced HTN (eg, preeclampsia, eclampsia). Not for inhibition/suppression of postpartum lactation. Use caution with respiratory or cardiac disorders linked to fibrotic tissue as risk of valvulopathy/fibrosis is possible; patient should be informed to notify physician if he/she develops cough.

**ADVERSE REACTIONS:** Nausea, constipation, abdominal pain, headache, dizziness, postural hypotension, fatigue, somnolence, depression, asthenia.

**INTERACTIONS:** Avoid with $D_2$-antagonists (eg, phenothiazines, butyrophenones, thioxanthines, metoclopramide). Caution with other drugs that lower BP.

**PREGNANCY:** Category B, not for use in nursing.

## DOVONEX RX

calcipotriene (Warner Chilcott/Bristol-Myers Squibb)

**THERAPEUTIC CLASS:** Vitamin $D_3$ derivative

**INDICATIONS:** Treatment of plaque psoriasis.

**DOSAGE:** *Adults:* (Cream) Apply bid up to 8 weeks. (Oint) Apply qd-bid. Rub in gently. Wash hands after application.

**HOW SUPPLIED:** Cre, Oint: 0.005% [60g, 120g]

**CONTRAINDICATIONS:** Hypercalcemia or vitamin D toxicity. Do not use on the face.

**WARNINGS/PRECAUTIONS:** Avoid face and eyes. Discontinue if irritation or hypercalcemia occurs; may continue once calcium levels are normal.

**ADVERSE REACTIONS:** Local irritation, rash, pruritus, dermatitis, erythema, itching, worsening of psoriasis.

**PREGNANCY:** Category C, caution in nursing.

## DOVONEX SCALP

RX

calcipotriene (Warner Chilcott/Bristol-Myers Squibb)



**THERAPEUTIC CLASS:** Vitamin $D_3$ derivative

**INDICATIONS:** Topical treatment of chronic, moderately severe psoriasis of the scalp.

**DOSAGE:** *Adults:* Comb hair to remove debris. Part hair and apply bid up to 8 weeks. Rub in gently. Avoid uninvolved skin. Wash hands after application.

**HOW SUPPLIED:** Sol: 0.005% [60mL]

**CONTRAINDICATIONS:** Acute psoriatic eruptions, hypercalcemia, vitamin D toxicity.

**WARNINGS/PRECAUTIONS:** Avoid mucous membranes and eyes. Discontinue if irritation, sensitivity reaction, or hypercalcemia occurs; may continue once calcium levels are normal.

**ADVERSE REACTIONS:** Transient burning, stinging, tingling, rash, dry skin, peeling, pruritus, dermatitis, worsening of psoriasis.

**PREGNANCY:** Category C, caution in nursing.

## DOXEPIN

RX

doxepin HCl (Various)

**Antidepressants increased the risk of suicidal thinking and behavior (suicidality) in short-term studies in children and adolescents with Major Depressive Disorder (MDD) and other psychiatric disorders. Doxepin is not approved for use in pediatric patients.**

**OTHER BRAND NAMES:** Sinequan (Pfizer)

**THERAPEUTIC CLASS:** Tricyclic antidepressant

**INDICATIONS:** Depression and/or anxiety.

**DOSAGE:** *Adults:* Very Mild Illness: Usual: 25-50mg/day. Mild to Moderate Severity: Initial: 75mg/day. Usual: 75-150mg/day. Severely Ill: May increase up to 300mg/day. Dilute solution with 120mL of water, milk or juice. Give once daily or in divided doses. Divide dose if >150mg. Elderly: Use lower doses and monitor closely.

**HOW SUPPLIED:** Cap: 10mg, 25mg, 50mg, 75mg, 100mg, 150mg; Sol, Concentrate: 10mg/mL [120mL]

**CONTRAINDICATIONS:** Glaucoma, urinary retention.

**WARNINGS/PRECAUTIONS:** Monitor for suicidal tendencies and increased symptoms of psychosis. Avoid abrupt discontinuation.

**ADVERSE REACTIONS:** Drowsiness, dry mouth, blurred vision, constipation, urinary retention, hypotension, tachycardia, rash, edema, photosensitization, pruritus, eosinophilia, nausea, dizziness.

**INTERACTIONS:** Caution with drugs metabolized by CYP2D6. Potentiated by inhibitors (eg, cimetidine, quinidine, SSRIs) and substrates (other antidepressants, phenothiazines, propafenone, flecainide) of CYP2D6. Increased danger of overdose with alcohol. Hypoglycemia reported with tolazamide. Avoid within 2 weeks of MAOI therapy. Increased side effects with anticholinergics. Caution when switching from TCAs to SSRIs (≥5 weeks may be needed before initiating TCA treatment after withdrawal from fluoxetine).

**PREGNANCY:** Safety in pregnancy and nursing not known.

# DOXIL

RX

doxorubicin HCl liposome (Ortho Biotech)

D

**Myocardial damage may lead to CHF when cumulative doses approach 550mg/m². May lead to cardiac toxicity, consider prior use of anthracyclines or anthracenediones in cumulative dose calculations. Cardiac toxicity may occur at lower cumulative doses with prior mediastinal irradiation or cyclophosphamide therapy. Acute infusion-associated reactions reported. Severe myelosuppression, myocardial toxicity may occur. Reduce dose with hepatic dysfunction. Severe side effects reported with accidental substitution for doxorubicin HCl. Only administer to cardiovascular disease patients when benefit outweighs risk.**

**THERAPEUTIC CLASS:** Anthracycline

**INDICATIONS:** Treatment of AIDS-related Kaposi's sarcoma (KS). Treatment of metastatic ovary carcinoma refractory to paclitaxel- and platinum-based therapy. In combination with bortezomib for the treatment of Multiple Myeloma in patients who have not previously received bortezomib and have received at least one prior therapy.

**DOSAGE:** *Adults:* KS: 20mg/m² IV over 30 minutes, once every 3 weeks. Ovarian Cancer: 50mg/m² IV once every 4 weeks. Multiple Myeloma: bortezomib, 1.3mg/m² bolus on days 1, 4, 8 and 11, every 3 weeks (patient may be treated up to 8 cycles depending on disease progression or unaccepable toxicity); Doxil, 30mg/m² IV on day 4 following bortezomib dose. Initiate at 1mg/mL to minimize infusion reactions; may increase rate if no reactions to complete infusion at 1 hr. Minimum 4 courses is recommended. Hepatic Dysfunction: If serum bilirubin 1.2-3mg/dL, give 50% of normal dose. If serum bilirubin >3mg/dL, give 25% of normal dose. Stomatitis/PPE Toxicity: Grade 1: Redose unless patient had previous Grade 3 or 4 toxicity. If so, delay up to 2 weeks and decrease dose by 25%. Return to original dose interval. Grade 2: Delay dose up to 2 weeks or until resolved to Grade 0-1. If no resolution after 2 weeks, discontinue. Grade 3 or 4: Delay dose up to 2 weeks or until resolved to Grade 0-1. Decrease dose by 25% and return to original dose interval. If no resolution after 2 weeks, discontinue. Hematological Toxicity: Grade 1: Resume therapy with no dose reduction. Grade 2 or 3: Wait until ANC >1500 and platelets >75,000; redose with no dose reduction. Grade 4: Wait until ANC >1500 and platelets >75,000; redose at 25% dose reduction or continue full dose with cytokine support. MM dosage adjustment for doxil + bortezomib: Fever ≥38°C & ANC <1000/mm³; do not dose this cycle if before day 4, if after day 4, reduce next dose for both by 25%. After day 1 of each cycle (platelet count < 25,000/mm³, Hgb <8g/dL, ANC <500/mm³): do not dose this cycle if before day 4; if after day 4, reduce next dose by 25% in the following cycles if borte

**HOW SUPPLIED:** Inj: 2mg/mL

**CONTRAINDICATIONS:** Nursing mothers.

**WARNINGS/PRECAUTIONS:** Monitor cardiac function. Cardiac toxicity may occur after discontinuation. Recall of skin reaction due to radiotherapy reported. Obtain CBC, including platelets, frequently and at a minimum before each dose. Secondary AML reported with anthracyclines. Evaluate hepatic function before therapy. Avoid extravasation. Can cause fetal harm. Palmar-plantar erythrodysestheia (PPE) reported.

**ADVERSE REACTIONS:** Neutropenia, leukopenia, anemia, thromobocytopenia, stomatitis, nausea, asthenia, vomiting, rash, alopecia, diarrhea, constipation, PPE.

**INTERACTIONS:** May potentiate toxicity of other anticancer therapies. May exacerbate cyclophosphamide-induced hemorrhagic cystitis. May enhance hepatotoxicity of 6-mercaptopurine. May increase radiation induced toxicity of the myocardium, mucosae, skin, and liver. Hematological toxicity may be more severe with agents that cause bone marrow suppression. See Black Box Warning.

**PREGNANCY:** Category D, not for use in nursing.

## DRISDOL RX

ergocalciferol (Sanofi-Aventis)

**THERAPEUTIC CLASS:** Vitamin D analog

**INDICATIONS:** Treatment of hypoparathyroidism, refractory rickets (vitamin D resistant rickets), and familial hypophosphatemia.

**DOSAGE:** *Adults:* Vitamin D Resistant Rickets: 12,000-500,000 IU qd. Hypoparathyroidism: 50,000-200,000 IU qd given concomitantly with calcium lactate 4g six times/day. Individualize dosage.

**HOW SUPPLIED:** Cap: 1.25mg (50,000 IU vitamin D)

**CONTRAINDICATIONS:** Hypercalcemia, malabsorption syndrome, abnormal sensitivity to the toxic effects of vitamin D, hypervitaminosis D.

**WARNINGS/PRECAUTIONS:** Avoid in infants with idiopathic hypercalcemia. Monitor serum calcium and phosphorous levels every 2 weeks or more frequently if necessary. X-rays of bones should be taken every month until condition is corrected and stabilized. IV calcium, parathyroid hormone, and/or dihydrotachysterol may be needed when treating hypoparathyroidism. Maintain normal serum phosphorous levels when treating hyperphosphatemia to prevent metastatic calcification. Maintain adequate dietary calcium. Contains FD&C Yellow No. 5 (tartrazine). Protect from light.

**ADVERSE REACTIONS:** Anemia, anorexia, constipation, nausea, bone demineralization, stiffness, weakness, calcification of soft tissues, impaired renal function, polyuria, nocturia, polydipsia, hypercalciuria, azotemia, HTN, nephrocalcinosis.

**INTERACTIONS:** Impaired absorption with mineral oil. Thiazide diuretics may cause hypercalcemia.

**PREGNANCY:** Category C, caution in nursing.

## DROXIA RX

hydroxyurea (Bristol-Myers Squibb)

**Mutagenic, carcinogenic, clastogenic, and causes cellular transformation to tumorigenic phenotypes. May develop secondary leukemia with long-term therapy for myeloproliferative disorders.**

**THERAPEUTIC CLASS:** Ribonucleotide reductase inhibitor

**INDICATIONS:** To reduce the frequency of painful crises and the need for blood transfusions in sickle cell anemia with recurrent moderate to severe painful crises.

**DOSAGE:** *Adults:* Initial: 15mg/kg/day as single dose. If blood counts are in acceptable range, increase by 5mg/kg/day every 12 weeks until maximum tolerated dose or 35mg/kg/day. If blood counts are toxic, discontinue until hematologic recovery. May resume treatment after dose reduction by 2.5mg/kg/day from dose associated with hematologic toxicity. May increase every 12 weeks by 2.5mg/kg/day until reaching a stable dose that does not result in toxicity for 24 weeks.

**HOW SUPPLIED:** Cap: 200mg, 300mg, 400mg

**WARNINGS/PRECAUTIONS:** Avoid in marked bone marrow depression. Caution with renal dysfunction. Severe, life-threatening myelosuppression reported. Monitor hematologic, liver, kidney function before therapy and repeatedly thereafter. Interrupt therapy if neutrophils <2000/mm$^3$ or platelets <80,000/mm$^3$, Hgb <4.5g/dL or reticulocytes <80,000/mm$^2$ with Hgb <9g/dL. Monitor blood counts every 2 weeks. Cutaneous vasculitic toxicities, including vasculitic ulcerations and gangrene, reported; d/c if cutaneous vasculitic ulcerations develop.

**ADVERSE REACTIONS:** Neutropenia, low reticulocyte and platelet levels, hair loss, fever, GI disturbances, weight gain, bleeding, melanonychia, dermatological reactions, cutaneous vasculitic toxicities.

**INTERACTIONS:** Monitor for hepatoxicity and pancreatitis with didanosine, stavudine.

**PREGNANCY:** Category D, not for use in nursing.



## DRYSOL RX
aluminum chloride (Person & Covey)

**THERAPEUTIC CLASS:** Antiperspirant

**INDICATIONS:** Aid in the management of hyperhidrosis.

**DOSAGE:** *Adults:* Apply qhs to dry area. Wash area the following morning. Maint: After excessive sweating stops, apply once or twice weekly or as needed.

**HOW SUPPLIED:** Sol: 20% [35mL, 37.5mL, 60mL]

**WARNINGS/PRECAUTIONS:** Avoid broken, irritated or recently shaved skin. Avoid eye contact. D/C if irritation or sensitization occurs. May be harmful to certain metals and fabrics. Keep away from open flame.

**ADVERSE REACTIONS:** Transient stinging or itching.

**PREGNANCY:** Safety in pregnancy and nursing not known.

## DRYVAX RX
smallpox vaccine, dried (Wyeth)

**Acute myopericarditis has been observed after administration. Encephalitis and progressive vaccinia have occured following smallpox immunization, almost always in immunocompromised patients. Severe vaccinal skin infections have occured among persons with eczema. Do not administer in persons with eczema, cardiac disease and immunocompromised.**

**THERAPEUTIC CLASS:** Vaccine

**INDICATIONS:** For active immunization against smallpox disease.

**DOSAGE:** *Adults:* Give IM into deltoid muscle or posterior aspect of arm over triceps muscle. Use 2 or 3 needle punctures for primary vaccination and 15 punctures for revaccination. May cover vaccination site with a porous bandage, until scab separates and underlying skin has healed. Inspect vaccination site 6-8 days later to interpret response.
*Pediatrics:* >12 months: Give IM into deltoid muscle or posterior aspect of arm over triceps muscle. Use 2 or 3 needle punctures for primary vaccination and 15 punctures for revaccination. May cover vaccination site with a porous bandage, until scab separates and underlying skin has healed. Inspect vaccination site 6-8 days later to interpret response.

**HOW SUPPLIED:** Inj: 100 million PFU

**CONTRAINDICATIONS:** (Routine non-emergency use) Hypersensitivity to polymyxin B sulfate, dihydrostreptomycin sulfate, chlortetracycline HCl, and neomycin sulfate; infants <12 months of age; eczema, history of eczema, or other acute, chronic, or exfoliative skin conditions (including household contacts of such persons); systemic corticosteroid use at doses >2mg/kg or >20mg/day of prednisone for >2 weeks, or immunosuppressive use (eg, alkylating agents, antimetabolites), or radiation (including household contacts of such persons); congenital or acquired immune deficiencies (including household contacts of such persons); immunosuppressed individuals (including household contacts of such persons); pregnancy (including household contacts of such persons).

**WARNINGS/PRECAUTIONS:** Vial stopper contains dry natural rubber; caution with latex sensitivity. Patients susceptible to adverse effects of caccinia virus should avoid contact with persons with active vaccination lesions. Vaccinia virus may be cultured from site of primary vaccine from time of papule development until scab separates from skin lesion. Not recommended for elderly in non-emergency conditions.

**ADVERSE REACTIONS:** Fever, rash, secondary pyogenic infections at vaccination site, inadvertent inoculation at other sites, regional lymphadenopathy, malaise.

**INTERACTIONS:** Avoid salves or ointments on vaccination site.

**PREGNANCY:** Category C, not for use in nursing in non-emergency conditions.



## DTIC-DOME RX
dacarbazine (Bayer)

**Hemopoietic toxicity and hepatotoxicity reported.**

**THERAPEUTIC CLASS:** Purine precursor analog

**INDICATIONS:** Treatment of metastatic malignant melanoma and 2nd line combination therapy for Hodgkin's disease.

**DOSAGE:** *Adults:* Malignant Melanoma: 2-4.5mg/kg/day for 10 days. May repeat every 4 weeks. Alternate Dosage: 250mg/m²/day IV for 5 days. May repeat every 3 weeks. Hodgkin's Disease: 150mg/m²/day for 5 days. May repeat every 4 weeks. Alternate Dosage: 375mg/m²/day on day 1. May repeat every 15 days.

**HOW SUPPLIED:** Inj: 200mg

**WARNINGS/PRECAUTIONS:** Hematopoietic depression, anemia, anaphylactic reactions reported. Hepatotoxicity with hepatic vein thrombosis and hepatocellular necrosis may result in death. Extravasation may result in tissue damage and severe pain.

**ADVERSE REACTIONS:** Nausea, vomiting, anorexia, diarrhea, flu-like syndromes, alopecia, renal or hepatic dysfunction, rash.

**PREGNANCY:** Category C, safety in nursing not known.

## DUAC RX
clindamycin - benzoyl peroxide (Stiefel)

**THERAPEUTIC CLASS:** Antibacterial/keratolytic

**INDICATIONS:** Topical treatment of inflammatory acne vulgaris.

**DOSAGE:** *Adults:* Wash face and pat dry. Apply qd in the evening. *Pediatrics:* >12 yrs: Wash face and pat dry. Apply qd in the evening.

**HOW SUPPLIED:** Gel: (Clindamycin-Benzoyl Peroxide) 1%-5% [45g]

**CONTRAINDICATIONS:** Hypersensitivity to lincomycin. History of regional enteritis, ulcerative colitis, pseudomembranous colitis, or antibiotic-associated colitis.

**WARNINGS/PRECAUTIONS:** Severe colitis reported with oral and parenteral clindamycin. Discontinue if severe diarrhea occurs. Avoid contact with eyes and mucous membranes. May bleach hair or colored fabric. Limit sunlight exposure.

**ADVERSE REACTIONS:** Dry skin, erythema, peeling, burning.

**INTERACTIONS:** Cumulative irritancy possible with other topical acne agents. Avoid erythromycin agents.

**PREGNANCY:** Category C, not for use in nursing.

## DUET STUARTNATAL RX
minerals - folic acid - multiple vitamin (Xanodyne)

**THERAPEUTIC CLASS:** Prenatal vitamin

**INDICATIONS:** Vitamin and mineral supplementation for before, during, and after pregnancy.

**DOSAGE:** *Adults:* 1 tab qd.

**HOW SUPPLIED:** Tab: Calcium 200mg-Copper 2mg-Folic Acid 1mg-Iron 29mg-Magnesium 25mg-Niacinamide 20mg-Vitamin A 3000IU-Vitamin $B_1$ 1.8mg-Vitamin $B_2$ 4mg-Vitamin $B_6$ 25mg-Vitamin $B_{12}$ 0.012mg-Vitamin C 120mg-Vitamin D 400IU-Vitamin E 30mg-Zinc 25mg; Tab, Chewable: Calcium 100mg-Copper 2mg-Folic Acid 1mg-Iron 29mg-Magnesium 25mg-Niacinamide 20mg-Vitamin A 3000IU-Vitamin $B_1$ 1.8mg-Vitamin $B_2$ 4mg-Vitamin $B_6$ 25mg-Vitamin $B_{12}$ 0.012mg-Vitamin C 120mg-Vitamin D 400IU-Vitamin E 30mg-Zinc 25mg



**WARNINGS/PRECAUTIONS:** Accidental overdose of iron-containing products is a leading cause of fatal poisoning in children <6 yrs. Not for the treatment of pernicious anemia and other megaloblastic anemias where vitamin $B_{12}$ is deficient. Folic acid >0.1mg/day may obscure pernicious anemia. Chewable tabs contain phenylalanine.

## DUETACT RX

glimepiride - pioglitazone HCl (Takeda)

**THERAPEUTIC CLASS:** Thiazolidinedione/sulfonylurea

**INDICATIONS:** Adjunct to diet and exercise to improve glycemic control in type 2 diabetes already being treated with combination of pioglitazone and sulfonylurea, with inadequate control on sulfonylurea alone, or with initial response to pioglitazone alone requiring additional glycemic control.

**DOSAGE:** *Adults:* Base recommended starting dose on current regimen of pioglitazone and/or sulfonylurea. Give with first meal of day. Current Glimepiride Monotherapy or Prior Therapy of Pioglitazone plus Glimepiride Separately: Initial: 30mg-2mg or 30mg-4mg qd. Current Pioglitazone or Different Sulfonylurea Monotherapy or Combination of Both: Initial: 30mg-2mg qd. Adjust dose based on response. Max: Once-daily at any dosage strength. Elderly/Debilitated/Malnourished/Renal or Hepatic Insufficiency (ALT ≤2.5x ULN): Initial: 1mg glimepiride prior to prescribing Duetact. Systolic Dysfunction: Initial: 15-30mg of pioglitazone; titrate carefully to lowest Duetact dose.

**HOW SUPPLIED:** Tab: (Pioglitazone-Glimepiride) 30mg-2mg, 30mg-4mg

**CONTRAINDICATIONS:** Diabetic ketoacidosis, with or without coma.

**WARNINGS/PRECAUTIONS:** (Glimepiride): Increased CV mortality. Hypoglycemia risk if debilitated, malnourished, or with adrenal, pituitary, renal or hepatic insufficiency. Hypoglycemia may be masked in elderly. May lose blood glucose control with stress. Secondary failure may occur. D/C if skin reactions persist or worsen. (Pioglitiazone): May cause fluid retention and exacerbation/initiation of heart failure; d/c if cardiac status deteriorates. Avoid if NYHA Class III or IV cardiac status. Not for use in type 1 DM or diabetic ketoacidosis treatment. Caution with edema. Dose-related weight gain reported. Ovulation in premenopausal anovulatory patient may occur; risk of pregnancy with inadequate contraception. May decrease Hgb and Hct. Avoid with active liver disease, if ALT levels >2.5x ULN, or if jaundice occurred. Check LFTs before therapy, every 2 months for 1 yr, and periodically thereafter, or if hepatic dysfunction symptoms occur. D/C if ALT >3x ULN on therapy. Mascular edema has been reported.

**ADVERSE REACTIONS:** Hypoglycemia, upper respiratory tract infection, increased weight, lower limb edema/pain, headache, UTI, diarrhea,nausea and a new onset or worsening diabetic macular edema with decreased visualacuity.

**INTERACTIONS:** (Pioglitiazone): CYP3A4 inducer. May decrease levels of ethinyl estradiol and midazolam. CYP2C8 inhibitor. May significantly increase the AUC levels of pioglitiazone. CYP2C8 inducer. May significantly decrease the AUC levels of pioglitiazone.(Glimepiride): Risk of hyperglycemia with thiazides, corticosteroids, phenothiazines, thyroid products, estrogens, oral contraceptives, phenytoin, nicotinic acid, sympathomimetics, and isoniazid.

Hypoglycemia may be potentiated with β-blockers, MAOIs, salicylates, sulfonamides, and coumarins. Risk of severe hypoglycemia with oral miconazole.

**PREGNANCY:** Category C, do not use in nursing.



## DULCOLAX OTC

bisacodyl (Boehringer Ingelheim)

**THERAPEUTIC CLASS:** Stimulant laxative

**INDICATIONS:** Relief of occasional constipation and irregularity. For bowel cleansing regimen for surgery or endoscopic exam.

**DOSAGE:** *Adults:* (Tab) Take 2-3 tabs qd. Do not crush/chew. (Sup) Insert 1 sup rectally; retain for 15-20 minutes. May coat tip with petroleum jelly with anal fissures or hemorrhoids. X-Ray Endoscopy For Barium Enema: Avoid food after tab administration. Insert 1 sup rectally 1-2 hrs before exam. *Pediatrics* >12 yrs: (Tab) 2-3 tabs qd. 6-12 yrs: 1 tab qd. Do not crush/chew. (Sup) >12 yrs: Insert 1 sup rectally; retain for 15-20 minutes. 6-12 yrs: Insert 1/2 sup rectally qd. May coat tip with petroleum jelly with anal fissures or hemorrhoids. X-Ray Endoscopy For Barium Enema: >6 yrs: Avoid food after tab administration. Insert 1 sup 1-2 hrs before exam. <6 yrs: Avoid tab. Insert 1/2 sup rectally 1-2 hrs before exam.

**HOW SUPPLIED:** Sup: 10mg; Tab, Delayed Release: 5mg

**CONTRAINDICATIONS:** Acute abdominal surgery, appendicitis, rectal bleeding, gastroenteritis, intestinal obstruction.

**WARNINGS/PRECAUTIONS:** Avoid with abdominal pain, nausea, or vomiting. Not for long-term use ( >7 days). D/C with rectal bleeding or fail to have bowel movement.

**ADVERSE REACTIONS:** Abdominal discomfort.

**INTERACTIONS:** Avoid tabs within 1 hr after antacids or milk.

**PREGNANCY:** Safety in pregnancy and nursing not known.

## DUONEB RX

albuterol sulfate - ipratropium bromide (Dey)

**THERAPEUTIC CLASS:** $Beta_2$ agonist/anticholinergic

**INDICATIONS:** Treatment of bronchospasm in COPD in patients requiring more than one bronchodilator.

**DOSAGE:** *Adults:* 3mL qid via nebulizer. May give 2 additional doses/day.

**HOW SUPPLIED:** Sol, Inhalation: (Albuterol-Ipratropium) 3mg-0.5mg/3mL [3mL, $30^s$ $60^s$]

**CONTRAINDICATIONS:** Hypersensitivity to atropine and its derivatives.

**WARNINGS/PRECAUTIONS:** Paradoxical bronchospasm and hypersensitivity reactions reported. Caution with cardiovascular disorders, convulsive disorders, hyperthyroidism, DM, narrow angle glaucoma, prostatic hypertrophy, and bladder-neck obstruction.

**ADVERSE REACTIONS:** Pain, chest pain, diarrhea, dyspepsia, nausea, leg cramps, bronchitis, lung disease, pharyngitis, pneumonia.

**INTERACTIONS:** Additive interactions with anticholinergic agents. Increased risk of cardiovascular side effects with sympathomimetics. Use $\beta_1$-selective blockers with hyperactive airways. Caution with or within 2 weeks of discontinuation of MAOIs or TCAs.

**PREGNANCY:** Category C, not for use in nursing.

## DURAGESIC

fentanyl (Ortho-McNeil)

CII

D

**Life-threatening hypoventilation can occur. Contraindicated for acute or post-op pain, mild/intermittent pain responsive to PRN or non-opioids, or in doses >25mcg/hr at initiation of opioid therapy. Avoid in patients <12 yrs or if <18 yrs and weigh <50kg. Only for use in opioid tolerant patients. Concomitant use with potent CYP450 3A4 inhibitors may result in an increase in fentanyl plasma concentrations which may cause potentially fatal respiratory depression. Monitor patients receiving potent CYP450 3A4 inhibitors.**

**THERAPEUTIC CLASS:** Opioid analgesic

**INDICATIONS:** Management of chronic pain when continuous opioid analgesia is required and cannot be managed by lesser means.

**DOSAGE:** *Adults:* Individualize dose. Determine dose based on opioid tolerance. Initial: 25mcg/hr for 72 hr.
*Pediatrics:* >12 yrs: Individualize dose. Determine dose based on opioid tolerance. Initial: 25mcg/hr for 72 hr.

**HOW SUPPLIED:** Patch: 12.5mcg/hr, 25mcg/hr, 50mcg/hr, 75mcg/hr, 100mcg/hr [5[s]]

**CONTRAINDICATIONS:** Management of acute/post-op pain, mild/intermittent pain responsive to PRN or non-opioid therapy. Doses >25mcg/hr at initiation. Hypersensitivity to adhesives. Diagnosis or suspicion of paralytic ileus.

**WARNINGS/PRECAUTIONS:** Monitor patients with adverse events for at least 12 hrs after removal. Avoid exposing application site to direct external heat. Hypoventilation may occur; caution with chronic pulmonary diseases. Caution with brain tumors, bradyarrhythmias, renal/hepatic impairment. Avoid with increased intracranial pressure, impaired consciousness, or coma. May obscure clinical course of head injury. Tolerance and physical dependence can occur.

**ADVERSE REACTIONS:** Hypoventilation, hypotension, HTN, nausea, vomiting, constipation, dry mouth, somnolence, confusion, asthenia, sweating.

**INTERACTIONS:** See Black Box Warning. Concomitant use with CNS depressants (opioids, sedatives, hypnotics, tranquilizers, general anesthetics, phenothiazines, skeletal muscle relaxants, alcohol) may cause respiratory depression, hypotension, profound sedation, or potentially coma or death. May increase clearance with CYP3A4 inducers (eg, rifampin, carbamazepine, phenytoin). Avoid use within 14 days of MAOI.

**PREGNANCY:** Category C, not for use in nursing.

## DURAMORPH

morphine sulfate (Baxter)

CII

**THERAPEUTIC CLASS:** Opioid analgesic

**INDICATIONS:** Management of pain unresponsive to non-narcotic analgesics.

**DOSAGE:** *Adults:* IV: Initial: 2-10mg/70kg. Epidural Injection: Initial: 5mg in lumbar region. Titrate: If inadequate pain relief within 1 hr, increase by 1-2mg. Max: 10mg/24hrs. Continuous Epidural: Initial: 2-4mg/24hrs. Give additional 1-2mg if needed. Intrathecal: 0.2-1mg single dose, do not repeat; may follow with 0.6mg/hr naloxone infusion to reduce incidence of side effects.

**HOW SUPPLIED:** Inj: 0.5mg/mL, 1mg/mL, 5mg/mL

**CONTRAINDICATIONS:** Allergy to opiates, acute bronchial asthma, upper airway obstruction. Severe hypotension may occur in volume depleted patients or with concurrent administration of phenothiazines or general anesthetics.

**WARNINGS/PRECAUTIONS:** Have resuscitation equipment, oxygen, and antidote (eg, naloxone) available; severe respiratory depression may occur. Avoid rapid administration. May be habit-forming. Caution with head injury, increased intracranial/intraocular pressure, decreased respiratory reserve, hepatic/renal dysfunction, elderly, debilitated. High doses may cause seizures.

Smooth muscle hypertonicity may cause biliary colic, urinary difficulty or retention. Orthostatic hypotension may occur with hypovolemia or myocardial dysfunction. Acute respiratory failure reported with COPD or acute asthmatic attack. Limit epidural/intrathecal route to lumbar area.

**ADVERSE REACTIONS:** Respiratory depression, convulsions, dysphoric reactions, pruritis, urinary retention, constipation, lumbar puncture-type headache, toxic psychoses.

**INTERACTIONS:** CNS depressants (eg, alcohol, sedatives, antihistamines) and psychotropics potentiate CNS depression. Neuroleptics may increase respiratory depression.

**PREGNANCY:** Category C, safety in nursing not known.



## DURATUSS

RX

guaifenesin - pseudoephedrine HCl (Victory)

**THERAPEUTIC CLASS:** Expectorant/decongestant

**INDICATIONS:** Relief of nasal congestion due to the common cold, hay fever, sinusitis, or other upper respiratory allergies. Relief of eustachian tube congestion and cough. Adjunct therapy in serious otitis media.

**DOSAGE:** *Adults:* 1 tab q12h.
*Pediatrics:* >12 yrs: 1 tab q12h. 6-12 yrs: 1/2 tab q12h.

**HOW SUPPLIED:** Tab, Extended Release: (Guaifenesin-Pseudoephedrine) 600mg-120mg* *scored

**CONTRAINDICATIONS:** Hypersensitivity to sympathomimetics, severe HTN, with MAOIs.

**WARNINGS/PRECAUTIONS:** Do not crush or chew tabs. Caution with HTN, hyperthyroidism, DM, heart disease, peripheral vascular disease, glaucoma, prostatic hypertrophy.

**ADVERSE REACTIONS:** Nervousness, insomnia, restlessness, headache.

**INTERACTIONS:** Avoid MAOIs. May reduce effects of antihypertensive drugs which interfere with sympathetic activity (eg, methyldopa, mecamylamine, reserpine). Increased ectopic pacemaker activity with digitalis. Caution with concomitant sympathomimetic amines.

**PREGNANCY:** Category C, not for use in nursing.

## DURATUSS DM

RX

guaifenesin - dextromethorphan hydrobromide (Victory)

**THERAPEUTIC CLASS:** Cough suppressant/expectorant

**INDICATIONS:** Relief of cough due to minor throat and bronchial irritation complicated by viscous mucus.

**DOSAGE:** *Adults:* 5mL q4h. Max: 30mL/24 hrs.
*Pediatrics:* >12 yrs: 5mL q4h. Max: 30mL/24 hrs. 6-12 yrs: 2.5mL q4h. Max: 15mL/24 hrs. 2-6 yrs: 1.25mL q4h. Max: 7.5mL/24 hrs.

**HOW SUPPLIED:** Elixir: (Dextromethorphan-Guaifenesin) 25mg-225mg/5mL

**CONTRAINDICATIONS:** Within 14 days of MAOI therapy.

**WARNINGS/PRECAUTIONS:** Re-evaluate if cough persists >1 week or recurs.

**ADVERSE REACTIONS:** Nausea, GI disturbances, dizziness, drowsiness, vomiting, headache, rash.

**INTERACTIONS:** Avoid use within 14 days of MAOI therapy; may cause serotonin syndrome. Additive CNS depressant effects with alcohol, antihistamines, psychotropics, other CNS depressants.

**PREGNANCY:** Category C, caution in nursing.

## DURATUSS G
RX
guaifenesin (Victory)

**OTHER BRAND NAMES:** Guaifenex G (Ethex) - Muco-Fen 1200 (Ivax) - Liquibid-D (Capellon) - Guaifenesin ER (Amide)



**THERAPEUTIC CLASS:** Expectorant

**INDICATIONS:** Temporary relief of symptoms associated with respiratory tract infections and related conditions. Loosens phlegm and thins bronchial secretions

**DOSAGE:** *Adults:* 1 tab q12h. Max: 2 tabs/24 hrs. May break tabs in half; do not crush or chew.
*Pediatrics:* >12 yrs: 1 tab q12h. Max: 2 tabs/24 hrs. 6-12 yrs: 1/2 tab q12h. Max: 1 tab/24 hrs. May break tabs in half; do not crush or chew.

**HOW SUPPLIED:** Tab, Extended Release: 1200mg* *scored

**ADVERSE REACTIONS:** Nausea, vomiting.

**PREGNANCY:** Category C, caution in nursing.

## DURICEF
RX
cefadroxil monohydrate (Warner Chilcott)

**THERAPEUTIC CLASS:** Cephalosporin (1st generation)

**INDICATIONS:** Skin and skin structure (SSSI) and urinary tract infection (UTI), pharyngitis, and tonsillitis.

**DOSAGE:** *Adults:* Uncomplicated Lower UTI: 1-2g/day given qd or bid. Other UTI: 1gm bid. SSSI: 1g qd or 500mg bid. Group A β-hemolytic Strep Pharyngitis/Tonsillitis: 1g qd or 500mg bid for 10 days. CrCl <50mL/min: Initial: 1g. Maint: CrCl 25-50mL/min: 500mg q12h; CrCl 10-25mL/min: 500mg q24h; CrCl 0-10mL/min: 500mg q36h.
*Pediatrics:* UTI/SSSI: 15mg/kg q12h. Pharyngitis/Tonsillitis/Impetigo: 30mg/kg qd or 15mg/kg q12h. Treat β-hemolytic strep infections for at least 10 days.

**HOW SUPPLIED:** Cap: 500mg; Sus: 250mg/5mL [50mL, 100mL], 500mg/5mL [50mL, 75mL, 100mL]; Tab: 1g* *scored

**WARNINGS/PRECAUTIONS:** Caution with markedly impaired renal function, history of GI disease. Cross-sensitivity with cephalosporins and penicillins. False (+) direct Coombs' tests, pseudomembranous colitis reported.

**ADVERSE REACTIONS:** Diarrhea, rash, hypersensitivity reactions, pruritus, hepatic dysfunction, genital moniliasis, vaginitis, fever, superinfection (prolonged use).

**PREGNANCY:** Category B, caution in nursing.

## DYAZIDE
RX
triamterene - hydrochlorothiazide (GlaxoSmithKline)

**THERAPEUTIC CLASS:** $K^+$-sparing diuretic/thiazide diuretic

**INDICATIONS:** For hypertension or edema if hypokalemia occurs on HCTZ alone, or when a thiazide diuretic is required and cannot risk hypokalemia.

**DOSAGE:** *Adults:* 1-2 caps qd.

**HOW SUPPLIED:** Cap: (Triamterene-HCTZ) 37.5mg-25mg

**CONTRAINDICATIONS:** Hyperkalemia, anuria, acute or chronic renal insufficiency, sulfonamide hypersensitivity, diabetic neuropathy, $K^+$-sparing agents (eg, diuretics), $K^+$ supplements (except with severe hypokalemia), $K^+$ salt substitutes, $K^+$-rich diet.

**WARNINGS/PRECAUTIONS:** Risk of hyperkalemia (>5.5mEq/L) especially with renal impairment, elderly, DM or severely ill; monitor levels frequently. Caution in severely ill in whom respiratory or metabolic acidosis may occur;

monitor acid-base balance frequently. May manifest DM. Caution with hepatic dysfunction, history of renal stones. Increases uric acid levels, BUN, creatinine. May decrease PBI levels. D/C before parathyroid function tests. May potentiate electrolyte imbalance with heart failure, renal disease, cirrhosis.

**ADVERSE REACTIONS:** Muscle cramps, GI effects, weakness, blood dyscrasias, arrhythmia, impotence, dry mouth, jaundice, paresthesia, renal stones, hypersensitivity reactions.



**INTERACTIONS:** Hyperkalemia risk with ACE inhibitors, blood from blood bank, low-salt milk, $K^+$-containing agents (eg, parenteral penicillin G potassium), salt substitutes. Increased risk of hyponatremia with chlorpropamide. Possible renal dysfunction with NSAIDs. Risk of lithium toxicity. Decreases arterial responsiveness to norepinephrine. ACTH, amphotericin B, and corticosteroids intensify electrolyte depletion. Adjust oral anticoagulants, antigout, and antidiabetic drugs. Increases effects of nondepolarizing muscle relaxants, antihypertensives. Overuse of laxatives or sodium polystyrene sulfonate reduces $K^+$ levels. Reduces methenamine effects.

**PREGNANCY:** Category C, not for use in nursing.

## DYNACIN

minocycline HCl (Medicis) RX

**THERAPEUTIC CLASS:** Tetracycline derivative

**INDICATIONS:** Treatment of inclusion conjunctivitis, nongonococcal urethritis, and other infections (eg, respiratory tract, endocervical, rectal, urinary tract, skin and skin structure) caused by susceptible strains of microorganisms. Alternative treatment in certain other infections (eg, urethritis, gonococcal, syphilis, anthrax). Adjunctive therapy in acute intestinal amebiasis and severe acne. Treatment of *Mycobacterium marinum* and asymptomatic carriers of *Neisseria meningitidis*.

**DOSAGE:** *Adults:* Usual: 200mg initially, then 100mg q12h; alternative is 100-200mg initially, then 50mg qid. Uncomplicated Gonococcal Infection (Men, other than urethritis and anorectal infections): 200mg initially, then 100mg q12h for minimum 4 days. Uncomplicated Gonococcal Urethritis (Men): 100mg q12h for 5 days. Syphilis: Administer usual dose for 10-15 days. Meningococcal Carrier State: 100mg q12h for 5 days. *Mycobacterium marinum:* 100mg q12h for 6-8 weeks. Uncomplicated urethral, endocervical, or rectal infection: 100mg q12h for at least 7 days. Renal Dysfunction: Reduce dose and/or extend dose intervals.
*Pediatrics:* >8 yrs: 4mg/kg initially followed by 2mg/kg q12h. Take with plenty of fluids.

**HOW SUPPLIED:** Cap: 50mg, 75mg, 100mg; Tab: 50mg, 75mg, 100mg

**WARNINGS/PRECAUTIONS:** May cause fetal harm during pregnancy. Use during tooth development (last half of pregnancy, infancy, <8yrs) may cause permanent discoloration of the teeth or enamel hypoplasia; avoid use during this period. Renal toxicity, hepatotoxicity, photosensitivity, increased BUN, superinfection, pseudotumor cerebri may occur; perform hematopoietic, renal, and hepatic monitoring. May impair mental/physical abilities. Use alternate form of contraception other than oral contraceptives. May decrease bone growth in premature infants.

**ADVERSE REACTIONS:** Anorexia, nausea, vomiting, diarrhea, dysphagia, enterocolitis, pancreatitis, increased LFTs, hepatitis, liver failure, renal toxicity, rash, exfoliative dermatitis, Stevens-Johnson syndrome, skin and mucous membrane pigmentation, blood dyscrasias, headache, tooth discoloration.

**INTERACTIONS:** May require downward adjustments of anticoagulant dosage. May interfere with bactericidal action of penicillin; avoid concurrent use when possible. May decrease efficacy of oral contraceptives. Impaired absorption with antacids containing aluminum, calcium, or magnesium and iron-containing products. Fatal renal toxicity with methoxyflurane has been reported.

**PREGNANCY:** Category D, not for use in nursing.

## DynaCirc RX
isradipine (Reliant)



**OTHER BRAND NAMES:** DynaCirc CR (Reliant)

**THERAPEUTIC CLASS:** Calcium channel blocker (dihydropyridine)

**INDICATIONS:** Management of hypertension.

**DOSAGE:** *Adults:* Initial: (Cap) 2.5mg bid or (Tab, CR) 5mg qd alone or with a thiazide diuretic. Titrate: May adjust by 5mg/day at 2-4 week intervals. Max: 20mg/day. Swallow CR tabs whole.

**HOW SUPPLIED:** Cap: 2.5mg, 5mg; Tab, Controlled Release: (CR) 5mg, 10mg.

**WARNINGS/PRECAUTIONS:** May produce symptomatic hypotension. Caution in CHF, especially with concomitant β-blockers. Caution with CR tab in pre-existing severe GI narrowing. Peripheral edema reported. Increased bioavailability in elderly.

**ADVERSE REACTIONS:** Headache, edema, dizziness, constipation, fatigue, flushing, abdominal discomfort.

**INTERACTIONS:** Additive effects with HCTZ. Severe hypotension possible with fentanyl and β-blockers. Increases AUC and Cmax of propranolol. Decreased levels with rifampicin.

**PREGNANCY:** Category C, not for use in nursing.

## Dyrenium RX
triamterene (WellSpring)

**THERAPEUTIC CLASS:** $K^+$-sparing diuretic

**INDICATIONS:** Treatment of edema associated with congestive heart failure, liver cirrhosis, and nephrotic syndrome. Treatment of steroid induced edema, idiopathic edema and edema due to secondary hyperaldosteronism.

**DOSAGE:** *Adults:* Initial: 100mg bid pc. Max: 300mg/day.

**HOW SUPPLIED:** Cap: 50mg, 100mg

**CONTRAINDICATIONS:** Anuria, severe or progressive kidney disease or dysfunction (except with nephrosis), severe hepatic disease, hyperkalemia, $K^+$ supplements, $K^+$ salt substitutes, $K^+$-sparing agents (eg, diuretics).

**WARNINGS/PRECAUTIONS:** Risk of hyperkalemia (>5.5mEq/L) especially with renal impairment, elderly, DM or severely ill; monitor levels frequently. Check ECG if hyperkalemia occurs. May cause decreased alkali reserve with possibility of metabolic acidosis, mild nitrogen retention. Monitor BUN periodically. May contribute to megaloblastosis in folic acid deficiency. Caution with gouty arthritis; may elevate uric acid levels. May aggravate or cause electrolyte imbalances in CHF, renal disease, or cirrhosis. Caution with history of renal stones.

**ADVERSE REACTIONS:** Hypersensitivity reactions, hyper- or hypokalemia, azotemia, renal stones, jaundice, nausea, vomiting, diarrhea, weakness, dizziness.

**INTERACTIONS:** Increased risk of hyperkalemia with ACE inhibitors. Indomethacin may cause renal failure; caution with NSAIDs. Risk of lithium toxicity. Avoid $K^+$-sparing diuretics, $K^+$ supplements, $K^+$-containing agents or salt substitutes, low-salt milk, and blood from blood bank; may potentiate serum $K^+$ levels. May cause hyperglycemia; adjust antidiabetic agents. Chlorpropamide may increase risk of severe hyponatremia. May potentiate nondepolarizing muscle relaxants, antihypertensives, other diuretics, preanesthetics, and anesthetics.

**PREGNANCY:** Category C, not for use in nursing.

## E.E.S. RX
erythromycin ethylsuccinate (Abbott)

**THERAPEUTIC CLASS:** Macrolide antibiotic

**INDICATIONS:** Mild to moderate upper and lower respiratory tract and skin and skin structure infections, listeriosis, pertussis, diphtheria, erythrasma, intestinal amebiasis, acute pelvic inflammatory disease (PID) (*N.gonorrhea*), primary syphilis in PCN allergy, Legionnaires' disease, chlamydial infections (eg, newborn conjunctivitis urethral, endocervical, or rectal, etc), and nongonococcal urethritis. Prophylaxis of endocarditis or rheumatic fever.

**DOSAGE:** *Adults:* Usual: 1600mg/day given q6h, q8h or q12h. Max: 4g/day. Treat strep infections for 10 days. Streptococcal Infection Prophylaxis with Rheumatic Heart Disease: 400mg bid. Urethritis (*C.trachomatis* or *U.urealyticum*): 800mg tid for 7 days. Primary Syphilis: 48-64g in divided doses over 10-15 days. Intestinal Amebiasis: 400mg qid for 10-14 days. Pertussis: 40-50mg/kg/day in divided doses for 5-14 days. Legionnaires' Disease: 1.6-4g/day in divided doses.
*Pediatrics:* Usual: 30-50mg/kg/day in divided doses q6h, q8h or q12h. Double dose for more severe infections. Treat strep infections for 10 days. Intestinal Amebiasis: 30-50mg/kg/day in divided doses for 10-14 days. Pertussis: 40-50mg/kg/day in divided doses for 5-14 days.

**HOW SUPPLIED:** Sus: 200mg/5mL, 400mg/5mL (100mL, 480mL), Tab: 400mg

**CONTRAINDICATIONS:** Concomitant terfenadine, astemizole, cisapride, pimozide.

**WARNINGS/PRECAUTIONS:** Pseudomembranous colitis, hepatic dysfunction reported. May aggravate myasthenia gravis.

**ADVERSE REACTIONS:** Nausea, vomiting, abdominal pain, diarrhea, anorexia, hepatic dysfunction, abnormal LFTs, allergic reactions, superinfection (prolonged use).

**INTERACTIONS:** Rhabdomyolysis reported with lovastatin. May increase levels of theophylline, digoxin, drugs metabolized by CYP450 (eg, carbamazepine, cyclosporine, tacrolimus, phenytoin, alfentanil, disopyramide, lovastatin, bromocriptine, valproate, etc). Increases effects of oral anticoagulants, triazolam, midazolam. Risk of acute ergot toxicity with ergotamine or dihydroergotamine. May potentiate sildenafil. Avoid terfenadine, astemizole, cisapride, pimozide.

**PREGNANCY:** Category B, caution in nursing.

## ECOTRIN OTC
aspirin (GlaxoSmithKline Consumer)

**THERAPEUTIC CLASS:** Salicylate

**INDICATIONS:** To reduce the risk of death and nonfatal stroke with previous ischemic stroke or transient ischemia of the brain. To reduce risk of vascular mortality with suspected acute MI. To reduce risk of death and nonfatal MI with previous MI or unstable angina. To reduce risk of MI and sudden death in chronic stable angina. Indicated for patients who have undergone revascularization procedures with a pre-existing condition for which ASA is indicated. Relief of signs of rheumatoid arthritis (RA), juvenile rheumatoid arthritis (JRA), osteoarthritis (OA), spondyloarthropathies, arthritis, and pleurisy associated with SLE.

**DOSAGE:** *Adults:* Ischemic Stroke/TIA: 50-325mg qd. Suspected Acute MI: Initial: 160-162.5mg qd as soon as suspect MI. Maint: 160-162.5mg for 30 days post-infarction, consider further therapy for prevention/recurrent MI.

Prevention or Recurrent MI/Unstable Angina/Chronic Stable Angina: 75-325mg qd. CABG: 325mg qd, start 6 hrs post-surgery. Continue for 1 year. PTCA: Initial: 325mg, 2 hrs pre-surgery. Maint: 160-325mg qd. Carotid Endarterectomy: 80mg qd to 650mg bid, start pre-surgery. RA/Arthritis/SLE Pleurisy: Initial: 3g qd in divided doses. Increase for anti-inflammatory efficacy to 150-300 mcg/mL plasma salicylate level. Spondyloarthropathies: Up to 4g/day in divided doses. OA: Up to 3g/day in divided doses.
*Pediatrics:* JRA: Initial: 90-130 mg/kg/day in divided doses. Increase for anti-inflammatory efficacy to 150-300 mcg/mL plasma salicylate level.



**HOW SUPPLIED:** Tab, Delayed Release: 81mg, 325mg, 500mg

**CONTRAINDICATIONS:** NSAID allergy, children or teenagers for viral infections with or without fever, syndrome of asthma, rhinitis, and nasal polyps.

**WARNINGS/PRECAUTIONS:** Increased risk of bleeding with heavy alcohol use (>3 drinks/day). May inhibit platelet function; can adversely affect inherited (hemophilia) or acquired (hepatic disease, vitamin K deficiency) bleeding disorders. Monitor for bleeding and ulceration. Avoid in history of active peptic ulcer, severe renal failure, severe hepatic insufficiency, and sodium restricted diets. Associated with elevated LFTs, BUN, and serum creatinine; hyperkalemia; proteinuria; and prolonged bleeding time. Avoid one week before and during labor.

**ADVERSE REACTIONS:** Fever, hypothermia, dysrhythmias, hypotension, agitation, cerebral edema, dehydration, hyperkalemia, dyspepsia, GI bleed, hearing loss, tinnitus, problems in pregnancy.

**INTERACTIONS:** Diminished hypotensive and hyponatremic effects of ACE inhibitors. May increase levels of acetazolamide, valproic acid. Increased risk of bleeds with heparin, warfarin. Decreased levels of phenytoin. Decreased hypotensive effects of β-blockers. Decreased diuretic effects with renal or cardiovascular disease. Decreased methotrexate clearance; increased risk of bone marrow toxicity. Avoid NSAIDs. Increased effects of hypoglycemic agents. Antagonizes uricosuric agents.

**PREGNANCY:** Avoid in 3rd trimester of pregnancy and nursing.

## EDECRIN RX

ethacrynic acid (Merck)

**THERAPEUTIC CLASS:** Aryloxyacetic acid derivative

**INDICATIONS:** Treatment of edema when agent of greater diuretic potential is required. Treatment of edema in CHF, hepatic cirrhosis, and renal disease. Short term management of ascites due to malignancy, idiopathic edema, lymphedema; congenital heart disease and nephrotic syndrome in hospitalized pediatrics.

**DOSAGE:** *Adults:* Initial: 50-100mg qd. Titrate: 25-50mg increments. Usual: 50-200mg/day. After diuresis achieved, give smallest effective dose continuously or intermittently.
*Pediatrics:* Initial: 25mg. Titrate: Increase by 25mg increments. Maint: Reduce dose and frequency once dry weight achieved; may give intermittently.

**HOW SUPPLIED:** Tab: 25mg*, 50mg* *scored

**CONTRAINDICATIONS:** Anuria, infants. Discontinue if increasing electrolyte imbalance, azotemia, or oliguria develops during treatment of severe, progressive renal disease. Discontinue if severe, watery diarrhea occurs.

**WARNINGS/PRECAUTIONS:** Caution in advanced liver cirrhosis. Monitor serum electrolytes, CO2, BUN early in therapy and periodically during active diuresis. Vigorous diuresis may induce acute hypotensive episode and in elderly cardiac patients, hemoconcentration resulting in thromboembolic disorders. Ototoxicity reported with severe renal dysfunction. Hypomagnesemia and transient increase in serum urea nitrogen may occur. Reduce dose or withdraw if excessive electrolyte loss occurs. Initiate therapy in the hospital for cirrhotic patients with ascites. Liberalize salt intake and supplement with $K^+$ if needed. Reduced responsiveness in renal edema with hypoproteinemia; use salt poor albumin.

**ADVERSE REACTIONS:** Anorexia, malaise, abdominal discomfort, gout, deafness, tinnitus, vertigo, headache, fatigue, rash, chills.

**INTERACTIONS:** Risk of lithium toxicity. May increase ototoxic potential of aminoglycosides and some cephalosporins. Displaces warfarin from plasma protein; may need dose reduction. NSAIDs may decrease effects. Orthostatic hypotension may occur with antihypertensives. Increased risk of gastric hemorrhage with corticosteroids. Excessive $K^+$ loss may precipitate digitalis toxicity. Caution with $K^+$-depleting steroids.



**PREGNANCY:** Category B, not for use in nursing.

## EDECRIN SODIUM

RX

ethacrynate sodium (Merck)

**THERAPEUTIC CLASS:** Aryloxyacetic acid derivative

**INDICATIONS:** For rapid onset of diuresis (eg, acute pulmonary edema, impaired GI absorption, oral medication not practicable).

**DOSAGE:** *Adults:* 50mg or 0.5-1mg/kg IV single dose. May give 2nd dose if necessary.

**HOW SUPPLIED:** Inj: 50mg

**CONTRAINDICATIONS:** Anuria, infants. Discontinue if increasing electrolyte imbalance, azotemia, or oliguria develops during treatment of severe, progressive renal disease. Discontinue if severe, watery diarrhea occurs.

**WARNINGS/PRECAUTIONS:** Caution in advanced liver cirrhosis. Monitor serum electrolytes, CO2, BUN early in therapy and periodically during active diuresis. Vigorous diuresis may induce acute hypotensive episode and in elderly cardiac patients, hemoconcentration resulting in thromboembolic disorders. Ototoxicity reported with severe renal dysfunction. Hypomagnesemia and transient increase in serum urea nitrogen may occur. Reduce dose or withdraw if excessive electrolyte loss occurs. Initiate therapy in the hospital for cirrhotic patients with ascites. Liberalize salt intake and supplement with $K^+$ if needed. Reduced responsiveness in renal edema with hypoproteinemia; use salt poor albumin.

**ADVERSE REACTIONS:** Anorexia, malaise, abdominal discomfort, gout, deafness, tinnitus, vertigo, headache, fatigue, rash, chills.

**INTERACTIONS:** Risk of lithium toxicity. May increase ototoxic potential of aminoglycosides and some cephalosporins. Displaces warfarin from plasma protein; may need dose reduction. NSAIDs may decrease effects. Orthostatic hypotension may occur with antihypertensives. Increased risk of gastric hemorrhage with corticosteroids. Excessive $K^+$ loss may precipitate digitalis toxicity. Caution with $K^+$-depleting steroids.

**PREGNANCY:** Category B, not for use in nursing.

## EFFEXOR

RX

venlafaxine HCl (Wyeth)

**Antidepressants increased the risk of suicidal thinking and behavior (suicidality) in short-term studies in children and adolescents with Major Depressive Disorder (MDD) and other psychiatric disorders. Venlafaxine is not approved for use in pediatric patients.**

**THERAPEUTIC CLASS:** Serotonin and norepinephrine reuptake inhibitor

**INDICATIONS:** Treatment of MDD

**DOSAGE:** *Adults:* ≥18 yrs: Initial: 75mg/day given bid-tid with food. Titrate: Increase by 75mg/day at no less than 4 day intervals. Max: 375mg/day. Hepatic Impairment (moderate): Reduce dose by 50%. Renal Impairment (mild to moderate): Reduce dose by 25%. Hemodialysis: Reduce dose by 50%.

Withhold dose until after hemodialysis treatment completed. If drug used 6 weeks or longer, taper gradually (over 2 weeks or more) when discontinuing treatment.

**HOW SUPPLIED:** Tab: 25mg*, 37.5mg*, 50mg*, 75mg*, 100mg* *scored

**CONTRAINDICATIONS:** Concomitant MAOIs.

**WARNINGS/PRECAUTIONS:** May cause sustained increases in BP. Treatment-emergent anxiety, nervousness, insomnia, and anorexia reported. Caution with history of mania or seizures and conditions affecting hemodynamic responses. Monitor with increased IOP or if at risk of acute narrow angle glaucoma. Activation of mania/hypomania reported. Risk of hyponatremia, SIADH, skin and mucous membrane bleeding. Caution with hyperthyroidism, heart failure, recent MI, renal or hepatic impairment. Serotonin syndrome may occur. Caution with concomitant serotonergic drugs. Patients who present with progressive dyspnea, cough or chest discomfort should consider the possibility of interstitial lung disease and eosinophilic pneumonia.

**ADVERSE REACTIONS:** Asthenia, sweating, nausea, constipation, anorexia, vomiting, insomnia, somnolence, dry mouth, dizziness, nervousness, anxiety, tremor, blurred vision, abnormal ejaculation/orgasm, impotence in men.

**INTERACTIONS:** See Contraindications. Avoid within 14 days of MAOI therapy. Upon discontinuation, wait at least 7 days before starting MAOI therapy. Caution with cimetidine in elderly, HTN, hepatic dysfunction. Caution with diuretics. Decreases clearance of haloperidol. Increases risperidone and desipramine plasma levels. Decreases indinavir plasma levels. Caution with potent inhibitors of CYP3A4 and CYP2D6, CNS-active drugs (eg, triptans, SSRIs, lithium), and serotonergic drugs (eg, tramadol, tryptophans, SNRIs). Avoid alcohol.

**PREGNANCY:** Category C, not for use in nursing.

## EFFEXOR XR

RX

venlafaxine HCl (Wyeth)

**Antidepressants increased the risk of suicidal thinking and behavior (suicidality) in short-term studies in children and adolescents with Major Depressive Disorder (MDD) and other psychiatric disorders. Venlafaxine is not approved for use in pediatric patients.**

**THERAPEUTIC CLASS:** Serotonin and norepinephrine reuptake inhibitor

**INDICATIONS:** Treatment of major depressive disorder (MDD), generalized anxiety disorder (GAD), social anxiety disorder (SAD), panic disorder (PD).

**DOSAGE:** *Adults:* MDD/GAD/SAD: Initial: 75mg qd, or 37.5mg qd increase to 75mg qd after 4-7 days. Titrate: May increase by 75mg/day at no less than 4 day intervals. Max: 225mg/day. PD: Initial: 37.5mg qd for 7 days. Titrate: May increase 75mg/day, as needed at no less than 7 day intervals. Max: 225mg/day. Moderate Hepatic Impairment: Reduce initial dose by 50%. Renal Impairment: Reduce total daily dose by 25-50%. Hemodialysis: Reduce total daily dose by 50%. Withhold dose until after hemodialysis treatment completed. If drug used 6 weeks or longer, taper gradually (over 2 weeks or more) when discontinuing treatment. Periodically reassess need for maintenance therapy. Take with food in the am or pm, the same time each day. May sprinkle on spoonful of applesauce. Do not divide, crush, chew or place in water.

**HOW SUPPLIED:** Cap, Extended Release: 37.5mg, 75mg, 150mg

**CONTRAINDICATIONS:** Concomitant MAOI therapy.

**WARNINGS/PRECAUTIONS:** May cause sustained increases in BP; monitor BP regularly. Treatment-emergent nervousness, insomnia and anorexia reported. Caution with seizures, conditions affecting hemodynamic responses or metabolism, volume-depletion, the elderly. Risk of mydriasis; monitor those with raised IOP or risk of acute narrow angle glaucoma. Abnormal bleeding (eg, ecchymosis) and activation of mania/hypomania reported. Risk of hyponatremia, SIADH. Caution with recent MI, hyperthyroidism, heart failure, renal or hepatic impairment. Serotonin syndrome may occur; caution with concomitant use of serotonergic drugs. Patients who present with progressive dyspnea, cough or chest discomfort should consider the possibility of interstitial lung disease and eosinophilic pneumonia.

**ADVERSE REACTIONS:** Asthenia, sweating, headache, nausea, constipation, anorexia, dry mouth, dizziness, insomnia, nervousness, somnolence, abnormal ejaculation, abnormal dreams.

**INTERACTIONS:** See Contraindications. Avoid within 14 days of MAOI therapy. Upon discontinuation, wait at least 7 days before starting MAOI therapy. Caution with cimetidine in elderly, hepatic dysfunction or pre-existing HTN. Caution with diuretics. Decreases clearance of haloperidol. Increases risperidone and desipramine plasma levels. Decreases indinavir plasma levels. Caution with potent inhibitors of CYP3A4 and CYP2D6, CNS-active drugs (eg, triptans, SSRIs, lithium), and with serotonergic drugs. Avoid alcohol.

**PREGNANCY:** Category C, not for use in nursing.



## EFUDEX — RX

fluorouracil (Valeant)

**OTHER BRAND NAMES:** Efudex-40 (Valeant)

**THERAPEUTIC CLASS:** Antimetabolite

**INDICATIONS:** (2%, 5%) Topical treatment of actinic or solar keratoses. (5%) Treatment of superficial basal cell carcinomas when conventional methods are impractical.

**DOSAGE:** *Adults:* Actinic or Solar Keratosis: Apply bid until erosion occurs, usually for 2-4 weeks. Superficial Basal Cell Carcinoma: Apply 5% bid for 3-6 weeks; may use up to 10-12 weeks to obliterate lesion.

**HOW SUPPLIED:** Cre: 5% [25g, 40g]; Sol: 2%, 5% [10mL]

**CONTRAINDICATIONS:** Pregnancy.

**WARNINGS/PRECAUTIONS:** Avoid mucous membranes, UV light. Caution with occlusive dressings; may increase absorption. Use a porous gauze dressing for treatment of basal cell carcinoma if necessary. Ulcerations, miscarriage, and birth defects reported when applied to mucous membranes. Increased absorption with ulcerated or inflamed skin. Confirm diagnosis with biopsy.

**ADVERSE REACTIONS:** Burning, crusting, allergic contact dermatitis, erosions, erythema, hyperpigmentation, irritation, pain, photosensitivity, pruritus, scarring, rash, soreness, ulceration, leukocytosis.

**PREGNANCY:** Category X, not for use in nursing.

## ELDEPRYL — RX

selegiline HCl (Somerset)

**THERAPEUTIC CLASS:** Monoamine oxidase inhibitor (Type B)

**INDICATIONS:** Adjunct to levodopa/carbidopa for management of Parkinson's disease.

**DOSAGE:** *Adults:* 5mg bid, at breakfast and lunch. Max: 10mg/day. May reduce levodopa/carbidopa by 10-30% after 2-3 days of therapy. May reduce further with continued therapy.

**HOW SUPPLIED:** Cap: 5mg

**CONTRAINDICATIONS:** Concomitant meperidine, other opioids.

**WARNINGS/PRECAUTIONS:** Do not exceed 10mg/day due to non-selective MAO inhibition. Decrease levodopa/carbidopa by 10-30% to prevent exacerbation of levodopa side effects.

**ADVERSE REACTIONS:** Nausea, dizziness, lightheadedness, fainting, abdominal pain, confusion, hallucinations, dry mouth.

**INTERACTIONS:** See Contraindications. Stupor, muscular rigidity, severe agitation, and elevated temperature reported with meperidine; avoid concomitant use. Avoid SSRIs and TCAs; severe toxicity reported. Allow 2 weeks between discontinuation of selegiline and initiation of TCAs or SSRIs. Allow 5 weeks for fluoxetine due to a longer half-life. Caution with sympathomimetics, tyramine-containing food.

**PREGNANCY:** Category C, not for use in nursing.



## ELDOPAQUE FORTE RX

hydroquinone (Valeant)

**OTHER BRAND NAMES:** Eldoquin Forte (Valeant)

**THERAPEUTIC CLASS:** Depigmenting agent

**INDICATIONS:** For the gradual bleaching of hyperpigmented skin conditions (eg, chloasma, melasma, freckles, senile lentigines).

**DOSAGE:** *Adults:* Apply bid. Do not rub in Eldopaque Forte. Use sunscreen with Eldoquin Forte.
*Pediatrics:* >12 yrs: Apply bid. Do not rub in Eldopaque Forte. Use sunscreen with Eldoquin Forte.

**HOW SUPPLIED:** Cre: 4% [28.4g]

**WARNINGS/PRECAUTIONS:** Avoid sun exposure on bleached skin. Eldopaque Forte contains sunblock; use sunscreen. May produce unwanted cosmetic effects if not used as directed. Test for skin sensitivity. D/C if no lightening effect after 2 months. Contains sodium metabisulfite; may cause serious allergic type reactions. Limit treatment to small areas of body at one time. Avoid contact with eyes.

**ADVERSE REACTIONS:** Cutaneous hypersensitivity (contact dermatitis).

**PREGNANCY:** Category C, caution in nursing.

## ELESTAT RX

epinastine HCl (Allergan)

**THERAPEUTIC CLASS:** $H_1$ antagonist

**INDICATIONS:** For the prevention of itching associated with allergic conjunctivitis.

**DOSAGE:** *Adults:* 1 drop in each eye bid.
*Pediatrics:* ≥3 yrs: 1 drop in each eye bid.

**HOW SUPPLIED:** Sol: 0.05% [5mL]

**WARNINGS/PRECAUTIONS:** Not for contact lens related irritation. May reinsert contact lens 10 minutes after dosing if eye is not red.

**ADVERSE REACTIONS:** Burning sensation in the eye, folliculosis, hyperemia, pruritus.

**PREGNANCY:** Category C, caution in nursing.

## ELESTRIN RX

estradiol (Kenwood Therapeutics)

> **Estrogens increase the risk of endometrial cancer. Estrogens, with or without progestins, should not be used for the prevention of cardiovascular disease or dementia. Increased risks of MI, stroke, invasive breast cancer, PE, and DVT in postmenopausal women reported.**

**THERAPEUTIC CLASS:** Estrogen

**INDICATIONS:** Treatment of moderate to severe vasomotor symptoms associated with menopause.

**DOSAGE:** *Adults:* Individualize dose.Apply 1 pump (0.87g) qd to upper arm. Use lowest effective dose consistent with treatment goals and risks. Re-evaluate periodically.

**HOW SUPPLIED:** Gel: 0.06% (0.87g [0.52g estradiol] per pump actuation) [144g]

**CONTRAINDICATIONS:** Undiagnosed abnormal genital bleeding, breast cancer, estrogen-dependent neoplasia, DVT or PE, active or recent (within 1 year) arterial thromboembolic disease (eg, stroke, MI), liver dysfunction or disease, pregnancy.

**WARNINGS/PRECAUTIONS:** May increase risk of cardiovascular events (eg, MI, stroke, venous thrombosis, and PE); d/c immediately if any of these events occur or are suspected. May increase risk of breast/endometrial cancer, and gallbladder disease. May lead to severe hypercalcemia with breast cancer and bone metastases; monitor and d/c if hypercalcemia occurs. Retinal vascular thrombosis reported; monitor and d/c if papilledema or retinal vascular lesions occur. Consider addition of a progestin if no hysterectomy. May elevate BP; monitor at regular intervals. May cause elevations of plasma triglycerides with pre-existing hypertriglyceridemia. Caution with history of cholestatic jaundice associated with past estrogen use or with pregnancy; d/c with recurrence. May lead to increased thyroid-binding globulin levels; monitor thyroid function. May cause fluid retention; monitor closely with cardiac/renal dysfunction. Caution with severe hypocalcemia. May increase risk of ovarian cancer. May exacerbate endometriosis, asthma, DM, epilepsy, migraine, porphyria, SLE, and hepatic hemangiomas; use with caution. Sunscreen may increase absorption; avoid applying sunscreen to application site for ≥25 minutes or for extended period of ≥7 days. Alcohol-based gels are flammable; avoid fire, flame, or smoking until the gel dried.

**ADVERSE REACTIONS:** Nausea, breast tenderness, metorrhagia, vaginal discharge, nasopharyngitis, upper respiratory infection, headache.

**INTERACTIONS:** CYP3A4 inducers (eg, St. John's wort, phenobarbital, carbamazepine, rifampin) may decrease levels which may decrease therapeutic effects and/or change uterine bleeding profile. CYP3A4 inhibitors (eg, erythromycin, clarithromycin, ketoconazole, itraconazole, ritonavir, grapefruit juice) may increase levels and result in unwanted side effects.

**PREGNANCY:** Contraindicated in pregnancy, caution in nursing.

## ELIDEL RX

pimecrolimus (Novartis)

**THERAPEUTIC CLASS:** Macrolactam ascomycin derivative

**INDICATIONS:** Short-term and intermittent long-term therapy of moderate to severe atopic dermatitis in non-immunocompromised patients intolerant to or unresponsive to conventional therapy.

**DOSAGE:** *Adults:* Apply bid. Re-evaluate if symptoms persist after 6 weeks. *Pediatrics:* >2 yrs: Apply bid. Re-evaluate if symptoms persist after 6 weeks.

**HOW SUPPLIED:** Cre: 1% [30g, 60g, 100g]

**WARNINGS/PRECAUTIONS:** Increased risk of varicella zoster infection, herpes simplex virus infection or eczema herpeticum. Lymphadenopathy reported; discontinue if unknown etiology of lymphadenopathy or acute mononucleosis presents. Skin papilloma or warts reported; consider discontinuation if worsening or unresponsive skin papilloma. Minimize or avoid natural or artificial sunlight exposure. Avoid with Netherton's syndrome, areas of active cutaneous viral infections, or occlusive dressings. Long-term safety has not been established. Rare cases of malignancy (eg, skin and lymphoma) have been reported with topical calcineurin inhibitors; therefore, continuous long-term use should be avoided and application limited to areas of involvement. Not indicated for use in children <2 yrs.

**ADVERSE REACTIONS:** Application site burning, headache, nasopharyngitis, influenza, pharyngitis, viral infection, pyrexia, cough.

**INTERACTIONS:** Caution with CYP3A4 inhibitors (eg, erythromycin, itraconazole, ketoconazole, fluconazole, calcium channel blockers, cimetidine) in widespread and/or erythrodermic disease.

**PREGNANCY:** Category C, not for use in nursing.

## ELIGARD RX
leuprolide acetate (Sanofi-Aventis)



**THERAPEUTIC CLASS:** Synthetic gonadotropin releasing hormone analog

**INDICATIONS:** Palliative treatment of advanced prostate cancer.

**DOSAGE:** *Adults:* 7.5mg SQ monthly, 22.5mg SQ every 3 months, 30mg SQ every 4 months, or 45mg SQ every 6 months. Rotate injection sites.

**HOW SUPPLIED:** Inj: 7.5mg, 22.5mg, 30mg, 45mg

**CONTRAINDICATIONS:** Women, pregnancy, pediatrics.

**WARNINGS/PRECAUTIONS:** Transient worsening of symptoms or onset of new signs/symptoms may occur during 1st few weeks of therapy. Closely monitor patients with metastatic vertebral lesions and/or urinary tract obstruction during 1st few weeks of therapy. Ureteral obstruction and spinal cord decompression reported. Monitor serum testosterone, PSA.

**ADVERSE REACTIONS:** Hot flashes, pain/burning/stinging/erythema/bruising at injection site, malaise/fatigue, atrophy of testes.

**PREGNANCY:** Category X, safety in nursing not known.

## ELIMITE RX
permethrin (Allergan)

**THERAPEUTIC CLASS:** Pyrethroid scabicidal agent

**INDICATIONS:** Treatment of scabies.

**DOSAGE:** *Adults:* Massage into skin from head to soles of feet. Wash off after 8-14 hrs. One treatment should be adequate. Retreat if living mites present after 14 days.
*Pediatrics:* >2 months: Massage into skin from head (scalp, temples and forehead) to soles of feet. Wash off after 8-14 hrs. One treatment should be adequate. Retreat if living mites present after 14 days.

**HOW SUPPLIED:** Cre: 5% [60g]

**CONTRAINDICATIONS:** Allergy to synthetic pyrethroid or pyrethrin.

**WARNINGS/PRECAUTIONS:** May temporarily exacerbate infection (eg, pruritus, edema, erythema). Avoid eyes. D/C if hypersensitivity occurs.

**ADVERSE REACTIONS:** Burning, stinging, pruritus, erythema, numbness, tingling, rash.

**PREGNANCY:** Category B, not for use in nursing.

## ELITEK RX
rasburicase (Sanofi-Aventis)

**May cause serious hypersensitivity reactions including anaphylaxis; discontinue if this occurs. Hemolysis may occur in G6PD deficiency; discontinue with hemolysis. Before initiate, screen patients at high risk for G6PD deficiency. Discontinue if develop methemoglobinemia. Causes enzymatic degradation of uric acid within blood samples left at room temperature. Collect blood in pre-chilled tubes containing heparin; immediately immerse and maintain in ice water bath and assay sample within 4 hrs of collection.**

**THERAPEUTIC CLASS:** Recombinant urate-oxidase enzyme

**INDICATIONS:** Initial management of plasma uric acid levels in pediatrics with leukemia, lymphoma, and solid tumor malignancies who are receiving anticancer therapy expected to result in tumor lysis and subsequent elevation of plasma uric acid.

**DOSAGE:** *Pediatrics:* 1 month-17 yrs: 0.15 or 0.2mg/kg IV as a single daily dose for 5 days. Administer over 30 minutes, not as a bolus infusion. Dosing >5 days or >1 course is not recommended. Initiate chemotherapy 4-24 hrs after 1st dose.

**HOW SUPPLIED:** Inj: 1.5mg

**CONTRAINDICATIONS:** G6PD deficiency, history of anaphylaxis or hypersensitivity reactions, hemolytic or methemoglobinemia reactions to rasburicase or any of the excipients.

**WARNINGS/PRECAUTIONS:** Screen patients at high risk for G6PD deficiency (eg, African or Mediterranean ancestry) prior to initiation. Administer IV hydration.

**ADVERSE REACTIONS:** Vomiting, fever, nausea, headache, abdominal pain, constipation, diarrhea, mucositis, rash, respiratory distress, sepsis, neutropenia with or without fever.

**PREGNANCY:** Category C, not for use in nursing.

## ELMIRON RX

pentosan sodium (Ortho-McNeil)

**THERAPEUTIC CLASS:** Analgesic, urinary

**INDICATIONS:** Relief of bladder pain/discomfort associated with interstitial cystitis.

**DOSAGE:** *Adults:* Take 1 hr before or 2 hrs after meals with water. 100mg tid for 3 months. Re-evaluate after 3 months; may continue for another 3 months.
*Pediatrics:* >16 yrs: Take 1 hr before or 2 hrs after meals with water. 100mg tid for 3 months. Re-evaluate after 3 months; may continue for another 3 months.

**HOW SUPPLIED:** Cap: 100mg

**WARNINGS/PRECAUTIONS:** Bleeding complications (eg, ecchymosis, epistaxis, gum hemorrhage), alopecia, increased PT/PTT reported. Caution with invasive procedures, coagulopathy, aneurysms, thrombocytopenia, hemophilia, GI ulcers, polyps, diverticula, history of heparin-induced thrombocytopenia, and hepatic impairment. Transient liver enzyme elevation reported.

**ADVERSE REACTIONS:** Nausea, diarrhea, alopecia, headache, rash, dyspepsia, abdominal pain.

**INTERACTIONS:** Increased risk of bleeding with anticoagulants, heparin, t-PA streptokinase, or high dose aspirin.

**PREGNANCY:** Category B, caution in nursing.

## ELOCON RX

mometasone furoate (Schering)

**THERAPEUTIC CLASS:** Corticosteroid

**INDICATIONS:** Corticosteroid responsive dermatoses.

**DOSAGE:** *Adults:* (Cre, Oint) Apply qd. (Lot) Apply a few drops qd. Reassess if no improvement within 2 weeks.
*Pediatrics:* (Cre, Oint) >2 yrs: Apply qd for up to 3 weeks if needed. Avoid in diaper area. Reassess if no improvement within 2 weeks.

**HOW SUPPLIED:** Cre, Oint: 0.1% [15g, 45g]; Lot: 0.1% [30mL, 60mL]

**WARNINGS/PRECAUTIONS:** May produce reversible HPA axis suppression, manifestations of Cushing's syndrome, hyperglycemia and glucosuria. Discontinue if irritation occurs. Use appropriate antifungal or antibacterial agent with dermatological infections. Pediatrics may be more susceptible to systemic toxicity. Caution when applied to large surface areas or with occlusive dressings.

**ADVERSE REACTIONS:** Burning, pruritus, skin atrophy, rosacea, acneiform reaction, tingling, stinging, furunculosis, folliculitis.

**PREGNANCY:** Category C, caution (Cre, Oint) or not for use (Lot) in nursing.



## ELOXATIN

RX

oxaliplatin (Sanofi-Aventis)

**Anaphylactic-like reactions may occur within minutes of administration.**

**THERAPEUTIC CLASS:** Organoplatinum complex

**INDICATIONS:** In combination with infusional 5-fluorouracil (5-FU) and leucovorin (LV), for treatment of advanced metastatic carcinoma of colon or rectum and adjuvant treatment of stage III colon cancer patients who have undergone complete resection of the primary tumor.

**DOSAGE:** *Adults:* Previously Untreated/Treated Advanced Colorectal Cancer: Day 1: 85mg/m$^2$ IV with LV 200mg/m$^2$; give over 120 min in separate bags using a Y-line; followed by 5-FU 400mg/m$^2$ bolus over 2-4 min, then 5-FU 600mg/m$^2$ as a 22 hr infusion. Day 2: LV 200mg/m$^2$ over 120 min; followed by 5-FU 400mg/m$^2$ bolus over 2-4 minutes, then 5-FU 600mg/m$^2$ as a 22 hr infusion. Repeat cycle every 2 weeks. Persistent Grade 2 Neurosensory Events: Reduce oxaliplatin to 65mg/m$^2$. Grade 3 Neurosensory Events: Consider discontinuation. After Recovery From Grade 3/4 GI or Grade 4 Hematologic Toxicity: Reduce oxaliplatin to 65mg/m$^2$ and 5-FU by 20%. Adjuvant Therapy Stage III Colon Cancer: Recommended cycle every 2 weeks for 6 months. Persistent Grade 2 Neurosensory Events: Reduce oxaliplatin to 75mg/m$^2$. Persistent Grade 3 Neurosensory Events: Consider discontinuation. After Recovery From Grade 3/4 GI or Grade 3/4 Hematologic Toxicity: Reduce oxaliplatin to 75mg/m$^2$ and 5-FU to 300mg/m$^2$ bolus and 500mg/m$^2$ 22 hr infusion.

**HOW SUPPLIED:** Inj: 50mg, 100mg

**CONTRAINDICATIONS:** Hypersensitivity to platinum compounds.

**WARNINGS/PRECAUTIONS:** Acute and persistent neuropathy reported. Cold may exacerbate acute neurological symptoms; avoid ice for mucositis prophylaxis. Potentially fatal pulmonary fibrosis reported. If unexplained respiratory symptoms develop, discontinue until interstitial lung disease or pulmonary fibrosis is ruled out. Monitor WBC with differential, Hgb, platelets, and blood chemistries (including ALT, AST, bilirubin, creatinine) before each cycle. Caution with renal impairment.

**ADVERSE REACTIONS:** Neuropathy, fatigue, nausea, neutropenia, emesis, diarrhea.

**INTERACTIONS:** Increased 5-FU plasma levels with doses of 130mg/m$^2$ oxaliplatin dosed every 3 weeks; clearance may be decreased with nephrotoxic agents.

**PREGNANCY:** Category D, not for use in nursing.

## EMADINE

RX

emedastine difumarate (Alcon)

**THERAPEUTIC CLASS:** $H_1$ receptor antagonist

**INDICATIONS:** Temporary relief of signs and symptoms of allergic conjunctivitis.

**DOSAGE:** *Adults:* 1 drop in affected eye up to qid.
*Pediatrics:* >3 yrs: 1 drop in affected eye up to qid.

**HOW SUPPLIED:** Sol: 0.05% [5mL]

**WARNINGS/PRECAUTIONS:** Wait at least 10 minutes after application to insert contact lens ( if eye is not red). Not for irritation due to contact lens.

**ADVERSE REACTIONS:** Headache, abnormal dreams, asthenia, bad taste, blurred vision, burning, stinging, corneal infiltrates, corneal staining, dermatitis, discomfort, dry eye, foreign body sensation, hyperemia, keratitis, pruritus, rhinitis, sinusitis, tearing.

**PREGNANCY:** Category B, caution in nursing.



## EMBELINE E

RX

clobetasol propionate (Healthpoint)

**THERAPEUTIC CLASS:** Corticosteroid

**INDICATIONS:** Corticosteroid responsive dermatoses.

**DOSAGE:** *Adults:* Apply bid. Limit to 2 consecutive weeks. Max: 50g/week. Moderate-Severe Psoriasis: Apply to 5%-10% BSA up to 4 weeks. Max: 50g/week.
*Pediatrics:* >12 yrs: Apply bid. Limit to 2 consecutive weeks. Max: 50g/week. Moderate-Severe Psoriasis: >16 yrs: Apply to 5%-10% BSA up to 4 weeks. Max: 50g/week.

**HOW SUPPLIED:** Cre: 0.05% [15g, 30g, 60g]

**WARNINGS/PRECAUTIONS:** Not for use on the face, groin, or axillae, or for treatment of rosacea or perioral dermatitis. May produce reversible HPA axis suppression, manifestations of Cushing's syndrome, hyperglycemia, and glucosuria. Reassess if no improvement after 2 weeks. D/C if irritation occurs. Peds may be more susceptible to systemic toxicity. Avoid occlusive dressings.

**ADVERSE REACTIONS:** Burning/stinging, pruritus, irritation, erythema, folliculitis, cracking/fissuring of skin, numbness of fingers, tenderness in elbows, telangiectasia, skin atrophy.

**PREGNANCY:** Category C, caution in nursing.

## EMBREX 600

RX

minerals - folic acid - multiple vitamin (Andrx)

**THERAPEUTIC CLASS:** Prenatal vitamin

**INDICATIONS:** Vitamin and mineral supplementation for before, during, and after pregnancy.

**DOSAGE:** *Adults:* 1 tab qd with 1 chewable tab qd.

**HOW SUPPLIED:** Tab: Copper 2mg-Docusate Sodium 50mg-Folic Acid 1mg-Iron 90mg-Magnesium 25mg-Vitamin A 3500 IU-Vitamin $B_1$ 2mg-Vitamin $B_2$ 3mg-Vitamin $B_6$ 3mg-Vitamin $B_{12}$ 0.012mg-Vitamin C 60mg-Vitamin D 400 IU-Vitamin E 30 IU-Zinc 20mg; Tab, Chewable: Calcium Carbonate 600mg

**WARNINGS/PRECAUTIONS:** Accidental overdose of iron-containing products is a leading cause of fatal poisoning in children <6 yrs. Not for the treatment of pernicious anemia and other megaloblastic anemias where vitamin $B_{12}$ is deficient. Folic acid >0.1mg/day may obscure pernicious anemia.

**ADVERSE REACTIONS:** Allergic sensitization.

## EMCYT

RX

estramustine phosphate sodium (Pharmacia & Upjohn)

**THERAPEUTIC CLASS:** Estradiol/nornitrogen mustard

**INDICATIONS:** Palliative treatment of metastatic and/or progressive prostate carcinoma.

**DOSAGE:** *Adults:* Usual: 14mg/kg/day given tid-qid. Take with water at least 1 hr before or 2 hrs after meals.

**HOW SUPPLIED:** Cap: 140mg

**CONTRAINDICATIONS:** Active thrombophlebitis, thromboembolic disorders; except when the tumor mass is causing the thromboembolic phenomenon and therapy benefits outweigh risks.

**WARNINGS/PRECAUTIONS:** Increased risk of thrombosis and MI. Caution with CVD, CAD, metabolic bone disease associated with hypercalcemia, hepatic or renal dysfunction, or with history of thrombophlebitis, thrombosis, or thromboembolic disorders. May decrease glucose tolerance. HTN may occur; monitor BP periodically. May exacerbate pre-existing peripheral edema or CHF. Allergic reactions, angioedema reported. Gynecomastia, impotence may occur.



**ADVERSE REACTIONS:** Edema, dyspnea, leg cramps, nausea, diarrhea, GI upset, breast tenderness/enlargement, increased hepatic enzymes.

**INTERACTIONS:** Milk, milk products, and calcium-rich foods or drugs may impair absorption.

**PREGNANCY:** Safety in pregnancy and nursing not known.

## EMEND RX

aprepitant (Merck)

**THERAPEUTIC CLASS:** Substance P/neurokinin 1 receptor antagonist

**INDICATIONS:** In combination with other antiemetics for prevention of acute and delayed nausea and vomiting associated with initial and repeat courses of highly emetogenic cancer chemotherapy (eg, high-dose cisplatin) and for moderately emetogenic cancer chemotherapy. For the prevention of postoperative nausea and vomiting.

**DOSAGE:** *Adults:* Prevention of Chemo-Induced N/V: Day 1: 125mg 1 hr prior to chemotherapy. Days 2 and 3: 80mg qam. Regimen should include a corticosteroid and a 5-$HT_3$ antagonist. Concomitant Corticosteroid: Reduce dexamethasone PO or methylprednisolone PO by 50% and methylprednisolone IV by 25%. Prevention of Post-Op N/V: 40mg within 3 hrs prior to induction of anesthesia.

**HOW SUPPLIED:** Cap: 40mg, 80mg, 125mg; Tri-Pak: (one 125mg & two 80mg caps)

**CONTRAINDICATIONS:** Concurrent treatment with pimozide, terfenadine, astemizole, or cisapride.

**WARNINGS/PRECAUTIONS:** Chronic continuous use is not recommended. Caution with severe hepatic insufficiency.

**ADVERSE REACTIONS:** Asthenia/fatigue, nausea, constipation, diarrhea, hiccups, anorexia, headache, vomiting, dizziness, dehydration, heartburn, abdominal pain, epigastric discomfort, gastritis, tinnitis, neutropenia.

**INTERACTIONS:** See Contraindications. May increase levels of drugs metabolized by CYP3A4 including chemotherapy agents (eg, docetaxel, paclitaxel, etoposide, irinotecan, ifosfamide, imatinib, vinorelbine, vinblastine, and vincristine), dexamethasone and methylprednisolone, certain benzodiazepines (eg, midazolam, alprazolam, triazolam). May reduce efficacy of oral contraceptives; use alternative contraception during treatment and for 1 month after last dose. May decrease levels of warfarin, tolbutamide, phenytoin or other drugs metabolized by CYP2C9. Caution with strong CYP3A4 inhibitors (eg, ketoconazole, itraconazole, nefazodone, troleandomycin, clarithromycin, ritonavir, nelfinavir and moderate CYP3A4 inhibitors (eg, diltiazem). Decreased efficacy with CYP3A4 inducers (eg, rifampin, carbamazepine, phenytoin). Concomitant paroxetine may decrease levels of both drugs.

**PREGNANCY:** Category B, not for use in nursing.

## EMLA

RX

lidocaine - prilocaine (AstraZeneca LP)

**OTHER BRAND NAMES:** EMLA Anesthetic Disc (AstraZeneca LP)

**THERAPEUTIC CLASS:** Acetamide local anesthetic

**INDICATIONS:** Topical anesthetic for use on normal intact skin or on genital mucous membranes for minor surgery. Pretreatment for infiltration anesthesia.

**DOSAGE:** *Adults:* Apply 1 disc or thick layer of cream to intact skin and cover with occlusive dressing. Minor Dermal Procedure: Apply 2.5g (1/2 tube) over 20-25cm² of skin surface or 1 disc for 1 hr. Major Dermal Procedure: Apply 2g/10cm² of skin for 2 hrs. Adult Male Genital Skin: Apply 1g/10cm² of skin surface for 15 minutes. Female External Genitalia: Apply 5-10g for 5-10 minutes. *Pediatrics:* All following doses are Max: 0-3 months or <5kg: 1g/10cm² for up to 1 hr. 3-12 months and >5 kg: 2g/20 cm² for up to 4 hrs. 1-6 yrs and >10 kg: 10g/100cm² for up to 4 hrs. 7-12 yrs and >20kg: 20g/200cm² for up to 4 hrs.

**HOW SUPPLIED:** (Lidocaine-Prilocaine) Cre: 2.5%-2.5%; Disc: 2.5%-2.5%

**WARNINGS/PRECAUTIONS:** Avoid application for longer than recommended times or large areas. Avoid with methemoglobinemia. Risk of methemoglobinemia in very young or with G6P deficiency. Avoid eye contact, use in ear. Caution with severe hepatic disease, acutely ill, debilitated, elderly, history of drug sensitivities. Avoid in neonates with a gestational age <37 weeks and infants <12 months receiving treatment with methemoglobin-inducing agents.

**ADVERSE REACTIONS:** Local reactions such as: erythema, edema, abnormal sensations, paleness (pallor or blanching), altered temperature sensations, itching, rash.

**INTERACTIONS:** Caution with Class I antiarrhythmics (eg, tocainide, mexiletine). Avoid drugs associated with drug-induced methemoglobinemia (eg, sulfonamides, APAP, nitrates/nitrites, nitrofurantoin, phenobarbital, phenytoin, quinine). Caution with other products containing local anesthetics; consider the amount absorbed from all formulations.

**PREGNANCY:** Category B, caution in nursing.

## EMSAM

RX

selegiline (Bristol-Myers Squibb)

**Antidepressants increased the risk of suicidal thinking and behavior (suicidality) in short-term studies in children and adolescents with Major Depressive Disorder and other psychiatric disorders. Selegiline transdermal system is not approved for use in pediatric patients.**

**THERAPEUTIC CLASS:** Monoamine oxidase inhibitor (Type B)

**INDICATIONS:** Treatment of major depressive disorder.

**DOSAGE:** *Adults:* Apply to dry, intact skin on the upper torso, upper thigh, or outer surface of upper arm once every 24 hrs. Initial/Target Dose: 6mg/24hrs. Titrate: May increase in increments of 3mg/24hrs at intervals no less than 2 weeks. Max: 12mg/24hrs. Elderly: 6mg/24hrs. Increase dose cautiously and monitor closely.

**HOW SUPPLIED:** Patch: 6mg/24hrs, 9mg/24hrs, 12mg/24hrs [30s]

**CONTRAINDICATIONS:** Pheochromocytoma. Concomitant SSRIs (eg, fluoxetine, sertraline, paroxetine), dual serotonin and norepinephrine reuptake inhibitors (eg, venlafaxine, duloxetine), TCAs (eg, imipramine, amitriptyline), bupropion, buspirone, meperidine, analgesic agents (eg, tramadol, methadone, and propoxyphene), dextromethorphan, St. John's wort, mirtazapine, cyclobenzaprine, carbamazepine, oxcarbazepine, sympathetic amines (including amphetamines), cold products and weight-reducing preparations that contain vasoconstrictors (eg, pseudoephedrine, phenylephrine, phenylpropanolamine, ephedrine), oral selegiline, other MAOIs(eg, isocarboxazid, phenelzine, tranylcypromine), general anesthesia agents, cocaine, or local anesthesia containing sympathomimetic vasoconstrictors. Dietary modifications required with 9mg/24hrs and 12mg/24hrs systems.

**WARNINGS/PRECAUTIONS:** Hypertensive crisis may occur with ingestion of foods with a high concentration of tyramine. Postural hypotension may occur; consider dosage adjustment with orthostatic symptoms. Activation of mania/hypomania may occur; caution with history of mania. Caution with disorders or conditions that can produce altered metabolism or hemodynamic responses. Avoid elective surgery requiring general anesthesia.



**ADVERSE REACTIONS:** Headache, diarrhea, dyspepsia, insomnia, dry mouth, pharyngitis, sinusitis, application site reaction, rash.

**INTERACTIONS:** Avoid alcohol. See Contraindications.

**PREGNANCY:** Category C, caution in nursing.

## EMTRIVA RX

emtricitabine (Gilead)

**Lactic acidosis and severe hepatomegaly with steatosis, including fatal cases, reported with nucleoside analogs alone or with concomitant antiretrovirals. Not indicated for the treatment of chronic HBV infection; severe acute exacerbations of hepatitis B reported in patients co-infected with HBV and HIV upon discontinuation of emtricitabine.**

**THERAPEUTIC CLASS:** Nucleoside analogue

**INDICATIONS:** Treatment of HIV-1 infection in combination with other antivirals.

**DOSAGE:** *Adults:* ≥18 yrs: Cap: 200mg qd. CrCl 30-49mL/min: 200mg q48h. CrCl 15-29mL/min: 200mg q72h. CrCl <15mL/min (including hemodialysis): 200mg q96h. Sol: 240mg (24mL) qd. CrCl 30-49mL/min: 120mg (12mL) qd. CrCl 15-29mL/min: 80mg (8mL) qd. CrCl <15mL/min (including hemodialysis): 60mg (6mL) qd.
*Pediatrics:* 0-3 months: Sol: 3mg/kg qd. 3 months-17 yrs: Cap: >33kg: 200mg qd. Sol: 6mg/kg qd. Max: 240mg (24mL).

**HOW SUPPLIED:** Cap: 200mg; Sol: 10mg/mL

**WARNINGS/PRECAUTIONS:** Test for chronic hepatitis B prior to initiation; post-treatment exacerbations reported. Monitor hepatic function for several months in patients who discontinue the drug and are co-infected with HIV and HBV. Reduce dose with renal dysfunction. Monitor changes in fasting cholesterol, serum amylase, creatinine kinase, and neutrophil count. Redistribution/accumulation of body fat reported. Immune reconstitution syndrome reported.

**ADVERSE REACTIONS:** Headache, diarrhea, nausea, rash, vomiting, dyspepsia, asthenia, abdominal pain, dizziness, insomnia, neuropathy, paresthesia, increased cough, rhinitis.

**INTERACTIONS:** Avoid co-administration with Atripla, Truvada, or lamivudine-containing products.

**PREGNANCY:** Category B, not for use in nursing.

## ENABLEX RX

darifenacin (Novartis)

**THERAPEUTIC CLASS:** Muscarinic antagonist

**INDICATIONS:** Treatment of overactive bladder with symptoms of urge urinary incontinence, urgency and frequency.

**DOSAGE:** *Adults:* Initial: 7.5mg qd with liquid. Max: 15mg qd. Moderate Hepatic Impairment/Concomitant Potent CYP3A4 Inhibitors: Do not exceed 7.5mg/d. Severe Hepatic Impairment: Avoid use. Tabs should be swallowed whole; do not chew, divide or crush.

**HOW SUPPLIED:** Tab, Extended-Release: 7.5mg, 15mg

**CONTRAINDICATIONS:** Urinary retention, gastric retention, uncontrolled narrow-angle glaucoma.

**WARNINGS/PRECAUTIONS:** Risk of urinary retention; caution with significant bladder outflow obstruction. Risk of gastric retention; caution with GI obstructive disorders. May decrease GI motility; caution with severe constipation, ulcerative colitis, and myasthenia gravis. Caution with moderate hepatic impairment and narrow-angle glaucoma. Avoid use with severe hepatic impairment. May produce blurred vision or dizziness.

**ADVERSE REACTIONS:** Dry mouth, constipation, dyspepsia, abdominal pain, nausea, diarrhea, UTI, dizziness, asthenia, dry eyes.

**INTERACTIONS:** Do not exceed 7.5mg/day with concomitant potent CYP3A4 inhibitors. Caution with medications metabolized by CYP2D6. Additive effects with other anticholinergic agents.

**PREGNANCY:** Category C, caution in nursing.

## ENBREL RX

etanercept (Amgen)

**THERAPEUTIC CLASS:** TNF receptor blocker

**INDICATIONS:** To reduce signs/symptoms, induce major clinical response, improve physical function, and inhibit progression of structural damage in moderate to severe rheumatoid arthritis (RA) (may be initiated in combination with methotrexate [MTX] or alone). To reduce signs/symptoms, inhibit progression of structural damage of active arthritis, and improve physical function in psoriatic arthritis (may be used with MTX in patients not responding to MTX alone). To reduce signs/symptoms of moderate to severe polyarticular-course juvenile rheumatoid arthritis (JRA) unresponsive to one or more DMARDs. To reduce signs/symptoms of active ankylosing spondylitis (AS). Chronic moderate to severe plaque psoriasis for candidates of systemic therapy or phototherapy.

**DOSAGE:** *Adults:* ≥18 yrs: RA/Psoriatic Arthritis/AS: 50mg SQ per week, given as one SQ injection. May continue MTX, glucocorticoids, salicylates, NSAIDs, or analgesics. Psoriasis: Initial: 50mg SQ twice weekly given 3 or 4 days apart for 3 months. May begin with 25-50mg/week. Maint: 50mg/week.
*Pediatrics:* 4-17 yrs: JRA: 0.8mg/kg SQ per week. Max: 50mg/week. Max per injection site: 25mg. ≤31kg: One SQ injection once weekly. >31kg: Two SQ injections on same day or 3 or 4 days apart. May continue glucocorticoids, NSAIDs, or analgesics.

**HOW SUPPLIED:** Inj: 25mg [vial], 50mg/mL [syringe]

**CONTRAINDICATIONS:** Sepsis.

**WARNINGS/PRECAUTIONS:** D/C if severe allergic reaction or infection (eg, sepsis) occurs. May cause autoimmune antibodies. Serious, fatal infections including sepsis reported. Avoid with active infections. Monitor closely if develop new infection. JRA patients should be brought up to date with current immunization guidelines prior to initiating therapy. D/C temporarily with significant varicella virus exposure and consider prophylaxis. Avoid with Wegener's granulomatosis.

**ADVERSE REACTIONS:** (Adults/Pediatrics) Injection site reactions, infections, headache. (Pediatrics) Varicella, gastroenteritis, depression, cutaneous ulcer, esophagitis.

**INTERACTIONS:** Do not give live vaccines. Avoid with cyclophosphamide.

**PREGNANCY:** Category B, not for use in nursing.

## ENDURON
RX

methyclothiazide (Abbott)

**THERAPEUTIC CLASS:** Thiazide diuretic

**INDICATIONS:** Adjunct therapy in edema associated with CHF, hepatic cirrhosis, renal dysfunction, corticosteroid and estrogen therapy. Management of hypertension.

E

**DOSAGE:** *Adults:* Edema: 2.5-10mg qd. Max: 10mg/dose. HTN: 2.5-5mg qd.

**HOW SUPPLIED:** Tab: 5mg* *scored

**CONTRAINDICATIONS:** Anuria, sulfonamide hypersensitivity.

**WARNINGS/PRECAUTIONS:** Caution in severe renal disease, liver dysfunction, electrolyte/fluid imbalance. Monitor electrolytes. Hyperuricemia, hyperglycemia, hypokalemia, hyponatremia, hypomagnesemia, hypercalcemia may occur. Increases in cholesterol and triglyceride levels reported. May exacerbate SLE. Sensitivity reactions reported. D/C prior to parathyroid test. Enhanced effects in post-sympathectomy patient.

**ADVERSE REACTIONS:** Headache, cramping, weakness, orthostatic hypotension, pancreatitis, hyperglycemia, hyperuricemia, electrolyte imbalance, blood dyscrasias, hypersensitivity reactions.

**INTERACTIONS:** Hypokalemia may develop with steroids or ACTH. May affect insulin requirements. May decrease arterial responsiveness to norepinephrine. May increase responsiveness to tubocurarine. Lithium toxicity. May potentiate other antihypertensives.

**PREGNANCY:** Category B, not for use in nursing.

## ENJUVIA
RX

conjugated estrogens (Duramed)

**Estrogens increase the risk of endometrial cancer. Estrogens and progestins should not be used for the prevention of cardiovascular disease or dementia. Increased risks of MI, stroke, invasive breast cancer, PE, and DVT in postmenopausal women (50 to 79 years of age) reported. Increased risk of developing probable dementia in postmenopausal women ≥65 yrs of age reported.**

**THERAPEUTIC CLASS:** Estrogen

**INDICATIONS:** Treatment of moderate to severe vasomotor symptoms associated with menopause. Treatment of symptoms of vulvar and vaginal atrophy associated with menopause. Treatment of moderate to severe vaginal dryness and pain with intercourse; if used solely for this purpose, topical vaginal products should be considered.

**DOSAGE:** *Adults:* Individualize dosing. Initial: 0.3mg qd. Adjust dose based on response.

**HOW SUPPLIED:** Tab: 0.3mg, 0.45mg, 0.625mg, 0.9mg, 1.25mg

**CONTRAINDICATIONS:** Pregnancy, undiagonosed abnormal genital bleeding, breast cancer, estrogen-dependent neoplasia, DVT/PE, arterial thromboembolic disease (eg, stroke, MI), liver dysfunction.

**WARNINGS/PRECAUTIONS:** Increased risk of retinal vascular thrombosis, severe hypercalcemia in patients with breast cancer and bone metastases, gallbladder disease and breast and ovarian cancers. Elavated BP reported; monitor BP at regular intervals. May elevate plasma triglycerides resulting in pancreatitis. Caution in patients with impaired liver function or history of cholestic jaundice. May increase TBG; monitor thyroid function of patients dependent on thyroid hormone replacement therapy and adjust dosage if needed. May cause fluid retention; caution with cardiac or renal dysfunction. Caution in individuals with severe hypocalcemia. May cause exacerbation of asthma, diabetes mellitus, epilepsy, migraine or porphyria, systemic lupus erythematosus, and hepatic hemangiomas.

**ADVERSE REACTIONS:** Abdominal pain, accidental injury, flu-syndrome, headache, pain, flatulence, nausea, dizziness, paresthesia, bronchitis, rhinitis, sinusitis, breast pain, dysmenorrhea, vaginitis.

**INTERACTIONS:** CYP3A4 inducers (eg, St. John's wort, phenobarbital, carbamazepine, rifampin) may decrease levels which may decrease therapeutic effects and/or uterine bleeding profile. CYP3A4 inhibitors (eg, erythromycin, clarithromycin, ketoconazole, itraconazole, ritonavir, grapefruit juice) may increase levels which may result in side effects.

**PREGNANCY:** Category X, caution in nursing.



## ENTEX HC

**CIII**

guaifenesin - phenylephrine HCl - hydrocodone bitartrate (Andrx)

**THERAPEUTIC CLASS:** Opioid antitussive

**INDICATIONS:** Temporary relief of nonproductive cough.

**DOSAGE:** *Adults:* 5-10mL q4-6h. Max 40mL/24 hrs.
*Pediatrics:* >12 yrs: 5-10mL q4-6h. Max 40mL/24 hrs. 6-12 yrs: 5mL q4-6h. Max 20mL/24 hrs. 2-6 yrs: 2.5mL q4-6h. Max 10mL/24 hrs.

**HOW SUPPLIED:** Liq: (Guaifenesin-Hydrocodone-Phenylephrine) 100mg-5mg-7.5mg/5mL [473mL]

**CONTRAINDICATIONS:** Infants, newborns, severe HTN or CAD, hyperthyroidism, or MAOI therapy.

**WARNINGS/PRECAUTIONS:** May be habit-forming. May cause respiratory depression or increase CSF pressure in the presence of other intracranial pathology. May obscure head injuries or acute abdominal conditions. Caution in elderly, debilitated, hepatic/renal dysfunction, Addison's disease, hypothyroidism, postoperative use, prostatic hypertrophy, pulmonary disease, and urethral stricture. Suppresses cough reflex.

**ADVERSE REACTIONS:** CNS stimulation, constipation, drowsiness, dizziness, excitability, headache, insomnia, lightheadedness, nausea, vomiting, nervousness, respiratory depression, restlessness, tachycardia, tremors, urinary retention, weakness, arrhythmias, and cardiovascular.

**INTERACTIONS:** Additive CNS effects with alcohol, antianxiety agents, antihistamines, antipsychotics, narcotics, tranquilizers, or other CNS depressants. Increased sympathomimetic effects with MAOIs or beta blockers. Sympathomimetics may reduce antihypertensive effects of methyldopa, mecamylamine, reserpine, veratrum alkaloids. May enhance the effects of TCAs, barbiturates, alcohol, other CNS depressants.

**PREGNANCY:** Category C, not for use in nursing.

## ENTEX LA

RX

guaifenesin - phenylephrine HCl (Andrx)

**THERAPEUTIC CLASS:** Expectorant/sympathomimetic

**INDICATIONS:** Temporary relief of symptoms associated with upper respiratory tract disorders and cough associated with respiratory tract infections and related disorders when complicated by tenacious mucous or mucous plugs and congestion.

**DOSAGE:** *Adults:* 1 tab q12h. Max: 2 tabs/24hrs.
*Pediatrics:* >12 yrs: 1 tab q12h. Max: 2 tabs/24hrs. 6-12 yrs: 1/2 tab q12h. Max: 1 tab/24hrs.

**HOW SUPPLIED:** Tab, Extended Release: (Guaifenesin-Phenylephrine) 400mg-30mg* *scored

**CONTRAINDICATIONS:** HTN, ventricular tachycardia, MAOI use within 14 days. Extreme caution in elderly, hyperthyroidism, bradycardia, partial heart block, myocardial disease, severe arteriosclerosis.

**WARNINGS/PRECAUTIONS:** Caution in HTN, DM, ischemic heart disease, increase IOP, hyperthyroidism, or prostatic hypertrophy. May produce CNS stimulation with convulsions or cadiovascular collapse with hypotension. Adverse effects occur more often in elderly.

**ADVERSE REACTIONS:** Palpitations, headache, dizziness, nausea, anxiety, restlessness, tremor, weakness, pallor, dysuria, respiratory difficulty.

**INTERACTIONS:** β-blockers and MAOIs may potentiate pressor response. Increased risk of arrhythmias with digitalis glycosides and halothane anesthesia. May reduce hypotensive effects of guanethidine, mecamylamine, methyldopa, reserpine, and veratrum alkaloids. TCAs may antagonize effects.

**PREGNANCY:** Category C, not for use in nursing.

## ENTEX PSE

RX

guaifenesin - pseudoephedrine HCl (Andrx)

**OTHER BRAND NAMES:** Ami-Tex PSE (Amide) - Guaifenex PSE 120 (Ethex)

**THERAPEUTIC CLASS:** Expectorant/decongestant

**INDICATIONS:** Relief of nasal congestion due to common cold, hay fever, upper respiratory allergies, and nasal congestion associated with sinusitis. To promote nasal or sinus drainage. For symptomatic relief of respiratory conditions characterized by dry nonproductive cough and in the presence of tenacious mucous plugs in the respiratory tract.

**DOSAGE:** *Adults:* 1 tab q12h.
*Pediatrics:* >12 yrs: 1 tab q12h. 6 to <12 yrs: 1/2 tab q12h.

**HOW SUPPLIED:** Tab, Extended Release: (Guaifenesin-Pseudoephedrine) 400mg-120mg* *scored

**CONTRAINDICATIONS:** Nursing, severe HTN, severe CAD, prostatic hypertrophy, concomitant MAOIs.

**WARNINGS/PRECAUTIONS:** Caution in HTN, DM, heart disease, peripheral vascular disease, increased IOP, hyperthyroidism, or prostatic hypertrophy.

**ADVERSE REACTIONS:** Nausea, vomiting, nervousness, dizziness, sleeplessness, lightheadedness, tremor, palpitations, tachycardia, weakness, respiratory difficulties.

**INTERACTIONS:** MAOI and β-blockers increase sympathomimetic effects. May reduce antihypertensive effects of methyldopa, guanethidine, mecamylamine, reserpine, and veratrum alkaloids.

**PREGNANCY:** Category C, contraindicated in nursing.

## ENTOCORT EC

RX

budesonide (Prometheus)

**THERAPEUTIC CLASS:** Corticosteroids

**INDICATIONS:** Treatment of mild to moderate active Crohn's disease involving the ileum and/or ascending colon. Maintenance of clinical remission of mild to moderate Crohn's disease involving the ileum and/or ascending colon for up to 3 months.

**DOSAGE:** *Adults:* Usual: 9mg qd, in the am for up to 8 weeks. Recurring Episodes: Repeat therapy for 8 weeks. Maint: 6mg qd for 3 months, then taper to complete cessation. Moderate to Severe Hepatic Insufficiency/Concomitant CYP3A4 Inhibitors: Reduce dose. Swallow whole; do not chew or break.

**HOW SUPPLIED:** Cap, Delayed Release: 3mg

**WARNINGS/PRECAUTIONS:** May reduce response of HPA axis to stress. Supplement with systemic glucocorticosteroids if undergoing surgery or other stressful situations. Increased risk of infection avoid exposure to chickenpox and measles. Caution with TB, HTN, DM, osteoporosis, peptic ulcer, glaucoma, cirrhosis, cataracts, family history of DM or glaucoma. Replacement of systemic glucocorticosteroids may unmask allergies. Chronic use may cause hypercorticism and adrenal suppression.

**ADVERSE REACTIONS:** Headache, respiratory infection, nausea, back pain, dyspepsia, dizziness, abdominal pain, diarrhea, flatulence, vomiting, sinusitis, viral infection, arthralgia.

**INTERACTIONS:** Increased levels with CYP3A4 inhibitors (eg, ketoconazole, itraconazole, saquinavir, erythromycin, grapefruit, grapefruit juice); reduce budesonide dose.

**PREGNANCY:** Category C, not for use in nursing.



## EPIFOAM

RX

pramoxine HCl - hydrocortisone acetate (Schwarz)

**THERAPEUTIC CLASS:** Corticosteroid

**INDICATIONS:** Corticosteroid responsive dermatoses.

**DOSAGE:** *Adults:* Apply tid-qid. Use occlusive dressings for management of psoriasis or recalcitrant conditions.
*Pediatrics:* Use least amount necessary for effective regimen. Use occlusive dressings for management of psoriasis or recalcitrant conditions.

**HOW SUPPLIED:** Foam: (Hydrocortisone-Pramoxine) 1%-1% [10g]

**WARNINGS/PRECAUTIONS:** Avoid prolonged use. Discontinue use if irritation persists. May produce reversible HPA axis suppression, manifestations of Cushing's syndrome, hyperglycemia, glucosuria. Pediatrics more susceptible to systemic toxicity.

**ADVERSE REACTIONS:** Burning, itching, irritation, dryness, folliculitis, hypertrichosis, acneiform eruptions, hypopigmentation, perioral dermatitis, maceration, secondary infection, skin atrophy, striae, miliaria.

**PREGNANCY:** Category C, caution in nursing.

## EPIPEN

RX

epinephrine (Dey)

**OTHER BRAND NAMES:** EpiPen Jr. (Dey)

**THERAPEUTIC CLASS:** Sympathomimetic catecholamine

**INDICATIONS:** Emergency treatment of allergic reactions (anaphylaxis) to insect stings or bites, foods, drugs, other allergens, and idiopathic or exercise-induced anaphylaxis.

**DOSAGE:** *Adults:* 0.3mg IM in thigh. May repeat with severe anaphylaxis.
*Pediatrics:* 0.15mg or 0.3mg (0.01mg/kg) IM in thigh. May repeat with severe anaphylaxis.

**HOW SUPPLIED:** Inj: (Epipen Jr) 0.5mg/mL, (Epipen) 1mg/mL

**WARNINGS/PRECAUTIONS:** Not for IV use. Contains sulfites. Extreme caution with heart disease. Anginal pain may be induced with coronary insufficiency. Increased risk of adverse reactions with hyperthyroidism, CVD, HTN, DM, elderly, pregnancy, pediatrics <30kg with Epipen and <15kg with Epipen, Jr.

**ADVERSE REACTIONS:** Palpitations, tachycardia, sweating, nausea, vomiting, respiratory difficulty, pallor, dizziness, weakness, tremor, headache, apprehension, anxiety.

**INTERACTIONS:** Potentiated by TCAs and MAOIs. Increased risk of arrhythmias with digitalis, mercurial diuretics, or quinidine. Pressor effects may be counteracted by rapidly acting vasodilators.

**PREGNANCY:** Category C, safety in nursing not known.

## EPIQUIN MICRO

RX

hydroquinone (SkinMedica)

**THERAPEUTIC CLASS:** Depigmenting agent

**INDICATIONS:** Gradual treatment of ultraviolet induced dyschromia and discoloration resulting from the use of oral contraceptives, pregnancy, hormone replacement therapy, or skin trauma.



**DOSAGE:** *Adults:* Apply bid (am and hs). Use sunscreen.
*Pediatrics:* ≥12yrs: Apply bid (am and hs). Use sunscreen.

**HOW SUPPLIED:** Cre: 4% [30g]

**WARNINGS/PRECAUTIONS:** Avoid sun exposure on bleached skin. Use sunscreen. May produce unwanted cosmetic effects if not used as directed. Test for skin sensitivity. Discontinue if no lightening effect after 2 months of therapy, if blue-black darkening of the skin occurs, or if itching, vesicle formation, or excessive inflammatory reactions occur. Contains sodium metabisulfite, may cause serious allergic type reactions. Avoid contact with eyes.

**ADVERSE REACTIONS:** Cutaneous hypersensitivity (contact dermatitis).

**PREGNANCY:** Category C, caution in nursing.

## EPIVIR

RX

lamivudine (GlaxoSmithKline)

**Lactic acidosis and severe, possibly fatal hepatomegaly reported. Tablets and solution have higher dose of active ingredient than Epivir-HBV; only dose with appropriate forms for HIV.**

**THERAPEUTIC CLASS:** Nucleoside analogue

**INDICATIONS:** Treatment of HIV infection in combination with other antiretrovirals.

**DOSAGE:** *Adults:* 150mg bid or 300mg qd, concomitantly with other antiretrovirals. CrCl 30-49mL/min: 150mg qd. CrCl 15-29mL/min: 150mg first dose, then 100mg qd. CrCl 5-14mL/min: 150mg first dose, then 50mg qd. CrCl <5mL/min: 50mg first dose, then 25mg qd.
*Pediatrics:* 3 months-16 yrs: 4mg/kg bid, concomitantly with other antiretrovirals. Max: 150mg bid. Adolescents: CrCl 30-49mL/min: 150mg qd. CrCl 15-29mL/min: 150mg first dose, then 100mg qd. CrCl 5-14mL/min: 150mg first dose, then 50mg qd. CrCl <5mL/min: 50mg first dose, then 25mg qd.

**HOW SUPPLIED:** Sol: 10mg/mL [240mL]; Tab: 150mg, 300mg

**WARNINGS/PRECAUTIONS:** Caution in peds with history of prior antiretroviral nucleoside exposure, history of pancreatitis, or other significant risk factors for developing pancreatitis. D/C if pancreatitis develops. Post-treatment exacerbations of hepatitis reported. Lactic acidosis and severe, fatal hepatomegaly reported. Hepatic decompensation occured when used with interferon alfa w/ or w/o ribavirin. Reduce dose in renal dysfunction. Possible redistribution or accumulation of body fat. Suspend therapy if develop lactic acidosis or pronounced hepatotoxicity. Immune reconstitution syndrome reported.

**ADVERSE REACTIONS:** Headache, malaise, fatigue, fever, chills, nausea, diarrhea, vomiting, anorexia, abdominal pain, neuropathy, dizziness, skin rash, musculoskeletal pain, cough, pancreatitis.

**INTERACTIONS:** TMP/SMX increases levels of lamivudine. Avoid with zalcitabine, zidovudine, lamivudine, and fixed-dose combinations of abacavir, lamivudine, and zidovudine.

**PREGNANCY:** Category C, not for use in nursing.

## EPIVIR-HBV RX
lamivudine (GlaxoSmithKline)

**Lactic acidosis and severe, possibly fatal, hepatomegaly reported. If prescribed for patients with unrecognized or untreated HIV infection, rapid emergence of HIV resistance is likely. Reports of severe acute exacerbations of hepatitis B upon discontinuation of therapy. Follow up liver function monitoring required.**

**THERAPEUTIC CLASS:** Nucleoside analogue

**INDICATIONS:** Treatment of chronic hepatitis B associated with viral replication and active liver inflammation.

**DOSAGE:** *Adults:* 100mg qd. CrCl 30-49mL/min: 100mg day 1, then 50mg qd. CrCl: 15-29mL/min: 100mg day 1, then 25mg qd. CrCl 5-14mL/min: 35mg day 1, then 15mg qd. CrCl <5mL/min: 35mg day 1, then 10mg qd.
*Pediatrics:* 2-17 yrs: 3mg/kg qd. Max: 100mg/day.

**HOW SUPPLIED:** Sol: 5mg/mL [240mL]; Tab: 100mg

**WARNINGS/PRECAUTIONS:** Reduce dose in renal dysfunction. Caution in elderly. This formulation is not appropriate in both HBV and HIV infections. Posttreatment exacerbations of hepatitis reported. Pancreatitis reported, especially in HIV-infected pediatrics with prior nucleoside exposure. Monitor patient regularly during treatment. Safety and efficacy with treatment after 1 yr is not known. Suspend therapy if develop lactic acidosis or pronounced hepatotoxicity.

**ADVERSE REACTIONS:** Pancreatitis, lactic acidosis, severe hepatomegaly, GI complaints, sore throat, infections, elevated LFTs, arthralgia.

**INTERACTIONS:** TMP/SMX may increase lamivudine levels. Avoid with zalcitabine.

**PREGNANCY:** Category C, not for use in nursing.

## EPOGEN RX
epoetin alfa (Amgen)

**Erythropoiesis-stimulating agents (ESAs) may increase risk for death and/or serious cardiovascular events when administered to a target Hgb >12g/dL. Use lowest dose that will gradually increase Hgb concentration to lowest level sufficient to avoid need for RBC transfusion. When ESAs are used preoperatively for reduction of allogenic RBC transfusions, a higher incidence of DVT was reported in patients not receiving prophylactic anticoagulation. Antithrombotic prophylaxis should be strongly considered when ESAs are used to reduce allogenic RBC transfusions.**

**THERAPEUTIC CLASS:** Erythropoiesis stimulator

**INDICATIONS:** Treatment of anemia of chronic renal failure (CRF), anemia related to zidovudine in HIV, chemotherapy-induced anemia in patients with non-myeloid malignancies (serum erythropoietin ≤200mU/mL), and reduction of allogeneic blood transfusions in anemic (≤13 to >10 g/dL) patients scheduled for elective, noncardiac, nonvascular surgery.

**DOSAGE:** *Adults:* CRF: Initial: 50-100 U/kg IV/SQ 3x/week. IV is preferred route in dialysis patients. Reduce dose when Hct approaches 36% or increase by >4 points in any 2 week period. Increase dose if Hct does not increase by 5-6 points after 8 weeks of therapy and Hct is below target range. Maint: Individually titrate. Zidovudine-Treated HIV Patients: Serum erythropoietin ≤500 mU/mL and zidovudine dose ≤4200mg/week: 100 U/kg IV/SQ 3x/week for 8 weeks. Max: 300 U/kg 3x/week. Maint: Individualize dose to maintain Hct within 30%-36%. Chemotherapy-Induced Anemia: Initial: 150 U/kg SQ 3x/week. Titrate: May increase to 300U/kg 3x/week after 8 weeks of therapy. Surgery: 300 U/kg/day SQ for 10 days before, on day of, and 4 days after surgery; or 600 U/kg SQ once weekly on 21, 14, and 7 days before surgery, and a 4th dose on day of surgery.
*Pediatrics:* CRF: Initial: 50 U/kg 3x/week IV/SQ. Reduce dose when Hct

approaches 36% or increase by >4 points in any 2 week period. Increase dose if Hct does not increase by 5-6 points after 8 weeks of therapy and Hct is below target range. Maint: Individually titrate.

**HOW SUPPLIED:** Inj: 2000 U/mL, 3000 U/mL, 4000 U/mL, 10,000 U/mL, 20,000 U/mL, 40,000 U/mL

**CONTRAINDICATIONS:** Uncontrolled HTN. Hypersensitivity to mammalian cell-derived products and Albumin (human).

**WARNINGS/PRECAUTIONS:** Pure red cell aplasia and severe anemia (with or without other cytopenias) may occur. Caution with porphyria, HTN or a history of seizures. Evaluate iron stores prior to and during therapy. Most patients need iron supplementation. Monitor Hct, BP, iron levels, serum chemistry, and CBC. Menses may resume. Multidose formulation contains benzyl alcohol.

E

**ADVERSE REACTIONS:** HTN, headache, fatigue, arthralgias, nausea, vomiting, diarrhea, edema, rash, pyrexia, clotted vascular access, respiratory congestion, dyspnea, asthenia, dizziness, seizures, thrombotic events.

**INTERACTIONS:** Adjust anticoagulant dose in dialysis patients.

**PREGNANCY:** Category C, caution in nursing.

## EPZICOM RX

lamivudine - abacavir sulfate (GlaxoSmithKline)

**Fatal hypersensitivity reactions reported with abacavir sulfate; discontinue if hypersensitivity reaction suspected and do not restart. Lactic acidosis and severe hepatomegaly with steatosis, including fatal cases, have been reported with nucleoside analogs alone or in combination with other antivirals. Severe acute exacerbations of hepatitis B reported in patients co-infected with HBV and HIV and who have discontinued lamivudine.**

**THERAPEUTIC CLASS:** Nucleoside analog combination

**INDICATIONS:** Treatment of HIV infection in combination with other antiretrovirals.

**DOSAGE:** *Adults:* ≥18 yrs: CrCl >50mL/min: 1 tab qd.

**HOW SUPPLIED:** Tab: (Abacavir Sulfate-Lamivudine) 600mg-300mg

**CONTRAINDICATIONS:** Hepatic impairment.

**WARNINGS/PRECAUTIONS:** Serious hypersensitivity reactions reported. Register abacavir hypersensitive patients at 1-800-270-0425. Suspend therapy if lactic acidosis or pronounced hepatotoxicity develops. Avoid with CrCl <50mL/min. Redistribution/accumulation of body fat reported. Hepatic decompensation has occurred in HIV/HCV co-infected patients receiving combination antiretroviral therapy for HIV and interferon alfa with or without ribavir. Immune reconstitution syndrome has been reported.

**ADVERSE REACTIONS:** Hypersensitivity, insomnia, depression, headache, fatigue, dizziness, nausea, diarrhea, rash, pyrexia, abdominal pain, abnormal dreams, anxiety.

**INTERACTIONS:** May increase methadone clearance. Decreased elimination with ethanol. TMP/SMX and/or nelfinavir may increase lamivudine exposure. Avoid with zalcitabine.

**PREGNANCY:** Category C, not for use in nursing.

## EQUAGESIC CIV

aspirin - meprobamate (Wyeth/Women First)

**THERAPEUTIC CLASS:** Carbamate derivative/salicylate

**INDICATIONS:** Adjunct in short-term treatment of pain accompanied by tension and/or anxiety in patients with musculoskeletal disease.

**DOSAGE:** *Adults:* 1-2 tabs tid-qid prn. Elderly/Debilitated: Use lowest effective dose.
*Pediatrics:* >12 yrs: 1-2 tabs tid-qid prn.

**HOW SUPPLIED:** Tab: (Meprobamate-ASA) 200mg-325mg* *scored

**CONTRAINDICATIONS:** Acute intermittent porphyria.

**WARNINGS/PRECAUTIONS:** Extreme caution with peptic ulcer, asthma, coagulation abnormalities, hypoprothrombinemia, or vitamin K deficiency. Abuse, physical and psychological dependence reported. Abrupt withdrawal after prolonged and excessive use may precipitate recurrence of pre-existing symptoms. May impair mental and physical abilities. Caution with hepatic or kidney dysfunction. May precipitate seizures in epileptic patients. Prescribe cautiously and in small amounts to suicidal patients.



**ADVERSE REACTIONS:** Epigastric discomfort, nausea, vomiting, drowsiness, ataxia, dizziness, slurred speech, headache, vertigo, weakness.

**INTERACTIONS:** Additive CNS suppression with alcohol or other psychotropic drugs. May antagonize uricosuric activity of probenecid and sulfinpyrazone. Extreme caution with anticoagulants. May enhance hypoglycemic effects of sulfonylureas.

**PREGNANCY:** Safety in pregnancy or nursing not known.

## EQUETRO

carbamazepine (Shire US)

RX

**Aplastic anemia and agranulocytosis reported. Obtain complete pretreatment hematological testing as baseline. Discontinue if evidence of bone marrow depression develops.**

**THERAPEUTIC CLASS:** Carboxamide

**INDICATIONS:** Treatment of acute manic and mixed episodes associated with Bipolar I Disorder.

**DOSAGE:** *Adults:* Initial: 400mg/day, given in divided doses, bid. Titrate: 200mg qd. Max: 1600mg/day. Do not crush or chew.

**HOW SUPPLIED:** Cap, Extended Release: 100mg, 200mg, 300mg

**CONTRAINDICATIONS:** Avoid in patients with a history of previous bone marrow depression, hypersensitivity to the drug, or known sensitivity to any of the tricyclic compounds. Use of MAOIs is not recommended and MAOIs should be discontinued for a minimum of 14 days prior to use.

**WARNINGS/PRECAUTIONS:** Monitor blood levels. Avoid use with any other medication containing carbamazepine. May cause fetal harm during pregnancy. Severe dermatologic reactions, including toxic epidermal necrolysis (Lyell's syndrome) and Stevens-Johnson syndrome, reported with carbamazepine. Avoid abrupt discontinuation with seizure disorder. Carbamazepine has mild anticholinergic activity; observe closely with increased IOP. Caution in patients with a history of cardiac, hepatic, or renal damage; adverse hematologic reaction to other drugs; or interrupted courses of therapy with carbamazepine. Closely monitor patients at high-risk for suicide attempts. May cause activate latent psychosis. May cause confusion/agitation in elderly. Perform eye exam and monitor LFTs and renal function at baseline and periodically.

**ADVERSE REACTIONS:** Dizziness, somnolence, nausea, vomiting, ataxia, pruritus, dry mouth, headache, infection, pain, rash, diarrhea, dyspepsia, asthenia, amnesia.

**INTERACTIONS:** See Contraindications. CYP3A4 inhibitors may increase plasma levels. CYP3A4 inducers may decrease plasma levels. May induce CYP1A2 and CYP3A4; may interact with any agent metabolized by these enzymes. May increase plasma levels of clomipramine, phenytoin, and primidone. May increase risk of neurotoxic side effects of lithium. Decreases levels of trazodone with concomitant administration. Anti-malarial drugs may antagonize the activity of carbamazepine. Caution with other centrally acting drugs and/or alcohol. Co-administration with delavirdine may lead to loss of virologic response and possible resistance to non-nucleoside reverse transcriptase inhibitors.

**PREGNANCY:** Category D, not for use in nursing.

## ERAXIS RX
anidulafungin (Pfizer)

**THERAPEUTIC CLASS:** Echinocandin
**INDICATIONS:** Treatment of candidemia and other forms of *Candida* infections (intra-abdominal abscess and peritonitis); esophageal candidiasis.
**DOSAGE:** *Adults:* Candidemia/*Candida* Infections: Loading Dose: 200mg on Day 1. Follow with 100mg qd thereafter. Continue therapy for at least 14 days after last positive culture. Esophageal Candidiasis: Loading Dose: 100mg on Day 1. Follow with 50mg qd thereafter. Treat for minimum of 14 days and for at least 7 days after symptoms resolve.
**HOW SUPPLIED:** Inj: 50mg, 100mg
**WARNINGS/PRECAUTIONS:** Hepatic abnormalities may occur; monitor hepatic function if abnormal LFTs develop during therapy.
**ADVERSE REACTIONS:** Diarrhea, nausea, rash, hypokalemia, headache, increased LFTs, neutropenia.
**INTERACTIONS:** Slightly increased levels with cyclosporine.
**PREGNANCY:** Category C, caution in nursing.

## ERBITUX RX
cetuximab (Bristol-Myers Squibb)

**Severe infusion reactions have occurred; discontinue if these reactions develop. Cardiopulmonary arrest and/or sudden death occurred in patients with squamous cell carcinoma of the head and neck.**

**THERAPEUTIC CLASS:** Epidermal growth factor receptor (EGFR) antagonist
**INDICATIONS:** In combination with irinotecan for the treatment of EGFR-expressing, metastatic colorectal carcinoma in patients who are refractory to irinotecan-based chemotherapy. As monotherapy, for the treatment of EGFR-expressing, metastatic colorectal carcinoma in patients who are intolerant to irinotecan-based chemotherapy. In combination with radiation therapy for the treatment of locally or regionally advanced squamous cell carcinoma of the head and neck. As monotherapy, for the treatment of patients with recurrent or metastatic squamous cell carcinoma of the head and neck for whom prior platinum-based therapy has failed.
**DOSAGE:** *Adults:* Pre-medication with $H_1$ antagonist (eg, diphenhydramine 50mg IV) is recommended. Colorectal Cancer: LD: 400mg/m² IV infusion over 120 min. Maint: 250mg/m² IV infusion over 60 min once weekly. Max Infusion Rate: 5mL/min. Squamous Cell Carcinoma of Head and Neck: Combination Therapy: Initial: 400mg/m² IV over 120 min 1 week prior to initiation of a course of radiation treatment. Maint: 250mg/m² over 60 min weekly for duration of radiation therapy. Max Infusion Rate: 5mL/min. Recurrent/Metastatic Squamous Cell Carcinoma of Head and Neck: Monotherapy: Initial: 400mg/m². Maint: 250mg/m² until disease progression or unacceptable toxicity. Mild-Moderate (Grade 1 or 2) Infusion Reactions: Reduce rate by 50%. Severe (Grade 3 or 4) Infusion Reactions: Discontinue. Development of Severe Acneform Rash: Delay infusion 1-2 weeks for first three occurrences. First Occurrence: If improvement seen, continue at 250mg/m². Second Occurrence: If improvement seen, reduce dose to 200mg/m². Third Occurrence: If improvement seen, reduce dose to 150mg/m². Fourth Occurrence/No improvement After Delaying Therapy: Discontinue.
**HOW SUPPLIED:** Inj: 2mg/mL [50mL]
**WARNINGS/PRECAUTIONS:** Infusion reactions reported; observe closely for 1 hr post-infusion. Dermatologic (eg, acneform rash, skin drying/fissuring,

inflammatory and infectious sequelae) or pulmonary toxicities may occur. Discontinue if interstitial lung disease is confirmed. Adjust dose in cases of severe acneform rash. Apply sunscreen and limit sun exposure. Caution with hypersensitivity to murine proteins. Potential for immunogenicity. Caution with radiation therapy and cisplatin therapy.

**ADVERSE REACTIONS:** Acneform rash, mucositis, asthenia/malaise, diarrhea, nausea, abdominal pain, vomiting, fever, constipation, infusion reactions, dermatologic toxicities, infection, headache, anorexia, dyspnea.

**PREGNANCY:** Category C, not for use in nursing.



## ERGOLOID MESYLATES RX

ergoloid mesylates (Various)

**THERAPEUTIC CLASS:** Ergot derivative dopamine agonist

**INDICATIONS:** Treatment of symptomatic decline in mental capacity of unknown etiology (eg, Alzheimer's dementia, multi-infarct dementia).

**DOSAGE:** *Adults:* Usual: 1mg tid.

**HOW SUPPLIED:** Tab: 1mg; Tab, Sublingual: 1mg

**CONTRAINDICATIONS:** Acute or chronic psychosis.

**WARNINGS/PRECAUTIONS:** Since symptoms are of unknown etiology, careful diagnosis should be attempted before prescribing.

**ADVERSE REACTIONS:** Transient nausea, gastric disturbances.

**PREGNANCY:** Safety in pregnancy and nursing is not known.

## ERTACZO RX

sertaconazole nitrate (Ortho Neutrogena)

**THERAPEUTIC CLASS:** Azole antifungal

**INDICATIONS:** Treatment of interdigital tinea pedis in immunocompetent patients caused by *Trichophyton rubrum*, *Trichophyton mentagrophytes*, and *Epidermophyton floccosum*.

**DOSAGE:** *Adults:* Apply bid to affected areas between toes and adjacent areas for 4 weeks. Re-evaluate if no clinical improvement after 2 weeks.
*Pediatrics:* ≥12 yrs: Apply bid to affected areas between toes and adjacent areas for 4 weeks. Re-evaluate if no clinical improvement after 2 weeks.

**HOW SUPPLIED:** Cre: 2% [30g]

**WARNINGS/PRECAUTIONS:** Not for ophthalmic, oral, or intravaginal use. Discontinue if irritation or sensitivity occurs.

**ADVERSE REACTIONS:** Contact dermatitis, dry skin, burning skin, application site reaction, skin tenderness.

**PREGNANCY:** Category C, caution in nursing.

## ERYC RX

erythromycin (Warner Chilcott)

**THERAPEUTIC CLASS:** Macrolide antibiotic

**INDICATIONS:** Mild-to-moderate upper and lower respiratory tract and skin and soft tissue infections, pertussis, diphtheria, erythrasma, intestinal amebiasis, acute pelvic inflammatory disease (PID) (*N. gonorrhea*), Listeria monocytogenes infections, primary syphilis in PCN allergy, Legionnaires' disease, chlamydial infections (eg, newborn conjunctivitis, urethral, endocervical, or rectal, etc), and nongonococcal urethritis. Prophylaxis of endocarditis or rheumatic fever in PCN allergy.

E

**DOSAGE:** *Adults:* Usual: 250mg q6h or 500mg q12h. Max: 4g/day. Treat strep infections for 10 days. Chlamydial Urogenital Infection During Pregnancy: 500mg qid for at least 7 days or 250mg qid for 14 days. Urethral/Endocervical/Rectal Chlamydial Infections: 500mg qid for 7 days. Primary Syphilis: 30-40g in divided doses for 10-15 days. Acute PID: 500mg (erythromycin lactobionate) IV q6h for 3 days, then 250mg PO q6h for 7 days. Streptococcal Infection Long-Term Prophylaxis of Rheumatic Fever: 250mg bid. Intestinal Amebiasis: 250mg qid for 10-14 days. Pertussis: 40-50mg/kg/day in divided doses for 5-14 days. Legionnaires' Disease: 1-4g/day in divided doses. Bacterial Endocarditis Prophylaxis: 1g 1 hr before procedure, then 500mg 6 hrs later.
*Pediatrics:* Usual: 30-50mg/kg/day in divided doses without food. Max: 4g/day. Severe Infections: Double dose up to 4g/day. Treat strep infections for 10 days. Intestinal Amebiasis: 30-50mg/kg/day in divided doses for 10-14 days. Bacterial Endocarditis Prophylaxis: 20mg/kg 1 hr before procedure, then 10mg/kg 6 hrs later.

**HOW SUPPLIED:** Cap, Delayed Release: 250mg

**CONTRAINDICATIONS:** Concomitant terfenadine or cisapride.

**WARNINGS/PRECAUTIONS:** Pseudomembranous colitis, hepatic dysfunction reported.

**ADVERSE REACTIONS:** Nausea, vomiting, abdominal pain, diarrhea, anorexia, abnormal LFTs, allergic reaction, superinfection (prolonged use).

**INTERACTIONS:** May increase levels of theophylline, digoxin, drugs metabolized by CYP450 (eg, carbamazepine, cyclosporine, phenytoin, tacrolimus, hexobarbital). Increases effects of oral anticoagulants and triazolam. Risk of acute ergot toxicity with ergotamine or dihydroergotamine. Avoid terfenadine and cisapride.

**PREGNANCY:** Category B, caution in nursing.

## ERYGEL — RX
erythromycin (Merz)

**THERAPEUTIC CLASS:** Macrolide antibiotic

**INDICATIONS:** Acne vulgaris.

**DOSAGE:** *Adults:* Apply a thin film qd-bid after skin is cleansed and patted dry. Discontinue if no improvement occurs after 6-8 weeks, or if condition worsens.

**HOW SUPPLIED:** Gel: 2% [30g, 60g]

**WARNINGS/PRECAUTIONS:** Avoid contact with eyes and all mucous membranes. Discontinue if overgrowth of antibiotic-resistant organisms occurs. Pseudomembranous colitis reported.

**ADVERSE REACTIONS:** Burning, peeling, dryness, itching, erythema, oiliness.

**INTERACTIONS:** Caution with other topical acne therapy; cumulative irritancy effect may occur with peeling, desquamating or abrasive agents;

**PREGNANCY:** Category B, caution in nursing.

## ERYPED — RX
erythromycin ethylsuccinate (Abbott)

**THERAPEUTIC CLASS:** Macrolide antibiotic

**INDICATIONS:** Treatment of mild to moderate upper and lower respiratory tract and skin and skin structure infections, listeriosis, pertussis, diphtheria, erythrasma, intestinal amebiasis, acute pelvic inflammatory disease (PID) (*N.gonorrhea*), primary syphilis in PCN allergy, Legionnaires' disease, chlamydial infections (eg, newborn conjunctivitis, urethral, endocervical, or rectal, etc.), and nongonococcal urethritis. Prophylaxis of endocarditis or rheumatic fever.

**DOSAGE:** *Adults:* Usual: 1600mg/day given q6h, q8h or q12h. Max: 4g/day. Treat strep infections for 10 days. Streptococcal Infection Prophylaxis with Rheumatic Heart Disease: 400mg bid. Urethritis (*C.trachomatis* or *U.urealyticum*): 800mg tid for 7 days. Primary Syphilis: 48-64g in divided doses over 10-15 days. Intestinal Amebiasis: 400mg qid for 10-14 days. Pertussis: 40-50mg/kg/day in divided doses for 5-14 days. Legionnaires' Disease: 1.6-4g/day in divided doses.
*Pediatrics:* Usual: 30-50mg/kg/day in divided doses q6h, q8h or q12h. Double dose for more severe infections. Treat strep infections for 10 days. Intestinal Amebiasis: 30-50mg/kg/day in divided doses for 10-14 days. Pertussis: 40-50mg/kg/day in divided doses for 5-14 days.



**HOW SUPPLIED:** Sus: 100mg/2.5mL [50mL], 200mg/5mL, 400mg/5mL [5mL, 100mL, 200mL]; Tab, Chewable: 200mg* *scored

**CONTRAINDICATIONS:** Concomitant terfenadine, astemizole, cisapride, pimozide.

**WARNINGS/PRECAUTIONS:** Pseudomembranous colitis, hepatic dysfunction reported. May aggravate myasthenia gravis.

**ADVERSE REACTIONS:** Nausea, vomiting, abdominal pain, diarrhea, anorexia, hepatic dysfunction, abnormal LFTs, allergic reactions, superinfection (prolonged use).

**INTERACTIONS:** Rhabdomyolysis reported with lovastatin. May increase levels of theophylline, digoxin, drugs metabolized by CYP450 (eg, carbamazepine, cyclosporine, tacrolimus, phenytoin, alfentanil, disopyramide, lovastatin, bromocriptine, valproate, etc). Increases effects of oral anticoagulants, triazolam, midazolam. Risk of acute ergot toxicity with ergotamine or dihydroergotamine. May potentiate sildenafil. Avoid terfenadine, astemizole, cisapride, pimozide.

**PREGNANCY:** Category B, caution in nursing.

## ERY-TAB RX

erythromycin (Abbott)

**THERAPEUTIC CLASS:** Macrolide antibiotic

**INDICATIONS:** Mild-to-moderate upper and lower respiratory tract and skin and skin structure infections, listeriosis, pertussis, diphtheria, erythrasma, intestinal amebiasis, acute pelvic inflammatory disease (PID) (*N.gonorrhea*), primary syphilis in PCN allergy, Legionnaires' disease, chlamydial infections (eg, newborn conjunctivitis urethral, endocervical, rectal, etc), and nongonococcal urethritis. Prophylaxis of rheumatic fever.

**DOSAGE:** *Adults:* Usual: 250mg qid, 333mg q8h or 500mg q12h without food. Max: 4g/day. Do not take bid when dose is >1g/day. Treat strep infections for 10 days. Chlamydial Urogenital Infection During Pregnancy: 500mg qid or 666mg q8h for 7 days, or 500mg q12h, 333mg q8h or 250mg qid for 14 days. Urethral/Endocervical/Rectal Chlamydial Infections and Nongonococcal Urethritis: 500mg qid or 666mg q8h for at least 7 days. Primary Syphilis: 30-40g in divided doses for 10-15 days. Acute PID: 500mg (erythromycin lactobionate) IV q6h for 3 days, then 500mg PO q12h or 333mg q8h for 7 days. Streptococcal Infection Long-Term Prophylaxis of Rheumatic Fever: 250mg bid. Intestinal Amebiasis: 500mg q12h, 333mg q8h or 250mg q6h for 10-14 days. Pertussis: 40-50mg/kg/day in divided doses for 5-14 days. Legionnaires' Disease: 1-4g/day in divided doses.
*Pediatrics:* Usual: 30-50mg/kg/day in divided doses without food. Max: 4g/day. Severe Infections: Double dose up to 4g/day. Treat strep infections for 10 days. Chlamydial Conjunctivitis of Newborns and Chlamydial Pneumonia in Infancy: 12.5mg/kg qid for 2 weeks and 3 weeks, respectively. Intestinal Amebiasis: 30-50mg/kg/day in divided doses for 10-14 days. Long-Term Prophylaxis of Rheumatic Fever: 250mg bid. Intestinal Amebiasis: 30-50mg/kg/day in divided doses for 10-14 days. Pertussis: 40-50mg/kg/day in divided doses for 5-14 days. Legionnaire's Disease: 1-4g/day in divided doses.

**HOW SUPPLIED:** Tab, Delayed Release: 250mg, 333mg, 500mg

**CONTRAINDICATIONS:** Concomitant terfenadine, astemizole, or cisapride.

**WARNINGS/PRECAUTIONS:** Pseudomembranous colitis, hepatic dysfunction reported. May aggravate myasthenia gravis. Erythromycin does not reach adequate concentrations in fetus to prevent congenital syphilis.

**ADVERSE REACTIONS:** Nausea, vomiting, abdominal pain, diarrhea, anorexia, abnormal LFTs, allergic reactions, superinfection (prolonged use).



**INTERACTIONS:** Rhabdomyolysis reported with lovastatin. May increase levels of theophylline, digoxin, drugs metabolized by CYP450 (eg, carbamazepine, cyclosporine, phenytoin, alfentanil, disopyramide, lovastatin, bromocriptine, valproate, etc). Increases effects of oral anticoagulants, triazolam, midazolam. Risk of acute ergot toxicity with ergotamine or dihydroergotamine. Avoid terfenadine, astemizole, or cisapride.

**PREGNANCY:** Category B, caution in nursing.

## ERYTHROCIN RX

erythromycin stearate (Abbott)

**THERAPEUTIC CLASS:** Macrolide antibiotic

**INDICATIONS:** Mild-to-moderate upper and lower respiratory tract, and skin and skin structure infections, listeriosis, pertussis, diphtheria, erythrasma, intestinal amebiasis, acute pelvic inflammatory disease (PID) (*N.gonorrhea*), primary syphilis in PCN allergy, Legionnaires' disease, chlamydial infections (eg, newborn conjunctivitis urethral, endocervical, or rectal, etc), and nongonococcal urethritis. Prophylaxis of rheumatic fever.

**DOSAGE:** *Adults:* Usual: 250mg q6h or 500mg q12h without food. Max: 4g/day. Treat strep infections for 10 days. Streptococcal Infection Prophylaxis of Rheumatic Fever: 250mg bid. Chlamydial Urogenital Infection During Pregnancy: 500mg qid for 7 days or 250mg qid for 14 days. Urethral/Endocervical/Rectal Chlamydial Infections and Nongonococcal Urethritis: 500mg qid for at least 7 days. Primary Syphilis: 30-40g in divided doses over 10-15 days. Acute PID: 500mg (erythromycin lactobionate) IV q6h for 3 days, then 500mg PO q12h for 7 days. Intestinal Amebiasis: 250mg qid for 10-14 days. Pertussis: 40-50mg/kg/day in divided doses for 5-14 days. Legionnaires' Disease: 1-4g/day in divided doses.
*Pediatrics:* Usual: 30-50mg/kg/day in divided doses without food. Severe Infections: Double dose up to 4g/day. Treat strep infections for 10 days. Streptococcal Infection Prophylaxis of Rheumatic Fever: 250mg bid. Chlamydial Conjunctivitis of Newborns/Chlamydial Pneumonia in Infancy: 12.5mg/kg qid for 2 weeks and 3 weeks, respectively. Intestinal Amebiasis: 30-50mg/kg/day in divided doses for 10-14 days. Pertussis: 40-50mg/kg/day in divided doses for 5-14 days.

**HOW SUPPLIED:** Tab: 250mg, 500mg

**WARNINGS/PRECAUTIONS:** Hepatic dysfunction, pseudomembranous colitis reported.

**ADVERSE REACTIONS:** Nausea, vomiting, abdominal pain, diarrhea, anorexia, abnormal LFTs, superinfection (prolonged use).

**INTERACTIONS:** Rhabdomyolysis reported with lovastatin. May increase levels of theophylline, digoxin, drugs metabolized by CYP450 (eg, carbamazepine, cyclosporine, phenytoin, etc). Increases effects of oral anticoagulants, triazolam. Risk of acute ergot toxicity with ergotamine or dihydroergotamine.

**PREGNANCY:** Category B, caution in nursing.

## ERYTHROMYCIN

erythromycin (Various) RX

**THERAPEUTIC CLASS:** Macrolide antibiotic

**INDICATIONS:** Mild to moderate upper and lower respiratory tract and skin and skin structure infections, listeriosis, pertussis, diphtheria, erythrasma, intestinal amebiasis, primary syphilis in PCN allergy, Legionnaires' disease, chlamydial infections (eg, newborn conjunctivitis urethral, endocervical, rectal, etc), and nongonococcal urethritis. Prophylaxis of endocarditis or rheumatic fever.

**DOSAGE:** *Adults:* Usual: 250mg q6h or 500mg q12h without food. Max: 4g/day. Treat strep infections for 10 days. Streptococcal Infection Prophylaxis of Rheumatic Fever: 250mg bid. Chlamydial Urogenital Infection During Pregnancy: 500mg qid for 7 days or 250mg qid for 14 days. Urethral/Endocervical/Rectal Chlamydial Infections: 500mg qid for at least 7 days. Primary Syphilis: 30-40g in divided doses over 10-15 days. Intestinal Amebiasis: 250mg q6h for 10-14 days. Pertussis: 40-50mg/kg/day in divided doses for 5-14 days. Legionnaires' Disease: 1-4g/day in divided doses. Bacterial Endocarditis Prophylaxis: 1g 1 hr before procedure, then 500mg 6 hrs later.
*Pediatrics:* Usual: 30-50mg/kg/day in divided doses without food. Severe Infections: Double dose up to 4g/day. Treat strep infections for 10 days. Streptococcal Infection Prophylaxis of Rheumatic Fever: 250mg bid. Intestinal Amebiasis: 30-50mg/kg/day in divided doses for 10-14 days. Pertussis: 40-50mg/kg/day in divided doses for 5-14 days. Bacterial Endocarditis Prophylaxis: 20mg/kg 1 hr before procedure, then 10mg/kg 6 hrs later.

**HOW SUPPLIED:** Cap, Delayed Release: 250mg

**WARNINGS/PRECAUTIONS:** Caution with hepatic dysfunction.

**ADVERSE REACTIONS:** Nausea, vomiting, abdominal pain, diarrhea, anorexia, hepatic dysfunction, abnormal LFTs, superinfection (prolonged use).

**INTERACTIONS:** Rhabdomyolysis reported with lovastatin. May increase levels of theophylline, digoxin, drugs metabolized by CYP450 (eg, carbamazepine, cyclosporine, phenytoin, etc). Increases effects of oral anticoagulants, triazolam. Risk of acute ergot toxicity with ergotamine or dihydroergotamine. Extreme caution with terfenadine.

**PREGNANCY:** Category B, caution in nursing.

## ERYTHROMYCIN BASE

erythromycin (Various) RX

**THERAPEUTIC CLASS:** Macrolide antibiotic

**INDICATIONS:** Mild to moderate upper and lower respiratory tract and skin and skin structure infections, listeriosis, pertussis, diphtheria, erythrasma, intestinal amebiasis, acute pelvic inflammatory disease (PID) (*N.gonorrhea*), primary syphilis in PCN allergy, Legionnaires' disease, chlamydial infections (eg, newborn conjunctivitis urethral, endocervical, rectal, etc), and nongonococcal urethritis. Prophylaxis of rheumatic fever.

**DOSAGE:** *Adults:* Usual: 250mg q6h or 500mg q12h without food. Max: 4g/day. Treat strep infections for 10 days. Streptococcal Infection Prophylaxis of Rheumatic Fever: 250mg bid. Chlamydial Urogenital Infection During Pregnancy: 500mg qid for 7 days or 250mg qid for 14 days. Urethral/Endocervical/Rectal Chlamydial Infections and Nongonococcal Urethritis: 500mg qid for at least 7 days. Primary Syphilis: 30-40g in divided doses over 10-15 days. Acute PID: 500mg (erythromycin lactobionate) IV q6h for 3 days, then 500mg PO q12h for 7 days. Intestinal Amebiasis: 250mg qid for 10-14 days. Pertussis: 40-50mg/kg/day in divided doses for 5-14 days. Legionnaires' Disease: 1-4g/day in divided doses.
*Pediatrics:* Usual: 30-50mg/kg/day in divided doses without food. Severe Infections: Double dose up to 4g/day. Treat strep infections for 10 days.

Streptococcal Infection Prophylaxis of Rheumatic Fever: 250mg bid. Chlamydial Conjunctivitis of Newborns and Chlamydial Pneumonia in Infancy: 12.5mg/kg qid for 2 weeks and 3 weeks, respectively. Intestinal Amebiasis: 30-50mg/kg/day in divided doses for 10-14 days. Pertussis: 40-50mg/kg/day in divided doses for 5-14 days.

**HOW SUPPLIED:** Tab: 250mg

**CONTRAINDICATIONS:** Concomitant terfenadine, astemizole, or cisapride.

**WARNINGS/PRECAUTIONS:** Pseudomembranous colitis, hepatic dysfunction reported. May aggravate myasthenia gravis.

E

**ADVERSE REACTIONS:** Nausea, vomiting, abdominal pain, diarrhea, anorexia, abnormal LFTs, allergic reactions, superinfection (prolonged use).

**INTERACTIONS:** Rhabdomyolysis reported with lovastatin. May increase levels of theophylline, digoxin, drugs metabolized by CYP450 (eg, carbamazepine, cyclosporine, phenytoin, etc). Increases effects of oral anticoagulants, triazolam. Risk of acute ergot toxicity with ergotamine or dihydroergotamine. Extreme caution with terfenadine.

**PREGNANCY:** Category B, caution in nursing.

## ERYTHROMYCIN OPHTHALMIC RX

erythromycin (Various)

**THERAPEUTIC CLASS:** Macrolide

**INDICATIONS:** Superficial ocular infections of the conjunctiva and/or cornea. Prophylaxis of ophthalmia neonatorum due to N.gonorrhoeae or C.trachomatis.

**DOSAGE:** *Adults:* Superficial Ocular Infections: Apply 1 cm to eye up to 6 times/day, depending on severity. Do not flush ointment from eye. *Pediatrics:* Superficial Ocular Infections: Apply 1 cm to eye up to 6 times/day, depending on severity. Neonatal Gonococcal or Chlamydial Ophthalmia Prophylaxis: Apply 1 cm into lower conjunctival sac. Do not flush ointment from eye.

**HOW SUPPLIED:** Oint: 5mg/g [1g, 3.5g]

**ADVERSE REACTIONS:** Minor ocular irritations, redness, hypersensitivity reactions, superinfection (prolonged use).

**PREGNANCY:** Category B, caution in nursing.

## ERYTHROMYCIN SWAB RX

erythromycin (Various)

**THERAPEUTIC CLASS:** Macrolide antibiotic

**INDICATIONS:** Topical treatment of acne vulgaris.

**DOSAGE:** *Adults:* Wash and dry area. Rub over area bid.

**HOW SUPPLIED:** Swab: 2% [60s]

**WARNINGS/PRECAUTIONS:** Topical use only. Superinfection may occur. Avoid eyes, nose, mouth, and mucous membranes.

**ADVERSE REACTIONS:** Peeling, dryness, itching, erythema, oiliness.

**INTERACTIONS:** Additive irritation with other topical acne agents, especially abrasive or desquamating agents.

**PREGNANCY:** Category B, caution in nursing.

## ESCLIM
estradiol (Women First)

RX

**Estrogens increase risk of endometrial cancer in postmenopausal women. Avoid during pregnancy.**

**THERAPEUTIC CLASS:** Estrogen

**INDICATIONS:** Treatment of moderate to severe vasomotor symptoms associated with menopause and/or vulvar/vaginal atrophy. Treatment of hypoestrogenism due to hypogonadism, castration, or primary ovarian failure.

**DOSAGE:** *Adults:* Initial: 0.025mg twice weekly (q3-4 days). Titrate: Increase/decrease dose depending upon clinical response. Apply to clean, dry area of skin on buttocks, femoral triangle (upper inner thigh), or upper arm; avoid breasts and waistline. Rotate sites; allow 1 week between same site. Discontinue or taper at 3-6 month intervals. Wait 1 week after withdrawal of oral therapy before initiating therapy. Give continuously without intact uterus and cyclically (3 weeks on, 1 week off) with intact uterus.

**HOW SUPPLIED:** Patch: 0.025mg/24 hrs, 0.0375mg/24hrs, 0.05mg/24 hrs, 0.075mg/24 hrs, 0.1mg/24 hrs [8[s]]

**CONTRAINDICATIONS:** Pregnancy, undiagnosed abnormal genital bleeding, breast cancer except in appropriately selected patients being treated for metastatic disease, estrogen-dependent neoplasia, thrombophlebitis, thromboembolic disorders.

**WARNINGS/PRECAUTIONS:** Risk of gallbladder disease, breast and endometrial cancer, elevated BP. Possible risk of cardiovascular disease. Caution with liver dysfunction, asthma, epilepsy, migraine, and cardiac or renal dysfunction. Increase in HDL, triglycerides, thyroid binding globulin. Acceleration of PT, PTT. Impaired glucose tolerance. Consider adding progestin in patient with intact uterus. Risk of fetal congenital reproductive tract disorder, hypercalcemia with breast cancer and bone metastases, hypercoagulability effects. Uterine bleeding and mastodynia reported.

**ADVERSE REACTIONS:** Breast pain, headache, infection, anxiety, emotional lability, pruritus, abdominal pain, monilia vagina, nausea, sinusitis, asthenia, diarrhea, leukorrhea.

**PREGNANCY:** Category X, caution in nursing.

## ESGIC
caffeine - butalbital - acetaminophen (Forest)

RX

**THERAPEUTIC CLASS:** Barbiturate/analgesic

**INDICATIONS:** Tension or muscle contraction headaches.

**DOSAGE:** *Adults:* 1-2 caps/tabs q4h prn. Max: 6 caps/tabs/day.
*Pediatrics:* >12 yrs: 1-2 caps/tabs q4h prn. Max: 6 caps/tabs/day.

**HOW SUPPLIED:** Cap/Tab: (Butalbital-APAP-Caffeine) 50mg-325mg-40mg*
*scored

**CONTRAINDICATIONS:** Porphyria.

**WARNINGS/PRECAUTIONS:** May be habit-forming; potential for abuse. Not for long-term use. Caution in elderly, debilitated, severe renal or hepatic impairment, acute abdominal conditions, suicidal tendencies, history of drug abuse.

**ADVERSE REACTIONS:** Drowsiness, lightheadedness, dizziness, sedation, shortness of breath, nausea, vomiting, abdominal pain, intoxicated feeling.

**INTERACTIONS:** Enhanced CNS effects with MAOIs. May enhance CNS depressant effects of other narcotic analgesics, alcohol, general anesthetics, tranquilizers, sedative hypnotics, or other CNS depressants.

**PREGNANCY:** Category C, not for use in nursing.

## ESGIC-PLUS RX

caffeine - butalbital - acetaminophen (Forest)

**THERAPEUTIC CLASS:** Barbiturate/analgesic

**INDICATIONS:** Tension or muscle contraction headaches.

**DOSAGE:** *Adults:* 1 cap/tab q4h prn. Max: 6 caps/tabs/day.
*Pediatrics:* >12 yrs: 1 cap/tab q4h prn. Max: 6 caps/tabs/day.



**HOW SUPPLIED:** Cap/Tab: (Butalbital-APAP-Caffeine) 50mg-500mg-40mg* *scored

**CONTRAINDICATIONS:** Porphyria.

**WARNINGS/PRECAUTIONS:** May be habit-forming; potential for abuse. Not for long-term use. Caution in elderly, debilitated, severe renal or hepatic impairment, acute abdominal conditions, suicidal tendencies, history of drug abuse.

**ADVERSE REACTIONS:** Drowsiness, lightheadedness, dizziness, sedation, shortness of breath, nausea, vomiting, abdominal pain, intoxicated feeling.

**INTERACTIONS:** Enhanced CNS effects with MAOIs. May enhance CNS depressant effects of other narcotic analgesics, alcohol, general anesthetics, tranquilizers, sedative hypnotics, or other CNS depressants.

**PREGNANCY:** Category C, not for use in nursing.

## ESKALITH RX

lithium carbonate (GlaxoSmithKline)

**Lithium toxicity is related to serum levels, and can occur at doses close to therapeutic levels.**

**OTHER BRAND NAMES:** Eskalith CR (GlaxoSmithKline)

**THERAPEUTIC CLASS:** Antimanic agents

**INDICATIONS:** Treatment of manic episodes of manic-depressive illness.

**DOSAGE:** *Adults:* (Cap) 300mg tid-qid. (Tab, Extended-Release) 450mg q12h. Monitor every 1-2 weeks and adjust dose if needed. When stable, monitor every 2 months to achieve levels of 0.6-1.2mEq/L. Maint: 900-1200mg/day. Acute Mania: 1800mg/day in divided doses. Monitor levels twice weekly to achieve 1-1.5mEq/L. When switching to extended-release tabs, give same total daily dose when possible.
*Pediatrics:* >12 yrs: (Cap) 300mg tid-qid. (Tab, Extended-Release) 450mg q12h. Monitor every 1-2 weeks and adjust dose if needed. When stable, monitor every 2 months to achieve levels of 0.6-1.2 mEq/L. Maint: 900-1200mg/day. Acute Mania: 1800mg/day in divided doses. Monitor levels twice weekly to achieve 1-1.5mEq/L. When switching to extended-release tabs, give same total daily dose when possible.

**HOW SUPPLIED:** Cap: (Eskalith) 300mg; Tab, Extended Release: (Eskalith CR) 450mg* *scored

**WARNINGS/PRECAUTIONS:** Avoid with significant renal or cardiovascular disease, severe debilitation, dehydration, or sodium depletion. Risk of encephalopathic syndrome (eg, weakness, lethargy, fever, tremulousness, confusion, EPS); discontinue therapy. Maintain normal diet, adequate salt/fluid intake. Reduce dose or discontinue with sweating, diarrhea, infection with elevated temperatures. Caution with hypothyroidism; may need supplemental therapy. Chronic therapy associated with diminution of renal concentrating ability, glomerular and interstitial fibrosis, and nephron atrophy.

**ADVERSE REACTIONS:** Fine hand tremor, polyuria, mild thirst, nausea, general discomfort, diarrhea, vomiting, drowsiness, muscular weakness.

**INTERACTIONS:** Increased risk of neurotoxicity with calcium channel blockers. Increased risk of toxicity with diuretics, metronidazole. Increased plasma levels with indomethacin, piroxicam, other NSAIDs, COX-2 inhibitors, ACE inhibitors, angiotensin II receptor antagonists. Caution with SSRIs. Decreased levels with acetazolamide, urea, xanthine agents, alkalinizing agents. Interacts with methyldopa, phenytoin, carbamazepine. May prolong effects of neuromuscular blockers.

**PREGNANCY:** Safety in pregnancy not known, not for use in nursing.

## ESTRACE
estradiol (Warner Chilcott)

RX



**Estrogens increase risk of endometrial cancer in postmenopausal women. Avoid during pregnancy.**

**THERAPEUTIC CLASS:** Estrogen

**INDICATIONS:** (Cre/Tab) Treatment of vulval and vaginal atrophy. (Tab) Treatment of moderate to severe vasomotor symptoms associated with menopause. Treatment of hypoestrogenism due to hypogonadism, castration, or primary ovarian failure. Palliative treatment of metastatic breast cancer and advanced androgen-dependent prostate carcinoma. Prevention of osteoporosis.

**DOSAGE:** *Adults:* (Cre) Vulval/Vaginal Atrophy: Initial: 2-4g/day for 1-2 weeks, then decrease to 1-2g/day for 1-2 weeks. Maint: 1g, 1-3x/week. Discontinue or taper at 3-6 month intervals. (Tab) Vasomotor Symptoms/Vulval/Vaginal Atrophy: Initial: 1-2mg/day (3 weeks on, 1 week off). Maint: Minimum effective dose. Discontinue or taper at 3-6 month intervals. Hypoestrogenism: 1-2mg/day. Maint: Minimum effective dose. Metastatic Breast Cancer: 10mg tid for at least 3 months. Prostate Carcinoma: 1-2mg tid. Osteoporosis Prevention: 0.5mg qd cyclically (23 days on and 5 days off).

**HOW SUPPLIED:** Cre, Vaginal: 0.1mg/g [12g, 42.5g]; Tab: 0.5mg*, 1mg*, 2mg* *scored

**CONTRAINDICATIONS:** Pregnancy, undiagnosed abnormal genital bleeding, breast cancer unless being treated for metastatic disease, estrogen-dependent neoplasia, thrombophlebitis, or thromboembolic disorders.

**WARNINGS/PRECAUTIONS:** Risk of gallbladder disease, cardiovascular disease, endometrial and breast carcinoma, fetal congenital reproductive tract disorder, elevated BP, and hypercalcemia with breast cancer and bone metastases. Caution in liver dysfunction, asthma, epilepsy, migraine, and cardiac or renal dysfunction. Increase in HDL, triglycerides, thyroid binding globulin. Acceleration of PT, PTT. Hypercoagulability effects. Impaired glucose tolerance. Consider adding progestin in patient with intact uterus.

**ADVERSE REACTIONS:** Altered vaginal bleeding, vaginal candidiasis, breast tenderness/enlargement, GI effects, melasma, CNS effects, weight changes, edema, altered libido.

**PREGNANCY:** Category X, caution in nursing.

## ESTRADERM
estradiol (Novartis)

RX

**Estrogens increase the risk of endometrial cancer. Estrogens, with or without progestins, should not be used for the prevention of cardiovascular disease or dementia. Increased risks of MI, stroke, invasive breast cancer, PE, and DVT in postmenopausal women (50-79 yrs of age) reported. Increased risk of developing probable dementia in postmenopausal women ≥65 yrs of age reported.**

**THERAPEUTIC CLASS:** Estrogen

**INDICATIONS:** Treatment of moderate-to-severe vasomotor symptoms and/or vulvar/vaginal atrophy associated with menopause. Treatment of hypoestrogenism due to hypogonadism, castration, or primary ovarian failure. Prevention of postmenopausal osteoporosis.

**DOSAGE:** *Adults:* Apply to clean, dry area on trunk of body. Do not apply to breast or waistline. Replace twice weekly. Rotate application sites. May give continuously without intact uterus. May give cyclically (3 weeks on, 1 week off) with intact uterus. Vasomotor Symptoms/Vulvar/Vaginal Atrophy: Initial: Apply 0.05mg/day twice weekly. Discontinue/Taper at 3-6 month intervals. Start 1 week after discontinuing oral hormone therapy. Osteoporosis Prevention: Initial: 0.05mg/day.

**HOW SUPPLIED:** Patch: 0.05mg/24 hrs, 0.1mg/24 hrs [$8^s$, $24^s$]



**CONTRAINDICATIONS:** Pregnancy, undiagnosed abnormal genital bleeding, breast cancer unless being treated for metastatic disease, estrogen-dependent neoplasia, DVT/PE, active or recent (eg, within past year) arterial thromboembolic disease (eg, stroke, MI), liver dysfunction or disease.

**WARNINGS/PRECAUTIONS:** May increase risk of cardiovascular events (eg, MI, stroke), venous thrombosis, and PE; d/c immediately if any of these events occur or are suspected. May increase risk of breast/endometrial cancer, and gallbladder disease. May lead to severe hypercalcemia with breast cancer and bone metastases; monitor and d/c if hypercalcemia occurs. Retinal vascular thrombosis reported; monitor and d/c if papilledema or retinal vascular lesions occur. Consider addition of a progestin if no hysterectomy. May elevate BP; monitor at regular intervals. May cause elevations of plasma triglycerides with pre-existing hypertriglyceridemia. Caution with history of cholestatic jaundice associated with past estrogen use or with pregnancy; d/c with recurrence. May lead to increased thyroid-binding globulin levels; monitor thyroid function. May cause fluid retention; caution with cardiac/renal dysfunction. Caution with severe hypocalcemia. May increase risk of ovarian cancer. May exacerbate endometriosis, asthma, DM, epilepsy, migraine, porphyria, SLE, and hepatic hemangiomas; use with caution.

**ADVERSE REACTIONS:** Redness/irritation at application site, altered vaginal bleeding, vaginal candidiasis, breast tenderness/enlargement, GI effects, melasma, CNS effects, retinal vascular thrombosis, weight changes, edema, altered libido.

**INTERACTIONS:** CYP3A4 inducers (eg, St. John's wort, phenobarbital, carbamazepine, rifampin) may decrease levels resulting in decreased therapeutic effects and/or changes in uterine bleeding profile. CYP3A4 inhibitors (eg, erythromycin, clarithromycin, ketoconazole, itraconazole, ritonavir, grapefruit juice) may increase levels and result in side effects.

**PREGNANCY:** Category X, caution in nursing.

## ESTRASORB RX

estradiol (Esprit)

**Estrogens increase the risk of endometrial cancer. Estrogens, with or without progestins, should not be used for the prevention of cardiovascular disease or dementia. Increased risks of MI, stroke, invasive breast cancer, PE, and DVT in postmenopausal women (50-79 yrs of age) reported. Increased risk of developing probable dementia in postmenopausal women ≥65 yrs of age reported.**

**THERAPEUTIC CLASS:** Estrogen

**INDICATIONS:** Treatment of moderate to severe vasomotor symptoms associated with menopause.

**DOSAGE:** *Adults:* Apply 2 pouches (0.05mg/day) qAM. Apply one pouch to each leg from the upper thigh to the calf. Rub in for 3 minutes.

**HOW SUPPLIED:** Emulsion, Topical: 2.5mg/g

**CONTRAINDICATIONS:** Undiagnosed abnormal genital bleeding, breast cancer (unless being treated for metastatic disease), estrogen-dependent neoplasia, DVT/PE, active or recent (eg, within 1 year) arterial thromboembolic disease (eg, stroke, MI), liver dysfunction or disease, pregnancy.

**WARNINGS/PRECAUTIONS:** Limit use to the shortest duration consistent with goals and risks; re-evaluate periodically. Increased risk of cardiovascular events (eg, MI, stroke, venous thromboembolism, pulmonary embolism), gallbladder disease, breast and endometrial cancer. D/C 4-6 weeks before surgery associated with an increased risk of thromboembolism or during prolonged immobilization. Possible increased risk of ovarian cancer. May lead to severe hypercalcemia in patients with breast cancer and bone metastases. Consider adding progestin in patients with intact uterus to avoid endometrial hyperplasia. Increased thyroid-binding globulin levels (may need higher doses of thyroid hormone). May cause fluid retention; caution in cardiac or renal dysfunction. Retinal vascular thrombosis and elevated BP reported. May lead to severe hypercalcemia with breast cancer and bone metastases; monitor and d/c if hypercalcemia occurs. May exacerbate endometriosis, asthma, diabetes mellitus, epilepsy, migraine, porphyria, SLE, or hepatic hemangiomas; use with caution. Avoid use in close proximity to sunscreen application; may increase absorption. Potential for estradiol transfer through physical contact; wash application site 8 hours post-application. May cause elevations of plasma triglycerides with pre-existing hypertriglyceridemia. Caution with history of cholestatic jaundice associated with past estrogen use or with pregnancy; d/c with recurrence.

**ADVERSE REACTIONS:** Headache, infection, sinusitis, pruritus, breast pain, endometrial disorder.

**INTERACTIONS:** CYP3A4 inducers (eg, St. John's wort, phenobarbital, carbamazepine, rifampin) may decrease levels which may decrease therapeutic effects and/or change uterine bleeding profile. CYP3A4 inhibitors (eg, erythromycin, clarithromycin, ketoconazole, itraconazole, ritonavir, grapefruit juice) may increase levels which may result in side effects.

**PREGNANCY:** Contraindicated in pregnancy, caution in nursing.

## ESTRATEST

methyltestosterone - esterified estrogens (Solvay)

RX

**Estrogens increase risk of endometrial cancer in postmenopausal women. Avoid during pregnancy. Estrogens, with or without progestins, should not be used for the prevention of cardiovascular disease. Increased risks of MI, stroke, invasive breast cancer, PE, and DVT in postmenopausal women reported.**

**OTHER BRAND NAMES:** Estratest H.S. (Solvay)

**THERAPEUTIC CLASS:** Estrogen/androgen combination

**INDICATIONS:** Treatment of moderate-severe vasomotor symptoms associated with menopause.

**DOSAGE:** *Adults:* Vasomotor Symptoms: 0.625-1.25mg or 1.25-2.5mg qd cyclically (3 weeks on, 1 week off). Discontinue/taper at 3-6 month intervals.

**HOW SUPPLIED:** (Esterified Estrogens-Methyltestosterone) Tab: (Estratest HS) 0.625-1.25mg, (Estratest) 1.25-2.5mg

**CONTRAINDICATIONS:** Pregnancy, nursing, severe liver damage, undiagnosed abnormal genital bleeding, breast cancer except in selected patients treated for metastatic disease, estrogen-dependent neoplasia, and thrombophlebitis or thromboembolic disease (active disease or past history associated with estrogen use, except when used in treatment of breast malignancy).

**WARNINGS/PRECAUTIONS:** Risk of gallbladder disease, endometrial carcinoma, thromboembolic disease, hepatic dysfunction/adenoma/neoplasm, peliosis hepatis, elevated BP, impaired glucose tolerance, hypercalcemia with breast cancer and bone metastases. Caution with metabolic bone disease associated with hypercalcemia or renal insufficiency. May increase size of pre-existing uterine leiomyomata. Caution in liver dysfunction, family history of breast cancer, breast nodules, fibrocystic disease, abnormal mammograms, diabetes, asthma, epilepsy, migraine, depression, and cardiac or renal dysfunction. D/C if cholestatic hepatitis And/or jaundice occurs, or if LFTs are abnormal. D/C 4 weeks prior to surgery if prolonged immobilization required. Increased risk of jaundice with history of jaundice during pregnancy. May effect epiphyseal closure; caution in young patients. D/C if virilization occurs. Increase in triglycerides, thyroid binding globulin, PT.

**ADVERSE REACTIONS:** Breakthrough bleeding, amenorrhea, virilization, inhibition of gonadotropin secretion, breast tenderness and enlargement, nausea, hirsutism, abdominal cramps, bloating, altered libido, cholestatic jaundice, weight gain, edema.

**INTERACTIONS:** May decrease insulin and anticoagulant requirements. May increase levels of oxyphenbutazone.

**PREGNANCY:** Category X, contraindicated in nursing.



## ESTRING

RX

estradiol (Pharmacia & Upjohn)

**Estrogens increase risk of endometrial cancer in postmenopausal women. Avoid during pregnancy.**

**THERAPEUTIC CLASS:** Estrogen

**INDICATIONS:** Treatment of urogenital symptoms associated with postmenopausal atrophy of vagina or lower urinary tract.

**DOSAGE:** *Adults:* Insert ring deeply into upper 1/3 of vaginal vault. Remove and replace after 90 days. Reassess at 3 or 6 month intervals.

**HOW SUPPLIED:** Vaginal Ring: 0.0075mg/24 hrs

**CONTRAINDICATIONS:** Pregnancy, undiagnosed abnormal vaginal bleeding, breast cancer, estrogen-dependent carcinoma.

**WARNINGS/PRECAUTIONS:** Breast cancer, congenital lesions with malignant potential, gallbladder or cardiovascular disease, elevated BP, and hypercalcemia may occur. Abnormal uterine bleeding, mastodynia reported. Caution with hepatic impairment, vaginal stenosis, narrow vagina, prolapse, or vaginal infections. Expulsions from vagina reported. Hypercoagulation, hyperlipidemia, and fluid retention may occur.

**ADVERSE REACTIONS:** Headache, leukorrhea, back pain, genital moniliasis, sinusitis, vaginitis, vaginal discomfort, vaginal hemorrhage, arthralgia, insomnia, abdominal pain.

**INTERACTIONS:** Remove during treatment with other vaginally administered agents.

**PREGNANCY:** Category X, not for use in nursing.

## ESTROGEL

RX

estradiol (Solvay)

**Estrogens increase the risk of endometrial cancer. Estrogens, with or without progestins, should not be used for the prevention of cardiovascular disease. Increased risks of MI, stroke, invasive breast cancer, PE, and DVT in postmenopausal women reported.**

**THERAPEUTIC CLASS:** Estrogen

**INDICATIONS:** Moderate to severe vasomotor symptoms and/or vulvar/vaginal atrophy associated with menopause.

**DOSAGE:** *Adults:* Apply one compression (1.25g) to one arm from wrist to shoulder once daily.

**HOW SUPPLIED:** Gel: 0.06% (1.25g (0.75mg estradiol) of gel per compression) [93g]

**CONTRAINDICATIONS:** Undiagnosed abnormal genital bleeding, breast cancer, estrogen-dependent neoplasia, DVT or PE, active or recent (within 1 year) arterial thromboembolic disease (eg, stroke, MI), liver dysfunction or disease, pregnancy.

**WARNINGS/PRECAUTIONS:** May increase risk of cardiovascular events (eg, MI, stroke), venous thrombosis, and PE; d/c immediately if any of these events occur or are suspected. May increase risk of breast/endometrial cancer, and gallbladder disease. May lead to severe hypercalcemia with breast cancer and bone metastases; monitor and d/c if hypercalcemia occurs. Retinal vascular thrombosis reported; monitor and d/c if papilledema or retinal vascular lesions occur. Consider addition of a progestin if no hysterectomy. May elevate BP; monitor at regular intervals. May cause elevations of plasma triglycerides with pre-existing hypertriglyceridemia. Caution with history of cholestatic jaundice associated with past estrogen use or with pregnancy; d/c with recurrence. May lead to increased thyroid-binding globulin levels; monitor thyroid function. May cause fluid retention; caution with cardiac/renal dysfunction. Caution with severe hypocalcemia. May increase risk of ovarian cancer. May exacerbate endometriosis, asthma, DM, epilepsy, migraine, porphyria, SLE, and hepatic hemangiomas; use with caution. Alcohol-based gels are flammable; avoid fire, flame, or smoking until the gel dried.

**ADVERSE REACTIONS:** Headache, infection, breast pain, vaginitis, abdominal pain, rash, nausea, pruritus, diarrhea.

**INTERACTIONS:** CYP3A4 inducers (eg, St. John's wort, phenobarbital, carbamazepine, rifampin) may decrease levels which may decrease therapeutic effects and/or change uterine bleeding profile. CYP3A4 inhibitors (eg, erythromycin, clarithromycin, ketoconazole, itraconazole, ritonavir, grapefruit juice) may increase levels which may result in side effects. May require higher doses of thyroid hormone.

**PREGNANCY:** Contraindicated in pregnancy, caution in nursing.

## ESTROSTEP FE — RX

ethinyl estradiol - norethindrone acetate (Warner Chilcott)

**THERAPEUTIC CLASS:** Estrogen/progestogen combination

**INDICATIONS:** Prevention of pregnancy. Treatment of acne vulgaris in females >15 yrs who want contraception (for at least 6 months), have achieved menarche and are unresponsive to topical acne agents.

**DOSAGE:** *Adults:* Contraception/Acne: 1 tab qd for 28 days, then repeat. Start 1st Sunday after menses begin or the 1st day of menses.
*Pediatrics:* >15 yrs: Contraception (Postpubertal Adolescents)/Acne: 1 tab qd for 28 days, then repeat. Start 1st Sunday after menses begin or the 1st day of menses.

**HOW SUPPLIED:** Tab: (Ethinyl Estradiol-Norethindrone) 0.035mg-1mg, 0.030mg-1mg, 0.020mg-1mg and 75mg ferrous fumarate

**CONTRAINDICATIONS:** Thrombophlebitis, history of DVT, active or history of thromboembolic disorders, pregnancy, cerebrovascular disease, CAD, undiagnosed abnormal genital bleeding, cholestatic jaundice of pregnancy, jaundice with prior pill use, hepatic adenoma or carcinoma, breast carcinoma, endometrium or other estrogen-dependent neoplasia.

**WARNINGS/PRECAUTIONS:** Cigarette smoking increases risk of serious cardiovascular side effects. This risk increases with age (especially >35 yrs) and heavy smoking. Increased risk of MI, vascular disease, thromboembolism, stroke, and gallbladder disease. Retinal thrombosis, hepatic neoplasia reported. May cause glucose intolerance. May increase BP, elevate LDL levels or cause other lipid changes, fluid retention, breakthrough bleeding, and spotting. May cause or exacerbate migraine. May develop visual changes with contact lens. Increased risk of MI with HTN, hyperlipidemia, obesity, and diabetes. D/C if jaundice, significant depression or ophthalmic irregularities develop. Perform annual physical exam. Use before menarche is not indicated. May affect certain endocrine, LFTs and blood components.

**ADVERSE REACTIONS:** Nausea, vomiting, breakthrough bleeding, spotting, amenorrhea, migraine, depression, vaginal candidiasis, edema, weight changes.

**INTERACTIONS:** Reduced effects, increased breakthrough bleeding, and menstrual irregularities with rifampin, barbiturates, phenylbutazone, phenytoin, carbamazepine, St. John's wort, and possibly with griseofulvin, ampicillin, and tetracyclines. Increased plasma levels with atorvastatin. Ascorbic acid and APAP may increase plasma levels. Decreased plasma levels of APAP. Increased clearance of temazepam, salicylic acid, morphine, and clofibric acid. Increased plasma levels of cyclosporine, prednisolone, and theophylline.

**PREGNANCY:** Category X, not for use in nursing.



## ETODOLAC

RX

etodolac (Various)

**NSAIDs may cause an increased risk of serious cardiovascular thrombotic events, MI, stroke and serious GI adverse events including bleeding, ulceration, and perforation of the stomach or intestines. Contraindicated for the treatment of peri-operative pain in the setting of coronary artery bypass graft (CABG) surgery.**

**THERAPEUTIC CLASS:** NSAID (pyranocarboxylic acid derivative)

**INDICATIONS:** Management of osteoarthritis (OA), rheumatoid arthritis (RA), and pain.

**DOSAGE:** *Adults:* Acute Pain: Usual: 200-400mg q6-8h. Max: 1200mg/day. OA/RA: Usual: 300mg bid-tid, or 400-500mg bid. Max: 1200mg/day.

**HOW SUPPLIED:** Cap: 200mg, 300mg

**CONTRAINDICATIONS:** ASA or other NSAID allergy that precipitates asthma, urticaria or other allergic type reactions. Treatment of peri-operative pain in the setting of CABG surgery.

**WARNINGS/PRECAUTIONS:** May lead to onset of new HTN or worsening of pre-existing HTN; monitor BP closely. Fluid retention and edema reported; caution with fluid retention or heart failure. Renal papillary necrosis and other renal injury reported after long-term use. Not recommended for use with advanced renal disease; if therapy must be initiated, monitor renal function. Anaphylactoid reactions may occur. May cause serious skin adverse events (eg, exfoliative dermatitis, Stevens-Johnson syndrome, and toxic epidermal necrolysis). Avoid in late pregnancy; may cause premature closure of ductus arteriosis. May cause elevations of LFTs; d/c if liver disease develops or systemic manifestations occur. Caution in elderly. Anemia may occur; with long-term use, monitor Hgb/Hct if signs or symptoms of anemia develop. May inhibit platelet aggregation and prolong bleeding time; monitor with coagulation disorders. Caution with asthma and avoid with aspirin-sensitive asthma.

**ADVERSE REACTIONS:** Dyspepsia, abdominal pain, diarrhea, flatulence, nausea, constipation, gastritis, asthenia, malaise, dizziness.

**INTERACTIONS:** May elevate digoxin, lithium, and methotrexate serum levels. May enhance nephrotoxicity associated with cyclosporine. Avoid with phenylbutazone and ASA. Increased adverse effect potential with ASA. Caution with warfarin. Diuretics may increase risk of renal toxicity.

**PREGNANCY:** Category C, not for use in nursing.

## ETODOLAC ER

RX

etodolac (Various)

**NSAIDs may cause an increased risk of serious cardiovascular thrombotic events, MI, stroke and serious GI adverse events including bleeding, ulceration, and perforation of the stomach or intestines. Contraindicated for the treatment of peri-operative pain in the setting of coronary artery bypass graft (CABG) surgery.**

**THERAPEUTIC CLASS:** NSAID (pyranocarboxylic acid derivative)

**INDICATIONS:** Relief of signs and symptoms of osteoarthritis (OA), rheumatoid arthritis (RA), and juvenile rheumatoid arthritis (JRA).

**DOSAGE:** *Adults:* Usual: 400-1000mg qd. Max: 1200mg/day. Pediatrics: 6-16 yrs: JRA: >60kg: 1000mg. 46-60kg: 800mg. 31-45kg: 600mg. 20-30kg: 400mg.

**HOW SUPPLIED:** Tab, Extended Release: 400mg, 500mg, 600mg

**CONTRAINDICATIONS:** ASA or other NSAID allergy that precipitates asthma, urticaria or allergic reaction. Treatment of peri-operative pain in the setting of CABG surgery.

**WARNINGS/PRECAUTIONS:** May lead to onset of new HTN or worsening of pre-existing HTN; monitor BP closely. Fluid retention and edema reported; caution with fluid retention or heart failure. Renal papillary necrosis and other renal injury reported after long-term use. Not recommended for use with advanced renal disease; if therapy must be initiated, monitor renal function. Anaphylactoid reactions may occur. May cause serious skin adverse events (eg, exfoliative dermatitis, Stevens-Johnson syndrome, and toxic epidermal necrolysis). Avoid in late pregnancy; may cause premature closure of ductus arteriosis. May cause elevations of LFTs; d/c if liver disease develops or systemic manifestations occur. Caution in elderly. Anemia may occur; with long-term use, monitor Hgb/Hct if signs or symptoms of anemia develop. May inhibit platelet aggregation and prolong bleeding time; monitor with coagulation disorders. Caution with asthma and avoid with aspirin-sensitive asthma.

**ADVERSE REACTIONS:** Dyspepsia, abdominal pain, diarrhea, flatulence, nausea, constipation, vomiting, GI ulcers, gross bleeding/perforation.

**INTERACTIONS:** May elevate digoxin, lithium, and methotrexate serum levels. May enhance nephrotoxicity associated with cyclosporine. Avoid with phenylbutazone. Increased adverse effect potential with ASA. Caution with warfarin. May decrease antihypertensive effects with ACE inhibitors. May reduce natriuretic effect of furosemide and thiazides.

**PREGNANCY:** Category C, not for use in nursing.

## ETOPOPHOS RX

etoposide phosphate (Bristol-Myers Squibb)

**Severe myelosuppression with bleeding or infection may occur.**

**THERAPEUTIC CLASS:** Podophyllotoxin derivative

**INDICATIONS:** Adjunct therapy for management of refractory testicular tumors. First line combination therapy for management of small cell lung cancer (SCLC).

**DOSAGE:** *Adults:* Testicular Cancer: Range: 50-100mg/m$^2$/day on days 1-5 to 100mg/m$^2$/day on days 1, 3, and 5. SCLC: Range: 35mg/m$^2$/day for 4 days to 50mg/m$^2$/day for 5 days. After adequate recovery from toxicity, repeat course for either therapy at 3-4 week intervals. CrCl 15-50mL/min: 75% of dose.

**HOW SUPPLIED:** Inj: 100mg

**WARNINGS/PRECAUTIONS:** Observe for myelosuppression during and after therapy. Risk of anaphylactic reaction manifested by chills, fever, tachycardia, bronchospasm, dyspnea, and hypotension. Increased risk of toxicity with a low serum albumin. Perform CBC before each dose, during, and after therapy. May cause fetal harm in pregnancy.

**ADVERSE REACTIONS:** Myelosuppression, nausea, vomiting, anaphylactic-like reactions, BP changes, alopecia, anorexia.

**INTERACTIONS:** Caution with drugs known to inhibit phosphatase activities (eg, levamisole). High dose oral cyclosporine reduces clearance.

**PREGNANCY:** Category D, not for use in nursing.

## ETOPOSIDE
RX

etoposide (Various)

**Severe myelosuppression with bleeding or infection may occur.**

**THERAPEUTIC CLASS:** Podophyllotoxin derivative

**INDICATIONS:** Adjunct therapy for management of refractory testicular tumors. First line combination therapy for management of small cell lung cancer (SCLC).

**DOSAGE:** *Adults:* Testicular Cancer: Range: 50-100mg/m²/day IV on days 1-5 to 100mg/m²/day on days 1, 3, and 5. SCLC: Range: 35mg/m²/day IV for 4 days to 50mg/m²/day for 5 days. After adequate recovery from toxicity, repeat course for either therapy at 3-4 week intervals.

**HOW SUPPLIED:** Inj: 20mg/mL

**WARNINGS/PRECAUTIONS:** Observe for myelosuppression during and after therapy. Risk of anaphylactic reaction manifested by chills, fever, tachycardia, bronchospasm, dyspnea, and hypotension. Perform CBC before each dose, during, and after therapy. May cause fetal harm in pregnancy.

**ADVERSE REACTIONS:** Myelosuppression, nausea, vomiting, anaphylactic-like reactions, hypotension (after rapid IV use), alopecia, anorexia.

**PREGNANCY:** Category D, not for use in nursing.

## EUFLEXXA
RX

hyaluronan (Ferring)

**THERAPEUTIC CLASS:** Hyaluronan

**INDICATIONS:** Treatment of pain in osteoarthritis of the knee with inadequate response to conservative non-pharmacologic therapy and simple analgesics (eg, APAP).

**DOSAGE:** *Adults:* Inject 2mL intra-articularly into the knee weekly for 3 weeks, for a total of 3 injections.

**HOW SUPPLIED:** Inj: 1% [2mL]

**CONTRAINDICATIONS:** Avoid use with knee joint infections, infections or skin diseases in the area of injection site.

**WARNINGS/PRECAUTIONS:** Precipitation may occur when mixing with quaternary ammonium salts (eg, benzalkonium chloride). Potential for immune response with repeated exposure. Do not inject intravascularly; systemic adverse events may occur. Remove any joint effusion before injecting.

**ADVERSE REACTIONS:** Arthralgia, back pain, BP increase, joint effusion/swelling, tendonitis, nausea, skin irritation, headache, paresthesia, rhinitis.

**PREGNANCY:** Safety in pregnancy and nursing is not known.

## EURAX
RX

crotamiton (Westwood-Squibb)

**THERAPEUTIC CLASS:** Scabicide/antipruritic

**INDICATIONS:** Treatment of scabies and pruritus.

**DOSAGE:** *Adults:* Shake lotion well before use. Scabies: Thoroughly massage into cleansed skin from the chin down to the toes. Re-apply in 24 hrs. Take cleansing bath 48 hrs after last application. Pruritus: Massage into affected area. Repeat prn.

**HOW SUPPLIED:** Cre: 10% [60g]; Lot: 10% [60mL, 480mL]

**WARNINGS/PRECAUTIONS:** Avoid eyes, mouth, acutely inflamed skin or raw or weeping surfaces. Discontinue if severe irritation or sensitization develops.

**ADVERSE REACTIONS:** Allergic sensitivity, irritation.

**PREGNANCY:** Category C, safety in nursing not known.

## EVISTA RX
raloxifene HCl (Lilly)

**THERAPEUTIC CLASS:** Selective estrogen receptor modulator

**INDICATIONS:** Treatment and prevention of osteoporosis in postmenopausal women.

**DOSAGE:** *Adults:* 60mg qd with or without meals.

**HOW SUPPLIED:** Tab: 60mg

**CONTRAINDICATIONS:** Nursing, pregnancy, venous thromboembolic events (eg, DVT, pulmonary embolism, retinal vein thrombosis).

**WARNINGS/PRECAUTIONS:** Increases risk of venous thromboembolism. D/C 72 hrs prior to and during prolonged immobilization. Lowers total and LDL cholesterol. Not for use in premenopausal women. Serum levels increase with hepatic dysfunction. Not for use with systemic estrogens.

**ADVERSE REACTIONS:** Hot flashes, leg cramps, abdominal pain, vaginal bleeding, arthralgia, rhinitis, headache.

**INTERACTIONS:** Avoid concomitant use with anion exchange resins; cholestyramine decreases absorption. Monitor PT/INR with warfarin and other anticoagulants. Caution with other highly protein-bound drugs (eg, diazepam, diazoxide, lidocaine).

**PREGNANCY:** Category X, contraindicated in nursing.

## EVOCLIN RX
clindamycin phosphate (Stiefel)

**THERAPEUTIC CLASS:** Lincomycin derivative

**INDICATIONS:** Treatment of acne vulgaris.

**DOSAGE:** *Adults*: Apply to affected area once daily.
*Pediatrics:* ≥12 yrs: Apply to affected area once daily.

**HOW SUPPLIED:** Foam: 1% [50g, 100g]

**CONTRAINDICATIONS:** History of regional enteritis, ulcerative colitis, or antibiotic-associated colitis.

**WARNINGS/PRECAUTIONS:** Diarrhea, bloody diarrhea, and colitis (including pseudomembranous colitis) reported with the use of topical and systemic clindamycin. Discontinue if significant diarrhea occurs. Caution in atopic individuals. Avoid eye contact.

**ADVERSE REACTIONS:** Headache, application site burning/pruritus/dryness, pseudomembranous colitis (rare).

**INTERACTIONS:** May potentiate neuromuscular blockers; caution with concomitant use.

**PREGNANCY:** Category B, caution in nursing.

## EVOXAC RX
cevimeline HCl (Daiichi)

**THERAPEUTIC CLASS:** Cholinergic agonist

**INDICATIONS:** Treatment of symptoms of dry mouth in patients with Sjogren's syndrome.

**DOSAGE:** *Adults:* 30mg tid.

**HOW SUPPLIED:** Cap: 30mg

**CONTRAINDICATIONS:** Uncontrolled asthma, when miosis in undesirable (eg, acute iritis, narrow-angle glaucoma).

**WARNINGS/PRECAUTIONS:** May alter cardiac conduction and/or HR; caution with angina or MI. Potential to increase airway resistance, bronchial smooth muscle tone, and bronchial secretions; caution with controlled asthma, chronic bronchitis, or COPD. Toxicity characterized by exaggerated parasympathomimetic effects (eg, headache, visual disturbance, lacrimation, sweating, respiratory distress, GI spasm, nausea, vomiting, cardiac abnormalities, mental confusion, tremors). Caution with history of nephrolithiasis, cholelithiasis. Ophthalmic formulations decrease visual acuity; caution while night driving or hazardous activities in reduced lighting. Risk of cholecystitis.

**ADVERSE REACTIONS:** Excessive sweating, nausea, rhinitis, diarrhea, cough, sinusitis, upper respiratory infection.

**INTERACTIONS:** CYP450 2D6 and CYP450 3A3/4 inhibitors also inhibit metabolism of cevimeline. Caution with CYP450 2D6 deficiency. Possible conduction disturbances with beta antagonists. Additive effects with parasympathomimetics. May interefere with drugs with antimuscarinic effects.

**PREGNANCY:** Category C, not for use in nursing.

## EXCEDRIN MIGRAINE — OTC

aspirin - caffeine - acetaminophen (Bristol-Myers Squibb)

**THERAPEUTIC CLASS:** Analgesic combination

**INDICATIONS:** Treatment of migraine.

**DOSAGE:** *Adults:* Take 2 tabs with water. Max: 2 tabs/day.

**HOW SUPPLIED:** Tab: (APAP-ASA-Caffeine) 250mg-250mg-65mg

**WARNINGS/PRECAUTIONS:** Children and teenagers should not use for viral illnesses. APAP and ASA may cause liver damage and GI bleeding.

**INTERACTIONS:** Limit caffeine containing medications, foods, or beverages. Caution with alcohol.

**PREGNANCY:** Safety in pregnancy and nursing not known.

## EXELON — RX

rivastigmine tartrate (Novartis)

**THERAPEUTIC CLASS:** Acetylcholinesterase inhibitor

**INDICATIONS:** Treatment of mild to moderate dementia of the Alzheimer's type and mild to moderate dementia associated with Parkinson's disease.

**DOSAGE:** *Adults:* Alzheimer's Dementia: Initial: 1.5mg bid. Titrate: May increase by 1.5mg bid every 2 weeks. Max: 12mg/day. If not tolerating, suspend therapy for several doses and restart at same or next lower dose. If interrupted longer than several days, reinitiate with lowest daily dose and titrate as above. Dementia Associated with Parkinson's Disease: Initial: 1.5mg bid. Titrate: May increase by 1.5mg every 4 weeks. Take with food in am and pm. May mix solution with water, cold fruit juice or soda.

**HOW SUPPLIED:** Cap: 1.5mg, 3mg, 4.5mg, 6mg; Sol: 2mg/mL [120mL]

**CONTRAINDICATIONS:** Hypersensitivity to carbamate derivatives.

**WARNINGS/PRECAUTIONS:** Significant GI intolerance (eg, nausea, vomiting, anorexia, and weight loss); always follow dosing guidelines. Vagotonic effect on HR (bradycardia), especially in"sick sinus syndrome" or supraventricular conduction abnormalities. May cause urinary obstruction and seizures. Monitor for peptic ulcers/GI bleeds. Caution in asthma and COPD. May exacerbate or induce extrapyramidal symptoms.

**ADVERSE REACTIONS:** Nausea, vomiting, abdominal pain, dyspepsia, constipation, somnolence, anorexia, dyspepsia, asthenia, headache, dizziness, fatigue, diarrhea, tremor.

**INTERACTIONS:** May block effects of anticholinergics. May be synergistic with succinylcholine, similar neuromuscular blockers, or cholinergic agonists (eg, bethanechol). May exaggerate succinylcholine-type muscle relaxation during anesthesia.

**PREGNANCY:** Category B, not for use in nursing.



## EXJADE RX
deferasirox (Novartis)

**THERAPEUTIC CLASS:** Iron Chelating Agent

**INDICATIONS:** Treatment of chronic iron overload due to blood transfusions (transfusional hemosiderosis).

**DOSAGE:** *Adults:* Initial: 20mg/kg/day. Titrate: May increase 5-10mg/kg q 3-6 months. Max: 30mg/kg/day. Take on empty stomach at least 30 minutes before food at same time each day. Tablets should be completely dispersed in 3.5oz of liquid if dose <1g or in 7oz if dose >1g. If serum ferritin falls below 500µg/L, consider interrupting therapy.
*Pediatrics:* ≥2 yrs: Initial: 20mg/kg/day. Titrate: May increase 5-10mg/kg q 3-6 months. Max: 30mg/kg/day. Take on empty stomach at least 30 minutes before food at same time each day. Tablets should be completely dispersed in 3.5oz of liquid if dose <1g or in 7oz if dose >1g. If serum ferritin falls below 500µg/L, consider interrupting therapy.

**HOW SUPPLIED:** Tab: 125mg, 250mg, 500mg

**WARNINGS/PRECAUTIONS:** Assess SCr before therapy and monitor monthly therafter; reduce dose, interrupt or d/c therapy if necessary. Intermittent proteinuria reported; monitor closely. Acute renal failure and cytopenias reported. Use caution and monitor SCr in those at risk of complications, having preexisting renal or comorbid conditions, receiving medicinal products that depress renal function, or elderly. Caution with pre-existing hematologic disorders; monitor CBC regularly. Hepatic abnormalities, increased transaminases reported; monitor LFTs monthly; modify dose for severe or persistent elevations. Reports of auditory (high frequency hearing loss, decreased hearing) and ocular distrubances (lens opacities, cataracts, elevated IOP, retinal disorders); initial and yearly auditory and ophthalmic testing recommended. Reports of skin rashes; d/c if severe, may reinitiate with short period of oral steriod.

**ADVERSE REACTIONS:** Diarrhea, vomiting, nausea, headache, abdominal pain, pyrexia, cough, increased SCr, rash, b-thalassemia, rare anemias, sicke cell disease.

**INTERACTIONS:** Avoid with aluminum-containing antacids or other iron chelator therapies.

**PREGNANCY:** Category B, caution in nursing.

## EXUBERA RX
insulin human, rdna origin (Pfizer)

**THERAPEUTIC CLASS:** Insulin

**INDICATIONS:** Treatment of adult patients with diabetes mellitus for the control of hyperglycemia.

**DOSAGE:** *Adults:* Individualize dose. Approximate Guidelines: Initial, Pre-Meal Dose: 120-139.9kg: 6mg/meal; 100-119.9kg: 5mg/meal; 80-99.9kg: 4mg/meal; 60-79.9kg: 3mg/meal; 40-59.9kg: 2mg/meal; 30-39.9kg: 1mg/meal. Adjust dose based on patient's need and titrate to optimal dosage based on blood glucose monitoring results.

**HOW SUPPLIED:** Pow, Inhalation: 1mg, 3mg [90[s]]

**CONTRAINDICATIONS:** Patients who smoke or have discontinued smoking <6 months prior to starting therapy (if patient starts/resumes smoking, discontinue immediately and utilize alternative treatment); safety and efficacy in smokers has not been established. Patients with unstable or poorly controlled lung disease; wide variations in lung function that could affect the absorption and increase risk of hypoglycemia/hyperglycemia.

**WARNINGS/PRECAUTIONS:** When used at mealtime, give 10 min before meal. Hypoglycemic reactions may occur. Type 1 diabetes also requires a longer-acting insulin. Change insulin cautiously and consider adjusting oral antidiabetic treatment. Glucose monitoring recomended. Assess pulmonary function prior to initiation of therapy, after first 6 months, and annually thereafter. Presence of pulmonary symptoms and declines in pulmonary function may require more frequent monitoring of pulmonary function and/or consideration of discontinuation. Use with underlying lung disease, such as asthma or COPD, is not recommended. Insulin requirements may be altered during intercurrent conditions such as illness, emotional disturbances, or stress. Dose reductions with renal or hepatic impairment. Rare generalized allergy to insulin may occur. Insulin antibodies may develop during treatment. Bronchospasm rarely reported; discontinue immediately. During intercurrent respiratory illness, close monitoring of blood glucose concentrations and dose adjustment may be required.

**ADVERSE REACTIONS:** Hypoglycemia, chest pain, dry mouth, respiratory tract infection, increased cough, pharyngitis, rhinitis, sinusitis, respiratory disorders, dyspnea, increased sputum, bronchitis.

**INTERACTIONS:** Corticosteroids, danazol, diazoxide, diuretics, sympathomimetic agents (eg, epinephrine, albuterol, terbutaline), glucagon, isoniazid, phenothiazine derivatives, somatropin, thyroid hormones, estrogens, progestogens (eg, oral contraceptives), protease inhibitors, and atypical antipsychotics (eg, olanzapine and clozapine) may reduce the blood glucose-lowering effect of insulin that may result in hyperglycemia. Oral antidiabetic products, ACE inhibitors, disopyramide, fibrates, fluoxetine, MAOIs, pentoxifylline, propoxyphene, salicylates, and sulfonamide antibiotics may increase the blood glucose-lowering effect of insulin and susceptibility to hypoglycemia. β-blockers, clonidine, lithium salts, and alcohol may either increase or reduce the blood glucose-lowering effect of insulin. Pentamidine may cause hypoglycemia, which may sometimes be followed by hyperglycemia. In addition, under the influence of sympatholytic medicinal products such as β-blockers, clonidine, guanethidine, and reserpine, the signs and symptoms of hypoglycemia may be reduced or absent. Bronchodilators and other inhaled products may alter absorption; consistent timing of dosing of bronchodilators, close monitoring of blood glucose concentrations and dose titration as appropriate are recommended.

**PREGNANCY:** Category C, caution in nursing.

## EYE WASH SOLUTION OTC

boric acid - sodium borate - sodium chloride (Bausch & Lomb)

**THERAPEUTIC CLASS:** Eye wash

**INDICATIONS:** For emergency use to flush irritants from eyes. For everyday to cleanse and refresh eyes

**DOSAGE:** *Adults:* Fill eye cup with sol and apply cup to affected eye, press tightly to prevent escape of liquid and tilt head backwards. Open eyelids wide and rotate eyeball to ensure thorough bathing with wash. If not using cup, flush affected eye prn.

**HOW SUPPLIED:** Sol: [120mL]

**WARNINGS/PRECAUTIONS:** Do not touch container tip to any surface to avoid contamination. D/C if eye pain or vision changes occur, if redness or irritation continues, or if condition worsens or persists.

**PREGNANCY:** Safety in pregnancy or nursing not known.

## FACTIVE
gemifloxacin mesylate (Oscient)

RX

**THERAPEUTIC CLASS:** Fluoroquinolone

**INDICATIONS:** Treatment of community-acquired pneumonia (CAP), including multi-drug resistant *Streptococcus pneumoniae* (MDRSP), and acute bacterial exacerbation of chronic bronchitis (ABECB).

**DOSAGE:** *Adults:* ≥18 yrs: ABECB: 320mg qd for 5 days. CAP: 320mg qd for 5 days (*S.pneumoniae,H.influenzae*, *M.pneumoniae*, or *C.pneumoniae*) or 7 days (MDRSP, *K.pneumoniae*, or *M.catarrhalis*). Renal Impairment: CrCl ≤ 40mL/min or Dialysis: 160mg qd. Take with fluids.

**HOW SUPPLIED:** Tab: 320mg

**WARNINGS/PRECAUTIONS:** May prolong QT interval; avoid in patients with a history of prolonged QTc interval, uncontrolled electrolyte disorders. Caution with proarrhythmic conditions, epilepsy, or if predisposed to convulsions. Discontinue at first sign of hypersensitivity (eg, rash). CNS effects, photosensitivity reactions, hypersensitivity reactions (some fatal) reported; discontinue if any of these occur. Pseudomembranous colitis, Achilles and other tendon rupture reported. Stop therapy if rash, pain, inflammation, or ruptured tendon occurs. Avoid excessive sunlight and UV light. Maintain hydration. Increases of the International Normalized Ratio (INR), or prothrombin time (PT), and/or clinical episodes of bleeding have been noted with concurrent administration with warfarin orits derivatives. Patients should notify their physicians if they are taking warfarin or its derivatives.

**ADVERSE REACTIONS:** Diarrhea, rash, nausea.

**INTERACTIONS:** Magnesium or aluminum containing antacids, Videx® (didanosine) chewable/buffered tablets or pediatric powder, and products containing iron, and zinc, or other metal cations decrease absorption, space doses at least 3 hrs before or 2 hrs after administration. Space dosing of sucralfate by 2 hrs. Potentiated by probenecid. Monitor PT. Avoid Class IA (eg, quinidine, procainamide) or III (eg, amiodarone, sotalol) antiarrhythmics. Caution with drugs that prolong the QTc interval (eg, erythromycin, antipsychotics, TCAs).

**PREGNANCY:** Category C, not for use in nursing.

## FAMVIR
famciclovir (Novartis)

RX

**THERAPEUTIC CLASS:** Nucleoside analogue

**INDICATIONS:** Treatment of acute herpes zoster (shingles). Treatment or suppression of recurrent genital herpes; or treatment of recurrent herpes labialis (cold sores) in immunocompetent patients. Treatment of recurrent mucocutaneous herpes simplex infections in HIV-infected patients;

**DOSAGE:** *Adults:* >18 yrs: Herpes Zoster: Usual: 500mg q8h for 7 days; start within 72 hrs after rash onset. CrCl 40-59mL/min: 500mg q12h. CrCl 20-39mL/min: 500mg q24h. CrCl <20mL/min: 250mg q24h. Hemodialysis: 250mg following dialysis. Recurrent Genital Herpes: 1000mg bid for 1 day; start within 6 hrs of onset of symptom. CrCl 40-59mL/min: 500mg q12h; CrCl 20-39mL/min 500mg as single dose; CrCl <20mL/min 250mg as a single dose; Hemodialysis: 250mg following dialysis. Suppression of Recurrent Genital Herpes: 250mg bid for up to 1 year. CrCl 20-39mL/min: 125mg q12h. CrCl <20mL/min: 125mg q24h. Hemodialysis: 125mg following dialysis. Recurrent Orolabial or Genital Herpes in HIV: 500mg bid for 7 days. CrCl <20mL/min: 250mg q24h. Hemodialysis: 250mg following dialysis. Recurrent Herpes Labialis: 1500mg as a single dose; CrCl 40-59mL/min: 750mg single dose; CrCl

20-39mL/min: 500mg single dose; CrCl <20mL/min: 20mg single dose; Hemodialysis: 250mg following dialysis

**HOW SUPPLIED:** Tab: 125mg, 250mg, 500mg

**CONTRAINDICATIONS:** Hypersensitivity to penciclovir cream.

**WARNINGS/PRECAUTIONS:** Prodrug of penciclovir. Dose adjustment in renal disease. Not indicated for initial episode of genital herpes infection, ophthalmic zoster, disseminated zoster or in immunocompromised patients with herpes zoster.

**ADVERSE REACTIONS:** Headache, migraine, nausea, diarrhea, vomiting, fatigue, urticaria, hallucinations, confusion.



**INTERACTIONS:** Increased plasma levels of penciclovir with probenecid and other drugs significantly eliminated by active renal tubular secretion. Potential interaction with drugs metabolized by aldehyde oxidase.

**PREGNANCY:** Category B, safety not known in nursing.

## FARESTON RX
toremifene citrate (GTx)

**THERAPEUTIC CLASS:** Nonsteroidal triphenylethylene derivative

**INDICATIONS:** Treatment of metastatic breast cancer in postmenopausal women with estrogen-receptor positive or unknown tumors.

**DOSAGE:** *Adults:* Usual: 60mg qd. Treat until disease progression is evident.

**HOW SUPPLIED:** Tab: 60mg

**WARNINGS/PRECAUTIONS:** Hypercalcemia and tumor flare reported with bone metastases. Endometrial hyperplasia reported. Avoid with history of thromboembolic disease. Do not treat long-term in pre-existing endometrial hyperplasia. Leukopenia and thrombocytopenia reported (rarely). May cause fetal harm with pregnancy.

**ADVERSE REACTIONS:** Hot flashes, sweating, nausea, vaginal discharge, dizziness, edema, vomiting, vaginal bleeding.

**INTERACTIONS:** Increased risk of hypercalcemia with drugs that decrease calcium excretion (eg, thiazide diuretics). CYP450 3A4 inducers (eg, phenobarbital, phenytoin, carbamazepine) decrease serum levels. Increased PT with coumarin-type anticoagulants. CYP450 3A4-6 inhibitors (eg, ketoconazole, erythromycin) may inhibit metabolism.

**PREGNANCY:** Category D, safety in nursing not known.

## FASLODEX RX
fulvestrant (AstraZeneca LP)

**THERAPEUTIC CLASS:** Estrogen receptor antagonist

**INDICATIONS:** For the treatment of hormone receptor positive metastatic breast cancer in postmenopausal women with disease progression following anti-estrogen therapy.

**DOSAGE:** *Adults:* 250mg IM into the buttock once monthly as either a single 5mL injection or two concurrent 2.5mL injections. The injection should be administered slowly.

**HOW SUPPLIED:** Inj: 50mg/mL [2.5mL, 5mL]

**CONTRAINDICATIONS:** Pregnancy.

**WARNINGS/PRECAUTIONS:** May cause fetal harm during pregnancy; women of childbearing age should be advised not to become pregnant and pregnancy should be ruled out prior to initiating therapy. Avoid in patients with bleeding diatheses or thrombocytopenia. Safety and efficacy have not been studied in patients with moderate or severe hepatic impairment.

**ADVERSE REACTIONS:** Nausea, vomiting, constipation, diarrhea, abdominal pain, headache, back pain, vasodilatation (hot flushes), pharyngitis, injection site reactions, asthenia, pain, dyspnea, increased cough.

**INTERACTIONS:** Avoid with concurrent anticoagulants.

**PREGNANCY:** Category D, not for use in nursing.

## FAZACLO

clozapine (Avanir)

RX



**Risk of agranulocytosis, seizures, myocarditis, and other cardiovascular and respiratory effects. Obtain baseline WBC and ANC before initiation of therapy, regularly during treatment, and for 4 weeks after discontinuation. Increased mortality in elderly patients with dementia-related psychosis.**

**THERAPEUTIC CLASS:** Dibenzapine derivative

**INDICATIONS:** Management of severe schizophrenia when response to standard schizophrenia treatment fails.

**DOSAGE:** *Adults:* Initial: 12.5mg qd-bid. Titrate: Increase by 25-50mg/day, up to 300-450mg/day by end of 2 weeks, then increase weekly or bi-weekly by increments up to 100mg. Usual 100-900mg/day given tid. Max: 900mg/day. To d/c, gradually reduce dose over 1-2 weeks. Monitor for psychotic symptoms if abrupt discontinuation warranted (eg, leukopenia).

**HOW SUPPLIED:** Tab, Disintegrating: 12.5mg, 25mg*, 50mg, 100mg* *scored

**CONTRAINDICATIONS:** Myeloproliferative disorders, uncontrolled epilepsy, history of clozapine-induced agranulocytosis or severe granulocytopenia, severe CNS depression, coma, or with other agents with potential to cause agranulocytosis or suppress bone marrow function.

**WARNINGS/PRECAUTIONS:** Reserve treatment for severely ill patients unresponsive to other schizophrenia therapies. Monitor for hyperglycemia, worsening of glucose control with DM and FBG levels with diabetes risk. Significant risk of orthostatic hypotension and tachycardia. May impair alertness with initial doses. May cause high fever or pulmonary embolism. Cardiomyopathy reported; discontinue unless benefit outweighs risk. Caution with prostatic enlargement, narrow angle glaucoma and renal, hepatic, or cardiac/pulmonary disease. NMS, tardive dyskinesias, impaired intestinal peristalsis and ECG changes reported. Obtain WBC and ANC at baseline, then weekly for 1st 6 months of therapy, then every 2 weeks for next 6 months, and then every 4 weeks thereafter if counts are acceptable. Avoid treatment if WBCs <3500/mm$^3$ or ANC <2000/mm$^3$, history of myeloproliferative disorder, previous clozapine-induced agranulocytosis, or granulocytopenia. Discontinue mtreatment if WBCs <3000/mm$^3$, ANC <1500/mm$^3$, eosinophils >4000/mm$^3$, or if myocarditis develops. Discontinue over 1-2 weeks.

**ADVERSE REACTIONS:** Drowsiness, vertigo, headache, tremor, salivation, sweating, dry mouth, visual disturbances, tachycardia, hypotension, syncope, constipation, nausea, fever.

**INTERACTIONS:** Avoid with other bone marrow suppressants, epinephrine, and carbamazepine. Caution with CNS-active drugs, anesthesia, alcohol, paroxetine, fluoxetine, fluvoxamine, sertraline, benzodiazepines, other psychotropics, or inhibitors/inducers of CYP1A2, 2D6, 3A4. Dosage reduction may be needed with drugs metabolized by CYP2D6 (eg, antidepressants, phenothiazines, carbamazepine, Type 1C antiarrhythmics). May potentiate hypotensive effects of antihypertensives and anticholinergic effects of atropine-type drugs. Caution with general anesthesia. CYP450 inducers (eg, phenytoin, nicotine, carbamazepine, rifampin) may decrease plasma levels. CYP450 inhibitors (eg, cimetidine, caffeine, fluvoxamine, erythromycin) may increase plasma levels.

**PREGNANCY:** Category B, not for use in nursing.

## FELBATOL
felbamate (MedPointe)

RX

**Associated with aplastic anemia and fatal hepatic failure. Monitor blood, LFTs. Avoid in history of hepatic dysfunction.**

**THERAPEUTIC CLASS:** Dicarbamate anticonvulsant

**INDICATIONS:** Not for 1st line therapy. Monotherapy or adjunct therapy in partial seizures with and without generalization in adults. Adjunct therapy for partial and generalized seizures with Lennox-Gastaut syndrome in children.



**DOSAGE:** *Adults:* Initial Monotherapy: 300mg qid or 400mg tid. Titrate: Increase by 600mg every 2 weeks to 2.4g/day. Max: 3.6g/day. Initial Monotherapy Conversion/Adjunct Therapy: 300mg qid or 400mg tid while reducing present AED (see literature). Titrate: For conversion, increase at week 2 to 2.4g/day, at week 3 up to 3.6g/day. Adjunct Therapy: Increase by 1.2g/day every week up to 3.6mg/day. Renal Dysfunction: May need to reduce dose with concomitant AEDs.
*Pediatrics:* >14 yrs: Initial Monotherapy: 300mg qid or 400mg tid. Titrate: Increase by 600mg every 2 weeks to 2.4g/day. Max: 3.6g/day. Initial Monotherapy Conversion/Adjunct Therapy: 300mg qid or 400mg tid while reducing present AED (see literature). Titrate: For conversion, increase at week 2 to 2.4g/day, at week 3 up to 3.6g/day. Adjunct Therapy: Increase by 1.2g/day every week up to 3.6mg/day. 2-14 yrs: Lennox-Gastaut Adjunct Therapy: Initial: 15mg/kg/day in 3-4 divided doses. Titrate: Increase by 15mg/kg/day every week to 45mg/kg/day. Renal Dysfunction: May need to reduce dose with concomitant AEDs.

**HOW SUPPLIED:** Sus: 600mg/5mL [240mL, 960mL]; Tab: 400mg*, 600mg* *scored

**CONTRAINDICATIONS:** History of blood dyscrasias, hepatic dysfunction.

**WARNINGS/PRECAUTIONS:** Avoid abrupt discontinuation. Caution with renal dysfunction. Obtain written, informed consent. Obtain full hematologic evaluations and LFTs before, during and after discontinuation. Discontinue if bone marrow depression or liver abnormalities occur.

**ADVERSE REACTIONS:** Anorexia, vomiting, insomnia, nausea, headache, anemias, hepatic failure.

**INTERACTIONS:** Increases plasma levels of phenytoin, valproate, active carbamazepine metabolite and phenobarbital. Decreases carbamazepine levels. Decreased felbamate levels with phenytoin, carbamazepine, and phenobarbital. Caution with OCs.

**PREGNANCY:** Category C, safety in nursing not known.

## FELDENE
piroxicam (Pfizer)

RX

**NSAIDs may cause an increased risk of serious cardiovascular thrombotic events, MI, stroke and serious GI adverse events including bleeding, ulceration, and perforation of the stomach or intestines. Contraindicated for the treatment of peri-operative pain in the setting of coronary artery bypass graft (CABG) surgery.**

**THERAPEUTIC CLASS:** NSAID

**INDICATIONS:** Relief of signs and symptoms of osteoarthritis and rheumatoid arthritis.

**DOSAGE:** *Adults:* 20mg qd or 10mg bid. Elderly: Start at lower end of dosing range.

**HOW SUPPLIED:** Cap: 10mg, 20mg

**CONTRAINDICATIONS:** ASA or other NSAID allergy that precipitates asthma, urticaria, or other allergic type reactions. Treatment of peri-operative pain in the setting of CABG surgery.

**WARNINGS/PRECAUTIONS:** May lead to onset of new HTN or worsening of pre-existing HTN; monitor BP closely. Fluid retention and edema reported; caution with fluid retention or heart failure. Renal papillary necrosis and other renal injury reported after long-term use. Not recommended for use with advanced renal disease; if therapy must be initiated, monitor renal function. Anaphylactoid reactions may occur. May cause serious skin adverse events (eg, exfoliative dermatitis, Stevens-Johnson syndrome, and toxic epidermal necrolysis). Avoid in late pregnancy; may cause premature closure of ductus arteriosis. May cause elevations of LFTs; d/c if liver disease develops or systemic manifestations occur. Caution in elderly. Anemia may occur; with long-term use, monitor Hgb/Hct if signs or symptoms of anemia develop. May inhibit platelet aggregation and prolong bleeding time; monitor with coagulation disorders. Caution with asthma and avoid with aspirin-sensitive asthma. Adverse eye findings reported. Dermatological and/or allergic signs and symptoms suggestive of serum sickness have occurred.

**ADVERSE REACTIONS:** Edema, dyspepsia, elevated liver enzymes, dizziness, rash, tinnitus, renal dysfunction, dry mouth, weight changes.

**INTERACTIONS:** Synergistic GI bleeding effects with warfarin. Diminished effect with ASA and may increase adverse effects. May decrease antihypertensive effects of ACE inhibitors. May reduce natriuretic effect of furosemide and thiazides. May increase lithium and methotrexate levels; monitor for toxicity. May displace other protein bound drugs.

**PREGNANCY:** Category C, not for use in nursing.

## FEMARA

RX

letrozole (Novartis)

**THERAPEUTIC CLASS:** Nonsteroidal aromatase inhibitor

**INDICATIONS:** First-line treatment of hormone receptor positive or hormone receptor unknown locally advanced or metastatic breast cancer in postmenopausal women. Treatment of advanced breast cancer with disease progression following antiestrogen therapy in postmenopausal women. Extended adjuvant treatment of early breast cancer in postmenopausal women who have received 5 years of adjuvant tamoxifen therapy. Adjuvant treatment of postmenopausal women with hormone receptor positive early breast cancer.

**DOSAGE:** *Adults:* 2.5mg qd. Continue until tumor progression is evident. Cirrhosis/Severe Liver Dysfunction: Reduce dose.

**HOW SUPPLIED:** Tab: 2.5mg

**CONTRAINDICATIONS:** Women of premenopausal endocrine status.

**WARNINGS/PRECAUTIONS:** May cause fetal harm in pregnancy. May elevate LFTs. Reduce dose in cirrhosis and severe liver dysfunction. May cause fatigue and dizziness; caution when driving or using machinery.

**ADVERSE REACTIONS:** Bone pain, back pain, nausea, arthralgia, dyspnea, fatigue, chest pain, decreased weight, hot flushes, peripheral edema, HTN, vomiting, constipation, diarrhea, musculoskeletal pain, insomnia, cough, alopecia.

**INTERACTIONS:** Co-administration with tamoxifen may reduce letrozole plasma levels; if co-administered, give letrozole immediately after tamoxifen.

**PREGNANCY:** Category D, caution in nursing.

## FEMHRT RX
ethinyl estradiol - norethindrone acetate (Warner Chilcott)

**Estrogens and progestins should not be used for prevention of cardiovascular disease or dementia. Increased risks of MI, stroke, invasive breast cancer, PE, and DVT in postmenopausal women (50-79 yrs of age) reported. Increased risk of developing probable dementia in postmenopausal women ≥65 yrs of age reported.**

**THERAPEUTIC CLASS:** Estrogen/progestogen combination

**INDICATIONS:** In women with an intact uterus, treatment of moderate to severe vasomotor symptoms associated with menopause and prevention of postmenopausal osteoporosis.

**DOSAGE:** *Adults:* Vasomotor Symptoms: 1 tab qd. Re-evaluate at 3-6 month intervals. Osteoporosis Prevention: 1 tab qd. Assess response by measuring bone mineral density.

**HOW SUPPLIED:** Tab: (Ethinyl Estradiol-Norethindrone) 2.5mcg-0.5mg, 5mcg-1mg

**CONTRAINDICATIONS:** Pregnancy, undiagnosed abnormal genital bleeding, breast cancer, estrogen-dependent neoplasia, DVT/PE, thrombophlebitis, thromboembolic disorders, active or recent (eg, within past year) arterial thromboembolic disease (eg, stroke, MI).

**WARNINGS/PRECAUTIONS:** Risk of gallbladder disease, endometrial and breast carcinoma, elevated BP, visual disturbances, thromboembolism, and hypercalcemia with breast cancer or bone metastases. Possible risk of cardiovascular disease, ovarian cancer. Caution with liver dysfunction, asthma, epilepsy, migraine, depression, and cardiac or renal dysfunction. Increase in HDL, triglycerides, thyroxine binding globulin. Hypercoagulability effects. Impaired glucose tolerance. D/C if sudden onset of visual abnormalities or migraine. May exacerbate endometriosis.

**ADVERSE REACTIONS:** Headache, back pain, abdominal pain, nausea, vomiting, breast pain, nervousness, depression, rhinitis, sinusitis, UTI, vaginitis.

**INTERACTIONS:** Increases plasma levels of cyclosporine, prednisolone, and theophylline. May decrease plasma levels of acetaminophen. May increase clearance of temazapam, salicylic acid, morphine, and clofibric acid. CYP3A4 inducers (eg, St. John's wort, phenobarbital, carbamazepine, rifampin) may decrease levels which may decrease therapeutic effects and/or change uterine bleeding profile. CYP3A4 inhibitors (eg, erythromycin, clarithromycin, ketoconazole, itraconazole, ritonavir, grapefruit juice) may increase levels which may result in side effects.

**PREGNANCY:** Contraindicated in pregnancy, caution in nursing.

## FEMRING RX
estradiol acetate (Warner Chilcott)

**Estrogens increase the risk of endometrial cancer. Estrogens, with or without progestins, should not be used for the prevention of cardiovascular disease or dementia. Increased risks of MI, stroke, invasive breast cancer, PE, and DVT in postmenopausal women (50-79 yrs of age) reported. Increased risk of developing probable dementia in postmenopausal women ≥65 yrs of age reported.**

**THERAPEUTIC CLASS:** Estrogen

**INDICATIONS:** Treatment of moderate to severe vasomotor symptoms and vulvar/vaginal atrophy associated with menopause. Consider other vaginal products if treating solely vulvar/vaginal symptoms.

**DOSAGE:** *Adults:* Initial: Use lowest effective dose. Insert ring vaginally. Replace every 3 months. Re-evaluate periodically.

**HOW SUPPLIED:** Vaginal Ring: 0.05mg/day, 0.1mg/day

**CONTRAINDICATIONS:** Undiagnosed abnormal genital bleeding, known/suspected/history of breast cancer (except in appropriately selected patients being treated for metastatic disease), estrogen-dependent neoplasia, active or history of DVT or pulmonary embolism, active or recent (within 1 yr) arterial thromboembolic disease (eg, stroke, MI), pregnancy.

**WARNINGS/PRECAUTIONS:** May increase risk of cardiovascular events (eg, MI, stroke), venous thrombosis, and PE; d/c immediately if any of these events occur or are suspected. May increase risk of breast/endometrial cancer, and gallbladder disease. Retinal vascular thrombosis reported; monitor and d/c if papilledema or retinal vascular lesions occur. Consider addition of a progestin if no hysterectomy. May elevate BP; monitor at regular intervals. May cause elevations of plasma triglycerides with pre-existing hypertriglyceridemia. Caution with history of cholestatic jaundice associated with past estrogen use or with pregnancy; d/c with recurrence. May lead to increased thyroid-binding globulin levels; monitor thyroid function. May cause fluid retention; caution with cardiac/renal dysfunction. Caution with severe hypocalcemia. May increase risk of ovarian cancer. May exacerbate endometriosis, asthma, DM, epilepsy, migraine, porphyria; use with caution. Few cases of toxic shock syndrome reported.



**ADVERSE REACTIONS:** Headache, intermenstrual bleeding, vaginal candidiasis, breast tenderness, back pain, abdominal distension, nausea, vulvovaginitis, uterine pain.

**INTERACTIONS:** CYP3A4 inducers (eg, St. John's wort, phenobarbital, carbamazepine, rifampin) may decrease levels which may decrease therapeutic effects and/or change uterine bleeding profile. CYP3A4 inhibitors (eg, erythromycin, clarithromycin, ketoconazole, itraconazole, ritonavir, grapefruit juice) may increase levels which may result in side effects. May require higher doses of thyroid hormone.

**PREGNANCY:** Contraindicated in pregnancy, caution in nursing.

## FEMTRACE

RX

estradiol acetate (Warner Chilcott)

**Estrogens increase risk of endometrial cancer. Estrogens, with or without progestins, should not be used for the prevention of cardiovascular disease. Increased risks of MI, stroke, invasive breast cancer, PE, and DVT in postmenopausal women (50-79 yrs of age) reported.**

**THERAPEUTIC CLASS:** Estrogen

**INDICATIONS:** Treatment of moderate to severe vasomotor symptoms associated with menopause.

**DOSAGE:** *Adults:* 1 tab qd. Use lowest effective dose for shortest duration. Re-evaluate menopausal symptoms at 3-6 month intervals.

**HOW SUPPLIED:** Tab: 0.45mg, 0.9mg, 1.8mg

**CONTRAINDICATIONS:** Pregnancy, undiagnosed abnormal genital bleeding, breast cancer, estrogen-dependent neoplasia, DVT/PE, active or recent (eg, within past year) arterial thromboembolic disease (eg, stroke, MI), liver dysfunction or disease.

**WARNINGS/PRECAUTIONS:** May increase risk of cardiovascular events (eg, MI, stroke), venous thrombosis, and PE; d/c immediately if any of these events occur or are suspected. May increase risk of breast/endometrial cancer, and gallbladder disease. Retinal vascular thrombosis reported; monitor and d/c if papilledema or retinal vascular lesions occur. Consider addition of a progestin if no hysterectomy. May elevate BP; monitor at regular intervals. May cause elevations of plasma triglycerides with pre-existing hypertriglyceridemia. Caution with history of cholestatic jaundice associated with past estrogen use or with pregnancy; d/c with recurrence. May lead to increased thyroid-binding globulin levels; monitor thyroid function. May cause fluid retention; caution with cardiac/renal dysfunction. Caution with severe hypocalcemia. May increase risk of ovarian cancer. May exacerbate endometriosis, asthma, DM, epilepsy, migraine, porphyria; use with caution.

**ADVERSE REACTIONS:** Vaginal and intermenstrual bleeding, breast tenderness, influenza, vaginal discharge, fungal infection, abdominal and back pain, headache.

**INTERACTIONS:** CYP3A4 inducers (eg, St. John's wort, phenobarbital, carbamazepine, rifampin) may decrease levels which may decrease therapeutic effects and/or change uterine bleeding profile. CYP3A4 inhibitors (eg, erythromycin, clarithromycin, ketoconazole, itraconazole, ritonavir, grapefruit juice) may increase levels which may result in side effects.

**PREGNANCY:** Contraindicated in pregnancy, caution in nursing



## FENOPROFEN RX

fenoprofen calcium (Various)

**NSAIDs may cause an increased risk of serious cardiovascular thrombotic events, MI, stroke and serious GI adverse events including bleeding, ulceration, and perforation of the stomach or intestines. Contraindicated for the treatment of peri-operative pain in the setting of coronary artery bypass graft (CABG) surgery.**

**OTHER BRAND NAMES:** Nalfon (Pedinol)

**THERAPEUTIC CLASS:** NSAID

**INDICATIONS:** Management of rheumatoid arthritis (RA) and osteoarthritis (OA). Relief of mild-to-moderate pain.

**DOSAGE:** *Adults:* RA/OA: 300-600mg tid-qid. Max: 3200mg/day. Pain: 200mg q4-6h prn. Take with food or milk with GI upset.

**HOW SUPPLIED:** Cap: 200mg, 300mg; Tab: 600mg

**CONTRAINDICATIONS:** Significantly impaired renal function. ASA or other NSAID allergy that precipitates asthma, rhinitis, or urticaria. Treatment of peri-operative pain in the setting of CABG surgery.

**WARNINGS/PRECAUTIONS:** May lead to onset of new HTN or worsening of pre-existing HTN; monitor BP closely. Fluid retention and edema reported; caution with fluid retention, compromised cardia function, or heart failure. Renal papillary necrosis and other renal injury reported after long-term use. Not recommended for use with advanced renal disease. Anaphylactoid reactions may occur. May cause serious skin adverse events (eg, exfoliative dermatitis, Stevens-Johnson syndrome, and toxic epidermal necrolysis). Avoid in late pregnancy; may cause premature closure of ductus arteriosis. May cause elevations of LFTs; d/c if liver disease develops or systemic manifestations occur. Caution in elderly. Anemia may occur; with long-term use, monitor Hgb/Hct if signs or symptoms of anemia develop. May inhibit platelet aggregation and prolong bleeding time; monitor with coagulation disorders. Caution with asthma and avoid with aspirin-sensitive asthma. Perform eye exams if visual disturbances occur. Caution with activities requiring mental alertness. With long-term use, monitor auditory function in hearing impaired patients.

**ADVERSE REACTIONS:** Dyspepsia, constipation, nausea, somnolence, dizziness, vomiting, abdominal pain, headache, diarrhea.

**INTERACTIONS:** ASA or chronic phenobarbital may decrease effects. Avoid salicylates. May potentiate hydantoins, sulfonamides, and sulfonylureas. May prolong PT with coumarin-type anticoagulants. May cause resistance to the effects of loop diuretics.

**PREGNANCY:** Category C, not for use in nursing.

## Fentora

fentanyl citrate (Cephalon)

CII

**Abuse liability. May cause life-threatening respiratory depression in opioid non-tolerant patients. Contraindicated in the management of acute or postoperative pain. Do not use in opioid non-tolerant patients. Adjust dose appropriately when converting from other oral fentanyl products. See Indications.**

**THERAPEUTIC CLASS:** Narcotic agonist analgesic

**INDICATIONS:** Management of breakthrough pain in patients with cancer who are already receiving and who are tolerant to opioid therapy for their underlying persistent cancer pain.

**DOSAGE:** *Adults:* Initial: Breakthrough Pain: 100mcg. Repeat once (30 min after starting dose) during a single pain episode. Titration Above 100mcg: Use two 100mcg tabs (one on each side of buccal cavity), if not controlled use two 100mcg tabs on each side (total four 100mcg tabs). Titration Above 400mcg: Use 200mcg tab increments. Max: Not more than 4 tabs simultaneously. Re-evaluate maintenance (around-the-clock) opioid dose if >4 episodes of breakthrough pain per day occured. Do not chew, crush, swallow, or dissolve; consume over 14-25 min. *Please see the PI for more information on conversion of dosage.*

**HOW SUPPLIED:** Tab, Buccal: 100mcg, 200mcg, 400mcg, 600mcg, 800mcg

**CONTRAINDICATIONS:** Opioid non-tolerant patients and management of acute or postoperative pain.

**WARNINGS/PRECAUTIONS:** Caution with concomitant use of other CNS depressants may cause hypoventilation, hypotension, and profound sedation. Caution wtih COPD, bradyarrhythmias, and hepatic or renal impairment. May cause physical dependence, respiratory depression. Extreme caution with evidence of increased intracranial pressure or impaired consciousness. May cause paresthesia, ulceration, or bleeding at application site.

**ADVERSE REACTIONS:** Respiratory depression, circulatory depression, headache, hypotension, shock, nausea, vomiting, constipation, dizziness, dyspnea, anxiety, somnolence.

**INTERACTIONS:** Dangerous increases in plasma concentration with potent inhibitors of CYP3A4 (eg, ketoconazole, itraconazole, clarithromycin, nelfinavir, nefazadone, ritonavir), moderate inhibitors of CYP3A4 (eg, amprenavir, diltiazem, fluconazole). CYP3A4 inducers may reduce efficacy. Increased depressant effects with other CNS depressants, including opioids, sedatives, hypnotics, general anesthetics, phenothiazines, tranquilizers, skeletal muscle relaxants, sedating antihistamines. Avoid within 14 days of MAOIs.

**PREGNANCY:** Category C, not for use in nursing.

## FeoGen Forte

vitamin C - folic acid - vitamin B12 - ferrous fumarate (Rising)

RX

**THERAPEUTIC CLASS:** Iron/vitamin

**INDICATIONS:** Treatment of all anemias responsive to oral iron therapy.

**DOSAGE:** *Adults:* 1-2 caps qd. Elderly: Start at low end of dosing range.

**HOW SUPPLIED:** (Ferrous Fumarate-Folic Acid-Vitamin $B_{12}$ -Vitamin C) Cap: 460mg-1mg-0.01mg-60mg

**CONTRAINDICATIONS:** Hemochromatosis, hemosiderosis, pernicious anemia.

**WARNINGS/PRECAUTIONS:** Accidental overdose of iron-containing products is a leading cause of fatal poisoning in children <6 yrs.

**ADVERSE REACTIONS:** Nausea, rash, vomiting, diarrhea, precordial pain, flushing of face or extremities.

**PREGNANCY:** Safety in pregnancy and nursing is not known.

## FEOSOL

OTC

iron carbonyl - ferrous sulfate (GlaxoSmithKline Consumer)

**THERAPEUTIC CLASS:** Iron supplement

**INDICATIONS:** Treatment of iron deficiency and iron deficiency anemia.

**DOSAGE:** *Adults:* 1 tab qd with food.
*Pediatrics:* >12 yrs: 1 tab qd with food.

**HOW SUPPLIED:** Tab: Feosol Caplet (Iron Carbonyl) 50mg (45mg elemental iron), Feosol Tablet (Ferrous Sulfate) 200mg (65mg elemental iron)



**WARNINGS/PRECAUTIONS:** Keep product out of reach of children. Accidental overdose of iron-containing products is a leading cause of fatal poisoning in children <6 yrs.

**ADVERSE REACTIONS:** Nausea, GI disturbance, constipation, diarrhea.

**INTERACTIONS:** Decreases absorption of tetracycline; space dose by 2 hrs.

**PREGNANCY:** Safety in pregnancy and nursing not known.

## FERO-FOLIC 500

RX

vitamin C - folic acid - ferrous sulfate (Abbott)

**THERAPEUTIC CLASS:** Iron/vitamin

**INDICATIONS:** Prevention and treatment of iron and folic acid deficiencies.

**DOSAGE:** *Adults:* 1 tab qd.

**HOW SUPPLIED:** (Ferrous Sulfate-Folic Acid-Vitamin C) Tab, Extended Release: 525mg-0.8mg-500mg

**CONTRAINDICATIONS:** Pernicious anemia.

**WARNINGS/PRECAUTIONS:** May mask pernicious anemia.

**ADVERSE REACTIONS:** Gastric intolerance, allergic sensitization.

**INTERACTIONS:** Absorption may be inhibited by eggs, milk, magnesium trisilicate or antacids containing carbonates. May interfere with the absorption of tetracyclines.

**PREGNANCY:** Category A, safety in nursing not known.

## FERO-GRAD-500

OTC

vitamin C - ferrous sulfate (Abbott)

**THERAPEUTIC CLASS:** Iron/vitamin

**INDICATIONS:** Iron supplementation.

**DOSAGE:** *Adults:* 1 tab qd.
*Pediatrics:* >4 yrs: 1 tab qd.

**HOW SUPPLIED:** Tab, Extended Release: Ferrous Sulfate 105mg-Vitamin C 500mg

## FERRLECIT

RX

sodium ferric gluconate complex (Watson)

**THERAPEUTIC CLASS:** Hematinic

**INDICATIONS:** Treatment of iron deficiency anemia in patients ≥6 yrs old undergoing chronic hemodialysis and receiving supplemental epoetin therapy.

**DOSAGE:** *Adults:* 10mL (125mg) as IV infusion (diluted) or as slow IV injection (undiluted). Minimum Cumulative Dose: 1g elemental iron over 8 sequential dialysis sessions.

*Pediatrics:* ≥6 yrs: 0.12mL/kg (1.5mg/kg) as IV infusion over 1 hr at 8 sequential dialysis sessions. Max: 125mg/dose.

**HOW SUPPLIED:** Inj: 62.5mg elemental iron/5mL

**CONTRAINDICATIONS:** Anemia not associated with iron deficiency. Iron overload.

**WARNINGS/PRECAUTIONS:** Hypersensitivity reactions and hypotension reported. Iron overload is more common in patients with hemoglobinopathies and other refractory anemia. Should not be administered to patients with iron overload.

**ADVERSE REACTIONS:** Injection site reactions, nausea, vomiting, diarrhea, hypotension, cramps, HTN, dizziness, dyspnea, abnormal erythrocytes, leg cramps, pain, chest pain, hypoesthesia, dysgeusia.

**PREGNANCY:** Category B, caution in nursing.



## FERRO-SEQUELS OTC

docusate sodium - ferrous fumarate (Inverness)

**THERAPEUTIC CLASS:** Iron supplement/stool softener

**INDICATIONS:** Iron deficiency.

**DOSAGE:** *Adults:* 1 tab qd.

**HOW SUPPLIED:** Tab, Extended Release: (Ferrous Fumarate-Docusate Sodium) 50mg-40mg

**WARNINGS/PRECAUTIONS:** Fatal poisoning reported in children <6 yrs with accidental overdose of iron-containing products.

**PREGNANCY:** Safety in pregnancy and nursing not known.

## FERTINEX RX

urofollitropin (Serono)

**THERAPEUTIC CLASS:** Follicle stimulating hormone

**INDICATIONS:** Sequentially with hCG, to stimulate follicular recruitment and development, and the induction of ovulation in polycystic ovary syndrome and infertility, after failed clomiphene therapy. With hCG, to stimulate development of multiple follicles in ovulatory patients undergoing Assisted Reproductive Technologies (ART).

**DOSAGE:** *Adults:* Individualize dose. Polycystic Ovary Syndrome: Initial: 75 IU SQ qd. Titrate: May increase after 5-7 days. Do not increase >2 times/cycle or >75 IU/adjustment. Maint: 75-300 IU/day. Give hCG 5000-10,000 U one day after last dose. Subsequent Cycles: Individualize dose based on response to previous cycle. ART: Initial: 150 IU SQ qd at cycle Day 2 or 3 (early follicular phase). Max: 10 days for most cases.

**HOW SUPPLIED:** Inj: 75 IU

**CONTRAINDICATIONS:** High FSH levels indicating primary ovarian failure, uncontrolled thyroid or adrenal dysfunction, organic intracranial lesions (eg, pituitary tumor), any cause of infertility other than anovulation (unless candidate for ART), abnormal bleeding of undetermined origin, ovarian cysts or enlargement not due to polycystic ovary syndrome, pregnancy.

**WARNINGS/PRECAUTIONS:** Exclude primary ovarian failure. Ovarian enlargement may occur; monitor ovarian response. Ovarian hyperstimulation syndrome (OHSS), multiple births, serious pulmonary and vascular complications reported. Avoid hCG if ovaries abnormally enlarged last day of therapy. Monitor follicular maturation by measuring estradiol levels and through vaginal ultrasound.

**ADVERSE REACTIONS:** Pulmonary and vascular complications, OHSS, adnexal torsion, ovarian enlargement, abdominal pain, ovarian cysts, GI and dermatological symptoms, injection site reactions, breast tenderness.

**PREGNANCY:** Category X, caution in nursing.

## FEVERALL

OTC

acetaminophen (Alpharma)

**THERAPEUTIC CLASS:** Analgesic

**INDICATIONS:** Treatment of pain and fever in patients who cannot tolerate oral meds due to nausea and vomiting.

**DOSAGE:** *Pediatrics:* Insert sup rectally. 3-11 months: 80mg q6h. Max: 480mg/24hrs. 12-36 months: 80mg q4h. Max: 480mg/24hrs. 3-6 yrs: 120mg q4-6h. Max: 720mg/24hrs. 6-12 yrs: 325mg q4-6h. Max: 2600mg/24hrs.

**HOW SUPPLIED:** Sup: 80mg, 120mg, 325mg, 650mg

**PREGNANCY:** Safety in pregnancy or nursing not known.



## FINACEA

RX

azelaic acid (Intendis)

**THERAPEUTIC CLASS:** Dicarboxylic acid antimicrobial

**INDICATIONS:** Topical treatment of inflammatory papules and pustules of mild to moderate rosacea.

**DOSAGE:** *Adults:* Wash and dry skin. Massage gently into affected area bid (am and pm) for up to 12 weeks.

**HOW SUPPLIED:** Gel: 15% [30g]

**CONTRAINDICATIONS:** Hypersensitivity to propylene glycol.

**WARNINGS/PRECAUTIONS:** Avoid the mouth, eyes, mucous membranes, occlusive dressings, or wrappings. Hypopigmentation reported. Discontinue if sensitivity or severe irritation occurs. Use only very mild soap or soapless cleansing lotion for facial cleansing. Avoid foods and beverages (eg, spicy foods, alcohol, thermally hot drinks) that may provoke erythema, flushing, and/or blushing.

**ADVERSE REACTIONS:** Burning, stinging, tingling, pruritus, scaling, dry skin.

**INTERACTIONS:** Avoid alcoholic cleansers, tinctures, astringents, abrasives and peeling agents.

**PREGNANCY:** Category B, caution in nursing.

## FINEVIN

RX

azelaic acid (Berlex)

**THERAPEUTIC CLASS:** Dicarboxylic acid antimicrobial

**INDICATIONS:** Mild-to-moderate inflammatory acne vulgaris.

**DOSAGE:** *Adults:* Wash and dry skin. Massage gently into affected area bid (am and pm).

*Pediatrics:* >12 yrs: Wash and dry skin. Massage gently into affected area bid (am and pm).

**HOW SUPPLIED:** Cre: 20% [30g, 50g]

**WARNINGS/PRECAUTIONS:** Hypopigmentation reported after use. Avoid the mouth, eyes, mucous membranes, occlusive dressings, or wrappings.

**ADVERSE REACTIONS:** Pruritus, burning, stinging, tingling.

**PREGNANCY:** Category B, caution in nursing.

## FIORICET

RX

caffeine - butalbital - acetaminophen (Watson)

**THERAPEUTIC CLASS:** Barbiturate/analgesic

**INDICATIONS:** Tension or muscle contraction headaches.

**DOSAGE:** *Adults:* 1-2 tabs q4h prn. Max: 6 tabs/day. Not for extended use. *Pediatrics:* >12 yrs: 1-2 tabs q4h prn. Max: 6 tabs/day. Not for extended use.

**HOW SUPPLIED:** Tab: (Butalbital-APAP-Caffeine) 50mg-325mg-40mg

**CONTRAINDICATIONS:** Porphyria.

**WARNINGS/PRECAUTIONS:** May be habit forming. Not for extended use. Caution in elderly, debilitated, severe renal or hepatic impairment, acute abdominal conditions. Caution in mentally depressed and suicidal tendencies, history of drug abuse.

**ADVERSE REACTIONS:** Drowsiness, lightheadedness, dizziness, sedation, shortness of breath, nausea, vomiting, abdominal pain, intoxicated feeling.

**INTERACTIONS:** Enhanced CNS effects with MAOIs. May enhance CNS depressant effects of other narcotic analgesics, alcohol, general anesthetics, tranquilizers, sedative hypnotics, or other CNS depressants.

**PREGNANCY:** Category C, not for use in nursing.

## FIORICET WITH CODEINE

CIII

caffeine - butalbital - acetaminophen - codeine phosphate (Watson)

**THERAPEUTIC CLASS:** Barbiturate/analgesic

**INDICATIONS:** Tension or muscle contraction headaches.

**DOSAGE:** *Adults:* 1-2 caps q4h prn. Max: 6 caps/day. Not for extended use.

**HOW SUPPLIED:** Cap: (Butalbital-APAP-Caffeine-Codeine) 50mg-325mg-40mg-30mg

**CONTRAINDICATIONS:** Porphyria.

**WARNINGS/PRECAUTIONS:** May be habit forming. Not for extended use. Respiratory depression and cerebrospinal fluid pressure enhanced with head injury or intracranial lesions. Caution in elderly, debilitated, severe renal or hepatic impairment, hypothyroidism, urethral stricture, Addison's disease, BPH, and history of drug abuse. May mask signs of acute abdominal conditions.

**ADVERSE REACTIONS:** Drowsiness, lightheadedness, dizziness, sedation, shortness of breath, nausea, vomiting, abdominal pain, intoxicated feeling.

**INTERACTIONS:** Enhanced CNS effects with MAOIs. May enhance CNS depressant effects of other narcotic analgesics, alcohol, general anesthetics, tranquilizers, sedative hypnotics, or other CNS depressants.

**PREGNANCY:** Category C, not for use in nursing.

## FIORINAL

CIII

aspirin - caffeine - butalbital (Watson)

**OTHER BRAND NAMES:** Lanorinal (Lannett)

**THERAPEUTIC CLASS:** Barbiturate/analgesic

**INDICATIONS:** Tension or muscle contraction headache.

**DOSAGE:** *Adults:* 1-2 caps or tabs q4h prn. Max: 6 caps or tabs/day. Not for extended use.

**HOW SUPPLIED:** Cap/Tab: (Butalbital-ASA-Caffeine) 50mg-325mg-40mg

**CONTRAINDICATIONS:** Porphyria, peptic ulcer disease, serious GI lesions, hemorrhagic diathesis. Syndrome of nasal polyps, angioedema and bronchospastic reactivity to ASA or NSAIDs.

**WARNINGS/PRECAUTIONS:** May be habit-forming. Not for extended use. Caution in elderly, debilitated, severe renal or hepatic impairment, hypothyroidism, urethral stricture, head injuries, elevated intracranial pressure, acute abdominal conditions, Addison's disease, prostatic hypertrophy, peptic ulcer, coagulation disorders. Avoid with ASA allergy. Risk of ASA hypersensitivity with nasal polyps and asthma. Caution in children with chickenpox or flu. Preoperative ASA may prolong bleeding time.

**ADVERSE REACTIONS:** Drowsiness, lightheadedness, dizziness, sedation, shortness of breath, nausea, vomiting, abdominal pain, intoxicated feeling.

**INTERACTIONS:** CNS effects enhanced by MAOIs. Additive CNS depression with alcohol, other narcotic analgesics, general anesthetics, tranquilizers (eg, chloral hydrate), sedatives/hypnotics, other CNS depressants. May enhance effects of anticoagulants. May cause hypoglycemia with oral antidiabetic agents and insulin. May cause bone marrow toxicity and blood dyscrasias with 6-MP and methotrexate. Increased risk of peptic ulceration and bleeding with NSAIDs. Decreased effects of uricosuric agents (eg, probenecid, sulfinpyrazone). Withdrawal of corticosteroids may cause salicylism with chronic ASA use.

**PREGNANCY:** Category C, not for use in nursing.

## FIORINAL WITH CODEINE CIII

aspirin - caffeine - butalbital - codeine phosphate (Watson)

**THERAPEUTIC CLASS:** Barbiturate/analgesic

**INDICATIONS:** Tension or muscle contraction headache.

**DOSAGE:** *Adults:* 1-2 caps q4h prn. Max: 6 caps/day. Not for extended use.

**HOW SUPPLIED:** Cap: (Butalbital-ASA-Caffeine-Codeine) 50mg-325mg-40mg-30mg

**CONTRAINDICATIONS:** Porphyria, peptic ulcer disease, serious GI lesions, hemorrhagic diathesis. Syndrome of nasal polyps, angioedema and bronchospastic reactivity to ASA or NSAIDs.

**WARNINGS/PRECAUTIONS:** May be habit-forming. Not for extended use. Respiratory depression and cerebrospinal fluid pressure may be enhanced with head injury or intracranial lesions. Caution in elderly, debilitated, severe renal or hepatic impairment, hypothyroidism, urethral stricture, head injuries, elevated intracranial pressure, acute abdominal conditions, Addison's disease, prostatic hypertrophy, peptic ulcer, coagulation disorders. Caution in children with chickenpox or flu. May obscure acute abdominal conditions. Preoperative ASA may prolong bleeding time. Avoid with ASA allergy. Risk of ASA hypersensitivity with nasal polyps and asthma.

**ADVERSE REACTIONS:** Drowsiness, lightheadedness, dizziness, sedation, shortness of breath, nausea, vomiting, abdominal pain, intoxicated feeling.

**INTERACTIONS:** CNS effects enhanced by MAOIs. Additive CNS depression with alcohol, other narcotic analgesics, general anesthetics, tranquilizers (eg, chloral hydrate), sedatives/hypnotics, other CNS depressants. May enhance effects of anticoagulants. May cause hypoglycemia with oral antidiabetic agents, insulin. May cause bone marrow toxicity, blood dyscrasias with 6-MP and methotrexate. Increased risk of peptic ulceration, bleeding with NSAIDs. Decreased effects of uricosuric agents (eg, probenecid, sulfinpyrazone). Withdrawal of corticosteroids may cause salicylism with chronic ASA use.

**PREGNANCY:** Category C, not for use in nursing.

## FLAGYL RX

metronidazole (Pharmacia & Upjohn)

**THERAPEUTIC CLASS:** Nitroimidazole

**INDICATIONS:** Treatment of symptomatic/asymptomatic trichomoniasis, amebic dysentery, amebic liver abscess, and anaerobic infections. Following IV metronidazole therapy, treatment of intra-abdominal, skin and skin structure, bone and joint, CNS, lower respiratory tract, and gynecologic infections, septicemia, and endocarditis.

**DOSAGE:** *Adults:* Trichomoniasis (Female and Male Sex Partner): (Cap/Tab) 375mg bid or 250mg tid for 7 days. One-day Therapy: (Tab) 2gm as single or divided doses. If repeat course needed, reconfirm diagnosis and allow 4-6 weeks between courses. Abscess: 500mg or 750mg tid for 5-10 days. Dysentery: 750mg tid for 5-10 days. Anaerobic Bacterial Infection: Usually IV therapy initially if serious, 7.5mg/kg q6h for 7-10 days or longer. Max: 4g/24 hrs. Elderly: Adjust dose based on serum levels. Hepatic Disease: Give lower dose cautiously; monitor levels.
*Pediatrics:* Amebiasis: 35-50mg/kg/24hrs given tid for 10 days.

**HOW SUPPLIED:** Cap: 375mg; Tab: 250mg, 500mg

**CONTRAINDICATIONS:** Treatment during 1st trimester of pregnancy.

**WARNINGS/PRECAUTIONS:** Seizures and peripheral neuropathy reported. Discontinue if abnormal neurological signs occur. Caution with severe hepatic impairment, blood dyscrasias, or CNS diseases. Monitor leukocytes before and after therapy.

**ADVERSE REACTIONS:** Seizures, peripheral neuropathy, nausea, vomiting, headache, anorexia, urticaria, rash, metallic taste, dysuria, vaginal candidiasis, vaginitis, dizziness, leukopenia.

**INTERACTIONS:** Avoid alcohol during and for 3 days after use. Avoid within 2 weeks of disulfiram use; increased possibility of psychotic reactions. Potentiates anticoagulant effects of warfarin; monitor PT. Increased elimination with phenytoin, phenobarbital and other hepatic enzyme inducers. May impair phenytoin clearance. Potentiated by cimetidine and other hepatic enzyme inhibitors. Increased lithium levels.

**PREGNANCY:** Category B, not for use in nursing.

## FLAGYL ER RX

metronidazole (Pharmacia & Upjohn)

**THERAPEUTIC CLASS:** Nitroimidazole antibacterial/antiprotozoal agent

**INDICATIONS:** Treatment of bacterial vaginosis.

**DOSAGE:** *Adults:* 750mg qd for 7 days; take 1 hr before or 2 hrs after meals. Elderly: Adjust dose based on serum levels. Hepatic Disease: Give lower dose cautiously; monitor levels.

**HOW SUPPLIED:** Tab, Extended Release: 750mg

**CONTRAINDICATIONS:** Treatment during 1st trimester of pregnancy.

**WARNINGS/PRECAUTIONS:** Seizures and peripheral neuropathy reported. D/C if abnormal neurological signs occur. Caution with severe hepatic impairment, blood dyscrasias, or CNS diseases. Monitor leukocytes before and after therapy.

**ADVERSE REACTIONS:** Headache, vaginitis, nausea, metallic taste, dizziness, seizures, peripheral neuropathy, vomiting, leukopenia, urticaria, rash, dysuria, vaginal candidiasis.

**INTERACTIONS:** Avoid alcohol during and for 3 days after use. Avoid within 2 weeks of disulfiram; increased possibility of psychotic reactions. Potentiates anticoagulant effects of warfarin; monitor PT. Increased elimination with phenytoin, phenobarbital. May impair phenytoin clearance. Potentiated by cimetidine. Increased lithium levels.

**PREGNANCY:** Category B, not for use in nursing.

# FLAGYL I.V. RX

metronidazole HCl (Various)

**OTHER BRAND NAMES:** Flagyl I.V. (RTU) (Baxter)

**THERAPEUTIC CLASS:** Nitroimidazole antibacterial/antiprotozoal agent

**INDICATIONS:** Treatment of anaerobic intra-abdominal, skin and skin structure, gynecologic, bone and joint, CNS, lower respiratory tract infections, endocarditis, and septicemia.

**DOSAGE:** *Adults:* LD: 15mg/kg IV. Maint: 6 hrs later, 7.5mg/kg IV q6h for 7-10 days or more. Max: 4g/24 hrs.



**HOW SUPPLIED:** Inj: 500mg; 500mg (RTU)

**WARNINGS/PRECAUTIONS:** Seizures and peripheral neuropathy reported. Discontinue if abnormal neurological signs occur. Caution with severe hepatic impairment, blood dyscrasias, or central nervous system disease. Monitor leukocytes before and after therapy. Metronidazole IV is effective in *B.fragilis* infections resistant to clindamycin, chloramphenicol, and penicillin.

**ADVERSE REACTIONS:** Convulsive seizures, peripheral neuropathy, nausea, vomiting, headache, leukopenia, rash, vaginal candidiasis, thrombophlebitis.

**INTERACTIONS:** Avoid alcohol during and for 3 days after use. Avoid within 2 weeks of disulfiram; increased possibility of psychotic reactions. Potentiates warfarin. Increased elimination with phenytoin, phenobarbital. May impair phenytoin clearance. Potentiated by cimetidine. Increased lithium levels.

**PREGNANCY:** Category B, not for use in nursing.

# FLECTOR RX

diclofenac epolamine (IBSA)

**NSAIDs may cause an increased risk of serious cardiovascular thrombotic events, MI, stroke and serious GI adverse events including bleeding, ulceration, and perforation of the stomach or intestines. Contraindicated for the treatment of peri-operative pain in the setting of coronary artery bypass graft (CABG) surgery.**

**THERAPEUTIC CLASS:** NSAID (benzeneacetic acid derivative)

**INDICATIONS:** Topical treatment of acute pain due to minor strains, sprains, and contusions.

**DOSAGE:** *Adults:* Apply 1 patch to the most painful area bid.

**HOW SUPPLIED:** Patch: 180mg [5$^s$]

**CONTRAINDICATIONS:** ASA or other NASID allergy that precipitates asthma, urticaria, or allergic-type reactions. Treatment of peri-operative pain in the setting of CABG surgery. Application to non-intact or damage skin (eg, exudative dermatitis, eczema, infected lesion, burns or wounds).

**WARNINGS/PRECAUTIONS:** See Black Box Warning. May lead to onset of new HTN or worsening of pre-existing HTN; monitor BP closely. Fluid retention and edema reported; caution with fluid retention or heart failure. Renal papillary necrosis and other renal injury reported after long-term use. Not recommended for use with advanced renal disease; if therapy must be initiated, monitor renal function. Anaphylactoid reactions may occur. May cause serious skin adverse events (eg, exfoliative dermatitis, Stevens-Johnson syndrome, and toxic epidermal necrolysis). Avoid in late pregnancy; may cause premature closure of ductus arteriosis. May cause elevations of LFTs; discontinue if liver disease develops or systemic manifestations occur. Rare cases of severe hepatic reactions (eg, jaundice, fatal fulminant hepatitis, liver necrosis, hepatic failure) reported. Anemia may occur; with long-term use, monitor Hgb/Hct if signs or symptoms of anemia develop. May inhibit platelet aggregation and prolong bleeding time; monitor with coagulation disorders.

Caution with asthma and avoid with aspirin-sensitive asthma. Wash hands after applying, handling or removing patch. Avoid contact with eye and mucosa.

**ADVERSE REACTIONS:** Pruritus, dermatitis, burning, nausea, dysgeusia, dyspepsia, headache, paresthesia, somnolence.

**INTERACTIONS:** May diminish the antihypertensive effect of ACE-inhibitors. Increased adverse effects with ASA; avoid use. May reduce natriuretic effect of furosemide and thiazides; monitor for renal failure. May enhance lithium and methotrexate toxicity; caution when co-administering. Synergistic effects on GI bleeding with warfarin.

**PREGNANCY:** Category C, not for use in nursing.



## FLEET BISACODYL

OTC

bisacodyl (Fleet)

**THERAPEUTIC CLASS:** Stimulant laxative

**INDICATIONS:** Relief of occasional constipation. For bowel cleansing for X-ray and endoscopic exam. Laxative in postoperative, antepartum, or postpartum care.

**DOSAGE:** *Adults:* (Enema) Use 1 rectally single dose qd. (Sup) Insert 1 rectally qd. Retain for 15-20 minutes. (Tab) 2-3 tabs single dose qd. Swallow tabs whole; do not chew or crush.
*Pediatrics:* >12 yrs: (Enema) Use 1 rectally single dose qd. (Sup) Insert 1 rectally qd. Retain for 15-20 minutes. (Tab) 2-3 tabs single dose qd. 6-11 yrs: (Sup) Insert 1/2 suppository rectally qd. Retain for 15-20 minutes. (Tab) 1 tab qd. Swallow tabs whole; do not chew or crush.

**HOW SUPPLIED:** Enema: 10mg; Sup: 10mg; Tab, Delayed Release: 5mg

**WARNINGS/PRECAUTIONS:** Do not use with nausea, vomiting, or abdominal pain. Rectal bleeding or failure to have a bowel movement after use may indicate a serious condition. Should not be used longer than 1 week.

**ADVERSE REACTIONS:** Abdominal discomfort, faintness, cramps.

**INTERACTIONS:** Do not administer tabs within 1 hr after taking an antacid, milk, or milk products.

**PREGNANCY:** Safety in pregnancy and nursing is not known.

## FLEET GLYCERIN LAXATIVES

OTC

glycerin (Fleet)

**THERAPEUTIC CLASS:** Laxative

**INDICATIONS:** Relief of constipation.

**DOSAGE:** *Adults:* 1 enema (5.6g) or 1 suppository (2g or 3g) rectally.
*Pediatrics:* 2-5 yrs: 1 enema (2.3g) or 1 suppository (1g) rectally. > 6 yrs: 1 enema (5.6g) or 1 suppository (2g or 3g) rectally.

**HOW SUPPLIED:** Enema: (Babylax) 2.3g, (Liquid Glycerin) 5.6g; Sup: 1g, 2g, 3g

**WARNINGS/PRECAUTIONS:** Rectal irritation may occur. Do not use with nausea, vomiting, or abdominal pain. Rectal bleeding or failure to have a bowel movement after use may indicate a serious condition. Do not use longer than 1 week.

**ADVERSE REACTIONS:** Rectal discomfort, burning sensation.

**PREGNANCY:** Safety in pregnancy and nursing in not known.

## FLEXERIL
RX

cyclobenzaprine HCl (McNeil Consumer)

**THERAPEUTIC CLASS:** Skeletal muscle relaxant (central-acting)

**INDICATIONS:** Relief of muscle spasm associated with acute, painful musculoskeletal conditions.

**DOSAGE:** *Adults:* Usual: 5mg tid. Titrate: May increase to 10mg tid. Mild Hepatic Dysfunction/Elderly: Initial: 5mg qd, then slowly increase. Moderate/Severe Hepatic Dysfunction: Avoid use. Treatment should not exceed 2-3 weeks.



*Pediatrics:* >15 yrs: Usual: 5mg tid. Titrate: May increase to 10mg tid. Mild Hepatic Dysfunction/Elderly: Initial: 5mg qd, then slowly increase. Moderate/Severe Hepatic Dysfunction: Avoid use. Treatment should not exceed 2-3 weeks.

**HOW SUPPLIED:** Tab: 5mg, 10mg

**CONTRAINDICATIONS:** Acute recovery phase of MI, arrhythmias, heart block or conduction disturbances, CHF, hyperthyroidism, MAOI use during or within 14 days.

**WARNINGS/PRECAUTIONS:** Caution with history of urinary retention, angle-closure glaucoma, increased IOP, hepatic dysfunction. Caution in elderly due to increased risk of CNS effects. May produce arrhythmias, sinus tachycardia and conduction time prolongation. May impair ability to drive.

**ADVERSE REACTIONS:** Drowsiness, dry mouth, headache, fatigue.

**INTERACTIONS:** Enhances effects of alcohol, barbiturates, and other CNS depressants. May block antihypertensive action of guanethidine and similar compounds. May enhance seizure risk with tramadol. Contraindicated with MAOIs. Caution with anticholinergic medication.

**PREGNANCY:** Category B, caution in nursing.

## FLOLAN
RX

epoprostenol sodium (GlaxoSmithKline)

**THERAPEUTIC CLASS:** Pulmonary and systemic vasodilator

**INDICATIONS:** Long-term treatment of primary pulmonary hypertension and pulmonary hypertension associated with the scleroderma spectrum of disease in NYHA Class III and IV patients inadequately responding to conventional therapy.

**DOSAGE:** *Adults:* Initial: 2ng/kg/min IV chronic infusion. Titrate: Increase by 2ng/kg/min every 15 minutes until no further increases are clinically warranted. May use a lower initial infusion rate if not tolerated.

**HOW SUPPLIED:** Inj: 0.5mg, 1.5mg

**CONTRAINDICATIONS:** Chronic use in CHF due to left ventricular systolic dysfunction, chronic therapy in patients who develop pulmonary edema during dose initiation.

**WARNINGS/PRECAUTIONS:** Abrupt withdrawal or large dose reductions may result in symptoms associated with rebound pulmonary HTN (eg, dyspnea, dizziness, and asthenia); avoid abrupt withdrawal. Unless contraindicated, administer anticoagulant therapy to reduce risk of pulmonary thromboembolism or systemic embolism through a patent foramen ovale. Monitor standing and supine BP and HR for several hours after dose adjustments.

**ADVERSE REACTIONS:** Flushing, headache, nausea, vomiting, hypotension, anxiety, nervousness, agitation, chest pain, dizziness, bradycardia, abdominal pain.

**INTERACTIONS:** Potentiates BP reduction with diuretics, antihypertensives, vasodilators. Increased risk of bleeding with antiplatelets or anticoagulants.

**PREGNANCY:** Category B, caution in nursing.

## FLOMAX

RX

tamsulosin HCl (Boehringer Ingelheim)

**THERAPEUTIC CLASS:** Alpha$_{1a}$ antagonist

**INDICATIONS:** Treatment of the signs and symptoms of benign prostatic hyperplasia.

**DOSAGE:** *Adults:* Initial: 0.4mg qd, 1/2 hr after the same meal each day. Titrate: May increase to 0.8mg qd after 2-4 weeks. If therapy is interrupted, restart with 0.4mg qd.

**HOW SUPPLIED:** Cap: 0.4mg

**WARNINGS/PRECAUTIONS:** Rule out prostate cancer. Orthostasis/syncope may occur. May cause priapism (rare). Intraoperative Floppy Iris Syndrome (IFIS) has been observed during cataract surgery. Do not crush, chew or open capsules.

**ADVERSE REACTIONS:** Headache, dizziness, somnolence, diarrhea, asthenia, back pain, pharyngitis, rhinitis, abnormal ejaculation.

**INTERACTIONS:** Avoid use with other α-blockers. Decreased clearance with cimetidine; caution with concomitant use especially with doses higher than 0.4mg. Caution with warfarin. Concomitant administration of flomax and an inhibitor of CYP2D6 or CYP3A4 may lead to increased flomax plasma exposure.

**PREGNANCY:** Category B, not for use in women.

## FLONASE

RX

fluticasone propionate (GlaxoSmithKline)

**THERAPEUTIC CLASS:** Corticosteroid

**INDICATIONS:** Management of the nasal symptoms of seasonal and perennial allergic rhinitis, and nonallergic rhinitis.

**DOSAGE:** *Adults:* Initial: 2 sprays per nostril qd or 1 spray per nostril bid. Maint: 1 spray per nostril qd. May dose as 2 sprays per nostril qd as needed for seasonal allergic rhinitis.
*Pediatrics:* ≥4 yrs: Initial: 1 sprays per nostril qd. If inadequate response, may increase to 2 sprays per nostril. Maint: 1 spray per nostril qd. Max: 2 sprays per nostril/day. ≥12 yrs: May dose as 2 sprays per nostril qd as needed for seasonal allergic rhinitis.

**HOW SUPPLIED:** Spray: 50mcg/spray [16g]

**WARNINGS/PRECAUTIONS:** Risk of adrenal insufficiency and withdrawal symptoms when replacing systemic corticosteroids with a topical corticosteroids. Caution with active or quiescent TB, ocular herpes simplex, or untreated bacterial, fungal and systemic viral infections. Avoid with recent nasal trauma, surgery or septum ulcers. Risk for more severe/fatal course of infections (eg, chickenpox, measles); avoid exposure in patients who have not had disease or been properly immunized. Candida infection of nose and pharynx reported (rare). Potential for growth velocity reduction in pediatrics. Excessive use may cause signs of hypercorticism or HPA suppression.

**ADVERSE REACTIONS:** Headache, pharyngitis, epistaxis, nasal burning/irritation, asthma symptoms, nausea/vomiting, cough.

**INTERACTIONS:** Caution with ketoconazole or other potent CYP3A4 inhibitors, may increase serum fluticasone levels. Concomitant inhaled corticosteroids increases risk of hypercorticism and/or HPA axis suppression. Increased levels with ritonavir; avoid use.

**PREGNANCY:** Category C, caution in nursing.

## FLOVENT HFA

RX

fluticasone propionate (GlaxoSmithKline)

**THERAPEUTIC CLASS:** Corticosteroid

**INDICATIONS:** Maintenance treatment of asthma as prophylactic therapy in patients ≥4 years; to reduce or eliminate the need for oral corticosteroidal therapy.

**DOSAGE:** *Adults:* Previous Bronchodilator Only: Initial: 88mcg bid. Max: 440mcg bid. Previous Inhaled Corticosteroids: Initial: 88-220mcg bid. Max: 440mcg bid. Previous Oral Corticosteroids: Initial: 440mcg bid. Max: 880mcg bid. Reduce PO prednisone no faster than 2.5 to 5mg/day weekly, beginning at least 1 week after starting fluticasone. Rinse mouth after use.
*Pediatrics:* ≥12 yrs: Previous Bronchodilator Only: Initial: 88mcg bid. Max: 440mcg bid. Previous Inhaled Corticosteroids: Initial: 88-220mcg bid. Max: 440mcg bid. Previous Oral Corticosteroids: Initial: 440mcg bid. Max: 880mcg bid. 4-11 yrs: Initial/Max: 88mcg bid. Reduce PO prednisone no faster than 2.5 to 5mg/day weekly, beginning at least 1 week after starting fluticasone. Rinse mouth after use.

**HOW SUPPLIED:** MDI: 44mcg/inh [10.6g], 110mcg/inh [12g], 220mcg/inh [12g]

**CONTRAINDICATIONS:** Primary treatment of status asthmaticus or other acute asthma attacks.

**WARNINGS/PRECAUTIONS:** Deaths due to adrenal insufficiency have occurred with transfer from systemic corticosteroids to inhaled corticosteroids. Resume oral corticosteroids during stress or severe asthma attack. Wean slowly from systemic corticosteroid therapy. Observe for adrenal insufficiency, systemic corticosteroid withdrawal effects, hypercorticism, adrenal suppression (including adrenal crisis), reduction in growth velocity (children and adolescents). May increase susceptibility to infections. Not for acute bronchospasm. D/C if bronchospasm occurs after dosing. Caution with TB of respiratory tract; untreated systemic fungal, bacterial, viral or parasitic infections; or ocular herpes simplex. *Candida* infection of mouth and pharynx reported. Glaucoma, increased IOP and cataracts reported. Rare cases of eosinophilic conditions.

**ADVERSE REACTIONS:** Pharyngitis, cough, bronchitis, nasal congestion, sinusitis, dysphonia, oral candidiasis, upper respiratory infection, influenza, headache, nasal discharge, allergic rhinitis, fever, paradoxical bronchospasm..

**INTERACTIONS:** Increased levels with ritonavir; avoid use. Caution with ketoconazole and other potent CYP3A4 inhibitors; may increase serum fluticasone levels.

**PREGNANCY:** Category C, caution in nursing.

## FLOXIN

RX

ofloxacin (Ortho-McNeil)

**THERAPEUTIC CLASS:** Fluoroquinolone

**INDICATIONS:** Treatment of acute urinary tract (UTI) and uncomplicated skin and skin structure infection (SSSI), acute bacterial exacerbation of chronic bronchitis (ABECB), community acquired pneumonia (CAP), acute uncomplicated urethral and cervical gonorrhea, nongonococcal urethritis and cervicitis, mixed infections of the urethra and cervix, acute pelvic inflammatory disease (PID), uncomplicated cystitis, prostatitis.

**DOSAGE:** *Adults:* >18 yrs: ABECB/CAP/SSSI: 400mg q12h for 10 days. Cervicitis/Urethritis: 300mg q12h for 7 days. Gonorrhea: 400mg single dose. PID: 400mg q12h for 10-14 days. Uncomplicated Cystitis: 200mg q12h for 3 days (*E.coli* or *K.pneumoniae*) or 7 days (other pathogens). Complicated UTI: 200mg q12h for 10 days. Prostatitis: *(E.coli)* 300mg q12h for 6 weeks. CrCl 20-50mL/min: Dose q24h. CrCl <20mL/min: After regular initial dose, give 50% of normal dose q24h. Severe Hepatic Impairment: Max: 400mg/day.

**HOW SUPPLIED:** Tab: 200mg, 300mg, 400mg

**WARNINGS/PRECAUTIONS:** Convulsions, increased intracranial pressure, toxic psychosis and CNS stimulation reported; d/c if any occur. Serious, fatal hypersensitivity reactions reported. Pseudomembranous colitis and ruptures of shoulder, hand, and Achilles tendon reported. Not shown to be effective for syphilis. Safety and efficacy unknown in patients <18 yrs old, pregnancy, and nursing. Maintain adequate hydration. Caution with renal or hepatic dysfunction, risk for seizures, CNS disorder with predisposition to seizures. Avoid excessive sunlight. Monitor blood, renal and hepatic function with prolonged therapy.

**ADVERSE REACTIONS:** Nausea, insomnia, headache, dizziness, diarrhea, vomiting, external genital pruritus in women, vaginitis.

**INTERACTIONS:** Decreased absorption with antacids, sucralfate, zinc, didanosine; separate dosing by 2 hrs. NSAIDs may increase risk of seizures. May potentiate theophylline, warfarin. May potentiate insulin, oral hypoglycemics; discontinue if hypoglycemia occurs. May increase half-life of drugs metabolized by CYP450.

**PREGNANCY:** Category C, not for use nursing.

## FLOXIN OTIC — RX

ofloxacin (Daiichi)

**OTHER BRAND NAMES:** Floxin Otic Singles (Daiichi)

**THERAPEUTIC CLASS:** Fluoroquinolone

**INDICATIONS:** Otitis externa in patients >6 mos. Chronic suppurative otitis media in patients >12 yrs with perforated tympanic membranes. Acute otitis media in patients >1 yr with tympanostomy tubes.

**DOSAGE:** *Adults:* Otitis Externa: 10 drops or 2 single-dispensing containers (SDCs) once daily for 7 days. Chronic Suppurative Otitis Media with Perforated Tympanic Membrane: 10 drops or 2 SDCs bid for 14 days.
*Pediatrics:* Otitis Externa: 6 mos-13 yrs: 5 drops or 1 single-dispensing container (SDC) once daily for 7 days. ≥13 yrs: 10 drops or 2 SDCs once daily for 7 days. Chronic Suppurative Otitis Media with Perforated Tympanic Membrane: ≥12 yrs: 10 drops or 2 SDCs bid for 14 days. Acute Otitis Media with Tympanostomy Tubes: 1-12 yrs: 5 drops or 1 SDC bid for 10 days.

**HOW SUPPLIED:** Sol: 0.3% [5mL, 10mL], (Singles) 0.3% [20$^{s}$]

**WARNINGS/PRECAUTIONS:** D/C if hypersensitivity reaction occurs. Re-evaluate if no improvement after one week.

**ADVERSE REACTIONS:** Pruritus, application site reaction, taste perversion.

**PREGNANCY:** Category C, not for use in nursing.

## FLUDARA — RX

fludarabine phosphate (Berlex)

> **Can severely suppress bone marrow function. High doses associated with severe neurologic effects, including blindness, coma, and death. Autoimmune hemolytic anemia reported. Monitor closely for hemolysis. High incidence of fatal pulmonary toxicity with pentostatin.**

**THERAPEUTIC CLASS:** Antimetabolite

**INDICATIONS:** Treatment of B-cell chronic lymphocytic leukemia (CLL) unresponsive to or with disease progression during treatment with at least on standard alkylating-agent containing regimen.

**DOSAGE:** *Adults:* 25mg/m$^2$ over 30 minutes qd for 5 days. Repeat course every 28 days. Administer 3 additional courses after achievement of maximum response. May decrease or delay dose based on hematologic or nonhematologic toxicity. Consider delaying or discontinuing if neurotoxicity occurs. CrCl 30-70mL/min: Reduce dose by 20%. CrCl <30mL/min: Not recommended.

**HOW SUPPLIED:** Inj: 50mg

**WARNINGS/PRECAUTIONS:** Severe bone marrow suppression reported. Predisposition to increased toxicity with advanced age, renal insufficiency, and bone marrow impairment; monitor for toxicity. Caution with renal insufficiency. Tumor lysis syndrome associated with large tumor burdens. Monitor hematologic profile regularly. Can cause fetal harm during pregnancy. Use irradiated blood products if transfusion required.

**ADVERSE REACTIONS:** Myelosuppression, fever, chills, infection, nausea, vomiting, malaise, fatigue, anorexia, weakness, serious opportunistic infections.



**INTERACTIONS:** Avoid pentostatin due to the risk of severe pulmonary toxicity.

**PREGNANCY:** Category D, not for use in nursing.

## FLUDROCORTISONE

fludrocortisone acetate (Various)

RX

**THERAPEUTIC CLASS:** Corticosteroid

**INDICATIONS:** Partial replacement therapy for adrenocortical insufficiency in Addison's disease. Treatment of salt-losing adrenogenital syndrome.

**DOSAGE:** *Adults:* Addison's Disease: Usual: 0.1mg/day with concomitant cortisone 10-37.5mg/day or hydrocortisone 10-30mg/day in divided doses. Dose Range: 0.1mg three times weekly to 0.2mg/day. If HTN develops, reduce to 0.05mg/day. Salt-Losing Adrenogenital Syndrome: 0.1-0.2mg/day.

**HOW SUPPLIED:** Tab: 0.1mg* *scored

**CONTRAINDICATIONS:** Systemic fungal infections.

**WARNINGS/PRECAUTIONS:** May to increase dose before, during, and after stressful situations. Caution with hypothyroidism, cirrhosis, ocular herpes simplex, HTN, ulcerative colitis, diverticulitis, peptic ulcer, osteoporosis, myasthenia gravis, renal impairment, and elderly. May mask signs of infection or cause new infection. Avoid exposure to chickenpox or measles. Marked effect on sodium retention; monitor electrolytes. May need salt restriction and potassium supplements. Monitor for psychic disturbances. Risk of glaucoma, cataracts, and eye infections. Avoid abrupt withdrawal.

**ADVERSE REACTIONS:** HTN, CHF, edema, convulsions, hypokalemia, hypokalemic alkalosis, muscle weakness, impaired wound healing, menstrual irregularities, cataracts, suppression of growth, hyperglycemia, HPA suppression, acne, rash.

**INTERACTIONS:** Decreases serum salicylate levels. Enhanced hypokalemia with amphotericin B and potassium-depleting diuretics (eg, furosemide, ethacrynic acid). Increased risk of digitalis toxicity and arrhythmias with hypokalemia. Decreased effects with rifampin, barbiturates, and hydantoins. Monitor PT with oral anticoagulants. Decreases effects of oral hypoglycemics, insulin. Enhanced edema with other anabolic steroids (eg, oxymethalone, norethandrolone). Adjust dose with initiation or termination of estrogen. Avoid live virus vaccines (including small pox) and other immunizations. Caution with ASA.

**PREGNANCY:** Category C, caution in nursing.

## FLULAVAL

influenza virus vaccine (GlaxoSmithKline)

RX

**THERAPEUTIC CLASS:** Vaccine

**INDICATIONS:** Active immunization against influenza disease caused by influenza virus subtypes A and B contained in the vaccine.

**DOSAGE:** *Adults:* ≥18 yrs: 0.5mL IM in deltoid.

**HOW SUPPLIED:** Inj: 15mcg/0.5mL [5mL]

**CONTRAINDICATIONS:** Delay immunization with acute evolving, neurologic disorder.

**WARNINGS/PRECAUTIONS:** Guillain-Barre syndrome reported within 6 weeks of administration. Avoid with bleeding disorders or concomitant anticoagulants. May reduce immune response in the immunocompromised.

**ADVERSE REACTIONS:** Pain, redness, and/or swelling at injection site, headache, fatigue, myalgia, low grade fever, malaise.

**INTERACTIONS:** Do not mix with any other vaccine in same syringe or vial; administer other vaccines at different injection sites. May increase blood levels of warfarin, theophylline, phenytion. Immunosuppressive therapies (eg, irradiation, antimetabolites, alkylating agents, cytotoxic drugs, corticosteroids) may reduce effectiveness.

**PREGNANCY:** Category C, caution in nursing.

F

## FLUMADINE RX

rimantadine HCl (Forest)

**THERAPEUTIC CLASS:** Adamantane class antiviral

**INDICATIONS:** Prophylaxis and treatment of influenza A virus.

**DOSAGE:** *Adults:* Prophylaxis/Treatment: 100mg bid. Elderly/Severe Hepatic Dysfunction/CrCl <10mL/min: 100mg qd. Initiate treatment within 48 hrs of onset of symptoms. Treat for 7 days from initial onset of symptoms. *Pediatrics:* Prophylaxis: 1-9 yrs: 5mg/kg qd. Max: 150mg qd. >10 yrs: 100mg bid.

**HOW SUPPLIED:** Syrup: 50mg/5mL [240mL]; Tab: 100mg

**WARNINGS/PRECAUTIONS:** Caution with a history of epilepsy. D/C if seizures develop. Caution with renal or hepatic dysfunction.

**ADVERSE REACTIONS:** Insomnia, dizziness, nervousness, nausea, vomiting, anorexia, dry mouth, abdominal pain, asthenia.

**INTERACTIONS:** May be potentiated by cimetidine. APAP and ASA may decrease levels of rimantadine. Avoid use of Live Influenza Virus Vaccine within 2 weeks before or 48 hrs after use.

**PREGNANCY:** Category C, not for use in nursing.

## FLUMIST RX

influenza virus vaccine live (MedImmune)

**THERAPEUTIC CLASS:** Vaccine

**INDICATIONS:** Active immunization for the prevention of disease caused by influenza A and B viruses in healthy children and adolescents, 5-17 years of age, and healthy adults, 18-49 years of age.

**DOSAGE:** *Adults:* 0.25mL per nostril.
*Pediatrics:* ≥9 yrs: 0.25mL per nostril. 5-8 yrs: Not Previously Vaccinated With FluMist: 0.25mL per nostril for 2 doses 60 days (+/- 14 days) apart. Previously Vaccinated With FluMist: 0.25mL per nostril.

**HOW SUPPLIED:** Nasal Spray: 0.5mL [10s]

**CONTRAINDICATIONS:** Parenteral use. Hypersensitivity to eggs or egg products. Children and adolescents 5-17 years of age receiving aspirin or aspirin-containing therapy. History of Guillain-Barre syndrome. Immune deficiency diseases such as combined immuno immunodeficiency, agammaglobulinemia, and thymic abnormalities, and conditions such as HIV infection, malignancy, leukemia, or lymphoma. Immunosuppressed or altered/compromised immune status due to treatment with systemic corticosteroids, alkylating drugs, antimetabolites, radiation, or other immunosuppressive therapies.

**WARNINGS/PRECAUTIONS:** Avoid with history of asthma or reactive airways disease, chronic disorders of the cardiovascular and pulmonary systems, second or third trimester of pregnancy, chronic metabolic diseases (including diabetes), renal dysfunction, hemoglobinopathies, congenital or acquired immunosuppression. Avoid close contact with immunocompromised individuals for at least 21 days. Have epinephrine available. Delay administration until after the acute phase (at least 72 hrs) of febrile and/or respiratory illnesses.

**ADVERSE REACTIONS:** Runny nose, congestion, cough, irritability, headache, sore throat, fever, chills, muscle aches, vomiting, tiredness/weakness.



**INTERACTIONS:** Avoid concurrent use with other vaccines and within 48 hrs after cessation of antiviral therapy; antiviral agents until 2 weeks after vaccination unless medically indicated; aspirin or aspirin-containing products in children and adolescents 5-17 yrs.

**PREGNANCY:** Category C, caution in nursing.

## FLUNISOLIDE NASAL SPRAY RX

flunisolide (Various)

**THERAPEUTIC CLASS:** Corticosteroid

**INDICATIONS:** Relief of seasonal or perennial rhinitis.

**DOSAGE:** *Adults:* Initial: 2 sprays per nostril bid. Titrate: May increase to 2 sprays per nostril tid. Max: 8 sprays per nostril/day.
*Pediatrics:* 6-14 yrs: Initial: 1 spray per nostril tid or 2 sprays per nostril bid. Max: 4 sprays per nostril/day.

**HOW SUPPLIED:** Spray: 25mcg/spray [25mL]

**CONTRAINDICATIONS:** Untreated localized infection of the nasal mucosa.

**WARNINGS/PRECAUTIONS:** Risk of adrenal insufficiency and withdrawal symptoms when replacing systemic corticosteroids with a topical corticosteroids. Caution with active or quiescent TB, ocular herpes simplex, or untreated bacterial, fungal and systemic viral infections. Avoid with recent nasal trauma, surgery or septum ulcers. Risk for more severe/fatal course of infections (eg, chickenpox, measles) and for *Candida* infections of the nose and pharynx.

**ADVERSE REACTIONS:** Nasal congestion, sneezing, epistaxis, bloody mucous, nasal irritation, watery eyes, sore throat, nausea, vomiting, headache.

**INTERACTIONS:** Concomitant systemic corticosteroids increases risk of hypercorticism and/or HPA axis suppression.

**PREGNANCY:** Category C, caution in nursing.

## FLUOROPLEX RX

fluorouracil (Allergan)

**THERAPEUTIC CLASS:** Antimetabolite

**INDICATIONS:** Topical treatment of multiple actinic (solar) keratoses.

**DOSAGE:** *Adults:* Apply bid for 2-6 weeks. Increased frequency and longer treatment periods may be required for areas other than the head and neck. Wash hands immediately after application.

**HOW SUPPLIED:** Cre: 1% [30g]; Sol: 1% [30mL]

**CONTRAINDICATIONS:** Pregnancy.

**WARNINGS/PRECAUTIONS:** Avoid mucous membranes. Caution with occlusive dressings. Avoid prolonged sun/UV light exposure. Increased absorption with ulcerated or inflamed skin. Confirm diagnosis with biopsy. Skin reactions such as erosion, ulceration, and necrosis occur before re-epithelization; d/c therapy at this point. Delayed hypersensitivity reported.

**ADVERSE REACTIONS:** Pain, pruritus, burning, irritations, inflammation, allergic contact dermatitis, telangiectasia, hyperpigmentation, scarring.

**PREGNANCY:** Category X, not for use in nursing.

## FLUPHENAZINE

RX

fluphenazine HCl (Various)

**OTHER BRAND NAMES:** Prolixin Decanoate (Sandoz) - Prolixin (Bristol-Myers Squibb)

**THERAPEUTIC CLASS:** Piperazine phenothiazine

**INDICATIONS:** (HCl) Management of psychotic disorders. (Decanoate) Long-acting formulation for prolonged parenteral neuroleptic therapy.

**DOSAGE:** *Adults:* (PO) Initial: 2.5-10mg/day in divided doses q6-8h. Titrate: May increase up to 40mg/day. Maint: 1-5mg qd. Elderly: Initial: 1-2.5mg/day. (Inj, HCl) Initial: 1.25mg IM q6-8h. Max: 10mg/day. (Decanoate) Initial: 12.5-25mg IM/SQ every 4-6 weeks. Max: 100mg/dose. For doses >50mg, succeeding doses should be increased in increments of 12.5mg.

**HOW SUPPLIED:** (HCl) Inj: 2.5mg/mL; Elixir: 2.5mg/5mL; Sol, Concentrate: 5mg/mL; Tab: 1mg, 5mg, 10mg; (Decanoate) Inj: 25mg/mL.

**CONTRAINDICATIONS:** Comatose state, severe depression, concomitant large dose hypnotics, blood dyscrasia, hepatic impairment, subcortical brain damage, cross-sensitivity to phenothiazine derivatives.

**WARNINGS/PRECAUTIONS:** May develop tardive dyskinesia, NMS. Caution with history of cholestatic jaundice, dermatoses or allergic reactions to phenothiazine derivatives. Elevated prolactin levels reported. Avoid abrupt withdrawal. Caution if exposed to extreme heat or phosphorous insecticides, seizure disorder, cardiovascular disease, pheochromocytoma. May develop liver damage, pigmentary retinopathy, lenticular and corneal dyskinesias with prolonged therapy. Monitor for hypotension in patients on large doses undergoing surgery.

**ADVERSE REACTIONS:** Extrapyramidal symptoms, tardive dyskinesia, HTN, hypotension, allergic reactions, nausea, loss of appetite, dry mouth, headache, constipation, perspiration, salivation, polyuria, hepatic dysfunction.

**INTERACTIONS:** Potentiates alcohol effects. Reduce dose of anesthetics or CNS depressants prior to surgery. May potentiate anticholinergics.

**PREGNANCY:** Safety in pregnancy or nursing not known.

## FLUTAMIDE

RX

flutamide (Various)

**Hepatic injury reported; discontinue if jaundice occurs or if ALT >2X ULN. Monitor LFTs monthly for first 4 months and periodically thereafter.**

**THERAPEUTIC CLASS:** Nonsteroidal antiandrogen

**INDICATIONS:** In combination with lutenizing hormone releasing hormone (LHRH) agonist for treatment of locally confined Stage $B_2$-C and Stage $D_2$ metastatic prostate carcinoma.

**DOSAGE:** *Adults:* 250mg q8h.

**HOW SUPPLIED:** Cap: 125mg

**CONTRAINDICATIONS:** Severe hepatic impairment.

**WARNINGS/PRECAUTIONS:** Monitor PSA regularly. If disease progression is evident, discontinue therapy and continue LHRH agonist. Monitor methemoglobin levels in G6PD deficiency, hemoglobin M disease, or smokers.

**ADVERSE REACTIONS:** Hot flashes, loss of libido, impotence, diarrhea, nausea, vomiting, gynecomastia, other GI disturbances, anemia, edema, hepatitis, jaundice, skin rash.

**INTERACTIONS:** May increase PT; monitor warfarin.

**PREGNANCY:** Category D, safety in nursing is not known.

## FLUVIRIN RX
influenza virus vaccine (Chiron)

**THERAPEUTIC CLASS:** Vaccine

**INDICATIONS:** Immunization against influenza viruses containing antigens related to those in the vaccine.

F

**DOSAGE:** *Adults:* 0.5mL IM in deltoid or thigh single dose. Shake well. *Pediatrics:* >4 yrs: 0.5mL IM. <9 yrs (Not Previously Vaccinated): Repeat dose minimum 1 month apart. Administer in deltoid muscle to older children and thigh muscle in infants and young children.

**HOW SUPPLIED:** Inj: 45mcg/0.5mL

**CONTRAINDICATIONS:** Allergy to chicken eggs, chicken, chicken feathers, chicken dander, or thimerosal (a mercury derivative). Delay administration to patients with an active neurological disorder or an acute febrile illness until disease stabilizes or symptoms subside. History of any neurological signs or symptoms following administration of any vaccine is contraindicated to further use.

**WARNINGS/PRECAUTIONS:** Do not administer in children younger than 6 months. Caution in children between the ages of 6 months through 4 years. Caution with thrombocytopenia, coagulation disorders, and impaired immune responses.

**ADVERSE REACTIONS:** Soreness at the injection site, fever, malaise, myalgia.

**INTERACTIONS:** Immunosuppressive therapies (eg, irradiation, corticosteroids, antimetabolites, alkylating and cytotoxic agents) may reduce effectiveness. May inhibit clearance of warfarin and theophylline.

**PREGNANCY:** Category C, safe for use in nursing.

## FLUVOXAMINE MALEATE RX
fluvoxamine maleate (Various)

**Antidepressants increased the risk of suicidal thinking and behavior (suicidality) in short-term studies in children and adolescents with Major Depressive Disorder (MDD) and other psychiatric disorders. Fluvoxamine is not approved for use in pediatric patients except for pateints with Obsessive Compulsive Disorder (OCD).**

**THERAPEUTIC CLASS:** Selective serotonin reuptake inhibitor

**INDICATIONS:** Treatment of OCD.

**DOSAGE:** *Adults:* Initial: 50mg qhs. Titrate: Increase by 50mg every 4-7 days. Maint: 100-300mg/day. Give bid if total dose >100mg daily. Max: 300mg/day. Elderly/Hepatic Impairment: Modify initial dose and titration.
*Pediatrics:* 8-17 yrs: Initial: 25mg qhs. Titrate: Increase by 25mg every 4-7 days. Maint: 50-200mg/day. Max: 8-11 yrs: 200mg/day. Adolescents: 300mg/day. Give bid if total dose >50mg daily.

**HOW SUPPLIED:** Tab: 25mg, 50mg*, 100mg* *scored

**CONTRAINDICATIONS:** Co-administration of thioridazine, terfenadine, astemizole, cisapride, pimozide, alosetron, tizanidine.

**WARNINGS/PRECAUTIONS:** Activation of mania/hypomania, SIADH, and hyponatremia reported. Close supervision with high risk suicide patients. Caution with history of seizures, hepatic dysfunction, with conditions altering metabolism or hemodynamic responses. Smoking increases metabolism.

**ADVERSE REACTIONS:** Headache, asthenia, nausea, diarrhea, vomiting, anorexia, dyspepsia, insomnia, somnolence, nervousness, agitation, dizziness, anxiety, dry mouth, sweating, tremor, abnormal ejaculation.

**INTERACTIONS:** See Contraindications. May potentiate metoprolol, propranolol. Avoid alcohol, diazepam, terfenadine, astemizole, cisapride, primozide. Increases serum levels of theophylline, warfarin, clozapine, carbamazepine, methadone. Bradycardia with diltiazem. Potential for serious, fatal interactions with MAOIs. Lithium may increase serotonergic effects. Reduces clearance of mexiletine and benzodiazepines metabolized by hepatic oxidation (eg, alprazolam, midazolam, triazolam). Caution with sumatriptan, TCAs, tryptophan. Avoid thioridazine; produces dose-related QTc interval prolongation. Increases tacrine serum levels.

**PREGNANCY:** Category C, not for use in nursing.



## FLUZONE RX

influenza virus vaccine (Sanofi Pasteur)

**THERAPEUTIC CLASS:** Vaccine

**INDICATIONS:** Active immunization against influenza disease caused by influenza virus types A and B contained in vaccine in subjects from 6 months of age and older.

**DOSAGE:** *Adults:* 0.5mL IM in the deltoid muscle.
*Pediatrics:* ≥9 yrs: 0.5mL IM. 3-8 yrs: 0.5mL IM. 6-35 months: 0.25mL IM. Children <9 yrs who have not previously been vaccinated should recevie two doses of vaccine ≥1 month apart. Older children should be given the IM injection in deltoid muscle, infants and young children should receive the IM injection in the anterolateral aspect of the thigh.

**HOW SUPPLIED:** Inj: 0.25mL, 0.5mL

**CONTRAINDICATIONS:** Hypersensitivity reactions to egg proteins or to chicken proteins. Vaccination may be postponed in case of febrile or acute disease. Immunization should be delayed in patients with an active neurologic disorder.

**WARNINGS/PRECAUTIONS:** Avoid in individuals who have a prior history of Guillain-Barre syndrome and in patients with bleeding disorders, such as hemophilia or thrombocytopenia or if patients is on anticoagulant therapy. Immunosuppressed patients may not obtain expected antibody response. Have epinephrine injection (1:1000) available.

**ADVERSE REACTIONS:** Local: soreness, pain, swelling. Systemic: fever, malaise, myalgia.

**PREGNANCY:** Category C, safety in nursing not known.

## FML RX

fluorometholone (Allergan)

**OTHER BRAND NAMES:** FML Forte (Allergan)

**THERAPEUTIC CLASS:** Corticosteroid

**INDICATIONS:** Treatment of inflammation of the palpebral and bulbar conjunctiva, cornea, and anterior segment of the globe.

**DOSAGE:** *Adults:* (Sus) 1 drop bid-qid or (Oint) apply 1/2 inch qd-tid. May give 0.1% q4h during initial 24-48 hrs. Re-evaluate after 2 days if no improvement.
*Pediatrics:* >2 yrs: (Sus) 1 drop bid-qid or (Oint) apply 1/2 inch qd-tid. May give 0.1% q4h during initial 24-48 hrs. Re-evaluate after 2 days if no improvement.

**HOW SUPPLIED:** Oint: (S.O.P.) 0.1% [3.5g]; Sus: 0.1% [5mL, 10mL, 15mL]; (Forte) 0.25% [2mL, 5mL, 10mL, 15mL]

**CONTRAINDICATIONS:** Viral diseases of the cornea and conjunctiva including epithelial herpes simplex keratitis, vaccinia, and varicella. Mycobacterial infection and fungal diseases of the eye.

**WARNINGS/PRECAUTIONS:** Caution with glaucoma, herpes simplex, diseases causing thinning of cornea/sclera and other ocular viral infections. Prolonged use can cause glaucoma or secondary ocular infections (eg, fungal). Monitor IOP after 10 days of therapy. Re-evaluate if no response after 2 days. Ointment may retard corneal healing. May delay healing and increase incidence of bleb formation after cataract surgery. Avoid abrupt withdrawal with chronic use.

**ADVERSE REACTIONS:** Elevation of IOP, glaucoma, infrequent optic nerve damage, posterior subcapsular cataract formation, delayed wound healing, burning/stinging upon instillation, ocular irritation, taste perversion, visual disturbance.

**PREGNANCY:** Category C, not for use in nursing.



## FOCALIN

**CII**

dexmethylphenidate HCl (Novartis)

**THERAPEUTIC CLASS:** Sympathomimetic amine

**INDICATIONS:** Treatment of attention deficit hyperactivity disorder (ADHD).

**DOSAGE:** *Adults:* Take bid at least 4 hrs apart. Methylphenidate Naive: Initial: 2.5mg bid. Titrate: Increase weekly by 2.5-5mg/day. Max: 20mg/day. Currently on Methylphenidate: Initial: Take 1/2 of methylphenidate dose. Max: 20mg/day. Reduce or discontinue if paradoxical aggravation of symptoms. Discontinue if no improvement after appropriate dosage adjustments over 1 month.
*Pediatrics:* >6 yrs: Take bid at least 4 hrs apart. Methylphenidate Naive: Initial: 2.5mg bid. Titrate: Increase weekly by 2.5-5mg/day. Max: 20mg/day. Currently on Methylphenidate: Initial: Take 1/2 of methylphenidate dose. Max: 20mg/day. Reduce or discontinue if paradoxical aggravation of symptoms. Discontinue if no improvement after appropriate dosage adjustments over 1 month.

**HOW SUPPLIED:** Tab: 2.5mg, 5mg, 10mg

**CONTRAINDICATIONS:** Marked anxiety, tension, and agitation; glaucoma; motor tics or family history or diagnosis of Tourette's syndrome; during or within 14 days of MAOI use.

**WARNINGS/PRECAUTIONS:** Caution in drug dependence or alcoholism. Avoid with known serious structural cardiac abnormalities, cardiomyopathy, serious heart rhythm abnormalities, CAD, or other serious cardiac problems. May cause modest increase in BP; caution with HTN, heart failure, recent MI, or ventricular arrhythmia. May exacerbate symptoms of behavior disturbance and thought disorder with pre-existing psychotic disorder. Caution when using stimulants to treat patients with comorbid bipolar disorder becuase of concern for possible induction of mixed/manic episodes in such patients. Stimulants at usual doses may cause treatment-emergent psychotic or manic symptoms (eg, hallucinations, delusional thinking, mania) in children and adolescents without prior history of psychotic illness or mania. Aggressive behavior or hostility reported in clinical trials and the postmarketing experience of some medications indicated for the treatment of ADHD. Suppression of growth reported with long-term use; monitor growth. May lower convulsive threshold; d/c in the presence of seizures. Visual disturbances reported. Monitor CBC, differential, and platelets with prolonged therapy.

**ADVERSE REACTIONS:** Abdominal pain, fever, anorexia, nausea, nervousness, insomnia. (Pediatrics) Loss of appetite, weight loss, tachycardia.

**INTERACTIONS:** See Contraindications. May decrease the effectiveness of antihypertensives. Caution with pressor agents. May inhibit metabolism of coumarin anticoagulants, anticonvulsants, and some antidepressants; adjust dose. Adverse events reported with clonidine.

**PREGNANCY:** Category C, caution in nursing.

## FOCALIN XR

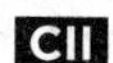

dexmethylphenidate HCl (Novartis)

**THERAPEUTIC CLASS:** Sympathomimetic amine

**INDICATIONS:** Treatment of attention deficit hyperactivity disorder (ADHD) in patients aged 6 yrs and older.

**DOSAGE:** *Adults:* Methylphenidate Naive: Initial: 10mg/day. Titrate: May adjust weekly by 10mg/day. Max: 20mg/day. Currently on Methylphenidate: Initial: Take 1/2 of methylphenidate dose. Max: 20mg/day. Reduce or discontinue if paradoxical aggravation of symptoms. Swallow capsule whole or sprinkle contents on applesauce. Contents should not be crushed, chewed or divided. Discontinue if no improvement after appropriate dosage adjustments over 1 month.

*Pediatrics:* ≥6 yrs: Methylphenidate Naive: Initial: 5mg/day. Titrate: May adjust weekly by 5mg/day. Max: 20mg/day. Currently on Methylphenidate: Initial: Take 1/2 of methylphenidate dose. Max: 20mg/day. Reduce or discontinue if paradoxical aggravation of symptoms. Swallow capsule whole or sprinkle contents on applesauce: contents should not be crushed, chewed or divided. Discontinue if no improvement after appropriate dosage adjustments over 1 month.

**HOW SUPPLIED:** Cap, Extended Release: 5mg, 10mg, 15mg, 20mg

**CONTRAINDICATIONS:** Marked anxiety, tension, and agitation; glaucoma; motor tics or family history or diagnosis of Tourette's syndrome; during or within 14 days of MAOI use.

**WARNINGS/PRECAUTIONS:** Caution in drug dependence or alcoholism. Avoid with known serious structural cardiac abnormalities, cardiomyopathy, serious heart rhythm abnormalities, CAD, or other serious cardiac problems. May cause modest increase in BP; caution with HTN, heart failure, recent MI, or ventricular arrhythmia. May exacerbate symptoms of behavior disturbance and thought disorder with pre-existing psychotic disorder. Caution when using stimulants to treat patients with comorbid bipolar disorder becuase of concern for possible induction of mixed/manic episodes in such patients. Stimulants at usual doses may cause treatment-emergent psychotic or manic symptoms (eg, hallucinations, delusional thinking, mania) in children and adolescents without prior history of psychotic illness or mania. Aggressive behavior or hostility reported in clinical trials and the postmarketing experience of some medications indicated for the treatment of ADHD. Suppression of growth reported with long-term use; monitor growth. May lower convulsive threshold; d/c in the presence of seizures. Visual disturbances reported. Monitor CBC, differential, and platelets with prolonged therapy.

**ADVERSE REACTIONS:** Dyspepsia, headache, anxiety. (Adults) dry mouth, pharyngolaryngeal pain, feeling jittery, dizziness. (Pediatrics) decreased appetite, nausea.

**INTERACTIONS:** See Contraindications. May decrease the effectiveness of antihypertensives. Caution with pressor agents. May inhibit metabolism of coumarin anticoagulants, anticonvulsants, and tricyclic drugs; adjust dose. Adverse events reported with clonidine. Antacids or acid supressants could alter the release of dexmethylphenidate.

**PREGNANCY:** Category C, caution in nursing.

## FOLGARD RX 2.2

RX

folic acid - vitamin B6 - vitamin B12 (Upsher-Smith)

**THERAPEUTIC CLASS:** Folic acid/vitamin combination

**INDICATIONS:** For nutritional support and folic acid supplementation.

**DOSAGE:** *Adults:* 1 tab qd.

**HOW SUPPLIED:** Tab: Folic Acid 2.2mg-Vitamin $B_6$ 25mg-Vitamin $B_{12}$ 0.5mg*
*scored

**WARNINGS/PRECAUTIONS:** Folic acid >0.1mg/day may obscure pernicious anemia.

**ADVERSE REACTIONS:** Allergic sensitization.

**PREGNANCY:** Safety in pregnancy and nursing is not known.

## FOLIC ACID RX

folic acid (Various)

F

**THERAPEUTIC CLASS:** Erythropoiesis agent

**INDICATIONS:** Treatment of megaloblastic anemia due to folic acid deficiency and in anemias of nutritional origin, pregnancy, infancy or childhood.

**DOSAGE:** *Adults:* Usual: Up to 1mg/day. Maint: 0.4mg qd. Pregnancy/Nursing: Maint: 0.8mg qd. Max: 1mg/day. Increase maintenance dose with alcoholism, hemolytic anemia, anticonvulsant therapy, chronic infection.
*Pediatrics:* Usual: Up to 1mg/day. Maint: Infants: 0.1mg qd. <4 yrs: 0.3mg qd. >4 yrs: 0.4mg qd.

**HOW SUPPLIED:** Inj: 5mg/mL; Tab: (OTC) 0.4mg, 0.8mg. (RX) 1mg

**WARNINGS/PRECAUTIONS:** Not for monotherapy in pernicious anemia and other megaloblastic anemias with $B_{12}$ deficiency. May obscure pernicious anemia in dosage >0.1 mg/day. Decreased $B_{12}$ serum levels with prolonged therapy.

**ADVERSE REACTIONS:** Allergic sensitization.

**INTERACTIONS:** Antagonizes phenytoin effects. Methotrexate, phenytoin, primidone, barbiturates, alcohol, alcoholic cirrhosis, nitrofurantoin, and pyrimethamine increase loss of folate. Increased seizures with phenytoin, primidone and phenobarbital reported. Tetracycline may cause false low serum and red cell folate due to suppression of Lactobacillus casei.

**PREGNANCY:** Category A, requirement increases during nursing.

## FOLLISTIM AQ RX

follitropin beta (Organon)

**OTHER BRAND NAMES:** Follistim AQ Cartridge (Organon)

**THERAPEUTIC CLASS:** Follicle stimulating hormone

**INDICATIONS:** For the development of multiple follicles in ovulatory patients participating in Assisted Reproductive Technology (ART). For the induction of ovulation and pregnancy in anovulatory infertile patients in whom the cause of infertility is functional and not due to primary ovarian failure.

**DOSAGE:** *Adults:* Ovulation Induction: Cartridge: 75 IU for 7 days. Titrate: Adjust dose at weekly intervals. Inj: 75 IU for 14 days. Titrate: increase by 37.5 IU weekly. Administer hCG 5000-10,000 U when pre-ovulatory conditions are equivalent to or greater than a normal individual. ART: Initial 150 to 225 IU for 5 days (cartridge) or 4 days (inj). Titrate: Adjust based upon ovarian response. Administer hCG 5000-10,000 U when a sufficient number of follicles of adequate size are present.

**HOW SUPPLIED:** Cartridge: 150 IU, 300 IU, 600 IU, 900 IU. Inj: 75 IU, 150 IU

**CONTRAINDICATIONS:** High FSH level indicating primary ovarian failure, uncontrolled thyroid or adrenal dysfunction, pregnancy, heavy or irregular vaginal bleeding of undetermined origin, ovarian cysts or enlargement not due to polycystic ovary syndrome; or tumor of the ovary, breast, uterus, hypothalamus or pituitary gland. Hypersensitivity to streptomycin or neomycin and to recombinant hFSH products.

**WARNINGS/PRECAUTIONS:** Exclude primary ovarian failure. Ovarian enlargement may occur; use the lowest effective dose and monitor ovarian response. Ovarian hyperstimulation syndrome (OHSS), multiple births, serious pulmonary and vascular complications reported. Avoid hCG if ovaries abnormally enlarged last day of therapy. Monitor follicular maturation by measuring estradiol levels and through sonographic visualization.

**ADVERSE REACTIONS:** Abdominal pain, flatulence, nausea, breast pain, injection site reaction, enlarged abdomen, back pain, constipation, headache, ovarian pain, OHSS, sinusitis, upper respiratory tract infection.

**PREGNANCY:** Category X, not for use in nursing.

## FOLTX

RX

folic acid - vitamin B6 - vitamin B12 (PamLab)

**THERAPEUTIC CLASS:** Folic acid/vitamin combination

**INDICATIONS:** To supply nutritional requirements for those with end stage renal failure, dialysis, hyperhomocystenimia, homocystinuria, nutrient malabsorption.

**DOSAGE:** *Adults:* 1-2 tabs qd.

**HOW SUPPLIED:** Tab: Folic Acid 2.5mg-Vitamin $B_6$ 25mg-Vitamin $B_{12}$ 2mg

**WARNINGS/PRECAUTIONS:** Folic acid >0.1mg/day may obscure pernicious anemia (may be alleviated by $B_{12}$ component).

**ADVERSE REACTIONS:** Allergic sensitization, paresthesia, somnolence, mild diarrhea, polycythemia vera, peripheral vascular thrombosis, itching, transitory exanthema, feeling of body swelling.

**INTERACTIONS:** Pyridoxine may antagonize levodopa; avoid concomitant use. May be used with carbidopa/levodopa. Decreases effect of phenytoin.

## FORADIL

RX

formoterol fumarate (Schering)

**Long-acting $\beta_2$-agonists may increase the risk of asthma-related death.**

**THERAPEUTIC CLASS:** $Beta_2$ agonist

**INDICATIONS:** Long-term maintenance treatment of asthma and prevention of bronchospasm with reversible obstructive airway disease (including nocturnal asthma) in patients who require regular treatment with inhaled short acting $\beta_2$-agonists. Maintenance treatment of bronchoconstriction in chronic obstructive pulmonary disease (COPD). Acute prevention of excercise-induced bronchospasm (EIB).

**DOSAGE:** *Adults:* Do not swallow cap; give only by inhalation with Aerolizer Inhaler. Asthma/COPD: 12mcg q12h. Max: 24mcg/day. EIB: 12mcg 15 minutes before exercise (do not give added dose if already on q12h dose).
*Pediatrics:* >5 yrs: Do not swallow cap; give only by inhalation with Aerolizer™ Inhaler. Asthma/COPD: 12mcg q12h. Max: 24mcg/day. ≥12 yrs: EIB: 12mcg 15 minutes before exercise (do not give added dose if already on q12h dose).

**HOW SUPPLIED:** Cap (Inhalation): 12mcg [$12^s$, $60^s$]

**WARNINGS/PRECAUTIONS:** Do not discontinue inhaled corticosteroids. Only use short-acting $\beta_2$-agonist inhaler for acute symptoms. Discontinue if paradoxical bronchospasm occurs. Discontinue if ECG changes, QT interval increases, or ST depression occurs. Caution with cardiovascular disorders (eg, HTN, arrhythmias), thyrotoxicosis and convulsive disorders. Anaphylactic and other allergic reactions reported. Not for use in acute asthmatic conditions. Should not be used with other long-acting $\beta_2$-agonist medications. May cause hypokalemia.

**ADVERSE REACTIONS:** Viral infection, dyspnea, chest pain, tremor, HTN, hypotension, tachycardia, arrhythmias, headache, nausea, vomiting, fatigue, hypokalemia, hyperglycemia, exacerbation of asthma.

**INTERACTIONS:** Potentiates other sympathomimetics. Hypokalemia potentiated by xanthine derivatives (eg, theophylline), steroids and nonpotassium sparing diuretics. Extreme caution with MAOIs, TCAs, and drugs known to prolong QT interval. Antagonized effect with β-blockers.

**PREGNANCY:** Category C, caution in nursing.

## FORTAMET
RX

metformin HCl (Sciele)

**THERAPEUTIC CLASS:** Biguanide

**INDICATIONS:** Adjunct to diet or with a sulfonylurea or insulin, to improve glycemic control in type 2 diabetes mellitus.

F

**DOSAGE:** *Adults:* ≥17 yrs: Take with evening meal. Initial: 500-1000mg qd. With Insulin: Initial: 500mg qd. Titrate: May increase by 500mg/week. Max: 2500mg/day. Decrease insulin dose by 10-25% if FPG <120mg/dL. Elderly/Debilitated/Malnourished: Conservative dosing; do not titrate to max.

**HOW SUPPLIED:** Tab, Extended Release: 500mg, 1000mg

**CONTRAINDICATIONS:** Renal disease/dysfunction (SrCr ≥1.5mg/dL [males], ≥1.4mg/dL [females], abnormal CrCl), CHF, metabolic acidosis, diabetic ketoacidosis. Discontinue temporarily (48 hrs) for radiologic studies with intravascular iodinated contrast materials.

**WARNINGS/PRECAUTIONS:** Lactic acidosis reported (rare); increased risk with renal dysfunction, increased age, DM, CHF, and other conditions with risk of hypoperfusion and hypoxemia. Avoid use in patients ≥80 yrs unless renal function is normal. Monitor renal function and for ketoacidosis and metabolic acidosis. Avoid in renal/hepatic impairment. Discontinue in hypoxic states (eg, CHF, shock, acute MI), loss of blood glucose control due to stress (give insulin), acidosis, dehydration, sepsis. Temporarily discontinue prior to surgery (due to restricted food intake) and procedures requiring intravascular iodinated contrast materials. May decrease serum vitamin $B_{12}$ levels. Increased risk of hypoglycemia in elderly, debilitated/malnourished, adrenal or pituitary insufficiency, or alcohol intoxication.

**ADVERSE REACTIONS:** Diarrhea, nausea, dyspepsia, flatulence, abdominal pain.

**INTERACTIONS:** Furosemide, nifedipine, cimetidine, cationic drugs (eg, digoxin, amiloride, procainamide, quinidine, quinine, ranitidine, trimethoprim, vancomycin, triamterene, morphine) may increase metformin levels. Thiazides, other diuretics, corticosteroids, phenothiazines, thyroid products, estrogens, oral contraceptives, phenytoin, nicotinic acid, sympathomimetics, calcium channel blockers, isoniazid may cause hyperglycemia. Risk of hypoglycemia with alcohol. Excess alcohol may increase potential for lactic acidosis. May decrease furosemide levels.

**PREGNANCY:** Category B, not for use in nursing.

## FORTAZ
RX

ceftazidime (GlaxoSmithKline)

**THERAPEUTIC CLASS:** Cephalosporin (3rd generation)

**INDICATIONS:** Treatment of lower respiratory tract (eg, pneumonia), skin and skin structure (SSSI), bone and joint, gynecologic, CNS (eg, meningitis), intra-abdominal, and urinary tract infections (UTI), and septicemia. For use in sepsis.

**DOSAGE:** *Adults:* Usual: 1g IM/IV q8-12h. Uncomplicated UTI: 250mg IM/IV q12h. Complicated UTI: 500mg IM/IV q8-12h. Bone and Joint Infection: 2g IV q12h. Uncomplicated Pneumonia/SSSI: 500mg-1g IM/IV q8h. Gynecological/Intra-Abdominal/Meningitis/Severe Life-Threatening Infection: 2g IV q8h. Lung Infection Caused by *Pseudomonas* spp. in Cystic Fibrosis (normal renal function): 30-50mg/kg IV q8h. Max: 6g/day. CrCl 31-50mL/min: 1g q12h. CrCl 16-30mL/min: 1g q24h. CrCl 6-15mL/min: 500mg q24h. CrCl <5mL/min: 500mg q48h. For severe infections (6g/day), increase renal

impairment dose by 50% or increase dosing interval. Apply reduced dosage recommendations after initial 1g LD is given. Hemodialysis: Give 1g before then 1g after each hemodialysis. Intra-Peritoneal Dialysis/Continuous Ambulatory Peritoneal Dialysis: Give 1g followed by 500mg q24h, or add to fluid at 250mg/2L.
*Pediatrics:* 1 month-12 yrs: 30-50mg/kg IV q8h. Max: 6g/day. Neonates (0-4 weeks): 30mg/kg IV q12h. Higher doses for cystic fibrosis or meningitis. CrCl 31-50mL/min: 1g q12h. CrCl 16-30mL/min: 1g q24h. CrCl 6-15mL/min: 500mg q24h. CrCl <5mL/min: 500mg q48h. For severe infections (6g/day), increase renal impairment dose by 50% or increase dosing interval. Apply reduced dosage recommendations after initial 1g LD is given. Hemodialysis: Give 1g before then 1g after each hemodialysis. Intra-Peritoneal Dialysis/Continuous Ambulatory Peritoneal Dialysis: Give 1g followed by 500mg q24h, or add to fluid at 250mg/2L.



**HOW SUPPLIED:** Inj: 500mg, 1g, 1g/50mL, 2g, 2g/50mL, 6g

**WARNINGS/PRECAUTIONS:** Monitor renal function; potential for nephrotoxicity. Prolonged use may result in overgrowth of nonsusceptible organisms. Possible cross-sensitivity between penicillins, cephalosporins, and other β-lactam antibiotics. Pseudomembranous colitis reported. Elevated levels with renal insufficiency can lead to seizures, encephalopathy, coma, asterixis and neuromuscular excitability. Possible decrease in PT; caution with renal or hepatic impairment, poor nutritional state; monitor PT and give vitamin K if needed. Caution with colitis, other GI diseases, and the elderly. Distal necrosis can occur after inadvertent intra-arterial administration. Continue therapy for 2 days after the signs and symptoms of infection have disappeared, but in complicated infections longer therapy may be required. False positive for urine glucose with Benedict's solution, Fehling's solution, and Clinitest tablets.

**ADVERSE REACTIONS:** Phlebitis and inflammation at injection site, pruritus, rash, fever, diarrhea.

**INTERACTIONS:** Nephrotoxicity reported with cephalosporins or potent diuretics (eg, furosemide). Avoid with chloramphenicol; may decrease effect of β-lactam antibiotics. Possible decrease in PT; caution with a protracted course of antimicrobial therapy; monitor PT and give vitamin K if needed. May reduced efficacy of oral contraceptives.

**PREGNANCY:** Category B, caution in nursing.

## FORTEO

RX

teriparatide (Lilly)

**Increased incidence of osteosarcoma seen in rats. Only prescribe when benefits outweigh risks. Not for those at increased baseline risk for osteosarcoma, including Paget's disease or unexplained alkaline phosphatase elevations, open epiphyses, or prior radiation therapy involving the skeleton.**

**THERAPEUTIC CLASS:** Recombinant human parathyroid hormone

**INDICATIONS:** Treatment of postmenopausal women with osteoporosis who are at high risk for fracture. To increase bone mass in men with primary or hypogonadal osteoporosis who are at high risk for fracture.

**DOSAGE:** *Adults:* 20mcg qd SQ into thigh or abdominal wall. Administer initially under circumstances where patient can sit or lie down if symptoms of orthostatic hypotension occur. Discard pen after 28 days. Use for >2 yrs is not recommended.

**HOW SUPPLIED:** Inj: 250mcg/mL [3mL pen]

**WARNINGS/PRECAUTIONS:** Avoid in pediatrics, or with bone metastases, or history of skeletal malignancies, metabolic bone diseases other than osteoporosis, or pre-existing hypercalcemia (eg, primary hyperparathyroidism). Potential exacerbation of active or recent urolithiasis.

Transient episodes of symptomatic orthostatic hypotension observed infrequently. Increases serum uric acid levels. Transient calcium increases.

**ADVERSE REACTIONS:** Pain, arthralgia, asthenia, nausea, rhinitis, dizziness, headache, HTN, increased cough, pharyngitis, constipation, diarrhea, dyspepsia.

**INTERACTIONS:** Hypercalcemia may predispose to digitalis toxicity; caution with concomitant use.

**PREGNANCY:** Category C; not for use in nursing.

## FORTICAL RX

calcitonin-salmon (rdna origin) (Upsher-Smith)



**THERAPEUTIC CLASS:** Hormonal bone resorption inhibitor

**INDICATIONS:** Treatment of postmenopausal osteoporosis in females >5 yrs postmenopause in conjunction with an adequate calcium and vitamin D intake.

**DOSAGE:** *Adults:* 200 IU qd intranasally. Alternate nostrils daily.

**HOW SUPPLIED:** Nasal Spray: 200 IU/inh

**CONTRAINDICATIONS:** Clinical allergy to calcitonin-salmon.

**WARNINGS/PRECAUTIONS:** Possibility of systemic allergic reactions. Consider skin testing if sensitivity suspected. If nasal mucosa ulceration occurs, discontinue until healed. Discontinue if severe ulceration of the nasal mucosa occurs. Perform periodic nasal exams. The incidence of rhinitis, irritation, erythema, and excoriation was higher in geriatric patients.

**ADVERSE REACTIONS:** Rhinitis, nasal symptoms, back pain, arthralgia, epistaxis, headache

**PREGNANCY:** Category C, not for use in nursing.

## FORTOVASE RX

saquinavir (Roche Labs)

**THERAPEUTIC CLASS:** Protease inhibitor

**INDICATIONS:** Treatment of HIV infection in combination with other antiretrovirals.

**DOSAGE:** *Adults:* 1200mg tid with meals or up to 2 hrs after meals. *Pediatrics:* >16 yrs: 1200mg tid with meals or up to 2 hrs after meals.

**HOW SUPPLIED:** Cap: 200mg

**CONTRAINDICATIONS:** Concomitant terfenadine, cisapride, astemizole, triazolam, midazolam, or ergot derivatives.

**WARNINGS/PRECAUTIONS:** Not interchangeable with saquinavir mesylate formulation. New onset DM, exacerbation of pre-existing DM, and hyperglycemia may occur. Exacerbation of chronic liver dysfunction reported with hepatitis or cirrhosis. Spontaneous bleeding may occur with hemophilia A and B. Possible redistribution or accumulation of body fat. Caution with hepatic dysfunction. Interrupt therapy if serious toxicity occurs.

**ADVERSE REACTIONS:** Nausea, diarrhea, abdominal discomfort, dyspepsia, flatulence, headache, fatigue.

**INTERACTIONS:** Avoid terfenadine, cisapride, astemizole, triazolam, midazolam, ergot derivatives, lovastatin, St. John's wort, and simvastatin. Decreased plasma levels with nevirapine. Consider alternatives to rifampin, rifabutin. Ritonavir increases adverse effects. Delavirdine increases plasma levels; monitor LFTs frequently. Ketoconazole, nelfinavir, indinavir increase plasma levels. Increased plasma levels of both clarithromycin and saquinavir. Increased sildenafil plasma levels; consider 25mg as initial sildenafil dose. Carbamazepine, phenobarbital, phenytoin, dexamethasone may decrease plasma levels.

**PREGNANCY:** Category B, not for use in nursing.

## FOSAMAX

RX

alendronate sodium (Merck)

**THERAPEUTIC CLASS:** Bisphosphonate

**INDICATIONS:** Treatment and prevention of osteoporosis in postmenopausal women. Treatment to increase bone mass in men with osteoporosis. Treatment of glucocorticoid-induced osteoporosis. Treatment of Paget's disease.

**DOSAGE:** *Adults:* Osteoporosis: Treatment: 70mg once weekly or 10mg qd. Prevention: 35mg once weekly or 5mg qd. Glucocorticoid-Induced: 5mg qd; 10mg qd for postmenopausal women not on estrogen. Paget's Disease: 40mg qd for 6 months. Take at least 30 minutes before the first food, beverage (other than water), or medication (Take tabs with 6-8 oz plain water or 2 oz with oral sol). Do not lie down for at least 30 minutes and until after the first food of the day.

**HOW SUPPLIED:** Sol: 70mg [75mL]; Tab: 5mg, 10mg, 35mg, 40mg, 70mg

**CONTRAINDICATIONS:** Esophagus abnormalities which delay esophageal emptying such as stricture or achalasia; inability to stand or sit upright for at least 30 minutes; hypocalcemia.

**WARNINGS/PRECAUTIONS:** Caution with active upper GI problems. May cause local irritation of the upper GI mucosa. Correct hypocalcemia or other mineral metabolism disturbances before initiating therapy. Supplement calcium and vitamin D if needed. Not recommended with renal insufficiency (CrCl <35mL/min). D/C if symptoms of esophageal disease develop. When combined with glucocorticoids, perform BMD test at initiation and 6-12 months later. Reports of severe, incapacitating bone, joint, and/or muscle pain.

**ADVERSE REACTIONS:** Abdominal pain, nausea, dyspepsia, constipation, diarrhea, flatulence, acid regurgitation, musculoskeletal pain, gastric ulcers, joint swelling, asthenia, dizziness/vertigo, and rarely peripheral edema.

**INTERACTIONS:** Calcium supplements, antacids, other oral medications may interfere with absorption; dose at least one-half hour after alendronate. Increased GI irritation with ASA and alendronate >10mg. Caution with NSAIDs, other GI irritants.

**PREGNANCY:** Category C, caution in nursing.

## FOSAMAX PLUS D

RX

cholecalciferol - alendronate sodium (Merck)

**THERAPEUTIC CLASS:** Bisphosphonate/vitamin D analog

**INDICATIONS:** Treatment of osteoporosis in postmenopausal women. Treatment to increase bone mass in men with osteoporosis.

**DOSAGE:** *Adults:* 1 tab (70mg/5600 IU or 70mg/2800 IU) once weekly. Take at least 30 minutes before the first food, beverage (other than water), or medication. Do not lie down for at least 30 minutes and until after first food of the day.

**HOW SUPPLIED:** Tab: (Alendronate Sodium-Cholecalciferol) 70mg-2800 IU, 70mg-5600 IU

**CONTRAINDICATIONS:** Esophagus abnormalities which delay esophageal emptying such as stricture or achalasia; inability to stand or sit upright for at least 30 minutes; hypocalcemia.

**WARNINGS/PRECAUTIONS:** Caution with active upper GI problems. May cause local irritation of the upper GI mucosa. Correct hypocalcemia or other mineral metabolism disturbances before initiating therapy. Do not use to treat vitamin D deficiency. May worsen hypercalcemia and/or hypercalciuria. Supplement calcium if needed. Not recommended with renal insufficiency

(CrCl <35mL/min). Discontinue if symptoms of esophageal disease develop. Reports of severe, incapacitating bone, joint, and/or muscle pain.

**ADVERSE REACTIONS:** Abdominal pain, nausea, dyspepsia, constipation, diarrhea, flatulence, acid regurgitation, musculoskeletal pain, gastric ulcers, joint swelling, asthenia, dizziness/vertigo, and rarely peripheral edema.

**INTERACTIONS:** Calcium supplements, antacids, other oral medications may interfere with absorption; dose at least one-half hour after alendronate. Caution with NSAIDs, other GI irritants. Olestra, mineral oils, orlistat, bile acid sequestrants may impair absorption. Anticonvulsants, cimetidine, thiazides may increase catabolism.

**PREGNANCY:** Category C, caution in nursing.



## FOSCAVIR RX

foscarnet (AstraZeneca LP)

**Renal impairment, seizures reported. Monitor serum creatinine and dose adjust for any changes in renal function. Use in immunocompromised patients with CMV retinitis and mucocutaneous acyclovir-resistant HSV infections.**

**THERAPEUTIC CLASS:** Pyrophosphate binding inhibitor

**INDICATIONS:** Treatment of cytomegalovirus (CMV) retinitis in AIDS patients; combination therapy with ganciclovir in patients that have relapsed from monotherapy. Treatment of mucocutaneous acyclovir-resistant HSV infections in immunocompromised patients.

**DOSAGE:** *Adults:* Induction: CMV retinitis: 90mg/kg q12h or 60mg/kg q8h for 2-3 weeks. Maint: 90-120mg/kg/day. Acyclovir-Resistant HSV: 40mg/kg q8-12h for 2-3 weeks or until healed. Administer 750-1000mL of normal saline or 5% dextrose with 1st infusion to establish diuresis. Then, 750-1000mL with 90-120 mg/kg dose and 500mL with 40-60 mg/kg dose. Use infusion pump to control rate of infusion. See labeling for renal adjustment details.

**HOW SUPPLIED:** Inj: 24mg/mL

**WARNINGS/PRECAUTIONS:** Hydration reduces risk of nephrotoxicity. Anemia, granulocytopenia, serum electrolyte alterations, decrease in ionized serum calcium reported. Infuse into veins with adequate blood flow to avoid local irritation. Avoid rapid administration.

**ADVERSE REACTIONS:** Fever, nausea, vomiting, diarrhea, anemia, renal impairment, hypocalcemia, hypophosphatemia, hyperphosphatemia, hypomagnesemia, hypokalemia, seizures, paresthesia, fatigue.

**INTERACTIONS:** Possible hypocalcemia with pentamidine. Caution with drugs that affect plasma calcium levels. Avoid potentially nephrotoxic drugs (eg, aminoglycosides, amphotericin B). Renal dysfunction reported with ritonavir, saquinavir.

**PREGNANCY:** Category C, safety in nursing not known.

## FOSRENOL RX

lanthanum carbonate (Shire US)

**THERAPEUTIC CLASS:** Phosphate binder

**INDICATIONS:** Reduction of serum phosphate in patients with end-stage renal disease.

**DOSAGE:** *Adults:* Initial: 750-1500mg/day in divided doses. Titrate: Every 2-3 weeks in increments of 750mg/day until acceptable serum phosphate level is reached. Take with meals and chew tablets completely before swallowing. Usual range: 1500-3000mg/day. Usual max: 3750mg/day.

**HOW SUPPLIED:** Tab, Chewable: 250mg, 500mg, 750mg, 1000mg

**WARNINGS/PRECAUTIONS:** Caution with acute peptic ulcer, ulcerative colitis, Crohn's disease or bowel obstruction.

**ADVERSE REACTIONS:** Nausea, vomiting, dialysis graft occulsion, abdominal pain.

**INTERACTIONS:** Should not be taken within 2 hrs of antacids.

**PREGNANCY:** Category C, caution in nursing.

## FRAGMIN

dalteparin sodium (Eisai/Pfizer)

RX

**Risk of paralysis by spinal/epidural hematoma with neuraxial anesthesia or spinal puncture. Increased risk with indwelling epidural catheters for analgesia, drugs affecting hemostasis (eg, NSAIDs, platelet inhibitors, anticoagulants), and traumatic or repeated epidural or spinal puncture.**

**THERAPEUTIC CLASS:** Low molecular weight heparin

**INDICATIONS:** Prevention of ischemic complications in unstable angina and non-Q-wave MI with concurrent ASA therapy. Prophylaxis of DVT in hip replacement surgery, abdominal surgery in patients who are at high risk for thromboembolic complications, and for those at risk for thromboembolic complications due to severely restricted mobility during acute illness. Extended treatment of symptomatic VTE (proximal DVT and/or PE), to reduce the recurrence of VTE in patients with cancer.

**DOSAGE:** *Adults:* Administer SQ. Unstable Angina/Non-Q-Wave MI: 120 IU/kg up to 10,000 IU q12h with ASA (75-165mg/day) for 5-8 days. Hip Surgery: Pre-Op Start: Initial (if start 2 hrs pre-op): 2500 IU within 2 hrs pre-op, then 2500 IU 4-8 hrs post-op. Initial (if start 10-14 hrs pre-op): 5000 IU 10-14 hrs pre-op, then 5000 IU 4-8 hrs post-op. Maint (for either initial dose): 5000 IU SQ qd for 5-10 days post-op (up to 14 days). Post-Op Start: 2500 IU 4-8 hrs post-op. Maint: 5000 IU qd. Abdominal Surgery: 2500 IU 1-2 hrs pre-op. Maint: 2500 IU qd for 5-10 days post-op. Abdominal Surgery with High Risk: 5000 IU evening before surgery. Maint: 5000 IU qd for 5-10 days post-op. Abdominal Surgery with Malignancy: Initial: 2500 IU 1-2 hrs pre-op, then 2500 IU 12 hrs later. Maint: 5000 IU qd for 5-10 days post-op. Severely Restricted Mobility During Acute Illness: 5000 IU qd for 12-14 days. Symptomatic VTE in Cancer Patients: 200 IU/kg qd for first 30 days, then 150 IU/kg qd for months 2-6. Max: 18,000 IU/day. Platelet Count 50,000-100,000/$mm^3$: Reduce dose by 2500 IU until platelet count ≥100,000/$mm^3$. Platelet Count <50,000/$mm^3$: D/C therapy until platelet count >50,000/$mm^3$. Renal Impairment (CrCl <30mL/min): Monitor anti-Xa levels to determine appropriate dose.

**HOW SUPPLIED:** Inj: (Syringe) 2500 IU/0.2mL, 5000 IU/0.2mL, 7500 IU/0.3mL, 10,000 IU/0.4mL, 10,000 IU/mL, 12,500 IU/0.5mL, 15,000 IU/0.6mL, 18,000 IU/0.72mL; (MDV) 25,000 IU/mL [3.8mL], 10,000 IU/mL [9.5mL]

**CONTRAINDICATIONS:** Heparin or pork allergy, regional anesthesia with unstable angina or non-Q-wave MI, active major bleeding, thrombocytopenia with a positive in vitro test for antiplatelet antibody.

**WARNINGS/PRECAUTIONS:** Not for IM injection. Cannot use interchangeably unit for unit with heparin or other low molecular weight heparins. Extreme caution with HIT, conditions with increased risk of hemorrhage (eg, bacterial endocarditis, hemorrhagic stroke, etc). Hemorrhage, thrombocytopenia, HIT may occur. Caution with bleeding diathesis, platelet defects, severe hepatic/kidney dysfunction, hypertensive or diabetic retinopathy, recent GI bleeding or in elderly with low body weight (<45kg) and predisposed to decreased renal function. D/C if thromboembolic event occurs. Perform periodic CBC, platelets, stool occult blood test. Multiple dose vial contains benzyl alcohol.

**ADVERSE REACTIONS:** Hemorrhage, injection site pain, allergic reactions, thrombocytopenia.

**INTERACTIONS:** Caution with oral anticoagulants, platelet inhibitors, thrombolytic agents due to increased risk of bleeding.

**PREGNANCY:** Category B, caution in nursing.

## FROVA

RX

frovatriptan succinate (Endo)

**THERAPEUTIC CLASS:** 5-$HT_{1D,1B}$ agonist

**INDICATIONS:** Acute treatment of migraine with or without aura.

**DOSAGE:** *Adults:* ≥18 yrs: 2.5mg with fluids. If headache recurs after initial relief, may repeat after 2 hrs. Max: 7.5mg/day. Safety of treating >4 headaches/30 days not known.

**HOW SUPPLIED:** Tab: 2.5mg



**CONTRAINDICATIONS:** Ischemic heart disease, coronary artery vasospasm (eg, Prinzmetal's angina), significant cardiovascular disease, cerebrovascular syndromes, peripheral vascular disease, uncontrolled HTN, hemiplegic or basilar migraine, use within 24 hrs of treatment with another 5-$HT_1$ agonist or ergot-type agent.

**WARNINGS/PRECAUTIONS:** Confirm diagnosis. Supervise 1st dose and monitor cardiac function in those at risk of CAD (eg, HTN, hypercholesterolemia, smoker, obesity, diabetes, CAD family history, postmenopausal women, males >40 yrs). Serious adverse cardiac events, cerebrovascular events, vasospastic reactions reported with 5-$HT_1$ agonists. May bind to melanin in the eye; possibility of long-term effects.

**ADVERSE REACTIONS:** Dizziness, headache, paresthesia, dry mouth, dyspepsia, fatigue, hot or cold sensation, chest pain, skeletal pain, flushing.

**INTERACTIONS:** Prolonged vasospastic reactions reported with ergot-containing drugs; avoid use within 24 hours. Avoid within 24 hours of other 5-$HT_{1B/1D}$ agonists. Weakness, hyperreflexia, and incoordination reported with SSRIs (rare).

**PREGNANCY:** Category C, caution in nursing.

## FUDR (STERILE)

RX

floxuridine (Mayne Pharma)

**Hospitalize for 1st course of therapy due to possible severe toxic reactions.**

**THERAPEUTIC CLASS:** Antimetabolite

**INDICATIONS:** Palliative management of GI adenocarcinoma metastatic to the liver.

**DOSAGE:** *Adults:* 0.1-0.6mg/kg/day continuous arterial infusion. Use higher dose (0.4-0.6mg) for hepatic artery infusion. Continue therapy until adverse reactions appear and resume when reactions subside. Maintain on therapy as long as response continues.

**HOW SUPPLIED:** Inj: 0.5g

**CONTRAINDICATIONS:** Poor nutritional state, depressed bone marrow function, potentially serious infections.

**WARNINGS/PRECAUTIONS:** Highly toxic drug with narrow margin of safety. Extreme caution in poor risk patients with renal or hepatic dysfunction, history of high-dose pelvic irradiation, or previous use of alkylating agents. Not intended as an adjuvant to surgery. D/C promptly if myocardial ischemia, stomatitis or esophagopharyngitis, leukopenia, intractable vomiting, diarrhea, GI ulceration and bleeding, thrombocytopenia, or if hemorrhage from any site occur. May cause fetal harm during pregnancy. Carefully monitor WBCs and platelets.

**ADVERSE REACTIONS:** Nausea, vomiting, diarrhea, enteritis, stomatitis, localized erythema, anemia, leukopenia, thrombocytopenia, LFT elevation, alopecia.

**INTERACTIONS:** Increased toxicity with therapies that add stress to patients, interfere with nutrition, or depress bone marrow function.

**PREGNANCY:** Category D, not for use in nursing.

## FURADANTIN RX

nitrofurantoin (Sciele)

**THERAPEUTIC CLASS:** Imidazolidinedione antibacterial

**INDICATIONS:** Treatment of urinary tract infection (UTI).

**DOSAGE:** *Adults:* Usual: 50-100mg qid with food for 1 week or at least 3 days after sterility of urine. Use lower doses for uncomplicated UTI. Long-Term Suppressive Therapy: 50-100mg qhs.
*Pediatrics:* >1 month: Usual: 5-7mg/kg/day given qid with food for 1 week or at least 3 days after sterility of urine. Long-Term Suppressive Therapy: 1mg/kg/day qd or bid.

**HOW SUPPLIED:** Sus: 25mg/5mL

**CONTRAINDICATIONS:** Anuria, oliguria, CrCl <60 mL/min, pregnancy at term (38-42 weeks gestation), during labor and delivery, neonates <1 month of age.

**WARNINGS/PRECAUTIONS:** Acute, subacute or chronic pulmonary reactions have occurred. Enhanced occurrence of peripheral neuropathy with anemia, DM, renal dysfunction, electrolyte imbalance, vitamin B deficiency, and debilitating disease. D/C therapy with acute and chronic pulmonary reactions, hepatic disorders, hemolysis, or peripheral neuropathy. Monitor renal function, LFTs and pulmonary function periodically during long-term therapy. Pseudomembranous colitis reported.

**ADVERSE REACTIONS:** Pulmonary disorders, hepatic damage, peripheral neuropathy, nausea, emesis, anorexia, dizziness, exfoliative dermatitis, Stevens-Johnson syndrome, anaphylaxis, blood dyscrasias.

**INTERACTIONS:** Antacids, especially magnesium trisilicate, decrease rate and extent of absorption. Probenecid and sulfinpyrazone increase nitrofurantoin levels.

**PREGNANCY:** Category B, not for use in nursing.

## FUROSEMIDE RX

furosemide (Various)

**Can lead to profound water and electrolyte depletion with excessive use.**

**OTHER BRAND NAMES:** Lasix (Sanofi-Aventis)

**THERAPEUTIC CLASS:** Loop diuretic

**INDICATIONS:** (Inj, PO) Treatment of edema associated with CHF, liver cirrhosis, and renal disease including nephrotic syndrome. (PO) Treatment of hypertension. (Inj) Adjunct therapy for acute pulmonary edema.

**DOSAGE:** *Adults:* (PO) HTN: Initial: 40mg bid. Edema: Initial: 20-80mg PO. May repeat or increase by 20-40mg after 6-8 hrs. Max: 600mg/day. Alternative Regimen: Dose on 2-4 consecutive days each week. Closely monitor if on >80mg/day. (Inj) Edema: Initial: 20-40mg IV/IM. May repeat or increase by 20mg after 2 hrs. Acute Pulmonary Edema: Initial: 40mg IV. May increase to 80mg IV after 1 hr.
*Pediatrics:* Edema: (PO) Initial: 2mg/kg single dose. May increase by 1-2mg/kg after 6-8 hrs. Max: 6mg/kg. (Inj) Initial: 1mg/kg IV/IM single dose. May increase by 1mg/kg IV/IM after 2 hrs. Max: 6mg/kg.

**HOW SUPPLIED:** Inj: 10mg/mL; Sol: 10mg/mL, 40mg/5mL; Tab: 20mg, 40mg*, 80mg *scored

**CONTRAINDICATIONS:** Anuria.

**WARNINGS/PRECAUTIONS:** Monitor for fluid/electrolyte imbalance (eg, hypokalemia), renal or hepatic dysfunction. Initiate in hospital with hepatic cirrhosis and ascites. Tinnitus, hearing impairment, hyperglycemia, hyperuricemia reported. May activate SLE. Cross-sensitivity with sulfonamide allergy. Avoid excessive diuresis, especially in elderly.

**ADVERSE REACTIONS:** Pancreatitis, jaundice, anorexia, paresthesias, ototoxicity, blood dyscrasias, dizziness, rash, urticaria, photosensitivity, fever, thrombophlebitis, restlessness.

**INTERACTIONS:** Ototoxicity with aminoglycosides, ethacrynic acid. Caution with high dose salicylates. Lithium toxicity. Antagonizes tubocurarine. Potentiates antihypertensives, succinylcholine, ganglionic or peripheral adrenergic blockers. Decreases arterial response to norepinephrine. Separate sucralfate dose by 2 hrs. Indomethacin may decrease effects. Hypokalemia with ACTH, corticosteroids. Renal changes with NSAIDs. Orthostatic hypotension may be aggravated by alcohol, barbiturates, or narcotics.

**PREGNANCY:** Category C, caution in nursing.



## FUZEON RX
enfuvirtide (Roche Labs)

**THERAPEUTIC CLASS:** Fusion inhibitor

**INDICATIONS:** Treatment of HIV-1 infection in combination with other antiretroviral agents in treatment-experienced patients with evidence of HIV-1 replication despite ongoing antiretroviral therapy.

**DOSAGE:** *Adults:* 90mg SQ bid. Inject SQ into the upper arm, anterior thigh, or abdomen. Do not inject into moles, scar tissue, bruises, the navel, or near any blood vessels. Rotate sites; do not give if injection site reaction occurred from an earlier dose.
*Pediatrics:* 6-16 yrs: 2mg/kg SQ bid. Max: 90mg bid. 11-15.5kg: 27mg bid. 15.6-20.0kg: 36mg bid. 20.1-24.5kg: 45mg bid. 24.6-29.0kg: 54mg bid. 29.1-33.5kg: 63mg bid. 33.6-38.0kg: 72mg bid. 38.1-42.5kg: 81mg bid. ≥ 42.6kg: 90mg bid. Inject SQ into the upper arm, anterior thigh, or abdomen. Do not inject into moles, scar tissue, bruises, or the navel. Rotate sites; do not give if injection site reaction occurred from an earlier dose.

**HOW SUPPLIED:** Inj: 90mg ($60^s$)

**WARNINGS/PRECAUTIONS:** Monitor for signs and symptoms of pneumonia, cellulitis, or local infection. Discontinue if hypersensitivity reactions occur. Theoretically may lead to production of anti-enfuvirtide antibodies; may result in false positive HIV test with an ELISA assay. Immune reconstitution syndrome reported. Increased risk of bleeding or bruising in patients with coagulation disorders.

**ADVERSE REACTIONS:** Diarrhea, nausea, fatigue, local injection site reactions, peripheral neuropathy, insomnia, depression, anxiety, cough, sinusitis, herpes simplex, decreased weight/appetite, pancreatitis, asthenia, pruritus, myalgia, nerve pain, bruising, hematomas.

**PREGNANCY:** Category B, not for use in nursing.

## GABITRIL RX
tiagabine HCl (Cephalon)

**THERAPEUTIC CLASS:** Nipecotic acid derivative

**INDICATIONS:** Adjunctive therapy in the treatment of partial seizures.

**DOSAGE:** *Adults:* Initial: 4mg qd. Titrate: May increase weekly by 4-8mg until clinical response. Max: 56mg/day given bid-qid. Take with food.
*Pediatrics:* ≥12 yo: Initial: 4mg qd. Titrate: May increase to 8mg qd at beginning of Week 2, then increase weekly by 4-8mg until clinical response. Max: 32mg/day. Take with food.

**HOW SUPPLIED:** Tab: 2mg, 4mg, 6mg, 8mg, 10mg, 12mg, 16mg

**WARNINGS/PRECAUTIONS:** Reports of new onset seizure or status epilepticus in patients without epilepsy. D/C and evaluate for underlying seizure disorder. Avoid abrupt withdrawal. Monitor during initial titration for impaired concentration, speech problem, somnolence, fatigue; may require hospitalization if reaction is severe. May exacerbate EEG abnormalities; adjust dose. Status epilepticus and sudden death reported. Reduce dose or d/c if generalized weakness occurs. Reduce dose with hepatic impairment. Serious skin rash reported.

**ADVERSE REACTIONS:** Dizziness, asthenia, somnolence, nausea, vomiting, nervousness, tremor, abdominal pain, abnormal thinking, depression, confusion, pharyngitis, rash.

**INTERACTIONS:** May reduce valproate levels. Diminished effects with carbamazepine, phenytoin. Additive CNS depression with alcohol, triazolam, CNS depressants.

**PREGNANCY:** Category C, caution in nursing.



## GAMMAR-P
immune globulin (ZLB Behring) RX

**THERAPEUTIC CLASS:** Immunoglobulin

**INDICATIONS:** Patients with primary defective antibody synthesis (eg, agammaglobulinemia or hypogammaglobulinemia), who are at increased risk of infection.

**DOSAGE:** *Adults:* 200-400mg/kg IV every 3-4 weeks. Adjust dose to maintain desired IgG levels and clinical response.
*Pediatrics/Adolescents:* 200mg/kg IV every 3-4 weeks. Adjust dose to maintain desired IgG levels and clinical response.

**HOW SUPPLIED:** Inj: 5g, 10g

**CONTRAINDICATIONS:** History of allergic reactions to human albumin, anaphylactic or severe systemic response to IM/IV immune globulin, isolated IgA deficiency.

**WARNINGS/PRECAUTIONS:** Make sure patient is not volume depleted before administration. Caution if predisposed to acute renal failure (eg, any degree of pre-existing renal insufficiency, DM, >65 yrs, volume depletion, sepsis, paraproteinemia, with nephrotoxic drugs). Monitor renal function and infusion rate. Aseptic meningitis syndrome reported. Made from human blood; risk of transmitting infection.

**ADVERSE REACTIONS:** Acute renal failure, acute tubular necrosis, proximal tubular nephropathy, osmotic nephrosis, chills, headache, backache, neck pain.

**INTERACTIONS:** May interfere with response to live viral vaccines (eg, measles, mumps, rubella).

**PREGNANCY:** Category C, safety in nursing not known.

## GAMUNEX
immune globulin intravenous (human) (Bayer) RX

**THERAPEUTIC CLASS:** Immune Globulin

**INDICATIONS:** Primary humoral immunodeficiency (PI) states. Idiopathic thrombocytopenic purpura (ITP).

**DOSAGE:** *Adults:* PI: 300-600mg/kg IV every 3-4 weeks. ITP: 2g/kg IV, given as 2 doses of 1g/kg IV on 2 consecutive days (not if fluid volume is a concern) or 5 doses of 0.4g/kg IV on 5 consecutive days. May withhold 2nd dose if platelet count is adequate 24 hrs after the first 1g/kg daily dose. Infusion Rates: PI/ITP: Initial: 0.01mL/kg/min for first 30 min. Max: 0.08mL/kg/min. Risk of Renal Dysfunction/Acute Renal Failure: Reduce dose, concentration, and/or rate (<0.08mL/kg/min).

**HOW SUPPLIED:** Inj: 10% [10mL, 25mL, 50mL, 100mL, 200mL]

**CONTRAINDICATIONS:** Extreme caution in severe, selective IgA deficiences.

**WARNINGS/PRECAUTIONS:** Caution with pre-existing renal insufficiency, DM, elderly (≥65 yrs), volume depletion, sepsis, paraproteinemia; use minimum concentration/rate. Assess renal function prior to initial infusion and at appropriate intervals thereafter; discontinue if renal fuction worsens. Risk of transmitting infectious agents. Aseptic meningitis syndrome reported with high doses and/or rapid infusion.

**ADVERSE REACTIONS:** Increased cough, rhinitis, pharyngitis, headache, fever, diarrhea, nausea, asthma, asthenia, ear pain, injection site reaction, ecchymosis (purpura), hemorrhage, epistaxis, petechiae, thrombocytopenia.

**INTERACTIONS:** Caution with concomitant nephrotoxic agents. Decreases effect of live, viral vaccines (eg, measles, mumps, rubella); separate use by 6 months.

**PREGNANCY:** Category C, safety in nursing not known.



## GANIRELIX ACETATE RX

ganirelix acetate (Organon)

**THERAPEUTIC CLASS:** GnRH antagonist

**INDICATIONS:** For inhibition of premature LH surges in women undergoing controlled ovarian stimulation.

**DOSAGE:** *Adults:* 250mcg SQ qd during the mid to late follicular phase. Continue until HCG administration.

**HOW SUPPLIED:** Inj: 250mcg/0.5mL

**CONTRAINDICATIONS:** Pregnancy.

**WARNINGS/PRECAUTIONS:** Exclude pregnancy before initiate therapy. Contains natural rubber latex.

**ADVERSE REACTIONS:** Abdominal pain (gynecological), fetal death, headache, ovarian hyperstimulation syndrome.

**PREGNANCY:** Category X, not for use in nursing.

## GANITE RX

gallium nitrate (Genta)

**Increased risk of severe renal insufficiency with concurrent use of other potentially nephrotoxic drugs (eg, aminoglycosides, amphotericin B). Discontinue if use of potentially nephrotoxic drug is indicated; hydrate for several days after administration. Discontinue if SCr >2.5mg/dL.**

**THERAPEUTIC CLASS:** Calcium regulator

**INDICATIONS:** Treatment of symptomatic cancer-related hypercalcemia unresponsive to adequate hydration.

**DOSAGE:** *Adults:* 200mg/m² IV infusion over 24 hours for 5 days. May consider 100mg/m²/day with mild cases. May stop early if serum calcium levels are WNL in <5 days.

**HOW SUPPLIED:** Inj: 500mg [20mL]

**CONTRAINDICATIONS:** Severe renal impairment (SCr >2.5mg/dL).

**WARNINGS/PRECAUTIONS:** Monitor renal function (SCr, BUN), serum calcium (daily) and phosphorous (twice weekly). Establish and maintain adequate hydration before and after initiation. Avoid overhydration with compromised cardiovascular status. Avoid diuretics prior to correction of hypovolemia. Discontinue if SCr >2.5mg/dL or if hypocalcemia occurs.

**ADVERSE REACTIONS:** Elevated BUN/SCr, hypocalcemia, transient hypophosphatemia, decreased serum bicarbonate, anemia (with high doses), decrease in BP, nausea, vomiting, tachycardia, lethargy, confusion, diarrhea, constipation.

**INTERACTIONS:** Avoid use with nephrotoxic drugs (eg, aminoglycosides, amphotericin B). Caution with cyclophosphamide, prednisone.

**PREGNANCY:** Category C, not for use in nursing.

## GANTRISIN PEDIATRIC RX

sulfisoxazole (Roche Labs)

**THERAPEUTIC CLASS:** Sulfonamide

**INDICATIONS:** Treatment of acute, recurrent or chronic urinary tract infection. Treatment and prophylaxis in meningococcal meningitis. Adjunct treatment of Haemophilus influenzae meningitis, acute otitis media, malaria, and toxoplasmosis. Treatment of trachoma, inclusion conjunctivitis, nocardiosis, chancroid.

**DOSAGE:** Pediatrics: >2 months: Initial: 1/2 of 24hr dose. Maint: 150mg/kg/24hr or 4g/m²/24hr given q4-6h. Max: 6g/24hr.

**HOW SUPPLIED:** Sus: 500mg/5mL

**CONTRAINDICATIONS:** Infants <2 months (except in congenital toxoplasmosis treatment), pregnancy at term, mothers nursing infants <2 months old.

**WARNINGS/PRECAUTIONS:** Fatalities reported due to Stevens-Johnson syndrome, toxic epidermal necrolysis, fulminant hepatic necrosis, agranulocytosis, aplastic anemia and other blood dyscrasias. Discontinue if develop skin rash or sign of an adverse reaction. Hypersensitivity reactions of the respiratory tract reported. Do not use in group A β-hemolytic streptococcal infections. Pseudomembranous colitis reported. Caution with renal/hepatic impairment, severe allergy or bronchial asthma. Hemolysis may occur in G6PD-deficient patients.

**ADVERSE REACTIONS:** Anaphylaxis, erythema multiforme, toxic epidermal necrolysis, tachycardia, hepatitis, nausea, anorexia, hematuria, crystalluria, BUN and creatinine elevations, blood dyscrasias, dizziness, psychosis, cough.

**INTERACTIONS:** May prolong PT with anticoagulants. May require less thiopental for anesthesia. May potentiate hypoglycemia effects of sulfonylureas. May displace methotrexate from plasma proteins.

**PREGNANCY:** Category C, not for use in nursing.

## GARDASIL RX

human papillomavirus recombinant vaccine, quadrivalent (Merck)

**THERAPEUTIC CLASS:** Vaccine

**INDICATIONS:** Vaccination of girls and women ages 9-26 yrs for the prevention of cervical cancer, genital warts, cervical adenocarcinoma *in situ*, cervical intraepithelial neoplasia grades 2 and 3, vulvar intraepithelial neoplasia grades 2 and 3, vaginal intraepithelial neoplasia grades 2 and 3, and cervical intraepithelial neoplasia grade 1 caused by Human Papillomavirus types 6, 11, 16, and 18.

**DOSAGE:** *Adults:* Give 3 separate 0.5mL IM doses in the deltoid region of upper arm or higher anterolateral area of the thigh. First dose: At elected date; Second dose: 2 months after first dose; Third dose: 6 months after first dose. *Pediatrics:* ≥9 yrs: Give 3 separate 0.5mL IM doses in the deltoid region of upper arm or higher anterolateral area of the thigh. First dose: At elected date; Second dose: 2 months after first dose; Third dose: 6 months after first dose.

**HOW SUPPLIED:** Inj: Vial/Syringe: 0.5mL

**WARNINGS/PRECAUTIONS:** Should not be administered with bleeding disorders or anticoagulant therapy unless the potential benefits outweight the risk. Patients with impaired immune responsiveness may have reduced antibody response to active immunization. Medical treatment should be readily available in case of rare anaphylactic reactions.

**ADVERSE REACTIONS:** Local site reactions, fever, pyrexia, nausea, nasopharyngitis, dizziness, diarrhea.

**INTERACTIONS:** Immunosuppressive therapies, including irradiation, antimetabolites, alkylating agents, cytotoxic drugs, and corticosteroids (used in greater than physiologic doses) may reduce the immune responses to vaccines.

**PREGNANCY:** Category B, caution in nursing.

## GELCLAIR RX

sodium hyaluronate - glycyrrhetinic acid - polyvinylpyrrolidone

(OSI/Helsinn Healthcare)



**THERAPEUTIC CLASS:** Oral analgesic

**INDICATIONS:** Relief of oral pain from various etiologies, including oral mucositis/stomatitis, irritation from oral surgery, traumatic ulcers from braces/ill-fitting dentures, diffuse aphthous ulcers.

**DOSAGE:** *Adults:* Mix one packet with 1-3 tablespoons of water. Gargle for 1 minute then spit out. Use tid or prn. Do not eat or drink for 1 hour after treatment. May be used undiluted.

**HOW SUPPLIED:** Gel: 15mL/packet [21[s]]

**PREGNANCY:** Safety not known in pregnancy or nursing.

## GEMZAR RX

gemcitabine HCl (Lilly)

**THERAPEUTIC CLASS:** Nucleoside analogue antimetabolite

**INDICATIONS:** Adjunct with cisplatin for 1st-line treatment of inoperable, locally advanced (Stage IIIA or IIIB) or metastatic (Stage IV) non-small cell lung cancer. If previously treated with 5-FU, 1st-line treatment of locally advanced (nonresectable Stage II or Stage III) or metastatic (Stage IV) pancreatic adenocarcinoma. Adjunct with paclitaxel for 1st-line treatment of metastatic breast cancer after failure of prior anthracycline-containing adjuvant chemotherapy, unless anthracyclines were clinically contraindicated. Combination with carboplatin for the treatment of advanced ovarian cancer that has relapsed at least 6 months after completion of platinum-based therapy.

**DOSAGE:** *Adults:* Pancreatic Cancer: 1000mg/m$^2$ IV weekly up to 7 weeks, then 1 week off. Give subsequent cycles as weekly infusions for 3 out of every 4 weeks. Lung Cancer: 4 Week Cycle: 1000mg/m$^2$ IV days 1, 8, and 15 of each 28-day cycle. Give cisplatin 100mg/m$^2$ IV on day 1 after infusion. 3 Week Cycle: 1250mg/m$^2$ on days 1 and 8 of each 21-day cycle. Give cisplatin 100mg/m$^2$ IV on day 1 after infusion. Breast Cancer: 1250mg/m$^2$ IV on days 1 and 8 of each 21-day cycle. Give paclitaxel 175mg/m$^2$ IV on day 1 before gemcitabine. Ovarian Cancer: 1000mg/m$^2$ IV on days 1 and 8 of each 21-day cycle. Give carboplatin AUC 4 IV on day 1 after gemcitabine. Adjust dose based on hematologic toxicity.

**HOW SUPPLIED:** Inj: 200mg, 1g

**WARNINGS/PRECAUTIONS:** Increased toxicity with infusion time >60 minutes and more than once weekly dosing. Hemolytic-Uremic syndrome, hepatotoxicity, pulmonary toxicity, renal failure, leukopenia, thrombocytopenia, and anemia reported. Myelosuppression is dose-limiting toxicity. D/C if severe lung toxicity occurs. Caution with significant renal or hepatic impairment. Pattern of tissue injury typically associated with radiation toxicity reported with concurrent and non-concurrent use. Greater tendency for older women to not preceed to next cycle and experience grade 3/4 neutropenia and thrombocytopenia. Perform CBC, differential, and platelets before each dose. Decreased clearance in women and elderly.

**ADVERSE REACTIONS:** Myelosuppression, nausea, vomiting, diarrhea, stomatitis, elevated serum transaminases, proteinuria, hematuria, fever, rash, dyspnea, edema, flu-syndrome, infection, alopecia, paresthesia.

**INTERACTIONS:** Monitor serum creatinine, $K^+$, calcium, and magnesium with cisplatin. Serious hepatotoxicity reported with hepatotoxic drugs.

**PREGNANCY:** Category D, not for use in nursing.

## GENOPTIC RX

gentamicin sulfate (Allergan)

**OTHER BRAND NAMES:** Genoptic S.O.P. (Allergan)

**THERAPEUTIC CLASS:** Aminoglycoside

**INDICATIONS:** Treatment of ocular bacterial infections including conjunctivitis, keratitis, keratoconjunctivitis, corneal ulcers, blepharitis, blepharoconjunctivitis, acute meibomianitis and dacryocystitis.

**DOSAGE:** *Adults:* Usual: 1-2 drops q4h or apply 1/2 inch of ointment bid-tid. Severe Infection: 2 drops every hour.

**HOW SUPPLIED:** Oint: (S.O.P.) 0.3% [3.5g]; Sol: 0.3% [1mL, 5mL]

**WARNINGS/PRECAUTIONS:** D/C if irritation, hypersensitivity, purulent discharge, inflammation, or pain develops. Prolonged use may result in superinfection. Ointment may retard corneal healing.

**ADVERSE REACTIONS:** Bacterial and fungal corneal ulcers, burning, irritation, conjunctivitis, conjunctival epithelial defects, conjunctival hyperemia.

**PREGNANCY:** Category C, unknown use in nursing.

## GENOTROPIN RX

somatropin (Pharmacia & Upjohn)

**OTHER BRAND NAMES:** Genotropin MiniQuick (Pharmacia & Upjohn)

**THERAPEUTIC CLASS:** Human growth hormone

**INDICATIONS:** Long-term treatment of pediatrics with growth failure due to growth hormone deficiency (GHD) or Prader-Willi syndrome (PWS) or who are born small for gestational age (SGA) and fail to catch-up by age 2. Long-term replacement therapy in adults with GHD of either childhood- or adult-onset etiology. Long-term treatment of growth failure associated with Turner Syndrome (TS) in patients who have open epiphyses.

**DOSAGE:** *Adults:* Individualize dose: GHD: Initial: Up to 0.04mg/kg/week. May increase at 4-8 week intervals. Max: 0.08mg/kg/week. Divide dose into 6-7 SQ injections. Elderly patients should receive a lower starting dose. *Pediatrics:* Individualize dose. GHD: 0.16-0.24mg/kg/week. PWS: 0.24mg/kg/week. SGA: 0.48mg/kg/week. TS: 0.33mg/kg/week. Divide doses into 6-7 SQ injections.

**HOW SUPPLIED:** Inj: 1.5mg, 5.8mg, 13.8mg; Inj, MiniQuick: 0.2mg, 0.4mg, 0.6mg, 0.8mg, 1mg, 1.2mg, 1.4mg, 1.6mg, 1.8mg, 2mg

**CONTRAINDICATIONS:** Evidence of neoplastic activity. Pediatrics with closed epiphyses. Patients with diabetic retinopathy or active malignancy. Acute critical illness due to complications after open heart or abdominal surgery, multiple accidental trauma, or with acute respiratory failure. Patients with PWS who are severely obese or have severe respiratory impairment.

**WARNINGS/PRECAUTIONS:** In PWS, evaluate for upper airway obstruction prior to initiation; monitor weight, for sleep apnea, signs of upper airway obstruction (eg, suspend therapy with onset of or increased snoring), respiratory infections (treat early and aggressively if occur). Monitor GHD secondary to intracranial lesion for progression/recurrence. Monitor gait, glucose intolerance because insulin sensitivity is decreased, for malignant transformation of skin lesions, scoliosis progression, intracranial HTN (perform fundoscopic exam at start and periodically). Caution with DM, endocrine disorders, hypopituitarism, and Turner syndrome. Tissue atrophy may occur (rotate injection site).

**ADVERSE REACTIONS:** Peripheral swelling/edema, arthralgia, pain/stiffness in extremities, myalgia, upper respiratory infection, paresthesia.

**INTERACTIONS:** Antagonized by glucocorticoids. May alter clearance of CYP450 substrates (eg, corticosteroids, sex steroids, anticonvulsants, cyclosporine). May need dose adjustment if taking oral estrogen replacement. May need insulin dose adjustment.

**PREGNANCY:** Category B, caution in nursing.



## GENTAMICIN OPHTHALMIC RX

gentamicin sulfate (Various)

**THERAPEUTIC CLASS:** Aminoglycoside

**INDICATIONS:** Treatment of ocular bacterial infections including conjunctivitis, keratitis, keratoconjunctivitis, corneal ulcers, blepharitis, blepharoconjunctivitis, acute meibomianitis and dacryocystitis.

**DOSAGE:** *Adults:* Usual: 1-2 drops q4h or apply 1/2 inch of ointment bid-tid. Severe Infection: 2 drops every hour.
*Pediatrics:* Usual: 1-2 drops q4h or apply half-inch of ointment bid-tid. Severe Infection: 2 drops every hour.

**HOW SUPPLIED:** Oint: 0.3% [3.5g]; Sol: 0.3% [5mL]

**WARNINGS/PRECAUTIONS:** Discontinue if develop irritation, hypersensitivity, purulent discharge, inflammation or pain. Prolonged use may result in superinfection. Ointment may retard corneal healing.

**ADVERSE REACTIONS:** Bacterial and fungal corneal ulcers, burning, irritation, conjunctivitis, conjunctival epithelial defects, conjunctival hyperemia.

**PREGNANCY:** Category C. Safety in nursing is not known.

## GENTAMICIN SULFATE INJECTION RX

gentamicin sulfate (Various)

**Potential nephrotoxicity, neurotoxicity, ototoxicity. Risk of toxicity is greater with impaired renal function, high dosage, or prolonged therapy. Monitor serum concentrations closely. Avoid prolonged peak levels >12mcg/mL and trough levels >2mcg/mL. Monitor renal and eight cranial nerve function, urine, BUN, serum creatinine, and CrCl. Obtain serial audiograms. Advanced age and dehydration increase risk of toxicity. Adjust dose or discontinue use with evidence of ototoxicity or nephrotoxicity. May cause fetal harm during pregnancy. Avoid concurrent and/or sequential systemic or topical use of other potentially neurotoxic and/or nephrotoxic drugs, such as cisplatin, cephaloridine, kanamycin, amikacin, neomycin, polymyxin B, colistin, paromomycin, streptomycin, tobramycin, vancomycin, and viomycin. Avoid concurrent use with potent diuretics, such as ethacrynic acid or furosemide.**

**THERAPEUTIC CLASS:** Aminoglycoside

**INDICATIONS:** Treatment of bacterial neonatal sepsis, bacterial septicemia, and serious bacterial infections of the CNS (meningitis), urinary tract, respiratory tract, gastrointestinal tract (including peritonitis), skin, bone and soft tissue (including burns) caused by susceptible strains of microorganisms.

**DOSAGE:** *Adults:* IM/IV: Serious Infections: 3mg/kg/day given q8h. Life-Threatening Infections: 5mg/kg/day tid-qid; reduce to 3mg/kg/day as soon as clinically indicated. Treat for 7-10 days; may need longer course in difficult and complicated infections. Renal Impairment: Reduced dose given q8h or usual dose given at prolonged intervals based on either CrCl or serum creatinine. Dialysis: 1-1.7mg/kg, depending on severity of infection, at end of each dialysis period. Obese Patients: Calculate dose based on estimated lean body mass.
*Pediatrics:* Children: 6-7.5mg/kg/day (2-2.5mg/kg given q8h). Infants and Neonates: 7.5mg/kg/day (2.5mg/kg given q8h). Premature and Full-Term

Neonates ≤1 week: 5mg/kg/day (2.5mg/kg given q12h). Treat for 7-10 days; may need longer course in difficult and complicated infections. Renal Impairment: Reduced dose given q8h or usual dose given at prolonged intervals based on either CrCl or serum creatinine. Dialysis: 2mg/kg at end of each dialysis period. Obese Patients: Calculate dose based on estimated lean body mass.

**HOW SUPPLIED:** Inj: 10mg/mL, 40mg/mL

**WARNINGS/PRECAUTIONS:** Contains metabisulfite. Neuromuscular blockade, respiratory paralysis, ototoxicity, and nephrotoxicity may occur after local irrigation or topical application during surgical procedures. Caution with neuromuscular disorders (eg, myasthenia gravis, parkinsonism). Caution in elderly; monitor renal function. Keep patients well-hydrated during treatment. May cause fetal harm when administered to pregnant women.

**ADVERSE REACTIONS:** Nephrotoxicity, neurotoxicity, rash, fever, urticaria, nausea, vomiting, headache, lethargy, confusion, depression, decreased appetite, weight loss, BP changes, blood dyscrasias, elevated LFTs.

**INTERACTIONS:** Increased nephrotoxicity with cephalosporins. Do not premix with other drugs; administer separately. Neuromuscular blockade and respiratory paralysis may occur in anesthetized patients or those receiving neuromuscular blockers (eg, succinylcholine, tubocurarine, decamethonium). See Black Box Warning.

**PREGNANCY:** Category D, safety not known in nursing.

## GENTAMICIN TOPICAL RX

gentamicin sulfate (Various)

**THERAPEUTIC CLASS:** Aminoglycoside

**INDICATIONS:** Treatment of primary skin infections such as impetigo contagiosa, folliculitis, ecthyma, furunculosis, sycosis barbae, and pyoderma gangrenosum; and secondary skin infections such as infectious eczematoid dermatitis, pustular acne, pustular psoriasis, infected seborrheic dermatitis, infected contact dermatitis, infected excoriations, and bacterial superinfections.

**DOSAGE:** *Adults:* Apply gently tid-qid. May apply gauze dressing. *Pediatrics:* >1 yr: Apply gently tid-qid. May apply gauze dressing.

**HOW SUPPLIED:** Cre, Oint: 0.1% [15g, 30g]

**WARNINGS/PRECAUTIONS:** Discontinue if irritation, sensitization, or superinfection develops.

**ADVERSE REACTIONS:** Irritation (erythema and pruritus).

**PREGNANCY:** Unknown use in pregnancy and nursing.

## GENTEAL OTC

hydroxypropyl methylcellulose (Novartis Ophthalmics)

**OTHER BRAND NAMES:** GenTeal Mild (Novartis Ophthalmics)

**THERAPEUTIC CLASS:** Lubricant

**INDICATIONS:** Relief of dry eye (Sol 0.2% for mild, Sol 0.3% for moderate, Gel 0.3% for severe). Temporary relief of discomfort due to minor irritations of eye from exposure to wind, sun, or other irritants and to protect against further irritation.

**DOSAGE:** *Adults:* 1-2 drops in affected eye prn.

**HOW SUPPLIED:** Gel: 0.3% [10mL]; Sol: (Mild) 0.2% [15mL, 25mL]; Sol: 0.3% [15mL, 25mL]

**WARNINGS/PRECAUTIONS:** Do not touch container tip to any surface. D/C if eye pain, vision changes, redness, or irritation continue >72 hrs; or if condition worsens.

**PREGNANCY:** Safety in pregnancy or nursing not known.

## GEOCILLIN
RX

carbenicillin disodium (Pfizer)

**THERAPEUTIC CLASS:** Semisynthetic penicillin

**INDICATIONS:** Treatment of acute and chronic infections of the upper and lower urinary tract (UTI) and asymptomatic bacteriuria.

**DOSAGE:** *Adults:* UTI: (*E.coli, Proteus,* and *Enterobacter*) 1-2 tabs qid. (*Pseudomonas, Enterococcus*) 2 tabs qid. Prostatitis: (*E.coli, Proteus, Enterococcus,* and *Enterobacter*) 2 tabs qid. CrCl 10-20mL/min: Adjust dose.

**HOW SUPPLIED:** Tab: 382mg

**WARNINGS/PRECAUTIONS:** Fatal hypersensitivity reactions reported. Long term use may cause superinfection. Patients with severe renal impairment (CrCl <10mL/min) will not achieve therapeutic urine levels. Adjust dose with CrCl 10-20mL/min. Monitor renal, hepatic, and hematopoietic systems periodically with prolonged use. Possible allergic response in hypersensitive patients.



**ADVERSE REACTIONS:** Nausea, bad taste, diarrhea, vomiting, flatulence, glossitis, rash, urticaria, SGOT elevations.

**INTERACTIONS:** Increased and prolonged levels with probenecid.

**PREGNANCY:** Category B, caution in nursing.

## GEODON
RX

ziprasidone HCl (Pfizer)

**Elderly patients with dementia-related psychosis treated with atypical antipsychotic drugs are at an increased risk of death; most appeared to be cardiovascular (eg, heart failure, sudden death) or infectious (eg, pneumonia) in nature. Ziprasidone is not approved for the treatment of patients with dementia-related psychosis.**

**OTHER BRAND NAMES:** Geodon for Injection (Pfizer)

**THERAPEUTIC CLASS:** Benzisoxazole derivative

**INDICATIONS:** Treatment of schizophrenia. Treatment of acute manic or mixed episodes associated with bipolar disorder, with or without psychotic features. (Inj) Treatment of acute agitation in schizophrenic patients who need IM medication for rapid control of agitation.

**DOSAGE:** *Adults:* Schizophrenia: (Cap) Initial: 20mg bid with food. Titrate: May increase up to 80mg bid; adjust dose at intervals of not less than 2 days. Maint: 20-80mg bid for up to 52 weeks. (Inj) 10-20mg IM up to max 40mg/day. May give 10mg q2h or 20mg q4h up to 40mg/day for 3 days. Bipolar Mania: (Cap) Initial: 40mg bid with food. Titrate: Increase to 60-80mg bid on 2nd day of treatment. Maint: 40-80mg bid.

**HOW SUPPLIED:** Cap: (HCl) 20mg, 40mg, 60mg, 80mg; Inj: (Mesylate) 20mg/mL

**CONTRAINDICATIONS:** Concomitant dofetilide, sotalol, quinidine, Class Ia/III antiarrhythmics, mesoridazine, thioridazine, chlorpromazine, droperidol, pimozide, sparfloxacin, gatifloxacin, moxifloxacin, halofantrine, mefloquine, pentamidine, arsenic trioxide, levomethadyl acetate, dolasetron, probucol, tacrolimus, and drugs that prolong QT interval. History of QT prolongation, recent acute MI, uncompensated heart failure.

**WARNINGS/PRECAUTIONS:** Discontinue if persistent QTc measurements >500 msec, NMS, tardive dyskinesia occurs. Monitor for hyperglycemia in patients with DM or at risk for DM. Avoid with congenital long QT syndrome, history of arrhythmia. Caution in history of seizures. Esophageal dysmotility and aspiration reported. May elevate prolactin levels. Orthostatic hypotension reported; caution with cardiovascular or cerebrovascular disease, conditions predisposed to hypotension (eg, dehydration, hypovolemia). Caution with IM use in renal dysfunction.

**ADVERSE REACTIONS:** Asthenia, nausea, constipation, dyspepsia, diarrhea, dry mouth, rash, somnolence, akathisia, dizziness, EPS, dystonia, hypertonia, respiratory disorder, upper respiratory infection, vomiting, headache, injection site pain.

**INTERACTIONS:** See Contraindications. Caution with centrally acting drugs. May enhance effects of antihypertensives. May antagonize effects of levodopa and dopamine agonists. Carbamazepine may decrease levels. CYP3A4 inhibitors may increase levels.

**PREGNANCY:** Category C, not for use in nursing.

## GLEEVEC

imatinib mesylate (Novartis)

RX



**THERAPEUTIC CLASS:** Protein-tyrosine kinase inhibitor

**INDICATIONS:** Treatment of Philadelphia chromosome positive chronic myeloid leukemia (CML) in blast crisis, accelerated phase, or in chronic phase after failure of interferon-alpha therapy or in newly adult diagnosed patients. Treatment of pediatric patients with Ph+ chronic phase CML whose disease has recurred after stem cell transplant or who are resistant to interferon-alpha therapy. Treatment of Kit (CD117) positive unresectable and/or metastatic malignant gastrointestinal stromal tumors (GIST).

**DOSAGE:** *Adults:* >18 yrs: CML: Chronic Phase: 400mg qd, may increase to 600 mg qd. Accelerated Phase/Blast Crisis: 600mg qd, may increase to 400 mg bid. See labeling for dose increase with CML. GIST: 400mg qd or 600mg qd. Hepatotoxicity/Non-Hematologic Adverse Reaction: If bilirubin >3X ULN or transaminases >5X ULN, hold drug until bilirubin <1.5X ULN and transaminases <2.5X ULN. Continue at reduced dose.
Neutropenia/Thrombocytopenia: See labeling for dose adjustment. Take with food and water.
*Pediatrics:* ≥3 yrs: CML: Chronic Phase: 260mg/m$^2$/day given qd or split into 2 doses (morning and evening). Neutropenia/Thrombocytopenia: See labeling for dose adjustment. Take with food and water.

**HOW SUPPLIED:** Tab: 100mg, 400mg

**WARNINGS/PRECAUTIONS:** Fluid retention/edema reported; monitor weight. Neutropenia/thrombocytopenia reported; monitor CBC weekly during 1st month, biweekly during 2nd month, and periodically thereafter. May be hepatotoxic; monitor LFTs at baseline, then monthly or as needed. Avoid becoming pregnant. Interrupt treatment if severe non-hematologic adverse reaction develops (eg, severe hepatotoxicity or severe fluid retention); resume if appropriate. GI bleeds reported. Severe congestive heart failure and left ventricular dysfunction. Hypereosinophilic cardiac toxicity.

**ADVERSE REACTIONS:** Nausea, vomiting, fluid retention, neutropenia, thrombocytopenia, diarrhea, hemorrhage, pyrexia, rash, headache, fatigue, abdominal pain, elevated transaminases or bilirubin, edema, muscle cramps, musculoskeletal pain, flatulence, nasopharyngitis, insomnia, anemia, anorexia, rhinitis.

**INTERACTIONS:** Increased levels with CYP3A4 inhibitors (eg, ketoconazole, erythromycin, clarithromycin, itraconazole). Decreased levels with CYP3A4 inducers (eg, dexamethasone, phenytoin, carbamazepine, rifampin, phenobarbital, St. John's Wort). Caution with CYP3A4 substrates with narrow therapeutic windows (eg, cyclosporine, pimozide). Increases levels of drugs metabolized by CYP3A4 (eg, dihydropyridines, triazolo-benzodiazepines, HMG-CoA reductase inhibitors). Switch patients on warfarin to low molecular weight or standard heparin.

**PREGNANCY:** Category D, not for nursing.

## GLIADEL
carmustine (Guilford)

RX

**THERAPEUTIC CLASS:** Nitrosourea oncolytic agent

**INDICATIONS:** Adjunct to surgery in patients with recurrent glioblastoma multiforme. Adjunct to surgery and radiation in patients with newly-diagnosed high grade malignant glioma.

**DOSAGE:** *Adults:* Place 8 wafers in resection cavity if size and shape allows; if not, place maximum number of wafers allowed. Max: 8 wafers per surgical procedure.

**HOW SUPPLIED:** Implant: (Polifeprosan 20 with Carmustine) 7.7mg

**WARNINGS/PRECAUTIONS:** Avoid communication between the surgical resection cavity and ventricular system. May cause CT and MRI enhancement due to edema and inflammation. Monitor closely for known complications of craniotomy. May cause fetal harm. Risk of possible cyst formation.



**ADVERSE REACTIONS:** Fever, pain, abnormal healing, nausea, vomiting, brain edema, confusion, somnolence, UTI, seizures, headache, intracranial infection.

**PREGNANCY:** Category D, not for use in nursing.

## GLOFIL-125
sodium iothalamate i-125 (Questcor)

RX

**THERAPEUTIC CLASS:** Radiopharmaceutical agent

**INDICATIONS:** For evaluation of glomerular filtration in the diagnosis or monitoring of patients with renal disease.

**DOSAGE:** *Adults:* 70kg: 20-100microcuries continuous IV or 10-30microcuries single IV injection.

**HOW SUPPLIED:** Inj: 1mg/mL (250-300microcuries/mL)

**WARNINGS/PRECAUTIONS:** Minimize radiation exposure to patient. Avoid rapid or bolus-like injections.

**PREGNANCY:** Category C, not for use in nursing.

## GLUCAGON
glucagon (Lilly)

RX

**THERAPEUTIC CLASS:** Glucagon

**INDICATIONS:** Treatment for severe hypoglycemia. Diagnostic aid for radiologic examination of the stomach, duodenum, small bowel, and colon.

**DOSAGE:** *Adults:* Severe Hypoglycemia: 1mg (1U) SQ/IM/IV. May give another dose after 15 minutes if patient does not respond, but IV glucose would be a better alternative. Use immediately after reconstitution; discard unused portion. Diagnostic Aid: Stomach/Duodenum/Small Bowel: 0.5mg (0.5U) IV or 2mg (2U) IM before procedure. Colon: 2mg (2U) IM 10 minutes before procedure.

*Pediatrics:* Severe Hypoglycemia: >20kg: 1mg (1U) SQ/IM/IV. <20kg: 0.5mg (0.5U) or 20-30mcg/kg. May give another dose after 15 minutes if patient does not respond, but IV glucose would be a better alternative. Use immediately after reconstitution; discard unused portion.

**HOW SUPPLIED:** Inj: 1mg

**CONTRAINDICATIONS:** Pheochromocytoma.

**WARNINGS/PRECAUTIONS:** Caution with history suggestive of insulinoma and/or pheochromocytoma. Glucagon can cause pheochromocytoma tumor to release catecholamines, which may result in a sudden and marked increase in BP. Effective in treating hypoglycemia only if sufficient liver glycogen is present. Glucagon is not effective in states of starvation, adrenal insufficiency, or chronic hypoglycemia; use glucose to treat instead.

**ADVERSE REACTIONS:** Nausea, vomiting, allergic reactions, urticaria, respiratory distress, hypotension.

**PREGNANCY:** Category B, caution in nursing.

## GLUCOPHAGE XR

RX

metformin HCl (Bristol-Myers Squibb)

**OTHER BRAND NAMES:** Riomet (Ranbaxy) - Glucophage (Bristol-Myers Squibb)

**THERAPEUTIC CLASS:** Biguanide

**INDICATIONS:** Adjunct to diet or with a sulfonylurea or insulin, to improve glycemic control in type 2 diabetes mellitus.

**DOSAGE:** *Adults:* (Sol, Tab) Initial: 500mg bid or 850mg qd with meals. Titrate: Increase by 500mg/week, or 850mg every 2 weeks, or may increase from 500mg bid to 850mg bid after 2 weeks. Max: 2550mg/day. Give in 3 divided doses with meals if dose is >2g/day. (Tab, Extended Release) Initial: >17 yrs: 500mg qd with evening meal. Titrate: Increase by 500mg/week. Max: 2000mg/day. With Insulin: Initial: 500mg qd. Titrate: Increase by 500mg/week. Max: 2500mg/day and 2000mg/day (XR). Decrease insulin dose by 10-25% when FPG <120mg/dL. Swallow whole; do not crush or chew. Elderly/Debilitated/Malnourished: Conservative dosing; do not titrate to Max. *Pediatrics:* 10-16 yrs: (Sol, Tab) Initial: 500mg bid with meals. Titrate: Increase by 500mg/week. Max: 2000mg/day.

**HOW SUPPLIED:** Sol: (Riomet) 500mg/5mL; Tab: 500mg, 850mg, 1000mg*; Tab, Extended Release: 500mg, 750mg *scored

**CONTRAINDICATIONS:** Renal disease/dysfunction (SrCr >1.5mg/dL [males], >1.4mg/dL [females], abnormal CrCl), CHF, metabolic acidosis, diabetic ketoacidosis. Discontinue temporarily (48 hrs) for radiologic studies with intravascular iodinated contrast materials.

**WARNINGS/PRECAUTIONS:** Lactic acidosis reported (rare); increased risk with renal dysfunction, increased age, DM, CHF, and other conditions with risk of hypoperfusion and hypoxemia. Avoid use in patients >80 yrs unless renal function is normal. Monitor renal function and for ketoacidosis and metabolic acidosis. Avoid in renal/hepatic impairment. D/C in hypoxic states (eg, CHF, shock, acute MI), loss of blood glucose control due to stress (give insulin), acidosis, dehydration, sepsis. Temporarily d/c prior to surgery (due to restricted food intake) and procedures requiring intravascular iodinated contrast materials. May decrease serum vitamin $B_{12}$ levels. Increased risk of hypoglycemia in elderly, debilitated/malnourished, adrenal or pituitary insufficiency, or alcohol intoxication. Monitor renal function.

**ADVERSE REACTIONS:** Lactic acidosis, diarrhea, nausea, vomiting, flatulence, abdominal discomfort, abnormal stools, hypoglycemia, myalgia, dizziness, dyspnea, nail disorder, rash, sweating, taste disorder, chest discomfort, chills, flu syndrome, palpitations, asthenia, indigestion, headache.

**INTERACTIONS:** Furosemide, nifedipine, cimetidine, cationic drugs (eg, digoxin, amiloride, procainamide, quinidine, quinine, ranitidine, trimethoprim, vancomycin, triamterene, morphine) may increase metformin levels. Thiazides, other diuretics, corticosteroids, phenothiazines, thyroid products, estrogens, oral contraceptives, phenytoin, nicotinic acid, sympathomimetics, calcium channel blockers, isoniazid may cause hyperglycemia. Risk of hypoglycemia with alcohol. Excess alcohol may increase potential for lactic acidosis. May decrease furosemide levels.

**PREGNANCY:** Category B, not for use in nursing.

## GLUCOTROL XL

RX

glipizide (Pfizer)

**OTHER BRAND NAMES:** Glucotrol (Pfizer) - Glipizide ER (Watson)

**THERAPEUTIC CLASS:** Sulfonylurea (2nd generation)

**INDICATIONS:** Adjunct to diet and exercise, to improve glycemic control in type 2 diabetes mellitus.

**DOSAGE:** *Adults:* (Glucotrol XL) Do not chew, divide, or crush. Initial: 5mg qd with breakfast. Use lower doses if sensitive to hypoglycemics. Usual: 5-10mg qd. Max: 20mg/day. Combination Therapy: Initial: 5mg qd. (Glucotrol): Initial: 5mg qd 30 minutes before breakfast. Geriatric/Hepatic Impairment: Initial 2.5mg qd. Titrate: Increase by 2.5-5mg after several days. Max: 40mg/day. Divide doses >15mg and give 30 min before a meal. (Glucotrol XL, Glucotrol) Switch From Insulin: If on <20 U/day: Stop insulin; start Glucotrol XL or Glucotrol 5mg qd. If on >20 U/day: Reduce insulin dose by 50% and add Glucotrol XL or Glucotrol 5mg qd. Further insulin reductions depend on response.



**HOW SUPPLIED:** Tab: (Glucotrol) 5mg*, 10mg*; Tab, Extended Release: (XL) 2.5mg, 5mg, 10mg *scored

**CONTRAINDICATIONS:** Diabetic ketoacidosis.

**WARNINGS/PRECAUTIONS:** Increased risk of hypoglycemia with the elderly, debilitated, malnourished, renal and hepatic disease, adrenal or pituitary insufficiency. Increased risk of cardiovascular mortality. Loss of blood glucose control when exposed to stress (fever, trauma, infection, or surgery); d/c therapy and start insulin. Secondary failure can occur over a period of time. (XL) GI disease will reduce retention time of the drug. Caution with pre-existing severe GI narrowing.

**ADVERSE REACTIONS:** Hypoglycemia, nausea, diarrhea, allergic skin reactions, disulfiram-like reactions, dizziness, drowsiness, asthenia, headache.

**INTERACTIONS:** Potentiated hypoglycemia with alcohol, NSAIDs, some azoles (eg, miconazole, fluconazole), highly protein bound drugs, salicylates, sulfonamides, chloramphenicol, probenecid, coumarins, MAOIs and β-blockers. Risk of hyperglycemia with diuretics, corticosteroids, phenothiazines, thyroid products, estrogens, oral contraceptives, phenytoin, nicotinic acid, sympathomimetics, calcium channel blockers and isoniazid. β-blockers may mask signs of hypoglycemia.

**PREGNANCY:** Category C, not for use in nursing.

## GLUCOVANCE

RX

glyburide - metformin HCl (Bristol-Myers Squibb)

**THERAPEUTIC CLASS:** Sulfonylurea/biguanide

**INDICATIONS:** Adjunct to diet and exercise, to improve glycemic control in type 2 diabetes mellitus. As second-line therapy when treatment with a sulfonylurea or metformin alone is inadequate. May add a thiazolidinedione (TZD) for additional glycemic control.

**DOSAGE:** *Adults:* Take with meals. Initial: 1.25mg-250mg qd. If $HbA_{1c}$ >9% or FPG >200mg/dL, give 1.25mg-250mg bid. Titrate: Increase by 1.25mg-250mg/day every 2 weeks. Do not use 50mg-500mg tab for initial therapy. Second-Line Therapy: Initial: 2.5mg-500mg or 5mg-500mg bid. Starting dose should not exceed daily doses of glyburide (or sulfonylurea equivalent) or metformin already being taken. Titrate: Increase by no more than 5mg-500mg/day. Max: 20mg-2000mg/day. With Concomitant TZD: Initiate and titrate TZD as recommended. If hypoglycemia occurs, reduce glyburide component. Elderly/Debilitated/Malnourished: Conservative dosing; do not titrate to max.

**HOW SUPPLIED:** Tab: (Glyburide-Metformin) 1.25mg-250mg, 2.5mg-500mg, 5mg-500mg

**CONTRAINDICATIONS:** Renal disease/dysfunction (SrCr >1.5mg/dL [males], >1.4mg/dL [females], abnormal CrCl), CHF, metabolic acidosis, diabetic ketoacidosis. Discontinue temporarily (48 hrs) for radiologic studies with IV iodinated contrast materials.

**WARNINGS/PRECAUTIONS:** Lactic acidosis reported (rare); increased risk with renal dysfunction, increased age, DM, CHF, and other conditions with risk of hypoperfusion and hypoxemia. Avoid use in patients >80 yrs unless renal function is normal. Increased risk of cardiovascular mortality. Increased risk of hypoglycemia in elderly, debilitated/malnourished, adrenal or pituitary insufficiency, or alcohol intoxication. Discontinue in hypoxic states (eg, CHF, shock, acute MI), loss of blood glucose control due to stress (give insulin), acidosis and prior to surgical procedures (due to restricted food intake). Monitor renal function and for ketoacidosis and metabolic acidosis. Avoid in renal/hepatic impairment. May decrease serum vitamin $B_{12}$ levels. When used with a TZD, monitor LFTs and for weight gain. Withhold treatment with any condition associated with hypoxemia, dehydration, or sepsis.

G

**ADVERSE REACTIONS:** Hypoglycemia, nausea, vomiting, abdominal pain, upper respiratory infection, headache, dizziness, diarrhea.

**INTERACTIONS:** Furosemide, nifedipine, cimetidine and cationic drugs (eg, digoxin, amiloride, procainamide, quinidine, quinine, ranitidine, trimethoprim, vancomycin, triamterene, morphine) may increase metformin levels. Potentiated hypoglycemia with alcohol, ciprofloxacin, miconazole, NSAIDs, salicylates, sulfonamides, chloramphenicol, probenecid, coumarins, MAOIs, TZDs (eg, rosiglitazone), and β-blockers. Thiazides and other diuretics, corticosteroids, phenothiazines, thyroid products, estrogens, oral contraceptives, phenytoin, nicotinic acid, sympathomimetics, calcium channel blockers, and isoniazid may cause hyperglycemia. Excess alcohol may increase potential for lactic acidosis. May decrease furosemide levels.

**PREGNANCY:** Category B, not for use in nursing.

## GLUMETZA

metformin HCl (Biovail) RX

**THERAPEUTIC CLASS:** Biguanide

**INDICATIONS:** Adjunct to diet and exercise or with a sulfonylurea or insulin, to improve glycemic control in type 2 diabetes mellitus.

**DOSAGE:** *Adults:* ≥18 yrs:Take with evening meal. Initial: 1000mg qd. With Insulin: Initial: 500mg qd. Titrate: May increase by 500mg/week. Max: 2000mg/day. Decrease insulin dose by 10-25% if FPG <120mg/dL. Elderly/Debilitated/Malnourished: Conservative dosing; do not titrate to Max. Swallow whole; do not crush or chew.

**HOW SUPPLIED:** Tab, Extended-Release: 500mg, 1000mg

**CONTRAINDICATIONS:** Renal disease/dysfunction (SrCr ≥1.5mg/dL [males], ≥1.4mg/dL [females], abnormal CrCl), CHF, metabolic acidosis, diabetic ketoacidosis. Discontinue temporarily (48 hrs) for radiologic studies with intravascular iodinated contrast materials.

**WARNINGS/PRECAUTIONS:** Lactic acidosis reported (rare); increased risk with renal dysfunction, increased age, DM, CHF, and other conditions with risk of hypoperfusion and hypoxemia. Avoid use in patients ≥80 yrs unless renal function is normal. Monitor renal function and for ketoacidosis and metabolic acidosis. Avoid in renal/hepatic impairment. Discontinue in hypoxic states (eg, CHF, shock, acute MI), loss of blood glucose control due to stress (give insulin), acidosis, dehydration, sepsis. Temporarily discontinue prior to surgery (due to restricted food/fluid intake) and procedures requiring intravascular iodinated contrast materials. May decrease serum vitamin B12 levels. Increased risk of hypoglycemia in elderly, debilitated/malnourished, adrenal or pituitary insufficiency, or alcohol intoxication.

**ADVERSE REACTIONS:** Hypoglycemia, diarrhea, nausea.

**INTERACTIONS:** Furosemide, nifedipine, cimetidine, cationic drugs (eg, digoxin, amiloride, procainamide, quinidine, quinine, ranitidine, trimethoprim, vancomycin, triamterene, morphine) may increase metformin levels. Thiazides, other diuretics, corticosteroids, phenothiazines, thyroid products, estrogens, oral contraceptives, phenytoin, nicotinic acid, sympathomimetics, calcium channel blockers, isoniazid may cause hyperglycemia. Risk of hypoglycemia with alcohol. Excess alcohol may increase potential for lactic acidosis. May decrease furosemide levels.

**PREGNANCY:** Category B, not for use in nursing.

## GLYNASE PRESTAB — RX

glyburide (Pharmacia & Upjohn)



**THERAPEUTIC CLASS:** Sulfonylurea (2nd generation)

**INDICATIONS:** Adjunct to diet and exercise, to improve glycemic control in type 2 diabetes mellitus. May use in combination with metformin.

**DOSAGE:** *Adults:* Initial: 1.5-3mg qd with breakfast or 1st main meal. Renal/Hepatic Disease/Elderly/Debilitated/Malnourished/Adrenal or Pituitary Insufficiency: Initial: 0.75mg qd. Titrate: Increase by no more than 1.5mg/day at weekly intervals. Maint: 0.75-12mg qd or in divided doses. Max: 12mg/day given qd or bid. Transfer from Other Sulfonylureas: Starting dose should not exceed 3mg/day. Switch from Insulin: If <20 U/day, substitute with 1.5-3mg qd. If 20-40 U/day, give 3mg qd. If >40 U/day, decrease insulin dose by 50% and give 3mg qd. Titrate: Progressive withdrawal of insulin and increase by 0.75-1.5mg every 2-10 days.

**HOW SUPPLIED:** Tab: 1.5mg*, 3mg*, 6mg* *scored

**CONTRAINDICATIONS:** Diabetic ketoacidosis, and as sole therapy of type 1 DM.

**WARNINGS/PRECAUTIONS:** Increased risk of cardiovascular mortality. Risk of hypoglycemia, especially with renal and hepatic disease, elderly, debilitated, malnourished, and adrenal or pituitary insufficiency. Loss of blood glucose control when exposed to stress (eg, fever, trauma, infection or surgery); d/c therapy and start insulin. Secondary failure can occur over a period of time. D/C if cholestatic jaundice or hepatitis occur. Retitrate when transferring from other glyburide products.

**ADVERSE REACTIONS:** Hypoglycemia, nausea, epigastric fullness, heartburn, allergic skin reactions, disulfiram-like reactions (rarely), hyponatremia, blood dyscrasias, LFT abnormalities, photosensitivity reactions.

**INTERACTIONS:** Hypoglycemia potentiated by alcohol, NSAIDs, miconazole, ciprofloxacin, highly protein bound drugs, salicylates, sulfonamides, chloramphenicol, probenecid, coumarins, MAOIs, and β-blockers. Risk of hyperglycemia with diuretics, corticosteroids, phenothiazines, thyroid products, estrogens, oral contraceptives, phenytoin, nicotinic acid, sympathomimetics, calcium channel blockers, and isoniazid. β-Blockers may mask hypoglycemia.

**PREGNANCY:** Category B, not for use in nursing.

## GLYSET — RX

miglitol (Pharmacia & Upjohn)

**THERAPEUTIC CLASS:** Alpha-glucosidase inhibitor

**INDICATIONS:** Adjunct to diet and exercise, to improve glycemic control in type 2 diabetes mellitus. May use in combination with a sulfonylurea.

**DOSAGE:** *Adults:* Initial: 25mg tid. May give 25mg qd (to minimize GI side effects) and gradually increase to tid. Titrate: After 4-8 weeks, increase to 50mg tid. Maint: 50mg tid. After 3 months may increase to 100mg tid if needed. Max: 100mg tid. Take with first bite of each main meal.

**HOW SUPPLIED:** Tab: 25mg, 50mg, 100mg

**CONTRAINDICATIONS:** Ketoacidosis, inflammatory bowel disease, colonic ulceration, partial intestinal obstruction or if predisposed to intestinal obstruction. Chronic intestinal diseases with digestion or absorption disorders/conditions may deteriorate with increased gas formation in the intestine.

**WARNINGS/PRECAUTIONS:** Use glucose (dextrose) not sucrose (cane sugar) to treat mild-moderate hypoglycemia. Temporary insulin therapy may be necessary at times of stress such as fever, trauma, infection, or surgery. Not recommended with renal impairment (SrCr >2mg/dL).

**ADVERSE REACTIONS:** Flatulence, diarrhea, abdominal pain, skin rash, decreased serum iron.

**INTERACTIONS:** Intestinal absorbents (eg, charcoal) and digestive enzyme preparations (eg, amylase, pancreatin) may reduce effects. May reduce bioavailability of ranitidine and propranolol. May interact with glyburide, metformin, and digoxin.

**PREGNANCY:** Category B, not for use in nursing.



## GoLYTELY RX

sodium sulfate - sodium chloride - potassium chloride - sodium bicarbonate - polyethylene glycol 3350 (Braintree)

**THERAPEUTIC CLASS:** Bowel cleanser

**INDICATIONS:** Bowel cleansing prior to colonoscopy or barium enema X-ray.

**DOSAGE:** *Adults:* Oral: 240mL every 10 minutes until fecal discharge is clear or 4L is consumed. Nasogastric Tube: 20-30mL/minute (1.2-1.8L/hr). Patient should fast at least 3-4 hours before administration.

**HOW SUPPLIED:** Sol: (Polyethylene Glycol-Potassium Chloride-Sodium Bicarbonate-Sodium Chloride-Sodium Sulfate) 236g-2.97g-6.74g-5.86g-22.74g [4000mL]

**CONTRAINDICATIONS:** GI obstruction, gastric retention, bowel perforation, toxic colitis, toxic megacolon, ileus.

**WARNINGS/PRECAUTIONS:** Do not add additional ingredients (eg, flavorings). Caution with severe ulcerative colitis. Monitor therapy with impaired gag reflex, unconsciousness/semiconsciousness and patients prone to regurgitation or aspiration. Slow administration or temporarily discontinue if severe bloating, distention, or abdominal pain develops.

**ADVERSE REACTIONS:** Nausea, abdominal fullness, cramping, bloating, vomiting, anal irritation.

**INTERACTIONS:** Oral medications taken within 1 hr of start of administration may not be absorbed from GI tract.

**PREGNANCY:** Category C, caution in nursing.

## GONAL-F RX

follitropin alfa (Serono)

**THERAPEUTIC CLASS:** Follicle stimulating hormone

**INDICATIONS:** For development of multiple follicles in ovulatory patients participating in Assisted Reproductive Technology (ART). (Men) For induction of spermatogenesis in primary and secondary hypogonadotropic hypogonadism not due to primary testicular failure.

**DOSAGE:** *Adults:* Individualize dose. Oligo-Anovulation: Initial: 75 IU/day SQ. Titrate: Increase up to 37.5 IU/day after 14 days and further increase after 7 days if needed. Give hCG 5000 U 1 day after last dose. Do not exceed 35 days of therapy unless an E2 rise indicates imminent follicular development. Max: 300 IU/day. ART: Initial: 150 IU/day SQ on cycle Day 2 or 3 (early follicular phase). If gonadotropins suppressed, initiate at 225 IU/day. Titrate: Adjust after 5 days if needed, then at intervals no less than 3-5 days and not exceeding 75-150 IU/adjustment. Max: 450 IU/day. Once follicular development is evident, give hCG 5000-10,000 U. Hypogonadotropic Hypogonadism: Pretreat with hCG 1000-2250 U 2-3x/week to achieve normal serum testosterone levels. When normal, give 150 IU SQ and hCG 1000 U 3x/week. Max: 300 IU 3x/week.

**HOW SUPPLIED:** Inj: 75 IU, 450 IU, 300 IU/0.5mL, 450 IU/0.75mL, 900 IU/1.5mL

**CONTRAINDICATIONS:** (Men, Women) High FSH levels indicating gonadal failure, uncontrolled thyroid or adrenal dysfunction, sex hormone dependent tumors of the reproductive tract and accessory organs, organic intracranial lesions (eg, pituitary tumor). (Women) Aabnormal uterine bleeding of undetermined origin, ovarian cyst or enlargement, pregnancy.

G

**WARNINGS/PRECAUTIONS:** Ovarian enlargement may occur; monitor ovarian response. Ovarian hyperstimulation syndrome, multiple births, serious pulmonary and vascular complications reported. Avoid hCG if ovaries abnormally enlarged last day of therapy. Monitor follicular maturation by measuring estradiol levels and through ultrasonography.

**ADVERSE REACTIONS:** (Women) Intermenstrual bleeding, breast pain, ovarian hyperstimulation, abdominal pain, nausea, diarrhea, flatulence, headache, ovarian cysts, pain, upper respiratory tract infection. (Men) Breast pain, acne, gynecomastia, injection site pain, fatigue.

**PREGNANCY:** Category X, not for use in nursing.

## GRANULEX RX

trypsin - castor oil - peruvian balsam (Mylan Bertek)

**THERAPEUTIC CLASS:** Debriding agent

**INDICATIONS:** Treatment of decubitus ulcers, varicose ulcers, debridement of eschar, dehiscent wounds and sunburn.

**DOSAGE:** *Adults:* Spray wound at least bid or more often prn.
*Pediatrics:* Spray wound at least bid or more often prn.

**HOW SUPPLIED:** Spray: (Castor Oil-Peruvian Balsam-Trypsin) 650mg-72.5mg-0.1mg/0.82mL [60mL, 120mL]

**WARNINGS/PRECAUTIONS:** Do not spray on fresh arterial clots. Avoid spraying in eyes. Wound may be left open or a wet bandage may be applied.

**PREGNANCY:** Safety in pregnancy and nursing is not known.

## GRIFULVIN V RX

griseofulvin (Ortho Neutrogena)

**THERAPEUTIC CLASS:** *Penicillium*-derived antifungal

**INDICATIONS:** Management of tinea capitis, tinea corporis, tinea pedis, tinea unguium, tinea barbae, and tinea cruris.

**DOSAGE:** *Adults:* Tinea Capitis: 500mg qd for 4-6 weeks. Tinea Corporis: 500mg qd for 2-4 weeks. Tinea Pedis: 1g qd for 4-8 weeks. Tinea Cruris: 500mg qd. Tinea Unguium: 1g qd for at least 4 months (fingernail) or at least 6 months (toenails).
*Pediatrics:* Usual: 5mg/lb/day. 30-50lb: 125-250mg qd. >50lb: 250-500mg qd. Tinea Capitis: Treat for 4-6 weeks. Tinea Corporis: Treat for 2-4 weeks. Tinea Pedis: Treat for 4-8 weeks. Tinea Unguium: Treat for at least 4 months (fingernail) or at least 6 months (toenails).

**HOW SUPPLIED:** Sus: 125mg/5mL [120mL]; Tab: 500mg

**CONTRAINDICATIONS:** Porphyria, hepatocellular failure, pregnancy.

**WARNINGS/PRECAUTIONS:** Confirm diagnosis. Not for prophylactic use. Monitor renal, hepatic, and hematopoietic functions periodically with prolonged therapy. Cross-sensitivity with penicillin may exist. Photosensitivity reported. D/C if granulocytopenia occurs.

**ADVERSE REACTIONS:** Rash, urticaria, oral thrush, nausea, vomiting, epigastric distress, diarrhea, headache, dizziness, insomnia, mental confusion.

**INTERACTIONS:** Oral anticoagulants may need adjustment. Barbiturates decrease effects. Decreases effects of oral contraceptives; may increase incidence of breakthrough bleeding.

**PREGNANCY:** Not for use in pregnancy and in nursing.

## GRIS-PEG

RX

griseofulvin (Pedinol)

**THERAPEUTIC CLASS:** *Penicillium*-derived antifungal

**INDICATIONS:** Treatment of tinea capitis, t.corporis, t.pedis, t.unguium, t.barbae and t.cruris.

**DOSAGE:** *Adults:* T.capitis: 375mg qd in single or divided doses for 4-6 weeks. T.corporis: 375mg qd in single or divided doses for 2-4 weeks. T.pedis: 375mg bid for 4-8 weeks. T.cruris: 375mg qd in single or divided doses. T.unguium: 375mg bid for at least 4 months (fingernail) or at least 6 months (toenails). *Pediatrics:* Usual: 3.3mg/lb/day. 35-60lb: 125-187.5mg qd. >60lb: 187.5-375mg qd. T.capitis: Treat for 4-6 weeks. T.corporis: Treat for 2-4 weeks. T.pedis: Treat for 4-8 weeks. T.unguium: Treat for at least 4 months (fingernail) or at least 6 months (toenails).

**HOW SUPPLIED:** Tab: 125mg*, 250mg* *scored

**CONTRAINDICATIONS:** Porphyria, hepatocellular failure, pregnancy.

**WARNINGS/PRECAUTIONS:** Not for prophylactic use. Periodically monitor renal, hepatic, and hematopoietic functions in prolonged therapy. Cross-sensitivity with penicillin may exist. Photosensitivity reported. D/C if granulocytopenia occurs.

**ADVERSE REACTIONS:** Rash, urticaria, oral thrush, nausea, vomiting, epigastric distress, diarrhea, headache, dizziness, insomnia, mental confusion.

**INTERACTIONS:** Oral anticoagulants may need dose adjustments. Decreased effects with barbiturates. Decreased effects of oral contraceptives. Increased alcohol effects.

**PREGNANCY:** Not for use in pregnancy and in nursing.

## GUAIFED-PD

RX

guaifenesin - phenylephrine HCl (Victory)

**THERAPEUTIC CLASS:** Nasal decongestant and expectorant

**INDICATIONS:** Temporary relief of nasal congestion and dry nonproductive cough associated with the common cold and other respiratory allergies.

**DOSAGE:** *Adults:* 1-2 caps q12h.
*Pediatrics:* >12 yrs: 1-2 caps q12h. 6 to <12yrs: 1 cap q12h.

**HOW SUPPLIED:** Cap: (Guaifenesin-Phenylephrine) 200mg-7.5mg

**CONTRAINDICATIONS:** Severe HTN, severe CAD, concomitant MAOIs, pregnancy, nursing mothers.

**WARNINGS/PRECAUTIONS:** Caution with HTN, DM, ischemic heart disease, hyperthyroidism, increased IOP, prostatic hypertrophy, and the elderly. Not for persistent or chronic cough such as occurs with smoking, asthma, emphysema, or where cough is accompanied by excessive secretions.

**ADVERSE REACTIONS:** Nausea, cardiac palpitations, increased irritability, headache, dizziness, tachycardia, diarrhea, drowsiness, stomach pain, seizures, slowed heart rate, shortness of breath.

**INTERACTIONS:** MAOIs and β-adrenergic blockers may increase the effect of sympathomimetics. Sympathomimetics may reduce the antihypertensive effects of methyldopa, mecamylamine, reserpine and veratrum alkaloids. Pseudoephedrine may increase the possibility of cardiac arrhythmias with digitalis glycosides.

**PREGNANCY:** Category B, not for use in nursing.

## GUAIFENESIN-HYDROCODONE BITARTRATE CIII

guaifenesin - hydrocodone bitartrate (Various)

**OTHER BRAND NAMES:** Codiclear DH (Victory)

G

**THERAPEUTIC CLASS:** Opioid antitussive

**INDICATIONS:** Nonproductive cough.

**DOSAGE:** *Adults:* Initial: 5mL pc and qhs (at least 4 hrs apart). Max: 30mL/day, and 15mL/single dose.
*Pediatrics:* >12 yrs: Initial: 5mL pc and qhs (at least 4 hrs apart); up to 10mL/single dose. 6-12 yrs: Initial: 2.5mL pc and qhs (at least 4 hrs apart); up to 5mL/single dose.

**HOW SUPPLIED:** Syrup: (Hydrocodone-Guaifenesin) 5mg-100mg/5mL

**WARNINGS/PRECAUTIONS:** May obscure diagnosis or clinical course of acute abdominal conditions or head injuries. May produce dose-related respiratory depression. Monitor for tolerance.

**ADVERSE REACTIONS:** Respiratory depression, nausea, vomiting, HTN, postural hypotension, palpitations, ureteral spasm, vesical sphinctor spasms, urinary retention, sedation, drowsiness, nausea, vomiting.

**INTERACTIONS:** Additive CNS depression with other narcotic analgesics, general anesthetics, phenothiazines, tranquilizers, sedative hypnotics, alcohol, CNS depressants.

**PREGNANCY:** Category C, not for use in nursing.

## GUIATUSS DAC CV

guaifenesin - codeine phosphate - pseudoephedrine HCl (Scientific Labs)

**THERAPEUTIC CLASS:** Cough suppressant/expectorant/ decongestant

**INDICATIONS:** Relief of nasal congestion and cough due to throat and bronchial irritation from a cold or inhaled irritants. Loosens phlegm and thins bronchial secretions to make coughs more productive.

**DOSAGE:** *Adults:* 10mL q4h. Max: 40mL/24 hrs.
*Pediatrics:* >12 yrs: 10mL q4h. Max: 40mL/24 hrs. 6 to <12 yrs: 5mL q4h. Max: 20mL/24 hrs.

**HOW SUPPLIED:** Syrup: (Codeine-Guaifenesin-Pseudoephedrine) 10mg-100mg-30mg/5mL

**WARNINGS/PRECAUTIONS:** Use caution with persistent/chronic cough, cough with excessive phlegm, chronic pulmonary disease, high BP, heart disease, DM, thyroid disease, or shortness of breath. May cause or aggravate constipation.

**ADVERSE REACTIONS:** Constipation, sedation.

**INTERACTIONS:** Caution with antidepressants, especially MAOIs.

**PREGNANCY:** Safety in pregnancy and nursing not known.

## GYNAZOLE-1
RX

butoconazole nitrate (Ther-Rx)

**THERAPEUTIC CLASS:** Azole antifungal

**INDICATIONS:** Local treatment of vulvovaginal infections caused by *Candida albicans*.

**DOSAGE:** *Adults:* 1 applicatorful intravaginally once.

**HOW SUPPLIED:** Cre: 2% [5g]

**WARNINGS/PRECAUTIONS:** Do not rely on condoms or diaphragm within 72 hrs after last use. Confirm diagnosis by KOH smears and/or cultures; reconfirm if no response.

**ADVERSE REACTIONS:** Vulvar/vaginal burning, itching, soreness, swelling, pelvic or abdominal pain, cramping.

**PREGNANCY:** Category C, caution in nursing.



## GYNE-LOTRIMIN
OTC

clotrimazole (Schering)

**OTHER BRAND NAMES:** Gyne-Lotrimin 3 (Schering) - Gyne-Lotrimin Combination Pack (Schering) - Gyne-Lotrimin 3 Combination Pack (Schering)

**THERAPEUTIC CLASS:** Azole antifungal

**INDICATIONS:** Treatment of vaginal candidiasis.

**DOSAGE:** *Adults:* 200mg sup or 2% cream intravaginally qhs for 3 days, or 100mg sup or 1% cream intravaginally qhs for 7 days. Apply 1% cream externally qd-bid prn.
*Pediatrics:* >12 yrs: 200mg sup or 2% cream intravaginally qhs for 3 days, or 100mg sup or 1% cream intravaginally qhs for 7 days. Apply 1% cream externally qd-bid prn.

**HOW SUPPLIED:** (Gyne-Lotrimin) Cre: 1% [5g, 45g]; Sup: 100mg [7s]; (Combination Pack) Cre: 1% [7g]; Sup: 100mg [7s]; (Gyne-Lotrimin 3) Sup: 200mg [3s]; (3 Combination Pack) Cre: 1% [7g]; Sup: 200mg [3s]

**WARNINGS/PRECAUTIONS:** Do not use if fever (>100°F), foul smelling vaginal discharge or abdominal, back or shoulder pain. Do not use with douches, spermicide or tampons. Do not rely on condoms or diaphragm to prevent STDs or pregnancy while using these products.

## GYNODIOL
RX

estradiol (Novavax)

**Estrogens increase risk of endometrial cancer in postmenopausal women. Avoid during pregnancy.**

**THERAPEUTIC CLASS:** Estrogen

**INDICATIONS:** Treatment of moderate to severe vasomotor symptoms associated with menopause. Treatment of vulval/vaginal atrophy. Treatment of hypoestrogenism due to hypogonadism, castration, or primary ovarian failure. Palliative treatment of breast cancer in patients with metastatic disease and/or advanced androgen-dependent carcinoma of the prostate. Prevention of osteoporosis.

**DOSAGE:** *Adults:* Vasomotor Symptoms/Vulval/Vaginal Atrophy: Initial: 1-2mg/day (3 weeks on, 1 week off). Maint: Minimum effective dose. Discontinue or taper at 3-6 month intervals. Hypoestrogenism: 1-2mg/day. Maint: Minimum effective dose. Metastatic Breast Cancer: 10mg tid for at least 3 months. Prostate Carcinoma: 1-2mg tid. Osteoporosis Prevention: 0.5mg qd (23 days on and 5 days off).

**HOW SUPPLIED:** Tab: 0.5mg*, 1mg*, 1.5mg*, 2mg* *scored

**CONTRAINDICATIONS:** Pregnancy, undiagnosed abnormal genital bleeding, breast cancer unless being treated for metastatic disease, estrogen-dependent neoplasia, thrombophlebitis, thromboembolic disorders.

**WARNINGS/PRECAUTIONS:** Risk of endometrial and breast cancer, fetal congenital reproductive tract disorder gallbladder disease, cardiovascular disease, elevated BP, and hypercalcemia with breast cancer and bone metastases. Caution in liver dysfunction, asthma, epilepsy, migraine, and cardiac or renal dysfunction. May develop uterine bleeding and mastodynia. Accelerated PT, PTT, and platelet aggregation time. Hypercoagulability effects. Impaired glucose tolerance. Consider addition of a progestin in patient with intact uterus. Increase in HDL, triglycerides, thyroid-binding globulin.

**ADVERSE REACTIONS:** Altered vaginal bleeding, vaginal candidiasis, breast tenderness/enlargement, GI effects, CNS effects, chloasma, melasma, weight changes, edema, altered libido.

**PREGNANCY:** Category X, not for use in nursing.

H

## HALCION CIV

triazolam (Pharmacia & Upjohn)

**THERAPEUTIC CLASS:** Benzodiazepine

**INDICATIONS:** Short-term treatment of insomnia.

**DOSAGE:** *Adults:* 0.25mg qhs. Max: 0.5mg. Elderly/Debilitated: Initial: 0.125mg. Max: 0.25mg.

**HOW SUPPLIED:** Tab: 0.125mg, 0.25mg* *scored

**CONTRAINDICATIONS:** Pregnancy. With ketoconazole, itraconazole, nefazodone, medications that impair CYP3A.

**WARNINGS/PRECAUTIONS:** Worsening or failure of response after 7-10 days may indicate other medical conditions. Increased daytime anxiety, abnormal thinking and behavioral changes have occurred. May impair mental/physical abilities. Anterograde amnesia reported with therapeutic doses. Caution with baseline depression, suicidal tendencies, history of drug dependence, elderly/debilitated, renal/hepatic impairment, chronic pulmonary insufficiency, and sleep apnea. Withdrawal symptoms after discontinuation; avoid abrupt withdrawal.

**ADVERSE REACTIONS:** Drowsiness, dizziness, lightheadedness, headache, nausea, vomiting, coordination disorders, ataxia.

**INTERACTIONS:** See Contraindications. Avoid the concomitant use with inhibitors of the CYP3A (eg, ketoconazole, itraconazole, all azole-type antifungals, nefazodone). Potentiated by the coadministration of isoniazid, OCs, grapefruit juice, ranitidine. Caution with fluvoxamine, diltiazem, verapamil, cimetidine, ergotamine, cyclosporine, amiodarone, nicardipine, nifedipine, sertraline, paroxetine, macrolides. Additive CNS depression with psychotropics, anticonvulsants, antihistamines, and alcohol.

**PREGNANCY:** Category X, not for use in nursing.

## HALFLYTELY RX

bisacodyl - sodium chloride - potassium chloride - sodium bicarbonate - polyethylene glycol 3350 (Braintree)

**THERAPEUTIC CLASS:** Bowel cleanser/stimulant laxative

**INDICATIONS:** Bowel cleansing prior to colonoscopy.

**DOSAGE:** *Adults:* Consume only clear liquids on day of preparation. Swallow all 4 bisacodyl tablets at noon (do not chew or crush). After first bowel movement (or maximum of 6 hours) begin drinking solution, 240mL every 10 minutes (approx. 8 glasses). Drink ALL solution.

**HOW SUPPLIED:** Kit: Tab, Delayed-Release: (Bisacodyl) 5mg [4s]. Sol: (Polyethylene Glycol 3350-Potassium Chloride-Sodium Bicarbonate-Sodium Chloride) 210g-0.74g-2.86g-5.60g [2000mL].

**CONTRAINDICATIONS:** Ileus, GI obstruction, gastric retention, bowel perforation, toxic colitis, toxic megacolon.

**WARNINGS/PRECAUTIONS:** Do not add additional ingredients (eg, flavorings). Caution with severe ulcerative colitis. Monitor with impaired gag reflex, prone to regurgitation or aspiration. Slow administration or temporarily discontinue if severe bloating, distention, or abdominal pain develops. Avoid large quantities of water during or after preparation or colonoscopy. Monitor closely with impaired water handling.

**ADVERSE REACTIONS:** Nausea, abdominal fullness, cramping, vomiting, overall discomfort.

**INTERACTIONS:** Oral medications taken within 1 hr of start of administration start may not be absorbed from GI tract. Avoid bisacodyl delayed release tablets within 1 hr of taking an antacid.

**PREGNANCY:** Category C, caution in nursing.



## HALFPRIN
aspirin (Kramer) OTC

**THERAPEUTIC CLASS:** Salicylate

**INDICATIONS:** To reduce the risk of vascular mortality and fatal and nonfatal cardiovascular and cerebrovascular events in patients with a suspected acute MI.

**DOSAGE:** *Adults:* 162mg as soon as MI suspected; continue qd for 30 days. May need to continue as prophylaxis for recurrent MI. Crush, chew, or suck the 1st dose.

**HOW SUPPLIED:** Tab, Delayed Release: 81mg, 162mg

**WARNINGS/PRECAUTIONS:** Caution with marked HTN or renal dysfunction; monitor renal function with long-term therapy.

**ADVERSE REACTIONS:** Stomach pain, heartburn, nausea, vomiting, GI bleeding, small increases in BP.

**PREGNANCY:** Safety in pregnancy and nursing is not known.

## HALOG
halcinonide (Westwood-Squibb) RX

**OTHER BRAND NAMES:** Halog-E (Westwood-Squibb)

**THERAPEUTIC CLASS:** Corticosteroid

**INDICATIONS:** Corticosteroid responsive dermatoses.

**DOSAGE:** *Adults:* (Cre, Oint, Sol) Apply bid-tid. (Cre in hydrophilic base) Apply qd-tid. May use occlusive dressings for psoriasis and recalcitrant conditions. *Pediatrics:* Limit to least amount compatible with an effective therapeutic regimen.

**HOW SUPPLIED:** (Halog) Cre, Oint: 0.1% [15g, 30g, 60g, 240g]; Sol: 0.1% [20mL, 60mL]; (Halog-E) Cre: 0.1% in a hydrophilic vanishing cream [30g, 60g]

**WARNINGS/PRECAUTIONS:** May produce reversible HPA axis suppression, manifestations of Cushing's syndrome, hyperglycemia and glucosuria. Occlusive dressings and application to large surface areas may augment systemic absorption. Pediatrics may be more susceptible to systemic toxicity. Discontinue if irritation occurs.

**ADVERSE REACTIONS:** Burning, itching, irritation, dryness, folliculitis, hypertrichosis, acneiform eruptions, hypopigmentation, perioral dermatitis, contact dermatitis, skin maceration, secondary infection.

**PREGNANCY:** Category C, caution in nursing.

## HALOPERIDOL
RX

haloperidol (Various)

**OTHER BRAND NAMES:** Haldol (Ortho-McNeil) - Haldol Decanoate (Ortho-McNeil)

**THERAPEUTIC CLASS:** Butyrophenone

**INDICATIONS:** (Immediate-Release) Treatment of psychosis, Tourette's disorder, severe childhood behavioral problems. Short-term treatment of hyperactivity in children. (Decanoate) Prolonged management of psychosis.

**DOSAGE:** *Adults:* Psychosis: (Immediate Release) PO: Moderate Symptoms/Elderly/Debilitated: 0.5-2mg bid-tid. Severe Symptoms/Resistant Patients: 3-5mg bid-tid. Max: 100mg/day. IM: Acute Agitation: 2-5mg every 4-8 hrs or hourly as needed for moderately severe to very severe symptoms. Max: 100mg/day. (Decanoate) Give every 4 weeks or monthly. Initial: 10-20 times daily oral dose up to 100mg. Give remainder of dose 3-7 days later if initial dose >100mg. Usual: 10-15 times daily oral dose. Max: 450mg/month. Elderly/Debilitated: Initial: 10-15 times daily oral dose.
*Pediatrics:* 3-12 yrs (15-40 kg): PO: Psychosis: 0.05-0.15mg/kg/day given bid-tid. Nonpsychotic Disorder/Tourette's: 0.05-0.075mg/kg/day given bid-tid. Max: 6mg/day.

**HOW SUPPLIED:** Inj: 5mg/mL; Inj: (Decanoate) 50mg/mL, 100mg/mL; Sol: 2mg/mL; Tab: 0.5mg*, 1mg*, 2mg*, 5mg*, 10mg*, 20mg* *scored

**CONTRAINDICATIONS:** Comatose states, severe toxic CNS depression, Parkinson's disease.

**WARNINGS/PRECAUTIONS:** Risk of tardive dyskinesia, especially in elderly. NMS, hyperpyrexia, heat stroke, bronchopneumonia reported. Decreased cholesterol, cutaneous and/or ocular changes may occur. Neurotoxicity may occur with thyrotoxicosis. Caution with cardiovascular disease, seizures, EEG abnormalities, elderly.

**ADVERSE REACTIONS:** Extrapyramidal symptoms, tardive dyskinesia, tardive dystonia, ECG changes, gynecomastia, insomnia, drowsiness, skin reactions, anorexia, anticholinergic effects, laryngospasm, cataracts.

**INTERACTIONS:** Caution with rifampin, anticonvulsants, anticoagulants, anticholinergics, antiparkinson agents. May potentiate CNS depression with alcohol, opiates, anesthetics and other CNS depressants. Antagonizes epinephrine. Monitor for neurological toxicity with lithium.

**PREGNANCY:** Category C, not for use in nursing.

## HALOTESTIN
CIII

fluoxymesterone (Pharmacia & Upjohn)

**THERAPEUTIC CLASS:** Androgen

**INDICATIONS:** Testosterone replacement therapy in males with primary hypogonadism or hypogonadotrophic hypogonadism. To stimulate puberty in males with delayed puberty. Palliation of androgen-responsive recurrent mammary cancer in females who are >1 to <5yrs postmenopausal or who have a hormone-dependent tumor as shown by previous beneficial response to castration.

**DOSAGE:** *Adults:* Male Replacement Therapy: 5-20mg/day, qd or in divided doses tid-qid. Breast Cancer: 10-40mg/day in divided doses tid-qid. Continue therapy for at least 1 month for a satisfactory subjective response, and for 2-3 months for an objective response.
*Pediatrics:* Male Replacement Therapy: 5-20mg/day, qd or in divided doses tid-qid. Delayed Puberty: Initial: Use low dose, titrate carefully; use for 4-6 months. Caution in children.

**HOW SUPPLIED:** Tab: 2mg*, 5mg*, 10mg* *scored

**CONTRAINDICATIONS:** Males with breast or prostate cancer, pregnancy, serious cardiac, hepatic or renal disease.

**WARNINGS/PRECAUTIONS:** Discontinue if hypercalcemia occurs in breast cancer or immobilized patients; monitor calcium levels. Risk of hepatic adenomas, hepatocellular carcinoma, and peliosis hepatitis with prolonged high doses. Discontinue if jaundice, cholestatic hepatitis occurs. Caution in the elderly; increased risk of prostatic hypertrophy and prostatic carcinoma. Risk of edema; caution with pre-existing cardiac, renal, or hepatic disease. Risk of compromised stature in children; monitor bone growth every 6 months. Should not be used for enhancement of athletic performance. Monitor for virilization in females. Patients with BPH may develop acute urethral obstruction. If priapism occurs, discontinue and if restarted use lower dose. Contains tartrazine; may cause allergic type reactions especially in those with aspirin hypersensitivity. Monitor LFTs, Hct, Hgb periodically.

**ADVERSE REACTIONS:** Amenorrhea, virilization, menstrual irregularities, gynecomastia, excessive frequency/duration of penile erections, male pattern baldness, increased/decreased libido, oligospermia, hirsutism, acne, fluid and electrolyte disturbances, nausea, hypercholesterolemia, clotting factor suppression, polycythemia, altered LFTs, oligospermia, priapism, anxiety, depression.

**INTERACTIONS:** Potentiates oral anticoagulants and oxyphenbutazone. May decrease blood glucose and insulin requirements.

**PREGNANCY:** Category X, not for use in nursing.

## HALOTHANE

RX

halothane (Various)

**THERAPEUTIC CLASS:** Inhalation anesthetic

**INDICATIONS:** Induction and maintenance of general anesthesia.

**DOSAGE:** *Adults:* Individualize dose. Maint: 0.5-1.5%.

**HOW SUPPLIED:** Liq: [125mL, 250mL]

**CONTRAINDICATIONS:** Obstetrical anesthesia except when uterine relaxation is required.

**WARNINGS/PRECAUTIONS:** Not for use in women where pregnancy is possible and particularly during early pregnancy unless potential benefits outweigh unknown hazards to fetus. Increases CSF pressure; caution with raised intracranial pressure.

**ADVERSE REACTIONS:** Hepatic necrosis, cardiac arrest, hypotension, respiratory arrest, cardiac arrhythmias, hyperpyrexia, shivering, nausea, emesis.

**INTERACTIONS:** Simultaneous use with epinephrine or norepinephrine may induce ventricular tachycardia or fibrillation. May augment actions of nondepolarizing relaxants and ganglionic blocking agents; use with caution. Use with succinylcholine may trigger malignant hyperthermic crisis in genetically susceptible individuals

**PREGNANCY:** Safety in pregnancy and nursing not known.

## HAVRIX

RX

hepatitis A vaccine (inactivated) (GlaxoSmithKline)

**THERAPEUTIC CLASS:** Vaccine

**INDICATIONS:** Active immunization in persons ≥12 months against hepatitis A virus.

**DOSAGE:** *Adults:* ≥18 yrs: 1440 EL U IM (deltoid), then booster after 6-12 months.
*Pediatrics:* 1-18 yrs: 720 EL U IM (deltoid), then booster after 6-12 months.

**HOW SUPPLIED:** Inj: 720 EL U/0.5mL, 1440 EL U/mL

**CONTRAINDICATIONS:** Hypersensitivity to any component, including neomycin.

**WARNINGS/PRECAUTIONS:** Have epinephrine available for anaphylaxis. Delay with febrile illness. Caution with thrombocytopenia or bleeding disorders. Immunosuppressed may show suboptimal response. May not prevent hepatitis A in patients already infected.

**ADVERSE REACTIONS:** Injection site soreness, induration, redness, swelling, fever, fatigue, malaise, anorexia, nausea, headache.

**INTERACTIONS:** Caution with anticoagulant therapy and IM injection. Give immunoglobulins and other vaccines in different syringe and injection site.

**PREGNANCY:** Category C, caution in nursing.



## HECTOROL RX

doxercalciferol (Bone Care)

**THERAPEUTIC CLASS:** Vitamin D analog

**INDICATIONS:** (Cap) Secondary hyperparathyroidism in patients with chronic kidney disease on dialysis or with Stage 3 or 4 chronic kidney disease. (Inj) Secondary hyperparathyroidism in patients with chronic kidney disease on dialysis.

**DOSAGE:** *Adults:* (Cap) Dialysis: Initial: 10mcg 3x/week (TTW) approximately qod at dialysis. Titrate: Adjust to obtain iPTH of 150-300 pg/mL. May increase by 2.5mcg at 8-week intervals if iPTH is not lowered by 50% and fails to reach target range. Max: 20mcg TIW (60mcg/week). Suspend therapy if iPTH <100pg/mL; restart after 1 week with dose at least 2.5mcg lower than last dose. Hypercalcemia/Hyperphosphatemia/Ca x P product >55mg²/dL²: Decrease or suspend therapy and/or adjust dose of phosphate binders; if suspended, restart at a dose at least 2.5mcg lower. Pre-dialysis: Initial: 1mcg qd. Titrate: May increase by 0.5mcg at 2-week intervals to achieve target iPTH range. Max: 3.5mcg qd. Hypercalcemia/Hyperphosphatemia/Ca x P product >55mg²/dL²: Decrease or suspend therapy and/or adjust dose of phosphate binders; if suspended, restart at a dose at least 0.5mcg lower. (Inj) Initial: 4mcg bolus TIW at the end of dialysis. Titrate: Adjust to obtain iPTH of 150-300pg/mL. May increase at 8-week intervals by 1-2mcg if iPTH is not lowered by 50% and fails to reach target range. Max: 18mcg/week. Suspend therapy if iPTH <100pg/mL; restart after 1 week with a dose at least 1mcg lower than last dose. Hypercalcemia/Hyperphosphatemia/Ca x P product >55mg²/dL²: Decrease or suspend therapy and/or adjust dose of phosphate binders; if suspended, restart at a dose at least 1mcg lower.

**HOW SUPPLIED:** Cap: 0.5mcg, 2.5mcg; Inj: 2mcg/mL [2mL]

**CONTRAINDICATIONS:** Tendency to develop hypercalcemia or vitamin D toxicity.

**WARNINGS/PRECAUTIONS:** Acute hypercalcemia may exacerbate arrythmias, seizures. Use oral Ca-based or non-aluminum containing antacids to control serum phosphate. Chronic hypercalcemia can cause calcification of soft tissues. Risk of hypercalcemia and hyperphospatemia. Maintain serum calcium times serum phosphorus at <55mg²/dL² in patients with chronic kidney disease. Avoid with recent history of hypercalcemia, hyperphosphatemia, or vitamin D toxicity. Caution with hepatic dysfunction. Monitor iPTH, serum calcium, and serum phosphorus initially then weekly during dose titration. Oversuppression of iPTH can cause adynamic bone syndrome.

**ADVERSE REACTIONS:** Headache, malaise, bradycardia, nausea, vomiting, edema, dizziness, dyspnea, pruritus, abscess, anorexia, constipation, dyspepsia, arthralgia, weight increase, sleep disorder.

**INTERACTIONS:** (Cap, Inj) Magnesium-containing antacids may cause hypermagnesemia especially with chronic renal dialysis. Enzyme inducers may affect metabolism; consider adjusting dose. CYP450 inhibitors (eg, ketoconazole, erythromycin) may prevent active moiety formation. Avoid vitamin D products and derivatives during treatment. Acute hypercalcemia may affect digitalis activity. (Cap) Colestyramine, mineral oil may impair absorption.

**PREGNANCY:** Category B, not for use in nursing.

## HELIDAC

RX

metronidazole - bismuth subsalicylate - tetracycline HCl (Prometheus)

**THERAPEUTIC CLASS:** Antimicrobial

**INDICATIONS:** In combination with an $H_2$ antagonist for eradication of *H.pylori* and for treatment of *H.pylori* infection and duodenal ulcer disease.

**DOSAGE:** *Adults:* (Bismuth) 2 tabs (525mg) qid + (Metronidazole) 250mg qid + (Tetracycline) 500mg qid, all for 14 days with an $H_2$ antagonist. Take with meals and hs. Take metronidazole and tetracycline with a full glass of water; swallow whole.

**HOW SUPPLIED:** Cap: (Tetracycline) 500mg; Tab: (Metronidazole) 250mg; Tab, Chewable: (Bismuth Subsalicylate) 262.4mg

**CONTRAINDICATIONS:** Pregnancy, nursing, pediatrics, nitroimidazole hypersensitivity, ASA or salicylate hypersensitivity, renal/hepatic impairment.

**WARNINGS/PRECAUTIONS:** Do not use to treat nausea and vomiting in children or teenagers who have or are recovering from chickenpox or flu. Rare reports of neurotoxicity with excessive bismuth doses. Seizures and peripheral neuropathy reported with metronidazole; caution with CNS disease; discontinue with abnormal neurological signs. Caution with blood dyscrasias. Unrecognized candidiasis may be unmasked. Avoid exposure to sunlight/UV light. Caution in elderly.

**ADVERSE REACTIONS:** Nausea, diarrhea, abdominal pain, melena, constipation, anorexia, asthenia, vomiting, discolored tongue, headache, dyspepsia, dizziness. Temporary, harmless darkening of tongue and black stool with bismuth. Tetracycline may cause permanent discoloration of teeth during tooth development, enamel hypoplasia, photosensitivity reactions, BUN increase, breakthrough bleeding, pseudotumor cerebri.

**INTERACTIONS:** Monitor anticoagulants; possible risk of bleeding and/or decreased prothrombin activity. Bismuth subsalicylate: Caution with antidiabetic agents, ASA, probenecid, and sulfinpyrazone. Tetracycline: Impaired absorption with antacids containing aluminum, calcium, magnesium; agents containing iron, zinc, sodium bicarbonate. Possible reduced absorption with dairy products, bismuth, or calcium carbonate. May interfere with bactericidal action of penicillin; avoid concomitant use. May antagonize oral contraceptive effects. Fatal renal toxicity with methoxyflurane reported. Metronidazole (MET): Decreased plasma clearance with drugs that decrease metabolism (eg, cimetidine). Increased elimination with drugs that induce metabolism (eg, phenytoin, phenobarbital). May impair phenytoin clearance. May increase lithium levels. Avoid alcohol during and at least 1 day after MET. Psychotic reactions reported in alcoholics with concomitant disulfiram and MET; space MET and disulfiram dosing by 2 weeks.

**PREGNANCY:** Category D, not for use in nursing.

## HEMABATE

RX

carboprost tromethamine (Pharmacia & Upjohn)

**THERAPEUTIC CLASS:** Prostaglandin analogue

**INDICATIONS:** Termination of pregnancy between 13th to 20th week of gestation. Termination of pregnancy in 2nd trimester if expulsion of fetus fails with other methods; premature, inadvertent, or spontaneous rupture of membranes occurs in previable fetus; or expulsion requires repeat intrauterine instillation. Treatment of postpartum hemorrhage due to uterine atony unresponsive to conventional methods.

**DOSAGE:** *Adults:* Consider pretreatment or concurrent use of antidiarrheals and antiemetics. Abortion/Fetal Expulsion Failure/Ruptured Membranes: May give initial optional test dose of 100mcg. Initial: 250mcg IM. Repeat 250mcg dose at 1.5-3.5 hr intervals, depending on uterine response. May increase to 500mcg if inadequate response after several doses of 250mcg. Max: 12mg total dose or continuous use for >2 days. Refractory Postpartum Uterine Bleeding: Initial: 250mcg IM. Determine additional doses and intervals based on clinical events. Max: 2mg total dose.

**HOW SUPPLIED:** Inj: 250mcg/mL

**CONTRAINDICATIONS:** Active pelvic inflammatory disease; active cardiac, pulmonary, renal or hepatic disease.

**WARNINGS/PRECAUTIONS:** Use in facility able to provide immediate intensive care and acute surgery. Adhere strictly to recommended dosages. Not indicated if fetus in utero is viable. If abortion fails, complete by other means. Contains benzyl alcohol. Caution with history of asthma, hypo- or hypertension, cardiovascular, renal, or hepatic disease, anemia, jaundice, diabetes, epilepsy, or with compromised uteri. Transient pyrexia reported. Increased BP in postpartum hemorrhage. Use with chorioamnionitis may inhibit uterine response.

**ADVERSE REACTIONS:** Vomiting, diarrhea, nausea, increased temperature, flushing.

**INTERACTIONS:** May augment activity of other oxytocic agents; avoid concurrent use.

**PREGNANCY:** Category C, safety in nursing not known.

## HEMATINIC PLUS — RX

minerals - folic acid - multiple vitamin - ferrous fumarate (Cypress)

**THERAPEUTIC CLASS:** Iron/vitamin

**INDICATIONS:** Iron and folate deficiency anemia. Iron and Vitamin C deficiencies with increased need for B-complex vitamins.

**DOSAGE:** *Adults:* 1 tab qd between meals.

**HOW SUPPLIED:** Ferrous Fumarate 324mg-Vit C 200mg, Vit $B_1$ 10mg-Vit $B_2$ 6mg-Vit $B_6$ 5mg-Vit $B_{12}$ 15mcg-Folic Acid 1mg- Niacinamide 30mg-Calcium 10mg-Zinc 18.2mg-Magnesium 6.9mg-Manganese 1.3mg-Copper 0.8mg.

**CONTRAINDICATIONS:** Hemochromatosis, hemosiderosis, hemolytic anemia, pernicious anemia.

**WARNINGS/PRECAUTIONS:** May mask pernicious anemia. May aggravate existing GI diseases. Ineffective in patients with steatorrhea and partial gastrectomy.

**ADVERSE REACTIONS:** Anorexia, nausea, diarrhea, constipation.

## HEMOCYTE — OTC

ferrous fumarate (US Pharmaceutical)

**THERAPEUTIC CLASS:** Iron Supplement

**INDICATIONS:** Iron deficiency anemia.

**DOSAGE:** *Adults:* 1 tab up to bid, between meals.

**HOW SUPPLIED:** Tab: 324mg (106mg elemental iron)

**CONTRAINDICATIONS:** Hemochromatosis, hemosiderosis, hemolytic anemia.

**WARNINGS/PRECAUTIONS:** May aggravate existing GI disorders. Ineffective with steatorrhea, partial gastrectomy.

**ADVERSE REACTIONS:** Anorexia, nausea, diarrhea, constipation.

## HEMOCYTE F

RX

folic acid - ferrous fumarate (US Pharmaceutical)

**THERAPEUTIC CLASS:** Iron/vitamin

**INDICATIONS:** Treatment and prevention of iron and/or folate deficiency, and treatment of iron and/or folate deficiency anemia.

**DOSAGE:** *Adults:* 1 tab qd. Elderly: Start at low end of dosing range.

**HOW SUPPLIED:** Tab: (Ferrous Fumarate-Folic Acid) 324mg-1mg

**CONTRAINDICATIONS:** Hemochromatosis, hemosiderosis, pernicious anemia.

**WARNINGS/PRECAUTIONS:** Toxic when overdoses are ingested by children. Not for the treatment of pernicious anemia and other megaloblastic anemias where vitamin $B_{12}$ is deficient. Folic acid >0.1mg-0.4mg/day may obscure pernicious anemia. Caution with peptic ulcer, regional enteritis, ulcerative colitis.

**ADVERSE REACTIONS:** GI disturbances, abdominal cramps, diarrhea, constipation, heartburn, nausea, vomiting, black stools, allergic sensitization.



## HEMOCYTE PLUS

RX

minerals - folic acid - multiple vitamin - ferrous fumarate (US Pharmaceutical)

**THERAPEUTIC CLASS:** Vitamin/mineral

**INDICATIONS:** Iron and folate deficiency anemia. Iron and Vitamin C deficiencies with increased need for B-complex vitamins.

**DOSAGE:** *Adults:* 1 tab qd between meals.

**HOW SUPPLIED:** Tab: Ferrous Fumarate 324mg-Vit C 200mg-Vit $B_1$ 10mg-Vit $B_2$ 6mg-Vit $B_6$ 5mg -Vit $B_{12}$ 15mcg - Folic acid 1mg - Niacinamide 30mg - Pantothenic acid 10mg- Zinc 18.2mg - Magnesium 6.9mg - Manganese 1.3mg - Copper 0.8mg

**CONTRAINDICATIONS:** Hemochromatosis, hemosiderosis, hemolytic anemia, pernicious anemia.

**WARNINGS/PRECAUTIONS:** May mask pernicious anemia.

**ADVERSE REACTIONS:** Allergic sensitization, anorexia, nausea, diarrhea, constipation.

## HEPARIN SODIUM

RX

heparin sodium (Wyeth)

**THERAPEUTIC CLASS:** Glycosaminoglycan

**INDICATIONS:** Prophylaxis and treatment of venous thrombosis and its extension, PE in atrial fibrillation, and peripheral arterial embolism. Prevention of postoperative DVT and PE. Diagnosis and treatment of acute and chronic consumptive coagulopathies, for prevention of clotting in arterial and cardiac surgery.

**DOSAGE:** *Adults:* Based on 68kg: Initial: 5000U IV, then 10,000-20,000U SQ. Maint: 8000-10,000U q8h or 15,000-20,000U q12h. Intermittent IV Injection: Initial: 10,000U. Maint: 5000-10,000U q4-6h. Continuous IV Infusion: Initial: 5000U. Maint: 20,000-40,000U/24 hours. Adjust to coagulation test results. See labeling for details in specific disease states.
*Pediatrics:* Initial: 50U/kg IV drip. Maint: 100U/kg IV drip q4h or 20,000U/$m^2$/24 hrs continuously.

**HOW SUPPLIED:** Inj: 1000U/mL, 2500U/mL, 5000U/mL, 7500U/mL, 10,000U/mL

**CONTRAINDICATIONS:** Severe thrombocytopenia, if cannot perform appropriate blood-coagulation tests (with full-dose heparin), uncontrollable active bleeding state (except in DIC).

**WARNINGS/PRECAUTIONS:** Not for IM use. Hemorrhage can occur at any site; caution with increased danger of hemorrhage (severe HTN, bacterial endocarditis, surgery, etc.). Monitor blood coagulation tests frequently. Thrombocytopenia reported; discontinue if platelets <100,000mm$^3$ or if recurrent thrombosis develops. Contains benzyl alcohol."White-clot syndrome" reported. Monitor platelets, Hct, and occult blood in the stool. Increased heparin resistance with fever, thrombosis, thrombophlebitis, infections with thrombosing tendencies, MI, cancer, and post-op. Higher bleeding incidence in women >60 yrs.

**ADVERSE REACTIONS:** Hemorrhage, local irritation, erythema, mild pain, hematoma, chills, fever, urticaria.



**INTERACTIONS:** Wait >5 hrs after last IV dose or 24 hrs after last SQ dose before measure PT for dicumarol or warfarin. Platelet inhibitors (eg, acetylsalicylic acid, dextran, phenylbutazone, ibuprofen, indomethacin, dipyridamole, hydroxychloroquine) may induce bleeding. Digitalis, tetracyclines, nicotine, or antihistamines may counteract anticoagulant action.

**PREGNANCY:** Category C, safe in nursing.

## HEPSERA

RX

adefovir dipivoxil (Gilead Sciences)

**Discontinuation may result in severe acute exacerbations of hepatitis. Chronic use may result in nephrotoxicity in patients at risk of or having underlying renal dysfunction. Lactic acidosis and severe hepatomegaly with steatosis reported. Emergence of HIV resistance may occur with unrecognized or untreated HIV infection.**

**THERAPEUTIC CLASS:** Acyclic nucleotide analog

**INDICATIONS:** Treatment of chronic hepatitis B with evidence of active viral replication and either evidence of persistent elevations in serum aminotransferases (ALT or AST) or histologically active disease.

**DOSAGE:** *Adults:* 10mg qd. CrCl 20-49mL/min: 10mg q48h. CrCl 10-19mL/min: 10mg q72h. Hemodialysis: 10mg every 7 days following dialysis.

**HOW SUPPLIED:** Tab: 10mg

**WARNINGS/PRECAUTIONS:** Monitor hepatic function at repeated intervals upon discontinuation. Monitor renal function during therapy, especially with pre-existing or risk factors for renal dysfunction. Offer HIV antibody testing to all patients prior to initiation. Suspend therapy if develop lactic acidosis or pronounced hepatotoxicity.

**ADVERSE REACTIONS:** Asthenia, headache, abdominal pain, nausea, flatulence, diarrhea, dyspepsia, elevated LFTs.

**INTERACTIONS:** Caution with nephrotoxic drugs (eg, cyclosporine, tacrolimus, aminoglycosides, vancomycin, NSAIDs). Administration with drugs that reduce renal function or compete for active tubular secretion may increase serum levels of adefovir or co-administered drugs.

**PREGNANCY:** Category C, not for use in nursing.

## HERCEPTIN
trastuzumab (Genentech)

RX

**May cause ventricular dysfunction, CHF. Evaluate left ventricular function (LVF) prior to and during therapy; d/c with significant decrease in LVF. Increased incidence/severity of cardiac dysfunction when used in combination with anthracyclines and cyclophosphamide. Hypersensitivity reactions, infusion reactions, pulmonary events reported. Interrupt infusion if dyspnea or clinically significant hypotension develops. D/C with anaphylaxis, angioedema, or acute respiratory distress syndrome.**

**THERAPEUTIC CLASS:** Monoclonal antibody/HER2-blocker

**INDICATIONS:** Part of a treatment regimen containing doxorubicin, cyclophosphamide, and paclitaxel for the adjuvant treatment of patients with HER2-overexpressing, node-positive breast cancer. Single agent for the treatment of patients with metastatic breast cancer whose tumors overexpress the HER2 protein and have received 1 or more chemotherapies. In combination with paclitaxel for the treatment of patients with metastatic breast cancer whose tumors overexpress the HER2 protein and who have not received previous chemotherapy.

**DOSAGE:** *Adults:* IV infusion: LD: 4mg/kg over 90 minutes. Maint: 2mg/kg/week over 30 minutes. Metastatic Breast Cancer: Administer until tumor progression. Adjuvant Therapy: Following completion of doxorubicin and cyclophosphamide, give weekly for 52 weeks; administer with paclitaxel for first 12 weeks.

**HOW SUPPLIED:** Inj: 440mg

**WARNINGS/PRECAUTIONS:** Obtain baseline cardiac assessment and monitor cardiac function frequently. D/C with development of significant CHF. Extreme caution with pre-existing cardiac dysfunction. May exacerbate chemotherapy-induced neutropenia. HER2 testing is necessary to detect HER2 protein overexpression which is needed to select patients for transtuzumab therapy.

**ADVERSE REACTIONS:** Pain, asthenia, fever, nausea, chills, headache, increased cough, diarrhea, vomiting, abdominal pain, back pain, dyspnea, infection, rash, tachycardia, anemia, peripheral edema.

**INTERACTIONS:** Paclitaxel may increase serum levels. Concomitant anthracyclines and cyclophosphamide may increase incidence/severity of cardiac dysfunction.

**PREGNANCY:** Category B, not for use in nursing.

## HEXALEN
altretamine (MGI Pharma)

RX

**Monitor peripheral blood counts at least monthly, before each course of therapy, and as clinically indicated. Possible neurotoxicity; perform neurologic exam regularly.**

**THERAPEUTIC CLASS:** S-triazine derivative

**INDICATIONS:** Monotherapy for palliative treatment of persistent or recurrent ovarian cancer following 1st-line therapy with cisplatin and/or alkylating agent-based combination.

**DOSAGE:** *Adults:* 260 mg/m$^2$/day in 4 divided doses for 14 or 21 consecutive days in 28 day cycle. Take after meals and qhs. Temporarily discontinue for >14 days and restart at 200 mg/m$^2$/day if any of the following occur: GI intolerance unresponsive to symptomatic measures; WBC <2000/mm$^3$ or granulocytes <1000/mm$^3$; platelets <75,000/mm$^3$; progressive neurotoxicity. Permanently discontinue if neurological symptoms don't stabilize.

**HOW SUPPLIED:** Cap: 50mg

**CONTRAINDICATIONS:** Pre-existing severe bone marrow depression or severe neurologic toxicity.

H

**WARNINGS/PRECAUTIONS:** Can cause mild to moderate myelosuppression and neurotoxicity. Perform blood counts and neurologic exam before each course of therapy and adjust dose as indicated.

**ADVERSE REACTIONS:** Nausea, vomiting, peripheral neuropathy, CNS symptoms (mood disorders, consciousness disorders, ataxia, dizziness, vertigo), leukopenia, thrombocytopenia, anemia, increased alkaline phosphatase.

**INTERACTIONS:** Severe orthostatic hypotension may occur with MAOIs. Avoid pyridoxine; possible adverse response duration effects. Cimetidine may increase levels.

**PREGNANCY:** Category D, not for use in nursing.



## HIPREX RX

methenamine hippurate (Sanofi-Aventis)

**THERAPEUTIC CLASS:** Hippuric acid salt

**INDICATIONS:** Prophylaxis or suppression of recurrent urinary tract infections when long-term therapy is necessary. For use only after infection is eradicated by other appropriate antimicrobials.

**DOSAGE:** *Adults:* 1g bid.
*Pediatrics:* >12 yrs: 1g bid. 6 to 12 yrs: 0.5g-1g bid.

**HOW SUPPLIED:** Tab: 1g* *scored

**CONTRAINDICATIONS:** Renal insufficiency, severe hepatic insufficiency, severe dehydration, concomitant sulfonamides.

**WARNINGS/PRECAUTIONS:** Maintain acid urine. Doses of 8g/day may cause bladder irritation, painful and frequent micturition, albuminuria, gross hematuria. Monitor LFTs and repeated urine cultures. Contains tartrazine.

**ADVERSE REACTIONS:** Nausea, upset stomach, dysuria, rash.

**INTERACTIONS:** Avoid alkalinizing agents or foods. Sulfonamides may precipitate in the urine; avoid concomitant use.

**PREGNANCY:** Safety in pregnancy and nursing unknown.

## HISTA-VENT DA RX

phenylephrine HCl - methscopolamine nitrate - chlorpheniramine maleate (Ethex)

**THERAPEUTIC CLASS:** Antihistamine/anticholinergic/sympathomimetic

**INDICATIONS:** Temporary relief of symptoms of allergic rhinitis, vasomotor rhinitis, sinusitis, and the common cold.

**DOSAGE:** *Adults:* 1 tab q12h. Do not crush or chew.
*Pediatrics:* >12 yrs: 1 tab q12h. 6 to <12 yrs: 1/2 tab q12h. May cut in 1/2; do not crush or chew.

**HOW SUPPLIED:** Tab, Extended Release: (Chlorpheniramine-Methscopolamine-Phenylephrine) 8mg-2.5mg-20mg* *scored.

**CONTRAINDICATIONS:** Severe HTN, severe CAD, MAOI therapy, narrow angle glaucoma, urinary retention, PUD, during asthma attack.

**WARNINGS/PRECAUTIONS:** Caution in HTN, DM, ischemic heart disease, hyperthyroidism, increased IOP, prostatic hypertrophy. May produce CNS stimulation, convulsions, or cardiovascular collapse with accompanying hypotension; more common in the elderly. May cause excitability in children. May impair ability to operate machinery.

**ADVERSE REACTIONS:** Tachycardia, palpitations, nervousness, insomnia, restlessness, headache, gastric irritation, irritability, fear, anxiety, tenseness, restlessness, tremor.

**INTERACTIONS:** Increased effect of sympathomimetic amines with MAOI and β-blockers. May reduce antihypertensive effect of methyldopa, mecamylamine, and reserpine. Additive effect with alcohol, TCAs, barbiturates, other CNS depressants.

**PREGNANCY:** Category C, not for use in nursing.

## HIVID

RX

zalcitabine (Roche Labs)

**Severe peripheral neuropathy, pancreatitis (rare), hepatic failure (rare), lactic acidosis, and severe hepatomegaly with steatosis, reported. Extreme caution with pre-existing neuropathy.**

**THERAPEUTIC CLASS:** Reverse transcriptase inhibitor

**INDICATIONS:** Treatment of HIV infection in combination with other antiretrovirals.

**DOSAGE:** *Adults:* 0.75mg q8h. CrCl 10-40mL/min: 0.75mg q12h. CrCl <10mL/min: 0.75mg q24h.
*Pediatrics:* >13 yrs: 0.75mg q8h.

**HOW SUPPLIED:** Tab: 0.375mg, 0.75mg

**WARNINGS/PRECAUTIONS:** Decreased CD4 counts increase risk of adverse effects including peripheral neuropathy, pancreatitis, lactic acidosis, severe hepatomegaly with steatosis, hepatic toxicity, oral/esophageal ulcers, cardiomyopathy and CHF. Caution in elderly. Reduce dose in renal impairment. Increased risk of lymphoma with high doses. D/C if moderate peripheral neuropathy develops; may reintroduce at 50% of dose if improve to mild symptoms. Interrupt or reduce dose if serious toxicities occur (eg, peripheral neuropathy, severe oral ulcers, pancreatitis, elevated LFTs). Monitor CBC and clinical chemistry tests before therapy and at appropriate intervals thereafter. Monitor hematologic indices frequently with poor bone marrow reserve. Interrupt therapy if severe anemia or granulocytopenia occurs; reduce dose if less severe. Possible redistribution or accumulation of body fat.

**ADVERSE REACTIONS:** Peripheral neuropathy, oral lesions/stomatitis, headache, elevated amylase, fatigue, abdominal pain, nausea, vomiting, hepatic dysfunction, blood dyscrasias, rash, urticaria, redistribution/accumulation of body fat.

**INTERACTIONS:** Avoid drugs associated with peripheral neuropathy. Monitor renal function and neuropathy development with amphotericin, foscarnet, aminoglycosides. Cimetidine and probenecid decrease clearance. Metoclopramide, aluminum- and magnesium-containing antacids reduce absorption. Interrupt therapy with pancreatitis causing agents (eg, intravenous pentamidine).

**PREGNANCY:** Category C, not for use in nursing.

## HUMALOG

RX

insulin lispro (Lilly)

**THERAPEUTIC CLASS:** Insulin

**INDICATIONS:** To control hyperglycemia in diabetes.

**DOSAGE:** *Adults:* Individualize dose. Inject SQ within 15 minutes before or immediately after a meal. May use with external insulin pump; do not dilute or mix with other insulin when used with pump.
*Pediatrics:* >3 yrs: Individualize dose. Inject SQ within 15 minutes before or immediately after a meal. May use with external insulin pump; do not dilute or mix with other insulin when used with pump.

**HOW SUPPLIED:** Cartridge: 100 U/mL; Inj: 100 U/mL; Pen: 100 U/mL

**CONTRAINDICATIONS:** Hypoglycemia.

H

**WARNINGS/PRECAUTIONS:** Any change of insulin should be made cautiously. Changes in strength, manufacturer, type or method of manufacture may result in the need for a change in dosage. Hypoglycemia may occur with taking too much insulin, missing or delaying meals, exercising or working more than usual. An infection or illness (especially with diarrhea or vomiting) may change insulin requirements. With type 1 DM a longer-acting insulin is usually required to maintain glucose control; not required with type 2 DM if regimen includes sulfonylureas. May be diluted with sterile diluent.

**ADVERSE REACTIONS:** Hypoglycemia, hypokalemia, allergic reaction, injection site reaction, lipodystrophy, pruritus, rash.

**INTERACTIONS:** Increased insulin requirements with corticosteroids, isoniazid, niacin, estrogens, oral contraceptives, phenothiazines, thyroid replacement therapy. Decreased insulin requirements with oral hypoglycemics, salicylates, sulfa antibiotics, MAOIs, ACEIs, β-blockers, octreotide and alcohol. β-blockers may mask symptoms of hypoglycemia.Caution with potassium-lowering drugs or drugs sensitive to serum potassium levels.



**PREGNANCY:** Category B, caution in nursing.

## HUMALOG MIX 75/25 RX

insulin lispro - insulin lispro protamine (Lilly)

**THERAPEUTIC CLASS:** Insulin

**INDICATIONS:** To control hyperglycemia in diabetes.

**DOSAGE:** *Adults:* Individualize dose. Inject SQ within 15 minutes before a meal. May need to reduce/adjust dose with renal/hepatic impairment.

**HOW SUPPLIED:** (Insulin Lispro Protamine, Human-Insulin Lispro, Human) Inj: 75U-25U/mL; Pen: 75U-25U/mL

**CONTRAINDICATIONS:** Hypoglycemia.

**WARNINGS/PRECAUTIONS:** Any change of insulin should be made cautiously. Changes in strength, manufacturer, type or method of manufacture may result in the need for a change in dosage. Hypoglycemia may occur with taking too much insulin, missing or delaying meals, exercising or working more than usual. An infection or illness (especially with diarrhea or vomiting) may change insulin requirements.

**ADVERSE REACTIONS:** Hypoglycemia, hypokalemia, allergic reaction, injection site reaction, lipodystrophy, pruritus, rash.

**INTERACTIONS:** Increased insulin requirements with corticosteroids, isoniazid, niacin, estrogens, oral contraceptives, phenothiazines, thyroid replacement therapy. Decreased insulin requirements with oral hypoglycemics, salicylates, sulfa antibiotics, MAOIs, ACEIs, β-blockers, octreotide and alcohol. β-blockers may mask symptoms of hypoglycemia.

**PREGNANCY:** Category B, caution in nursing.

## HUMATROPE RX

somatropin (Lilly)

**THERAPEUTIC CLASS:** Human growth hormone

**INDICATIONS:** Long-term treatment of pediatrics with growth failure due to growth hormone deficiency (GHD). For short stature associated with Turner syndrome if epiphyses are not closed. Long-term treatment of idiopathic short stature in pediatrics. Replacement therapy in adults.

**DOSAGE:** *Adults:* GHD: Up to 0.006mg/kg SQ qd. Titrate: Increase by individual requirements. Max: 0.0125mg/kg/day.
*Pediatrics:* GHD: 0.18mg/kg weekly SQ/IM. Max: 0.3mg/kg weekly in equally divided doses given either on 3 alternate days, 6 times per week or daily. Turner Syndrome: Up to 0.375mg/kg SQ weekly equally divided given either

daily or on 3 alternate days. Idiopathic Short Stature: Up to 0.37mg/kg SQ weekly given 6 to 7 times per week equally divided.

**HOW SUPPLIED:** Inj: 5mg, 6mg, 12mg, 24mg

**CONTRAINDICATIONS:** Pediatrics with closed epiphyses. Active malignancy. Hypersensitivity to Metacresol or glycerin. Acute critical illness due to complications after open heart or abdominal surgery, multiple accidental trauma. Acute respiratory failure.

**WARNINGS/PRECAUTIONS:** If sensitivity to diluent occurs reconstitute with bacteriostatic (contains benzyl alcohol; avoid in newborns) or sterile water for injection. Monitor GHD secondary to intracranial lesion for progression/recurrence. Monitor gait, glucose intolerance, for malignant transformation of skin lesions, scoliosis progression, intracranial HTN (perform fundoscopic exam at start and periodically). Caution with DM, endocrine disorders, hypopituitarism. With Turner syndrome monitor for otic or cardiovascular disorders, autoimmune thyroid disease. Caution with endocrine disorders, monitor for otic and cardiovascular disorder.

**ADVERSE REACTIONS:** Injection site pain, headache, edema, myalgia, pain, rhinitis. (Adults) arthralgia, paresthesia, HTN, back pain. (Pediatrics) flu-syndrome, AST/ALT increases, pharyngitis, gastritis, respiratory disorder.

**INTERACTIONS:** Antagonized by glucocorticoids. May alter clearance of CYP450 substrates (eg, corticosteroids, sex steroids, anticonvulsants, antipyrine, cyclosporine).

**PREGNANCY:** Category C, caution in nursing.

## HUMIBID — OTC
guaifenesin (Adams)

**THERAPEUTIC CLASS:** Expectorant

**INDICATIONS:** Help loosen phlegm and thin bronchial secretions to rid the bronchial passageways of bothersome mucus and make coughs more productive.

**DOSAGE:** *Adults*: 1200mg q12h. Max: 2400mg/24hrs. Do not crush, chew, or break tablet. Take with full glass of water.
*Pediatrics:* ≥12 yrs: 1200mg q12h. Max: 2400mg/24hrs. Do not crush, chew, or break tablet. Take with full glass of water.

**HOW SUPPLIED:** Tab, Extended-Release: 1200mg

**WARNINGS/PRECAUTIONS:** Stop use if cough lasts >7 days, comes back, or occurs with fever, rash, or persistent headache.

**PREGNANCY:** Safety in pregnancy and nursing is not known.

## HUMIRA — RX
adalimumab (Abbott)

**Reports of TB, invasive fungal infections, and other opportunistic infections. Evaluate for latent TB and treat if necessary prior to initiation of therapy.**

**THERAPEUTIC CLASS:** Monoclonal antibody/TNF-blocker

**INDICATIONS:** For reducing signs and symptoms, inducing major clinical response, inhibiting structural damage progression, and improving physical function in moderate to severe active rheumatoid arthritis (RA). Can use alone or in combination with methotrexate (MTX) or other disease-modifying antirheumatic drugs (DMARDs). For reducing signs and symptoms of active arthritis, inhibiting the progression of structural damage and improving physical function in patients with psoriatic arthritis. Can use alone or in combination with DMARDs. For reducing signs and symptoms in patients with active alkylosing spondylitis (AS). Reducing signs and symptoms and inducing and maintaining clinical remission of moderate-severe Crohn's disease who have had an inadequate response to conventional therapy. Reducing signs and symptoms and inducing clinical remission in patients who have lost response or are intolerant to infliximab.

**DOSAGE:** *Adults:* 40mg SQ every other week. Some patients with RA not taking concomitant MTX may derive additional benefit from increasing the dosing frequency to 40mg every week. Crohn's Disease: Initial: 160mg (may be given as 4 injections on Day 1, or 2 injections/day for 2 consecutive days); 80mg at Week 2. Maint: 40mg every other week beginning at Week 4.

**HOW SUPPLIED:** Inj: 40mg/0.8mL

**WARNINGS/PRECAUTIONS:** Serious infections including sepsis and tuberculosis reported. Monitor for signs of infection during and after therapy; d/c if serious infection develops. Avoid with active infection. Monitor HBV carriers as reactivation may occur; if reactivation occurs, stop Humira and start antiviral therapy. Caution with history of recurrent infections or underlying conditions predisposing to infections or in areas where TB and histoplasmosis are endemic. Caution with pre-existing or recent-onset CNS demyelinating disorders. Lymphomas, allergic reactions observed. May affect host defenses against infections and malignancies. May result in autoantibody formation; d/c if lupus-like syndrome develops. Rare possibility of anaphylaxis and pancytopenia including aplastic anemia.

**ADVERSE REACTIONS:** URI, injection site pain/reactions, headache, rash, sinusitis, nausea, UTI, flu syndrome, abdominal pain, hyperlipidemia, hypercholesterolemia, back pain, hematuria, alkaline phosphatase increased, HTN, immunogenicity.

**INTERACTIONS:** Do not give concurrently with live vaccines. Reduced clearance with MTX. Do not use concurrently with anakinra due to increased risk of serious infections.

**PREGNANCY:** Category B, not for use in nursing.

## HUMULIN OTC

insulin, human regular - insulin, human isophane - insulin human, rdna origin (Lilly)

**OTHER BRAND NAMES:** Humulin N (Lilly) - Humulin R (Lilly)

**THERAPEUTIC CLASS:** Insulin

**INDICATIONS:** To control hyperglycemia in diabetes.

**DOSAGE:** *Adults:* Individualize dose.
*Pediatrics:* Individualize dose.

**HOW SUPPLIED:** Inj: 100U/mL (Humulin N, Humulin R), 500U/mL (Humulin R U-500); Pen: 100U/mL (Humulin N).

**WARNINGS/PRECAUTIONS:** Human insulin differs from animal source insulin. Any change of insulin should be made cautiously. Changes in strength, manufacturer, type or method of manufacture may result in the need for a change in dosage. Hypoglycemia may occur with taking too much insulin, missing or delaying meals, exercising or working more than usual. An infection or illness (especially with diarrhea or vomiting) may change insulin requirements. Administration of insulin SQ can result in lipoatrophy.

**ADVERSE REACTIONS:** Hypoglycemia, sweating, dizziness, palpitation, tremor, hunger, restlessness, lightheadedness, inability to concentrate, headache, injection site reaction, allergic reaction.

**INTERACTIONS:** Increased insulin requirements with oral contraceptives, corticosteroids, or thyroid replacement therapy. Reduced insulin requirements with oral hypoglycemics, salicylates, sulfa antibiotics, and certain antidepressants. Alcoholic beverages may change insulin requirements. β-blockers may mask symptoms of hypoglycemia.

**PREGNANCY:** Pregnancy category is not known.

## HUMULIN 70/30 OTC

insulin human, rdna origin - insulin, human (isophane/regular) (Lilly)

**OTHER BRAND NAMES:** Humulin 50/50 (Lilly)

**THERAPEUTIC CLASS:** Insulin

**INDICATIONS:** To control hyperglycemia in diabetes.

**DOSAGE:** *Adults:* Individualize dose. Administer SQ.
*Pediatrics:* Individualize dose. Administer SQ.

**HOW SUPPLIED:** (Isophane-Regular) Inj: (Humulin 70/30) 70U-30U/mL, (Humulin 50/50) 50U-50U/mL

**WARNINGS/PRECAUTIONS:** Human insulin differs from animal source insulin. Make any change of insulin cautiously. Changes in strength, manufacturer, type, or method of manufacture may result in the need for a change in dosage. Hypoglycemia may occur with too much insulin, missing or delaying meals, exercising, or working more than usual. Infection or illness (especially with diarrhea or vomiting) may change insulin requirements. Administration of insulin SQ can result in lipoatrophy.

**ADVERSE REACTIONS:** Hypoglycemia, sweating, dizziness, palpitation, tremor, hunger, restlessness, lightheadedness, inability to concentrate, headache, injection site reaction, allergic reaction.

**INTERACTIONS:** Increased insulin requirements with oral contraceptives, corticosteroids, or thyroid replacement therapy. Reduced insulin requirements with oral hypoglycemics, salicylates, sulfa antibiotics, and certain antidepressants. Alcoholic beverages may change insulin requirements. β-blockers may mask symptoms of hypoglycemia.

**PREGNANCY:** Pregnancy category is not known.

## HYCAMTIN RX

topotecan HCl (GlaxoSmithKline)

**Do not give if baseline neutrophils <1500cells/mm³. Monitor peripheral blood cell counts frequently due to risk of bone marrow suppression, primarily neutropenia.**

**THERAPEUTIC CLASS:** Topoisomerase I inhibitor

**INDICATIONS:** Treatment of refractory metastatic ovarian carcinoma after failure of initial or subsequent chemotherapy and small cell lung cancer sensitive disease after 1st-line chemotherapy failure. Treatment of stage IV-B, recurrent, or persistent carcinoma of the cervix which is not amenable to curative treatment with surgery and/or radiation therapy, in combination with cisplatin.

**DOSAGE:** *Adults:* Ovarian and Small Cell Lung Cancer: 1.5mg/m² IV qd over 30 minutes for 5 days, starting on day 1 of 21-day course. Minimum of 4 courses is recommended in absence of tumor progression. Severe Neutropenia During Therapy: Reduce dose by 0.25mg/m², or give G-CSF following subsequent course (before dose reduction) starting from day 6 of the course (24 hrs after completion of topotecan administration). Renal Impairment: CrCl 39-20mL/min: 0.75mg/m². CrCl <20mL/min: Insufficient data to provide recommendation. Cervical Cancer: 0.75mg/m² IV qd over 30 minutes on days 1, 2 , and 3; followed by cisplatin 50mg/m² IV on day 1 of every 21-day course. Severe Febrile Neutropenia (<1000 cells/mm³ & temperature of 38°C): Reduce dose by 20% to 0.60mg/m² for subsequent courses (doses should be similarly reduced if the platelet count falls below 10,000 cells/mm³) or give G-CSF following subsequent course (before dose reduction) starting from day 4 of the course (24 hrs after completion of topotecan administration); if febrile neutropenia occurs despite the use of G-CSF, reduce dose by another 20% to 0.45mg/m² for subsequent courses. Renal Impairment: CrCl 39-20mL/min: 0.75mg/m². CrCl <20mL/min: Insufficient data to provide recommendation.

**HOW SUPPLIED:** Inj: 4mg

**CONTRAINDICATIONS:** Pregnancy, nursing, severe bone marrow depression

**WARNINGS/PRECAUTIONS:** Bone marrow suppression (thrombocytopenia, anemia and primarily neutropenia) is dose-limiting toxicity. Baseline neutrophils >1500 cells/mm³ and platelets >100,000cells/mm³ required. Neutrophils >1000 cells/mm³, platelets >100,000cells/mm³, and HgB ≥9g/dL required before subsequent courses. May cause fetal harm during pregnancy.

**ADVERSE REACTIONS:** Neutropenia, leukopenia, thrombocytopenia, anemia, sepsis/fever/infection, nausea, vomiting, diarrhea, constipation, abdominal pain, anorexia, fatigue, pain, asthenia, alopecia.

**INTERACTIONS:** Concomitant G-CSF can prolong duration of neutropenia; should not initiate until day 6 of therapy course, 24 hrs after treatment completion with topotecan. Increased severity of myelosuppression with other cytotoxic agents, cisplatin or carboplatin.

**PREGNANCY:** Category D, contraindicated in nursing.

H

## HYCOTUSS CIII

guaifenesin - hydrocodone bitartrate (Endo)

**OTHER BRAND NAMES:** Vi-Q-Tuss (Vintage)

**THERAPEUTIC CLASS:** Cough suppressant/expectorant

**INDICATIONS:** Symptomatic relief of irritating nonproductive cough associated with upper and lower respiratory tract congestion.

**DOSAGE:** *Adults:* Initial: 5mL after meals and hs, not less than 4 hrs apart. Titrate: May increase up to 15mL after meals and hs. Max: 30mL/24 hrs. *Pediatrics:* >12 yrs: Initial: 5mL after meals and hs, not less than 4 hrs apart. Max Single Dose: 10mL. 6-12 yrs: Initial: 2.5mL after meals and hs, not less than 4 hrs apart. Max Single Dose: 5mL.

**HOW SUPPLIED:** Syrup: (Hydrocodone-Guaifenesin) 5mg-100mg/5mL

**CONTRAINDICATIONS:** Cross sensitivity to other opioids. Intracranial lesion associated with increased intracranial pressure and whenever ventilatory function is depressed.

**WARNINGS/PRECAUTIONS:** May be habit forming. Risk of psychic dependence, physical dependence, tolerance, and potential for abuse. Dose-related respiratory depression. Caution with head injury, other intracranial lesions or a pre-existing increase in intracranial pressure. May obscure the clinical course head injuries, acute abdominal conditions.

**ADVERSE REACTIONS:** Respiratory depression, HTN, postural hypotension, palpitations, urinary retention, sedation, drowsiness, mental clouding, lethargy.

**INTERACTIONS:** Additive CNS depression with other narcotics, analgesics, general anesthetics, phenothiazines, other tranquilizers, sedative hypnotics or other CNS depressants (including alcohol).

**PREGNANCY:** Category C, not for use in nursing.

## HYDRALAZINE RX

hydralazine HCl (Various)

**THERAPEUTIC CLASS:** Vasodilator

**INDICATIONS:** Management of hypertension.

**DOSAGE:** *Adults:* Initial: 10mg qid for 2-4 days. Titrate: Increase to 25mg qid for the rest of the week, then increase to 50mg qid. Maint: Use lowest effective dose. Resistant Patients: 300mg/day or titrate to lower dose combined with thiazide diuretic and/or reserpine, or β-blocker.
*Pediatrics:* Initial: 0.75mg/kg/day given qid. Titrate: Increase gradually over 3-4 weeks to a max of 7.5mg/kg/day or 200mg/day.

**HOW SUPPLIED:** Inj: 20mg/mL; Tab: 10mg, 25mg, 50mg, 100mg

**CONTRAINDICATIONS:** CAD and mitral valvular rheumatic heart disease.

**WARNINGS/PRECAUTIONS:** Discontinue if SLE symptoms occur. May cause angina and ECG changes of MI. Caution with suspected CAD, CVA, advanced renal impairment. May increase pulmonary artery pressure in mitral valvular disease. Postural hypotension reported. Add pyridoxine if develop peripheral neuritis. Monitor CBC and ANA titer before and periodically during therapy.

**ADVERSE REACTIONS:** Headache, anorexia, nausea, vomiting, diarrhea, tachycardia, angina.

**INTERACTIONS:** Caution with MAOIs. Profound hypotension with potent parenteral antihypertensives (eg, diazoxide). May reduce pressor response to epinephrine.

**PREGNANCY:** Category C, safety in nursing not known.

## HYDREA

RX

hydroxyurea (Bristol-Myers Squibb)



**THERAPEUTIC CLASS:** Ribonucleotide reductase inhibitor

**INDICATIONS:** Significant tumor response demonstrated in melanoma, resistant chronic myelocytic leukemia (CML), and recurrent, metastatic, or inoperable carcinoma of the ovary. Adjunct therapy with irradiation therapy for local control of primary squamous cell carcinomas of the head and neck, excluding the lip.

**DOSAGE:** *Adults:* Solid Tumors: Intermittent: 80mg/kg single dose every 3rd day. Continuous: 20-30mg/kg qd. Head and Neck Carcinoma: 80mg/kg single dose every 3rd day. Start at least 7 days before irradiation. Resistant CML: 20-30mg/kg qd. Elderly/Renal Impairment: May need dose reduction.

**HOW SUPPLIED:** Cap: 500mg

**CONTRAINDICATIONS:** Marked bone marrow depression (leukopenia, thrombocytopenia or severe anemia).

**WARNINGS/PRECAUTIONS:** Patients with previous irradiation therapy may have exacerbation of post-irradiation erythema. Bone marrow suppression, erythrocytic abnormalities may occur. Correct severe anemia before initiating therapy. Caution with marked renal dysfunction. May develop secondary leukemia with long-term therapy for myeloproliferative disorders. Monitor CBC, bone marrow, hepatic and kidney function before therapy and repeatedly thereafter. Interrupt therapy if WBC <2500/$mm^3$ or platelets <100,000/$mm^3$. Cutaneous vasculitic toxicities, including vasculitic ulcerations and gangrene, reported; d/c if cutaneous vasculitic ulcerations develop.

**ADVERSE REACTIONS:** Bone marrow depression (leukopenia, anemia, thrombocytopenia), GI effects (stomatitis, anorexia, nausea, vomiting, diarrhea, constipation), and dermatological reactions (maculopapular rash, skin ulceration, dermatomyositis-like skin changes, peripheral and facial erythema), cutaneous vasculitic toxicities.

**INTERACTIONS:** Increased risk of bone marrow depression with other myelosuppressants or radiation therapy. Uricosurics may need dose adjustments. Pancreatitis and peripheral neuropathy reported in HIV patients with concomitant didanosine. Hepatotoxicity and hepatic failure reported in HIV patients with antiretrovirals (eg, stavudine, didanosine).

**PREGNANCY:** Category D, not for use in nursing.

## HYDROCHLOROTHIAZIDE

RX

hydrochlorothiazide (Various)

**THERAPEUTIC CLASS:** Thiazide diuretic

**INDICATIONS:** Adjunct therapy in edema associated with CHF, hepatic cirrhosis, corticosteroid and estrogen therapy, renal dysfunction. Management of hypertension.

**DOSAGE:** *Adults:* Edema: 25-100mg qd or in divided doses. May give every other day or 3-5 days/week. HTN: Initial: 25mg qd. Titrate: May increase to 50mg/day.
*Pediatrics:* Diuresis/HTN: 1-2mg/kg/day given qd-bid. Max: Infants up to 2 yrs: 37.5mg/day. 2-12 yrs: 100mg/day. <6 months: Up to 1.5mg/kg bid may be required.

**HOW SUPPLIED:** Tab: 25mg*, 50mg* *scored

**CONTRAINDICATIONS:** Anuria, sulfonamide hypersensitivity.

**WARNINGS/PRECAUTIONS:** Caution in severe renal disease, liver dysfunction, electrolyte/fluid imbalance. Monitor electrolytes. Hyperuricemia, hyperglycemia, hypokalemia, hyponatremia, hypomagnesemia, hypercalcemia may occur. Increases in cholesterol and triglyceride levels reported. May exacerbate SLE. Sensitivity reactions reported. D/C prior to parathyroid test. Enhanced effects in post-sympathectomy patients.

**ADVERSE REACTIONS:** Weakness, hypotension, pancreatitis, jaundice, diarrhea, vomiting, blood dyscrasias, rash, photosensitivity, electrolyte imbalance, impotence.

**INTERACTIONS:** May potentiate orthostatic hypotension with alcohol, barbiturates, narcotics. Adjust antidiabetic drugs. Possible decreased response to pressor amines. Corticosteroids, ACTH increase electrolyte depletion. May potentiate nondepolarizing skeletal muscle relaxants, antihypertensives. Lithium toxicity. NSAIDs decrease effects. Decreased PO absorption with cholestyramine, colestipol.

**PREGNANCY:** Category B, not for use in nursing.

## HYDROCORTISONE ACETATE RX

hydrocortisone acetate (Truxton)

**THERAPEUTIC CLASS:** Corticosteroid

**INDICATIONS:** By intra-articular or soft tissue injection as adjunctive therapy for short-term administration in: synovitis of osteoarthritis, rheumatoid arthritis, bursitis, gouty arthritis, epicondylitis, nonspecific tenosynovitis, and post-traumatic osteoarthritis. By intralesional injection in: keloids, localized inflammatory lesions, discoid lupus erythematosus, necrobiosis lipoidica diabeticorum, alopecia areata, and cystic tumors of an aponeurosis or tendon.

**DOSAGE:** *Adults:* Usual: Large joints: 25-37.5mg. Max: 50mg. Small joints: 10-25mg. Bursae: 25-37.5mg. Tendon Sheaths: 5-12.5mg. Soft Tissue Infiltration: 25-50mg, occasionally 75mg. Ganglia: 12.5-25mg. For intra-articular, intralesional, and soft tissue injection only. Injection given once every 2-3 weeks; once a week for more severe conditions.
*Pediatrics:* Usual: Large joints: 25-37.5mg. Max: 50mg. Small joints: 10-25mg. Bursae: 25-37.5mg. Tendon Sheaths: 5-12.5mg. Soft Tissue Infiltration: 25-50mg, occasionally 75mg. Ganglia: 12.5-25mg. For intra-articular, intralesional, and soft tissue injection only. Injection given once every 2-3 weeks; once a week for more severe conditions.

**HOW SUPPLIED:** Inj: 25mg/mL.

**CONTRAINDICATIONS:** Systemic fungal infections.

**WARNINGS/PRECAUTIONS:** May need to increase dose before, during, and after stressful situations. May mask signs of infection or cause new infections. Avoid with cerebral malaria. May activate latent amebiasis. Prolonged use may produce glaucoma, optic nerve damage, secondary ocular infections. Increases BP, salt/water retention, potassium excretion. More severe/fatal course of infections reported with chickenpox, measles. Caution with Strongyloides, latent TB, recent MI, hypothyroidism, cirrhosis, ocular herpes simplex, HTN, diverticulitis, fresh intestinal anastomosis, ulcerative colitis, osteoporosis, myasthenia gravis, renal insufficiency, peptic ulcer disease. May increase or decrease sperm count. Growth and development of children on prolonged therapy should be monitored. Monitor for psychic disturbances.

Avoid abrupt withdrawal. Avoid injection into an infected site or unstable joint. Frequent intra-articular injections may cause joint tissue damage.

**ADVERSE REACTIONS:** Fluid and electrolyte disturbances, HTN, osteoporosis, muscle weakness, cushingoid state, menstrual irregularities, nervousness, insomnia, impaired wound healing, DM, ulcerative esophagitis, excessive sweating, increases intracranial pressure, carbohydrate intolerance, glaucoma, cataracts, weight gain, nausea, malaise.

**INTERACTIONS:** Reduced efficacy and increased clearance with hepatic enzyme inducers (eg, phenobarbital, phenytoin, ephedrine, and rifampin). Caution with ASA in hypoprothrombinemia. Effects on oral anticoagulants are variable; monitor PT. Increased insulin and oral hypoglycemic requirements in DM. Avoid live vaccines with immunosuppressive doses. Possible decreased vaccine response with killed or inactivated vaccines with immunosuppressive doses. Monitor for hypokalemia with potassium-depleting diuretics.

**PREGNANCY:** Safety in pregnancy not known, not for use in nursing.



## HYDROXYZINE HCL — RX

hydroxyzine HCl (Various)

**OTHER BRAND NAMES:** Atarax (Pfizer)

**THERAPEUTIC CLASS:** Piperazine antihistamine

**INDICATIONS:** (PO) Relief of anxiety associated with psychoneurosis and as adjunct in organic disease states with anxiety. As a sedative when used as premedication and following general anesthesia. Management of allergic pruritus. (Inj) Management of anxiety, tension, and psycomotor agitation in conditions of emotional stress. As pre-/postoperative and pre-/postpartum adjunctive medication to permit reduction in narcotic dosage, allay anxiety, and control emesis. To control nausea and vomiting, excluding pregnancy.

**DOSAGE:** *Adults:* PO: Anxiety: 50-100mg qid. Pruritus: 25mg tid-qid. Sedation: 50-100mg. IM: Nausea/Vomiting: 25-100mg. Pre-/Postoperative and Pre-/Postpartum Adjunct: 25-100mg. Psychiatric/Emotional Emergencies: 50-100mg q4-6h prn.
*Pediatrics:* PO: Anxiety/Pruritus: <6 yrs: 50mg/day in divided doses. >6 yrs: 50-100mg in divided doses. Sedation: 0.6mg/kg. IM: Nausea/Vomiting: 0.5mg/lb. Pre-/Postoperative Adjunct: 0.5mg/lb.

**HOW SUPPLIED:** Inj: 25mg/mL, 50mg/mL; Syrup: 10mg/5mL; Tab: 10mg, 25mg, 50mg, 100mg

**CONTRAINDICATIONS:** Early pregnancy. Inj is intended only for IM administration and should not, under any circumstances, be injected subcutaneously, intra-arterially, or IV.

**WARNINGS/PRECAUTIONS:** Caution in elderly. May impair mental/physical abilities. Effectiveness as an antianxiety agent for long term use (>4 months) has not been established.

**ADVERSE REACTIONS:** Dry mouth, drowsiness, involuntary motor activity.

**INTERACTIONS:** Potentiates CNS depression with other CNS depressants (eg, narcotics, non-narcotic analgesics, barbiturates, alcohol). May increase alcohol effects.

**PREGNANCY:** Not for use in pregnancy or nursing.

## HYDROXYZINE PAMOATE — RX

hydroxyzine pamoate (Various)

**OTHER BRAND NAMES:** Vistaril (Pfizer)

**THERAPEUTIC CLASS:** Piperazine antihistamine

**INDICATIONS:** Relief of anxiety. Allergic pruritus. For sedation as premedication and following anesthesia.

**DOSAGE:** *Adults:* Anxiety: 50-100mg qid. Pruritus: 25mg tid-qid. Sedation: 50-100mg.
*Pediatrics:* Anxiety/Pruritus: >6 yrs: 50-100mg/day in divided doses. <6 yrs: 50mg/day in divided doses. Sedation: 0.6mg/kg.

**HOW SUPPLIED:** Cap: 25mg, 50mg, 100mg; Sus: 25mg/5mL [120mL, 480mL]

**CONTRAINDICATIONS:** Early pregnancy.

**WARNINGS/PRECAUTIONS:** Caution in elderly. May impair mental/physical abilities. Effectiveness as an antianxiety agent for long term use (>4 months) has not been established.

**ADVERSE REACTIONS:** Dry mouth, drowsiness, involuntary motor activity.

**INTERACTIONS:** Potentiated by CNS depressants(eg, narcotics, non-narcotic analgesics, barbiturates); reduce dose.

**PREGNANCY:** Safety unknown in pregnancy and is contraindicated in early pregnancy, not for use in nursing.



## HYTONE RX
hydrocortisone (Dermik)

**THERAPEUTIC CLASS:** Corticosteroid

**INDICATIONS:** Corticosteroid responsive dermatoses.

**DOSAGE:** *Adults:* Apply bid-qid depending on the severity. May use occlusive dressings for psoriasis or recalcitrant conditions. Discontinue dressings if infection develops.
*Pediatrics:* Apply bid-qid depending on the severity. May use occlusive dressings for psoriasis or recalcitrant conditions. Discontinue dressings if infection develops.

**HOW SUPPLIED:** Cre: 2.5% [30g, 60g]; Lot: 2.5% [60mL]; Oint: 2.5% [30g]

**WARNINGS/PRECAUTIONS:** May produce reversible HPA axis suppression, manifestations of Cushing's syndrome, hyperglycemia, and glucosuria. Caution when applied to large surface areas or under occlusive dressings. Use appropriate antifungal or antibacterial agent with dermatological infections; discontinue if infection does not clear. Pediatrics may be more susceptible to systemic toxicity. Avoid eyes. Discontinue if irritation occurs.

**ADVERSE REACTIONS:** Burning, itching, irritation, dryness, folliculitis, hypertrichosis, acneiform eruptions, hypopigmentation, perioral dermatitis, allergic contact dermatitis, skin maceration, secondary infection, skin atrophy, striae, miliaria.

**PREGNANCY:** Category C, caution in nursing.

## HYTONE 1% OTC
hydrocortisone (Dermik)

**THERAPEUTIC CLASS:** Corticosteroid

**INDICATIONS:** Relief of itching associated with minor skin irritation, inflammation and rashes due to eczema, insect bites, poison ivy/oak/sumac, soaps/detergents, cosmetics, jewelry, seborrheic dermatitis, psoriasis, and/or external feminine and external anal itching.

**DOSAGE:** *Adults:* Apply up to tid-qid. External Anal Itching: Clean and dry area before applying.
*Pediatrics:* >2 yrs: Apply up to tid-qid. External Anal Itching: >12 yrs: Clean and dry area before applying.

**HOW SUPPLIED:** Lot: 1% [30mL, 120mL]

**WARNINGS/PRECAUTIONS:** Avoid eyes. Discontinue use if condition worsens, if symptoms persist for more than 7 days, or if symptoms recur after clearing up. Not for diaper rash. For external feminine itching, avoid use with vaginal discharge. For external anal itching, do not insert into rectum with fingers or applicator.

**PREGNANCY:** Safety in pregnancy and nursing is not known.

## HYTRIN RX
terazosin HCl (Abbott)

**THERAPEUTIC CLASS:** Alpha$_1$-blocker (quinazoline)

**INDICATIONS:** Treatment of hypertension. Treatment of symptomatic benign prostatic hyperplasia.

**DOSAGE:** *Adults:* HTN: Initial: 1mg hs, then slowly increase dose. Usual: 1-5mg/day. Max: 20mg/day. If response is substantially diminished at 24 hrs, may increase dose or give in 2 divided doses. BPH: Initial: 1mg qhs. Titrate: Increase stepwise as needed. Usual: 10mg/day. May increase to 20mg/day after 4-6 weeks. Max: 20mg/day. If discontinue for several days, restart at initial dose.

**HOW SUPPLIED:** Cap: 1mg, 2mg, 5mg, 10mg

**WARNINGS/PRECAUTIONS:** Monitor for orthostatic hypotension and syncope initially and with dose increase. Rule out prostate cancer. Priapism (rare) reported. Possibility of hemodilution.

**ADVERSE REACTIONS:** Asthenia, postural hypotension, headache, dizziness, dyspnea, nasal congestion/rhinitis, somnolence, impotence, blurred vision, palpitations, nausea, peripheral edema, priapism, thrombocytopenia, atrial fibrillation.

**INTERACTIONS:** Increased levels with verapamil. Possibility of significant hypotension with other antihypertensives; may need dose reduction or retitration of either agent.

**PREGNANCY:** Category C, caution with nursing.

## HYZAAR RX
hydrochlorothiazide - losartan potassium (Merck)

**Can cause death/injury to developing fetus during 2nd and 3rd trimesters. Discontinue if pregnancy detected.**

**THERAPEUTIC CLASS:** Angiotensin II receptor antagonist/thiazide diuretic

**INDICATIONS:** Treatment of hypertension. Initial treatment of severe hypertension only when the value of acheiving prompt BP control exceeds the risk. To reduce risk of stroke in patients with hypertension and left ventricular hypertrophy (may not apply to African-American patients).

**DOSAGE:** *Adults:* HTN: If BP uncontrolled on losartan monotherapy, HCTZ alone or controlled with HCTZ 25mg/day but hypokalemic: 50mg-12.5mg tab qd. Titrate/Max: If uncontrolled after 3 weeks, increase to 2 tabs of 50mg-12.5mg qd or 1 tab of 100mg-25mg qd. If uncontrolled on losartan 100mg monotherapy, may switch to 100mg-12.5mg qd. Severe HTN: Initial: 50mg-12.5mg qd. Titrate/Max: If inadequate response after 2-4 weeks, increase to 1 tab of 100mg-25mg qd. HTN With Left Ventricular Hypertrophy: Initial: Losartan 50mg qd. If BP reduction inadequate, add HCTZ 12.5 mg or substitute losartan/HCTZ 50-12.5. If additional BP reduction is needed, losartan 100mg and HCTZ 12.5mg or losartan/HCTZ 100-12.5 may be substituted, followed by losartan 100mg and HCTZ 25mg or losartan/HCTZ 100-25.

**HOW SUPPLIED:** Tab: (Losartan-HCTZ) 50mg-12.5mg, 100-12.5mg, 100mg-25mg

**CONTRAINDICATIONS:** Anuria, sulfonamide hypersensitivity.

**WARNINGS/PRECAUTIONS:** Can cause fetal injury/death. Correct volume or salt depletion before therapy. Caution with hepatic or renal dysfunction, renal artery stenosis, severe CHF, history of allergies, asthma. May exacerbate or activate SLE. Monitor serum electrolytes. Avoid if CrCl ≤30mL/min. Observe for signs of fluid or electrolyte imbalance. May precipitate hyperuricemia or gout. Enhanced effects in post-sympathectomy patient. May increase cholesterol, TG levels. Angioedema reported. Not recommended with hepatic dysfunction requiring losartan titration.

**ADVERSE REACTIONS:** Dizziness, upper respiratory infection, back pain, cough.

**INTERACTIONS:** Decreased levels with rifampin. Increased levels with fluconazole. Avoid $K^+$-sparing diuretics (eg, spironolactone, triamterene, amiloride), $K^+$ supplements, $K^+$-containing salt substitutes. Potentiates orthostatic hypotension with alcohol, barbiturates, narcotics. Adjust insulin, antidiabetic drugs. Cholestyramine, colestipol impair absorption. Corticosteroids, ACTH deplete electrolytes. May decrease response to pressor amines (eg, norepinephrine). Potentiates other antihypertensives, skeletal muscle relaxants (eg, tubocurarine). Risk of lithium toxicity. NSAIDs, including COX-2 inhibitors, may decrease effects and may result in a further deterioration of renal function in the renally impaired.

**PREGNANCY:** Category C (1st trimester) and D (2nd and 3rd trimesters), not for use in nursing.



## IBERET-FOLIC-500 RX

folic acid - multiple vitamin - ferrous sulfate (Abbott)

**THERAPEUTIC CLASS:** Iron/vitamin

**INDICATIONS:** Prevention and treatment of iron and folic acid deficiencies.

**DOSAGE:** *Adults:* 1 tab qd on empty stomach.

**HOW SUPPLIED:** Tab, Extended Release: Ferrous Sulfate 105mg-Folic Acid 0.8mg-Vitamin $B_1$ 6mg-Vitamin $B_2$ 6mg-Vitamin $B_3$ 30mg-Vitamin $B_5$ 10mg-Vitamin $B_6$ 5mg-Vitamin $B_{12}$ 25mcg-Vitamin C 500mg

**CONTRAINDICATIONS:** Pernicious anemia.

**WARNINGS/PRECAUTIONS:** May mask pernicious anemia.

**ADVERSE REACTIONS:** Allergic sensitization.

**INTERACTIONS:** Iron absorption is inhibited by magnesium trisilicate, eggs, milk, carbonate-containing antacids. May interfere with absorption of tetracyclines. Pyridoxine may reverse antiparkinsonism effects of levodopa.

**PREGNANCY:** Category A, caution in nursing.

## IB-STAT RX

hyoscyamine sulfate (InKine)

**THERAPEUTIC CLASS:** Anticholinergic

**INDICATIONS:** Adjunct treatment of peptic ulcer, irritable bowel syndrome, functional GI disorders, neurogenic bladder, neurogenic bowel disturbances. Management of functional intestinal disorders (eg, mild dysenteries, diverticulitis). To control gastric secretion, visceral spasm, and hypermotility in spastic colitis, spastic bladder, cystitis, pylorospasm, and associated abdominal cramps. Symptomatic relief of biliary and renal colic with concomitant morphine or other narcotics."Drying agent" for symptomatic relief of acute rhinitis. To reduce rigidity and tremors of Parkinson's disease and control associated sialorrhea and hyperhidrosis. For anticholinesterase poisoning.

**DOSAGE:** *Adults:* 1-2 sprays q4h or prn. Max: 12 sprays/24hrs.
*Pediatrics:* ≥12 yrs: 1-2 sprays q4h or prn. Max: 12 sprays/24hrs.

**HOW SUPPLIED:** Sol: 0.125mg/mL [30mL]

**CONTRAINDICATIONS:** Glaucoma, obstructive uropathy, GI tract obstructive disease, paralytic ileus, intestinal atony of elderly/debilitated, unstable cardiovascular status in acute hemorrhage, severe ulcerative colitis, toxic megacolon, myasthenia gravis.

**WARNINGS/PRECAUTIONS:** Risk of heat prostration with high environmental temperature. May impair mental/physical abilities. Psychosis has been reported. Caution with diarrhea, autonomic neuropathy, hyperthyroidism, coronary heart disease, CHF, arrhythmias/tachycardia, HTN, renal disease, hiatal hernia with reflux esophagitis.

**ADVERSE REACTIONS:** Drowsiness, dizziness, blurred vision, mouth dryness, urinary hesitancy and retention, tachycardia, palpitations.

**INTERACTIONS:** Additive effects with other antimuscarinics, amantadine, haloperidol, phenothiazines, MAOIs, TCAs, or some antihistamines. Antacids interfere with absorption; take ac and antacids pc.

**PREGNANCY:** Category C, caution in nursing.

## IC-GREEN RX
indocyanine green (Akorn)

**THERAPEUTIC CLASS:** Diagnostic dye

**INDICATIONS:** To determine cardiac output, hepatic function and liver blood flow, and for ophthalmic angiography.

**DOSAGE:** *Adults:* For Dilution Curves: 5mg. Max: 2 mg/kg. Refer to prescribing information for further instructions for dilution curves and administration depending on study being conducted.
*Pediatrics:* For Dilution Curves: 2.5mg. Infants: 1.25mg. Max: 2 mg/kg. Refer to prescribing information for further instructions for dilution curves and administration depending on study being conducted.

**HOW SUPPLIED:** Inj: 25mg

**CONTRAINDICATIONS:** Caution with allergy to iodides.

**WARNINGS/PRECAUTIONS:** Use solvent provided for dissolution. Use aqueous solution within 6 hrs.

**ADVERSE REACTIONS:** Anaphylactic or urticarial reactions.

**INTERACTIONS:** Do not use with heparin preparations containing sodium bisulfate; may reduce absorption. Do not perform radioactive iodine uptake studies for at least 1 week following use.

**PREGNANCY:** Category C, caution in nursing.

## IFEX RX
ifosfamide (Bristol-Myers Squibb)

**Risk of urotoxic side effects, especially hemorrhagic cystitis, and CNS toxicities (eg, confusion, coma); may require discontinuation of therapy. Severe myelosuppression reported.**

**THERAPEUTIC CLASS:** Cyclophosphamide analog

**INDICATIONS:** Third line chemotherapy of germ cell testicular cancer.

**DOSAGE:** *Adults:* 1.2g/m²/day slow IV infusion over a minimum of 30 minutes for 5 consecutive days. Repeat treatment every 3 weeks or after recovery from hematologic toxicity (platelets ≥100,000/µL, WBC ≥4000/µL). Give with extensive hydration (eg, 2L fluid/day) and protector (eg, mesna) to prevent bladder toxicity/hemorrhagic cystitis.

**HOW SUPPLIED:** Inj: 1g, 3g

**CONTRAINDICATIONS:** Severely depressed bone marrow function.

**WARNINGS/PRECAUTIONS:** Obtain urinalysis before each dose. Withhold dose until complete resolution of microscopic hematuria. Monitor WBCs, platelets, Hgb before each dose and at appropriate intervals. Avoid with WBC <2000/µL and/or platelets <50,000/µL. D/C if somnolence, confusion, hallucinations, and/or coma occur. Caution with impaired renal function, compromised bone marrow reserve, prior radiation therapy. May interfere with normal wound healing.

**ADVERSE REACTIONS:** Alopecia, nausea, vomiting, hematuria, CNS toxicity, infection, renal impairment, liver dysfunction.

**INTERACTIONS:** Severe myelosuppression with other chemotherapeutic agents. Caution with other cytotoxic agents.

**PREGNANCY:** Category D, not for use in nursing.

## IMDUR RX
isosorbide mononitrate (Schering)

**THERAPEUTIC CLASS:** Nitrate vasodilator

**INDICATIONS:** Prevention of angina pectoris. Not for acute attack.

**DOSAGE:** *Adults:* Initial: 30-60mg qd in the am. Titrate: May increase after several days to 120mg/day. Swallow whole with fluids. Elderly: Start at lower end of dosing range.

I

**HOW SUPPLIED:** Tab, Extended Release: 30mg*, 60mg*, 120mg *scored

**WARNINGS/PRECAUTIONS:** Not for use with acute MI or CHF. Severe hypotension may occur; caution with volume depletion and hypotension. Hypotension may increase angina pectoris. May aggravate angina caused by hypertrophic cardiomyopathy. Monitor for tolerance. May interfere with cholesterol test.

**ADVERSE REACTIONS:** Headache, dizziness, hypotension.

**INTERACTIONS:** Severe hypotension with sildenafil. Orthostatic hypotension with calcium channel blockers. Additive vasodilation with other vasodilators (eg, alcohol).

**PREGNANCY:** Category B, caution with nursing.

## IMITREX RX
sumatriptan (GlaxoSmithKline)

**THERAPEUTIC CLASS:** 5-$HT_1$ agonist

**INDICATIONS:** (Inj, Spray, Tab) Acute treatment of migraine with or without aura. (Inj) Acute treatment of cluster headaches.

**DOSAGE:** *Adults:* ≥18 yrs: (Inj) Initial: 6mg SQ; may repeat after 1 hr. Max: 12mg/24 hrs. (Spray) 5mg, 10mg, or 20mg single dose; may repeat after 2 hrs. Max: 40mg/24 hrs. (Tab) Initial: 25-100mg; may repeat after 2 hrs. Max: 200mg/24 hrs. May give up to 100mg/day of tabs after initial inj dose. Hepatic Disease: Max: 50mg/single dose. Safety of treating >4 headaches/30 days not known.

**HOW SUPPLIED:** Inj: 6mg/0.5mL; Nasal Spray: 5mg, 20mg [0.1mL $6^s$]; Tab: 25mg, 50mg, 100mg [$9^s$]

**CONTRAINDICATIONS:** History, symptoms, or signs of ischemic cardiac, cerebrovascular, or peripheral vascular syndromes. Other significant CVD, uncontrolled HTN, hemiplegic or basilar migraine, severe hepatic impairment, MAOIs during or within 2 weeks of use, within 24 hrs of ergotamine-containing agents, ergot-type agents, or other 5-$HT_1$ agonists.

**WARNINGS/PRECAUTIONS:** Confirm diagnosis. Supervise first dose and monitor cardiac function in those at risk of CAD (eg, HTN, hypercholesterolemia, smoker, obesity, diabetes, CAD family history, postmenopausal women, males >40 yrs). Monitor cardiac function in intermittent long-term users with CAD risk factors. Serious adverse cardiac events, cerebrovascular events, vasospastic reactions reported. Avoid in elderly. Caution with hepatic or renal impairment, history of seizures or brain lesions. Possible long-term ophthalmic effects. Reconsider diagnosis before 2nd dose.

**ADVERSE REACTIONS:** Tingling, burning sensation, flushing, chest/mouth/tongue discomfort, injection site reaction, numbness, weakness, neck pain/stiffness.

**INTERACTIONS:** Prolonged vasospastic reactions with ergot-containing drugs; avoid use within 24 hrs. Weakness, hyperreflexia, and incoordination reported with SSRIs (rare). Avoid MAOIs and other 5-$HT_1$ agonists.

**PREGNANCY:** Category C, caution in nursing.

## IMODIUM A-D

OTC

loperamide HCl (McNeil Consumer)

**THERAPEUTIC CLASS:** Anti-peristalsis agent

**INDICATIONS:** Management of diarrhea and traveler's diarrhea.

**DOSAGE:** *Adults:* >12 yrs: Initial: 4mg after the first loose bowel movement then 2mg after each additional loose bowel with plenty of liquid. Max: 8mg/day for no more than 2 days.
*Pediatrics:* 9-11 yrs (60-95 lbs): 2mg after the first loose bowel movement then 1mg after each additional loose bowel with plenty of liquid. Max: 6mg/day for no more than 2 days. 6-8 yrs (48-59 lbs): 2mg after the first loose bowel movement then 1mg after each additional loose bowel. Max: 4mg/day for no more than 2 days. 2-5 yrs (24-47 lbs): 1mg after the first loose bowel movement then 1mg after each additional loose bowel. Max: 3mg/day

**HOW SUPPLIED:** Sol: 1mg/5mL; Tab: 2mg

**WARNINGS/PRECAUTIONS:** Do not use if diarrhea is accompanied with high fever, blood, or mucus in stool. Caution with history of liver disease.

**PREGNANCY:** Safety in pregnancy and nursing is not known.

## IMOGAM RABIES-HT

RX

rabies immune globulin (Sanofi Pasteur)

**THERAPEUTIC CLASS:** Immunoglobulin

**INDICATIONS:** Suspected exposure to rabies, particularly severe exposure, except persons previously immunized with HDCV Rabies Vaccine in a pre- or post-exposure.

**DOSAGE:** *Adults:* 20IU/kg IM. Infiltrate as much of dose around wound, if feasible, with remaining portion given IM in gluteal region.
*Pediatrics:* 20IU/kg IM. Infiltrate as much of dose around wound, if feasible, with remaining portion given IM in gluteal region.

**HOW SUPPLIED:** Inj: 150IU/mL

**CONTRAINDICATIONS:** Do not repeat dose once vaccine treatment has started.

**WARNINGS/PRECAUTIONS:** Do not give in same syringe or into same site as vaccine. Made from human plasma, risk of infection. Patients with IgA deficiency could have anaphylactic reaction to IgA containing blood products. Have epinephrine (1:1000) available.

**ADVERSE REACTIONS:** Local reactions: tenderness, pain, soreness, stiffness. Systemic reactions: headache, malaise.

**INTERACTIONS:** Wait 3 months before giving live vaccines.

**PREGNANCY:** Category C, safety in nursing not known.

## IMOVAX RABIES VACCINE RX
rabies vaccine (Sanofi Pasteur)

**THERAPEUTIC CLASS:** Vaccine

**INDICATIONS:** Pre-exposure immunization and postexposure treatment of rabies.

**DOSAGE:** *Adults:* Pre-exposure: 3 doses of 1mL IM on days 0, 7, and either 21 or 28. 1mL booster every 2 yrs (see labeling for details). Post-exposure: 1mL IM on days 0, 3, 7, 14, 30 (ACIP recommendations; 5 doses) and 90 ( WHO recommendations; 6 doses). Give 1st dose with rabies immune globulin (RIG) or antirabies serum (ARS). If possible, infiltrate half of RIG or ARS into wound. Previously Immunized: 2 doses; immediately after exposure and 3 days later (no RIG needed).
*Pediatrics:* Pre-exposure: 3 doses of 1mL IM on days 0, 7, and either 21 or 28. 1mL booster every 2 yrs (see labeling for details). Post-exposure: 1mL IM on days 0, 3, 7, 14, 30 ( ACIP recommendations; 5 doses), and 90 (WHO recommendations; 6 doses). Give 1st dose with rabies immune globulin (RIG) or antirabies serum (ARS). If possible, infiltrate half of the RIG or ARS into the wound. Previously Immunized: 2 doses; immediately after exposure and 3 days later (no RIG needed).

I

**HOW SUPPLIED:** Inj: 2.5IU

**WARNINGS/PRECAUTIONS:** Postpone preexposure immunization during acute febrile illness. Neurologic illness resembling Guillain-Barre syndrome reported. May give antihistamines with history of hypersensitivity. Have epinepherine (1:1000) available. Suboptimal response may occur in immunocompromised patients.

**ADVERSE REACTIONS:** Local reactions: pain, erythema, swelling, itching. Systemic reactions: headache, nausea, abdominal pain, muscle aches, dizziness.

**INTERACTIONS:** Immunosuppressants can interfere with development of active immunity.

**PREGNANCY:** Category C, safety in nursing not known.

## IMURAN RX
azathioprine (Prometheus)

**Increased risk of neoplasia with chronic therapy. Mutagenic potential and possible hematological toxicities.**

**THERAPEUTIC CLASS:** Purine antagonist antimetabolite

**INDICATIONS:** Adjunct therapy for prevention of rejection in renal homotransplantation. Management of severe, active rheumatoid arthritis (RA) unresponsive to rest, aspirin, NSAIDs, or gold.

**DOSAGE:** *Adults:* Renal Homo Transplantation: Initial: 3-5mg/kg/day, start at time of transplant. Maint: 1-3mg/kg/day. Rheumatoid Arthritis: Initial: 1mg/kg/day given qd-bid. Titrate: Increase by 0.5mg/kg/day after 6-8 weeks, then at 4 week intervals. Max: 2.5mg/kg/day. Maint: Lowest effective dose. Decrease by 0.5mg/kg/day or 25mg/day every 4 weeks. If no response by week 12, then considered refractory. Renal Dysfunction: Lower dose.

**HOW SUPPLIED:** Tab: 50mg* *scored

**CONTRAINDICATIONS:** Pregnancy in RA treatment. Previous treatment of RA with alkylating agents (eg, cyclophosphamide, chlorambucil, melphalan) may increase risk of neoplasia.

**WARNINGS/PRECAUTIONS:** Dose-related leukopenia, thrombocytopenia, macrocytic anemia, pancytopenia and severe bone marrow suppression may occur. Monitor CBCs, including platelets, weekly during the 1st month, twice monthly for the 2nd and 3rd months, then monthly or more frequently if dose/therapy changes. Monitor for infections.

**ADVERSE REACTIONS:** Leukopenia, thrombocytopenia, infections, nausea, vomiting, hepatotoxicity.

**INTERACTIONS:** Reduce dose by 1/3-1/4 with allopurinol. Drugs affecting leukocyte production (eg, co-trimazole) may exaggerate leukopenia. ACE inhibitors may induce anemia, leukopenia. Inhibited anticoagulant effects of warfarin.

**PREGNANCY:** Category D, not for use in nursing.

## INAPSINE RX

droperidol (Akorn)

**QT prolongation, torsade de pointes, arrhythmias reported. Use in patients resistant or intolerant to other therapies. Monitor ECG before and 2-3 hrs after treatment. Extreme caution if at risk for developing prolonged QT syndrome.**

**THERAPEUTIC CLASS:** Neuroleptic butyrophenone

**INDICATIONS:** To reduce incidence of nausea and vomiting associated with surgical and diagnostic procedures.

**DOSAGE:** *Adults:* Initial (Max): 2.5mg IM/IV. May give additional 1.25mg cautiously to achieve desired effect. Lower initial doses in elderly, debilitated, poor-risk patients.

*Pediatrics:* 2-12 yrs: Initial (Max): 0.1 mg/kg IM/IV. May give additional dose cautiously. Lower initial doses in debilitated, poor-risk patients.

**HOW SUPPLIED:** Inj: 2.5mg/mL

**CONTRAINDICATIONS:** Known or suspected QT prolongation, including congenital long QT syndrome.

**WARNINGS/PRECAUTIONS:** Caution with renal/hepatic impairment. HTN, tachycardia reported with pheochromocytoma. Risk of prolonged QT syndrome with CHF, cardiac disease, bradycardia, cardiac hypertrophy, electrolyte imbalances (eg, hypokalemia, hypomagnesemia), >65 yrs, alcohol abuse. NMS reported; give dantrolene with increased temperature, HR, or carbon dioxide production. May decrease pulmonary arterial pressure.

**ADVERSE REACTIONS:** QT interval prolongation, torsade de pointes, cardiac arrest, hypotension, tachycardia, dysphoria, post-op drowsiness, restlessness, hyperactivity, anxiety, depression, syncope, irregular cardiac rhythm.

**INTERACTIONS:** Avoid drugs that prolong the QT interval (eg, antimalarials, calcium channel blockers, antidepressants, Class I and III antiarrhythmics, certain antihistamines, neuroleptics). Caution with MAOIs, alcohol, diuretics and drugs that induce hypokalemia, hypomagnesemia. May potentiate and be potentiated by CNS depressants (eg, barbiturates, benzodiazepines, tranquilizers, opioids, general anesthetics); use lower doses. Caution with conduction anesthesia (eg, spinal, peridural). Increased BP with fentanyl citrate or other parenteral analgesics. Epinephrine may paradoxically decrease BP.

**PREGNANCY:** Category C, caution in nursing.

## INDERAL RX

propranolol HCl (Wyeth)

**THERAPEUTIC CLASS:** Nonselective beta-blocker

**INDICATIONS:** (Tab) Management of hypertension, angina pectoris, hypertrophic subaortic stenosis. Migraine prophylaxis. (Inj/Tab) For cardiac arrhythmias (supraventricular, ventricular tachycardia, tachyarrhythmia of digitalis intoxication, resistant tachyarrhythmia), reduction of cardiovascular mortality post-MI, essential tremor, and pheochromocytoma.

**DOSAGE:** *Adults:* HTN: (Tab) Initial: 40mg bid. Titrate: Increase gradually. Maint: 120-240mg/day. Angina: (Tab) 80-320mg/day, given bid-qid.

Arrhythmia: (Inj) 1-3mg IV at 1 mg/min. (Tab) 10-30mg tid-qid ac and qhs. MI: (Tab) 180-240mg/day, given bid-tid. Migraine: (Tab) Initial: 80mg/day in divided doses. Usual: 160-240mg/day in divided doses. Tremor: (Tab) Initial: 40mg bid. Maint: 120mg/day. Max: 320mg/day. Hypertrophic Subaortic Stenosis: (Tab) 20-40mg tid-qid, ac and qhs. Pheochromocytoma: (Tab) 60mg/day in divided doses for 3 days before surgery with alpha-blocker. Inoperable Tumor: (Tab) 30mg/day in divided doses.
*Pediatrics:* HTN (Tab): Initial: 1mg/kg/day PO. Usual: 1-2mg/kg bid. Max: 16mg/kg/day.

**HOW SUPPLIED:** Inj: 1mg/mL; Tab: 10mg*, 20mg*, 40mg*, 60mg*, 80mg* *scored

**CONTRAINDICATIONS:** Cardiogenic shock, sinus bradycardia and >1st-degree block, bronchial asthma, CHF (unless failure is secondary to tachyarrhythmia treatable with propranolol).

**WARNINGS/PRECAUTIONS:** Caution with well-compensated cardiac failure, nonallergic bronchospasm, Wolff-Parkinson-White syndrome, hepatic or renal dysfunction. Withdrawal before surgery is controversial. May mask hypoglycemia or hyperthyroidism symptoms. Avoid abrupt discontinuation. May reduce IOP. Can cause cardiac failure.

I

**ADVERSE REACTIONS:** Bradycardia, CHF, hypotension, lightheadedness, mental depression, nausea, vomiting, allergic reactions, agranulocytosis.

**INTERACTIONS:** Bradycardia/hypotension with catecholamine-depleting drugs. Potentiated by chlorpromazine, cimetidine. Antagonized by NSAIDs, phenytoin, phenobarbital, rifampin. May increase cardiac effects of calcium channel blockers. Reduces clearance of antipyrine, lidocaine, and theophylline. Aluminum hydroxide gel reduces intestinal absorption. Alcohol decreases absorption rate. May block epinephrine, thyroxine effects. Hypotension and cardiac arrest reported with haloperidol. May increase warfarin concentration; monitor prothrombin time. Concomitant use with alcohol may increase plasma levels of propranolol.

**PREGNANCY:** Category C, caution in nursing. Intrauterine growth retardation, small placenta, and congenital abnormalities have been reported in neonates whose mothers received propranolol during pregnancy. Neonates whose mothers received propranolol at parturition have exhibited bradycardia, hypoglycemia, and/or respiratory depression.

## INDERAL LA

propranolol HCl (Wyeth) RX

**THERAPEUTIC CLASS:** Nonselective beta-blocker

**INDICATIONS:** Management of hypertension, angina pectoris, hypertrophic subaortic stenosis. Migraine prophylaxis.

**DOSAGE:** *Adults:* HTN: Initial: 80mg qd. Maint: 120-160mg qd. Angina: Initial: 80mg qd. Titrate: Increase gradually every 3-7 days. Maint: 160mg qd. Max: 320mg/day. Migraine: Initial: 80mg qd. Maint: 160-240mg qd. Discontinue gradually if no response within 4-6 weeks. Hypertrophic Subaortic Stenosis: 80-160mg qd.

**HOW SUPPLIED:** Cap, Extended Release: 60mg, 80mg, 120mg, 160mg

**CONTRAINDICATIONS:** Cardiogenic shock, sinus bradycardia and >1st-degree block, bronchial asthma, CHF (unless failure is secondary to tachyarrhythmia treatable with propranolol).

**WARNINGS/PRECAUTIONS:** Caution with well-compensated cardiac failure, nonallergic bronchospasm, Wolff-Parkinson-White syndrome, hepatic or renal dysfunction. Withdrawal before surgery is controversial. May mask hypoglycemia or hyperthyroidism symptoms. Avoid abrupt discontinuation. May reduce IOP. Can cause cardiac failure.

**ADVERSE REACTIONS:** Bradycardia, CHF, hypotension, lightheadedness, mental depression, nausea, vomiting, allergic reactions, agranulocytosis.

**INTERACTIONS:** Bradycardia/hypotension with catecholamine-depleting drugs. Potentiated by chlorpromazine, cimetidine. Antagonized by NSAIDs, phenytoin, phenobarbital, rifampin. May increase cardiac effects of calcium channel blockers. Reduces clearance of antipyrine, lidocaine, and theophylline. Aluminum hydroxide gel reduces intestinal absorption. Alcohol decreases absorption rate. May block epinephrine, thyroxine effects. Hypotension and cardiac arrest reported with haloperidol. Concomitant use with alcohol may increase plasma levels of propranolol.

**PREGNANCY:** Category C, caution in nursing.

## INDERIDE

RX

hydrochlorothiazide - propranolol HCl (Wyeth)

**OTHER BRAND NAMES:** Inderide LA (Wyeth)

**THERAPEUTIC CLASS:** Nonselective beta-blocker/thiazide diuretic

**INDICATIONS:** Management of hypertension. Not for initial therapy.

**DOSAGE:** *Adults:* Initial: 80-160mg propranolol/day; 25mg-50mg HCTZ/day. Max: (propranolol-HCTZ) 160mg-50mg/day. Elderly: Start at low end of dosing range. Do not substitute mg-for-mg of extended release cap for immediate release tab plus HCTZ. Dose tab bid and extended release cap qd.

**HOW SUPPLIED:** (Propranolol-HCTZ) Tab: (Inderide) 40mg-25mg*, 80mg-25mg*; Cap, Extended Release: (Inderide LA) 80mg-50mg *scored

**CONTRAINDICATIONS:** Cardiogenic shock, sinus bradycardia and >1st-degree block, bronchial asthma, CHF (unless failure is secondary to tachyarrhythmia treatable with propranolol), anuria, sulfonamide hypersensitivity.

**WARNINGS/PRECAUTIONS:** Caution with well-compensated cardiac failure, nonallergic bronchospasm, Wolff-Parkinson-White Syndrome, hepatic or renal dysfunction. Withdrawal before surgery is controversial. May mask hypoglycemia or hyperthyroidism symptoms. Avoid abrupt discontinuation. May reduce IOP. Can cause cardiac failure, hypokalemia, hyperuricemia, hypercalcemia, hypophosphatemia. May exacerbate or activate SLE. Monitor for fluid/electrolyte imbalance. May manifest latent DM. Enhanced effect in postsympathectomy patient. Concomitant use with alcohol may increase plasma levels of propranolol

**ADVERSE REACTIONS:** Bradycardia, CHF, hypotension, lightheadedness, mental depression, nausea, vomiting, allergic reactions, blood dyscrasias, pancreatitis.

**INTERACTIONS:** Bradycardia/hypotension with catecholamine-depleting drugs. Potentiated by chlorpromazine, cimetidine. Antagonized by NSAIDs, phenytoin, phenobarbital, rifampin. May increase cardiac effects of calcium channel blockers. Reduces clearance of antipyrine, lidocaine, and theophylline. Aluminum hydroxide gel reduces intestinal absorption. Alcohol decreases absorption rate. May block epinephrine, thyroxine effects. Hypotension and cardiac arrest reported with haloperidol. May increase response to tubocurarine. May decrease arterial response to norepinephrine. Insulin dose may need adjustment. Risk of hypokalemia with corticosteroids, ACTH. Alcohol, barbiturates, or narcotics may aggravate orthostatic hypotension. Monitor digoxin. Potentiation with ganglionic or peripheral adrenergic-blockers. Concomitant use with alcohol may increase plasma levels of propranolol

**PREGNANCY:** Category C, not for use in nursing. Intrauterine growth retardation, small placenta, and congenital abnormalities have been reported in neonates whose mothers received propranolol during pregnancy. Neonates whose mothers received propranolol at parturition have exhibited bradycardia, hypoglycemia, and/or respiratory depression.

## INDOCIN I.V. RX

indomethacin sodium trihydrate (Merck)

**THERAPEUTIC CLASS:** NSAID (indole derivative)

**INDICATIONS:** To close hemodynamically significant patent ductus arteriosus in premature infants weighing between 500-1750g after 48 hrs of ineffective medical management.

**DOSAGE:** *Pediatrics:* Neonates 500-1750g: Therapy includes 3 doses at 12-24 hr intervals. <48 hrs old: 0.2mg/kg IV followed by 0.1mg/kg IV then 0.1mg/kg IV. 2-7 days old: 0.2mg/kg IV for 3 doses. >7 days old: 0.2mg/kg IV followed by 0.25mg/kg IV then 0.25mg/kg IV. If anuria or marked oliguria (urinary output <0.6mL/kg/hr) occurs at scheduled time of second or third dose, hold doses until renal function normalizes. May repeat course if ductus arteriosus reopens. Surgery may be needed if unresponsive after 2 courses.

**HOW SUPPLIED:** Inj: 1mg

**CONTRAINDICATIONS:** Untreated infection, bleeding, thrombocytopenia, coagulation defects, necrotizing enterocolitis, significant renal impairment, congenital heart disease when patency of ductus arteriosus is necessary for pulmonary or systemic blood flow.



**WARNINGS/PRECAUTIONS:** Risk of minor GI bleeding, intraventricular bleeding. May reduce urine output, CrCl, glomerular filtration rate and may increase serum creatinine, BUN. May cause renal insufficiency, including acute renal failure; caution with extracellular volume depletion, CHF, sepsis, hepatic dysfunction. Monitor renal function and serum electrolytes. May mask signs of infection. D/C if liver disease develops. Avoid extravascular injection or leakage.

**ADVERSE REACTIONS:** Intracranial bleeding, GI bleeding, hyponatremia, elevated serum potassium, retrolental fibroplasia.

**INTERACTIONS:** May prolong half-life of digitalis; monitor ECG and serum digitalis levels. May elevate gentamicin and amikacin levels. May decrease natriuretic effect of furosemide. May reduce renal function; consider reducing dosage of medications that rely on adequate renal function for elimination. Increased risk of renal insufficiency with nephrotoxic drugs. Increased risk of bleeding with anticoagulants.

**PREGNANCY:** Safety in pregnancy or nursing not known.

## INDOMETHACIN RX

indomethacin (Various)

> **NSAIDs may cause an increased risk of serious cardiovascular thrombotic events, MI, stroke and serious GI adverse events including bleeding, ulceration, and perforation of the stomach or intestines. Contraindicated for the treatment of perioperative pain in the setting of coronary artery bypass graft (CABG) surgery.**

**OTHER BRAND NAMES:** Indocin (Merck)

**THERAPEUTIC CLASS:** NSAID (indole derivative)

**INDICATIONS:** Management of moderate to severe rheumatoid arthritis (RA), ankylosing spondylitis, osteoarthritis (OA), acute painful shoulder (bursitis and/or tendinitis) and/or acute gouty arthritis.

**DOSAGE:** *Adults:* RA/Ankylosing Spondylitis/OA: Initial: 25mg PO bid-tid. Titrate: May increase by 25-50mg/day at weekly intervals. Max: 200mg/day. Bursitis/Tendinitis: 75-150mg/day given tid-qid for 7-14 days. Acute Gouty Arthritis: 50mg PO tid until pain is tolerable, then d/c. Take with food. *Pediatrics:* >14 yrs: RA/Ankylosing Spondylitis/OA: Initial: 25mg PO bid-tid. Titrate: May increase by 25-50mg/day at weekly intervals. Max: 200mg/day. Bursitis/Tendinitis: 75-150mg/day given tid-qid for 7-14 days. Acute Gouty Arthritis: 50mg PO tid until pain is tolerable, then d/c. 2-14 yrs (safety and effectiveness not established): Initial: 1-2mg/kg/day in divided doses. Max: 3mg/kg/day or 150-200mg/day. Take with food.

**HOW SUPPLIED:** Cap: 25mg, 50mg; Sus: 25mg/5mL [237mL]

**CONTRAINDICATIONS:** ASA or other NSAID allergy that precipitates acute asthmatic attack, urticaria or rhinitis. Do not give suppositories with history of proctitis or recent rectal bleeding. Treatment of perioperative pain in the setting of CABG surgery.

**WARNINGS/PRECAUTIONS:** May lead to onset of new HTN or worsening of pre-existing HTN; monitor BP closely. Fluid retention and edema reported; caution with fluid retention or heart failure. Renal papillary necrosis and other renal injury reported after long-term use. Not recommended for use with advanced renal disease; if therapy must be initiated, monitor renal function. Anaphylactoid reactions may occur. May cause serious skin adverse events (eg, exfoliative dermatitis, Stevens-Johnson syndrome, and toxic epidermal necrolysis). Avoid in late pregnancy; may cause premature closure of ductus arteriosis. May cause elevations of LFTs; d/c if liver disease develops or systemic manifestations occur. Caution in elderly. Anemia may occur; with long-term use, monitor Hgb/Hct if signs or symptoms of anemia develop. May inhibit platelet aggregation and prolong bleeding time; monitor with coagulation disorders. Caution with asthma and avoid with aspirin-sensitive asthma. Corneal deposits and retinal disturbances reported with prolonged therapy; perform eye exams at periodic intervals during prolonged therapy. May aggravate depression or other psychiatric disturbances, epilepsy, and parkinsonism; use with caution. D/C if severe CNS adverse reactions develop. May impair mental/physical abilities.

**ADVERSE REACTIONS:** Headache, dizziness, nausea, vomiting, dyspepsia, diarrhea, abdominal pain, constipation, vertigo, somnolence, depression, fatigue.

**INTERACTIONS:** Avoid salicylates, diflunisal, other NSAIDs and triamterene. Potassium sparing diuretics may cause hyperkalemia. Increase toxicity of methotrexate, cyclosporine, lithium and digoxin. Probenecid increases levels. Caution with antihypertensives and anticoagulants. May decrease effects of diuretics, β-blockers, captopril.

**PREGNANCY:** Category C, not for use in nursing.

## INFANRIX

RX

tetanus toxoid - diphtheria toxoid - pertussis vaccine, acellular

(GlaxoSmithKline)

**THERAPEUTIC CLASS:** Vaccine/toxoid combination

**INDICATIONS:** Active immunization against diphtheria, tetanus, and pertussisas a 5-dose series in infants and children 6wks-7yrs old.

**DOSAGE:** *Pediatrics:* >6 weeks up to 7 yrs: 3 doses of 0.5mL IM at 4-8 week intervals. Start at 2 months or as early as 6 weeks if necessary. 2 Booster doses: Give at 15-20 months and at 4 to 6 years. Do not start series over again, regardless of time elapsed between doses. May use to complete primary series in infants who received 1-2 doses of whole-cell DTP vaccine.

**HOW SUPPLIED:** Inj: (Diphtheria-Tetanus-Pertussis) 25Lf-10Lf-25mcg/0.5mL

**CONTRAINDICATIONS:** Hypersensitivity to any component; serious allergic (eg, anaphylaxis) associated with previous dose. Encephalopathy not due to an identifiable cause within 7 days prior to pertussis immunization and progressive neurologic disorder, uncontrolled epilepsy, or progressive encephalopathy. Not contraindicated in individuals with HIV infection.

**WARNINGS/PRECAUTIONS:** Caution if within 48 hrs of previous whole-cell DTP or acellular DTP vaccine, fever >105°F not due to another identifiable cause, collapse or shock-like state, or inconsolable crying lasting >3 hrs occurs, or if convulsions occur within 3 days. For high seizure risk, give APAP at time of vaccination and q4-6h for 24 hrs. Caution with neurologic or CNS disorders.

Avoid with coagulation disorders. Have epinephrine available. Suboptimal response may occur in immunocompromised patients.

**ADVERSE REACTIONS:** Local reactions, fever, irritability, drowsiness, anorexia, vomiting, diarrhea, crying.

**INTERACTIONS:** Avoid with anticoagulants. Immunosuppressive therapy (eg, irradiation, antimetabolites, alkylating agents, cytotoxic drugs, corticosteroids) may decrease response. Administer tetanus immune globulin, diphtheria antitoxin, hepatitis B vaccine, and *Haemophilus influenzae* type B vaccine at separate site.

**PREGNANCY:** Category C, safety in nursing not known.

## INFED RX
iron dextran (Watson)

**Anaphylactic-type reactions and death possible. Only use when indication clearly established and lab investigations confirm iron deficient state not amenable to oral therapy.**

I

**THERAPEUTIC CLASS:** Iron supplement

**INDICATIONS:** Treatment of iron deficiency when oral administration is not possible.

**DOSAGE:** *Adults:* Iron Deficiency Anemia: Dose (mL)=0.0442 (desired Hgb-observed Hgb) x LBW + (0.26 x LBW); LBW=lean body weight (kg). See labeling for more details. Blood Loss: Replace equivalent amount of iron in blood loss.
*Pediatrics:* >4 months: >15kg: Iron Deficiency Anemia: Dose (mL)=0.0442 (desired Hgb-observed Hgb) x LBW + (0.26 x LBW); LBW=lean body weight (kg). 5-15kg: Dose (mL)=0.0442 (desired Hgb-observed Hgb) x weight + (0.26 x weight). See labeling for more details. Blood Loss: Replace equivalent amount of iron in blood loss.

**HOW SUPPLIED:** Inj: 50mg/mL

**CONTRAINDICATIONS:** Anemia not associated with iron deficiency.

**WARNINGS/PRECAUTIONS:** Large IV doses associated with increased incidence of adverse effects. Caution with serious hepatic impairment, significant allergies, asthma. Avoid during acute phase of infectious kidney disease. May exacerbate cardiovascular complications in pre-existing cardiovascular disease and joint pain or swelling in rheumatoid arthritis. Hypersensitivity reactions reported after uneventful test doses. Unwarranted therapy can cause exogenous hemosiderosis. Have epinephrine (1:1000) available. Risk of carcinogenesis with IM use. Give 0.5mL test dose before IM/IV administration.

**ADVERSE REACTIONS:** Anaphylactic reactions, chest pain/tightness, urticaria, pruritus, abdominal pain, nausea, arthralgia, convulsions, respiratory arrest, hematuria, febrile episodes.

**INTERACTIONS:** Discontinue oral iron before use.

**PREGNANCY:** Category C, caution in nursing.

## INFERGEN RX
interferon alfacon-1 (InterMune)

**May cause or aggravate fatal or life-threatening neuropsychiatric, autoimmune, ischemic, and infectious disorders. Monitor closely with periodic clinical and laboratory evaluations.**

**THERAPEUTIC CLASS:** Biological response modifier

**INDICATIONS:** Treatment of chronic hepatitis C virus (HCV) with compensated liver disease in patients with anti-HCV antibodies and/or presence of HCV RNA.

**DOSAGE:** *Adults:* >18 yrs: 9mcg 3x/week (TIW) SQ for 24 weeks, wait 48 hrs between doses. If No Response or Relapse: 15mcg TIW for up to 48 weeks. Hold dose temporarily in severe adverse effects and reduce to 7.5mcg.

**HOW SUPPLIED:** Inj: 30mcg/mL

**CONTRAINDICATIONS:** Hypersensitivity to *E.coli*-derived products.

**WARNINGS/PRECAUTIONS:** Severe psychiatric adverse events (eg, depression, suicidal ideation, suicide attempt) may occur. Avoid in decompensated hepatic disease. Monitor CBC, platelets, and clinical chemistry tests before therapy and periodically thereafter. D/C if severe decrease in neutrophils or platelets, or serious hypersensitivity reaction occurs. Caution with cardiac disease, history of endocrine disorders, or low peripheral blood cell counts. Decrease/loss of vision and retinopathy reported; perform eye examination at baseline, if any ocular symptoms develop, and periodically with pre-existing disorder. May exacerbate autoimmune disorders. Neutropenia, thrombocytopenia, hypertriglyceridemia, and thyroid disorders reported. Caution in elderly.

**ADVERSE REACTIONS:** Flu-like symptoms, depression, leukopenia, granulocytopenia, hot flushes, malaise, insomnia, dizziness, headache, myalgia, abdominal pain, nausea, diarrhea, anorexia, vomiting, thrombocytopenia, nervousness.

**INTERACTIONS:** Caution with agents that cause myelosuppression or are metabolized by CYP450.

**PREGNANCY:** Category C, caution in nursing.

## INFLAMASE — RX

prednisolone sodium phosphate (Novartis Ophthalmics)

**OTHER BRAND NAMES:** AK-Pred (Akorn) - Inflamase Forte (Novartis Ophthalmics)

**THERAPEUTIC CLASS:** Corticosteroid

**INDICATIONS:** Treatment of inflammation of the palpebral and bulbar conjunctiva, cornea, and anterior segment of the globe.

**DOSAGE:** *Adults:* Initial: 1-2 drops every hr (day) and q2h (night). Maint: 1 drop q4h, reduce to 1 drop tid-qid to control symptoms.

**HOW SUPPLIED:** Sol: (Inflamase) 0.125% [5mL, 10mL], (Forte) 1% [10mL, 15mL], (AK-Pred) 1% [5mL, 15mL]

**CONTRAINDICATIONS:** Viral diseases of the cornea and conjunctiva including superficial herpes simplex keratitis, vaccinia, and varicella. Tuberculosis and fungal diseases of the eye. After uncomplicated removal of corneal foreign body.

**WARNINGS/PRECAUTIONS:** Prolonged use can cause optic nerve damage, visual defects, cataracts, glaucoma or secondary ocular infections (eg, fungal). Check IOP frequently. Caution with diseases causing thinning of cornea/sclera. May mask or enhance infection with acute purulent conditions. Discontinue if develop irritation.

**ADVERSE REACTIONS:** Secondary infection, visual defects, glaucoma, cataract formation.

**PREGNANCY:** Category C, caution in nursing.

## INFUMORPH — CII

morphine sulfate (Baxter)

**THERAPEUTIC CLASS:** Opioid analgesic

**INDICATIONS:** Treatment of intractable chronic pain in microinfusion devices.

**DOSAGE:** *Adults:* Lumbar Intrathecal: Opioid Intolerant: 0.2-1mg/day. Opioid Tolerant: 1-10mg/day. Max: Must be individualized. Caution with >20mg/day.

Epidural: Opioid Intolerant: 3.5-7.5mg/day. Opioid tolerant: 4.5-10mg/day. May increase to 20-30mg/day. Max: Must be individualized. Starting dose must be based on in-hospital evaluation of response to serial single-dose intrathecal/epidural bolus injections of regular morphine sulfate.

**HOW SUPPLIED:** Inj: 10mg/mL (200mg), 25mg/mL (500mg)

**CONTRAINDICATIONS:** For neuraxial analgesia: Infection at injection site, anticoagulants, uncontrolled bleeding diathesis, any therapy or condition that may render intrathecal or epidural administration hazardous.

**WARNINGS/PRECAUTIONS:** Have resuscitation equipment, oxygen, and antidote (eg, naloxone) available; severe respiratory depression may occur. Use only if less invasive means of controlling pain fail. Not for single-dose IV, IM, or SQ administration. May be habit-forming. Observe patient for 24 hours following test dose, and for the first several days after catheter implantation. Caution with determining refill frequency. Make sure needle is properly placed in the filling port of device. Myoclonic-like spasm of the lower extremities reported if dose >20mg/day; may need detoxification. Caution with head injury, increased intracranial pressure, decreased respiratory reserve, hepatic/renal dysfunction (epidural injection), elderly. Avoid with chronic asthma, upper airway obstruction, other chronic pulmonary disorders. Biliary colic reported. May cause micturition disturbances especially with BPH. Increased risk of orthostatic hypotension with reduced circulating blood volume and impaired myocardial function. Avoid abrupt withdrawal. Risk of withdrawal in patients maintained on parenteral/oral narcotics. Not for routine use in obstetric labor/delivery.



**ADVERSE REACTIONS:** Respiratory depression, myoclonus convulsions, dysphoric reactions, pruritus, urinary retention, constipation, lumbar puncture-type headache, peripheral edema, orthostatic hypotension.

**INTERACTIONS:** Depressant effect may be potentiated by CNS depressants (eg, alcohol, sedatives, antihistamines, psychotropics). Increased risk of respiratory depression with neuroleptics. Contraindicated with anticoagulants. Risk of withdrawal with narcotic antagonists. Increased risk of orthostatic hypotension with sympatholytic drugs.

**PREGNANCY:** Category C, safety in nursing not known.

## INNOHEP RX

tinzaparin sodium (Pharmion)

**Risk of paralysis by spinal/epidural hematoma with neuraxial anesthesia or spinal puncture. Increased risk with indwelling epidural catheters for analgesia, drugs affecting hemostasis (eg, NSAIDs, platelet inhibitors, anticoagulants), and traumatic or repeated epidural or spinal puncture.**

**THERAPEUTIC CLASS:** Low molecular weight heparin

**INDICATIONS:** Treatment of acute symptomatic DVT with or without PE with concomitant warfarin.

**DOSAGE:** *Adults:* 175 anti-Xa IU/kg SQ qd for at least 6 days and until anticoagulated with warfarin (INR is at least 2 for 2 days). Begin warfarin within 1-3 days of therapy.

**HOW SUPPLIED:** Inj: 20,000 anti-Xa IU/mL

**CONTRAINDICATIONS:** Heparin, sulfite, benzoyl alcohol, or pork allergy. Active major bleeding, with or history of heparin-induced thrombocytopenia (HIT).

**WARNINGS/PRECAUTIONS:** Not for IM injection. Cannot use interchangeably unit for unit with heparin or other low molecular weight heparins. Extreme caution in conditions with an increased risk of hemorrhage (eg, bacterial endocarditis, hemorrhagic stroke, etc). Bleeding can occur at any site during therapy. Discontinue if severe hemorrhage occurs. Perform periodic CBC, platelets, and stool occult blood test. Asymptomatic increase in AST and ALT. Priapism reported (rare). Thrombocytopenia can occur; discontinue if platelets <100,000/$mm^3$. Multiple dose vial contains benzyl alcohol. Contains sodium metabisulfite. Caution with bleeding diathesis, uncontrolled arterial HTN, recent GI ulceration, diabetic retinopathy, hemorrhage. Reduced elimination with elderly or in renal dysfunction; use with caution.

**ADVERSE REACTIONS:** Hemorrhage, thrombocytopenia, elevated LFTs, local reactions (ecchymosis, hematoma), hypersensitivity reactions.

**INTERACTIONS:** Increased risk of bleeding with anticoagulants, platelet inhibitors (eg, salicylates, dipyridamole, sulfinpyrazone, dextran, NSAIDs, ticlopidine, clopidogrel), and thrombolytics; monitor closely if co-administered.

**PREGNANCY:** Category B, caution use in nursing.

## INNOPRAN XL

RX

propranolol HCl (Reliant)

**THERAPEUTIC CLASS:** Nonselective beta-blocker

**INDICATIONS:** For the management of hypertension.

**DOSAGE:** *Adults:* Initial: 80mg qhs (approximately 10 PM) consistently either on an empty stomach or with food. Titrate: Based on response may titrate to a dose of 120mg.

**HOW SUPPLIED:** Cap, Extended Release: 80mg, 120mg

**CONTRAINDICATIONS:** Cardiogenic shock, sinus bradycardia and >1st-degree block, bronchial asthma.

**WARNINGS/PRECAUTIONS:** Caution with well-compensated cardiac failure, nonallergic bronchospasm (eg, chronic bronchitis, emphysema), Wolff-Parkinson-White syndrome, hepatic or renal dysfunction or with history of severe anaphylactic reactions. Withdrawal before surgery is controversial. May mask hypoglycemia or hyperthyroidism symptoms. Avoid abrupt discontinuation. May reduce IOP. Can cause cardiac failure.

**ADVERSE REACTIONS:** Fatigue, dizziness (except vertigo), constipation.

**INTERACTIONS:** Caution with drugs that effect CYP2D6, 1A2, or 2C19 or that slow down AV conduction (eg, digitalis, lidocaine, calcium channel blockers). ACE inhibitors can cause hypotension and certain ACE inhibitors may increase bronchial hyperactivity. May antagonize clonidine effects; caution when withdrawing from clonidine. Potentiated by alpha-blockers (eg, prazosin, terazosin, doxazosin), antiarrhythmics (eg, propafenone, quinidine, amiodarone), CYP2D6 substrates or inhibitors (eg, cimetidine, delavudin, fluoxetine, paroxetine, quinidine, ritonavir), CYP1A2 substrates or inhibitors (eg, imipramine, cimetidine, ciprofloxacin, fluvoxamine, isoniazid, theophylline, zileuton, zolmitriptan, rizatriptan), CYP2C19 substrates or inhibitors (eg, fluconazole, fluoxetine, fluvoxamine, teniposide, tolbutamide). Severe bradycardia, asystole, and heart failure associated with concomitant disopyramide. Decreases clearance of lidocaine and theophylline. Uncontrolled HTN may develop with concurrent epinephrine. Closely monitor for excessive reduction of resting sympathetic nervous activity (eg, hypotension, bradycardia, vertigo, orthostatic hypotension, syncopy) with concurrent reserpine; reserpine may also potentiate depression. Anesthetics (eg, methoxyflurane, trichloroethylene) may depress myocardial contractility. Effects may be reversed by β-agonists (eg, dobutamine, isoproterenol). May exacerbate hypotensive effects of MAOIs or tricyclic antidepressants. Hypotension and cardiac arrest reported with haloperidol. Antagonized by NSAIDs. May result in lower than expected $T_3$ level with concomitant thyroxin. Increases level of warfarin, diazepam, zolmitriptan, rizatriptan, thioridazine. Decreased levels with aluminum hydroxide gel (1200mg), cholestyramine, colestipol, rifampin, ethanol, and cigarette smoking. Co-administration with chlorpromazine may increase levels of both drugs. Decreases levels of lovastatin and pravastatin.

**PREGNANCY:** Category C; caution in nursing.

## INSPRA RX
eplerenone (Pfizer)

**THERAPEUTIC CLASS:** Aldosterone blocker

**INDICATIONS:** To improve survival with left ventricular systolic dysfunction and congestive heart failure (CHF) post-MI. Treatment of hypertension, alone or with other antihypertensives.

**DOSAGE:** *Adults:* CHF Post-MI: Initial: 25mg qd. Titrate: To 50mg qd within 4 weeks. Maint: 50mg qd. Adjust dose based on $K^+$ level: See labeling. HTN: Initial: 50mg qd. May increase to 50mg bid if inadequate effect on BP. Max: 100mg/day. With Weak CYP3A4 Inhibitors: Initial: 25mg qd.

**HOW SUPPLIED:** Tab: 25mg, 50mg

**CONTRAINDICATIONS:** All: Serum $K^+$ >5.5mgEq/L at initiation, CrCl ≤30mL/min, with potent CYP3A4 inhibitors (eg, ketoconazole, itraconazole, nefazodone, troleandomycin, clarithromycin, ritonavir, nelfinavir). When treating HTN: Type 2 diabetes with microalbuminuria, SCr >2mg/dL (males) or >1.8mg/dL (females), CrCl <50mg/min, with $K^+$ supplements or $K^+$-sparing diuretics (eg, amiloride, spironolactone, triamterene).

**WARNINGS/PRECAUTIONS:** Risk of hyperkalemia (>5.5mEq/L); monitor periodically. With CHF post-MI use caution with SCr >2mg/dL (males) or >1.8mg/dL (females), CrCl ≤50mL/min, and in diabetics (also with proteinuria).

**ADVERSE REACTIONS:** Headache, dizziness, hyperkalemia, increased SCr/triglycerides/GGT, angina/MI.

**INTERACTIONS:** Avoid with potent CYP3A4 inhibitors (eg, ketoconazole, itraconazole, nefazodone, troleandomycin, clarithromycin, ritonavir, nelfinavir). Increased levels with other CYP3A4 inhibitors (eg, erythromycin, verapamil, saquinavir, fluconazole). In HTN, use caution, with ACE inhibitors and angiotensin II receptor antagonists; increased risk of hyperkalemia especially with diabetics with microalbuminuria. Monitor lithium levels. Monitor antihypertensive effect with NSAIDs.

**PREGNANCY:** Category B, not for use in nursing.

## INTAL RX
cromolyn sodium (King)

**THERAPEUTIC CLASS:** Mast cell stabilizer

**INDICATIONS:** Prophylactic treatment of bronchial asthma and of acute bronchoconstriction due to exercise, environmental agents, and known antigens.

**DOSAGE:** *Adults:* Asthma: (Inhaler) Usual/Max: 2 inh qid. (Sol) 20mg nebulized qid. Acute Bonchospasm Prevention: (Inhaler) Usual: 2 inh 10-60 minutes before exposure to precipitant. (Sol) 20mg nebulized shortly before exposure to precipitant. Renal/Hepatic Dysfunction: Decrease inhaler dose. *Pediatrics:* Asthma: (Inhaler) >5 yrs: Usual/Max: 2 inh qid. (Sol) >2 yrs: 20mg nebulized qid. Acute Bronchospasm Prevention: (Inhaler) >5 yrs: Usual: 2 inh 10-60 minutes before exposure to precipitant. (Sol) >2 yrs: 20mg nebulized shortly before exposure to precipitant. Renal/Hepatic Dysfunction: Decrease inhaler dose.

**HOW SUPPLIED:** MDI: 0.8mg/inh [8.1g, 14.2g]; Sol (neb): 10mg/mL [2mL, 10s 60s]

**WARNINGS/PRECAUTIONS:** Not for treatment of acute attack. Severe anaphylaxis may occur. D/C if eosinophilic pneumonia or pulmonary infiltrates with eosinophilia develop. May experience cough and/or bronchospasm. Caution with inhaler in CAD or history of cardiac arrhythmias. Decrease dose or d/c with renal/hepatic dysfunction.

**ADVERSE REACTIONS:** Throat irritation/dryness, bad taste, cough, nausea, bronchospasm, sneezing, wheezing.

**INTERACTIONS:** Avoid with isoproterenol during pregnancy.

**PREGNANCY:** Category B, caution in nursing.

## INTEGRILIN RX
eptifibatide (Schering)

**THERAPEUTIC CLASS:** Glycoprotein IIb/IIIa inhibitor

**INDICATIONS:** Treatment of acute coronary syndrome (ACS) in patients being medically managed or undergoing percutaneous coronary intervention (PCI) including intracoronary stenting.

**DOSAGE:** *Adults:* ACS: SCr <2mg/dL: 180mcg/kg IV bolus, then 2mcg/kg/min IV infusion until discharge, initiation of CABG, or up to 72 hrs. If undergoing PCI, continue until discharge or 18-24 hrs post-PCI. SCr 2-4 mg/dL: 180mcg/kg IV bolus, then 1mcg/kg/min IV infusion. PCI: SCr <2mg/dL: 180mcg/kg IV bolus immediately before PCI, then 2mcg/kg/min IV infusion. Give 2nd bolus of 180mcg/kg 10 minutes after 1st bolus. Continue until discharge or 18-24 hrs post-PCI. SCr: 2-4 mg/dL: 180mcg/kg IV bolus immediately before PCI, then 1mcg/kg/min IV infusion. Give 2nd bolus of 180mcg/kg 10 minutes after 1st bolus. ACS/PCI: >121kg: SCr <2mg/dL: Max: 22.6mg IV bolus, then 15mg/hr IV infusion. SCr 2-4mg/dL: Max: 22.6mg IV bolus, then 7.5mg/hr IV infusion. See labeling for concomitant ASA and heparin doses.

**HOW SUPPLIED:** Sol: 0.75mg/mL, 2mg/mL

**CONTRAINDICATIONS:** Active abnormal bleeding, history of bleeding diathesis, or stroke within past 30 days. Severe HTN uncontrolled with antihypertensives, major surgery within preceding 6 weeks, history of hemorrhagic stroke, concomitant parenteral glycoprotein IIb/IIIa inhibitor, renal dialysis dependency.

**WARNINGS/PRECAUTIONS:** Bleeding reported. Caution with renal dysfunction, platelets <100,000$mm^3$, femeral access site in PCI. Minimize vascular and other trauma. D/C if thrombocytopenia occurs. Monitor Hct, Hgb, platelets, serum creatinine (SCr), and PT/aPTT before therapy (and activated clotting time before PCI). D/C before CABG surgery.

**ADVERSE REACTIONS:** Bleeding, thrombocytopenia, hypotension.

**INTERACTIONS:** Caution with other drugs that affect hemostasis (eg, thrombolytics, anticoagulants, NSAIDs, dipyridamole). Avoid other glycoprotein IIb/IIIa inhibitors. Cerebral, pulmonary, GI hemorrhage reported with ASA and heparin.

**PREGNANCY:** Category B, caution in nursing.

## INTRON A RX
interferon alfa-2b (Schering)

**May cause or aggravate fatal or life-threatening neuropsychiatric, autoimmune, ischemic, and infectious disorders. Monitor closely with periodic clinical and laboratory evaluations.**

**THERAPEUTIC CLASS:** Biological response modifier

**INDICATIONS:** Treatment of hairy cell leukemia, malignant melanoma, follicular lymphoma, condylomata acuminata, AIDS-related Kaposi's sarcoma, chronic hepatitis C and B.

**DOSAGE:** *Adults:* >18 yrs: Hairy Cell Leukemia: 2MIU/$m^2$ IM/SQ 3x/week up to 6 months. Reduce dose by 50% or stop therapy with severe reactions. Malignant Melanoma: Initial: 20MIU/$m^2$ IV for 5 consecutive days/week for 4 weeks. Maint: 10MIU/$m^2$ SQ 3x/week for 48 weeks. Follicular Lymphoma: 5MIU SQ 3x/week up to 18 months. Condylomata Acuminata: 1MIU into lesion 3x/week alternating days for 3 weeks. Kaposi's Sarcoma: 30MIU/$m^2$ 3x/week IM/SQ. Hepatitis C: 3MIU IM/SQ 3x/week for 18-24 months. Hepatitis B: IM/SC: 5MIU qd or 10MIU IM/SQ 3x/week for 16 weeks.

*Pediatrics:* >1 yr: Hepatitis B: 3MIU/m² SQ 3x/week for 1 week, then 6MIU/m² 3x/week for total therapy of 16-24 weeks. Max: 10MIU/m² 3x/week. Reduce dose by 50% or stop therapy with severe reactions. Adjust based on WBC, granulocyte, and/or platelet counts.

**HOW SUPPLIED:** Inj: 10MIU, 18MIU, 50MIU, 10MIU/mL, 3MIU/0.2mL, 5MIU/0.2mL, 10MIU/0.2mL

**WARNINGS/PRECAUTIONS:** Do not give IM if platelet count is less than 50,000/mm³. Hepatotoxicity, retinal hemorrhages, autoimmune diseases, pulmonary infiltrates, pneumonitis, thyroid abnormalities and pneumonia reported. Avoid with immunosuppressed transplant, autoimmune disorders, decompensated liver disease. Caution with cardiac disease, coagulation disorders, severe myelosuppression, pulmonary disease, thyroid disorders, or DM prone to ketoacidosis. Avoid with pre-existing psychiatric condition; depression and suicidal behavior reported. May exacerbate psoriasis or sarcoidosis. Do not interchange brands.

**ADVERSE REACTIONS:** Fever, headache, chills, fatigue, myalgia, GI disturbances, alopecia, dyspnea, depression.

**INTERACTIONS:** Increases theophylline levels by 100%. Caution with myelosuppressive agents (eg, zidovudine). Antidiabetics and thyroid agents may need adjustments. Increased risk of hemolytic anemia when coadministered with ribavirin.

**PREGNANCY:** Category C, Category X when used with ribavirn, not for use in nursing.

## INVANZ RX

ertapenem sodium (Merck)

**THERAPEUTIC CLASS:** Carbapenem

**INDICATIONS:** Treatment of complicated intra-abdominal infections; skin and skin structure infections (SSSI), including diabetic foot infections without osteomyelitits; community acquired pneumonia (CAP); complicated urinary tract infections (UTI) including pyelonephritis; acute pelvic infections including postpartum endomyometritis, septic abortion, and post surgical gynecologic infections; prophylaxis of surgical site infection following elective colorectal surgery.

**DOSAGE:** *Adults:* Treatment: 1g IM/IV qd. Duration: Intra-Abdominal Infections: 5-14 days. SSSI: 7-14 days. CAP/UTI: 10-14 days. Pelvic Infection: 3-10 days. May administer IV for up to 14 days and IM for up to 7 days. CrCl <30mL/min/1.73m²: 500mg IM/IV qd. Hemodialysis: Give 150mg IM/IV after dialysis only if 500mg dose was given within 6 hrs prior to dialysis. Prophylaxis: 1g IV as single dose given 1 hr prior to surgical incision. *Pediatrics:* ≥13 years: 1g IM/IV qd. 3 mo-12 yrs: 15mg/kg IM/IV bid (not to exceed 1g/day). Treatment Duration: Intra-Abdominal Infections: 5-14 days. SSSI: 7-14 days. CAP/UTI: 10-14 days. Pelvic Infections: 3-10 days. May administer IV for up to 14 days and IM for up to 7 days. CrCl <30mL/min/1.73 m²: 500mg IM/IV qd.

**HOW SUPPLIED:** Inj: 1g

**CONTRAINDICATIONS:** Hypersensitivity to drugs in same class, anaphylactic reactions to beta-lactams, hypersensitivity to local anesthetics of the amide type (due to lidocaine diluent).

**WARNINGS/PRECAUTIONS:** Anaphylactic reactions reported with beta-lactam therapy; increased incidence with sensitivity to multiple allergens. Seizures, CNS adverse experiences, pseudomembranous colitis reported. Increased risk of seizures with CNS disorders and/or compromised renal function. Use lidocaine HCl as the diluent; avoid dextrose-containing diluents. Monitor renal, hepatic, hematopoietic functions during prolonged therapy. Do not inject into blood vessel.

**ADVERSE REACTIONS:** Diarrhea, infused vein complication, nausea, headache, vaginitis, edema/swelling, fever, abdominal pain, constipation, altered mental status, headache, insomnia, phlebitis/thrombophlebitis, vomiting.

**INTERACTIONS:** Decreased clearance with probenecid. Do not mix or co-infuse with other drugs.

**PREGNANCY:** Category B, caution in nursing.

## INVEGA
paliperidone (Janssen) RX

**Elderly patients with dementia-related psychosis treated with atypical antipsychotic drugs are at an increased risk of death; most appeared to be cardiovascular (eg, heart failure, sudden death) or infectious (eg, pneumonia) in nature. Paliperidone is not approved for the treatment of patients with dementia-related psychosis.**

**THERAPEUTIC CLASS:** Benzisoxazole derivative

**INDICATIONS:** Acute and maintenance treatment of schizophrenia.

**DOSAGE:** *Adults:* 6mg qd in am. Range: 3-12mg/day. Titrate: May increase by 3mg/day at intervals of >5 days. Max: 12mg/day. Swallow whole; do not chew, divide, or crush. CrCl 50 to <80mL/min: Max of 6mg/day. CrCl 10 to <50mL/min: Max of 3mg/day. Evaluate periodically for long-term use.

**HOW SUPPLIED:** Tab, Extended-Release: 3mg, 6mg, 9mg

**WARNINGS/PRECAUTIONS:** May increase QTc interval; avoid with congenital long QT syndrome and with a history of cardiac arrhythmias. Neuroleptic malignant syndrome and tardive dyskinesia may occur. Monitor for hyperglycemia; perform fasting blood glucose testing if symptoms develop or with risk factors for DM. Avoid with pre-existing severe GI narrowing. Cerebrovascular events (eg, stroke, TIA) reported in elderly with dementia-related psychosis. Not approved for the treatment of dementia-related psychosis. May induce priapism. May induce orthostatic hypotension and syncope; monitor closely in those vulnerable to hypotension. Caution with history of seizures or other conditions that may lower seizure threshold. May elevate prolactin levels. May cause esophageal dysmotility and aspiration; caution in those at risk for aspiration pneumonia. May disrupt body's ability to reduce core body temperature; caution in those who may experience conditions which may contribute to an elevation in core body temperature. Caution with known suicidal tendencies, cardiovascular disease, elderly, and renal impairment. Re-evaluate periodically.

**ADVERSE REACTIONS:** Tachycardia, nausea, akathisia, dizziness, extrapyramidal disorder, headache, somnolence, anxiety, parkinsonism, dyskinesia, hyperkinesia.

**INTERACTIONS:** Caution with other CNS drugs, alcohol. May antagonize the effect of levodopa and other dopamine agonists. Because of its potential for inducing orthostatic hypotension, additive effect may be observed when administered with other agents that have this potential. Avoid in combination with other drugs known to prolong QTc interval including Class 1A (eg, quinidine, procainamide) or Class III (eg, amiodarone, sotalol) antiarrhythmics, antipsychotic medications (eg, chlopromazine, thioridazine), antibiotics (eg, gatifloxacin, moxifloxacin), or any other class of drugs known to prolong the QTc interval.

**PREGNANCY:** Category C, not for use in nursing.

## INVERSINE
mecamylamine HCl (Targacept) RX

**THERAPEUTIC CLASS:** Ganglionic blocker

**INDICATIONS:** Management of moderately severe to severe essential hypertension and in uncomplicated cases of malignant hypertension.

**DOSAGE:** *Adults:* Initial: 2.5mg bid after meals. Titrate: Increase by 2.5mg/day at intervals of not less than 2 days. Usual: 25mg/day given tid. Give larger doses at noontime and evening. Reduce dose by 50% with thiazides.

**HOW SUPPLIED:** Tab: 2.5mg

**CONTRAINDICATIONS:** Coronary insufficiency, recent MI, uremia, glaucoma, organic pyloric stenosis, uncooperative patients, mild to moderate or labile HTN, with antibiotics or sulfonamides. Administer with great discretion in renal insufficiency.

**WARNINGS/PRECAUTIONS:** Caution with renal, cerebral, or cardiovascular dysfunction, marked cerebral or coronary insufficiency, prostatic hypertrophy, bladder neck obstruction, urethral stricture. Large doses in cerebral or renal insufficiency may produce CNS effects. Withdraw gradually and add other antihypertensives. May be potentiated by excessive heat, fever, infection, hemorrhage, pregnancy, anesthesia, surgery, vigorous exercise, other antihypertensive drugs, alcohol, salt depletion. D/C if paralytic ileus occurs.

**ADVERSE REACTIONS:** Ileus, constipation, vomiting, nausea, anorexia, dryness of mouth, syncope, postural hypotension, convulsions, tremor, interstitial pulmonary edema, urinary retention, impotence, blurred vision.



**INTERACTIONS:** Avoid with antibiotics and sulfonamides. Anesthesia, alcohol or other antihypertensives may potentiate effect.

**PREGNANCY:** Category C, not for use in nursing.

## INVIRASE RX

saquinavir mesylate (Roche Labs)

**Not interchangeable with Fortovase®.**

**THERAPEUTIC CLASS:** Protease inhibitor

**INDICATIONS:** Treatment of HIV infection in combination with other antiretrovirals.

**DOSAGE:** *Adults:* 1000mg bid with ritonavir 100mg bid. Take within 2 hrs after a full meal.
*Pediatrics:* >16 yrs: 1000mg bid with ritonavir 100mg bid. Take within 2 hrs after a full meal.

**HOW SUPPLIED:** Cap: 200mg; Tab: 500mg

**CONTRAINDICATIONS:** Concomitant amiodarone, bepridil, flecainide, propafenone, quinidine, rifampin, pimozide, terfenadine, cisapride, astemizole, triazolam, midazolam, ergot derivatives.

**WARNINGS/PRECAUTIONS:** New onset DM, exacerbation of pre-existing DM, hyperglycemia may occur. Exacerbation of chronic liver dysfunction reported with hepatitis or cirrhosis. Spontaneous bleeding may occur with hemophilia A, B. Possible redistribution or accumulation of body fat. Caution with hepatic dysfunction. Interrupt therapy if serious toxicity occurs.

**ADVERSE REACTIONS:** Diarrhea, abdominal discomfort, nausea, dyspepsia, mucosa damage, headache, paresthesia, extremity numbness, asthenia, myalgia.

**INTERACTIONS:** See contraindications. Avoid lovastatin, simvastatin, St. John's wort. Decreased plasma levels with nevirapine. Consider alternatives to CYP3A4 inducers (eg, phenobarbital, phenytoin, dexamethasone, carbamazepine). Ritonavir increases adverse effects. Risk of toxicity with substrates of CYP3A4 substrates (eg, calcium channel blockers, clindamycin, dapsone, quinidine, triazolam). Delavirdine increases plasma levels; monitor LFTs frequently.

**PREGNANCY:** Category B, not for use in nursing.

## IONAMIN

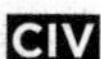

phentermine (Celltech)

**THERAPEUTIC CLASS:** Anorectic sympathomimetic amine

**INDICATIONS:** Short term adjunct for exogenous obesity if initial BMI >30kg/m² or >27kg/m² with other risk factors (eg, HTN, diabetes hyperlipidemia).

**DOSAGE:** *Adults:* 15-30mg before breakfast or 10-14 hrs before bedtime. Swallow caps whole.
*Pediatrics:* >16 yrs: 15-30mg prior to breakfast or 10-14 hrs before bedtime. Swallow caps whole.

**HOW SUPPLIED:** Cap: 15mg, 30mg

**CONTRAINDICATIONS:** Advanced arteriosclerosis, CVD, moderate to severe HTN, hyperthyroidism, glaucoma, agitated states, history of drug abuse, within 14 days of MAOI use.

**WARNINGS/PRECAUTIONS:** Primary pulmonary HTN and valvular heart disease reported. D/C if tolerance occurs. Abuse potential. Caution with mild HTN.

**ADVERSE REACTIONS:** Primary pulmonary HTN, palpitations, tachycardia, BP elevation, restlessness, dizziness, insomnia, headache, diarrhea, constipation, impotence.

**INTERACTIONS:** See Contraindications. May alter insulin requirements. Avoid with weight loss products including SSRIs. Valvular heart disease and primary pulmonary hypertension reported with fenfluramine and dexfenfluramine. May decrease effects of adrenergic neuron blocking agents.

**PREGNANCY:** Safety in pregnancy and nursing not known.

## IOPIDINE

RX

apraclonidine HCl (Alcon)

**THERAPEUTIC CLASS:** Alpha adrenergic agonist

**INDICATIONS:** (0.5%) Short-term adjunct in patients on maximally tolerated medical therapy who require additional IOP reduction. (1%) To control or prevent postsurgical IOP elevations that occur after laser surgery.

**DOSAGE:** *Adults:* (0.5%) 1-2 drops tid. Space dosing of other ophthalmic drugs by 5 minutes. (1%) 1 drop 1 hr pre-op, then 1 drop immediately post-op.

**HOW SUPPLIED:** Sol: 0.5% [5mL, 10mL], 1% [0.1mL 24[s]]

**CONTRAINDICATIONS:** Hypersensitivity to clonidine, concomitant MAOIs.

**WARNINGS/PRECAUTIONS:** Vasovagal attacks may occur during laser surgery. Monitor visual fields periodically. Monitor CV parameters with renal or hepatic dysfunction. Caution with severe cardiovascular disease, HTN, coronary insufficiency, recent MI, cerebrovascular disease, chronic renal failure, Raynaud's disease, depression, or thromboangitis obliterans. D/C if allergic-like symptoms occur. May cause dizziness or somnolence.

**ADVERSE REACTIONS:** Hyperemia, ocular pruritus, tearing, ocular discomfort, dry mouth, taste perversion, conjunctival blanching, mydriasis.

**INTERACTIONS:** (0.5%, 1%) Avoid MAOIs. (0.5%) May potentiate CNS depressants. TCAs may decrease effects. May have additive hypotensive effects with neuroleptics. Caution with β-blockers, antihypertensives, and cardiac glycosides. May potentiate the risk of insulin-induced hypoglycemia. Wait 5 minutes before administering other drops.

**PREGNANCY:** Category C, (0.5%) caution in nursing, and (1%) not for use in nursing.

## IQUIX

RX

levofloxacin (Vistakon)

**THERAPEUTIC CLASS:** Fluoroquinolone

**INDICATIONS:** Bacterial corneal ulcer.

**DOSAGE:** *Adults:* Days 1-3: 1-2 drops q30min-2h while awake and 4-6 hrs after retiring. Days 4-completion: 1-2 drops q1-4h while awake.
*Pediatrics:* ≥6 yrs: Days 1-3: 1-2 drops q30min-2h while awake and 4-6 hrs after retiring. Days 4-completion: 1-2 drops q1-4h while awake.

**HOW SUPPLIED:** Sol: 1.5% [5mL]

**WARNINGS/PRECAUTIONS:** Discontinue if hypersensitivity or superinfection occurs. Avoid contact lenses with corneal ulcer.

**ADVERSE REACTIONS:** Headache, taste disturbance.

**INTERACTIONS:** Systemic quinolone therapy increases theophylline levels, interferes with caffeine metabolism, enhances warfarin effects, and elevates SCr with cyclosporine.



**PREGNANCY:** Category C, caution in nursing.

## IRESSA

RX

gefitinib (AstraZeneca LP)

**THERAPEUTIC CLASS:** Anilinoquinazoline

**INDICATIONS:** Monotherapy for treatment of locally advanced or metastatic non-small cell lung cancer (NSCLC) after failure of both platinum-based and docetaxel chemotherapies who are benefiting or have benefited from gefitinib.

**DOSAGE:** *Adults:* 250mg qd. Tolerated Diarrhea/Skin Adverse Reactions: Provide brief (up to 14 days) therapy interruption followed by re-instatement of 250mg daily dose. Concomitant Potent CYP3A4 Inducers (eg, rifampin, phenytoin): Consider increasing dose to 500mg qd, in the absence of severe adverse reactions. Difficulty Swallowing Solids/NG tube: Dissolve tablet in half a glass of water and drink (do not crush), rinse glass with water and drink.

**HOW SUPPLIED:** Tab: 250mg

**WARNINGS/PRECAUTIONS:** Interstitial lung disease reported; interrupt treatment with acute onset or worsening of pulmonary symptoms (dyspnea, cough, fever) and investigate cause. If interstitial lung disease confirmed, d/c. May cause fetal harm. Asymptomatic increases in liver transaminases observed; consider periodic liver function testing. Hepatic dysfunction may increase gefitinib exposure. Caution with severe renal impairment.

**ADVERSE REACTIONS:** Diarrhea, rash, acne, dry skin, nausea, vomiting, pruritus, anorexia, asthenia, weight loss, eye pain, corneal erosion/ulcer.

**INTERACTIONS:** CYP3A4 inducers (eg, rifampicin, phenytoin) may decrease levels. Caution with potent CYP3A4 inhibitors (eg, ketoconazole, itraconazole); may increase levels. INR increases and/or bleeding reported with warfarin. Drugs causing significant sustained elevation in gastric pH (eg, ranitidine, cimetidine) may reduce efficacy.

**PREGNANCY:** Category D, not for use in nursing.

## IROFOL

RX

folic acid - polysaccharide iron complex (Dayton)

**THERAPEUTIC CLASS:** Iron/vitamin

**INDICATIONS:** Prevention and treatment of iron and folic acid deficiencies.

**DOSAGE:** *Adults:* 1-2 tabs or 5-10mL qd.
*Pediatrics:* >12 yrs: 1-2 tabs or 5-10mL qd.

**HOW SUPPLIED:** (Folic Acid-Polysaccharide Iron Complex) Liquid: 1mg-100mg/5mL; Tab: 1mg-150mg

**WARNINGS/PRECAUTIONS:** Not for the treatment of pernicious anemia and other megaloblastic anemias. Folic acid >0.1mg/day may obscure pernicious anemia.

**ADVERSE REACTIONS:** Gastric intolerance, allergic sensitization.

**INTERACTIONS:** Absorption may be inhibited by eggs, milk, magnesium trisilicate or antacids containing carbonates.

**PREGNANCY:** Safety in pregnancy and nursing not known.

## ISMO RX

isosorbide mononitrate (ESP Pharma)

**THERAPEUTIC CLASS:** Nitrate vasodilator

**INDICATIONS:** Prevention of angina pectoris. Not for acute attack.

**DOSAGE:** *Adults:* 20mg bid; 1st dose on awakening then 7 hrs later.

**HOW SUPPLIED:** Tab: 20mg* *scored

**WARNINGS/PRECAUTIONS:** Not for use with acute MI or CHF. Severe hypotension may occur. May aggravate angina caused by hypertrophic cardiomyopathy. Caution with volume depletion, elderly. Monitor for tolerance.

**ADVERSE REACTIONS:** Headache, dizziness, nausea, vomiting.

**INTERACTIONS:** Severe hypotension with sildenafil. Marked orthostatic hypotension with calcium channel blockers. Additive vasodilation with other vasodilators (eg, alcohol).

**PREGNANCY:** Category C, caution in nursing.

## ISOFLURANE RX

isoflurane (Various)

**THERAPEUTIC CLASS:** Inhalation anesthetic

**INDICATIONS:** For induction and maintenance of general anesthesia.

**DOSAGE:** *Adults:* Induction: 1.5-3%. Maint: 1-2.5% with concomitant nitrous oxide or an additional 0.5-1% may be required when used with oxygen.

**HOW SUPPLIED:** Liq: [100mL, 250mL]

**CONTRAINDICATIONS:** Genetic susceptibility to malignant hyperthermia.

**WARNINGS/PRECAUTIONS:** Hypotension and respiratory depression increase as anesthesia is deepened. Increased blood loss comparable to that seen with halothane reported in patients undergoing abortions. May cause a reversible rise in CSF pressure. May cause sensitivity hepatitis in patients sensitized by previous exposure to halogenated anesthetics. May cause a slight decrease in intellectual function for 2-3 days post-anesthesia. May cause small mood changes and symptoms may persist for up to 6 days post-administration. Transient increases in BSP retention, blood glucose, and serum creatinine with decrease in BUN, serum cholesterol, and alkaline phosphatase reported.

**ADVERSE REACTIONS:** Respiratory depression, hypotension, arrhythmias, shivering, nausea, vomiting, ileus.

**INTERACTIONS:** May potentiate the muscle relaxant effect of all muscle relaxants, most notably nondepolarizing muscle relaxants. Minimum alveolar concentration is reduced by concomitant administration of nitrous oxide.

**PREGNANCY:** Category C, caution in nursing.

## ISONIAZID

RX

isoniazid (Various)

**Severe, fatal hepatitis may develop. Monitor LFTs monthly.**

**OTHER BRAND NAMES:** Nydrazid (Sandoz)

**THERAPEUTIC CLASS:** Isonicotinic acid hydrazide

**INDICATIONS:** Prevention and treatment of tuberculosis (TB).

**DOSAGE:** *Adults:* Active TB: 5mg/kg single dose. Max: 300mg/day. Use with other antituberculosis agents. Prevention: 300mg qd single dose.
*Pediatrics:* Active TB: 10-20mg/kg single dose. Max: 300mg qd. Use with other antituberculosis agents. Prevention: 10mg/kg qd single dose. Max: 300mg qd.

**HOW SUPPLIED:** Inj: 100mg/mL; Syrup: 50mg/5mL; Tab: 100mg, 300mg

**CONTRAINDICATIONS:** Severe hypersensitivity reactions including drug-induced hepatitis, previous INH-associated hepatic injury, severe adverse effects to INH (eg, drug fever, chills, arthritis), acute liver disease.

**WARNINGS/PRECAUTIONS:** Discontinue if hypersensitivity occurs. Monitor closely with liver or renal disease. Take with vitamin $B_6$ in malnourished and those predisposed to neuropathy.

**ADVERSE REACTIONS:** Peripheral neuropathy, nausea, vomiting, epigastric distress, elevated serum transaminases, bilirubinemia, jaundice, hepatitis, skin eruptions, pyridoxine deficiency.

**INTERACTIONS:** Alcohol is associated with hepatitis. May increase phenytoin, theophylline, and valproate serum levels. Do not take with food. Severe acetaminophen toxicity reported. Decreases carbamazepine metabolism and AUC of ketoconazole.

**PREGNANCY:** Safety in pregnancy and nursing is not known.

## ISOPTIN SR

RX

verapamil HCl (FSC Laboratories)

**THERAPEUTIC CLASS:** Calcium channel blocker (nondihydropyridine)

**INDICATIONS:** Management of hypertension.

**DOSAGE:** *Adults:* Initial: 180mg qam. Titrate: If inadequate response, increase to 240mg qam, then 180mg bid; or 240mg qam plus 120mg qpm, then 240mg q12h. Elderly/Small Stature: Initial: 120mg qam. Take with food.

**HOW SUPPLIED:** Tab, Extended Release: 120mg, 180mg*, 240mg* *scored

**CONTRAINDICATIONS:** Severe ventricular dysfunction, hypotension, cardiogenic shock, sick sinus syndrome or 2nd- or 3rd-degree AV block (except with functioning ventricular pacemaker), A-Fib/Flutter with an accessory bypass tract.

**WARNINGS/PRECAUTIONS:** Avoid with moderate to severe cardiac failure, and ventricular dysfunction if taking a β-blocker. May cause hypotension, AV block, transient bradycardia, PR interval prolongation. Monitor LFTs periodically; hepatocellular injury reported. Give 30% of normal dose with severe hepatic dysfunction. Caution with hypertrophic cardiomyopathy, renal or hepatic dysfunction. Decrease dose in those with decreased neuromuscular transmission.

**ADVERSE REACTIONS:** Constipation, dizziness, nausea, hypotension, headache, edema, CHF, pulmonary edema, fatigue, dyspnea, bradycardia, AV block, rash, flushing.

**INTERACTIONS:** CYP3A4 inhibitors (eg, erythromycin, ritonavir) or grapefruit juice may increase levels. CYP3A4 inducers (eg, rifampin) may decrease levels. Bleeding time may increase with ASA use. May prolong effects of alcohol. Additive effects on HR, AV conduction, and contractility with β-blockers. Potentiates other antihypertensives. May increase digoxin, carbamazepine, theophylline, and cyclosporine levels. Avoid disopyramide within 48 hrs before or 24 hrs after verapamil. Additive negative inotropic effects and AV conduction prolongation with flecainide. Avoid quinidine with hypertrophic cardiomyopathy. Monitor lithium levels. Increased clearance with phenobarbital. May potentiate neuromuscular blockers; both agents may need dose reduction. Caution with inhalation anesthetics.

**PREGNANCY:** Category C, not for use in nursing.

## ISOPTO CARBACHOL

RX

carbachol (Alcon)

**THERAPEUTIC CLASS:** Cholinergic agent

**INDICATIONS:** To lower IOP in glaucoma treatment.

**DOSAGE:** *Adults:* 2 drops in eye up to tid.

**HOW SUPPLIED:** Sol: 1.5% [15mL], 3% [15mL, 30mL]

**CONTRAINDICATIONS:** Conditions where constriction is undesirable (eg, acute iritis).

**WARNINGS/PRECAUTIONS:** For topical use only. Caution with corneal abrasion; excessive penetration may produce systemic toxicity. Caution with acute cardiac failure, asthma, active peptic ulcer, hyperthyroidism, GI spasm, urinary tract obstruction, Parkinson's disease, recent MI, HTN, or hypotension. Retinal detachment reported. Caution in night driving or hazardous activity in poor light. Do not touch container tip to any surface to avoid contamination.

**ADVERSE REACTIONS:** Burning, stinging, headache, ciliary spasm, visual acuity decrease, salivation, syncope, arrhythmia, GI cramping, vomiting, asthma, hypotension, diarrhea, frequent urge to urinate, increased sweating, eye irritation.

**PREGNANCY:** Category C, caution in nursing.

## ISOSORBIDE DINITRATE

RX

isosorbide dinitrate (Various)

**OTHER BRAND NAMES:** Isordil (Biovail) - Isordil Titradose (Biovail)

**THERAPEUTIC CLASS:** Nitrate vasodilator

**INDICATIONS:** Prevention and treatment of angina pectoris.

**DOSAGE:** *Adults:* Prevention: Initial: 5-20mg bid-tid. Maint: 10-40mg bid-tid. Allow a dose-free interval of at least 14 hrs for both formulations. Elderly: Start at low end of dosing range.

**HOW SUPPLIED:** Tab: 2.5mg, 5mg*, 10mg*, 20mg*, 30mg*, 40mg* *scored

**WARNINGS/PRECAUTIONS:** Not for use with acute MI or CHF. Severe hypotension may occur. May aggravate angina caused by hypertrophic cardiomyopathy. Caution with volume depletion, hypotension, elderly. Monitor for tolerance.

**ADVERSE REACTIONS:** Headache, lightheadedness, hypotension.

**INTERACTIONS:** Severe hypotension with sildenafil. Additive vasodilation with other vasodilators (eg, alcohol).

**PREGNANCY:** Category C, caution in nursing.

## ISTALOL

RX

timolol maleate (Ista)

**THERAPEUTIC CLASS:** Nonselective beta-blocker

**INDICATIONS:** Treatment of elevated IOP in patients with open-angle glaucoma or ocular hypertension.

**DOSAGE:** *Adults:* 1 drop in affected eye qam.

**HOW SUPPLIED:** Sol: 0.5% [5mL]

**CONTRAINDICATIONS:** Bronchial asthma, history of bronchial asthma, severe COPD, sinus bradycardia, 2nd- or 3rd-degree AV block, overt cardiac failure, cardiogenic shock.

**WARNINGS/PRECAUTIONS:** Caution with cardiac failure, DM and cerebrovascular insufficiency. Severe cardiac and respiratory reactions reported. May mask symptoms of hypoglycemia and hyperthyroidism. Reinsert contact lenses 15 minutes after applying drops. Avoid with COPD, bronchospastic disease. Not for use alone in angle-closure glaucoma. May potentiate muscle weakness. Discontinue at first sign of cardiac failure. Withdrawal before surgery is controversial.

**ADVERSE REACTIONS:** Ocular burning, ocular stinging, blurred vision, cataract, conjunctival injection, headache, HTN, infection, itching, decreased visual acuity.

**INTERACTIONS:** May potentiate systemic/ophthalmic β-blockers and catecholamine-depleting drugs (eg, reserpine). Oral/IV calcium antagonists can cause AV conduction disturbances, left ventricular failure, or hypotension. Digitalis can cause additive effects in prolonging AV conduction time. Quinidine may potentiate β-blockade. May antagonize epinephrine. May exacerbate rebound HTN following clonidine withdrawal.



**PREGNANCY:** Category C, not for use in nursing.

## JANUMET RX

sitagliptin - metformin HCl (Merck)

**Lactic acidosis may occur due to metformin accumulation. If acidosis suspected, d/c drug and hospitalize patient immediately.**

**THERAPEUTIC CLASS:** Dipeptidyl peptidase-4 inhibitor/biguanide

**INDICATIONS:** Adjunct to diet and exercise to improve glycemic control in adult patients with type 2 diabetes mellitus who are not adequately controlled on metformin or sitagliptin alone or in patients already being treated with the combination of sitagliptin and metformin. Not for use in patients with type 1 diabetes or for treatment of diabetic ketoacidosis.

**DOSAGE:** *Adults:* Individualize dosing. Patient Not Controlled on Metformin Monotherapy: Initial: 100mg/day (50mg bid) of sitagliptin + metformin dose. Patient on Metformin 850mg BID: Initial: 50mg-1000mg tab bid. Patient Not Controlled on Sitagliptin Monotherapy: Initial: 50mg-500mg tab bid. Titrate: Gradual increase to 50mg-1000mg tab bid. Max: 100mg of sitagliptin and 2000mg of metformin. Take with meals

**HOW SUPPLIED:** Tab: (Sitagliptin-Metformin) 50mg-500mg, 50mg-1000mg.

**CONTRAINDICATIONS:** Renal disease (SrCR ≥1.5mg/dL [males], ≥1.4mg/dL [females], or abnormal CrCl). Acute or chronic metabolic acidosis, including diabetic ketoacidosis, with or without coma. D/C for 48 hrs in patients undergoing radiologic studies with intravascular iodinated contrast materials.

**WARNINGS/PRECAUTIONS:** Lactic acidosis reported (rare), increased risk with renal dysfunction. Assess renal function prior to initiation and during treatment; caution in elderly. Avoid in renal/hepatic impairment. May decrease vitamin $B_{12}$ levels; monitor hematologic parameters. May cause hypoglycemia in elderly, debilitated/malnourished, adrenal or pituitary insufficiency, or alcohol intoxication. D/C in hypoxic states (eg, CHF, shock, acute MI), prior to surgical procedures (due to restricted food and fluid intake), and procedures requiring use of intravascular iodinated contrast materials.

**ADVERSE REACTIONS:** (Metformin) Diarrhea, nausea/vomiting, flatulence, abdominal discomfort, indigestion, asthenia, and headache. (Sitagliptin) Nasopharyngitis.

**INTERACTIONS:** Furosemide, nifedipine, and cationic drugs (eg, digoxin, amiloride, procainamide, quinidine, quinine, rantidine, trimethoprim, vancomycin, triamterene, morphine) may increase metformin levels. Caution with concomitant medications affecting renal function or metformin disposition. Thiazides and other diuretics, corticosteroids, phenothiazines, thyroid products, estrogens, oral contraceptives, phenytoin, nicotinic acid, sympathomimetics, CCB, and isoniazid may cause hyperglycemia. Alcohol may potentiate effect of metformin on lactate metabolism; avoid excessive alcohol intake. May decrease furosemide levels. Monitor digoxin levels

**PREGNANCY:** Category B, caution in nursing.

## JANUVIA

RX

sitagliptin phosphate (Merck)

**THERAPEUTIC CLASS:** Dipeptidyl peptidase-4 inhibitor

**INDICATIONS:** Adjunct to diet and exercise to improve glycemic control in patients with type 2 diabetes mellitus. May be used as monotherapy or combination therapy with metformin or a peroxisome proliferator-activated receptor gamma agonist (eg, thiazolidinediones) when the single agent does not provide adequate glycemic control.

**DOSAGE:** *Adults:* Monotherapy/Combination Therapy: 100mg qd. CrCl ≥30 to <50mL/min: 50mg qd. CrCl: <30mL/min: 25mg qd.

**HOW SUPPLIED:** Tab: 25mg, 50mg, 100mg

**WARNINGS/PRECAUTIONS:** Assess renal function prior to initiation of treatment.

**ADVERSE REACTIONS:** Upper respiratory tract infection, nasopharyngitis, headache.

**INTERACTIONS:** May slightly increase digoxin levels; monitor appropriately.

**PREGNANCY:** Category B, caution in nursing.

## KADIAN

**CII**

morphine sulfate (Alpharma)

**Contains morphine sulfate, an opioid agonist and Schedule II controlled substance, with an abuse liability similar to other opioid analgesics. Indicated for management of moderate-to-severe pain when a continuous, around-the-clock opioid analgesic is needed for an extended period of time. Not for use as a prn analgesic. The 100mg and 200mg capsules are for use in opioid-tolerant patients only. Swallow capsules whole or sprinkle contents on apple sauce. Do not crush, chew, or dissolve pellets in capsules.**

**THERAPEUTIC CLASS:** Opioid analgesic

**INDICATIONS:** Management of moderate to severe pain.

**DOSAGE:** *Adults:* Individualize dose. Conversion from other Oral Morphine: Give 50% of daily oral morphine dose q12h or give 100% oral morphine dose q24h. Do not give more frequently than q12h. Conversion from Parenteral Morphine: Oral morphine 3x the daily parenteral morphine dose may be sufficient in chronic use settings. Conversion from Other Parenteral or Oral Opioids: Initial: Give 50% of estimated daily morphine demand and supplement with immediate-release morphine. May sprinkle contents on small amount of applesauce or in water for gastrostomy tube. Do not chew, crush or dissolve pellets. Avoid administration through NG-tube.

**HOW SUPPLIED:** Cap, Extended Release: 10mg, 20mg, 30mg, 50mg, 60mg, 80mg, 100mg, 200mg

**CONTRAINDICATIONS:** Respiratory depression in the absence of resuscitative equipment, acute or severe bronchial asthma, paralytic ileus.

**WARNINGS/PRECAUTIONS:** Respiratory depression possible; caution in COPD, cor pulmonale, decreased respiratory reserve. May obscure neurologic signs in head injuries, intracranial lesions, or a pre-existing increase in intracranial pressure. May cause severe hypotension. Avoid with GI obstruction. Caution in biliary tract disease, elderly, debilitated, renal/hepatic insufficiency, Addison's disease, myxedema, hypothyroidism, prostatic hypertrophy, urethral stricture, CNS depression, toxic psychosis, acute alcoholism, delirium tremens, and convulsive disorders. Depresses cough reflex. Decreases gastric, biliary, and pancreatic secretions. D/C 24 hrs before procedure that interrupts pain transmission pathways (eg, cordotomy); give short-acting parenteral opioid.

**ADVERSE REACTIONS:** Drowsiness, dizziness, constipation, nausea, anxiety.

**INTERACTIONS:** Increased risk of respiratory depression, hypotension, profound sedation or coma with CNS depressants (eg, sedatives, hypnotics, general anesthetics, antiemetics, phenothiazines, tranquilizers, alcohol); reduce initial dose of one or both agents by 50%. May enhance neuromuscular blocking action of skeletal relaxants. Mixed agonist/antagonist analgesics may reduce analgesic effects or precipitate withdrawal symptoms. Avoid MAOIs during or within 14 days of use. May reduce diuretic effects.

**PREGNANCY:** Category C, not for use in nursing.

## KALETRA RX

lopinavir - ritonavir (Abbott)

K

**THERAPEUTIC CLASS:** Protease inhibitor

**INDICATIONS:** Treatment of HIV infection in combination with other antiretrovirals.

**DOSAGE:** *Adults:* Therapy-Naive: 400/100mg (2 tabs or 5mL) bid or 800/200mg qd (4 tabs or 10mL). Therapy-Experienced: 400/100mg (2 tabs or 5mL) bid. Once daily administration not recommended. Concomitant Efavirenz, Nevirapine, Fosamprenavir, Nelfinavir: Therapy-Naive: 400/100mg (2 tabs) bid. Concomitant Efavirenz, Nevirapine, Amprenavir or Nelfinavir: 533/133mg (6.5mL) bid. Concomitant Efavirenz, Nevirapine, Fosamprenavir without Ritonavir, or Nelfinavir: Treatment-Experienced with Decreased Susceptibility to Lopinavir: 600/150mg (3 tabs) bid. Tablets can be taken with or without food. Oral solution must be taken with food.
Pediatrics: >12 yrs: Therapy-Naive: 400/100mg (2 tabs or 5mL) bid or 800/200mg qd (4 tabs or 10mL). Therapy-Experienced: 400/100mg (2 tabs or 5mL) bid. Once daily administration not recommended. Concomitant Efavirenz, Nevirapine, Fosamprenavir, Nelfinavir: Therapy-Naive: 400/100mg (2 tabs) bid. Concomitant Efavirenz, Nevirapine, Amprenavir or Nelfinavir: 533/133mg (6.5mL) bid. Concomitant Efavirenz, Nevirapine, Fosamprenavir without Ritonavir, or Nelfinavir: Treatment-Experienced with Decreased Susceptibility to Lopinavir: 600/150mg (3 tabs) bid. 6 months-12 yrs: >40kg: 400/100mg (2 tabs or 5 mL) bid. 15-40kg: (Sol) 10/2.5mg/kg bid. 7-<15kg: (Sol) 12/3mg/kg bid. Concomitant Efavirenz, Nevirapine, Amprenavir: >45kg: 533/133mg (2 tabs or 6.5mL) bid. 15-45kg: (Sol) 11/2.75mg/kg bid. 7-<15kg: (Sol) 13/3.25mg/kg bid. Tablets can be taken with or without food. Oral solution must be taken with food.

**HOW SUPPLIED:** Tab: (Lopinavir-Ritonavir) 200mg-50mg; Sol: (Lopinavir-Ritonavir) 80mg-20mg/mL [160mL]

**CONTRAINDICATIONS:** Concomitant drugs dependent on CYP3A or CYP2D6 for clearance (eg, flecainide, propafenone, astemizole, terfenadine, dihydroergotamine, ergonovine, ergotamine, methylergonovine, cisapride, pimozide, midazolam, triazolam).

**WARNINGS/PRECAUTIONS:** May elevate triglyceride and total cholesterol levels; monitor levels at baseline then periodically. Possible redistribution or accumulation of body fat. Discontinue if symptoms of pancreatitis occur. May exacerbate DM or cause hyperglycemia. Caution in hepatic impairment. Increased bleeding may occur with hemophilia A and B. Risk of further transaminase elevation or hepatic decompensation in patients with underlying hepatitis B or C or marked transaminase elevation prior to treatment; monitor ALT/AST more frequently during first several months of therapy.

**ADVERSE REACTIONS:** Abdominal pain, asthenia, headache, diarrhea, nausea, vomiting, dyspepsia, flatulence.

**INTERACTIONS:** See Contraindications. Avoid use with rifampin, St. John's wort; may cause loss of virologic response and resistance. Avoid use with lovastatin and simvastatin; risk of myopathy and rhabdomyolysis. May increase levels of antiarrhythmics (eg, amiodarone, bepridil, systemic lidocaine, quinidine), dihydropyridine calcium channel blockers (eg, felodipine, nifedipine, nicardipine), immunosuppressants (eg, cyclosporine, tacrolimus, rapamycin); monitoring recommended. May increase levels of trazodone; use with caution and consider lower trazodone dose. May increase levels of fluticasone; coadministration not recommended. CYP3A inducers may decrease lopinavir levels. CYP3A inhibitors may increase lopinavir levels. May increase levels of drugs primarily metabolized by CYP3A. May increase levels of amprenavir, indinavir, saquinavir. May increase levels of clarithromycin with renal impairment; reduce clarithromycin dose by 50% if CrCl 30-60mL/min and by 75% if CrCl <30mL/min. Decreased effect with dexamethasone, carbamazepine, phenobarbital, phenytoin. Monitor PT/INR with warfarin. Space dosing with didanosine; give 1 hr before or 2 hrs after lopinavir/ritonavir. Increased levels with delavirdine. Efavirenz and nevirapine may decrease levels; adjust dose. May increase levels of ketoconazole or itraconazole; avoid ketoconazole or itraconazole doses >200mg/day. May increase rifabutin levels; reduce usual rifabutin dose by 75%. Decreases atovaquone levels. Oral solution contains alcohol; disulfiram reaction may occur with disulfiram or metronidazole. May increase sildenafil, tadalafil, vardenafil levels; reduce dose of sildenafil (eg, 25mg q48h); reduce dose of tadalafil (eg, 10mg q72h); reduce dose of vardenafil (eg, 2.5mg q72h). May decrease methadone levels; may need to increase methadone dose. May decrease ethinyl estradiol levels; use alternate/additional contraception. Increased atorvastatin levels; use lowest atorvastatin dose or consider alternate HMG-

**PREGNANCY:** Category C, not for use in nursing.

## KAYEXALATE RX

sodium polystyrene sulfonate (Sanofi-Aventis)

**THERAPEUTIC CLASS:** Cation-exchange resin

**INDICATIONS:** Treatment of hyperkalemia.

**DOSAGE:** *Adults:* Oral: 15g qd-qid. Rectal Enema: 30-50g q6h.
*Pediatrics:* Oral: Use 1g per 1mEq of potassium as basis of calculation.

**HOW SUPPLIED:** Sus: 15g/60mL

**CONTRAINDICATIONS:** Hypokalemia.

**WARNINGS/PRECAUTIONS:** May be insufficient for emergency correction of hyperkalemia. Monitor for electrolyte disturbances. Caution in those intolerant to sodium increases (eg, severe CHF or HTN, or marked edema). Treat constipation with sorbital.

**ADVERSE REACTIONS:** Anorexia, nausea, vomiting, constipation, hypokalemia, hypocalcemia, sodium retention, diarrhea, (elderly) fecal impaction.

**INTERACTIONS:** Avoid nonabsorbable cation-donating antacids and laxatives; systemic alkalosis may occur (eg, magnesium hydroxide, aluminum carbonate). Hypokalemia exaggerates toxic effects of digitalis. Intestinal obstruction reported with aluminum hydroxide.

**PREGNANCY:** Category C, caution in nursing.

## K-DUR

RX

potassium chloride (Schering)

**THERAPEUTIC CLASS:** $K^+$ supplement

**INDICATIONS:** (For those unable to tolerate liquid or effervescent potassium preparations). Treatment and prevention of hypokalemia with or without metabolic alkalosis. Treatment of digitalis intoxication and hypokalemic familial periodic paralysis.

**DOSAGE:** *Adults:* Prevention: 20mEq/day. Hypokalemia: 40-100mEq/day. Divide dose if >20mEq. Take with meals and a full glass of water or liquid. Tab can be broken in half or dissolved in water.

**HOW SUPPLIED:** Tab, Extended Release: 10mEq, 20mEq* *scored

**CONTRAINDICATIONS:** Hyperkalemia, esophageal ulceration, delay in GI passage (from structural, pathological, pharmacologic causes), cardiac patients with esophageal compression due to enlarged left atrium.

**WARNINGS/PRECAUTIONS:** Potentially fatal hyperkalemia may occur. Extreme caution with acidosis, cardiac and renal disease; monitor ECG and electrolytes. Hypokalemia with metabolic acidosis should be treated with an alkalinizing potassium salt (eg, potassium bicarbonate, potassium citrate). May produce ulcerative or stenotic GI lesions.

K

**ADVERSE REACTIONS:** Hyperkalemia, GI effects (obstruction, bleeding, ulceration), nausea, vomiting, abdominal pain, flatulence, diarrhea.

**INTERACTIONS:** Risk of hyperkalemia with ACE inhibitors (eg, captopril, enalapril), $K^+$-sparing diuretics and $K^+$ supplements. Contraindicated with anticholinergic agents due to possible delay in tablet passage through GI tract.

**PREGNANCY:** Category C, safe for use in nursing.

## KEFLEX

RX

cephalexin (Advancis)

**THERAPEUTIC CLASS:** Cephalosporin (1st generation)

**INDICATIONS:** Treatment of otitis media and skin and skin structure (SSSI), bone, genitourinary tract, and respiratory tract infections.

**DOSAGE:** *Adults:* Usual: 25-50mg/kg/day in divided doses. Streptococcal Pharyngitis/SSSI/Uncomplicated Cystitis (>15 yrs): 500mg q12h. Treat cystitis for 7-14 days. Max: 4g/day.
*Pediatrics:* Usual: 25-50mg/kg/day in divided doses. Streptococcal Pharyngitis (>1 yr)/SSSI: May divide dose and give q12h. Otitis Media: 75-100mg/kg/day in divided doses. Administer for ≥10 days in β-hemolytic streptococcal infections.

**HOW SUPPLIED:** Cap: 250mg, 333mg, 500mg, 750mg; Sus: 125mg/5ml, 250mg/5ml [100ml, 200ml]

**WARNINGS/PRECAUTIONS:** Caution with markedly impaired renal function, history of GI disease. Cross-sensitivity with cephalosporins and penicillins. Pseudomembranous colitis reported. False (+) direct Coombs' tests reported. False (+) for urine glucose with Benedict's, Fehling's solution, and Clinitest tablets.

**ADVERSE REACTIONS:** Diarrhea, allergic reactions, dyspepsia, gastritis, abdominal pain, superinfection (prolonged use).

**INTERACTIONS:** Probenecid inhibits excretion.

**PREGNANCY:** Category B, caution in nursing.

## KENALOG
triamcinolone acetonide (Apothecon)

RX

**THERAPEUTIC CLASS:** Corticosteroid

**INDICATIONS:** Corticosteroid responsive dermatoses.

**DOSAGE:** *Adults:* (Cre, Lot, Oint) Apply 0.025% bid-qid. Apply 0.1% or 0.5% bid-tid. (Spray) Apply tid-qid. May use occlusive dressings for psoriasis or recalcitrant conditions. Discontinue dressings if infection develops.

**HOW SUPPLIED:** Cre: 0.1% [15g, 60g, 80g], 0.5% [20g]; Lot: 0.025%, 0.1% [60mL]; Oint: 0.1% [15g, 60g]; Spray: 0.147mg/g [63g]

**WARNINGS/PRECAUTIONS:** May produce reversible HPA axis suppression, manifestations of Cushing's syndrome, hyperglycemia, and glucosuria. Discontinue if irritation occurs. Pediatrics may be more susceptible to systemic toxicity. Monitor for HPA suppression if apply to large surface areas or under occlusive dressings. Avoid eyes.

**ADVERSE REACTIONS:** Burning, itching, irritation, dryness, folliculitis, hypertrichosis, acneiform eruptions, hypopigmentation, perioral dermatitis, allergic contact dermatitis.

**PREGNANCY:** Category C, caution in nursing.

## KEPIVANCE
palifermin (Amgen)

RX



**THERAPEUTIC CLASS:** Keratinocyte growth factor

**INDICATIONS:** Decrease the incidence and duration of severe oral mucositis in patients with hematologic malignancies receiving myelotoxic therapy requiring hematopoietic stem cell support.

**DOSAGE:** *Adults:* 60mcg/kg/day IV bolus 3 consecutive days before and after myelotoxic therapy.

**HOW SUPPLIED:** Inj: 6.25mg

**CONTRAINDICATIONS:** Known hypersensitivity to *E.coli*-derived proteins, palifermin, or any other component of the product.

**WARNINGS/PRECAUTIONS:** Potential for stimulation of tumor growth. Safety and efficacy have not been established in patients with non-hematologic malignancies.

**ADVERSE REACTIONS:** Rash, erythema, edema, pruritus, dysesthesia, tongue discoloration, tongue thickening, alteration of taste, pain arthralgias.

**INTERACTIONS:** Do not administer 24 hrs before, during infusion, or 24 hrs after administration of myelotoxic chemotherapy due to risk of increased severity and duration of oral mucositis.

**PREGNANCY:** Category C, caution in nursing.

## KEPPRA
levetiracetam (UCB Pharma)

RX

**THERAPEUTIC CLASS:** Pyrrolidine derivative

**INDICATIONS:** (PO) Adjunctive therapy for partial onset seizures in adults and children ≥4 yrs of age. Adjunctive therapy in the treatment of myoclonic seizures in adults and children ≥12 yrs with juvenile myoclonic epilepsy (JME). Adjunctive therapy in the treatment of primary generalized tonic-clonic (PGTC) seizures in adults and children ≥6 yrs with idiopathic generalized epilepsy. (Inj) Adjunctive therapy for partial onset seizures in adults and as alternative when oral administration is temporarily not feasible.

**DOSAGE:** *Adults:* Inj/PO: Initial: 500mg bid. Titrate: Increase by 1000mg/day every 2 weeks. Max: 3000mg/day. Inj: Replacement Therapy: Initial total daily

dosage and frequency should equal total daily dosage and frequency of oral therapy. Dilute injection in 100mL of compatible diluent and give as 15-min IV infusion. CrCl 50-80mL/min: 500-1000mg q12h. CrCl 30-50mL/min: 250-750mg q12h. CrCl <30mL/min: 250-500mg q12h. ESRD with Dialysis: 500-1000mg q24h; supplemental 250-500mg after dialysis.
*Pediatrics:* PO: Partial Onset Seizures/PGTC: ≥16 yrs or JME: ≥ 12 yrs: Initial: 500mg bid. Titrate: Increase by 1000mg/day every 2 weeks. Max: 3000mg/day. Partial Onset Seizures: 4 to <16 yrs or PGTC: 6-16 yrs: Initial: 10mg/kg bid: Titrate: Increase by 20mg/kg/day every 2 weeks. Max: 60mg/kg/day. Inj: Partial Onset Seizures: Initial: 500mg bid. Titrate: Increase by 1000mg/day every 2 weeks. Max: 3000mg/day. Replacement Therapy: Initial total daily dosage and frequency should equal total daily dosage and frequency of oral therapy. Dilute injection in 100mL of compatible diluent and give as 15-min IV infusion. CrCl 50-80mL/min: 500-1000mg q12h. CrCl 30-50mL/min: 250-750mg q12h. CrCl <30mL/min: 250-500mg q12h. ESRD with Dialysis: 500-1000mg q24h; supplemental 250-500mg after dialysis.

**HOW SUPPLIED:** Inj: 500mg/5mL; Sol: 100mg/mL; Tab: 250mg*, 500mg*, 750mg*, 1000mg* *scored

**WARNINGS/PRECAUTIONS:** Associated with somnolence, fatigue, coordination difficulties, and behavioral abnormalities. Avoid abrupt withdrawal. Hematologic abnormalities reported. Caution in renal dysfunction.

**ADVERSE REACTIONS:** Somnolence, asthenia, headache, infection, pain, anorexia, dizziness, nervousness, vertigo, ataxia, vertigo, pharyngitis, rhinitis, irritability.



**PREGNANCY:** Category C, caution in nursing.

## KETAMINE

CIII

ketamine HCl (Various)

**THERAPEUTIC CLASS:** Nonbarbiturate anesthetic

**INDICATIONS:** Sole anesthetic agent for diagnostic and surgical procedures that do not require skeletal muscle relaxation. Induction of anesthesia prior to the administration of other general anesthetic agents. To supplement low-potency agents (eg, nitrous oxide).

**DOSAGE:** *Adults:* Initial: IV: 1-4.5mg/kg. Infuse slowly over 60 seconds. May administer with 2-5mg doses of diazepam over 60 seconds. IM: 6.5-13mg/kg. Maint: Adjust according to anesthetic needs. May increase in increments of one-half to full induction dose.
*Pediatrics:* Initial: IV: 1-4.5mg/kg. Infuse slowly over 60 seconds. IM: 6.5-13mg/kg. Maint: Adjust according to anesthetic needs. May increase in increments of one-half to full induction dose.

**HOW SUPPLIED:** Inj: 50mg/mL

**CONTRAINDICATIONS:** Patients in whom a significant elevation in blood pressure would constitute a serious hazard.

**WARNINGS/PRECAUTIONS:** Monitor cardiac function in patients with hypertension or cardiac dysfunction. Postoperative confusional states may occur during recovery. Respiratory depression may occur; maintain airway and respiration. Do not use alone in pharynx, larynx, or bronchial tree procedures. Use with caution in chronic alcoholics and acutely intoxicated patients. May increase cerebrospinal fluid pressure, use with extreme caution in patients with preanesthetic cerebrospinal fluid pressure. Use with agent that obtunds visceral pain when surgical procedure involving visceral pain.

**ADVERSE REACTIONS:** Nausea, vomiting, anorexia, elevated blood pressure and pulse, hypotension, bradycardia, arrhythmia, respiratory depression, apnea, airway obstruction, diplopia, nystagmus, slight elevation of IOP, enhanced skeletal muscle tone.

**INTERACTIONS:** Prolonged recovery time with barbiturates and/or narcotics.

**PREGNANCY:** Not recommended with pregnancy, use in nursing unknown.

## KETEK

telithromycin (Sanofi-Aventis)

RX

**Contraindicated with myasthenia gravis.**

**THERAPEUTIC CLASS:** Ketolide antibiotic

**INDICATIONS:** Treatment of mild to moderate community-acquired pneumonia (CAP).

**DOSAGE:** *Adults:* 800mg qd for 7-10 days. Severe Renal Impairment (CrCl <30mL/min): 600mg qd. Hemodialysis: Give after dialysis session on dialysis days. Severe Renal Impairment (CrCl <30mL/min) with Hepatic Impairment: 400mg qd.

**HOW SUPPLIED:** Tab: 300mg [20s], 400mg [60s, Ketek Pak, 100s]

**CONTRAINDICATIONS:** Myasthenia gravis. History of hepatitis And/or jaundice associated with the use of telithromycin or any macrolide antibiotic. Hypersensitivity to macrolide antibiotics, concomitant use with cisapride or pimozide.

**WARNINGS/PRECAUTIONS:** Acute hepatic failure and severe liver injury, including fulminant hepatitis And hepatic necrosis, reported. Discontinue if hepatitis occurs. Visual disturbances and loss of consciousness reported, minimize hazardous activities such as driving and operating heavy machinery. Pseudomembranous colitis, hepatic dysfunction reported. May prolong QTc interval; avoid with congenital prolongation, ongoing proarrhythmic conditions (eg, uncorrected hypokalemia or hypomagnesemia), significant bradycardia.

**ADVERSE REACTIONS:** Diarrhea, nausea, headache, dizziness, loss of consciousness, and vomiting.

**INTERACTIONS:** Increases levels of drugs metabolized by the CYP450 system (eg, carbamazepine, cyclosporine, tacrolimus, sirolimus, hexobarbital, phenytoin, triazolam, metoprolol) especially CYP3A4. Avoid cisapride, pimozide, simvastatin, lovastatin, atorvastatin, rifampin, ergot alkaloid derivatives, Class IA (eg, quinidine, procainamide) or Class III (eg, dofetilide) antiarrhythmics. Increased levels with itraconazole, ketoconazole. Monitor with midazolam, digoxin. Decreased effects with CYP3A4 inducers (eg, phenytoin, carbamazepine, phenobarbital). Decreases levels of sotalol. Space dosing of theophylline by 1 hr to reduce GI effects. Concomitant administration with oral anticoagulants may potentiate effects of the oral anticoagulants.

**PREGNANCY:** Category C, caution in nursing.

## KETOCONAZOLE TOPICAL

ketoconazole (Various)

RX

**THERAPEUTIC CLASS:** Azole antifungal

**INDICATIONS:** (Cre) T.corporis, t.cruris, t.pedis, t.versicolor, cutaneous candidiasis, seborrheic dermatitis. (Shampoo) T.versicolor.

**DOSAGE:** *Adults:* (Cre) Cutaneous candidiasis/T.corporis/T.cruris/T.versicolor: Apply qd for 2 weeks. T.pedis: Apply qd for 6 weeks. Seborrheic Dermatitis: Apply bid for up to 4 weeks. Re-evaluate if no improvement after treatment period. (Shampoo) Apply to damp skin and lather. Rinse with water after 5 minutes. One application should be sufficient.

**HOW SUPPLIED:** Cre: 2% [15g, 30g, 60g]; Shampoo: 2% [120mL]

**WARNINGS/PRECAUTIONS:** Cream contains sulfites. Shampoo may remove curl from permanently waved hair. Avoid eyes.

**ADVERSE REACTIONS:** (Cre) Irritation, pruritus, stinging. (Shampoo) Abnormal hair texture, scalp pustules, mild skin dryness, pruritus, increase in normal hair loss, oily or dry scalp and hair.

**PREGNANCY:** Category C, (cre) not for use in nursing; (shampoo) caution in nursing.

## KETOPROFEN RX

ketoprofen (Various)

**THERAPEUTIC CLASS:** NSAID (propionic acid derivative)

**INDICATIONS:** Management of osteoarthritis (OA), rheumatoid arthritis (RA), pain and primary dysmenorrhea.

**DOSAGE:** *Adults:* OA/RA: 75mg tid or 50mg qid. Max: 300mg/day. Pain/Dysmenorrhea: 25-50mg q6-8h. Max: 300mg. Small Patients/Debilitated/Elderly/Hepatic or Renal Dysfunction: Reduce dose.

**HOW SUPPLIED:** Cap: 25mg, 50mg, 75mg

**CONTRAINDICATIONS:** ASA or other NSAID allergy that precipitates acute asthmatic attack, urticaria or allergic-type reactions.

**WARNINGS/PRECAUTIONS:** Risk of GI ulceration, bleeding, and perforation. Caution with heart failure, HTN, fluid retention, liver or renal dysfunction, hypoalbuminemia, elderly.

**ADVERSE REACTIONS:** Dyspepsia, nausea, abdominal pain, diarrhea, constipation, flatulence, headache, renal dysfunction, LFT abnormalities, CNS effects.

K

**INTERACTIONS:** Avoid aspirin and probenecid. Renal toxicity potentiated by diuretics. Monitor anticoagulants. Increases levels of methotrexate and lithium.

**PREGNANCY:** Category B, not for use in nursing.

## KETOROLAC RX

ketorolac tromethamine (Various)

**For short-term use only (≤5 days). Contraindicated with peptic ulcer disease, GI bleeding/perforation, perioperative pain in coronary artery bypass graft (CABG) surgery, advanced renal impairment, risk of renal failure due to volume depletion, CV bleeding, hemorrhagic diathesis, incomplete hemostasis, high-risk of bleeding, intraoperatively when hemostasis is critical, intrathecal/epidural use, L&D, nursing, and with ASA, NSAIDs, or probenecid. Caution greater risk of GI events with elderly patients. NSAIDs may cause an increased risk of CV thrombotic events (MI, stroke).**

**OTHER BRAND NAMES:** Toradol (Roche Labs)

**THERAPEUTIC CLASS:** NSAID (pyrrolo-pyrrole derivative)

**INDICATIONS:** Short-term (≤5 days) management of moderately severe, acute pain.

**DOSAGE:** *Adults:* >16 to <65 yrs: Single-Dose: 60mg IM or 30mg IV. Multiple-Dose: 30mg IM/IV q6h. Max: 120mg/day. Transition from IM/IV to PO: 20mg PO single dose, then 10mg PO q4-6h. Max: 40mg/24 hrs. ≥65 yrs/Renal Impairment/<50kg: Single-Dose: 30mg IM or 15mg IV. Multiple-Dose: 15mg IM/IV q6h. Max: 60mg/day. Transition from IM/IV to PO: 10mg PO q4-6h. Max: 40mg/24 hrs.

*Pediatrics:* 2-16 yrs: Single-Dose: IM: 1mg/kg. Max: 30mg. IV: 0.5mg/kg. Max: 15mg.

**HOW SUPPLIED:** Inj: 15mg/mL, 30mg/mL; Tab: 10mg

**CONTRAINDICATIONS:** Active or history of peptic ulcer, GI bleeding, perioperative pain in CABG surgery, advanced renal impairment or risk of renal failure due to volume depletion, labor/delivery, nursing mothers, ASA or NSAID allergy, preoperatively or intraoperatively when hemostasis is critical, cerebrovascular bleeding, hemorrhagic diathesis, incomplete hemostasis, if high risk of bleeding, neuraxial (epidural or intrathecal) administration, and concomitant ASA, NSAIDs, probenecid, or pentoxifylline.

**WARNINGS/PRECAUTIONS:** Do not exceed 5 days of therapy. Risk of GI ulcerations, bleeding and perforation. Caution with renal or liver dysfunction, dehydration, HTN, congestive heart failure, coagulation disorders, debilitated and elderly, pre-existing asthma. Preoperative use prolongs bleeding. CV thrombotic events, fluid retention, edema, NaCl retention, oliguria, anaphylactic reactions, elevated BUN and serum creatinine, anemia reported. Correct hypovolemia before therapy.

**ADVERSE REACTIONS:** Nausea, dyspepsia, GI pain, diarrhea, edema, headache, drowsiness, dizziness.

**INTERACTIONS:** May increase risk of bleeding with anticoagulants. May reduce diuretic response to furosemide. Increased serum levels with salicylates. Avoid ASA, NSAIDs and probenecid. Increased lithium and methotrexate levels. May increase risk of renal impairment with ACE inhibitors. May increase seizures with phenytoin and carbamazepine. Hallucinations reported with fluoxetine, thiothixene and alprazolam. Do not mix in the same syringe as morphine. May have adverse effects with nondepolarizing muscle relaxants.

**PREGNANCY:** Category C, not for use in nursing.

## KINERET — RX

anakinra (Amgen)

**THERAPEUTIC CLASS:** Interleukin-1 receptor antagonist

**INDICATIONS:** As sole or adjunct therapy with DMARDs (except TNF blockers) to reduce the signs/symptoms and slow the progression of moderate to severe rheumatoid arthritis unresponsive to one or more DMARDs.

**DOSAGE:** *Adults:* >18 yrs: 100mg SQ qd at approximately the same time every day. CrCl <30mL/min: 100mg SQ qod.

**HOW SUPPLIED:** Inj: 100mg/0.67mL

**WARNINGS/PRECAUTIONS:** Increased incidence of serious infections alone and with coadministration with etanercept. Discontinue if serious infection or hypersensitivity reaction occurs. Do not initiate with active infection. Obtain neutrophil count before therapy, monthly for 3 months, quarterly thereafter for up to one year.

**ADVERSE REACTIONS:** Injection site reactions, headache, nausea, diarrhea, infections, abdominal pain, arthralgia, flu-like symptoms.

**INTERACTIONS:** Neutropenia and higher rate of infections reported with etanercept. Vaccines may be ineffective; avoid live vaccines. Concurrent therapy with etanercept is not recommended.

**PREGNANCY:** Category B, caution in nursing.

## KLARON — RX

sulfacetamide sodium (Dermik)

**THERAPEUTIC CLASS:** Sulfonamide

**INDICATIONS:** Topical treatment of acne vulgaris.

**DOSAGE:** *Adults:* Apply thin film bid.
*Pediatrics:* >12 yrs: Apply thin film bid.

**HOW SUPPLIED:** Lot: 10% [118mL]

**WARNINGS/PRECAUTIONS:** D/C if irritation, rash, or hypersensitivity reaction occurs. Avoid eyes. Contains sulfites. Caution with denuded or abraded skin.

**ADVERSE REACTIONS:** Erythema, itching, edema, stinging, burning, local irritation.

**PREGNANCY:** Category C, caution in nursing.

## KLONOPIN

CIV

clonazepam (Roche Labs)

**OTHER BRAND NAMES:** Klonopin Wafers (Roche Labs)

**THERAPEUTIC CLASS:** Benzodiazepine

**INDICATIONS:** Adjunct or monotherapy in Lennox-Gastaut syndrome, akinetic and myoclonic seizures. Absence seizures refractory to succinimides. Panic disorder with or without agoraphobia.

**DOSAGE:** *Adults:* Seizure Disorders: Initial: Not to exceed 1.5mg/day given tid. Titrate: May increase by 0.5-1mg every 3 days. Max: 20mg qd. Panic Disorder: Initial: 0.25mg bid. Titrate: Increase to 1mg/day after 3 days, then may increase by 0.125-0.25mg bid every 3 days. Max: 4mg/day. Wafer: Dissolve in mouth with or without water.
*Pediatrics:* <10 yrs or 30kg: Seizure Disorders: Initial: 0.01-0.03mg/kg/day up to 0.05mg/kg/day given bid-tid. Titrate: Increase by no more than 0.25-0.5mg every 3 days. Maint: 0.1-0.2mg/kg/day given tid. Wafer: Dissolve in mouth with or without water.

**HOW SUPPLIED:** Tab: 0.5mg*, 1mg, 2mg; Tab, Disintegrating (Wafer): 0.125mg, 0.25mg, 0.5mg, 1mg, 2mg *scored

**CONTRAINDICATIONS:** Significant liver disease, acute narrow angle glaucoma, untreated open angle glaucoma.

K

**WARNINGS/PRECAUTIONS:** May increase incidence of generalized tonic-clonic seizures. Monitor blood counts and LFT's periodically with long-term therapy. Caution with renal dysfunction, chronic respiratory depression. Increased fetal risks during pregnancy. Avoid abrupt withdrawal. Hypersalivation reported.

**ADVERSE REACTIONS:** Somnolence, depression, ataxia, CNS depression, upper respiratory tract infection, fatigue, dizziness, sinusitis, colpitis.

**INTERACTIONS:** Decreased serum levels with CYP450 inducers (eg, phenytoin, carbamazepine, phenobarbital). Caution with CYP3A inhibitors (eg, oral antifungals). Alcohol, narcotics, barbiturates, nonbarbiturate hypnotics, antianxiety agents, phenothiazines, thioxanthene and butyrophenone antipsychotics, MAOIs, TCAs and other anticonvulsant drugs potentiate CNS-depressant effects.

**PREGNANCY:** Category D, not for use in nursing.

## KLOR-CON M

RX

potassium chloride (Upsher-Smith)

**OTHER BRAND NAMES:** Klor-Con (Upsher-Smith)

**THERAPEUTIC CLASS:** $K^+$ supplement

**INDICATIONS:** (For those unable to tolerate liquid or effervescent potassium preparations). Treatment of hypokalemia with or without metabolic alkalosis, in digitalis intoxication and with hypokalemic familial periodic paralysis. Prevention of hypokalemia in patients at risk (eg, digitalized, cardiac arrhythmias).

**DOSAGE:** *Adults:* Prevention: 20mEq/day. Hypokalemia: 40-100mEq/day. Divide dose if >20mEq. Take with meals and fluids. Swallow tabs whole; may break Klor-Con M in half or mix with 4 ounces of water.

**HOW SUPPLIED:** (Klor-Con M) Tab, Extended Release: 10mEq, 15mEq, 20mEq; (Klor-Con) Pow: 20mEq, 25mEq; Tab, Extended Release: 8mEq, 10mEq

**CONTRAINDICATIONS:** Hyperkalemia, esophageal ulceration, delay in GI passage (from structural, pathological, pharmacologic causes), cardiac patients with esophageal compression due to enlarged left atrium.

**WARNINGS/PRECAUTIONS:** Potentially fatal hyperkalemia may occur. Extreme caution with acidosis, cardiac and renal disease; monitor ECG and electrolytes. Hypokalemia with metabolic acidosis should be treated with an alkalinizing potassium salt (eg, potassium bicarbonate, potassium citrate). May produce ulcerative or stenotic GI lesions.

**ADVERSE REACTIONS:** Hyperkalemia, GI effects (obstruction, bleeding, ulceration), nausea, vomiting, abdominal pain, flatulence, diarrhea.

**INTERACTIONS:** Risk of hyperkalemia with ACE inhibitors (eg, captopril, enalapril), $K^+$-sparing diuretics, and $K^+$ supplements. Contraindicated with anticholinergics or other agents that decrease GI motility.

**PREGNANCY:** Category C, safe for use in nursing.

## K-LYTE

RX

potassium citrate - potassium bicarbonate (Bristol-Myers Squibb)

**OTHER BRAND NAMES:** K-Lyte DS (Bristol-Myers Squibb)

**THERAPEUTIC CLASS:** $K^+$ Supplement

**INDICATIONS:** For treatment or prophylaxis of potassium deficiency. Treatment of digitalis intoxication.

**DOSAGE:** *Adults:* Usual: (K-Lyte) Dissolve 25meq in 3-4 oz cold/ice water and drink bid-qid. (K-Lyte DS) Dissolve 50meq in 6-8 oz cold/ice water and drink qd-bid. Dose according to patient's requirements. Take with food.

**HOW SUPPLIED:** Tab, Effervescent: (K-Lyte) 25meq, (K-Lyte DS) 50meq

**CONTRAINDICATIONS:** Hyperkalemia.

**WARNINGS/PRECAUTIONS:** Risk of hyperkalemia and cardiac arrest with impaired $K^+$ excretion (eg, chronic renal disease). Potentially fatal hyperkalemia may occur rapidly and may be asymptomatic. Monitor serum $K^+$ levels carefully with condtions that impair $K^+$ excretion. Monitor acid-base balance, serum electrolytes, ECG, and clinical status when treating $K^+$ depletion.

**ADVERSE REACTIONS:** Nausea, vomiting, diarrhea, abdominal discomfort.

**INTERACTIONS:** Risk of hyperkalemia with $K^+$ sparing diuretics, and $K^+$-containing salt substitutes.

**PREGNANCY:** Category C, not for use in nursing.

## K-LYTE/CL

RX

potassium chloride (Bristol-Myers Squibb)

**OTHER BRAND NAMES:** K-Lyte/CL 50 (Bristol-Myers Squibb)

**THERAPEUTIC CLASS:** $K^+$ Supplement

**INDICATIONS:** Treatment or prophylaxis of potassium deficiency. Management of hypokalemia with metabolic alkalosis and hypochloremia. Treatment of digitalis intoxication.

**DOSAGE:** *Adults:* Usual: (K-Lyte/CL) Dissolve 25meq in 3-4 oz cold/ice water and drink bid-qid. (K-Lyte/CL 50) Dissolve 50meq in 6-8 oz cold/ice water and drink qd-bid. Dose according to patient's requirements. Take with food.

**HOW SUPPLIED:** Tab, Effervescent: (K-Lyte/CL) 25meq, (K-Lyte/CL 50) 50meq

**CONTRAINDICATIONS:** Hyperkalemia.

**WARNINGS/PRECAUTIONS:** Risk of hyperkalemia and cardiac arrest with impaired $K^+$ excretion (eg, chronic renal disease). Potentially fatal hyperkalemia may occur rapidly and may be asymptomatic. Monitor serum $K^+$ levels carefully with condtions that impair $K^+$ excretion. Monitor acid-base balance, serum electrolytes, ECG, and clinical status when treating $K^+$ depletion.

**ADVERSE REACTIONS:** Nausea, vomiting, diarrhea, abdominal discomfort.

**INTERACTIONS:** Risk of hyperkalemia with $K^+$ sparing diuretics, and $K^+$-containing salt substitutes.

**PREGNANCY:** Category C, not for use in nursing.

## KOGENATE FS

RX

antihemophilic factor (Bayer)

**THERAPEUTIC CLASS:** Antihemophilic Factor (Recombinant)

**INDICATIONS:** Treatment of hemophilia A in which there is a deficiency of activity of clotting factor FVIII.

**DOSAGE:** *Adults:* Minor hemorrhage: 10-20 IU/kg IV; repeat if evidence of further bleeding. Moderate to major hemorrhage/surgery (minor): 15-30 IU/kg IV; repeat one dose at 12-24 hrs if needed. Major to life-threatening hemorrhage/fractures/head trauma: Initial: 40-50 IU/kg IV; repeat dose 20-25 IU/kg IV q 8-12 hrs. Surgery (major): Preoperative dose: 50 IU/kg IV (verify 100% FVIII activity prior to surgery); repeat as necessary after 6-12 hrs initially, and for 10-14 days until healing is complete.
*Pediatrics:* Minor hemorrhage: 10-20 IU/kg IV; repeat if evidence of further bleeding. Moderate to major hemorrhage/surgery (minor): 15-30 IU/kg IV; repeat one dose at 12-24 hrs if needed. Major to life-threatening hemorrhage/fractures/head trauma: Initial: 40-50 IU/kg IV; repeat dose 20-25 IU/kg IV q 8-12 hrs. Surgery (major): Preoperative dose: 50 IU/kg IV (verify 100% FVIII activity prior to surgery); repeat as necessary after 6-12 hrs initially, and for 10-14 days until healing is complete.

**HOW SUPPLIED:** Inj: 250 IU, 500 IU, 1000 IU



**CONTRAINDICATIONS:** Known hypersensitivity to mouse or hamster protein.

**WARNINGS/PRECAUTIONS:** Development of circulating neutralizing antibodies to FVIII may occur; monitor by appropriate clinical observation and laboratory tests. Hypotension, urticaria, and chest tightness in association with hypersensitivity reported.

**ADVERSE REACTIONS:** Local injection site reactions, dizziness, rash, unusual taste, mild increase in BP, pruritus, depersonalization, nausea, rhinitis.

**PREGNANCY:** Category C, safety not known in nursing.

## KRISTALOSE

RX

lactulose (Cumberland)

**THERAPEUTIC CLASS:** Osmotic laxative

**INDICATIONS:** Treatment of constipation.

**DOSAGE:** *Adults:* 10-20g/day. Max 40g/day. Dissolve packet contents in 4oz of water.

**HOW SUPPLIED:** Powder (crystals for suspension): 10g/packet, 20g/packet [1s, 30s]

**CONTRAINDICATIONS:** Patients who require a low galactose diet.

**WARNINGS/PRECAUTIONS:** Caution in DM due to galactose and lactose content. Monitor electrolytes periodically in elderly or debilitated if used for >6 months. Potential for explosive reaction with electrocautery procedures during proctoscopy or colonoscopy.

**ADVERSE REACTIONS:** Flatulence, intestinal cramps, diarrhea, nausea, vomiting.

**INTERACTIONS:** Nonabsorbable antacids may decrease effects.

**PREGNANCY:** Category B, caution in nursing.

## K-TAB
RX

potassium chloride (Abbott)

**OTHER BRAND NAMES:** Klotrix (Apothecon)

**THERAPEUTIC CLASS:** $K^+$ supplement

**INDICATIONS:** (For those unable to tolerate liquid or effervescent potassium preparations). Treatment and prevention of hypokalemia with or without metabolic alkalosis. Treatment of digitalis intoxication and hypokalemic familial periodic paralysis.

**DOSAGE:** *Adults:* Prevention: 20mEq/day. Hypokalemia: 40-100mEq/day. Divide dose if >20mEq. Take with meals and full glass of water or liquid. Do not cut, crush or chew tab.

**HOW SUPPLIED:** Tab, Extended Release: 10mEq

**CONTRAINDICATIONS:** Hyperkalemia, esophageal ulceration, delay in GI passage (from structural, pathological, pharmacologic causes), cardiac patients with esophageal compression due to enlarged left atrium.

**WARNINGS/PRECAUTIONS:** Potentially fatal hyperkalemia may occur. Extreme caution with acidosis, cardiac and renal disease; monitor ECG and electrolytes. Hypokalemia with metabolic acidosis should be treated with an alkalinizing potassium salt (eg, potassium bicarbonate, potassium citrate). May produce ulcerative or stenotic GI lesions. Use with caution in elderly due to decreased renal function, start dose at low end of dosing range.

**ADVERSE REACTIONS:** Hyperkalemia, GI effects (obstruction, bleeding, ulceration), nausea, vomiting, abdominal pain, flatulence, diarrhea.

**INTERACTIONS:** Risk of hyperkalemia with ACE inhibitors (eg, captopril, enalapril), potassium-sparing diuretics and potassium supplements. Contraindicated with anticholinergic agents due to possible delay in tablet passage through GI tract.

**PREGNANCY:** Category C, safe for use in nursing.



## KYTRIL
RX

granisetron HCl (Roche Labs)

**THERAPEUTIC CLASS:** 5-$HT_3$ antagonist

**INDICATIONS:** (Inj, Sol, Tab) Prevention of nausea and vomiting associated with chemotherapy. (Sol, Tab) Prevention of nausea and vomiting associated with radiation. (Inj) Prevention and treatment of post-op nausea and vomiting.

**DOSAGE:** *Adults:* Prevention with Chemotherapy: (PO) 2mg qd up to 1 hr before chemotherapy or 1mg bid (up to 1 hr before chemotherapy and 12 hrs later). (IV) 10mcg/kg within 30 minutes before chemotherapy. Prevention with Radiation: (PO) 2mg within 1 hr of radiation. Post-Op Prevention: (IV) Administer 1 mg over 30 seconds before induction of anesthesia or immediately before anesthesia reversal. Post-Op Treatment: (IV) Administer 1mg over 30 seconds.
*Pediatrics:* 2-16 yrs: Prevention with Chemotherapy: 10mcg/kg IV within 30 minutes before chemotherapy.

**HOW SUPPLIED:** Inj: 0.1mg/ml, 1mg/mL; Sol: 2mg/10mL; Tab: 1mg

**WARNINGS/PRECAUTIONS:** (Inj) Does not stimulate gastric or intestinal peristalsis. Do not use instead of nasogastric suction. May mask progressive ileus or gastric distension.

**ADVERSE REACTIONS:** Headache, asthenia, somnolence, diarrhea, constipation, abdominal pain, dizziness, insomnia, decreased appetite, fever.

**INTERACTIONS:** Hepatic CYP450 enzyme inducers or inhibitors may alter clearance.

**PREGNANCY:** Category B, caution in nursing.

## LABETALOL HCL

RX

labetalol HCl (Various)

**THERAPEUTIC CLASS:** Nonselective beta-blocker/alpha$_1$ blocker

**INDICATIONS:** (Tab) Management of hypertension. (Inj) Management of severe hypertension.

**DOSAGE:** *Adults:* (Tab) HTN: Initial: 100mg bid. Titrate: 100mg bid every 2-3 days. Maint: 200-400mg bid. Severe HTN: 1200-2400mg/day given bid-tid. Increments should not exceed 200mg bid for titration. (Inj) Severe HTN: Administer in supine position. Repeated IV Infusion: Initial: 20mg over 2 minutes. Titrate: Give additional 40-80mg at 10 minute intervals if needed. Max: 300mg. Slow Continuous Infusion: 200mg at a rate of 2mg/min. May adjust dose according to BP. Switch to tabs when BP is stable while in hospital. Initial: 200mg, then 200-400mg 6-12 hrs later on Day 1. Titrate: May increase at 1 day interval.

**HOW SUPPLIED:** Inj: 5mg/mL; Tab: 100mg*, 200mg*, 300mg *scored

**CONTRAINDICATIONS:** Bronchial asthma, obstructive airway disease, overt cardiac failure, >1st-degree heart block, cardiogenic shock, severe bradycardia, other conditions associated with severe and prolonged hypotension.

**WARNINGS/PRECAUTIONS:** Severe hepatocellular injury reported; caution with hepatic dysfunction. Monitor LFTs periodically; discontinue at 1st sign of hepatic injury. Caution with well-compensated heart failure. Can cause heart failure. Exacerbation of ischemic heart disease with abrupt withdrawal. Caution in nonallergic bronchospasm patients refractory to or intolerant to other antihypertensives. May mask hypoglycemia symptoms. Withdrawal before surgery is controversial. Paradoxical HTN may occur with pheochromocytoma. Death reported during surgery. Avoid injection with low cardiac indices and elevated systemic vascular resistance.

**ADVERSE REACTIONS:** Fatigue, dizziness, dyspepsia, nausea, nasal stuffiness.

**INTERACTIONS:** Increased tremors with TCAs. Potentiated by cimetidine. Blunts reflex tachycardia of NTG without preventing hypotensive effect. Caution with calcium antagonists. Antagonizes bronchodilator effect of β-agonists. Antidiabetic agents may need dose adjustment. May block epinephrine effects. (Inj) Synergistic with halothane; do not use >3% halothane.

**PREGNANCY:** Category C, caution in nursing.



## LAC-HYDRIN

RX

ammonium lactate (Westwood-Squibb)

**THERAPEUTIC CLASS:** Emollient

**INDICATIONS:** Treatment of ichthyosis vulgaris and xerosis.

**DOSAGE:** *Adults:* Apply bid and rub thoroughly.
*Pediatrics:* (Lot) Infants/Children: (Cre) >2 yrs: Apply bid and rub in thoroughly.

**HOW SUPPLIED:** Cre: 12% [140g, 385g]; Lot: 12% [225g, 400g]

**WARNINGS/PRECAUTIONS:** Avoid sun exposure to treated skin. Avoid eyes, lips, mucous membranes, intravaginal use and oral use. Caution if used on face; potential for irritation Stinging, burning may occur if applied to fissures, erosions, or abrasions. Discontinue if skin condition worsens.

**ADVERSE REACTIONS:** Burning, stinging, itching, erythema.

**PREGNANCY:** Category B, caution in nursing.

## LACRISERT
hydroxypropyl cellulose (Merck)

RX

**THERAPEUTIC CLASS:** Lubricant

**INDICATIONS:** Treatment of moderate to severe dry eye syndromes (eg, keratoconjunctivitis sicca) and in patients not responsive to artificial tear solutions. Treatment of exposure keratitis, decreased corneal sensitivity, and recurrent corneal erosions.

**DOSAGE:** *Adults:* One insert in each eye qd, up to bid.

**HOW SUPPLIED:** Insert: 5mg [60s]

**WARNINGS/PRECAUTIONS:** May result in corneal abrasion if improperly placed. May cause blurred vision; use caution while operating machinery.

**ADVERSE REACTIONS:** Transient blurred vision, ocular discomfort/irritation, matting/stickiness of eyelashes, photophobia, hypersensitivity, eyelid edema, hyperemia.

**PREGNANCY:** Safety in pregnancy and nursing not known.

## LACTULOSE
lactulose (Various)

RX

**OTHER BRAND NAMES:** Constilac (Alra) - Enulose (Alpharma) - Constulose (Alpharma) - Generlac (Morton Grove)

**THERAPEUTIC CLASS:** Osmotic laxative

**INDICATIONS:** Treatment of constipation.

**DOSAGE:** *Adults:* 15-30mL qd. Max 60mL/day. May mix with fruit juice, water, or milk.

**HOW SUPPLIED:** Sol: 10g/15mL

**CONTRAINDICATIONS:** Patients who require a low galactose diet.

**WARNINGS/PRECAUTIONS:** Caution in DM due to galactose and lactose content. Monitor electrolytes periodically in elderly or debilitated if used >6 months. Potential for explosive reaction with electrocautery procedures during proctoscopy or colonoscopy.

**ADVERSE REACTIONS:** Flatulence, intestinal cramps, diarrhea, nausea, vomiting.

**INTERACTIONS:** Decreased effect with nonabsorbable antacids.

**PREGNANCY:** Category B, caution in nursing.

## LAMICTAL
lamotrigine (GlaxoSmithKline)

RX

**Serious life threatening rash including Stevens-Johnson syndrome and toxic epidermal necrolysis reported. Occurs more often in peds than adults. D/C at 1st sign of rash.**

**OTHER BRAND NAMES:** Lamictal CD (GlaxoSmithKline)

**THERAPEUTIC CLASS:** Phenyltriazine

**INDICATIONS:** Adjunctive therapy in patients (>2 yrs) with partial seizures and for generalized seizures of Lennox-Gastaut syndrome. For conversion to monotherapy in adults (>16 yrs) with partial seizures receiving a single enzyme-inducing antiepileptic drug (EIAED) or valproate (VPA). Maintenance treatment of Bipolar I Disorder to delay the time to occurrence of mood episodes (depression, mania, hypomania, mixed episodes) in patients treated for acute mood episodes with standard therapy.

**DOSAGE:** *Adults:* Epilepsy: Concomitant AEDs with valproate (VPA): Weeks 1 and 2: 25mg every other day. Weeks 3 and 4: 25mg qd. Titrate: Increase every 1-2 weeks by 25-50mg/day. Maint: 100-400mg/day, given qd or bid; 100-

L

200mg/day when added to VPA alone. Concomitant EIAEDs without VPA: Weeks 1 and 2: 50mg qd. Weeks 3 and 4: 50mg bid. Titrate: Increase every 1-2 weeks by 100mg/day. Maint: 150-250mg bid. Conversion to Monotherapy From Single EIAED: >16 yrs: Weeks 1 and 2: 50mg qd. Weeks 3 and 4: 50mg bid. Titrate: Increase every 1-2 weeks by 100mg/day. Maint: 250mg bid. Withdraw EIAED over 4 weeks. Conversion to Monotherapy From VPA: ≥16 yrs: Step 1: Follow Concomitant AEDs with VPA dosing regimen to achieve Lamictal dose of 200mg/day. Maintain previous VPA dose. Step 2: Maintain Lamictal 200mg/day. Decrease VPA to 500mg/day by decrements of ≤500mg/day per week. Maintain VPA 500mg/day for 1 week. Step 3: Increase to Lamictal 300mg/day for 1 week. Decrease VPA simultaneously to 250mg/day for 1 week. Step 4: D/C VPA. Increase Lamictal 100mg/day every week to maint dose of 500mg/day. Bipolar Disorder: Patients not taking carbamazepine, other enzyme-inducing drugs (EIDs) or VPA: Weeks 1 and 2: 25mg qd. Weeks 3 and 4: 50mg qd. Week 5: 100mg qd. Weeks 6 and 7: 200mg qd. Patients taking VPA: Weeks 1 and 2: 25mg every other day. Weeks 3 and 4: 25mg qd. Week 5: 50mg qd. Weeks 6 and 7: 100mg qd. Patients taking carbamazepine (or other EIDs) and not taking VPA: Weeks 1 and 2: 50mg qd. Weeks 3 and 4: 100mg qd (divided doses). Week 5: 200mg qd (divided doses). Week 6: 300mg qd (divided doses). Week 7: up to 400mg qd (divided doses). After d/c of psychotropic drugs excluding VPA, carbamazepine, or other EIDs: Maintain current dose. After d/c of VPA and current lamotrigine dose of 100mg qd: Week 1: 150mg qd. Week 2 and onward: 200mg qd. After d/c of carbamazepine or other EIDs and current lamotrigine dose of 400mg qd: Week 1: 400mg qd. Week 2: 300mg qd

L

*Pediatrics:* Round dose down to nearest whole tab. 2-12 yrs: >6.7kg: Lennox-Gastaut/Partial Seizures: Concomitant AEDs with VPA: Weeks 1 and 2: 0.15mg/kg/day given qd-bid. Weeks 3 and 4: 0.3mg/kg/day given qd or bid. Titrate: Increase every 1-2 weeks by 0.3mg/kg/day. Maint: 1-5mg/kg/day given qd or bid; 1-3mg/kg/day when added to VPA alone. Max: 200mg/day. Concomitant EIAEDs without VPA: Weeks 1 and 2: 0.3mg/kg bid. Weeks 3 and 4: 0.6mg/kg bid. Titrate: Increase every 1-2 weeks by 1.2mg/kg/day. Maint: 2.5-7.5mg/kg bid. Max: 400mg/day. >12 yrs: Concomitant AEDs with VPA: Weeks 1 and 2: 25mg every other day. Weeks 3 and 4: 25mg qd. Titrate: Increase every 1-2 weeks by 25-50mg/day. Maint: 100-400mg/day, given qd or bid; 100-200mg/day when added to VPA alone. Concomitant EIAEDs without VPA: Weeks 1 and 2: 50mg qd. Weeks 3 and 4: 50mg bid. Titrate: Increase every 1-2 weeks by 100mg/day. Maint: 150-250mg bid. Hepatic Impairment: Initial/Titrate/Maint: Reduce by 50% for moderate (Child-Pugh Grade B) and 75% for severe (Child-Pugh Grade C) impairment. Significant Renal Impairment: Maint: Reduce dose.

**HOW SUPPLIED:** Tab: 25mg*, 100mg*, 150mg*, 200mg*; Tab, Chewable: (Lamictal CD) 2mg, 5mg, 25mg *scored

**WARNINGS/PRECAUTIONS:** Risk of serious life-threatening rash; d/c if rash occurs. Multiorgan failure, sudden unexplained death, hypersensitivity reactions, and pure red cell aplasia reported. Avoid abrupt withdrawal. Caution with renal, hepatic, or cardiac functional impairment. May cause ophthalmic toxicity. Do not exceed recommended initial dose and dose escalations. Caution in elderly. Chewable tabs may be swallowed whole, chewed (with water/diluted fruit juice) or dispersed in water/diluted fruit juice; do administer partial quantities.

**ADVERSE REACTIONS:** Serious rash, dizziness, ataxia, somnolence, headache, diplopia, blurred vision, nausea, vomiting, insomnia, back/abdominal pain, fatigue, xerostomia, rhinitis.

**INTERACTIONS:** Decreased levels with phenytoin, carbamazepine, phenobarbital, primidone, rifampin, estrogen-containing oral contraceptives. Risk of life-threatening rash with valproic acid. Lamotrigine decreases valproic acid levels; valproic acid increases lamotrigine levels. Inhibits dihydrofolate reductase; may potentiate folate inhibitors.

**PREGNANCY:** Category C, not for use in nursing.

## LAMISIL

terbinafine HCl (Novartis) RX

**THERAPEUTIC CLASS:** Allylamine antifungal

**INDICATIONS:** Treatment of onychomycosis of toenail or fingernail due to dermatophytes (tinea unguium).

**DOSAGE:** *Adults:* Fingernail: 250mg qd for 6 weeks. Toenail: 250mg qd for 12 weeks.

**HOW SUPPLIED:** Tab: 250mg

**WARNINGS/PRECAUTIONS:** Liver disease and serious skin reactions reported; stop therapy if these develop. Avoid with liver disease or renal impairment (CrCl <50 mL/min). Check serum transaminases before therapy. Monitor CBC if immunocompromised and taking terbinafine >6 weeks. Stop therapy if neutrophil count <1,000 cells/mm$^3$. Changes in ocular lens and retina reported (unknown significance).

**ADVERSE REACTIONS:** Headache, diarrhea, dyspepsia, rash, liver enzyme abnormalities.

**INTERACTIONS:** Increased clearance of cyclosporine. May potentiate levels of drugs metabolized by CYP2D6 (eg, TCAs, β-blockers, SSRIs, MAOIs-type B). Decreased clearance of IV caffeine. Clearance increased by rifampin and decreased by cimetidine.

**PREGNANCY:** Category B, not for use in nursing.

## LAMISIL AT

terbinafine HCl (Novartis Consumer) OTC

**THERAPEUTIC CLASS:** Allylamine antifungal

**INDICATIONS:** Treatment of tinea pedis, tinea cruris, tinea corporis.

**DOSAGE:** *Adults:* Wash and dry area. Tinea pedis: Apply bid for 1 week (interdigital) or for 2 weeks (bottom or sides of foot). Tinea cruris/corporis: Apply qd for 1 week.
*Pediatrics:* >12 yrs: Wash and dry area. Tinea pedis: Apply bid for 1 week (interdigital) or for 2 weeks (bottom or sides of foot). Tinea cruris/corporis: Apply qd for 1 week.

**HOW SUPPLIED:** Cre: 1% [12g, 24g]; Spray: 1% [30mL]

**WARNINGS/PRECAUTIONS:** Do not use on nails, scalp, in or near the mouth or eyes, or for vaginal yeast infections.

**PREGNANCY:** Not rated in pregnancy or nursing.

## LANOXIN

digoxin (GlaxoSmithKline) RX

**OTHER BRAND NAMES:** Digitek (Mylan Bertek) - Lanoxicaps (GlaxoSmithKline)

**THERAPEUTIC CLASS:** Cardiac glycoside

**INDICATIONS:** Treatment of mild to moderate heart failure and to control ventricular response rate with chronic atrial fibrillation.

**DOSAGE:** *Adults:* Rapid Digitalization: LD: (Cap/Inj) 0.4-0.6mg PO/IV or (Tab) 0.5-0.75mg PO, may give additional (Cap/Inj) 0.1-0.3mg or (Tab) 0.125-0.375mg at 6-8 hr intervals until clinical effect. Maint: (Tab) 0.125-0.5mg qd. Elderly (>70 yrs)/Renal Dysfunction: Initial: 0.125mg qd. Marked Renal Dysfunction: Initial: 0.0625mg qd. Titrate: Increase every 2 weeks based on response. A-Fib: Titrate to minimum effective dose for desired response.
*Pediatrics:* (Ped Sol) Oral Digitalizing Dose: Premature Infants: 20-30mcg/kg. Full-Term Infants: 25-35mcg/kg. 1-24 months: 35-60mcg/kg. 2-5 yrs: 30-

40mcg/kg. 5-10 yrs: 20-35mcg/kg. >10 yrs: 10-15mcg/kg. Maint: Premature Infants: 20-30% of PO digitalizing dose/day. Full-Term Infants to >10 yrs: 25-35% of PO digitalizing dose. (Ped Inj) IV Digitalizing Dose: Premature Infants: 15-25mcg/kg. Full-Term Infants: 20-30mcg/kg. 1-24 months: 30-50mcg/kg. 2-5 yrs: 25-35mcg/kg. 5-10 yrs: 15-30mcg/kg. >10 yrs: 8-12mcg/kg. Maint: Premature Infants: 20-30% of IV digitalizing dose. Full-Term Infants to >10 yrs: 25-35% of IV digitalizing dose/day. (Cap) Oral Digitalizing Dose: 2-5 yrs: 25-35mcg/kg. 5-10 yrs: 15-30mcg/kg. >10 yrs: 8-12mcg/kg. Maint: >2 yrs: 25-25% of PO or IV digitalizing dose. (Tab) Maint: 2-5 yrs: 10-15mcg/kg. 5-10 yrs: 7-10mcg/kg. >10 yrs: 3-5mcg/kg. A-Fib: Titrate to minimum effective dose for desired response.

**HOW SUPPLIED:** Cap: (Lanoxicaps) 0.1mg, 0.2mg; Inj: (Pediatric Inj) 0.1mg/mL, 0.25mg/mL; Sol: (Pediatric Sol) 0.05mg/mL [60mL]; Tab: 0.125mg*, 0.25mg* *scored

**CONTRAINDICATIONS:** Ventricular fibrillation, digitalis hypersensitivity.

**WARNINGS/PRECAUTIONS:** May cause severe sinus bradycardia or sinoatrial block with pre-existing sinus node disease. May cause advanced or complete heart block with pre-existing incomplete AV block. May cause very rapid ventricular response or ventricular fibrillation. Caution with thyroid disorders, AMI, hypermetabolic states, restrictive cardiomyopathy, constrictive pericarditis, amyloid heart disease, elderly, acute cor pulmonale, and idiopathic hypertrophic subaortic stenosis. Caution with renal dysfunction; high risk for toxicity. Caution with hypokalemia, hypomagnesemia, or hypercalcemia; toxicity may occur. Hypocalcemia can nullify effects of digoxin. Monitor electrolytes and renal function periodically. Risk of ventricular arrhythmia with electrical cardioversion. Bioavailability is different between dosage forms.



**ADVERSE REACTIONS:** Heart block, rhythm disturbances, anorexia, nausea, vomiting, diarrhea, visual disturbances, headache, weakness, dizziness, mental disturbances.

**INTERACTIONS:** Risk of toxicity with $K^+$-depleting diuretics. Increased risk of arrhythmias with calcium, sympathomimetics, and succinylcholine. Increased serum levels with quinidine, verapamil, amiodarone, propafenone, indomethacin, itraconazole, alprazolam, and spironolactone; monitor for toxicity. Increased absorption with propantheline, diphenoxylate, macrolides, and tetracycline; monitor for toxicity. Decreased intestinal absorption with antacids, kaolin-pectin, sulfasalazine, neomycin, cholestyramine, certain anticancer drugs, and metoclopramide. Decreased serum levels with rifampin. Increased digoxin dose requirement with thyroid supplements. Additive effects on AV node conduction with β-blockers or calcium channel blockers. Caution with drugs that deteriorate renal function.

**PREGNANCY:** Category C, caution in nursing.

## LANTUS — RX

insulin glargine, human (Sanofi-Aventis)

**THERAPEUTIC CLASS:** Insulin

**INDICATIONS:** Treatment of adults and pediatrics with type 1 diabetes mellitus. Treatment of adults with type 2 diabetes mellitus who require basal (long-acting) insulin.

**DOSAGE:** *Adults:* Individualize dose. For SQ injection only. Administer qd at same time each day. Insulin naive patients on oral antidiabetic drugs, start with 10U qd. Switching from once-daily NPH or Ultralente does not require initial dose change. Switching from bid NPH, reduce initial dose by 20%. Maint: 2-100U/day.

*Pediatrics:* >6 yrs: Individualize dose. For SQ injection only. Administer qd at same time each day. Insulin naive patients on oral antidiabetic drugs, start with 10U qd. Switching from once-daily NPH or Ultralente does not require initial dose change. Switching from bid NPH, reduce initial dose by 20%. Maint: 2-100U/day.

**HOW SUPPLIED:** Inj: 100U/mL; OptiPen: 100U/mL

**WARNINGS/PRECAUTIONS:** Human insulin differs from animal source insulin. Any change of insulin should be made cautiously. Changes in strength, manufacturer, type or method of manufacture may result in the need for a change in dosage. Hypoglycemia may occur with taking too much insulin, missing or delaying meals, exercising or working more than usual. An infection or illness (especially with diarrhea or vomiting) may change insulin requirements. Administration of insulin SQ can result in lipodystrophy. Not for IV use. Do not mix with other insulins. May cause sodium retention and edema.

**ADVERSE REACTIONS:** Hypoglycemia, allergic reactions, injection site reactions, lipodystrophy, pruritus, rash.

**INTERACTIONS:** Increased glucose lowering effects with ACE inhibitors, disopyramide, fibrates, fluoxetine, MAOIs, propoxyphene, salicylates, somatostatin analog, sulfonamide antibiotics, and other antidiabetic agents. Decreased blood glucose lowering effects with corticosteroids, danazol, diuretics, sympathomimetic amines, isoniazid, phenothiazine derivatives, somatropin, thyroid hormones, estrogens, progestogens. Pentamidine may cause hypoglycemia, followed by hyperglycemia. β-blockers, clonidine, lithium salts, and alcohol may potentiate or weaken glucose lowering effect. β-blockers, clonidine, guanethidine, and reserpine may reduce or mask signs of hypoglycemia.

**PREGNANCY:** Category C, caution in nursing.

## LARIAM

RX

mefloquine HCl (Roche Labs)

**THERAPEUTIC CLASS:** Quinolinemethanol derivative

**INDICATIONS:** Treatment and prophylaxis of mild to moderate acute malaria caused by *P.falciparum* or *P.vivax.*

**DOSAGE:** *Adults:* Treatment: 1250mg single dose. Prophylaxis: 250mg/week. Start 1 week before arrival in endemic area and continue weekly (same day of week) while in area. Continue for 4 weeks after leaving the area. Take with food and 8 oz of water.

*Pediatrics:* >6 months: Treatment: Usual: 20-25mg/kg, split in 2 doses. Take 6-8 hrs apart. If vomiting occurs <30 minutes after dose, give a 2nd full dose. If vomiting occurs 30-60 minutes after dose, give additional half-dose. Prophylaxis: >3 months: 3-5mg/kg/week. >45kg: 250mg/week. 31-45kg: 3/4 tab/week. 21-30kg: 125mg/week. 5-20kg: 1/4 tab/week. Take with food and water. May crush and mix with water.

**HOW SUPPLIED:** Tab: 250mg* *scored

**CONTRAINDICATIONS:** Hypersensitivity to related compounds (eg, quinine, quinidine). Use as prophylaxis with active or recent history of depression, generalized anxiety disorder, psychosis or schizophrenia, or other major psychiatric disorder, or with a history of convulsions.

**WARNINGS/PRECAUTIONS:** In life-threatening malaria infection due to *P.falciparum*, use IV antimalarials. High risk of relapse seen with acute *P.vivax*; after initial treatment, subsequently treat with 8-aminoquinoline (eg, primaquine). May cause psychiatric symptoms. During prophylaxis, d/c if symptoms of acute anxiety, depression, restlessness, or confusion occur. In long-term therapy, monitor LFTs and perform ophthalmic exams. May impair mental/physical abilities. Increase risk of convulsions in epileptic patients. Caution with cardiac disease, hepatic dysfunction and elderly.

**ADVERSE REACTIONS:** Nausea, vomiting, myalgia, fever, dizziness, headache, somnolence, sleep disorders, loss of balance, chills, diarrhea, abdominal pain, fatigue, tinnitus, pruritus, skin rash.

**INTERACTIONS:** Avoid halofantrine; may prolong QTc interval. Concomitant administration with other related compounds (eg, quinine, quinidine, chloroquine) may cause ECG abnormalities and increased risk of convulsions;

delay mefloquine dose for 12 hrs after last dose of these drugs. Avoid propranolol; cardiopulmonary arrest reported. Drugs that may alter cardiac conduction (eg, anti-arrhythmic or β-blockers, calcium channel blockers, antihistamines, $H_1$-blockers, TCAs, and phenothiazines) may prolong $QT_c$ interval. May lower plasma levels of anticonvulsants (eg, valproic acid, carbamazepine, phenobarbital, phenytoin); monitor blood levels and adjust dosage accordingly. Complete vaccinations with live, attenuated vaccines (eg, typhoid vaccine) at least 3 days before mefloquine therapy. Caution with anticoagulants, antidiabetic agents.

**PREGNANCY:** Category C, not for use in nursing.

## LESCOL XL — RX

fluvastatin sodium (Novartis)

**OTHER BRAND NAMES:** Lescol (Novartis)

**THERAPEUTIC CLASS:** HMG-CoA reductase inhibitor

**INDICATIONS:** Adjunct to diet, to reduce total cholesterol (Total-C), LDL-C, TG, and Apo B levels, and to increase HDL-C in primary hypercholesterolemia and mixed dyslipidemia (Types IIa and IIb) when response to nonpharmacological measures is inadequate. To slow coronary atherosclerosis progression in coronary heart disease by lowering Total-C and LDL-C. To reduce risk of undergoing coronary revascularization procedures in patients with coronary heart disease. Adjunct to diet to reduce Total-C, LDL-C, and Apo B levels in adolescent boys and girls who are at least one year post-menarche, 10-16 years of age, with heterozygous familial hypercholesterolemia when response to dietary restriction is inadequate and LDL-C remains ≥190mg/dL or if LDL-C remains ≥160mg/dL and there is positive family history of premature CV disease or 2 or more other CV disease risk factors are present.

**DOSAGE:** *Adults:* ≥18 yrs: (For LDL-C reduction of ≥25%) Initial: 40mg cap qpm or 80mg XL tab at anytime of day (or 40mg cap bid). (For LDL-C reduction of <25%) Initial: 20mg cap qpm. Usual: 20-80mg/day. Severe Renal Impairment: Caution with dose >40mg/day. Take 2 hrs after bile-acid resins qhs.

*Pediatrics:* Heterozygous Familial Hypercholesterolemia: 10-16 yrs (≥1 yr post-menarche): Individualize dose: Initial: 20mg cap. Titrate: Adjust dose at 6 week intervals. Max: 40mg cap bid or 80mg XL tab qd.

**HOW SUPPLIED:** Cap: (Lescol) 20mg, 40mg; Tab, Extended-Release: (Lescol XL) 80mg

**CONTRAINDICATIONS:** Active liver disease, unexplained persistent elevations of serum transaminases, pregnancy, nursing mothers.

**WARNINGS/PRECAUTIONS:** Monitor LFTs prior to therapy, at 12 weeks or with dose elevation. D/C if AST or ALT >3X ULN on 2 consecutive occasions. Risk of myopathy and/or rhabdomyolysis reported. D/C if markedly elevated CPK levels occur, if myopathy is diagnosed or suspected, or if predisposition to renal failure secondary to rhabdomyolysis. Less effective with homozygous familial hypercholesterolemia. Caution with heavy alcohol use and/or history of hepatic disease. Evaluate if endocrine dysfunction develops.

**ADVERSE REACTIONS:** Dyspepsia, abdominal pain, headache, nausea, diarrhea, abnormal LFTs, myalgia, flu-like symptoms.

**INTERACTIONS:** Rifampicin significantly decreases serum levels. Increases levels of glyburide, diclofenac, and phenytoin. Increase serum levels with glyburide, phenytoin, cimetidine, ranitidine, and omeprazole. Caution with drugs that decrease levels of endogenous steroid hormones (eg, ketoconazole, spironolactone, cimetidine). Avoid fibrates. Cyclosporine, gemfibrozil, erythromycin, or niacin may increase risk of myopathy/rhabdomyolysis. Cholestyramine given within 4 hrs decreases serum levels but has additive effects when given 4 hrs after fluvastatin (immediate-release). Monitor digoxin, anticoagulants.

**PREGNANCY:** Category X, not for use in nursing.

## LEUCOVORIN CALCIUM

leucovorin calcium (Various) RX

**THERAPEUTIC CLASS:** Cytoprotective agent

**INDICATIONS:** (Inj, Tab) Rescue therapy after high-dose methotrexate (MTX) therapy in osteosarcoma. To reduce toxicity of impaired MTX elimination or overdose of folic acid antagonists. Adjunct to 5-fluorouracil (5-FU) for palliative treatment of advanced colorectal cancer. Treatment of megaloblastic anemia due to folic acid deficiency.

**DOSAGE:** *Adults:* Colorectal Cancer: 200mg/m$^2$ slow IV push over 3 min. followed by 5-FU 370mg/m$^2$ IV qd for 5 days, or 20mg/m$^2$ IV qd followed by 5-FU 425mg/m$^2$ IV qd for 5 days. May repeat at 4 week intervals for 2 courses then at 4-5 week intervals. May increase 5-FU dose by 10% if no toxicity. Reduce 5-FU dose by 20% with moderate GI/hematologic toxicity and by 30% with severe toxicity. Leucovorin Rescue: 15mg q6h for 10 doses starting 24 hrs after start of MTX until serum MTX is <5x10$^{-8}$M. Give IV/IM with GI toxicity. See labeling for leucovorin adjustments and extended therapy. Impaired MTX Elimination/Overdose: 10mg/m$^2$ IV/IM/PO q6h until serum MTX is <10$^{-8}$M. Increase to 100mg/m$^2$ q3h if 24-hr serum creatinine is 50% over baseline, or if 24-hr serum MTX is >5x10$^{-6}$M, or the 48-hr level is >9x10$^{-7}$M. Give IV/IM with GI toxicity. Start ASAP after overdose and within 24 hrs of MTX with delayed excretion. Megaloblastic Anemia: Up to 1mg/day. Elderly: Caution with dose selection.

**HOW SUPPLIED:** Inj: 10mg/mL, 50mg, 100mg, 200mg, 350mg, 500mg; Tab: 5mg, 10mg, 15mg, 25mg

**CONTRAINDICATIONS:** Improper therapy for pernicious anemia and other megaloblastic anemias secondary to lack of vitamin $B_{12}$.

**WARNINGS/PRECAUTIONS:** Do not administer >160mg/min. Do not give intrathecally. Monitor serum MTX. Higher than recommended PO doses must be given IV. Increased risk of severe toxicity in elderly/debilitated colorectal cancer patients taking 5-FU with leucovorin. Monitor renal function in elderly.

**ADVERSE REACTIONS:** Allergic sensitization.

**INTERACTIONS:** Folic acid in large amounts may antagonize phenobarbital, phenytoin, and primidone, and increase seizure frequency in children. May enhance 5-FU toxicity. May reduce MTX efficacy. Increased treatment failure and morbidity in TMP-SMZ-treated HIV patients with PCP.

**PREGNANCY:** Category C, caution use in nursing.

## LEUKERAN

chlorambucil (GlaxoSmithKline) RX

**Risk of bone marrow suppression. Potentially carcinogenic, mutagenic, and teratogenic. Produces human infertility.**

**THERAPEUTIC CLASS:** Nitrogen mustard alkylating agent

**INDICATIONS:** Treatment of chronic lymphatic (lymphocytic) leukemia (CLL), malignant lymphomas, and Hodgkin's disease.

**DOSAGE:** *Adults:* Usual: 0.1-0.2mg/kg qd for 3-6 weeks. Adjust according to response; reduce with abrupt WBC decline. Lymphocytic Infiltration of Bone Marrow/Hypoplastic Bone Marrow: Max: 0.1mg/kg/day. Caution within 4 weeks of full course of radiation or chemotherapy.

**HOW SUPPLIED:** Tab: 2mg

**CONTRAINDICATIONS:** Prior resistance to therapy.

**WARNINGS/PRECAUTIONS:** Convulsions, infertility, leukemia and secondary malignancies observed. Shown to cause chromatid or chromosome damage and sterility. Skin rash progressing to erythema multiforme, toxic epidermal necrolysis, or Stevens-Johnson syndrome reported. Avoid becoming pregnant. Lymphopenia reported, usually returns to normal upon completion. Monitor Hgb, leukocyte count and differential, platelet counts weekly. Avoid live vaccines in the immunocompromised.

**ADVERSE REACTIONS:** Bone marrow suppression, nausea, vomiting, diarrhea, tremors, muscular twitching, confusion, agitation, ataxia, urticaria, angioneurotic syndrome, pulmonary fibrosis, hepatotoxicity, jaundice.

**INTERACTIONS:** Cross-hypersensitivity may occur with other alkylating agents.

**PREGNANCY:** Category D, not for use in nursing.

## LEUKINE RX

sargramostim (Berlex)

**THERAPEUTIC CLASS:** Granulocyte-macrophage colony stimulating factor

**INDICATIONS:** Acute myelogenous leukemia (AML) following induction chemotherapy in older adults (≥55 yrs) to shorten time to neutrophil recovery and to reduce incidence of severe and life-threatening infections and infections resulting in death. For mobilization of hematopoietic progenitor cells into peripheral blood for collection by leukopheresis. Myeloid recovery after autologous bone marrow transplantation (BMT) in non-Hodgkin's lymphoma (NHL), acute lymphoblastic leukemia (ALL) and Hodgkin's disease. Myeloid recovery after allogeneic BMT. BMT (allogeneic or autologous) failure or engraftment delay.

L

**DOSAGE:** *Adults:* Myeloid Reconstitution After BMT: 250mcg/m²/day IV over 2 hrs 2-4 hrs post bone marrow infusion and not less than 24 hrs after last dose of chemo- or radiotherapy. Do not give until ANC <500 cells/mm³. Continue until ANC >1500 cells/mm³ for 3 consecutive days. May reduce dose by 50% or temporarily discontinue if severe adverse reaction occurs. Discontinue immediately if blast cells appear or disease progression occurs. BMT Failure/Engraftment Delay: 250mcg/m²/day IV over 2 hrs for 14 days. May repeat after 7 days if needed. Give third course after another 7 days of 500mcg/m²/day IV for 14 days if needed. May reduce dose by 50% or temporarily discontinue if severe adverse reaction occurs. Discontinue immediately if blast cells appear or disease progression occurs. Reduce dose by 50% or interrupt treatment if ANC >20,000 cells/mm³. Post Peripheral Blood Progenitor Cell Transplant: 250mcg/m²/day IV over 24 hrs or SC once daily. Begin immediately after infusion of progenitor cells and continue until ANC >1500 cells/mm³ for 3 consecutive days. Mobilization of Peripheral Blood Progenitor Cells (PBPC): 250mcg/m²/day IV over 24 hrs or SC once daily. Continue through PBPC collection period. Reduce dose by 50% if WBC >50,000 cells/mm³. Neutrophil Recovery Post-Chemo in AML: ≥55 yrs: Hypoplastic Bone Marrow With <5% Blasts: 250mcg/m²/day IV over 4 hrs starting on day 11 or 4 days after completion of induction chemo. If 2nd cycle of induction chemo is needed, give 4 days after completion of chemo. Continue until ANC >1500 cells/mm³ for 3 consecutive days or max of 42 days. Discontinue immediately if leukemi

**HOW SUPPLIED:** Inj: 250mcg/vial, 500mcg/mL

**CONTRAINDICATIONS:** Excessive leukemic myeloid blasts in bone marrow or peripheral blood (≥10%), concomitant chemotherapy or radiotherapy.

**WARNINGS/PRECAUTIONS:** Contains benzyl alcohol; avoid use in neonates. Caution with pre-existing fluid retention, pulmonary infiltrate, CHF, hypoxia, cardiac disease, renal/hepatic dysfunction, or myeloid malignancies. Monitor CBC twice weekly and renal/hepatic function every other week with pre-existing dysfunction.

**ADVERSE REACTIONS:** Fever, nausea, diarrhea, vomiting, alopecia, rash, headache, stomatitis, anorexia, mucous membrane disorder, asthenia, malaise, abdominal pain, edema, HTN.

**INTERACTIONS:** Caution with drugs that may potentiate myeloproliferative effects (eg, lithium, corticosteroids).

**PREGNANCY:** Category C, caution in nursing.

## LEVAQUIN
levofloxacin (Ortho-McNeil)

RX

**THERAPEUTIC CLASS:** Fluoroquinolone

**INDICATIONS:** Uncomplicated and complicated skin and skin structure (SSSI), and urinary tract infections (UTI), acute bacterial sinusitis, acute bacterial exacerbation of chronic bronchitis (ABECB), community acquired pneumonia (CAP), including multi-drug resistant *Streptococcus pneumoniae*, nosocomial pneumonia, chronic bacterial prostatitis (CBP), and acute pyelonephritis caused by susceptible strains of microorganisms. Prevention of inhalational anthrax following exposure to *Bacillus anthracis*.

**DOSAGE:** *Adults:* ≥18 yrs: IV/PO: ABECB: 500mg qd for 7 days. CAP: 500mg qd for 7-14 days or 750mg qd for 5 days. Sinusitis: 500mg qd for 10-14 days or 750mg qd for 5 days. CBP: 500mg qd for 28 days. Uncomplicated SSSI: 500mg qd for 7-10 days. Complicated SSSI/Nosocomial Pneumonia: 750mg qd for 7-14 days. Inhalational Anthrax: 500mg qd for 60 days. Complicated SSSI/Nosocomial Pneumonia/CAP/Sinusitis: CrCl 20-49mL/min: 750mg, then 750mg q48h. CrCl 10-19mL/min/Hemodialysis/CAPD: 750mg, then 500mg q48h. ABECB/CAP/Sinusitis/Uncomplicated SSSI/CBP/Inhalational Anthrax: CrCl 20-49mL/min: 500mg, then 250mg q24h. CrCl 10-19mL/min/Hemodialysis/CAPD: 500mg, then 250mg q48h. Complicated UTI/Acute Pyelonephritis: 250mg qd for 10 days. CrCl 10-19mL/min: 250mg, then 250mg q48h. Uncomplicated UTI: 250mg qd for 3 days. Take oral solution 1 hr before or 2 hrs after eating.

**HOW SUPPLIED:** Inj: 5mg/mL, 25mg/mL; Sol: 25mg/mL; Tab: 250mg, 500mg, 750mg [Leva-pak, 5[s]]

**WARNINGS/PRECAUTIONS:** Only administer injection via IV infusion over a period of not less than 60 or 90 minutes depending on dosage. Convulsions, toxic psychoses, increased ICP, CNS stimulation reported; D/C if any occur. Caution with CNS disorders that may predispose to seizures/lower seizure threshold (eg, epilepsy, renal insufficiency, drug therapy). Hyper- or hypoglycemia with insulin or oral hypoglycemics. Moderate to severe phototoxicity can occur. Serious/fatal hypersensitivity reactions; d/c at first sign of rash. Pseudomembranous colitis and torsade de pointes (rare) have been reported. May permit overgrowth of clostridia. Caution in renal insufficiency. Stop therapy if pain, inflammation, or ruptured tendon occurs.

**ADVERSE REACTIONS:** Nausea, diarrhea, headache, insomnia, constipation.

**INTERACTIONS:** Decreased levels with antacids, sucralfate, didanosine, metal cations (eg, iron), and multivitamins with zinc; separate dosing by 2 hrs. Concomitant NSAIDs may increase seizure risk and CNS stimulation. Blood glucose changes with concomitant antidiabetic agents. Monitor theophylline levels. Increases PT with warfarin; monitor closely.

**PREGNANCY:** Category C, not for use in nursing.

## LEVATOL
penbutolol sulfate (Schwarz)

RX

**THERAPEUTIC CLASS:** Nonselective beta-blocker

**INDICATIONS:** Treatment of mild to moderate arterial hypertension.

**DOSAGE:** *Adults:* 20mg qd.

**HOW SUPPLIED:** Tab: 20mg* *scored

**CONTRAINDICATIONS:** Cardiogenic shock, sinus bradycardia, 2nd- and 3rd-degree AV block, bronchial asthma.

L

**WARNINGS/PRECAUTIONS:** Caution with well-compensated heart failure, elderly, nonallergic bronchospasm, renal impairment. Can cause cardiac failure. Avoid abrupt withdrawal. Withdrawal before surgery is controversial. May mask hypoglycemia or hyperthyroidism symptoms.

**ADVERSE REACTIONS:** Diarrhea, nausea, dyspepsia, dizziness, fatigue, headache, insomnia, cough.

**INTERACTIONS:** Increases volume of distribution of lidocaine; may need larger LD. Synergistic hypotensive effects, bradycardia, and arrhythmias with oral calcium channel blockers. Avoid catecholamine-depleting drugs. Caution with alcohol, anesthetics that depress the myocardium. May antagonize epinephrine.

**PREGNANCY:** Category C, caution in nursing.

## LEVBID RX

hyoscyamine sulfate (Schwarz)

**OTHER BRAND NAMES:** Levsin (Schwarz) - Levsinex (Schwarz)

**THERAPEUTIC CLASS:** Anticholinergic

**INDICATIONS:** Adjunct treatment of peptic ulcer, irritable bowel syndrome, neurogenic bladder, and neurogenic bowel disturbances. Management of functional intestinal disorders (eg, mild dysenteries, diverticulitis). To control gastric secretion, visceral spasm, and hypermotility in spastic colitis, spastic bladder, cystitis, pylorospasm, and associated abdominal cramps. Symptomatic relief of biliary and renal colic with concomitant morphine or other narcotics."Drying agent" for symptomatic relief of acute rhinitis. To reduce rigidity and tremors of Parkinson's disease and control associated sialorrhea and hyperhidrosis. For anticholinesterase poisoning. To reduce pain and hypersecretion in pancreatitis. For certain cases of partial heart block associated with vagal activity. (Elixir, Drops) Treatment of infant colic. (Inj) Facilitates GI diagnostic procedures. In anesthesia as a pre-op antimuscarinic. In urology to improve radiologic visibility of kidneys.

**DOSAGE:** *Adults:* May also chew or swallow SL tab. (Drops, Eli, Tab, and Tab, SL) 0.125-0.25mg q4h or prn. Max: 1.5mg/24hrs. (Cap and Tab, Extended Release) 0.375-0.75mg q12h; or 1 cap q8h. Max: 1.5mg/24hrs. Do not crush or chew. (Inj) GI Disorders: 0.25-0.5mg IM/IV/SQ as single dose or up to qid at 4 hr intervals. Diagnostic Procedures: 0.25-0.5mg IV 5-10 minutes before procedure. Anesthesia: 5mcg/kg IM/IV/SQ 30-60 minutes before anesthesia or with narcotic/sedative administration. Drug-Induced Bradycardia (Surgery): Increments of 0.25mL IV; repeat prn. Neuromuscular Blockade Reversal: 0.2mg for every 1mg neostigmine or equal dose of physostigmine or pyridostigmine.
*Pediatrics:* May also chew or swallow SL tab. >12 yrs: (Drops, Eli, Tab, and Tab, SL) 0.125-0.25mg q4h or prn. Max: 1.5mg/24hrs. (Cap and Tab, Extended Release) 0.375-0.75mg q12h; or 1 cap may be given q8h. Max: 1.5mg/24hrs. Do not crush or chew. 2 to <12 yrs: (Tab and Tab, SL) 0.0625-0.125mg q4h or prn. Max: 0.75mg/24hrs. (Eli) Give q4h or prn. 10kg: 1.25mL. 20kg: 2.5mL. 40kg: 3.75mL. 50kg: 5mL. Max: 30mL/24hrs. (Drops) 0.25-1mL q4h or prn. Max: 6mL/24 hrs. <2 yrs: (Drops) Give q4h or prn. 3.4kg: 4 drops. Max: 24 drops/24hrs. 5kg: 5 drops. Max: 30 drops/24hrs. 7kg: 6 drops. Max: 36 drops/24hrs. 10kg: 8 drops. Max: 48 drops/24hrs. >2 yrs: Anesthesia: (Inj) 5mcg/kg IM/IV/SQ 30-60 minutes before anesthesia or with narcotic/sedative administration.

**HOW SUPPLIED:** (Levbid) Tab, Extended Release: 0.375mg*. (Levsin) Drops: 0.125mg/mL [15mL]; Elixir: 0.125mg/5mL [473mL]; Inj: 0.5mg/mL; Tab: 0.125mg*; Tab, SL: 0.125mg*. (Levsinex) Cap, Extended Release: 0.375mg *scored

**CONTRAINDICATIONS:** Glaucoma, obstructive uropathy, GI tract obstruction, paralytic ileus; intestinal atony of elderly/debilitated, unstable cardiovascular status in acute hemorrhage, toxic megacolon complicating ulcerative colitis, myasthenia gravis.

**WARNINGS/PRECAUTIONS:** Risk of heat prostration with high environmental temperature. Avoid activities requiring mental alertness. Psychosis has been reported. Caution with diarrhea, autonomic neuropathy, hyperthyroidism, coronary heart disease, CHF, arrhythmias/tachycardia, HTN, renal disease, and hiatal hernia associated with reflux esophagitis.

**ADVERSE REACTIONS:** Anticholinergic effects, drowsiness, headache, nervousness.

**INTERACTIONS:** Additive effects with other antimuscarinics, amantadine, haloperidol, phenothiazines, MAOIs, TCAs, and some antihistamines. Antacids interfere with absorption; take ac and antacids pc.

**PREGNANCY:** Category C, caution in nursing.

## LEVEMIR

RX

insulin detemir, rdna origin (Novo Nordisk)

**THERAPEUTIC CLASS:** Insulin

**INDICATIONS:** Treatment of adults and pediatrics with type 1 diabetes or adults with type 2 diabetes who require basal (long acting) insulin for the control of hyperglycemia.

**DOSAGE:** *Adults:* Individualize dose. Administer SQ qd or bid. Once-Daily Dosing: Administer with evening meal or bedtime. Twice-Daily Dosing: Administer evening dose with evening meal, at bedtime, or 12 hrs after morning dose. Type 1/Type 2 Diabetes on Basal-Bolus Treatment or Patients Only on Basal Insulin: Change on a unit-to-unit basis. Insulin-Naive with Type 2 Diabetes Inadequately Controlled on Oral Antidiabetics: Initial: 0.1-0.2 U/kg in evening or 10 U qd or bid.

*Pediatrics:* Individualize dose. Administer SQ qd or bid. Once-Daily Dosing: Administer with evening meal or bedtime. Twice-Daily Dosing: Administer evening dose with evening meal, at bedtime, or 12 hrs after morning dose. Type 1 Diabetes on Basal-Bolus Treatment or Patients Only on Basal Insulin: Change on a unit-to-unit basis.

**HOW SUPPLIED:** Inj: 100 U/mL [3mL, 10mL]

**WARNINGS/PRECAUTIONS:** Monitor glucose; may cause hypoglycemia. Not for use in an insulin infusion pump. Should not be diluted or mixed with any other insulin preparations. May cause lipodystrophy or hypersensitivity. Dose adjustment may be needed in renal or hepatic impairment and during intercurrent conditions such as illness, emotional distrubances, or other stresses.

**ADVERSE REACTIONS:** Allergic reactions, injection site reactions, lipodystrophy, pruritus, rash, hypoglycemia, weight gain.

**INTERACTIONS:** Avoid mixing with other insulins. Increased glucose lowering effects with ACE inhibitors, disopyramide, fibrates, fluoxetine, MAOIs, propoxyphene, salicylates, somatostatin analog, sulfonamide antibiotics, and other antidiabetic agents. Decreased blood glucose lowering effects with corticosteroids, danazol, diuretics, sympathomimetic agents, isoniazid, phenothiazine derivates, somatotropin, thyroid hormones, estrogens, progestogens. Pentamidine may cause hypoglycemia, followed by hyperglycemia. β-blockers, clonidine, lithium salts, and alcohol may potentiate or weaken glucose lowering effect. β-blockers, clonidine, guanethidine, and reserpine may reduce or mask signs of hypoglycemia.

**PREGNANCY:** Category C, caution in nursing.

## LEVITRA

RX

vardenafil HCl (Schering)

**THERAPEUTIC CLASS:** Phosphodiesterase type 5 inhibitor

**INDICATIONS:** Treatment of erectile dysfunction.

**DOSAGE:** *Adults:* Initial: 10mg one hour prior to sexual activity at frequency of up to once daily. Titrate: May decrease to 5mg or increase to max of 20mg based on response. Elderly: ≥65 yrs: Initial: 5mg. Moderate Hepatic Impairment: Initial: 5mg; Max: 10mg. Concomitant Ritonavir: Max: 2.5mg/72 hrs. Concomitant Indinavir, Ketoconazole 400mg daily/Itraconazole 400mg daily: Max: 2.5mg/24 hrs. Concomitant Ketoconazole 200mg daily/Itraconazole 200mg daily/Erythromycin: Max: 5mg/24 hrs.

**HOW SUPPLIED:** Tab: 2.5mg, 5mg, 10mg, 20mg

**CONTRAINDICATIONS:** Concomitant nitrates or nitric oxide donors.

**WARNINGS/PRECAUTIONS:** Avoid when sexual activity is inadvisable due to underlying CV status. Increased sensitivity to vasodilation effects with left ventricular outflow obstruction. Decrease in supine BP reported. Avoid with unstable angina, hypotension (SBP<90 mmHg), uncontrolled HTN(>170/100 mmHg), recent history of stroke, life-threatening arrhythmia, myocardial infarction (within last 6 months), severe cardiac failure, severe hepatic impairment (Child-Pugh C), end-stage renal disease requiring dialysis, hereditary degenerative retinal disorders including retinitis pigmentosa, congenital QT prolongation. Caution with bleeding disorders, peptic ulcers, anatomical deformation of the penis, or predisposition to priapism. Rare reports of non-arteritic anterior ischemic optic neuropathy (NAION) with PDE5 inhibitors.

**ADVERSE REACTIONS:** Headache, flushing, rhinitis, dyspepsia, sinusitis, flu syndrome.

**INTERACTIONS:** Avoid use with alpha-blockers, nitrates, Class IA (eg, quinidine, procainamide) or Class III (eg, amiodarone, sotalol) antiarrhythmics, and other agents for erectile dysfunction. Increased levels with ritonavir, indinavir, ketoconazole, erythromycin. May have additive hypotensive effect with nifedipine. Increased levels with CYP3A4 inhibitors.

**PREGNANCY:** Category B, not for use in nursing.

L

## LEVLEN

RX

levonorgestrel - ethinyl estradiol (Berlex)

**THERAPEUTIC CLASS:** Estrogen/progestogen combination

**INDICATIONS:** Prevention of pregnancy.

**DOSAGE:** *Adults*: Start 1st Sunday after menses begin. *21-day*: 1 tab qd for 21 days, stop for 7 days, then repeat. *28-day*: 1 tab qd for 28 days, then repeat.

**HOW SUPPLIED:** Tab: (Ethinyl Estradiol-Levonorgestrel) 0.03mg-0.15mg

**CONTRAINDICATIONS:** Thrombophlebitis, DVT or thromboembolic disorders, pregnancy, cerebrovascular or coronary artery disease, undiagnosed abnormal genital bleeding, cholestatic jaundice of pregnancy or jaundice with prior pill use, hepatic adenomas or carcinomas, breast cancer or other estrogen-dependent neoplasia.

**WARNINGS/PRECAUTIONS:** Cigarette smoking increases risk of serious cardiovascular side effects. This risk increases with age (especially >35 yrs) and heavy smoking. Increased risk of MI, vascular disease, thromboembolism, stroke and gallbladder disease. Retinal thrombosis, hepatic neoplasia, carcinoma of breast and reproductive organs reported. May cause glucose intolerance. May increase BP, elevate LDL levels or cause other lipid changes, fluid retention, breakthrough bleeding, and spotting. May cause or exacerbate migraine. May develop visual changes with contact lens. Increased risk of MI with HTN, hyperlipidemia, obesity, and diabetes. Discontinue if develop jaundice, significant depression or ophthalmic irregularities. Perform annual physical exam. Use before menarche is not indicated. May affect certain endocrine, LFTs and blood components.

**ADVERSE REACTIONS:** Nausea, vomiting, breakthrough bleeding, spotting, amenorrhea, migraine, depression, vaginal candidiasis, edema, weight changes.

**INTERACTIONS:** Reduced effects, increased breakthrough bleeding, and menstrual irregularities with rifampin, barbiturates, phenylbutazone, phenytoin, and possibly with griseofulvin, ampicillin, and tetracyclines.

**PREGNANCY:** Category X, not for use in nursing.

## LEVLITE RX

levonorgestrel - ethinyl estradiol (Berlex)

**THERAPEUTIC CLASS:** Estrogen/progestogen combination

**INDICATIONS:** Prevention of pregnancy.

**DOSAGE:** *Adults:* Start 1st Sunday after menses begins or the 1st day of menses. 1 tab qd for 28 days, then repeat.

**HOW SUPPLIED:** Tab: (Ethinyl Estradiol-Levonorgestrel) 0.02mg-0.1mg

**CONTRAINDICATIONS:** Thrombophlebitis, DVT or thromboembolic disorders, pregnancy, cerebrovascular or CAD, undiagnosed abnormal genital bleeding, cholestatic jaundice of pregnancy or jaundice with prior pill use, hepatic adenomas or carcinomas, active liver disease (as long as liver function has not returned to normal), breast cancer or other estrogen-dependent neoplasia, thrombogenic valvulopathies, thrombogenic rhythm disorders, diabetes with vascular involvement, uncontrolled HTN.

**WARNINGS/PRECAUTIONS:** Cigarette smoking increases risk of serious cardiovascular side effects. This risk increases with age (especially >35 yrs) and heavy smoking. Increased risk of MI, vascular disease, thromboembolism, stroke and gallbladder disease. Retinal thrombosis, hepatic neoplasia, carcinoma of breast and reproductive organs reported. May cause glucose intolerance. May increase BP, elevate LDL levels or cause other lipid changes, fluid retention, breakthrough bleeding, and spotting. May cause or exacerbate migraine. May develop visual changes with contact lens. Diarrhea and/or vomiting may reduce absorption. Increased risk of MI with HTN, hyperlipidemia, obesity, and diabetes. Discontinue if develop jaundice, significant depression or ophthalmic irregularities. Perform annual physical exam. Use before menarche is not indicated. May affect certain endocrine, LFTs and blood components.

**ADVERSE REACTIONS:** Nausea, vomiting, breakthrough bleeding, spotting, amenorrhea, migraine, depression, vaginal candidiasis, edema, weight changes.

**INTERACTIONS:** Reduced effects, increased breakthrough bleeding, and menstrual irregularities with rifampin, barbiturates, phenylbutazone, phenytoin, griseofulvin, topiramate, some protease inhibitors, modafinil, ampicillin, tetracyclines, and possibly with St. John's wort. Troleandomycin may increase risk of intrahepatic cholestasis. Ascorbic acid, APAP, CYP3A4 inhibitors (eg, indinavir, fluconazole, troleandomycin), atorvastatin may increase plasma levels. Increased plasma levels of cyclosporine, theophylline, and corticosteroids.

**PREGNANCY:** Category X, not for use in nursing.

## LEVOTHROID RX

levothyroxine sodium (Forest)

**THERAPEUTIC CLASS:** Thyroid replacement hormone

**INDICATIONS:** Hypothyroidism. As a pituitary TSH suppressant for nonendemic goiter and for chronic lymphocytic thyroiditis. Diagnostic agent in suppression tests to differentiate mild hyperthyroidism or thyroid gland autonomy. Adjunct therapy with antithyroid drugs to treat thyrotoxicosis. Adjunct to surgery and radioiodine therapy for TSH-dependent thyroid cancer.

**DOSAGE:** *Adults:* Hypothyroidism: Usual: 100-200mcg/day. Endocrine/Cardiovascular Complications: Initial: 50mcg/day. Titrate: Increase by 50mcg/day every 2-4 weeks until euthyroid. Hypothyroid with Angina: Initial: 25mcg/day. Titrate: Increase by 25-50mcg every 2-4 weeks until euthyroid.

*Pediatrics:* Hypothyroidism: >12 yrs: Usual: 100-200mcg/day. 6-12 yrs: 4-5mcg/kg/day. 1-5 yrs: 5-6mcg/kg/day. 6-12 months: 6-8mcg/kg/day. 0-6 months: 10-15mcg/kg/day. May crush tab and sprinkle over food (applesauce) or mix with 5-10mL water, formula (non-soy), or breast milk.

**HOW SUPPLIED:** Tab: 25mcg*, 50mcg*, 75mcg*, 88mcg*, 100mcg*, 112mcg*, 125mcg*, 137mcg*, 150mcg*, 175mcg*, 200mcg*, 300mcg* *scored

**CONTRAINDICATIONS:** Untreated thyrotoxicosis, acute MI, and uncorrected adrenal insufficiency.

**WARNINGS/PRECAUTIONS:** Do not use in the treatment of obesity; larger doses in euthyroid patients can cause serious or even life threatening toxicity. Caution with cardiovascular disease, HTN. May aggravate diabetes mellitus or insipidus and adrenal cortical insufficiency. Excessive doses in infants may produce craniosynostosis. Add glucocorticoid with myxedema coma.

**ADVERSE REACTIONS:** Lactose hypersensitivity, transient partial hair loss in children.

**INTERACTIONS:** Monitor insulin and oral hypoglycemic requirements. May potentiate anticoagulant effects of warfarin; adjust warfarin dose and monitor PT/INR. Increased adrenergic effects of catecholamines; caution with CAD. Decreased absorption with cholestyramine and colestipol; space dosing by 4-5 hrs. Estrogens increase thyroxine-binding globulin; increase in thyroid dose may be needed. Large dose may cause life-threatening toxicities with sympathomimetic amines. Avoid mixing crushed tabs with foods/formula with large amounts of iron, soybean or fiber.



**PREGNANCY:** Category A, caution in nursing.

## LEVOXYL
levothyroxine sodium (King)

RX

**THERAPEUTIC CLASS:** Thyroid replacement hormone

**INDICATIONS:** Hypothyroidism. As a pituitary TSH suppressant in the treatment and prevention of euthyroid goiters, including thyroid nodules, lymphocytic thyroiditis, and multinodular goiter. Adjunct to surgery and radioiodine therapy for thyrotropin-dependent well-differentiated thyroid cancer.

**DOSAGE:** *Adults:* Take in the AM at least one-half hour before food. Hypothyroid: Usual: 1.7mcg/kg/day. >200mcg/day (seldom). >50 yrs/<50 yrs with Cardiac Disease: Initial: 25-50mcg/day. Titrate: Increase by 12.5-25mcg/day every 6-8 weeks until euthyroid. Elderly with Cardiac Disease: Initial: 12.5-25mcg/day. Titrate: Increase by 12.5-25mcg/day every 4-6 weeks until euthyroid. Severe Hypothyroidism: Initial: 12.5-25mcg/day. Titrate: Increase by 25mcg/day every 2-4 weeks until euthyroid. Pregnancy: May increase dose requirements. Subclinical Hypothyroidism: Lower doses required.

*Pediatrics:* Take in the AM at least one-half hour before food. Hypothyroidism: 0-3 months: 10-15mcg/kg/day. 3-6 months: 8-10mcg/kg/day. 6-12 months: 6-8mcg/kg/day. 1-5 yrs: 5-6mcg/kg/day. 6-12 yrs: 4-5mcg/kg/day. >12 yrs: 2-3mcg/kg/day. Growth/Puberty Complete: 1.7mcg/kg/day. Cardiac Risk: Initial: Use lower dose. Titrate: Increase dose every 4-6 weeks until euthyroid. Infants with Serum $T_4$ <5mcg/dL: Initial: 50mcg/day. Chronic/Severe Hypothyroidism: Children: Initial: 25mcg/day. Titrate: Increase by 25mcg/day every 2-4 weeks until desired effect. Minimize Hyperactivity in Older Children: Initial: Give 1/4 of full replacement dose. Titrate: Increase by same amount weekly until full dose achieved. May crush tab and mix with 5-10mL water.

**HOW SUPPLIED:** Tab: 25mcg*, 50mcg*, 75mcg*, 88mcg*, 100mcg*, 112mcg*, 125mcg*, 137mcg*, 150mcg*, 175mcg*, 200mcg*, 300mcg* *scored

**CONTRAINDICATIONS:** Untreated thyrotoxicosis, acute MI, and uncorrected adrenal insufficiency.

**WARNINGS/PRECAUTIONS:** Do not use in the treatment of obesity; larger doses in euthyroid patients can cause serious or even life threatening toxicity. Caution with cardiovascular disease, CAD, adrenal insufficiency, and the elderly with risk of occult cardiac disease. Carefully titrate dose to avoid over or under treatment. Decreased bone mineral density with long term use. Caution with nontoxic diffuse goiter or nodular thyroid disease. With adrenal insufficiency supplement with glucocorticoids before therapy.

**ADVERSE REACTIONS:** Pseudotumor cerebri in children reported. Seizures (rare), hypersensitivity reactions, dysphagia, choking, gagging, hyperthyroidism (increased appetite, weight loss, heat intolerance, hyperactivity, tremors, palpitations, tachycardia, diarrhea, vomiting, hair loss).

**INTERACTIONS:** Sympathomimetics may increase risk of coronary insufficiency with CAD. Upward dose adjustments needed for insulin and oral hypoglycemic agents. Decreased absorption with soybean flour (infant formula), cottonseed meal, walnuts, and fiber. May potentiate oral anticoagulant effects; adjust dose and monitor PT/INR. May decrease levels and effects of digitalis glycosides. Cholestyramine, colestipol, ferrous sulfate, aluminum hydroxide, sodium polystyrene, soybean flour, sucralfate may decrease absorption. Reduced TSH secretion with dopamine/dopamine agonists, glucocorticoids, octreotide. Decreased thyroid hormone secretion with aminoglutethimide, amiodarone, iodine (including iodine-containing radiographic contrast agents), lithium, methimazole, PTU, sulfonamides, tolbutamide. Increased thyroid hormone secretion with amiodarone, iodide (including iodine-containing radiographic contrast agents). Decreased $T_4$ absorption with antacids (aluminum & magnesium hydroxides), simethicone, bile acid sequestrants (cholestyramine, colestipol), calcium carbonate, cation exchange resins (kayexalate), ferrous sulfate, sucralfate. Increased serum TBG concentration with clofibrate, estrogens, heroin/methadone, 5-FU, mitotane, tamoxifen. Decreased serum TBG concentration with androgens/anabolic steroids, asparaginase, glucocorticoids, nicotinic acid (slow-release). Protein-binding site displacement with furosemide, heparin, hydantoins, NSAIDs, salicylates. Increased hepatic metabolism with carbamazepine, hydantoins, phenobarbital, rifampin. Decreased conversion of $T_4$ to $T_3$ levels with amiodarone, β-adrenergic antagonists (propranolol >160mg/day), glucocorticoids (dexamethasone >4mg/day), PTU. Additive effects of both agents with antidepressants. Interferon-(alpha) may cause development of antithyroid microsomal antibodies causing transient hypothyroidism, hyperthyroidism, or both. Interleukin

**PREGNANCY:** Category A, caution in nursing.

## LEVULAN KERASTICK RX

aminolevulinic acid (Dusa)

**THERAPEUTIC CLASS:** Protoporphyrin precursor

**INDICATIONS:** Adjunct to BLU-U blue light photodynamic therapy illuminator, for treatment of non-hyperkeratotic actinic keratoses of the face or scalp.

**DOSAGE:** *Adults:* Apply directly to target lesion. After 14-18 hrs, expose area to BLU-U blue light photodynamic illumination. May repeat treatment after 8 weeks if lesions not completely resolved.

**HOW SUPPLIED:** Sol: 20% [1 app, 6 app]

**CONTRAINDICATIONS:** Cutaneous photosensitivity at wavelengths of 400-450nm, porphyria, allergy to porphyrins.

**WARNINGS/PRECAUTIONS:** After application, avoid sunlight or bright indoor light. Application to perilesional areas of photodamaged skin may cause photosensitization. Avoid eyes, periorbital area, and mucous membranes.

**ADVERSE REACTIONS:** Scaling/crusting, erythema, itching, edema, stinging, ulceration, bleeding, vesiculation, hypo/hyperpigmentation, pustules, erosion.

**INTERACTIONS:** Possible increased photosensitivity with photosensitizers (eg, griseofulvin, thiazide diuretics, sulfonylureas, phenothiazines, sulfonamides, tetracyclines).

**PREGNANCY:** Category C, caution in nursing.

## LEXAPRO RX

escitalopram oxalate (Forest)

**Antidepressants increased the risk of suicidal thinking and behavior (suicidality) in short-term studies in children and adolescents with Major Depressive Disorder (MDD) and other psychiatric disorders. Escitalopram is not approved for use in pediatric patients.**

**THERAPEUTIC CLASS:** Selective serotonin reuptake inhibitor

**INDICATIONS:** Treatment of MDD and generalized anxiety disorder (GAD).

**DOSAGE:** *Adults:* Initial: 10mg qd, in am or pm. Titrate: May increase to 20mg after a minimum of 1 week. Elderly/Hepatic Impairment: 10mg qd. Re-evaluate periodically.

**HOW SUPPLIED:** Sol: 5mg/5mL [240mL]; Tab: 5mg, 10mg*, 20mg* *scored

**CONTRAINDICATIONS:** Concomitant MAOI or pimozide therapy.

**WARNINGS/PRECAUTIONS:** Avoid abrupt withdrawal. Activation of mania/hypomania, hyponatremia reported. SIADH reported with citalopram. Caution with history of mania or seizures, hepatic impairment, severe renal impairment, conditions that alter metabolism or hemodynamic responses, suicidal tendencies. May impair mental/physical abilities. Consider tapering dose during 3rd trimester of pregnancy.

**ADVERSE REACTIONS:** Nausea, insomnia, ejaculation disorder, increased sweating, somnolence, fatigue, diarrhea.

**INTERACTIONS:** See Contraindications. Avoid alcohol, citalopram, or within 14 days of MAOI therapy. Caution with other CNS drugs, lithium, carbamazepine, cimetidine, drugs metabolized by CYP2D6 (eg, desipramine). Increased risk of bleeding with NSAIDs, aspirin, warfarin. May increase metoprolol levels which leads to decreased cardioselectivity. Rare reports of weakness, hyperreflexia, incoordination with an SSRI and sumatriptan. Serotonin syndrome reported with linezolid.

**PREGNANCY:** Category C, not for use in nursing.

## LEXXEL RX

felodipine - enalapril maleate (AstraZeneca LP)

**ACE inhibitors can cause death/injury to developing fetus during 2nd and 3rd trimesters. Stop therapy if pregnancy detected.**

**THERAPEUTIC CLASS:** ACE inhibitor/calcium channel blocker (dihydropyridine)

**INDICATIONS:** Treatment of hypertension; not for initial therapy.

**DOSAGE:** *Adults:* For Combination Therapy from Monotherapy (felodipine or enalapril): Initial: One 5mg-5mg tab qd. Titrate: If inadequate control, may increase after 1-2 weeks to two 5mg-5mg tabs qd, and then to four 5mg-2.5mg tabs qd. If receiving both felodipine and enalapril separately, may give same component doses. Elderly/Hepatic Impairment: Initial: 2.5mg felodipine qd. CrCl <30mL/min: Initial: 2.5mg enalapril qd. Take without food or with light meal. Swallow tab whole.

**HOW SUPPLIED:** Tab, Extended Release: (Enalapril-Felodipine) 5mg-5mg

**CONTRAINDICATIONS:** History of ACE inhibitor associated angioedema and hereditary or idiopathic angioedema.

**WARNINGS/PRECAUTIONS:** D/C if angioedema, jaundice, or if marked LFT elevation occur. Risk of hyperkalemia with DM, renal dysfunction. ACE inhibitor-induced cough reported. Monitor WBCs in renal or collagen vascular disease. Anaphylactoid reactions reported. Fetal/neonatal morbidity and death reported. Monitor for hypotension in high risk patients (heart failure, surgery/anesthesia, hyponatremia, high dose diuretic therapy, severe volume and/or salt depletion, etc.). Caution with CHF, obstruction to left ventricle outflow tract, renal dysfunction, and renal artery stenosis. More reports of angioedema in blacks than non-blacks. Peripheral edema reported with felodipine. Caution with hepatic dysfunction or elderly; increased felodipine levels. Mild gingival hyperplasia reported.

**ADVERSE REACTIONS:** Edema, headache, dizziness, cough.

**INTERACTIONS:** May increase lithium levels. Hypotension risk with diuretics. May further decrease renal function with NSAIDs. Risk of hyperkalemia with $K^+$-sparing diuretics, $K^+$-containing salt substitutes, or $K^+$ supplements. Augmented effect by antihypertensives that cause renin release (eg, diuretics). CYP3A4 inhibitors (eg, itraconazole, ketoconazole, erythromycin, grapefruit juice, cimetidine) may increase plasma levels. Levels decreased with long-term anticonvulsant therapy. May increase metoprolol levels. Peak levels doubled and trough levels halved when taken with food.

**PREGNANCY:** Category C (1st trimester) and D (2nd and 3rd trimesters), not for use in nursing.

## LIALDA

mesalamine (Shire) — RX

**THERAPEUTIC CLASS:** Anti-Inflammatory Agent

**INDICATIONS:** Induction of remission in adult patients with active, mild to moderate ulcerative colitis.

**DOSAGE:** *Adults:* 2-4 tabs qd with meals for up to 8 weeks. Max: 2.4g or 4.8g per day.

**HOW SUPPLIED:** Tab, Delayed Release: 1.2g

**WARNINGS/PRECAUTIONS:** Prolonged gastric retention with pyloric stenosis, delaying mesalamine release in the colon. Caution with sulfasalazine allergy. May cause acute intolerance syndrome, if suspected prompt withdrawal is required. Caution with cardiac hypersensitivity reactions, myocarditis and pericarditis reported. Renal impairment, including minimal change nephropathy, and acute or chronic interstitial nephritis reported; caution with known renal dysfunction. Monitor renal function prior to therapy and periodically after.

**ADVERSE REACTIONS:** Headache, flatulence.

**INTERACTIONS:** Concurrent use with nephrotoxic agents (eg, NSAIDs) may increase risk of renal reactions. Concurrent azathioprine or 6-mercaptopurine can increase potential for blood disorders.

**PREGNANCY:** Category B, caution in nursing.

## LIBRAX

clidinium bromide - chlordiazepoxide HCl (Valeant) — RX

**THERAPEUTIC CLASS:** Benzodiazepine/anticholinergic

**INDICATIONS:** Adjunct treatment of irritable bowel syndrome (IBS), acute enterocolitis and peptic ulcer.

**DOSAGE:** *Adults:* Usual/Maint: 1-2 caps tid-qid ac and hs. Elderly/Debilitated: Initial: 2 caps/day and increase gradually, if needed.

**HOW SUPPLIED:** Cap: (Chlordiazepoxide-Clidinium) 5mg-2.5mg

**CONTRAINDICATIONS:** Glaucoma, prostatic hypertrophy, benign bladder neck obstruction.

**WARNINGS/PRECAUTIONS:** Risk of congenital malformations during first trimester of pregnancy; avoid use. Avoid abrubt withdrawal. Paradoxical reactions reported in psychiatric patients. Caution with depression, renal or hepatic dysfunction, the elderly. Inhibition of lactation may occur.

**ADVERSE REACTIONS:** Drowsiness, ataxia, confusion, skin eruptions, extrapyramidal symptoms, dry mouth, nausea, constipation, altered libido, blood dyscrasias, jaundice, hepatic dysfunction.

**INTERACTIONS:** Avoid with other psychotropics; if combination is indicated, use caution especially with MAOIs and phenothiazines. Caution with alcohol, other CNS depressants. Altered coagulation effects with oral anticoagulants.

**PREGNANCY:** Not for use in pregnancy; safety in nursing is not known.

## LIBRIUM

chlordiazepoxide HCl (Valeant)

CIV

**THERAPEUTIC CLASS:** Benzodiazepine

**INDICATIONS:** Management of anxiety disorders and short-term relief of anxiety symptoms, withdrawal symptoms of acute alcoholism, and preoperative apprehension and anxiety.

**DOSAGE:** *Adults:* Mild-Moderate Anxiety: 5-10mg tid-qid. Severe Anxiety: 20-25mg tid-qid. Alcohol Withdrawal: 50-100mg; repeat until agitation controlled. Max: 300mg/day. Preoperative Anxiety: 5-10mg PO tid-qid on days prior to surgery. Elderly/Debilitated: 5mg bid-qid.
*Pediatrics:* > 6 yrs: 5mg bid-qid. May increase to 10mg bid-tid.

**HOW SUPPLIED:** Cap: 5mg, 10mg, 25mg

**WARNINGS/PRECAUTIONS:** Avoid in pregnancy. Paradoxical reactions reported in psychiatric patients and in hyperactive aggressive pediatrics. Caution with porphyria, renal or hepatic dysfunction. Reduce dose in elderly, debilitated. Avoid abrupt withdrawal after extended therapy.

**ADVERSE REACTIONS:** Drowsiness, ataxia, confusion, skin eruptions, edema, nausea, constipation, extrapyramidal symptoms, libido changes, EEG changes.

**INTERACTIONS:** Additive effects with CNS depressants and alcohol. Avoid other psychotropic agents.

**PREGNANCY:** Not for use in pregnancy, safety in nursing not known.

## LIDEX

fluocinonide (Medicis)

RX

**OTHER BRAND NAMES:** Lidex-E (Medicis)

**THERAPEUTIC CLASS:** Corticosteroid

**INDICATIONS:** Corticosteroid responsive dermatoses.

**DOSAGE:** *Adults:* Apply bid-qid. May use occlusive dressing for psoriasis or recalcitrant conditions; discontinue dressings if infection develops.
*Pediatrics:* Apply bid-qid. May use occlusive dressing for psoriasis or recalcitrant conditions; discontinue dressings if infection develops.

**HOW SUPPLIED:** (Lidex) Cre, Gel, Oint: 0.05% [15g, 30g, 60g]; Sol: 0.05% [60mL]; (Lidex-E) Cre: 0.05% [15g, 30g, 60g]

**WARNINGS/PRECAUTIONS:** May produce reversible HPA axis suppression, manifestations of Cushing's syndrome, hyperglycemia, and glucosuria. Caution when applied to large surface areas or under occlusive dressings. Use appropriate antifungal or antibacterial agent with dermatological infections; discontinue if infection does not clear. Pediatrics may be more susceptible to systemic toxicity. Avoid eyes. Discontinue if irritation occurs.

**ADVERSE REACTIONS:** Burning, itching, irritation, dryness, folliculitis, hypertrichosis, acneiform eruptions, hypopigmentation, perioral dermatitis, allergic contact dermatitis, skin maceration, secondary infection, skin atrophy, striae, miliaria.

**PREGNANCY:** Category C, caution in nursing.

## LIDOCAINE OINTMENT
lidocaine (Fougera)

RX

**THERAPEUTIC CLASS:** Acetamide local anesthetic

**INDICATIONS:** Topical anesthesia of the oropharynx. Anesthetic lubricant for intubation. Temporary relief of pain associated with minor burns, abrasions, and insect bites.

**DOSAGE:** *Adults:* Apply up to 5g (6 inches)/application. Max: 17-20g/day. *Pediatrics:* Determine dose by age and weight. Max: 4.5mg/kg.

**HOW SUPPLIED:** Oint: 5% [35g]

**WARNINGS/PRECAUTIONS:** Reduce dose in elderly, debilitated, acutely ill, and children. Avoid excessive dosage or too frequent administration; may result in serious adverse effects requiring resuscitative measures. Caution with heart block and severe shock. Extreme caution if mucosa is traumatized or sepsis is present in the area of application; risk of rapid systemic absorption.

**ADVERSE REACTIONS:** Lightheadedness, nervousness, confusion, euphoria, dizziness, drowsiness, blurred vision, tremors, convulsions, respiratory depression, bradycardia, hypotension, urticaria, edema, anaphylactoid reactions.

**PREGNANCY:** Category B, caution in nursing.



## LIDODERM PATCH
lidocaine (Endo)

RX

**THERAPEUTIC CLASS:** Acetamide local anesthetic

**INDICATIONS:** Relief of pain associated with postherpetic neuralgia.

**DOSAGE:** *Adults:* Apply to intact skin, cover most painful area. Apply up to 3 patches, once for up to 12 hrs within 24-hr period. May cut patches into smaller sizes before removal of the release liner. Debilitated/Impaired Elimination: Treat smaller areas. Remove if irritation or burning occurs; may reapply when irritation subsides.

**HOW SUPPLIED:** Patch: 5% [30s]

**WARNINGS/PRECAUTIONS:** Serious adverse events may occur in children or pets if ingested. Increased risk of toxicity in severe hepatic disease. Avoid broken or inflamed skin, eye contact, larger area or longer duration than recommended. Increased levels with application of >3 patches, small patients.

**ADVERSE REACTIONS:** Application site reactions such as: erythema, edema, bruising, papules, vesicles, discoloration, depigmentation, burning sensation, pruritus, dermatitis, petechia, blisters, exfoliation, abnormal sensation, irritation.

**INTERACTIONS:** Additive toxic effects with concomitant Class I antiarrhythmics (eg, tocainide, mexiletine). Consider total amount absorbed from all formulations with other local anesthetics.

**PREGNANCY:** Category B, caution in nursing.

## LIMBITROL
chlordiazepoxide - amitriptyline HCl (Valeant)

CIV

**Antidepressants increased the risk of suicidal thinking and behavior (suicidality) in short-term studies in children and adolescents with Major Depressive Disorder (MDD) and other psychiatric disorders. Chlordiazepoxide-Amitriptyline is not approved for use in pediatric patients.**

**OTHER BRAND NAMES:** Limbitrol DS (Valeant)

**THERAPEUTIC CLASS:** Benzodiazepine/tricyclic antidepressant

**INDICATIONS:** Moderate to severe depression associated with moderate to severe anxiety.

**DOSAGE:** *Adults:* Initial: 3-4 tabs/day in divided doses. Max: (Limbitrol DS) 6 tabs/day. Elderly: Start at low end of dosing range.

**HOW SUPPLIED:** (Chlordiazepoxide-Amitriptyline) Tab: (Limbitrol) 5mg-12.5mg, (Limbitrol DS) 10mg-25mg

**CONTRAINDICATIONS:** MAOI use during or within 14 days, acute recovery period following MI.

**WARNINGS/PRECAUTIONS:** Caution with urinary retention, angle-closure glaucoma, cardiovascular disorder, history of seizures, hyperthyroidism, renal or hepatic dysfunction. May produce arrhythmia, sinus tachycardia, and conduction time prolongation. May impair mental alertness. Caution in elderly. Avoid abrupt withdrawal. Monitor blood and LFT's periodically with long-term therapy.

**ADVERSE REACTIONS:** Drowsiness, dry mouth, constipation, blurred vision, dizziness, bloating, anorexia, fatigue, weakness, restlessness, lethargy.

**INTERACTIONS:** May antagonize antihypertensives (eg, guanethidine). Caution with thyroid agents. Additive effects may occur with psychotropics. Increased levels with CYP2D6 inhibitors (eg, quinidine, cimetidine, SSRIs) and enzyme substrates (eg, phenothiazines, propafenone, flecainide). Avoid within 5 weeks of fluoxetine use. Additive sedative effects with alcohol and CNS depressants. Severe constipation with anticholinergics.



**PREGNANCY:** Not for use in pregnancy or nursing.

## LIMBREL RX
flavocoxid (Primus)

**THERAPEUTIC CLASS:** Flavonoid

**INDICATIONS:** Clinical dietary management of the metabolic processes of osteoarthritis.

**DOSAGE:** *Adults*: 250-500mg q12h for total daily dose of 500-1000mg/day. May increase to 2 or more caps q12h under physician supervision.

**HOW SUPPLIED:** Cap: 250mg, 500mg

**CONTRAINDICATIONS:** Hypersensitivity to flavocoxid or flavonoids (eg, colored fruits and vegetables, dark chocolate, tea, red wine, Brazil nuts).

**ADVERSE REACTIONS:** Varicose veins, hypertension, fluid accumulation in knee, psoriasis, nausea, vomiting, rash, itching, synovitis, joint pain, fever.

**PREGNANCY:** Not recommended for pregnant or lactating patients..

## LINCOCIN RX
lincomycin HCl (Pharmacia & Upjohn)

**Diarrhea, colitis, pseudomembranous colitis reported; may begin up to several weeks after discontinuation. Reserve for serious infections where less toxic antimicrobials are inappropriate.**

**THERAPEUTIC CLASS:** *Streptomyces lincolnensis* derivative

**INDICATIONS:** Treatment of serious infections due to streptococci, pneumococci, and staphylococci. Reserve for PCN allergy or if PCN is inappropriate.

**DOSAGE:** *Adults:* IM: Serious Infection: 600mg q24h. More Severe Infection: 600mg q12h or more often. IV: Dose depends on severity. Serious Infection: 600mg-1g q8-12h. More Severe Infection: Increase dose. Infuse over >1 hr. Life-Threatening Situation: Up to 8g/day has been given. Max: 8g/day. Severe Renal Dysfunction: 25-30% of normal dose.

*Pediatrics:* >1 month: IM: Serious Infection: 10mg/kg q24h. More Severe Infection: 10mg/kg q12h or more often. IV: 10-20mg/kg/day, depending on severity infused in divided doses as described for adults. Severe Renal Dysfunction: 25-30% of normal dose.

**HOW SUPPLIED:** Inj: 300mg/mL

**CONTRAINDICATIONS:** Clindamycin hypersensitivity.

**WARNINGS/PRECAUTIONS:** May be inadequate for meningitis treatment. Contains benzyl alcohol. Monitor elderly for change in bowel frequency. Caution with severe renal/hepatic dysfunction, or with history of GI disease (eg, colitis), asthma, significant allergies. Superinfections may occur. Perform periodic CBC, LFTs, and renal function tests with prolonged therapy. Do not administer undiluted as IV bolus. Cardiopulmonary arrest and hypotension with too rapid IV administration.

**ADVERSE REACTIONS:** Glossitis, stomatitis, nausea, vomiting, diarrhea, colitis, pruritus, blood dyscrasias, hypersensitivity reactions, rash, urticaria, vaginitis, tinnitus, vertigo.

**INTERACTIONS:** Caution with neuromuscular blockers; may enhance effects. Possible antagonism with erythromycin; avoid concomitant use. Kaolin-pectin inhibits oral lincomycin.

**PREGNANCY:** Category C, not for use in nursing.

## LINDANE

RX

lindane (Alpharma)

L

**Only for patients who are intolerant or have failed 1st-line therapy with safer agents. Seizures and deaths reported with repeat or prolonged use. Caution in infants, children, elderly, those with other skin conditions, and those <50kg due to increased risk of neurotoxicity. Contraindicated in premature infants or those with uncontrolled seizure disorders. Instruct patients on proper use and inform that itching occurs after successful killing of scabies or lice.**

**THERAPEUTIC CLASS:** Ectoparasiticide/ovicide

**INDICATIONS:** (Lot) Treatment of *Sarcoptes scabiei* (scabies) resistant to other therapies. (Shampoo) Treatment of head and pubic lice resistant to or if intolerant to other therapies.

**DOSAGE:** *Adults:* (Lot) Apply 1-2oz to dry skin; rub in thoroughly. Apply to whole body from neck down. Wash off after 8-12 hrs. Apply only once. (Shampoo) Wash and dry hair with regular shampoo. Apply Lindane to hair without water. Add water after 4 minutes; lather then rinse immediately. Towel briskly. Remove nits with comb or tweezers. Use 1oz for short hair, 1.5oz for medium length hair, and 2oz for long hair. Max: 2oz/application. Retreat if lice remain after 7 days.
*Pediatrics:* (Lot) Apply (>6 yrs) 1-2oz or 1oz (<6 yrs) to dry skin; rub in thoroughly. Apply to whole body from neck down. Wash off after 8-12 hrs. Apply only once. (Shampoo) Wash and dry hair with regular shampoo. Apply Lindane to hair without water. Add water after 4 minutes; lather then rinse immediately. Towel briskly. Remove nits with comb or tweezers. Use 1oz for short hair, 1.5oz for medium length hair, and 2oz for long hair. Max: 2oz/application. Retreat if lice remain after 7 days.

**HOW SUPPLIED:** Lot, Shampoo: 1% [60mL, 480mL]

**CONTRAINDICATIONS:** Premature infants, Norwegian (crusted) scabies, skin conditions (eg, atopic dermatitis, psoriasis) that increase systemic absorption of the drug, uncontrolled seizure disorders.

**WARNINGS/PRECAUTIONS:** Adverse events with serious outcomes reported. Caution in those at increased risk of seizure (eg, HIV, head trauma, prior seizure, CNS tumor, severe hepatic cirrhosis, excessive alcohol use, abrupt alchol or sedative withdrawal). Give Medication Guide to each patient when dispensing. Avoid eyes and mouth. Do not use with open wounds, cuts, or scores. Use rubber gloves to apply.

**ADVERSE REACTIONS:** CNS stimulation, dizziness, convulsions.

**INTERACTIONS:** Avoid creams, ointments, oils, oil based hair dressings or conditioners; may enhance absorption. Caution with drugs that may lower seizure threshold (eg, antipsychotics, antidepressants, theophylline, cyclosporine, mycophenolate, tacrolimus, penicillins, imipenem, quinolones, chloroquine sulfate, pyrimethamine, isoniazid, meperidine, radiographic contrast agents, centrally active anticholinesterases, methocarbamol).

**PREGNANCY:** Category C, not for use in nursing.

## LIPITOR RX

atorvastatin calcium (Parke-Davis/Pfizer)

**THERAPEUTIC CLASS:** HMG-CoA reductase inhibitor

**INDICATIONS:** Adjunct to diet, to reduce total cholesterol (total-C), LDL-C, TG, and Apo B levels, and to increase HDL-C in primary hypercholesterolemia (heterozygous familial and nonfamilial) and mixed dyslipidemia (Types IIa and IIb). Adjunct to diet for elevated serum TG levels (Type IV). Treatment of primary dysbetalipoproteinemia (Type III) inadequately responding to diet. Adjunct to other lipid-lowering treatments or if treatments are unavailable, to reduce total-C and LDL-C in homozygous familial hypercholesterolemia. Adjunct to diet to lower total-C, LDL-C and apolipoprotein B in postmenarchal adolescents with heterozygous familial hypercholesterolemia. To reduce the risk of MI, revascularization procedures, and angina in adults without clinically evident CHD but with multiple risk factors for CHD. To reduce the risk of MI and stroke in patients with Type II DM, and without clinically evident CHD, but with multiple risk factors for CHD. In patients with clinically evident CHD to reduce the risk of non-fatal MI, fatal and non-fatal stroke, revascularization procedures, hospitalization for CHF, and angina.



**DOSAGE:** *Adults:* Hypercholesterolemia/Mixed Dyslipidemia: Initial: 10-20mg qd (or 40mg qd for LDL-C reduction >45%). Titrate: Adjust dose if needed at 2-4 week intervals. Usual: 10-80mg qd. Homozygous Familial Hypercholesterolemia: 10-80mg qd.
*Pediatrics:* Heterozygous Familial Hypercholesterolemia: 10-17 yrs (postmenarchal): Initial: 10mg/day. Titrate: Adjust dose if needed at intervals of ≥4 weeks. Max: 20mg/day.

**HOW SUPPLIED:** Tab: 10mg, 20mg, 40mg, 80mg

**CONTRAINDICATIONS:** Active liver disease, unexplained persistent elevations of serum transaminases, pregnancy, nursing mothers.

**WARNINGS/PRECAUTIONS:** Monitor LFTs prior to therapy, at 12 weeks or with dose elevation, and periodically thereafter. Reduce dose or withdraw if AST or ALT ≥3x ULN persist. Caution with heavy alcohol use and/or history of hepatic disease. D/C if markedly elevated CPK levels occur, if myopathy is diagnosed or suspected, or if predisposition to renal failure secondary to rhabdomyolysis. Caution in patients with recent stroke or TIA.

**ADVERSE REACTIONS:** Constipation, flatulence, dyspepsia, abdominal pain, transaminase and CK elevation in higher doses.

**INTERACTIONS:** Increases levels with erythromycin. Increases levels of oral contraceptives (norethindrone, ethinyl estradiol), digoxin. Monitor digoxin. Cyclosporine, fibric acid derivatives, niacin, erythromycin, and azole antifungals may increase risk of myopathy. Caution with drugs that decrease levels or activity of endogenous steroid hormones (eg, ketoconazole, spironolactone, cimetidine). Decreases levels with Maalox TC, but LDL-C reduction not altered. Colestipol decreases levels when coadministered, but greater LDL-C reduction with coadministration than when each given alone. Avoid fibrates.

**PREGNANCY:** Category X, not for use in nursing.

## LITHIUM CARBONATE

RX

lithium carbonate (Roxane)

**Lithium toxicity is related to serum lithium levels and can occur at doses close to therapeutic levels.**

**THERAPEUTIC CLASS:** Antimanic agents

**INDICATIONS:** Treatment of manic episodes of bipolar disorder and maintenance treatment of bipolar disorder.

**DOSAGE:** *Adults:* Acute Mania: 600mg tid to achieve effective serum levels of 1-1.5mEq/L; monitor levels twice a week until stabilized. Maint: 300mg tid-qid to maintain serum levels of 0.6-1.2 mEq/L; monitor levels every 2 months. Elderly: Reduce dose.
*Pediatrics:* >12 yrs: Acute Mania: 600mg tid. Effective serum levels are 1-1.5mEq/L; monitor levels twice a week until stabilized. Maint: 300mg tid-qid to maintain serum levels of 0.6-1.2mEq/L; monitor levels every 2 months.

**HOW SUPPLIED:** Cap: 150mg, 300mg, 600mg; Tab: 300mg

**CONTRAINDICATIONS:** Renal or cardiovascular disease, severe debilitation or dehydration, sodium depletion, and diuretic use.

**WARNINGS/PRECAUTIONS:** May cause fetal harm; if possible withdraw for at least the 1st trimester of pregnancy. Caution in the elderly. Maintain normal diet, adequate salt/fluid intake. Assess kidney function prior to and during therapy. May impair mental/physical abilities. Reduce dose or d/c with sweating, diarrhea, infection with elevated temperatures. Caution with thyroid disorders; monitor thyroid function. Chronic therapy associated with diminution of renal concentrating ability (eg, diabetes insipidus), glomerular and interstitial fibrosis, and nephron atrophy.

**ADVERSE REACTIONS:** Fine hand tremor, polyuria, mild thirst, nausea, incoordination, diarrhea, vomiting, drowsiness, muscular weakness.

**INTERACTIONS:** Risk of encephalopathic syndrome (eg, weakness, lethargy, fever, tremulousness, confusion, EPS) with haloperidol and other antipsychotics; discontinue therapy if such signs occur. May prolong effects of neuromuscular blockers. Increased levels with indomethacin, piroxicam and other NSAIDs. Increased risk of toxicity due to decreased clearance with diuretics and ACE inhibitors; contraindicated with diuretics.

**PREGNANCY:** Category D, not for use in nursing.

## LITHOBID

RX

lithium carbonate (JDS)

**Lithium toxicity is related to serum levels, and can occur at doses close to therapeutic levels.**

**THERAPEUTIC CLASS:** Antimanic agent

**INDICATIONS:** Treatment of manic episodes of manic-depressive illness.

**DOSAGE:** *Adults:* Acute Mania: Initial: 900mg bid or 600mg tid to achieve effective serum levels of 1-1.5mEq/L; monitor levels twice weekly until stabilized. Maint: 900-1200mg/day, given bid-tid to maintain serum levels of 0.6-1.2mEq/L; monitor levels every 2 months.
*Pediatrics:* >12 yrs: Acute Mania: Initial: 900mg bid or 600mg tid to achieve effective serum levels of 1-1.5mEq/L; monitor levels twice weekly until stabilized. Maint: 900-1200mg/day, given bid-tid to maintain serum levels of 0.6-1.2 mEq/L; monitor levels every 2 months.

**HOW SUPPLIED:** Tab, Extended Release: 300mg

**WARNINGS/PRECAUTIONS:** Avoid with significant renal or cardiovascular disease, severe debilitation, dehydration, or sodium depletion. Assess kidney function prior to and during therapy. Risk of encephalopathic syndrome (eg, weakness, lethargy, fever, tremulousness, confusion, EPS); discontinue therapy. May impair mental/physical abilities. Reduce dose or discontinue with

L

sweating, diarrhea, infection with elevated temperatures. Caution with hypothyroidism; may need supplemental therapy. Chronic therapy associated with diminution of renal concentrating ability, glomerular and interstitial fibrosis, and nephron atrophy.

**ADVERSE REACTIONS:** Fine hand tremor, polyuria, mild thirst, nausea, general discomfort, diarrhea, vomiting, drowsiness, muscular weakness.

**INTERACTIONS:** Avoid diuretics and ACE inhibitors; risk of lithium toxicity due to reduced renal clearance. May prolong effects of neuromuscular blockers. Decreased levels with acetazolamide, urea, xanthine preparations, and alkalinizing agents. May produce hypothyroidism with iodide preparations. Increased plasma levels with indomethacin, piroxicam, other NSAIDs. Increased risk of neurotoxic effects with carbamazepine and calcium channel blockers. Reduced renal clearance with metronidazole. Fluoxetine may increase and/or decrease lithium levels.

**PREGNANCY:** Category D, not for use in nursing.

## LIVOSTIN — RX

levocabastine HCl (Novartis Ophthalmics)

**THERAPEUTIC CLASS:** $H_1$ antagonist

**INDICATIONS:** Relief of signs and symptoms of seasonal allergic conjunctivitis.

**DOSAGE:** *Adults:* 1 drop qid.
*Pediatrics:* >12 yrs: 1 drop qid.

**HOW SUPPLIED:** Sus: 0.05% [5mL, 10mL]

**CONTRAINDICATIONS:** Do not use while wearing soft contact lenses.

**WARNINGS/PRECAUTIONS:** For topical use only.

**ADVERSE REACTIONS:** Transient stinging/burning, headache.

**PREGNANCY:** Category C, safety in nursing not known.

## LO/OVRAL — RX

norgestrel - ethinyl estradiol (Wyeth)

**OTHER BRAND NAMES:** Cryselle (Duramed) - Low-Ogestrel (Watson)

**THERAPEUTIC CLASS:** Estrogen/progestogen combination

**INDICATIONS:** Prevention of pregnancy.

**DOSAGE:** *Adults:* Start 1st Sunday after menses begins or the 1st day of menses. *21-day:* 1 tab qd for 21 days, stop 7 days, then repeat. *28-day:* 1 tab qd for 28 days, then repeat.

**HOW SUPPLIED:** Tab: (Ethinyl Estradiol-Norgestrel) 0.03mg-0.3mg

**CONTRAINDICATIONS:** Thrombophlebitis, DVT or thromboembolic disorders, pregnancy, cerebrovascular or coronary artery disease, undiagnosed abnormal genital bleeding, cholestatic jaundice of pregnancy or jaundice with prior pill use, hepatic adenomas or carcinomas, breast cancer or other estrogen-dependent neoplasia, thrombogenic valvulopathies, thrombogenic rhythm disorders, diabetes with vascular involvement, uncontrolled HTN, endometrium carcinoma, active liver disease if liver function has not returned to normal.

**WARNINGS/PRECAUTIONS:** Cigarette smoking increases risk of serious cardiovascular side effects. This risk increases with age (especially >35 yrs) and heavy smoking. Increased risk of MI, vascular disease, thromboembolism, stroke and gallbladder disease. Retinal thrombosis, hepatic neoplasia reported. May cause glucose intolerance. May increase BP, elevate LDL levels or cause other lipid changes, fluid retention, breakthrough bleeding, and spotting. May cause or exacerbate migraine. May develop visual changes with contact lens. Increased risk of MI with HTN, hyperlipidemia, obesity, and diabetes. Discontinue if develop jaundice, significant depression or ophthalmic irregularities. Perform annual physical exam. Use before menarche is not indicated. May affect certain endocrine, LFTs and blood components.

**ADVERSE REACTIONS:** Nausea, vomiting, breakthrough bleeding, spotting, amenorrhea, migraine, depression, vaginal candidiasis, edema, weight changes.

**INTERACTIONS:** Reduced effects, increased breakthrough bleeding, and menstrual irregularities with rifampin, rifabutin, barbiturates, phenylbutazone, phenytoin, griseofulvin, topiramate, some protease inhibitors, modafinil and possibly with St. John's wort, some penicillins, ampicillin and tetracylines. Increased levels with ascorbic acid and acetaminophen, indinavir, fluconazole, troleandomycin, and atorvastatin. May affect cyclosporine, theophylline and corticosteroid levels.

**PREGNANCY:** Category X, not for use in nursing.

## LOCOID RX
hydrocortisone butyrate (Ferndale)

**THERAPEUTIC CLASS:** Corticosteroid

**INDICATIONS:** (Cre, Oint) Corticosteroid responsive dermatoses. (Sol) Seborrheic dermatitis.

**DOSAGE:** *Adults:* (Cre, Oint) Apply bid-tid. May use occlusive dressings for psoriasis or recalcitrant conditions. D/C dressings if infection develops. (Sol) Apply bid-tid.
*Pediatrics:* (Cre, Oint) Apply bid-tid. May use occlusive dressings for psoriasis or recalcitrant conditions. D/C dressings if infection develops. (Sol) Apply bid-tid.

**HOW SUPPLIED:** Cre, Oint: 0.1% [15g, 45g]; Sol: 0.1% [20mL, 60mL]

**WARNINGS/PRECAUTIONS:** May produce reversible HPA axis suppression, manifestations of Cushing's syndrome, hyperglycemia, and glucosuria. D/C if irritation occurs. Use appropriate antifungal or antibacterial agent with dermatological infections. Peds may be more susceptible to systemic toxicity. Caution when applied to large surface areas. Avoid contact with eyes. Limit to least amount compatible with an effective therapeutic regimen. Chronic corticosteroid therapy may interfere with the growth and development of children.

**ADVERSE REACTIONS:** Burning, itching, irritation, dryness, folliculitis, hypertrichosis, acneiform eruptions, hypopigmentation, perioral dermatitis, allergic dermatitis, skin maceration, secondary infection, skin atrophy, striae, miliaria.

**PREGNANCY:** Category C, caution in nursing.

## LODRANE 24 RX
brompheniramine maleate (ECR)

**THERAPEUTIC CLASS:** Alkylamine Antihistamine

**INDICATIONS:** Temporary relief of seasonal and perennial allergic rhinitis and vasomotor rhinitis.

**DOSAGE:** *Adults:* 12-24mg qd.
*Pediatrics:* ≥12 yrs: 12-24mg qd. 6-12 yrs: 12mg qd.

**HOW SUPPLIED:** Cap, Extended Release: 12mg

**CONTRAINDICATIONS:** Nursing mothers, patients taking MAOIs, narrow angle glaucoma, urinary retention, peptic ulcer, and during an asthmatic attack.

**WARNINGS/PRECAUTIONS:** Caution with HTN, DM, ischemic heart disease, hyperthyroidism, bronchial asthma, increased IOP, prostatic hypertrophy, CVD, and elderly. May impair mental/physical abilities.

**ADVERSE REACTIONS:** Drowsiness, confusion, restlessness, nausea, vomiting, rash, vertigo, palpitation, anorexia, dizziness, headache, insomnia, anxiety, tension, excitability.

**INTERACTIONS:** See Contraindications. MAOIs and TCA's may prolong and intensify the anticholinergic effects of antihistamines. Concomitant use of antihistamines with alcohol, TCA's, barbiturates, other CNS depressants may have an additive effect.

**PREGNANCY:** Category C, not for use in nursing.

## LOESTRIN RX

ferrous fumarate - ethinyl estradiol - norethindrone acetate

(Duramed/Warner Chilcott)

**OTHER BRAND NAMES:** Junel 1/20 (Barr) - Junel 1.5/30 (Barr) - Junel Fe 1/20 (Barr) - Junel Fe 1.5/30 (Barr) - Microgestin Fe 1/20 (Watson) - Microgestin Fe 1.5/30 (Watson) - Loestrin 1/20 (Duramed/Warner Chilcott) - Loestrin 1.5/30 (Duramed/Warner Chilcott) - Loestrin Fe 1/20 (Duramed/Warner Chilcott) - Loestrin Fe 1.5/30 (Duramed/Warner Chilcott)

**THERAPEUTIC CLASS:** Estrogen/progestogen combination

**INDICATIONS:** Prevention of pregnancy.

**DOSAGE:** *Adults:* Start 1st Sunday after menses begin or the 1st day of menses. *21-day:* 1 tab qd for 21 days, stop 7 days, then repeat. *28-day:* 1 tab qd for 28 days, then repeat.

**HOW SUPPLIED:** (Ethinyl Estradiol-Norethindrone) Tab: (1/20) 20mcg-1mg, (1.5/30) 30mcg-1.5mg; (Fe 1/20) 20mcg-1mg and 75mg ferrous fumarate, (Fe 1.5/30) 30mcg-1.5mg and 75mg ferrous fumarate

**CONTRAINDICATIONS:** Thrombophlebitis, DVT or thromboembolic disorders, pregnancy, cerebrovascular or coronary artery disease, undiagnosed abnormal genital bleeding, cholestatic jaundice of pregnancy or jaundice with prior pill use, hepatic adenomas or carcinomas, breast cancer or other estrogen-dependent neoplasia.

**WARNINGS/PRECAUTIONS:** Cigarette smoking increases risk of serious cardiovascular side effects. This risk increases with age (especially >35 yrs) and heavy smoking. Increased risk of MI, vascular disease, thromboembolism, stroke, and gallbladder disease. Retinal thrombosis, hepatic neoplasia, carcinoma of breast and reproductive organs reported. May cause glucose intolerance. May increase BP, elevate LDL levels or cause other lipid changes, fluid retention, breakthrough bleeding, and spotting. May cause or exacerbate migraine. May develop visual changes with contact lens. Increased risk of MI with HTN, hyperlipidemia, obesity, and diabetes. D/C if jaundice, significant depression or ophthalmic irregularities develop. Perform annual physical exam. Use before menarche is not indicated. May affect certain endocrine, LFTs, and blood components.

**ADVERSE REACTIONS:** Nausea, vomiting, breakthrough bleeding, spotting, amenorrhea, migraine, depression, vaginal candidiasis, edema, weight changes.

**INTERACTIONS:** Reduced effects, increased breakthrough bleeding, and menstrual irregularities with rifampin, barbiturates, phenylbutazone, phenytoin, carbamazepine, and possibly with griseofulvin, ampicillin, and tetracyclines. Increased levels with atorvastatin, ascorbic acid, and APAP. Increased plasma levels of cyclosporine, prednisolone, and theophylline. Decreased levels of APAP. Increased clearance of temazepam, salicylic acid, morphine, and clofibric acid. Troglitazone reduces plasma levels of hormones.

**PREGNANCY:** Category X, not for use in nursing.

## LOFIBRA
fenofibrate (Gate)

RX

**THERAPEUTIC CLASS:** Fibric acid derivative

**INDICATIONS:** Adjunct to diet, for treatment of hypertriglyceridemia (Types IV and V). Adjunct to diet, for reduction of total-C, LDL-C, Apo B, and TG in primary hypercholesterolemia or mixed dyslipidemia (Types IIa and IIb).

**DOSAGE:** *Adults:* Hypercholesterolemia/Mixed Dyslipidemia: Initial: Cap: 200mg qd. Hypercholeserolemia/Mixed Hyperlipidemia: Tab: 160mg qd. Hypertriglyceridemia: Initial: Cap: 67-200mg/day. Tab: 54-160mg qd. Titrate: Adjust if needed after repeat lipid levels at 4-8 week intervals. Max: Cap: 200mg/day. Tab: 160mg/day. Renal Dysfunction/Elderly: Initial: Cap: 67mg/day. Tab: 54mg/day. Take with meals.

**HOW SUPPLIED:** Cap: 67mg, 134mg, 200mg; Tab: 54mg, 160mg

**CONTRAINDICATIONS:** Pre-existing gallbladder disease, unexplained persistent hepatic function abnormality, hepatic or severe renal dysfunction (including primary biliary cirrhosis).

**WARNINGS/PRECAUTIONS:** Monitor LFTs regularly; discontinue if >3X ULN. May cause cholelithiasis; discontinue if gallstones found. Discontinue if myopathy or marked CPK elevation occurs. Decreased Hgb, Hct, WBCs, thrombocytopenia, and agranulocytosis reported; monitor CBCs during 1st 12 months of therapy. Acute hypersensitivity reactions (rare) and pancreatitis reported. Monitor lipids periodically initially, discontinue if inadequate response after 2 months on 200mg/day. Minimize dose in severe renal impairment. Caution in elderly.

**ADVERSE REACTIONS:** Abdominal pain, back pain, headache, abnormal LFTs, increased creatine phosphokinase, respiratory disorder.

**INTERACTIONS:** May potentiate coumarin anticoagulants; reduce anticoagulant dose and monitor PT/INR. Avoid HMG-CoA reductase inhibitors unless benefits outweigh risks. Bile acid sequestrants may impede absorption; take at least 1 hr before or 4-6 hrs after the resin. Evaluate benefits/risks with immunosuppressants (eg, cyclosporine) and other nephrotoxic agents.

**PREGNANCY:** Category C, not for use in nursing.

## LOMOTIL
atropine sulfate - diphenoxylate HCl (Pharmacia & Upjohn)

CV

**OTHER BRAND NAMES:** Lonox (Sandoz)

**THERAPEUTIC CLASS:** Opioid/anticholinergic

**INDICATIONS:** Adjunctive therapy for management of diarrhea.

**DOSAGE:** *Adults:* Initial: 2 tabs or 10mL qid. Titrate: Reduce dose after symptoms are controlled. Maint: 2 tabs or 10mL qd. Max: 20mg/day diphenoxylate. Discontinue if symptoms are not controlled after 10 days of max dose 20mg/day (diphenoxylate).
*Pediatrics:* 2-12 yrs: Initial: 0.3-0.4mg/kg/day of solution given qid. 13-16 yrs: Initial: 2 tabs or 10mL tid. Titrate: Reduce dose after symptoms are controlled. Maint: 25% of initial dose. Discontinue if no improvement within 48 hrs.

**HOW SUPPLIED:** (Diphenoxylate-Atropine) Sol: 2.5mg-0.025/5mL [60mL]; Tab: 2.5mg-0.025mg

**CONTRAINDICATIONS:** Obstructive jaundice, diarrhea associated with pseudomembranous enterocolitis or enterotoxin-producing bacteria.

**WARNINGS/PRECAUTIONS:** May induce toxic megacolon in ulcerative colitis; discontinue if abdominal distention occurs. May cause intestinal fluid retention. Avoid use with diarrhea associated with organisms that penetrate the intestinal mucosa, and with pseudomembranous enterocolitis. Caution in pediatrics, especially with Down's syndrome. Extreme caution advanced hepatorenal disease and liver dysfunction. Do not use with severe dehydration or electrolyte imbalance until corrective therapy is initiated.

**ADVERSE REACTIONS:** Numbness of extremities, dizziness, anaphylaxis, hyperthermia, tachycardia, urinary retention, flushing, drowsiness, toxic megacolon, nausea, vomiting.

**INTERACTIONS:** May potentiate barbiturates, tranquilizers and alcohol. MAOIs may precipitate hypertensive crisis.

**PREGNANCY:** Category C, caution in nursing.

## LOPID — RX

gemfibrozil (Parke-Davis)

**THERAPEUTIC CLASS:** Fibric acid derivative

**INDICATIONS:** Types IV and V hyperlipidemia with risk of pancreatitis not responding to dietary management (usually TG >2000mg/dL). May consider therapy if TG 1000-2000mg/dL with history of pancreatitis or recurrent abdominal pain typical of pancreatitis. Risk reduction of CAD in Type IIb patients without history or symptoms of existing coronary heart disease inadequately responding to weight loss, dietary therapy, exercise, other pharmacologic agents; with triad of low HDL, and elevated LDL and TG levels.

**DOSAGE:** *Adults:* 600mg bid. Give 30 minutes before morning and evening meals.

**HOW SUPPLIED:** Tab: 600mg* *scored

L

**CONTRAINDICATIONS:** Hepatic or severe renal dysfunction, including primary biliary cirrhosis; pre-existing gallbladder disease, concomitant cerivastatin.

**WARNINGS/PRECAUTIONS:** Abnormal LFTs reported; monitor periodically. Only use if indicated and d/c if significant lipid response not obtained. Associated with myositis. D/C if suspect or diagnose myositis, if abnormal LFTs persists, or develop gallstones. Cholelithiasis reported. Monitor blood counts periodically during first 12 months. May worsen renal insufficiency.

**ADVERSE REACTIONS:** Dyspepsia, abdominal pain, diarrhea, fatigue, bacterial and viral infections, musculoskeletal symptoms, abnormal LFTs, hematologic changes, hypesthesia, paresthesia, taste perversion.

**INTERACTIONS:** Caution with anticoagulants; reduce dose and monitor PT. Increased risk of myopathy and rhabdomyolysis with HMG-CoA reductase inhibitors. Benefit with concomitant HMG-CoA reductase inhibitors does not outweigh risks. Avoid initiating therapy with repaglinide. If already on repaglinide therapy, monitor levels and adjust repaglinide dose. Avoid itraconazole in patients taking gemfibrozil and repaglinide.

**PREGNANCY:** Category C, not for use in nursing.

## LOPRESSOR — RX

metoprolol tartrate (Novartis)

**THERAPEUTIC CLASS:** Selective beta$_1$-blocker

**INDICATIONS:** Management of hypertension. Long-term management of angina pectoris. To reduce cardiovascular mortality in hemodynamically stable patients with definite or suspected AMI.

**DOSAGE:** *Adults:* HTN: Initial: 100mg/day in single or divided doses. Titrate: May increase weekly. Usual: 100-450mg/day. Max: 450mg/day. Angina: Initial: 50mg bid. Titrate: May increase weekly. Usual: 100-400mg/day. Max: 400mg/day. MI (Early Phase): 5mg IV every 2 minutes for 3 doses (monitor BP, HR, and ECG). If tolerated, give 50mg PO q6h (25-50mg q6h depending on IV dose intolerance) for 48 hrs. PO dose should be initiated 15 min after last IV dose. MI (Late Phase): 100mg bid for at least 3 months. Take with meals.

**HOW SUPPLIED:** Inj: 1mg/mL; Tab: 50mg*, 100mg* *scored

**CONTRAINDICATIONS:** (HTN, Angina) Sinus bradycardia, >1st-degree heart block, cardiogenic shock, overt cardiac failure, sick-sinus syndrome, severe peripheral arterial circulatory disorders, pheochromocytoma. (MI) Significant 1st degree heart block, 2nd- and 3rd-degree heart block, moderate-to-severe cardiac failure, HR <45 beats/min, and SBP <100mmHg.

**WARNINGS/PRECAUTIONS:** Caution in patients with ischemic heart disease, avoid abrupt withdrawal; taper over 1-2 weeks. Withdrawal before surgery is controversial. May mask hyperthyroidism and of hypoglycemia symptoms. May exacerbate cardiac failure. Caution with hepatic dysfunction, CHF controlled by digitalis. Avoid in bronchospastic disease. May decrease sinus HR and/or slow AV conduction. DC if heart block or hypotension occurs.

**ADVERSE REACTIONS:** Bradycardia, shortness of breath, fatigue, dizziness, depression, diarrhea, pruritus, rash, heart block, hypotension.

**INTERACTIONS:** Additive effects with catecholamine-depleting drugs (eg, reserpine). May block epinephrine effects. Caution with digitalis; both agents slow AV conduction. Potent CYP2D6 inhibitors may increase levels. Stop lopressor several days before clonidine discontinuation when both agents given concurrently.

**PREGNANCY:** Category C, caution in nursing.

## LOPRESSOR HCT

RX

hydrochlorothiazide - metoprolol tartrate (Novartis)

**THERAPEUTIC CLASS:** Selective $beta_1$-blocker/thiazide diuretic

**INDICATIONS:** Treatment of hypertension. Not for initial therapy.

**DOSAGE:** *Adults:* Usual: 100-450mg metoprolol/day and 12.5-50mg HCTZ/day. Max: 50mg HCTZ/day.

**HOW SUPPLIED:** Tab: (Metoprolol-HCTZ) 50mg-25mg*, 100-25mg*, 100mg-50mg* *scored

**CONTRAINDICATIONS:** Sinus bradycardia, >1st-degree heart block, cardiogenic shock, overt cardiac failure, sick-sinus syndrome, severe peripheral arterial circulatory disorders, pheochromocytoma, anuria, sulfonamide hypersensitivity.

**WARNINGS/PRECAUTIONS:** Avoid abrupt withdrawal; taper over 1-2 weeks. Withdrawal before surgery is controversial. May mask hyperthyroidism and of hypoglycemia symptoms. May cause cardiac failure. Caution with hepatic dysfunction, CHF controlled by digitalis, severe renal disease, allergy or asthma history. Avoid in bronchospastic disease. Monitor for fluid/electrolyte imbalance. May manifest latent DM. Hypokalemia, hyperuricemia, hypercalcemia, hypophosphatemia, and hypomagnesemia may occur. May exacerbate SLE. Enhanced effects in post-sympathectomy patient.

**ADVERSE REACTIONS:** Fatigue, dizziness, flu syndrome, drowsiness, hypokalemia, headache, bradycardia.

**INTERACTIONS:** Additive effects with catecholamine-depleting drugs (eg, reserpine). May block epinephrine effects. Caution with digitalis; both agents slow AV conduction. Potent CYP2D6 inhibitors may increase levels. Stop lopressor several days before clonidine discontinuation when both agents given concurrently. Corticosteroids, ACTH may increase risk of hypokalemia. Risk of lithium toxicity. NSAIDs can reduce effects. Insulin may need adjustment. Impaired absorption with cholestyramine, colestipol. Additive effects with other antihypertensives. May increase responsiveness to tubocurarine. Alcohol, barbiturates, or narcotics may potentiate orthostatic hypotension. May decrease arterial responsiveness to norepinephrine.

**PREGNANCY:** Category C, not for use in nursing.

## LOPROX

RX

ciclopirox (Medicis)

**OTHER BRAND NAMES:** Loprox TS (Medicis)

**THERAPEUTIC CLASS:** Broad-spectrum antifungal

**INDICATIONS:** (Cre/Sus) Treatment of dermal infections of tinea pedis, tinea cruris, tinea corporis, cutaneous candidiasis and tinea versicolor. (Gel) Treatment of interdigital tinea pedis and tinea corporis. (Gel/Shampoo) Treatment of seborrheic dermatitis of the scalp.

**DOSAGE:** *Adults:* (Cre/Gel/Sus) Massage affected and surrounding areas bid (am and pm) up to 4 weeks. (Shampoo) Apply about 5mL (up to 10mL for long hair) to wet scalp. Lather and rinse off after 3 minutes. Repeat twice weekly for 4 weeks, at least 3 days apart.
*Pediatrics:* >10 yrs: (Cre/Sus) Massage affected and surrounding areas bid (am and pm) up to 4 weeks. Gel or Shampoo not recommended in pediatrics <16 yrs.

**HOW SUPPLIED:** Cre: 0.77% [15g, 30g, 90g]; Gel: 0.77% [30g, 45g, 100g]; Shampoo: 1% [120mL]; Sus: Loprox TS 0.77% [30mL, 60mL]

**WARNINGS/PRECAUTIONS:** Avoid eyes, mucous membranes, occlusive wrappings or dressings. D/C if sensitization or chemical irritation occurs. Hair discoloration reported in patients with lighter hair color.

**ADVERSE REACTIONS:** Contact dermatitis, pruritus, burning.

**PREGNANCY:** Pregnancy B, caution in nursing.



## LORCET

CIII

acetaminophen - hydrocodone bitartrate (Forest)

**OTHER BRAND NAMES:** Lorcet HD (Forest) - Lorcet Plus (Forest) - Lorcet 10/650 (Forest)

**THERAPEUTIC CLASS:** Opioid analgesic

**INDICATIONS:** Relief of moderate to moderately severe pain.

**DOSAGE:** *Adults:* (Plus, 10/650) Usual: 1 cap/tab q4-6h prn pain. Max: 6 tabs/caps/day. (HD) 1-2 caps q4-6h prn pain. Max: 8 caps/day.

**HOW SUPPLIED:** (Hydrocodone-APAP) Cap: (HD) 5mg-500mg; Tab: (Plus) 7.5mg-650mg*, (10/650) 10mg-650mg* *scored

**WARNINGS/PRECAUTIONS:** May produce dose-related respiratory depression. May obscure acute abdominal conditions or head injuries. Caution in elderly, debilitated, severe hepatic or renal dysfunction, hypothyroidism, Addison's disease, prostatic hypertrophy, urethral stricture, pulmonary disease and postoperative use. May be habit-forming. Suppresses cough reflex.

**ADVERSE REACTIONS:** Dizziness, drowsiness, nausea, vomiting, dysphoria, urinary retention, urethral spasm, dyspnea, shortness of breath, rash.

**INTERACTIONS:** May potentiate CNS depression with narcotics, alcohol, antianxiety agents, antihistamines, antipsychotics, other CNS depressants. Increased effect of antidepressant or hydrocodone with MAOIs or TCAs.

**PREGNANCY:** Category C, not for use in nursing.

## LORTAB

CIII

acetaminophen - hydrocodone bitartrate (UCB Pharma)

**THERAPEUTIC CLASS:** Opioid analgesic

**INDICATIONS:** Relief of moderate-to-moderately severe pain.

**DOSAGE:** *Adults:* (2.5/500, 5/500) 1-2 tabs q4-6h prn. Max: 8 tabs/day. (7.5/500, 10/500) 1 tab q4-6h prn. Max: 6 tabs/day. (Sol) 15mL q4-6h prn. Max: 90mL/day.

*Pediatrics:* >2 yrs: (Sol) 12-15kg: 3.75mL. 16-22kg: 5mL. 23-31kg: 7.5mL. 32-45kg: 10mL. >46kg: 15mL. May repeat q4-6h prn.

**HOW SUPPLIED:** (Hydrocodone-APAP) Sol: 7.5mg-500mg/15mL; Tab: 2.5mg-500mg*, 5mg-500mg*, 7.5mg-500mg*, 10mg-500mg* *scored

**WARNINGS/PRECAUTIONS:** May produce dose-related respiratory depression. May obscure acute abdominal conditions or head injuries. Caution in elderly, debilitated, severe hepatic or renal dysfunction, hypothyroidism, Addison's disease, prostatic hypertrophy, urethral stricture, pulmonary disease, postoperative use. May be habit-forming. Suppresses cough reflex.

**ADVERSE REACTIONS:** Lightheadedness, dizziness, sedation, nausea, vomiting.

**INTERACTIONS:** Additive CNS depression with other narcotics, antihistamines, antipsychotics, antianxiety agents, alcohol, CNS depressants. Increased effect of antidepressant or hydrocodone with MAOIs or TCAs.

**PREGNANCY:** Category C, not for use in nursing.

## LOTEMAX RX

loteprednol etabonate (Bausch & Lomb)

**THERAPEUTIC CLASS:** Corticosteroid

**INDICATIONS:** Treatment of inflammation of the palpebral and bulbar conjunctiva, cornea and anterior segment of the globe. Management of post-operative inflammation.

**DOSAGE:** *Adults:* Steroid-Responsive Disease: 1-2 drops qid, may increase up to 1 drop every hr within the 1st week of treatment. Re-evaluate after 2 days if no improvement. Postoperative: 1-2 drops qid starting 24 hrs post-op and continue for 2 weeks.

**HOW SUPPLIED:** Sus: 0.5% [2.5mL, 5mL, 10mL, 15mL]

**CONTRAINDICATIONS:** Viral diseases of the cornea and conjunctiva including epithelial herpes simplex keratitis, vaccinia, and varicella. Mycobacterial infection and fungal diseases of the eye.

**WARNINGS/PRECAUTIONS:** Caution with glaucoma, history of herpes simplex, and diseases causing thinning of cornea/sclera. Prolonged use can cause glaucoma, optic nerve damage, defects in visual acuity and fields of vision, cataracts, or secondary ocular infections (eg, fungal). Monitor IOP after 10 days of therapy. Re-evaluate if no response after 2 days. May delay healing and increase incidence of bleb formation after cataract surgery. May mask or enhance existing infection in acute, purulent conditions.

**ADVERSE REACTIONS:** Elevated IOP, abnormal vision, chemosis, discharge, dry eyes, burning on instillation, epiphora, itching, photophobia, foreign body sensation, optic nerve damage, visual field defects.

**PREGNANCY:** Category C, caution in nursing.

## LOTENSIN RX

benazepril HCl (Novartis)

**Avoid use in pregnancy, ACE inhibitors can cause injury and even death to the developing fetus. Discontinue when pregnancy is detected.**

**THERAPEUTIC CLASS:** ACE inhibitor

**INDICATIONS:** Treatment of hypertension.

**DOSAGE:** *Adults:* If possible, discontinue diuretic 2-3 days prior to therapy. Initial: 10mg qd, 5mg with concomitant diuretic. Maint: 20-40mg/day given qd-bid. Resume diuretic if BP not controlled. Max: 80mg/day. CrCl <30mL/min: Initial: 5mg qd. Max: 40mg/day.
*Pediatrics:* ≥6 yrs: Initial: 0.2mg/kg qd. Max: 0.6mg/kg.

**HOW SUPPLIED:** Tab: 5mg, 10mg, 20mg, 40mg

**WARNINGS/PRECAUTIONS:** Discontinue if angioedema, jaundice, or if marked LFT elevation occurs. Risk of hyperkalemia with DM, renal dysfunction. Persistent nonproductive cough reported. Monitor WBCs in renal and collagen vascular disease. Anaphylactoid reactions reported. Fetal/neonatal morbidity and death reported. Monitor for hypotension in high risk patients (eg, surgery/anesthesia, prolonged diuretic therapy, heart failure, volume and/or salt depletion, etc). Caution with CHF, renal dysfunction, and renal artery stenosis. Less effective on BP in blacks and more reports of angioedema than nonblacks.

**ADVERSE REACTIONS:** Cough, dizziness, headache, fatigue, somnolence, postural dizziness, nausea.

**INTERACTIONS:** May increase lithium levels. Hypotension risk with diuretics. Increase risk of hyperkalemia with $K^+$-sparing diuretics, $K^+$-containing salt substitutes, or $K^+$ supplements.

**PREGNANCY:** Category C (1st trimester) and D (2nd and 3rd trimesters), not for use in nursing.

## LOTENSIN HCT

hydrochlorothiazide - benazepril HCl (Novartis) RX

**Avoid use in pregnancy, ACE inhibitors can cause injury and even death to the developing fetus. Discontinue when pregnancy is detected.**

L

**THERAPEUTIC CLASS:** ACE inhibitor/thiazide diuretic

**INDICATIONS:** Treatment of hypertension. Not for initial therapy.

**DOSAGE:** *Adults:* Initial (if not controlled on benazepril monotherapy): 10mg-12.5mg tab or 20mg-12.5mg tab. Titrate: May increase after 2-3 weeks. Initial (if controlled on 25mg HCTZ/day with hypokalemia): 5mg-6.25mg tab. Replacement Therapy: Substitute combination for titrated components.

**HOW SUPPLIED:** Tab: (Benazepril-HCTZ) 5mg-6.25mg*, 10mg-12.5mg*, 20mg-12.5mg*, 20mg-25mg* *scored

**CONTRAINDICATIONS:** Anuria, sulfonamide hypersensitivity.

**WARNINGS/PRECAUTIONS:** Avoid if CrCl <30mL/min/1.73m². Discontinue if angioedema, jaundice, or if marked LFT elevation occurs. Risk of hyperkalemia with DM, renal dysfunction. May cause persistent nonproductive cough, hypokalemia, hyperuricemia, hypomagnesemia, hypercalcemia, hypophosphatemia. Monitor WBCs in renal and collagen vascular disease. Anaphylactoid reactions reported. Fetal/neonatal morbidity and death reported. Monitor for hypotension in high risk patients (eg, surgery/anesthesia, prolonged diuretic therapy, heart failure, volume and/or salt depletion, etc). Caution with CHF, renal dysfunction, and renal artery stenosis. More reports of angioedema in blacks than nonblacks. Monitor for fluid/electrolyte imbalance. May increase cholesterol and TG levels. May exacerbate/activate SLE.

**ADVERSE REACTIONS:** Cough, dizziness/postural dizziness, headache, fatigue.

**INTERACTIONS:** Increase risk of hyperkalemia with $K^+$ supplements and $K^+$-sparing diuretics. Risk of lithium toxicity. May increase responsiveness to tubocurarine. NSAIDs reduce effects. Cholestyramine, colestipol decrease absorption. Insulin may need adjustment. May decrease arterial responsiveness to norepinephrine.

**PREGNANCY:** Category C (1st trimester) and D ( 2nd and 3rd trimesters). Not for use in nursing.

## LOTREL

RX

benazepril HCl - amlodipine besylate (Novartis)

**When use in pregnancy, ACE inhibitors can cause injury and even death to the developing fetus. D/C when pregnancy detected.**

**THERAPEUTIC CLASS:** Calcium channel blocker (dihydropyridine)/ACE inhibitor

**INDICATIONS:** Treatment of hypertension. Not for initial therapy.

**DOSAGE:** *Adults:* Usual: 2.5-10mg amlodipine and 10-80mg benazepril per day. Small/Elderly/Frail/Hepatic Impairment: Initial: 2.5mg amlodipine.

**HOW SUPPLIED:** Cap: (Amlodipine-Benazepril) 2.5mg-10mg, 5mg-10mg, 5mg-20mg, 5mg-40mg, 10mg-20mg, 10mg-40mg

**WARNINGS/PRECAUTIONS:** D/C if angioedema, jaundice, or if marked LFT elevation occurs. Risk of hyperkalemia with DM, renal dysfunction. Persistent nonproductive cough reported. Monitor WBCs in collagen vascular disease. Anaphylactoid reactions reported. Fetal/neonatal morbidity and death reported. Monitor for hypotension in high risk patients (heart failure, surgery/anesthesia, volume and/or salt depletion,etc.). Caution with CHF, severe hepatic or renal dysfunction, and renal artery stenosis. Avoid if CrCl ≤30mL/min.

**ADVERSE REACTIONS:** Cough, headache, dizziness, edema.

**INTERACTIONS:** May increase lithium levels. Hypotension risk with diuretics. Increase risk of hyperkalemia with $K^+$-sparing diuretics, $K^+$ supplements, or $K^+$-containing salt substitutes. Caution with other peripheral vasodilators.

**PREGNANCY:** Category C (1st trimester) and D (2nd and 3rd trimesters), not for use in nursing.

L

## LOTRIMIN

RX

clotrimazole (Schering)

**THERAPEUTIC CLASS:** Azole antifungal

**INDICATIONS:** Topical treatment of candidiasis caused by *Candida albicans* and tinea versicolor caused by *Malassezia furfur*.

**DOSAGE:** *Adults:* Apply bid (am and pm). Re-evaluate if no improvement after 4 weeks.
*Pediatrics:* Apply bid (am and pm). Re-evaluate if no improvement after 4 weeks.

**HOW SUPPLIED:** Cre: 1% [15g, 30g, 45g]; Lot: 1% [30mL]; Sol: 1% [10mL, 30mL]

**WARNINGS/PRECAUTIONS:** Discontinue if irritation or sensitivity occurs. Not for opthalmic use.

**ADVERSE REACTIONS:** Erythema, stinging, blistering, peeling, edema, pruritus, urticaria, burning, irritation.

**PREGNANCY:** Category B, caution in nursing.

## LOTRIMIN AF

OTC

clotrimazole (Schering)

**THERAPEUTIC CLASS:** Azole antifungal

**INDICATIONS:** Tinea pedis, t.cruris, t.corporis.

**DOSAGE:** *Adults:* Cleanse skin with soap and water and dry thoroughly. Apply to affected area am and pm. Athlete's Foot and Ringworm: Treat for 4 weeks. Jock Itch: Treat for 2 weeks.
*Pediatrics:* >2 yrs: Cleanse skin with soap and water and dry thoroughly. Apply

to affected area am and pm. Athlete's Foot and Ringworm: Treat for 4 weeks. Jock Itch: Treat for 2 weeks.

**HOW SUPPLIED:** Cre: 1% [24g]; Lot: 1% [20mL]; Sol: 1% [10mL]

**WARNINGS/PRECAUTIONS:** Discontinue if irritation occurs or no improvement in 4 weeks (t.pedis or t. corporis) or 2 weeks (t. cruris). Avoid eye contact. Not effective on scalp or nails.

**PREGNANCY:** Safety in pregnancy and nursing not known.

## LOTRIMIN AF SPRAY POWDER OTC

miconazole nitrate (Schering)

**THERAPEUTIC CLASS:** Azole antifungal

**INDICATIONS:** To treat and relieve the itching, cracking, burning, and scaling of athlete's foot (tinea pedis), jock itch, (tinea cruris), and ringworm (tinea corporis). Powder aids in the drying of moist areas.

**DOSAGE:** *Adults:* Cleanse skin with soap and water and dry thoroughly. (Powder) Sprinkle a thin layer over affected area am and pm. (Spray) Spray a thin layer over affected area am and pm. Athlete's Foot and Ringworm: Treat for 4 weeks. Jock Itch: Treat for 2 weeks.

*Pediatrics:* >2 yrs: Cleanse skin with soap and water and dry thoroughly. (Powder) Sprinkle a thin layer over affected area am and pm. (Spray) Spray a thin layer over affected area am and pm. Athlete's Foot and Ringworm: Treat for 4 weeks. Jock Itch: Treat for 2 weeks.



**HOW SUPPLIED:** Powder: 2% [90g]; Spray, Powder: 2% [100g]; Spray: 2% [113g]

**WARNINGS/PRECAUTIONS:** Avoid eye contact. Discontinue if irritation occurs or no improvement in 4 weeks (athlete's foot or ringworm) or 2 weeks (jock itch). Avoid while smoking or near heat/flame.

**PREGNANCY:** Safety in pregnancy and nursing not known.

## LOTRIMIN ULTRA OTC

butenafine HCl (Schering)

**THERAPEUTIC CLASS:** Benzylamine antifungal

**INDICATIONS:** To cure and relieve itching, cracking, burning, and scaling of athlete's foot (tinea pedis), jock itch, (tinea cruris), and ringworm (tinea corporis).

**DOSAGE:** *Adults:* Wash and dry area. Tinea Pedis: Apply between toes bid (am and pm) for 1 week, or qd for 4 weeks. Tinea Cruris/Corporis: Apply qd for 2 weeks.

*Pediatrics:* >12 yrs: Wash and dry area. Tinea Pedis: Apply between toes bid (am and pm) for 1 week, or qd for 4 weeks. Tinea Cruris/Corporis: Apply qd for 2 weeks.

**HOW SUPPLIED:** Cre: 1% [12g]

**WARNINGS/PRECAUTIONS:** Avoid nails, scalp, mouth, and eyes. Discontinue if too much irritation occurs. Not for vaginal yeast infections. Effectiveness on bottom of foot is unknown.

**PREGNANCY:** Safety in pregnancy and nursing not known.

## LOTRISONE

RX

clotrimazole - betamethasone dipropionate (Schering)

**THERAPEUTIC CLASS:** Corticosteroid/azole antifungal

**INDICATIONS:** Topical treatment of tinea pedis, tinea cruris, and tinea corporis caused by *Trichophyton rubrum*, *Trichophyton mentagrophytes*, and *Epidermophyton floccosum*.

**DOSAGE:** *Adults:* >17 yrs: Massage sufficient amount bid (am and pm) to area for 2 weeks for t.cruris and t.corporis and 4 weeks for t.pedis. Discontinue if condition persists after 2 weeks for t.cruris and t.corporis, and after 4 weeks for t.pedis.

**HOW SUPPLIED:** (Betamethasone-Clotrimazole) Cre: 0.05-1% [15g, 45g]; Lot: 0.05-1% [30mL]

**WARNINGS/PRECAUTIONS:** May produce reversible HPA axis suppression, Cushing's syndrome, hyperglycemia, and glucosuria. Discontinue if irritation develops. Pediatrics may be more susceptible to systemic toxicity. Not for use with occlusive dressing.

**ADVERSE REACTIONS:** Paresthesia, rash, edema, secondary infection.

**PREGNANCY:** Category C, caution in nursing.

## LOTRONEX

RX

alosetron HCl (GlaxoSmithKline)

**Serious GI adverse events, some fatal, reported (eg, ischemic colitis, serious constipation complications). Physicians must enroll in the Prescribing Program for Lotronex and patients must sign the Patient-Physician Agreement. Discontinue immediately if constipation or symptoms of ischemic colitis develop (rectal bleeding, bloody diarrhea, abdominal pain); do not resume therapy.**

**THERAPEUTIC CLASS:** 5-$HT_3$ antagonist

**INDICATIONS:** Treatment for women with severe diarrhea-predominant IBS who have chronic symptoms (>6 months), exclusion of anatomic or biochemical abnormalities of GI tract, failure to respond to conventional therapy, frequent and severe abdominal pain/discomfort, frequent bowel urgency/fecal incontinence, and disability/restriction of daily activities due to IBS.

**DOSAGE:** *Adults:* Initial: 1mg qd for 4 weeks. Titrate: If tolerated and IBS symptoms not controlled, may increase to 1mg bid. Discontinue after 4 weeks if symptoms not controlled on 1mg bid.

**HOW SUPPLIED:** Tab: 0.5mg, 1mg

**CONTRAINDICATIONS:** Current constipation. History of chronic/severe constipation or sequelae of constipation, intestinal obstruction/stricture, toxic megacolon, GI perforation/adhesions, ischemic colitis, impaired intestinal circulation, thrombophlebitis, hypercoagulable state, Crohn's disease, ulcerative colitis, diverticulitis, severe hepatic impairment. Inability to understand/comply with Patient-Physician Agreement.

**WARNINGS/PRECAUTIONS:** Increased risk of constipation and ischemic colitis. Caution with mild or moderate hepatic impairment.

**ADVERSE REACTIONS:** Constipation, abdominal discomfort/pain, nausea, GI discomfort/pain.

**INTERACTIONS:** Increased risk of constipation with medications that decrease GI motility. Inducers and inhibitors of hepatic CYP drug-metabolizing enzymes may change the clearance of alosetron. Fluvoxamine increases AUC, concomitant administration is contraindicated. Avoid with quinolone antibiotics and cimetidine. Caution with ketoconazole, clarithromycin, telithromycin, protease inhibitors, voriconazole, itraconazole.

**PREGNANCY:** Category B, caution in nursing.

# LOVENOX

RX

enoxaparin sodium (Sanofi-Aventis)

**Risk of paralysis by spinal/epidural hematoma with neuraxial anesthesia or spinal puncture. Increased risk with indwelling epidural catheters for analgesia, drugs affecting hemostasis (eg, NSAIDs, platelet inhibitors, anticoagulants), and traumatic or repeated epidural or spinal puncture.**

**THERAPEUTIC CLASS:** Low molecular weight heparin

**INDICATIONS:** Prevention of DVT in hip or knee replacement surgery, abdominal surgery, or with severely restricted mobility during acute illness. With concomitant warfarin, inpatient treatment of acute DVT with or without PE and outpatient treatment of DVT without PE. Prevention of ischemic complications in unstable angina and non-Q-wave MI with concurrent ASA therapy. Treatment of acute ST-segment elevation MI managed medically or with subsequent percutaneous coronary intervention.

**DOSAGE:** *Adults:* Hip/Knee Surgery: 30mg SQ q12h, starting 12-24 hrs post-op, for 7-10 days (up to 14 days) or 40mg SQ qd for hip surgery for 3 weeks. Abdominal Surgery: 40mg SQ qd, starting 2 hrs pre-op, for 7-10 days (up to 14 days). DVT with or without PE treatment: (inpatient/outpatient) 1mg/kg SQ q12h or (inpatient) 1.5mg/kg qd with warfarin (start within 72 hrs) for 7 days (up to 17 days). Acute Illness: 40mg SQ qd for 6-11 days (up to 14 days).

Unstable Angina/Non-Q-Wave MI: 1mg/kg SQ q12h with 100-325mg/day of ASA for 2-8 days (up to 12.5 days). Acute STEMI (patients <75 years): 30mg single IV bolus plus a 1mg/kg SQ followed by 1mg/kg SQ q12h with aspirin. Acute STEMI (patients ≥75 years of age): 0.75mg/kg SQ q12h. CrCl <30mL/min: Surgery/Acute Illness: 30mg SQ qd. DVT with or without PE treatment (inpatient/outpatient)/Unstable Angina/Non-Q-Wave MI: 1mg/kg SQ qd. Acute STEMI (<75 yrs) 30mg single IV bolus plus a 1mg/kg SC dose followed by 1mg/kg SQ qd. Acute STEMI(≥75yrs): 1mg/kg SQ qd.

**HOW SUPPLIED:** Inj: (MDV) 300mg/3mL; (Syringe) 30mg/0.3mL, 40mg/0.4mL, 60mg/0.6mL, 80mg/0.8mL, 100mg/mL, 120mg/0.8mL, 150mg/mL

**CONTRAINDICATIONS:** Heparin or pork allergy, active major bleeding, thrombocytopenia with a positive *in vitro* test for anti-platelet antibody. Hypersensitivity to benzyl alcohol (multi-dose formulation).

**WARNINGS/PRECAUTIONS:** Not for IM injection. Cannot use interchangeably unit for unit with heparin or other low molecular weight heparins. Extreme caution with HIT, conditions with an increased risk of hemorrhage (eg, bacterial endocarditis, hemorrhagic stroke, etc). Major hemorrhages (eg, retroperitoneal, intracranial), thrombocytopenia reported. D/C if platelets <100,000/mm³. Perform periodic CBC, platelets, and stool occult blood test. Caution with bleeding diathesis, uncontrolled arterial HTN, recent GI ulceration, diabetic retinopathy, hemorrhage. Delayed elimination with elderly or in renal dysfunction. Monitor elderly with low body weight (<45 kg) and predisposition to decreased renal function. Higher risk of thromboembolism in pregnant women with prosthetic heart valves. Not for thromboprophylaxis in prosthetic heart valve patients. Obtain homeostasis at the puncture site before sheath removal after percutaneous coronary revascularisation.

**ADVERSE REACTIONS:** Hemorrhage, thrombocytopenia, local reactions (ecchymosis, erythema), anemia.

**INTERACTIONS:** D/C agents that increase risk of hemorrhage (eg, anticoagulants, acetylsalicylic acid, salicylates, NSAIDs, dipyridamole, sulfinpyrazone), unless really needed; monitor closely if co-administered.

**PREGNANCY:** Category B, caution in nursing.

## LOXITANE

RX

loxapine succinate (Watson)

**OTHER BRAND NAMES:** Loxitane C (Watson) - Loxitane IM (Watson)

**THERAPEUTIC CLASS:** Dibenzapine derivative

**INDICATIONS:** Treatment of schizophrenia.

**DOSAGE:** *Adults:* (PO) Initial: 10mg bid, up to 50mg/day for severely disturbed. Titrate: Increase rapidly over 7-10 days. Maint: 60-100mg/day. Max: 250mg/day. Mix concentrate with orange or grapefruit juice; use dropper to dose. (IM) 12.5-50mg q4-6h. Individualize dose.

**HOW SUPPLIED:** Cap: 5mg, 10mg, 25mg, 50mg; Inj: 50mg/mL; Sol, Concentrate: (Loxitane C) 25mg/mL [120mL]

**CONTRAINDICATIONS:** Comatose states, severe drug-induced depressed states (eg, alcohol, barbiturates, narcotics).

**WARNINGS/PRECAUTIONS:** Extrapyramidal symptoms, tardive dyskinesia, NMS can occur. May lower seizure threshold. May mask symptoms of overdose of other drugs. May obscure diagnosis of intestinal obstruction, brain tumor. Ocular toxicity reported. Caution in cardiovascular disease, glaucoma, urinary retention. Elevates prolactin levels. Caution with activities requiring alertness.

**ADVERSE REACTIONS:** Drowsiness, weakness, NMS, tachycardia, hypotension, HTN, syncope, edema, dry mouth, constipation, blurred vision.

**INTERACTIONS:** Significant respiratory depression and hypotension reported with lorazepam (rare). Caution with CNS-active drugs, including alcohol. Antagonizes epinephrine.

**PREGNANCY:** Safety in pregnancy not known. Not for use in nursing.



## LOZOL

RX

indapamide (Sanofi-Aventis)

**THERAPEUTIC CLASS:** Indoline diuretic

**INDICATIONS:** Treatment of hypertension and salt/fluid retention associated with congestive heart failure.

**DOSAGE:** *Adults:* HTN: 1.25mg qam. Titrate: May increase to 2.5mg qd after 4 weeks, then to 5mg qd after another 4 weeks. Max: 5mg/day. CHF: 2.5mg qam. Titrate: May increase to 5mg qd after 1 week. Max: 5mg/day.

**HOW SUPPLIED:** Tab: 1.25mg, 2.5mg

**CONTRAINDICATIONS:** Anuria, sulfonamide hypersensitivity.

**WARNINGS/PRECAUTIONS:** Caution in severe renal disease, liver dysfunction. May exacerbate or activate SLE. Monitor for fluid/electrolyte imbalance. Hyperuricemia, hypercalcemia, hypokalemia, hypophosphatemia, and hyperglycemia may occur. Monitor renal function, serum uric acid levels periodically. May precipitate gout. May manifest latent DM. Enhanced effects in post-sympathectomy patient.

**ADVERSE REACTIONS:** Headache, infection, pain, back pain, dizziness, rhinitis, fatigue, muscle cramps, nervousness, numbness of extremities, electrolyte imbalance, anxiety, agitation.

**INTERACTIONS:** May decrease arterial responsiveness to norepinephrine. May potentiate other antihypertensives. Risk of lithium toxicity. Increases risk of hypokalemia with ACTH, corticosteroids. Antidiabetic agents may need adjustment.

**PREGNANCY:** Category B, not for use in nursing.

## LUCENTIS
RX

ranibizumab (Genentech)

**THERAPEUTIC CLASS:** Monoclonal antibody/VEGF-A blocker

**INDICATIONS:** Treatment of patients with neovascular (wet) age-related macular degeneration.

**DOSAGE:** *Adults:* Administer 0.5mg (0.05mL) by intravitreal injection once a month. May reduce to 1 injection every 3 months after the first 4 injections if monthly injections not feasible.

**HOW SUPPLIED:** Inj: 10mg/mL

**CONTRAINDICATIONS:** Ocular or periocular infections.

**WARNINGS/PRECAUTIONS:** Intravitreal injections have been associated with endophthalmitis and retinal detachments. Increased IOP noted within 60 minutes of intravitreal injection. Arterial thromboembolic events were observed.

**ADVERSE REACTIONS:** Conjunctival hemorrhage, eye pain, vitreous floaters, increase IOP, intraocular inflammation.

**INTERACTIONS:** May develop serious intraocular inflammation when used adjunctively with Verteporfin photodynamic therapy.

**PREGNANCY:** Category C, caution in nursing.

## LUNESTA
CIV

eszopiclone (Sepracor)

L

**THERAPEUTIC CLASS:** Nonbenzodiazepine hypnotic agent

**INDICATIONS:** Treatment of insomnia.

**DOSAGE:** *Adults:*Initial: 2mg qhs. Max: 3mg qhs. Elderly: Difficulty Falling Asleep: Initial: 1mg qhs. Max: 2mg qhs. Difficulty Staying Asleep: Initial/Max: 2mg qhs. Avoid high-fat meal.

**HOW SUPPLIED:** Tab: 1mg, 2mg, 3mg

**WARNINGS/PRECAUTIONS:** Abnormal thinking and behavioral changes reported. Amnesia and other neuropsychiatric symptoms may occur. Worsening of depression including suicidal thinking reported in primarily depressed patients. Avoid rapid dose decrease or abrupt discontinuation. Should only be taken immediately prior to bed or after gonig to bed and experiencing difficulty falling asleep. Avoid hazardous occupations. Caution in elderly, debilitated, or conditions affecting metabolism or hemodynamic responses. Reduce dose with severe hepatic impairment or concurrent use of potent CYP3A4 inhibitors. Caution with signs and symptoms of depression or suicidal tendencies.

**ADVERSE REACTIONS:** Headache, unpleasant taste, somnolence, dry mouth, dizziness, infection, rash, chest pain, peripheral edema, migraine.

**INTERACTIONS:** Possible additive effect on psychomotor performance with ethanol. Coadministration with olanzapine produced a decrease in DSST score. Strong inhibitors of CYP3A4 may significantly increase the AUC of eszopiclone.

**PREGNANCY:** Category C, caution in nursing.

## LUPRON
RX

leuprolide acetate (TAP)

**THERAPEUTIC CLASS:** Synthetic gonadotropin releasing hormone analog

**INDICATIONS:** Palliative treatment of advanced prostate cancer.

**DOSAGE:** *Adults:* 1mg SQ qd. Rotate injection sites.

**HOW SUPPLIED:** Inj: 5mg/mL

**CONTRAINDICATIONS:** Pregnancy.

**WARNINGS/PRECAUTIONS:** Transient worsening of symptoms may occur during 1st few weeks of therapy. Closely monitor patients with metastatic vertebral lesions and/or urinary tract obstruction during 1st few weeks of therapy; may cause neurological problems or increase obstruction. Monitor serum testosterone, acid phosphatase levels. Contains benzyl alcohol.

**ADVERSE REACTIONS:** General pain, headache, hot flashes, urinary disorders, dizziness/vertigo, ECG changes/ischemia, peripheral edema, HTN, asthenia, constipation, anorexia, insomnia.

**PREGNANCY:** Category X, safety in nursing not known.

## LUPRON DEPOT (GYN) RX

leuprolide acetate (TAP)

**OTHER BRAND NAMES:** Lupron Depot 3.75 mg (TAP) - Lupron Depot-3 Month 11.25mg (TAP)

**THERAPEUTIC CLASS:** Synthetic gonadotropin releasing hormone analog

**INDICATIONS:** Management of endometriosis alone or with norethindrone acetate 5mg, including pain relief and reduction of endometriotic lesions. Retreatment of endometriosis with norethindrone acetate 5mg daily. Adjunct with iron for preoperative hematologic improvement of anemia caused by uterine leiomyomata.

**DOSAGE:** *Adults:* Endometriosis: 11.25mg IM every 3 months or 3.75mg IM monthly, alone or with norethindrone acetate 5mg/day. Max: 6 months of therapy. If symptoms recur after course of therapy, may retreat with the combination (leuprolide + norethindrone) up to 6 months. Uterine Leiomyomata: 11.25mg IM single dose or 3.75mg IM monthly up to 3 months. Assess bone density before retreatment.

**HOW SUPPLIED:** Inj: (1 month) 3.75mg, (3 month) 11.25mg

**CONTRAINDICATIONS:** Undiagnosed abnormal vaginal bleeding, pregnancy, nursing.

**WARNINGS/PRECAUTIONS:** Exclude pregnancy before therapy. Use nonhormonal methods of contraception. D/C if pregnancy occurs. Retreatment is not recommended with endometriosis. Limit to 6 months of therapy. Use if require hormonal suppression for at least 3 months. Transient worsening of symptoms may occur during initial days of therapy. Breakthrough bleeding with skipped doses. May develop or worsen depression and cause memory disorders.

**ADVERSE REACTIONS:** Hot flashes, sweating, dizziness, headache, vaginitis, depression, emotional lability, general pain, asthenia, decreased libido, joint disorder, breast tenderness/pain, GI upset, edema, bone density loss.

**PREGNANCY:** Category X, not for use in nursing.

## LUPRON DEPOT (ONCOLOGY) RX

leuprolide acetate (TAP)

**OTHER BRAND NAMES:** Lupron Depot 7.5mg (TAP) - Lupron Depot-4 Month (TAP) - Lupron Depot-3 Month 22.5 mg (TAP)

**THERAPEUTIC CLASS:** Synthetic gonadotropin releasing hormone analog

**INDICATIONS:** Palliative treatment of advanced prostate cancer.

**DOSAGE:** *Adults:* 7.5mg IM as single dose monthly, 22.5mg IM single dose every 3 months, or 30mg IM single dose every 4 months. Rotate injection site.

**HOW SUPPLIED:** Inj: (1 month) 7.5mg, (3 month) 22.5mg, (4 month) 30mg

**CONTRAINDICATIONS:** Pregnancy.

**WARNINGS/PRECAUTIONS:** Transient worsening of symptoms may occur during 1st few weeks of therapy. Closely monitor patients with metastatic vertebral lesions and/or urinary tract obstruction during 1st few weeks of therapy. Monitor serum testosterone, PSA. (7.5mg, 30mg) Temporary increase in bone pain. Ureteral obstruction and spinal cord compression reported; may initiate with SQ formulation for 1st 2 weeks to facilitate withdrawal if needed.

**ADVERSE REACTIONS:** Injection site reactions, general pain, headache, hot flashes, sweating, edema, urinary disorders, dizziness/vertigo, asthenia, GI disorders, impotence.

**PREGNANCY:** Category X, safety in nursing not known.

## LUPRON PEDIATRIC — RX
leuprolide acetate (TAP)

**OTHER BRAND NAMES:** Lupron Depot-Ped (TAP)

**THERAPEUTIC CLASS:** Synthetic gonadotropin releasing hormone analog

**INDICATIONS:** Treatment of central precocious puberty.

**DOSAGE:** *Pediatrics:* Initial: 50mcg/kg/d as single SQ dose or (depot) 0.3mg/kg every 4 weeks (minimum 7.5mg) as single IM dose. Depot Start Dose: ≤25kg: 7.5mg; >25-37.5kg: 11.25mg; >37.5kg: 15mg. Titrate: Increase by 10 mcg/kg/day SQ or (depot) 3.75mg IM every 4 weeks if downregulation not achieved. Maint: Dose that produces adequate downregulation. Verify adequate downregulation with significant weight increase.

**HOW SUPPLIED:** Inj: 5mg/mL, (Depot) 7.5mg, 11.25mg, 15mg

**CONTRAINDICATIONS:** Pregnancy.

**WARNINGS/PRECAUTIONS:** Monitor hormonal effects after 1-2 months of therapy. Measure bone age every 6-12 months. Increase in clinical signs and symptoms may occur in early phase of therapy due to rise in gonadotropins and sex steroids. Discontinue before age 11 in females and age 12 in males.

**ADVERSE REACTIONS:** Initial exacerbation of signs and symptoms, injection site reactions, pain, acne/seborrhea, rash, urogenital bleeding/discharge, vaginitis.

**PREGNANCY:** Category X, not for use in nursing.

## LURIDE — RX
sodium fluoride (Colgate Oral)

**THERAPEUTIC CLASS:** Fluoride supplement

**INDICATIONS:** To prevent dental caries in areas where drinking water fluoride content is <0.6ppm.

**DOSAGE:** *Pediatrics:* (Drops) <0.3ppm: 6 months-3 yrs: 0.5mL qd. 3-6 yrs: 1mL qd. 6-16 yrs: 2mL qd. 0.3-0.6ppm: 3-6 yrs: 0.5mL qd. 6-16 yrs: 1mL qd. (Tab) <0.3ppm: 6 months-<3 yrs: 0.25mg qd. 3-6 yrs: 0.5mg qd. 6-16 yrs: 1mg qd. 0.3-0.6ppm: 3-6 yrs: 0.25mg qd. 6-16 yrs: 0.5mg qd. Dissolve tab in mouth or chew tab before swallowing. Take at bedtime after brushing teeth.

**HOW SUPPLIED:** Drops: 0.5mg/mL [50mL]; Tab, Chewable: 0.25mg, 0.5mg, 1mg

**CONTRAINDICATIONS:** (Drips) Areas where drinking water fluoride is >0.6 ppm, pediatrics <6 months. (Tab) 1mg: Water fluoride is >0.3ppm, pediatrics <6 yrs. 0.5mg: Water fluoride is >0.6ppm, pediatrics <6 yrs. 0.25mg: Water fluoride is >0.6ppm.

**WARNINGS/PRECAUTIONS:** Dental fluorosis may result from daily ingestion of excessive fluoride in pediatrics <6 yrs especially if water fluoride is >0.6ppm.

**ADVERSE REACTIONS:** Allergic rash.

**INTERACTIONS:** Do not eat or drink dairy products within 1 hour of administration.

**PREGNANCY:** Safety in pregnancy not known. Caution in nursing.

## LUSTRA RX
hydroquinone (Taro)

**OTHER BRAND NAMES:** Lustra-AF (Taro)

**THERAPEUTIC CLASS:** Depigmenting agent

**INDICATIONS:** Gradual treatment of ultraviolet induced dyschromia and discoloration resulting from use of oral contraceptive, pregnancy, hormone replacement therapy, or skin trauma.

**DOSAGE:** *Adults:* Apply bid (am and hs). Use sunscreen with Lustra. *Pediatrics:* >12 yrs: Apply bid (am and hs). Use sunscreen with Lustra.

**HOW SUPPLIED:** Cre: 4% [56.8g]

**WARNINGS/PRECAUTIONS:** Avoid sun exposure on bleached skin. Lustra-AF contains sunscreen; use sunscreen with Lustra. May produce unwanted cosmetic effects if not used as directed. Test for skin sensitivity. D/C if no lightening effect after 2 months of therapy, if blue-black darkening of the skin occurs, or if itching, vesicle formation, or excessive inflammatory reactions occur. Contains sodium metabisulfite, may cause serious allergic type reactions. Avoid contact wtih eyes.

**ADVERSE REACTIONS:** Cutaneous hypersensitivity (contact dermatitis).

**PREGNANCY:** Category C, caution in nursing.



## LUVERIS RX
lutropin alfa (Serono)

**THERAPEUTIC CLASS:** Recombinant Human Luteinizing Hormore

**INDICATIONS:** Used in combination with Gonal-f (follitropin alfa) for stimulation of follicular development in infertile hypogonadotropic hypogonadal women with profound luteinizing hormone deficiency (LH<1.2 IU/L).

**DOSAGE:** *Adults:* Initial: 75 IU with 75-150 IU of Gonal-f qd SQ as two separate injections. Give hCG 1 day after last dose. Do not exceed 14 days of therapy unless signs of imminent follicular development. Do not exceed 225 IU/day of Gonal-f.

**HOW SUPPLIED:** Inj: 75 IU.

**CONTRAINDICATIONS:** Primary ovarian failure, uncontrolled thyroid or adrenal dysfunction, uncontrolled organic intracranial lesion (eg, pituitary tumor), abnormal uterine bleeding of undetermined origin, ovarian cyst or enlargement of undetermined origin, sex hormone dependent tumors of the reproductive tract and accessory organs, and pregnancy.

**WARNINGS/PRECAUTIONS:** Ovarian enlargement may occur; monitor ovarian response. Ovarian hyperstimulation syndrome (OHSS), multiple births, serious pulmonary and vascular complications reported. Do not administer hCG dose if evidence of OHSS. Monitor follicular maturation through ultrasonography and serum estradiol levels.

**ADVERSE REACTIONS:** Headache, nausea, ovarian hyperstimulation, breast pain (female), abdominal pain, ovarian cyst, flatulence, injection site reaction, dysmenorrhea, ovarian disorder, diarrhea, constipation, pain, fatigue, upper respiratory tract infection.

**PREGNANCY:** Category X, caution in nursing.

## LUXIQ
betamethasone valerate (Stiefel)

RX

**THERAPEUTIC CLASS:** Corticosteroid

**INDICATIONS:** Corticosteroid responsive dermatoses of the scalp.

**DOSAGE:** *Adults:* Place foam onto saucer or other cool surface first, then apply in small amounts to scalp. Gently massage into affected area bid (am and pm) until foam disappears. Reassess if no improvement after 2 weeks.

**HOW SUPPLIED:** Foam: 0.12% [50g, 100g]

**WARNINGS/PRECAUTIONS:** May produce reversible HPA axis suppression, manifestations of Cushing's syndrome, hyperglycemia, and glucosuria. Caution when applied to large surface areas, for prolonged use, or under occlusive dressings. Use appropriate antifungal or antibacterial agent with dermatological infections; discontinue if infection does not clear. Pediatrics may be more susceptible to systemic toxicity. Avoid eyes. Discontinue if irritation occurs.

**ADVERSE REACTIONS:** Burning, stinging, pruritus, paresthesia, acne, alopecia, conjunctivitis.

**PREGNANCY:** Category C, caution in nursing.

## LYRICA
pregabalin (Pfizer)

CV



**THERAPEUTIC CLASS:** GABA analog

**INDICATIONS:** Adjunct therapy for adult patients with partial onset seizures. Management of neuropathic pain associated with diabetic peripheral neuropathy. Management of post-herpetic neuralgia and fibromyalgia.

**DOSAGE:** *Adults:* Neuropathic Pain: Initial: 50mg tid (150mg/day). Titrate: May increase to 300mg/day within 1 week. Max: 100mg tid (300mg/day). Post-Herpetic Neuralgia: Initial: 150mg/day divided bid or tid. Max: 600mg/day divided bid or tid. Epilepsy: Initial: 150mg/day divided bid-tid. Max: 600mg/day. Fibromyalgia: Initial: 75mg bid (150mg/day). Titrate: May increase to 150mg bid (300mg/day) within 1 week based on efficacy and tolerability. May further increase to 225mg bid (450mg/day) if needed. Max: 450mg/day. Renal Impairment: CrCl 30-60 mL/min: 75-300mg/day divided bid or tid. CrCl 15-30 mL/min: 25-150mg/day divided qd or bid. CrCl <15mL/min: 25-75mg/day given qd. Give supplemental dose (25-150mg) immediately after every 4-hour hemodialysis treatment. Refer to prescribing information. D/C over 1 week.

**HOW SUPPLIED:** Cap: 25mg, 50mg, 75mg, 100mg, 150mg, 200mg, 225mg, 300mg

**WARNINGS/PRECAUTIONS:** Avoid abrupt withdrawal. Gradually taper over 1 week. Possible tumorigenic potential. May impair physical/mental abilities. May cause weight gain; blurred vision, monitor for ophthalmic changes; peripheral edema, caution in heart failure; elevated creatine kinase, discontinue if myopathy or markedly elevated creatine kinase levels occur; decreased platelet count; and mild PR interval prolongation.

**ADVERSE REACTIONS:** Somnolence, dizziness, dry mouth, edema, blurred vision, weight gain, abnormal thinking (difficulty with concentration/attention).

**INTERACTIONS:** Additive CNS side effects with CNS depressants (eg, opiates, benzodiazepines). May potentiate the impairment of motor skills and sedation of alcohol; avoid consumption of alcohol during therapy.

**PREGNANCY:** Category C, not for use in nursing.

## LYSODREN

RX

mitotane (Bristol-Myers Squibb)

**Temporarily discontinue immediately following shock or severe trauma and administer exogenous steroids.**

**THERAPEUTIC CLASS:** Adrenal cytotoxic agent

**INDICATIONS:** Treatment of inoperable adrenal cortical carcinoma of both functional and nonfunctional types.

**DOSAGE:** *Adults:* Initial: 2-6g/day given tid-qid. Titrate: Increase up to 9-10g/day. If severe side effects occur, reduce to max tolerated dose (MTD). MTD varies from 2-16g/day.

**HOW SUPPLIED:** Tabs: 500mg* *scored

**WARNINGS/PRECAUTIONS:** Caution with liver disease other than metastatic lesions from the adrenal cortex. Surgically remove all possible tumor tissues from large metastatic masses before administration. Perform behavioral and neurological assessments at regular intervals when continuous treatment >2 yrs. Monitor for signs of adrenal insufficiency and institute steroid replacement where appropriate. May impair mental/physical abilities.

**ADVERSE REACTIONS:** GI disturbances, depression, lethargy, somnolence, dizziness, vertigo, skin toxicity.

**INTERACTIONS:** May increase dosage requirements with warfarin; monitor with coumarin-type anticoagulants. Caution with drugs susceptible to hepatic enzyme induction.

**PREGNANCY:** Category C, not for use in nursing.



## MACROBID

RX

nitrofurantoin monohydrate (Procter & Gamble)

**THERAPEUTIC CLASS:** Imidazolidinedione antibacterial

**INDICATIONS:** Treatment of acute uncomplicated urinary tract infections (acute cystitis).

**DOSAGE:** *Adults:* 100mg every 12 hrs for 7 days. Take with food.
*Pediatrics:* >12 yrs: 100mg every 12 hrs for 7 days. Take with food.

**HOW SUPPLIED:** Cap: 100mg

**CONTRAINDICATIONS:** Anuria, oliguria, CrCl <60mL/min, pregnancy at term (38-42 weeks gestation), labor and delivery, and neonates <1 month of age.

**WARNINGS/PRECAUTIONS:** Acute, subacute, or chronic pulmonary reactions have occurred. Anemia, diabetes mellitus, renal dysfunction, electrolyte imbalance, vitamin B deficiency, and debilitating disease enhance occurrence of peripheral neuropathy. Stop therapy with acute and chronic pulmonary reactions, hepatic disorders, hemolysis, or peripheral neuropathy. Monitor renal function, LFTs and pulmonary function periodically during long-term therapy. Optic neuritis and hepatic reactions reported.

**ADVERSE REACTIONS:** Pulmonary disorders, hepatic damage, peripheral neuropathy, nausea, headache, flatulence, anorexia, diarrhea, dizziness, alopecia, exfoliative dermatitis, Stevens-Johnson syndrome, anaphylaxis, blood dyscrasias, aplastic anemia.

**INTERACTIONS:** Antacids, especially magnesium trisilicate, decrease rate and extent of absorption. Uricosuric drugs (eg, probenecid and sulfinpyrazone) increase nitrofurantoin levels.

**PREGNANCY:** Category B, not for use in nursing.

## MACRODANTIN RX

nitrofurantoin macrocrystals (Procter & Gamble)

**THERAPEUTIC CLASS:** Imidazolidinedione antibacterial

**INDICATIONS:** Treatment of urinary tract infection.

**DOSAGE:** *Adults:* 50-100mg qid for at least 7 days. Take with food. Long-term Suppressive Use: 50-100mg at bedtime.
*Pediatrics:* >1 month: 5-7mg/kg/day given qid for at least 7 days. Take with food. Long-term Suppressive Use: 1mg/kg/day given qd-bid.

**HOW SUPPLIED:** Cap: 25mg, 50mg, 100mg

**CONTRAINDICATIONS:** Anuria, oliguria, CrCl <60mL/min, pregnancy at term (38-42 weeks gestation), labor and delivery, neonates <1 month of age.

**WARNINGS/PRECAUTIONS:** Acute, subacute or chronic pulmonary reactions have occurred. Anemia, diabetes mellitus, renal dysfunction, electrolyte imbalance, vitamin B deficiency, and debilitating disease enhance occurrence of peripheral neuropathy. Stop therapy with acute and chronic pulmonary reactions, hepatic disorders, hemolysis, or peripheral neuropathy. Monitor renal function, LFT's and pulmonary function periodically during long-term therapy. Optic neuritis and hepatic reactions reported.

**ADVERSE REACTIONS:** Pulmonary disorders, hepatic damage, peripheral neuropathy, nausea, emesis, anorexia, dizziness, alopecia, exfoliative dermatitis, Stevens-Johnson syndrome, anaphylaxis, blood dyscrasias, aplastic anemia.

**INTERACTIONS:** Antacids, especially magnesium trisilicate, decrease rate and extent of absorption. Uricosuric drugs (eg, probenecid and sulfinpyrazone) increase nitrofurantoin levels.



**PREGNANCY:** Category B, not for use in nursing

## MACUGEN RX

pegaptanib sodium (Eyetech/Pfizer)

**THERAPEUTIC CLASS:** VEGF antagonist

**INDICATIONS:** Treatment of neovascular (wet) age-related macular degeneration.

**DOSAGE:** *Adults*: 0.3mg by intravitreous injection once every 6 weeks.

**HOW SUPPLIED:** Inj: 0.3mg

**CONTRAINDICATIONS:** Ocular or periocular infections.

**WARNINGS/PRECAUTIONS:** Rare post-marketing cases of anaphylaxis/anaphylactoid reactions, including angioedema, reported. Endophthalmitis associated with intravitreous injections. Use proper aseptic injection technique. Monitor for increased IOP. For ophthalmic intravitreal injection only.

**ADVERSE REACTIONS:** Anterior chamber inflammation, blurred vision, cataract, conjunctival hemorrhage, corneal edema, eye discharge, eye irritation, eye pain, HTN, increased IOP, ocular discomfort, punctate keratitis, reduced visual acuity, visual disturbance, vitreous floaters, and vitreous opacities.

**PREGNANCY:** Category B, caution in nursing

## MAG-OX OTC

magnesium oxide (Blaine)

**THERAPEUTIC CLASS:** Magnesium supplement

**INDICATIONS:** To increase magnesium intake. For relief of acid indigestion and upset stomach.

**DOSAGE:** *Adults:* Supplement: 1-2 tabs qd. Antacid: 1 tab bid. Max: 2 tabs/day or 2 weeks of therapy.

**HOW SUPPLIED:** Tab: 400mg

**WARNINGS/PRECAUTIONS:** Not for use in amounts over the Recommended Daily Intake (RDI). May have a laxative effect.

**INTERACTIONS:** May interact with certain prescription drugs.

**PREGNANCY:** Safety in pregnancy and nursing not known.

## MALARONE

RX

atovaquone - proguanil HCl (GlaxoSmithKline)

**OTHER BRAND NAMES:** Malarone Pediatric (GlaxoSmithKline)

**THERAPEUTIC CLASS:** Pyrimidine synthesis inhibitor

**INDICATIONS:** Prophylaxis or treatment of malaria caused by *P.falciparum.*

**DOSAGE:** *Adults:* Prevention: Begin 1-2 days before entering endemic area, continue during stay and for 7 days after return. 1 tab qd. Treatment: 4 tabs qd for 3 days. Repeat dose if vomiting occurs within 1 hr after dosing. Take as single dose with food or milky drink.
*Pediatrics:* Prevention: Begin 1-2 days before entering endemic area, continue during stay and for 7 days after return. 11-20kg: 1 pediatric tab qd. 21-30kg: 2 pediatric tabs qd. 31-40kg: 3 pediatric tabs qd. >40kg: Dose as adult. Treatment: Treat for 2 consecutive days. 5-8kg: 2 pediatric tabs qd. 9-10kg: 3 pediatric tabs. 11-20kg: 1 tab qd. 21-30kg: 2 tabs qd. 31-40kg: 3 tabs. >40kg: Dose as adult. Repeat dose if vomiting occurs within 1 hr after dosing. Take as single dose with food or milky drink.

**HOW SUPPLIED:** (Atovaquone-Proguanil) Tab: 250mg-100mg; Tab, Pediatric: 62.5mg-25mg

**CONTRAINDICATIONS:** For prophylaxis in severe renal impairment (CrCl <30mL/min).

**WARNINGS/PRECAUTIONS:** Not for cerebral malaria. Patients with severe malaria are not candidates for oral therapy. Rare cases of anaphylaxis have been reported.

**ADVERSE REACTIONS:** Vomiting, pruritus, elevation of LFTs.

**INTERACTIONS:** Rifampin, rifabutin may decrease levels; concomitant use is not recommended. Reduced bioavailability with metoclopramide and tetracycline.

**PREGNANCY:** Category C, caution in nursing.



## MARCAINE

RX

bupivacaine HCl (Hospira)

**THERAPEUTIC CLASS:** Local anesthetic

**INDICATIONS:** Production of local or regional anesthesia for surgery, dental, or oral surgery procedures, diagnostic and therapeutic procedures, and for obstetrical procedures. Only 0.25% and 0.5% are indicated for obstetrical anesthesia.

**DOSAGE:** *Adults:* Individualize dose. Dosage varies depending on procedure, area to be anesthetized. vascularity of tissues, number of neural segments to be blocked, depth and duration of anesthesia, degree of muscle relaxation required, and patient tolerance and physical condition. Single Dose Max: 175mg. May repeat once every 3 hrs. Total Daily Dose Max: 400mg. Epidural Anesthesia: 0.5% or 0.75% in 3-5mL increments. In obstetrics, use only 0.25% or 0.5%. Use 3-5mL increments of 0.5% solution not to exceed 50-100mg at any dosing interval. Test dose using 0.5% with 1:200,000 epinephrine recommended prior to caudal and lumbar epidural blocks.
Elderly/Debilitated/Cardiac or Liver Disease: Reduce dose.

*Pediatrics:* ≥12 yrs: Individualize dose. Dosage varies depending on procedure, area to be anesthetized, vascularity of tissues, number of neural segments to be blocked, depth and duration of anesthesia, degree of muscle relaxation required, and patient tolerance and physical condition. Single Dose Max: 175mg. May repeat once every 3 hrs. Total Daily Dose Max: 400mg. Epidural Anesthesia: 0.5% or 0.75% in 3-5mL increments. In obstetrics, use only 0.25% or 0.5%. Use 3-5mL increments of 0.5% solution not to exceed 50-100mg at any dosing interval. Test dose using 0.5% with 1:200,000 epinephrine recommended prior to caudal and lumbar epidural blocks.

**HOW SUPPLIED:** Inj: 0.25%, 0.5%, 0.75%

**CONTRAINDICATIONS:** Obstetrical paracervical block anesthesia.

**WARNINGS/PRECAUTIONS:** The 0.75% strength is not recommended for obstetrical anesthesia. Acidosis, cardiac arrest, death reported from delay in toxicity management. Local anesthetic solutions containing antimicrobial preservatives should not be used for epidural or caudal anesthesia. Not recommended for IV regional anesthesia. Monitor cardiovascular and respiratory vital signs and state of consciousness after each injection. Caution with hepatic disease and impaired cardiovascular function. Monitor circulation and respiration with injections into head and neck area. Respiratory arrest following local anesthetic injection during retrobulbar blocks has been reported.

**ADVERSE REACTIONS:** Restlessness, anxiety, dizziness, tinnitus, blurred vision, tremors, convulsions, nausea, vomiting, chills, hypotension, bradycardia, ventricular arrhythmias, urticaria, pruritus, erythema, edema.

**INTERACTIONS:** Avoid use with any other local anesthetics.

**PREGNANCY:** Category C, not for use in nursing.



## MARCAINE WITH EPINEPHRINE RX

epinephrine - bupivacaine HCl (Hospira)

**THERAPEUTIC CLASS:** Local anesthetic

**INDICATIONS:** Production of local or regional anesthesia for surgery, dental, or oral surgery procedures, diagnostic and therapeutic procedures, and for obstetrical procedures. Only 0.25% and 0.5% are indicated for obstetrical anesthesia.

**DOSAGE:** *Adults:* Individualize dose. Dosage varies depending on procedure, area to be anesthetized, vascularity of tissues, number of neural segments to be blocked, depth and duration of anesthesia, degree of muscle relaxation required, and patient tolerance and physical condition. Single Dose Max: 225mg. May repeat once every 3 hrs. Total Daily Dose Max: 400mg. Epidural Anesthesia: 0.5% or 0.75% in 3-5mL increments. In obstetrics, use only 0.25% or 0.5%. Use 3-5mL increments of 0.5% solution not to exceed 50-100mg at any dosing interval. Test dose using 0.5% with 1:200,000 epinephrine recommended prior to caudal and lumbar epidural blocks. Dentistry: 0.5% with epinephrine. Average Dose: 1.8mL (9mg) per injection site. May repeat after 2-10 minutes if necessary. Max: 90mg total dose for all sites. Elderly/Debilitated/Cardiac or Liver Disease: Reduce dose.
*Pediatrics:* ≥12 yrs: Individualize dose. Dosage varies depending on procedure, area to be anesthetized, vascularity of tissues, number of neural segments to be blocked, depth and duration of anesthesia, degree of muscle relaxation required, and patient tolerance and physical condition. Single Dose Max: 225mg. May repeat once every 3 hrs. Total Daily Dose Max: 400mg. Epidural Anesthesia: 0.5% or 0.75% in 3-5mL increments. In obstetrics, use only 0.25% or 0.5%. Use 3-5mL increments of 0.5% solution not to exceed 50-100mg at any dosing interval. Test dose using 0.5% with 1:200,000 epinephrine recommended prior to caudal and lumbar epidural blocks. Dentistry: 0.5% with epinephrine. Average Dose: 1.8mL (9mg) per injection site. May repeat after 2-10 minutes if necessary. Max: 90mg total dose for all sites.

**HOW SUPPLIED:** Inj: (Bupivacaine-Epinephrine) 0.25%/1:200,000, 0.5%/1:200,000

**CONTRAINDICATIONS:** Obstetrical paracervical block anesthesia.

**WARNINGS/PRECAUTIONS:** The 0.75% strength is not recommended for obstetrical anesthesia. Acidosis, cardiac arrest, death reported from delay in toxicity management. Local anesthetic solutions containing antimicrobial preservatives should not be used for epidural or caudal anesthesia. Not recommended for IV regional anesthesia. Bupivacaine with epinephrine solutions contain sodium metabisulfite which may cause allergic-type reactions in susceptible people. Monitor cardiovascular and respiratory vital signs and state of consciousness after each injection. Caution when local anesthetic solutions containing a vasoconstrictor are used in areas of the body supplied by end arteries or having otherwise compromised blood supply; ischemic injury or necrosis may result with hypertensive vascular disease. Caution with hepatic disease and impaired cardiovascular function. Monitor circulation and respiration with injections into head and neck area. Respiratory arrest following local anesthetic injection during retrobulbar blocks has been reported.

**ADVERSE REACTIONS:** Restlessness, anxiety, dizziness, tinnitus, blurred vision, tremors, convulsions, nausea, vomiting, chills, hypotension, bradycardia, ventricular arrhythmias, urticaria, pruritus, erythema, edema.

**INTERACTIONS:** Avoid use with any other local anesthetics. Anesthetic solutions containing epinephrine or norepinephrine with MAOIs or TCAs may produce severe, prolonged HTN; avoid concurrent use or monitor closely if concurrent use is necessary. Concurrent administration of vasopressors and ergot-type oxytocic drugs may cause severe, persistent HTN or CVA. Phenothiazines and butyrophenones may reduce or reverse the pressor effect of epinephrine. Serious dose-related cardiac arrhythmias may occur with use during or following administration of potent inhalation anesthetics.

**PREGNANCY:** Category C, not for use in nursing.



## MARINOL — CIII

dronabinol (Unimed)

**THERAPEUTIC CLASS:** Cannabinoid

**INDICATIONS:** Treatment of anorexia associated with weight loss in AIDS patients and nausea and vomiting associated with chemotherapy when conventional treatment has failed.

**DOSAGE:** *Adults:* Appetite Stimulation: Initial: 2.5mg bid before lunch and supper or 2.5mg qpm or qhs if 5mg/day is intolerable. Max: 20mg/day in divided doses. Antiemetic: Initial: 5mg/m$^2$ given 1-3 hrs before chemotherapy, then q2-4h after chemotherapy, up to 4-6 doses/day. Titrate: May increase by 2.5mg/m$^2$ increments. Max: 15mg/m$^2$ /dose.

**HOW SUPPLIED:** Cap: 2.5mg, 5mg, 10mg

**CONTRAINDICATIONS:** Hypersensitivity to sesame oil and cannabinoids.

**WARNINGS/PRECAUTIONS:** Do not engage in any hazardous activity till ability to tolerate drug is established. Caution with cardiac disorders due to possible HTN/hypotension, syncope, tachycardia. Caution with history of substance abuse. Monitor with mania, depression, schizophrenia; may exacerbate illness. Caution in elderly due to increased sensitivity to the psychoactive, neurological, and postural hypotensive effects. Initial dose and adjustments should be supervised by responsible adult. Caution with history of seizure disorders, may lower seizure threshold.

**ADVERSE REACTIONS:** Euphoria, dizziness, paranoid reaction, somnolence, abnormal thinking, abdominal pain, nausea, vomiting, diarrhea, conjunctivitis, hypotension, flushing.

**INTERACTIONS:** Highly protein bound drugs may require dosage changes. Additive effects with alcohol, sedatives, hypnotics, or other psychoactive drugs. Additive HTN, tachycardia, and possible cardiotoxicity with amphetamines, cocaine, and sympathomimetics. Increased tachycardia, and drowsiness with anticholinergic agents. Potentiates effects of TCAs and CNS depressants. Decreases clearance of antipyrine and barbiturates.

**PREGNANCY:** Category C, not for use in nursing.

## MATULANE RX
procarbazine HCl (Sigma-Tau)

**THERAPEUTIC CLASS:** Hydrazine derivative

**INDICATIONS:** In combination with other antineoplastics for the treatment of Stage III/IV Hodgkin's disease.

**DOSAGE:** *Adults:* 2-4mg/kg/day as single or divided doses for first week then increase to 4-6mg/kg/day until maximum response or WBC <4000mm³ or platelets <100,000/mm³. Maint: 1-2mg/kg/day. In MOPP: 100mg/m² qd for 14 days. Adjust dose for combination regimens.
*Pediatrics:* 50mg/m²/day for first week then increase to 100mg/m²/day until response is obtained or leukopenia or thrombocytopenia occurs. Maint: 50mg/m²/day. Adjust dose for combination regimens.

**HOW SUPPLIED:** Cap: 50mg

**CONTRAINDICATIONS:** Inadequate marrow reserve.

**WARNINGS/PRECAUTIONS:** Toxicity may occur in renal or hepatic impairment. Wait one month or longer with prior use of bone marrow suppressing radiation or chemotherapy. Discontinue if CNS symptoms (paresthesias, neuropathies, confusion), leukopenia, thrombocytopenia, hypersensitivity, stomatitis, diarrhea, hemorrhage or bleeding tendencies occur. Bone marrow depression often occurs 2-8 weeks after initiation. Monitor urinalysis, transaminases, LFTs weekly, hematologic status every 3-4 days.



**ADVERSE REACTIONS:** Leukopenia, anemia, thrombopenia, nausea, vomiting.

**INTERACTIONS:** Avoid sympathomimetics, TCAs, tyramine-containing drugs/foods, alcohol (may cause disulfiram-type reaction), tobacco. Caution with barbiturates, antihistamines, narcotics, hypotensives, phenothiazines.

**PREGNANCY:** Category D, not for use in nursing.

## MAVIK RX
trandolapril (Abbott)

**ACE inhibitors can cause death/injury to developing fetus during 2nd and 3rd trimesters. Stop therapy if pregnancy detected.**

**THERAPEUTIC CLASS:** ACE inhibitor

**INDICATIONS:** Treatment of hypertension. To decrease risk of hospitalization and mortality in stable patients with signs of left-ventricular systolic dysfunction or CHF post-MI.

**DOSAGE:** *Adults:* HTN: If possible, d/c diuretic 2-3 days before therapy. Initial: 1mg qd in non-black patients; 2mg qd in black patients; 0.5mg with concomitant diuretic. Titrate: Adjust at 1 week intervals. Usual: 2-4mg qd. Resume diuretic if not controlled. Max: 8mg/day. Post-MI: Initial: 1mg qd. Titrate: Increase to target dose of 4mg qd as tolerated. CrCl <30mL/min/Hepatic Cirrhosis for HTN or Post-MI: Initial: 0.5mg qd.

**HOW SUPPLIED:** Tab: 1mg*, 2mg, 4mg *scored

**CONTRAINDICATIONS:** History of ACE inhibitor associated angioedema.

**WARNINGS/PRECAUTIONS:** D/C if angioedema or jaundice occurs. Risk of hyperkalemia with DM, renal dysfunction. Persistent nonproductive cough reported. Monitor WBCs in renal impairment and/or collagen vascular disease. Anaphylactoid reactions reported. Fetal/neonatal morbidity and death reported. Monitor for hypotension in high risk patients (heart failure, surgery/anesthesia, prolonged diuretic therapy, volume and/or salt depletion, etc.). Caution with CHF, renal dysfunction, and renal artery stenosis. More reports of angioedema in blacks than nonblacks.

**ADVERSE REACTIONS:** Cough, dizziness, hypotension, elevated serum uric acid, elevated BUN, elevated creatinine, asthenia, syncope, myalgia, gastritis, hypocalcemia, hyperkalemia, dyspepsia.

**INTERACTIONS:** May increase lithium levels. Hypotension risk with diuretics. Increase risk of hyperkalemia with $K^+$-sparing diuretics, $K^+$-containing salt substitutes or $K^+$ supplements.

**PREGNANCY:** Category C (1st trimester) and D (2nd and 3rd trimesters), not for use in nursing.

## MAXAIR

RX

pirbuterol acetate (Graceway)

**OTHER BRAND NAMES:** Maxair Autohaler (Graceway)

**THERAPEUTIC CLASS:** $Beta_2$ agonist

**INDICATIONS:** Prevention and reversal of bronchospasm in reversible bronchospasm (eg, asthma).

**DOSAGE:** *Adults:* 1-2 inh q4-6h. Max: 12 inh/day.
*Pediatrics:* ≥12 yrs: 1-2 inh q4-6h. Max: 12 inh/day.

**HOW SUPPLIED:** Autohaler: 0.2mg/inh [14g, 25.6g]; MDI: 0.2mg/inh [14g]

**WARNINGS/PRECAUTIONS:** Caution with cardiovascular disorders, (eg, ischemic heart disease, HTN, arrhythmias), hyperthyroidism, diabetes, convulsive disorders. Fatalities reported with excessive use. Can produce paradoxical bronchospasm. Monitor BP.

**ADVERSE REACTIONS:** Nervousness, tremor, headache, dizziness, palpitations, tachycardia, cough, nausea.

**INTERACTIONS:** Avoid other aerosol $\beta_2$ agonists. Vascular effects may be potentiated by MAOIs, TCAs, and sympathomimetics. ECG changes and/or hypokalemia may occur with non-potassium sparing diuretics. Decreased effect with β-blockers.

**PREGNANCY:** Category C, caution in nursing.

## MAXALT

RX

rizatriptan benzoate (Merck)

**OTHER BRAND NAMES:** Maxalt-MLT (Merck)

**THERAPEUTIC CLASS:** $5\text{-}HT_{1D,1B}$ agonist

**INDICATIONS:** Acute treatment of migraine attacks with or without aura.

**DOSAGE:** *Adults:* >18 yrs: 5-10mg, may repeat q2h. Max: 30mg/24 hrs. Safety of treating >4 headaches/30 days not known. MLT: Dissolve on tongue without water. Concomitant Propranolol: 5mg, up to 3 doses/24 hrs.

**HOW SUPPLIED:** Tab: 5mg, 10mg; Tab, Disintegrating: (MLT) 5mg, 10mg

**CONTRAINDICATIONS:** Ischemic heart disease, coronary artery vasospasm (eg, Prinzmetal's angina), uncontrolled HTN, significant cardiovascular disease, hemiplegic or basilar migraine, MAOI use within 14 days, other $5\text{-}HT_1$ agonist or ergot-type agent use within 24 hrs.

**WARNINGS/PRECAUTIONS:** Confirm diagnosis. Supervise 1st dose and monitor cardiac function in those at risk of CAD (eg, HTN, hypercholesterolemia, smoker, obesity, diabetes, CAD family history, postmenopausal women, males >40 yrs). Serious adverse cardiac events, cerebrovascular events, vasospastic reactions, hypertensive crisis, and fatalities reported with $5\text{-}HT_1$ agonists. Disintegrating tabs contain phenylalanine. Caution with renal dialysis and hepatic dysfunction.

**ADVERSE REACTIONS:** Paresthesia, dry mouth, nausea, dizziness, somnolence, asthenia/fatigue.

**INTERACTIONS:** Increased plasma levels with propranolol. Prolonged vasospastic reactions with ergot-type agents and other 5-$HT_1$ agonists. SSRIs may cause weakness, hyperreflexia, and incoordination (rare). Avoid MAOIs during or within 14 days.

**PREGNANCY:** Category C, caution in nursing.

## MAXAQUIN RX
lomefloxacin HCl (Pharmacia)

**THERAPEUTIC CLASS:** Fluoroquinolone

**INDICATIONS:** Treatment of acute bacterial exacerbation of chronic bronchitis (ABECB) and uncomplicated/complicated urinary tract infections (UTI). Preoperatively for the prevention of infections from transrectal prostate biopsy (TRPB) and in transurethral surgical procedures (TUSP).

**DOSAGE:** *Adults:* >18 yrs: ABECB: 400mg qd for 10 days. Uncomplicated Cystitis: 400mg qd for 3 days (*E.coli*) or 10 days (*K.pneumoniae, P.mirabilis, or S.saprophyticus*). Complicated UTI: 400mg qd for 14 days. Hemodialysis/CrCl >10 to <40mL/min: LD: 400mg. Maint: 200mg qd. Preoperative Prevention: TRPB: 400mg single dose 1-6 hrs before procedure. TUSP: 400mg single dose 2-6 hrs before procedure.

**HOW SUPPLIED:** Tab: 400mg* *scored

**WARNINGS/PRECAUTIONS:** Moderate to severe phototoxicity, convulsions, pseudomembranous colitis, serious fatal hypersensitivity reactions reported. Avoid in pregnancy and nursing. Not for empiric treatment of Pseudomonas bacteremia or ABECB caused by *S.pneumoniae*. Caution with CNS disorder or those predisposed to seizures. Adjust dose in renal impairment. Discontinue if pain, inflammation, or tendon rupture occurs. Increased risk of tendon rupture in patients receiving concomitant corticosteriods. Maintain adequate hydration. Rare cases of sensory or sensorimotor axonal polyneuropathy have been reported; discontinue if symptoms of neuropathy occur.

**ADVERSE REACTIONS:** Headache, nausea, photosensitivity, dizziness, diarrhea, abdominal pain.

**INTERACTIONS:** Decreased bioavailability with sucralfate, divalent or trivalent cations (didanosine), and magnesium- or aluminum-containing antacids; take 4 hrs before or 2 hrs after lomefloxacin. Cimetidine may increase effects. Probenecid slows the renal elimination. May enhance cyclosporine, warfarin effects.

**PREGNANCY:** Category C, not for use in nursing.

## MAXIPIME RX
cefepime HCl (Elan)

**THERAPEUTIC CLASS:** Cephalosporin (4th generation)

**INDICATIONS:** Treatment of uncomplicated/complicated urinary tract (UTI), uncomplicated skin and skin structure (SSSI), and complicated intra-abdominal infections, and pneumonia. Emperic therapy for febrile neutropenia.

**DOSAGE:** *Adults:* Moderate-Severe Pneumonia: 1-2g IV q12h for 10 days. Febrile Neutropenia Emperic Therapy: 2g IV q8h for 7 days or until neutropenia resolved. Mild-Moderate UTI: 0.5-1g IM/IV q12h for 7-10 days. Severe UTI/Moderate-Severe SSSI: 2g IV q12h for 10 days. Complicated Intra-Abdominal Infections: 2g IV q12h for 7-10 days. CrCl <60mL/min: Initial: Same dose as normal renal function. Maint: Refer to prescribing information for dose-adjustment.
*Pediatrics:* 2 months-16 yrs: <40kg: UTI/SSSI/Pneumonia: 50mg/kg IV q12h. Febrile Neutropenia: 50mg/kg IV q8h. Max: Do not exceed adult dose. CrCl

<60mL/min: Initial: Same dose as normal renal function. Maint: Refer to prescribing information for dose-adjustment.

**HOW SUPPLIED:** Inj: 500mg, 1g, 2g

**WARNINGS/PRECAUTIONS:** Caution with penicillin sensitivity; cross hypersensitivity may occur. Pseudomembranous colitis reported. Treatment may result in overgrowth of nonsusceptible organisms. Caution with renal impairment or history of GI disease especially colitis. Encephalopathy, myoclonus, seizures, and/or renal failure reported. D/C if seizure occurs. Associated with a fall in PT; monitor PT with renal or hepatic impairment, poor nutritional state, and protracted course of antimicrobials; give vitamin K as indicated.

**ADVERSE REACTIONS:** Local reactions (eg, phlebitis) rash, diarrhea.

**INTERACTIONS:** Increased risk of nephrotoxicity and ototoxicity with aminoglycosides. Risk of nephrotoxicity with potent diuretics (eg, furosemide).

**PREGNANCY:** Category B, caution in nursing.

## MAXZIDE — RX

triamterene - hydrochlorothiazide **(Mylan Bertek)**

**OTHER BRAND NAMES:** Maxzide-25 (Mylan Bertek)

**THERAPEUTIC CLASS:** $K^+$-sparing diuretic/thiazide diuretic

**INDICATIONS:** For hypertension or edema if hypokalemia occurs on HCTZ alone, or when a thiazide diuretic is required and cannot risk hypokalemia.

**DOSAGE:** *Adults:* (37.5mg-25mg tab) 1-2 tabs qd. (75mg-50mg tab) 1 tab qd.

M

**HOW SUPPLIED:** (Triamterene-HCTZ) Tab: (Maxzide) 75mg-50mg*, (Maxzide-25) 37.5mg-25mg* *scored

**CONTRAINDICATIONS:** Hyperkalemia, anuria, acute or chronic renal insufficiency, sulfonamide hypersensitivity, diabetic neuropathy, $K^+$-sparing agents (eg, diuretics), $K^+$ supplements, $K^+$ salt substitutes, $K^+$-rich diet.

**WARNINGS/PRECAUTIONS:** Risk of hyperkalemia (>5.5mEq/L) especially with renal impairment, elderly, DM or severely ill; monitor levels frequently. Check ECG if hyperkalemia occurs. Caution with history of renal lithiasis, hepatic dysfunction. Monitor BUN and creatinine periodically. D/C if azotemia increases. May contribute to megaloblastosis in folic acid deficiency. Hyperuricemia, hypercalcemia, hypophosphatemia, hypokalemia may occur. May manifest latent DM. May decrease serum PBI levels. Monitor for fluid/electrolyte imbalance.

**ADVERSE REACTIONS:** Jaundice, pancreatitis, nausea, vomiting, taste alteration, drowsiness, dry mouth, depression, anxiety, tachycardia, blood dyscrasias, electrolyte disturbances.

**INTERACTIONS:** May potentiate other antihypertensives. Risk of lithium toxicity. Indomethacin may cause renal failure; caution with NSAIDs. Increased risk of hyperkalemia with ACE inhibitors. May increase responsiveness to tubocurarine. May decrease arterial responsiveness to norepinephrine. May alter insulin requirements. Alcohol, barbiturates, or narcotics may potentiate orthostatic hypotension.

**PREGNANCY:** Category C, not for use in nursing.

## MEBARAL — CIV

mephobarbital **(Ovation)**

**THERAPEUTIC CLASS:** Barbiturate

**INDICATIONS:** As a sedative for relief of anxiety, tension, and apprehension. Treatment of grand mal and petit mal epilepsy.

**DOSAGE:** *Adults:* Epilepsy: 400-600mg/day. Start with small dose, gradually increase over 4-5 days until optimum dose. Elderly/Debilitated/Renal or Hepatic Dysfunction: Reduce dose. Concomitant Phenobarbital: Give 50% of each drug. Concomitant Phenytoin: Reduce phenytoin dose. Sedation: 32-100mg tid-qid. Optimum Dose: 50mg tid-qid.
*Pediatrics:* Epilepsy: >5 yrs: 32-64mg tid-qid. <5 yrs: 16-32mg tid-qid. Start with small dose, gradually increase over 4-5 days until optimum dose. Sedation: 16-32mg tid-qid.

**HOW SUPPLIED:** Tab: 32mg, 50mg, 100mg

**CONTRAINDICATIONS:** Manifest or latent porphyria.

**WARNINGS/PRECAUTIONS:** May be habit forming; tolerance and dependence may occur with continued use. Avoid abrupt withdrawal. Caution in acute/chronic pain; paradoxical excitement may occur or symptoms masked. Can cause fetal damage. May cause marked excitement, depression and confusion in elderly or debilitated. Reduce initial dose with hepatic damage. Careful adjustment in impaired renal, cardiac, or respiratory function, myasthenia gravis, and myxedema. May increase vitamin D requirements. Caution with depression, suicidal tendencies and history of drug abuse.

**ADVERSE REACTIONS:** Somnolence, agitation, confusion, hyperkinesia, ataxia, CNS depression, hypoventilation, apnea, bradycardia, hypotension, syncope, nausea, vomiting, headache.

**INTERACTIONS:** MAOIs may prolong effects. Additive CNS depression with alcohol and other CNS depressants. Decreases effects of oral anticoagulants, oral contraceptives. Increases corticosteroid metabolism. Interferes with griseofulvin absorption. Decreases half-life of doxycycline. May alter phenytoin metabolism. Sodium valproate and valproic acid decrease metabolism.

**PREGNANCY:** Category D, caution with nursing.



## MEBENDAZOLE — RX

mebendazole (Various)

**THERAPEUTIC CLASS:** Broad-spectrum anthelmintic

**INDICATIONS:** Treatment of Enterobiasis (pinworm), Trichuriasis (whipworm), Ascariasis (common roundworm), *Ancylostoma duodenale* (common hookworm), *Necator americanus* (American hookworm).

**DOSAGE:** *Adults:* Pinworm: 100mg single dose. Other Parasites: 100mg bid for 3 days. May repeat in 3 weeks if needed. Chew, swallow, crush or mix tab with food.
*Pediatrics:* >2 yrs: Pinworm: 100mg single dose. Other Parasites: 100mg bid for 3 days. May repeat in 3 weeks if needed. Chew, swallow, crush or mix tab with food.

**HOW SUPPLIED:** Tab, Chewable: 100mg

**WARNINGS/PRECAUTIONS:** Neutropenia, agranulocytosis reported with prolonged use. Periodically assess organ system functions with prolonged use.

**ADVERSE REACTIONS:** Abdominal pain, diarrhea.

**INTERACTIONS:** Cimetidine may increase plasma levels.

**PREGNANCY:** Category C, caution in nursing.

## MECLOFENAMATE — RX

meclofenamate sodium (Various)

**THERAPEUTIC CLASS:** NSAID

**INDICATIONS:** Relief of mild to moderate pain, primary dysmenorrhea, and idiopathic heavy menstrual blood loss. Symptomatic treatment of acute and chronic rheumatoid arthritis (RA) and osteoarthritis (OA).

**DOSAGE:** *Adults:* Mild to Moderate Pain: 50mg q4-6h. Max: 400mg/day. Excessive Menstrual Blood Loss/Primary Dysmenorrhea: 100mg tid for up to 6 days starting at onset of menstrual flow. RA/OA: 200-400mg/day in 3-4 divided doses. Max: 400mg/day.
*Pediatrics:* >14 yrs: Mild to Moderate Pain: 50mg q4-6h. Max: 400mg/day. Excessive Menstrual Blood Loss/Primary Dysmenorrhea: 100mg tid for up to 6 days starting at onset of menstrual flow. RA/OA: 200-400mg/day in 3-4 divided doses. Max: 400mg/day.

**HOW SUPPLIED:** Cap: 50mg, 100mg

**CONTRAINDICATIONS:** ASA or other NSAID allergy that precipitates bronchospasm, allergic rhinitis or urticaria.

**WARNINGS/PRECAUTIONS:** Risk of GI ulcerations, bleeding, and perforation. Borderline LFT elevations may occur. Renal and hepatic toxicity. Extreme caution in the elderly. If visual symptoms occur, discontinue.

**ADVERSE REACTIONS:** Diarrhea, nausea, vomiting, abdominal pain, edema, urticaria, pruritis, headache, dizziness, tinnitus, pyrosis, flatulence, anorexia, constipation, peptic ulcer.

**INTERACTIONS:** Enhanced effects of warfarin. ASA may lower levels.

**PREGNANCY:** Safety in pregnancy is not known. Not for use in nursing.

## MEDROL

RX

methylprednisolone (Pharmacia & Upjohn)

**OTHER BRAND NAMES:** Medrol Dose Pack (Pharmacia & Upjohn)

**THERAPEUTIC CLASS:** Glucocorticoid

**INDICATIONS:** Steroid responsive disorders.

**DOSAGE:** *Adults:* Initial: 4-48mg/day depending on disease and response. Maint: Decrease dose by small amounts to lowest effective dose. MS: Initial: 160mg/day for 1 week. Maint: 64mg every other day for 1 month. Alternate Day Therapy: Twice the usual dose every other day for long-term therapy.
*Pediatrics:* Initial: 4-48mg/day depending on disease and response. Maint: Decrease dose by small amounts to lowest effective dose. MS: Initial: 160mg/day for 1 week. Maint: 64mg every other day for 1 month. Alternate Day Therapy: Twice the usual dose every other day for long-term therapy.

**HOW SUPPLIED:** Tab: 2mg*, 4mg*, 8mg*, 16mg*, 32mg*; (Dose-Pak) 4mg* [21$^{s}$] *scored

**CONTRAINDICATIONS:** Systemic fungal infections.

**WARNINGS/PRECAUTIONS:** May need to increase dose before, during, and after stressful situations. May mask signs of infection or or cause new infections. Prolonged use may produce glaucoma, optic nerve damage, secondary ocular infections. Increases BP, salt/water retention, potassium excretion. More severe/fatal course of infections reported with chickenpox, measles. Caution with Strongyloides, latent TB, hypothyroidism, cirrhosis, ocular herpes simplex, HTN, diverticulitis, fresh intestinal anastomoses, ulcerative colitis, osteoporosis, myasthenia gravis, renal insufficiency, peptic ulcer disease. Kaposi's sarcoma reported. Growth and development of children on prolonged therapy should be monitored. Monitor for psychic disturbances. Avoid abrupt withdrawal. The 24mg tabs contain tartrazine; caution with tartrazine sensitivity.

**ADVERSE REACTIONS:** Fluid and electrolyte disturbances, HTN, osteoporosis, muscle weakness, cushingoid state, menstrual irregularities, nervousness, insomnia, impaired wound healing, DM, ulcerative esophagitis, excessive sweating, increases intracranial pressure, carbohydrate intolerance, glaucoma, cataracts, weight gain, nausea, malaise.

**INTERACTIONS:** Reduced efficacy with hepatic enzyme inducers (eg, phenobarbital, phenytoin, and rifampin). Increases clearance of chronic high dose ASA. Caution with ASA in hypoprothrombinemia. Effects on oral anticoagulants are variable; monitor PT. Increased insulin and oral hypoglycemic requirements in DM. Avoid live vaccines with immunosuppressive doses. Possible decreased vaccine response with killed or inactivated vaccines with immunosuppressive doses. Mutual inhibition of metabolism with cyclosporine; convulsions reported. Potentiated by ketoconazole and troleandomycin.

**PREGNANCY:** Safety in pregnancy and nursing not known.

## MEGACE ES

megestrol acetate (Par)

RX

**OTHER BRAND NAMES:** Megace Suspension (Bristol-Myers Squibb)

**THERAPEUTIC CLASS:** Progesterone

**INDICATIONS:** Management of anorexia, cachexia, or unexplained significant weight loss in AIDS patients.

**DOSAGE:** *Adults:* (Megace) Initial: 800mg/day (20mL/day). Usual: 400-800mg/day. Shake well before use. Elderly: Start at lower end of dosing range. (Megace ES) Initial/Usual: 625mg/day (5mL/day).

**HOW SUPPLIED:** Sus: 40mg/mL [240mL], (ES) 125mg/mL [150mL]

**CONTRAINDICATIONS:** Pregnancy.

**WARNINGS/PRECAUTIONS:** May cause fetal harm; avoid in pregnancy. New onset or exacerbation of diabetes or Cushing's syndrome reported. Risk of adrenal suppression if taking or withdrawing from chronic therapy; monitor for hypotension, nausea, vomiting, dizziness, or weakness. Caution with history of thromboembolic diseases. Experience is limited in HIV-infected women. Do not use as prophylactic to avoid weight loss.



**ADVERSE REACTIONS:** Abdominal pain, chest pain, cardiomyopathy, palpitation, constipation, dry mouth, edema, confusion, convulsion, dyspnea, cough, alopecia, pruritus, thromboembolic phenomena.

**INTERACTIONS:** May increase insulin requirements. Decrease in pharmacokinetic parameters of indinavir, higher dose should be considered.

**PREGNANCY:** Category X, not for use in nursing.

## MEGESTROL

megestrol acetate (Various)

RX

**THERAPEUTIC CLASS:** Progesterone

**INDICATIONS:** Palliative treatment of advanced breast carcinoma or endometrial carcinoma (eg, recurrent, inoperable or metastatic disease).

**DOSAGE:** *Adults:* Breast Carcinoma: 40mg qid for a minimum of 2 months. Endometrial Carcinoma: 40-320mg/day in divided doses for a minimum of 2 months. Elderly: Start at lower end of dosing range.

**HOW SUPPLIED:** Tab: 20mg*, 40mg* *scored

**WARNINGS/PRECAUTIONS:** May cause fetal harm; avoid in pregnancy. May cause adrenal suppression; monitor for Cushing's syndrome or new onset/exacerbation of DM. Risk of adrenal suppression if taking or withdrawing from chronic therapy; monitor for hypotension, nausea, vomiting, dizziness, weakness. Caution with history of thromboembolic diseases.

**ADVERSE REACTIONS:** Heart failure, nausea, vomiting, edema, breakthrough menstrual bleeding, dyspnea, glucose intolerance, alopecia, HTN, carpal tunnel syndrome, mood changes, hot flashes, malaise, weight gain.

**INTERACTIONS:** May increase insulin requirements.

**PREGNANCY:** Category D, not for use in nursing.

## MENACTRA RX

meningococcal polysaccharide diptheria toxoid conjugate vaccine
(Sanofi Pasteur)

**THERAPEUTIC CLASS:** Vaccine

**INDICATIONS:** Active immunization of adolescents and adults 11-55 yrs of age for the prevention of invasive menigococcal disease caused by N.meningitidis serogroups A, C, Y and W-135.

**DOSAGE:** *Adults:* ≤55 yo: 0.5 mL IM into the deltoid region. *Pediatrics:* ≥11 yo: 0.5mL IM into the deltoid region.

**HOW SUPPLIED:** Inj: 0.5mL

**CONTRAINDICATIONS:** Life-threatening reaction after previous administration of vaccine with similar contents. Known hypersensitivity to dry natural rubber latex.

**WARNINGS/PRECAUTIONS:** Guillain-Barre syndrome (GBS) has been reported. Avoid with bleeding disorders (eg. hemophilia, thrombocytopenia, anticoagulant therapy). Do not administer IV, SC, or intradermally. Have epinephrine injection (1:1000) available, in case of anaphylatic reaction.

**ADVERSE REACTIONS:** Redness, swelling, induration, pain, headache, fatigue, malaise, arthralgia, anorexia, chills, fever.

**INTERACTIONS:** Caution with anticoagulants. Immunosuppressive therapies may reduce immune response to vaccines.

**PREGNANCY:** Category C, caution in nursing.

## MENEST RX

esterified estrogens (King)

**Estrogens increase the risk of endometrial cancer. Estrogens, with or without progestins, should not be used for the prevention of cardiovascular disease. Increased risks of MI, stroke, invasive breast cancer, PE, and DVT in postmenopausal women (50-79 yrs of age) reported. Increased risk of developing probable dementia in postmenopausal women ≥65 yrs of age reported.**

**THERAPEUTIC CLASS:** Estrogen

**INDICATIONS:** Treatment of moderate to severe vasomotor symptoms associated with menopause, atrophic vaginitis, kraurosis vulvae, female hypogonadism, female castration, primary ovarian failure. Palliative therapy for metastatic breast cancer in selected men and women, and of advanced prostatic carcinoma.

**DOSAGE:** *Adults:* Vasomotor Symptoms: 1.25mg qd cyclically (3 weeks on, 1 week off). Start arbitrarily if not menstruating, or on day 5 of bleeding. Atrophic Vaginitis/Kraurosis Vulvae: 0.3-1.25mg qd cyclically (3 weeks on, 1 week off). Discontinue/Taper at 3-6 month intervals. Female Hypogonadism: 2.5-7.5mg/day in divided doses for 20 days, then 10 days off therapy; repeat until menses occurs. If bleeding occurs before the end of the 10 day period, begin a 20 day estrogen-progestin cyclic regimen with Menest 2.5-7.5mg/day in divided doses, for 20 days. During the last 5 days of estrogen therapy, give an oral progestin. If bleeding occurs before this regimen is concluded, therapy is discontinued and may be resumed on the fifth day of bleeding. Female Castration/Primary Ovarian Failure: 1.25mg qd cyclically (3 weeks on, 1 week off). Maint: Lowest effective dose. Prostate Cancer: 1.25-2.5mg tid. Breast Cancer: 10mg tid for at least 3 months.

**HOW SUPPLIED:** Tab: 0.3mg, 0.625mg, 1.25mg, 2.5mg

**CONTRAINDICATIONS:** Pregnancy, undiagnosed abnormal genital bleeding, breast cancer unless being treated for metastatic disease, estrogen-dependent neoplasia, DVT/PE, active or recent (eg, within past year) arterial thromboembolic disease (eg, stroke, MI), liver dysfunction or disease.

**WARNINGS/PRECAUTIONS:** May increase risk of cardiovascular events (eg, MI, stroke), venous thrombosis, and PE; d/c immediately if any of these events occur or are suspected. May increase risk of breast/endometrial cancer, and gallbladder disease. May lead to severe hypercalcemia with breast cancer and bone metastases; monitor and d/c if hypercalcemia occurs. Retinal vascular thrombosis reported; monitor and d/c if papilledema or retinal vascular lesions occur. Consider addition of a progestin if no hysterectomy. May elevate BP; monitor at regular intervals. May cause elevations of plasma triglycerides with pre-existing hypertriglyceridemia. Caution with history of cholestatic jaundice associated with past estrogen use or with pregnancy; d/c with recurrence. May lead to increased thyroid-binding globulin levels; monitor thyroid function. May cause fluid retention; caution with cardiac/renal dysfunction. Caution with severe hypocalcemia. May increase risk of ovarian cancer. May exacerbate endometriosis, asthma, DM, epilepsy, migraine, porphyria, SLE, and hepatic hemangiomas; use with caution.

**ADVERSE REACTIONS:** Altered vaginal bleeding, vaginal candidiasis, breast tenderness/enlargement, GI effects, melasma, CNS effects, weight changes, edema, altered libido.

**INTERACTIONS:** CYP3A4 inducers (eg, St. John's wort, phenobarbital, carbamazepine, rifampin) may decrease levels which may decrease therapeutic effects and/or change uterine bleeding profile. CYP3A4 inhibitors (eg, erythromycin, clarithromycin, ketoconazole, itraconazole, ritonavir, grapefruit juice) may increase levels which may result in side effects.

**PREGNANCY:** Contraindicated in pregnancy, caution in nursing.



## MENOPUR

RX

menotropins (Ferring)

**THERAPEUTIC CLASS:** Follicle stimulating hormone/luteinizing hormone

**INDICATIONS:** Development of multiple follicles and pregnancy in the ovulatory patients participating in an ART program.

**DOSAGE:** *Adults:* Initial: 225 IU SQ. Titrate: Adjust subsequent dosing to individual response at intervals no less than every 2 days and not exceeding 150 IU/adjustment. Max: 450 IU/day. Dosing >20 days not recommended. If adequate response, administer hCG. Withhold hCG if ovaries abnormally enlarged last day of therapy.

**HOW SUPPLIED:** Inj: (FSH-LH) 75 IU-75 IU

**CONTRAINDICATIONS:** High FSH level indicating primary ovarian failure; uncontrolled thyroid and adrenal dysfunction; organic intracranial lesion (pituitary tumor); sex hormone dependent tumor of the reproductive tract and accessory organs; abnormal uterine bleeding of undetermined origin; ovarian cysts or enlargement not due to polycystic ovary syndrome; pregnant women.

**WARNINGS/PRECAUTIONS:** Ovarian hyperstimulation syndrome (OHSS) with or without pulmonary or vascular complications. Mild to moderate uncomplicated ovarian enlargement with abdominal distention and/or abdominal pain may occur. Reports of serious pulmonary conditions (eg, atelectasis, acute respiratory distress syndrome) and thromboembolic events (intravascular thrombosis, embolism, venous thrombophlebitis, pulmonary embolism, pulmonary infarction, cerebral vascular occlusion, arterial occlusion) which may lead to death. Potential risk of multiple births.

**ADVERSE REACTIONS:** Headache, abdominal pain, injection site reaction, nausea, abdominal cramps, abdominal fullness, OHSS, respiratory disorder, vomiting.

**PREGNANCY:** Category X, caution in nursing.

## MENOSTAR RX
estradiol (Berlex)

**Estrogens increase the risk of endometrial cancer. Estrogens, with or without progestins, should not be used for the prevention of cardiovascular disease. Increased risks of MI, stroke, invasive breast cancer, PE, and DVT in postmenopausal women (50-79 yrs of age) reported. Increased risk of developing probable dementia in postmenopausal women ≥65 yrs of age reported.**

**THERAPEUTIC CLASS:** Estrogen

**INDICATIONS:** Prevention of postmenopausal osteoporosis.

**DOSAGE:** *Adults:* Apply 1 patch weekly to lower abdomen (avoid breasts, waistline, and areas where sitting would dislodge the patch). Rotate application sites.

**HOW SUPPLIED:** Patch: 14mcg/day [4s]

**CONTRAINDICATIONS:** Pregnancy, undiagnosed abnormal genital bleeding, breast cancer, estrogen-dependent neoplasia, DVT/PE, active or recent (eg, within past year) arterial thromboembolic disease (eg, stroke, MI), liver dysfunction or disease.

**WARNINGS/PRECAUTIONS:** May increase risk of cardiovascular events (eg, MI, stroke), venous thrombosis, and PE; discontinue immediately if any of these events occur or are suspected. May increase risk of breast/endometrial cancer, and gallbladder disease. May lead to severe hypercalcemia with breast cancer and bone metastases; monitor and discontinue if hypercalcemia occurs. Retinal vascular thrombosis reported; monitor and discontinue if papilledema or retinal vascular lesions occur. Consider addition of a progestin if no hysterectomy. May elevate BP; monitor at regular intervals. May cause elevations of plasma triglycerides with pre-existing hypertriglyceridemia. Caution with history of cholestatic jaundice associated with past estrogen use or with pregnancy; discontinue with recurrence. May lead to increased thyroid-binding globulin levels; monitor thyroid function. May cause fluid retention; caution with cardiac/renal dysfunction. Caution with severe hypocalcemia. May increase risk of ovarian cancer. May exacerbate endometriosis, asthma, DM, epilepsy, migraine, porphyria, SLE, and hepatic hemangiomas; use with caution.

**ADVERSE REACTIONS:** Pain, leukorrhea, arthralgia, application site reaction, bronchitis, cervical polyps, constipation, dyspepsia, myalgia, dizziness, breast pain.

**INTERACTIONS:** CYP3A4 inducers (eg, St. John's wort, phenobarbital, carbamazepine, rifampin) may reduce effects. CYP3A4 inhibitors (eg, erythromycin, clarithromycin, ketoconazole, itraconazole, ritonavir, grapefruit juice) may increase levels. May require higher doses of thyroid hormone.

**PREGNANCY:** Contraindicated in pregnancy, caution in nursing.

## MENTAX RX
butenafine HCl (Mylan Bertek)

**THERAPEUTIC CLASS:** Benzylamine antifungal

**INDICATIONS:** Interdigital tinea pedis, tinea corporis, tinea cruris, and tinea versicolor.

**DOSAGE:** *Adults:* T.pedis: Apply bid for 7 days or qd for 4 weeks. T.corporis/T.cruris/T.versicolor: Apply qd for 2 weeks.
*Pediatrics:* >12 yrs: T.pedis: Apply bid for 7 days or qd for 4 weeks. T.corporis/T.cruris/T.versicolor: Apply qd for 2 weeks.

**HOW SUPPLIED:** Cre: 1% [15g, 30g]

**WARNINGS/PRECAUTIONS:** Avoid eyes, nose, mouth, and other mucous membranes. D/C if irritation or sensitivity develops. Confirm diagnosis. Caution if sensitive to other allylamine antifungals.

M

**ADVERSE REACTIONS:** Burning, stinging, itching, contact dermatitis, irritation, erythema, worsening of condition.

**PREGNANCY:** Category B, caution in nursing.

## MEPERIDINE/PROMETHAZINE CII

meperidine HCl - promethazine HCl (Ethex)

**THERAPEUTIC CLASS:** Opioid analgesic/phenothiazine

**INDICATIONS:** Management of moderate pain and sedation for postoperative and postpartum use, and pain associated with malignancies.

**DOSAGE:** *Adults:* 1 cap q4-6h prn.

**HOW SUPPLIED:** Cap: (Meperidine-Promethazine) 50mg-25mg

**CONTRAINDICATIONS:** During or within 14 days of MAOIs.

**WARNINGS/PRECAUTIONS:** May cause tolerance and dependence; potential for abuse. Extreme caution with head injury, increased intracranial pressure, intracranial lesions, acute asthma, COPD, cor pulmonale, decreased respiratory reserve, respiratory depression, hypoxia, hypercapnia. Severe hypotension may occur with depleted blood volume. Orthostatic hypotension may occur. Caution with atrial flutter and other supraventricular tachycardias. May obscure diagnosis or clinical course of acute abdominal conditions. Reduce initial dose in elderly, debilitated, severe hepatic or renal dysfunction, hypothyroidism, Addison's disease, prostatic hypertrophy, urethral stricture. May aggravate seizure disorders. Not for use in pregnant women prior to labor.

**ADVERSE REACTIONS:** Lightheadedness, dizziness, sedation, nausea, vomiting, sweating.



**INTERACTIONS:** See Contraindications. Additive sedative effects with CNS depressants (eg, narcotics, anesthetics, phenothiazines, tranquilizers, sedative-hypnotics, TCAs, alcohol). Reduce analgesic depressant dose by 25-50% and dose of barbiturates by 50%. Severe hypotension possible with concurrent phenothiazines, certain anesthetics.

**PREGNANCY:** Safety in pregnancy and nursing not known.

## MEPHYTON RX

phytonadione (Merck)

**THERAPEUTIC CLASS:** Vitamin K derivative

**INDICATIONS:** For coagulation disorders caused by vitamin K deficiency or interference with vitamin K activity, including anticoagulant-induced prothrombin deficiency caused by coumarin or indanedione derivatives; and hypoprothrombinemia secondary to antibacterials, salicylates, obstructive jaundice, or biliary fistulas.

**DOSAGE:** *Adults:* Anticoagulant-Induced Prothrombin Deficiency: Initial: 2.5-10mg up to 25mg (rarely 50mg). May repeat if PT is still elevated 12-48 hrs after initial dose. Hypoprothrombinemia Due to Other Causes: 2.5-25mg or more (rarely up to 50mg). Give bile salts when endogenous bile supply to GIT is deficient.

**HOW SUPPLIED:** Tab: 5mg* *scored

**WARNINGS/PRECAUTIONS:** Does not produce an immediate coagulant effect. Maintain lowest possible dose to prevent original thromboembolic events. Avoid repeated large doses with hepatic disease. Failure to respond may indicate a congenital coagulation defect or a condition unresponsive to vitamin K. Avoid large doses in liver disease. Monitor PT regularly.

**ADVERSE REACTIONS:** Severe hypersensitivity reactions (anaphylactoid reactions, death), flushing, peculiar taste sensations, dizziness, rapid and weak pulse, profuse sweating, hypotension, dyspnea, cyanosis.

**INTERACTIONS:** Does not counteract anticoagulant effects of heparin. Temporary resistance to prothrombin-depressing anticoagulants, especially with large doses.

**PREGNANCY:** Category C, caution in nursing.

## MEPRON

RX

atovaquone (GlaxoSmithKline)

**THERAPEUTIC CLASS:** Napthoquinone antiprotozoal

**INDICATIONS:** Prevention and treatment of mild to moderate *Pneumocystis carinii* pneumonia (PCP) in those intolerant to trimethoprim-sulfamethoxazole.

**DOSAGE:** *Adults:* Take with food. Prevention: 1500mg qd. Treatment: 750mg bid for 21 days.
*Pediatrics:* 13-16 yrs: Take with food. Prevention: 1500mg qd. Treatment: 750mg bid for 21 days.

**HOW SUPPLIED:** Sus: 750mg/5mL [5mL, 42[s]; 210mL]

**WARNINGS/PRECAUTIONS:** Monitor with severe hepatic impairment. Absorption significantly increased with food.

**ADVERSE REACTIONS:** Rash, nausea, GI effects, cough increased, rhinitis, asthenia, infection, dyspnea, insomnia, asthenia, pruritus.

**INTERACTIONS:** Significantly decreased plasma levels with rifampin. Caution with other highly protein-bound drugs.

**PREGNANCY:** Category C, caution in nursing.

M

## MEPROZINE

CII

meperidine HCl - promethazine HCl (Vintage)

**THERAPEUTIC CLASS:** Narcotic analgesic/phenothiazine

**INDICATIONS:** For sedation or analgesia in moderate pain.

**DOSAGE:** *Adults:* 1 cap q4-6h prn.

**HOW SUPPLIED:** Cap: (Meperidine-Promethazine) 50-25mg

**CONTRAINDICATIONS:** Intra-arterial or subcutaneous route of administration, during or within 14 days of MAOI therapy.

**WARNINGS/PRECAUTIONS:** May be habit-forming. May produce hypotension. Decrease dose with severe hepatic or renal impairment, hypothyroidism, elderly, debilitated, Addison's disease, prostatic hypertrophy and urethral stricture. May aggravate convulsive disorders. May obscure clinical course of head injury patients and diagnosis of acute abdominal conditions. Caution with atrial flutter, supraventricular tachycardias. Extreme caution in acute asthmatic attack, COPD, cor pulmonale, head injuries, increased intracranial pressure and pre-existing respiratory depression.

**ADVERSE REACTIONS:** Dizziness, sedation, nausea, vomiting, respiratory depression, sweating.

**INTERACTIONS:** Contraindicated with MAOIs. Additive sedative effects with alcohol, CNS depressants. Caution and reduce dose with other narcotics, general anesthetics, phenothiazines, tranquilizers, sedative-hypnotics, TCAs and CNS depressants.

**PREGNANCY:** Safety in pregnancy and nursing not known.

## MERIDIA

CIV

sibutramine HCl monohydrate (Abbott)

**THERAPEUTIC CLASS:** Dopamine/norepinephrine/serotonin reuptake inhibitor

**INDICATIONS:** To induce and maintain weight loss in obese patients with an initial BMI >30kg/$m^2$ or >27kg/$m^2$ with risk factors (eg, HTN, diabetes, dyslipidemias)

**DOSAGE:** *Adults:* Initial: 10mg qd. Titrate: May increase after 4 weeks to 15mg qd. Max: 15mg/day. Use 5mg/day in patients unable to tolerate 10mg/day. May continue for up to 2 yrs.
*Pediatrics:* >16 yrs: Initial: 10mg qd. Titrate: May increase after 4 weeks to 15mg qd. Use 5mg/day in patients unable to tolerate 10mg/day. Max: 15mg/day. May continue for up to 2 yrs.

**HOW SUPPLIED:** Cap: 5mg, 10mg, 15mg

**CONTRAINDICATIONS:** Concomitant MAOIs or centrally acting appetite suppressants, anorexia nervosa.

**WARNINGS/PRECAUTIONS:** May increase BP and/or pulse. Avoid with uncontrolled or poorly controlled HTN, CAD, CHF, arrhythmias, stroke, severe hepatic or renal dysfunction. Monitor BP and pulse before therapy and regularly thereafter. Caution with narrow angle glaucoma, mild-moderate renal impairment, seizures and if predisposed to bleeding. Exclude organic causes of obesity. Gallstones precipitated with weight loss.

**ADVERSE REACTIONS:** Anorexia, constipation, increased appetite, nausea, dyspepsia, dry mouth, insomnia, dizziness, nervousness, HTN, tachycardia, dysmenorrhea, headache.



**INTERACTIONS:** Avoid excess alcohol, CNS-active drugs, other serotonergic agents (eg, SSRIs, migraine therapy agents, certain opioids), within 14 days of MAOI use. Caution with drugs affecting hemostasis or platelet function, ephedrine, pseudoephedrine, and other agents that increase BP, heart rate. Possible decreased metabolism with ketoconazole and erythromycin.

**PREGNANCY:** Category C, not for use in nursing

## MERREM

RX

meropenem (AstraZeneca LP)

**THERAPEUTIC CLASS:** Carbapenem

**INDICATIONS:** Treatment of intra-abdominal infections, bacterial meningitis, and complicated skin and skin structure infections (cSSSI).

**DOSAGE:** *Adults:* IV: Intra-abdominal: 1g q8h. CrCl 26-50mL/min: 1g q12h. CrCl 10-25mL/min: 500mg q12h. CrCl <10mL/min: 500mg q24h. SSSI: 500mg q8h. CrCl 26-50mL/min: 500mg q12h. CrCl 10-25mL/min: 250mg q12h. CrCl <10mL/min: 250mg q24h.
*Pediatrics:* IV: >3 months: >50kg: Intra-abdominal: 1g q8h. Meningitis: 2g q8h. SSSI: 500mg q8h. <50kg: Intra-abdominal: 20mg/kg q8h. Max: 1g q8h. Meningitis: 40mg/kg q8h. Max: 2g q8h. SSSI: 10mg/kg q8h. Max: 500mg q8h.

**HOW SUPPLIED:** Inj: 500mg, 1g

**CONTRAINDICATIONS:** Hypersensitivity to beta-lactams.

**WARNINGS/PRECAUTIONS:** Severe and fatal hypersensitivity reactions reported; increased risk with allergens and/or penicillin sensitivity. Pseudomembranous colitis reported. Seizures and other CNS effects reported particularly with pre-existing CNS disorders, bacterial meningitis, and renal dysfunction. Thrombocytopenia reported with severe renal impairment. Prolonged use may result in superinfection. Use as monotherapy for meningitis caused by penicillin nonsusceptible strains of *Streptococcus pneumoniae* has not been established.

**ADVERSE REACTIONS:** Headache, rash, local reactions, diarrhea, nausea, vomiting, constipation.

**INTERACTIONS:** Probenecid inhibits renal excretion; avoid concomitant use. May reduce valproic acid levels.

**PREGNANCY:** Category B, caution in nursing.

## MERUVAX II — RX

rubella vaccine live (Merck)

**THERAPEUTIC CLASS:** Vaccine

**INDICATIONS:** Vaccination against rubella.

**DOSAGE:** *Adults:* 0.5mL SQ in outer aspect of upper arm.
*Pediatrics:* Primary Vaccination at 12-15 months: 0.5mL SQ in outer aspect of upper arm. Revaccinate with MMR II prior to elementary school entry.

**HOW SUPPLIED:** Inj: 1000 $TCID_{50}$

**CONTRAINDICATIONS:** Avoid pregnancy for 3 months after vaccine, anaphylactic reaction to neomycin, febrile/active respiratory illness, immunosuppressive therapy (except corticosteroids as replacement therapy), blood dyscrasias, leukemia, lymphoma, malignant neoplasms affecting bone marrow or lymphatic system, immunodeficiency states.

**WARNINGS/PRECAUTIONS:** May worsen thrombocytopenia. Defer vaccination for at least 3 months after blood or plasma transfusions, immune globulin (except susceptible postpartum patients with follow-up HI titer after 6-8 weeks). Do not vaccinate with active untreated TB. Temperature elevation may occur after vaccination. Contains albumin, remote risk of viral infection transmission. Have epinephrine (1:1000) available.

**ADVERSE REACTIONS:** Fever, syncope, headache, dizziness, malaise, irritability, thrombocytopenia, arthritis, vasculitis, diarrhea, local reactions.

**INTERACTIONS:** Do not give with immune globulin. May depress TB skin sensitivity, administer test either simultaneously or before. Do not give <1 month before or after other live viral vaccines. Do not give simultaneously with DTP or oral poliovirus vaccine.

**PREGNANCY:** Category C, contraindicated in pregnancy and caution in nursing.

## MESNEX — RX

mesna (Baxter/Bristol-Myers Squibb Oncology/Immunology)

**THERAPEUTIC CLASS:** Sodium 2-mercaptoethane sulfonate

**INDICATIONS:** Prophylactic agent to reduce incidence of ifosfamide-induced hemorrhagic cystitis.

**DOSAGE:** *Adults:* (IV) IV bolus as 20% of ifosfamide dose given concurrently, and 4 and 8 hrs after each ifosfamide dose. Max: 60% of ifosfamide dose/day. (IV/PO) IV bolus as 20% of ifosfamide dose given concurrently, then give tabs as 40% of ifosfamide dose 2 and 6 hrs after each ifosfamide dose. Max: 100% of ifosfamide dose/day.

**HOW SUPPLIED:** Inj: 100mg/mL; Tab: 400mg

**CONTRAINDICATIONS:** Hypersensitivity to thiol compounds.

**WARNINGS/PRECAUTIONS:** Allergic reaction reported; higher incidence with autoimmune disorders. Does not prevent hemorrhagic cystitis in all patients. Hematuria reported; examine morning urine specimen daily prior to therapy. Multi-dose vial contains benzyl alcohol. False positive test for urinary ketones may occur.

**ADVERSE REACTIONS:** Nausea, vomiting, constipation, leukopenia, fatigue, fever, anorexia, thrombocytopenia, anemia, granulocytopenia, asthenia, abdominal pain, alopecia.

**PREGNANCY:** Category B, not for use in nursing.

## MESTINON RX

pyridostigmine bromide (Valeant)

**THERAPEUTIC CLASS:** Cholinesterase inhibitor

**INDICATIONS:** Treatment of myasthenia gravis.

**DOSAGE:** *Adults:* Adjust dose and frequency based on the needs of the individual patient. (Syrup, Tab) 600mg qd in divided doses. (Tab, Extended Release) 180-540mg given qd-bid. Dosing interval should be at least 6 hrs apart.

**HOW SUPPLIED:** Syrup: 60mg/5mL; Tab: 60mg*; Tab, Extended Release: 180mg* *scored

**CONTRAINDICATIONS:** Mechanical intestinal or urinary obstruction.

**WARNINGS/PRECAUTIONS:** Caution with bronchial asthma. Cholinergic crisis or myasthenic crisis may occur; it is important to differentiate. May need dose adjustment with renal disease.

**ADVERSE REACTIONS:** Nausea, vomiting, diarrhea, abdominal cramps, increased peristalsis, increased salivation, increased bronchial secretions, miosis, diaphoresis.

**INTERACTIONS:** Effects may be antagonized by atropine; caution when counteracting side effects.

**PREGNANCY:** Safety in pregnancy and nursing not known.

## METADATE CD CII

methylphenidate HCl (Celltech)



**THERAPEUTIC CLASS:** Sympathomimetic amine

**INDICATIONS:** Treatment of attention deficit hyperactivity disorder (ADHD).

**DOSAGE:** *Pediatrics:* >6 yrs: Usual: 20mg qam before breakfast. Titrate: Increase weekly by 20mg depending on tolerability/efficacy. Max: 60mg/day. Reduce dose or discontinue if paradoxical aggravation of symptoms occur. Discontinue if no improvement after appropriate dose adjustments over 1 month. Swallow whole with liquids or open and sprinkle on 1 tbs applesauce followed by water. Do not crush, chew, or divide.

**HOW SUPPLIED:** Cap, Extended-Release: 10mg, 20mg, 30mg

**CONTRAINDICATIONS:** Marked anxiety, tension, and agitation; glaucoma; motor tics, family history or diagnosis of Tourette's syndrome, severe hypertension, angina pectoris, cardiac arrhythmias, heart failure, recent MI, hyperthyroidism or thyrotoxicosis; during or within 14 days of MAOI use.

**WARNINGS/PRECAUTIONS:** Monitor growth in children. Not for severe depression or fatigue. May exacerbate symptoms of behavior disturbance and thought disorder in psychotic patients. Caution when using stimulants to treat patients with comorbid bipolar disorder because of concern for possible induction of mixed/manic episode in such patients. Stimulants at usual doses can cause treatment emergent psychotic or manic symptoms (eg, hallucinations, delusional thinking, mania) in children and adolescents without prior history of psychotic illness. Aggressive behavior or hostility reported in clinical trials and postmarketing experience of some medications indicated for the treatment of ADHD. May lower seizure threshold, especially in known EEG abnormalities. Caution with HTN, conditions affected by BP or HR elevation, history of drug abuse or alcoholism. Monitor during withdrawal from abusive use. Visual disturbances may occur (rare). Monitor CBC, differential, and platelets with prolonged use. Avoid with serious structural cardiac abnormalities, cardiomyopathy, serious heart rhythm abnormalities, CAD, or other serious cardiac problems.

**ADVERSE REACTIONS:** Headache, abdominal pain, anorexia, insomnia.

**INTERACTIONS:** See Contraindications. Potentiates anticoagulants, anticonvulsants (eg, phenobarbital, phenytoin, primidone), TCAs, and SSRIs. Caution with alpha$a_2$-agonist (eg, clonidine) and pressor agents.

**PREGNANCY:** Category C, caution in nursing.

## METADATE ER

methylphenidate HCl (Celltech)

CII

**THERAPEUTIC CLASS:** Sympathomimetic amine

**INDICATIONS:** Treatment of attention deficit disorder and narcolepsy.

**DOSAGE:** *Adults:* (Immediate-Release Methylphenidate) 10-60mg/day given bid-tid 30-45 minutes ac. Take last dose before 6 pm if insomnia occurs. (Tab, Extended Release) May use in place of immediate release tabs when the 8 hr dose corresponds to the titrated 8 hr immediate release dose. Swallow whole; do not chew or crush.
*Pediatrics:* >6 yrs: (Immediate-Release Methylphenidate) Initial: 5mg bid before breakfast and lunch. Titrate: Increase gradually by 5-10mg weekly. Max: 60mg/day. (Tab, Extended Release) May use in place of immediate release tabs when the 8 hr dose corresponds to the titrated 8 hr immediate release dose. Swallow whole; do not chew or crush. Reduce dose or discontinue if paradoxical aggravation of symptoms occur. Discontinue if no improvement after appropriate dose adjustment over 1 month.

**HOW SUPPLIED:** Tab, Extended Release: 10mg, 20mg

**CONTRAINDICATIONS:** Marked anxiety, tension, and agitation; glaucoma; motor tics or family history or diagnosis of Tourette's syndrome; during or within 14 days of MAOI use.

**WARNINGS/PRECAUTIONS:** Monitor growth in children. Not for severe depression or fatigue. May exacerbate symptoms of behavior disturbance and thought disorder in psychotic children. May lower seizure threshold, especially in known EEG abnormalities. Caution with HTN, emotionally-unstable patients. Monitor during withdrawal. Visual disturbances may occur (rare). Monitor CBC, differential, and platelets with prolonged use. Periodically d/c to assess condition.

**ADVERSE REACTIONS:** Nervousness, insomnia, hypersensitivity reactions, anorexia, nausea, dizziness, palpitations, headache, dyskinesia, drowsiness, BP and pulse changes, tachycardia, angina, arrhythmia, abdominal pain.

**INTERACTIONS:** See Contraindications. May decrease hypotensive effect of guanethidine. Caution with pressor agents. Potentiates anticoagulants, anticonvulsants (eg, phenobarbital, phenytoin, primidone), phenylbutazone, TCAs (eg, imipramine, clomipramine, desipramine).

**PREGNANCY:** Safety in pregnancy and nursing not known.

## METAGLIP

glipizide - metformin HCl (Bristol-Myers Squibb)

RX

**THERAPEUTIC CLASS:** Sulfonylurea/biguanide

**INDICATIONS:** Adjunct to diet and exercise, as initial therapy to improve glycemic control in type 2 diabetes, and as second-line therapy when treatment with a sulfonylurea or metformin is inadequate.

**DOSAGE:** *Adults:* Initial: 2.5mg-250mg qd. If FBG 280-320mg/dL, give 2.5mg-500mg bid. Titrate: Increase by 1 tab/day every 2 weeks. Max: 10mg-1g/day or 10mg-2g/day given in divided doses. Second-Line Therapy: Initial: 2.5mg-500mg or 5mg-500mg bid (with morning and evening meals). Starting dose should not exceed daily dose of metformin or glipizide already being taken. Titrate: Increase by no more than 5mg-500mg/day. Max: 20mg-2g/day. Elderly/Debilitated/Malnourished: Do not titrate to max dose. Take with meals.

**HOW SUPPLIED:** Tab: (Glipizide-Metformin) 2.5mg-250mg, 2.5mg-500mg, 5mg-500mg

**CONTRAINDICATIONS:** Renal disease/dysfunction (SrCr >1.5mg/dL [males], >1.4mg/dL [females], abnormal CrCl), CHF, metabolic acidosis, diabetic ketoacidosis. Discontinue temporarily (48 hrs) for radiologic studies with intravascular iodinated contrast materials.

**WARNINGS/PRECAUTIONS:** Lactic acidosis reported (rare); increased risk with renal dysfunction, increased age, DM, CHF, and other conditions with risk of hypoperfusion and hypoxemia. Avoid use in patients >80 yrs unless renal function is normal. Increased risk of cardiovascular mortality. Increased risk of hypoglycemia in elderly, debilitated/malnourished, adrenal or pituitary insufficiency, or alcohol intoxication. Discontinue in hypoxic states (eg, CHF, shock, acute MI) and prior to surgical procedures (due to restricted food intake). Avoid in renal/hepatic impairment. May decrease serum vitamin $B_{12}$ levels. Impaired renal and/or hepatic function may slow glipizide excretion. Withhold treatment with any condition associated with dehydration or sepsis. Monitor renal function.

**ADVERSE REACTIONS:** Upper respiratory tract infection, HTN, headache, diarrhea, dizziness, musculoskeletal pain, nausea, vomiting, abdominal pain.

**INTERACTIONS:** Furosemide, nifedipine, cimetidine and cationic drugs (eg, digoxin, amiloride, procainamide, quinidine, quinine, ranitidine, trimethoprim, vancomycin, triamterene, morphine) may increase metformin levels. Potentiated hypoglycemia with alcohol, NSAIDs, some azoles, and other highly protein bound drugs, salicylates, sulfonamides, chloramphenicol, probenecid, coumarins, MAOIs, and β-blockers. Severe hypoglycemia reported with concomitant oral miconazole. Thiazides and other diuretics, corticosteroids, phenothiazines, thyroid products, estrogens, oral contraceptives, phenytoin, nicotinic acid, sympathomimetics, calcium channel blockers, and isoniazid may cause hyperglycemia. Alcohol potentiates effect of metformin on lactate metabolism. May decrease furosemide levels.

**PREGNANCY:** Category C, not for use in nursing.



## METANX — RX

vitamin B6 - vitamin B12 - l-methylfolate (PamLab)

**THERAPEUTIC CLASS:** Folate/vitamin combination

**INDICATIONS:** Dietary management of endothelial dysfunction or hyperhomocysteinemia with particular emphasis for individuals with or at risk for atherosclerotic vascular disease in the coronary, peripheral, or cerebral vessels; C677T mutation of the MTHFR gene; or Vitamin $B_{12}$ deficiency.

**DOSAGE:** *Adults:* 1-2 tabs qd.

**HOW SUPPLIED:** Tab: L-methylfolate 2.8mg-Vitamin $B_6$ 25mg-Vitamin $B_{12}$ 2mg

**WARNINGS/PRECAUTIONS:** Folates >0.1mg/day may obscure pernicious anemia (may be alleviated by $B_{12}$ component).

**ADVERSE REACTIONS:** Paresthesia, somnolence, nausea, headache, diarrhea, polycythemia vera, itching, transitory exanthema, feeling of body swelling.

**INTERACTIONS:** Pyridoxal 5'-phosphate may antagonize levodopa; avoid concomitant use. May be used with carbidopa/levodopa.

## METAPROTERENOL — RX

metaproterenol sulfate (Various)

**OTHER BRAND NAMES:** Alupent (Boehringer Ingelheim)

**THERAPEUTIC CLASS:** $Beta_2$ agonist

**INDICATIONS:** For bronchial asthma and reversible bronchospasm. (Sol, Inhalation 5%) Treatment of acute asthmatic attacks in children >6 years.

**DOSAGE:** *Adults:* (MDI) 2-3 inh q3-4h. Max: 12 inh/day. (Sol 5%) Nebulizer or IPPB: 0.2-0.3mL (dilute in 2.5mL saline) tid-qid. Hand-bulb Nebulizer: 5-15 inh (undiluted) tid-qid. (Sol 0.4%, 0.6%) 2.5mL by IPPB tid-qid, up to q4h. (Syr, Tab) 20mg tid-qid.
*Pediatrics:* (MDI) >12 yrs: 2-3 inh q3-4h. Max: 12 inh/day. (Sol 5%) >12 yrs: Nebulizer or IPPB: 0.2-0.3mL (dilute in 2.5mL saline) tid-qid. Hand-bulb Nebulizer: 5-15 inh (undiluted) tid-qid. 6-12 yrs: Nebulizer: 0.1-0.2mL (dilute in 3mL saline) tid-qid. (Sol 0.4%, 0.6%) >12 yrs: 2.5mL by IPPB tid-qid, up to q4h. (Syr, Tab) >9 yrs or >60 lbs: 20mg tid-qid. 6-9 yrs or <60 lbs: 10mg tid-qid.

**HOW SUPPLIED:** MDI: 0.65mg/inh [14g]; Sol, Inhalation: 0.4% [2.5mL], 0.6% [2.5mL]; Syrup: 10mg/5mL [480mL]; Tab: 10mg, 20mg

**CONTRAINDICATIONS:** Cardiac arrhythmias associated with tachycardia.

**WARNINGS/PRECAUTIONS:** Caution with cardiovascular disorders, (eg, ischemic heart disease, HTN, arrhythmias), hyperthyroidism, diabetes, convulsive disorders. Fatalities reported with excessive use. Can produce paradoxical bronchospasm. Monitor BP. Nebulized solution single dose may not abort an asthma attack.

**ADVERSE REACTIONS:** Headache, dizziness, HTN, GI distress, throat irritation, cough, asthma exacerbation, nervousness, tremor, nausea, vomiting.

**INTERACTIONS:** Avoid other aerosol $\beta_2$ agonists. Vascular effects may be potentiated by MAOIs, TCAs, and sympathomimetics.

**PREGNANCY:** Category C, caution in nursing.

## METHADOSE

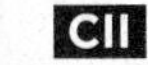

methadone HCl (Mallinckrodt)

**Only approved hospitals and pharmacies can dispense oral methadone for the treatment of narcotic addiction. Methadone can be dispensed in any licensed pharmacy when used as an analgesic.**

**THERAPEUTIC CLASS:** Opioid analgesic

**INDICATIONS:** (Concentrate/Tab, Dispersible) Detoxification and maintenance treatment of narcotic addiction (heroin or other morphine-like drugs). (Tab) Relief of severe pain. Detoxification and temporary maintenance treatment of narcotic addiction.

**DOSAGE:** *Adults:* Detoxification: Initial: 15-20mg/day (up to 40mg/day may be required). Stabilize for 2-3 days, then may decrease every 1-2 days depending on patient symptoms. Max: 21 days. May not repeat earlier than 4 weeks after completing previous course. Maintenance Treatment: >18 yrs: (see literature for ages 16 to <18) individualized 20-120mg/day. Pain: Usual: 2.5-10mg q3-4h prn.

**HOW SUPPLIED:** Concentrate: 10mg/mL; Tab: 5mg, 10mg; Tab, Dispersible: 40mg

**WARNINGS/PRECAUTIONS:** Do not inject agent. Extreme caution if use narcotic antagonists in patients physically dependent on narcotics. Can cause respiratory depression and elevate CSF pressure. Caution with head injuries, acute asthma attacks, COPD, cor pulmonale, decreased respiratory reserve, pre-existing respiratory depression, hypoxia, or hypercapnia. Reduce initial dose in elderly, debilitated, severe hepatic or renal impairment, hypothyroidism, Addison's disease, prostatic hypertrophy, or urethral stricture. Risk of tolerance, dependence, and abuse may occur. Impairs physical and mental abilities. Ineffective in relieving anxiety. May mask symptoms of acute abdominal conditions. May produce hypotension.

**ADVERSE REACTIONS:** Lightheadedness, dizziness, sedation, sweating, nausea, vomiting.

**INTERACTIONS:** Pentazocine may precipitate withdrawal. Decreased serum levels with rifampin. Caution and reduce dose with CNS depressants (eg, tranquilizers, sedative-hypnotics, phenothiazines, TCAs, alcohol). MAOIs may cause severe reactions.

**PREGNANCY:** Safety in pregnancy and nursing not known.

## METHERGINE
methylergonovine maleate (Novartis) RX

**THERAPEUTIC CLASS:** Ergot alkaloid

**INDICATIONS:** Management after delivery of the placenta. To treat postpartum atony and hemorrhage. For subinvolution.

**DOSAGE:** *Adults:* (Inj) 0.2mg IM/IV after delivery of the anterior shoulder, placenta, or during puerperium. May be repeated q2-4h. (Tab) 0.2mg PO tid-qid in the puerperium. Max: 1 week.

**HOW SUPPLIED:** Inj: 0.2mg/mL; Tab: 0.2mg

**CONTRAINDICATIONS:** HTN, toxemia, pregnancy.

**WARNINGS/PRECAUTIONS:** Risk of hypertensive or cerebrovascular accidents with IV administration. Caution in sepsis, obliterative vascular disease, hepatic/renal involvement, and during second stage of labor.

**ADVERSE REACTIONS:** Seizures, headache, hypotension, nausea, vomiting, acute MI, dyspnea, hematuria, thrombophlebitis, water intoxication, hallucinations, leg cramps, dizziness, nasal congestion, diarrhea.

**INTERACTIONS:** Caution with vasoconstrictors or ergot alkaloids.

**PREGNANCY:** Category C, caution in nursing.

## METHOTREXATE SODIUM
methotrexate sodium (Various) RX

**Only for life-threatening neoplastic disease, or in severe RA, and psoriasis unresponsive to other therapies. Death, fetal death/congenital anomalies, lung disease, tumor lysis syndrome, fatal skin reactions, PCP reported. Monitor for bone marrow, liver, lung, and kidney toxicities. Bone marrow suppression, aplastic anemia and GI toxicity reported with NSAIDs. Hepatotoxicity, fibrosis, and cirrhosis with prolonged use. Interrupt therapy with diarrhea, ulcerative stomatitis. Reduced elimination with renal dysfunction, ascites, or pleural effusion. Increased risk of soft tissue necrosis and osteonecrosis with radiotherapy. Malignant lymphoma may occur. Extreme caution with high dose regimen for osteosarcoma. Do not use formulations/diluents with preservatives for intrathecal or high dose therapy.**

**OTHER BRAND NAMES:** Rheumatrex (Stada)

**THERAPEUTIC CLASS:** Dihydrofolic acid reductase inhibitor

**INDICATIONS:** Treatment of neoplastic diseases (eg, acute lymphocytic leukemia, gestational choriocarcinoma, chorioadenoma destruens, hydatidiform mole, breast cancer, epidermoid cancer of the head and neck, advanced mycosis fungoides, lung cancer, advanced stage non-Hodgkin's lymphomas). Prophylaxis and treatment of meningeal leukemia, and maintenance with other chemotherapeutics. For prolonging relapse-free survival in non-metastatic osteosarcoma followed by leucovorin. Symptomatic control of severe, recalcitrant, disabling psoriasis, and management of rheumatoid arthritis (RA) or polyarticular-course juvenile rheumatoid arthritis (JRA) unresponsive to other therapies.

**DOSAGE:** *Adults:* Choriocarcinoma/Trophoblastic disease: 15-30mg qd PO/IM for 5 days. May repeat 3-5 times as required with rest period of >1 week. Leukemia: Induction: 3.3mg/m$^2$ with prednisone 60mg/m$^2$ qd. Remission Maintenance: 15mg/m$^2$ PO/IM twice weekly or 2.5mg/kg IV every 14 days. Burkitt's Tumor: Stages I-II: 10-25mg/day PO for 4-8 days. Administer several courses with rest periods of 7-10 days in between. Lymphosarcoma: Stage III: 0.625-2.5mg/kg/day with other antitumor agents. Mycosis Fungoides: 5-50mg once weekly. If poor response, give 15-37.5mg twice weekly. Adjust dose based on response and hematologic monitoring. Osteosarcoma: Initial: 12g/m$^2$ IV, increase to 15g/m$^2$ if peak serum levels of 1000 micromolar not reached at end of infusion. Meningeal Leukemia: Dilute preservative free MTX

to 1mg/mL. Give 12mg intrathecally at 2-5 day intervals. Psoriasis: Initial: 10-25mg weekly until response or use divided oral dose schedule, 2.5mg at 12 hr intervals for 3 doses. Titrate: Increase gradually until optimal response. Maint: Reduce to lowest effective dose. Max: 30mg/week. Rheumatoid Arthritis: Initial: 7.5mg PO once weekly, or 2.5mg q12h for 3 doses given as a course once weekly. Titrate: Gradual increase. Max: 20mg weekly. After response, reduce dose to lowest effective amount of drug.
*Pediatrics:* Meningeal Leukemia: Dilute preservative free MTX to 1mg/mL. <1 yr: 6mg. 1 yr: 8mg. 2 yrs: 10mg. > 3yrs: 12mg. Give intrathecally at 2-5 day intervals. JRA: 2-16 yrs: Initial: 10mg/m$^2$ once weekly. Adjust dose gradually to achieve optimal response.

**HOW SUPPLIED:** Inj: (Generic) 20mg, 25mg/mL, 1g; Tab: (Rheumatrex) 2.5mg* [Dose Pack 15mg, 4 x 6 tabs; 12.5mg, 4 x 5 tabs; 10mg, 4 x 4 tabs; 7.5mg, 4 x 3 tabs; 5mg, 4 x 2 tabs] *scored

**CONTRAINDICATIONS:** Pregnancy, nursing. Psoriasis or RA patients with alcoholism, alcoholic liver disease, chronic liver disease, immunodeficiency syndrome, and pre-existing blood dyscrasias.

**WARNINGS/PRECAUTIONS:** Monitor closely; toxicity may be related to dose and frequency of administration. When reactions do occur, doses should be reduced or discontinued and corrective measures should be taken. Avoid pregnancy if either partner is receiving therapy. Avoid intrathecal administration or high-dose therapy. Injection contains benzyl alcohol; avoid use in neonates (<1 month), may cause gasping syndrome.

**ADVERSE REACTIONS:** Ulcerative stomatitis, leukopenia, nausea, abdominal distress, malaise, fatigue, chills, fever, dizziness, decreased resistance to infection.

**INTERACTIONS:** Avoid NSAIDs with high doses. Caution with nephrotoxic agents (eg, cisplatin), NSAIDs, probenecid, and highly protein bound drugs (eg, sulfonamides, phenytoin, phenylbutazone, salicylates). Oral antibiotics (eg, tetracycline, chloramphenicol) may decrease absorption or interfere with enterohepatic circulation. Penicillins may decrease clearance. Closely monitor with hepatotoxins (eg, azathioprine, retinoids, sulfasalazine). Folic acid may decrease response to MTX. TMP/SMZ may increase bone marrow suppression. Decreased theophylline clearance.

**PREGNANCY:** Category X, contraindicated in nursing.



## METHYLDOPA — RX

methyldopa (Various)

**THERAPEUTIC CLASS:** Central alpha-adrenergic agonist

**INDICATIONS:** Treatment of hypertension.

**DOSAGE:** *Adults:* Initial: 250mg bid-tid for 48 hrs. Adjust dose at intervals of not less than 2 days. Maint: 500mg-2g/day given bid-qid. Max: 3g/day. Concomitant Antihypertensives (other than thiazides): Initial: Limit to 500mg/day. Renal Impairment: May respond to lower doses.
*Pediatrics:* Initial: 10mg/kg/day given bid-qid. Max: 65mg/kg/day or 3g/day, whichever is less.

**HOW SUPPLIED:** Tab: 125mg, 250mg, 500mg

**CONTRAINDICATIONS:** Active hepatic disease, history of methyldopa associated liver disorder, concomitant MAOIs.

**WARNINGS/PRECAUTIONS:** Positive Coombs test, hemolytic anemia, and liver disorders may occur. Fever reported within the 1st 3 weeks of therapy. HTN has recurred after dialysis. Caution with liver disease or dysfunction. D/C if signs of heart failure, or involuntary choreoathetotic movements develop. Edema and weight gain reported. Blood count, Coombs test and LFTs prior to therapy and periodically thereafter.

**ADVERSE REACTIONS:** Sedation, headache, asthenia, edema/weight gain, hepatic disorders, vomiting, diarrhea, nausea, sore or"black" tongue, blood dyscrasias, BUN increase, gynecomastia, impotence.

**INTERACTIONS:** See Contraindications. May potentiate other antihypertensives. Anesthetics may need dose reduction. Monitor for lithium toxicity. Ferrous sulfate and ferrous gluconate may decrease bioavailability; avoid coadministration.

**PREGNANCY:** Category B, caution in nursing.

## METHYLDOPA/HCTZ RX

methyldopa - hydrochlorothiazide (Various)

**Not for initial therapy of HTN.**

**THERAPEUTIC CLASS:** Central alpha-adrenergic agonist/thiazide diuretic

**INDICATIONS:** Treatment of HTN. Not for initial treatment.

**DOSAGE:** *Adults:* Initial: 250mg-15mg tab bid-tid, 250mg-25mg tab bid, or 500mg-30mg qd. Max: 50mg HCTZ/day or 3g methyldopa/day.

**HOW SUPPLIED:** Tab: (HCTZ-Methyldopa) 15mg-250mg, 25-250mg, 30mg-500mg

**CONTRAINDICATIONS:** Active hepatic disease, anuria, sulfonamide allergy, concomitant MAOIs, history of methyldopa associated liver disorder.

**WARNINGS/PRECAUTIONS:** Positive Coombs test, hemolytic anemia, liver disorders, sensitivity reactions, hypokalemia, hyperuricemia, hyperglycemia, hypomagnesemia, hypercalcemia may occur. Fever reported within the 1st 3 weeks of therapy. HTN has recurred after dialysis. Caution with liver disease or dysfunction, severe renal disease. D/C if signs of heart failure, progressive renal dysfunction, or involuntary choreoathetotic movements develop. Edema and weight gain reported. Blood count, Coombs test and LFTs before therapy and periodically thereafter. Monitor electrolytes. May exacerbate or activate SLE. May increase cholesterol and TG levels. Enhanced effects in postsympathectomy patient.



**ADVERSE REACTIONS:** Weakness, asthenia, headache, pancreatitis, diarrhea, vomiting, constipation, nausea, blood dyscrasias, rash, electrolyte imbalance, renal failure, impotence, vertigo.

**INTERACTIONS:** See Contraindications. Potentiates orthostatic hypotension with alcohol, barbiturates, narcotics. Lithium toxicity. Adjust antidiabetic drugs. NSAIDs decrease diuretic effects. Reduce dose of anesthetics. Ferrous sulfate and ferrous gluconate may decrease bioavailability; avoid coadministration. May potentiate nondepolarizing skeletal muscle relaxants, antihypertensives. May decrease response to pressor amines. Corticosteroids, ACTH intensify electrolyte depletion. Impaired absorption with cholestyramine, colestipol.

**PREGNANCY:** Category C, not for use in nursing.

## METHYLDOPATE HCL RX

methyldopate HCl (American Regent)

**THERAPEUTIC CLASS:** Central alpha-adrenergic agonist

**INDICATIONS:** Treatment of hypertension and hypertensive crises.

**DOSAGE:** *Adults:* 250-500mg IV q6h as needed. Max: 1gm q6h. Elderly/Renal Dysfunction: May reduce dose. Switch to oral therapy once BP is controlled. *Pediatrics:* 20-40mg/kg/day IV given q6h. Max: 65mg/kg/day or 3 g/day, whichever is less. Switch to oral therapy once BP is controlled.

**HOW SUPPLIED:** Inj: 50mg/mL

**CONTRAINDICATIONS:** Hypersensitivity to sulfites, active hepatic disease, liver disorders previously associated with methyldopa therapy, concomitant MAOIs.

**WARNINGS/PRECAUTIONS:** Positive Coombs test, hemolytic anemia, and liver disorders may occur. Fever reported within the first 3 weeks of therapy. HTN has recurred after dialysis. Caution with liver disease or dysfunction. D/C if signs of heart failure develop. Edema and weight gain reported. Blood count, Coombs test and LFTs prior to therapy and periodically thereafter. Caution with cerebrovascular disease.

**ADVERSE REACTIONS:** Sedation, headache, asthenia, weakness, edema, weight gain, liver disorders, vomiting, diarrhea, nausea, sore or"black" tongue, blood dyscrasias, BUN increase, gynecomastia, impotence.

**INTERACTIONS:** See Contraindications. May potentiate other antihypertensives. Anesthetics may need dose reduction. May increase lithium levels. Ferrous sulfate and ferrous gluconate may decrease bioavailability; avoid coadministration.

**PREGNANCY:** Category C, caution in nursing.

## METHYLIN **CII**

methylphenidate HCl (Mallinckrodt)

**OTHER BRAND NAMES:** Methylin ER (Mallinckrodt)

**THERAPEUTIC CLASS:** Sympathomimetic amine

**INDICATIONS:** Treatment of attention deficit disorder and narcolepsy.

**DOSAGE:** *Adults:* (Sol/Tab/Tab, Chewable) 10-60mg/day given bid-tid 30-45 min ac. Take last dose before 6 pm if insomnia occurs. (Tab, Extended-Release) May use in place of immediate release tabs when the 8 hr dose corresponds to the titrated 8 hr immediate release dose. Swallow whole; do not chew or crush.

*Pediatrics:* >6 yrs: (Sol/Tab/Tab, Chewable) Initial: 5mg bid before breakfast and lunch. Titrate: Increase gradually by 5-10mg weekly. Max: 60mg/day. (Tab, Extended-Release) May be used in place of immediate release tabs when the 8 hr dose corresponds to the titrated 8 hr immediate release dose. Swallow whole; do not chew or crush. Reduce dose or discontinue if paradoxical aggravation of symptoms occur. Discontinue if no improvement after appropriate dose adjustment over 1 month.

**HOW SUPPLIED:** Sol: 5mg/5mL [500mL], 10mg/5mL [500mL]; Tab: 5mg, 10mg, 20mg; Tab, Chewable: 2.5mg, 5mg, 10mg; Tab, Extended-Release: 10mg, 20mg

**CONTRAINDICATIONS:** Marked anxiety, tension, and agitation; glaucoma; motor tics or family history or diagnosis of Tourette's syndrome, during or within 14 days of MAOI use.

**WARNINGS/PRECAUTIONS:** Monitor growth in children. Not for severe depression or fatigue. May exacerbate symptoms of behavior disturbance or thought disorder in psychotic children. Caution when using stimulants to treat patients with comorbid bipolar disorder because of concern for possible induction of mixed/manic episode in such patients. Stimulants at usual doses can cause treatment emergent psychotic or manic symptoms (hallucinations, delusional thinking, mania) in children and adolescents without prior history of psychotic illness. Aggressive behavior or hostility has been reported in clinical trials and the postmarketing experience of some medications indicated for the treatment of ADHD. May lower seizure threshold, especially in known EEG abnormalities. Caution with HTN, heart failure, recent MI, ventricular arrhythmia, or emotionally-unstable patients. Monitor during withdrawal. Visual disturbances may occur (rare). Monitor CBC, differential, and platelets with prolonged use. Periodically d/c to assess condition. Avoid with serious structural cardiac abnormalities, cardiomyopathy, serious heart rhythm abnormalities, CAD, or other serious cardiac problems. Caution in emotionally unstable patients with history of drug dependence or alcoholism.

**ADVERSE REACTIONS:** Nervousness, insomnia, hypersensitivity reactions, anorexia, nausea, dizziness, palpitations, headache, dyskinesia, drowsiness, BP and pulse changes, tachycardia, angina, arrhythmia, abdominal pain.

**INTERACTIONS:** May decrease hypotensive effect of guanethidine. Caution with pressor agents. Avoid during or within 14 days of MAOI use. Potentiates anticoagulants, anticonvulsants (phenobarbital, diphenylhydantoin, primidone), phenylbutazone, TCAs (imipramine, clomipramine, desipramine).

**PREGNANCY:** Safety in pregnancy and nursing not known.

## METOCLOPRAMIDE — RX

metoclopramide HCl (Various)

**OTHER BRAND NAMES:** Reglan (Schwarz) - Reglan Injection (Baxter)

**THERAPEUTIC CLASS:** Dopamine antagonist/prokinetic

**INDICATIONS:** (PO) Symptomatic treatment of gastroesophageal reflux in patients who fail to respond to conventional therapy. (Inj, PO) Symptomatic relief of diabetic gastroparesis. (Inj) Prevention of post-op or chemo-induced nausea/vomiting. Diagnostic aid during radiological examination and facilitates intubation of small intestine.

**DOSAGE:** *Adults:* GERD: PO: 10-15mg qid 30 minutes ac and hs. Elderly: 5 mg qid. Max: 12 weeks of therapy. Intermittent Symptoms: Up to 20mg single dose prior to provoking situation. Gastroparesis: 10mg PO 30 minutes ac and hs for 2-8 weeks. Severe Gastroparesis: May give same doses IV/IM for up to 10 days if needed. Antiemetic: (Postoperative) 10-20mg IM near end of surgery. (Chemotherapy-Induced) 1-2mg/kg 30 minutes before chemotherapy then q2h for two doses, then q3h for three doses. Give 2mg/kg for highly emetogenic drugs for initial 2 doses. Small Bowel Intubation/Radiological Exam: 10mg IV single dose. CrCl <40mL/min: 50% of normal dose. *Pediatrics:* Small Bowel Intubation: 6-14 yrs: 2.5-5mg IV single dose. <6 yrs: 0.1mg/kg IV single dose. CrCl <40mL/min: 50% of normal dose.



**HOW SUPPLIED:** Inj: 5mg/mL; Syr: 5mg/5mL; Tab: 5mg, 10mg* *scored

**CONTRAINDICATIONS:** Where GI mobility stimulation is dangerous (eg, perforation, obstruction, hemorrhage), pheochromocytoma, seizure disorder, concomitant drugs that cause EPS effects.

**WARNINGS/PRECAUTIONS:** Caution with HTN, Parkinson's disease, depression. EPS, tardive dyskinesia, Parkinsonian-like symptoms, neuroleptic malignant syndrome reported. Administer IV injection slowly. Risk of developing fluid retention and volume overload especially with cirrhosis or CHF; d/c if these occur. May increase pressure of suture lines.

**ADVERSE REACTIONS:** Restlessness, drowsiness, fatigue, EPS effects (acute dystonic reactions), galactorrhea, hyperprolactinemia, hypotension, arrhythmia, diarrhea, dizziness, urinary frequency.

**INTERACTIONS:** See Contraindications. May decrease gastric absorption of drugs (eg, digoxin) and increase intestinal absorption of drugs (eg, APAP, tetracycline, levodopa, ethanol, and cyclosporine). Additive sedation with alcohol, hypnotics, narcotics, or tranquilizers. Caution with MAOIs. Antagonized by anticholinergics, narcotics. Insulin dose or timing of dose may need adjustment to prevent hypoglycemia.

**PREGNANCY:** Category B, caution with nursing.

## METROGEL — RX

metronidazole (Galderma)

**OTHER BRAND NAMES:** MetroCream (Galderma) - MetroLotion (Galderma)

**THERAPEUTIC CLASS:** Imidazole antibiotic

**INDICATIONS:** Treatment of inflammatory papules and pustules of rosacea.

**DOSAGE:** *Adults:* (Cre, Gel 0.75%, Lot) Wash affected area(s) then apply bid, am and pm. (Cre 1%) Wash affected area(s) then apply qd.

**HOW SUPPLIED:** Cre: 0.75% [45g]; Gel: 0.75%, 1% [45g]; Lot 0.75% [59mL]

**CONTRAINDICATIONS:** Hypersensitivity to parabens.

**WARNINGS/PRECAUTIONS:** Avoid eye contact. Decrease frequency or d/c if skin irritation occurs. Caution with blood dyscrasias.

**ADVERSE REACTIONS:** Burning, skin irritation, dryness, redness, metallic taste, tingling/numbness of extremities, nausea.

**INTERACTIONS:** Oral metronidazole may potentiate warfarin; unknown effect with topical formulation.

**PREGNANCY:** Category B, not for use in nursing.

## METROGEL-VAGINAL RX

metronidazole (Graceway)

**THERAPEUTIC CLASS:** Imidazole antibacterial

**INDICATIONS:** Treatment of bacterial vaginosis.

**DOSAGE:** *Adults:* One applicatorful intravaginally qd-bid for 5 days. For once daily dosing, administer at bedtime .

**HOW SUPPLIED:** Gel: 0.75% [70g]

**CONTRAINDICATIONS:** Hypersensitivity to other nitroimidazole derivatives.

**WARNINGS/PRECAUTIONS:** Caution with CNS or severe hepatic disease. D/C if abnormal neurologic signs appear. Avoid vaginal intercourse during therapy. May develop *Candida* vaginitis. May interfere with lab tests (ALT, SGPT, AST, SGOT, LDH, triglycerides, and glucose hexokinase).

**ADVERSE REACTIONS:** *Candida* cervicitis/vaginitis, vaginal discharge, pelvic discomfort, nausea, vomiting, headache, vulva/vaginal irritation, GI discomfort, change in WBC count.

**INTERACTIONS:** May potentiate warfarin, other anticoagulants, and lithium. Cimetidine may potentiate metronidazole. Avoid alcohol; possible disulfiram-like reaction may occur. Do not administer gel within 2 weeks of discontinuing disulfiram therapy.

**PREGNANCY:** Category B, not for use in nursing.

## MEVACOR RX

lovastatin (Merck)

**THERAPEUTIC CLASS:** HMG-CoA reductase inhibitor

**INDICATIONS:** To reduce risk of MI, unstable angina, and coronary revascularization procedures in patients without symptomatic coronary disease, average to moderately elevated total-C and LDL-C, and below average HDL-C. To slow coronary atherosclerosis progression in patients with coronary heart disease to reduce total-C and LDL-C. Adjunct to diet to lower total-C and LDL-C in primary hypercholesterolemia (Types IIa and IIb). Adjunct to diet to lower total-C, LDL-C and apolipoprotein B in adolescents at least 1-yr postmenarchal with heterozygous familial hypercholesterolemia.

**DOSAGE:** *Adults:* Initial: 20mg qd at dinner (10mg/day if need LDL-C reduction <20%). Usual: 10-80mg/day given qd or bid. May adjust every 4 weeks. Max: 80mg/day. Concomitant Cyclosporine: Initial: 10mg/day. Max: 20mg/day. Fibrates/Niacin (≥1g/day): Max: 20mg/day. Concomitant Amiodarone/Verapamil: Max: 40mg/day. CrCl <30mL/min: Consider dose increase of >20mg/day carefully and implement cautiously.
*Pediatrics:* Heterozygous Familial Hypercholesterolemia: 10-17 yrs (at least 1-yr postmenarchal): Initial: If <20% LDL-C Reduction Needed: 10mg qd. If >20% LDL-C Reduction Needed: 20mg qd. May adjust every 4 weeks. Max: 40mg/day. Concomitant Cyclosporine: Initial: 10mg/day. Max: 20mg/day. Fibrates/Niacin (≥1g/day): Max: 20mg/day. Concomitant Amiodarone/Verapamil: Max: 40mg/day. CrCl <30mL/min: Consider dose increase of >20mg/day carefully and implement cautiously.

**HOW SUPPLIED:** Tab: 20mg, 40mg

**CONTRAINDICATIONS:** Active liver disease, unexplained persistent elevations of serum transaminases, pregnancy, nursing mothers.

**WARNINGS/PRECAUTIONS:** May increase serum transaminases and CPK levels; consider in differential diagnosis of chest pain. D/C if AST or ALT >3X ULN persist, or if myopathy diagnosed or suspected. Monitor LFTs prior to therapy, at 6 weeks, 12 weeks, then periodically or with dose elevation. Caution with heavy alcohol use and/or history of hepatic disease. Caution with dose escalation in renal insufficiency. Less effective with homozygous familial hypercholesterolemia. Rhabdomyolysis (rare), myopathy reported. D/C a few days before elective major surgery and when any major acute medical or surgical condition supervenes.

**ADVERSE REACTIONS:** Headache, constipation, flatulence, dizziness, rash, elevated transaminases or CK levels, GI upset, blurred vision.

**INTERACTIONS:** Increased risk of myopathy with CYP3A4 inhibitors (eg, cyclosporine, itraconazole, ketoconazole, erythromycin, clarithromycin, telithromycin, protease inhibitors, nefazodone, >1 quart/day of grapefruit juice), verapamil, amiodarone, fibrates (eg, gemfibrozil), danazol, and >1g/day of niacin. Monitor anticoagulants. Caution with drugs that diminish levels or activity of steroid hormones (eg, ketoconazole, spironolactone, cimetidine).

**PREGNANCY:** Category X, not for use in nursing.

## MEXILETINE — RX

mexiletine HCl (Various)



**THERAPEUTIC CLASS:** Class IB antiarrhythmic

**INDICATIONS:** Treatment of life-threatening ventricular arrhythmias.

**DOSAGE:** *Adults:* Initial: 200mg q8h when rapid control is not essential. Titrate: Adjust by 50-100mg, not less than every 2-3 days. Usual: 200-300mg q8h. Max: 1200mg/day. If control with <300mg q8h, then may divide daily dose and give q12h. Max: 450mg q12h. For Rapid Control: LD: 400mg, then 200mg in 8 hrs. Transfer from Class I Oral Agents: Initial: 200mg and titrate as above, 6-12 hrs after last quinidine sulfate or disopyramide dose, 3-6 hrs after last procainamide dose, or 8-12 hrs after last tocainide dose. Severe Hepatic Disease: May need lower dose. Take with food or antacid.

**HOW SUPPLIED:** Cap: 150mg, 200mg, 250mg

**CONTRAINDICATIONS:** Cardiogenic shock, pre-existing 2nd- or 3rd-degree AV block (without a pacemaker).

**WARNINGS/PRECAUTIONS:** Reserve for life-threatening arrhythmias. May treat patients with 2nd- or 3rd-degree AV block with a pacemaker; monitor continuously. Can worsen arrhythmias. Caution with hypotension, severe CHF, seizure disorder, hepatic impairment, sinus node dysfunction, or intraventricular conduction abnormalities. Leukopenia, agranulocytosis, and abnormal LFTs reported. Monitor ECG.

**ADVERSE REACTIONS:** Coordination difficulties, tremor, GI distress, lightheadedness.

**INTERACTIONS:** Avoid drugs or diet regimens that may alter urinary pH. Enzyme inducers (eg, rifampin, phenobarbital, phenytoin) lower plasma levels. May increase theophylline levels. Decreases caffeine clearance. Cimetidine may alter levels.

**PREGNANCY:** Category C, not for use in nursing.

## MIACALCIN RX
calcitonin-salmon (Novartis)

**THERAPEUTIC CLASS:** Hormonal bone resorption inhibitor

**INDICATIONS:** (Inj) Treatment of Paget's disease, hypercalcemia, and postmenopausal osteoporosis. (Spray) Treatment of postmenopausal osteoporosis in females >5yrs postmenopause.

**DOSAGE:** *Adults:* (Inj) Paget's Disease: Usual: 100 IU IM/SQ qd. Hypercalcemia: Initial: 4 IU/kg IM/SQ q12h. Titrate: May increase to 8 IU/kg q12h after 1-2 days, then to 8 IU/kg q6h after 2 days if unsatisfactory response. Osteoporosis: (Inj) 100 IU IM/SQ every other day. If >2mL, use IM injection. (Spray) 200 IU qd intranasally. Alternate nostrils daily. Take with supplemental calcium and vitamin D for postmenopausal osteoporosis.

**HOW SUPPLIED:** Inj: 200 IU/mL; Nasal Spray: 200 IU/inh [2mL 2[s]]

**WARNINGS/PRECAUTIONS:** Possibility of systemic allergic reactions. Monitor urine sediment periodically with chronic use. If nasal mucosa ulceration occurs, discontinue until healed. D/C if severe ulceration of the nasal mucosa occurs. Perform periodic nasal exams. Monitor drug effects.

**ADVERSE REACTIONS:** (Inj) Nausea, vomiting, injection site inflammation, flushing of face or hands, nocturia, ear lobe pruritus, poor appetite, abdominal pain. (Spray) Nasal symptoms, back pain, headache, arthralgia.

**PREGNANCY:** Category C, not for use in nursing.

## MICARDIS RX
telmisartan (Boehringer Ingelheim)

**Can cause death/injury to developing fetus during 2nd and 3rd trimesters. Stop therapy if pregnancy detected.**

**THERAPEUTIC CLASS:** Angiotensin II receptor antagonist

**INDICATIONS:** Treatment of hypertension, alone or with other antihypertensives.

**DOSAGE:** *Adults:* Initial: 40mg qd. Usual: 20-80mg/day. May add diuretic if need additional BP reduction after 80mg/day.

**HOW SUPPLIED:** Tab: 20mg, 40mg*, 80mg* *scored

**WARNINGS/PRECAUTIONS:** Can cause fetal injury/death. Correct volume or salt depletion before therapy. Changes in renal function may occur; caution with renal artery stenosis, severe CHF. Closely monitor with biliary obstructive disorders or hepatic dysfunction.

**ADVERSE REACTIONS:** Upper respiratory infection, back pain, diarrhea, bradycardia, eosinophilia, thrombocytopenis, uric acid increased, abnormal hepatic funtion/liver disorder, renal impairment including acute renal failure, anemia, increased CPK, cases of alopecia, aggression and psychotic disorder.

**INTERACTIONS:** Increases digoxin levels. May alter warfarin levels.

**PREGNANCY:** Category C (1st trimester) and D (2nd and 3rd trimesters), not for use in nursing.

## MICARDIS HCT RX
telmisartan - hydrochlorothiazide (Boehringer Ingelheim)

**Can cause death/injury to developing fetus during 2nd and 3rd trimesters. Stop therapy if pregnancy detected.**

**THERAPEUTIC CLASS:** Angiotensin II receptor antagonist/thiazide diuretic

**INDICATIONS:** Treatment of hypertension. Not for initial therapy.

M

**DOSAGE:** *Adults:* If BP not controlled on 80mg telmisartan, or 25mg HCTZ/day, or controlled on 25mg HCTZ/day but serum $K^+$ decreased, 80mg-12.5mg tab qd. Titrate/Max: If uncontrolled after 2-4 weeks, increase to 160mg-25mg. Biliary Obstruction/Hepatic Dysfunction: Initial: 40mg-12.5mg tab qd; monitor closely.

**HOW SUPPLIED:** Tab: (HCTZ-Telmisartan) 12.5mg-40mg, 12.5mg-80mg, 25mg-80mg

**CONTRAINDICATIONS:** Anuria, sulfonamide hypersensitivity.

**WARNINGS/PRECAUTIONS:** Can cause fetal injury/death. Correct volume or salt depletion before therapy. Caution with hepatic or renal dysfunction, biliary obstructive disorders, renal artery stenosis, severe CHF, history of allergies, and asthma. May exacerbate or activate SLE. Monitor serum electrolytes. Avoid if CrCl <30mL/min. Hyperuricemia, hyperglycemia, hypokalemia, hypomagnesemia, hypercalcemia may occur. Enhanced effects in post-sympathectomy patient. May increase cholesterol and triglyceride levels.

**ADVERSE REACTIONS:** Dizziness, fatigue, sinusitis, upper respiratory infection, diarrhea, bradycardia, eosinophilia, thrombocytopenia,uric acid increased, abnormal hepatic function/liver disorder, renal impairment including acute renal failure, anemia, and increased CPK.

**INTERACTIONS:** Potentiates orthostatic hypotension with alcohol, barbiturates, and narcotics. Adjust insulin and antidiabetic drugs. Impaired absorption with cholestyramine, colestipol. Corticosteroids and ACTH deplete electrolytes. May decrease response to pressor amines. Potentiates other antihypertensives. May increase responsiveness to skeletal muscle relaxants. Risk of lithium toxicity. NSAIDs decrease diuretic effects. Increases digoxin levels. May alter warfarin levels.

**PREGNANCY:** Category C (1st trimester) and D (2nd and 3rd trimesters), not for use in nursing.



## MICRO-K

RX

potassium chloride (Ther-Rx)

**THERAPEUTIC CLASS:** $K^+$ supplement

**INDICATIONS:** (For those unable to tolerate liquid or effervescent potassium preparations). Treatment and prevention of hypokalemia with or without metabolic alkalosis. Treatment of digitalis intoxication and hypokalemic familial periodic paralysis.

**DOSAGE:** *Adults:* Prevention: 20mEq/day. Hypokalemia: 40-100mEq/day. Divide dose if >20mEq. Take with meal and full glass of water or liquid. May sprinkle on soft food; swallow without chewing.

**HOW SUPPLIED:** Cap, Extended Release: 8mEq, 10mEq

**CONTRAINDICATIONS:** Hyperkalemia, esophageal ulceration, delay in GI passage (from structural, pathological, pharmacologic causes), cardiac patients with esophageal compression due to enlarged left atrium.

**WARNINGS/PRECAUTIONS:** Potentially fatal hyperkalemia may occur. Extreme caution with acidosis, cardiac and renal disease; monitor ECG and electrolytes. Hypokalemia with metabolic acidosis should be treated with an alkalinizing potassium salt (eg, potassium bicarbonate, potassium citrate). May produce ulcerative or stenotic GI lesions.

**ADVERSE REACTIONS:** Hyperkalemia, GI effects (obstruction, bleeding, ulceration), nausea, vomiting, abdominal pain, diarrhea.

**INTERACTIONS:** Risk of hyperkalemia with ACE inhibitors (eg, captopril, enalapril), $K^+$-sparing diuretics, and $K^+$ supplements. Contraindicated with anticholinergic agents due to possible delay in tablet passage through GI tract.

**PREGNANCY:** Category C, safe for use in nursing.

## MICRONASE RX
glyburide (Pharmacia & Upjohn)

**THERAPEUTIC CLASS:** Sulfonylurea (2nd generation)

**INDICATIONS:** Adjunct to diet and exercise, to improve glycemic control in type 2 diabetes mellitus. May use in combination with metformin.

**DOSAGE:** *Adults:* Initial: 2.5-5mg qd with breakfast or 1st main meal; give 1.25mg if sensitive to hypoglycemia. Titrate: Increase by no more than 2.5mg/day at weekly intervals. Maint: 1.25-20mg given qd or in divided doses. Max: 20mg/day. May give bid with >10mg/day. Renal or Hepatic Disease/Elderly/Debilitated/Malnourished/Adrenal or Pituitary Insufficiency: Initial: 1.25mg qd. Transfer From Other Oral Antidiabetic Agents: Initial: 2.5-5mg/day. Switch From Insulin: If >40 U/day, decrease dose by 50% and give 5mg qd. Titrate: Progressive withdrawal of insulin, and increase by 1.25-2.5mg/day every 2-10 days. Concomitant Metformin: Add glyburide gradually to max dose of metformin monotherapy after 4 weeks if needed.

**HOW SUPPLIED:** Tab: 1.25mg*, 2.5mg*, 5mg* *scored

**CONTRAINDICATIONS:** Diabetic ketoacidosis, and as sole therapy for type 1 DM.

**WARNINGS/PRECAUTIONS:** Increased risk of cardiovascular mortality. Risk of hypoglycemia, especially with renal and hepatic disease, elderly, debilitated or malnourished patients, and those with adrenal or pituitary insufficiency. May need to d/c and give insulin with stress (eg, fever, trauma). Secondary failure may occur. D/C if jaundice, hepatitis, or persistent skin reaction occur. Hematologic reactions and hyponatremia reported.

**ADVERSE REACTIONS:** Hypoglycemia, nausea, epigastric fullness, heartburn, allergic skin reactions, disulfiram-like reactions (rarely), hyponatremia, liver function abnormalities, photosensitivity reactions.

**INTERACTIONS:** Hypoglycemia potentiated by alcohol, NSAIDs, miconazole, fluoroquinolones, highly protein bound drugs, salicylates, sulfonamides, chloramphenicol, probenecid, coumarins, MAOIs, and β-blockers. Risk of hyperglycemia with diuretics, corticosteroids, phenothiazines, thyroid products, estrogens, oral contraceptives, phenytoin, nicotinic acid, sympathomimetics, calcium channel blockers, and INH. β-blockers may mask hypoglycemia. Disulfiram-like reactions (rarely) with alcohol.

**PREGNANCY:** Category B, not for use in nursing.

## MICRONOR RX
norethindrone (Ortho-McNeil)

**OTHER BRAND NAMES:** Errin (Barr)

**THERAPEUTIC CLASS:** Progestogen

**INDICATIONS:** Prevention of pregnancy.

**DOSAGE:** *Adults:* 1 tab qd without interruption (continuous regimen) on 1st day of menstrual period. If fully nursing, start 6 weeks postpartum. If partially nursing, start 3 weeks postpartum.

**HOW SUPPLIED:** Tab: 0.35mg

**CONTRAINDICATIONS:** Pregnancy, breast carcinoma, undiagnosed abnormal genital bleeding, benign or malignant liver tumors, acute liver disease.

**WARNINGS/PRECAUTIONS:** Avoid smoking. Perform annual physical exam. Not for use before menarche. May affect certain endocrine tests (eg, sex hormone binding globulin, thyroxine binding globulin). Monitor glucose tolerance in prediabetics and diabetics. May alter lipid metabolism. May increase risk of breast cancer and hepatic adenomas. May cause irregular menstrual patterns. Delayed follicular atresia/ovarian cysts and ectopic pregnancy may occur. D/C with recurrent migraines or severe headaches.

**ADVERSE REACTIONS:** Menstrual irregularities, frequent or irregular bleeding, headache, breast tenderness, nausea, dizziness, androgenic effects (rare).

**INTERACTIONS:** Reduced efficacy with hepatic enzyme inducers (eg, rifampin, phenytoin, carbamazepine, barbiturates).

**PREGNANCY:** Not for use in pregnancy, caution use in nursing.

## MICROZIDE RX
hydrochlorothiazide (Watson)

**THERAPEUTIC CLASS:** Thiazide diuretic

**INDICATIONS:** Management of hypertension.

**DOSAGE:** *Adults:* Initial: 12.5mg qd. Max: 50mg/day.

**HOW SUPPLIED:** Cap: 12.5mg

**CONTRAINDICATIONS:** Anuria, sulfonamide hypersensitivity.

**WARNINGS/PRECAUTIONS:** Caution in severe renal disease, liver dysfunction, electrolyte/fluid imbalance. Monitor electrolytes. Hyperuricemia, hyperglycemia, hypokalemia, hyponatremia, hypomagnesemia, hypercalcemia may occur. Increases in cholesterol and triglyceride levels reported. May exacerbate SLE. Sensitivity reactions reported. Discontinue prior to parathyroid test. Enhanced effects in post-sympathectomy patient.

**ADVERSE REACTIONS:** Weakness, hypotension, pancreatitis, jaundice, diarrhea, vomiting, blood dyscrasias, rash, photosensitivity, electrolyte imbalance, impotence.

**INTERACTIONS:** May potentiate orthostatic hypotension with alcohol, barbiturates, narcotics. Adjust antidiabetic drugs. Possible decreased response to pressor amines. Corticosteroids, ACTH increase electrolyte depletion. May potentiate nondepolarizing skeletal muscle relaxants, antihypertensives. Lithium toxicity. NSAIDs decrease effects. Decreased PO absorption with cholestyramine, colestipol.

**PREGNANCY:** Category B, not for use in nursing.

## MIDAMOR RX
amiloride HCl (Merck)

**THERAPEUTIC CLASS:** $K^+$-sparing diuretic

**INDICATIONS:** Adjunct therapy in CHF or hypertension to help restore normal serum $K^+$ levels and to prevent hypokalemia.

**DOSAGE:** *Adults:* Initial: 5mg qd. Titrate: Increase to 10mg/day. If hyperkalemia persists, may increase to 15mg/day then to 20mg/day with careful monitoring. Take with food.

**HOW SUPPLIED:** Tab: 5mg

**CONTRAINDICATIONS:** Hyperkalemia, anuria, acute or chronic renal insufficiency, diabetic neuropathy, $K^+$-sparing agents (eg, diuretics), and $K^+$ supplements, $K^+$ salt substitutes, $K^+$-rich diet (except with severe hypokalemia).

**WARNINGS/PRECAUTIONS:** Risk of hyperkalemia (>5.5 mEq/L) especially with renal impairment, elderly, DM; monitor levels frequently. D/C if hyperkalemia occurs. Caution in severely ill in whom respiratory or metabolic acidosis may occur; monitor acid-base balance frequently. Hepatic encephalopathy reported with severe hepatic disease. Increased BUN reported. D/C at least 3 days before glucose tolerance test. Monitor electrolytes and renal function in DM.

**ADVERSE REACTIONS:** Headache, nausea, anorexia, vomiting, elevated serum potassium, diarrhea.

**INTERACTIONS:** Increased risk of hyperkalemia with ACE inhibitors, angiotensin II receptor antagonists, indomethacin, cyclosporine, and tacrolimus. Risk of lithium toxicity. Decreased effects with NSAIDs. Hyponatremia and hypochloremia with other diuretics.

**PREGNANCY:** Category B, not for use in nursing.

## MIDRIN

CIV

acetaminophen - dichloralphenazone - isometheptene mucate

(Women First)

**OTHER BRAND NAMES:** Amidrine (Amide) - Duradrin (Duramed) - Migquin (Qualitest) - Migrazone (Various)

**THERAPEUTIC CLASS:** Analgesic/sedative/sympathomimetic

**INDICATIONS:** Relief of tension and vascular headaches. FDA has classified this agent as"possibly" effective in the treatment of migraine headache.

**DOSAGE:** *Adults:* Migraine: 2 caps, then 1 cap every hr until relieved. Max: 5 caps/12hrs. Tension Headache: 1-2 caps q4h. Max: 8 caps/day.

**HOW SUPPLIED:** Cap: (APAP-Dichloralphenazone-Isometheptene) 325mg-100mg-65mg

**CONTRAINDICATIONS:** Glaucoma, severe renal disease, HTN, organic heart disease, hepatic disease, concomitant MAOI therapy.

**WARNINGS/PRECAUTIONS:** Caution with HTN, peripheral vascular disease, or recent cardiovascular attacks.

**ADVERSE REACTIONS:** Transient dizziness, skin rash.

**PREGNANCY:** Safety in pregnancy and nursing are not known.

## MIFEPREX

RX

M

mifepristone (Danco Laboratories)

**Serious and sometimes fatal infections and bleeding occur very rarely following spontaneous, surgical, and medical abortions, including following Mifeprex use. Before prescribing Mifeprex, inform the patient about the risk of these serious events and discuss the Medication Guide and Patient Agreement. Ensure that the patient knows whom to call and what to do, including going to the Emergency Room if none of the provided contacts are reachable, if she experiences sustained fever, severe abdominal pain, prolonged heavy bleeding, or syncope.**

**THERAPEUTIC CLASS:** Abortifacient

**INDICATIONS:** Medical termination of intrauterine pregnancy through 49 days of pregnancy.

**DOSAGE:** *Adults:* Day 1: 600mg single dose. Day 3: Unless abortion is confirmed, give 400mcg PO of misoprostol. Day 14: Assess if complete termination of pregnancy has occurred. Perform surgical termination if mifeprex and misoprostol fail.

**HOW SUPPLIED:** Tab: 200mg

**CONTRAINDICATIONS:** Ectopic pregnancy, undiagnosed adnexal mass, IUD in place, chronic adrenal failure, concurrent long-term corticosteroid therapy, hemorrhagic disorders, concurrent anticoagulant therapy, inherited porphyrias, prostaglandin hypersensitivity. Patients who do not have access to medical facilities or who are unable to understand the treatment or comply with regimen.

**WARNINGS/PRECAUTIONS:** Vaginal bleeding lasts for average 9-16 days. Infection and sepsis, including rare cases of fatal septic shock. Conduct follow-up visit 14 days after initial dose to confirm pregnancy termination. Preventive measures required to prevent rhesus immunization. Patients should review medication guide and patient agreement prior to procedure. Caution with women >35 yrs who smoke ≥10 cigarettes daily. Risk of fetal malformation if treatment fails. May cause decreases in Hgb, Hct and RBCs. Very rare cases of fatal septic shock have been reported.

**ADVERSE REACTIONS:** Abdominal pain, uterine cramping, nausea, headache, vomiting, diarrhea, dizziness, fatigue, back pain, uterine hemorrhage, fever, viral infections, vaginitis.

**INTERACTIONS:** Ketoconazole, itraconazole, erythromycin, and grapefruit juice may inhibit metabolism. Rifampin, dexamethasone, St. John's wort and certain anticonvulsants may induce metabolism.

**PREGNANCY:** Not for use in pregnancy or nursing.

## MIGRANAL RX

dihydroergotamine mesylate (Xcel Pharm)

**Serious and life-threatening peripheral ischemia reported with potent CYP3A4 inhibitors (eg, protease inhibitors, macrolides). Elevated levels of dihydroergotamine increases risk of vasospasm leading to cerebral ischemia or ischemia of the extremities. Concomitant use with CYP3A4 inhibitors is contraindicated.**

**THERAPEUTIC CLASS:** Ergot alkaloid

**INDICATIONS:** Acute treatment of migraine headache with or without aura.

**DOSAGE:** *Adults:* 1 spray per nostril, repeat in 15 minutes. Max: 6 sprays/24 hrs or 8 sprays/week.

**HOW SUPPLIED:** Nasal Spray: 0.5mg/inh [4mL]

**CONTRAINDICATIONS:** Ischemic heart disease (angina, history of MI, documented silent ischemia), coronary artery vasospasm (Prinzmetal's variant angina), uncontrolled HTN, known peripheral artery disease, sepsis, following vascular surgery, severe renal or hepatic dysfunction, hemiplegic or basilar migraine, pregnancy, or nursing, with potent CYP3A4 inhibitors (eg, ritonavir, nelfinavir, indinavir, erythromycin, clarithromycin, troleandomycin, ketoconazole, itraconazole). Do not use with peripheral and central vasoconstrictors or within 24 hrs of 5-$HT_1$ agonists, ergot-type drugs, or methysergide.

**WARNINGS/PRECAUTIONS:** Confirm diagnosis. Monitor and consider ECG with 1st dose in patients with CAD risk factors (eg, HTN, hypercholesterolemia, smoker, obesity, DM, strong family history, postmenopausal women, men >40 yrs). Risk of elevated BP, MI and other adverse cardiac or vasospastic effects. Monitor cardiovascular function with intermittent long-term use.

**ADVERSE REACTIONS:** Rhinitis, altered taste, application site reactions, dizziness, nausea, vomiting, pharyngitis, somnolence.

**INTERACTIONS:** Greater ischemic response to ergots with nicotine. Increased BP with peripheral vasoconstrictors. Potentiation of vasoconstriction with propranolol and macrolides. May have additive coronary artery vasospasms with sumatriptan. Do not use with peripheral and central vasoconstrictors or within 24 hrs of 5-$HT_1$ agonists, ergot-type drugs, or methysergide. Contraindicated with CYP3A4 inhibitors (eg, macrolides, protease inhibitors). Caution with less potent CYP3A4 inhibitors (eg, saquinavir, nefazodone, fluconazole, grapefruit juice, fluoxetine, fluvoxamine, zileuton, clotrimazole).

**PREGNANCY:** Category X, not for use in nursing.

## MILTOWN CIV

meprobamate (MedPointe)

**THERAPEUTIC CLASS:** Carbamate derivative

**INDICATIONS:** Management of anxiety disorders or short-term relief of symptoms of anxiety.

**DOSAGE:** *Adults:* Usual: 1200-1600mg/day given tid-qid. Max: 2400mg/day. Elderly: >65 yrs: Start at low end of dosing range.
*Pediatrics:* 6-12 yrs: 200-600mg/day given bid-tid.

**HOW SUPPLIED:** Tab: 200mg, 400mg

**CONTRAINDICATIONS:** Porphyria, allergic or idiosyncratic reactions to carisoprodol, mebutamate, tybamate, carbromal.

**WARNINGS/PRECAUTIONS:** Physical and psychological dependence reported. Avoid abrupt withdrawal after prolonged or excessive use. Increased risk of congenital malformations with use during 1st trimester of pregnancy. Caution with liver or renal dysfunction, and in elderly. May precipitate seizures in epileptic patients. Prescribe small quantities in suicidal patients.

**ADVERSE REACTIONS:** Drowsiness, ataxia, slurred speech, vertigo, weakness, nausea, vomiting, diarrhea, tachycardia, transient ECG changes, rash, leukopenia, petechiae.

**INTERACTIONS:** Administration with other CNS depressants, alcohol, psychotropics have additive effects.

**PREGNANCY:** Safety in pregnancy and nursing not known.

## MINIPRESS

RX

prazosin HCl (Pfizer)

**THERAPEUTIC CLASS:** Alpha$_1$-blocker (quinazoline)

**INDICATIONS:** Treatment of hypertension.

**DOSAGE:** *Adults:* Initial: 1mg bid-tid. Maint: 6-15mg/day in divided doses. Max: 40mg/day. Concomitant Diuretic/Antihypertensive: Reduce to 1-2mg tid, then retitrate.

**HOW SUPPLIED:** Cap: 1mg, 2mg, 5mg

**WARNINGS/PRECAUTIONS:** Syncope may occur, usually after initial dose or dose increase. Excessive postural hypotensive effects. Avoid driving for 24 hrs after 1st dose or dose increase. Always start on 1mg cap. False (+) for pheochromocytoma.

**ADVERSE REACTIONS:** Dizziness, headache, drowsiness, lack of energy, weakness, palpitations, nausea.

**INTERACTIONS:** Additive hypotensive effects with diuretics, β-blockers, or other antihypertensives. Dizziness or syncope may occur with alcohol.

**PREGNANCY:** Category C, caution in nursing.

## MINIZIDE

RX

polythiazide - prazosin HCl (Pfizer)

**Not for initial therapy of HTN.**

**THERAPEUTIC CLASS:** Diuretic/alpha$_1$-blocker

**INDICATIONS:** Treatment of HTN.

**DOSAGE:** *Adults:* 1 cap bid-tid. Determine strength by individual component titration.

**HOW SUPPLIED:** Cap: (Polythiazide-Prazosin) 0.5mg-1mg, 0.5mg-2mg, 0.5mg-5mg

**CONTRAINDICATIONS:** Anuria, thiazide or sulfonamide sensitivity.

**WARNINGS/PRECAUTIONS:** Syncope may occur, usually after initial dose or dose increase. Excessive postural hypotensive effects. Avoid driving for 24 hrs after 1st dose or dose increase. Always start on 1mg prazosin. Caution with severe renal disease, hepatic dysfunction, or progressive liver disease. Sensitivity reactions may occur with history of allergy or bronchial asthma. May exacerbate or activate SLE. Hyperuricemia, hypokalemia or frank gout may occur. Monitor electrolytes. May manifest latent DM. Enhanced effects in the post-sympathectomy patient. May decrease serum protein-bound iodine levels. False (+) for pheochromocytoma.

**ADVERSE REACTIONS:** Dizziness, headache, drowsiness, lack of energy, weakness, palpitations, nausea, blood dyscrasias, rash.

**INTERACTIONS:** Additive effects with other antihypertensives. Potentiation with ganglionic or peripheral adrenergic blockers. Increased risk of hypokalemia with ACTH, corticosteroids. May increase responsiveness to tubocurarine. May alter insulin requirements. May decrease arterial responsiveness to norepinephrine. Orthostatic hypotension aggravated by alcohol, barbiturates, or narcotics.

**PREGNANCY:** Category C, not for use in nursing.

## MINOCIN — RX

minocycline HCl (Triax)

**THERAPEUTIC CLASS:** Tetracycline derivative

**INDICATIONS:** Treatment of inclusion conjunctivitis, nongonococcal urethritis, and other infections (eg, respiratory tract, endocervical, rectal, urinary tract, skin and skin structure) caused by susceptible strains of microorganisms. Alternative treatment, when penicillin is contraindicated, in certain other infections (eg, urethritis, gonococcal, syphilis, anthrax). Adjunctive therapy in acute intestinal amebiasis and severe acne. Treatment of *Mycobacterium marinum* and asymptomatic carriers of *Neisseria meningitidis*.

**DOSAGE:** *Adults:* Usual: 200mg initially, then 100mg q12h; alternative is 100-200mg initially, then 50mg qid. Uncomplicated Gonococcal Infection (Men, other than urethritis and anorectal infections): 200mg initially, then 100mg q12h for minimum 4 days. Uncomplicated Gonococcal Urethritis (Men): 100mg q12h for 5 days. Syphilis: Administer usual dose for 10-15 days. Meningococcal Carrier State: 100mg q12h for 5 days. *Mycobacterium marinum:* 100mg q12h for 6-8 weeks. Uncomplicated Urethral, Endocervical, or Rectal Infection Caused by *Chlamydia trachomatis* or *Ureaplasma urealyticum*: 100mg q12h for at least 7 days. Gonorrhea in Patients Sensitive to PCN: 200mg initially, then 100mg q12h for at least 4 days, with post-therapy cultures within 2-3 days. Take with plenty of fluids. Renal Dysfunction: Max: 200mg/24hrs.
*Pediatrics:* >8 yrs: 4mg/kg initially followed by 2mg/kg q12h, not to exceed adult dose. Take with plenty of fluids. Renal Dysfunction: Max: 200mg/24hrs.

**HOW SUPPLIED:** Cap: 50mg, 100mg; Inj: 100mg; Sus: 50mg/5mL [60mL]

**WARNINGS/PRECAUTIONS:** May cause fetal harm during pregnancy. Use during tooth development (last half of pregnancy, infancy, <8yrs) may cause permanent discoloration of the teeth or enamel hypoplasia; avoid use during this period. Renal toxicity, hepatotoxicity, photosensitivity, increased BUN, superinfection, pseudotumor cerebri may occur; perform hematopoietic, renal, and hepatic monitoring. Caution with hepatic dysfunction. Caution in renal impairment; may lead to azotemia, hyperphosphatemia, and acidosis. Use alternate form of contraception other than oral contraceptives. May decrease bone growth in premature infants. If *clostridium difficile* associated diarrhea (CDAD) develops, appropriate therapy should be initiated.

**ADVERSE REACTIONS:** Anorexia, nausea, vomiting, diarrhea, dysphagia, enterocolitis, pancreatitis, increased LFTs, renal toxicity, rash, exfoliative dermatitis, Stevens-Johnson syndrome, skin and mucous membrane pigmentation, blood dyscrasias, headache, tooth discoloration.

**INTERACTIONS:** May require downward adjustments of anticoagulant dosage. May interfere with bactericidal action of penicillin; avoid concurrent use when possible. May decrease efficacy of oral contraceptives. Impaired absorption with antacids containing aluminum, calcium, or magnesium and iron-containing products. Fatal renal toxicity with methoxyflurane has been reported. Avoid isotretinoin shortly before, during and after therapy. Caution with other hepatotoxic drugs. Risk of ergotism with ergot alkaloids.

**PREGNANCY:** Category D, not for use in nursing.

M

## MINOXIDIL

minoxidil (Par)

RX

**May cause pericardial effusion, occasionally progressing to tamponade, and angina pectoris may be exacerbated. Only for nonresponders to maximum therapeutic doses of two other antihypertensives and a diuretic. Administer under supervision with a β-blocker and diuretic. Monitor in hospital for a decrease in BP in those receiving guanethidine with malignant hypertension.**

**THERAPEUTIC CLASS:** Peripheral vasodilator

**INDICATIONS:** Treatment of hypertension that is symptomatic or associated with target organ damage and is not manageable with maximum therapeutic doses of diuretic plus two other antihypertensive drugs.

**DOSAGE:** *Adults:* Initial: 5mg qd. Titrate: Increase by no less than 3 days; may increase every 6 hrs if closely monitored. Usual: 10-40mg/day. Max: 100mg/day. Frequency: Give qd if diastolic BP is reduced to <30 mmHg and if reduced to >30 mmHg give bid. Give with a diuretic (eg, HCTZ 50mg bid, furosemide 40mg bid) and a β-blocker (equivalent to propranolol 80-160mg/day) or methyldopa (250-750mg bid starting 24 hrs before therapy). Renal Failure/Dialysis: Reduce dose.
*Pediatrics:* >12 yrs: Initial: 5mg qd. Titrate: Increase by no less than 3 days; may increase every 6 hrs if closely monitored. Usual: 10-40mg/day. Max: 100mg/day. Frequency: Give qd if diastolic BP is reduced to <30 mmHg and if reduced to >30 mmHg give bid. Give with a diuretic (eg, HCTZ 50mg bid, furosemide 40mg bid) and a β-blocker (equivalent to propranolol 80-160mg/day) or methyldopa (250-750mg bid starting 24 hrs before therapy). <12 yrs: 0.2mg/kg qd. Titrate: May increase by 50-100% increments. Usual: 0.25-1mg/kg/day. Max: 50mg/day. Renal Failure/Dialysis: Reduce dose.

**HOW SUPPLIED:** Tab: 2.5mg*, 10mg* *scored

**CONTRAINDICATIONS:** Pheochromocytoma.

**WARNINGS/PRECAUTIONS:** Administer with a diuretic and β-blocker. Pericarditis, pericardial effusion and tamponade reported. With renal failure or dialysis, reduce dose to prevent renal failure exacerbation and precipitation of cardiac failure. Avoid rapid control with severe HTN. Monitor body weight, fluid and electrolyte balance. Extreme caution with post-MI. Hypersensitivity reactions reported.

**ADVERSE REACTIONS:** Salt and water retention, pericarditis, pericardial effusion, tamponade, hypertrichosis, nausea, vomiting, rash, ECG changes, hemodilution effects.

**INTERACTIONS:** Severe orthostatic hypotension with guanethidine.

**PREGNANCY:** Category C, not for use in nursing.

## MINTEZOL

thiabendazole (Merck)

RX

**THERAPEUTIC CLASS:** Vermicidal and/or vermifugal agent

**INDICATIONS:** Treatment of strongyloidiasis (threadworm), cutaneous larva migrans (creeping eruption), visceral larva migrans, and trichinosis. Second line or adjunct treatment for uncinariasis, trichuriasis, ascariasis (intestinal roundworms).

**DOSAGE:** *Adults:* 100 lbs: 1g or 10mL bid. 125 lbs: 1.25g or 12.5mL bid. >150 lbs: 1.5g or 15mL bid. Max: 3g/day. Take with meals. Treatment Duration: Strongyloidiasis/Cutaneous Larva Migrans/Intestinal Roundworms: 2 days. Trichinosis: 2-4 days. Visceral Larva Migrans: 7 days.
*Pediatrics:* 30 lbs: 250mg or 2.5mL bid. 50 lbs: 500mg or 5mL bid. 75 lbs: 750mg or 7.5mL bid. Max: 3g/day. Take with meals. Treatment Duration: Strongyloidiasis/Cutaneous Larva Migrans/Intestinal Roundworms: 2 days. Trichinosis: 2-4 days. Visceral Larva Migrans: 7 days.

**HOW SUPPLIED:** Sus: 500mg/5mL [120mL]; Tab, Chewable: 500mg* *scored

**CONTRAINDICATIONS:** Prophylactic treatment for pinworm infestation.

**WARNINGS/PRECAUTIONS:** D/C if hypersensitivity reactions occurs. Erythema multiforme and Stevens-Johnson syndrome, jaundice, cholestasis, and parenchymal hepatic damage reported. Prolonged use may cause abnormal sensation in eyes, xanthopsia, and blurred vision. Not for mixed infections with ascaris, prophylaxis, or first line treatment of enterobiasis. Monitor with hepatic or renal dysfunction.

**ADVERSE REACTIONS:** Anorexia, nausea, vomiting, diarrhea, weariness, drowsiness, dizziness, abnormal sensation in eyes, xanthopsia, hypotension, hyperglycemia, leukopenia, hematuria, pruritus, fever.

**INTERACTIONS:** Decreases metabolism of xanthine derivatives; monitor blood levels and/or reduce dose.

**PREGNANCY:** Category C, not for use in nursing.

## MIOCHOL-E RX

acetylcholine chloride (Novartis Ophthalmics)

**THERAPEUTIC CLASS:** Cholinergic agent

**INDICATIONS:** To obtain miosis of iris seconds after delivery of lens in cataract surgery, in penetrating keratoplasty, iridectomy, and other anterior segment surgery when rapid miosis may be required.

**DOSAGE:** *Adults:* Draw up 0.5-2mL using an 18-20 gauge needle. Replace needle with atraumatic cannulae for intraocular irrigation. Instill acetylcholine into anterior chamber before or after securing one or more sutures. Instill gently and parallel to iris face and tangential to pupil border.



**HOW SUPPLIED:** Inj: 20mg [2mL]

**WARNINGS/PRECAUTIONS:** Do not gas sterilize. Open under aseptic conditions only. Release any anatomical hindrances to miosis (eg, anterior/posterior synechiae) prior to administration. Use only after lens delivery in cataract surgery. Prepare solution immediately prior to use.

**ADVERSE REACTIONS:** Corneal edema, corneal clouding, corneal decompensation.

**INTERACTIONS:** May be ineffective in patients treated with topical NSAIDs.

**PREGNANCY:** Safety in pregnancy or nursing not known.

## MIRALAX OTC

polyethylene glycol 3350 (Schering-Plough)

**THERAPEUTIC CLASS:** Osmotic laxative

**INDICATIONS:** Treatment of occasional constipation.

**DOSAGE:** *Adults:* Stir and dissolve 17g in 4-8 oz of beverage and drink qd. Use no more than 7 days.
*Pediatrics:* ≥17 yrs: Stir and dissolve 17g in 4-8 oz of beverage and drink qd. Use no more than 7 days.

**HOW SUPPLIED:** Powder: 17g/dose [119g, 238g]

**WARNINGS/PRECAUTIONS:** Avoid in kidney disease; talk to your doctor before use if you have nausea, vomiting, abdominal pain, sudden change in bowel habits for ≥2 weeks, or IBS.

## MIRAPEX

RX

pramipexole dihydrochloride (Boehringer Ingelheim)

**THERAPEUTIC CLASS:** Non-ergot dopamine agonist

**INDICATIONS:** Treatment of signs and symptoms of idiopathic Parkinson's disease. Treatment of moderate-to-severe primary Restless Legs Syndrome (RLS).

**DOSAGE:** *Adults:* Parkinson's: Initial: 0.125mg tid. Titrate: May increase every 5-7 days (eg, Week 2: 0.25mg tid; Week 3: 0.5mg tid; Week 4: 0.75mg tid; Week 5: 1mg tid; Week 6: 1.25mg tid; Week 7: 1.5mg tid). Maint: 0.5-1.5mg tid. Max: 1.5mg tid. CrCl >60mL/min: Initial: 0.125mg tid. Max: 1.5mg tid. CrCl 35-59mL/min: Initial: 0.125mg bid. Max: 1.5mg bid. CrCl 15-34mL/min: Initial: 0.125mg qd. Max: 1.5mg qd. RLS: Initial: 0.125mg once daily, 2-3 hours before bedtime. Titrate: May double dose every 4-7 days up to 0.5mg/day.

**HOW SUPPLIED:** Tab: 0.125mg, 0.25mg*, 0.5mg*, 1mg*, 1.5mg* *scored

**WARNINGS/PRECAUTIONS:** Somnolence, symptomatic hypotension, hallucinations and rhabdomyolysis reported. Caution with renal insufficiency. May potentiate dyskinesia. May cause retinal pathology, fibrotic complications, withdrawal-emergent hyperpyrexia and confusion. Consider discontinuation if significant daytime sleepiness or sudden onset of sleep occurs during daily activities. Cases of pathological gambling, hypersexuality, and compulsive eating reported. Rebound and augmentation in RLS reported. Falling asleep during activities of daily living.

**ADVERSE REACTIONS:** Nausea, dizziness, somnolence, insomnia, constipation, asthenia, hallucination, vision abnormalities, peripheral edema, arthritis, dry mouth, postural hypotension, chest pain, malaise

**INTERACTIONS:** Cimetidine, ranitidine, diltiazem, triamterene, verapamil, quinidine, and quinine may decrease clearance. Dopamine antagonists (eg, phenothiazines, butyrophenones, thioxanthenes, metoclopramide) may decrease effects.

**PREGNANCY:** Category C, not for use in nursing.



## MIRCETTE

RX

desogestrel - ethinyl estradiol (Organon)

**OTHER BRAND NAMES:** Kariva (Barr)

**THERAPEUTIC CLASS:** Estrogen/progestogen combination

**INDICATIONS:** Prevention of pregnancy.

**DOSAGE:** *Adults:* Start 1st Sunday after menses begins or 1st day of menses. *28-day:* 1 tab qd for 28 days, then repeat.

**HOW SUPPLIED:** Tab: (Ethinyl Estradiol-Desogestrel) 0.02mg-0.15mg and 0.01mg-NA

**CONTRAINDICATIONS:** Thrombophlebitis, DVT or thromboembolic disorders, pregnancy, cerebrovascular or coronary artery disease, undiagnosed abnormal genital bleeding, cholestatic jaundice of pregnancy or jaundice with prior pill use, hepatic adenomas or carcinomas, breast cancer or other estrogen-dependent neoplasia.

**WARNINGS/PRECAUTIONS:** Cigarette smoking increases risk of serious cardiovascular side effects. This risk increases with age (especially >35 yrs) and heavy smoking. Increased risk of MI, vascular disease, thromboembolism, stroke and gallbladder disease. Retinal thrombosis, hepatic neoplasia, carcinoma of breast and reproductive organs reported. May cause glucose intolerance. May increase BP, elevate LDL levels or cause other lipid changes, fluid retention, breakthrough bleeding, and spotting. May cause or exacerbate migraine. May develop visual changes with contact lens. Increased risk of MI with HTN, hyperlipidemia, obesity, and diabetes. D/C if jaundice, significant depression, or ophthalmic irregularities develop. Perform annual physical exam. Use before menarche is not indicated. May affect certain endocrine, LFTs and blood components.

**ADVERSE REACTIONS:** Nausea, vomiting, breakthrough bleeding, spotting, amenorrhea, migraine, depression, vaginal candidiasis, edema, weight changes.

**INTERACTIONS:** Reduced effects, increased breakthrough bleeding, and menstrual irregularities with rifampin, barbiturates, phenylbutazone, phenytoin, carbamazepine, and possibly with griseofulvin, ampicillin, and tetracyclines.

**PREGNANCY:** Category X, not for use in nursing.

## MIRENA — RX

levonorgestrel (Berlex)

**THERAPEUTIC CLASS:** Progestogen

**INDICATIONS:** For intrauterine contraception.

**DOSAGE:** *Adults:* Insert intravaginally for contraception. Initial insertion is recommended within 7 days of the onset of menses. Replacement may be done at any time in the cycle. May insert 6 weeks postpartum or until involution of uterus is complete, and immediately after 1st trimester abortion. Reexamine within 3 months after insertion. Replace every 5 yrs.

**HOW SUPPLIED:** Intrauterine Insert: 52mg

**CONTRAINDICATIONS:** Pregnancy, congenital or acquired uterine anomaly, acute or history of PID, postpartum endometriosis, infected abortion in the past 3 months, uterine or cervical neoplasia, abnormal Pap smear, genital bleeding of unknown etiology, untreated acute cervicitis or vaginitis, acute liver disease, liver tumor, women or partner with multiple sexual partners, conditions associated with increased susceptibility to microorganisms, genital actinomycosis, previously inserted IUD that is not removed, breast carcinoma, and predisposition to ectopic pregnancy.

**WARNINGS/PRECAUTIONS:** Risk of ectopic pregnancy, glucose intolerance. Pregnancy with IUD in place, increases risk of septic abortion, congenital anomalies, premature labor, miscarriage. Increased risk of PID, sepsis, ovarian cysts. Can alter bleeding patterns. Partial penetration or embedment in myometrium may decrease effectiveness. May perforate the uterus or cervix during insertion. Displacement may occur.

**ADVERSE REACTIONS:** Abdominal pain, leukorrhea, headache, vaginitis, back pain, breast pain, acne, depression, HTN, upper respiratory infection, nausea, dysmenorrhea, weight increase, skin disorder, decreased libido, abnormal pap smear.

**INTERACTIONS:** Enzyme inducers may decrease effectiveness.

**PREGNANCY:** Category X, not for use in nursing.

## MOBAN — RX

molindone HCl (Endo)

**THERAPEUTIC CLASS:** Dihydroindolone

**INDICATIONS:** Management of psychotic disorders.

**DOSAGE:** *Adults:* Initial: 50-75mg/day. Titrate: Increase to 100mg/day in 3-4 days; adjust to patient response. Maint: Mild: 5-15mg tid-qid. Moderate: 10-25mg tid-qid. Severe: 225mg/day.
*Pediatrics:* >12 yrs: Initial: 50-75mg/day. Titrate: Increase to 100mg/day in 3-4 days; adjust to patient response. Maint: Mild: 5-15mg tid-qid. Moderate: 10-25mg tid-qid. Severe: 225mg/day.

**HOW SUPPLIED:** Tab: 5mg, 10mg, 25mg*, 50mg* *scored

**CONTRAINDICATIONS:** Severe CNS depression (alcohol, barbiturates, narcotics), comatose states.

**WARNINGS/PRECAUTIONS:** Tardive dyskinesia, NMS may occur. Concentrate contains sulfites. Caution with activities requiring alertness. Convulsions, increased activity reported. May obscure signs of intestinal obstruction or brain tumor. May elevate prolactin levels.

**ADVERSE REACTIONS:** Drowsiness, depression, hyperactivity, euphoria, extrapyramidal reactions, akathisia, Parkinson's syndrome, blurred vision, nausea, dry mouth.

**INTERACTIONS:** Tabs contain calcium sulfate; may interfere with phenytoin sodium and tetracycline absorption.

**PREGNANCY:** Safety in pregnancy and nursing not known.

## MOBIC

meloxicam (Boehringer Ingelheim)

RX

**NSAIDs may cause an increased risk of serious cardiovascular thrombotic events, MI, stroke and serious GI adverse events including bleeding, ulceration, and perforation of the stomach or intestines. Contraindicated for the treatment of peri-operative pain in the setting of coronary artery bypass graft (CABG) surgery.**

**THERAPEUTIC CLASS:** NSAID

**INDICATIONS:** Relief of signs and symptoms of osteoarthritis (OA) and rheumatoid arthritis (RA). Relief of the signs and symptoms of pauciarticular or polyarticular course juvenile rheumatoid arthritis (JRA) in patients >2 yrs.

**DOSAGE:** *Adults:* ≥18 yrs: OA/RA: Initial/Maint: 7.5mg qd. Max: 15mg/day. *Pediatrics:* >2 yrs: JRA: 0.125mg/kg qd. Max: 7.5mg/day.

**HOW SUPPLIED:** Sus: 7.5mg/5mL; Tab: 7.5mg, 15mg

**CONTRAINDICATIONS:** ASA or other NSAID allergy that precipitates asthma, urticaria, or allergic-type. Treatment of peri-operative pain in the setting of CABG surgery.

**WARNINGS/PRECAUTIONS:** May lead to onset of new HTN or worsening of pre-existing HTN; monitor BP closely. Fluid retention and edema reported; caution with fluid retention, HTN, or heart failure. Renal papillary necrosis, renal insufficiency, acute renal failure, and other renal injury reported after long-term use. Not recommended for use with advanced renal disease; if therapy must be initiated, monitor renal function. Anaphylactoid reactions may occur. May cause serious skin adverse events (eg, exfoliative dermatitis, Stevens-Johnson syndrome, and toxic epidermal necrolysis). Avoid in late pregnancy; may cause premature closure of ductus arteriosis. May cause elevations of LFTs; d/c if liver disease develops or systemic manifestations occur. Caution with considerable dehydration and in elderly. Anemia may occur; with long-term use, monitor Hgb/Hct if signs or symptoms of anemia develop. May inhibit platelet aggregation and prolong bleeding time; monitor with coagulation disorders. Caution with asthma and avoid with aspirin-sensitive asthma.

**ADVERSE REACTIONS:** Abdominal pain, constipation, diarrhea, dyspepsia, nausea, vomiting, headache, anemia, arthralgia, insomnia, upper respiratory tract infection, UTI.

**INTERACTIONS:** May decrease antihypertensive effects of ACE inhibitors. Potentiates GI bleeds with ASA; avoid concomitant use. Increased clearance with cholestyramine. May decrease natriuretic effects of furosemide, thiazides. Decreased lithium clearance/increased serum levels. Monitor PT/INR with warfarin. Caution with methotrexate.

**PREGNANCY:** Category C, not for use in nursing.

## MODICON RX
norethindrone - ethinyl estradiol (Ortho-McNeil)

**OTHER BRAND NAMES:** Brevicon (Watson) - Necon 0.5/35 (Watson) - Nortrel 0.5/35 (Barr)

**THERAPEUTIC CLASS:** Estrogen/progestogen combination

**INDICATIONS:** Prevention of pregnancy.

**DOSAGE:** *Adults:* Start 1st Sunday after onset of menstruation or the 1st day of menstruation. *21-day:* 1 tab qd for 21 days, stop 7 days, then repeat. *28-day:* 1 tab qd for 28 days continuously, then repeat.

**HOW SUPPLIED:** Tab: (Ethinyl Estradiol-Norethindrone) 0.035mg-0.5mg

**CONTRAINDICATIONS:** Thrombophlebitis, DVT or thromboembolic disorders, pregnancy, cerebrovascular or coronary artery disease, undiagnosed abnormal genital bleeding, cholestatic jaundice of pregnancy or jaundice with prior pill use, hepatic adenomas or carcinomas, breast cancer or other estrogen-dependent neoplasia.

**WARNINGS/PRECAUTIONS:** Cigarette smoking increases risk of serious cardiovascular side effects. This risk increases with age (especially >35 yrs) and heavy smoking. Increased risk of MI, vascular disease, thromboembolism, stroke, and gallbladder disease. Retinal thrombosis, hepatic neoplasia, carcinoma of breast and reproductive organs reported. May cause glucose intolerance. May increase BP, elevate LDL levels or cause other lipid changes, fluid retention, breakthrough bleeding, and spotting. May cause or exacerbate migraine. May develop visual changes with contact lens. Increased risk of MI with HTN, hyperlipidemia, obesity, and diabetes. Discontinue if develop jaundice, significant depression or ophthalmic irregularities. Perform annual physical exam. Use before menarche is not indicated. May affect certain endocrine, LFTs, and blood components.



**ADVERSE REACTIONS:** Nausea, vomiting, breakthrough bleeding, spotting, amenorrhea, migraine, depression, vaginal candidiasis, edema, weight changes.

**INTERACTIONS:** Reduced effects, increased breakthrough bleeding, and menstrual irregularities with rifampin, barbiturates, phenylbutazone, phenytoin, carbamazepine, griseofulvin, topiramate, St. John's wort, and possibly with ampicillin and tetracyclines.

**PREGNANCY:** Category X, not for use in nursing.

## MOISTURE EYES OTC
glycerin - propylene glycol (Bausch & Lomb)

**THERAPEUTIC CLASS:** Lubricant

**INDICATIONS:** Temporary relief of burning and irritation due to dryness of the eye. To prevent further irritation or to relieve dryness of the eye.

**DOSAGE:** *Adults:* 1-2 drops in affected eye prn.

**HOW SUPPLIED:** Sol: (Glycerin-Propylene Glycol) 0.3%-1% [15mL, 30mL]

**WARNINGS/PRECAUTIONS:** Remove contact lenses before use. Do not touch container tip to any surface to avoid contamination. D/C if eye pain or vision changes occur, if redness or irritation continues, or if condition worsens or continues >72 hrs.

**PREGNANCY:** Safety in pregnancy or nursing not known.

## MOISTURE EYES PM PRESERVATIVE FREE OTC
mineral oil - white petrolatum (Bausch & Lomb)

**THERAPEUTIC CLASS:** Lubricant

**INDICATIONS:** To prevent further irritation or to relieve dryness of the eye.

**DOSAGE:** *Adults:* Apply a small amount to inside of lower eyelid.

**HOW SUPPLIED:** Oint: (Mineral Oil-White Petrolatum ) 20%-80% [3.5g]

**WARNINGS/PRECAUTIONS:** Not for use with contact lenses. Do not touch container tip to any surface to avoid contamination. D/C if eye pain or vision changes occur, if redness or irritation continues, or if condition worsens or continues >72 hrs.

**PREGNANCY:** Safety in pregnancy or nursing not known.

## MOISTURE EYES PRESERVATIVE FREE OTC
propylene glycol (Bausch & Lomb)

**THERAPEUTIC CLASS:** Lubricant

**INDICATIONS:** Temporary relief of burning and irritation due to dryness of the eye. To prevent further irritation or to relieve dryness of the eye.

**DOSAGE:** *Adults:* 1-2 drops in affected eye prn.

**HOW SUPPLIED:** Sol: 0.95% [6mL 32s]

**WARNINGS/PRECAUTIONS:** Do not touch container tip to any surface to avoid contamination. D/C if eye pain or vision changes occur, if redness or irritation continues, or if condition worsens or continues >72 hrs. Do not reuse once opened; discard.

**PREGNANCY:** Safety in pregnancy or nursing not known.

## MONISTAT OTC
miconazole nitrate (Personal Products Company)

M

**OTHER BRAND NAMES:** Monistat 3 (Personal Products Company) - Monistat 7 (Personal Products Company)

**THERAPEUTIC CLASS:** Azole antifungal

**INDICATIONS:** Treatment of vaginal yeast infections.

**DOSAGE:** *Adults:* 100mg sup or 2% cream intravaginally qhs for 7 days or 200mg sup or 4% cream intravaginally qhs for 3 days.
*Pediatrics:* >12 yrs: 100mg sup or 2% cream intravaginally qhs for 7 days or 200mg sup or 4% cream intravaginally qhs for 3 days.

**HOW SUPPLIED:** (Monistat 3) Cre: 4% [15g, 25g]; Sup: 200mg [3s]; (Monistat 7) Cre: 2% [35g, 45g]; Sup: 100mg [7s]

**WARNINGS/PRECAUTIONS:** Avoid or d/c if abdominal pain, fever (>100°F), shoulder pain, back pain, or foul smelling discharge occurs. Do not use with tampons. Do not rely on condoms or diaphragm to prevent STDs or pregnancy.

**ADVERSE REACTIONS:** Vulvovaginal burning.

**PREGNANCY:** Safety in pregnancy and nursing not known.

## MONISTAT 1 COMBINATION PACK OTC
miconazole nitrate (Personal Products Company)

**THERAPEUTIC CLASS:** Azole antifungal

**INDICATIONS:** (Cre) Relief of external vulvular itching and irritation associated with a yeast infection. (Sup) Topical treatment of vulvovaginal candidiasis.

**DOSAGE:** *Adults:* 1200mg intravaginally qhs for 1 day. Apply 2% cream bid for up to 7 days for external itching.
*Pediatrics:* >12 yrs: 1200mg intravaginally qhs for 1 day. Apply 2% cream bid for up to 7 days for external itching.

**HOW SUPPLIED:** Cre: 2% [9g]; Sup: 1200mg

**WARNINGS/PRECAUTIONS:** Do not rely on condoms or diaphragm to prevent STDs or pregnancy until 3 days after last use. Do not use tampons, douches, or spermicides until 7 days after last use. Confirm diagnosis by KOH smears and/or cultures; reconfirm if no response.

**ADVERSE REACTIONS:** Female genitalia burning and irritation, external female genitalia pruritus, female genitalia discharge.

**PREGNANCY:** Category C, caution in nursing.

## MONISTAT-DERM RX

miconazole nitrate (Ortho-McNeil)

**THERAPEUTIC CLASS:** Azole antifungal

**INDICATIONS:** Treatment of tinea pedis, tinea cruris, tinea corporis, tinea versicolor, cutaneous candidiasis.

**DOSAGE:** *Adults:* T.pedis/T.cruris/T.corporis/Candidiasis: Apply bid (am and pm). T.versicolor: Apply qd. Treat t. pedis for 1 month and other infections for 2 weeks.

**HOW SUPPLIED:** Cre: 2% [15g, 30g, 85g]

**WARNINGS/PRECAUTIONS:** D/C if irritation occurs. If no improvement after a month, reassess diagnosis. Avoid eyes.

**ADVERSE REACTIONS:** Irritation, burning, skin maceration, allergic contact dermatitis.

**PREGNANCY:** Safety in pregnancy and nursing not known.



## MONOCAL OTC

fluoride - calcium carbonate (Mericon)

**THERAPEUTIC CLASS:** Mineral supplement

**INDICATIONS:** Fluoride and calcium supplementation.

**DOSAGE:** *Adults:* 1 tab qd.

**HOW SUPPLIED:** Tab: (Calcium-Fluoride) 250mg-3mg

**PREGNANCY:** Safety in pregnancy and nursing not known.

## MONODOX RX

doxycycline monohydrate (Watson)

**THERAPEUTIC CLASS:** Tetracycline derivative

**INDICATIONS:** Treatment of respiratory tract, urinary tract, skin and skin structure, uncomplicated urethral/endocervical/rectal infection caused by *C.trachomatis*, nongonococcal urethritis caused by *C.trachomatis* and *U.urealyticum*, lymphogranuloma, psittacosis, trachoma, chancroid, plague, cholera, brucellosis. Treatment of uncomplicated gonorrhea, syphilis, listeriosis, anthrax, *Clostridium* species when PCN is contraindicated. Adjunct therapy for amebicides and severe acne.

**DOSAGE:** *Adults:* Usual: 100mg q12h or 50mg q6h for 1 day, then 100mg/day. Severe Infection: 100mg q12h. Uncomplicated Gonococcal Infections (except anorectal infections in men): 100mg bid for 7 days or 300mg stat, then repeat in 1 hr. Acute Epididymo-Orchitis caused by *N.gonorrhea* or *C.trachomatis:* 100mg bid for at least 10 days. Primary/Secondary Syphilis: 300mg/day in divided dose for at least 10 days. Uncomplicated Urethral/Endocervical/Rectal Infection caused by *C.trachomatis:* 100mg bid for at least 7 days. Nongonococcal Urethritis caused by *C.trachomatis* and*U.urealyticum:* 100mg bid for at least 7 days. Take with full glass of water. Take with food if GI upset occurs.
*Pediatrics:* >8 yrs:<100 lbs: 2mg/lb divided in 2 doses for 1 day, then 1mg/lb

daily in single or 2 divided doses. Severe Infection: May use up to 2mg/lb/day. >100 lbs: 100mg q12h or 50mg q6h for 1 day, then 100mg/day. Severe Infection: 100mg q12h. Take with a full glass of water. Take with food if GI upset occurs.

**HOW SUPPLIED:** Cap: 50mg, 100mg

**WARNINGS/PRECAUTIONS:** Avoid direct sunlight or UV light. May cause permanent tooth discoloration during tooth development (last half of pregnancy and children <8 years). Monitor renal/hepatic function, and blood with long-term therapy. May increase BUN. Photosensitivity, pseudotumor cerebri reported. D/C if superinfection occurs. Bulging fontanels in infants and intracranial HTN in adults reported.

**ADVERSE REACTIONS:** GI effects, photosensitivity, rash, blood dyscrasias, hypersensitivity reactions.

**INTERACTIONS:** Carbamazepine, barbiturates, phenytoin decrease half-life of doxycycline. May decrease PT; adjust anticoagulants. May decrease bactericidal agents (eg, penicillin). May decrease effects of oral contraceptives. Take 1 hr before or 2 hrs after dairy products. Aluminum-, calcium-, iron- and magnesium-containing products impair absorption. Fatal renal toxicity may occur with methoxyflurane.

**PREGNANCY:** Category D, not for use in nursing.

## MONOKET RX
isosorbide mononitrate (Schwarz)

**THERAPEUTIC CLASS:** Nitrate vasodilator

**INDICATIONS:** Prevention and treatment of angina pectoris. Not for acute attack.

**DOSAGE:** *Adults:* 20mg bid (space doses 7 hours apart). Small Patients: Initial: 5mg per dose for 1 day, then increase to 10mg by 2nd or 3rd day.

**HOW SUPPLIED:** Tab: 10mg*, 20mg* *scored

**WARNINGS/PRECAUTIONS:** Not for use with acute MI or CHF. Severe hypotension may occur; caution with volume depletion or hypotension. May aggravate angina caused by hypertrophic cardiomyopathy. Monitor for tolerance.

**ADVERSE REACTIONS:** Headache, dizziness, fatigue, GI upset.

**INTERACTIONS:** Severe hypotension with sildenafil. Marked orthostatic hypotension with calcium channel blockers. Additive vasodilation with other vasodilators (eg, alcohol).

**PREGNANCY:** Category B, caution with nursing.

## MONOPRIL RX
fosinopril sodium (Bristol-Myers Squibb)

**ACE inhibitors can cause death/injury to developing fetus during 2nd and 3rd trimesters. Stop therapy if pregnancy detected.**

**THERAPEUTIC CLASS:** ACE inhibitor

**INDICATIONS:** Treatment of hypertension. Adjunct therapy for heart failure.

**DOSAGE:** *Adults:* If possible, d/c diuretic 2-3 days before therapy. Initial: 10mg qd, monitor carefully if cannot d/c diuretic. Maint: 20-40mg/day. Resume diuretic if BP not controlled. Max: 80mg/day. Heart Failure: Initial: 10mg qd, 5mg with moderate to severe renal failure or vigorous diuresis. Titrate: Increase over several weeks. Maint: 20-40mg qd. Max: 40mg qd. Elderly: Start at low end of dosing range.

**HOW SUPPLIED:** Tab: 10mg*, 20mg, 40mg *scored

**CONTRAINDICATIONS:** History of ACE inhibitor associated angioedema.

**WARNINGS/PRECAUTIONS:** D/C if angioedema, jaundice, or if marked LFT elevation occur. Risk of hyperkalemia with DM, renal dysfunction. Persistent non-productive cough reported. Monitor WBCs in renal and collagen vascular disease. Anaphylactoid reactions reported. Fetal/neonatal morbidity and death reported. Monitor for hypotension in high risk patients (heart failure, volume and/or salt depletion, surgery/anesthesia, etc.). Less effective on BP in blacks and more reports of angioedema than nonblacks. Caution with CHF, renal or hepatic dysfunction, renal artery stenosis. May cause false low measurement of serum digoxin level.

**ADVERSE REACTIONS:** Dizziness, cough, hypotension, musculoskeletal pain.

**INTERACTIONS:** May increase lithium levels. Hypotension risk with diuretics. Increase risk of hyperkalemia with $K^+$-sparing diuretics, $K^+$-containing salt substitutes or $K^+$ supplements. Decreased absorption with antacids; space dosing by 2 hrs.

**PREGNANCY:** Category C (1st trimester) and D (2nd and 3rd trimesters), not for use in nursing.

## MONOPRIL HCT RX

hydrochlorothiazide - fosinopril sodium (Bristol-Myers Squibb)

**ACE inhibitors can cause death/injury to developing fetus during 2nd and 3rd trimesters. Stop therapy if pregnancy detected.**

**THERAPEUTIC CLASS:** ACE inhibitor/thiazide diuretic

**INDICATIONS:** Hypertension. Not for initial therapy.

**DOSAGE:** *Adults:* Initial (if not controlled with fosinopril/HCTZ monotherapy): 12.5mg-10mg tab or 12.5mg-20mg tab qd.

M

**HOW SUPPLIED:** Tab: (Fosinopril-HCTZ) 10mg-12.5mg, 20mg-12.5mg

**CONTRAINDICATIONS:** Anuria, sulfonamide hypersensitivity.

**WARNINGS/PRECAUTIONS:** Discontinue if angioedema, jaundice, or if marked LFT elevation occurs. Risk of hyperkalemia with DM, renal dysfunction. Persistent nonproductive cough reported. Monitor WBCs in renal and collagen vascular disease. Anaphylactoid reactions reported. Fetal/neonatal morbidity and death reported. Monitor for hypotension in high risk patients (eg, surgery/anesthesia, volume/salt depletion). Caution with CHF, renal or hepatic dysfunction. More reports of angioedema in blacks than nonblacks. May exacerbate or activate SLE. Monitor electrolytes. Avoid if CrCl $<30mL/min/1.7m^2$. May increase cholesterol, TG. Hypercalcemia, hypomagnesemia, hyperuricemia may occur.

**ADVERSE REACTIONS:** Headache, cough, fatigue, dizziness, upper respiratory infection, musculoskeletal pain.

**INTERACTIONS:** Increase risk of hyperkalemia with $K^+$-sparing diuretics, $K^+$ supplements, or $K^+$-containing salt substitutes. Risk of lithium toxicity. Antacids may impair absorption; separate dose by 2 hrs. May alter insulin requirements. May increase responsiveness to tubocurarine. NSAIDs reduce effects. May decrease effects of methenamine. Reduced absorption with cholestyramine, colestipol. Caution with other antihypertensives. May decrease response to norepinephrine.

**PREGNANCY:** Category C (1st trimester) and D (2nd and 3rd trimesters), not for use in nursing.

## MONUROL RX

fosfomycin tromethamine (Forest)

**THERAPEUTIC CLASS:** Phosphonic acid derivative

**INDICATIONS:** Uncomplicated urinary tract infection (acute cystitis) in women.

**DOSAGE:** *Adults:* >18 yrs: 1 single-dose sachet. Mix with 3-4oz of water before ingesting.

**HOW SUPPLIED:** Powder: 3g/sachet

**WARNINGS/PRECAUTIONS:** Maximum of 1 dose per episode.

**ADVERSE REACTIONS:** Diarrhea, headache, vaginitis, nausea.

**INTERACTIONS:** Metoclopramide and other drugs that increase GI motility may decrease serum levels and urinary excretion.

**PREGNANCY:** Category B, not for use in nursing.

## MORPHINE SULFATE IMMEDIATE RELEASE CII

morphine sulfate (Various)

**THERAPEUTIC CLASS:** Opioid analgesic

**INDICATIONS:** Relief of severe pain.

**DOSAGE:** *Adults:* (Sol) 10-20mg q4h. (Tab) 15-30mg q4h.

**HOW SUPPLIED:** Sol: 10mg/5mL, 20mg/5mL [100mL, 500mL]; Tab: 15mg*, 30mg* *scored

**CONTRAINDICATIONS:** Respiratory insufficiency or depression; severe CNS depression; attack of bronchial asthma; heart failure secondary to chronic lung disease; cardiac arrhythmias; increased intracranial or cerebrospinal pressure; head injuries; brain tumor; acute alcoholism; delirium tremens; convulsive disorders; after biliary tract surgery; suspected surgical abdomen; surgical anastomosis; concomitantly with MAOIs or within 14 days of such treatment.

**WARNINGS/PRECAUTIONS:** May cause tolerance, psychological/physical dependence; avoid abrupt withdrawal. Caution with head injury, increased intracranial pressure, acute asthma attack, chronic COPD or cor pulmonale, decreased respiratory reserve, pre-existing respiratory depression, hypoxia, hypercapnia, elderly, debilitated, severe hepatic/renal impairment, hypothyroidism, Addison's disease, prostatic hypertrophy, or urethral stricture. May cause severe hypotension. May obscure diagnosis or clinical course with abdominal conditions. May impair mental/physical abilities.

**ADVERSE REACTIONS:** Respiratory depression, lightheadedness, dizziness, sedation, nausea, vomiting, sweating.

**INTERACTIONS:** See Contraindications. Effects may be potentiated by alkalinizing agents and antagonized by acidifying agents. Analgesic effect may be potentiated by chlorpromazine and methocarbamol. Depressant effects may be enhanced by other CNS depressants (eg, anesthetics, sedatives, hypnotics, TCAs, barbiturates, phenothiazines, chloral hydrate, glutethimide, antihistamines, β-blockers (propranolol), alcohol, furazolidone, and other narcotic analgesics). May increase anticoagulant activity of coumarin and other anticoagulants.

**PREGNANCY:** Category C, caution in nursing.

## MOTRIN RX

ibuprofen (Pharmacia & Upjohn)

**NSAIDs may cause an increased risk of serious cardiovascular thrombotic events, MI, stroke and serious GI adverse events including bleeding, ulceration, and perforation of the stomach or intestines. Contraindicated for the treatment of peri-operative pain in the setting of coronary artery bypass graft (CABG) surgery.**

**THERAPEUTIC CLASS:** NSAID

**INDICATIONS:** Adults: Relief of mild-to-moderate pain. Dysmenorrhea. Rheumatoid arthritis (RA) Osteoarthritis (OA). Pediatrics: Fever. Relief of mild-to-moderate pain. Juvenile arthritis (JA).

**DOSAGE:** *Adults:* Pain: 400mg q4-6h prn. Dysmenorrhea: 400mg q4h prn. RA/OA: 300mg qid or 400mg, 600mg or 800mg tid-qid. Max: 3200mg/day.

M

Take with meals/milk. Renal Impairment: Reduce dose.
*Pediatrics:* Fever: 6 months-12 yrs: 5mg/kg for temp <102.5°F; 10mg/kg if temp >102.5°F q6-8h. Max: 40mg/kg/day. Pain: 6 months-12 yrs: 10mg/kg q6-8h. Max: 40mg/kg/day. JA: 30-40mg/kg/day divided into 3 or 4 doses. Milder disease may use 20mg/kg/day.

**HOW SUPPLIED:** Sus: 100mg/5mL [120mL, 480mL]; Tab: 400mg, 600mg, 800mg

**CONTRAINDICATIONS:** Syndrome of nasal polyps, angioedema, and bronchospastic reactions to ASA or other NSAIDs. Treatment of peri-operative pain in the setting of CABG surgery.

**WARNINGS/PRECAUTIONS:** May lead to onset of new HTN or worsening of pre-existing HTN; monitor BP closely. Fluid retention and edema reported; caution with fluid retention or heart failure. Renal papillary necrosis and other renal injury reported after long-term use. Not recommended for use with advanced renal disease; if therapy must be initiated, monitor renal function. Anaphylactoid reactions may occur. May cause serious skin adverse events (eg, exfoliative dermatitis, Stevens-Johnson syndrome, and toxic epidermal necrolysis). Avoid in late pregnancy; may cause premature closure of ductus arteriosis. May cause elevations of LFTs; d/c if liver disease develops or systemic manifestations occur. Caution in elderly. Anemia may occur; with long-term use, monitor Hgb/Hct if signs or symptoms of anemia develop. May inhibit platelet aggregation and prolong bleeding time; monitor with coagulation disorders. Caution with asthma and avoid with aspirin-sensitive asthma. D/C if visual disturbances occur. Aseptic meningitis with fever and coma reported.

**ADVERSE REACTIONS:** Nausea, epigastric pain, heartburn, dizziness, rash.

**INTERACTIONS:** Use caution with anticoagulants. May enhance methotrexate toxicity. May decrease the natriuretic effects of furosemide or thiazides. Avoid use with aspirin. Decrease lithium clearance; monitor for toxicity.



**PREGNANCY:** Category C, not for use in nursing.

## MOTRIN IB — OTC
ibuprofen (McNeil Consumer)

**THERAPEUTIC CLASS:** NSAID

**INDICATIONS:** Temporary relief of headache, muscular aches, minor pain of arthritis, toothache, backache, minor aches and pains. Fever.

**DOSAGE:** *Adults:* 200mg q4-6h. 400mg if symptoms do not respond. Max: 1200mg/24hrs.
*Pediatrics:* >12 yrs: 200mg q4-6h. 400mg if symptoms do not respond. Max: 1200mg/24hrs.

**HOW SUPPLIED:** Tab: 200mg

**WARNINGS/PRECAUTIONS:** Do not take for >10 days for pain or >3 days for fever. May cause severe allergic reaction. Do not use if history of allergic reaction to other pain relievers/fever reducers.

**INTERACTIONS:** Avoid other ibuprofen-containing products.

**PREGNANCY:** Safety in pregnancy and nursing not known.

## MOTRIN MIGRAINE — OTC
ibuprofen (McNeil Consumer)

**THERAPEUTIC CLASS:** NSAID

**INDICATIONS:** Treatment of migraine headache.

**DOSAGE:** *Adults:* >18 yrs: 1-2 tabs with water. Max: 2 tabs/24hrs.

**HOW SUPPLIED:** Tab: 200mg

**WARNINGS/PRECAUTIONS:** May cause severe allergic reactions.

**INTERACTIONS:** Increased risk of GI bleed with alcohol.

**PREGNANCY:** Do not use in last 3 months of pregnancy, safety in nursing not known.

## Motrin, Children's OTC

ibuprofen (McNeil Consumer)

**OTHER BRAND NAMES:** Motrin, Junior (McNeil Consumer) - Motrin, Infants (McNeil Consumer)

**THERAPEUTIC CLASS:** NSAID

**INDICATIONS:** To temporarily reduce fever, relief of minor aches and pains associated with the common cold, flu, sore throat, headaches and toothaches.

**DOSAGE:** *Pediatrics:* Infant Drops: 6-11 months (12-17lbs): 1.25mL q6-8h. 12-23 months (18-23lbs): 1.875mL q6-8h. Use only with enclosed dropper. Sus: 2-3 yrs (24-35lbs): 5mL q6-8h. 4-5 yrs (36-47lbs): 7.5mL q6-8h. 6-8 yrs (48-59lbs): 10mL q6-8h. 9-10 yrs (60-71lbs): 12.5mL q6-8h. 11 yrs (72-95lbs): 15mL q6-8h. Use only with enclosed measuring cup. Children's Chewable Tab: 4-5 yrs (36-47lbs): 150mg q6-8h. 6-8 yrs (48-59lbs): 200mg q6-8h. 9-10 yrs (60-71lbs): 250mg q6-8h. 11 yrs (72-95lbs): 300mg q6-8h. Junior Tab/Chewable Tab: 6-8 yrs (48-59lbs): 200mg q6-8h. 9-10 yrs (60-71lbs): 250mg q6-8h. 11 yrs (72-95lbs): 300mg q6-8h. Max: 4 doses/24hrs. Take with food/milk to avoid upset stomach. Take chewable tabs with food/water to avoid mouth/throat burning.

**HOW SUPPLIED:** Infant Drops: 50mg/1.25mL [15mL]; Children's Sus: 100mg/5mL [60mL, 120mL]; Children's Tab, Chewable: 50mg; Junior Tab/Tab, Chewable: 100mg

**WARNINGS/PRECAUTIONS:** May cause severe allergic reaction (eg, hives, facial swelling, wheezing, shock). Avoid with history of allergic reaction to any other pain reliever/fever reducer. Not for use >2-3 days.

**INTERACTIONS:** Caution with other products that contain ibuprofen or any other pain reliever/fever reducer.

**PREGNANCY:** Safety in pregnancy and nursing not known.



## MoviPrep RX

ascorbic acid - sodium sulfate - sodium chloride - sodium ascorbate - potassium chloride - polyethylene glycol 3350 (Salix)

**THERAPEUTIC CLASS:** Bowel Cleanser

**INDICATIONS:** Colon cleansing as a preparation for colonoscopy in adults ≥18 yrs of age.

**DOSAGE:** *Adults:* ≥18 yrs: Split-Dose Regimen: 8oz every 15 min (first liter) followed by 0.5 liters of clear liquid the evening prior, then another liter over 1 hr followed by 0.5 liters of clear liquid in the morning at least 1 hr prior to colonoscopy. Evening-Only Regimen: Around 6 pm take 8oz every 15 min (first liter), then 1.5 hrs later take second liter over one hour, additionally take 1 liter of clear liquid.

**HOW SUPPLIED:** Pow: (PEG 3350-Sodium Sulfate-Sodium Chloride-Potassium Chloride-Ascorbic Acid-Sodium Ascorbate) 100g-7.5g-2.69g-1.015g-4.7g-5.9g

**WARNINGS/PRECAUTIONS:** Rare reports of generalized tonic-clonic seizures with use of PEG colon preparations. Caution with concomitant medications that increase risk of electrolyte abnormalities (eg, diuretics, ACEIs) or in patients with hyponatremia; consider baseline and post-colonoscopy lab tests (eg, sodium, potassium, calcium, creatinine, BUN).

**ADVERSE REACTIONS:** Abdominal distension, anal discomfort, thirst, nausea, abdominal pain, sleep disorder, rigors, hunger, malaise, vomiting, dizziness.

**INTERACTIONS:** Oral medications given within 1 hour of administration may be flushed from GI and may not be absorbed.

**PREGNANCY:** Category C, caution in nursing.

## MS CONTIN

CII

morphine sulfate (Purdue Pharma)

**THERAPEUTIC CLASS:** Opioid analgesic

**INDICATIONS:** Relief of moderate to severe pain over periods of more than a few days.

**DOSAGE:** *Adults:* Conversion from MSIR: Give 1/2 of total daily MSIR dose as MS Contin q12h or give 1/3 of total daily MSIR dose as MS Contin q8h. Conversion from Parenteral Morphine: Initial: If daily morphine dose <120mg/day, give MS Contin 30mg. Titrate: Switch to 60mg or 100mg MS Contin. Swallow whole; do not crush, chew, or break. Taper dose; do not discontinue abruptly.

**HOW SUPPLIED:** Tab, Extended Release: 15mg, 30mg, 60mg, 100mg, 200mg

**CONTRAINDICATIONS:** Paralytic ileus, respiratory depression in the absence of resuscitative equipment, acute or severe bronchial asthma.

**WARNINGS/PRECAUTIONS:** Extreme caution with COPD, cor pulmonale, decreased respiratory reserve, hypoxia, hypercapnia, respiratory depression. Caution with elderly, debilitated, head injury, increased intracranial pressure, circulatory shock, severe hepatic/renal/pulmonary dysfunction, myxedema, hypothyroidism, adrenocortical insufficiency, CNS depression, coma, toxic psychosis, prostatic hypertrophy, urethral stricture, alcoholism, delirium tremens, kyphoscoliosis, inability to swallow, convulsive disorder, acute abdominal problems, biliary tract surgery, acute pancreatitis secondary to biliary tract disease. May cause hypotension and drug dependence. Reserve 200mg tabs for opioid tolerant patients requiring >400mg/day of morphine.

**ADVERSE REACTIONS:** Constipation, lightheadedness, dizziness, sedation, nausea, vomiting, sweating, dysphoria, euphoria, respiratory depression.



**INTERACTIONS:** Additive depressant effects with other CNS depressants (eg, sedatives, hypnotics, general anesthetics, phenothiazines, tranquilizers, alcohol). Enhances neuromuscular blocking effects and increases respiratory depression with skeletal muscle relaxants. Avoid agonist/antagonist analgesics (eg, pentazocine, nalbuphine, butorphanol, buprenorphine); may reduce analgesic effect or cause withdrawal symptoms. Risk of hypotension with phenothiazines or general anesthetics.

**PREGNANCY:** Category C, not for use in nursing.

## MUCINEX

OTC

guaifenesin (Adams)

**THERAPEUTIC CLASS:** Expectorant

**INDICATIONS:** To help loosen phlegm, thin bronchial secretions and make coughs more productive.

**DOSAGE:** *Adults:* 1-2 tabs every 12hrs. Max: 4 tabs/24hrs. Take with a full glass of water. Do not crush, chew, or break tab.
*Pediatrics:* >12 yrs: 1-2 tabs every 12hrs. Max: 4 tabs/24hrs. Take with a full glass of water. Do not crush, chew, or break tab.

**HOW SUPPLIED:** Tab, Extended Release: 600mg

**WARNINGS/PRECAUTIONS:** Discontinue if cough lasts >7 days, recurs, or occurs with fever, rash, or persistent headache.

**PREGNANCY:** Safety in pregnancy or nursing not known.

## MUCINEX D

OTC

guaifenesin - pseudoephedrine HCl (Adams)

**THERAPEUTIC CLASS:** Expectorant/nasal decongestant

**INDICATIONS:** Help loosen phlegm and thin bronchial secretions. Temporarily relieve nasal congestion due to common cold, hay fever, or upper respiratory allergies. Promote nasal and sinus drainage. Temporarily relieve sinus congestion and pressure.

**DOSAGE:** *Adults:* 2 tabs every 12hrs. Max: 4 tabs/24hrs. Do not crush, chew, or break.

*Pediatrics:* ≥12 yrs: 2 tabs every 12hrs. Max: 4 tabs/24hrs. Do not crush, chew, or break.

**HOW SUPPLIED:** Tab, Extended Release: (Guaifenesin-Pseudoephedrine HCl) 600mg-60mg

**WARNINGS/PRECAUTIONS:** Avoid use during or for 2 weeks after stopping MAOI therapy. Caution with heart disease, high BP, thyroid disease, diabetes, difficulty urinating due to enlarged prostate, persistent or chronic cough. D/C if cough lasts >7 days, or occurs with fever, rash or persistent headache.

**INTERACTIONS:** See Warnings and Precautions.

**PREGNANCY:** Safety in pregnancy and nursing not known.

## MUCINEX DM

OTC

guaifenesin - dextromethorphan hydrobromide (Adams)

**THERAPEUTIC CLASS:** Cough suppressant/expectorant

**INDICATIONS:** To help loosen phlegm, thin bronchial secretions and makes coughs more productive. Temporarily relieves cough.

**DOSAGE:** *Adults:* 1-2 tabs q12hrs. Max: 4 tabs/24hrs. Take with a full glass of water. Do not crush, chew, or break tab.

*Pediatrics:* ≥12 yrs: 1-2 tabs q12hrs. Max: 4 tabs/24hrs. Take with a full glass of water. Do not crush, chew, or break tab.

**HOW SUPPLIED:** Tab: (Dextromethorphan-Guaifenesin) 30mg-600mg

**WARNINGS/PRECAUTIONS:** Discontinue if cough lasts >7 days, recurs, or occurs with fever, rash, or persistent headache. Avoid during or within 14 days of MAOIs.

**INTERACTIONS:** See Warnings and Precautions.

**PREGNANCY:** Safety in pregnancy or nursing not known.

## MUCOMYST

RX

acetylcysteine (Sandoz)

**THERAPEUTIC CLASS:** Acetaminophen antidote/Mucolytic

**INDICATIONS:** Adjunctive mucolytic therapy in acute and chronic bronchopulmonary disease; pulmonary complications of cystic fibrosis and surgery; tracheostomy care; during anesthesia; post-traumatic chest conditions; atelectasis; diagnostic bronchial studies. Antidote for acute acetaminophen (APAP) toxicity.

**DOSAGE:** *Adults:* Antidote: Empty stomach by lavage or emesis before administration. Administer immediately, regardless of quantity, if APAP ingestion ≤24hrs. LD: 140mg/kg PO then 70mg/kg PO q4h for 17 doses starting 4 hours after LD. Discontinue if predetoxification APAP level is in the nontoxic range and overdose occurred at least 4 hrs before assay. Obtain 2nd plasma level if range is nontoxic and time of ingestion is unknown or <4 hrs. Mucolytic: Nebulization (face mask, mouth piece, tracheostomy): 1-10mL of 20% or 2-10mL of 10% q2-6h. Usual: 3-5mL of 20% or 6-10mL of 10% 3-4

times/day. Closed Tent or Croupette: Up to 300mL of 10% or 20%. Direct Instillation: 1-2 mL of 10% or 20% q1-4h. Percutaneous Intratracheal Catheter: 1-2mL of 20% or 2-4mL of 10% q1-4h. Diagnostic Bronchograms: Give before procedure. 2-3 doses of 1-2mL of 20% or 2-4mL of 10%.
*Pediatrics:* Antidote: Empty stomach by lavage or emesis before administration. Administer immediately, regardless of quantity, if APAP ingestion ≤24hrs. LD: 140mg/kg PO then 70mg/kg PO q4h for 17 doses starting 4 hours after LD. Discontinue if predetoxification APAP level is in the nontoxic range and overdose occurred at least 4 hrs before assay. Obtain 2nd plasma level if range is nontoxic and time of ingestion is unknown or <4 hrs. Mucolytic: Nebulization (face mask, mouth piece, tracheostomy): 1-10mL of 20% or 2-10mL of 10% q2-6h. Usual: 3-5mL of 20% or 6-10mL of 10% 3-4 times/day. Closed Tent or Croupette: Up to 300mL of 10% or 20%. Direct Instillation: 1-2 mL of 10% or 20% q1-4h. Percutaneous Intratracheal Catheter: 1-2mL of 20% or 2-4mL of 10% q1-4h. Diagnostic Procedures: Give before procedure. 2-3 doses of 1-2mL of 20% or 2-4mL of 10%.

**HOW SUPPLIED:** Sol: 10%, 20%

**WARNINGS/PRECAUTIONS:** (Oral) Discontinue if generalized urticaria or encephalopathy due to hepatic failure develops. May aggravate vomiting; evaluate with risk of gastric hemorrhage. (Inhalation) Monitor asthmatics. Discontinue if bronchospasm progresses.

**ADVERSE REACTIONS:** (Oral) Nausea, vomiting, other GI symptoms. (Inhalation) Stomatitis, nausea, vomiting, fever, rhinorrhea, drowsiness, clamminess, chest tightness, bronchoconstriction.

**PREGNANCY:** Category B, caution in nursing.



## MUMPSVAX RX

mumps virus vaccine live (Merck)

**THERAPEUTIC CLASS:** Vaccine

**INDICATIONS:** Vaccination against mumps.

**DOSAGE:** *Adults:* 0.5mL SQ into outer aspect of upper arm.
*Pediatrics:* >12 mos: 0.5mL SQ in outer aspect of upper arm. Give primary vaccine at 12-15 months. Revaccinate prior to elementary school.

**HOW SUPPLIED:** Inj: 20,000 $TCID_{50}$

**CONTRAINDICATIONS:** Avoid pregnancy for 3 months after vaccine, anaphylactic reaction to neomycin, febrile/active respiratory illness, immunosuppressive therapy (except corticosteroids as replacement therapy), blood dyscrasias, leukemia, lymphoma, malignant neoplasms affecting bone marrow or lymphatic system, immunodeficiency states.

**WARNINGS/PRECAUTIONS:** Caution with hypersensitivity to eggs and neomycin. May worsen thrombocytopenia. Defer vaccine for at least 3 months after blood or plasma transfusion and immune globulin. Do not revaccinate with active untreated TB. Monitor for temperature elevation after administration. Contains albumin, remote risk of viral infection transmission. Have epinephrine (1:1000) available.

**ADVERSE REACTIONS:** Fever, syncope, irritability, diarrhea, diabetes, purpura, cough, febrile seizures, local site reactions.

**INTERACTIONS:** Do not give with immune globulin. May depress TB skin sensitivity, administer test either simultaneously or before. Do not give <1 month before or after other live viral vaccines. Do not give simultaneously with DTP or oral poliovirus vaccine.

**PREGNANCY:** Category C, caution in nursing.

## MURINE TEARS

OTC

povidone - polyvinyl alcohol (Ross)

**THERAPEUTIC CLASS:** Lubricant

**INDICATIONS:** Temporary relief or prevention of further discomfort due to minor irritations and symptoms related to dry eyes.

**DOSAGE:** *Adults:* 1-2 drops in affected eye prn.

**HOW SUPPLIED:** Sol: (Polyvinyl Alcohol-Povidone) 0.5%-0.6% [15mL, 30mL]

**WARNINGS/PRECAUTIONS:** Do not touch container tip to any surface to avoid contamination. D/C if eye pain or vision changes occur, if redness or irritation continues, or if condition worsens or persists >72 hrs.

**PREGNANCY:** Safety in pregnancy and nursing not known.

## MURINE TEARS PLUS

OTC

povidone - polyvinyl alcohol - tetrahydrozoline HCl (Ross)

**THERAPEUTIC CLASS:** Decongestant/lubricant

**INDICATIONS:** Temporary relief or prevention of further discomfort due to minor irritations and symptoms related to dry eyes plus removal of redness.

**DOSAGE:** *Adults:* 1-2 drops in affected eye up to qid.

**HOW SUPPLIED:** Sol: (Tetrahydrozoline-Polyvinyl alcohol-Povidone) 0.05%-0.5%-0.6% [15mL, 30mL]

**WARNINGS/PRECAUTIONS:** May temporarily enlarge pupils. Overuse may cause increased eye redness. Do not touch container tip to any surface to avoid contamination. D/C if eye pain or vision changes occur, if redness or irritation continues, or if condition worsens or persists >72 hrs. Supervision required in patients with narrow angle glaucoma.

**PREGNANCY:** Safety in pregnancy and nursing not known.



## MURO 128

OTC

sodium chloride (Bausch & Lomb)

**THERAPEUTIC CLASS:** Hypertonic agent

**INDICATIONS:** Temporary relief of corneal edema.

**DOSAGE:** *Adults:* (Sol) 1-2 drops q3-4h. (Oint) Apply 1/4 inch q3-4h.

**HOW SUPPLIED:** Oint: 5% [3.5g]; Sol: 2% [15mL], 5% [15mL, 30mL]

**WARNINGS/PRECAUTIONS:** Temporary burning and irritation may occur. Do not use if solution becomes cloudy or changes color.

**ADVERSE REACTIONS:** Burning, irritation.

**PREGNANCY:** Safety in pregnancy and nursing not known.

## MUSE

RX

alprostadil (Vivus)

**THERAPEUTIC CLASS:** Prostaglandin $E_1$

**INDICATIONS:** Treatment of erectile dysfunction.

**DOSAGE:** *Adults:* Supervise dose determination. Insert in urethra after urination. Initial: 125-250mcg. Titrate: Adjust in a stepwise manner. Max: 2 sup/24hrs.

**HOW SUPPLIED:** Sup: 125mcg, 250mcg, 500mcg, 1000mcg

**CONTRAINDICATIONS:** Urethral stricture, balanitis, severe hypospadias and curvature, urethritis, venous thrombosis predisposition (eg, sickle cell anemia or trait, thrombocythemia, polycythemia, multiple myeloma), hyperviscosity syndrome, men when sexual activity is not advisable, and sexual intercourse with a pregnant woman without a condom.

**WARNINGS/PRECAUTIONS:** Use condoms with pregnant women. Symptomatic hypotension and syncope reported. Exclude reversible causes before therapy. Monitor cardiac function. Priapism reported (infrequently).

**ADVERSE REACTIONS:** Penile pain, urethral burning and/or bleeding, testicular pain, flu symptoms, headache, pain, infection.

**INTERACTIONS:** May potentiate hypotension with antihypertensives. Drugs that attenuate erectile function may influence response to alprostadil. Increased risk of penile bleeding with anticoagulants.

**PREGNANCY:** Category C, not for use in nursing.

## MUTAMYCIN RX

mitomycin (Bristol-Myers Squibb)

**Bone marrow suppression (eg, thrombocytopenia, leukopenia) may occur. Hemolytic Uremic Syndrome (HUS) reported, mostly with high doses (≥60mg). Blood product transfusion may exacerbate HUS.**

**THERAPEUTIC CLASS:** DNA synthesis inhibitor

**INDICATIONS:** Disseminated adenocarcinoma of the stomach or pancreas as an adjunct to other chemotherapeutic agents or as palliative treatment when other modalities have failed. Not recommended as single-agent.

**DOSAGE:** *Adults:* Usual: (after full hematological recovery): 20mg/m² IV single dose q6-8 weeks. Dosage Adjustments: Leukocytes 2000-2999/mm³, Platelets 25,000-74,999/mm³: Give 70% of prior dose. Leukocytes <2000/mm³, Platelets <25,000/mm³: Give 50% of prior dose. No repeat dosage should be given until leukocyte count has returned to 4000/mm³ and platelet count to 100,000/mm³.

M

**HOW SUPPLIED:** Inj: 5mg, 20mg, 40mg

**CONTRAINDICATIONS:** Thrombocytopenia, coagulation disorder, increased bleeding tendency due to other causes.

**WARNINGS/PRECAUTIONS:** See Black Box Warning, Drug Interactions. Monitor platelets, WBCs, differential and Hgb repeatedly during therapy and for at least 8 weeks after. May cause renal toxicity, avoid if serum creatinine is >1.7mg %. Bladder fibrosis/contraction reported with intravesical administration.

**ADVERSE REACTIONS:** Bone marrow toxicity, integument and mucous membrane toxicity (eg, cellulitis, stomatitis, alopecia, skin necrosis), renal/pulmonary/cardiac toxicity, fever, anorexia, nausea, vomiting.

**INTERACTIONS:** Acute shortness of breath and bronchospasm reported following concomitant vinca alkaloids use. Adult respiratory distress syndrome reported with concomitant chemotherapy; monitor oxygen and fluid balance.

**PREGNANCY:** Safety in pregnancy unknown, not for use in nursing.

## MYAMBUTOL RX

ethambutol HCl (Elan)

**THERAPEUTIC CLASS:** Cell metabolism inhibitor

**INDICATIONS:** Adjunct treatment of pulmonary tuberculosis (TB) with at least one other anti-TB drug.

**DOSAGE:** *Adults:* Initial: 15mg/kg q24h. Retreatment: 25mg/kg q24h. After 60 days, decrease to 15mg/kg q24h. Renal Dysfunction: Reduce dose. *Pediatric:* >13 yrs: Initial: 15mg/kg q24h. Retreatment: 25mg/kg q24h. After 60 days, decrease to 15mg/kg q24h. Renal Dysfunction: Reduce dose.

**HOW SUPPLIED:** Tab: 100mg, 400mg* *scored

**CONTRAINDICATIONS:** Optic neuritis. Patients unable to appreciate and report visual side effects or changes in vision.

**WARNINGS/PRECAUTIONS:** Test visual acuity before and periodically during therapy; monthly with dose >15mg/kg/day. Liver toxicity reported; monitor hepatic function at baseline and periodically. Evaluate renal and hematopoietic functions periodically.

**ADVERSE REACTIONS:** Decreased visual acuity, optic neuropathy, anaphylactic reactions, dermatitis, pruritus, joint pain, GI effects, malaise, dizziness, elevated uric acid levels, pulmonary infiltrates, abnormal LFTs, eosinophilia.

**PREGNANCY:** Category C, safety in nursing not known.

## MYCAMINE

RX

micafungin sodium (Fujisawa)

**THERAPEUTIC CLASS:** Glucan synthesis inhibitor

**INDICATIONS:** Treatment of esophageal candidiasis and prophylaxis of *Candida* infections in patients undergoing hematopoietic stem cell transplantation (HSCT).

**DOSAGE:** *Adults:* Esophageal Candidiasis: 150mg/day IV infusion over 1 hour (usual range 10-30 days). *Candida* Infection Prophylaxis in HSCT: 50mg/day IV infusion over 1 hour (usual range 6-51 days). Do not mix or co-infuse with other drugs.

**HOW SUPPLIED:** Inj: 50mg

**WARNINGS/PRECAUTIONS:** Report of serious hypersensitivity (eg, anaphylaxis, anaphylactoid, shock). LFT abnormalities, monitor for evidence of worsening. Reports of significant renal dysfunction, acute renal failure, and elevations in BUN and creatinine. Reports of acute intravascular hemolysis and hemoglobinuria. May precipitate when mixed or co-infused with other drugs.

**ADVERSE REACTIONS:** Hyperbilirubinemia, leukopenia, headache, rash, phlebitis, nausea.

**INTERACTIONS:** Monitor for sirolimus or nifedipine toxicity; reduce sirolimus/nifedipine dose if toxicity occurs.

**PREGNANCY:** Category C, caution in nursing.

## MYCELEX TROCHE

RX

clotrimazole (Ortho-McNeil)

**THERAPEUTIC CLASS:** Triazole antifungal

**INDICATIONS:** Treatment of oropharyngeal candidiasis. To prevent oropharyngeal candidiasis in immunocompromised conditions (eg, chemotherapy, radiotherapy or steroid therapy).

**DOSAGE:** *Adults:* Treatment: Slowly dissolve 1 troche in mouth 5 times/day for 14 days. Prophylaxis: Slowly dissolve 1 troche in mouth tid for duration of chemotherapy or until steroids are reduced.
*Pediatrics:* >3 yrs: Treatment: Slowly dissolve 1 troche in mouth 5 times/day for 14 days.

**HOW SUPPLIED:** Loz/Troche: 10mg [70 loz, 140 loz]

**WARNINGS/PRECAUTIONS:** Not for systemic mycoses. May cause abnormal LFTs; monitor hepatic function. Only use in patients mentally and physically able to dissolve the troche. Confirm diagnosis by KOH smear and/or culture.

**ADVERSE REACTIONS:** Abnormal LFTs, nausea, vomiting, unpleasant mouth sensations, pruritus.

**PREGNANCY:** Category C, safety in nursing is not known.

## MYCELEX-3 OTC

butoconazole nitrate (Bayer Healthcare)

**THERAPEUTIC CLASS:** Azole antifungal

**INDICATIONS:** Treatment of vaginal yeast infection.

**DOSAGE:** *Adults:* Insert 1 applicatorful vaginally qhs for 3 days.
*Pediatrics:* >12 yrs: Insert 1 applicatorful vaginally qhs for 3 days.

**HOW SUPPLIED:** Cre: 2% [5g, 20g]

**WARNINGS/PRECAUTIONS:** Do not use if abdominal pain, fever, foul smelling discharge, pregnancy, diabetes, HIV positive and AIDS patients. Avoid tampons. Do not rely on condoms or diaphragms to prevent STDs or pregnancy while on therapy; use alternate birth control method.

**PREGNANCY:** Safety in pregnancy or nursing not known.

## MYCELEX-7 OTC

clotrimazole (Bayer Healthcare)

**THERAPEUTIC CLASS:** Azole antifungal

**INDICATIONS:** (Cre, Combination Pack) Treatment of vaginal yeast infection. (Combination Pack) For relief of external vulvar itching and irritation associated with vaginal yeast infections.

**DOSAGE:** *Adults:* (Cre) Insert 1 applicatorful vaginally qhs for 7 days. (Combination Pack) 1 insert vaginally qhs for 7 days. Apply small amount of cream onto irritated area of vulva qd-bid for up to 7 days.
*Pediatrics:* >12 yrs: (Cre) Insert 1 applicatorful vaginally qhs for 7 days. (Combination Pack) 1 insert vaginally qhs for 7 days. Apply small amount of cream onto irritated area of vulva qd-bid for up to 7 days.

**HOW SUPPLIED:** Cre: 1% [45g]; (Combination Pack) Cre: 1% [7g], Vaginal Insert: 100 mg [7s]

**WARNINGS/PRECAUTIONS:** Do not use if abdominal pain, fever, foul smelling discharge, during pregnancy. Avoid tampons. May reduce effectiveness of condoms, diaphragm or vaginal spermicides.

**PREGNANCY:** Safety in pregnancy or nursing not known.

## MYCOBUTIN RX

rifabutin (Pharmacia & Upjohn)

**THERAPEUTIC CLASS:** Semisynthetic ansamycin (RNA polymerase inhibitor)

**INDICATIONS:** Prevention of disseminated *Mycobacterium avium* complex (MAC) in advanced HIV.

**DOSAGE:** *Adults:* 300mg qd; give 150mg bid with food if intolerant to GI side effects. Concomitant Nelfinavir/Indinavir or CrCl <30mL/min: Reduce dose by 50%.

**HOW SUPPLIED:** Cap: 150mg

**WARNINGS/PRECAUTIONS:** Avoid with active TB. Neutropenia and thrombocytopenia may occur; obtain hematologic studies periodically. May permanently stain soft contact lenses. May cause discoloration of body fluids and skin. Caution in elderly.

**ADVERSE REACTIONS:** Rash, GI intolerance (eg, abdominal pain, nausea), neutropenia, rash, urine discoloration, taste perversion.

**INTERACTIONS:** May reduce levels of drugs metabolized by CYP3A enzymes (eg, itraconazole, clarithromycin, saquinavir). Increased levels with CYP3A inhibitors (eg, fluconazole, clarithromycin). Avoid delavirdine; rifabutin levels increase and delavirdine levels decrease. Avoid ritonavir; increased risk of adverse effects. Increased levels with nelfinavir, indinavir. May decrease efficacy of oral contraceptives.

**PREGNANCY:** Category B, not for use in nursing.

## MYCOLOG-II
nystatin - triamcinolone acetonide (Apothecon)

RX

**THERAPEUTIC CLASS:** Polyene antifungal/corticosteroid

**INDICATIONS:** Topical treatment of cutaneous candidiasis.

**DOSAGE:** *Adults:* Apply bid (am and pm). Max: 25 days of treatment.
*Pediatrics:* Apply bid (am and pm). Max: 25 days of treatment.

**HOW SUPPLIED:** Cre, Oint: (Nystatin-Triamcinolone) 100,000 U/g-0.1% [15g, 30g, 60g]

**WARNINGS/PRECAUTIONS:** Avoid occlusive dressing. Monitor periodically for HPA axis suppression with prolonged use or when applied over a large area. Discontinue if develop hypersensitivity or irritation. Systemic absorption with topical corticosteroids reported; children are more prone to systemic toxicity. May cause Cushing's syndrome, hyperglycemia, and glucosuria.

**ADVERSE REACTIONS:** Acneform eruption, burning, itching, irritation, secondary infection.

**PREGNANCY:** Category C, caution in nursing.

## MYCOSTATIN TOPICAL
nystatin (Westwood-Squibb)

RX

M

**THERAPEUTIC CLASS:** Polyene antifungal

**INDICATIONS:** Treatment of cutaneous or mucocutaneous mycotic infections caused by susceptible *Candida* species.

**DOSAGE:** *Adults:* (Cre) Apply to affected area bid until healing is complete. (Powder) Apply to lesions bid-tid until healing is complete. For fungal infections of the feet, dust powder on feet and in shoes also.
Pediatrics: Neonates and Older: (Cre) Apply to affected area bid until healing is complete. (Powder) Apply to lesions bid-tid until healing is complete. For fungal infections of the feet, dust powder on feet and in shoes also.

**HOW SUPPLIED:** Cre: 100,000 U/g [30g]; Powder, Topical: 100,000 U/g [15g]

**WARNINGS/PRECAUTIONS:** Discontinue if irritation or sensitization occurs. Confirm diagnosis. Not for systemic, oral, intravaginal, or ophthalmic use. For fungal infections of the feet, dust powder on feet as well as in all footwear. Moist lesions are best treated with topical dusting powder.

**ADVERSE REACTIONS:** Allergic reactions, burning, itching, rash, eczema, pain at application site.

**PREGNANCY:** Category C, caution in nursing.

## MYFORTIC
mycophenolic acid (Novartis)

RX

**Increased susceptibility to infection. Possible development of lymphoma and other neoplasms.**

**THERAPEUTIC CLASS:** Inosine monophosphate dehydrogenase inhibitor

**INDICATIONS:** Prophylaxis of organ rejection in patients receiving allogeneic renal transplants, administered in combination with cyclosporine and corticosteroids.

**DOSAGE:** *Adults:* 720mg bid on empty stomach, 1 hr before or 2 hrs after food intake.
*Pediatrics:* 400mg/m$^2$ bid. Max: 720mg bid. BSA 1.19-1.58m$^2$: 540mg bid. BSA

>1.58m²: 720mg bid. BSA <1.19m² cannot be accurately adminsitered with current formulations.

**HOW SUPPLIED:** Tab, Delayed Release: 180mg, 360mg

**WARNINGS/PRECAUTIONS:** Risk of lymphomas and other malignancies, especially of the skin. Avoid sunlight to decrease risk of skin cancer. May cause fetal harm during pregnancy. Must have negative serum/urine pregnancy test within 1 week before therapy. Two reliable forms of contraception required before and during therapy, and 6 weeks following discontinuation. Monitor for bone marrow suppression. Risk of GI ulceration, hemorrhage, and perforation; caution with active digestive system disease. Caution with delayed renal graft function post-transplant. Oral suspension contains phenylalanine; caution with phenylketonurics. Monitor CBC weekly during the 1st month, twice monthly for the 2nd and 3rd months, and then monthly through 1st year. Avoid with rare hereditary deficiency of hypoxanthine-guanine phosphoribosyl-transferase (eg, Lesch-Nyhan and Kelley-Seegmiller syndrome).

**ADVERSE REACTIONS:** Infections, diarrhea, leukopenia, sepsis, vomiting, GI bleeding, pain, abdominal pain, fever, headache, asthenia, chest pain, back pain, anemia, leukopenia, thrombocytopenia.

**INTERACTIONS:** Additive bone marrow suppression with azathioprine; avoid use. Reduced efficacy with drugs that interfere with enterohepatic recirculation (eg, cholestyramine). Efficacy/safety with other immunosuppressive agents not determined. Avoid live attenuated vaccines. Increased levels of both drugs with acyclovir, ganciclovir. Decreased levels with magnesium- and aluminum-containing antacids; space dosing. Decreased effects of oral contraceptives. Increased levels with probenecid. Other drugs that compete for renal tubular secretion may raise levels of both drugs.

**PREGNANCY:** Category C, not for use in nursing.

M

## MYLANTA GAS MAXIMUM STRENGTH OTC

simethicone (J&J – Merck)

**OTHER BRAND NAMES:** Mylanta Gas Maximum Strength Softgels (J&J – Merck) - Mylanta Gas Regular Strength Chewable Tablets (J&J - Merck)

**THERAPEUTIC CLASS:** Antigas

**INDICATIONS:** For the relief of bloating, pressure, and discomfort of gas caused by food or air swallowing.

**DOSAGE:** *Adults:* (Maximum Strength) Softgels or Chewable Tabs: 1-2 prn. Max: 4 per day. (Regular Strength) Chewable Tabs: 2-4 prn. Max: 6 per day. Take after meals and at bedtime.

**HOW SUPPLIED:** Softgels, Maximum Strength: 125mg; Tab, Maximum Strength Chewable: 125mg; Tab, Regular Strength Chewable: 80mg

## MYLANTA MAXIMUM STRENGTH LIQUID OTC

simethicone - aluminum hydroxide - magnesium hydroxide (J&J – Merck)

**OTHER BRAND NAMES:** Mylanta Regular Strength Liquid (J&J – Merck)

**THERAPEUTIC CLASS:** Antacid/antigas

**INDICATIONS:** For the relief of heartburn, acid indigestion, sour stomach, upset stomach, pressure and bloating.

**DOSAGE:** *Adults:* ≥12 yrs: 2-4 tsp between meals or at bedtime. Max: 24 tsp/day for 2 weeks. Shake well.
*Pediatrics:* ≥12 yrs: 2-4 tsp between meals or at bedtime. Max: 24 tsp/day for 2 weeks. Shake well.

**HOW SUPPLIED:** Liq: (Aluminum Hydroxide-Magnesium Hydroxide-Simethicone) Maximum Strength: 400mg/5mL-400mg/5mL-40mg/5mL. Regular Strength: 200mg/5mL-200mg/5mL-20mg/5mL

## MYLANTA SUPREME

OTC

calcium carbonate - magnesium hydroxide (J&J - Merck)

**OTHER BRAND NAMES:** Mylanta Ultra Tabs (J&J - Merck) - Mylanta Gelcaps Antacid (J&J - Merck)

**THERAPEUTIC CLASS:** Antacid

**INDICATIONS:** For the relief of acid indigestion, heartburn, sour and upset stomach associated with these symptoms.

**DOSAGE:** *Adults:* (Gelcaps) 2-4 caps prn. Max: 12 caps/24hrs. (Ultra Tabs) Chew 2-4 tabs between meals or at bedtime. Max: 10 tabs/24hrs. (Supreme Liquid) 2-4 tsp between meals or at bedtime. Max: 18 tsp/24hrs. Shake well.

**HOW SUPPLIED:** Cap: (Calcium Carbonate-Magnesium Hydroxide) 550mg-125mg. Tab: 700mg-300mg. Liq: 400mg/5mL-135mg/5mL

**WARNINGS/PRECAUTIONS:** Caution with kidney disease.

**INTERACTIONS:** Antacids may interact with other prescription drugs.

## MYLERAN

RX

busulfan (GlaxoSmithKline)

**Do not use unless CML diagnosis is established. May induce severe bone marrow hypoplasia. Reduce dose or discontinue if unusual depression occurs.**

**THERAPEUTIC CLASS:** Alkylating agent

**INDICATIONS:** Palliative treatment of chronic myelogenous leukemia (CML).

**DOSAGE:** *Adults:* 60mcg/kg/day or 1.8mg/m$^2$/day. Range: 4-8mg/day. Reserve dose >4mg/day for the most compelling symptoms.
*Pediatrics:* 60mcg/kg/day or 1.8mg/m$^2$/day. Range: 4-8mg/day. Reserve dose >4mg/day for the most compelling symptoms.

**HOW SUPPLIED:** Tab: 2mg* *scored

**CONTRAINDICATIONS:** Lack of definitive diagnosis of CML.

**WARNINGS/PRECAUTIONS:** Induction of bone marrow failure resulting in severe pancytopenia reported. Bronchopulmonary dysplasia with pulmonary fibrosis, cellular dysplasia, malignant tumors, acute leukemias, hepatic veno-occlusive disease reported. Ovarian suppression and amenorrhea with menopausal symptoms have occurred. Cardiac tamponade in patients with thalassemia and seizures reported. Caution with compromised bone marrow reserve from prior irradiation/chemotherapy.

**ADVERSE REACTIONS:** Myelosuppression, pulmonary fibrosis, cardiac tamponade, hyperpigmentation, weakness, fatigue, weight loss, nausea, vomiting, melanoderma, hyperuricemia, myasthenia gravis, hepatic veno-occlusive disease.

**INTERACTIONS:** Additive myelosuppression with myelosuppressive drugs. Additive pulmonary toxicity with myelotoxic drugs. Reduced clearance with cyclophosphamide. Reduced clearance with itraconazole; monitor for signs of toxicity.

**PREGNANCY:** Category D, not for use in nursing.

## MYLOCEL

RX

hydroxyurea (MGI Pharma)

**THERAPEUTIC CLASS:** Ribonucleotide reductase inhibitor

**INDICATIONS:** Significant tumor response demonstrated in melanoma, resistant chronic myelocytic leukemia (CML), and recurrent, metastatic, or inoperable carcinoma of the ovary. Adjunct therapy with irradiation therapy for local control of primary squamous cell carcinomas of the head and neck, excluding the lip.

**DOSAGE:** *Adults:* Solid Tumors: Intermittent: 80mg/kg single dose every 3rd day. Continuous: 20-30mg/kg qd. Head and Neck Carcinoma: 80mg/kg single dose every 3rd day. Start at least 7 days before irradiation. Resistant CML: 20-30mg/kg qd. Elderly/Renal Impairment: May need dose reduction.

**HOW SUPPLIED:** Tab: 1g* *scored

**CONTRAINDICATIONS:** Marked bone marrow depression (leukopenia, thrombocytopenia or severe anemia).

**WARNINGS/PRECAUTIONS:** Patients with previous irradiation therapy may have exacerbation of post-irradiation erythema. Bone marrow suppression, erythrocytic abnormalities may occur. Correct severe anemia before initiating therapy. Caution with marked renal dysfunction. May develop secondary leukemia with long-term therapy for myeloproliferative disorders. Monitor CBC, bone marrow, hepatic and kidney function before therapy and repeatedly thereafter. Interrupt therapy if WBC <2500/mm$^3$ or platelets <100,000/mm$^3$.

**ADVERSE REACTIONS:** Bone marrow depression, GI effects, maculopapular rash, skin ulceration, dermatomyositis-like skin changes, peripheral and facial erythema.

**INTERACTIONS:** Increased risk of bone marrow depression with other myelosuppressants or radiation therapy. Uricosurics may need dose adjustments.

**PREGNANCY:** Category D, not for use in nursing.



## MYOBLOC RX

botulinum toxin type B (Solstice)

**THERAPEUTIC CLASS:** Purified neurotoxin complex

**INDICATIONS:** Treatment of cervical dystonia to decrease severity of abnormal head position and neck pain.

**DOSAGE:** *Adults:* Initial: 2500-5000U divided among affected muscles with history of tolerating the toxin. Use lower dose without history of tolerance. Adjust dose to patient response.

**HOW SUPPLIED:** Inj: 2500U/0.5mL, 5000U/mL

**WARNINGS/PRECAUTIONS:** Do not exceed dosing recommendations. Caution with peripheral motor neuropathic diseases (eg, amyotrophic lateral sclerosis, motor neuropathy), neuromuscular junctional disorders (eg, myasthenia gravis, Lambert-Eaton syndrome); increased risk of dysphagia and respiratory compromise. Contains albumin.

**ADVERSE REACTIONS:** Dry mouth, dysphagia, dyspepsia, injection site pain, infection, pain.

**INTERACTIONS:** May be potentiated with aminoglycosides, agents interfering with neuromuscular transmission (eg, curare-like compounds). Potentiated by coadministration or overlapping administration of different botulinum toxin serotypes.

**PREGNANCY:** Category C, caution in nursing.

## MYOZYME RX

alglucosidase alfa (Genzyme)

**Risk of hypersensitivity reactions. Life threatening anaphylactic reactions, including anaphylactic shock observed during infusion. Appropriate medical support should be readily available when administered.**

**THERAPEUTIC CLASS:** Enzyme

**INDICATIONS:** Treatment of Pompe Disease.

**DOSAGE:** *Adults:* 20 mg/kg IV every 2 weeks. Administer over 4 hrs.
*Pediatrics:* 20 mg/kg IV every 2 weeks. Administer over 4 hrs.

**HOW SUPPLIED:** Inj: 50 mg

**WARNINGS/PRECAUTIONS:** See Black Box Warning. Risk of cardiac arrhythmia, sudden cardiac death during general anesthesia for central venous catheter placement, and acute cardiorespiratory failure. Infusion reactions observed. Caution with acutely ill patients.

**ADVERSE REACTIONS:** Pyrexia, cough, respiratory distress/failure, pneumonia, otitis media, upper respiratory tract infection, gastroenteritis, pharyngitis, diarrhea, vomiting, rash, decreased oxygen saturation, anemia, oral candidiasis.

**PREGNANCY:** Category B, caution in nursing.

## MYSOLINE
primidone (Valeant)

RX

**THERAPEUTIC CLASS:** Pyrimidinedione derivative

**INDICATIONS:** For control of grand mal, psychomotor, and focal epileptic seizures.

**DOSAGE:** *Adults:* Initial: Day 1-3: 100-125mg qhs. Day 4-6: 100-125mg bid. Day 7-9: 100-125mg tid. Day 10-Maint: 250mg tid. Max: 500mg qid. Effective serum level is 5-12mcg/mL. Prior Anticonvulsant Therapy: Initial: 100-125mg qhs. Titrate: Increase gradually to maintenance dose as other drug is discontinued over 2 weeks.
*Pediatrics:* >8 yrs: Initial: Day 1-3: 100-125mg qhs. Day 4-6: 100-125mg bid. Day 7-9: 100-125mg tid. Day 10-Maint: 250mg tid. Max: 500mg qid. <8 yrs: Day 1-3: 50mg qhs. Day 4-6: 50mg bid. Day 7-9: 100mg bid. Day 10-Maint: 125-250mg tid or 10-25mg/kg/day in divided doses. Effective serum level is 5-12mcg/mL. Prior Anticonvulsant Therapy: Initial: 100-125mg qhs. Titrate: Increase gradually to maintenance dose as other drug is discontinued over 2 weeks.

**HOW SUPPLIED:** Tab: 50mg*, 250mg* *scored

**CONTRAINDICATIONS:** Porphyria, phenobarbital hypersensitivity.

**WARNINGS/PRECAUTIONS:** Avoid abrupt withdrawal. May take several weeks to assess therapeutic efficacy. Pregnant women should receive prophylactic vitamin $K_1$ therapy for one month prior to, and during delivery. Perform CBC and a SMA-12 test every 6 months. Phenobarbital is a metabolite of primidone.

**ADVERSE REACTIONS:** Ataxia, vertigo, nausea, anorexia, vomiting, fatigue, hyperirritability, emotional disturbances, sexual impotency, diplopia, nystagmus, drowsiness, morbilliform skin eruptions.

**PREGNANCY:** Safety in pregnancy not known, caution in nursing.

## NABUMETONE
nabumetone (Various)

RX

**NSAIDs may cause an increased risk of serious cardiovascular thrombotic events, MI, stroke and serious GI adverse events including bleeding, ulceration, and perforation of the stomach or intestines. Contraindicated for the treatment of peri-operative pain in the setting of coronary artery bypass graft (CABG) surgery.**

**THERAPEUTIC CLASS:** NSAID (naphthylalkanone derivative)

**INDICATIONS:** Relief of signs and symptoms of osteoarthritis and rheumatoid arthritis.

**DOSAGE:** *Adults:* Initial: 1000mg qd. Max: 2000mg/day.

**HOW SUPPLIED:** Tab: 500mg, 750mg

**CONTRAINDICATIONS:** Allergy to ASA or other NSAID that precipitates asthma, urticaria or other allergic-type reaction. Treatment of peri-operative pain in the setting of CABG surgery.

**WARNINGS/PRECAUTIONS:** May lead to onset of new HTN or worsening of pre-existing HTN; monitor BP closely. Fluid retention and edema reported; caution with fluid retention or heart failure. Renal papillary necrosis and other renal injury reported after long-term use. Not recommended for use with advanced renal disease; if therapy must be initiated, monitor renal function. Anaphylactoid reactions may occur. May cause serious skin adverse events (eg, exfoliative dermatitis, Stevens-Johnson syndrome, and toxic epidermal necrolysis). Avoid in late pregnancy; may cause premature closure of ductus arteriosis. May cause elevations of LFTs; d/c if liver disease develops or systemic manifestations occur. Caution in elderly. Anemia may occur; with long-term use, monitor Hgb/Hct if signs or symptoms of anemia develop. May inhibit platelet aggregation and prolong bleeding time; monitor with coagulation disorders. Caution with asthma and avoid with aspirin-sensitive asthma. May induce photosensitivity.

**ADVERSE REACTIONS:** Diarrhea, dyspepsia, abdominal pain, constipation, flatulence, nausea, positive stool guaiac, dizziness, headache, pruritus, rash, tinnitus, edema.

**INTERACTIONS:** Caution with warfarin, other protein bound drugs. Nephrotoxicity risk with diuretics.

**PREGNANCY:** Category C, not for use in nursing.

## NAFTIN RX

naftifine HCl (Merz)



**THERAPEUTIC CLASS:** Allylamine antifungal

**INDICATIONS:** Topical treatment of tinea pedis, tinea cruris, and tinea corporis caused by *Trichophyton rubrum*, *Trichophyton mentagrophytes*, and *Epidermophyton floccosum*.

**DOSAGE:** *Adults:* Massage into affected and surrounding areas (Cre) qd or (Gel) bid (am and pm). Wash hands after use. Re-evaluate if no improvement after 4 weeks.

**HOW SUPPLIED:** Cre: 1% [15g, 30g, 60g]; Gel: 1% [20g, 40g, 60g]

**WARNINGS/PRECAUTIONS:** Stop therapy if irritation develops. Avoid eyes, nose, and mucous membranes.

**ADVERSE REACTIONS:** Burning/stinging, rash, erythema, itching, dryness, skin tenderness.

**PREGNANCY:** Category B, caution in nursing.

## NALOXONE RX

naloxone HCl (Various)

**OTHER BRAND NAMES:** Narcan (Endo)

**THERAPEUTIC CLASS:** Opioid antagonist

**INDICATIONS:** For complete or partial opioid depression reversal induced by natural and synthetic opioids. Diagnosis of suspected opioid tolerance or acute opioid overdose. Adjunct in management of septic shock to increase blood pressure.

**DOSAGE:** *Adults:* Opioid Overdose: Initial: 0.4-2mg IV every 2-3 minutes up to 10mg. IM/SQ if IV route not available. Post-op Opioid Depression: 0.1-0.2mg IV every 2-3 minutes to desired response. May repeat in 1-2 hr intervals. Supplemental IM doses last longer. Narcan Challenge Test: IV: 0.1-0.2mg, observe 30 secs for signs of withdrawal, then 0.6mg, observe for 20 minutes.

SQ: 0.8mg, observe for 20 minutes.
*Pediatrics:* Opioid Overdose: Initial: 0.01mg/kg IV. Inadequate Response: repeat 0.01mg/kg once. IM/SQ in divided doses if IV route not available. Post-op Opioid Depression: 0.005-0.01mg IV every 2-3 minutes to desired response. May repeat in 1-2 hr intervals. Supplemental IM doses last longer. Neonates: Opioid-induced Depression: 0.01mg/kg IV/IM/SQ, may repeat every 2-3 minutes until desired response.

**HOW SUPPLIED:** Inj: 0.4mg/mL, 1mg/mL

**WARNINGS/PRECAUTIONS:** Caution in patients including newborns of mothers known or suspected of opioid physical dependence. May precipitate acute withdrawal syndrome. Have other resuscitative measures available. Caution with cardiac, renal, or hepatic disease. Monitor patients satisfactorily responding due to extended opioid duration of action. Abrupt postoperative opioid depression reversal may result in serious adverse effects leading to death.

**ADVERSE REACTIONS:** HTN, hypotension, ventricular tachycardia and fibrillation, dyspnea, pulmonary edema, cardiac arrest, nausea, vomiting, sweating, seizures, body aches, fever, nervousness.

**INTERACTIONS:** Caution using drugs with potential adverse cardiac effects. Reversal of buprenorphine-induced respiratory depression may be incomplete.

**PREGNANCY:** Category B, caution in nursing.

## NAMENDA — RX

memantine HCl (Forest)

**THERAPEUTIC CLASS:** NMDA receptor antagonist

**INDICATIONS:** Treatment of moderate to severe dementia of the Alzheimer's type.

**DOSAGE:** *Adults:* Initial: 5mg qd. Titrate: Increase at intervals of at least one week to 5mg bid, then 5mg and 10mg as separate doses, then to 10mg bid. Severe Renal Impairment: Reduce dose.

**HOW SUPPLIED:** Sol: 2mg/mL; Tab: 5mg, 10mg; Titration-Pak: 5mg [28s], 10mg [21s].

**WARNINGS/PRECAUTIONS:** Use not evaluated with seizure disorders. Alkalinized urine (eg, renal tubular acidosis, severe urinary tract infections) may increase levels. Reduce dose with severe renal impairment. Should be administered with caution to patients with severe hepatic impairment.

**ADVERSE REACTIONS:** Dizziness, confusion, headache, constipation, coughing, HTN, pain, vomiting, somnolence, hallucinations.

**INTERACTIONS:** Caution with other NMDA antagonists (eg, amantadine, ketamine, dextromethorphan), urinary alkalinizers (eg, carbonic anhydrase inhibitors, sodium bicarbonate). Other renally-excreted drugs (eg, HCTZ, triamterene, metformin, cimetidine, ranitidine, quinidine, nicotine) may alter levels of both agents.

**PREGNANCY:** Category B, caution in nursing.

## NAPHCON-A — OTC

naphazoline HCl - pheniramine maleate (Alcon)

**THERAPEUTIC CLASS:** $H_1$ antagonist/alpha-agonist (imidazoline)

**INDICATIONS:** Temporary relief of ocular itching and redness caused by ragweed, pollen, grass, animal hair and dander.

**DOSAGE:** *Adults:* 1-2 drops up to 4 times daily.
*Pediatrics:* >6 yrs: 1-2 drops up to 4 times daily.

**HOW SUPPLIED:** Sol: (Pheniramine-Naphazoline) 0.3%-0.025% [15mL]

**CONTRAINDICATIONS:** Heart disease, high BP, enlargement of the prostate, narrow-angle glaucoma.

**WARNINGS/PRECAUTIONS:** Do not use if solution changes color or becomes cloudy. D/C with eye pain, changes in vision, continued redness or irritation, and if the condition worsens or persists for more than 72 hrs. Remove contact lenses before use. Supervision required with heart disease, high BP, difficulty in urination due to prostate enlargement or narrow angle glaucoma.

**PREGNANCY:** Safety in pregnancy and nursing not known.

## NAPRELAN RX

naproxen sodium (Elan)

> **NSAIDs may cause an increased risk of serious cardiovascular thrombotic events, MI, stroke and serious GI adverse events including bleeding, ulceration, and perforation of the stomach or intestines. Contraindicated for the treatment of peri-operative pain in the setting of coronary artery bypass graft (CABG) surgery.**

**THERAPEUTIC CLASS:** NSAID (arylacetic acid derivative)

**INDICATIONS:** Treatment of rheumatoid arthritis (RA), osteoarthritis (OA), ankylosing spondylitis (AS), tendinitis, bursitis, primary dysmenorrhea and acute gout. Relief of mild-to-moderate pain.

**DOSAGE:** *Adults:* RA/OA/AS: Usual: 750mg-1g qd. Max: 1.5g/day. Pain/Primary Dysmenorrhea/Tendinitis/Bursitis: 1q/day or 1.5g for a limited period. Max: 1g/day thereafter. Acute Gout: 1-1.5g qd for 1 day, then 1g qd until attack subsides.

**HOW SUPPLIED:** Tab, Extended Release: 375mg, 500mg

**CONTRAINDICATIONS:** History of angioedema, urticaria, bronchospastic reactivity, nasal polyps. NSAID allergy that precipitates asthma, nasal polyps, urticaria, and hypotension. Treatment of peri-operative pain in the setting of CABG surgery.

N

**WARNINGS/PRECAUTIONS:** May lead to onset of new HTN or worsening of pre-existing HTN; monitor BP closely. Fluid retention and edema reported; caution with fluid retention or heart failure. Renal papillary necrosis and other renal injury reported after long-term use. Not recommended for use with advanced renal disease; if therapy must be initiated, monitor renal function. Anaphylactoid reactions may occur. May cause serious skin adverse events (eg, exfoliative dermatitis, Stevens-Johnson syndrome, and toxic epidermal necrolysis). Avoid in late pregnancy; may cause premature closure of ductus arteriosis. May cause elevations of LFTs; d/c if liver disease develops or systemic manifestations occur. Caution in elderly. Anemia may occur; with long-term use, monitor Hgb/Hct if signs or symptoms of anemia develop. May inhibit platelet aggregation and prolong bleeding time; monitor with coagulation disorders. Caution with asthma and avoid with aspirin-sensitive asthma.

**ADVERSE REACTIONS:** Headache, dyspepsia, flu syndrome, pain, infection, nausea, diarrhea, constipation, abdominal pain, heartburn, drowsiness, edema, skin rash, ecchymoses.

**INTERACTIONS:** Avoid with other products containing naproxen. May inhibit natriuretic effect of furosemide. Probenecid increases plasma levels and extends its plasma half-life. May increase methotrexate toxicity. Avoid ASA. Caution with coumarin-type anticoagulants, hydantoins, sulfonamides or sulfonylureas; monitor for toxicity. ACE inhibitors may potentiate renal disease states. May displace albumin-bound drugs. May reduce antihypertensive effect of β-blockers. May increase lithium levels.

**PREGNANCY:** Category C, not for use in nursing.

# NAPROSYN

RX

naproxen (Roche Labs)

**NSAIDs may cause an increased risk of serious cardiovascular thrombotic events, MI, stroke and serious GI adverse events including bleeding, ulceration, and perforation of the stomach or intestines. Contraindicated for the treatment of peri-operative pain in the setting of coronary artery bypass graft (CABG) surgery.**

**OTHER BRAND NAMES:** EC-Naprosyn (Roche Labs)

**THERAPEUTIC CLASS:** NSAID

**INDICATIONS:** (Naprosyn, EC-Naprosyn) Relief of signs and symptoms of rheumatoid arthritis (RA), osteoarthritis (OA), ankylosing spondylitis and juvenile arthritis (JA). (Naprosyn) Relief of signs and symtoms of tendinitis, bursitis, and acute gout. Management of pain and primary dysmenorrhea. EC-Naprosyn is not recommended for initial treatment of acute pain.

**DOSAGE:** *Adults:* RA/OA/Ankylosing Spondylitis: Naprosyn: 250, 375, or 500mg bid; EC-Naprosyn: 375 or 500mg bid. Max: 1500mg/day. Acute Gout: Naprosyn: 750mg followed by 250mg q8h until attack subsides. Pain/Dysmenorrhea/Tendinitis/Bursitis: Naprosyn: 500mg followed by 500mg q12h or 250mg q6-8h prn. Max: 1250mg day 1, then 1000mg/day. EC-Naprosyn should not be chewed, crushed, or broken.
*Pediatrics:* >2 yrs: JA: (Sus) 5mg/kg bid. Max: 15mg/kg/day.

**HOW SUPPLIED:** (Naproxen) Sus: 25mg/mL; Tab: 250mg*, 375mg, 500mg*; Tab, Delayed Release: (EC-Naprosyn) 375mg, 500mg *scored

**CONTRAINDICATIONS:** History of ASA or NSAID allergy that cause symptoms of asthma, rhinitis, nasal polyps, and hypotension. Treatment of peri-operative pain in the setting of CABG surgery.

**WARNINGS/PRECAUTIONS:** May lead to onset of new HTN or worsening of pre-existing HTN; monitor BP closely. Fluid retention, edema, and peripheral edema reported; caution with fluid retention, HTN, or heart failure. Renal papillary necrosis and other renal injury reported after long-term use. Not recommended for use with advanced renal disease; if therapy must be initiated, monitor renal function. Anaphylactoid reactions may occur. May cause serious skin adverse events (eg, exfoliative dermatitis, Stevens-Johnson syndrome, and toxic epidermal necrolysis). Avoid in late pregnancy; may cause premature closure of ductus arteriosis. Monitor Hgb levels with long-term therapy if initial Hgb ≤10g. Monitor for visual changes or disturbances. May cause elevations of LFTs; d/c if liver disease develops or systemic manifestations occur. Caution with high doses in chronic alcoholic liver disease and elderly. Anemia may occur; with long-term use, monitor Hgb/Hct if signs or symptoms of anemia develop. May inhibit platelet aggregation and prolong bleeding time; monitor with coagulation disorders. Caution with asthma and avoid with aspirin-sensitive asthma.

**ADVERSE REACTIONS:** Edema, drowsiness, dizziness, constipation, heartburn, abdominal pain, nausea, headache, tinnitus, dyspnea, pruritus, skin eruptions, ecchymoses.

**INTERACTIONS:** (Naprosyn, EC-Naprosyn) Avoid with other products containing naproxen. Decreased plasma levels with ASA. May reduce tubular secretion of methotrexate; monitor for toxicity. May increase nephrotoxicity of cyclosporine; caution when co-administering. May diminish antihypertensive effect and potentiate renal disease with ACE inhibitors. May reduce natriuretic effect of furosemide and thiazides; monitor for renal failure. May increase lithium levels; monitor for toxicity. Synergistic effects on GI bleeding with warfarin. Observe for dose adjustment with hydantoins, sulfonamides, or sulfonylureas. May reduce antihypertensive effects of propranolol and other β-blockers. Probenecid may increase half-life. (EC-Naprosyn) Avoid with $H_2$-blockers, sucralfate, or intensive antacid therapy.

**PREGNANCY:** Category C, not for use in nursing.

## NARDIL RX
phenelzine sulfate (Parke-Davis)

**Antidepressants increased the risk of suicidal thinking and behavior (suicidality) in short-term studies in children and adolescents with Major Depressive Disorder (MDD) and other psychiatric disorders. Phenelzine is not approved for use in pediatric patients.**

**THERAPEUTIC CLASS:** Monoamine oxidase inhibitor

**INDICATIONS:** Treatment of atypical, nonendogenous or neurotic depression not responsive to other antidepressants.

**DOSAGE:** *Adults:* Initial: 15mg tid. Titrate: Increase to 60-90mg/day at a fairly rapid pace until maximum benefit. Maint: Reduce slowly over several weeks to 15mg qd or 15mg every other day.

**HOW SUPPLIED:** Tab: 15mg

**CONTRAINDICATIONS:** Pheochromocytoma, CHF, history of liver disease, abnormal LFT's, severe renal impairment or renal disease, meperidine, MAOIs, dextromethorphan, CNS depressants, alcohol, certain narcotics, sympathomimetic drugs (eg, amphetamines, cocaine, methylphenidate, dopamine, epinephrine, norepinephrine), or related compounds (eg, methyldopa, L-dopa, L-tryptophan, L-tyrosine, phenylalanine), high tyramine-containing food (eg, cheese, pickled herring, beer, wine, yeast extract, salami, yogurt), excessive caffeine and chocolate, dextromethorphan, CNS depressants, buspirone, serotoninergic agents (eg, dexfenfluramine, fluoxetine, fluvoxamine, paroxetine, sertraline, venlafaxine), bupropion, guanethidine.

**WARNINGS/PRECAUTIONS:** Hypertensive crisis, postural hypotension reported; monitor BP frequently. Caution with epilepsy, asthma, DM, or psychosis. D/C if palpitations or headache occur. Excessive stimulation in schizophrenics. D/C 10 days prior to elective surgery. Avoid abrupt withdrawal.

N

**ADVERSE REACTIONS:** Dizziness, headache, drowsiness, sleep disturbances, constipation, dry mouth, GI disturbances, elevated serum transaminases, weight gain, edema, sexual disturbances.

**INTERACTIONS:** See Contraindications. Hypertensive crisis with other MAOIs, sympathomimetics, high tyramine-containing foods. Allow 10 days between starting another MAOI, or antidepressant or buspirone. Serious reactions reported with serotoninergic agents. Allow 5 weeks after discontinuing fluoxetine before starting therapy. Allow 2 weeks after discontinuing therapy before starting bupropion. Avoid cocaine, local, general, and spinal anesthesia. Reduce dose of barbiturates. Caution with rauwolfia alkaloids. Exaggerated hypotensive effects with antihypertensives. Excitation, seizures, delirium, hyperpyrexia, circulatory collapse, coma, and death have been reported with meperidine.

**PREGNANCY:** Safety in pregnancy and nursing not known.

## NAROPIN RX
ropivacaine HCl (Abraxis)

**THERAPEUTIC CLASS:** Local anesthetic

**INDICATIONS:** Production of local or regional anesthesia in surgery. Management of acute pain.

**DOSAGE:** *Adults:* Dose may vary by procedure, area to be anesthetized, tissue vascularity, duration and depth of anesthesia needed. Administer test dose of 3-5mL before induction of complete block. Surgical: Lumbar Epidural: Usual: 75-200mg in 15-30mL. Thoracic Epidural for Surgery: 25-113mg in 5-15mL. Lumbar Epidural in Cesarean: 100-150mg in 15-30mL. Major Nerve Block: 75-300mg in 10-50mL. Field Block: 5-200mg in 1-40mL Labor: Lumbar Epidural:

Initial: 20-40mg. Maint: 12-28mg/h. Postoperative: Lumbar/Thoracic Epidural: 12-28mg/hr. Infiltration: 2-200mg in 1-100mL.

**HOW SUPPLIED:** Inj: 2mg/mL, 5mg/mL, 7.5mg/mL, 10mg/mL

**WARNINGS/PRECAUTIONS:** Administer in incremental doses. High risk of arrhythmias, circulatory arrest, and death reported in pregnant patients. Not for production of obstetrical paracervical block, retrobulbar block, or spinal anesthesia. Use lowest effective dose. Perform syringe aspiration to avoid extravasation and subarachnoid injection. Administer test dose with epidural anesthesia. Anxiety, dizziness, blurred vision, tremors, depression, and tinnitus are early signs of CNS toxicity. Caution in hepatic impairment, cardiovascular disorders, hypotension, hypovolemia, heart block. Should cardiac arrest occur, prolonged resuscitative efforts may be required to improve the probability of a successful outcome.

**ADVERSE REACTIONS:** Hypotension, bradycardia, nausea, vomiting, paresthesia, back pain, fever, chills, headache, pain, urinary retention, dizziness, pruritus, HTN, anemia, headache, paresthesia.

**INTERACTIONS:** Caution with other local anesthetics, amide-type anesthetics; additive toxic effects may occur. Caution with class III antiarrhythmics. Increased levels with inhibitors of CYP450 1A2 (eg, fluvoxamine) and CYP450 3A4 (eg, ketoconazole).

**PREGNANCY:** Category B, caution in nursing.

## NASACORT AQ RX

triamcinolone acetonide (Sanofi-Aventis)

**OTHER BRAND NAMES:** Nasacort HFA (Sanofi-Aventis)

**THERAPEUTIC CLASS:** Corticosteroid

**INDICATIONS:** Nasal treatment of seasonal and perennial allergic rhinitis symptoms.

**DOSAGE:** *Adults:* (AQ Spray) Initial/Max: 2 sprays per nostril qd. With improvement, may reduce dose to 1 spray per nostril qd. (HFA Aerosol) Initial: 2 sprays per nostril qd. Max: 4 sprays per nostril qd.
*Pediatrics:* ≥12 yrs: (AQ Spray) Initial/Max: 2 sprays per nostril qd. With improvement, may reduce dose to 1 spray per nostril qd. (HFA Aerosol) Initial: 2 sprays per nostril qd. Max: 4 sprays per nostril qd. 6-12 yrs: (AQ Spray) Initial: 1 spray per nostril qd. Max: 2 sprays per nostril qd. 6-11 yrs: (HFA Aerosol) 2 sprays per nostril qd.

**HOW SUPPLIED:** AQ Spray: 55mcg/spray [16.5g]; HFA Aerosol: 55mcg/spray [9.3g]

**WARNINGS/PRECAUTIONS:** Risk of adrenal insufficiency and withdrawal symptoms when replacing systemic corticosteroid with a topical corticosteroids. Caution with active or quiescent TB, ocular herpes simplex, or untreated bacterial, fungal and systemic viral infections. Avoid with recent nasal trauma, surgery or septum ulcers. Risk for more severe/fatal course of infections (eg, chickenpox, measles) and for *Candida* infections of the nose and pharynx. Potential for growth velocity reduction in pediatrics.

**ADVERSE REACTIONS:** Pharyngitis, epistaxis, infection, otitis media, headache, sneezing, rhinitis, nasal irritation, cough, sinusitis, vomiting.

**PREGNANCY:** Category C, caution in nursing.

## NASAREL RX

flunisolide (Ivax)

**THERAPEUTIC CLASS:** Corticosteroid

**INDICATIONS:** Relief of seasonal or perennial rhinitis.

**DOSAGE:** *Adults:* Initial: 2 sprays per nostril bid. Titrate: May increase to 2 sprays per nostril tid. Max: 8 sprays per nostril/day.
*Pediatrics:* 6-14 yrs: Initial: 1 spray per nostril tid or 2 sprays per nostril bid. Max: 4 sprays per nostril/day.

**HOW SUPPLIED:** Spray: 29mcg/spray [25mL]

**CONTRAINDICATIONS:** Untreated localized infection of the nasal mucosa.

**WARNINGS/PRECAUTIONS:** Risk of adrenal insufficiency and withdrawal symptoms when replacing systemic corticosteroids with a topical corticosteroids. Caution with active or quiescent TB, ocular herpes simplex, or untreated bacterial, fungal and systemic viral infections. Avoid with recent nasal trauma, surgery or septum ulcers. Risk for more severe/fatal course of infections (eg, chickenpox, measles) and for *Candida* infections of the nose and pharynx. Potential for growth velocity reduction in pediatrics.

**ADVERSE REACTIONS:** Aftertaste, nasal burning/stinging, cough, epistaxis, nasal dryness.

**INTERACTIONS:** Concomitant systemic corticosteroids increases risk of hypercorticism and/or HPA axis suppression.

**PREGNANCY:** Category C, caution in nursing.

## NASCOBAL RX

cyanocobalamin (Questcor)

**THERAPEUTIC CLASS:** Synthetic Vitamin $B_{12}$

**INDICATIONS:** Maintenance of hematologic status of patients in remission following IM vitamin $B_{12}$ therapy for the following conditions: pernicious anemia; dietary deficiency in vegetarians; malabsorption resulting from structural/functional damage to the stomach (eg, HIV, AIDS, Crohn's disease); lesions that destroy gastric mucosa and conditions associated with gastric atrophy (eg, MS, HIV, AIDS); intestinal parasites; and inadequate utilization of vitamin $B_{12}$ (antimetabolites used to treat neoplasia).



**DOSAGE:** *Adults:* 500mcg intranasally once weekly. Patients should be in hematologic remission before treatment.

**HOW SUPPLIED:** Gel, Spray: 500mcg/0.1mL (per actuation) [2.3mL]

**CONTRAINDICATIONS:** Sensitivity to cobalt.

**WARNINGS/PRECAUTIONS:** Severe and swift optic atrophy reported with Leber's disease. Hypokalemia and sudden death may occur in severe megaloblastic anemia treated intensely. Folic acid is not a substitute for vitamin $B_{12}$-deficient anemia. Perform intradermal test dose if sensitivity suspected. Vitamin $B_{12}$ deficiency may suppress signs of polycythemia vera. Hypokalemia and thrombocytosis may occur upon conversion of severe megaloblastic to normal erythropoiesis. Avoid use with nasal congestion, allergic rhinitis, upper respiratory infection. Monitor vitamin $B_{12}$ levels and peripheral blood counts prior to and periodically during therapy.

**ADVERSE REACTIONS:** Nausea, headache, rhinitis.

**INTERACTIONS:** Antibiotics, MTX, pyrimethamine invalidate folic acid and vitamin $B_{12}$ blood assays. Colchicine, para-aminosalicylic acid and heavy alcohol intake for >2 weeks may produce vitamin $B_{12}$ malabsorption.

**PREGNANCY:** Category C, consume recommended amount by the Food and Nutrition Board during nursing.

## NASONEX RX

mometasone furoate monohydrate (Schering)

**THERAPEUTIC CLASS:** Corticosteroid

**INDICATIONS:** Treatment of the nasal symptoms of seasonal and perennial allergic rhinitis. Prophylaxis of the nasal symptoms of seasonal allergic rhinitis. Treatment of nasal polyps in patients 18 years of age and older.

**DOSAGE:** *Adults:* Allergic Rhinitis: Treatment/Prophylaxis: 2 sprays per nostril qd. For prophylaxis, start 2-4 weeks before allergy season. Nasal Polyps: 2 sprays per nostril bid.
*Pediatrics:* >12 yrs: Treatment/Prophylaxis: 2 sprays per nostril qd. For prophylaxis, start 2-4 weeks before allergy season. 2-11 yrs: Treatment: 1 spray per nostril qd.

**HOW SUPPLIED:** Spray: 50mcg/spray [17g]

**WARNINGS/PRECAUTIONS:** Risk of adrenal insufficiency and withdrawal symptoms when replacing systemic corticosteroids with a topical corticosteroids. Caution with active or quiescent TB, ocular herpes simplex, or untreated bacterial, fungal and systemic viral infections. Avoid with recent nasal trauma, surgery or septum ulcers. Risk for more severe/fatal course of infections (eg, chickenpox, measles) and for *Candida* infections of the nose and pharynx. Potential for growth velocity reduction in pediatrics.

**ADVERSE REACTIONS:** Headache, viral infection, pharyngitis, epistaxis, cough, upper respiratory tract infection, dysmenorrhea, myalgia, sinusitis.

**PREGNANCY:** Category C, caution with nursing.

## NATACHEW — RX
minerals - folic acid - multiple vitamin (Warner Chilcott)

**THERAPEUTIC CLASS:** Prenatal vitamin

**INDICATIONS:** Vitamin and mineral supplementation for before, during, and after pregnancy.

**DOSAGE:** *Adults:* 1 tab qd.

**HOW SUPPLIED:** Tab, Chewable: Folic Acid 1mg-Iron 29mg-Niacinamide 20mg-Vitamin A 1000 IU-Vitamin $B_1$ 2mg-Vitamin $B_2$ 3mg-Vitamin $B_6$ 10mg-Vitamin $B_{12}$ 0.012mg-Vitamin C 120mg-Vitamin D 400 IU-Vitamin E 11 IU*
*scored

**WARNINGS/PRECAUTIONS:** Accidental overdose of iron-containing products is a leading cause of fatal poisoning in children <6 yrs. Folic acid may partially correct hematological damage due to vitamin $B_{12}$ deficiency of pernicious anemia, while neurological damage progresses.

## NATACYN — RX
natamycin (Alcon)

**THERAPEUTIC CLASS:** Tetraene polyene antifungal

**INDICATIONS:** Treatment of fungal blepharitis, conjunctivitis, and keratitis. Not recommended as monotherapy for fungal endophthalmitis.

**DOSAGE:** *Adults:* Keratitis: 1 drop q1-2h for 3-4 days, then 1 drop 6-8 times daily for 14-21 days or until the resolution of infection. Reduce dose at 4-7 day intervals. Blepharitis/Conjunctivitis: 1 drop 4-6 times daily.

**HOW SUPPLIED:** Sus: 5% [15mL]

**WARNINGS/PRECAUTIONS:** Re-evaluate if no improvement after 7-10 days. Monitor twice weekly for toxicity.

**ADVERSE REACTIONS:** Conjunctival chemosis, hyperemia.

**PREGNANCY:** Category C, caution in nursing.

## NATAFORT — RX
iron - folic acid - multiple vitamin (Warner Chilcott)

**THERAPEUTIC CLASS:** Prenatal vitamin

**INDICATIONS:** Vitamin and mineral supplementation for before, during, and after pregnancy.

**DOSAGE:** *Adults:* 1 tab qd.

**HOW SUPPLIED:** Tab: Folic Acid 1mg-Iron 60mg-Niacinamide 20mg-Vitamin A 1000 IU-Vitamin $B_1$ 2mg-Vitamin $B_2$ 3mg-Vitamin $B_6$ 10mg-Vitamin $B_{12}$ 12mcg-Vitamin C 120mg-Vitamin D3 400 IU-Vitamin E 11 IU

**WARNINGS/PRECAUTIONS:** Accidental overdose of iron-containing products is leading cause of fatal poisoning in children <6 yrs. Folic acid may partially correct hematological damage due to vitamin $B_{12}$ deficiency of pernicious anemia, while neurological damage progresses.

## NATALCARE CFE 60 RX

minerals - folic acid - multiple vitamin (Ethex)

**THERAPEUTIC CLASS:** Prenatal vitamin

**INDICATIONS:** Vitamin and mineral supplementation for before, during, and after pregnancy.

**DOSAGE:** *Adults:* 1 tab qd.

**HOW SUPPLIED:** Tab: Folic Acid 1mg-Iron 60mg-Niacinamide 20mg-Vitamin A 1000 IU-Vitamin $B_1$ 2mg-Vitamin $B_2$ 3mg-Vitamin $B_6$ 10mg-Vitamin $B_{12}$ 0.012mg-Vitamin C 120mg-Vitamin D 400 IU-Vitamin E 11 IU

**WARNINGS/PRECAUTIONS:** Accidental overdose of iron-containing products is a leading cause of fatal poisoning in children <6 yrs. Folic acid may partially correct hematological damage due to vitamin $B_{12}$ deficiency of pernicious anemia, while neurological damage progresses.

**ADVERSE REACTIONS:** Allergic hypersensitivity.

N

## NATRECOR RX

nesiritide (Scios Inc.)

**THERAPEUTIC CLASS:** Human B-type natriuretic peptide

**INDICATIONS:** Treatment of acutely decompensated congestive heart failure with dyspnea at rest or with minimal activity.

**DOSAGE:** *Adults:* 2mcg/kg IV bolus over 60 seconds, then 0.01mcg/kg/min IV infusion. Reduce dose or discontinue if hypotension occurs.

**HOW SUPPLIED:** Inj: 1.5mg

**CONTRAINDICATIONS:** Primary therapy with cardiogenic shock or systolic BP <90mmHg.

**WARNINGS/PRECAUTIONS:** Avoid with low cardiac filling pressures. Use precautions for parenteral administration of protein pharmaceuticals or E. coli-derived products; may cause allergic reaction. Avoid when vasodilators are inappropriate (eg, significant valvular stenosis, restrictive/obstructive cardiomyopathy, constrictive pericarditis, pericardial tamponade, conditions where cardiac output is dependent on venous return). May affect renal function; azotemia reported. Monitor BP closely; hypotension reported. Caution with BP <100 mmHg at baseline. Reduce dose or discontinue if hypotension occurs.

**ADVERSE REACTIONS:** Hypotension, ventricular tachycardia, ventricular extrasystoles, headache, back pain, dizziness, anxiety, nausea, abdominal pain, insomnia

**INTERACTIONS:** Increased risk of hypotension with drugs that cause hypotension such as oral ACE inhibitors. Do not co-administer through the same IV catheter with heparin, insulin, ethacrynate sodium, bumetamide, enalaprilat, hydralazine, furosemide, or injectable drugs containing sodium metabisulfite. Flush catheter between uses with incompatible drugs.

**PREGNANCY:** Category C, caution in nursing.

## NAVANE
thiothixene (Pfizer)

RX

**THERAPEUTIC CLASS:** Thioxanthene

**INDICATIONS:** Management of schizophrenia.

**DOSAGE:** *Adults:* Mild Condition: Initial: 2mg tid. Titrate: May increase to 15mg/day. Severe Condition: Initial: 5mg bid. Usual: 20-30mg/day. Max: 60mg/day.
*Pediatrics:* >12yrs: Mild Condition: Initial: 2mg tid. Titrate: May increase to 15mg/day. Severe Condition: Initial: 5mg bid. Usual: 20-30mg/day. Max: 60mg/day.

**HOW SUPPLIED:** Cap: 2mg, 5mg, 10mg, 20mg

**CONTRAINDICATIONS:** Circulatory collapse, comatose states, CNS depression, blood dyscrasias.

**WARNINGS/PRECAUTIONS:** May develop tardive dyskinesia, NMS. May mask symptoms of overdose of toxic drugs. May obscure conditions such as intestinal obstruction and brain tumor. May lower seizure threshold. Monitor for pigmentary retinopathy and lenticular pigmentation. Caution with cardiovascular disease, extreme heat exposure, activities requiring alertness. May elevate prolactin levels.

**ADVERSE REACTIONS:** Tachycardia, hypotension, lightheadedness, syncope, drowsiness, agitation, insomnia, hyperreflexia, cerebral edema, pseudoparkinsonism, LFT elevation, blood dyscrasias, rash, photosensitivity, dry mouth, blurred vision.

**INTERACTIONS:** Possible additive effects including hypotension with CNS depressants, alcohol. Caution with atropine or related drugs. Paradoxical effects with pressor agents.

**PREGNANCY:** Safety in pregnancy and nursing not known.

N

## NAVELBINE
vinorelbine tartrate (GlaxoSmithKline)

RX

**For IV use only; fatal if given intrathecally. Severe granulocytopenia may occur; granulocyte counts should be >1000cells/mm³ prior to administration. Use extreme caution to prevent extravasation; if this occurs, d/c and restart in another vein.**

**THERAPEUTIC CLASS:** Vinca alkaloid

**INDICATIONS:** Single agent or in combination with cisplatin for 1st-line treatment of unresectable, advanced nonsmall cell lung cancer (NSCLC), including Stage IV NSCLC. For use in combination with cisplatin for Stage III NSCLC .

**DOSAGE:** *Adults:* Single-Agent: 30mg/m² IV weekly over 6-10 minutes. With Cisplatin: 25mg/m² weekly with cisplatin 100mg/m² every 4 weeks, or 30mg/m² weekly with cisplatin 120mg/m² on days 1 and 29, then every 6 weeks. Adjustments Based on Granulocytes: If 1000-1499cells/mm³ give 50% starting dose. If <1000cells/mm³, hold dose and repeat count in 1 week. D/C if hold 3 consecutive weekly doses because granulocyte <1000cells/mm³. If fever and/or sepsis occurs while granulocytopenic or if hold 2 consecutive weekly doses due to granulocytopenia; give 75% of the starting dose if granulocytes >1500cells/mm³, and 37.5% of the starting dose if granulocytes 1000-1499cells/mm³. Hepatic Insufficiency: (bilirubin 2.1-3mg/dL) 50% of the starting dose or (bilirubin >3mg/dL) 25% of the starting dose. If both hematologic toxicity and hepatic insufficiency, use lowest dose. Neurotoxicity: D/C if Grade >2 develops.

**HOW SUPPLIED:** Inj: 10mg/mL

**CONTRAINDICATIONS:** Pretreatment granulocytes <1000cells/mm³.

**WARNINGS/PRECAUTIONS:** Monitor for myleosuppression during and after therapy, and for infection and/or fever with developing severe granulocytopenia. Interstitial pulmonary changes, ARDS, acute shortness of breath and severe bronchospasm reported. Extreme caution with compromised bone marrow reserve due to prior irradiation or chemotherapy. Radiation recall reactions may occur. Monitor for new or worsening signs/symptoms of neuropathy. D/C if moderate or severe neurotoxicity develops. Avoid contact with skin, mucosa, and eyes. Avoid pregnancy.

**ADVERSE REACTIONS:** Granulocytopenia, leukopenia, thrombocytopenia, anemia, asthenia, injection site reactions/pain, phlebitis, peripheral neuropathy, nausea, vomiting, diarrhea, severe constipation, paralytic ileus, intestinal obstruction, necrosis, and/or perforation, dyspnea, alopecia, chest pain, fatigue.

**INTERACTIONS:** Risk of acute pulmonary reactions with mitomycin. Increased incidence of granulocytopenia with cisplatin. Monitor for signs/symptoms of neuropathy with paclitaxel, either concomitantly or sequentially. Radiosensitizing effects may occur with prior or concomitant radiation therapy. Caution with CYP450 3A inhibitors, or with hepatic dysfunction; earlier onset and/or increased severity of side effects may occur.

**PREGNANCY:** Category D, not for use in nursing.

## NEFAZODONE RX

nefazodone HCl (Various)

**Antidepressants increased the risk of suicidal thinking and behavior (suicidality) in short-term studies in children and adolescents with Major Depressive Disorder (MDD) and other psychiatric disorders. Nefazodone is not approved for use in pediatric patients. Life-threatening hepatic failure reported. Avoid with active liver disease or elevated serum transaminases. Discontinue and do not retreat if symptoms of hepatic disease develop or if ALT/AST >3X ULN.**



**THERAPEUTIC CLASS:** Serotonin and norepinephrine reuptake inhibitor

**INDICATIONS:** Treatment of depression.

**DOSAGE:** *Adults:* Initial: 100mg bid. Usual: 300-600mg/day. Titrate: May increase by 100-200mg/day at intervals of no less than 1 week. Elderly/Debilitated: Initial: 50mg bid.

**HOW SUPPLIED:** Tab: 50mg, 100mg*, 150mg*, 200mg, 250mg *scored

**CONTRAINDICATIONS:** Coadministration of terfenadine, astemizole, cisapride, pimozide, carbamazepine, triazolam. Liver injury from previous treatment.

**WARNINGS/PRECAUTIONS:** May cause postural hypotension. Caution with cardiovascular or cerebrovascular disease that could be exacerbated by hypotension and conditions with predisposition to hypotension (eg, dehydration, hypotension). May activate mania/hypomania. Priapism reported. Caution with history of MI, unstable heart disease, seizures, liver cirrhosis. Avoid with active liver disease.

**ADVERSE REACTIONS:** Hepatic failure, somnolence, dry mouth, nausea, dizziness, insomnia, agitation, constipation, asthenia, lightheadedness, blurred vision, confusion, abnormal vision.

**INTERACTIONS:** Avoid MAOIs within 14 days of use. Avoid alcohol, terfenadine, astemizole, cisapride, pimozide. Reduce triazolam dose by 75% and avoid in elderly. Reduce alprazolam dose by 50%. Effects antagonized by carbamazepine. Caution with highly protein bound drugs, drugs metabolized by CYP3A4, CNS-active drugs. Discontinue prior to general anesthesia. Haloperidol may need dose adjustment. Increases plasma levels of cyclosporine, tacrolimus. Rhabdomyolysis (rare) reported with simvastatin and lovastatin. Monitor digoxin. Institute a wash-out period and lower doses if used after fluoxetine therapy. May increase buspirone levels; decrease buspirone dose to 2.5mg qd.

**PREGNANCY:** Category C, caution in nursing.

## NEGGRAM RX
nalidixic acid (Sanofi-Aventis)

**THERAPEUTIC CLASS:** Fluoroquinolone

**INDICATIONS:** Treatment of urinary tract infection.

**DOSAGE:** *Adults:* Initial: 1g qid with fluids for 1-2 weeks. Prolonged Therapy: Reduce to 2g/day after initial therapy.
*Pediatrics:* >12 yrs: Initial: 1g qid with fluids for 1-2 weeks. Prolonged Therapy: Reduce to 2g/day after initial therapy. 3 months-12 yrs: Initial: 25mg/lb/day given qid. Prolonged Therapy: Reduce dose to 15mg/lb/day after initial therapy. Use only in patients <18 yrs if potential benefit justifies the potential risk of cartilage erosion in weight-bearing joints and other signs of arthropathy.

**HOW SUPPLIED:** Sus: 250mg/5mL; Tab: 250mg*, 500mg*, 1g* *scored

**CONTRAINDICATIONS:** History of convulsive disorder.

**WARNINGS/PRECAUTIONS:** Convulsions, increased intracranial pressure, and toxic psychosis reported; caution with CNS disorders (eg, epilepsy, severe cerebral arteriosclerosis). May cause CNS stimulation (eg, tremor, lightheadedness, confusion, hallucinations). Pseudomembranous colitis and serious, fatal hypersensitivity reactions reported. If therapy >2 weeks, monitor blood counts and hepatic and liver function. Photosensitivity reaction reported; avoid excessive sunlight. D/C if phototoxicity occurs.

**ADVERSE REACTIONS:** Drowsiness, weakness, headache, dizziness, vertigo, abdominal pain, nausea, vomiting, diarrhea, rash, pruritus, angioedema.

**INTERACTIONS:** May potentiate theophylline, caffeine, oral anticoagulants, and cyclosporine. Diminished effects with nitrofurantoin, antacid containing magnesium, aluminum or calcium, sucralfate, iron, multivitamins containing zinc, didanosine; separate dose by 2 hrs.

**PREGNANCY:** Category C, not for use in nursing.



## NEMBUTAL SODIUM CII
pentobarbital sodium (Ovation)

**THERAPEUTIC CLASS:** Barbiturate

**INDICATIONS:** Short-term treatment of insomnia; sedation; preoperative anesthesia; anticonvulsant in the emergency control of certain acute convulsive episodes.

**DOSAGE:** *Adults:* Usual: 150-200mg as a single IM injection. IV: 100mg (commonly used initial dose for 70kg adult); if needed additional small increments may be given up to 200-500mg total dose. Rate of IV injection should not exceed 50mg/min. Elderly/Debilitated/Renal or Hepatic Impairment: Reduce dose.
*Pediatrics:* 2-6mg/kg as a single IM injection. Max: 100mg. IV: Proportional reduction in dosage. Slow IV injection is essential.

**HOW SUPPLIED:** Inj: 50mg/mL

**CONTRAINDICATIONS:** History of manifest or latent porphyria.

**WARNINGS/PRECAUTIONS:** May be habit forming; avoid abrupt cessation after prolonged use. Avoid rapid administration. Tolerance to hypnotic effect can occur. Prehepatic coma use not recommended. Use with caution in patients with chronic or acute pain, mental depression, suicidal tendencies, history of drug abuse or hepatic impairment. Monitor blood, liver and renal function. May impair mental/physical abilities. Avoid alcohol.

**ADVERSE REACTIONS:** Agitation, confusion, hyperkinesia, ataxia, CNS depression, somnolence, bradycardia, hypotension, nausea, vomiting, constipation, headache, hypersensitivity reactions, liver damage.

**INTERACTIONS:** May produce additive CNS depression with other CNS depressants (eg, other sedatives/hypnotics, antihistamines, tranquilizers, alcohol). May decrease levels of oral anticoagulants, corticosteroids, griseofulvin, and doxycycline. Dosage adjustments may be required for anticoagulants and corticosteroids. Variable effects on phenytoin and increased levels with valproic acid, sodium valproate; monitor blood levels and adjust dose appropriately. May decrease effects of estradiol; alternative contraceptive method should be suggested. Prolonged effect with MAOIs.

**PREGNANCY:** Category D, caution with nursing.

## NEORAL

RX

cyclosporine (Novartis)

**Increased susceptibility to infection, and development of neoplasia, HTN, nephrotoxicity. Monitor blood levels to avoid toxicity. Neoral is not bioequivalent to Sandimmune. Risk of skin malignancies if previously treated with PUVA, UVB, coal tar, radiation, MTX, or other immunosuppressives.**

**THERAPEUTIC CLASS:** Cyclic polypeptide immunosuppressant

**INDICATIONS:** Organ rejection prophylaxis in kidney, liver, and heart allogeneic transplants. Treatment of severe active, rheumatoid arthritis (RA) unresponsive to methotrexate (MTX). Treatment of nonimmunocompromised adults with severe, recalcitrant, plaque psoriasis unresponsive to at least 1 systemic therapy (eg, PUVA, retinoids, MTX) or when other systemic therapies are contraindicated/not tolerated.

**DOSAGE:** *Adults:* Transplant: Give initial oral dose 4-12 hrs before transplant or post-op. Dose bid. Initial: Renal Transplant: 9 3 3mg/kg/day. Liver Transplant: 834mg/kg/day. Heart Transplant: 7 3 3mg/kg/day. Give with corticosteroids initially. Conversion from Sandimmune: 1:1 dose conversion. Adjust to trough levels. Monitor every 4-7 days. RA: Initial: 1.25mg/kg bid. Titrate: May increase by 0.5-0.75mg/kg/day after 8 weeks, again after 12 weeks. Max: 4mg/kg/day. Discontinue if no benefit by week 16. Psoriasis: Initial: 1.25mg/kg bid for 4 weeks. Titrate: May increase by 0.5mg/kg/day every 2 weeks. Max: 4mg/kg/day. Decrease dose by 25-50% to control adverse events. Take at the same time every day. Dilute sol in orange or apple juice that is room temp.

**HOW SUPPLIED:** Cap: 25mg, 100mg; Sol: 100mg/mL [50mL]

**CONTRAINDICATIONS:** Abnormal renal function, uncontrolled HTN, malignancies. PUVA or UVB therapy, MTX, other immunosuppressants, coal tar, or radiation in psoriasis patients.

**WARNINGS/PRECAUTIONS:** Risk of hepatotoxicity and nephrotoxicity. Caution in elderly. Hyperkalemia, hyperuricemia, thrombocytopenia, microangiopathic hemolytic anemia, and encephalopathy reported in transplant patients. Monitor CBC and LFTs monthly with MTX. Monitor BP and renal function before therapy, every 2 weeks during 1st 3 months, then monthly if stable with RA or psoriasis. Monitor SCr after initiate or increase NSAID dose in RA. Monitor CBC, uric acid, $K^+$, lipids, and magnesium every 2 weeks during 1st 3 months, then monthly if stable in RA. Monitor LFTs repeatedly. Monitor CBC, SCr with transplants.

**ADVERSE REACTIONS:** Renal dysfunction, HTN, hirsutism, muscle cramps, acne, tremor, headache, gingival hyperplasia, diarrhea, nausea, vomiting, paresthesia, flushing, dyspepsia, hypertrichosis, stomatitis, hypomagnesemia.

**INTERACTIONS:** Phenytoin, phenobarbital, rifampin, nafcillin, carbamazepine, orlistat, ticlopidine, octreotide, St. John's wort decrease levels. Increases MTX levels. Potentiated by clarithromycin, diltiazem, fluconazole, erythromycin, itraconazole, ketoconazole, verapamil, nicardipine, quinupristin/dalfopristin, allopurinol, bromocriptine, danazol, metoclopramide, colchicine, amiodarone, grapefruit juice. Aminoglycosides, ciprofloxacin, vancomycin, SMZ/TMP, melphalan, ketoconazole, NSAIDs, colchicine, cimetidine, ranitidine, tacrolimus, amphotericin B, bezafibrate, fenofibrate may potentiate renal dysfunction. Digitalis toxicity reported. Myotoxicity with statins, frequent gingival hyperplasia with nifedipine, and convulsions with high dose methylprednisolone reported. Avoid potassium-sparing diuretics, grapefruit juice. Decreased clearance of prednisolone, digoxin, and lovastatin. Caution with HIV protease inhibitors, ACEIs, angiotensin II blockers. Decreased effects of vaccinations; avoid live attenuated vaccines.

**PREGNANCY:** Category C, not for use in nursing.

## NEOSAR RX

cyclophosphamide (Teva)

**THERAPEUTIC CLASS:** Nitrogen mustard alkylating agent

**INDICATIONS:** Treatment of malignant lymphomas, Hodgkin's disease, lymphocytic lymphoma, mixed-cell type or histiocytic lymphoma, Burkitt's lymphoma, multiple myeloma, chronic lymphocytic leukemia, chronic granulocytic leukemia, acute myelogenous and monocytic leukemia, acute lymphoblastic leukemia in children, mycosis fungoides, neuroblastoma, ovary adenocarcinoma, retinoblastoma, breast carcinoma. Treatment of biopsy proven"minimal change" nephrotic syndrome in children, but not as primary therapy.

**DOSAGE:** *Adults:* Malignant Diseases (Without Hematologic Deficiency): Monotherapy: Initial: 40-50mg/kg IV in divided doses over 2-5 days, or 10-15mg/kg IV given every 7-10 days, or 3-5mg/kg twice weekly. Oral Cyclophosphamide: Initial/Maint: 1-5mg/kg/day PO. Adjust dose according to antitumor activity and/or leukopenia. May need to reduce dose when combined with other cytotoxic drugs.
*Pediatrics:* Malignant Diseases (Without Hematologic Deficiency): Monotherapy: Initial: 40-50mg/kg IV in divided doses over 2-5 days, or 10-15mg/kg IV given every 7-10 days, or 3-5mg/kg twice weekly. Oral Cyclophosphamide: Initial/Maint: 1-5mg/kg/day PO. Adjust dose according to antitumor activity and/or leukopenia. May need to reduce dose when combined with other cytotoxic drugs. Nephrotic Syndrome: 2.5-3mg/kg/day PO for 60-90 days.

**HOW SUPPLIED:** Inj: 100mg, 200mg, 500mg, 1g, 2g

**CONTRAINDICATIONS:** Severely depressed bone marrow function.

**WARNINGS/PRECAUTIONS:** Second malignancies, cardiac dysfunction, testicular atrophy, urinary bladder and ovarian fibrosis reported. Force fluid intake to prevent hemorrhagic cystitis. May cause fetal harm in pregnancy. Serious, fatal infections may develop if severely immunosuppressed. Discontinue or reduce dose with infection. Monitor for toxicity with leukopenia, thrombocytopenia, tumor cell infiltration of bone marrow, previous X-ray therapy or cytotoxic therapy, and impaired hepatic and/or renal function. Monitor hematologic profile and examine urine for red blood cells. Possible cross-sensitivity with other alkylating agents. May cause sterility. May interfere with normal wound healing. Consider dose adjustment with adrenalectomy.

**ADVERSE REACTIONS:** Impairment of fertility, amenorrhea, nausea, vomiting, anorexia, abdominal discomfort, diarrhea, alopecia, leukopenia, thrombocytopenia, hemorrhagic ureteritis, interstitial pneumonitis, malaise, asthenia, renal tubular necrosis, skin rash, fever, SIADH, anaphylactic reactions.

**INTERACTIONS:** Increased metabolism and leukopenic activity with chronic, high doses of phenobarbital. Potentiates succinylcholine chloride effects and doxorubicin-induced cardiotoxicity. Alert anesthesiologist if treated within 10 days of general anesthesia.

**PREGNANCY:** Category D, not for use in nursing.

## NEOSPORIN + PAIN RELIEF MAXIMUM STRENGTH OTC

neomycin - bacitracin - polymyxin B - pramoxine HCl (McNeil)

**THERAPEUTIC CLASS:** Antibacterial/analgesic

**INDICATIONS:** To help prevent infection and provide temporary relief of pain or discomfort in minor cuts, scrapes, and burns.

**DOSAGE:** *Adults:* Clean area and apply a small amount qd-tid. May cover with sterile bandage.
*Pediatrics:* >2 yrs: Clean area and apply a small amount qd-tid. May cover with sterile bandage.

**HOW SUPPLIED:** Cre: (Neomycin-Polymyxin-Pramoxine) 3.5mg-10,000 U-10mg/g [15g]; Oint: (Bacitracin-Neomycin-Polymyxin-Pramoxine) 500 U-3.5mg-10,000 U-10mg/g [15g, 30g]

**WARNINGS/PRECAUTIONS:** Avoid eyes. Do not use over large areas. Discontinue if condition worsens, if develop rash or other allergic reaction, if symptoms persist >1 week, or if symptoms clear up and re-occur within a few days.

## NEOSPORIN OINTMENT — OTC

neomycin - bacitracin zinc - polymyxin B sulfate (McNeil)

**THERAPEUTIC CLASS:** Antibacterial combination

**INDICATIONS:** To help prevent infection in minor cuts, scrapes, and burns.

**DOSAGE:** *Adults:* Clean area and apply a small amount qd-tid. May cover with sterile bandage.
*Pediatrics:* Clean area and apply a small amount qd-tid. May cover with sterile bandage.

**HOW SUPPLIED:** Oint: (Neomycin-Polymyxin-Bacitracin) 3.5mg-5000 U-400 U/g [15g, 30g], [Neo To Go, 10 x 0.9g packets]

**WARNINGS/PRECAUTIONS:** Avoid eyes. Do not use over large areas. Discontinue if condition persists, worsens, or if a rash or other allergic reaction develops.

**PREGNANCY:** Safety in pregnancy and nursing not known.



## NEOSPORIN OPHTHALMIC — RX

bacitracin zinc - neomycin sulfate - polymyxin B sulfate (King)

**THERAPEUTIC CLASS:** Antibacterial combination

**INDICATIONS:** Superficial ocular infections including conjunctivitis, keratitis and keratoconjunctivitis, blepharitis and blepharoconjunctivitis.

**DOSAGE:** *Adults:* (Oint) Apply q3-4h for 7-10 days. (Sol) Instill 1-2 drops q4h for 7-10 days. Severe Infection: 2 drops q1h.

**HOW SUPPLIED:** Oint: (Bacitracin-Neomycin-Polymyxin B) 400U-3.5mg-10,000U/g [3.5g]; Sol: (Gramicidin-Neomycin-Polymixin B) 0.025mg-1.75mg-10,000U/mL [10mL]

**WARNINGS/PRECAUTIONS:** May cause cutaneous sensitization. Ointment may retard corneal wound healing.

**ADVERSE REACTIONS:** Itching, swelling, conjunctival erythema, local irritation, superinfection.

**PREGNANCY:** Category C, caution in nursing.

## NEO-SYNEPHRINE OPHTHALMIC — RX

phenylephrine HCl (Sanofi-Aventis)

**THERAPEUTIC CLASS:** Sympathomimetic

**INDICATIONS:** Use as a decongestant, vasoconstrictor, and pupil dilator in uveitis (posterior synechiae), wide angle glaucoma, before surgery, refraction, ophthalmoscopic exam, and diagnostic procedures.

**DOSAGE:** *Adults:* Vasoconstriction/Pupil Dilation: 1 drop 10% on upper limbus. May repeat after 1 hr. May precede by topical anesthetic. Uveitis: 1 drop 10% to upper surface of cornea. May repeat next day. Apply hot compresses tid for 5-

10 minutes, with 1 drop atropine sulfate before and after compresses. Glaucoma: 1 drop 10% on upper surface of cornea, repeat prn. Surgery: Apply 2.5% or 10% drops 30-60 minutes before surgery. Refraction: 1 drop of cycloplegic, then 1 drop 2.5% after 5 minutes, then repeat cycloplegic 10 minutes later. Eyes ready for refraction in 50-60 minutes."One Application Method": Combine 2.5% solution with cycloplegic for synergistic action. Consider increasing cycloplegic concentration. Ophthalmoscopic Exam: 1 drop 2.5% per eye. Diagnostic Procedures: Test for Angle Block with Glaucoma: Measure IOP before and after 2.5% solution. Shadow Test: Use 2.5% solution. Blanching Test: 1-2 drops 2.5% to injected eye.
*Pediatrics:* Refraction: 1 drop of atropine 1%, then 1 drop 2.5% after 10-15 minutes, then repeat 1 drop of atropine in 5-10 minutes. Eyes ready for refraction in 1-2 hrs.

**HOW SUPPLIED:** Sol: 2.5% [15mL], 10% [5mL]

**CONTRAINDICATIONS:** Narrow angle glaucoma, (10%) infants, (10%) aneurysm.

**WARNINGS/PRECAUTIONS:** (10%) Associated with cardiovascular reactions (eg, ventricular arrhythmias, MI) in elderly with pre-existing cardiovascular disease. May cause BP elevation; caution in low body weight children, elderly, insulin-dependent diabetes, HTN, hyperthyroidism, generalized arteriosclerosis, cardiovascular disease. (2.5%, 10%) Systemic vasopressor response may occur when exceed recommended doses or apply to instrumented, traumatized, diseased or postsurgical eye, adnexa, or in suppressed lacrimation.

**ADVERSE REACTIONS:** Rebound miosis (elderly), eye pain.

**INTERACTIONS:** TCAs, propranolol, reserpine, guanethidine, methyldopa, atropine-like drugs may potentiate pressor response. MAOIs during or up to 21 days after, may exaggerate adrenergic effects. Acute HTN and congenital cerebral aneurysm rupture reported with 10% solution and systemic β-blockers. May potentiate cardiovascular depressant effects of potent inhalation anesthetics.

**PREGNANCY:** Category C, caution in nursing.



## NEPHROCAPS RX

multiple vitamin (Fleming)

**THERAPEUTIC CLASS:** Vitamin supplement

**INDICATIONS:** Vitamin supplement for wasting syndrome in chronic renal failure, uremia, impaired metabolic functions of the kidney to maintain or replace depleted vitamins. Effective as a stress vitamin.

**DOSAGE:** *Adults:* 1 cap qd. Take after treatment if on dialysis.

**HOW SUPPLIED:** Cap: Biotin 0.15mg-Calcium Pantothenate 5mg-Folate 1mg-Niacin 20mg-Vitamin $B_1$ 1.5mg-Vitamin $B_2$ 1.7mg-Vitamin $B_6$ 10mg-Vitamin $B_{12}$ 0.006mg-Vitamin C 100mg

**WARNINGS/PRECAUTIONS:** Folic acid may mask symptoms of pernicious anemia.

**PREGNANCY:** Safety in pregnancy and nursing not known.

## NEPHRO-VITE RX RX

multiple vitamin (R&D)

**THERAPEUTIC CLASS:** Vitamin supplement

**INDICATIONS:** Vitamin supplement for dialysis patients and azotemic patients not on dialysis who eat poorly.

**DOSAGE:** *Adults:* 1 tab qd.

**HOW SUPPLIED:** Tab: Biotin 0.3mg-Calcium Pantothenic Acid 10mg-Folic Acid 1mg-Niacinamide 20mg-Vitamin $B_1$ 1.5mg-Vitamin $B_2$ 1.7mg-Vitamin $B_6$ 10mg-Vitamin $B_{12}$ 0.006mg-Vitamin C 60mg

**WARNINGS/PRECAUTIONS:** Folic acid may partially correct the hematological damage due to vitamin $B_{12}$ deficiency of pernicious anemia, while neurological damage progresses.

**PREGNANCY:** Safety in pregnancy and nursing not known.

## NESACAINE

chloroprocaine HCl (Abraxis) RX

**OTHER BRAND NAMES:** Nesacaine-MPF (Abraxis)

**THERAPEUTIC CLASS:** Local anesthetic

**INDICATIONS:** (Nesacaine) Production of local anesthesia by infiltration and peripheral nerve block. (Nesacaine-MPF) Production of local anesthesia by infiltration, peripheral and central nerve block, including lumbar and caudal epidural blocks.

**DOSAGE:** *Adults:* Dosage varies depending on procedure, vascularity of tissues, depth and duration of anesthesia, degree of muscle relaxation required, and patient physical condition. Max: 11mg/kg (800mg total dose) without epinephrine or 14mg/kg (1000mg total dose) with epinephrine. MPF: Caudal/Lumbar Epidural Block: Test dose: 3mL of 3% or 5mL of 2% prior to complete block. Caudal Epidural: 15-25mL of 2% or 3% solution. Repeat dose may be given at 40-60 minute intervals. Lumbar Epidural: 2-2.5mL/segment of 2% or 3% solution. Usual: 15-25mL. Repeat doses of 2-6mL less than original dose at 40-50 minute intervals. Elderly/Debilitated/Acutely Ill/Cardiac or Liver Disease: Reduce dose.
*Pediatrics:* >3 yrs: Max: 11mg/kg. Use 0.5-1% for infiltration and 1-1.5% for nerve block.



**HOW SUPPLIED:** Inj: 1%, 2%; (MPF) 2%, 3%

**CONTRAINDICATIONS:** Extreme caution with lumbar and caudal epidural anesthesia in existing neurological disease, spinal deformities, septicemia, severe HTN.

**WARNINGS/PRECAUTIONS:** Acidosis, cardiac arrest, death reported from delay in toxicity management. Nesacaine contains methylparaben and should not be used for lumbar or caudal epidural anesthesia. MPF formulation contains no preservative; discard any unused injection after initial use. Use lowest effective dose. Perform syringe aspiration to avoid intravascular injection. Caution with hepatic disease or impaired cardiovascular function. Monitor cardiovascular and respiratory vital signs and state of consciousness after each injection. Caution when local anesthetic injections containing a vasoconstrictor are used in areas of the body supplied by end arteries or having otherwise compromised blood supply; ischemic injury or necrosis may result with peripheral or hypertensive vascular disease due to exaggerated vasoconstrictor response. Do not rely on lack of corneal sensation after retrobulbar block to determine if patient is ready for surgery.

**ADVERSE REACTIONS:** Restlessness, anxiety, dizziness, tinnitus, blurred vision, tremors, convulsions, drowsiness, hypotension, bradycardia, ventricular arrhythmias, urticaria, pruritus, nausea, vomiting, loss of bladder/bowel control, loss of sexual function.

**INTERACTIONS:** Caution regarding toxic equivalence when using local anesthetic mixtures. Vasopressors, ergot-type oxytocic drugs may cause severe, persistent HTN or CVA. Anesthetic solutions containing epinephrine or norepinephrine with MAOIs, TCAs, or phenothiazines may produce severe, prolonged hypotension or HTN. Avoid sulfonamides.

**PREGNANCY:** Category C, caution in nursing.

## NESTABS CBF

RX

minerals - folic acid - multiple vitamin (Fielding)

**THERAPEUTIC CLASS:** Prenatal vitamin

**INDICATIONS:** Vitamin and mineral supplementation for before, during, and after pregnancy.

**DOSAGE:** *Adults:* 1 tab qd.

**HOW SUPPLIED:** Tab: Calcium 200mg-Folic Acid 1mg-Iodine 0.15mg-Iron 50mg-Niacin 20mg-Vitamin A 4000 IU-Vitamin $B_1$ 3mg-Vitamin $B_2$ 3mg-Vitamin $B_6$ 3mg-Vitamin $B_{12}$ 0.008mg-Vitamin C 120mg-Vitamin D 400 IU-Vitamin E 30 IU-Zinc 15mg* *scored

**WARNINGS/PRECAUTIONS:** Accidental overdose of iron-containing products is a leading cause of fatal poisoning in children <6 yrs. Not for the treatment of pernicious anemia and other megaloblastic anemias where vitamin $B_{12}$ is deficient. Folic acid >0.1mg/day may obscure pernicious anemia.

**ADVERSE REACTIONS:** Allergic sensitization.

## NESTABS FA

RX

minerals - folic acid - multiple vitamin (Fielding)

**THERAPEUTIC CLASS:** Prenatal vitamin

**INDICATIONS:** Vitamin and mineral supplementation for before, during, and after pregnancy.

**DOSAGE:** *Adults:* 1 tab qd.

**HOW SUPPLIED:** Tab: Calcium 200mg-Folic Acid 1mg-Iodine 0.15mg-Iron 29mg-Niacin 20mg-Vitamin A 4000 IU-Vitamin $B_1$ 3mg-Vitamin $B_2$ 3mg-Vitamin $B_6$ 3mg-Vitamin $B_{12}$ 0.008mg-Vitamin C 120mg-Vitamin D 400 IU-Vitamin E 30 IU-Zinc 15mg* *scored

**WARNINGS/PRECAUTIONS:** Accidental overdose of iron-containing products is a leading cause of fatal poisoning in children <6 yrs. Not for the treatment of pernicious anemia and other megaloblastic anemias where vitamin $B_{12}$ is deficient. Folic acid >0.1mg/day may obscure pernicious anemia.

**ADVERSE REACTIONS:** Allergic sensitization.



## NESTABS RX

RX

minerals - folic acid - multiple vitamin (Fielding)

**THERAPEUTIC CLASS:** Prenatal vitamin

**INDICATIONS:** Vitamin and mineral supplementation for before, during, and after pregnancy.

**DOSAGE:** *Adults:* 1 tab qd.

**HOW SUPPLIED:** Tab: Biotin 0.03mg-Calcium 200mg-Calcium Pantothenate 7mg-Copper 3mg-Folic Acid 1mg-Iodine 0.15mg-Iron 29mg-Magnesium 100mg-Niacinamide 20mg-Vitamin A 4000IU-Vitamin $B_1$ 3mg-Vitamin $B_2$ 3mg-Vitamin $B_6$ 3mg-Vitamin $B_{12}$ 0.008mg-Vitamin C 120mg-Vitamin D 400IU-Vitamin E 30IU-Zinc 15mg* *scored

**WARNINGS/PRECAUTIONS:** Accidental overdose of iron-containing products is a leading cause of fatal poisoning in children <6 yrs. Not for the treatment of pernicious anemia and other megaloblastic anemias where vitamin $B_{12}$ is deficient. Folic acid >0.1mg/day may obscure pernicious anemia.

**ADVERSE REACTIONS:** Allergic sensitization.

## NEULASTA RX
pegfilgrastim (Amgen)

**THERAPEUTIC CLASS:** Pegylated granulocyte colony stimulating factor

**INDICATIONS:** To decrease the incidence of infection, as manifested by febrile neutropenia, in patients with non-myeloid malignancies receiving myelosuppressive anti-cancer drugs.

**DOSAGE:** *Adults:* 6mg SQ, once per chemotherapy cycle. Do not administer in the period 14 days before and 24 hrs after chemotherapy.

**HOW SUPPLIED:** Inj: 6mg/0.6mL

**CONTRAINDICATIONS:** Hypersensitivity to *E coli*-derived proteins.

**WARNINGS/PRECAUTIONS:** Rare cases of splenic rupture reported, some fatal. Evaluate for enlarged spleen or splenic rupture if complaints of upper abdominal and/or shoulder tip pain. ARDS, allergic reactions (eg, anaphylaxis, rash) reported with filgrastim. Caution with sickle cell disease; monitor for sickle cell crises. Obtain CBC, platelets before chemotherapy. Monitor Hct, platelets regularly. Do not use in infants, children, and smaller adolescents <45kg.

**ADVERSE REACTIONS:** Medullary bone pain, nausea, fatigue, alopecia, diarrhea, vomiting, constipation, fever, anorexia, headache.

**INTERACTIONS:** Lithium may potentiate release of neutrophils; monitor neutrophil counts. Increased hematopoetic activity of the bone marrow in response to growth factor therapy has been associated with transient positive bone imaging changes. This should be considered when interpreting bone-imaging results.

**PREGNANCY:** Category C, caution in nursing.



## NEUMEGA RX
oprelvekin (Wyeth)

**THERAPEUTIC CLASS:** Thrombopoietic agent

**INDICATIONS:** Prevention of severe thrombocytopenia and reduction of the need for platelet transfusions following myelosuppressive chemotherapy in nonmyeloid malignancy patients at high risk.

**DOSAGE:** *Adults:* 50mcg/kg qd SQ. Initiate 6-24 hrs after chemotherapy completion. Monitor platelets to assess optimal duration of therapy. Continue therapy until post-nadir platelets >50,000 cells/mcL. D/C at least 2 days before next chemotherapy cycle. Max: 21 days of therapy.

**HOW SUPPLIED:** Inj: 5mg

**WARNINGS/PRECAUTIONS:** Fluid retention reported; caution in CHF, pleural or pericardial effusions, and patients receiving aggressive hydration. Monitor fluid and electrolyte balance with chronic diuretic therapy, renal dysfunction. Permanently d/c if significant allergic reactions occur. Moderate decreases in Hgb, Hct, and RBCs; transient, mild visual disturbances; papilledema; and rash reported. Caution with history of atrial arrhythmias. May develop antibodies to therapy. Obtain CBC before therapy, then regularly. Monitor platelets during expected nadir time and until adequate recovery.

**ADVERSE REACTIONS:** Edema, atrial fibrillation/flutter, oral moniliasis, tachycardia, palpitations, dyspnea, pleural effusion, conjunctival injection, asthenia, pain, chills, abdominal pain, infection, anorexia, constipation, alopecia, myalgia, dyspepsia, ecchymosis.

**PREGNANCY:** Category C, not for use in nursing.

## NEUPOGEN

RX

filgrastim (Amgen)

**THERAPEUTIC CLASS:** Granulocyte colony stimulating factor

**INDICATIONS:** To decrease incidence of infection, as manifested by febrile neutropenia, in nonmyeloid malignancies with myelosuppressive anti-cancer drugs (eg, bone marrow transplants). To reduce duration of neutropenia and fever in adults after induction or consolidation chemotherapy with acute myeloid leukemia. For peripheral blood progenitor cell collection (PBPC) and therapy. For severe chronic neutropenia.

**DOSAGE:** *Adults:* Myelosuppressive Chemotherapy: Initial: 5mcg/kg qd SQ bolus, short IV infusion, or continuous SQ/IV infusion. Monitor CBCs and platelets before therapy, twice weekly during therapy. Titrate: Increase 5mcg/kg for each chemotherapy cycle according to duration and severity of ANC nadir. Avoid 24 hours before through 24 hours after cytotoxic chemotherapy. Perform CBC twice weekly during therapy. Continue therapy after chemotherapy until the post nadir ANC =10,000/mm$^3$. BMT: Following BMT, 10mcg/kg/day by IV infusion of 4 or 24 hrs, or by continuous 24-hr SQ infusion. First dose at least 24 hrs after chemotherapy and at least 24 hrs after bone marrow infusion. Dose Adjustment: If ANC >1000/mm$^3$ for 3 days, 5mcg/kg/day; increase to 10mcg/kg/day if ANC <1000/mm$^3$. If ANC >1000/mm$^3$ for 3 more days, stop therapy. If ANC drops to <1000/mm$^3$, resume 5mcg/kg/day. PBPC: 10mcg/kg/day bolus or continuous SQ 4 days before and for 6-7 days with leukapheresis on days 5, 6 and 7. Monitor neutrophils after 4 days and adjust if WBC >100,000/mm$^3$. Chronic Neutropenia: Congenital Neutropenia: Initial: 6mcg/kg SQ bid. Idiopathic or Cyclic Neutropenia: Initial: 5mcg/kg SQ qd. Adjust dose based on clinical course and ANC.

**HOW SUPPLIED:** Inj: 300mcg/0.5mL, 300mcg/mL, 480mcg/0.8mL, 480mcg/1.6mL [10$^s$]

**CONTRAINDICATIONS:** Hypersensitivity to *E coli*-derived proteins.

**WARNINGS/PRECAUTIONS:** Allergic-type reactions may occur. Rare cases of splenic rupture reported, somet fatal. Evaluate for enlarged spleen or splenic rupture if complaints of left upper abdominal and/or shoulder tip pain. Adult respiratory distress syndrome reported with sepsis; d/c until resolved. Sickle cell crisis reported with sickle cell disease; keep patient well hydrated. Potential for immunogenicity. The patient may be at greater risk of thromobocytopenia, anemia, and nonhematologic consequences due to the potential of receiving higher doses of chemotherapy. Regular monitoring of Hct and platelet count recommended.

**ADVERSE REACTIONS:** Bone pain, nausea, vomiting, HTN, rash.

**INTERACTIONS:** Caution with drugs that may potentiate the release of neutrophils (eg, lithium). Transient positive bone imaging changes has been associated with increased hematopoetic activity of the bone marrow in response to growth factor therapy. This should be considered when interpreting bone-imaging results.

**PREGNANCY:** Category C, caution in nursing.

## NEUPRO

RX

rotigotine (Schwarz)

**THERAPEUTIC CLASS:** Non-ergolonic dopamine agonist

**INDICATIONS:** Treatment of signs and symptoms of early-stage idiopathic Parkinson's disease.

**DOSAGE:** *Adults*: Initial: 2mg/24hrs. Titrate: May increase weekly by 2mg/24hrs. Max: 6mg/24hrs. D/C Therapy: Reduce by 2mg/24hrs every other day. Apply to clean, dry, intact healthy skin; rotate application site.

**HOW SUPPLIED:** Patch: 2mg/24hrs, 4mg/24hrs, 6mg/24hrs [7$^s$, 30$^s$]

**WARNINGS/PRECAUTIONS:** Sulfite sensitivity may occur. Somnolence reported; d/c if significant daytime sleepiness or sleeping episodes develop during daily activities. Postural hypotension may occur, especially during dose escalation. Syncope, hallucinations, elevation of HR and BP, weight gain, and fluid retention reported. May cause or exacerbate dyskinesia. Application site reactions reported. May increase risk of melanoma, monitor skin periodically. Patch should be removed prior to MRI or cardioversion. Avoid heat application.

**ADVERSE REACTIONS:** Nausea, application site reactions, somnolence, dizziness, headache, vomiting, insomnia, fatigue, extremity edema, constipation, dyspepsia, back pain, increased sweating, arthralgia.

**INTERACTIONS:** Caution with dopamine antagonists (eg. antipsychotics, metoclopramide), may diminish effect. May inhibit CYP2C19 and CYP2D6 catalyzed metabolism of other drugs (low risk).

**PREGNANCY:** Category C, caution in nursing.

## NEURONTIN RX

gabapentin (Parke-Davis)

**THERAPEUTIC CLASS:** GABA analog

**INDICATIONS:** Adjunct therapy for partial seizures with or without secondary generalization in patients >12 yrs. Adjunct therapy for partial seizures in pediatrics 3-12 yrs. Management of postherpetic neuralgia (PHN).

**DOSAGE:** *Adults:* Epilepsy: Initial: 300mg tid. Titrate: Increase up to 1800mg/day. Max: 3600mg/day. PHN: 300mg single dose on Day 1, then 300mg bid on Day 2, and 300mg tid on Day 3. Increase further prn pain. Max: 600mg tid. Renal Impairment: CrCl 30-59mL/min: 400-1400 mg/day. CrCl 15-29mL/min: 200-700 mg/day. CrCl 15mL/min: 100-300mg/day. CrCl <15 mL/min: Reduce dose in proportion to CrCl. Hemodialysis: Maint: Base on CrCl. Give supplemental dose (125-350mg) after 4 hrs of hemodialysis. Refer to prescribing information for dose-adjustment.

*Pediatrics:* Epilepsy: >12 yrs: Initial: 300mg tid. Titrate: Increase up to 1800mg/day. Max: 3600mg/day. 3-12 yrs: Initial: 10-15mg/kg/day given tid. Titrate: Increase over 3 days. Usual: 3-4 yrs: 40mg/kg/day given tid. >5 yrs: 25-35mg/kg/day given tid. Max: 50mg/kg/day. Renal Impairment: >12 yrs: CrCl 30-59mL/min: 400-1400 mg/day. CrCl 15-29mL/min: 200-700 mg/day. CrCl 15mL/min: 100-300mg/day. CrCl <15 mL/min: Reduce dose in proportion to CrCl. Hemodialysis: Maint: Base on CrCl. Give supplemental dose (125-350 mg) after 4 hrs of hemodialysis. Refer to prescribing information for dose-adjustment.

**HOW SUPPLIED:** Cap: 100mg, 300mg, 400mg; Sol: 250mg/5mL; Tab: 600mg*, 800mg* *scored

**WARNINGS/PRECAUTIONS:** Avoid abrupt withdrawal. Possible tumorigenic potential. Sudden and unexplained deaths reported. Neuropsychiatric adverse events in pediatrics (3-12 yrs).

**ADVERSE REACTIONS:** Somnolence, dizziness, ataxia, nystagmus, fatigue, tremor, rhinitis, weight gain, nausea, vomiting, viral infection, fever, dysarthria, diplopia.

**INTERACTIONS:** Take 2 hrs after antacids. Increased levels with controlled-release morphine.

**PREGNANCY:** Category C, caution in nursing.

## NEVANAC RX

nepafenac (Alcon)

**THERAPEUTIC CLASS:** NSAID

**INDICATIONS:** Treatment of pain and inflammation associated with cataract surgery.

**DOSAGE:** *Adults:* 1 drop tid, start 24 hrs prior to surgery, continue to 2 weeks post-op.

**HOW SUPPLIED:** Sus: 0.1% [3mL]

**WARNINGS/PRECAUTIONS:** Possible cross-sensitivity to acetylsalicylic acid, phenylacetic acid derivatives, and other NSAIDs. May cause increased bleeding of ocular tissue; slowed or delayed healing; keratitis. With continued use, may cause epithelial breakdown, corneal thinning, erosion, ulceration, perforation. Caution with bleeding tendencies and in complicated ocular surgeries, corneal denervation, corneal epithelial defects, diabetes mellitus, ocular surface diseases, rheumatoid arthritis, or repeat ocular surgeries.

**ADVERSE REACTIONS:** Capsular opacity, decreased visual acuity, foreign body sensation, increased IOP, and sticky sensation.

**PREGNANCY:** Category C, caution in nursing.

## NEXAVAR RX

sorafenib (Bayer/Onyx)

**THERAPEUTIC CLASS:** Multikinase inhibitor

**INDICATIONS:** Treatment of advanced renal cell carcinoma.

**DOSAGE:** *Adults:* 400mg bid without food (1 hr before or 2 hrs after eating). Continue until no clinical benefit or unacceptable toxicity. Temporary interruption or dose reduction to 400mg qd or qod may be necessary if serious adverse events suspected.

**HOW SUPPLIED:** Tab: 200mg

**WARNINGS/PRECAUTIONS:** Shown to be teratogenic. May cause fetal harm when administered to a pregnant woman; use only if potential benefits justify potential risks to fetus. Discontinue if GI perforation occurs.

**ADVERSE REACTIONS:** HTN, fatigue, rash/desquamation, hand-foot skin reaction, alopecia, pruritus, diarrhea, nausea, anorexia, vomiting, constipation, hemorrhage, neuropathy-sensory, dyspnea, pain (bone, mouth).

**INTERACTIONS:** Caution with compounds metabolized/eliminated predominantly by the UGT1A1 pathway (eg, irinotecan). Caution with doxorubicin; increased AUC of doxorubicin. Sorafenib inhibits CYP2B6 and CYP2C8; caution with substrates of CYP2B6 and CYP2C8.

**PREGNANCY:** Category D, not for use in nursing.



## NEXIUM RX

esomeprazole magnesium (AstraZeneca LP)

**THERAPEUTIC CLASS:** Proton pump inhibitor

**INDICATIONS:** Symptomatic treatment of GERD; healing and maintenance treatment of erosive esophagitis. Reduction in the occurrence of gastric ulcers associated with continuous NSAID therapy in patients at risk for developing gastric ulcers. Adjunct therapy (with amoxicillin and clarithromycin) for *H. pylori* eradication to reduce the risk of duodenal ulcer recurrence. Long-term treatment of pathological hypersecretory conditions including Zollinger-Ellison Syndrome.

**DOSAGE:** *Adults:* Erosive Esophagitis: Healing: 20-40mg qd for 4-8 weeks; may extend treatment for 4-8 weeks if not healed. Maint: 20mg qd for up to 6 months. Risk Reduction of NSAID-Associated Gastric Ulcer: 20-40mg qd for up to 6 months. Symptomatic GERD: 20mg qd for 4 weeks; may extend treatment for 4 weeks if symptoms do not resolve. *H. pylori:* Triple Therapy: 40mg qd + amoxicillin 1000mg bid + clarithromycin 500mg bid, all for 10 days. Zollinger-Ellison Syndrome: 40mg bid. Severe Hepatic Dysfunction: Max: 20mg/day. Take 1 hr before meals. Swallow capsule whole. Contents may be mixed with soft food (eg, applesauce, yogurt) that does not require chewing. *Pediatrics:* 12-17 yrs: GERD: 20-40mg qd for up to 8 weeks. Severe Hepatic

Dysfunction: Max: 20mg/day. Take 1 hr before meals. Swallow capsule whole. Contents may be mixed with soft food (eg, applesauce, yogurt) that does not require chewing.

**HOW SUPPLIED:** Cap, Delayed Release: 20mg, 40mg; Sus, Delayed Release: 20mg, 40mg (granules/packet).

**CONTRAINDICATIONS:** Hypersensitivity to substituted benzimidazoles. Clarithromycin is contraindicated with pimozide.

**WARNINGS/PRECAUTIONS:** Atrophic gastritis may occur. Symptomatic response does not preclude gastric malignancy.

**ADVERSE REACTIONS:** Headache, diarrhea, abdominal pain, constipation, nausea, flatulence, dry mouth.

**INTERACTIONS:** Potentiates diazepam. May alter absorption of pH-dependent drugs (eg, ketoconazole, digoxin, and iron salts). May reduce levels of atazanavir when used concomitantly. Increased levels with amoxicillin and clarithromycin. Clarithromycin is contraindicated with pimozide.

**PREGNANCY:** Category B, not for use in nursing.

## NEXIUM IV — RX

esomeprazole sodium (AstraZeneca LP)

**THERAPEUTIC CLASS:** Proton pump inhibitor

**INDICATIONS:** Short-term treatment (up to 10 days) of GERD with history of erosive esophagitis when oral therapy not possible or appropriate.

**DOSAGE:** *Adults:* 20mg or 40mg qd IV injection (no less than 3 minutes) or infusion (10-30 minutes). Discontinue as soon as patient is able to resume oral therapy. Sever Hepatic Dysfunction: Max: 20mg/day.

**HOW SUPPLIED:** Inj: 20mg, 40mg



**CONTRAINDICATIONS:** Hypersensitivity to substituted benzimidazoles.

**WARNINGS/PRECAUTIONS:** Atrophic gastritis may occur. Symptomatic response does not preclude gastric malignancy. Discontinue and convert to oral therapy as soon as possible.

**ADVERSE REACTIONS:** Headache, flatulence, dyspepsia, nausea, abdominal pain, diarrhea, dry mouth,

**INTERACTIONS:** Potentiates diazepam. May alter absorption of gastric pH-dependent drugs (eg, ketoconazole, iron salts, digoxin).

**PREGNANCY:** Category B, not for use in nursing.

## NIASPAN — RX

niacin (Kos)

**THERAPEUTIC CLASS:** B-complex vitamin

**INDICATIONS:** Adjunct to diet, to reduce total cholesterol (total-C), LDL-C, TG, and Apo B levels, and to increase HDL-C in primary hypercholesterolemia (heterozygous familial and nonfamilial) and mixed dyslipidemia (Types IIa and IIb). With concomitant lovastatin, to further reduce LDL-C and TG, or increase HDL-C in primary hypercholesterolemia (heterozygous familial and nonfamilial) and mixed dyslipidemia (Types IIa and IIb). To reduce risk of recurrent nonfatal MI with history of MI and hypercholesterolemia. With concomitant bile acid binding resin, to slow progression/promote regression of atherosclerotic disease with history of CAD and hypercholesterolemia. Adjunct to diet with concomitant bile acid binding resin to reduce total-C and LDL-C in primary hypercholesterolemia (Type IIa) inadequately responding to diet or diet plus monotherapy. Adjunct for very high TG levels (Type IV and Type V hyperlipidemia) with risk of pancreatitis, inadequately responding to diet.

**DOSAGE:** *Adults:* Take qhs after low-fat snack. Initial: 500mg qhs. Titrate: Increase by 500mg every 4 weeks. Maint: 1-2g qhs. Max: 2g/day. Take ASA or NSAIDs 30 min before to reduce flushing. Do not chew, crush, or break; swallow whole. Women may respond to lower doses than men.

**HOW SUPPLIED:** Tab, Extended-Release: 500mg, 750mg, 1000mg

**CONTRAINDICATIONS:** Unexplained or significant hepatic dysfunction, active peptic ulcer disease, arterial bleeding.

**WARNINGS/PRECAUTIONS:** Do not substitute with equivalent doses of immediate-release niacin (severe hepatic toxicity may occur). Associated with abnormal LFTs; monitor LFTs before therapy, every 6-12 weeks during 1st year, then periodically thereafter. D/C if LFTs >3X ULN persists or develop signs of hepatotoxicity. Monitor for rhabdomyolysis. Observe closely with history of jaundice, hepatobiliary disease, and peptic ulcer; monitor LFTs and blood glucose frequently. Dose-related rise in glucose tolerance in diabetics. Caution with history of hepatic disease, heavy alcohol use, renal dysfunction, unstable angina, and acute phase of MI. Elevated uric acid levels reported. May reduce platelet and phosphorous levels.

**ADVERSE REACTIONS:** Flushing episodes (eg, warmth, redness, itching, tingling), dizziness, tachycardia, shortness of breath, sweating, chills, edema.

**INTERACTIONS:** Rhabdomyolysis may occur with HMG-CoA reductase inhibitors. May potentiate antihypertensives (eg, ganglionic blockers, vasoactive drugs). Separate dosing from bile acid resins by at least 4-6 hrs. Avoid concomitant alcohol or hot drinks; may increase flushing and pruritus. High dose niacin or nicotinamide may potentiate adverse effects. Caution with anticoagulants. Antidiabetic agents may need adjustment.

**PREGNANCY:** Category C, not for use in nursing.

## NICODERM CQ

OTC

nicotine (GlaxoSmithKline Consumer)



**THERAPEUTIC CLASS:** Nicotine

**INDICATIONS:** To reduce withdrawal symptoms associated with smoking cessation.

**DOSAGE:** *Adults:* Stop smoking completely. >10 cigarettes/day: 21mg qd for 6 weeks, then 14mg qd for 2 weeks, then 7mg qd for 2 weeks, then discontinue. <10 cigarettes/day: 14mg qd for 6 weeks, then 7mg qd for 2 weeks, then discontinue. Apply to clean, dry, hairless area; hold for 10 seconds; wash hands. Rotate application sites. Remove after 16 or 24 hours; if crave cigarettes when wake up, wear patch for 24 hrs. If vivid dreams occur, remove before sleep. Do not wear >1 patch at a time. Do not cut patch in half. Do not use same patch >24 hrs.

**HOW SUPPLIED:** Patch: 7mg/24hrs [14[s]], 14mg/24hrs [14[s]], 21mg/24hrs [7[s] 14[s]]

**WARNINGS/PRECAUTIONS:** Avoid with serious arrhythmias, severe or worsening angina, accelerated HTN, and immediately post-MI. Tachycardia, palpitations reported. Discontinue with irregular heartbeat, palpitations, symptoms of nicotine overdose (eg, nausea, vomiting, dizziness, weakness, rapid heartbeat), skin redness or swelling, or rash >4 days. Avoid creams or lotions at application site.

**ADVERSE REACTIONS:** Skin irritation, tobacco withdrawal symptoms, tachycardia.

**INTERACTIONS:** Antidepressants and antiasthmatic drugs may need adjustment. Avoid smoking, chewing tobacco, snuff, nicotine gum, or other nicotine products.

**PREGNANCY:** Safety in pregnancy and nursing not known.

## NICOMIDE — RX

folic acid - nicotinamide - zinc oxide (Sirus Laboratories)

**THERAPEUTIC CLASS:** Vitamin/Mineral combination

**INDICATIONS:** Treatment of acne vulgaris, acne rosacea, or other inflammatory skin disorders in nonpregnant patients.

**DOSAGE:** *Adults:* 1 tab qd-bid.

**HOW SUPPLIED:** Tab: (Nicotinamide-Folic Acid-Zinc) 750mg-500mcg-25mg

**WARNINGS/PRECAUTIONS:** Folic acid is improper treatment of pernicious anemia and other megaloblastic anemias with vitamin $B_{12}$-deficiency. Folic acid >0.1mg/day may obscure pernicious anemia. Caution with history of jaundice, liver disease, DM, or in elderly.

**ADVERSE REACTIONS:** Nausea, vomiting, transient LFT elevations, allergic sensitization.

**INTERACTIONS:** Reduced clearance of primidone and carbamazepine. Decreased absorption of quinolones and tetracyclines.

**PREGNANCY:** Avoid in pregnancy, caution in nursing.

## NICORETTE — OTC

nicotine polacrilex (GlaxoSmithKline Consumer)

**THERAPEUTIC CLASS:** Nicotine

**INDICATIONS:** To reduce withdrawal symptoms associated with smoking cessation.

**DOSAGE:** *Adults:* Stop smoking completely before use. <25 Cigarettes/Day: Use 2mg. >25 Cigarettes/Day: Use 4mg. Chew 1 piece for 30 minutes q1-2h for 6 weeks, then 1 piece q2-4h for 3 weeks, then 1 piece q4-8h for 3 weeks. Max 24 pieces/day and 12 weeks of therapy. Chew at least 9 pieces/day. Do not eat/drink for 15 minutes before or while chewing gum.

**HOW SUPPLIED:** Gum: 2mg, 4mg

**WARNINGS/PRECAUTIONS:** Do not use if continue to smoke, chew tobacco, use snuff, use a nicotine patch, or other nicotine products. Caution with heart disease, recent MI, irregular heartbeat, HTN, stomach ulcers. May increase BP and HR. D/C with mouth, teeth, or jaw problems, or with symptoms of nicotine overdose (nausea, vomiting, dizziness, weakness, palpitations). Use under medical supervision if <18 yrs of age.

**ADVERSE REACTIONS:** Headache, nausea, upset stomach, dizziness.

**INTERACTIONS:** Insulin, antidepressants, and asthma agents may need adjustment. Reduced effect with coffee, juices, wine, or soft drinks.

**PREGNANCY:** Safety in pregnancy and nursing is not known.

## NICOTROL INHALER — RX

nicotine (Pharmacia & Upjohn)

**THERAPEUTIC CLASS:** Nicotine

**INDICATIONS:** To reduce withdrawal symptoms associated with smoking cessation.

**DOSAGE:** *Adults:* Initial: At least 6 cartridges/day for 3-6 weeks. Usual: 6-16 cartridges/day. Max: 16 cartridges/day for 12 weeks. Best effect achieved by frequent continuous puffing (20 minutes). Continue for 3 months. Wean by gradual reduction of daily dose over the following 6-12 weeks. Do not treat >6 months.

**HOW SUPPLIED:** Inh: 4mg/inh

**CONTRAINDICATIONS:** Hypersensitivity or allergy to menthol.

**WARNINGS/PRECAUTIONS:** Can be toxic and addictive. Keep away from children and pets. Stop smoking completely before start therapy. May cause bronchospasm; caution with bronchospastic disease. Caution with coronary heart disease, arrhythmias, vasospastic diseases, renal/hepatic insufficiency, hyperthyroidism, pheochromocytoma, insulin-dependent diabetes, active peptic ulcers and in elderly. Tachycardia and palpitations reported; avoid in post-MI, severe arrhythmias, severe or worsening angina. Increased risk for malignant HTN with accelerated HTN.

**ADVERSE REACTIONS:** Mouth and throat local irritation, coughing, rhinitis, dizziness, anxiety, sleep disorder, depression, withdrawal syndrome, drug dependence, fatigue, dyspepsia, nausea, diarrhea.

**INTERACTIONS:** TCAs and theophylline may need dose adjustment.

**PREGNANCY:** Category D, not for use in nursing.

## NICOTROL NASAL SPRAY — RX

nicotine (Pharmacia & Upjohn)

**THERAPEUTIC CLASS:** Nicotine

**INDICATIONS:** To reduce withdrawal symptoms associated with smoking cessation.

**DOSAGE:** *Adults:* Initial: 2-4 sprays/hr, up to 10 sprays/hr, for up to 8 weeks. Minimum: 16 sprays/day. Max: 80 sprays/day. Elderly: Start at low end of the dosing range. May discontinue abruptly or over 4-6 weeks. Do not treat >3 months. Do not sniff, swallow, or inhale through nose as spray is being administered. Tilt head back slightly to administer.

**HOW SUPPLIED:** Nasal spray: 0.5mg/inh [10mL]

**WARNINGS/PRECAUTIONS:** Avoid with known chronic nasal disorders. Can be toxic and addictive. Keep away from children and pets. Stop smoking completely before start therapy. May cause bronchospasm; caution with bronchospastic disease. Caution with coronary heart disease, arrhythmias, vasospastic diseases, renal or hepatic insufficiency, hyperthyroidism, pheochromocytoma, insulin-dependent diabetes, active peptic ulcers, and elderly. Tachycardia and palpitations reported. Increased risk for malignant HTN with accelerated HTN.

**ADVERSE REACTIONS:** Local irritation, chest tightness, dyspepsia, numbness, constipation, stomatitis, anxiety, irritability, restlessness, cravings, dizziness, impaired concentration, weight increase, increased sweating, insomnia.

**INTERACTIONS:** May need dose reduction of APAP, caffeine, imipramine, oxazepam, pentazocine, theophylline, insulin, adrenergic antagonists, propranolol or other β-blockers after smoking cessation.

**PREGNANCY:** Category D, not for use in nursing.

## NICOTROL PATCH — OTC

nicotine (Pharmacia & Upjohn)

**THERAPEUTIC CLASS:** Nicotine

**INDICATIONS:** To reduce withdrawal symptoms associated with smoking cessation.

**DOSAGE:** *Adults:* >18 yrs: >10 cigarettes/day: Step 1 (weeks 1-6): 15mg patch qd. Step 2 (weeks 7 & 8): 10mg patch qd. Step 3 (weeks 9 & 10): 5mg patch qd. Apply onto clean, dry, hairless skin. Hold for 10 seconds. Wash hands. Wear patch for 16 hrs/day and remove qhs. Apply new patch at same time each day; rotate site.

**HOW SUPPLIED:** Patch: (Step 1) 15mg/16hrs [7[s], 14[s]], (Step 2) 10mg/16hrs [14[s]], (Step 3) 5mg/16hrs [14[s]]

**WARNINGS/PRECAUTIONS:** Do not use if continue to smoke, chew tobacco, use snuff, use a nicotine patch, or other nicotine products. Keep away from children and pets. Remove patch before bedtime to prevent sleep disruptions. Do not wear more than 1 patch at a time or cut patch in half/smaller pieces. Caution with heart disease, recent MI or irregular heartbeat; can increase HR and BP. Risk of skin rash with adhesive tape allergy or skin problems. D/C with irregular heartbeat, palpitations, symptoms of nicotine overdose (eg, nausea, vomiting, dizziness, weakness, rapid heartbeat), skin redness, swelling, or rash >4 days.

**ADVERSE REACTIONS:** Application site redness or rash, irregular heartbeat, palpitations, nausea, vomiting, dizziness, weakness.

**INTERACTIONS:** Antidepressants and antiasthmatic drugs may need dose adjustments.

**PREGNANCY:** Safety in pregnancy and nursing not known.

## NIFEDIPINE RX

nifedipine (Various)

**OTHER BRAND NAMES:** Procardia (Pfizer)

**THERAPEUTIC CLASS:** Calcium channel blocker (dihydropyridine)

**INDICATIONS:** Management of vasospastic angina and chronic stable angina.

**DOSAGE:** *Adults:* Initial: 10mg tid. Titrate over 7-14 days. Usual: 10-20mg tid. Max: 180mg/day. Elderly: Start at low end of dosing range.

**HOW SUPPLIED:** Cap: 10mg, 20mg

**WARNINGS/PRECAUTIONS:** May cause hypotension; monitor BP initially or with titration. May exacerbate angina from β-blocker withdrawal. CHF risk, especially with aortic stenosis or β-blockers. Peripheral edema reported. Not for acute reduction of BP or essential HTN. May increase angina or MI with severe obstructive CAD. Avoid with acute coronary syndrome or within 1-2 weeks of MI. Caution in elderly.

**ADVERSE REACTIONS:** Dizziness, lightheadedness, giddiness, flushing, muscle cramps, headache, weakness, nausea, peripheral edema, nervousness/mood changes.

**INTERACTIONS:** β-Blockers may increase risk of CHF, severe hypotension, or angina exacerbation. Possible hypotension with fentanyl. Potentiates digoxin. Monitor quinidine, coumarin. Potentiated by cimetidine and grapefruit juice. Avoid grapefruit juice.

**PREGNANCY:** Category C, unknown use in nursing.

## NIFEREX OTC

iron (Ther-Rx)

**THERAPEUTIC CLASS:** Iron supplement

**INDICATIONS:** Treatment of uncomplicated iron deficiency anemias.

**DOSAGE:** *Adults:* 1-2 tabs bid or 5-10mL qd.
*Pediatrics:* >6 yrs: 1-2 tabs qd or 5mL qd. <6 yrs: (Sol): Individualize dose.

**HOW SUPPLIED:** Cap: 60mg; Sol: 100mg/5mL

**WARNINGS/PRECAUTIONS:** Fatal poisoning reported in children <6 yrs with accidental overdose of iron-containing products.

**PREGNANCY:** Safety in pregnancy and nursing not known.

## NIFEREX-150

OTC

iron - vitamin C (Ther-Rx)

**OTHER BRAND NAMES:** Fe-Tinic 150 (Ethex)

**THERAPEUTIC CLASS:** Iron supplement

**INDICATIONS:** Treatment of uncomplicated iron deficiency anemias.

**DOSAGE:** *Adults:* 1-2 caps qd.

**HOW SUPPLIED:** Cap: (Iron-Vitamin C) 150mg-50mg

**WARNINGS/PRECAUTIONS:** Fatal poisoning reported in children <6 yrs with accidental overdose of iron-containing products.

**PREGNANCY:** Safety in pregnancy and nursing not known.

## NIFEREX-150 FORTE

RX

iron - vitamin C - folic acid - vitamin B12 (Ther-Rx)

**OTHER BRAND NAMES:** Fe-Tinic 150 Forte (Ethex)

**THERAPEUTIC CLASS:** Iron/vitamin

**INDICATIONS:** Prevention and treatment of iron deficiency anemia and/or nutritional megaloblastic anemias.

**DOSAGE:** *Adults:* 1 cap qd.

**HOW SUPPLIED:** Cap: (Folic Acid-Iron-Vitamin $B_{12}$-Vitamin C) 1mg-150mg-25mcg-60mg

**CONTRAINDICATIONS:** Hemochromatosis, hemosiderosis.

**WARNINGS/PRECAUTIONS:** Fatal poisoning reported in children <6 yrs with accidental overdose of iron-containing products. Determination of type, cause of anemia is recommended before starting therapy. Folic acid >0.1mg/day may obscure pernicious anemia.

**ADVERSE REACTIONS:** Constipation, diarrhea, nausea, vomiting, dark stools, abdominal pain.

**PREGNANCY:** Safety in pregnancy and nursing not known.

## NIFEREX-PN

RX

iron - folic acid - multiple vitamin (Ther-Rx)

**THERAPEUTIC CLASS:** Iron/vitamin/mineral

**INDICATIONS:** Prevention and treatment of dietary vitamin And mineral deficiencies associated with pregnancy and lactation.

**DOSAGE:** *Adults:* 1 tab qd.

**HOW SUPPLIED:** Tab: Calcium 125mg-Folic Acid 1mg-Iron 60mg-Niacinamide 10mg-Vitamin A 4000IU-Vitamin $B_1$ 2.43mg-Vitamin $B_2$ 3mg-Vitamin $B_6$ 1.64mg-Vitamin $B_{12}$ 0.003mg-Vitamin C 50mg-Vitamin D 400IU-Zinc 18mg

**CONTRAINDICATIONS:** Hemochromatosis, hemosiderosis.

**WARNINGS/PRECAUTIONS:** Fatal poisoning reported in children <6 yrs with accidental overdose of iron-containing products. Folic acid >0.1mg/day may obscure pernicious anemia. High doses of vitamin A may be associated with birth defects.

**ADVERSE REACTIONS:** Constipation, diarrhea, nausea, vomiting, dark stools, abdominal pain.

**PREGNANCY:** Safety in pregnancy and nursing not known.

## NIFEREX-PN FORTE RX
iron - minerals - folic acid - multiple vitamin (Ther-Rx)

**THERAPEUTIC CLASS:** Iron/vitamin/mineral

**INDICATIONS:** Prevention and treatment of dietary vitamin And mineral deficiencies associated with pregnancy and lactation.

**DOSAGE:** *Adults:* 1 tab qd.

**HOW SUPPLIED:** Tab: Calcium 250mg-Copper 2mg-Folic Acid 1mg-Iodine 0.2mg-Iron 60mg-Magnesium 10mg-Niacinamide 20mg-Vitamin A 5000IU-Vitamin $B_1$ 3mg-Vitamin $B_2$ 3.4mg-Vitamin $B_6$ 4mg-Vitamin $B_{12}$ 0.012mg-Vitamin C 80mg-Vitamin D 400IU-Vitamin E 30IU-Zinc 25mg

**CONTRAINDICATIONS:** Hemochromatosis, hemosiderosis.

**WARNINGS/PRECAUTIONS:** Fatal poisoning reported in children <6 yrs with accidental overdose of iron-containing products. Folic acid >0.1mg/day may obscure pernicious anemia. High doses of vitamin A may be associated with birth defects.

**ADVERSE REACTIONS:** Constipation, diarrhea, nausea, vomiting, dark stools, abdominal pain.

**PREGNANCY:** Safety in pregnancy and nursing not known.

## NILANDRON RX
nilutamide (Sanofi-Aventis)

> **Interstitial pneumonitis reported. Perform routine chest X-ray and baseline pulmonary function test before therapy. D/C if symptoms occur.**

**THERAPEUTIC CLASS:** Nonsteroidal antiandrogen

N

**INDICATIONS:** Treatment of metastatic prostatic cancer (Stage $D_2$) in combination with surgical castration.

**DOSAGE:** *Adults:* Initial: 300mg/day for 30 days. Maint: 150mg qd. Begin on the same day or the day after surgical castration.

**HOW SUPPLIED:** Tab: 150mg

**CONTRAINDICATIONS:** Severe hepatic impairment, respiratory insufficiency.

**WARNINGS/PRECAUTIONS:** Hepatotoxicity, aplastic anemia reported. D/C if develop jaundice or ALT >2x ULN. Delay in adaptation to dark; caution with driving at night or in tunnels; wear tinted glasses to alleviate effect. Evaluate baseline hepatic enzymes before therapy, at regular intervals for 1st 4 months, and periodically thereafter.

**ADVERSE REACTIONS:** Hot flushes, decreased libido, abnormal vision, increased LFTs, interstitial pneumonitis, dyspnea, GI effects, dry skin, sweating.

**INTERACTIONS:** May potentiate vitamin K antagonists, phenytoin, and theophylline. Intolerance to alcohol (eg, hypotension, malaise).

**PREGNANCY:** Category C. Safety in nursing is not known.

## NIMBEX RX
cisatracurium besylate (Abbott)

**THERAPEUTIC CLASS:** Skeletal muscle relaxant (nondepolarizing)

**INDICATIONS:** Adjunct to general anesthesia, to facilitate tracheal intubation, and to provide skeletal muscle relaxation during surgery/mechanical ventilation.

**DOSAGE:** *Adults:* Initial: 0.15mg/kg (3 x $ED_{95}$) or 0.20mg/kg (4 x $ED_{95}$) IV. Serious Cardiovascular Disease: Up to 8 x $ED_{95}$. Maint/Prolonged Surgical Procedures: 0.03mg/kg IV (for 20 minute blockade) 40-50 minutes after initial 0.15mg/kg, and 50-60 minutes after initial 0.20mg/kg. Operating Room

Infusion: After initial bolus dose, give 3mcg/kg/min to counteract recovery from bolus, then 1-2mcg/kg/min. ICU: 3mcg/kg/min IV; dose requirements may increase/decrease with time.
*Pediatrics:* >12 yrs: Initial: 0.15mg/kg (3 x $ED_{95}$) or 0.20mg/kg (4 x $ED_{95}$) IV. Serious Cardiovascular Disease: Up to 8 x $ED_{95}$. Maint/Prolonged Surgical Procedures: 0.03mg/kg IV (for 20 minute blockade) 40-50 minutes after initial 0.15mg/kg, and 50-60 minutes after initial 0.20mg/kg. 2-12 yrs: Initial: 0.10mg/kg over 5-10 seconds during halothane or opioid anesthesia. >2 yrs: Operating Room Infusion: After initial bolus dose, give 3mcg/kg/min to counteract recovery from bolus, then 1-2mcg/kg/min.

**HOW SUPPLIED:** Inj: 2mg/mL, 10mg/mL

**CONTRAINDICATIONS:** Hypersensitivity to bis-benzylisoquinolinium agents and benzyl alcohol.

**WARNINGS/PRECAUTIONS:** Avoid administration before unconsciousness has been induced. Use in facility with resuscitation and life support, and have antagonist available. Monitor neuromuscular function with peripheral nerve stimulator during administration. Multi-dose vials contain benzyl alcohol. Not for rapid sequence endotracheal intubation. May have profound effect with neuromuscular diseases (eg, myasthenia gravis, carcinomatosis); monitor neuromuscular function with peripheral nerve stimulator. Resistance may develop in burn victims; consider increasing dose. Resistance with hemiparesis or paraparesis. Acid-base and/or serum electrolyte abnormalities may potentiate or antagonize effect. Monitor for malignant hyperthermia.

**ADVERSE REACTIONS:** Bradycardia, hypotension, flushing, bronchospasm, rash, muscle weakness, myopathy, prolonged/inadequate neuromuscular blockade.

**INTERACTIONS:** Prolonged duration of action and required infusion rate decreased with isoflurane or enflurane with nitrous oxide/oxygen. Enhanced neuromuscular blocking action with certain antibiotics (eg, aminoglycosides, tetracyclines, bacitracin, polymyxins, lincomycin, clindamycin, colistin, sodium colistimethate), magnesium salts, lithium, local anesthetics, procainamide, and quinidine. Antagonized effect with phenytoin and carbamazepine. May not be compatible with pH >8.5 alkaline solutions (eg, barbiturate solutions).

**PREGNANCY:** Category B, caution in nursing.



## NIMOTOP
nimodipine (Bayer) RX

**Do not administer IV or by other parenteral routes. Deaths and serious, life-threatening adverse events have occurred when contents of capsules have been injected parenterally.**

**THERAPEUTIC CLASS:** Calcium channel blocker

**INDICATIONS:** Improvement of neurological outcome in patients with subarachnoid hemorrhage (SAH) from ruptured intracranial berry aneurysms regardless of their post-ictus neurological condition.

**DOSAGE:** *Adults:* 60mg q 4 hrs for 21 days, 1 hr before or 2 hrs after meals. Hepatic Cirrhosis: 30mg q 4 hrs for 21 days. Start therapy within 96 hrs of SAH. If cannot swallow cap, extract contents into syringe and empty into NG tube, then flush with 30mL of 0.9% NaCl.

**HOW SUPPLIED:** Cap: 30mg

**WARNINGS/PRECAUTIONS:** Carefully monitor BP. Monitor BP and HR closely with hepatic dysfunction. Do not administer IV or by other parenteral routes.

**ADVERSE REACTIONS:** Decreased BP, headache, rash, diarrhea, bradycardia, nausea, abnormal LFTs.

**INTERACTIONS:** May enhance cardiovascular effects of other calcium channel blockers. Increased serum levels with cimetidine. May intensify effects of antihypertensives.

**PREGNANCY:** Category C, not for use in nursing.

## NIRAVAM

CIV

alprazolam (Schwarz)

**THERAPEUTIC CLASS:** Benzodiazepine

**INDICATIONS:** Management of anxiety disorders and short-term relief of anxiety symptoms. Treatment of panic disorder with or without agoraphobia.

**DOSAGE:** *Adults:* Anxiety: Initial: 0.25-0.5mg tid. Titrate: May increase every 3-4 days. Max: 4mg/day. Panic Disorder: Initial: 0.5mg tid. Titrate: Increase by no more than 1mg/day every 3-4 days; slower titration if ≥4mg/day. Usual: 1-10mg/day. Decrease dose slowly (no more than 0.5mg every 3 days). Elderly/Advanced Liver Disease/Debilitated: Initial: 0.25mg bid-tid. Titrate: Increase gradually as tolerated.

**HOW SUPPLIED:** Tab, Orally Disintegrating: 0.25mg*, 0.5mg*, 1mg*, 2mg* *scored

**CONTRAINDICATIONS:** Acute narrow angle glaucoma, untreated open angle glaucoma, concomitant ketoconazole or itraconazole.

**WARNINGS/PRECAUTIONS:** Risk of dependence. Withdrawal symptoms, including seizure, reported with dose reduction or abrupt discontinuation; avoid abrupt withdrawal. Risk of CNS depression and impaired performance. May cause fetal harm. Caution with impaired renal, hepatic, or pulmonary function, severe depression, obesity, elderly and debilitated. Hypomania/mania reported with depression. Weak uricosuric effect.

**ADVERSE REACTIONS:** Drowsiness, fatigue/tiredness, impaired coordination, irritability, memory impairment, cognitive disorder, dysarthria, decreased libido, confusional state, light-headedness, dry mouth, hypotension, increased salivation.

**INTERACTIONS:** Avoid with potent CYP3A inhibitors (eg, azole antifungals). Potentiated by nefazodone, fluvoxamine, cimetidine, fluoxetine, oral contraceptives. Decreased plasma levels with propoxyphene and carbamazepine. Caution with diltiazem, isoniazid, macrolides, grapefruit juice, sertraline, paroxetine, ergotamine, cyclosporine, amiodarone, nicardipine, nifedipine and other CYP3A inhibitors. Increases levels of imipramine and desipramine. Additive CNS depressant effects with psychotropic agents, anticonvulsants, antihistamines, ethanol.

**PREGNANCY:** Category D, not for use in nursing.



## NITRO-BID

RX

nitroglycerin (Fougera)

**THERAPEUTIC CLASS:** Nitrate vasodilator

**INDICATIONS:** Prevention of angina pectoris. Not for acute attacks.

**DOSAGE:** *Adults:* Initial: Apply 0.5 inch bid (once in the am and 6 hrs later). Titrate: May increase to 1 inch bid, then to 2 inches bid. Should have 10-12 hr nitrate-free period.

**HOW SUPPLIED:** Oint: 2% (15mg/inch)

**WARNINGS/PRECAUTIONS:** Monitor with acute MI or CHF. Severe hypotension may occur; caution with volume depletion and hypotension. May aggravate angina caused by hypertrophic cardiomyopathy. Tolerance to other nitrates may decrese effects.

**ADVERSE REACTIONS:** Headache, lightheadedness, hypotension, flushing, syncope.

**INTERACTIONS:** Additive vasodilating effects with other vasodilators (eg, alcohol). Severe hypotension with sildenafil. Marked orthostatic hypotension reported with calcium channel blockers.

**PREGNANCY:** Category C, caution in nursing.

## NITRO-DUR

RX

nitroglycerin (Schering)

**OTHER BRAND NAMES:** Minitran (Graceway) - Nitrek (Mylan Bertek)

**THERAPEUTIC CLASS:** Nitrate vasodilator

**INDICATIONS:** Prevention of angina pectoris. Not for acute attack.

**DOSAGE:** *Adults:* Initial: 0.2-0.4mg/hr for 12-14 hrs. Remove for 10-12 hrs.

**HOW SUPPLIED:** Patch: (Minitran) 0.1mg/hr, 0.2mg/hr, 0.4mg/hr, 0.6mg/hr [30s]; (Nitrek) 0.2mg/hr, 0.4mg/hr, 0.6mg/hr [30s]; (Nitro-Dur) 0.1mg/hr, 0.2mg/hr, 0.3mg/hr, 0.4mg/hr, 0.6mg/hr, 0.8mg/hr [30s]

**CONTRAINDICATIONS:** Allergy to adhesives in NTG patches.

**WARNINGS/PRECAUTIONS:** Severe hypotension may occur; caution with volume depletion or hypotension. Vasodilatory effects with phosphodiesterase inhibitors (eg, sildenafil) can result in severe hypotension. May aggravate angina caused by hypertrophic cardiomyopathy. Tolerance to other nitrate forms may decrease effects. Monitor with acute MI or CHF. Do not discharge defibrillator/cardioverter through the patch.

**ADVERSE REACTIONS:** Headache, lightheadedness, hypotension, syncope.

**INTERACTIONS:** Additive vasodilating effects with other vasodilators (eg, alcohol). Marked orthostatic hypotension reported with calcium channel blockers. Severe hypotension with sildenafil.

**PREGNANCY:** Category C, caution in nursing.

## NITROLINGUAL SPRAY

RX

nitroglycerin (Sciele)

N

**OTHER BRAND NAMES:** NitroMist (NovaDel Pharma)

**THERAPEUTIC CLASS:** Nitrate vasodilator

**INDICATIONS:** For acute relief of angina attack. Prophylaxis of angina pectoris.

**DOSAGE:** *Adults:* Acute: 1-2 sprays at onset of attack onto or under tongue. Max: 3 sprays/15 minutes. Prophylaxis: 1-2 sprays onto or under tongue 5-10 minutes before activity that may cause acute attack. Do not expectorate medication or rinse mouth for 5-10 minutes after administration.

**HOW SUPPLIED:** Spray: 400mcg/spray

**CONTRAINDICATIONS:** Concomitant use with Phosphodiesterase type 5 (PDE5) inhibitors such as sildenafil, vardenafil, and tadalafil.

**WARNINGS/PRECAUTIONS:** Severe hypotension may occur; caution with volume depletion or hypotension. May aggravate angina caused by hypertrophic cardiomyopathy. Tolerance and cross-tolerance to other nitrates/nitrites may occur. Monitor during early days of AMI.

**ADVERSE REACTIONS:** Headache, hypotension, flushing, dizziness, weakness, rash, exfoliative dermatitis.

**INTERACTIONS:** Avoid PDE5 inhibitors (eg. sildenafil, vardenafil, tadalafil); severe hypotension may occur. Concomitant use w/ calcium channel blockers may cause orthostatic hypotension. Alcohol may cause hypotenion. (NitroMist) Increased hypotensive effects with beta-adrenergic blockers (eg. labetolol). Aspirin may increase levels. May decrease anticoagulant effect of heparin. Avoid ergotamine. Caution w/ tissue-type plasminogen activator.

**PREGNANCY:** Category C, caution in nursing.

## NITROSTAT

RX

nitroglycerin (Parke-Davis)

**OTHER BRAND NAMES:** Nitroquick (Ethex)

**THERAPEUTIC CLASS:** Nitrate vasodilator

**INDICATIONS:** For acute relief of angina attack. Prophylaxis of angina pectoris.

**DOSAGE:** *Adults:* Treatment: 1 tab SL or in buccal pouch at onset of attack. May repeat in 5 minutes. Max: 3 tabs in 15 minutes. Prophylaxis: Take 5-10 minutes before activity that may cause acute attack.

**HOW SUPPLIED:** Tab, Sublingual: 0.3mg, 0.4mg, 0.6mg

**CONTRAINDICATIONS:** Early MI, severe anemia, increased ICP, concomitant sildenafil.

**WARNINGS/PRECAUTIONS:** Do not swallow tabs. Severe hypotension may occur; caution with volume depletion or hypotension. May aggravate angina caused by hypertrophic cardiomyopathy. D/C if develop blurred vision or dry mouth. May interfere with cholesterol test. Monitor with acute MI or CHF. Tolerance to other nitrate forms may decrease effects. Caution in elderly.

**ADVERSE REACTIONS:** Headache, vertigo, dizziness, weakness, palpitation, syncope, flushing, postural hypotension, drug rash, exfoliative dermatitis.

**INTERACTIONS:** Additive hypotension with alcohol, β-blockers, phenothiazines, calcium channel blockers, other antihypertensives. Avoid ergotamine (related drugs), sildenafil. Vasodilatory and hemodynamic effects potentiated by ASA. Caution with alteplase. TCAs, anticholinergics may make sublingual dissolution difficult. Long-acting nitrates may decrease effects.

**PREGNANCY:** Category C, caution in nursing.



## NIX

OTC

permethrin (Insight Pharmaceuticals)

**THERAPEUTIC CLASS:** Pyrethroid pediculicide

**INDICATIONS:** (Liquid) Treatment of head lice and prophylactic use during epidemics (at least 20% of population are infested). (Spray) To kill lice on bedding and furniture. Not for use in humans.

**DOSAGE:** *Adults:* (Liquid) Treatment: Wash then towel dry hair. Apply liquid and saturate hair and scalp. Rinse with water after 10 minutes. Remove nits with comb provided. Repeat after 7 days if live lice is observed. Prophylaxis: Same as treatment. Repeat therapy after 2 weeks in epidemic setting. (Spray) Use from an 8-10 inch distance. Treat only garments, bedding, and furniture that cannot be washed or dry cleaned. Allow area to dry completely. *Pediatrics:* >2 months: (Liquid) Treatment: Wash and dry hair, then saturate hair and scalp. Rinse with water after 10 minutes. Remove nits with comb provided. Repeat after 7 days if observe lice. Prophylaxis: Same as treatment. Do not use nit comb.

**HOW SUPPLIED:** Liq: (Creme Rinse) 1% [60mL]; Spray: 0.25% [148mL]

**WARNINGS/PRECAUTIONS:** (Liquid) Protect from getting into eyes, inside nose, mouth, or vagina. May cause breathing difficulty or asthmatic episodes in susceptible persons. Discontinue if skin irritation persists or infection develops. (Spray) Do not use in food serving areas or while food is exposed. Do not apply in classrooms while in use.

**ADVERSE REACTIONS:** Itching, redness, swelling of the scalp.

**PREGNANCY:** Safety in pregnancy and nursing not known.

## NIZORAL
ketoconazole (Janssen)

RX

**Risk of fatal hepatotoxicity. Concomitant terfenadine, astemizole and cisapride are contraindicated due to serious cardiovascular adverse events.**

**THERAPEUTIC CLASS:** Azole antifungal

**INDICATIONS:** Treatment of systemic fungal infections including candidiasis, chronic mucocutaneous candidiasis, oral thrush, candiduria, blastomycosis, coccidioidomycosis, histoplasmosis, chromomycosis, and paracoccidioidomycosis. Treatment of severe recalcitrant cutaneous dermatophyte infections not responsive to topical therapy or oral griseofulvin. Not for treatment of fungal meningitis.

**DOSAGE:** *Adults:* Initial: 200mg qd. Max: 400mg qd.
*Pediatrics:* >2 yrs: 3.3-6.6mg/kg/day.

**HOW SUPPLIED:** Tab: 200mg* *scored

**CONTRAINDICATIONS:** Concomitant terfenadine, astemizole, cisapride or triazolam.

**WARNINGS/PRECAUTIONS:** Hepatotoxicity reported. Monitor LFTs prior to therapy and periodically thereafter. Serum testosterone levels may be lowered. Hypersensitivity reactions reported. Tablets require acidity for dissolution. Not for use in children unless benefit outweighs risk.

**ADVERSE REACTIONS:** Nausea, vomiting, abdominal pain, pruritus.

**INTERACTIONS:** Give antacids, anticholinergics, and $H_2$ blockers 2 hrs after ketoconazole. Contraindicated with terfenadine, astemizole, and cisapride due to cardiac adverse effects. May potentiate midazolam, triazolam, oral hypoglycemics. May enhance anticoagulant effect of coumarin-like drugs. Avoid rifampin, isoniazid. Monitor digoxin, phenytoin. May alter metabolism of cyclosporine, tacrolimus, methylprednisolone and drugs metabolized by CYP3A4.

**PREGNANCY:** Category C, not for use in nursing.



## NIZORAL A-D
ketoconazole (McNeil Consumer)

OTC

**THERAPEUTIC CLASS:** Azole antifungal

**INDICATIONS:** Controls flaking, scaling and itching associated with dandruff.

**DOSAGE:** *Adults:* Wet hair. Apply and lather. Rinse thoroughly and repeat. Apply every 3-4 days up to 8 weeks if needed.
*Pediatrics:* >12 yrs: Wet hair. Apply and lather. Rinse thoroughly and repeat. Apply every 3-4 days up to 8 weeks if needed.

**HOW SUPPLIED:** Shampoo: 1% [4 oz, 7 oz]

**CONTRAINDICATIONS:** Scalp that is broken or inflamed.

**WARNINGS/PRECAUTIONS:** Avoid eyes. D/C if rash appears, or if condition worsens or does not improve in 2-4 weeks.

**PREGNANCY:** Use in pregnancy and nursing not known.

## NIZORAL SHAMPOO
ketoconazole (McNeil Consumer)

RX

**THERAPEUTIC CLASS:** Azole antifungal

**INDICATIONS:** Tinea versicolor.

**DOSAGE:** *Adults:* Apply to damp skin and lather. Rinse with water after 5 minutes. One application should be sufficient.

**HOW SUPPLIED:** Shampoo: 2% [120mL]

**WARNINGS/PRECAUTIONS:** Shampoo may remove curl from permanently waved hair. Avoid eyes.

**ADVERSE REACTIONS:** Abnormal hair texture, scalp pustules, mild skin dryness, pruritus, increase in normal hair loss, oily or dry scalp and hair.

**PREGNANCY:** Category C, caution in nursing.

## NORCO

CIII

acetaminophen - hydrocodone bitartrate (Watson)

**THERAPEUTIC CLASS:** Opioid analgesic

**INDICATIONS:** Relief of moderate to moderately severe pain.

**DOSAGE:** *Adults:* Usual: (5/325) 1-2 tabs q4-6h prn pain. Usual: (7.5/325, 10/325)1 tab q4-6h prn pain. Max: 6 tabs/day.

**HOW SUPPLIED:** Tab: (Hydrocodone-APAP) 5mg-325mg*, 7.5mg-325mg*, 10mg-325mg* *scored

**WARNINGS/PRECAUTIONS:** May produce dose-related respiratory depression. May obscure diagnosis of acute abdominal conditions or head injuries. Caution in elderly, debilitated, severe hepatic or renal dysfunction, hypothyroidism, Addison's disease, prostatic hypertrophy, urethral stricture, pulmonary disease and postoperative use. May be habit-forming. Suppresses cough reflex.

**ADVERSE REACTIONS:** Lightheadedness, dizziness, sedation, nausea, vomiting.

**INTERACTIONS:** Additive CNS depression with narcotics, antipsychotics, antihistamines, antianxiety agents, alcohol, or other CNS depressants. Increased effect of antidepressant or hydrocodone with MAOIs or TCAs.

**PREGNANCY:** Category C, not for use in nursing.



## NORDETTE-28

RX

levonorgestrel - ethinyl estradiol (Duramed)

**OTHER BRAND NAMES:** Portia (Barr) - Levora (Watson)

**THERAPEUTIC CLASS:** Estrogen/progestogen combination

**INDICATIONS:** Prevention of pregnancy.

**DOSAGE:** *Adults:* Start 1st Sunday after menses begins. 1 tab qd for 28 days, then repeat.

**HOW SUPPLIED:** Tab: (Ethinyl Estradiol-Levonorgestrel) 0.03mg-0.15mg

**CONTRAINDICATIONS:** Thrombophlebitis, DVT or thromboembolic disorders, pregnancy, cerebrovascular or coronary artery disease, undiagnosed abnormal genital bleeding, cholestatic jaundice of pregnancy or jaundice with prior pill use, hepatic adenomas or carcinomas, breast cancer or other estrogen-dependent neoplasia.

**WARNINGS/PRECAUTIONS:** Cigarette smoking increases risk of serious cardiovascular side effects. This risk increases with age (especially >35 yrs) and heavy smoking. Increased risk of MI, vascular disease, thromboembolism, stroke and gallbladder disease. Retinal thrombosis, hepatic neoplasia, carcinoma of breast and reproductive organs reported. May cause glucose intolerance. May increase BP, elevate LDL levels or cause other lipid changes, fluid retention, breakthrough bleeding, and spotting. May cause or exacerbate migraine. May develop visual changes with contact lens. Increased risk of MI with HTN, hyperlipidemia, obesity, and diabetes. Discontinue if develop jaundice, significant depression or ophthalmic irregularities. Perform annual physical exam. Use before menarche is not indicated. May affect certain endocrine, LFTs and blood components.

**ADVERSE REACTIONS:** Nausea, vomiting, breakthrough bleeding, spotting, amenorrhea, migraine, depression, vaginal candidiasis, edema, weight changes.

**INTERACTIONS:** Reduced effects, increased breakthrough bleeding, and menstrual irregularities with rifampin, barbiturates, phenylbutazone, phenytoin, griseofulvin, topiramate, some protease inhibitors, modafinil, and possibly St. John's wort, penicillins, and tetracyclines. Increased plasma levels with ascorbic acid, APAP, indinavir, fluconazole, troleandomycin, and atorvastatin. May affect cyclosporine, theophylline, and corticosteroid levels.

**PREGNANCY:** Category X, not for use in nursing.

## NORDITROPIN

somatropin (Novo Nordisk)

RX

**OTHER BRAND NAMES:** Norditropin Nordiflex (Novo Nordisk)

**THERAPEUTIC CLASS:** Human growth hormone

**INDICATIONS:** (Adults) Replacement of endogenous growth hormone deficiency who meet either of the following criteria: (1) adult onset-patients with growth hormone deficiency, either alone or associated with multiple hormone deficiencies (hypopituitarism), as a result of pituitary disease, hypothalamic disease, surgery, radiation therapy, or trauma: or (2) childhood onset-patients who were growth hormone deficient during childhood should have growth hormone deficiency confirmed as an adult before replacement therapy is started. (Pediatrics) Long-term treatment of children with growth failure due to inadequate growth hormone secretion. Treatment of children with short stature associated with Noonan syndrome.

**DOSAGE:** *Adults*: Initial: No more than 0.004mg/kg/day. Increase to no more than 0.016mg/kg/day after 6 weeks.
*Pediatrics*: Growth Hormone Deficiency: 0.024-0.034mg/kg SQ 6-7x/week. Noonan Syndrome: Dose up to 0.066mg/kg/day.

**HOW SUPPLIED:** Inj: (Norditropin (cartridge) and Norditropin Nordiflex (prefilled pen)) 5mg/1.5mL, 10mg/1.5ml,15mg/1.5mL

**CONTRAINDICATIONS:** Presence of active neoplasia; acute critical illness due to complications following open heart or abdominal surgery, multiple accidental trauma or acute respiratory failure; proliferative or preproliferative diabetic retinopathy; closed epiphyses; and Prader-Willi syndrome with severe obesity or severe respiratory impairment.

**WARNINGS/PRECAUTIONS:** Monitor for recurrence or progression of underlying disease in growth hormone deficiency secondary to intracranial lesions. Hypothyroidism reported. May develop slipped capital epiphyses. Intracranial HTN with papilledema, visual changes, headache, nausea, and vomiting reported. Progression of scholiosis may occur in rapid growth. Monitor for any form of malignant skin lesion prior to and during therapy. May decrease insulin sensitivity; monitor blood sugar.

**ADVERSE REACTIONS:** *Pediatric*: Headache, injection site reaction, localized muscle pain, rash, weakness, mild hyperglycemia, glucosuria, arthralgia, leukemia. *Adults*: Edema, arthralgia, myalgia, infection, parasthesia, skeletal pain, headache, bronchitis.

**INTERACTIONS:** Diminished effects with glucocorticoid therapy. Insulin resistance reported. May reduce plasma levels of oral estrogens.

**PREGNANCY:** Category C, caution in nursing.

N

## NORGESIC RX

aspirin - caffeine - orphenadrine citrate (Graceway)

**OTHER BRAND NAMES:** Norgesic Forte (Graceway)

**THERAPEUTIC CLASS:** Muscular analgesic combination

**INDICATIONS:** Symptomatic relief of mild to moderate pain of acute musculoskeletal disorders.

**DOSAGE:** *Adults:* 1-2 tabs tid-qid. (Forte) 1/2-1 tab tid-qid.

**HOW SUPPLIED:** Tab: (Orphenadrine-ASA-Caffeine) 25mg-385mg-30mg; Tab: (Forte) 50mg-770mg-60mg* *scored

**CONTRAINDICATIONS:** Glaucoma, pyloric or duodenal obstruction, achalasia, prostatic hypertrophy, bladder neck obstruction, myasthenia gravis.

**WARNINGS/PRECAUTIONS:** Reye's syndrome may develop with chickenpox, influenza, or flu symptoms. Extreme caution with peptic ulcers and coagulation abnormalities. Monitor blood, urine, and LFT's periodically with prolonged use.

**ADVERSE REACTIONS:** Tachycardia, urinary hesitancy/retention, dry mouth, blurred vision, increased intraocular tension, nausea, vomiting, headache, dizziness, constipation, drowsiness, urticaria, GI hemorrhage.

**INTERACTIONS:** Confusion, tremor, anxiety reported with propoxyphene.

**PREGNANCY:** Safety in pregnancy and nursing not known.

## NORITATE RX

metronidazole (Dermik)

**THERAPEUTIC CLASS:** Imidazole antibiotic

N

**INDICATIONS:** Inflammatory lesions and erythema of rosacea.

**DOSAGE:** *Adults:* Apply thin film to clean area qd.

**HOW SUPPLIED:** Cre: 1% [30g, 60g]

**WARNINGS/PRECAUTIONS:** Conjunctivitis reported with use on face. Avoid eye contact. Caution with blood dyscrasias.

**ADVERSE REACTIONS:** Local irritation, condition aggravated.

**INTERACTIONS:** May potentiate anticoagulant effects of warfarin.

**PREGNANCY:** Category B, not for use in nursing.

## NOROXIN RX

norfloxacin (Merck)

**THERAPEUTIC CLASS:** Fluoroquinolone

**INDICATIONS:** Treatment of complicated and uncomplicated urinary tract infection (UTI), uncomplicated urethral and cervical gonorrhea, and prostatitis due to *E.coli*.

**DOSAGE:** *Adults:* >18 yrs: Uncomplicated UTI Due To *E.coli, K.pneumonia, P.mirabilis*: 400mg q12h for 3 days. Uncomplicated UTI Due To Other Organisms: 400mg q12h for 7-10 days. Complicated UTI: 400mg q12h for 10-21 days. CrCl <30mL/min: 400mg qd. Uncomplicated Gonorrhea: 800mg single dose. Acute/Chronic Prostatitis: 400mg q12h for 28 days. Take 1 hr before or 2 hrs after meals or milk/dairy products.

**HOW SUPPLIED:** Tab: 400mg

**CONTRAINDICATIONS:** History of tendinitis or tendon rupture associated with the use of quinolones.

**WARNINGS/PRECAUTIONS:** Pseudomembranous colitis, convulsions, phototoxicity and ruptures of the shoulder, hand, and Achilles tendons reported. Avoid in pregnancy and nursing mothers. Convulsions reported.

Caution with renal dysfunction. D/C if CNS stimulation, increase in intracranial pressure, or toxic psychoses occurs. Not effective for treatment of syphilis. May exacerbate myasthenia gravis. Hemolytic reactions reported with G6P deficiency. *Clostridium difficile*-associated diarrhea reported.

**ADVERSE REACTIONS:** Dizziness, nausea, headache, abdominal pain, asthenia.

**INTERACTIONS:** May increase theophylline and cyclosporine levels. May enhance effects of warfarin. Diminished urinary excretion with probenecid. Antagonized effects with nitrofurantoin. Iron- or zinc-containing products, antacids, or didanosine (chewable/buffered tabs, pediatric oral solution) may interfere with absorption; space dose by 2 hrs. May reduce clearance of caffeine. Coadminstration with a non-steroidal anti-inflammatory drug (NSAID) may increase the risk of CNS stimulation and convulsive seizures.

**PREGNANCY:** Category C, not for use in nursing.

## NORPACE

RX

disopyramide phosphate (Pharmacia & Upjohn)

**OTHER BRAND NAMES:** Norpace CR (Pharmacia & Upjohn)

**THERAPEUTIC CLASS:** Class I antiarrhythmic

**INDICATIONS:** Treatment of documented life-threatening ventricular arrhythmias.

**DOSAGE:** *Adults:* Usual: 400-800mg/day in divided dose. Recommended: 150mg q6h immediate-release (IR) or 300mg q12h extended-release (CR). Adjust dose with anticholinergic effects. Weight <110lbs/Moderate Hepatic or Renal Insufficiency (CrCl >40mL/min): 100mg q6h IR or 200mg q12h CR. Severe Renal Insufficiency (with or without initial 150mg LD): CrCl 30-40mL/min: 100mg q8h IR. CrCl 30-15mL/min: 100mg q12h IR. CrCl <15mL/min: 100mg q24h IR. Rapid Control of Ventricular Arrhythmia: LD: 300mg IR (200mg if <110lbs). Follow with maint dose. Cardiomyopathy/Cardiac Decompensation: Initial: 100mg q6-8h IR. Adjust gradually. See labeling if no response or toxicity occurs. Elderly: Start at low end of dosing range. *Pediatrics:* <1 yr: 10-30mg/kg/day. 1-4 yrs: 10-20mg/kg/day. 4-12 yrs: 10-15mg/kg/day. 12-18 yrs: 6-15mg/kg/day. Give in equally divided doses q6h. Hospitalize patient during initial therapy. Start dose titration at lower end of range.

N

**HOW SUPPLIED:** Cap: (Norpace) 100mg, 150mg; Cap, Extended Release: (Norpace CR) 100mg, 150mg

**CONTRAINDICATIONS:** Cardiogenic shock, 2nd- or 3rd-degree AV block (if no pacemaker present), congenital QT prolongation.

**WARNINGS/PRECAUTIONS:** Proarrhythmic; reserve for life-threatening ventricular arrhythmias. May cause or worsen CHF and produce hypotension due to negative inotropic properties. Reduce dose if 1st-degree heart block occurs. Avoid with urinary retention, glaucoma, and myasthenia gravis unless adequate overriding measures taken. Atrial flutter/fibrillation; digitalize first. Monitor closely or withdraw if QT prolongation >25% occurs and ectopy continues. Discontinue if QRS widening >25% occurs. Avoid LD with cardiomyopathy or cardiac decompensation. Correct $K^+$ abnormalities before therapy. Reduce dose with renal/hepatic dysfunction; monitor ECG. Avoid CR formulation with CrCl <40mL/min. Caution with sick sinus syndrome, Wolff-Parkinson-White syndrome, bundle branch block, in elderly. May significantly lower blood glucose.

**ADVERSE REACTIONS:** Dry mouth, urinary retention/frequency/urgency, constipation, blurred vision, GI effects, dizziness, fatigue, headache.

**INTERACTIONS:** Avoid type IA and IC antiarrhythmics, and propranolol except in unresponsive, life-threatening arrhythmias. Hepatic enzyme inducers may lower levels. Avoid within 48 hrs before or 24 hrs after verapamil. Possible fatal interactions with CYP3A4 inhibitors. Monitor blood glucose with β-blockers, alcohol.

**PREGNANCY:** Category C, not for use in nursing.

## NORPLANT
RX

levonorgestrel (Wyeth)

**THERAPEUTIC CLASS:** Progestogen

**INDICATIONS:** Long-term (up to 5 yrs) prevention of pregnancy.

**DOSAGE:** *Adults:* Implant 216mg (6 implants) in the midportion of the upper arm during 1st 7 days of onset of menses. Replace by end of 5th year.

**HOW SUPPLIED:** Implant: 36mg

**CONTRAINDICATIONS:** Active thrombophlebitis or thromboembolic disorders, undiagnosed abnormal genital bleeding, pregnancy, acute live disease or liver tumors, carcinoma of the breast, and idiopathic intracranial HTN.

**WARNINGS/PRECAUTIONS:** Complications related to insertion and removal of capsules reported. Bleeding irregularities have occurred. Retinal thrombosis leading to partial or complete loss of vision, hepatic neoplasia, carcinoma of breast and reproductive organs reported. Risk of thromboembolic and thrombotic diseases, MI, ectopic pregnancy, ovarian cysts, breast cancer, gall bladder and autoimmune diseases, cerebrovascular diseases. Cigarette smoking increases risk of serious cardiovascular side effects. This risk increases with age (especially >35 yrs) and the extent of smoking. Idiopathic intracranial HTN and increases in BP reported. Caution with fluid retention, contact lenses. May worsen depression, increase LDL levels. If jaundice develops, remove implants. Altered glucose tolerance; monitor diabetics. Rare reports of congenital anomalies with use during early pregnancy.

**ADVERSE REACTIONS:** Amenorrhea, irregular bleeding, pain/itching or infection at implant site, headache, nervousness, GI effects, dizziness, adnexal enlargement, rash, acne, change in appetite, mastalgia, weight gain, hirsutism, cervicitis, musculoskeletal pain.

**INTERACTIONS:** Decreased efficacy with phenytoin and carbamazepine.



**PREGNANCY:** Category X, safety in nursing is not known.

## NORPRAMIN
RX

desipramine HCl (Sanofi-Aventis)

**Antidepressants increased the risk of suicidal thinking and behavior (suicidality) in short-term studies in children and adolescents with Major Depressive Disorder (MDD) and other psychiatric disorders. Desipramine is not approved for use in pediatric patients.**

**THERAPEUTIC CLASS:** Tricyclic antidepressant

**INDICATIONS:** Treatment of depression.

**DOSAGE:** *Adults:* Usual: 100-200mg/day given qd or in divided doses. Max: 300mg/day. Elderly/Adolescents: Usual: 25-100mg/day given qd or in divided doses. Max: 150mg/day.

**HOW SUPPLIED:** Tab: 10mg, 25mg, 50mg, 75mg, 100mg, 150mg

**CONTRAINDICATIONS:** MAOI use within 14 days, acute recovery period following MI.

**WARNINGS/PRECAUTIONS:** Hypomania with manic-depressive disease. D/C prior to elective surgery. Do not withdraw abruptly. Extreme caution with urinary retention, glaucoma, seizure disorders, cardiovascular disease, thyroid disease, alcohol abuse. May exacerbate psychosis; caution with schizophrenia. May impair mental or physical abilities. May alter blood glucose levels.

**ADVERSE REACTIONS:** Arrhythmias, hypotension, HTN, tachycardia, confusion, hallucination, dizziness, anxiety, numbness, tingling, ataxia, tremors, dry mouth, urinary retention, urticaria, photosensitivity, SIADH, altered libido.

**INTERACTIONS:** See Contraindications. Additive sedative effects with benzodiazepines (eg, diazepam, chlordiazepoxide), other CNS depressants (eg, sedatives/hypnotics, psychotropics). Blocks antihypertensive effects of guanethidine. Exaggerates response to alcohol. Monitor with other anticholinergic or sympathomimetic drugs. Potentiated by CYP2D6 inhibitors (eg, quinidine, cimetidine, SSRIs) or substrates of CYP2D6 (eg, other antidepressants, phenothiazines, propafenone, flecainide). Caution with thyroid medications.

**PREGNANCY:** Safety in pregnancy and nursing not known.

## NOR-QD

norethindrone (Watson) RX

**OTHER BRAND NAMES:** Camila (Barr)

**THERAPEUTIC CLASS:** Progestogen

**INDICATIONS:** Prevention of pregnancy.

**DOSAGE:** *Adults:* 1 tab qd without interruption (continuous regimen) on 1st day of menstrual period. If fully nursing, start 6 weeks postpartum. If partially nursing, start 3 weeks postpartum.

**HOW SUPPLIED:** Tab: 0.35mg

**CONTRAINDICATIONS:** Pregnancy, breast carcinoma, undiagnosed abnormal genital bleeding, benign or malignant liver tumors, acute liver disease.

**WARNINGS/PRECAUTIONS:** Avoid smoking. Perform annual physical exam. Not for use before menarche. May affect certain endocrine tests (eg, sex hormone binding globulin, thyroxine binding globulin). Monitor glucose tolerance in prediabetics and diabetics. May alter lipid metabolism. May increase risk of breast cancer and hepatic adenomas. May cause irregular menstrual patterns. Delayed follicular atresia/ovarian cysts and ectopic pregnancy may occur. Discontinue with recurrent migraines or severe headaches.

**ADVERSE REACTIONS:** Menstrual irregularities, frequent or irregular bleeding, headache, breast tenderness, nausea, dizziness.

**INTERACTIONS:** Reduced effects with hepatic enzyme inducers (eg, rifampin, phenytoin, carbamazepine, barbiturates).

**PREGNANCY:** Category X, caution in nursing.



## NORVASC

amlodipine besylate (Pfizer) RX

**THERAPEUTIC CLASS:** Calcium channel blocker (dihydropyridine)

**INDICATIONS:** Treatment of hypertension and Coronary Artery Disease (CAD) including chronic stable or vasospastic angina (Prinzmetal's or Variant Angina).

**DOSAGE:** *Adults:* HTN: Initial: 5mg qd. Titrate over 7-14 days. Max: 10mg qd. Small, Fragile, or Elderly/Hepatic Dysfunction/Concomitant Antihypertensive: Initial: 2.5mg qd. Angina: 10mg qd. Elderly/Hepatic Dysfunction: 5mg qd. CAD: 5-10mg qd.
*Pediatrics:* 6-17 yrs: HTN: 2.5-5mg qd.

**HOW SUPPLIED:** Tab: 2.5mg, 5mg, 10mg

**WARNINGS/PRECAUTIONS:** May increase angina or MI with severe obstructive CAD. Caution with severe aortic stenosis, CHF, severe hepatic impairment, and in elderly.

**ADVERSE REACTIONS:** Edema, flushing, palpitation, dizziness, headache, fatigue.

**PREGNANCY:** Category C, not for use in nursing.

# NORVIR

RX

ritonavir (Abbott)

**Use with certain non-sedating antihistamines, sedative hypnotics, antiarrhythmics, or ergot alkaloids may result in life-threatening adverse events.**

**THERAPEUTIC CLASS:** Protease inhibitor

**INDICATIONS:** Treatment of HIV infection in combination with other antiretrovirals.

**DOSAGE:** *Adults:* Initial: 300mg bid. Titrate: Increase every 2-3 days by 100mg bid. Maint: 600mg bid. If combined with saquinavir, adjust dose to 400mg bid. Elderly: Start at low end of dosing range. Take with meals if possible. *Pediatrics:* >1 month: Initial: 250mg/$m^2$ po bid. Titrate: Increase by 50mg/$m^2$ every 2-3 days. Maint: 350-400mg/$m^2$ po bid or highest tolerated dose. Max: 600mg bid.

**HOW SUPPLIED:** Cap: 100mg; Sol: 80mg/mL [240mL]

**CONTRAINDICATIONS:** Alfuzosin, amiodarone, bepridil, flecainide, propafenone, quinidine, voriconazole, astemizole, terfenadine, ergot derivatives, midazolam, triazolam, cisapride, pimozide.

**WARNINGS/PRECAUTIONS:** Allergic reactions (eg, urticaria, mild skin eruptions, bronchospasm, and angioedema), pancreatitis, new onset/exacerbation of pre-existing diabetes mellitus, hyperglycemia, immune reconstitution syndrome, hepatic transaminase elevations and hepatic dysfunction reported. Caution with moderate to severe hepatic impairment and in elderly. Monitor LFTs, especially first 3 months. Increased bleeding may occur with hemophilia A and B. Possible redistribution or accumulation of body fat. May increase total triglyceride and cholesterol levels.

**ADVERSE REACTIONS:** Diarrhea, anorexia, vomiting, nausea, abdominal pain, taste perversion, circumoral, peripheral paresthesia.



**INTERACTIONS:** See Contraindications. Avoid use with rifampin, St. John's wort; may cause loss of virologic response and resistance. Avoid use with lovastatin and simvastatin; risk of myopathy and rhabdomyolysis. Neurologic and cardiac events reported with disopyramide, mexiletine, nefazodone, fluoxetine, and β-blockers. May increase levels of saquinavir, desipramine, indinavir, rifabutin. May increase levels of clarithromycin with renal impairment; reduce clarithromycin dose by 50% if CrCl 30-60mL/min and by 75% if CrCl<30mL/min. May increase ketoconazole levels; avoid ketoconazole doses >200mg/day. May increase sildenafil levels; do not exceed sildenafil 25mg/48hrs. May increase levels of tramadol, propoxyphene, disopyramide, lidocaine, mexilitene, carbamazepine, clonazepam, ethosuximide, bupropion, nefazodone, SSRIs, TCAs, dronabinol, itraconazole, quinine, metoprolol, timolol, diltiazem, nifedipine, verapamil, atorvastatin, cyclosporine, tacrolimus, sirolimus, perphenazine, risperidone, thioridazine, clorazepate, diazepam, estazolam, flurazepam, zolpidem, dexamethasone, fluticasone, prednisone, methamphetamine. May increase levels of trazodone; use with caution and consider lower trazodone dose. Decreases levels of theophylline, meperidine, methadone. May decrease levels of phenytoin, divalproex, lamotrigine, and atovaquone. Separate dosing with didanosine by 2.5 hrs. May increase plasma levels of drugs metabolized by CYP3A or CYP2D6. May decrease ethinyl estradiol levels; use alternative contraceptive measures. Monitor PT/INR with warfarin. Contains alcohol; may produce disulfiram-like reactions with disulfiram, metronidazole.

**PREGNANCY:** Category B, not for use in nursing.

## NOVACORT RX

pramoxine HCl - hydrocortisone acetate (Primus)

**THERAPEUTIC CLASS:** Corticosteroid/anesthetic

**INDICATIONS:** Relief of the inflammatory and pruritic manifestations of corticosteroid-responsive dermatoses.

**DOSAGE:** *Adults:* Apply to affected area(s) tid-qid. May use occlusive dressings for psoriasis or recalcitrant conditions. Discontinue dressings if infection develops.
*Pediatrics:* Apply to affected area(s) tid-qid. May use occlusive dressings for psoriasis or recalcitrant conditions. Discontinue dressings if infection develops.

**HOW SUPPLIED:** Gel: (Hydrocortisone-Pramoxine) 2%-1% [29g]

**WARNINGS/PRECAUTIONS:** May produce reversible HPA axis suppression, manifestations of Cushing's syndrome, hyperglycemia, and glucosuria. Caution when applied to large surface areas, under occlusive dressings, or with prolonged use. Use appropriate antifungal or antibacterial agent with dermatological infections; discontinue if infection does not clear. Pediatrics may be more susceptible to systemic toxicity. Discontinue if irritation develops. Avoid eyes.

**ADVERSE REACTIONS:** Burning, itching, irritation, dryness, folliculitis, hypertrichosis, acneiform eruptions, hypopigmentation, perioral dermatitis, allergic dermatitis, skin maceration, secondary infection, skin atrophy, striae, miliaria.

**PREGNANCY:** Category C, caution in nursing.

## NOVANTRONE RX

mitoxantrone (Serono)

**Severe local tissue damage with extravasation. Administer only as slow IV infusion; not for IM, SQ, intra-arterial, or intrathecal use. Should not be given to patients with baseline neutrophil count <1,500cells/mm$^3$. Cardiotoxicity can occur at any time and risk increases with cumulative dose; toxicity can occur during therapy or months to years after discontinuation. CHF may occur during or after termination of therapy. Secondary AML reported in MS and cancer patients treated with Novatrone.**

**THERAPEUTIC CLASS:** Topoisomerase II inhibitor (anthracenedione)

**INDICATIONS:** With corticosteroids, for initial treatment of advanced hormone-refractory prostate cancer with pain. Initial therapy of acute nonlymphocytic leukemia (ANLL) in combination with other agents. To reduce neurologic disability and/or frequency of clinical relapses in secondary (chronic) progressive, progressive relapsing, or worsening relapsing-remitting multiple sclerosis (MS).

**DOSAGE:** *Adults:* Prostate Cancer: 12-14mg/m$^2$/day IV every 21 days. ANLL: Induction: 12mg/m$^2$/day IV on days 1-3 and 100mg/m$^2$/day IV of cytarabine on days 1-7. Consolidation: 12mg/m$^2$/day on days 1-2 and cytarabine 100mg/m$^2$/day on days 1-5. MS: 12mg/m$^2$/day IV every 3 months.

**HOW SUPPLIED:** Inj: 2mg/mL

**WARNINGS/PRECAUTIONS:** Can cause myelosuppression at any dose. Severe myelosuppression with high doses (leukemia); assure full hematologic recovery before consolidation therapy. Avoid with pre-existing myelosuppression. Increased risk of cardiac toxicity with prior anthracyclines or mediastinal radiotherapy, or with pre-existing cardiovascular disease. Irreversible CHF has been reported. Avoid in MS when baseline left ventricular ejection fraction <50%. Caution in hepatic impairment. Risk of hyperuricemia in leukemia; monitor serum uric acid levels. Obtain CBC, platelet count, and LFTs before each course. May cause blue-green urine and bluish sclera 24 hrs after administration. Perform pregnancy test in women with MS before each dose. Caution in elderly.

**ADVERSE REACTIONS:** Nausea, alopecia, menstrual disorder, upper respiratory infection, UTI, stomatitis, arrhythmia, diarrhea, constipation, back pain, abnormal ECG, asthenia, headache, cardiac toxicity.

**INTERACTIONS:** Development of acute leukemia associated with other concomitant antineoplastics. Possible danger of cardiac toxicity if previously treated with anthracyclines.

**PREGNANCY:** Category D, not for use in nursing.

## NOVAREL RX

chorionic gonadotropin (Ferring)

**THERAPEUTIC CLASS:** Human chorionic gonadotropin

**INDICATIONS:** For prepubertal cryptorchidism not due to anatomic obstruction. For hypogonadotropic hypogonadism (secondary to a pituitary deficiency) in males. To induce ovulation (OI) and pregnancy in anovulatory, infertile women in whom anovulation is not due to primary ovarian failure and pretreated with human menotropins.

**DOSAGE:** *Adults:* Hypogonadism: 500-1000 U IM 3x/week (TIW) for 3 weeks, then twice weekly for 3 weeks; or 4000 U IM TIW for 6-9 months, then reduce to 2000 U TIW for 3 months. OI: 5000-10,000 U IM 1 day after last dose of menotropins.
*Pediatrics:* >4 yrs: Cryptorchidism: 4000 U IM TIW for 3 weeks; or 5000 U IM every 2nd day for 4 doses; or 15 doses of 500-1000 U over 6 weeks; or 500 U TIW for 4-6 weeks (if treatment fails, give 1000 U/injection starting 1 month later). Initiate therapy between 4-9 yrs. Hypogonadism: 500-1000 U IM TIW for 3 weeks, then twice weekly for 3 weeks; or 4000 U IM TIW for 6-9 months, then reduce to 2000 U TIW for 3 months.

**HOW SUPPLIED:** Inj: 10,000 U



**CONTRAINDICATIONS:** Precocious puberty, prostatic carcinoma or other androgen-dependent neoplasms, pregnancy.

**WARNINGS/PRECAUTIONS:** Potential ovarian hyperstimulation, enlargement or rupture of ovarian cysts, multiple births, and arterial thromboembolism with infertility treatment. D/C if precocious puberty occurs in cryptorchidism patients. Caution with cardiac or renal disease, epilepsy, migraine, asthma. Not effective treatment for obesity.

**ADVERSE REACTIONS:** Headache, irritability, restlessness, depression, fatigue, edema, precocious puberty, gynecomastia, injection site pain.

**PREGNANCY:** Category C, caution in nursing.

## NOVOLIN OTC

insulin, human regular - insulin, human isophane - insulin human, rdna origin (Novo Nordisk)

**OTHER BRAND NAMES:** Novolin N (Novo Nordisk) - Novolin R (Novo Nordisk)

**THERAPEUTIC CLASS:** Insulin

**INDICATIONS:** To control hyperglycemia in diabetes.

**DOSAGE:** *Adults:* Individualize dose.
*Pediatrics:* Individualize dose.

**HOW SUPPLIED:** Inj: 100U/mL (Novolin N, Novolin R); PenFill: 100U/mL (Novolin N, Novolin R); Prefilled: 100U/mL (Novolin N, Novolin R)

**WARNINGS/PRECAUTIONS:** Human insulin differs from animal source insulin. Any change of insulin should be made cautiously. Changes in strength, manufacturer, type or method of manufacture may result in the need for a change in dosage. Hypoglycemia may occur with taking too much insulin, missing or delaying meals, exercising or working more than usual. An infection or illness (especially with diarrhea or vomiting) may change insulin requirements. Administration of insulin SQ can result in lipoatrophy. Novolin R is not recommended for use in insulin pumps.

**ADVERSE REACTIONS:** Hypoglycemia, sweating, dizziness, palpitation, tremor, hunger, restlessness, lightheadedness, inability to concentrate, headache, injection site reaction, allergic reaction.

**INTERACTIONS:** Increased insulin requirements with oral contraceptives, corticosteroids, or thyroid replacement therapy. Reduced insulin requirements with oral hypoglycemics, salicylates, sulfa antibiotics, and certain antidepressants. Alcoholic beverages may change insulin requirements. β-blockers may mask symptoms of hypoglycemia.

**PREGNANCY:** Pregnancy category is not known.

## NOVOLIN 70/30 OTC

insulin human, rdna origin - insulin, human (isophane/regular)
(Novo Nordisk)

**THERAPEUTIC CLASS:** Insulin

**INDICATIONS:** To control hyperglycemia in diabetes.

**DOSAGE:** *Adults:* Individualize dose. Administer SQ.
*Pediatrics:* Individualize dose. Administer SQ.

**HOW SUPPLIED:** (Isophane/Regular) Inj: 70U-30U/mL; PenFill: 70U-30U/mL; Prefilled: 70U-30U/mL

**WARNINGS/PRECAUTIONS:** Human insulin differs from animal source insulin. Any change of insulin should be made cautiously. Changes in strength, manufacturer, type or method of manufacture may result in the need for a change in dosage. Hypoglycemia may occur with taking too much insulin, missing or delaying meals, exercising or working more than usual. An infection or illness (especially with diarrhea or vomiting) may change insulin requirements. Caution with diseases of adrenal, pituitary, or thyroid glands, or progression of kidney or liver disease. Administration of insulin SQ can result in lipoatrophy.

**ADVERSE REACTIONS:** Hypoglycemia, sweating, dizziness, palpitation, tremor, hunger, restlessness, lightheadedness, inability to concentrate, headache, injection site reaction, allergic reaction.

**INTERACTIONS:** Increased insulin requirements with oral contraceptives, corticosteroids, or thyroid replacement therapy. Reduced insulin requirements with oral hypoglycemics, salicylates, sulfa antibiotics, and certain antidepressants. Alcoholic beverages may change insulin requirements. β-blockers may mask symptoms of hypoglycemia.

**PREGNANCY:** Pregnancy category is not known.

## NOVOLOG RX

insulin aspart (Novo Nordisk)

**THERAPEUTIC CLASS:** Insulin

**INDICATIONS:** To control hyperglycemia in diabetes.

**DOSAGE:** *Adults:* Individualize dose. Inject SQ within 5-10 minutes before a meal. Draw first when mixing with NPH human insulin; inject immediately. Do not mix with crystalline zinc insulins, animal source insulins, or other manufacturer insulins. External Insulin Pump: Do not dilute or mix with other insulins.
*Pediatrics:* Individualize dose. Inject SQ within 5-10 minutes before a meal. Draw first when mixing with NPH human insulin; inject immediately. Do not mix with crystalline zinc insulins, animal source insulins, or other manufacturer insulins. External Insulin Pump: Do not dilute or mix with other insulins.

**HOW SUPPLIED:** Inj: 100 U/mL; PenFill: 100 U/mL; Prefilled: 100 U/mL

**CONTRAINDICATIONS:** Hypoglycemia.

**WARNINGS/PRECAUTIONS:** Any change of insulin should be made cautiously. Changes in strength, manufacturer, type or method of manufacture may result in the need for a change in dosage. Hypoglycemia may occur with taking too much insulin, missing or delaying meals, exercising or working more than usual, diseases of adrenal, pituitary, or thyroid glands, or progression of kidney or liver disease. Dosage adjustments may be needed with hepatic or renal dysfunction, during any infection, illness (especially with diarrhea or vomiting) or pregnancy. A longer-acting insulin is usually required to maintain adequate glucose control. Infusion sets and the insulin in the infusion sets should be changed q48h or sooner. Do not use in quick-release infusion sets or cartridge adapters.

**ADVERSE REACTIONS:** Hypoglycemia, hypokalemia, lipodystrophy, hypersensitivity reaction, injection site reactions, pruritus, rash.

**INTERACTIONS:** Increased glucose lowering effects with ACE inhibitors, disopyramide, fibrates, fluoxetine, MAOIs, propoxyphene, salicylates, somatostatin analog, sulfonamide antibiotics and other antidiabetic agents. Decreased blood glucose lowering effects with corticosteroids, niacin, danazol, diuretics, sympathomimetic agents, isoniazid, phenothiazine derivatives, somatropin, thyroid hormones, estrogens, progesterones. Pentamidine may cause hypoglycemia followed by hyperglycemia. β-blockers, clonidine, lithium salts, and alcohol may potentiate or weaken glucose lowering effect. Masked or reduced hypoglycemic symptoms with β-blockers, clonidine, guanethidine, and reserpine.

**PREGNANCY:** Category B, caution in nursing.

## NOVOLOG MIX 70/30 RX

insulin aspart - insulin aspart protamine (Novo Nordisk)

N

**THERAPEUTIC CLASS:** Insulin

**INDICATIONS:** To control hyperglycemia in diabetes.

**DOSAGE:** *Adults:* Individualize dose. For SQ injection only. Inject SQ bid within 15 minutes before breakfast and dinner. Do not mix with other insulins or use in insulin pumps.

**HOW SUPPLIED:** (Insulin Aspart Protamine-Insulin Aspart) Inj: 70U-30U/mL; PenFill: 70U-30U/mL; Prefilled: 70U-30U/mL

**CONTRAINDICATIONS:** Hypoglycemia.

**WARNINGS/PRECAUTIONS:** Any change of insulin should be made cautiously. Changes in strength, manufacturer, type or method of manufacture may result in the need for a change in dosage. Hypoglycemia and hypokalemia may occur; caution with fasting and autonomic neuropathy. Illness, stress, change in meals and exercise may change insulin requirements. Smoking, temperature, and exercise affect insulin absorption. Caution with liver or kidney disease. Administration of insulin SQ can result in lipoatrophy.

**ADVERSE REACTIONS:** Hypoglycemia, hypokalemia, lipodystrophy, hypersensitivity reaction, injection site reactions, pruritus, rash.

**INTERACTIONS:** Increased glucose lowering effects with ACE inhibitors, disopyramide, fibrates, fluoxetine, MAOIs, propoxyphene, salicylates, somatostatin analog, sulfonamide antibiotics and oral antidiabetics. Decreased blood glucose lowering effects with corticosteroids, niacin, danazol, diuretics, sympathomimetics, isoniazid, phenothiazine derivatives, somatropin, thyroid hormones, estrogens, progesterones. β-blockers, clonidine, lithium salts, and alcohol may potentiate or weaken glucose lowering effect. β-blockers, clonidine, guanethidine, and reserpine may reduce or mask signs of hypoglycemia. Do not mix with other insulin products. Caution with potassium-lowering drugs or drugs sensitive to serum potassium levels. Pentamidine may cause hypoglycemia, followed by hyperglycemia.

**PREGNANCY:** Category C, safety in nursing not known.

## NOXAFIL RX

posaconazole (Schering)

**THERAPEUTIC CLASS:** Triazole antifungal

**INDICATIONS:** Prophylaxis of invasive *Aspergillus* and *Candida* infections in patients, ≥13 yrs, who are at high risk of developing these infections due to being severely immunocompromised. Treatment of oropharyngeal candidiasis, including oropharyngeal candidiasis refractory to itraconazole and/or fluconazole.

**DOSAGE:** *Adults:* Prophylaxis of Invasive Fungal Infections: 200mg (5mL) tid. Base duration of therapy on recovery from neutropenia or immunosuppression. Oropharyngeal Candidiasis: LD: 100mg (2.5mL) bid on 1st day, then 100mg qd for 13 days. Oropharyngeal Candidiasis Refractory to Itraconazole and/or Fluconazole: 400mg (10mL) bid. Base duration of therapy on severity of underlying disease and clinical response. Give each dose with full meal or nutritional supplement.
*Pediatrics:* ≥13 yrs: Prophylaxis of Invasive Fungal Infections: 200mg (5mL) tid. Base duration of therapy on recovery from neutropenia or immunosuppression. Oropharyngeal Candidiasis: LD: 100mg (2.5mL) bid on 1st day, then 100mg qd for 13 days. Oropharyngeal Candidiasis Refractory to Itraconazole and/or Fluconazole: 400mg (10mL) bid. Base duration of therapy on severity of underlying disease and clinical response. Give each dose with full meal or nutritional supplement.

**HOW SUPPLIED:** Susp: 40mg/mL

**CONTRAINDICATIONS:** Concomitant ergot alkaloids, terfenadine, astemizole, cisapride, pimozide, halofantrine, or quinidine.

**WARNINGS/PRECAUTIONS:** Hepatic reactions (eg, mild-to-moderate elevations in ALT, AST, alkaline phosphatase, total bilirubin, and/or clinical hepatitis) reported; monitor LFTs at start of and during therapy. Caution with hepatic impairment. Monitor closely with severe renal impairment. Prolongation of QT interval reported; caution with potentially proarrhythmic conditions.

**ADVERSE REACTIONS:** Fever, headache, rigors, hypertension, anemia, neutropenia, diarrhea, nausea, vomiting, abdominal pain, constipation, hypokalemia, thrombocytopenia, coughing, dyspnea.

**INTERACTIONS:** See Contraindications. May elevate cyclosporine and tacrolimus levels; consider dose reduction and more frequent clinical monitoring of cyclosporine, tacrolimus, and sirolimus when therapy is initiated. Avoid use with drugs that are known to prolong the QTc interval and are metabolized through CYP3A4. Avoid concurrent use of cimetidine, rifabutin, and phenytoin unless benefits outweigh risks. If concomitant phenytoin is required, monitor closely and consider phenytoin dose reduction. If concomitant rifabutin is required, monitor CBC and adverse events. Monitor adverse events with concomitant benzodiazepines metabolized by CYP3A4; consider dose reduction of these benzodiazepines during co-administration. May increase levels of vinca alkaloids; consider dose adjustment of vinca alkaloid. Consider dose reduction of concomitant HMG-CoA reductase inhibitors (statins). Monitor for adverse events and toxicity with concomitant calcium channel blockers; dose reduction of calcium channel blockers may be needed.

**PREGNANCY:** Category C, not for use in nursing.

## NUBAIN RX

nalbuphine HCl (Endo)

**THERAPEUTIC CLASS:** Agonist-antagonist analgesic

**INDICATIONS:** Relief of moderate to severe pain. Adjunct to balanced anesthesia for pre- and postoperative analgesia, and for obstetrical analgesia during labor and delivery.

**DOSAGE:** *Adults:* ≥18 yrs: Pain: Initial: 10mg/70kg IV/IM/SQ q3-6h prn. Adjust according to severity, physical status and concomitant agents. Max: 20mg/dose or 160mg/day. Anesthesia Adjunct: Induction: 0.3-3mg/kg IV over 10-15 minutes. Maint: 0.25-0.5mg/kg IV.

**HOW SUPPLIED:** Inj: 10mg/mL, 20mg/mL

**WARNINGS/PRECAUTIONS:** Increased risk of respiratory depression with head injury, intracranial lesions, or pre-existing increased intracranial pressure. Only for use by specifically trained persons. Naloxone, resuscitative and intubation equipment, and oxygen should be readily available. Caution with emotionally unstable patients, narcotic abuse, impaired respiration, MI with nausea and vomiting, biliary tract surgery. May impair ability to drive or operate machinery. Caution with renal or hepatic dysfunction; reduce dose. Caution during labor and delivery; monitor newborns for respiratory depression, apnea, bradycardia, and arrhythmias.

**ADVERSE REACTIONS:** Sedation, sweating, nausea/vomiting, dizziness/vertigo, dry mouth, headache, injection site reactions.

**INTERACTIONS:** Possible additive effects with narcotic analgesics, general anesthetics, phenothiazines, tranquilizers, sedatives, hypnotics, or other CNS depressants. Incompatible with nafcillin and ketorolac.

**PREGNANCY:** Category B, caution in nursing.

## NUCOFED CIII

codeine phosphate - pseudoephedrine HCl (King)



**THERAPEUTIC CLASS:** Antitussive/decongestant

**INDICATIONS:** Relief of cough and congestion associated with respiratory infections, bronchitis, influenza, and sinusitis.

**DOSAGE:** *Adults:* 1 cap q6h. Max: 4 caps/24 hrs.
*Pediatrics:* >12 yrs: 1 cap q6h. Max: 4 caps/24 hrs.

**HOW SUPPLIED:** (Codeine-Pseudoephedrine) Cap: 20mg-60mg; Syrup: 20mg-60mg/5mL

**WARNINGS/PRECAUTIONS:** Not for cough associated with smoking, emphysema, asthma, or excessive secretions. May cause constipation. Caution with pulmonary disease, shortness of breath, HTN, heart disease, DM, thyroid disease, prostatic hypertrophy, Addison's disease, children, ulcerative colitis, drug dependence, liver or kidney dysfunction. May impair alertness.

**ADVERSE REACTIONS:** Nervousness, restlessness, insomnia, drowsiness, dysuria, dizziness, headache, nausea, vomiting, constipation, trembling, dyspnea, sweating, paleness, weakness, heart rate changes.

**INTERACTIONS:** β-blockers, MAOIs, sympathomimetics may increase the effects of pseudoephedrine. Avoid within 14 days of MAOI use. TCAs may antagonize effects of pseudoephedrine. Caution with CNS depressants, general anesthetics, alcohol. Anticholinergics may cause paralytic ileus. Digitalis glycosides may cause cardiac arrhythmias. Decreases effects of antihypertensive agents.

**PREGNANCY:** Category C, caution in nursing.

## NUCOFED PEDIATRIC EXPECTORANT

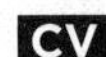


guaifenesin - codeine phosphate - pseudoephedrine HCl (King)

**OTHER BRAND NAMES:** Mytussin DAC (Morton Grove)

**THERAPEUTIC CLASS:** Antitussive/expectorant/decongestant

**INDICATIONS:** Relief of cough and congestion associated with respiratory infections, bronchitis, influenza, and sinusitis.

**DOSAGE:** *Adults:* 10mL q6h. Max: 40mL/24 hrs.
*Pediatrics:* >12 yrs: 10mL q6h. Max: 40mL/24hrs. 6 to <12 yrs: 5mL q6h. Max: 20mL/24hrs. 2 to <6 yrs: 2.5mL q6h. Max: 10mL/24hrs.

**HOW SUPPLIED:** (Codeine-Guaifenesin-Pseudoephedrine) Syrup: 10mg-100mg-30mg/5mL

**WARNINGS/PRECAUTIONS:** Not for cough associated with smoking, emphysema, asthma, or excessive secretions. May cause constipation. Caution with pulmonary disease, shortness of breath, HTN, heart disease, DM, thyroid disease, prostatic hypertrophy, Addison's disease, children, ulcerative colitis, drug dependence, liver or kidney dysfunction. May impair alertness.

**ADVERSE REACTIONS:** Nervousness, restlessness, insomnia, drowsiness, dysuria, dizziness, headache, nausea, vomiting, constipation, trembling, dyspnea, sweating, paleness, weakness, heart rate changes.

**INTERACTIONS:** β-blockers, MAOIs, sympathomimetics may increase the effects of pseudoephedrine. Avoid within 14 days of MAOI use. TCAs may antagonize effects of pseudoephedrine. Caution with CNS depressants, general anesthetics, alcohol. Anticholinergics may cause paralytic ileus. Digitalis glycosides may cause cardiac arrhythmias. Decreases effects of antihypertensive agents.

**PREGNANCY:** Category C, caution in nursing.

## NuLev — RX

hyoscyamine sulfate (Schwarz)

**THERAPEUTIC CLASS:** Anticholinergic

**INDICATIONS:** Adjunct treatment of peptic ulcer, irritable bowel syndrome, neurogenic bladder, and neurogenic bowel disturbances. Management of functional intestinal disorders (eg, mild dysenteries, diverticulitis). To control gastric secretion, visceral spasm, and hypermotility in spastic colitis, spastic bladder, cystitis, pylorospasm, and associated abdominal cramps. Symptomatic relief of biliary and renal colic with concomitant morphine or other narcotics."Drying agent" for symptomatic relief of acute rhinitis. To reduce rigidity and tremors of Parkinson's disease and control associated sialorrhea and hyperhidrosis. For anticholinesterase poisoning.

**DOSAGE:** *Adults:* 0.125-0.25mg q4h or prn. Max: 1.5mg/24hrs. Take with or without water.
*Pediatrics:* >12 yrs: 0.125-0.25mg q4h or prn. Max: 1.5mg/24hrs. 2 to <12 yrs: 0.0625-0.125mg q4h or prn. Max: 0.75mg/24hrs. Take with or without water.

**HOW SUPPLIED:** Tab, Disintegrating: 0.125mg

**CONTRAINDICATIONS:** Glaucoma, obstructive uropathy, GI tract obstruction, paralytic ileus; intestinal atony of elderly/debilitated, unstable cardiovascular status in acute hemorrhage, toxic megacolon complicating ulcerative colitis, myasthenia gravis.

**WARNINGS/PRECAUTIONS:** Risk of heat prostration with high environmental temperature. Avoid activities requiring mental alertness. Psychosis has been reported in sensitive patients. Caution with diarrhea, autonomic neuropathy, hyperthyroidism, coronary heart disease, CHF, arrhythmias/tachycardia, HTN, renal disease, and hiatal hernia associated with reflux esophagitis. Contains phenylalanine.

**ADVERSE REACTIONS:** Anticholinergic effects, drowsiness, headache, nervousness.

**INTERACTIONS:** Additive effects with other antimuscarinics, amantadine, haloperidol, phenothiazines, MAOIs, TCAs, and some antihistamines. Antacids interfere with absorption; take ac and antacids pc.

**PREGNANCY:** Category C, caution in nursing.

## NuLYTELY RX

sodium chloride - potassium chloride - sodium bicarbonate - polyethylene glycol 3350 (Braintree)

**OTHER BRAND NAMES:** Trilyte (Schwarz Pharma)

**THERAPEUTIC CLASS:** Bowel cleanser

**INDICATIONS:** Bowel cleansing prior to colonoscopy.

**DOSAGE:** *Adults:* Oral: 240mL every 10 minutes until fecal discharge is clear or 4L is consumed. Nasogastric Tube: 20-30mL/minute (1.2-1.8L/hr). Patient should fast at least 3-4 hours before administration.
*Pediatrics:* >6 months: Oral/Nasogastric Tube: 25mL/kg/hr until fecal discharge is clear. Patient should fast at least 3-4 hours before administration.

**HOW SUPPLIED:** Sol: (Polyethylene Glycol-Potassium Chloride-Sodium Bicarbonate-Sodium Chloride) 420g-1.48g-5.72g-11.2g [4000mL]

**CONTRAINDICATIONS:** GI obstruction, gastric retention, bowel perforation, toxic colitis, toxic megacolon, ileus.

**WARNINGS/PRECAUTIONS:** Do not add additional ingredients (eg, flavorings). Caution with severe ulcerative colitis. Monitor therapy with impaired gag reflex, unconsciousness/semiconsciousness and patients prone to regurgitation and aspiration. Temporarily d/c if develop severe bloating, distention, or abdominal pain. Monitor for hypoglycemia in pediatrics <2 yrs of age.

**ADVERSE REACTIONS:** Nausea, abdominal fullness/cramps, bloating, vomiting, anal irritation.

**INTERACTIONS:** Oral medications taken within 1 hr of start of administration may not be absorbed from GI tract.

**PREGNANCY:** Category C, caution in nursing.



## NUMORPHAN CII

oxymorphone HCl (Endo)

**THERAPEUTIC CLASS:** Opioid analgesic

**INDICATIONS:** (Inj, Sup) Relief of moderate to severe pain. (Inj) Indicated for preoperative medication, for anesthesia support, for obstetrical analgesia, and relief of anxiety with dyspnea associated with pulmonary edema secondary to acute left ventricular dysfunction.

**DOSAGE:** *Adults:* ≥18 yrs: (Inj) 1-1.5mg IM/SQ q4-6h prn or 0.5mg IV. Titrate: Non-Debilitated Patients: Increase cautiously until satisfactory pain relief obtained. Labor Analgesia: 0.5-1mg IM. (Sup) 5mg PR q4-6h. Titrate: Non-Debilitated Patients: Increase cautiously until satisfactory pain relief obtained. Debilitated/Elderly/Severe Liver Disease: Use smaller doses.

**HOW SUPPLIED:** Inj: 1mg/mL, 1.5mg/mL; Sup: 5mg

**CONTRAINDICATIONS:** Hypersensitivity to morphine analogs. Acute asthma attack, severe respiratory depression, upper airway obstruction, paralytic ileus, pulmonary edema secondary to chemical respiratory irritant.

**WARNINGS/PRECAUTIONS:** Extreme caution in conditions with hypoxia, hypercapnia and decreased respiratory reserve (eg, asthma, COPD, cor pulmonale, severe obesity, sleep apnea syndrome, myxedema, kyphoscoliosis, CNS depression, coma). Caution with head injury, intracranial lesions, or pre-existing increase in intracranial pressure; risk of increased CSF pressure and respiratory depression. May obscure clinical course of head injury and acute abdominal conditions. May produce tolerance and dependence. Caution in debilitated, elderly, cardiovascular/pulmonary disease, renal/hepatic disease, hypothyroidism, acute alcoholism, delirium tremens, convulsive disorders, Addison's disease, gallbladder disease, gallstones, prostatic hypertrophy, urethral strictures, GI or genitourinary tract surgery, inflammatory bowel disease, diarrhea from poisoning until toxin removed, diarrhea from pseudomembranous colitis, cardiac arrhythmias, increased IOP, and toxic psychosis. Risk of severe hypotension; caution with depleted blood volume and circulatory shock. Avoid abrupt withdrawal. Impaired mental/physical abilities.

**ADVERSE REACTIONS:** Lightheadedness, drowsiness, sedation, nausea, vomiting, dry mouth, hypotension, orthostatic hypotension, respiratory depression, atelectasis, ureteral spasm, urinary hesitancy, itching, sweating, injection site reaction.

**INTERACTIONS:** Additive CNS depression with other CNS depressants (eg, sedatives, hypnotics, tranquilizers, general anesthetics, phenothiazines, other opioids, TCAs, MAOIs, acohol); reduce dose of either/both agents. Anticholinergics may increase risk of urinary retention and/or severe constipation which may lead to paralytic ileus. Increased bradycardia reported with propofol. CNS toxicity (eg, confusion, disorientation, respiratory depression, apnea, seizures) reported with cimetidine. Increased risk of hypotension with general anesthetics and phenothiazines.

**PREGNANCY:** Category C, caution in nursing.

## NUTROPIN

RX

somatropin (Genentech)

**OTHER BRAND NAMES:** Nutropin AQ (Genentech)

**THERAPEUTIC CLASS:** Human growth hormone

**INDICATIONS:** (Adults) Replacement of endogenous growth hormone (GH) in GH deficiency (GHD). (Pediatrics) Long-term treatment of growth failure due to lack of adequate endogenous GH secretion, in short-stature associated with Turner Syndrome, and in idiopathic short stature (ISS). Treatment of growth failure associated with chronic renal insufficiency (CRI) up to the time of renal transplantation.

**DOSAGE:** *Adults:* GHD: Initial: Up to 0.006mg/kg/day SQ. Max: <35 yrs: 0.025mg/kg/day. ≥35 yrs: 0.0125mg/kg/day.
*Pediatrics:* GHD: Usual: 0.30mg/kg/week divided into daily SQ doses. Pubertal Patients: Up to 0.7mg/kg/week divided into daily SQ doses. CRI: 0.35mg/kg/week divided into daily SQ doses. Continue until renal transplantation. Hemodialysis: Give qhs or 3-4 hrs post dialysis. Chronic Cycling Peritoneal Dialysis: Give in am after dialysis. Chronic Ambulatory Peritoneal Dialysis: Give qhs during overnight exchange. Turner Syndrome: Up to 0.375mg/kg/week SQ in divided doses 3-7x/week. ISS: 0.3mg/kg/week divided into daily SQ doses.

**HOW SUPPLIED:** Inj: 5mg, 10mg, (AQ) 5mg/mL

**CONTRAINDICATIONS:** Acute critical illness after serious surgeries (eg, open heart or abdominal surgery, accidental trauma, acute respiratory failure), closed epiphyses in pediatrics, active neoplasia, evidence of recurrence or progression of an intracranial tumor, benzyl alcohol sensitivity. Prader-Willi syndrome (unless also diagnosed with GH deficiency) with severe obesity or respiratory impairment.

**WARNINGS/PRECAUTIONS:** Caution with epiphyseal closure in adults treated with GH-replacement therapy in childhood. Recurrence/progression reported with intracranial lesions. Renal osteodystrophy may occur with growth failure secondary to renal impairment. Scoliosis and slipped capital femoral epiphysis may develop in rapid growth. Caution with Turner syndrome and ISS.Intracranial hypertension with papilledema, visual changes, headache, nausea, and/or vomiting has beed reported. Funduscopic exam should be done before and during treatment. Slipped capital femoral epiphysis may occur. Monitor for malignant transformation of skin lesions.Injecting SQ in the same site over a long period of time may cause tissue atrophy. May decrease insulin sensitivity, monitor blood sugar.

**ADVERSE REACTIONS:** Antibodies to the protein, leukemia, transient peripheral edema, arthralgia, carpal tunnel syndrome, malignant transformations, gynecomastia, pancreatitis.

**INTERACTIONS:** Decreased effects with glucocorticoids. May reduce insulin sensitivity; may need insulin adjustment.

**PREGNANCY:** Category C, caution in nursing.

## NUVARING RX

etonogestrel - ethinyl estradiol (Organon)

**THERAPEUTIC CLASS:** Estrogen/progestogen combination

**INDICATIONS:** Prevention of pregnancy.

**DOSAGE:** *Adults:* Insert ring vaginally on or before the 5th day of cycle. Remove ring after 3 consecutive weeks. Insert new ring 1 week later on same day of the week and same time of day.

**HOW SUPPLIED:** Vaginal ring: (Ethinyl estradiol-Etonogestrel) 0.015mg-0.120mg/day

**CONTRAINDICATIONS:** Thrombophlebitis, active or history of thromboembolic disorders, history of DVT, cerebrovascular or coronary artery disease, valvular heart disease with complications, severe HTN, diabetes with vascular complications, headaches with focal neurological symptoms, major surgery with prolonged immobilization, breast carcinoma, endometrial carcinoma or other estrogen-dependent neoplasia, undiagnosed abnormal genital bleeding, cholestatic jaundice of pregnancy or jaundice with prior hormonal contraceptive use, hepatic tumors, active liver disease, pregnancy, heavy smoking and >35 yrs.

**WARNINGS/PRECAUTIONS:** Cigarette smoking increases risk of serious cardiovascular side effects. This risk increases with age (especially >35 yrs) and heavy smoking. Increases risk of MI, thromboembolism, stroke, and gallbladder disease. Retinal thrombosis and benign hepatic adenomas reported. May decrease glucose tolerance. May increase BP, PT, sex hormone-binding globulins, thyroid hormone, or LDL levels. May cause other lipid changes, fluid retention, breakthrough bleeding and spotting, or exacerbate migraines. May develop visual changes with contact lens. D/C if jaundice, significant depression, severe headaches or migraines develop. Toxic shock syndrome with tampon use reported.



**ADVERSE REACTIONS:** Vaginitis, headache, upper respiratory tract infection, leukorrhea, sinusitis, weight gain, nausea.

**INTERACTIONS:** Reduced effects with barbiturates, griseofulvin, rifampin, phenylbutazone, phenytoin, carbamazepine, felbamate, oxycarbazepine, topiramate, modafinil, St. John's Wort, and possibly with ampicillin and tetracyclines. Increases levels of cyclosporine, prednisolone, and theophylline. Protease inhibitors may affect efficacy. Increased levels of ethinyl estradiol with atorvastatin, ascorbic acid, APAP, and CYP3A4 inhibitors (eg, ketoconazole, itraconazole). Increased levels of etonogestrel and ethinyl estradiol with vaginal miconazole nitrate. Decreases levels of APAP and increases clearance of temazepam, salicylic acid, morphine, and clofibric acid.

**PREGNANCY:** Category X, not for use in nursing.

## NYSTATIN RX

nystatin (Various)

**THERAPEUTIC CLASS:** Polyene antifungal

**INDICATIONS:** (Loz, Sus) Treatment of oral candidiasis. (Tab) Treatment of non-esophageal mucous membrane GI candidiasis.

**DOSAGE:** *Adults:* Oral Candidiasis: (Loz) 200,000-400,000 U 4-5 times/day. Max: 14 days. Dissolve slowly in mouth. (Sus) 4-6mL qid. Retain in mouth as

long as possible before swallowing. GI Candidiasis: (Tab) 500,000-1,000,000 U tid.
*Pediatrics:* Oral Candidiasis: (Loz) 200,000-400,000 U 4-5 times/day. Max: 14 days. Dissolve slowly in mouth. (Sus) 4-6mL qid. Infants: 2mL qid. Retain in mouth as long as possible before swallowing.

**HOW SUPPLIED:** Loz: (Pastille) 200,000 U [30 loz]; Sus: 100,000 U/mL [60mL, 480mL]; Tab: 500,000 U

**WARNINGS/PRECAUTIONS:** Not for systemic mycoses. D/C if irritation/hypersensitivity occurs. Confirm diagnosis with KOH smear and/or cultures if symptoms persist after course of therapy. Continue at least 48 hrs after clinical response.

**ADVERSE REACTIONS:** Diarrhea, nausea, vomiting, GI distress, rash, urticaria, Stevens-Johnson syndrome, oral irritation.

**PREGNANCY:** Category C, caution in nursing.

## NYSTATIN VAGINAL — RX

nystatin (Odyssey)

**THERAPEUTIC CLASS:** Polyene antifungal

**INDICATIONS:** Local treatment of vulvovaginal candidiasis.

**DOSAGE:** *Adults:* Insert 1 tablet vaginally qd for 2 weeks. Deposit tablets high in the vagina by means of the applicator.

**HOW SUPPLIED:** Tab, Vaginal: 100,000U [15[s]]

**WARNINGS/PRECAUTIONS:** D/C if sensitization or irritation occurs. Confirm diagnosis by KOH smears and/or cultures.

**PREGNANCY:** Category A, safety in nursing not known.

## NYSTOP — RX

nystatin (Paddock)



**THERAPEUTIC CLASS:** Polyene antifungal

**INDICATIONS:** Treatment of cutaneous and mucocutaneous mycotic infections caused by susceptible *Candida* species.

**DOSAGE:** *Adults:* Apply to lesions bid-tid until healing is complete. For fungal infections of the feet, dust powder on feet and also in shoes.
*Pediatrics:* Neonates and Older: Apply to lesions bid-tid until healing is complete. For fungal infections of the feet, dust powder on feet and in shoes also.

**HOW SUPPLIED:** Powder, Topical: 100,000 U/g [15g, 30g, 60g]

**WARNINGS/PRECAUTIONS:** D/C if irritation or sensitization occurs. Confirm diagnosis. Not for systemic, oral, intravaginal, or ophthalmic use.

**ADVERSE REACTIONS:** Allergic reactions, burning, itching, rash, eczema, pain at application site.

**PREGNANCY:** Safety in pregnancy and nursing not known.

## OBEGYN — RX

minerals - folic acid - multiple vitamin (Fleming)

**THERAPEUTIC CLASS:** Prenatal vitamin

**INDICATIONS:** Vitamin and mineral supplementation for before, during, and after pregnancy.

**DOSAGE:** *Adults:* Mix 1 scoop or 4 tsp (8.25g) in 4-5 oz water and drink qhs, or take in divided doses. Drink immediately after mixing.

**HOW SUPPLIED:** Powder: (Per scoop or 4 tsp) Biotin 0.3mg-Calcium 455mg-Calcium Pantothenate 10mg-Copper 2mg-Folic Acid 1mg-Iron 18mg-Iodine-0.15mg-Magnesium 150mg-Niacin 20mg-Vitamin A 5000IU-Vitamin $B_1$ 1.7mg-Vitamin $B_2$ 2mg-Vitamin $B_6$ 10mg-Vitamin $B_{12}$ 0.012mg-Vitamin C 120mg-Vitamin D 400IU-Vitamin E 60IU-Zinc 25mg [$60^s$, 495g]

**WARNINGS/PRECAUTIONS:** Accidental overdose of iron-containing products is a leading cause of fatal poisoning in children <6 yrs. Folic acid may mask symptoms of pernicious anemia. Consider calcium content; caution with kidney stones. Contains phenylalanine.

**ADVERSE REACTIONS:** Allergic sensitization.

## OcuCoat RX

hydroxypropyl methylcellulose (Bausch & Lomb Surgical)

**THERAPEUTIC CLASS:** Surgical aid

**INDICATIONS:** Ophthalmic surgical aid in anterior segment surgical procedures (eg, cataract extraction, intraocular lens (IOL) implantation).

**DOSAGE:** *Adults:* Anterior Segment Surgery: Introduce into anterior chamber with 20 gauge or smaller cannula. Inject into chamber prior to or following delivery of crystalline lens. Injection prior to lens delivery provides protection to corneal endothelium and other ocular tissues. May use to coat IOL and tips of surgical instruments prior to implantation surgery. May inject during anterior segment surgery to maintain chamber or to replace fluid lost during procedure.

**HOW SUPPLIED:** Sol: 2% [1mL]

**WARNINGS/PRECAUTIONS:** Remove from anterior chamber at end of surgery. Administer appropriate therapy if post-op IOP above expected levels.

**ADVERSE REACTIONS:** Transient increased IOP.

**PREGNANCY:** Safety in pregnancy or nursing not known.



## OcuCoat PF Drops RX

dextran 70 - hydroxypropyl methylcellulose (Bausch & Lomb)

**OTHER BRAND NAMES:** OcuCoat Drops (Bausch & Lomb)

**THERAPEUTIC CLASS:** Lubricant

**INDICATIONS:** To prevent further irritation or to relieve dryness of the eye.

**DOSAGE:** *Adults:* 1-2 drops in affected eye prn.

**HOW SUPPLIED:** Sol: (Dextran 70-Hydroxypropyl Methylcellulose) 0.1%-0.8% [15mL, (PF) 0.5mL $28^s$] (PF is preservative free)

**WARNINGS/PRECAUTIONS:** Do not touch container tip to any surface to avoid contamination. D/C if eye pain or vision changes occur, if redness or irritation continues, or if condition worsens or persists >72 hrs.

**PREGNANCY:** Safety in pregnancy or nursing not known.

## Ocuflox RX

ofloxacin (Allergan)

**THERAPEUTIC CLASS:** Fluoroquinolone

**INDICATIONS:** Management of bacterial infections in conjunctivitis and corneal ulcers.

**DOSAGE:** *Adults:* Conjunctivitis: 1-2 drops q2-4h for 2 days, then 1-2 drops qid for 5 days. Corneal Ulcer: 1-2 drops every 30 minutes while awake and 1-2 drops 4-6 hrs after retiring for 2 days, then 1-2 drops q1h while awake for 5-7 days, then 1-2 drops qid for 2 days or until treatment completion.

*Pediatrics:* >1 yr: Conjunctivitis: 1-2 drops q2-4h for 2 days, then 1-2 drops qid for 5 days. Corneal Ulcer: 1-2 drops every 30 minutes while awake and 1-2 drops 4-6 hrs after retiring for 2 days, then 1-2 drops q1h while awake for 5-7 days, then 1-2 drops qid for 2 days or until treatment completion.

**HOW SUPPLIED:** Sol: 0.3% [5mL, 10mL]

**WARNINGS/PRECAUTIONS:** Not for injection into eye. Do not inject subconjunctivally nor into the eye's anterior chamber. Superinfection may result with prolonged use. Fatal hypersensitivity reactions reported after 1st dose of systemic quinolone therapy. Avoid allowing tip of container to contact fingers, eye or surrounding structures.

**ADVERSE REACTIONS:** Transient ocular burning or discomfort, stinging, redness, itching, keratitis, ocular periocular/facial edema, photophobia, blurred vision, tearing, dryness, eye pain.

**INTERACTIONS:** Systemic quinolone therapy may increase theophylline levels, interfere with caffeine metabolism, enhance warfarin effects, and elevate serum creatinine with cyclosporine.

**PREGNANCY:** Category C, not for use in nursing.

## OCUPRESS RX

carteolol HCl (Novartis Ophthalmics)

**THERAPEUTIC CLASS:** Nonselective beta-blocker

**INDICATIONS:** Reduction of IOP in chronic open-angle glaucoma and intraocular hypertension.

**DOSAGE:** *Adults:* 1 drop bid.

**HOW SUPPLIED:** Sol: 1% [5mL, 10mL, 15mL]

**CONTRAINDICATIONS:** Bronchial asthma, severe COPD, sinus bradycardia, 2nd- and 3rd-degree AV block, overt cardiac failure, cardiogenic shock.

**WARNINGS/PRECAUTIONS:** May be absorbed systemically. Caution with cardiac failure, bronchospasm, diminished pulmonary function, and DM. May mask symptoms of hypoglycemia and hyperthyroidism. Not for use alone in angle-closure glaucoma. May potentiate muscle weakness. D/C if cardiac failure develops. Withdrawal before surgery is controversial.



**ADVERSE REACTIONS:** Eye irritation, burning, tearing, conjunctival hyperemia, conjunctival edema, photophobia, decreased night vision, ptosis, bradycardia, decreased BP, dyspnea, asthenia, headache, dizziness, taste perversion.

**INTERACTIONS:** May potentiate systemic effects with oral β-blockers. Possible hypotension and bradycardia with catecholamine-depleting drugs (eg, reserpine). May antagonize epinephrine.

**PREGNANCY:** Category C, caution in nursing.

## OCUVITE LUTEIN OTC

zinc - copper - lutein - vitamin C - vitamin E (Bausch & Lomb)

**THERAPEUTIC CLASS:** Vitamin/mineral combination

**INDICATIONS:** To provide nutritional support for the eye.

**DOSAGE:** *Adults:* 1 cap qd-bid.

**HOW SUPPLIED:** Cap: Copper 2mg-Lutein 6mg-Vitamin C 60mg-Vitamin E 30IU-Zinc 15mg

**PREGNANCY:** Safety in pregnancy or nursing not known.

## OCUVITE PRESERVISION OTC

zinc - copper - vitamin A - vitamin C - vitamin E (Bausch & Lomb)

**THERAPEUTIC CLASS:** Vitamin/mineral combination

**INDICATIONS:** To help preserve eye health.

**DOSAGE:** *Adults:* 2 tabs bid.

**HOW SUPPLIED:** Tab: Copper 0.4mg-Vitamin A 7160IU-Vitamin C 113mg-Vitamin E 100IU-Zinc 17.4mg

**PREGNANCY:** Safety in pregnancy or nursing not known.

## OGEN RX

estropipate (Pharmacia & Upjohn)

**Estrogens increase the risk of endometrial cancer. Estrogens, with or without progestins, should not be used for the prevention of cardiovascular disease. Increased risks of MI, stroke, invasive breast cancer, PE, and DVT in postmenopausal women (50-79 yrs of age) reported. Increased risk of developing probable dementia in postmenopausal women ≥65 yrs of age reported.**

**THERAPEUTIC CLASS:** Estrogen

**INDICATIONS:** Treatment of moderate to severe vasomotor symptoms and/or vulval/vaginal atrophy associated with menopause. Treatment of hypoestrogenism due to hypogonadism, castration, or primary ovarian failure. Prevention of postmenopausal osteoporosis.

**DOSAGE:** *Adults:* Vasomotor Symptoms: 0.75-6mg/day (as estropipate). Start cyclic administration arbitrarily if not menstruating, or on day 5 of bleeding if menstruating. Vulval/Vaginal Atrophy: 0.75-6mg/day (as estropipate), administer cyclically. Discontinue/Taper over 3-6 month interval. Hypoestrogenism: 1.5-9mg/day (as estropipate) for 1st 3 weeks of cycle, then 8-10 days off. Maint: Lowest effective dose. For female hypogonadism, repeat dose if bleeding doesn't occur or add progestogen in 3rd week of cycle. Osteoporosis Prevention: 0.75mg (as estropipate) qd for 25 days of 31-day cycle.



**HOW SUPPLIED:** Tab: 0.625mg* (0.75mg estropipate), 1.25mg* (1.5mg estropipate), 2.5mg* (3mg estropipate) *scored

**CONTRAINDICATIONS:** Pregnancy, undiagnosed abnormal genital bleeding, breast cancer, estrogen-dependent neoplasia, DVT/PE, active or recent (eg, within past year) arterial thromboembolic disease (eg, stroke, MI), liver dysfunction or disease.

**WARNINGS/PRECAUTIONS:** May increase risk of cardiovascular events (eg, MI, stroke), venous thrombosis, and PE; d/c immediately if any of these events occur or are suspected. May increase risk of breast/endometrial cancer, and gallbladder disease. May lead to severe hypercalcemia with breast cancer and bone metastases; monitor and d/c if hypercalcemia occurs. Retinal vascular thrombosis reported; monitor and d/c if papilledema or retinal vascular lesions occur. Consider addition of a progestin if no hysterectomy. May elevate BP; monitor at regular intervals. May cause elevations of plasma triglycerides with pre-existing hypertriglyceridemia. Caution with history of cholestatic jaundice associated with past estrogen use or with pregnancy; d/c with recurrence. May lead to increased thyroid-binding globulin levels; monitor thyroid function. May cause fluid retention; caution with cardiac/renal dysfunction. Caution with severe hypocalcemia. May increase risk of ovarian cancer. May exacerbate endometriosis, asthma, DM, epilepsy, migraine, porphyria, SLE, and hepatic hemangiomas; use with caution.

**ADVERSE REACTIONS:** Altered vaginal bleeding, vaginal candidiasis, breast tenderness/enlargement, GI effects, melasma, CNS effects, weight changes, edema, altered libido.

**INTERACTIONS:** CYP3A4 inducers (eg, St. John's wort, phenobarbital, carbamazepine, rifampin) may decrease levels which may decrease therapeutic effects and/or change uterine bleeding profile. CYP3A4 inhibitors (eg, erythromycin, clarithromycin, ketoconazole, itraconazole, ritonavir, grapefruit juice) may increase levels which may result in side effects.

**PREGNANCY:** Contraindicated in pregnancy, caution in nursing

## OLUX
clobetasol propionate (Stiefel) RX

**THERAPEUTIC CLASS:** Corticosteroid

**INDICATIONS:** Short-term treatment of inflammatory and pruritic manifestations of moderate to severe corticosteroid responsive dermatoses of the scalp. Short-term treatment of mild to moderate plaque-type psoriasis of non-scalp regions excluding the face and intertriginous areas.

**DOSAGE:** *Adults:* Apply to affected area bid (am and pm). No more than 1.5 capfuls/application. Limit to 2 consecutive weeks. Do not use with occlusive dressings. Max 50g/week.
*Pediatrics:* >12 yrs: Apply to affected area bid (am and pm). No more than 1.5 capfuls/application. Limit to 2 consecutive weeks. Do not use with occlusive dressings. Max 50g/week.

**HOW SUPPLIED:** Foam: 0.05% [50g, 100g]

**WARNINGS/PRECAUTIONS:** May produce reversible HPA axis suppression, manifestations of Cushing's syndrome, hyperglycemia, and glucosuria. Caution when applied to large surface areas or under occlusive dressings. Use appropriate antifungal or antibacterial agent with dermatological infections; discontinue if infection does not clear. Pediatrics may be more susceptible to systemic toxicity. Avoid eyes. Discontinue if irritation occurs.

**ADVERSE REACTIONS:** Burning/stinging, pruritus, irritation, erythema, folliculitis, cracking/fissuring of skin, numbness of fingers, telangiectasia, skin atrophy.

**PREGNANCY:** Category C, caution in nursing.



## OLUX-E
clobetasol propionate (Stiefel) RX

**THERAPEUTIC CLASS:** Corticosteroid

**INDICATIONS:** Treatment of inflammatory and pruritic manifestations of corticosteroid-responsive dermatoses.

**DOSAGE:** *Adults:* Apply thin layer to affected area bid (am and pm). Limit to 2 consecutive weeks. Avoid with occlusive dressings. Max: 50g/week.
*Pediatrics:* ≥12 yrs: Apply thin layer to affected area bid (am and pm). Limit to 2 consecutive weeks. Avoid with occlusive dressings. Max: 50g/week.

**HOW SUPPLIED:** Foam: 0.05% [100g]

**WARNINGS/PRECAUTIONS:** May produce reversible HPA axis suppression, Cushing's syndrome, hyperglycemia, and glucosuria. Caution when applied to large surface area or under occlusive dressings. Use appropriate antifungal or antibacterial agent with dermatological infections; discontinue if infection does not clear. Pediatrics may be more susceptible to systemic toxicity. Discontinue if irritation occurs. Should not be used to treat rosacea or perioral dermatitis. Avoid use on face, groin, axillae, or other intertriginous areas.

**ADVERSE REACTIONS:** Folliculitits, acneiform eruptions, hypopigmentation, perioral dermatitis, allergic contact dermatitis, secondary infection, irritation, striae, miliaria.

**PREGNANCY:** Category C, caution in nursing.

## OMACOR
RX

omega-3-acid ethyl esters (Reliant)

**THERAPEUTIC CLASS:** Lipid-regulating agent

**INDICATIONS:** Adjunct to diet to reduce very high (≥ 500mg/dL) triglyceride levels in adult patients.

**DOSAGE:** *Adults:* 4g qd. Given as single 4-g dose (4 capsules) or as two 2-g doses (2 capsules bid).

**HOW SUPPLIED:** Cap: 1g

**WARNINGS/PRECAUTIONS:** Caution in patients with known sensitivity or allergy to fish. Possible increases in alanine aminotransferase levels without a concurrent increase in aspartate aminotransferase levels. Possible increased low-density lipoprotein cholesterol levels.

**ADVERSE REACTIONS:** Eructation, infection, flu-syndrome, dyspepsia.

**INTERACTIONS:** Possible prolongation of bleeding time with concomitant anticoagulants.

**PREGNANCY:** Category C, caution in nursing.

## OMNARIS
RX

ciclesonide (Altana)

**THERAPEUTIC CLASS:** Corticosteroid

**INDICATIONS:** Treatment of nasal symptoms associated with seasonal and perennial allergic rhinitis.

**DOSAGE:** *Adults:* 2 sprays (50mcg/spray) in each nostril qd. Max: 2 sprays/nostril/day (200mcg/day).
*Pediatrics:* ≥12 yrs: 2 sprays (50mcg/spray) in each nostril qd. Max: 2 sprays/nostril/day (200mcg/day).

**HOW SUPPLIED:** Spray: 50mcg/spray [12.5g]



**WARNINGS/PRECAUTIONS:** Risk of adrenal insufficiency and withdrawal symptoms when replacing systemic corticosteroids with a topical corticosteroids; monitor closely. Risk for more severe/fatal course of infections (eg, chickenpox, measles); avoid exposure in patients who have not had disease or been properly immunized. Potential for growth velocity reduction in pediatrics. Avoid with recent nasal septal ulcers, nasal surgery, or nasal trauma until healed. Symptoms of hypercorticism may occur with excessive use or in highly sensitive patients.

**ADVERSE REACTIONS:** Headache, epistaxis, nasopharyngitis, ear pain.

**INTERACTIONS:** Ketoconazole may increase levels of the pharmacologically active metabolite des-ciclesonide; co-administer with caution.

**PREGNANCY:** Category C, caution in nursing.

## OMNICEF
RX

cefdinir (Abbott)

**THERAPEUTIC CLASS:** Cephalosporin (3rd generation)

**INDICATIONS:** Community acquired pneumonia (CAP), acute exacerbations of chronic bronchitis (AECB), acute maxillary sinusitis, pharyngitis/tonsillitis, uncomplicated skin and structure infections (SSSI), and acute bacterial otitis media.

**DOSAGE:** *Adults:* (Cap) SSSI/CAP: 300mg q12h for 10 days.
AECB/Pharyngitis/Tonsillitis: 300mg q12h for 5-10 days or 600mg q24h for 10 days. Sinusitis: 300mg q12h or 600mg q24h for 10 days. CrCl <30mL/min: 300mg qd.
*Pediatrics:* (Sus) 6 months-12 yrs: Otitis Media/Pharyngitis/Tonsillitis: 7mg/kg

q12h for 5-10 days or 14mg/kg q24h for 10 days. Sinusitis: 7mg/kg q12h or 14mg/kg q24h for 10 days. SSSI: 7mg/kg q12h for 10 days. (Cap) >13 yrs: CAP/SSSI: 300mg q12h for 10 days. AECB/Pharyngitis/Tonsillitis: 300mg q12h for 5-10 days or 600mg q24h for 10 days. Sinusitis: 300mg q12h or 600mg q24h for 10 days. CrCl <30mL/min/1.73m²: 7mg/kg qd. Max: 300mg qd.

**HOW SUPPLIED:** Cap: 300mg; Sus: 125mg/5mL, 250mg/5mL [60mL, 100mL]

**WARNINGS/PRECAUTIONS:** Cross sensitivity to penicillins and other cephalosporins may occur. Pseudomembranous colitis reported. Positive direct Coombs' tests may occur. Caution with renal dysfunction, history of colitis. Suspension contains 2.86g/5mL of sucrose; caution in diabetes. False (+) for urine glucose with Clinitest® and Benedict's or Fehling's solution.

**ADVERSE REACTIONS:** Diarrhea, vaginal moniliasis, nausea, headache, abdominal pain, superinfection (prolonged use).

**INTERACTIONS:** Iron-fortified foods, iron supplements, and aluminum- or magnesium-containing antacids reduce absorption; separate doses by 2 hrs. Probenecid inhibits the renal excretion. Reddish stools reported with iron-containing products.

**PREGNANCY:** Category B, caution in nursing.

## OMNITROPE

somatropin (Sandoz) RX

**THERAPEUTIC CLASS:** Human growth hormone

**INDICATIONS:** Long-term treatment of pediatric patients who have growth failure due to an inadequate secretion of endogenous growth hormone. Long-term replacement therapy in adults with growth hormone deficiency (GHD) of either childhood- or adult-onset etiology.

**DOSAGE:** *Adults:* Individualize dose. GHD: ≤0.04mg/kg/week. May increase at 4-8 week intervals. Max: 0.08mg/kg/week. Divide dose into daily SQ injections (give preferably in the evening).
*Pediatrics:* Individualize dose. GHD: 0.16-0.24mg/kg/week. Divide dose into daily SQ injections (give preferably in the evening).



**HOW SUPPLIED:** Inj: 1.5mg, 5.8mg

**CONTRAINDICATIONS:** Evidence of neoplastic activity. Pediatrics with fused epiphyses. Acute critical illness due to complications after open heart or abdominal surgery, multiple accidental trauma, or with acute respiratory failure. Patients with Prader-Willi syndrome who are severely obese or have severe respiratory impairment.

**WARNINGS/PRECAUTIONS:** Contains benzyl alcohol; avoid use in newborns. Patients with GHD secondary to an intracranial lesion should be monitored closely for progression or recurrence of underlying disease process. Monitor closely for any malignant transformation of skin lesions, scoliosis progression, or gait abnormalities. Monitor closely with DM, glucose intolerance, hypopituitarism. Intracranial HTN reported. Funduscopic exam recomended at initiation, and periodically during course of therapy.

**ADVERSE REACTIONS:** Hypothyroidism, elevated HbA1c, eosinophilia, hematoma, headache, hypertriglyceridemia, leg pain.

**INTERACTIONS:** Growth promoting effects may be inhibited by glucocorticoids. May alter clearance of CYP450 substrates (eg, corticosteroids, sex steroids, anticonvulsants, cyclosporine); monitor closely. May need insulin dose adjustment.

**PREGNANCY:** Category B, caution in nursing.

## ONCASPAR RX
pegaspargase (Enzon)

**THERAPEUTIC CLASS:** Protein synthesis inhibitor

**INDICATIONS:** Acute lymphoblastic leukemia in patients who have developed hypersensitivity to the native forms of L-asparaginase. May be given as monotherapy if multi-agent therapy is inappropriate.

**DOSAGE:** *Adults:* Usual: 2500 IU/m² IM every 14 days.
*Pediatrics:* BSA ≥0.6m²: 2500 IU/m² every 14 days. BSA <0.6m²: 82.5 IU/kg every 14 days.

**HOW SUPPLIED:** Inj: 750 IU/mL [5mL]

**CONTRAINDICATIONS:** Pancreatitis. History of pancreatitis, significant hemorrhagic events, or serious thrombosis with prior L-asparaginase therapy.

**WARNINGS/PRECAUTIONS:** May be a contact irritant. Avoid inhalation or contact with skin or mucous membranes. Serious allergic reaction, pancreatitis, or glucose intolerance can occur. Increased prothrombin time, partial thromboplastin time, and hypofibrinogenemia can occur; monitor coagulation parameters. May predispose to infections, bleeding, thrombosis. D/C in patients with serious thrombotic event including sagittal sinus thrombosis.

**ADVERSE REACTIONS:** Allergic reactions, SGPT increase, nausea, vomiting, fever, malaise.

**INTERACTIONS:** May increase toxicity of protein bound drugs. May interfere with the action of drugs that require cell replication for their lethal effects (eg, methotrexate), and the enzymatic detoxification of other drugs, particularly in the liver. Caution with concomitant anticoagulants (eg, coumadin, heparin, dipyridamole, aspirin or NSAIDs), hepatotoxic agents.

**PREGNANCY:** Category C, not for use in nursing.



## ONTAK RX
denileukin diftitox (Ligand)

**THERAPEUTIC CLASS:** Fusion enzyme

**INDICATIONS:** Treatment of persistent or recurrent cutaneous T-cell lymphoma whose malignant cells express the CD25 component of the interleukin-2 (IL-2) receptor.

**DOSAGE:** *Adults:* Treatment Cycle: 9 or 18mcg/kg/day IV for 5 days every 21 days. Infuse over 15 min. Discontinue or reduce infusion rate (up to 80 min) if adverse reactions occur.

**HOW SUPPLIED:** Inj: 150mcg/mL

**CONTRAINDICATIONS:** Hypersensitivity to IL-2 or diphtheria toxin.

**WARNINGS/PRECAUTIONS:** Hypersensitivity reactions reported. Vascular leak syndrome reported; caution with pre-existing cardiovascular disease. Pre-existing low serum albumin may increase risk of syndrome; monitor weight, edema, BP, and serum albumin levels. Monitor for infection. Test malignant cells for CD25 expression prior to therapy. Perform CBC, blood chemistry panel, liver and renal function, and serum albumin prior to and weekly during therapy. Hypoalbuminemia reported; delay therapy until serum albumin >3g/L. Loss of visual acuity, usually with loss of color vision, with or without retinal pigment mottling.

**ADVERSE REACTIONS:** Chills/fever, asthenia, hypotension, nausea, vomiting, infection, pain, headache, anorexia, diarrhea, hypoalbuminemia, anemia, transaminase increase, myalgia, dizziness, dyspnea, cough increase, rash, infusion-associated reactions.

**PREGNANCY:** Category C, not for use in nursing.

# OPANA ER

oxymorphone HCl (Endo)

**(Tab, ER) Abuse liability and potential. For continuous analgesia only. To be swallowed whole; not to be broken, chewed, dissolved, or crushed. Must not be taken with alcohol.**

**OTHER BRAND NAMES:** Opana (Endo)

**THERAPEUTIC CLASS:** Opioid analgesic

**INDICATIONS:** (Tab) Relief of moderate to severe acute pain. (Tab, ER) Relief of moderate to severe pain in patients requiring continuous, around-the-clock opioid treatment for an extended period of time.

**DOSAGE:** *Adults:* Individualize dose. Opana: Opioid-Naive: Initial: 5-20mg q4-6h. Titrate based on response. Max: 20mg/dose. Conversion from Parenteral Oxymorphone: Give 10x total daily parenteral oxymorphone dose in 4 or 6 equally divided doses. Conversion from Other Oral Opioids: Give half of calculated total daily dose in 4-6 equally divided doses, q4-6h. Opana ER: Swallow whole; do not break, chew, crush, or dissolve. Opioid-Naive: Initial: 5mg q12h. Titrate based on response. Usual: Increase dose by 5-10mg q12h every 3-7 days. Conversion from Opana: Divide 24h Opana dose in half to obtain q12h dose. Conversion from Parenteral Oxymorphone: Give 10x total daily parenteral oxymorphone dose in 2 equally divided doses. Conversion from Other Oral Opioids: Divide calculated 24h Opana dose (refer to PI for conversion ratios) in half to obtain q12h dose. Mild Hepatic Impairment or Renal Impairment (CrCl <50mL/min): Start with lowest dose and titrate slowly while carefully monitoring side effects. With CNS Depressants: Start at 1/3 to 1/2 of usual dose. Elderly: Start at lower end of dosing range.

**HOW SUPPLIED:** Tab: (Opana) 5mg, 10mg; Tab, Extended Release: (Opana ER) 5mg, 10mg, 20mg, 40mg

**CONTRAINDICATIONS:** Respiratory depression (except in monitored settings with resuscitative equipment), acute/severe bronchial asthma or hypercarbia, paralytic ileus, moderate/severe hepatic impairment.

**WARNINGS/PRECAUTIONS:** Schedule II controlled substance with abuse liability. May have additive effects in conjunction with alcohol, other opioids, or illicit drugs that cause CNS depression; respiratory depression, hypotension, and profound sedation or coma may result. With head injury, intracranial lesions or a pre-existing increase in intracranial pressure, possible respiratory depressant effects and potential to elevate CSF pressure may be markedly exaggerated; effects on pupillary response and consciousness may obscure neurologic signs of further increases in intracranial pressure with head injuries. May cause severe hypotension with compromised ability to maintain BP due to depleted blood volume. Caution in elderly or debilitated patients sensitive to CNS depressants. Caution with circulatory shock, acute alcoholism, adrenocortical insufficiency (eg, Addison's disease), CNS depression or coma, delirium tremens, kyphoscoliosis associated with respiratory depression, myxedema or hypothyroidism, prostatic hypertrophy or urethral stricture, biliary tract disease (including acute pancreatitis), severe impairment of pulmonary or renal function, moderate impairment of hepatic function and toxic psychosis. May aggravate convulsions with convulsive disorders; may induce or aggravate seizures in some clinical settings. Monitor for decreased bowel motility in post-op patients. May cause spasm of the sphincter of Oddi; caution with biliary tract disease. May produce tolerance and dependence.

**ADVERSE REACTIONS:** Constipation, nausea, pyrexia, somnolence, headache, dizziness, vomiting, pruritis, increased sweating, xerostomia, sedation, diarrhea, insomnia, fatigue, tachycardia, miosis, biliary colic, hypotension.

**INTERACTIONS:** Additive CNS depression with other CNS depressants (eg, sedatives, hypnotics, tranquilizers, general anesthetics, phenothiazines, other opioids, alcohol); reduce dose of either/both agents. Caution with concomitant use of MAOIs; reduce dose of either/both agents. Anticholinergics may increase risk of urinary retention and/or severe constipation which may lead to paralytic ileus. CNS toxicity (eg, confusion, disorientation, respiratory depression, apnea, seizures) reported with cimetidine.

**PREGNANCY:** Category C, caution with nursing.

## OPCON-A OTC
naphazoline HCl - pheniramine maleate (Bausch & Lomb)

**THERAPEUTIC CLASS:** $H_1$ antagonist/alpha-agonist (imidazoline)

**INDICATIONS:** Temporary relief of redness and itching of the eye due to various allergens.

**DOSAGE:** *Adults:* 1-2 drops up to qid.
*Pediatrics:* >6 yrs: 1-2 drops up to qid.

**HOW SUPPLIED:** Sol: (Pheniramine-Naphazoline) 0.3%-0.027% [15mL]

**CONTRAINDICATIONS:** Cardiovascular disease, HTN, narrow angle glaucoma, BPH.

**WARNINGS/PRECAUTIONS:** D/C if pain, vision changes, no improvement, condition worsens or persists >72 hrs. Remove contact lens before use. Overuse may produce increased redness of eye. Supervision required with heart disease, high BP, difficulty in urination due to prostate enlargement, or narrow angle glaucoma.

**ADVERSE REACTIONS:** Brief tingling sensation.

**PREGNANCY:** Safety in pregnancy and nursing not known.

## OPHTHETIC RX
proparacaine HCl (Allergan)

**THERAPEUTIC CLASS:** Anesthetics

O

**INDICATIONS:** For procedures in which topical ophthalmic anesthesia are indicated: corneal anesthesia of short duration (eg, tonometry, gonioscopy, corneal foreign body removal, short corneal and conjunctival procedures).

**DOSAGE:** *Adults:* Tonometry/Removal of Foreign Bodies or Sutures: 1-2 drops in each eye before procedure. Deep Anesthesia: 1 drop in each eye every 5-10 minutes for 5-7 doses.

**HOW SUPPLIED:** Sol: 0.5% [15mL]

**WARNINGS/PRECAUTIONS:** Not for prolonged use. May produce permanent corneal opacification with accompanying visual loss.

**ADVERSE REACTIONS:** Temporary stinging, burning, or conjunctival redness.

**PREGNANCY:** Category C, caution in nursing.

## OPTICROM RX
cromolyn sodium (Allergan)

**THERAPEUTIC CLASS:** Mast cell stabilizer

**INDICATIONS:** Treatment of vernal keratoconjunctivitis, vernal conjunctivitis, and vernal keratitis.

**DOSAGE:** *Adults:* 1-2 drops 4-6x/day at regular intervals.
*Pediatrics:* >4 yrs: 1-2 drops 4-6x/day at regular intervals.

**HOW SUPPLIED:** Sol: 4% [10mL]

**WARNINGS/PRECAUTIONS:** Do not wear contacts during therapy. Do not exceed recommended frequency.

**ADVERSE REACTIONS:** Transient burning or stinging.

**PREGNANCY:** Category B, caution in nursing.

## OPTINATE RX

iron - minerals - folic acid - multiple vitamin (Sciele)

**THERAPEUTIC CLASS:** Prenatal vitamins

**INDICATIONS:** Vitamin and mineral supplementation for before, during, and after pregnancy.

**DOSAGE:** *Adults:* One tablet and one L-Vcaps capsule qd. Max: Do not exceed 1g/day of DHA.

**HOW SUPPLIED:** Cap: (L-Vcaps) Docosahexaenoic Acid (DHA) 250mg. Tab: Biotin 0.03mg-Calcium 200mg-Copper 2mg-Docusate Sodium 50mg-Folate 1mg-Iron 90mg-Magnesium 30mg-Niacinamide 20mg-Pantothenic Acid 6mg-Vitamin $B_1$ 3mg-Vitamin $B_2$ 3.4mg-Vitamin $B_6$ 20mg-Vitamin $B_{12}$ 0.012mg-Vitamin C 120mg-Vitamin $D_3$ 400 IU-Vitamin E 10 IU-Zinc 15mg

**WARNINGS/PRECAUTIONS:** Accidental overdose of iron-containing products is a leading cause of fatal poisoning in children <6 yrs. Omega-3 fatty acids >3g/day may increase bleeding time and INR; avoid in patients with inherited or acquired bleeding diathesis. Folic acid alone is improper treatment of pernicious anemia and other megaloblastic anemias with vitamin $B_{12}$-deficiency. Folic acid >0.1mg/day may obscure pernicious anemia.

**ADVERSE REACTIONS:** Allergic sensitization

**INTERACTIONS:** Avoid with anticoagulants. DHA component has potential antithrombotic effects.

## OPTIPRANOLOL RX

metipranolol (Bausch & Lomb)

**THERAPEUTIC CLASS:** Nonselective beta-blocker

**INDICATIONS:** Treatment of elevated intraocular pressure in ocular hypertension or open angle glaucoma.

**DOSAGE:** *Adults:* 1 drop in affected eye bid.

**HOW SUPPLIED:** Sol: 0.3% [5mL, 10mL]

**CONTRAINDICATIONS:** Bronchial asthma, severe COPD, symptomatic sinus bradycardia, greater than 1st-degree AV block, cardiogenic shock, overt cardiac failure.

**WARNINGS/PRECAUTIONS:** May be absorbed systemically. Severe respiratory and cardiac reactions may occur. Caution with heart failure, DM, cerebrovascular insufficiency, and in those with a history of anaphylactic reactions. May mask signs of hyperthyroidism; abrupt withdrawal may precipitate a thyroid storm. May cause muscle weakness. Withdraw gradually before surgery. Avoid with COPD.

**ADVERSE REACTIONS:** Abnormal vision, blepharitis, photophobia, uveitis, conjunctivitis, eyelid dermatitis, allergic reactions.

**INTERACTIONS:** Additive systemic blockade with oral β-blockers. Additive hypotension or bradycardia catecholamine-depleting agents (eg, reserpine). Calcium channel blockers may precipitate left ventricular dysfunction and hypotension. Digoxin and calcium channel blockers may prolong AV conduction. Caution with adrenergic psychotropics. Effects can be reversed by β-agonists. Use with miotic agent in angle-closure glaucoma.

**PREGNANCY:** Category C, caution in nursing.

## OPTIVAR RX

azelastine HCl (MedPointe)

**THERAPEUTIC CLASS:** $H_1$ antagonist

**INDICATIONS:** Treatment of itching of the eye associated with allergic conjunctivitis.

**DOSAGE:** *Adults:* 1 drop bid.
*Pediatrics:* >3 yrs: 1 drop bid.

**HOW SUPPLIED:** Sol: 0.05% [6mL]

**WARNINGS/PRECAUTIONS:** Not for injection or oral use. Do not wear contact lens if the eye is red. Not for treatment of contact lens irritation. Wait 10 minutes after instilling drops to insert contact lens.

**ADVERSE REACTIONS:** Transient eye burning/stinging, headaches, asthma, conjunctivitis, dyspnea, eye pain, fatigue, influenza like symptoms, pharyngitis, pruritus, rhinitis, temporary blurring.

**PREGNANCY:** Category C, caution in nursing.

## ORACEA — RX

doxycycline (CollaGenex)

**THERAPEUTIC CLASS:** Tetracycline derivatives

**INDICATIONS:** Treatment of only inflammatory lesions (papules and pustules) of rosacea.

**DOSAGE:** *Adults:* 40mg qd in am. Take on empty stomach.

**HOW SUPPLIED:** Cap: 40mg

**WARNINGS/PRECAUTIONS:** May cause fetal harm during pregnancy. Use during tooth development (last half of pregnancy, infancy, ≤8 yrs) may cause permanent discoloration of teeth or enamel hypoplasia. Pseudomembranous colitis reported. Caution in patients with renal impairment. May cause superinfection, photosensitivity, increase in BUN, bacterial resistance, autoimmune syndromes and hyperpigmentation. Bulging fontanels in infants and benign intracranial HTN in adults reported.

**ADVERSE REACTIONS:** Nasopharyngitis, sinusitis, fungal infection, influenza, diarrhea, HTN, pharyngolaryngeal pain, nasal congestion, abdominal pain, dry mouth, anxiety, sinus headache.



**INTERACTIONS:** May require downward adjustments of anticoagulant dosage. May interfere with bactericidal action of penicillin; avoid concurrent use when possible. Concomitant use with methoxyflurane may result in fatal renal toxicity. Bismuth subsalicylate, proton pump inhibitors, antacids containing aluminum, calcium or magnesium and iron-containing preparations may impair absorption. May interfere with the effectiveness of oral contraceptives. Avoid concurrent use with oral retinoids (eg, isotetinoin). False elevations of urinary catecholamine levels may occur.

**PREGNANCY:** Category D, not for use in nursing.

## ORAMORPH SR — CII

morphine sulfate (aaiPharma)

**This is a sustained release tablet. Swallow tablet whole; do not break in half, crush or chew.**

**THERAPEUTIC CLASS:** Opioid analgesic

**INDICATIONS:** Relief of pain in patients who require opioid analgesics for more than a few days.

**DOSAGE:** *Adults:* Conversion from Parenteral or Immediate Release Oral Morphine: Daily dose determined by the daily requirement of the immediate-release formulation. A single dose is half of the daily requirement given q12h. Initial: 30mg is recommended if daily morphine requirement is <120mg. Use 15mg for low daily morphine requirements. Titrate: increase to 60mg or 100mg after stable dose is reached.

**HOW SUPPLIED:** Tab, Extended Release: 15mg, 30mg, 60mg, 100mg

**CONTRAINDICATIONS:** Respiratory depression in the absence of resuscitative equipment, acute or severe bronchial asthma, paralytic ileus.

**WARNINGS/PRECAUTIONS:** Not for initial treatment. Caution with hepatic and renal dysfunction, increased intracranial pressure or with head injury, decreased respiratory reserve (eg, emphysema, severe obesity, kyphoscoliosis, or paralysis of the phrenic nerve), chronic asthma, upper airway obstruction, or in other chronic pulmonary disorders. Tolerance, psychological and physical dependence may develop. Avoid abrupt discontinuation. Not for pediatrics or for use in women during or immediately before labor.

**ADVERSE REACTIONS:** Constipation, nausea, vomiting, dizziness, sedation, dysphoria, euphoria, and sweating, respiratory depression.

**INTERACTIONS:** Potentiated depressant effects with CNS depressants, alcohol, sedatives, antihistaminics, or psychotropics. Increased risk of respiratory depression, hypotension, sedation and coma with neuroleptics. Mixed agonist/antagonist opioid analgesics (eg, pentazocine, nalbuphine, butorphanol, or buprenorphine) may alter effect or precipitate withdrawal symptoms.

**PREGNANCY:** Category C, not for use in nursing.

## ORAP

pimozide (Gate)

RX

**THERAPEUTIC CLASS:** Diphenylbutylperidine

**INDICATIONS:** Suppression of motor and phonic tics in Tourette's Syndrome in patients that failed standard therapy.

**DOSAGE:** *Adults:* Initial: 1-2mg/day in divided doses. May increase every other day. Maint: <0.2mg/kg/day or 10mg/day, whichever is less. Max: 0.2mg/kg/day or 10mg/day.
*Pediatrics:* >12 yrs: Initial: 0.05mg/kg qhs. Titrate: May increase every 3 days. Max: 0.2mg/kg/day or 10mg/day.

**HOW SUPPLIED:** Tab: 1mg*, 2mg* *scored

**CONTRAINDICATIONS:** Severe CNS depression, comatose states, congenital long QT syndrome, history of cardiac arrhythmias, hypokalemia, hypomagnesemia, simple tics or tics not associated with Tourette's Syndrome. CYP3A4 inhibitors (eg, nefazadone, macrolide antibiotics, azole antifungals, protease inhibitors), sertraline, and drugs that cause motor and phonic tics (eg, pemoline, methylphenidate, amphetamines) or prolong the QT interval.

**WARNINGS/PRECAUTIONS:** May cause tardive dyskinesia, NMS, hyperpyrexia. Caution with history of seizures, EEG abnormalities, severe hepatic/renal impairment. Perform ECG before therapy, periodically thereafter, with dose adjustment. Produces anticholinergic effects. Sudden death reported. May impair mental/physical abilities.

**ADVERSE REACTIONS:** Akinesia, QT prolongation, tardive dyskinesia, sedation, impotence, constipation, dry mouth, visual disturbances, headache, asthenia, increased salivation.

**INTERACTIONS:** May potentiate CNS depressants (eg, analgesics, sedatives, anxiolytics, alcohol). Bradycardia reported with fluoxetine. Avoid grapefruit juice, CYP3A4 inhibitors (eg, azole antifungal drugs, macrolides, protease inhibitors, zileuton, fluvoxamine), sertraline. May interact with CYP1A2 inhibitors. Avoid other drugs that may potentiate QT prolongation such as phenothiazines, TCAs, antiarrhythmics, sparfloxacin, gatifloxacin, moxifloxacin, halofantrine, mefloquine, pentamidine, arsenic trioxide, levomethadyl acetate, dolasetron mesylate, probucol, tacrolimus, ziprasidone.

**PREGNANCY:** Category C, not for use in nursing.

## ORAPRED
RX

prednisolone sodium phosphate (Biomarin)

**THERAPEUTIC CLASS:** Glucocorticoid

**INDICATIONS:** Steroid responsive dermatoses.

**DOSAGE:** *Adults:* Initial: 5-60mg/day depending on disease and response. Maint: Decrease dose by small amounts to lowest effective dose. MS Exacerbations: 200mg qd for 1 week, then 80mg every other day for 1 month. *Pediatrics:* Initial: 0.14-2mg/kg/day, depending on disease and response, given tid-qid. Nephrotic Syndrome: 20mg/m$^2$ tid for 4 weeks, then 40mg/m$^2$ every other day for 4 weeks. Uncontrolled Asthma: 1-2mg/kg/day in single or divided doses until peak expiratory flow rate of 80% is achieved (usually 3-10 days).

**HOW SUPPLIED:** Sol: 15mg/5mL [237mL]

**CONTRAINDICATIONS:** Systemic fungal infections.

**WARNINGS/PRECAUTIONS:** May produce reversible HPA axis suppression. Adjust dose during stress or change in thyroid status. May mask signs of infection or cause new infections. May activate latent amebiasis. Avoid with cerebral malaria. Avoid exposure to chickenpox or measles. Not for treatment of optic neuritis or active ocular herpes simplex. May cause elevation of BP or IOP, cataracts, glaucoma, optic nerve damage, Kaposi's sarcoma, psychic derangements, salt/water retention, increased excretion of potassium and/or calcium, osteoporosis, growth suppression in children, secondary ocular infections. Caution with Strongyloides, CHF, diverticulitis, HTN, renal insufficiency, fresh intestinal anastomoses, active or latent peptic ulcer, ulcerative colitis. Enhanced effect in hypothyroidism or cirrhosis. Avoid abrupt withdrawal.

**ADVERSE REACTIONS:** Edema, fluid/electrolyte disturbances, osteoporosis, muscle weakness, pancreatitis, peptic ulcer, impaired wound healing, increased intracranial pressure, cushingoid state, hirsutism, menstrual irregularities, growth suppression in children, glaucoma, nausea, weight gain.



**INTERACTIONS:** Enhanced metabolism with barbiturates, phenytoin, ephedrine, and rifampin. Use with cyclosporine may increase activity of both drugs; convulsions reported with concomitant use. Decreased metabolism with estrogens or ketoconazole. May inhibit response to warfarin. Increased risk of GI side effects with ASA or other NSAIDs. May increase clearance of salicylates. High doses or concurrent neuromuscular drugs may cause acute myopathy. Enhanced possibility of hypokalemia when given with potassium-depleting agents. May produce severe weakness in myasthenia gravis patients on anticholinesterase agents. Avoid live vaccines with immunosuppressive doses. Possible diminished response with killed or inactivated vaccines. May increase blood glucose; adjust antidiabetic agents. May suppress reactions to skin tests.

**PREGNANCY:** Category C, caution in nursing.

## ORENCIA
RX

abatacept (Bristol-Myers Squibb)

**THERAPEUTIC CLASS:** Selective costimulation modulator

**INDICATIONS:** Moderately to severely active rheumatoid arthritis with inadequate response to one or more disease modifying, anti-rheumatic drugs (DMARDs) (eg, MTX, TNF antagonists). May be used as monotherapy or concomitantly with DMARDs other than TNF antagonists.

**DOSAGE:** *Adults:* Initial: <60kg: 500mg; 60-100kg: 750mg; >100kg: 1g IV over 30 minutes. Maint: Give at 2 and 4 weeks after initial infusion, then q 4 weeks thereafter.

**HOW SUPPLIED:** Inj: 250mg

**WARNINGS/PRECAUTIONS:** Increased risk of infections and serious infections with concomitant TNF antagonist therapy; concurrent use is not recommended. Anaphylaxis or anaphylactoid reactions reported. Caution with history of recurrent infections; discontinue if serious infections develop. Screen for latent TB prior to initiation. Avoid live vaccines. Caution with COPD. Concurrent use with anakinra is not recommended. Cases of lung cancer and lymphoma reported.

**ADVERSE REACTIONS:** Headache, nasopharyngitis, dizziness, cough, back pain, HTN, dyspepsia, UTI, rash, pain in extremities.

**INTERACTIONS:** See Warnings/Precautions.

**PREGNANCY:** Category C, not for use in nursing.

## ORFADIN

RX

nitisinone (Rare Disease Therapeutics)

**THERAPEUTIC CLASS:** 4-hydroxyphenylpyruvate dioxygenase inhibitor

**INDICATIONS:** Adjunct to dietary restriction of tyrosine and phenylalanine in the treatment of hereditary tyrosinemia type I.

**DOSAGE:** *Adults:* Initial: 1mg/kg/day in divided doses, qam and qpm. Titrate: Increase to 1.5mg/kg/day if biochemical parameters (except plasma succinylacetone) are not normalized within 1 month. Max: 2mg/kg/day. Take at least 1 hr before a meal. May sprinkle contents of capsule in small amount of water, formula or apple sauce immediately before use.
*Pediatrics:* Initial: 1mg/kg/day in divided doses, qam and qpm. Titrate: Increase to 1.5mg/kg/day if biochemical parameters (except plasma succinylacetone) are not normalized within 1 month. Max: 2mg/kg/day. Take at least 1 hr before a meal. May sprinkle contents of capsule in small amount of water, formula or apple sauce immediately before use.

**HOW SUPPLIED:** Cap: 2mg, 5mg, 10mg

**WARNINGS/PRECAUTIONS:** Inadequate restriction of tyrosine and phenylalanine can result in elevated tyrosine levels. Maintain tyrosine levels <500µmol/L to avoid toxicity. Transient thrombocytopenia and leucopenia reported; monitor platelet and WBC count. Perform slit-lamp eye examination before initiation and if patient develops photophobia, eye pain or inflammation. Do not adjust dose further to lower tyrosine levels; may deteriorate patients condition; use diet restriction instead. Increased risk of porphyric crises, liver failure, or hepatic neoplasms; monitor liver by imaging and lab tests including serum alpha-fetoprotein. Monitor urine succinylacetone levels to guide dose-adjustment. Monitor serum phosphate to screen for renal involvement.



**ADVERSE REACTIONS:** Hepatic neoplasm, liver failure, conjunctivitis, corneal opacity, keratitis, photophobia, thrombocytopenia, leucopenia.

**PREGNANCY:** Category C, caution in nursing.

## ORPHENADRINE

RX

orphenadrine citrate (Various)

**THERAPEUTIC CLASS:** Muscular analgesic (central-acting)

**INDICATIONS:** Adjunct for acute, painful musculoskeletal conditions.

**DOSAGE:** *Adults:* (Tab) 100mg bid, in the am and pm. (Inj) 60mg IM/IV q12h.

**HOW SUPPLIED:** Inj: 30mg/mL; Tab, Extended Release: 100mg

**CONTRAINDICATIONS:** Glaucoma, pyloric or duodenal obstruction, stenosing peptic ulcers, prostatic hypertrophy, bladder neck obstruction, cardiospasm, myasthenia gravis.

**WARNINGS/PRECAUTIONS:** Caution with tachycardia, cardiac decompensation, coronary insufficiency, cardiac arrhythmias. Monitor blood, urine, and LFTs periodically with prolonged use. Injection contains sodium bisulfite.

**ADVERSE REACTIONS:** Dry mouth, tachycardia, palpitation, urinary hesitancy/retention, blurred vision, pupil dilation, increased ocular tension, weakness, dizziness, constipation.

**INTERACTIONS:** Confusion, anxiety, and tremors reported with propoxyphene.

**PREGNANCY:** Category C, safety in nursing not known.

## ORTHO DIAPHRAGM KITS — RX

diaphragm (Ortho-McNeil)

**THERAPEUTIC CLASS:** Contraceptive device

**INDICATIONS:** Prevention of pregnancy in conjunction with appropriate spermicide.

**DOSAGE:** *Adults:* Use with contraceptive cream/jelly; apply into cup of diaphragm and around the rim. May insert up to 6 hrs before intercourse. Insert additional contraceptive cream/jelly if more than 6 hrs has elapsed; do not remove diaphragm to do this. Keep diaphragm in place for 6 hrs after intercourse and remove as soon as possible thereafter. Cleanse diaphragm with mild, non-perfumed soap and warm water before initial use, and after each use. Rinse and dry carefully.

**HOW SUPPLIED:** ALL-FLEX Arcing Spring Diaphragm or ORTHO Coil Spring Diaphragm: 55mm, 60mm, 65mm, 70mm, 75mm, 80mm, 85mm, 90mm, 95mm

**CONTRAINDICATIONS:** History of toxic shock syndrome (TSS), hypersensitivity to dry natural rubber.



**WARNINGS/PRECAUTIONS:** Avoid continuous use for >24 hrs. Risk of TSS. Increased risk of vaginal tract infection with retention of diaphragm for any period of time. Increased risk of UTI if not properly fitted. Refit diaphragm if lose/gain >10 lbs, same diaphragm for >1 yr, or if have baby or abortion. D/C with spermicide sensitivity.

**INTERACTIONS:** Avoid petroleum jelly, mineral oil, vegetable oil, cold cream lubricants. Some vaginal drugs or lubricating agents may damage the diaphragm.

**PREGNANCY:** Safety in pregnancy and nursing not known.

## ORTHO EVRA — RX

norelgestromin - ethinyl estradiol (Ortho-McNeil)

**THERAPEUTIC CLASS:** Estrogen/progestogen combination

**INDICATIONS:** Prevention of pregnancy.

**DOSAGE:** *Adults:* Start 1st Sunday after menses begins or the 1st day of menses. Apply patch every week on the same day for 3 weeks. Week 4 is patch-free. Apply to clean, dry intact skin on buttock, abdomen, upper arm, or upper torso.

**HOW SUPPLIED:** Patch: (Ethinyl Estradiol-Norelgestromin): 0.02mg-0.15mg/24hrs [$1^s$, $3^s$]

**CONTRAINDICATIONS:** Thrombophlebitis, DVT, thromboembolic disorders, pregnancy, cerebrovascular or coronary artery disease, valvular heart disease with complications, undiagnosed abnormal genital bleeding, cholestatic jaundice of pregnancy or jaundice with prior pill use, hepatic adenomas or carcinomas, breast cancer or other estrogen-dependent neoplasia, severe HTN, diabetes with vascular involvement, headaches with focal neurological symptoms, major surgery with prolonged immobilization, acute/chronic hepatocellular disease with abnormal liver function.

**WARNINGS/PRECAUTIONS:** Cigarette smoking increases risk of serious cardiovascular side effects. This risk increases with age (especially >35 yrs) and heavy smoking. Increased risk of MI, vascular disease, thromboembolism, stroke and gallbladder disease. Retinal thrombosis, hepatic neoplasia reported. May cause glucose intolerance. May increase BP, elevate LDL levels or cause other lipid changes, fluid retention, breakthrough bleeding and spotting. May cause or exacerbate migraine. May develop visual changes with contact lens. Increased risk of MI with HTN, hyperlipidemia, and diabetes. D/C if jaundice or depression develops. Perform annual physical exam. Use before menarche is not indicated. May affect certain endocrine, LFTs, and blood components. May be less effective in women with body weight >198 lbs.

**ADVERSE REACTIONS:** Breast symptoms, headache, application site reaction, nausea, upper respiratory infection, menstrual cramps, abdominal pain.

**INTERACTIONS:** Reduced effects and increased breakthrough bleeding with rifampin, barbiturates, phenylbutazone, phenytoin, carbamazepine, topiramate, St. John's wort, griseofulvin, felbamate, oxycarbazepine, possibly with ampicillin. Protease inhibitors alter levels. Increased levels with atorvastatin, ascorbic acid, acetaminophen, and CYP3A4 inhibitors (eg, itraconazole, ketoconazole). May increase levels of cyclosporine, prednisolone, theophylline. May decrease levels of acetaminophen and increase clearance of temazepam, salicylic acid, morphine, and clofibric acid.

**PREGNANCY:** Category X, not for use in nursing.

## Ortho Tri-Cyclen RX

norgestimate - ethinyl estradiol (Ortho-McNeil)

**OTHER BRAND NAMES:** Tri-Previfem (Teva) - Tri-Sprintec (Barr)

**THERAPEUTIC CLASS:** Estrogen/progestogen combination

**INDICATIONS:** Prevention of pregnancy. Treatment of acne vulgaris in females >15 yrs who want contraception, have achieved menarche and are unresponsive to topical acne agents.

**DOSAGE:** *Adults:* Contraception/Acne: 28-day: 1 tab qd for 28 days, then repeat. Start 1st Sunday after menses begin or 1st day of menses.
*Pediatrics:* Contraception (postpubertal adolescents)/Acne: 28-day: 1 tab qd for 28 days, then repeat. Start 1st Sunday after menses begin or 1st day of menses.

**HOW SUPPLIED:** Tab: (Ethinyl Estradiol-Norgestimate) 0.035mg-0.18mg, 0.035mg-0.215mg, and 0.035mg-0.25mg

**CONTRAINDICATIONS:** Thrombophlebitis, deep vein thrombophlebitis, thromboembolic disorders, pregnancy, cerebrovascular or coronary artery disease, migraine with focal aura, acute or chronic hepatocellular disease with abnormal liver function, undiagnosed abnormal genital bleeding, cholestatic jaundice of pregnancy or jaundice with prior pill use, hepatic adenomas or carcinomas, breast cancer, endometrium carcinoma, or other estrogen-dependent neoplasia.

**WARNINGS/PRECAUTIONS:** Cigarette smoking increases risk of serious cardiovascular side effects. This risk increases with age (especially >35 yrs) and heavy smoking. Increased risk of MI, vascular disease, thromboembolism, stroke, and gallbladder disease. Retinal thrombosis, hepatic neoplasia, carcinoma of breast and reproductive organs reported. May cause glucose intolerance, fluid retention, breakthrough bleeding, and spotting. May increase BP, elevate LDL levels, or cause other lipid changes. May cause or exacerbate migraine. May develop visual changes with contact lens. Increased risk of morbidity and mortality with HTN, hyperlipidemia, obesity, and diabetes. D/C if jaundice, significant depression, or ophthalmic irregularities develop. Perform annual physical exam. Use before menarche is not indicated. May affect certain endocrine, LFTs, and blood components.

**ADVERSE REACTIONS:** Nausea, vomiting, breakthrough bleeding, spotting, amenorrhea, migraine, depression, vaginal candidiasis, edema, weight changes.

**INTERACTIONS:** Reduced effects, increased breakthrough bleeding, and menstrual irregularities with rifampin, barbiturates, phenylbutazone, phenytoin, carbamazepine, griseofulvin, topiramate, St. John's wort, and possibly with ampicillin and tetracyclines.

**PREGNANCY:** Category X, not for use in nursing.

## Ortho Tri-Cyclen Lo RX

norgestimate - ethinyl estradiol (Ortho-McNeil)

**THERAPEUTIC CLASS:** Estrogen/progestogen combination

**INDICATIONS:** Prevention of pregnancy.

**DOSAGE:** *Adults:* Start 1st Sunday after menses begins or the 1st day of menses. *28-day:* 1 tab qd for 28 days, then repeat.

**HOW SUPPLIED:** Tab: (Ethinyl Estradiol-Norgestimate) 0.025mg-0.18mg, 0.025mg-0.215mg, and 0.025mg-0.25mg

**CONTRAINDICATIONS:** Thrombophlebitis, deep vein thrombophlebitis, thromboembolic disorders, pregnancy, cerebrovascular or CAD, valvular heart disease with complications, severe HTN, DM with vascular involvement, headaches with focal neurological symptoms, major surgery with prolonged immobilization, undiagnosed abnormal genital bleeding, cholestatic jaundice of pregnancy or jaundice with prior pill use, hepatic adenomas or carcinomas, breast cancer, endometrial carcinoma, or other estrogen-dependent neoplasia.

**WARNINGS/PRECAUTIONS:** Cigarette smoking increases risk of serious CV side effects. This risk increases with age (especially >35 yrs) and heavy smoking. Increased risk of MI, vascular disease, thromboembolism, stroke, and gallbladder disease. Retinal thrombosis, hepatic neoplasia, carcinoma of breast and reproductive organs reported. May cause glucose intolerance, fluid retention, breakthrough bleeding, and spotting. May increase BP, elevate LDL levels or cause other lipid changes. May cause or exacerbate migraine. May develop visual changes with contact lens. Increased risk of morbidity and mortality with HTN, hyperlipidemia, obesity, and DM. Discontinue if develop jaundice, significant depression or ophthalmic irregularities. Perform annual physical exam. Use before menarche is not indicated. May affect certain endocrine, LFTs, and blood components.



**ADVERSE REACTIONS:** Nausea, vomiting, breakthrough bleeding, spotting, amenorrhea, migraine, depression, vaginal candidiasis, edema, weight changes.

**INTERACTIONS:** Reduced effects, increased breakthrough bleeding with rifampin, barbiturates, phenylbutazone, phenytoin, carbamazepine, felbamate, oxcarbazepine, griseofulvin, topiramate, St. John's wort, and possibly with ampicillin and tetracyclines. Atorvastatin, ascorbic acid, APAP, CYP3A4 inhibitors (eg, itraconazole, ketoconazole) may increase hormone levels. HIV protease inhibitors may increase or decrease levels. Increases levels of cyclosporine, prednisolone, theophylline. Decreases levels of APAP. Increases clearance of temazepam, salicylic acid, morphine, clofibric acid.

**PREGNANCY:** Category X, not for use in nursing.

## Ortho-Cept RX

desogestrel - ethinyl estradiol (Ortho-McNeil)

**THERAPEUTIC CLASS:** Estrogen/progestogen combination

**INDICATIONS:** Prevention of pregnancy.

**DOSAGE:** *Adults:* 1 tab qd for 28 days, then repeat. Start 1st Sunday after menses begin or 1st day of menses.

**HOW SUPPLIED:** Tab: (Ethinyl Estradiol-Desogestrel) 0.03mg-0.15mg

**CONTRAINDICATIONS:** Thrombophlebitis, DVT or thromboembolic disorders, pregnancy, cerebrovascular or coronary artery disease, undiagnosed abnormal genital bleeding, cholestatic jaundice of pregnancy or jaundice with prior pill use, hepatic adenomas or carcinomas, breast cancer or other estrogen-dependent neoplasia.

**WARNINGS/PRECAUTIONS:** Cigarette smoking increases risk of serious cardiovascular side effects. This risk increases with age (especially >35 yrs) and heavy smoking. Increased risk of MI, vascular disease, thromboembolism, stroke and gallbladder disease. Retinal thrombosis, hepatic neoplasia, carcinoma of breast and reproductive organs reported. May cause glucose intolerance. May increase BP, elevate LDL levels or cause other lipid changes, fluid retention, breakthrough bleeding, and spotting. May cause or exacerbate migraine. May develop visual changes with contact lens. Increased risk of MI with HTN, hyperlipidemia, obesity, and diabetes. D/C if jaundice, significant depression, or ophthalmic irregularities develop. Perform annual physical exam. Use before menarche is not indicated. May affect certain endocrine, LFTs and blood components.

**ADVERSE REACTIONS:** Nausea, vomiting, breakthrough bleeding, spotting, amenorrhea, migraine, depression, vaginal candidiasis, edema, weight changes.

**INTERACTIONS:** Reduced effects, increased breakthrough bleeding, and menstrual irregularities with rifampin, barbiturates, phenylbutazone, phenytoin, carbamazepine, griseofulvin, topiramate, St. John's wort, and possibly with ampicillin and tetracyclines.

**PREGNANCY:** Category X, not for use in nursing.

## ORTHO-CYCLEN RX

norgestimate - ethinyl estradiol (Ortho-McNeil)

**OTHER BRAND NAMES:** Sprintec (Barr) - MonoNessa (Watson)

**THERAPEUTIC CLASS:** Estrogen/progestogen combination

**INDICATIONS:** Prevention of pregnancy.

**DOSAGE:** *Adults:* Start 1st Sunday after menses begin or the 1st day of menses. *28-day:* 1 tab qd for 28 days, then repeat.

**HOW SUPPLIED:** Tab: (Ethinyl Estradiol-Norgestimate) 0.035mg-0.25mg

**CONTRAINDICATIONS:** Thrombophlebitis, deep vein thrombophlebitis, thromboembolic disorders, pregnancy, cerebrovascular or coronary artery disease, migraine with focal aura, acute or chronic hepatocellular disease with abnormal liver function, undiagnosed abnormal genital bleeding, cholestatic jaundice of pregnancy or jaundice with prior pill use, hepatic adenomas or carcinomas, breast cancer, endometrium carcinoma, or other estrogen-dependent neoplasia.

**WARNINGS/PRECAUTIONS:** Cigarette smoking increases risk of serious cardiovascular side effects. This risk increases with age (especially >35 yrs) and heavy smoking. Increased risk of MI, vascular disease, thromboembolism, stroke and gallbladder disease. Retinal thrombosis, hepatic neoplasia, carcinoma of breast and reproductive organs reported. May cause glucose intolerance. May increase BP, elevate LDL levels or cause other lipid changes, fluid retention, breakthrough bleeding, and spotting. May cause or exacerbate migraine. May develop visual changes with contact lens. Increased risk of MI with HTN, hyperlipidemia, obesity, and diabetes. Discontinue if develop jaundice, significant depression or ophthalmic irregularities. Perform annual physical exam. Use before menarche is not indicated. May affect certain endocrine, LFTs and blood components.

**ADVERSE REACTIONS:** Nausea, vomiting, breakthrough bleeding, spotting, amenorrhea, migraine, depression, vaginal candidiasis, edema, weight changes.

**INTERACTIONS:** Reduced effects, increased breakthrough bleeding, and menstrual irregularities with rifampin, barbiturates, phenylbutazone, phenytoin, carbamazepine, griseofulvin, topiramate, St. John's wort, and possibly with ampicillin and tetracyclines.

**PREGNANCY:** Category X, not for use in nursing.

## ORTHO-EST

RX

estropipate (Women First)

**Estrogens increase risk of endometrial cancer in postmenopausal women. Avoid during pregnancy.**

**THERAPEUTIC CLASS:** Estrogen

**INDICATIONS:** Treatment of moderate to severe vasomotor symptoms of menopause and/or vulval/vaginal atrophy. Treatment of hypoestrogenism due to hypogonadism, castration, or primary ovarian failure. Prevention of osteoporosis.

**DOSAGE:** *Adults:* Vasomotor Symptoms: 0.75-6mg/day (as estropipate). Start cyclic administration arbitrarily if not menstruating, or on day 5 of bleeding if menstruating. Vulval/Vaginal Atrophy: 0.75-6mg/day (as estropipate), administer cyclically. Discontinue/Taper over a 3-6 month interval. Female Hypogonadism/Castration/Primary Ovarian Failure: 1.5-9mg/day (as estropipate) for 1st 3 weeks of cycle, then 8-10 days off. For female hypogonadism, repeat dose if bleeding does not occur, or add progestogen in 3rd week of cycle. Maint: Lowest effective dose. Osteoporosis Prevention: 0.75mg (as estropipate) qd for 25 days of a 31-day cycle.

**HOW SUPPLIED:** Tab: 0.625mg* (0.75mg estropipate), 1.25mg* (1.5mg estropipate) *scored

**CONTRAINDICATIONS:** Pregnancy, undiagnosed abnormal genital bleeding, breast cancer unless being treated for metastatic disease, estrogen-dependent neoplasia, thrombophlebitis, or thromboembolic disorders.



**WARNINGS/PRECAUTIONS:** Risk of gallbladder disease, endometrial and breast carcinoma, fetal congenital reproductive tract disorder, elevated BP, and hypercalcemia with breast cancer and bone metastases. Possible risk of cardiovascular disease. Caution in liver dysfunction, asthma, epilepsy, migraine, and cardiac or renal dysfunction. Increase in HDL, triglycerides, thyroid binding globulin. Acceleration of PT, PTT. Hypercoagulability effects. Impaired glucose tolerance. Consider adding progestin in patient with intact uterus.

**ADVERSE REACTIONS:** Altered vaginal bleeding, vaginal candidiasis, breast tenderness/enlargement, GI effects, melasma, CNS effects, weight changes, edema, altered libido.

**PREGNANCY:** Category X, caution in nursing.

## ORTHO-NOVUM 1/35

RX

norethindrone - ethinyl estradiol (Ortho-McNeil)

**OTHER BRAND NAMES:** Necon 1/35 (Watson) - Nortrel 1/35 (Barr) - Norinyl 1/35 (Watson)

**THERAPEUTIC CLASS:** Estrogen/progestogen combination

**INDICATIONS:** Prevention of pregnancy.

**DOSAGE:** *Adults: 21-day*: 1 tab qd for 21 days, stop 7 days, then repeat. *28-day*: 1 tab qd for 28 days, then repeat. Start 1st Sunday after menses begin or 1st day of menses.

**HOW SUPPLIED:** (Ethinyl Estradiol-Norethindrone) Tab: 0.035mg-1mg

**CONTRAINDICATIONS:** Thrombophlebitis, DVT or thromboembolic disorders, pregnancy, cerebrovascular or coronary artery disease, undiagnosed abnormal genital bleeding, cholestatic jaundice of pregnancy or jaundice with prior pill use, hepatic adenomas or carcinomas, breast cancer or other estrogen-dependent neoplasia.

**WARNINGS/PRECAUTIONS:** Cigarette smoking increases risk of serious cardiovascular side effects. This risk increases with age (especially >35 yrs) and heavy smoking. Increased risk of MI, vascular disease, thromboembolism, stroke and gallbladder disease. Retinal thrombosis, hepatic neoplasia, carcinoma of breast and reproductive organs reported. May cause glucose intolerance. May increase BP, elevate LDL levels or cause other lipid changes, fluid retention, breakthrough bleeding, and spotting. May cause or exacerbate migraine. May develop visual changes with contact lens. Increased risk of MI with HTN, hyperlipidemia, obesity, and diabetes. D/C if jaundice, significant depression, or ophthalmic irregularities develop. Perform annual physical exam. Use before menarche is not indicated. May affect certain endocrine, LFTs and blood components.

**ADVERSE REACTIONS:** Nausea, vomiting, breakthrough bleeding, spotting, amenorrhea, migraine, depression, vaginal candidiasis, edema, weight changes.

**INTERACTIONS:** Reduced effects, increased breakthrough bleeding, and menstrual irregularities with rifampin, barbiturates, phenylbutazone, phenytoin, carbamazepine, griseofulvin, topiramate, St. John's wort, and possibly with ampicillin and tetracyclines.

**PREGNANCY:** Category X, not for use in nursing.

## ORTHO-NOVUM 1/50 RX

mestranol - norethindrone (Ortho-McNeil)

**OTHER BRAND NAMES:** Necon 1/50 (Watson) - Norinyl 1/50 (Watson)

**THERAPEUTIC CLASS:** Estrogen/progestogen combination

**INDICATIONS:** Prevention of pregnancy.

**DOSAGE:** *Adults: 21-day*: 1 tab qd for 21 days, stop 7 days, then repeat. *28-day:* 1 tab qd for 28 days, then repeat. Start 1st Sunday after menses begin or 1st day of menses.

**HOW SUPPLIED:** Tab: (Mestranol-Norethindrone) 0.05mg-1mg

**CONTRAINDICATIONS:** Thrombophlebitis, DVT or thromboembolic disorders, pregnancy, cerebrovascular or coronary artery disease, undiagnosed abnormal genital bleeding, cholestatic jaundice of pregnancy or jaundice with prior pill use, hepatic adenomas or carcinomas, breast cancer or other estrogen-dependent neoplasia.

**WARNINGS/PRECAUTIONS:** Cigarette smoking increases risk of serious cardiovascular side effects. This risk increases with age (especially >35 yrs) and heavy smoking. Increased risk of MI, vascular disease, thromboembolism, stroke and gallbladder disease. Retinal thrombosis, hepatic neoplasia, carcinoma of breast and reproductive organs reported. May cause glucose intolerance. May increase BP, elevate LDL levels or cause other lipid changes, fluid retention, breakthrough bleeding, and spotting. May cause or exacerbate migraine. May develop visual changes with contact lens. Increased risk of MI with HTN, hyperlipidemia, obesity, and diabetes. D/C if jaundice, significant depression, or ophthalmic irregularities develop. Perform annual physical exam. Use before menarche is not indicated. May affect certain endocrine, LFTs and blood components.

**ADVERSE REACTIONS:** Nausea, vomiting, breakthrough bleeding, spotting, amenorrhea, migraine, depression, vaginal candidiasis, edema, weight changes.

**INTERACTIONS:** Reduced effects, increased breakthrough bleeding, and menstrual irregularities with rifampin, barbiturates, phenylbutazone, phenytoin, carbamazepine, griseofulvin, topiramate, St. John's wort, and possibly with ampicillin and tetracyclines.

**PREGNANCY:** Category X, not for use in nursing.

## ORTHO-NOVUM 10/11 RX

norethindrone - ethinyl estradiol (Ortho-McNeil)

**OTHER BRAND NAMES:** Necon 10/11 (Watson)

**THERAPEUTIC CLASS:** Estrogen/progestogen combination

**INDICATIONS:** Prevention of pregnancy.

**DOSAGE:** *Adults:* Start 1st Sunday after menses begins or the 1st day of menses. *21-day:* 1 tab qd for 21 days, stop 7 days, then repeat. *28-day:* 1 tab qd for 28 days, then repeat.

**HOW SUPPLIED:** Tab: (Ethinyl Estradiol-Norethindrone) 0.035mg-0.5mg and 0.035mg-1mg

**CONTRAINDICATIONS:** Thrombophlebitis, DVT or thromboembolic disorders, pregnancy, cerebrovascular or coronary artery disease, undiagnosed abnormal genital bleeding, cholestatic jaundice of pregnancy or jaundice with prior pill use, hepatic adenomas or carcinomas, breast cancer or other estrogen-dependent neoplasia.

**WARNINGS/PRECAUTIONS:** Cigarette smoking increases risk of serious cardiovascular side effects. This risk increases with age (especially >35 yrs) and heavy smoking. Increased risk of MI, vascular disease, thromboembolism, stroke and gallbladder disease. Retinal thrombosis, hepatic neoplasia reported. May cause glucose intolerance. May increase BP, elevate LDL levels or cause other lipid changes, fluid retention, breakthrough bleeding, and spotting. May cause or exacerbate migraine. May develop visual changes with contact lens. Morbidity and mortality risk increased with HTN, hyperlipidemia, obesity, and diabetes. Discontinue if develop jaundice, significant depression or ophthalmic irregularities. Perform annual physical exam. Use before menarche is not indicated. May affect certain endocrine, LFTs and blood components.

**ADVERSE REACTIONS:** Nausea, vomiting, breakthrough bleeding, spotting, amenorrhea, migraine, depression, vaginal candidiasis, edema, weight changes.



**INTERACTIONS:** Reduced effects, increased breakthrough bleeding, and menstrual irregularities with rifampin, barbiturates, phenylbutazone, phenytoin, carbamazepine ,and possibly with griseofulvin, ampicillin, and tetracyclines.

**PREGNANCY:** Category X, not for use in nursing.

## ORTHO-NOVUM 7/7/7 RX

norethindrone - ethinyl estradiol (Ortho-McNeil)

**OTHER BRAND NAMES:** Nortrel 7/7/7 (Barr)

**THERAPEUTIC CLASS:** Estrogen/progestogen combination

**INDICATIONS:** Prevention of pregnancy.

**DOSAGE:** *Adults:* Start 1st Sunday after menses begins or the 1st day of menses. *21-day:* 1 tab qd for 21 days, stop 7 days, then repeat. *28-day:* 1 tab qd for 28 days, then repeat.

**HOW SUPPLIED:** Tab: (Ethinyl Estradiol-Norethindrone) 0.035mg-0.5mg, 0.035mg-0.75mg and 0.035mg-1mg

**CONTRAINDICATIONS:** Thrombophlebitis, DVT or thromboembolic disorders, pregnancy, cerebrovascular or coronary artery disease, undiagnosed abnormal genital bleeding, cholestatic jaundice of pregnancy or jaundice with prior pill use, hepatic adenomas or carcinomas, breast cancer or other estrogen-dependent neoplasia.

**WARNINGS/PRECAUTIONS:** Cigarette smoking increases risk of serious cardiovascular side effects. This risk increases with age (especially >35 yrs) and heavy smoking. Increased risk of MI, vascular disease, thromboembolism, stroke and gallbladder disease. Retinal thrombosis, hepatic neoplasia, carcinoma of breast and reproductive organs reported. May cause glucose intolerance. May increase BP, elevate LDL levels or cause other lipid changes, fluid retention, breakthrough bleeding, and spotting. May cause or exacerbate migraine. May develop visual changes with contact lens. Increased risk of MI with HTN, hyperlipidemia, obesity, and diabetes. Discontinue if develop jaundice, significant depression or ophthalmic irregularities. Perform annual physical exam. Use before menarche is not indicated. May affect certain endocrine, LFTs and blood components.

**ADVERSE REACTIONS:** Nausea, vomiting, breakthrough bleeding, spotting, amenorrhea, migraine, depression, vaginal candidiasis, edema, weight changes.

**INTERACTIONS:** Reduced effects, increased breakthrough bleeding, and menstrual irregularities with rifampin, barbiturates, phenylbutazone, phenytoin, carbamazepine, griseofulvin, topiramate, St. John's wort, and possibly with ampicillin and tetracyclines.

**PREGNANCY:** Category X, not for use in nursing.

## Ovace — RX

sulfacetamide sodium (Healthpoint)

**THERAPEUTIC CLASS:** Sulfonamide

**INDICATIONS:** Topical application for seborrheic dermatitis, seborrhea sicca (dandruff). Treatment of secondary bacterial infections of the skin.

**DOSAGE:** *Adults:* Seborrheic Dermatitis/Dandruff: (Cream/Gel/Foam) Apply to affected area bid for 8-10 days. (Wash) Wash affected area bid for 8-10 days. To prevent recurrence, apply once or twice weekly, or every other week. Bacterial Infection: (Cream/Gel) Apply to affected area bid for 8-10 days. (Foam) Apply to affected area qd for 8-10 days. (Wash) Wash affected area qd for 8-10 days.

**HOW SUPPLIED:** Cre: 10% [30g, 60g]; Gel: 10% [30g, 60g]; Foam: 10% [50g, 100g]; Wash: 10% [170mL, 340mL]

**CONTRAINDICATIONS:** Hypersensitivity to sulfonamides.

**WARNINGS/PRECAUTIONS:** Stevens-Johnson syndrome in hypersensitive individuals, and systemic lupus erythematous reported with sulfonamides. May cause proliferation of nonsusceptible organisms. Discontinue if hypersensitivity or untoward reactions occur. Greater systemic absorption in application to large, infected, abraded, denuded or severely burned area.

**ADVERSE REACTIONS:** Irritation, hypersensitivity.

**INTERACTIONS:** Incompatible with silver preparations.

**PREGNANCY:** Category C, caution in nursing.

## Ovcon-35 — RX

norethindrone - ethinyl estradiol (Warner Chilcott)

**OTHER BRAND NAMES:** Ovcon-50 (Warner Chilcott)

**THERAPEUTIC CLASS:** Estrogen/progestogen combination

**INDICATIONS:** Prevention of pregnancy.

**DOSAGE:** *Adults:* 1 tab qd for 28 days, then repeat. Start 1st Sunday after menses begin or the 1st day of menses.

**HOW SUPPLIED:** (Ethinyl Estradiol-Norethindrone) Tab: (Ovcon 35) 0.035mg-0.4mg; (Ovcon 50) 0.05mg-1mg

**CONTRAINDICATIONS:** Thrombophlebitis, DVT or thromboembolic disorders, pregnancy, cerebrovascular or coronary artery disease, valvular heart disease with thrombogenic complications, uncontrolled HTN, DM with vascular involvement, HA with focal neurological symptoms, major surgery with prolonged immobilization, undiagnosed abnormal genital bleeding, cholestatic jaundice of pregnancy or jaundice with prior pill use, hepatic adenomas or carcinomas, breast cancer, endometrial cancer or other estrogen-dependent neoplasia.

**WARNINGS/PRECAUTIONS:** Cigarette smoking increases risk of serious cardiovascular side effects. This risk increases with age (especially >35 yrs) and heavy smoking. Increased risk of MI, vascular disease, thromboembolism, stroke and gallbladder disease. Retinal thrombosis, hepatic neoplasia, carcinoma of breast and reproductive organs reported. May cause glucose intolerance. May increase BP, elevate LDL levels or cause other lipid changes, fluid retention, breakthrough bleeding, and spotting. May cause or exacerbate migraine. May develop visual changes with contact lens. Increased risk of MI with HTN, hyperlipidemia, obesity, and diabetes. D/C if develop jaundice, significant depression or ophthalmic irregularities. Perform annual physical exam. Use before menarche is not indicated. May affect certain endocrine, LFTs and blood components.

**ADVERSE REACTIONS:** Nausea, vomiting, breakthrough bleeding, spotting, amenorrhea, migraine, depression, vaginal candidiasis, edema, weight changes.

**INTERACTIONS:** Reduced effects, increased breakthrough bleeding, and menstrual irregularities with rifampin, barbiturates, phenylbutazone, phenytoin, carbamazepine, felbamate, oxcarbazepine, topiramate, griseofulvin, ampicillin, and tetracyclines. Anti-HIV PIs may change (increase or decrease) the levels of OCs. Herbal products, such as St. John's Wort may reduce the levels of OCs and result in breakthrough bleeding. Atorvastatin, ascorbic acid, acetaminophen, CYP3A4 inhibitors (itraconazole or ketoconazole) may increase the levels of ehinyl estradiol. Increased levels of cyclosporin, prednisolone, theophylline reported. Decreased levels of actaminophen and increased clearance of temazepam, salicylic acid, morphine, clofibric acid reported.



**PREGNANCY:** Category X, not for use in nursing.

## Ovcon-35 Fe RX

norethindrone - ferrous fumarate - ethinyl estradiol (Warner Chilcott)

**THERAPEUTIC CLASS:** Estrogen/progestogen combination

**INDICATIONS:** Prevention of pregnancy.

**DOSAGE:** *Adults:* 1 tab qd for 28 days, then repeat. Start 1st Sunday after menses begin or the 1st day of menses.

**HOW SUPPLIED:** Tab, Chewable: (Ethinyl Estradiol-Norethindrone) 0.035mg-0.4mg [21s], (Ferrous Fumarate) 75mg [7s]

**CONTRAINDICATIONS:** Thrombophlebitis, DVT or thromboembolic disorders, pregnancy, cerebrovascular or coronary artery disease, valvular heart disease with thrombogenic complications, uncontrolled HTN, DM with vascular involvement, HA with focal neurological symptoms, major surgery with prolonged immobilization, undiagnosed abnormal genital bleeding, cholestatic jaundice of pregnancy or jaundice with prior pill use, hepatic adenomas or carcinomas, breast cancer, endometrial cancer or other estrogen-dependent neoplasia.

**WARNINGS/PRECAUTIONS:** Cigarette smoking increases risk of serious cardiovascular side effects. This risk increases with age (especially >35 yrs) and heavy smoking. Increased risk of MI, vascular disease, thromboembolism, stroke and gallbladder disease. Retinal thrombosis, hepatic neoplasia, carcinoma of breast and reproductive organs reported. May cause glucose intolerance. May increase BP, elevate LDL levels or cause other lipid changes, fluid retention, breakthrough bleeding, and spotting. May cause or exacerbate migraine. May develop visual changes with contact lens. Increased risk of MI with HTN, hyperlipidemia, obesity, and diabetes. Discontinue if develop jaundice, significant depression or ophthalmic irregularities. Perform annual physical exam. Use before menarche is not indicated. May affect certain endocrine, LFTs and blood components.

**ADVERSE REACTIONS:** Nausea, vomiting, breakthrough bleeding, spotting, amenorrhea, migraine, depression, vaginal candidiasis, edema, weight changes.

**INTERACTIONS:** Reduced effects, increased breakthrough bleeding, and menstrual irregularities with rifampin, barbiturates, phenylbutazone, phenytoin, carbamazepine, felbamate, oxcarbazepine, topiramate, griseofulvin, ampicillin, and tetracyclines. Anti-HIV PIs may change (increase or decrease) the levels of OCs. Herbal products, such as St. John's Wort may reduce the levels of OCs and result in breakthrough bleeding. Atorvastatin, ascorbic acid, acetaminophen, CYP3A4 inhibitors (itraconazole or ketoconazole) may increase the levels of ehinyl estradiol. Increased levels of cyclosporin, prednisolone, theophylline reported. Decreased levels of actaminophen and increased clearance of temazepam, salicylic acid, morphine, clofibric acid reported.

**PREGNANCY:** Category X, not for use in nursing.

## OVIDE

malathion (Taro)

RX

**THERAPEUTIC CLASS:** Organophosphate/cholinesterase inhibitor

**INDICATIONS:** For infections of *Pediculus humanus capitis* (head lice and their ova) of scalp hair.

**DOSAGE:** *Adults:* Apply sufficient amount on dry hair to thoroughly wet hair and scalp. Allow hair to dry naturally. Shampoo after 8-12 hrs. Rinse and use a fine-toothed comb to remove dead lice and eggs. Repeat with 2nd application if lice present after 7-9 days.
*Pediatrics:* >6 yrs: Apply sufficient amount on dry hair to thoroughly wet hair and scalp. Allow hair to dry naturally. Shampoo after 8-12 hrs. Rinse and use a fine-toothed comb to remove dead lice and eggs. Repeat with 2nd application if lice present after 7-9 days.

**HOW SUPPLIED:** Lot: 0.5% [59mL]

**CONTRAINDICATIONS:** Neonates, infants.

**WARNINGS/PRECAUTIONS:** Lotion is flammable; do not expose lotion or wet hair to open flames or electric heat sources (eg, hair dryers, electric curlers). If contact with eyes, flush immediately with water. If skin irritation develops, d/c until irritation clears. Slight stinging sensations reported. Adult supervision is required with use in children.

**ADVERSE REACTIONS:** Skin and scalp irritation, mild conjunctivitis (with eye contact).

**PREGNANCY:** Category B, caution in nursing.

## OVIDREL

choriogonadotropin alfa (Serono)

RX

**THERAPEUTIC CLASS:** Recombinant human chorionic gonadotropin

**INDICATIONS:** For induction of final follicular maturation and early luteinization in infertile women who have undergone pituitary desensitization and pretreated with follicle stimulating hormone in an Assisted Reproductive Technology program. To induce ovulation and pregnancy in anovulatory, infertile women in whom anovulation is not due to primary ovarian failure.

**DOSAGE:** *Adults:* 250mcg SQ 1 day following the last dose of follicle stimulating agent. Withhold if excessive ovarian response.

**HOW SUPPLIED:** Inj: 250mcg/0.5mL

**CONTRAINDICATIONS:** Primary ovarian failure, uncontrolled thyroid or adrenal function, uncontrolled organic intracranial lesion (eg, pituitary tumor), abnormal uterine bleeding of undetermined origin, ovarian cyst or enlargement of undetermined origin, sex hormone dependent tumors of reproductive tract and accessory organs, pregnancy.

**WARNINGS/PRECAUTIONS:** Ovarian hyperstimulation syndrome (OHSS), multiple births, and elevated ALTs reported. Potential for arterial thromboembolism. Withhold hCG if ovarian enlargement or OHSS occurs. Administer when adequate follicular development indicated by serum estradiol and vaginal ultrasonography occurs.

**ADVERSE REACTIONS:** Injection site pain/bruising, abdominal pain, nausea, vomiting.

**PREGNANCY:** Category X, caution in nursing.

## OXANDRIN

CIII

oxandrolone (Savient)

**THERAPEUTIC CLASS:** Anabolic steroid

**INDICATIONS:** Adjunctive therapy to promote weight gain after weight loss following extensive surgery, chronic infections, severe trauma, and for those who fail to gain or maintain normal weight without pathophysiologic reasons, to offset protein catabolism associated with prolonged administration of corticosteroids, for the relief of osteoporotic bone pain.

**DOSAGE:** *Adults:* Usual: 2.5-20mg/day given bid-qid for 2-4 weeks. May repeat course intermittently as indicated. Elderly: 5mg bid.
*Pediatrics:* ≤0.1mg/kg/day. May repeat intermittently as indicated.



**HOW SUPPLIED:** Tab: 2.5mg*, 10mg *scored

**CONTRAINDICATIONS:** Carcinoma of the prostate or breast, carcinoma of the breast in females with hypercalcemia, pregnancy, nephrosis, hypercalcemia.

**WARNINGS/PRECAUTIONS:** D/C if peliosis hepatis, liver cell tumors, cholestatic hepatitis, jaundice, LFT abnormalities, hypercalcemia or signs of virilization (females) occur. Edema, with or without CHF, may occur with pre-existing cardiac, renal, or hepatic disease. Monitor bone growth in children every 6 months. Increased risk of prostatic hypertrophy/carcinoma in the elderly. May decrease levels of thyroxine-binding globulin, suppress clotting factors II, V, VII, and X and increase PT. Caution with CAD and history of MI. Lower dose recommended in elderly.

**ADVERSE REACTIONS:** Cholestatic jaundice, gynecomastia, edema, CNS effects, acne, phallic enlargement, increased frequency/persistence of erections, inhibition of testicular function, chronic priapism, epididymitis, impotence, testicular atrophy, oligospermia, bladder irritability, menstrual irregularities, virilization.

**INTERACTIONS:** Increased sensitivity to oral anticoagulants (eg, warfarin). May increase edema with adrenal cortical steroids or ACTH. May inhibit metabolism of oral hypoglycemics.

**PREGNANCY:** Category X, not for use in nursing.

## OXAZEPAM

CIV

oxazepam (Various)

**THERAPEUTIC CLASS:** Benzodiazepine

**INDICATIONS:** Management of anxiety and alcohol withdrawal.

**DOSAGE:** *Adults:* Anxiety: Mild-Moderate: 10-15mg tid-qid. Severe: 15-30mg tid-qid. Elderly: Initial: 10mg tid. Titrate: Increase to 15mg tid-qid. Alcohol Withdrawal: 15-30mg tid-qid.

**HOW SUPPLIED:** Cap: 10mg, 15mg, 30mg; Tab: 15mg

**CONTRAINDICATIONS:** Psychoses.

**WARNINGS/PRECAUTIONS:** May impair mental/physical abilities. Withdrawal symptoms with abrupt discontinuation. Caution in sensitivity to hypotension, elderly. Caution with tablets in tartrazine or ASA allergy. Risk of congenital malformations; avoid in pregnancy.

**ADVERSE REACTIONS:** Drowsiness, dizziness, vertigo, headache, paradoxical excitement, transient amnesia, memory impairment.

**INTERACTIONS:** Additive effects with alcohol and other CNS depressants.

**PREGNANCY:** Not for use in pregnancy or nursing.

## OXISTAT RX

oxiconazole nitrate (GlaxoSmithKline)

**THERAPEUTIC CLASS:** Azole antifungal

**INDICATIONS:** (Cre/Lot) Topical treatment of tinea pedis, tinea cruris and tinea corporis due to *Trichophyton rubrum*, *Trichophyton mentagrophytes* , or *Epidermophyton floccosum*. (Cre) Topical treatment of tinea versicolor due to *Malassezia furfur*.

**DOSAGE:** *Adults:* (Cre/Lot) T.pedis/T.corporis/T.cruris: Apply qd-bid. (Cre) T.versicolor: Apply qd. Treat t.pedis for 1 month and other infections for 2 weeks.
*Pediatrics:* >12 yrs: (Cream) T.pedis/T.corporis/T.cruris: Apply qd-bid. T.versicolor: Apply qd. Treat t.pedis for 1 month and other infections for 2 weeks.

**HOW SUPPLIED:** Cre: 1% [15g, 30g, 60g]; Lot: 1% [30mL]

**WARNINGS/PRECAUTIONS:** Not for ophthalmic or intravaginal use. D/C if irritation or sensitivity occurs.

**ADVERSE REACTIONS:** Pruritus, burning/stinging.

**PREGNANCY:** Category B, caution in nursing.

## OXSORALEN RX

methoxsalen (Valeant)

**THERAPEUTIC CLASS:** Psoralen

**INDICATIONS:** As a topical repigmenting agent in vitiligo with controlled doses of UVA (320-400nm) or sunlight.

**DOSAGE:** *Adults:* Apply to small well defined lesions before UVA exposure. Determine treatment intervals by erythema response; generally 1 week or less often.
*Pediatrics:* >12 yrs: Apply to small well defined lesions before UVA exposure. Determine treatment intervals by erythema response; generally 1 week or less often.

**HOW SUPPLIED:** Lot: 1% [30mL]

**CONTRAINDICATIONS:** Current or history of melanoma, invasive skin carcinoma, photosensitive diseases (eg, acute lupus erythematosus, porphyria, xeroderma pigmentosum), patients <12 yrs.

**WARNINGS/PRECAUTIONS:** May develop serious burns if exceed recommended dose or exposure. Protect treated areas from sunlight. Increased risk of skin cancer in fair-skinned patients or prior coal tar UVA treatment, ionizing radiation, or taken arsenical compounds. Protect treated areas from light by using protective clothing or sunscreen.

**ADVERSE REACTIONS:** Minor blistering, severe burns (from overexposure to UVA).

**INTERACTIONS:** Caution with photosensitizers such as anthralin, coal tar and its derivatives, griseofulvin, phenothiazines, nalidixic acid, halogenated salicylanilides, sulfonamides, tetracyclines, thiazides, and certain organic staining dyes (eg, methylene blue, toluidine blue, rose bengal, methyl orange).

**PREGNANCY:** Category C, caution in nursing.

## OXSORALEN-ULTRA

RX

methoxsalen (Valeant)

**Risk of ocular damage, aging skin, and skin cancer. Determine minimum phototoxic dose (MPD) and phototoxic peak time after drug administration and before photochemotherapy. Do not interchange with regular Oxsoralen® or 8-Mop®.**

**THERAPEUTIC CLASS:** Psoralen

**INDICATIONS:** Photochemotherapy (methoxsalen with long wave UVA radiation) is for symptomatic control of severe, recalcitrant, disabling psoriasis (supported by a biopsy).

**DOSAGE:** *Adults:* Initial: <30kg: 10mg. 30-50kg: 20mg. 51-65kg: 30mg. 66-80kg: 40mg. 81-90kg: 50mg. 91-115kg: 60mg. >115kg: 70mg. Take 1.5-2 hrs before UVA exposure with a low fat meal or milk. Titrate: May increase by 10mg after 15th treatment under certain conditions. Max: Do not treat more often than every other day.

**HOW SUPPLIED:** Cap: 10mg

**CONTRAINDICATIONS:** History of light sensitive diseases (eg, lupus erythematosus, porphyria cutanea tarda, erythropoietic protoporphyria, variegate porphyria, xeroderma pigmentosum, albinism), history/active melanoma, invasive squamous cell carcinoma, aphakia.



**WARNINGS/PRECAUTIONS:** May develop serious burns if exceed recommended dose or exposure. Increase risk of squamous cell carcinoma with pre-PUVA exposure to prolonged tar/UVB treatment, ionizing radiation, or arsenic. Diligently observe and treat basal cell carcinomas. Patients should wear UVA-absorbing, wrap-around sunglasses for 24 hrs after methoxsalen ingestion to avoid cataractogenicity. Sunlight/UV radiation exposure may cause premature skin aging. Monitor for carcinomas with history of x-ray, genz ray, or arsenic therapy. Caution with hepatic impairment. Avoid vertical UVA chamber with cardiac disease. Ophthalmologic exam before therapy, then yearly. Obtain routine lab test before therapy, regularly thereafter. Avoid sunbathing 24 hrs before or 48 hrs post treatment. Avoid sun exposure 8 hrs after ingestion. Protect eyes, abdominal skin, breasts, genitalia, and other sensitive areas during PUVA therapy.

**ADVERSE REACTIONS:** Nausea, nervousness, insomnia, depression, pruritus, erythema.

**INTERACTIONS:** Caution with photosensitizers such as anthralin, coal tar and its derivatives, griseofulvin, phenothiazines, nalidixic acid, halogenated salicylanilides, sulfonamides, tetracyclines, thiazides, and certain organic staining dyes (eg, methylene blue, toluidine blue, rose bengal, methyl orange).

**PREGNANCY:** Category C, not for use in nursing.

## OXYCONTIN

CII

oxycodone HCl (Purdue Pharma)

**For continuous analgesia. Abuse potential. 80mg and 160mg tabs are only for opioid-tolerant patients. Swallow tabs whole.**

**THERAPEUTIC CLASS:** Opioid analgesic

**INDICATIONS:** Management of moderate to severe pain when a continuous analgesic is needed for an extended period. Only for postoperative use in patients already receiving the drug before surgery or those expected to have moderate-severe postoperative pain for an extended period of time.

**DOSAGE:** *Adults:* >18 yrs: Opioid Naive: 10mg q12h. Titrate: May increase to 20mg q12h, then may increase the total daily dose by 25-50% of the current dose. Increase every 1-2 days. Conversion from Oxycodone: Divide 24 hr oxycodone dose in half to obtain the q12h dose. Round down to appropriate tab strength. Opioid Tolerant Patients: May use 80mg or 160mg tabs. Discontinue other around-the-clock opioids. With CNS depressants: Reduce dose by 1/3 or 1/2. Swallow whole; do not break, crush, or chew. High-fat meals increase peak levels with 160mg tab.

**HOW SUPPLIED:** Tab, Extended Release: 10mg, 20mg, 40mg, 80mg, 160mg

**CONTRAINDICATIONS:** Significant respiratory depression, acute or severe bronchial asthma, hypercarbia, paralytic ileus.

**WARNINGS/PRECAUTIONS:** Do not break, chew, or crush tabs. Extreme caution with COPD, cor pulmonale, decreased respiratory reserve, hypoxia, hypercapnia, pre-existing respiratory depression. Caution with circulatory shock, delirium tremens, acute alcoholism, adrenocortical insufficiency, CNS depression, myxedema or hypothyroidism, BPH, severe hepatic/renal/pulmonary impairment, toxic psychosis, biliary tract disease, increased intracranial pressure, or head injury, elderly or debilitated. May cause severe hypotension. May produce drug dependence; caution in known drug abuse. May aggravate convulsive disorders and mask abdominal disorders.

**ADVERSE REACTIONS:** Respiratory depression, constipation, nausea, somnolence, dizziness, vomiting, pruritus, headache, dry mouth, sweating, asthenia.

**INTERACTIONS:** Respiratory depression, hypotension and profound sedation with other CNS depressants (eg, sedatives, anesthetics, phenothiazines, alcohol). Mixed agonist/antagonist analgesics may reduce the analgesic effect and/or cause withdrawal. Risk of severe hypotension with phenothiazines, or other agents that compromise vasomotor tone. May enhance skeletal muscle relaxant effects and increase respiratory depression. May interact with CYP2D6 inhibitors (eg, amiodarone, quinidine, polycyclic antidepressants). Caution with MAOIs.

**PREGNANCY:** Category B, not for use in nursing.



## OxyFast CII

oxycodone HCl (Purdue Pharma)

**OTHER BRAND NAMES:** OxyIR (Purdue Pharma)

**THERAPEUTIC CLASS:** Opioid analgesic

**INDICATIONS:** Moderate to moderately-severe pain.

**DOSAGE:** *Adults:* Usual: 5mg q6h prn for pain. May add to 30mL of juice or other liquid, applesauce, pudding, or other semi-solid foods.

**HOW SUPPLIED:** Cap: (OxyIR) 5mg; Sol: (OxyFast) 20mg/mL [30mL]

**CONTRAINDICATIONS:** Respiratory depression, acute or severe bronchial asthma, hypercarbia, paralytic ileus, situations where opioids are contraindicated.

**WARNINGS/PRECAUTIONS:** Extreme caution with COPD, cor pulmonale, decreased respiratory reserve, hypoxia, hypercapnia, pre-existing respiratory depression. Caution with circulatory shock, delirium tremens, acute alcoholism, adrenocortical insufficiency, CNS depression, myxedema or hypothyroidism, BPH, severe hepatic/renal/pulmonary impairment, toxic psychosis, biliary tract disease, increased intracranial pressure, or head injury, elderly or debilitated. May cause severe hypotension. May produce drug dependence; caution in known drug abuse. May aggravate convulsive disorders and mask abdominal disorders.

**ADVERSE REACTIONS:** Lightheadedness, dizziness, nausea, vomiting, sedation.

**INTERACTIONS:** Respiratory depression, hypotension and profound sedation with other CNS depressants (eg, sedatives, anesthetics, phenothiazines, alcohol). Mixed agonist/antagonist analgesics may reduce the analgesic effect and/or cause withdrawal. Risk of severe hypotension with phenothiazines, or other agents that compromise vasomotor tone. May enhance skeletal muscle relaxant effects and increase respiratory depression. May interact with CYP2D6 inhibitors (eg, amiodarone, quinidine, polycyclic antidepressants). Caution with MAOIs.

**PREGNANCY:** Category B, not for use in nursing.

## OXYTROL RX
oxybutynin (Watson)

**THERAPEUTIC CLASS:** Anticholinergic

**INDICATIONS:** Treatment of overactive bladder with symptoms of urge urinary incontinence, urgency, and frequency.

**DOSAGE:** *Adults:* Apply to dry, intact skin on the abdomen, hip, or buttock twice weekly (every 3-4 days). Rotate sites.

**HOW SUPPLIED:** Patch: 3.9mg/day [8[s]]

**CONTRAINDICATIONS:** Urinary retention, gastric retention, uncontrolled narrow-angle glaucoma, and in patients at risk for these conditions.

**WARNINGS/PRECAUTIONS:** Caution with hepatic or renal impairment, bladder outflow obstruction, GI obstructive disorders, ulcerative colitis, intestinal atony, myasthenia gravis, and gastroesophageal reflux. Heat prostration may occur when used in a hot environment.

**ADVERSE REACTIONS:** Application site reactions, dry mouth, diarrhea, constipation, drowsiness, dizziness, blurred vision.

**INTERACTIONS:** Increased adverse events with other anticholinergics. Alcohol may enhance drowsiness effect. Caution with bisphosphonates or other drugs that may exacerbate esophagitis. May alter GI absorption of other drugs due to GI motility effects.



**PREGNANCY:** Category B, caution in nursing.

## PACERONE RX
amiodarone HCl (Upsher-Smith)

**THERAPEUTIC CLASS:** Class III antiarrhythmic

**INDICATIONS:** Treatment of documented, life-threatening recurrent ventricular fibrillation and recurrent hemodynamically unstable ventricular tachycardia.

**DOSAGE:** *Adults:* Give LD in hospital. LD: 800-1600mg/day in divided doses for 1-3 weeks. After control is achieved, then 600-800mg/day for 1 month. Maint: 400mg/day; up to 600mg/day if needed. Use lowest effective dose. Take with meals. Elderly: Start at low end of dosing range.

**HOW SUPPLIED:** Tab: 100mg, 200mg*, 300mg*, 400mg* *scored

**CONTRAINDICATIONS:** Severe sinus-node dysfunction causing marked sinus bradycardia; 2nd- and 3rd-degree AV block; when episodes of bradycardia have caused syncope (except when used with a pacemaker).

**WARNINGS/PRECAUTIONS:** Only for life-threatening arrhythmias due to its substantial toxicity (eg, pulmonary toxicity, hepatic injury, arrhythmia exacerbation). Hospitalize when giving LD. May cause a clinical syndrome of cough and progressive dyspnea. Discontinue if LFTs are 3X the normal or if an elevated baseline doubles; monitor LFTs regularly. Optic neuropathy, optic neuritis reported. Fetal harm in pregnancy. May develop reversible corneal micro deposits (eg, visual halos, blurred vision), photosensitivity, peripheral neuropathy (rare). May decrease $T_3$ levels, increase thyroxine levels, increase inactive reverse $T_3$ levels and can cause hypo- or hyperthyroidism. Adult Respiratory Distress Syndrome reported with surgery. Correct $K^+$ or magnesium deficiency before therapy. Caution in elderly.

**ADVERSE REACTIONS:** Pulmonary toxicity (inflammation, fibrosis), arrhythmia exacerbation, hepatic injury, malaise, fatigue, tremor, poor coordination, paresthesis, nausea, vomiting, constipation, anorexia, ophthalmic abnormalities, photosensitivity.

**INTERACTIONS:** Risk of interactions after discontinuation due to its long half-life. May increase sensitivity to myocardial depressant and conduction effects of halogenated inhalation anesthetics. Elevates cyclosporine plasma levels. Discontinue or reduce digoxin dose by 50%. Discontinue or decrease warfarin dose by 1/3-1/2. Caution with β-blockers, calcium blockers. May increase levels of quinidine, procainamide and phenytoin. Initiate added antiarrhythmic drug at lower than usual dose. Discontinue or decrease quinidine dose by 1/3-1/2. Discontinue or decrease procainamide dose by 1/3.

**PREGNANCY:** Category D, not for use in nursing.

## PALGIC RX
carbinoxamine maleate (PamLab)

**THERAPEUTIC CLASS:** $H_1$ antagonist

**INDICATIONS:** Seasonal and perennial allergic rhinitis, vasomotor rhinitis, allergic conjunctivitis, urticaria, angioedema, dermatographism, allergic reactions to blood or plasma. Adjunct in anaphylaxis.

**DOSAGE:** *Adults:* Usual: 4mg prn. Max: 24mg/day given q6-8h. *Pediatrics:* ≥6 yrs: Usual: 4mg prn. Max: 24mg/day given q6-8h. 1-6 yrs: Usual: 2mg prn. May increase to 0.2-0.4mg/kg/day given q6-8h.

**HOW SUPPLIED:** Sol: 4mg/5mL; Tab: 4mg* *scored

**CONTRAINDICATIONS:** Concomitant MAOIs, newborns, premature infants, lower respiratory tract disorders (eg, asthma), nursing mothers.

P

**WARNINGS/PRECAUTIONS:** Caution in narrow angle glaucoma, stenosing peptic ulcer, symptomatic prostatic hypertrophy, bladder neck or pyloroduodenal obstruction, history of bronchial asthma, increased IOP, hyperthyroidism, CVD, HTN, and elderly. May impair mental/physicial abilities.

**ADVERSE REACTIONS:** Sedation, sleepiness, dizziness, disturbed coordination, epigastric distress, thickening of bronchial secretions, excitation, diminished mental alertness.

**INTERACTIONS:** See Contraindications. Intensified anticholinergic effects with MAOIs; avoid concurrent use. Additive effects with alcohol, other CNS depressants (eg, hypnotics, sedatives, tranquilizers).

**PREGNANCY:** Category C, not for use in nursing.

## PAMELOR RX
nortriptyline HCl (Mallinckrodt)

**Antidepressants increased the risk of suicidal thinking and behavior (suicidality) in short-term studies in children and adolescents with Major Depressive Disorder and other psychiatric disorders. Nortriptyline is not approved for use in pediatric patients.**

**THERAPEUTIC CLASS:** Tricyclic antidepressant

**INDICATIONS:** Relief of symptoms of depression.

**DOSAGE:** *Adults:* 25mg tid-qid. Max: 150mg/day. Total daily dose may be given once a day. Monitor serum levels if dose >100mg/day. Elderly/Adolescents: 30-50mg/day in single or divided doses.

**HOW SUPPLIED:** Cap: 10mg, 25mg, 50mg, 75mg; Sol: 10mg/5mL

**CONTRAINDICATIONS:** MAOI use within 14 days, acute recovery period following MI.

**WARNINGS/PRECAUTIONS:** MI, arrhythmia, strokes have occurred. Caution with cardiovascular disease, glaucoma, history of urinary retention, hyperthyroidism. May lower seizure threshold, exacerbate psychosis or activate schizophrenia, cause symptoms of mania in bipolar disease, or alter glucose levels. Discontinue several days prior to elective surgery.

**ADVERSE REACTIONS:** Arrhythmias, hypotension, HTN, tachycardia, MI, heart block, stroke, confusion, hallucination, insomnia, tremors, ataxia, anxiety, dry mouth, blurred vision, skin rash, extrapyramidal symptoms, photosensitivity, SIADH, anorexia.

**INTERACTIONS:** See Contraindications. May block guanethidine effects. Arrhythmia risk with thyroid agents. Alcohol may potentiate effects."Stimulating" effect with reserpine. Monitor with anticholinergic and sympathomimetic drugs. Increased plasma levels with cimetidine. Hypoglycemia reported with chlorpropamide. SSRIs, antidepressants, phenothiazines, propafenone, flecainide and CYP2D6 inhibitors (eg, quinidine) may potentiate effects. Decreased clearance with quinidine.

**PREGNANCY:** Safety during pregnancy and nursing not known.

## PAMINE

RX

methscopolamine bromide (Kenwood Therapeutics)

**OTHER BRAND NAMES:** Pamine Forte (Kenwood Therapeutics)

**THERAPEUTIC CLASS:** Anticholinergic

**INDICATIONS:** Adjunctive therapy for the treatment of peptic ulcer.

**DOSAGE:** *Adults:* 2.5mg tid 30 minutes ac and 2.5-5mg qhs. Severe Symptoms: 5mg 30 minutes ac and qhs. Max: 30mg/day.



**HOW SUPPLIED:** Tab: 2.5mg; (Forte) 5mg

**CONTRAINDICATIONS:** Glaucoma, obstructive uropathy, obstructive GI disease, paralytic ileus, intestinal atony of the elderly or debilitated, unstable cardiovascular status in acute hemorrhage, severe ulcerative colitis, toxic megacolon, myasthenia gravis.

**WARNINGS/PRECAUTIONS:** Heat prostration may occur with high environmental temperatures. Avoid or discontinue use if diarrhea develops, especially with ileostomy or colostomy. Caution in elderly, autonomic neuropathy, hepatic/renal disease, ulcerative colitis, hyperthyroidism, coronary heart disease, CHF, tachyrhythmia, tachycardia, HTN, or prostatic hypertrophy. May impair mental/physical abilities.

**ADVERSE REACTIONS:** Constipation, decreased sweating, headache, drowsiness, dizziness.

**INTERACTIONS:** Additive anticholinergic effects with antipsychotics, TCAs, and other drugs with anticholinergic effects. Antacids may interfere with absorption.

**PREGNANCY:** Category C, caution in nursing.

## PANAFIL

RX

urea - papain - chlorophyllin copper complex sodium (Healthpoint)

**THERAPEUTIC CLASS:** Proteolytic enzyme (debriding/healing agent)

**INDICATIONS:** Treatment of acute and chronic lesions such as varicose, diabetic and decubitus ulcers, burns, postoperative wounds, pilonidal cyst wounds, carbuncles and other traumatic or infected wounds.

**DOSAGE:** *Adults:* (Oint, Spray) Clean wound, then apply qd-bid. Cover with dressing.

**HOW SUPPLIED:** Oint: (Chlorophyllin-Papain-Urea) 0.5%-10%-10% [6g, 30g]; Spray: (Chlorophyllin-Papain-Urea) 0.5%-10%-10% [33mL]

**WARNINGS/PRECAUTIONS:** Not for ophthalmic use.

**ADVERSE REACTIONS:** Transient burning, skin irritation.

**INTERACTIONS:** May be inactivated by hydrogen peroxide, salts of heavy metals (eg, lead, silver, mercury).

**PREGNANCY:** Safety in pregnancy and nursing not known.

## PANCREASE

RX

lipase - amylase - protease (McNeil Consumer)

**OTHER BRAND NAMES:** Pancrease MT (McNeil Consumer)

**THERAPEUTIC CLASS:** Pancreatic enzyme supplement

**INDICATIONS:** Treatment of steatorrhea secondary to pancreatic insufficiency such as cystic fibrosis (CF) and chronic alcoholic pancreatitis.

**DOSAGE:** *Adults:* Initial: 400 U lipase/kg/meal. Max: 2500 U lipase/kg/meal. Adjust dose based on 3-day fecal fat studies. Take with plenty of water. Do not chew/crush caps. May add capsule contents to soft food (pH <7.3) and swallow immediately without chewing.
*Pediatrics:* <12 months: 2000-4000 U lipase/120mL formula or per breast feeding. 13 months-3 yrs: Initial: 1000 U lipase/kg/meal. Max: 2500 U lipase/kg/meal. >4 yrs: Initial: 400U lipase/kg/meal. Max: 2500 U lipase/kg/meal. Adjust dose based on 3-day fecal fat studies. Take with plenty of water. Do not chew/crush caps. May add capsule contents to soft food (pH <7.3) and swallow immediately without chewing.

**HOW SUPPLIED:** Cap, Extended Release: (Amylase-Lipase-Protease) 20,000 U-4500 U-25,000 U, (MT 4) 12,000 U-4000 U-12,000 U, (MT 10) 30,000 U-10,000 U-30,000 U, (MT 16) 48,000 U-16,000 U-48,000 U, (MT 20) 56,000 U-20,000 U-44,000 U

**CONTRAINDICATIONS:** Pork protein hypersensitivity.

**WARNINGS/PRECAUTIONS:** May cause fibrotic strictures in colon of primarily CF patients. Caution when changing dose or brand of medication.

**ADVERSE REACTIONS:** Diarrhea, abdominal pain, intestinal obstruction, vomiting, flatulence, nausea, constipation, melena, perianal irritation, weight loss, pain.

**PREGNANCY:** Category B, safety in nursing not known.

## PANCURONIUM

RX

pancuronium bromide (Various)

**Administer by adequately trained individuals familiar with actions, characteristics, and hazards.**

**THERAPEUTIC CLASS:** Skeletal muscle relaxant (nondepolarizing)

**INDICATIONS:** Adjunct to general anesthesia, to facilitate endotracheal intubation, and to provide skeletal muscle relaxation during surgery or mechanical ventilation.

**DOSAGE:** *Adults:* Individualize dose. Initial: 0.04-0.1mg/kg IV. Late incremental doses of 0.01mg/kg may be used. Skeletal Muscle Relaxation For Endotracheal Intubation: 0.06-0.1mg/kg bolus.
*Pediatrics:* Individualize dose. Initial: 0.04-0.1mg/kg IV. Late incremental doses of 0.01mg/kg may be used. Skeletal Muscle Relaxation For Endotracheal Intubation: 0.06-0.1mg/kg bolus. Neonates: Use test dose of 0.02mg/kg.

**HOW SUPPLIED:** Inj: 1mg/mL, 2mg/mL

**WARNINGS/PRECAUTIONS:** May have profound effect in myasthenia gravis or myasthenic (Eaton Lambert) syndrome; use small test dose and monitor closely. Contains benzyl alcohol; caution in neonates. Use peripheral nerve stimulator to monitor neuromuscular blocking effect. Caution with pre-existing pulmonary, hepatic, or renal disease. Conditions associated with slower circulation time in cardiovascular disease, old age, and edematous states may delay onset time; dosage should not be increased. Possible slower onset, higher total dosage, and prolongation of neuromuscular blockade with hepatic and/or biliary tract disease. In ICU, long-term use may be associated with prolonged paralysis and/or skeletal muscle weakness; monitor closely. Severe obesity and neuromuscular disease may pose airway or ventilatory problems. Electrolyte imbalances may alter neuromuscular blockade.

**ADVERSE REACTIONS:** Skeletal muscle weakness and paralysis, salivation, rash.

**INTERACTIONS:** Prior administration of succinylcholine may enhance neuromuscular blocking effect. Avoid use with vercuronium, atracurium, d-tubocurarine, metocurine, gallamine. Enhanced neuromuscular blockade with enflurane, isoflurane, halothane, aminoglycosides, tetracyclines, bacitracin, polymyxin B, colistin, sodium colistimethate, and magnesium salts. Quinidine injection during recovery from use of other muscle relaxants suggests that recurrent paralysis may occur.

**PREGNANCY:** Category C, safety in nursing not known.

## PANDEL — RX

hydrocortisone probutate (CollaGenex)

P

**THERAPEUTIC CLASS:** Corticosteroid

**INDICATIONS:** Relief of the inflammatory and pruritic manifestations of corticosteroid-responsive dermatoses in patients ≥18 yrs.

**DOSAGE:** *Adults:* Apply qd-bid depending on severity of condition. Use occlusive dressing for refractory lesions of psoriasis and other deep-seated dermatoses.

**HOW SUPPLIED:** Cre: 0.1% [15g, 45g, 80g]

**WARNINGS/PRECAUTIONS:** May produce reversible HPA axis suppression, manifestations of Cushing's syndrome, hyperglycemia, glucosuria. Discontinue if irritation occurs. Use appropriate antifungal or antibacterial agent with dermatological infections. Pediatrics may be more susceptible to systemic toxicity. Caution when applied to large surface areas. Avoid eyes.

**ADVERSE REACTIONS:** Burning, stinging, moderate paresthesia, itching, dryness, folliculitis, hypertrichosis, acneiform eruptions, hypopigmentation, perioral dermatitis, skin atrophy, secondary infections, striae, millaria.

**PREGNANCY:** Category C, caution in nursing.

## PANIXINE — RX

cephalexin (Ranbaxy)

**THERAPEUTIC CLASS:** Cephalosporin (1st generation)

**INDICATIONS:** Skin and skin structure (SSSI), bone, genitourinary and respiratory tract infections, otitis media, acute prostatitis.

**DOSAGE:** *Adults*: ≥15 yrs:Usual: 250mg q6h. Streptococcal pharyngitis/SSSI: 500mg q12h. Cystitis: 500mg q12h for minimum of 7-14 days. Max: 4g/day. Do not crush, cut, or chew tab. Treat β-hemolytic streptococcal infections for ≥10 days.
*Pediatrics:* Usual: 25-50mg/kg/day in divided doses. Streptococcal Pharyngitis (>1 yr)/SSSI: May divide into 2 doses, give q12h. Otitis Media: 75-100mg/kg/day given qid. Treat β-hemolytic streptococcal infections for ≥10 days.

**HOW SUPPLIED:** Tab, Dispersible: 125mg, 250mg

**WARNINGS/PRECAUTIONS:** Caution with markedly impaired renal function, history of GI disease. Cross-sensitivity with cephalosporins and penicillins. Pseudomembranous colitis reported. False (+) direct Coombs' tests reported. False (+) for urine glucose with Benedict's, Fehling's solution, and Clinitest® tablets.

**ADVERSE REACTIONS:** Diarrhea, dyspepsia, gastritis, abdominal pain, allergic reactions, genital and anal pruritus, moniliasis, vaginitis, dizziness, fatigue, headache, superinfection (prolonged use).

**INTERACTIONS:** Probenecid inhibits excretion.Concomitant usage with metformin may require monitoring and dose adjustment.

**PREGNANCY:** Category B, caution in nursing.

## PANRETIN — RX

alitretinoin (Ligand)

**THERAPEUTIC CLASS:** Retinoid

**INDICATIONS:** Topical treatment of cutaneous lesions in patients with AIDS-related Kaposi's sarcoma (KS).

**DOSAGE:** *Adults:* Initial: Apply bid to lesions. Titrate: Gradually increase to tid-qid as tolerated. Allow to dry before covering with clothing. Reduce frequency if application site toxicity occurs. Discontinue temporarily if severe irritation occurs.

**HOW SUPPLIED:** Gel: 0.1% [60g]

**WARNINGS/PRECAUTIONS:** Avoid mucous membranes, normal skin. Not for use when systemic anti-KS therapy is required. Possible photosensitizing effects, treatment-limiting toxicities. Avoid occlusive dressings or in pregnancy.

**ADVERSE REACTIONS:** Rash, pain, pruritus, erythema, exfoliative dermatitis, skin disorder, paresthesia, edema.

**INTERACTIONS:** Avoid DEET-containing products (eg, insect repellents).

**PREGNANCY:** Category D, not for use in nursing.

## PARAFON FORTE DSC — RX

chlorzoxazone (Ortho-McNeil)

**THERAPEUTIC CLASS:** Muscular analgesic (central-acting)

**INDICATIONS:** Adjunct for relief of acute, painful musculoskeletal conditions.

**DOSAGE:** *Adults:* Usual: 500mg tid-qid. Titrate: May increase to 750mg tid-qid.

**HOW SUPPLIED:** Tab: 500mg* *scored

**WARNINGS/PRECAUTIONS:** Serious (including fatal) hepatocellular toxicity reported. D/C if signs of hepatotoxicity develop. Caution with history of drug allergies.

**ADVERSE REACTIONS:** Drowsiness, dizziness, malaise, lightheadedness, overstimulation.

**INTERACTIONS:** Additive effects with alcohol and CNS depressants.

**PREGNANCY:** Safety in pregnancy and nursing not known.

## PARCOPA
RX

levodopa - carbidopa (Schwarz)

**THERAPEUTIC CLASS:** Dopa-decarboxylase inhibitor/dopamine precursor

**INDICATIONS:** Treatment of symptoms of idiopathic Parkinson's disease, postencephalitic parkinsonism, and symptomatic parkinsonism.

**DOSAGE:** *Adults:* >18yrs: 25mg-100mg tab: Initial: 1 tab tid. Titrate: Increase by 1 tab qd or qod until 8 tabs/day. 10mg-100mg tab: Initial: 1 tab tid-qid. Titrate: Increase 1 tab qd or qod until 2 tabs qid. 70-100mg/day carbidopa required. Max 200mg/day carbidopa. Levodopa must be discontinued 12 hrs before starting carbidopa-levodopa.

**HOW SUPPLIED:** Tab, Disintegrating: (Carbidopa-Levodopa) 10mg-100mg*, 25mg-100mg*, 25mg-250mg* *scored

**CONTRAINDICATIONS:** MAOIs during or within 14 days of use, narrow-angle glaucoma, suspicious, undiagnosed skin lesions, history of melanoma.

**WARNINGS/PRECAUTIONS:** Dyskinesias and mental disturbances may occur. Caution with severe cardiovascular or pulmonary disease, bronchial asthma, renal or hepatic disease, endocrine disease, chronic wide-angle glaucoma, peptic ulcer, and MI with residual arrhythmias. NMS reported during dose reduction or withdrawal. Dark color may appear in saliva, urine, or sweat. May cause false (+) ketonuria or false (-) glucosuria (glucose-oxidase method).

**ADVERSE REACTIONS:** Dyskinesias, choreiform, dystonic, other involuntary movements, nausea.

**INTERACTIONS:** See Contraindications. Risk of postural hypotension with antihypertensives, selegiline. HTN and dyskinesia may occur with TCAs. Reduced effects with dopamine $D_2$ antagonists (eg, phenothiazines, butyrophenones, risperidone), isoniazid. Antagonized by phenytoin, papaverine, metoclopramide. Reduced bioavailability with iron salts, high-protein diets.

**PREGNANCY:** Category C, caution in nursing

## PAREMYD
RX

tropicamide - hydroxyamphetamine hbr (Akorn)

P

**THERAPEUTIC CLASS:** Adrenergic/anticholinergic agent

**INDICATIONS:** For mydriasis in routine diagnostic procedures and in conditions where short-term pupil dilation is desired.

**DOSAGE:** *Adults:* 1-2 drops in conjunctival sac.

**HOW SUPPLIED:** Sol: (Hydroxyamphetamine-Tropicamide) 1%-0.25% [15mL]

**CONTRAINDICATIONS:** Angle-closure glaucoma, patients with narrow angles in whom pupil dilation may precipitate angle-closure glaucoma attack.

**WARNINGS/PRECAUTIONS:** For topical ophthalmic use only. May produce transient IOP elevation in open-angle glaucoma. May cause CNS disturbances. Monitor patients with HTN, hyperthyroidism, DM, cardiac disease, elderly, and those who may encounter glaucoma/increased IOP.

**ADVERSE REACTIONS:** Increased IOP, transient stinging, dry mouth, blurred vision, photophobia, tachycardia, headache, allergic reactions, nausea, vomiting, pallor, muscle rigidity.

**PREGNANCY:** Category C, caution in nursing.

## PARLODEL RX

bromocriptine mesylate (Novartis)

**THERAPEUTIC CLASS:** Dopamine receptor agonist

**INDICATIONS:** Management of hyperprolactinemia including amenorrhea with or without galactorrhea, infertility, or hypogonadism. Treatment of prolactin-secreting adenomas, acromegaly, and symptoms of Parkinson's disease.

**DOSAGE:** *Adults:* Take with food. Parkinson's Disease: Initial: 1.25mg bid. Titrate: if needed, increase by 2.5mg/day every 2-4 weeks. Max: 100mg/day. Hyperprolactinemia: Initial: 1.25mg-2.5mg qd. Titrate: If needed, increase by 2.5mg every 2-7 days. Usual: 2.5-15mg/day. Acromegaly: Initial: 1.25-2.5mg qhs for 3 days. Titrate: Increase by 1.25-2.5mg every 3-7 days until optimal response. Usual: 20-30mg/day. Max: 100mg/day. Withdraw for 4-8 weeks every year in patients treated with pituitary irradiation.
*Pediatrics:* Take with food. 11-15 yrs: Prolactin-Secreting Pituitary Adenomas: Initial: 1.25-2.5mg/day. Titrate: Increase as tolerated. Usual: 2.5-10mg/day.

**HOW SUPPLIED:** Cap: 5mg; Tab: 2.5mg* *scored

**CONTRAINDICATIONS:** Uncontrolled HTN, ergot alkaloid sensitivity, postpartum with CVD unless withdrawal is medically contraindicated, pregnancy if treating hyperprolactinemia, HTN in pregnancy.

**WARNINGS/PRECAUTIONS:** Caution with renal or hepatic dysfunction, psychosis, CVD, peptic ulcer, dementia. Discontinue with macroadenomas associated with rapid regrowth of tumor and increased prolactin levels and if severe headache or HTN develops. Risk of pulmonary infiltrates, pleural effusion, thickening of pleura, and retroperitoneal fibrosis with long-term use. Not for prevention of physiological lactation. Monitor BP for symptomatic hypotension and HTN.

**ADVERSE REACTIONS:** Headache, dizziness, GI effects, orthostatic hypotension, fatigue, arrhythmia, insomnia, hallucinations, abnormal involuntary movements, depression, syncope.

**INTERACTIONS:** Decreased effects with dopamine antagonists (eg, butyrophenones, haloperidol, phenothiazines, pimozide, metoclopramide). Levodopa may cause hallucinations. Caution with antihypertensives. Alcohol may potentiate side effects. Not for use with other ergot alkaloids.

**PREGNANCY:** Category B, not for use in nursing.

P

## PARNATE RX

tranylcypromine sulfate (GlaxoSmithKline)

**Antidepressants increased the risk of suicidal thinking and behavior (suicidality) in short-term studies in children and adolescents with Major Depressive Disorder and other psychiatric disorders. Tranylcypromine is not approved for use in pediatric patients.**

**THERAPEUTIC CLASS:** Monoamine oxidase inhibitor

**INDICATIONS:** Treatment of major depressive episode without melancholia.

**DOSAGE:** *Adults:* Usual: 30mg/day in divided doses. Titrate: After 2 weeks, may increase by 10mg/day every 1-3 weeks depending on signs of improvement. Max: 60mg/day.

**HOW SUPPLIED:** Tab: 10mg

**CONTRAINDICATIONS:** Cardiovascular disorder, cerebrovascular disorder, HTN, history of headache, pheochromocytoma. Concomitant MAOIs, dibenzazepine derivatives, sympathomimetics (including amphetamines), some CNS depressants (including narcotics and alcohol), antihypertensives, diuretics, antihistamines, sedatives, anesthetics, bupropion, buspirone, meperidine, SSRIs, dexfenfluramine, dextromethorphan, foods with high tyramine content (cheese) and excessive quantities of caffeine. Elective surgery requiring general anesthesia. History of liver disease or abnormal LFTs. Caution with anti-parkinsonism drugs.

**WARNINGS/PRECAUTIONS:** Use in patients who are resistant to other therapies. Hypotension reported. Drug dependency possible in doses excessive of the therapeutic range. May suppress anginal pain in myocardial ischemia. Caution with hyperthyroidism, renal dysfunction, diabetes, elderly. May aggravate depression symptoms. May lower seizure threshold. Inhibits MAO 10 days after discontinuation. Discontinue at least 10 days before elective surgery. Discontinue if palpitations or frequent headaches occur.

**ADVERSE REACTIONS:** Restlessness, insomnia, weakness, drowsiness, nausea, diarrhea, tachycardia, anorexia, edema, tinnitis, muscle spasm, overstimulation, dizziness, dry mouth, blood dyscrasias.

**INTERACTIONS:** See Contraindications. Caution with disulfiram. Additive hypotensive effects with phenothiazines. Tryptophan may precipitate disorientation, memory impairment and other neurological and behavioral signs. Avoid metrizamide; discontinue 48hrs before myelography and may resume 24hrs post-procedure.

**PREGNANCY:** Safety in pregnancy and nursing not known.

## PASER RX

aminosalicylic acid (Jacobus)

**THERAPEUTIC CLASS:** Hydroxybenzoic acid derivative

**INDICATIONS:** Treatment of tuberculosis in combination with other agents.

**DOSAGE:** *Adults:* 4g tid. Sprinkle on apple sauce, yogurt, or mix with tomato or orange juice.
*Pediatrics:* Use correspondingly smaller doses to the adult dose.

**HOW SUPPLIED:** Packet: 4g

**CONTRAINDICATIONS:** Severe renal disease.

**WARNINGS/PRECAUTIONS:** Monitor for rash, or signs of intolerance during 1st 3 months. D/C if hypersensitivity occurs. Can desensitize by administering small, gradually increasing doses.

**ADVERSE REACTIONS:** Diarrhea, nausea, vomiting, abdominal pain, fever, dermatitis, lymphoma-like syndrome, agranulocytosis, thrombocytopenia, anemia, jaundice, hepatitis, hypoglycemia.

P

**INTERACTIONS:** Reduces acetylation of isoniazid, especially in rapid acetylators. Decreases vitamin $B_{12}$ absorption; consider vitamin $B_{12}$ maintenance treatment. Decreases digoxin levels.

**PREGNANCY:** Category C, safety in nursing not known.

## PATANOL RX

olopatadine HCl (Alcon)

**THERAPEUTIC CLASS:** $H_1$ antagonist and mast cell stabilizer

**INDICATIONS:** Allergic conjunctivitis.

**DOSAGE:** *Adults:* 1 drop bid, q6-8h.
*Pediatrics:* >3 yrs: 1 drop bid, q6-8h.

**HOW SUPPLIED:** Sol: 0.1% [5mL]

**WARNINGS/PRECAUTIONS:** May reinsert contact lens 10 minutes after dosing if eye is not red.

**ADVERSE REACTIONS:** Headache, asthenia, blurred vision, burning, stinging, cold syndrome, dry eye, foreign body sensation, hyperemia, hypersensitivity, keratitis, lid edema, nausea, pharyngitis, pruritus, rhinitis, sinusitis, taste perversion.

**PREGNANCY:** Category C, caution in nursing.

## PAXIL
paroxetine HCl (GlaxoSmithKline)

RX

**Antidepressants increased the risk of suicidal thinking and behavior (suicidality) in short-term studies in children and adolescents with Major Depressive Disorder (MDD) and other psychiatric disorders. Paroxetine is not approved for use in pediatric patients.**

**THERAPEUTIC CLASS:** Selective serotonin reuptake inhibitor

**INDICATIONS:** Treatment of major depressive disorder (MDD), panic disorder with or without agoraphobia. Treatment of obsessive compulsive disorder (OCD), social anxiety disorder (SAD), generalized anxiety disorder (GAD), and posttraumatic stress disorder (PTSD).

**DOSAGE:** *Adults:* Give qd, usually in the AM. MDD: Initial: 20mg/day. Max: 50mg/day. OCD: Initial: 20mg qd. Usual: 40mg qd. Max: 60mg/day. Panic Disorder: Initial: 10mg qd. Usual: 40mg/day. Max: 60mg/day. GAD: Initial: 20mg/day. Usual: 20-50mg/day. SAD: Initial/Usual: 20mg/day. PTSD: Initial: 20mg/day. Usual: 20-50mg/day. To titrate, may increase weekly by 10mg/day. Elderly/Debilitated/Severe Renal/Hepatic Impairment: Initial: 10mg qd. Max: 40mg/day.

**HOW SUPPLIED:** Sus: 10mg/5mL [250mL]; Tab: 10mg*, 20mg*, 30mg, 40mg *scored

**CONTRAINDICATIONS:** Concomitant MAOIs, thioridazine, or pimozide.

**WARNINGS/PRECAUTIONS:** Caution with history of mania or seizures, conditions that affect metabolism or hemodynamic responses, narrow angle glaucoma. Discontinue if seizures occur. Altered platelet function, hyponatremia, mydriasis reported. Avoid abrupt withdrawal. Re-evaluate periodically. Monitor for clinical worsening and/or suicidality, especially at initiation of therapy or dose changes.

**ADVERSE REACTIONS:** Somnolence, insomnia, nausea, asthenia, abnormal ejaculation, dry mouth, constipation, dizziness, diarrhea, decreased libido, sweating.

**INTERACTIONS:** See Contraindications. Avoid alcohol, tryptophan. May shift concentrations with plasma-bound drugs. Increased risk of bleeding with NSAIDs, aspirin, oral anticoagulants. May inhibit metabolism of TCAs. Rare reports of weakness, hyperreflexia, incoordination with an SSRI and sumatriptan. Caution with other agents that may affect the serotonergic neurotransmitter systems, such as triptans, serotonin reuptake inhibitors, linezolid, lithium, tramadol, or St. John's Wort. Monitor theophylline. Reduce procyclidine dose if anticholinergic effects occur. Caution with diuretics, digoxin, lithium, cimetidine, warfarin, phenobarbital, phenytoin, drugs metabolized by CYP2D6 (eg, antidepressants, phenothiazines, Type 1C antiarrhythmics), or drugs that inhibit CYP2D6 (eg, quinidine). May increase levels of risperidone. May increase levels of atomoxetine; dosage adjustment of atomoxetine may be necessary and initiate atomoxetine at reduced dose. Fosamprenavir/ritonavir may decrease levels.

**PREGNANCY:** Category D, caution in nursing.



## PAXIL CR
paroxetine HCl (GlaxoSmithKline)

RX

**Antidepressants increased the risk of suicidal thinking and behavior (suicidality) in short-term studies in children and adolescents with Major Depressive Disorder (MDD) and other psychiatric disorders. Paroxetine is not approved for use in pediatric patients.**

**THERAPEUTIC CLASS:** Selective serotonin reuptake inhibitor

**INDICATIONS:** Treatment of major depressive disorder (MDD), panic disorder with or without agoraphobia, social anxiety disorder (SAD), and premenstrual dysphoric disorder (PMDD).

**DOSAGE:** *Adults:* Give qd, usually in the AM. Swallow whole. MDD: Initial: 25mg/day. Titrate: May increase weekly by 12.5mg/day. Max: 62.5mg/day. Panic Disorder: Initial: 12.5mg/day. May increase weekly by 12.5mg/day. Max: 75mg/day. SAD: Initial: 12.5mg/day. May increase weekly by 12.5mg/day. Max: 37.5mg/day. PMDD: Initial: 12.5mg/day continuous or limited to luteal phase of cycle. May increase weekly by 12.5mg/day. Elderly/Debilitated/Severe Renal/Hepatic Impairment: Initial: 12.5mg/day. Max: 50mg/day.

**HOW SUPPLIED:** Tab, Controlled Release: 12.5mg, 25mg, 37.5mg

**CONTRAINDICATIONS:** Concomitant MAOIs, thioridazine, or pimozide.

**WARNINGS/PRECAUTIONS:** Caution with history of mania or seizures, conditions that affect metabolism or hemodynamic responses, narrow angle glaucoma. Discontinue if seizures occur. Hyponatremia, mydriasis reported. Avoid abrupt withdrawal. Re-evaluate periodically. Monitor for clinical worsening and/or suicidality, especially at initiation of therapy or dose changes.

**ADVERSE REACTIONS:** Somnolence, insomnia, nausea, asthenia, abnormal ejaculation, dry mouth, constipation, dizziness, diarrhea, decreased libido, sweating.

**INTERACTIONS:** See Contraindications. Avoid alcohol, tryptophan. May shift concentrations with plasma-bound drugs. May inhibit metabolism of TCAs. Rare reports of weakness, hyperreflexia, incoordination with an SSRI and sumatriptan. Caution with other drugs or agents that may affect the serotonergic neurotransmitter systems, such as tryptophan, triptans, serotonin reuptake inhibitors, linezolid, lithium, tramadol, or St. John's Wort. Monitor theophylline. Increased risk of bleeding with NSAIDs, aspirin, oral anticoagulants. Reduce procyclidine dose if anticholinergic effects occur. Caution with TCAs, diuretics, digoxin, lithium, cimetidine, warfarin, phenobarbital, phenytoin, drugs metabolized by CYP2D6 (eg, antidepressants, phenothiazines, Type 1C antiarrhythmics), or drugs that inhibit CYP2D6 (eg, quinidine). May increase levels of risperidone. May increase levels of atomoxetine; dosage adjustment of atomoxetine may be necessary and initiate atomoxetine at reduced dose. Fosamprenavir/ritonavir may decrease levels.

**PREGNANCY:** Category C, caution in nursing.



## PCE

RX

erythromycin (Abbott)

**THERAPEUTIC CLASS:** Macrolide antibiotic

**INDICATIONS:** Mild to moderate upper and lower respiratory tract and skin and skin structure infections, listeriosis, pertussis, diphtheria, erythrasma, intestinal amebiasis, acute pelvic inflammatory disease (PID) (*N.gonorrhea*), primary syphilis in PCN allergy, Legionnaires' disease, chlamydial infections (eg, newborn conjunctivitis urethral, endocervical, or rectal, etc), and nongonococcal urethritis. Prophylaxis of rheumatic fever.

**DOSAGE:** *Adults:* Usual: 333mg q8h or 500mg q12h without food. Max: 4g/day. Do not take bid when dose is >1g/day. Treat strep infections for 10 days. Chlamydial Urogenital Infection During Pregnancy: 500mg qid or 666mg q8h for 7 days, or 500mg q12h, 333mg q8h or 250mg qid for 14 days. Urethral/Endocervical/Rectal Chlamydial Infections and Nongonococcal Urethritis: 500mg qid or 666mg q8h for at least 7 days. Primary Syphilis: 30-40g in divided doses for 10-15 days. Acute PID: 500mg (erythromycin lactobionate) IV q6h for 3 days, then 500mg PO q12h or 333mg q8h for 7 days. Streptococcal Infection Long-Term Prophylaxis of Rheumatic Fever: 250mg bid. Intestinal Amebiasis: 500mg q12h, or 333mg q8h or 250mg q6h for 10-14 days. Pertussis: 40-50mg/kg/day in divided doses for 5-14 days. Legionnaires' Disease: 1-4g/day in divided doses.
*Pediatrics:* Usual: 30-50mg/kg/day in divided doses without food. Max: 4g/day. Severe Infections: Double dose up to 4g/day. Treat strep infections

for 10 days. Chlamydial Conjunctivitis of Newborns and Chlamydial Pneumonia in Infancy: 12.5mg/kg qid for 2 weeks and 3 weeks, respectively. Intestinal Amebiasis: 30-50mg/kg/day in divided doses for 10-14 days. Long-Term Prophylaxis of Rheumatic Fever: 250mg bid. Pertussis: 40-50mg/kg/day in divided doses for 5-14 days. Legionnaires' Disease: 1-4g/day in divided doses.

**HOW SUPPLIED:** Tab, Extended Release: 333mg, 500mg

**CONTRAINDICATIONS:** Concomitant terfenadine, astemizole, cisapride, pimozide.

**WARNINGS/PRECAUTIONS:** Pseudomembranous colitis, hepatic dysfunction reported. May aggravate myasthenia gravis. Erythromycin does not reach adequate concentrations in fetus to prevent congenital syphilis.

**ADVERSE REACTIONS:** Nausea, vomiting, abdominal pain, diarrhea, anorexia, hepatic dysfunction, abnormal LFTs, allergic reactions, superinfection (prolonged use).

**INTERACTIONS:** Rhabdomyolysis reported with lovastatin. May increase levels of theophylline, digoxin, drugs metabolized by CYP450 (eg, carbamazepine, cyclosporine, phenytoin, alfentanil, disopyramide, lovastatin, bromocriptine, valproate, etc). Increases effects of oral anticoagulants, triazolam, midazolam. Risk of acute ergot toxicity with ergotamine or dihydroergotamine. May potentiate sildenafil. Avoid terfenadine, astemizole, cisapride, pimozide.

**PREGNANCY:** Category B, caution in nursing.

## PEDIAPRED — RX

prednisolone sodium phosphate (Celltech)

**THERAPEUTIC CLASS:** Glucocorticoid

**INDICATIONS:** Steroid responsive dermatoses.

**DOSAGE:** *Adults:* Initial: 5-60mg/day depending on disease and response. Maint: Decrease dose by small amounts to lowest effective dose. MS Exacerbations: 200mg qd for 1 week, then 80mg every other day for 1 month. *Pediatrics:* Initial: 0.14-2mg/kg/day given tid-qid. Nephrotic Syndrome: $20mg/m^2$ tid for 4 weeks, then $40mg/m^2$ every other day for 4 weeks. Uncontrolled Asthma: 1-2mg/kg/day in single or divided doses peak expiratory rate of 80% is achieved (usually 3-10 days).

**HOW SUPPLIED:** Sol: 5mg/5mL [120mL]

**CONTRAINDICATIONS:** Systemic fungal infections.

**WARNINGS/PRECAUTIONS:** May produce reversible HPA axis suppression. Adjust dose during stress or change in thyroid status. May mask signs of infection or cause new infections. May activate latent amebiasis. Avoid with cerebral malaria. Avoid exposure to chickenpox or measles. Not for treatment of optic neuritis or active ocular herpes simplex. May cause elevation of BP or IOP, cataracts, glaucoma, optic nerve damage, Kaposi's sarcoma, psychic derangements, salt/water retention, increased excretion of potassium and/or calcium, osteoporosis, growth suppression in children, secondary ocular infections. Caution with Strongyloides, CHF, diverticulitis, HTN, renal insufficiency, fresh intestinal anastomoses, active or latent peptic ulcer, ulcerative colitis. Enhanced effect in hypothyroidism or cirrhosis. Avoid abrupt withdrawal. Use with caution in elderly, increased risk of corticosteroid-induced side effects; start at low end of dosing range; monitor bone mineral density.

**ADVERSE REACTIONS:** Edema, fluid/electrolyte disturbances, osteoporosis, muscle weakness, pancreatitis, peptic ulcer, impaired wound healing, increased intracranial pressure, cushingoid state, hirsutism, menstrual irregularities, growth suppression in children, glaucoma, nausea, weight gain.

**INTERACTIONS:** Enhanced metabolism with barbiturates, phenytoin, ephedrine, and rifampin. Use with cyclosporine may increase activity of both drugs; convulsions reported with concomitant use. Decreased metabolism with estrogens or ketoconazole. May inhibit response to warfarin. Increased risk of GI side effects with ASA or other NSAIDs. May increase clearance of salicylates. High doses or concurrent neuromuscular drugs may cause acute myopathy. Enhanced possibility of hypokalemia when given with potassium-depleting agents. May produce severe weakness in myasthenia gravis patients on anticholinesterase agents. Avoid live vaccines with immunosuppressive doses. Possible diminished response with killed or inactivated vaccines. May increase blood glucose; adjust antidiabetic agents. May suppress reactions to skin tests.

**PREGNANCY:** Category C, caution in nursing.

## PEDIARIX RX

tetanus toxoid - diphtheria toxoid - hepatitis B (recombinant) - pertussis vaccine, acellular - poliovirus vaccine, inactivated (GlaxoSmithKline)

**THERAPEUTIC CLASS:** Vaccine/toxoid combination

**INDICATIONS:** Active immunization against diphtheria, tetanus, pertussis, hepatitis B, and poliomyelitis (polioviruses Types 1, 2, and 3).

**DOSAGE:** *Pediatrics:* >6 weeks-up to 7 yrs: 3 doses of 0.5mL IM at 6-8 week intervals. Start at 2 months old or as early as 6 weeks old if necessary. May use to complete primary series in infants who have received 1 or 2 doses of Infanrix® or IPV or to complete a hepatitis B vaccine (Recombinant) series. Not recommended for completion of the first 3 doses of the DTaP vaccination series initiated with a DTaP vaccine from a different manufacturer.

**HOW SUPPLIED:** Inj: 0.5mL

**CONTRAINDICATIONS:** Hypersensitivity to yeast, neomycin, and polymyxin B. Anaphylaxis associated with previous dose or encephalopathy within 7 days of previous vaccine, progressive neurologic disorder (including infantile spasms, uncontrolled epilepsy, progressive encephalopathy).

**WARNINGS/PRECAUTIONS:** Higher rates of fever reported. Tip cap and plunger contains latex. Caution if within 48 hrs of previous whole-cell DTP or vaccine containing an acellular pertussis component, fever >105°F not due to another identifiable cause, collapse or shock-like state, or inconsolable crying lasting >3 hrs occurs, or if seizures occur within 3 days. Re-evaluate need if Guillain-Barre syndrome occurs within 6 weeks of receipt of tetanus toxoid-containing vaccine. Defer vaccination with moderate or severe illness, with or without fever. Administer antipyretic for initial 24 hours for those with higher risk for seizures. Caution with bleeding disorders (eg, hemophilia, thrombocytopenia). Have epinephrine available. Suboptimal response may occur in immunocompromised patients.



**ADVERSE REACTIONS:** Local injection-site reactions, fever, fussiness.

**INTERACTIONS:** Avoid with anticoagulants unless benefit outweighs risk. Immunosuppressive therapy (eg, irradiation, antimetabolites, alkylating agents, cytotoxic drugs, large doses of corticosteroids) may decrease response. Do not mix with other vaccines in same syringe/vial. Tetanus immune globulin or diphtheria antitoxin should be given at separate site with separate needle/syringe.

**PREGNANCY:** Category C, safety in nursing not known.

## PEDIAZOLE RX

sulfisoxazole acetyl - erythromycin ethylsuccinate (Ross)

**THERAPEUTIC CLASS:** Macrolide antibiotic/sulfonamide

**INDICATIONS:** Acute otitis media caused by *H.influenzae.*

**DOSAGE:** *Pediatrics:* >2 months: Dose based on 50mg/kg/day erythromycin or 150mg/kg/day sulfisoxazole given tid-qid for 10 days. Max: 6g/day sulfisoxazole.

**HOW SUPPLIED:** Sus: (Erythromycin Ethylsuccinate-Sulfisoxazole Acetyl) 200mg-600mg/5mL [100mL, 150mL, 200mL]

**CONTRAINDICATIONS:** Pediatrics <2 months old, pregnant women at term, mothers nursing infants <2 months old, concomitant terfenadine.

**WARNINGS/PRECAUTIONS:** Pseudomembranous colitis, hepatic dysfunction reported. Severe, fatal allergic reactions reported with sulfonamides. Caution with hepatic or renal dysfunction, bronchial asthma, and severe allergies. May aggravate myasthenia gravis. Erythromycin does not reach adequate concentrations in fetus' to prevent congenital syphilis. Hemolysis may occur in G6P-deficiency patients. Sulfonamides not for treatment of group A beta-hemolytic infections.

**ADVERSE REACTIONS:** Nausea, vomiting, abdominal pain, diarrhea, anorexia, hepatic dysfunction, abnormal LFTs, allergic reactions, tachycardia, syncope, blood dyscrasias, BUN elevation, edema, superinfection.

**INTERACTIONS:** Rhabdomyolysis reported with lovastatin. May increase levels of theophylline, digoxin, methotrexate, drugs metabolized by CYP450 (eg, carbamazepine, cyclosporine, tacrolimus, phenytoin, alfentanil, disopyramide, lovastatin, bromocriptine, valproate, etc). Increases effects of oral anticoagulants, triazolam, midazolam, sulfonylureas. Risk of acute ergot toxicity with ergotamine or dihydroergotamine. Avoid terfenadine. May require less thiopental for anesthesia. May have cross-sensitivity with thiazides, acetazolamide, and oral hypoglycemics.

**PREGNANCY:** Category C, not for use in nursing.

## PEDIOTIC — RX

hydrocortisone - neomycin sulfate - polymyxin B sulfate (King)

**THERAPEUTIC CLASS:** Antibacterial/corticosteroid combination

**INDICATIONS:** Superficial bacterial infections of the external auditory canal. Infections of mastoidectomy and fenestration cavities.

**DOSAGE:** *Adults:* Clean and dry ear canal. Instill 4 drops tid-qid. Max: 10 days. *Pediatrics:* Clean and dry ear canal. Instill 4 drops tid-qid. Max: 10 days.

**HOW SUPPLIED:** Sus: (Neomycin-Hydrocortisone-Polymyxin B) 0.35%-1%-10,000 U/mL [7.5mL]

**CONTRAINDICATIONS:** Herpes simplex, vaccinia, and varicella infections.

**WARNINGS/PRECAUTIONS:** Caution with perforated eardrum or chronic otitis media; ototoxicity may develop. Re-evaluate if no improvement after 10 days.

**ADVERSE REACTIONS:** Allergic sensitization, superinfection.

**INTERACTIONS:** Cross-reactivity with kanamycin, paromomycin, streptomycin, and gentamycin.

**PREGNANCY:** Category C, caution in nursing.



## PEGASYS — RX

peginterferon alfa-2a (Roche)

> **May cause or aggravate fatal or life-threatening neuropsychiatric, autoimmune, ischemic, and infectious disorders. Monitor closely with periodic clinical and laboratory evaluations. Discontinue with persistently severe or worsening signs or symptoms of these conditions. When used with ribavirin, refer to the individual monograph.**

**THERAPEUTIC CLASS:** Pegylated virus proliferation inhibitor

**INDICATIONS:** Treatment of chronic hepatitis C, alone or in combination with Copegus®, in adults with compensated liver disease not previously treated with interferon alfa. Patients in whom efficacy was demonstrated included patients with compensated liver disease and histological evidence of cirrhosis (Child-Pugh class A) and patients with HIV disease that is clinically stable.

Treatment, with Pegasys® alone, of adult patients with chronic hepatitis B who have compensated liver disease and evidence of viral replication and liver inflammation.

**DOSAGE:** *Adults:* ≥18 yrs: HCV: Monotherapy: 180mcg SQ (in abdomen or thigh) once weekly for 48 weeks. ANC <750cells/mm³/End-Stage Renal Disease Requiring Hemodialysis/Progressive ALT Increases Above Baseline/Moderate Depression: Reduce to 135mcg. ANC <500cells/mm³: Suspend therapy until ANC >1000cells/mm³. Reinstitute dose at 90mcg. Platelets <50,000cells/mm³: Reduce to 90mcg. Platelets <25,000cells/mm³/Continued ALT Increases/Increased Bilirubin/Hepatic Decompensation/Severe Depression: Discontinue therapy. Combination Therapy With Copegus®: 180mcg SQ once weekly for 24 weeks with genotypes 2 and 3 or 48 weeks with genotypes 1 and 4. HCV/HIV 48 weeks regardless of genotype. Consider discontinuing if no virological response after 12-24 weeks. HBV: Monotherapy: 180mcg SQ once weekly for 48 weeks. ALT Elevations (>5X ULN): Reduce dose to 135mcg or temporarily suspend therapy. Consider discontinuation if persistent, severe (ALT >10X ULN) hepatitis B flares.

**HOW SUPPLIED:** Inj: Syringe: 180mcg/0.5mL; Single Dose Vial: 180mcg/mL

**CONTRAINDICATIONS:** Autoimmune hepatitis, hepatic decompensation; neonates and infants (contains benzyl alcohol). Additionally, hemoglobinopathies, women who are pregnant, and men whose female partners are pregnant when used with ribavirin.

**WARNINGS/PRECAUTIONS:** Life-threatening neuropsychiatric reactions may occur; extreme caution with history of depression. Risk of bone marrow suppression; obtain CBCs prior to initiation and routinely thereafter. HTN, arrhythmias, chest pain, and MI reported; caution with pre-existing cardiac disease. Decrease/loss of vision and retinopathy reported; perform eye exam at baseline (periodically with pre-existing disorder); discontinue if patient develops new or worsening of ophthalmologic disorders. Monitor for signs/symptoms of toxicity with impaired renal function and caution with CrCl <50mL/min. Development or exacerbation of autoimmune disorders reported. Caution in elderly. May induce or aggravate dyspnea, pulmonary infiltrates, pneumonia, bronchiolitis obliterans, interstitial pneumonitis, and sarcoiditis; discontinue if persistent or unexplained pulmonary infiltrates or pulmonary function impairment. Discontinue if hypersensitivity reaction occurs. Hypersensitivity reactions, hemorrhagic/ischemic colitis, and pancreatitis reported; discontinue if any of these develop. May cause or aggravate hypothyroidism or hyperthyroidism. Hypoglycemia, hyperglycemia and DM reported. Avoid if failed other alpha interferon treatments, liver or other organ transplant recipients, or with HIV or HBV co-infection.



**ADVERSE REACTIONS:** Injection site reaction, fatigue/asthenia, pyrexia, rigors, nausea/vomiting, neutropenia, myalgia, headache, irritability/anxiety/nervousness, insomnia, depression, alopecia.

**INTERACTIONS:** May inhibit CYP1A2 and increase theophylline AUC; monitor theophylline serum levels. Hepatic decompensation can occur with concomitant use of NRTIs and peginterferon alpha-2a/ribavirin.

**PREGNANCY:** Category C (monotherapy) and Category X (with ribavirin), not for use in nursing.

## PEG-INTRON

RX

peginterferon alfa-2b (Schering)

**May cause or aggravate fatal or life-threatening neuropsychiatric, autoimmune, ischemic, and infectious disorders. Monitor closely with periodic clinical and laboratory evaluations. D/C with severe or worsening signs or symptoms of these conditions. When used with Rebetol, refer to the individual monograph.**

**THERAPEUTIC CLASS:** Pegylated virus proliferation inhibitor

**INDICATIONS:** Treatment of chronic hepatitis C alone or in combination with Rebetol®, in patients with compensated liver disease not previously treated with interferon alpha.

**DOSAGE:** *Adults:* >18 yrs: Administer SQ once weekly for 1 yr. Monotherapy: 1mcg/kg/week. Combination Therapy With Rebetol: 1.5mcg/kg/week. Monotherapy or With Rebetol: D/C if HCV levels remain high after 6 months. Hematologic Toxicity: If Hgb <10g/dL then decrease ribavirin by 200mg/day. Reduce peginterferon by 50% if WBC <1.5x$10^9$/L, neutrophils <0.75x$10^9$/L, or platelets <80x$10^9$/L. D/C peginterferon and ribavirin if Hgb <8.5 g/dL, WBC <1x$10^9$/L, neutrophils <0.5x$10^9$/L or platelets <50x$10^9$/L. Moderate Depression: Reduce peginterferon by 50%. Severe Depression: D/C peginterferon and ribavirin therapy. CrCl <50mL/min: D/C ribavirin.

**HOW SUPPLIED:** Inj: 50mcg/0.5mL, 80mcg/0.5mL, 120mcg/0.5mL, 150mcg/0.5mL

**CONTRAINDICATIONS:** Autoimmune hepatitis, decompensated liver disease. When used with Rebetol, refer to the individual monograph.

**WARNINGS/PRECAUTIONS:** Life-threatening neuropsychiatric reactions may occur; caution with history of depression or psychiatric symptoms/disorders. Risk of bone marrow suppression; monitor CBCs and blood chemistry at initiation and periodically thereafter. Hypotension, arrhythmia, tachycardia, angina pectoris, MI reported; caution with cardiovascular disease. Conduct baseline eye exam in all patients and periodical exams with pre-existing ophthalmologic disorders; discontinue if new or worsening ophthalmologic disorders occur. Caution with CrCl<50mL/min, autoimmune disorders, and the elderly. D/C if persistent or unexplained pulmonary infiltrates, or pulmonary dysfunction, or hypersensitivity reaction occurs, or if hemorrhagic/ischemic colitis or pancreatitis develops. May cause or aggravate hypothyroidism/hyperthyroidism. Hyperglycemia and DM reported. Avoid if failed other alpha interferon treatments, liver or other organ transplant recipients, or with HIV or HBV co-infection. Monitor renal impairment for toxicity.

**ADVERSE REACTIONS:** Headache, fatigue, rigors, dizziness, nausea, anorexia, depression, insomnia, irritability, myalgia, arthralgia, weight loss, alopecia, pruritus, decreased platelets/Hgb/neutrophils.

**INTERACTIONS:** Hemolytic anemia reported with ribavirin. May increase AUC of methadone, resulting in an increased narcotic effect.

**PREGNANCY:** Category C, safety in nursing not known.

## PENICILLIN VK

RX

penicillin V potassium (Various)

**OTHER BRAND NAMES:** Veetids (Sandoz)

**THERAPEUTIC CLASS:** Acid-stable penicillin

**INDICATIONS:** Mild to moderately severe bacterial infections including conditions of the respiratory tract, oropharynx, skin and soft tissue. Prevention of recurrence following rheumatic fever and/or chorea.

**DOSAGE:** *Adults:* Usual: Streptococcal Infections (Scarlet Fever, Erysipelas, Upper Respiratory Tract): 125-250mg q6-8h for 10 days. Pneumococcal Infections (Otitis media, Respiratory Tract): 250-500mg q6h until afebrile for at least 2 days. Staphylococcus Infections (Skin/Soft Tissue): 250-500mg q6-8h. Fusospirochetosis Infections (Oropharynx): 250-500mg q6-8h. Rheumatic Fever/Chorea Prevention: 125-250mg bid.
*Pediatrics:* >12 yrs: Usual: Streptococcal Infections (Scarlet fever, Erysipelas, Upper Respiratory Tract): 125-250mg q6-8h for 10 days. Pneumococcal Infections (Otitis media, Respiratory Tract): 250-500mg q6h until afebrile for at least 2 days. Staphylococcus Infections (Skin/Soft Tissue): 250-500mg q6-8h. Fusospirochetosis Infections (Oropharynx): 250-500mg q6-8h. Rheumatic Fever/Chorea Prevention: 125-250mg bid.

**HOW SUPPLIED:** Sus: 125mg/5mL, 250mg/5mL [100mL, 200mL]; Tab: 250mg, 500mg

**WARNINGS/PRECAUTIONS:** Not for severe pneumonia, empyema, bacteremia, pericarditis, meningitis and arthritis during the acute stage. Serious, fatal anaphylactic reactions reported. Pseudomembranous colitis reported. Oral administration may not be effective with severe illnesses, nausea, vomiting, gastric dilation, cardiospasm, intestinal hypermobility. Cross-sensitivity with cephalosporins. Caution with asthma and allergies.

**ADVERSE REACTIONS:** Nausea, vomiting, epigastric distress, diarrhea, hypersensitivity reactions, black hairy tongue, anaphylaxis, superinfection (prolonged use).

**PREGNANCY:** Category B, caution in nursing.

## PENLAC
ciclopirox (Dermik)

RX

**THERAPEUTIC CLASS:** Broad-spectrum antifungal

**INDICATIONS:** Mild to moderate onychomycosis of fingernails or toenails without lunula involvement due to *Trichophyton rubrum* (in immunocompetent patients).

**DOSAGE:** *Adults:* Apply qhs or 8 hrs before washing to nail bed, hyponychium, and under surface when it is free of nail bed. Apply daily over previous coat and remove with alcohol every 7 days. Repeat cycle up to 48 weeks.

**HOW SUPPLIED:** Sol: 8% [6.6mL]

**WARNINGS/PRECAUTIONS:** Only for use on nails and adjacent skin. Caution with removal of infected nail in insulin-dependent diabetes mellitus or diabetic neuropathy.

**ADVERSE REACTIONS:** Periungual erythema, erythema of proximal nail fold, nail shape change, nail irritation, ingrown toenail, nail discoloration.

**INTERACTIONS:** Avoid nail polish or other nail cosmetics on treated nails.

**PREGNANCY:** Category B, caution in nursing.



## PENTASA
mesalamine (Shire US)

RX

**THERAPEUTIC CLASS:** Anti-inflammatory agent

**INDICATIONS:** Induction of remission and for treatment of mild to moderate active ulcerative colitis.

**DOSAGE:** *Adults:* 1g qid. Can be given up to 8 weeks.

**HOW SUPPLIED:** Cap, Extended Release: 250mg, 500mg

**CONTRAINDICATIONS:** Hypersensitivity to salicylates.

**WARNINGS/PRECAUTIONS:** Caution with hepatic and renal dysfunction; monitor closely. D/C if acute intolerance syndrome develops (eg, cramping, bloody diarrhea, abdominal pain, headache). If rechallenge is considered, perform under careful observation.

**ADVERSE REACTIONS:** Diarrhea, headache, nausea, abdominal pain.

**PREGNANCY:** Category B, caution in nursing.

## PENTOTHAL
thiopental sodium (Hospira)

CIII

**THERAPEUTIC CLASS:** Thiobarbiturate

**INDICATIONS:** Sole anesthetic agent for brief (15 minute) procedures. For induction of anesthesia prior to administration of other anesthetic agents. To supplement regional anesthesia. To provide hypnosis during balanced anesthesia with other agents for analgesia or muscle relaxation. For the control of convulsive states during or following inhalation/local anesthesia or other causes. In neurosurgical patients with increased intracranial pressure, if adequate ventilation is provided. For narcoanalysis and narcosynthesis in psychiatric disorders.

**DOSAGE:** *Adults:* Individualize dose. IV: Test Dose: 25-75mg. Anesthesia: 50-75mg at 20-40 second intervals. Once anesthesia is established, additional injections of 25-50mg may be given whenever patient moves. Induction In Balanced Anesthesia: Initial: 3-4mg/kg. Convulsive States: Following anesthesia, give 75-125mg as soon as possible after convulsion begins.

Convulsions following use of local anesthetic may require 125-250mg over 10 minute period. Neurosurgical Patients With Increased Intracranial Pressure: 1.5-3.5mg/kg bolus. Psychiatric Disorders: After test dose, infuse at 100mg/min with patient counting backwards from 100; discontinue shortly after counting becomes confused but before actual sleep is produced.

**HOW SUPPLIED:** Inj: 20mg/mL, 25mg/mL

**CONTRAINDICATIONS:** Absolute: Absence of suitable veins for IV administration, variegate porphyria (South Africa) or acute intermittent porphyria. Relative: Severe cardiovascular disease, hypotension, shock, conditions in which the hypnotic effect may be prolonged or potentiated (excessive premedication, Addison's disease, hepatic/renal dysfunction, myxedema, increased blood urea, severe anemia, asthma, and myasthenia gravis), and status asthmaticus.

**WARNINGS/PRECAUTIONS:** Avoid extravasation or intra-arterial injection. May be habit forming. Reduce dose and administer slowly with relative contraindications. Caution with advanced cardiac disease, increased intracranial pressure, ophthalmoplegia plus, asthma, myasthenia gravis, and endocrine insufficiency (pituitary, thyroid, adrenal, pancreas).

**ADVERSE REACTIONS:** Respiratory/myocardial depression, cardiac arrhythmias, prolonged somnolence and recovery, sneezing, coughing, bronchospasm, laryngospasm, shivering, anaphylactic and anaphylactoid reactions.

**INTERACTIONS:** Prolonged action with probenecid. Hypotension with diazoxide. Antagonism with zimelidine or aminophylline. Decreased antinociceptive action with opioid analgesics. Synergism with midazolam.

**PREGNANCY:** Category C, caution in nursing.



## PEPCID
famotidine (Merck) RX

**OTHER BRAND NAMES:** Pepcid RPD (Merck)

**THERAPEUTIC CLASS:** $H_2$ blocker

**INDICATIONS:** (PO/Inj) Short term treatment of active duodenal ulcer (DU), active benign gastric ulcer (GU), gastroesophageal reflux disease (GERD) and esophagitis due to GERD. Maintenance therapy for DU. Treatment of hypersecretory conditions (eg, Zollinger-Ellison syndrome). (Inj) For hospitalized patients with hypersecretory conditions or intractable ulcers. As an alternative in patients unable to take oral forms.

**DOSAGE:** *Adults:* (PO) Acute DU: 40mg qhs or 20mg bid for 4-8 weeks. Maint DU: 20mg qhs. GU: 40mg qhs. GERD: 20mg bid up to 6 weeks. GERD with Esophagitis: 20-40mg bid up to 12 weeks. Hypersecretory Conditions: Initial: 20mg q6h. Max: 160mg q6h. (Inj) 20mg IV q12h, hypersecretory conditions may require higher doses. CrCl <50mL/min: Reduce to 1/2 dose, or increase interval to q36-48h.
*Pediatrics:* 1-16 yrs: (PO) DU/GU: Usual: 0.5mg/kg/day qhs or divided bid. Max: 40mg/day. GERD With or Without Esophagitis: 0.5mg/kg PO bid. Max: 40mg bid. (Inj) 0.25mg/kg IV q12h up to 40mg/day. Base duration of therapy on

clinical response, and/or pH, and endoscopy. (PO) GERD: 3 months-1yr: 0.5mg/kg bid for up to 8 weeks. <3 months: 0.5mg/kg qd for up to 8 weeks. CrCl <50mL/min: Reduce to 1/2 dose, or increase interval to q36-48h.

**HOW SUPPLIED:** Inj: 0.4mg/mL, 10mg/mL; Sus: 40mg/5mL [50mL]; Tab: 20mg, 40mg; Tab, Disintegrating: (RPD) 20mg, 40mg

**CONTRAINDICATIONS:** Hypersensitivity to other $H_2$ antagonists.

**WARNINGS/PRECAUTIONS:** CNS adverse effects reported with moderate to severe renal insufficiency; adjust dose. Disintegrating tabs contain phenylalanine; caution in phenylketonurics. Symptomatic response does not preclude the presence of gastric malignancy.

**ADVERSE REACTIONS:** Headache, dizziness, constipation, diarrhea.

**INTERACTIONS:** May give with antacids.

**PREGNANCY:** Category B, not for use in nursing.

## PEPCID AC — OTC

famotidine (J&J - Merck)

**THERAPEUTIC CLASS:** $H_2$ blocker

**INDICATIONS:** Relief and prevention of heartburn, acid indigestion, and sour stomach.

**DOSAGE:** *Adults:* Relief: 1 tab/cap prn. Max: 2 doses/24 hrs. Prevention: 1 tab/cap 15-60 minutes before food or beverages that cause heartburn. Max: 2 doses/24 hrs.
*Pediatrics:* >12yrs: 1 tab/cap prn. Max: 2 doses/24 hrs. Prevention: 1 tab/cap 15-60 minutes before food or beverages that cause heartburn. Max: 2 doses/24 hrs.

**HOW SUPPLIED:** Cap: 10mg; Tab: 10mg, 20mg; Tab, Chewable: 10mg

**INTERACTIONS:** Avoid with other acid reducers.

## PEPCID COMPLETE — OTC

famotidine - calcium carbonate - magnesium hydroxide (J&J - Merck)

**THERAPEUTIC CLASS:** $H_2$ blocker/antacid

**INDICATIONS:** To relieve heartburn associated with acid indigestion and sour stomach.

**DOSAGE:** *Adults:* Chew 1 tab to relieve symptoms. Max: 2 tabs/24hrs.
*Pediatrics:* >12 yrs: Chew 1 tab to relieve symptoms. Max: 2 tabs/24hrs.

**HOW SUPPLIED:** Tab, Chewable: (Famotidine-Calcium Carbonate-Magnesium Hydroxide) 10mg-800mg-165mg

**WARNINGS/PRECAUTIONS:** Not for use in those with trouble swallowing. Avoid use if allergic to other acid reducers.

**PREGNANCY:** Safety in pregnancy and nursing not known.

## PEPTO-BISMOL — OTC

bismuth subsalicylate (Procter & Gamble)

**OTHER BRAND NAMES:** Pepto-Bismol Maximum Strength (Procter & Gamble)

**THERAPEUTIC CLASS:** Antimicrobial

**INDICATIONS:** To control diarrhea within 24 hours, relieving associated abdominal cramps; soothes heartburn, and indigestion without constipation; and relieves nausea and upset stomach.

**DOSAGE:** *Adults:* (Sus) 30mL every 0.5-1 hr prn. Max: 8 doses/24hrs. (Sus, Max Strength) 30mL hourly prn. Max: 4 doses/24 hrs. (Tab; Tab, Chewable) 2 tabs every 0.5-1 hr prn. Max: 8 doses/24hrs. Drink plenty of clear fluids.

*Pediatrics:* (Sus) 9-12 yrs: 15mL every 0.5-1 hr prn. 6-9 yrs: 10mL every 0.5-1 hr prn. 3-6 yrs: 5mL every 0.5-1 hr. Max: 8 doses/24hrs. (Sus, Max Strength) 9-12 yrs: 15mL hourly prn. 6-9 yrs: 10mL hourly prn. 3-6 yrs: 5mL hourly prn. Max: 4 doses/24hrs. (Tab; Tab, Chewable) 9-12 yrs: 1 tab every 0.5-1 hr prn. 6-9 yrs: 2/3 tab every 0.5-1 hr prn. 3-6 yrs: 1/3 tab every 0.5-1 hr prn. Max: 8 doses/24 hrs. Drink plenty of clear fluids.

**HOW SUPPLIED:** Sus: 262mg/15mL; Sus, Maximum Strength: 525mg/15mL; Tab: 262mg; Tab, Chewable: 262mg

**WARNINGS/PRECAUTIONS:** Avoid in children and teenagers with or recovering from chickenpox or flu. Do not give with aspirin or non-aspirin salicylate allergy. May cause temporary darkening of tongue or stool. Product may contain small amounts of naturally occurring lead.

**INTERACTIONS:** May cause ringing in the ears with aspirin; discontinue if this occurs. Caution with anticoagulants, antidiabetic, and antigout agents.

**PREGNANCY:** Safety in pregnancy and nursing not known.

## PERCOCET

**CII**

acetaminophen - oxycodone HCl (Endo)

**OTHER BRAND NAMES:** Endocet (Endo)

**THERAPEUTIC CLASS:** Opioid analgesic

**INDICATIONS:** Relief of moderate to moderately severe pain.

**DOSAGE:** *Adults:* (2.5/325): 1-2 tabs q6h. Max: 12 tabs/day. (5/325): 1 tab q6h prn. Max: 12 tabs/day. (7.5/500): 1 tab q6h prn. Max: 8 tabs/day. (10-650) 1 tab q6h prn. Max: 6 tabs/day. (7.5/325): 1 tab q6h prn. Max: 8 tabs/day. (10/325): 1 tab q6h prn. Max: 6 tabs/day. Do not exceed APAP 4g/day.

**HOW SUPPLIED:** Tab: (Oxycodone-APAP) 2.5mg-325mg, 5mg-325mg, 7.5mg-325mg, 7.5mg-500mg, 10mg-325mg, 10mg-650mg

**WARNINGS/PRECAUTIONS:** May cause drug dependence and tolerance; potential for abuse. Risk of respiratory depression. Capacity to elevate CSF pressure may be exaggerated with head injury, other intracranial lesions or a pre-existing increase in intracranial pressure. May obscure the diagnosis or clinical course with head injuries or with acute abdominal conditions. Caution with severe hepatic impairment, renal dysfunction, hypothyroidism, Addison's disease, prostatic hypertrophy, urethral stricture, the elderly or debilitated.

**ADVERSE REACTIONS:** Lightheadedness, dizziness, sedation, nausea, vomiting, euphoria, dysphoria, constipation, skin rash, pruritus.

**INTERACTIONS:** Potentiates CNS depression with other opioid analgesics, general anesthetics, phenothiazines, tranquilizers, sedative-hypnotics, alcohol and other CNS depressants. Risk of paralytic ileus with anticholinergics.

**PREGNANCY:** Category C, caution in nursing.

## PERCODAN

**CII**

aspirin - oxycodone (Endo)

**OTHER BRAND NAMES:** Endodan (Endo)

**THERAPEUTIC CLASS:** Opioid analgesic

**INDICATIONS:** Relief of moderate to moderately severe pain.

**DOSAGE:** *Adults:* Usual: 1 tab q6h prn. Max: 12 tabs/day or ASA 4g/day.

**HOW SUPPLIED:** Tab: (Oxycodone HCl-Oxycodone Terephthalate-ASA) 4.5mg-0.38mg-325mg* *scored

**WARNINGS/PRECAUTIONS:** May cause drug dependence and tolerance; potential for abuse. Risk of respiratory depression. Capacity to elevate CSF pressure may be exaggerated with head injury, other intracranial lesions or a pre-existing increase in intracranial pressure. May obscure the diagnosis or clinical course with head injuries or with acute abdominal conditions. Caution with severe of hepatic impairment, renal dysfunction, hypothyroidism, Addison's disease, prostatic hypertrophy, urethral stricture, peptic ulcer, coagulation abnormalities, and the elderly or debilitated. May increase the risk of developing Reye's syndrome in children and teenagers.

**ADVERSE REACTIONS:** Lightheadedness, dizziness, sedation, nausea, vomiting, euphoria, dysphoria, constipation, pruritus.

**INTERACTIONS:** Additive CNS depression with other opioid analgesics, general anesthetics, phenothiazines, tranquilizers, sedative-hypnotics or other CNS depressants (including alcohol). ASA may enhance effect of anticoagulants and inhibit effects of uricosuric agents.

**PREGNANCY:** Safety in pregnancy and nursing is not known.

## PERGONAL RX

menotropins (Serono)

**THERAPEUTIC CLASS:** Follicle stimulating hormone/luteinizing hormone

**INDICATIONS:** (Women) Sequentially with hCG, to induce ovulation and pregnancy in functional anovulation not due to primary ovarian failure. With hCG, to stimulate development of multiple follicles in ovulatory patients for in vitro fertilization. (Men) With hCG, to stimulate spermatogenesis in primary or secondary hypogonadotropic hypogonadism.

**DOSAGE:** *Adults:* (Women) Follicle Maturation: Individualize dose. Initial: 75 IU IM qd for 7-12 days followed by hCG 5000-10,000U 1 day after last dose. If ovulation without pregnancy occurs, repeat at least twice before increasing to 150 IU qd for 7-12 days, followed by hCG. If ovulation without pregnancy occurs, repeat twice. In Vitro Fertilization: 150 IU qd, may repeat course twice if ovulation without pregnancy occurs. (Men) Pretreat with hCG 5000U 3x/week (TIW) until testosterone levels are within normal range and masculinization achieved. After pretreatment, 75 IU IM TIW and hCG 2000U twice weekly for at least 4 months. If insufficient response, continue with 75 IU TIW or increase to 150 IU TIW with hCG dose unchanged.

**HOW SUPPLIED:** Inj: 75 IU

P

**CONTRAINDICATIONS:** (Women) High FSH levels indicating primary ovarian failure, uncontrolled thyroid or adrenal dysfunction, organic intracranial lesions (eg, pituitary tumor), any cause of infertility other than anovulation (unless candidate for in vitro fertilization), abnormal bleeding of undetermined origin, ovarian cysts or enlargement not due to polycystic ovary syndrome, pregnancy. (Men) Normal or elevated gonadotropin levels, infertility disorders other than hypogonadotropic hypogonadism.

**WARNINGS/PRECAUTIONS:** Exclude primary ovarian failure. Ovarian enlargement may occur; monitor ovarian response. Ovarian hyperstimulation syndrome (OHSS), hypersensitivity/anaphylactic reactions, multiple births, serious pulmonary and vascular complications reported. Avoid hCG if ovaries abnormally enlarged last day of therapy. Monitor follicular maturation by measuring estradiol levels and through sonographic visualization.

**ADVERSE REACTIONS:** (Women) Pulmonary and vascular complications, OHSS, hemoperitoneum, adnexal torsion, ovarian enlargement, ovarian cysts, abdominal pain, GI symptoms, injection site reactions, rash. (Men) Gynecomastia, erythrocytosis.

**PREGNANCY:** Category X, caution in nursing.

## PERI-COLACE OTC

senna - docusate sodium (Purdue Products)

**THERAPEUTIC CLASS:** Stool softener/laxative combination

**INDICATIONS:** Management of constipation.

**DOSAGE:** *Adults:* 2-4 tabs daily
*Pediatrics:* ≥12yrs: 2-4 tabs daily. 6-<12yrs: 1-2 tabs daily. 2-<6yrs: Max of 1 tab daily.

**HOW SUPPLIED:** (Docusate Sodium-Sennosides) Tab: 50mg-8.6mg

**WARNINGS/PRECAUTIONS:** Caution with use >1 week.

**INTERACTIONS:** Caution with mineral oil.

**PREGNANCY:** Safety in pregnancy and nursing not known.

## PERIDEX
chlorhexidine gluconate (Zila) RX

**THERAPEUTIC CLASS:** Antimicrobial

**INDICATIONS:** For use between dental visits for treatment of gingivitis.

**DOSAGE:** *Adults:* Swish for 30 seconds and expectorate 15mL bid, am and hs, after brushing. Initiate after a dental prophylaxis. Max: 6 month intervals.

**HOW SUPPLIED:** Liq: 0.12%

**WARNINGS/PRECAUTIONS:** May stain oral surfaces and alter taste perception.

**ADVERSE REACTIONS:** Staining of teeth and other oral surfaces, calculus formation, taste perception alteration, minor gum irritation.

**PREGNANCY:** Category B, caution in nursing.

## PERIOGARD
chlorhexidine gluconate (Colgate Oral) RX

**THERAPEUTIC CLASS:** Antimicrobial

**INDICATIONS:** Treatment of gingivitis between dental visits, including gingival bleeding.

**DOSAGE:** *Adults:* Rinse with 15mL for 30 seconds bid, am and pm, after toothbrushing. Expectorate after rinsing; do not ingest. Do not rinse with water or other mouthwashes, brush teeth, or eat immediately after use.

**HOW SUPPLIED:** Liq: 0.12%

**WARNINGS/PRECAUTIONS:** Effect in periodontitis not known. May increase supraginigival calculus. Hypersensitivity, allergic reactions and altered taste reported. May stain tooth, oral surfaces and dorsum of the tongue. Caution with anterior facial restoration.

**ADVERSE REACTIONS:** Increases staining of teeth and other oral surfaces, increases calculus formation, alteration in taste perception, oral irritation, local allergy-type symptoms, stomatitis, gingivitis, glossitis, ulcer, dry mouth, hypesthesia, glossal edema, paresthesia.

**PREGNANCY:** Category B, caution in nursing.

## PERIOSTAT
doxycycline hyclate (CollaGenex) RX

**THERAPEUTIC CLASS:** Tetracycline derivative

**INDICATIONS:** Adjunct to scaling and root planing to promote attachment level gain and reduces pocket depth in patients with adult periodontitis.

**DOSAGE:** *Adults:* Following scaling and root planing, 20mg bid, 1 hour prior to morning and evening meals for up to 9 months. Maintain adequate fluid intake with caps to reduce risk of esophageal irritation and ulceration.

**HOW SUPPLIED:** Tab: 20mg

**WARNINGS/PRECAUTIONS:** Do not exceed recommended dosage. May cause permanent tooth discoloration during tooth development (last half of pregnancy and up to 8 years old). Risk of fetal harm in pregnancy. May increase BUN and vaginal candidiasis. Photosensitivity reported. Superinfection with nonsusceptible microorganism. Caution with history of oral candidiasis.

**ADVERSE REACTIONS:** Headache, nausea, vomiting, dyspepsia, diarrhea, joint pain, rash.

**INTERACTIONS:** Decreased effects with barbiturates, phenytoin and carbamazepine. Interferes with bactericidal effects of β-lactam (eg, penicillin) antibiotics. Depresses plasma PT activity; adjust oral anticoagulant dose. Absorption impaired by aluminum-, calcium- or magnesium-containing antacids, iron-containing products and bismuth subsalicylate. Decreases effects of oral contraceptives. Fatal renal toxicity reported with concurrent methoxyflurane.

**PREGNANCY:** Category D, contraindicated in nursing.

## PERMAPEN RX

penicillin G benzathine (Pfizer)

**THERAPEUTIC CLASS:** Penicillin

**INDICATIONS:** Treatment of microorganisms susceptible to low and very prolonged serum levels in upper respiratory tract infections (streptococci group A - without bacteremia), syphilis, yaws, bejel, and pinta. Prophylaxis for rheumatic fever and/or chorea. Follow-up prophylactic therapy for rheumatic heart disease and acute glomerulonephritis.

**DOSAGE:** *Adults:* Streptococcal Infection: 1.2MU IM single dose. Primary/Secondary/Latent Syphilis: 1MU IM single dose. Late (Tertiary/Neurosyphilis) Syphilis: 3MU IM every 7 days for total of 6-9MU. Yaws/Bejel/Pinta: 1.2MU IM single dose. Rheumatic Fever/Glomerulonephritis Prophylaxis: 1.2MU IM once monthly or 600,000U IM twice monthly. Use upper outer quadrant of buttock. Rotate injection site.
*Pediatrics:* <12 yrs: Adjust dose according to age and weight and severity of infection. Streptococcal Infection: 900,000U IM single dose in older children. Congenital Syphilis: <2 yrs: 50,000U/kg IM single dose. 2-12 yrs: Adjust dose based on adult schedule. Use midlateral aspect of thigh in infants and small children. May divide dose between 2 buttocks in peds <2 yrs. Rotate injection site.

**HOW SUPPLIED:** Inj: 600,000U/mL

**WARNINGS/PRECAUTIONS:** Caution in newborns; evaluate organ system function frequently. Evaluate renal, hepatic and hematopoietic systems with prolonged therapy. Serious, fatal anaphylactic reactions reported; increased risk with hypersensitivity to penicillins, cephalosporins, and other allergens. Avoid IV, intra-arterial administration, or injection into/near major peripheral nerves or blood vessels may cause severe neurovascular damage. May result in overgrowth of nonsusceptible organisms. Avoid subcutaneous and fat-layer injections. Take culture after therapy completion to determine streptococci eradication.

**ADVERSE REACTIONS:** Skin eruptions, urticaria, laryngeal edema, anaphylaxis, fever, eosinophilia.

**INTERACTIONS:** Bacteriostatic agents (eg, tetracycline, erythromycin) may diminish effects. Prolonged levels with probenecid.

**PREGNANCY:** Category B, caution in nursing.

## PERPHENAZINE
RX

perphenazine (Various)

**THERAPEUTIC CLASS:** Phenothiazine

**INDICATIONS:** Treatment of schizophrenia. To control severe nausea and vomiting.

**DOSAGE:** *Adults:* Moderately Disturbed Non-Hospitalized With Schizophrenia: Initial: 4-8mg tid. Maint: Reduce to minimum effective dose. Hospitalized Psychotic Patients With Schizophrenia: 8-16mg bid-qid. Max: 64mg/day. Severe Nausea/Vomiting: 8-16mg/day in divided doses. Max: 24mg/day. Elderly: Lower dosages recommended.
*Pediatrics:* >12 yrs: Use lowest limits of adult dose.

**HOW SUPPLIED:** Tab: 2mg, 4mg, 8mg, 16mg

**CONTRAINDICATIONS:** Comatose or greatly obtunded patients, large doses of CNS depressants (eg, barbiturates, alcohol, narcotics, analgesics, or antihistamines), blood dyscrasias, bone marrow depression, liver damage, subcortical brain damage with or without hypothalamic involvement.

**WARNINGS/PRECAUTIONS:** Tardive dyskinesia may develop. NMS, photosensitivity reported. May lower convulsive threshold; caution with alcohol withdrawal. Caution with psychic depression, renal impairment, respiratory impairment. May impair mental/physical abilities. May mask signs of overdosage to other drugs. May obsure diagnosis of intestinal obstruction, brain tumor. Severe hypotension may occur in surgery. May elevate prolactin levels. Monitor hepatic/renal functions, blood counts. Increased risk of liver damage, jaundice, corneal and lenticular deposits, and irreversible dyskinesias with long-term use.

**ADVERSE REACTIONS:** Aching/numbness of the limbs, motor restlessness, cerebral edema, seizures, drowsiness, dry mouth, salivation, nausea, vomiting, diarrhea, lactation, postural hypotension, tachycardia.

**INTERACTIONS:** See Contraindications. Additive effects with CNS depressants and phenothiazine; use reduced amount of added drug. Additive anticholinergic effects with atropine/atropine-like drugs, exposure to phosphorous insecticide. Additive effects and hypotension may occur with alcohol. Cytochrome P450 2D6 inhibitors (TCAs, SSRIs) may increase levels; lower doses may be required.

**PREGNANCY:** Safety in pregnancy and nursing not known.



## PERSANTINE
RX

dipyridamole (Boehringer Ingelheim)

**THERAPEUTIC CLASS:** Platelet inhibitor

**INDICATIONS:** Adjunct to coumarin anticoagulants for prevention of postoperative thromboembolic complications of cardiac valve replacement.

**DOSAGE:** *Adults:* 75-100mg qid.

**HOW SUPPLIED:** Tab: 25mg, 50mg, 75mg

**WARNINGS/PRECAUTIONS:** Caution with hypotension or severe CAD (eg, unstable angina or recent MI); may aggravate chest pain. Elevated hepatic enzymes and hepatic failure reported.

**ADVERSE REACTIONS:** Dizziness, abdominal distress.

**INTERACTIONS:** Increases levels of adenosine. May counteract effects of cholinesterase inhibitors.

**PREGNANCY:** Category B, caution in nursing.

## PEXEVA

RX

paroxetine mesylate (Synthon)

**Antidepressants increased the risk of suicidal thinking and behavior (suicidality) in short-term studies in children and adolescents with Major Depressive Disorder (MDD) and other psychiatric disorders. Pexeva is not approved for use in pediatric patients.**

**THERAPEUTIC CLASS:** Selective serotonin reuptake inhibitor

**INDICATIONS:** Treatment of MDD, obsessive compulsive disorder (OCD), and panic disorder with or without agoraphobia.

**DOSAGE:** *Adult:* MDD: Initial: 20mg/day. Max: 50mg/day. OCD: Initial: 40mg/day. Max: 60mg/day. Panic Disorder: Initial: 10mg/day. Titrate: 10mg/day increments at intervals of at least 1 week. Max: 60mg/day. Elderly/Debilitated/Severe Renal or Hepatic Impairment: Initial: 10mg qd. Max: 40mg/day.

**HOW SUPPLIED:** Tab: 10mg, 20mg, 30mg, 40mg

**CONTRAINDICATIONS:** Concomitant MAOIs, thioridazine, and pimozide.

**WARNINGS/PRECAUTIONS:** Caution with history of mania, seizures, history of suicidal thoughts or attempts(adolescents have an increased risk of suicidal thoughts and/or atempts), conditions that affect metabolism or hemodynamic responses, narrow angle glaucoma. Risk of serotonin syndrome with contomitant use of triptans, tramadol, and other serotonergic agents. Discontinue if seizures occur. Altered platelet function, hyponatremia, mydriasis reported. Avoid abrupt withdrawal. Re-evaluate periodically. Monitor for clinical worsening and/or suicidality, especially at initiation of therapy or dose changes.

**ADVERSE REACTIONS:** Asthenia, sweating, nausea, decreased appetite, somnolence, dizziness, insomnia, tremor, nervousness, abnormal ejaculation, dry mouth, constipation, decreased libido, impotence, headache, tinnitus.

**INTERACTIONS:** Avoid alcohol, tryptophan, thioridazine, and within 14 days of MAOI therapy. May shift concentrations with plasma-bound drugs. Increased risk of bleeding with NSAIDS, aspirin, oral anticoagulants. May inhibit metabolism of TCAs. Rare reports of weakness, hyperreflexia, incoordination with an SSRI and sumatriptan; avoid triptans unless necessary-carefully monitor patient when on paroxetine and triptan with initiation and dose changes. Monitor theophylline. Reduce procyclidine dose if anticholinergic effects occur. Caution with diuretics, digoxin, lithium, cimetidine, warfarin, phenobarbital, phenytoin, drugs metabolized by CYP2D6 (eg., antidepressants, phenothiazines, Type 1C antiarrhythmics), quinidine, avoid concomitant use with SSRI's and SNRI's. Fosamprenavir/ritonavir decreases paroxetine levels. Pimozide levels are increased with concomitant administration of paroxetine, which could result in QT prolongation.

**PREGNANCY:** Category D, increased risk of cardiovascular malformations(ventrciular/atrial septal defects) in newborns; avoid unless benefit outweighs risk.



## PFIZERPEN

RX

penicillin G potassium (Pfizer)

**THERAPEUTIC CLASS:** Penicillin

**INDICATIONS:** For therapy of severe infections when rapid and high blood levels of penicillin required. Management of streptococcal, pneumococcal, staphylococcal, clostridial, fusospirochetal, listeria, and gram negative bacillary, and pasteurella infections. For anthrax, actinomycosis, diphtheria, erysipeloid, meningitis, endocarditis, bacteremia, rat-bite fever, syphilis, and gonorrheal endocarditis and arthritis. With combined oral therapy, prophylaxis against endocarditis in patients with congenital heart disease, rheumatic, or other acquired valvular heart disease undergoing dental procedures or surgical procedures of upper respiratory tract.

**DOSAGE:** *Adults:* Anthrax/Gonorrheal Endocarditis/Severe Infections (Streptococci, Pneumococci, Staphylococci): Minimum of 5MU/day. Syphilis: Administer in hospital. Determine dose and duration based on age and weight. Meningococcic Meningitis: 1-2MU IM q2h or 20-30MU/day continuous IV. Actinomycosis: 1-6MU/day for cervicofacial cases; 10-20MU/day for thoracic and abdominal disease. Clostridial Infections: 20MU/day (adjunct to antitoxin). Fusospirochetal Severe Infections: 5-10MU/day for oropharynx, lower respiratory tract, and genital area infection. Rat-bite Fever: 12-15MU/day for 3-4 weeks. Listeria Endocarditis: 15-20MU/day for 4 weeks. Pasteurella Bacteremia/Meningitis: 4-6MU/day for 2 weeks. Erysipeloid Endocarditis: 2-20MU/day for 4-6 weeks. Gram Negative Bacillary Bacteremia: 20-80MU/day. Diphtheria (carrier state): 0.3-0.4MU/day in divided doses for 10-12 days. Endocarditis Prophylaxis: 1MU IM mixed with 0.6MU procaine penicillin G 0.5-1 hr before procedure. Renal/Cardiac/Vascular Dysfunction: Consider dose reduction. For streptococcal infection, treat for minimum 10 days.
*Pediatrics:* Listeria Infections: Neonates: 0.5-1MU/day. Congenital Syphilis: Administer in hospital. Determine dose and duration based on age and weight. Endocarditis Prophylaxis: 30,000U/kg IM mixed with 0.6MU procaine penicillin G 0.5-1 hr before procedure. For streptococcal infection, treat for minimum 10 days.

**HOW SUPPLIED:** Inj: 1MU, 5MU, 20MU

**WARNINGS/PRECAUTIONS:** Serious, fatal anaphylactic reactions reported; increased risk with hypersensitivity to penicillins, cephalosporins, and other allergens. Avoid IV, intra-arterial administration, or injection into/near major peripheral nerves or blood vessels; may cause severe neurovascular damage. Take culture after therapy completion to determine streptococci eradication. Caution with history of significant allergies or asthma. May result in overgrowth of nonsusceptible organisms. Evaluate renal, hepatic and hematopoietic systems with prolonged therapy. Administer slowly to avoid electrolyte imbalance from potassium or sodium content; monitor electrolytes and consider dose reductions with renal, cardiac, or vascular dysfunction. Caution in newborns; evaluate organ system function frequently.

**ADVERSE REACTIONS:** Skin rash (eg, maculopapular eruption, exfoliative dermatitis) urticaria, chills, fever, edema, arthralgia, prostration, anaphylaxis, arrhythmias, cardiac arrest, Jarisch-Herxheimer reaction.

**INTERACTIONS:** Bacteriostatic agents (eg, tetracycline, erythromycin) may diminish effects. Prolonged levels with probenecid.

**PREGNANCY:** Category B, caution in nursing.



## PHENERGAN INJECTION — RX

promethazine HCl (Baxter)

**THERAPEUTIC CLASS:** Phenothiazine derivative

**INDICATIONS:** For blood or plasma allergic reactions, allergic reactions where oral therapy is not possible, sedation, and special surgical situations (eg, repeated bronchoscopy). Adjunct for anaphylactic reactions and postoperative pain. Treatment of motion sickness. Prevention and control of nausea and vomiting in surgery.

**DOSAGE:** *Adults:* (IM/IV) IM is preferred. Allergy: Initial: 25mg, may repeat within 2 hrs. Sedation: 25-50mg qhs. Nausea/Vomiting: 12.5-25mg q4h. Preoperative/Postoperative: 25-50mg. Obstetrics: 50mg in early labor, 25-75mg in established labor, may repeat once or twice q4h. Max: 100mg/24 hrs of labor. Do not give IV administration >25mg/mL and at a rate >25mg/minute.
*Pediatrics:* >2 yrs: Dose should not exceed half of adult dose. Premedication: Usual: 0.5mg/lb. Do not give IV administration >25mg/mL and at a rate >25mg/minute.

**HOW SUPPLIED:** Inj: 25mg/mL, 50mg/mL

**CONTRAINDICATIONS:** Comatose states, intra-arterial or subcutaneous injection. Hypersensitivity to other phenothiazines.

**WARNINGS/PRECAUTIONS:** Caution in patients >2 yrs. Not recommended for uncomplicated vomiting in pediatrics. May cause marked drowsiness; caution with operating machinery. Fatal respiratory depression reported; avoid with respiratory dysfunction (eg, COPD, sleep apnea). Avoid prolonged sun exposure. May lower seizure threshold. Caution with bone marrow depression. NMS reported. Caution in acutely ill pediatric patients. Avoid in pediatrics with Reye's syndrome or hepatic disease. Avoid perivascular extravasation or inadvertent intra-arterial injection. Caution with narrow-angle glaucoma, prostatic hypertrophy, stenosing peptic ulcer, bladder-neck or pyloroduodenal obstruction, cardiovascular disease, hepatic dysfunction. Cholestatic jaundice reported. Alters HCG pregnancy test reading. May increase blood glucose.

**ADVERSE REACTIONS:** Drowsiness, dizziness, tinnitus, blurred vision, dry mouth, increased or decreased blood pressure, urticaria, nausea, vomiting, blood dyscrasia.

**INTERACTIONS:** Added sedative effects with CNS depressants (eg, alcohol, narcotics, narcotic analgesics, sedatives, hypnotics, general anesthetics, tranquilizers, TCAs); reduce dose or eliminate these agents. Reduce barbiturate dose by one-half and analgesic depressant dose by one-quarter to one-half. Caution with drugs that alter seizure threshold (eg, narcotics, local anesthetics). Do not use epinephrine for promethazine injection overdose. Caution with anticholinergics. Possible adverse reactions with MAOIs.

**PREGNANCY:** Category C, caution in nursing.

## PHENOBARBITAL

CIV

phenobarbital (Various)

**THERAPEUTIC CLASS:** Barbiturate

**INDICATIONS:** Treatment of generalized, tonic-clonic and cortical focal seizures. For relief of anxiety, tension and apprehension. Short-term treatment of insomnia.

P

**DOSAGE:** *Adults:* Sedation: 30-120mg/day given bid-tid. Max: 400mg/24h. Hypnotic: 100-200mg. Seizures: 60-200mg/day. Elderly/Debilitated/Renal or Hepatic Dysfunction: Reduce dosage.
*Pediatrics:* Seizures: 3-6mg/kg/day.

**HOW SUPPLIED:** Elixir: 20mg/5mL; Tab: 15mg, 30mg, 32.4mg, 60mg, 64.8mg, 100mg

**CONTRAINDICATIONS:** Respiratory disease with dyspnea or obstruction, porphyria, severe liver dysfunction. Large doses with nephritic patients.

**WARNINGS/PRECAUTIONS:** May be habit forming. Avoid abrupt withdrawal. Caution with acute or chronic pain; may mask symptoms or paradoxical excitement may occur. Cognitive deficits reported in children with febrile seizures. May cause excitement in children and excitement, depression or confusion in elderly, debilitated. Caution with hepatic dysfunction, borderline hypoadrenal function, depression.

**ADVERSE REACTIONS:** Drowsiness, residual sedation, lethargy, vertigo, somnolence, respiratory depression, hypersensitivity reactions, nausea, vomiting, headache.

**INTERACTIONS:** May be potentiated by MAOIs, antihistamines, alcohol, tranquilizers, sedative/hypnotics, other CNS depressants. Decreases effects of oral anticoagulants. Increases corticosteroid metabolism. Decreases effects of oral contraceptives. Decreases absorption of griseofulvin. Decreases half-life of doxycycline. May alter phenytoin metabolism. Increased levels with sodium valproate and valproic acid.

**PREGNANCY:** Category D, caution in nursing.

## PHENYTEK
RX

phenytoin sodium (Mylan Bertek)

**THERAPEUTIC CLASS:** Hydantoin

**INDICATIONS:** Control of generalized tonic-clonic (grand mal) and complex partial (psychomotor, temporal lobe) seizures. Prevention and treatment of neurosurgically induced seizures.

**DOSAGE:** *Adults:* No Previous Treatment: Initial: 100mg extended phenytoin sodium capsule tid. Titrate: May increase at 7-10 day intervals. Usual: 100mg tid-qid. May increase up to 200mg Phenytek tid. Once Daily Dosing: 300mg Phenytek qd may replace 100mg extended phenytoin sodium capsule tid if seizures are controlled. LD (clinic/hospital): 1g in 3 divided doses (400mg, 300mg, 300mg) given 2 hrs apart. Start maintenance 24 hrs later. Avoid LD with renal and hepatic disease.
*Pediatrics:* Initial: 5mg/kg/day given bid-tid. Titrate: May increase at 7-10 day intervals. Maint: 4-8mg/kg/day. Max: 300mg/day. >6 yrs: May require the minimum adult dose (300mg/day).

**HOW SUPPLIED:** Cap, Extended Release: 200mg, 300mg

**WARNINGS/PRECAUTIONS:** Avoid abrupt discontinuation. Caution with porphyria, hepatic dysfunction, elderly, diabetes, debilitated. Discontinue if rash occurs. Lymphadenopathy reported. Serum sickness may occur with lymph node involvement. Gingival hyperplasia reported; maintain proper dental hygiene. Hyperglycemia, birth defects and osteomalacia reported. Monitor levels. Confusional states reported with toxic levels. Increased seizure frequency during pregnancy. Neonatal coagulation defects reported within first 24 hrs of birth; give Vitamin K to mother before delivery and to neonate after birth. Avoid use with seizures due to hypoglycemia or other metabolic causes.

**ADVERSE REACTIONS:** Nystagmus, ataxia, slurred speech, decreased coordination, confusion, dizziness, insomnia, transient nervousness, motor twitchings, headaches, nausea, vomiting, constipation, rash, hypersensitivity reactions.

**INTERACTIONS:** Increased levels with acute alcohol intake, amiodarone, chloramphenicol, chlordiazepoxide, diazepam, dicumarol, disulfiram, estrogens, $H_2$-antagonists, halothane, isoniazid, methylphenidate, phenothiazines, phenylbutazone, salicylates, succinamides, sulfonamides, tolbutamide, trazodone. Decreased levels with chronic alcohol abuse, carbamazepine, reserpine, sucralfate. Decreases effects of corticosteroids, coumarin anticoagulants, digitoxin, doxycycline, estrogens, furosemide, oral contraceptives, quinidine, rifampin, theophylline, vitamin D. Phenobarbital, sodium valproate, valproic acid may increase or decrease levels. May increase or decrease levels of phenobarbital, sodium valproate, valproic acid. Calcium antacids decrease absorption; space dosing. Moban® contains calcium ions which interfere with absorption. TCAs may precipitate seizures. Increased risk of phenytoin hypersensitivity with barbiturates, succinamides, oxazolidinediones.

**PREGNANCY:** Possibly teratogenic, weigh benefits versus risk; not for use in nursing.

## PHISOHEX
RX

hexachlorophene (Sanofi-Aventis)

**THERAPEUTIC CLASS:** Detergent cleanser

**INDICATIONS:** As a surgical scrub and a bacteriostatic skin cleanser. Also to control outbreak of gram-positive infection, when other infection control methods failed.

**DOSAGE:** *Adults:* Surgical Scrub: Apply 5mL with water and lather over hands and forearms. Scrub well with a wet brush for 3 minutes, including nails and

P

interdigital spaces. Rinse thoroughly then repeat. Bacteriostatic Cleansing: Apply 5mL with water and lather, apply to areas that need cleansing. Rinse thoroughly.
*Pediatrics:* Bacteriostatic Cleansing: Apply 5mL with water and lather, apply to areas that need cleansing. Rinse thoroughly. Do not use routinely for bathing infants.

**HOW SUPPLIED:** Liq: 3% [150mL, 480mL, 3840mL]

**CONTRAINDICATIONS:** Burned/denuded skin. Should not use as wet pack, vaginal pack, tampon, occlusive dressing, lotion, on mucous membranes, or as a routine prophylactic bath. Light sensitivity to halogenated phenol derivatives.

**WARNINGS/PRECAUTIONS:** D/C promptly if cerebral irritability occurs. Infants are more susceptible to CNS toxicity. Avoid skin lesions; may cause toxic blood levels. Do not apply to burns; may cause neurotoxicity and death. Avoid eye contact.

**ADVERSE REACTIONS:** Dermatitis, photosensitivity, redness, mild scaling, dryness.

**INTERACTIONS:** Skin products containing alcohol may decrease efficacy.

**PREGNANCY:** Category C, not for use in nursing.

## PhosLo — RX

calcium acetate (Nabi)

**THERAPEUTIC CLASS:** Phosphate binder

**INDICATIONS:** Control of hyperphosphatemia in end stage renal failure (ESRF). Does not promote aluminum absorption.

**DOSAGE:** *Adults:* Initial: 2 caps/tabs with each meal. Titrate: Increase gradually until serum phosphate is <6mg/dL, as long as hypercalcemia does not develop. Maint: 3-4 caps/tabs with each meal.

**HOW SUPPLIED:** Cap: 667mg; Tab: 667mg

**CONTRAINDICATIONS:** Hypercalcemia.

P

**WARNINGS/PRECAUTIONS:** Increased risk of hypercalcemia when calcium given with meals in ESRF. Monitor serum calcium twice weekly during early dose adjustment period. If hypercalcemia develops, reduce dose or d/c depending on severity. Caution with arrhythmias.

**ADVERSE REACTIONS:** Hypercalcemia, constipation, anorexia, nausea, vomiting, confusion, delirium, stupor, coma.

**INTERACTIONS:** Decreased bioavailability of tetracyclines. Hypercalcemia may precipitate arrhythmia; avoid digitalis. Avoid other calcium supplements.

**PREGNANCY:** Category C, safety in nursing not known.

## Phospholine Iodide — RX

echothiophate iodide (Wyeth)

**THERAPEUTIC CLASS:** Cholinesterase inhibitor

**INDICATIONS:** Treatment of glaucoma and accommodative esotropias.

**DOSAGE:** *Adults:* Early Chronic Simple Glaucoma: (0.3%) 1 drop bid, am and hs. Advanced Chronic Simple Glaucoma/Glaucoma Secondary to Cataract Surgery: Initial: (0.3%) 1 drop bid, am and hs. Titrate: Increase to higher strengths as needed.
*Pediatrics:* Accommodative Esotropia: Diagnosis: (0.125%) 1 drop qhs for 2-3 weeks. Treatment: Decrease dose to 1 drop (0.125%) every other day or (0.6%) 1 drop qd. Titrate: Decrease strength gradually. Max: (0.125%) 1 drop qd.

**HOW SUPPLIED:** Sol: 0.125% [5mL]

**CONTRAINDICATIONS:** Active uveal inflammation, angle-closure glaucoma.

**WARNINGS/PRECAUTIONS:** Avoid with quiescent uveitis. Should hold nose for 1-2 minutes to prevent absorption. Discontinue with cardiac irregularities, salivation, urinary incontinence, diarrhea, profuse sweating, muscle weakness, or respiratory difficulties. Caution with vagotonia, bronchial asthma, spastic GI disturbance, peptic ulcer, bradycardia, hypotension, recent MI, epilepsy, parkinsonism, retinal detachment. Tolerance may develop.

**ADVERSE REACTIONS:** Stinging, burning, lacrimation, lid muscle twitching, conjunctival and ciliary redness, browache, induced myopia, visual blurring.

**INTERACTIONS:** Risk of respiratory or cardiovascular collapse with succinylcholine during general anesthesia. Potentiates effects of other cholinesterase inhibitors (eg, succinylcholine, organophosphate, carbamate insecticides, myasthenia gravis drugs).

**PREGNANCY:** Category C, not for use in nursing.

## PHRENILIN FORTE RX

butalbital - acetaminophen (Amarin)

**OTHER BRAND NAMES:** Phrenilin (Amarin)

**THERAPEUTIC CLASS:** Barbiturate/analgesic

**INDICATIONS:** Tension or muscle contraction headaches.

**DOSAGE:** *Adults:* (Phrenilin Forte) 1 cap q4h. (Phrenilin) 1-2 tabs q4h. Max: 6 caps/tabs/day.
*Pediatrics:* >12 yrs: (Phrenilin Forte) 1 cap q4h. (Phrenilin) 1-2 tabs q4h. Max: 6 caps/tabs/day.

**HOW SUPPLIED:** (Butalbital-APAP) Cap: (Phrenilin Forte) 50mg-650mg; Tab: (Phrenilin)50mg-325mg.

**CONTRAINDICATIONS:** Porphyria.

**WARNINGS/PRECAUTIONS:** Abuse potential. Caution in elderly/debilitated, severe renal/hepatic impairment, and acute abdominal conditions.

**ADVERSE REACTIONS:** Drowsiness, lightheadedness, dizziness, sedation, shortness of breath, nausea, vomiting, abdominal pain, intoxicated feeling.

**INTERACTIONS:** Enhanced CNS effects with MAOIs. May enhance CNS depression effects of narcotic analgesics, alcohol, general anesthetics, tranquilizers (eg, chlordiazepoxide, sedative hypnotics, CNS depressants).

**PREGNANCY:** Category C, not for use in nursing.



## PHYTONADIONE RX

phytonadione (Merck)

**Severe, fatal reactions reported during or immediately after IV or IM use. Only use IV or IM route when SC route is not feasible.**

**THERAPEUTIC CLASS:** Vitamin K derivative

**INDICATIONS:** For coagulation disorders caused by vitamin K deficiency or interference with vitamin K activity, including prophylaxis and therapy of hemorrhagic disease of the newborn; anticoagulant-induced prothrombin deficiency caused by coumarin or indanedione derivatives; and hypoprothrombinemia caused by antibacterials, secondary factors that limit absorption or synthesis of vitamin K (obstructive jaundice, biliary fistula), or by drugs that interfere with vitamin K metabolism (eg, salicylates).

**DOSAGE:** *Adults:* Administer SQ when possible. Anticoagulant-Induced PT Deficiency: Initial: 2.5-10mg up to 25mg (rarely 50mg). May repeat if PT is still elevated 6-8 hrs after initial dose. Hypoprothrombinemia Due to Other Causes: 2.5-25mg or more (rarely up to 50mg); route depends on severity of condition and response.
*Pediatrics:* Prophylaxis of Hemorrhagic Disease in Newborn: 0.5-1mg IM within

1 hr of birth. Treatment of Hemorrhagic Disease in Newborn: 1mg SQ/IM (may need higher dose if mother has received oral anticoagulants).

**HOW SUPPLIED:** Inj: 1mg/0.5 mL, 10mg/mL

**WARNINGS/PRECAUTIONS:** Contains benzyl alcohol; toxicity in newborns may occur. Takes 1-2 hrs to observe improvement in PT. Maintain lowest possible dose to prevent original thromboembolic events. Avoid repeated large doses with hepatic disease. Failure to respond may indicate a congenital coagulation defect or a condition unresponsive to vitamin K. Monitor PT regularly.

**ADVERSE REACTIONS:** Anaphylactoid reactions, flushing, peculiar taste sensations, dizziness, rapid and weak pulse, profuse sweating, hypotension, dyspnea, cyanosis, injection site tenderness or swelling, hyperbilirubinemia (in newborns).

**INTERACTIONS:** Does not counteract anticoagulant effects of heparin. Temporary resistance to prothrombin-depressing anticoagulants, especially with large doses.

**PREGNANCY:** Category C, caution in nursing.

## PILOCARPINE RX

pilocarpine HCl (Various)

**OTHER BRAND NAMES:** Isopto Carpine (Alcon)

**THERAPEUTIC CLASS:** Cholinergic agent

**INDICATIONS:** To control intraocular pressure.

**DOSAGE:** *Adults:* 2 drops tid-qid or more if needed. Heavily pigmented irises may require higher strengths.

**HOW SUPPLIED:** Sol: 0.5%, 1%, 2%, 3%, 4%, 6% [15mL]

**CONTRAINDICATIONS:** Where constriction is undesirable (eg, acute iritis) or pupillary block glaucoma.

**WARNINGS/PRECAUTIONS:** Difficulty adapting in the dark. Caution while night driving and in poor illumination. Risk of retinal detachment.



**ADVERSE REACTIONS:** Local irritation, ciliary spasm, conjunctival vascular congestion, temporal or supraorbital headache, induced myopia, reduced visual acuity in poor illumination (elderly), lens opacity (prolonged use).

**PREGNANCY:** Category C, caution in nursing.

## PILOPINE HS RX

pilocarpine HCl (Alcon)

**THERAPEUTIC CLASS:** Direct acting parasympathomimetic

**INDICATIONS:** To control intraocular pressure.

**DOSAGE:** *Adults:* Apply 1/2 inch into conjunctival sac at bedtime.

**HOW SUPPLIED:** Gel: 4% [4g]

**CONTRAINDICATIONS:** Situations where constriction is undesirable (eg, acute iritis).

**WARNINGS/PRECAUTIONS:** For topical use only. May cause difficulty in dark adaptation; caution in night driving and situations in poor illumination.

**ADVERSE REACTIONS:** Lacrimation, burning, discomfort, headache, ciliary spasm, conjunctival vascular congestion, superficial keratitis, myopia.

**PREGNANCY:** Category C, caution in nursing.

## PINDOLOL
pindolol (Various)

RX

**THERAPEUTIC CLASS:** Nonselective beta-blocker

**INDICATIONS:** Management of hypertension.

**DOSAGE:** *Adults:* Initial: 5mg bid. Titrate: May increase by 10mg/day after 3-4 weeks. Max: 60mg/day.

**HOW SUPPLIED:** Tab: 5mg, 10mg

**CONTRAINDICATIONS:** Bronchial asthma, overt cardiac failure, cardiogenic shock, 2nd- and 3rd-degree heart block, severe bradycardia.

**WARNINGS/PRECAUTIONS:** Caution with well-compensated heart failure, nonallergic bronchospasm, renal or hepatic impairment. Can cause cardiac failure. Avoid abrupt withdrawal. Withdrawal before surgery is controversial. May mask hypoglycemia or hyperthyroidism symptoms.

**ADVERSE REACTIONS:** Dizziness, fatigue, insomnia, nervousness, dyspnea, edema, joint pain, muscle cramps/pain.

**INTERACTIONS:** Additive hypotension and/or bradycardia with catecholamine-depleting drugs. Both thioridazine and pindolol levels may increase when used concomitantly.

**PREGNANCY:** Category B, not for use in nursing.

## PIPERACILLIN
piperacillin sodium (Various)

RX

**THERAPEUTIC CLASS:** Broad-spectrum penicillin

**INDICATIONS:** Treatment of serious intra-abdominal, urinary tract, gynecologic, lower respiratory tract, skin and skin structure, bone and joint, and gonococcal infections, septicemia, and perioperative surgical prophylaxis.

**DOSAGE:** *Adults:* Usual: 3-4g IM/IV q4-6h. Max: 24g/day; IM: 2g/site. Serious Infections: 200-300mg/kg/day IV divided q4-6h. Complicated UTI: 125-200mg/kg/day IV divided q6-8h. Uncomplicated UTI/Community Acquired Pneumonia: 100-125mg/kg/day IM/IV divided q6-12h. Uncomplicated Gonorrhea: 2g IM single dose with 1g PO probenecid 1/2 hr before injection. Surgical Prophylaxis: 2g IV 20-30 minute just prior to anesthesia (See labeling for follow-up dosing). C-section: 2g IV after cord is clamped, then 2g 4 hrs and 8 hrs after 1st dose. Renal Impairment: Uncomplicated/Complicated UTI: CrCl <20mL/min: 3g q12h. Complicated UTI: CrCl 20-40mL/min: 3g q8h. Serious Infection: CrCl 20-40mL/min: 4g q8h. CrCl <20mL/min: 4g q12h. Hemodialysis: Give 1g additional dose after each dialysis. Max: 2g q8h. Usual treatment is for 7-10 days; treat gynecologic infections for 3-10 days; treat *S.pyogenes* infections for at least 10 days.
*Pediatrics:* ≥12 yrs: Usual: 3-4g IM/IV q4-6h. Max: 24g/day; IM: 2g/site. Serious Infections: 200-300mg/kg/day IV divided q4-6h. Complicated UTI: 125-200mg/kg/day IV divided q6-8h. Uncomplicated UTI/Community Acquired Pneumonia: 100-125mg/kg/day IM/IV divided q6-12h. Uncomplicated Gonorrhea: 2g IM single dose with 1g PO probenecid 1/2 hr before injection. Surgical Prophylaxis: 2g IV 20-30 minute just prior to anesthesia (See labeling for follow-up dosing). C-section: 2g IV after cord is clamped, then 2g 4 hrs and 8 hrs after 1st dose. Renal Impairment: Uncomplicated/Complicated UTI: CrCl <20mL/min: 3g q12h. Complicated UTI: CrCl 20-40mL/min: 3g q8h. Serious Infection: CrCl 20-40mL/min: 4g q8h. CrCl <20mL/min: 4g q12h. Hemodialysis: Give 1g additional dose after each dialysis. Max: 2g q8h. Usual treatment is for 7-10 days; treat gynecologic infections for 3-10 days; treat *S.pyogenes* infections for at least 10 days.

**HOW SUPPLIED:** Inj: 2g, 3g, 4g

**CONTRAINDICATIONS:** Hypersensitivity to cephalosporins.

**WARNINGS/PRECAUTIONS:** Serious hypersensitivity reactions reported; increased risk with sensitivity to multiple allergens. Cross sensitivity to cephalosporins. Monitor renal, hepatic and hematopoietic functions with prolonged use. D/C if bleeding manifestations occur; increased risk with renal failure. Prolonged use may cause superinfections. May experience neuromuscular excitability or convulsions with higher than recommended doses. Contains 1.85mEq/g sodium; caution with salt restriction. Monitor electrolytes periodically with low potassium levels. May mask symptoms of syphilis. Increased incidence of rash and fever in cystic fibrosis. Continue treatment for at least 48-72 hrs after patient becomes asymptomatic.

**ADVERSE REACTIONS:** Thrombophlebitis, erythema and pain at injection site, diarrhea, headache, dizziness, anaphylaxis, rash, superinfections.

**INTERACTIONS:** Do not mix with aminoglycoside in a syringe or infusion bottle; may cause inactivation of aminoglycoside. May prolong neuromuscular blockade of non-depolarizing muscle relaxants (eg, vecuronium). Increased risk of hypokalemia with cytotoxic therapy or diuretics. May reduce methotrexate clearance. Probenecid may increase levels. Monitor coagulation parameters closely with concomitant anticoagulants.

**PREGNANCY:** Category B, caution in nursing.

## PITOCIN RX

oxytocin (King)

**THERAPEUTIC CLASS:** Uterine Stimulant

**INDICATIONS:** For induction, stimulation or reinforcement of labor. Adjunct for management of incomplete or inevitable abortion. To control postpartum bleeding or hemorrhage.

**DOSAGE:** *Adults:* Labor Induction or Stimulation: Initial: 0.5-1mU/min IV infusion. Titrate: Increase by 1-2mU/min every 30-60 minutes until desired contraction pattern established. Once 5-6cm dilation achieved, reduce dose by similar increments. Rates >9-10mU/min rarely required. Postpartum Bleeding: IV Infusion: Add 10-40U. Max: 40U/1000mL. Adjust infusion rate to sustain contraction and control uterine atony. IM: Give 10U after placenta delivery. Incomplete/Inevitable/Elective Abortion: Add 10U to 500mL physiologic saline IV solution or 5% dextrose-in-water IV solution after a suction or sharp curettage. Midtrimester Elective Abortion: 10-20mU/min IV. Max: 30U/12hrs.



**HOW SUPPLIED:** Inj: 10U/mL

**CONTRAINDICATIONS:** Significant cephalopelvic disproportion, unfavorable fetal positions or presentations, obstetrical emergencies, fetal distress if delivery is not imminent, unsatisfactory progress with adequate uterine activity, hyperactive or hypertonic uterus, when vaginal delivery is contraindicated (eg, invasive cervical carcinoma, active herpes genitalis, total placenta previa, vasa previa, cord presentation or prolapse).

**WARNINGS/PRECAUTIONS:** Continuously monitor by trained personnel. Not indicated for elective induction of labor. D/C if uterine hyperactivity or fetal distress occurs. Except in unusual circumstances, avoid with fetal distress, hydramnios, partial placenta previa, prematurity, borderline cephalopelvic disproportion, and with predisposition to uterine rupture. Hypertonic contractions can occur. Has intrinsic antidiuretic effect; water intoxication may occur.

**ADVERSE REACTIONS:** Mother: Anaphylaxis, postpartum hemorrhage, arrhythmias, fatal fibrinogenemia, nausea, vomiting, pelvic hematoma, subarachnoid hemorrhage, hypertensive episodes, uterine rupture. Fetus: Bradycardia, arrhythmias, CNS damage, seizures, low Apgar scores, jaundice, retinal hemorrhage.

**INTERACTIONS:** Severe HTN reported 3-4 hrs after prophylactic administration of a vasoconstrictor with caudal block anesthesia. Hypotension, maternal sinus bradycardia with abnormal AV rhythms reported with cyclopropane anesthesia.

## PLAN B
levonorgestrel (Duramed)

RX

**THERAPEUTIC CLASS:** Emergency contraceptive kit

**INDICATIONS:** To prevent pregnancy after known or suspected contraceptive failure or unprotected intercourse.

**DOSAGE:** *Adults:* 1 tab as soon as possible, within 72 hrs after unprotected intercourse, then 1 tab 12 hrs after 1st dose. May use during menstrual cycle.

**HOW SUPPLIED:** Tab: 0.75mg

**CONTRAINDICATIONS:** Pregnancy and undiagnosed abnormal genital bleeding.

**WARNINGS/PRECAUTIONS:** Not for routine use as a contraceptive. Risk of glucose intolerance; monitor women with DM. Not effective in terminating an existing pregnancy. Risk of ectopic pregnancy. Irregular menstrual bleeding may occur. Vomiting within 1 hr after doses may decrease effectiveness.

**ADVERSE REACTIONS:** Nausea, abdominal pain, fatigue, headache, menstrual changes, dizziness, breast tenderness, vomiting, diarrhea.

**INTERACTIONS:** Hepatic enzyme inducers (eg, phenytoin, carbamazepine, barbiturates, rifampin) may reduce effectiveness.

**PREGNANCY:** Pregnancy category unknown, caution in nursing.

## PLAQUENIL
hydroxychloroquine sulfate (Sanofi-Aventis)

RX

**Be familiar with complete prescribing information before prescribing hydroxychloroquine.**

**THERAPEUTIC CLASS:** Quinine derivative

**INDICATIONS:** Suppression and treatment of acute attacks of malaria in adults and children. Treatment of discoid and systemic lupus erythematosus and rheumatoid arthritis (RA) in adults.

**DOSAGE:** *Adults:* Malaria Suppression: 400mg weekly. Begin 2 weeks before exposure and continue for 8 weeks after leaving endemic area. Give 400mg q6h for 2 doses if therapy is not begun before exposure. Acute Attack: 800mg, then 400mg 6-8 hrs later, then 400mg for 2 more days. RA: Initial: 400-600mg qd with food or milk; increase until optimum response. Maint: After 4-12 weeks, 200-400mg qd with food or milk. Lupus Erythematosus: Initial: 400mg qd-bid for several weeks depending on response. Maint: 200-400mg/day.
*Pediatrics:* Malaria Suppression: 5mg/kg (base) weekly, max 400mg/dose. Begin 2 weeks before exposure and continue for 8 weeks after leaving endemic area. q6h for 2 doses if therapy is not begun before exposure. Acute Attack: 10mg base/kg, max 800mg/dose; then 5mg base/kg, max 400mg/dose at 6, 24 and 48 hrs after 1st dose.

**HOW SUPPLIED:** Tab: 200mg (200mg tab=155mg base)

**CONTRAINDICATIONS:** Long term therapy in children or if retinal/visual field changes due to 4-aminoquinoline compounds.

**WARNINGS/PRECAUTIONS:** Caution with hepatic disease, G6PD deficiency, alcoholism, psoriasis, and porphyria. Perform baseline and periodic (3 months) ophthalmologic exams and blood cell counts with prolonged therapy. Test periodically for muscle weakness. Discontinue if blood disorders occur. Avoid if possible in pregnancy. Discontinue after 6 months if no improvement in rheumatoid arthritis.

**ADVERSE REACTIONS:** Headache, dizziness, diarrhea, loss of appetite, muscle weakness, nausea, abdominal cramps, bleaching of hair, dermatitis, ocular toxicity, visual field defects.

**INTERACTIONS:** Caution with hepatotoxic drugs.

**PREGNANCY:** Safety in pregnancy and nursing not known.

## PLATINOL-AQ

RX

cisplatin (Bristol-Myers Squibb)

**Cumulative renal toxicity is severe. Myelosuppression, nausea, and vomiting are also dose-related toxicities. Ototoxicity is significant. Anaphylactic-like reactions reported. Avoid inadvertent confusion with carboplatin. Doses >100mg/m²/cycle once every 3-4 weeks are rarely used.**

**THERAPEUTIC CLASS:** Heavy-metal platinum complex

**INDICATIONS:** Combination therapy for metastatic testicular or ovarian tumors after surgery and/or radiotherapy. Monotherapy as secondary therapy for metastatic ovarian tumors refractory to standard treatment. Monotherapy for transitional cell bladder cancer no longer amenable to local treatments.

**DOSAGE:** *Adults:* Testicular Tumor: 20mg/m² IV qd for 5 days per cycle. Ovarian Tumor: Cyclophosphamide Combination Therapy: 75-100mg/m² IV per cycle once every 4 weeks. Monotherapy: 100mg/m² IV per cycle once every 4 weeks. Bladder Cancer: 50-70mg/m² IV per cycle every 3-4 weeks. Pretreatment hydration with 1-2L of fluid 8-12 hrs before therapy, and maintain adequate hydration and urinary output for the 24 hrs after infusion. Hold repeat course until SCr <1.5mg/100mL, BUN <25mg/100mL, platelets >100,000/mm³, WBC >4000/mm³. Hold subsequent doses until audiometric analysis is within normal limits.

**HOW SUPPLIED:** Inj: 50mg, 100mg

**CONTRAINDICATIONS:** Renal impairment, myelosuppression, hearing impairment, allergy to platinum-containing compounds.

**WARNINGS/PRECAUTIONS:** Severe neuropathies reported with higher doses or greater frequency than recommended. Loss of motor function reported. Perform audiometric testing and measure SCr, BUN, CrCl, magnesium, sodium, potassium, and calcium before each dose. Can cause fetal harm during pregnancy. Perform peripheral blood counts weekly, LFTs periodically, and neurologic exam regularly. Avoid aluminum containing IV sets; may cause precipitate. Caution in elderly.

**ADVERSE REACTIONS:** Nephrotoxicity, ototoxicity, vestibular toxicity, myelosuppression, Coombs' positive hemolytic anemia, immediate or delayed nausea and vomiting, serum electrolyte disturbances, hyperuricemia, neurotoxicity, hepatotoxicity.



**INTERACTIONS:** Cumulative nephrotoxicity potentiated with aminoglycosides. Anticonvulsant levels may become subtherapeutic. Response duration adversely affected with pyridoxine and altretamine.

**PREGNANCY:** Category D, not for use in nursing.

## PLAVIX

RX

clopidogrel bisulfate (Bristol-Myers Squibb/Sanofi-Aventis)

**THERAPEUTIC CLASS:** Platelet aggregation inhibitor

**INDICATIONS:** For reduction of thrombotic events in those with recent stroke or MI, established peripheral arterial disease (PAD); or with non-ST-segment elevation acute coronary syndrome (unstable angina/non-Q-wave MI); and patients with ST-segment elevation acute myocardial infarction (STEMI).

**DOSAGE:** *Adults:* MI/Stroke/PAD: 75mg qd. Acute Coronary Syndrome: Take with 75-325mg ASA qd. LD: 300mg. Maint: 75mg qd. STEMI: 75mg, with 75-325mg ASA, qd with or without LD.

**HOW SUPPLIED:** Tab: 75mg

**CONTRAINDICATIONS:** Active pathological bleeding (eg, peptic ulcer, intracranial hemorrhage).

**WARNINGS/PRECAUTIONS:** Caution with risk of increased bleeding, ulcers or lesions with a propensity to bleed, severe hepatic or renal impairment. D/C 5 days before surgery if antiplatelet effect is not desired. Monitor blood cell count and other appropriate tests if symptoms of bleeding or undesirable hematological effects arise. Thrombotic thrombocytopenic purpura (TTP) reported (rare).

**ADVERSE REACTIONS:** Chest pain, influenza-like symptoms, pain, edema, HTN, headache, dizziness, abdominal pain, dyspepsia, diarrhea, arthralgia, purpura, upper respiratory tract infection, back pain, dyspnea.

**INTERACTIONS:** Potentiates effect of aspirin on collagen-induced platelet aggregation. Caution with warfarin. Increased occult GI loss with NSAIDs. Inhibits CYP2C9; caution with phenytoin, tamoxifen, tolbutamide, warfarin, torsemide, fluvastatin, and many NSAIDs. Caution with drugs that may induce GI lesions.

**PREGNANCY:** Category B, not for use in nursing.

## PLENDIL

RX

felodipine (AstraZeneca LP)

**THERAPEUTIC CLASS:** Calcium channel blocker (dihydropyridine)

**INDICATIONS:** Treatment of hypertension.

**DOSAGE:** *Adults:* Initial: 5mg qd. Titrate: Adjust at no less than 2 week intervals. Maint: 2.5-10mg qd. Elderly/Hepatic Dysfunction: Initial: 2.5mg qd. Take without food or with a light meal. Swallow tab whole.

**HOW SUPPLIED:** Tab, Extended Release: 2.5mg, 5mg, 10mg

**WARNINGS/PRECAUTIONS:** May cause hypotension and lead to reflex tachycardia with precipitation of angina. Caution with heart failure or ventricular dysfunction, especially with concomitant β-blockers. Monitor dose adjustment with hepatic dysfunction or elderly. Peripheral edema reported. Maintain good dental hygiene; gingival hyperplasia reported.

**ADVERSE REACTIONS:** Peripheral edema, headache, flushing, dizziness.

**INTERACTIONS:** CYP3A4 inhibitors (eg, itraconazole, ketoconazole, erythromycin, grapefruit juice, cimetidine) may increase plasma levels. Levels decreased with long-term anticonvulsant therapy. May increase metoprolol levels.

**PREGNANCY:** Category C, not for use in nursing.



## PLETAL

RX

cilostazol (Otsuka America)

**Contraindicated with CHF of any severity due to possible decrease in survival.**

**THERAPEUTIC CLASS:** Phosphodiesterase III inhibitor

**INDICATIONS:** Reduction of symptoms with intermittent claudication.

**DOSAGE:** *Adults:* 100mg bid, 1/2 hr before or 2 hrs after breakfast and dinner. Concomitant CYP3A4 and CYP2C19 Inhibitors: Consider 50mg bid.

**HOW SUPPLIED:** Tab: 50mg, 100mg

**CONTRAINDICATIONS:** CHF of any severity.

**WARNINGS/PRECAUTIONS:** Risks not known in patients with severe underlying heart disease, moderate or severe hepatic impairment, or with long-term use. Rare cases of thrombocytopenia or leukopenia reported.

**ADVERSE REACTIONS:** Headache, palpitation, tachycardia, abnormal stool, diarrhea, peripheral edema, dizziness, infection.

**INTERACTIONS:** Caution with CYP3A4 inhibitors (eg, ketoconazole, diltiazem, erythromycin) or CYP2C19 inhibitors (eg, omeprazole); may increase cilostazol levels. Avoid grapefruit juice.

**PREGNANCY:** Category C, not for use in nursing.

## PLEXION RX
sulfur - sulfacetamide sodium (Medicis)

**OTHER BRAND NAMES:** Plexion TS (Medicis) - Plexion SCT (Medicis)

**THERAPEUTIC CLASS:** Sulfonamide/sulfur combination

**INDICATIONS:** Topical treatment of acne vulgaris, acne rosacea, and seborrheic dermatitis.

**DOSAGE:** *Adults:* (Cleanser) Wash qd-bid. Massage into skin for 10-20 seconds, then rinse and dry. (TS) Apply qd-tid. (Cre) Apply to wet skin. Rinse off with water after 10 minutes or if dry.
*Pediatrics:* >12 yrs: (Cleanser) Wash qd-bid. Massage into skin for 10-20 seconds, then rinse and dry. (TS) Apply qd-tid. (Cre) Apply to wet skin. Rinse off with water after 10 minutes or if dry.

**HOW SUPPLIED:** Cleanser: (Sulfacetamide-Sulfur) 10%-5% [170.3g, 340.2g]; Cre: (SCT) 10%-5% [120g]; Lot: (TS) 10%-5% [30g]; Pads: 10%-5% [30$^s$]

**CONTRAINDICATIONS:** Kidney disease.

**WARNINGS/PRECAUTIONS:** D/C if irritation occurs. Avoid eye contact or mucous membranes. Caution with denuded or abraded skin, patients prone to topical sulfonamide hypersensitivity. Can cause reddening and scaling of epidermis.

**ADVERSE REACTIONS:** Local irritation.

**PREGNANCY:** Category C, caution in nursing.

## PNEUMOVAX 23 RX
pneumococcal vaccine (Merck)

**THERAPEUTIC CLASS:** Vaccine

**INDICATIONS:** Immunization against pneumococcal disease caused by those pneumococcal types included in the vaccine.

**DOSAGE:** *Adults:* Usual: 0.5mL SQ/IM in deltoid muscle or lateral mid-thigh.
*Pediatrics:* >2 yrs: 0.5mL SQ/IM in deltoid muscle or lateral mid-thigh.

**HOW SUPPLIED:** Inj: 575mcg/0.5mL



**WARNINGS/PRECAUTIONS:** Vaccination timing is critical for chemotherapy or immunosuppressive therapy. Suboptimal response may occur in immunocompromised patients. Caution with severely compromised cardiovascular or pulmonary function where systemic reaction would be a significant risk. Delay vaccine with febrile respiratory illness or other active infection. Do not revaccinate immunocompetent patients. Continue prophylaxis pneumococcal antibiotics. May not prevent pneumococcal meningitis with chronic CSF leakage.

**ADVERSE REACTIONS:** Local injection site reactions (eg, soreness, warmth, erythema, swelling, induration), fever (<102°F).

**PREGNANCY:** Category C, caution use in nursing.

## PODOCON-25 RX
podophyllin (Paddock)

**THERAPEUTIC CLASS:** Cytotoxic agent

**INDICATIONS:** Removal of soft genital warts (condylomata acuminata).

**DOSAGE:** *Adults:* Cleanse area. Initial: Apply to lesion; remove after 30-45 minutes to determine sensitivity. Usual: Apply to lesion; remove with alcohol or soap and water when achieve desired result (1-4 hrs).

**HOW SUPPLIED:** Liq: 25% [15mL]

**CONTRAINDICATIONS:** Diabetes, steroid therapy, poor blood circulation, bleeding warts, moles, birthmarks, unusual warts with hair, pregnancy, nursing.

**WARNINGS/PRECAUTIONS:** Powerful caustic and severe irritant; avoid healthy tissue. Avoid inflamed or irritated tissue, eyes, bleeding warts, moles, birthmarks, or unusual warts with hair.

**ADVERSE REACTIONS:** Paresthesia, polyneuritis, paralytic ileus, pyrexia, leukopenia, thrombocytopenia, coma, death.

**PREGNANCY:** Contraindicated in pregnancy and nursing.

## POLYCITRA RX

citric acid - potassium citrate (Ortho-McNeil)

**THERAPEUTIC CLASS:** Alkalinizing agent

**INDICATIONS:** Alkalinizing agent for uric acid and cystine calculi of the urinary tract. Adjunct to uricosuric agents for gout. Correction of renal tubular acidosis.

**DOSAGE:** *Adults:* 15mL or 1 packet qid, pc and hs. Dilute in 6 oz of water or juice.

**HOW SUPPLIED:** Packet: 1002mg-3300mg/pack [100s]; Sol: (Citric Acid-Potassium Citrate) 334mg-550mg/5mL [480mL]

**CONTRAINDICATIONS:** Severe renal impairment with oliguria or azotemia, untreated Addison's disease, adynamia episodica hereditaria, acute dehydration, heat cramps, anuria, severe myocardial damage, hyperkalemia.

**WARNINGS/PRECAUTIONS:** Large doses can cause hyperkalemia and alkalosis. Caution with low urinary output. Dilute adequately in water to minimize GI injury.

**ADVERSE REACTIONS:** Diarrhea and other GI effects.

**INTERACTIONS:** Risk of toxicity with $K^+$-containing agents, $K^+$-sparing diuretics, ACE inhibitors, cardiac glycosides.

**PREGNANCY:** Safety in pregnancy and nursing not known.



## POLYSPORIN OPHTHALMIC RX

bacitracin zinc - polymyxin B sulfate (King)

**THERAPEUTIC CLASS:** Antibacterial combination

**INDICATIONS:** Superficial ocular infections involving the conjunctive and/or cornea caused by susceptible organisms.

**DOSAGE:** *Adults:* Apply q3-4h for 7-10 days, depending on severity.

**HOW SUPPLIED:** Oint: (Bacitracin-Polymyxin B) 500U-10,000U/g [3.5g]

**WARNINGS/PRECAUTIONS:** May retard corneal wound healing or cause cutaneous sensitization.

**ADVERSE REACTIONS:** Allergic reactions (eg, itching, swelling, conjunctival erythema), local irritation upon instillation, superinfection (prolonged use).

**PREGNANCY:** Category C, caution in nursing.

## POLYTRIM RX

polymyxin B sulfate - trimethoprim sulfate (Allergan)

**THERAPEUTIC CLASS:** Dihydrofolate reductase inhibitor/antibiotic

**INDICATIONS:** Surface ocular bacterial infections, including blepharoconjunctivitis, acute bacterial conjunctivitis.

**DOSAGE:** *Adults:* Mild-Moderate Infections: 1 drop q3h for 7-10 days. Max: 6 doses/day.
*Pediatrics:* >2 months: Mild-Moderate Infections: 1 drop q3h for 7-10 days. Max: 6 doses/day.

**HOW SUPPLIED:** Sol: (Trimethoprim-Polymyxin B) 1mg-10,000U/mL [10mL]

**WARNINGS/PRECAUTIONS:** Not indicated for the prophylaxis or treatment of ophthalmia neonatorum.

**ADVERSE REACTIONS:** Local irritation, lid edema, itching, increased redness, tearing, burning, stinging, circumocular rash, superinfection (prolonged use).

**PREGNANCY:** Category C, caution in nursing.

## POLY-VI-FLOR RX

sodium fluoride - multiple vitamin (Mead Johnson)

**THERAPEUTIC CLASS:** Multiple vitamin/fluoride supplement

**INDICATIONS:** Vitamin supplement. Fluoride supplement for caries prophylaxis in areas where water contains less than optimal fluoride levels.

**DOSAGE:** *Pediatrics:* (Sol) 6 months-3 yrs and <0.3 ppm Fluoride or 3-6 yrs and 0.3-0.6 ppm Fluoride: 1mL (0.25mg) qd. 3-6 yrs and <0.3 ppm Fluoride or >6 yrs and 0.3-0.6 ppm Fluoride: 1mL (0.5mg) qd. (Tab) 4-6 yrs and 0.3-0.6 ppm Fluoride: 0.25mg qd. 4-6 yrs and <0.3 ppm Fluoride or >6 yrs and 0.3-0.6 ppm Fluoride: 0.5mg qd. 6-16 yrs and <0.3 ppm Fluoride: 1mg qd.

**HOW SUPPLIED:** Sol: Vitamin A 1500 IU-Vitamin C 35mg-Vitamin D 400 IU-Vitamin E 5 IU-Thiamin 0.5mg-Riboflavin 0.6mg-Niacin 8mg-Vitamin $B_6$ 0.4mg-Vitamin $B_{12}$ 2mcg. 0.25mg drops contains 0.25mg Fluoride [50mL], 0.5mg drops contain 0.5mg Fluoride [50mL]; Tab, Chewable: Vitamin A 2500 IU-Vitamin C 60mg-Vitamin D 400 IU-Vitamin E 15 IU-Thiamin 1.05mg-Riboflavin 1.2mg-Niacin 13.5mg-Vitamin $B_6$ 1.05mg-Folate 0.3mg-Vitamin $B_{12}$ 4.5mcg. 0.25mg tabs contain 0.25mg Fluoride; 0.5mg tabs contain 0.5mg Fluoride; 1mg tabs contain 1mg Fluoride

**WARNINGS/PRECAUTIONS:** Must chew tab; not for pediatrics <4yrs. Risk of dental fluorosis from ingestion of large amounts of fluoride. Children up to 16 yrs, in areas where water contains less than optimal fluoride levels, should receive daily fluoride supplementation.

**ADVERSE REACTIONS:** Allergic rash.

**PREGNANCY:** Safety in pregnancy and nursing not known.

## PONSTEL RX

mefenamic acid (Sciele)

**NSAIDs may cause an increased risk of serious cardiovascular thrombotic events, MI, stroke and serious GI adverse events including bleeding, ulceration, and perforation of the stomach or intestines. Contraindicated for the treatment of peri-operative pain in the setting of coronary artery bypass graft (CABG) surgery.**

**THERAPEUTIC CLASS:** NSAID (fenamate derivative)

**INDICATIONS:** Relief of mild to moderate pain in patients >14 yrs, when therapy will not exceed 7 days. Treatment of primary dysmenorrhea.

**DOSAGE:** *Adults:* Acute Pain: Usual: 500mg, then 250mg q6h prn up to 1 week. Primary Dysmenorrhea: Usual: 500mg, then 250mg q6h up to 3 days. Take with food.
*Pediatrics:* >14 yrs: Acute Pain: Usual: 500mg, then 250mg q6h prn, up to 1 week. Primary Dysmenorrhea: Usual: 500mg, then 250mg q6h up to 3 days. Take with food.

**HOW SUPPLIED:** Cap: 250mg

**CONTRAINDICATIONS:** Pre-existing renal disease, active ulceration or chronic inflammation of the GI tract. Allergic-type reactions, including asthma and urticaria, after taking ASA or other NSAIDs. Treatment of peri-operative pain in the setting of CABG surgery.

**WARNINGS/PRECAUTIONS:** May lead to onset of new HTN or worsening of pre-existing HTN; monitor BP closely. Fluid retention and edema reported; caution with fluid retention or heart failure. Renal papillary necrosis and other renal injury reported after long-term use. Not recommended for use with advanced renal disease. Anaphylactoid reactions may occur. May cause serious skin adverse events (eg, exfoliative dermatitis, Stevens-Johnson syndrome, and toxic epidermal necrolysis). Avoid in late pregnancy; may cause premature closure of ductus arteriosis. May cause elevations of LFTs; d/c if liver disease develops or systemic manifestations occur. Caution in elderly. Anemia may occur; with long-term use, monitor Hgb/Hct if signs or symptoms of anemia develop. May inhibit platelet aggregation and prolong bleeding time; monitor with coagulation disorders. Caution with asthma and avoid with aspirin-sensitive asthma.

**ADVERSE REACTIONS:** Abdominal pain, constipation, diarrhea, dyspepsia, flatulence, gross bleeding/perforation, heartburn, nausea, GI ulcers, vomiting, abnormal renal function, anemia, dizziness, edema, elevated liver enzymes, headache, increased bleeding time, pruritus, rash, tinnitus.

**INTERACTIONS:** ASA may increase adverse effects; avoid use. Warfarin may increase GI bleeding. May prolong PT with oral anticoagulants. May enhance methotrexate toxicity. Decrease effects of ACE inhibitors, furosemide and thiazides; monitor for renal toxicity. Increase in lithium levels. Magnesium hydroxide may increase mefenamic acid levels. Caution with CYP2C9 inhibitors including fluconazole, lovastatin and trimethoprim.

**PREGNANCY:** Category C, not for use in nursing.

## POTABA RX

potassium p-aminobenzoate (Glenwood)

**THERAPEUTIC CLASS:** Vitamin B complex

**INDICATIONS:** Possibly effective for the treatment of Peyronie's disease, dermatomyositis, linear scleroderma, pemphigus.

**DOSAGE:** *Adults:* Usual: 12g/day, in 4 to 6 divided doses. Take with meals or snacks. Tabs should be taken with plenty of liquid. Dissolve powder in water or juice.
*Pediatrics:* 1g/day for each 10 lbs of body weight given in divided doses. Dissolve powder in water or juice. Take with food and plenty of liquid.

**HOW SUPPLIED:** Cap: 0.5g; Pow: 2g/envule [50$^s$]; Tab: 0.5g

**CONTRAINDICATIONS:** Concomitant sulfonamides.

**WARNINGS/PRECAUTIONS:** Suspend therapy if anorexia, nausea, occurs. D/C if hypersensitivity reaction develops. Caution with renal disease.

**ADVERSE REACTIONS:** Anorexia, nausea, fever, rash.

**PREGNANCY:** Safety in pregnancy or nursing not known.

## PRAMOSONE RX

pramoxine HCl - hydrocortisone acetate (Ferndale)

**THERAPEUTIC CLASS:** Corticosteroid/anesthetic

**INDICATIONS:** Relief of the inflammatory and pruritic manifestations of corticosteroid-responsive dermatoses.

**DOSAGE:** *Adults:* Apply tid-qid. May use occlusive dressings for psoriasis or recalcitrant conditions. D/C dressings if infection develops.
*Pediatrics:* Apply tid-qid. May use occlusive dressings for psoriasis or recalcitrant conditions. D/C dressings if infection develops.

**HOW SUPPLIED:** (Pramoxine-Hydrocortisone) Cre: 1%-1%, 1%-2.5% [30g, 60g]; Lot: 1%-1% [60mL, 120mL, 240mL], 1%-2.5% [60mL, 120mL]; Oint: 1%-1%, 1%-2.5% [30g]

**WARNINGS/PRECAUTIONS:** May produce reversible HPA axis suppression, manifestations of Cushing's syndrome, hyperglycemia, and glucosuria. Caution when applied to large surface areas or under occlusive dressings. Use appropriate antifungal or antibacterial agent with dermatological infections; d/c if infection does not clear. Peds may be more susceptible to systemic toxicity. Avoid eyes. D/C if irritation occurs.

**ADVERSE REACTIONS:** Burning, itching, irritation, dryness, folliculitis, hypertrichosis, acneiform eruptions, hypopigmentation, perioral dermatitis, allergic dermatitis, skin maceration, secondary infection, skin atrophy, striae, miliaria.

**PREGNANCY:** Category C, caution in nursing.

## PRANDIN RX

repaglinide (Novo Nordisk)

**THERAPEUTIC CLASS:** Meglitinide

**INDICATIONS:** Adjunct to diet and exercise, to improve glycemic control in type 2 diabetes mellitus. May use in combination with metformin or thiazolidinediones (TZDs).

**DOSAGE:** *Adults:* Take within 15-30 minutes before meals. Skip dose if skipping meal and add dose if adding meal. Initial: Treatment-Naive or $HbA_{1c}$ <8%: 0.5mg with each meal. Previous Oral Therapy/Combination Therapy and $HbA_{1c}$ >8%: 1-2mg with each meal. Titrate: May double preprandial dose up to 4mg (bid-qid) at no less than 1 week intervals. Maint: 0.5-4mg with meals. Max: 16mg/day. If hypoglycemia with combination metformin or TZD occurs, reduce repaglinide dose. Renal Dysfunction: CrCl 20-40mg/dL: Initial: 0.5mg with each meal; titrate carefully. Hepatic Dysfunction: Increase intervals between dose adjustments.

**HOW SUPPLIED:** Tab: 0.5mg, 1mg, 2mg

**CONTRAINDICATIONS:** Diabetic ketoacidosis and type 1 diabetes.

P

**WARNINGS/PRECAUTIONS:** Hypoglycemia risk especially with renal/hepatic insufficiency, elderly, malnourished and adrenal/pituitary insufficiency. Loss of blood glucose control when exposed to stress (fever, trauma, infection or surgery); d/c therapy and start insulin. Secondary failure can occur over a period of time. Caution with hepatic and renal dysfunction. Not indicated for use in combination with NPH insulin.

**ADVERSE REACTIONS:** Hypoglycemia, cardiovascular effects, respiratory infections, UTI, bronchitis, sinusitis, rhinitis, paresthesia, nausea, diarrhea, constipation, vomiting, dyspepsia, arthralgia, back pain, headache, chest pain.

**INTERACTIONS:** Increased metabolism with CYP3A4 inducers (eg, rifampin, barbiturates, carbamazepine). Ketoconazole, miconazole, and erythromycin (CYP3A4 inhibitors) may inhibit metabolism. Increased levels with gemfibrozil; use caution and monitor levels if already on both drugs, avoid initiation of concurrent use. Avoid itraconazole if already on gemfibrozil and repaglinide; synergistic effect may occur. Potentiated hypoglycemia with alcohol, β-blockers, NSAIDs, and other highly protein bound drugs, salicylates, sulfonamides, chloramphenicol, coumarins, probenecid, MAOIs. Risk of hyperglycemia with diuretics, corticosteroids, phenothiazines, thyroid products, estrogens, phenytoin, nicotinic acid, sympathomimetics, calcium channel blockers, and isoniazid. β-blockers may mask hypoglycemia. Increases levonorgestrel and ethinyl estradiol levels. Increased levels with simvastatin, levonorgestrel, and ethinyl estradiol.

**PREGNANCY:** Category C, not for use in nursing.

## PRAVACHOL RX

pravastatin sodium (Bristol-Myers Squibb)

**THERAPEUTIC CLASS:** HMG-CoA reductase inhibitor

**INDICATIONS:** As adjunct to diet, to reduce elevated total-C, LDL-C, Apo B, TG levels, and to increase HDL-C in primary hypercholesterolemia and mixed dyslipidemia (Type IIa and IIb). Treatment of primary dysbetalipoproteinemia (Type III) and heterozygous familial hypercholesterolemia. To reduce elevated serum TG levels (Type IV). In hypercholesterolemic patients without coronary heart disease, to reduce risk of: MI, undergoing myocardial revascularization procedures, and cardiovascular mortality with no increase in death from non-cardiovascular causes. In patients with coronary heart disease, to reduce risk of: mortality by reducing coronary death, undergoing myocardial revascularization procedures, MI, stroke, and TIA; and to slow progression of coronary atherosclerosis.

**DOSAGE:** *Adults:* >18 yrs: Initial: 40mg qd. Perform lipid tests within 4 weeks and adjust according to response and guidelines. Titrate: May increase to 80mg qd if needed. Significant Renal/Hepatic Dysfunction: Initial: 10mg qd. Concomitant Immunosuppressives (eg, Cyclosporine): Initial: 10mg qhs. Max: 20mg/day.
*Pediatrics:* Heterozygous Familial Hypercholesterolemia: 14-18 yrs: Initial: 40mg qd. 8-13 yrs: 20mg qd. Concomitant Immunosuppressives (eg, Cyclosporine): Initial: 10mg qhs. Max: 20mg/day.

**HOW SUPPLIED:** Tab: 10mg, 20mg, 40mg, 80mg

**CONTRAINDICATIONS:** Active liver disease, unexplained persistent elevations of LFTs, pregnancy, nursing mothers.

**WARNINGS/PRECAUTIONS:** Perform LFTs before therapy, before dose increases, and if clinically indicated. Risk of myopathy, myalgia, and rhabdomyolysis. D/C if AST or ALT >3X ULN persists, if elevated CPK levels occur, or if myopathy diagnosed or suspected. Less effective with homozygous familial hypercholesterolemia. Monitor for endocrine dysfunction. Closely monitor with heavy alcohol use, recent history or signs of hepatic disease, or renal dysfunction.

**ADVERSE REACTIONS:** Rash, nausea, vomiting, diarrhea, headache, chest pain, influenza, abdominal pain, dizziness, increases ALT, AST, CPK.

**INTERACTIONS:** Risk of myopathy with fibrates, niacin, cyclosporine, erythromycin. Increased levels with gemfibrozil, itraconazole. Avoid fibrates unless benefit outweighs drug combination risk. Decreased levels with concomitant cholestyramine/colestipol; take 1 hr before or 4 hrs after resins. Caution with drugs that diminish levels or activity of steroid hormones (eg, ketoconazole, spironolactone, cimetidine).

**PREGNANCY:** Category X, not for use in nursing.

## PRECARE CONCEIVE RX

minerals - folic acid - multiple vitamin (Ther-Rx)

**THERAPEUTIC CLASS:** Prenatal vitamin

**INDICATIONS:** Vitamin and mineral supplementation for before and during pregnancy.

**DOSAGE:** *Adults:* 1 tab qd.

**HOW SUPPLIED:** Tab: Calcium 200mg-Copper 2mg-Folic Acid 1mg-Iron 30mg-Magnesium 100mg-Niacin 20mg-Vitamin $B_1$ 3mg-Vitamin $B_2$ 3.4mg-Vitamin $B_6$ 50mg-Vitamin $B_{12}$ 0.012mg-Vitamin C 60mg-Vitamin E 30IU-Zinc 15mg

**WARNINGS/PRECAUTIONS:** Accidental overdose of iron-containing products is a leading cause of fatal poisoning in children <6 yrs. Not for the treatment of pernicious anemia and other megaloblastic anemias where vitamin $B_{12}$ is deficient. Folic acid >0.1mg/day may obscure pernicious anemia.

**ADVERSE REACTIONS:** Allergic sensitization.

P

## PRECARE PRENATAL RX

minerals - folic acid - multiple vitamin (Ther-Rx)

**THERAPEUTIC CLASS:** Prenatal vitamin

**INDICATIONS:** Vitamin and mineral supplementation for before, during, and after pregnancy.

**DOSAGE:** *Adults:* 1 tab qd.

**HOW SUPPLIED:** Tab: Calcium 250mg-Copper 2mg-Folic Acid 1mg-Iron 40mg-Magnesium 50mg-Niacin 20mg-Vitamin $B_1$ 3mg-Vitamin $B_2$ 3.4mg-Vitamin $B_6$ 50mg-Vitamin $B_{12}$ 0.012mg-Vitamin C 50mg-Vitamin D 0.006mg-Vitamin E 3.5mg-Zinc 15mg* *scored

**WARNINGS/PRECAUTIONS:** Accidental overdose of iron-containing products is a leading cause of fatal poisoning in children <6 yrs. Not for the treatment of pernicious anemia and other megaloblastic anemias where vitamin $B_{12}$ is deficient. Folic acid >0.1mg/day may obscure pernicious anemia.

**ADVERSE REACTIONS:** Allergic sensitization.

## PRECOSE RX

acarbose (Bayer)

**THERAPEUTIC CLASS:** Alpha-glucosidase inhibitor

**INDICATIONS:** Adjunct to diet and exercise, to improve glycemic control in type 2 diabetes mellitus. May use with insulin, metformin, or a sulfonylurea.

**DOSAGE:** *Adults:* Initial: 25mg tid with first bite of each main meal. To minimize GI effects: 25mg qd, increase gradually to 25mg tid. Titrate: After reaching 25mg tid, may increase at 4-8 week intervals. Maint: 50-100mg tid. Max: <60kg: 50mg tid. >60kg: 100mg tid. If no further reduction in post prandial or $HbA_{1c}$ with 100mg tid, consider reducing dose.

**HOW SUPPLIED:** Tab: 25mg, 50mg, 100mg

**CONTRAINDICATIONS:** Diabetic ketoacidosis, cirrhosis, inflammatory bowel disease, colonic ulceration, partial or predisposition to intestinal obstruction, chronic intestinal disease with marked disorders of digestion or absorption, and conditions that may deteriorate from increased intestinal gas formation.

**WARNINGS/PRECAUTIONS:** Avoid with significant renal dysfunction (SrCr >2mg/dL). May need to d/c and give insulin with stress (eg, fever, trauma). Dose related elevated serum transaminase levels reported. Monitor serum transaminases every 3 months for first year then periodically. Reduce dose or d/c if elevated serum transaminases persist. Use glucose (dextrose) instead of sucrose (sugar cane) to treat mild to moderate hypoglycemia.

**ADVERSE REACTIONS:** Transient flatulence, diarrhea, abdominal pain.

**INTERACTIONS:** Risk of hyperglycemia with diuretics, corticosteroids, phenothiazines, thyroid products, estrogens, oral contraceptives, phenytoin, nicotinic acid, sympathomimetics, calcium channel blockers, and isoniazid. Reduced effect with intestinal adsorbents (eg, charcoal) and digestive enzymes containing carbohydrate-splitting enzymes (eg, amylase, pancreatin); avoid concomitant use. May affect digoxin bioavailability; may require dose adjustment of digoxin. Monitor for hypoglycemia with insulin or sulfonylureas.

**PREGNANCY:** Category B, not for use in nursing.

## PRED FORTE

RX

prednisolone acetate (Allergan)

**THERAPEUTIC CLASS:** Corticosteroid

**INDICATIONS:** Treatment of inflammation of the palpebral and bulbar conjunctiva, cornea and anterior segment of the globe.

**DOSAGE:** *Adults:* 1-2 drops bid-qid. May dose more frequently during initial 24-48 hrs. Re-evaluate after 2 days if no improvement.

**HOW SUPPLIED:** Sus: 1% [1mL, 5mL, 10mL, 15mL]

**CONTRAINDICATIONS:** Viral diseases of the cornea and conjunctiva including epithelial herpes simplex keratitis, vaccinia, and varicella. Mycobacterial infection and fungal diseases of the eye.

**WARNINGS/PRECAUTIONS:** Caution with glaucoma, herpes simplex, diseases causing thinning of cornea/sclera and other ocular viral infections. Prolonged use can cause glaucoma or secondary ocular infections (eg, fungal). Monitor IOP after 10 days of therapy. Re-evaluate if no response after 2 days. May delay healing and increase incidence of bleb formation after cataract surgery. Avoid abrupt withdrawal with chronic use. Contains sodium bisulfite.

**ADVERSE REACTIONS:** Elevation of IOP, glaucoma, infrequent optic nerve damage, posterior subcapsular cataract formation, delayed wound healing, burning/stinging upon instillation, ocular irritation, secondary infection, visual disturbance.

**PREGNANCY:** Category C, not for use in nursing.

## PRED MILD

RX

prednisolone acetate (Allergan)

**THERAPEUTIC CLASS:** Corticosteroid

**INDICATIONS:** Treatment of noninfectious ocular inflammation.

**DOSAGE:** *Adults:* 1-2 drops bid-qid. May dose more frequently during initial 24-48 hrs. Re-evaluate after 2 days if no improvement.

**HOW SUPPLIED:** Sus: 0.12% [5mL, 10mL]

**CONTRAINDICATIONS:** Viral diseases of the cornea and conjunctiva including epithelial herpes simplex keratitis, vaccinia, and varicella. Mycobacterial infection and fungal diseases of the eye.

**WARNINGS/PRECAUTIONS:** Caution with glaucoma, herpes simplex, diseases causing thinning of cornea/sclera and other ocular viral infections. Prolonged use can cause glaucoma or secondary ocular infections (eg, fungal). Monitor IOP after 10 days of therapy. Re-evaluate if no response after 2 days. May delay healing and increase incidence of bleb formation after cataract surgery. Avoid abrupt withdrawal with chronic use. Contains sodium bisulfite.

**ADVERSE REACTIONS:** Elevation of IOP, glaucoma, infrequent optic nerve damage, posterior subcapsular cataract formation, delayed wound healing, burning/stinging upon instillation, ocular irritation, secondary infection, visual disturbance.

**PREGNANCY:** Category C, not for use in nursing.

## PRED-G

RX

gentamicin sulfate - prednisolone acetate (Allergan)

**OTHER BRAND NAMES:** Pred-G S.O.P. (Allergan)

**THERAPEUTIC CLASS:** Aminoglycoside/corticosteroid

**INDICATIONS:** Ocular inflammation associated with infection or risk of infection.

**DOSAGE:** *Adults:* (Sus) 1 drop bid-qid. May increase dose to every hour during initial 24-48 hrs. Max: 20mL for initial prescription. (Oint) Apply 1/2 inch in conjunctival sac qd-tid. Max: 8g for initial prescription.

**HOW SUPPLIED:** (Gentamicin-Prednisolone) Oint: (S.O.P.) 0.3%-0.6% [3.5g]; Sus: 0.3%-1% [2mL, 5mL, 10mL]

**CONTRAINDICATIONS:** Viral diseases of the cornea and conjunctiva including epithelial herpes simplex keratitis, vaccinia, and varicella. Mycobacterial infection and fungal diseases of the eye.

**WARNINGS/PRECAUTIONS:** Caution with glaucoma, herpes simplex, diseases causing thinning of cornea/sclera and other ocular viral infections. Prolonged use can cause glaucoma or secondary ocular infections (eg, fungal). Monitor IOP after 10 days of therapy. Re-evaluate if no response after 2 days. May delay healing and increase incidence of bleb formation after cataract surgery. Ocular irritation and punctate keratitis reported.

**ADVERSE REACTIONS:** Elevation of IOP, glaucoma, infrequent optic nerve damage, posterior subcapsular cataract formation, delayed wound healing, irritation upon instillation, ocular discomfort, secondary infection.

**PREGNANCY:** Category C, not for use in nursing.

## PREDNISONE

RX

prednisone (Roxane)

**OTHER BRAND NAMES:** Deltasone (Pharmacia & Upjohn)

**THERAPEUTIC CLASS:** Glucocorticoid

**INDICATIONS:** Steroid responsive disorders.

**DOSAGE:** *Adults:* Initial: 5-60mg/day depending on disease and response. Maint: Decrease dose by small amounts to lowest effective dose.
*Pediatrics:* Initial: 5-60mg/day depending on disease and response. Maint: Decrease dose by small amounts to lowest effective dose.

**HOW SUPPLIED:** Sol: 5mg/mL, 5mg/5mL; Tab: 1mg, 2.5mg*, 5mg*, 10mg*, 20mg*, 50mg* *scored



**CONTRAINDICATIONS:** Systemic fungal infections.

**WARNINGS/PRECAUTIONS:** May need to increase dose before, during, and after stressful situations. May mask signs of infection or cause new infections. Prolonged use may produce glaucoma, optic nerve damage, secondary ocular infections. Increases BP, salt/water retention, potassium excretion. More severe/fatal course of infections reported with chickenpox, measles. Caution with latent TB, hypothyroidism, cirrhosis, ocular herpes simplex, HTN, diverticulitis, fresh intestinal anastomosis, ulcerative colitis, osteoporosis, myasthenia gravis, renal insufficiency, peptic ulcer disease. Growth and development of children on prolonged therapy should be monitored. Monitor for psychic disturbances. Avoid abrupt withdrawal.

**ADVERSE REACTIONS:** Fluid and electrolyte disturbances, HTN, osteoporosis, muscle weakness, cushingoid state, menstrual irregularities, nervousness, insomnia, impaired wound healing, DM, ulcerative esophagitis, excessive sweating, increases intracranial pressure, carbohydrate intolerance, glaucoma, cataracts, weight gain, nausea, malaise.

**INTERACTIONS:** Increases clearance of high dose ASA; caution in hypoprothrombinemia. Increased insulin and oral hypoglycemic requirements in DM. Avoid small pox vaccine, and live vaccines with immunosuppressive doses. Possible decreased vaccine response with killed or inactivated vaccines with immunosuppressive doses. Increased clearance with hepatic enzyme inducers. Decreased metabolism with troleandomycin, ketoconazole. Variable effect on oral anticoagulants.

**PREGNANCY:** Safety in pregnancy and nursing not known.

## PREFEST RX
estradiol - norgestimate (King)

**Estrogens and progestins should not be used for the prevention of cardiovascular disease. Increased risks of MI, stroke, invasive breast cancer, PE, and DVT in postmenopausal women (50-79 yrs of age) reported. Increased risk of developing probable dementia in postmenopausal women ≥65 yrs of age reported.**

**THERAPEUTIC CLASS:** Estrogen/progestogen combination

**INDICATIONS:** In women with an intact uterus, treatment of moderate to severe vasomotor symptoms and/or vulvar/vaginal atrophy associated with menopause and prevention of postmenopausal osteoporosis.

**DOSAGE:** *Adults:* Vasomotor Symptoms/Vulvar/Vaginagil Atrophy/Osteoporosis Prevention: 1mg (estradiol) qd for 3 days followed by 1mg-0.09mg (estradiol-norgestimate) qd for 3 days. Repeat regimen continuously. Re-evaluate at 3-6 month intervals when treating menopausal symptoms.

**HOW SUPPLIED:** Tab: (Estradiol) 1mg and (Estradiol-Norgestimate) 1mg-0.09mg

**CONTRAINDICATIONS:** Pregnancy, undiagnosed abnormal genital bleeding, breast cancer, estrogen-dependent neoplasia, DVT/PE, active or recent (eg, within past year) arterial thromboembolic disease (eg, stroke, MI), liver dysfunction or disease.

**WARNINGS/PRECAUTIONS:** May increase risk of cardiovascular events (eg, MI, stroke), venous thrombosis, and PE; d/c immediately if any of these events occur or are suspected. May increase risk of breast/endometrial cancer, and gallbladder disease. May lead to severe hypercalcemia with breast cancer and bone metastases; monitor and d/c if hypercalcemia occurs. Retinal vascular thrombosis reported; monitor and d/c if papilledema or retinal vascular lesions occur. May elevate BP; monitor at regular intervals. May cause elevations of plasma triglycerides with pre-existing hypertriglyceridemia. Caution with history of cholestatic jaundice associated with past estrogen use or with pregnancy; d/c with recurrence. May lead to increased thyroid-binding globulin levels; monitor thyroid function. May cause fluid retention; caution with cardiac/renal dysfunction. Caution with severe hypocalcemia. May increase risk of ovarian cancer. May exacerbate endometriosis, asthma, DM, epilepsy, migraine, porphyria, SLE, and hepatic hemangiomas; use with caution.

**ADVERSE REACTIONS:** Altered vaginal bleeding, vaginal candidiasis, breast tenderness/enlargement, nausea, vomiting, melasma, headache, weight changes, edema, altered libido.

**INTERACTIONS:** CYP3A4 inducers (eg, St. John's wort, phenobarbital, carbamazepine, rifampin) may decrease levels which may decrease therapeutic effects and/or change uterine bleeding profile. CYP3A4 inhibitors (eg, erythromycin, clarithromycin, ketoconazole, itraconazole, ritonavir, grapefruit juice) may increase levels which may result in side effects.

**PREGNANCY:** Contraindicated in pregnancy, caution in nursing.



## PREGNYL RX
chorionic gonadotropin (Organon)

**THERAPEUTIC CLASS:** Human chorionic gonadotropin

**INDICATIONS:** For prepubertal cryptorchidism not due to anatomic obstruction. For hypogonadotropic hypogonadism (secondary to a pituitary deficiency) in males. To induce ovulation (OI) and pregnancy in anovulatory, infertile women in whom anovulation is not due to primary ovarian failure and pretreated with human menotropins.

**DOSAGE:** *Adults:* Hypogonadism: 500-1000 U IM 3x/week (TIW) for 3 weeks, then twice weekly for 3 weeks; or 4000 U IM TIW for 6-9 months, then reduce to 2000 U TIW for 3 months. OI: 5000-10,000 U IM 1 day after last dose of menotropins.
*Pediatrics:* Cryptorchidism: 4000 U IM TIW for 3 weeks; or 5000 U IM every 2nd day for 4 doses; or 15 doses of 500-1000 U over 6 weeks; or 500 U TIW for 4-6 weeks (if treatment fails, give 1000 U/injection starting 1 month later). Initiate therapy between 4-9 yrs. Hypogonadism: 500-1000 U IM TIW for 3 weeks, then twice weekly for 3 weeks; or 4000 U IM TIW for 6-9 months, then reduce to 2000 U TIW for 3 months.

**HOW SUPPLIED:** Inj: 10,000 U

**CONTRAINDICATIONS:** Precocious puberty, prostatic carcinoma or other androgen-dependent neoplasms, pregnancy.

**WARNINGS/PRECAUTIONS:** Potential ovarian hyperstimulation, enlargement or rupture of ovarian cysts, multiple births, and arterial thromboembolism with infertility treatment. D/C if precocious puberty occurs in cryptorchidism patients. Caution with cardiac or renal disease, epilepsy, migraine, asthma. Not effective treatment for obesity.

**ADVERSE REACTIONS:** Headache, irritability, restlessness, depression, fatigue, edema, precocious puberty, gynecomastia, injection site pain.

**PREGNANCY:** Safety in pregnancy and nursing not known.

## PRELONE

RX

prednisolone (Muro)

**THERAPEUTIC CLASS:** Glucocorticoid

**INDICATIONS:** Treatment of steroid responsive disorders.

**DOSAGE:** *Adults:* Initial: 5-60mg/day depending on disease and response. Maint: Decrease dose by small amounts to lowest effective dose.
*Pediatrics:* Initial: 5-60mg/day depending on disease and response. Maint: Decrease dose by small amounts to lowest effective dose.

**HOW SUPPLIED:** Syrup: 5mg/5mL [120mL], 15mg/5mL [240mL, 480mL]



**CONTRAINDICATIONS:** Systemic fungal infections.

**WARNINGS/PRECAUTIONS:** Adjust dose during stress or change in thyroid status. May mask signs of infection or or cause new infections. Prolonged use may produce glaucoma, optic nerve damage, secondary ocular infections. Increases BP, salt/water retention, potassium excretion. Avoid exposure to chickenpox, measles. Caution with latent TB, hypothyroidism, cirrhosis, ocular herpes simplex, HTN, diverticulitis, fresh intestinal anastomosis, ulcerative colitis, osteoporosis, myasthenia gravis, renal insufficiency, peptic ulcer disease. Growth and development of children on prolonged therapy should be monitored. Monitor for psychic disturbances. Avoid abrupt withdrawal.

**ADVERSE REACTIONS:** Fluid and electrolyte disturbances, osteoporosis, muscle weakness, cushingoid state, menstrual irregularities, nervousness, insomnia, impaired wound healing, excessive sweating, carbohydrate intolerance, glaucoma, cataracts, weight gain, nausea, malaise.

**INTERACTIONS:** Avoid ASA with hypoprothrombinemia. May increase blood glucose; adjust antidiabetic agents. Avoid smallpox vaccination, and live vaccines with immunosuppressive doses. Possible decreased vaccine response with killed or inactivated vaccines with immunosuppressive doses.

**PREGNANCY:** Safety in pregnancy and nursing not known.

# PREMARIN RX

conjugated estrogens (Wyeth)

**Estrogens increase the risk of endometrial cancer. Estrogens, with or without progestins, should not be used for the prevention of cardiovascular disease or dementia. Increased risks of MI, stroke, invasive breast cancer, PE, and DVT in postmenopausal women (50-79 yrs of age) reported. Increased risk of developing probable dementia in postmenopausal women ≥65 yrs of age reported.**

**THERAPEUTIC CLASS:** Estrogen

**INDICATIONS:** Treatment of moderate to severe vasomotor symptoms and/or vulvar/vaginal atrophy associated with menopause. Treatment of hypoestrogenism due to hypogonadism, castration, or primary ovarian failure. Palliative treatment of breast cancer in patients with metastatic disease and/or advanced androgen-dependent carcinoma of the prostate. Prevention of postmenopausal osteoporosis.

**DOSAGE:** *Adults:* Vasomotor Symptoms/Vulvar/Vaginal Atrophy: 0.3mg qd continuously or cyclically (eg, 25 days on, 5 days off). Adjust dose based on response. Re-evaluate at 3-6 month intervals. Osteoporosis Prevention: 0.3mg qd continuously or cyclically (eg, 25 days on, 5 days off). Female Hypogonadism: 0.3-0.625mg qd cyclically (eg, 3 weeks on, 1 week off). Titrate at 6-12 month intervals. Female Castration/Ovarian Failure: 1.25mg qd cyclically. Breast Cancer (palliation): 10mg tid for minimum 3 months. Prostate Cancer (palliation): 1.25-2.5mg tid.

**HOW SUPPLIED:** Tab: 0.3mg, 0.45mg, 0.625mg, 0.9mg, 1.25mg

**CONTRAINDICATIONS:** Pregnancy, undiagnosed abnormal genital bleeding, breast cancer unless being treated for metastatic disease, estrogen-dependent neoplasia, DVT/PE, active or recent (eg, within past year) arterial thromboembolic disease (eg, stroke, MI), liver dysfunction or disease.

**WARNINGS/PRECAUTIONS:** May increase risk of cardiovascular events (eg, MI, stroke), venous thrombosis, and PE; d/c immediately if any of these events occur or are suspected. May increase risk of breast/endometrial cancer, and gallbladder disease. May lead to severe hypercalcemia with breast cancer and bone metastases; monitor and d/c if hypercalcemia occurs. Retinal vascular thrombosis reported; monitor and d/c if papilledema or retinal vascular lesions occur. Consider addition of a progestin if no hysterectomy. May elevate BP; monitor at regular intervals. May cause elevations of plasma triglycerides with pre-existing hypertriglyceridemia. Caution with history of cholestatic jaundice associated with past estrogen use or with pregnancy; d/c with recurrence. May lead to increased thyroid-binding globulin levels; monitor thyroid function. May cause fluid retention; caution with cardiac/renal dysfunction. Caution with severe hypocalcemia. May increase risk of ovarian cancer. May exacerbate endometriosis, asthma, DM, epilepsy, migraine, porphyria, SLE, and hepatic hemangiomas; use with caution.

**ADVERSE REACTIONS:** Abdominal pain, back pain, headache, infection, pain, arthralgia, leg cramps, breast pain, vaginal hemorrhage, vaginitis

**INTERACTIONS:** CYP3A4 inducers (eg, St. John's wort, phenobarbital, carbamazepine, rifampin) may decrease levels which may decrease therapeutic effects and/or change uterine bleeding profile. CYP3A4 inhibitors (eg, erythromycin, clarithromycin, ketoconazole, itraconazole, ritonavir, grapefruit juice) may increase levels which may result in side effects.

**PREGNANCY:** Contraindicated in pregnancy, caution in nursing.

## PREMARIN INTRAVENOUS RX

conjugated estrogens (Wyeth)

**Estrogens increase the risk of endometrial cancer. Estrogens, with or without progestins, should not be used for the prevention of cardiovascular disease or dementia. Increased risks of MI, stroke, invasive breast cancer, PE, and DVT in postmenopausal women (50-79 yrs of age) reported. Increased risk of developing probable dementia in postmenopausal women ≥65 yrs of age reported.**

**THERAPEUTIC CLASS:** Estrogen

**INDICATIONS:** Treatment of abnormal uterine bleeding due to hormonal imbalance in the absence of organic pathology.

**DOSAGE:** *Adults:* 25mg IV or IM. Repeat in 6-12 hrs if needed.

**HOW SUPPLIED:** Inj: 25mg

**CONTRAINDICATIONS:** Pregnancy, undiagnosed abnormal genital bleeding, breast cancer, estrogen-dependent neoplasia, DVT/PE, active or recent (eg, within past year) arterial thromboembolic disease (eg, stroke, MI), liver dysfunction or disease.

**WARNINGS/PRECAUTIONS:** May increase risk of cardiovascular events (eg, MI, stroke), venous thrombosis, and PE; d/c immediately if any of these events occur or are suspected. May increase risk of breast/endometrial cancer, and gallbladder disease. May lead to severe hypercalcemia with breast cancer and bone metastases; monitor and d/c if hypercalcemia occurs. Retinal vascular thrombosis reported; monitor and d/c if papilledema or retinal vascular lesions occur. Consider addition of a progestin if no hysterectomy. May elevate BP; monitor at regular intervals. May cause elevations of plasma triglycerides with pre-existing hypertriglyceridemia. Caution with history of cholestatic jaundice associated with past estrogen use or with pregnancy; d/c with recurrence. May lead to increased thyroid-binding globulin levels; monitor thyroid function. May cause fluid retention; caution with cardiac/renal dysfunction. Caution with severe hypocalcemia. May increase risk of ovarian cancer. May exacerbate endometriosis, asthma, DM, epilepsy, migraine, porphyria, SLE, and hepatic hemangiomas; use with caution.

**ADVERSE REACTIONS:** Abnormal vaginal bleeding, vaginal candidiasis, nausea, vomiting, abdominal cramps, bloating, breast pain/tenderness/enlargement, erythema multiforme, headache, dizziness, nervousness, weight changes, libido changes.



**INTERACTIONS:** CYP3A4 inducers (eg, St. John's wort, phenobarbital, carbamazepine, rifampin) may decrease levels which may decrease therapeutic effects and/or change uterine bleeding profile. CYP3A4 inhibitors (eg, erythromycin, clarithromycin, ketoconazole, itraconazole, ritonavir, grapefruit juice) may increase levels which may result in side effects.

**PREGNANCY:** Contraindicated in pregnancy, caution in nursing.

## PREMARIN VAGINAL RX

conjugated estrogens (Wyeth)

**Estrogens increase risk of endometrial cancer. Estrogens, with or without progestins, should not be used for the prevention of cardiovascular disease or dementia. Increased risks of MI, stroke, invasive breast cancer, PE, and DVT in postmenopausal women (50-79 yrs of age) reported. Increased risk of developing probable dementia in postmenopausal women ≥65 yrs of age reported. Estrogens with or without progestins should be prescribed at the lowest effective dose and for the shortest duration consistent with treatment goals and risks for the individual woman.**

**THERAPEUTIC CLASS:** Estrogen

**INDICATIONS:** Treatment of atrophic vaginitis and kraurosis vulvae.

**DOSAGE:** *Adults:* Usual: 1/2-2g intravaginally qd cyclically (3 weeks on, 1 week off). Discontinue or taper at 3-6 month intervals.

**HOW SUPPLIED:** Cre: 0.625mg/g [42.5g]

**CONTRAINDICATIONS:** Pregnancy, undiagnosed abnormal genital bleeding, breast cancer, estrogen-dependent neoplasia, DVT/PE, active or recent (eg, within past year) arterial thromboembolic disease (eg, stroke, MI), liver dysfunction or disease.

**WARNINGS/PRECAUTIONS:** May increase risk of cardiovascular events (eg, MI, stroke), venous thrombosis, and PE; d/c immediately if any of these events occur or are suspected. Risk factors for arterial vascular disease and/or venous thromboembolism should be managed appropriately. May increase risk of breast/endometrial cancer, dementia and gallbladder disease. May lead to severe hypercalcemia with breast cancer and bone metastases; monitor and d/c if hypercalcemia occurs. Retinal vascular thrombosis reported; monitor and d/c if papilledema or retinal vascular lesions occur. Consider addition of a progestin if no hysterectomy. May elevate BP; monitor at regular intervals. May cause elevations of plasma triglycerides with pre-existing hypertriglyceridemia. Caution with history of cholestatic jaundice associated with past estrogen use or with pregnancy; d/c with recurrence. May lead to increased thyroid-binding globulin levels; monitor thyroid function. May cause fluid retention; caution with cardiac/renal dysfunction. Caution with severe hypocalcemia. May increase risk of ovarian cancer. May exacerbate endometriosis, asthma, DM, epilepsy, migraine, porphyria, SLE, and hepatic hemangiomas; use with caution. May weaken and contribute to the failure of condoms, diaphragms, or cervical caps made of latex or rubber.

**ADVERSE REACTIONS:** Breakthrough bleeding, vaginal candidiasis, change in cervical secretion, breast tenderness and enlargement, nausea, vomiting, abdominal cramps, bloating, chloasma, melasma, venous thromboembolism, pulmonary embolism, headache.

**INTERACTIONS:** CYP3A4 inducers (eg, St. John's wort, phenobarbital, carbamazepine, rifampin) may decrease levels which may decrease therapeutic effects and/or change uterine bleeding profile. CYP3A4 inhibitors (eg, erythromycin, clarithromycin, ketoconazole, itraconazole, ritonavir, grapefruit juice) may increase levels which may result in side effects.

**PREGNANCY:** Contraindicated in pregnancy, caution in nursing.

## PREMESIS RX — RX

minerals - folic acid - multiple vitamin (Ther-Rx)

**THERAPEUTIC CLASS:** Prenatal vitamin

**INDICATIONS:** Vitamin and mineral supplementation during pregnancy.

**DOSAGE:** *Adults:* 1 tab qd.

**HOW SUPPLIED:** Tab: Calcium 200mg-Folic Acid 1mg-Vitamin $B_6$ 75mg-Vitamin $B_{12}$ 0.012mg

**WARNINGS/PRECAUTIONS:** Not for the treatment of pernicious anemia and other megaloblastic anemias where vitamin $B_{12}$ is deficient. Folic acid >0.1mg/day may obscure pernicious anemia.

**ADVERSE REACTIONS:** Allergic sensitization.

## PREMPHASE — RX

conjugated estrogens - medroxyprogesterone acetate (Wyeth)

**Estrogens and progestins should not be used for prevention of cardiovascular disease or dementia. Increased risks of MI, stroke, invasive breast cancer, PE, and DVT in postmenopausal women (50-79 yrs of age) reported. Increased risk of developing probable dementia in postmenopausal women ≥65 yrs of age reported.**

**THERAPEUTIC CLASS:** Estrogen/progestogen combination

**INDICATIONS:** In women with intact uterus, treatment of moderate to severe vasomotor symptoms and/or vulvar/vaginal atrophy associated with menopause and prevention of postmenopausal osteoporosis.

**DOSAGE:** *Adults:* Vasomotor Symptoms/Vulvar/Vaginal Atrophy/Osteoporosis Prevention: 0.625mg tab qd on days 1-14 and 0.625mg-5mg tab qd on days 15-28. Re-evaluate after 3-6 months.

**HOW SUPPLIED:** Tab: 0.625mg (Estrogens, Conjugated) and 0.625mg-5mg (Estrogens, Conjugated-Medroxyprogesterone)

**CONTRAINDICATIONS:** Pregnancy, undiagnosed abnormal genital bleeding, breast cancer, estrogen dependent neoplasia, DVT/PE, active or recent (eg, within past year) arterial thromboembolic disease (eg, stroke, MI), liver dysfunction or disease.

**WARNINGS/PRECAUTIONS:** May increase risk of cardiovascular events (eg, MI, stroke), venous thrombosis, and PE; d/c immediately if any of these events occur or are suspected. May increase risk of breast/endometrial cancer, and gallbladder disease. May lead to severe hypercalcemia with breast cancer and bone metastases; monitor and d/c if hypercalcemia occurs. Retinal vascular thrombosis reported; monitor and d/c if papilledema or retinal vascular lesions occur. May elevate BP; monitor at regular intervals. May cause elevations of plasma triglycerides with pre-existing hypertriglyceridemia. Caution with history of cholestatic jaundice associated with past estrogen use or with pregnancy; d/c with recurrence. May lead to increased thyroid-binding globulin levels; monitor thyroid function. May cause fluid retention; caution with cardiac/renal dysfunction. Caution with severe hypocalcemia. May increase risk of ovarian cancer. May exacerbate endometriosis, asthma, DM, epilepsy, migraine, porphyria, SLE, and hepatic hemangiomas; use with caution.

**ADVERSE REACTIONS:** Abdominal pain, dysmenorrhea, vaginal moniliasis, breast pain, nausea, arthralgia, headache, depression, back pain, infection, pain, vaginal hemorrhage, vaginitis.

**INTERACTIONS:** CYP3A4 inducers (eg, St. John's wort, phenobarbital, carbamazepine, rifampin) may decrease levels which may decrease therapeutic effects and/or change uterine bleeding profile. CYP3A4 inhibitors (eg, erythromycin, clarithromycin, ketoconazole, itraconazole, ritonavir, grapefruit juice) may increase levels which may result in side effects.

**PREGNANCY:** Contraindicated in pregnancy, caution in nursing.



## PREMPRO RX

conjugated estrogens - medroxyprogesterone acetate (Wyeth)

**Estrogens and progestins should not be used for prevention of cardiovascular disease or dementia. Increased risks of MI, stroke, invasive breast cancer, PE, and DVT in postmenopausal women (50-79 yrs of age) reported. Increased risk of developing probable dementia in postmenopausal women ≥65 yrs of age reported.**

**THERAPEUTIC CLASS:** Estrogen/progestogen combination

**INDICATIONS:** In women with intact uterus, treatment of moderate to severe vasomotor symptoms and/or vulvar/vaginal atrophy associated with menopause and prevention of postmenopausal osteoporosis.

**DOSAGE:** *Adults:* Vasomotor Symptoms/Vulvar/Vaginal Atrophy/Osteoporosis Prevention: Initial: 0.3mg-1.5mg qd. Adjust dose based on response. Re-evaluate after 3-6 months.

**HOW SUPPLIED:** Tab: (Estrogens, Conjugated-Medroxyprogesterone) 0.3mg-1.5mg, 0.45mg-1.5mg, 0.625mg-2.5mg, 0.625mg-5mg

**CONTRAINDICATIONS:** Pregnancy, undiagnosed abnormal genital bleeding, breast cancer, estrogen dependent neoplasia, DVT/PE, active or recent (eg, within past year) arterial thromboembolic disease (eg, stroke, MI), liver dysfunction or disease.

**WARNINGS/PRECAUTIONS:** May increase risk of cardiovascular events (eg, MI, stroke), venous thrombosis, and PE; d/c immediately if any of these events occur or are suspected. May increase risk of breast/endometrial cancer, and gallbladder disease. May lead to severe hypercalcemia with breast cancer and bone metastases; monitor and d/c if hypercalcemia occurs. Retinal vascular thrombosis reported; monitor and d/c if papilledema or retinal vascular lesions occur. May elevate BP; monitor at regular intervals. May cause elevations of plasma triglycerides with pre-existing hypertriglyceridemia. Caution with history of cholestatic jaundice associated with past estrogen use or with pregnancy; d/c with recurrence. May lead to increased thyroid-binding globulin levels; monitor thyroid function. May cause fluid retention; caution with cardiac/renal dysfunction. Caution with severe hypocalcemia. May increase risk of ovarian cancer. May exacerbate endometriosis, asthma, DM, epilepsy, migraine, porphyria, SLE, and hepatic hemangiomas; use with caution.

**ADVERSE REACTIONS:** Abdominal pain, dysmenorrhea, vaginal moniliasis, breast pain, nausea, arthralgia, headache, depression, back pain, infection, pain, vaginal hemorrhage, vaginitis.

**INTERACTIONS:** CYP3A4 inducers (eg, St. John's wort, phenobarbital, carbamazepine, rifampin) may decrease levels which may decrease therapeutic effects and/or change uterine bleeding profile. CYP3A4 inhibitors (eg, erythromycin, clarithromycin, ketoconazole, itraconazole, ritonavir, grapefruit juice) may increase levels which may result in side effects.

**PREGNANCY:** Contraindicated in pregnancy, caution in nursing.

## PRENATE ADVANCE — RX

minerals - folic acid - multiple vitamin (Sciele)

**OTHER BRAND NAMES:** Advanced Natalcare (Ethex)

**THERAPEUTIC CLASS:** Prenatal vitamin

**INDICATIONS:** Vitamin and mineral supplementation for before, during, and after pregnancy.

**DOSAGE:** *Adults:* 1 tab qd.

**HOW SUPPLIED:** Tab: Calcium 200mg-Copper 2mg-Docusate Sodium 50mg-Folic Acid 1mg-Iron 90mg-Magnesium 30mg-Niacinamide 20mg-Vitamin A 2700 IU-Vitamin $B_1$ 3mg-Vitamin $B_2$ 3.4mg-Vitamin $B_6$ 20mg-Vitamin $B_{12}$ 0.012mg- Vitamin C 120mg-Vitamin $D_3$ 400 IU-Vitamin E 30 IU-Zinc 25mg

**WARNINGS/PRECAUTIONS:** Accidental overdose with iron-containing products is a leading cause of fatal poisoning in children <6 yrs. Not for the treatment of pernicious anemia and other megaloblastic anemias where vitamin $B_{12}$ is deficient. Folic acid >0.1mg/day may obscure pernicious anemia.

**ADVERSE REACTIONS:** Allergic sensitization.

## PRENATE ELITE — RX

iron - minerals - folic acid - multiple vitamin (Sciele)

**THERAPEUTIC CLASS:** Prenatal vitamin

**INDICATIONS:** Multivitamin/multimineral nutritional supplement for the use before, during, and after pregnancy.

**DOSAGE:** *Adults:* 1 tab qd.

**HOW SUPPLIED:** Tab: Biotin 0.03mcg-Calcium Carbonate 200mg-Calcium Pantothenate 6mg-Copper 2mg-Docusate Sodium 50mg-Folate 1mg-Iron 90mg-Magnesium 30mg-Niacinamide 20mg-Vitamin $B_1$ 3mg-Vitamin $B_2$ 3.4mg-Vitamin $B_6$ 20mg-Vitamin $B_{12}$ 0.012mg-Vitamin C 120mg-Vitamin $D_3$ 400 IU-Vitamin E 10 IU-Zinc 15mg

**WARNINGS/PRECAUTIONS:** Accidental overdose of iron-containing products is a leading cause of fatal poisoning in children <6 yrs. Not for the treatment of pernicious anemia and other megaloblastic anemias where vitamin $B_{12}$ is deficient. Folic Acid >0.1mg/day may obscure pernicious anemia.

**ADVERSE REACTIONS:** Allergic sensitization.

## PRENATE GT

RX

minerals - folic acid - multiple vitamin (Sciele)

**THERAPEUTIC CLASS:** Prenatal vitamin

**INDICATIONS:** Vitamin and mineral supplementation for before, during, and after pregnancy.

**DOSAGE:** *Adults:* 1 tab qd.

**HOW SUPPLIED:** Tab: Biotin 0.03mg-Calcium 200mg-Calcium Pantothenate 6mg-Copper 2mg-Docusate Sodium 50mg-Folic Acid 1mg-Iron 90mg-Magnesium 30mg-Niacinamide 20mg-Vitamin A 2700IU-Vitamin $B_1$ 3mg-Vitamin $B_2$ 3.4mg-Vitamin $B_6$ 20mg-Vitamin $B_{12}$ 0.012mg-Vitamin C 120mg-Vitamin D 400IU-Vitamin E 10IU-Zinc 15mg

**WARNINGS/PRECAUTIONS:** Accidental overdose of iron-containing products is a leading cause of fatal poisoning in children <6 yrs. Not for the treatment of pernicious anemia and other megaloblastic anemias where vitamin $B_{12}$ is deficient. Folic acid >0.1mg/day may obscure pernicious anemia.

**ADVERSE REACTIONS:** Allergic sensitization.

## PREPIDIL

RX

dinoprostone (Pharmacia & Upjohn)

**THERAPEUTIC CLASS:** Prostaglandin $E_2$ analog

**INDICATIONS:** For ripening of an unfavorable cervix in pregnant women at or near term with a medical or obstetrical need for labor induction.

**DOSAGE:** *Adults:* Bring to room temperature before administration. Choose appropriate length shielded catheter. Use 20mm endocervical catheter if no effacement present or 10mm catheter if cervix is 50% effaced. Patient should remain in supine position for 15-30 minutes after administration. May give repeat dose of 0.5mg with dosing interval of 6 hrs. Max: 1.5mg/24hrs.

**HOW SUPPLIED:** Gel: 0.5mg/3g [3g]

P

**CONTRAINDICATIONS:** Patients in whom oxytocic drugs are contraindicated or where prolonged contractions of the uterus are inappropriate (eg, history of cesarean section, major uterine surgery, history of difficult labor or traumatic delivery, cephalopelvic disproportion, grand multiparae with >6 previous term pregnancy cases with non-vertex presentation, hyperactive or hypertonic uterine patterns, fetal distress where delivery is not imminent, obstetric emergencies where benefit-to-risk ratio for fetus or mother favors surgical intervention). Placenta previa, unexplained vaginal bleeding during this pregnancy, vaginal delivery not indicated (eg, vasa previa, active herpes genitalia).

**WARNINGS/PRECAUTIONS:** Strictly adhere to recommended dosage. Monitor uterine activity, fetal status, and character of cervix. Continuously monitor uterine activity and fetal status with history of hypertonic uterine contractility or tetanic uterine contractions. Caution with asthma, glaucoma, increased IOP, renal/hepatic dysfunction, ruptured membranes. Avoid administration above level of internal os. Evaluate feto-pelvic relationship before therapy.

**ADVERSE REACTIONS:** (Maternal) Abnormal uterine contractility, GI effects, back pain, warm feeling in vagina, fever. (Fetal) Abnormal heart rate, bradycardia, altered deceleration.

**INTERACTIONS:** May augment activity of other oxytocic agents; avoid concomitant use. Use 6-12 hr dosing interval with sequential use of oxytocin.

**PREGNANCY:** Category C, safety in nursing not known.

# PREVACID

RX

lansoprazole (TAP)

**OTHER BRAND NAMES:** Prevacid IV (TAP) - Prevacid Solutab (TAP)

**THERAPEUTIC CLASS:** Proton pump inhibitor

**INDICATIONS:** (PO) Treatment of active duodenal ulcer (DU), active benign gastric ulcer (GU), erosive esophagitis, symptomatic GERD. Maintain healing of erosive esophagitis and duodenal ulcers. Treatment of pathological hypersecretory conditions (eg, Zollinger-Ellison syndrome). Combination therapy with amoxicillin +/- clarithromycin for *H.pylori* eradication in duodenal ulcer disease, to reduce risk of ulcer recurrence. Treatment and risk reduction in NSAID induced gastric ulcer. (Inj) Short-term treatment of erosive esophagitis.

**DOSAGE:** *Adults:* >17 yrs: (PO) DU: 15mg qd for 4 weeks. Maint: 15mg qd. GU: 30mg qd up to 8 weeks. GERD: 15mg qd up to 8 weeks. Erosive Esophagitis: 30mg qd up to 8 weeks. May repeat for 8 weeks if needed. Maint: 15mg qd. NSAID Induced GU: 30mg qd for 8 weeks. Reduce Risk of NSAID Induced GU: 15mg qd for 12 weeks. Hypersecretory Conditions: Initial: 60mg qd, then adjust. Max: 90mg bid. Divide dose if >120mg/day. *H.pylori*: Triple Therapy: 30mg + clarithromycin 500mg + amoxicillin 1000mg, all bid (q12h) for 10-14 days. Dual Therapy: 30mg + amoxicillin 1000mg both tid (q8h) for 14 days. Take before eating. Caps: Swallow whole or sprinkle cap contents on 1 tbsp of applesauce, ENSURE® pudding, cottage cheese, yogurt, strained pears, or in 60mL orange juice or tomato juice; swallow immediately. Sus: Do not chew or crush. Mix packet with 30mL of water; stir well and drink immediately; not for use with NG tube. Solutab: Place on tongue with or without water. Oral Syringe: (SoluTab) Place 15mg tab in oral syringe and draw up 4mL of water, or 30mg tab in oral syringe and draw up 10mL of water. Shake contents and administer after tablet has dispersed within 15 mins. Refill syringe with 2mL (5mL for 30mg tab) of water, shake, and give any remaining contents. NG Tube: (Cap) Mix cap contents with 40mL apple juice and inject into NG tube; flush with additional juice to clear tube. (SoluTab) Place 15mg tab and draw up 4mL of water, or 30mg tab and draw up 10mL of water. Shake contents and after tablet has dispersed, inject through NG tube into stomach within 15 mins. Refill syringe with 5mL of water, shake, and flush NG tube. (Inj) Erosive Esophagitis: 30mg IV qd over 30 mins for 7 days. May switch to PO formulation for total of 6 to 8 weeks of therapy once patient is able to take oral medications. Severe Hepatic Impairment: Adjust dose.

*Pediatrics:* 12-17 yrs: Short-Term Symptomatic GERD: 15mg qd for up to 8 weeks. Erosive Esophagitis: 30mg qd for up to 8 weeks. 1-11 yrs: Short-Term Symptomatic GERD/Erosive Esophagitis: <30kg: 15mg qd for up to 12 weeks. >30kg: 30mg qd for up to 12 weeks. Titrate: May increase up to 30mg bid after 2 weeks if symptomatic. Severe Hepatic Impairment: Adjust dose. Take before eating. Caps: Swallow whole or sprinkle contents on 1 tbsp of applesauce, ENSURE® pudding, cottage cheese, yogurt, strained pears, or in 60mL orange juice or tomato juice; swallow immediately. Sus: Do not chew or crush. Mix packet with 30mL water; stir well and drink immediately; not for use with NG tube. Solutab: Place on tongue with or without water. Oral Syringe: (SoluTab) Place 15mg tab in oral syringe and draw up 4mL of water, or 30mg tab in oral syringe and draw up 10mL of water. Shake contents and administer after tablet has dispersed within 15 mins. Refill syringe with 2mL (5mL for 30mg tab) of water, shake, and give any remaining contents. NG Tube: (Cap) Mix cap contents with 40mL apple juice and inject into NG tube; flush with additional juice to clear tube. (SoluTab) Place 15mg tab and draw up 4mL of water, or 30mg tab and draw up 10mL of water. Shake contents and after tablet has dispersed, inject through NG tube into stomach within 15 mins. Refill syringe with 5mL of water, shake, and flush NG tube.

**HOW SUPPLIED:** Cap, Delayed Release: 15mg, 30mg; Inj: 30mg; Sus, Delayed Release: 15mg, 30mg (granules/packet); Tab, Disintegrating (SoluTab): 15mg, 30mg.

**WARNINGS/PRECAUTIONS:** Symptomatic response does not preclude the presence of gastric malignancy. Adjust dose with hepatic impairment.

**ADVERSE REACTIONS:** Abdominal pain, constipation, diarrhea, nausea.

**INTERACTIONS:** May alter absorption of pH-dependent drugs (eg, ketoconazole, ampicillin esters, digoxin, and iron salts). Give at least 30 minutes prior to sucralfate. Theophylline may need dose adjustment. Concomitant use with warfarin may increase INR and prothrombin time.

**PREGNANCY:** Category B, not for use in nursing.

## PREVACID NAPRAPAC RX

naproxen - lansoprazole (TAP)

**NSAIDs may cause an increased risk of serious cardiovascular thrombotic events, myocardial infarction and stroke. Risk may increase with duration of use and in patients with cardiovascular disease or risk factors for cardiovascular disease. NSAIDs may cause an increasd risk of serious gastrointestinal events which may be fatal. Patients with a history of gastric and/or duodenal ulcers (especially patients with a history of bleeding or perforation) and geriatric patients are at greater risk for serious gastrointestinal events. Contraindicated for the treatment of peri-operative pain in the setting of coronary artery bypass graft (CABG) surgery.**

**THERAPEUTIC CLASS:** NSAID/Proton Pump Inhibitor

**INDICATIONS:** To reduce the risk of NSAID-associated gastric ulcers in patients with a history of documented gastric ulcers who require the use of an NSAID for treatment of rheumatoid arthritis, osteoarthritis, and ankylosing spondylitis.

**DOSAGE:** *Adults:* Take AM dose before eating. Lansoprazole 15mg qam + naproxen 250, 375, or 500mg bid in the AM and PM. Max: 1000mg naproxen/day. Swallow lansoprazole whole.

**HOW SUPPLIED:** Cap, Delayed-Release: (Naproxen-Lansoprazole): 250mg-15mg, 375mg-15mg, 500mg-15mg [14 tabs naproxen + 7 caps lansoprazole/weekly blister card; 4 cards/pkg]

P

**CONTRAINDICATIONS:** Presence or history of NSAID/ASA allergy that precipitates asthma, rhinitis, nasal polyps, hypotension. Peri-operative pain in the setting of CABG surgery.

**WARNINGS/PRECAUTIONS:** Risk of GI ulceration, bleeding, and perforation. Monitor for visual disturbances, fluid retention/edema, Hgb levels (if initial ≤10g), and LFTs with chronic use. Acute interstitial nephritis, hematuria, proteinuria, nephrotic syndrome and severe hepatic reactions reported. Caution with impaired renal (CrCl<20mL/min) or hepatic function, elderly, heart failure, and high doses with chronic alcoholic liver disease. Caution NSAIDs can lead to onset or worsening of pre-existing HTN.

**ADVERSE REACTIONS:** Nausea, abdominal pain, constipation, heartburn, headache, dizziness, drowsiness, pruritus, skin eruptions, ecchymoses, tinnitus, edema, dyspnea.

**INTERACTIONS:** Avoid other forms of naproxen, ASA. May potentiate renal disease with ACE inhibitors. Naproxen may displace other albumin-bound drugs. Caution with warfarin. Monitor for toxicity with hydantoin, sulfonamide, or sulfonylureas. Decreased plasma levels with ASA. May antagonize natriuretic effect of furosemide and thiazides. Decreases renal clearance of lithium and methotrexate. May decrease antihypertensive effects of propranolol and other β-blockers. Increased levels and half-life with probenecid. Take lansoprazole 30 minutes prior to sucralfate. Lansoprazole may alter absorption of pH-dependent drugs (eg, ketoconazole, ampicillin, iron, digoxin).

**PREGNANCY:** Category C, not for use in nursing.

## PREVIDENT — RX

sodium fluoride (Colgate Oral)

**OTHER BRAND NAMES:** PreviDent 5000 Plus (Colgate Oral)

**THERAPEUTIC CLASS:** Fluoride preparation

**INDICATIONS:** Prevention of dental caries.

**DOSAGE:** *Adults:* Apply thin ribbon to teeth with toothbrush or mouth tray qhs for at least 1 minute with the gel and 2 minutes with the cream after regular brushing. Expectorate after use. Do not eat, drink or rinse for 30 minutes. *Pediatrics:* 6-16 yrs: Apply thin ribbon to teeth with toothbrush or mouth tray qhs for at least 1 minute with the gel and 2 minutes with the cream after regular brushing. Expectorate and rinse mouth thoroughly after use.

**HOW SUPPLIED:** Gel: (PreviDent) 1.1%; Cre: (PreviDent 5000 Plus) 1.1%

**CONTRAINDICATIONS:** Not for children <6 years of age, unless recommended by dentist or physician.

**WARNINGS/PRECAUTIONS:** Prolonged ingestion may lead to dental fluorosis in children <6 years of age. Not for systemic treatment. Do not swallow.

**ADVERSE REACTIONS:** Allergic reactions.

**PREGNANCY:** Category B, caution in nursing.

## PREVPAC — RX

amoxicillin - lansoprazole - clarithromycin (TAP)

**THERAPEUTIC CLASS:** *H.pylori* treatment combination

**INDICATIONS:** Treatment of *H.pylori* infection associated with active duodenal ulcer and to reduce the risk of duodenal ulcer recurrence.

**DOSAGE:** *Adults:* 1g amoxicillin, 500mg clarithromycin and 30mg lansoprazole, all bid (am and pm) before meals for 10 or 14 days. Swallow each pill whole. Renal Impairment (with or without hepatic impairment): Decrease clarithromycin dose or prolong intervals. Avoid with CrCl <30mL/min.

**HOW SUPPLIED:** Cap: (Amoxicillin) 500mg, Tab: (Clarithromycin) 500mg, Cap, Delayed Release: (Lansoprazole) 30mg

**CONTRAINDICATIONS:** Concomitant cisapride, pimozide, astemizole, terfenadine, ergotamine or dihydroergotamine. Hypersensitivity to prevacid, macrolide or penicillin antibiotics.

**WARNINGS/PRECAUTIONS:** Avoid if CrCl <30mL/min. Caution with cephalosporin allergy. Pseudomembranous colitis reported. Possibility of superinfections. Caution in elderly. Clarithromycin may increase colchicine; monitor for toxicity. Do not use clarithromycin during pregnancy. Symptomatic response to lansoprazole does not preclude the presence of gastric malignancy.

**ADVERSE REACTIONS:** Diarrhea, taste perversion, headache, abdominal pain, dark stools, dry mouth, nausea, moniliasis, tongue discoloration, vomiting, confusion, dizziness, vaginitis.

**INTERACTIONS:** Contraindicated with cisapride, pimozide, astemizole, terfenadine, ergotamine or dihydroergotamine. May interfere with absorption of drugs dependent on gastric pH for bioavailability (eg, ketoconazole, ampicillin esters, iron salts, digoxin). Clarithromycin increases plasma levels of carbamazepine, digoxin. Clarithromycin potentiates oral anticoagulants and may decrease triazolam clearance. Erythromycin or Clarithromycin can cause acute ergot toxicity with ergotamine or dihydroergotamine. Clarithromycin increases levels of HMG CoA reductase inhibitors (eg, lovastatin, simvastatin). Theophylline may need dose adjustment. Take lansoprazole and other proton pump inhibitors 30 minutes before sucralfate. Caution with drugs metabolized by CYP450 (eg, cyclosporine, tacrolimus, phenytoin); monitor levels.

**PREGNANCY:** Category C, not for use in nursing.

## PREZISTA
darunavir (Tibotec)

RX

**THERAPEUTIC CLASS:** Protease inhibitor

**INDICATIONS:** For use with 100mg ritonavir, and other antiretroviral agents, for the treatment of HIV infection in antiretroviral treatment-experienced adult patients.

**DOSAGE:** *Adults*: 600mg bid with ritonavir 100mg bid. Take with food.

**HOW SUPPLIED:** Tab: 300mg

**CONTRAINDICATIONS:** Concomitant antihistamines (eg, astemizole, terfenadine), ergot derivatives (eg, dihydroergotamine, ergonovine, ergotamine, methylergonovine), cisapride, pimozide, sedative hypnotics (eg, midazolam, triazolam).

**WARNINGS/PRECAUTIONS:** Severe skin rash, including erythema multiforme and Stevens-Johnson syndrome reported. Fever and elevations of transaminases reported. Caution with sulfonamide allergy. New onset DM, exacerbation of pre-existing DM, and hyperglycemia reported. Caution with hepatic impairment. Increased frequency of liver function abnormalities reported with pre-existing liver dysfunction, including chronic active hepatitis. Increased bleeding, including spontaneous skin hematomas and hemarthrosis in hemophilia type A and B reported. Redistribution/accumulation of body fat, including central obesity, dorsocervical fat enlargement, peripheral wasting, facial wasting, breast enlargement, and cushingoid appearance observed with antiretroviral therapy.

**ADVERSE REACTIONS:** Diarrhea, vomiting, abdominal pain, constipation, headache.

**INTERACTIONS:** See Contraindications. Avoid with carbamazepine, phenobarbital, phenytoin, rifampin, St. John's wort; significant decreases in plasma concentrations may occur. Potential for serious reactions (eg, myopathy, rhabdomyolysis) with HMG-CoA reductase inhibitors. Concomitant darunavir/ritonavir and efavirenz may decrease darunavir and increase efavirenz levels; use with caution. Concentrations of antiarrhythmics (eg, bepridil, lidocaine, quinidine, amiodarone) may be increased with concomitant use; caution is warranted and therapeutic concentration monitoring recommended. Monitor INR with concomitant warfarin use. Trazadone concentrations may increase; use combination with caution. Therapeutic concentration monitoring recommended for concomitant immunosuppressants (eg, cyclosporine, tacrolimus, sirolimus). May decreased methadone concentrations. Alternative/additional measures of contraception should be used with concurrent use. Refer to Prescribing Information for a complete list of drug interactions.



**PREGNANCY:** Category B, not for use in nursing.

## PRIALT
ziconotide acetate (Elan)

RX

**Severe psychiatric symptoms and neurological impairment may occur during treatment. Patients with a pre-existing history of psychosis should not be treated with ziconotide. Monitor patients for evidence of cognitive impairment, hallucinations, or changes in mood or consciousness. Therapy can be interrupted or discontinued abruptly without evidence of withdrawal effects in the event of serious neurological or psychiatric signs or symptoms.**

**THERAPEUTIC CLASS:** N-type Calcium Channel Blocker

**INDICATIONS:** Management of severe chronic pain in patients for whom intrathecal (IT) therapy is warranted, and who are intolerant of or refractory to other treatment, such as systemic analgesics, adjunctive therapies, or IT morphine.

**DOSAGE:** *Adults*: Initial: No more than 2.4mcg/d IT (0.1mcg/hr). Titrate by 2.4mcg/d no more than 2-3x/week. Max: 19.2mcg/d (0.8mcg/hr) by Day 21.

**HOW SUPPLIED:** Sol: 25mcg/mL [20mL], 100mcg/mL [1mL, 2mL, 5mL]

**CONTRAINDICATIONS:** Pre-existing history of psychosis. Contraindications to the use of IT analgesia: presence of infection at the microinfusion injection site, uncontrolled bleeding diathesis, and spinal canal obstruction that impairs circulation of CSF.

**WARNINGS/PRECAUTIONS:** Caution against engaging in hazardous activity requiring complete mental alertness or motor coordination. Dosage adjustments may be necessary when combined with other CNS-depressants due to additive effects. Ziconotide is not an opiate and cannot prevent or relieve the symptoms associated with the withdrawal of opiates. Risk of meningitis due to inadvertent contamination of the microinfusion device. Monitor for signs and symptoms of meningitis. Reports of CNS-related adverse events: psychiatric symptoms, cognitive impairment, and decreased alertness/unresponsiveness. Discontinue if patient becomes unresponsive or stuporous. Monitor for elevations in serum creatine kinase levels.

**ADVERSE REACTIONS:** Dizziness, nausea, confusion, headache, somnolence, nystagmus, asthenia, pain.

**INTERACTIONS:** Coadministration with CNS depressants increases the risk of CNS adverse effects.

**PREGNANCY:** Category C, caution in nursing.

## PRIFTIN

rifapentine (Sanofi-Aventis) RX

**THERAPEUTIC CLASS:** Rifamycin derivative

**INDICATIONS:** Treatment of pulmonary tuberculosis. Do not use alone, as initial or retreatment.

**DOSAGE:** *Adults:* Intensive Phase: Initial: 600mg twice weekly with an interval of not <3 days (72 hrs) between doses. Continue for 2 months. Maint: 600mg once weekly for 4 months. Elderly: Start at low end of dosing range. *Pediatrics:* >12 yrs: Intensive Phase: Initial: 600mg twice weekly with an interval of not <3 days (72 hrs) between doses. Continue for 2 months. Maint: 600mg once weekly for 4 months.

**HOW SUPPLIED:** Tab: 150mg

**WARNINGS/PRECAUTIONS:** Give with pyridoxine in the malnourished, if predisposed to neuropathy (eg, alcoholics, diabetics), and adolescents. Caution with hepatic impairment; monitor LFTs before and every 2-4 weeks during therapy. May cause postnatal hemorrhages in mother and infant during last weeks of pregnancy; monitor clotting parameters; may need vitamin K. May produce a red-orange discoloration of body tissues, fluids. May stain/discolor contact lenses, breast milk or dentures. Pseudomembranous colitis reported. Avoid with porphyria. Caution in elderly.

**ADVERSE REACTIONS:** Hyperuricemia, increased ALT/AST, neutropenia, pyuria, proteinuria, lymphopenia, urinary casts, rash, pruritus, acne, anorexia, anemia.

**INTERACTIONS:** Antagonizes drugs metabolized by CYP3A4, CYP2C8, and CYP2C9 due to enzyme induction (eg, anticonvulsants, antiarrhythmics, oral anticoagulants, antibiotics, antifungals, barbiturates, benzodiazepines, β-blockers, calcium channel blockers, corticosteroids, cardiac glycosides, clofibrate, hormonal contraceptives, oral hypoglycemics, haloperidol, immunosuppressants, levothyroxine, narcotic analgesics, progestins, quinine, reverse transcriptase inhibitors, sildenafil, theophylline, TCAs). Increases indinavir metabolism; extreme caution with protease inhibitors. Avoid hormonal contraceptives. Consider hepatotoxic effects of other antituberculosis drug therapy (eg, isoniazid, pyrazinamide).

**PREGNANCY:** Category C, not for use in nursing.

P

## PRILOSEC

RX

omeprazole (AstraZeneca LP)

**THERAPEUTIC CLASS:** Proton pump inhibitor

**INDICATIONS:** Active duodenal ulcer, active benign gastric ulcer, erosive esophagitis, symptomatic GERD. Maintain healing of erosive esophagitis. Long-term treatment of pathological hypersecretory conditions (eg, Zollinger-Ellison syndrome). Combination therapy with clarithromycin +/- amoxicillin for *H.pylori* eradication in duodenal ulcer disease, and to reduce risk of ulcer recurrence.

**DOSAGE:** *Adults:* Duodenal Ulcer: 20mg qd for 4-8 weeks. Gastric Ulcer: 40mg qd for 4-8 weeks. GERD: 20mg qd up to 4 weeks without esophageal lesions and 4-8 weeks with erosive esophagitis. Treatment Erosive Esophagitis with GERD: 20mg qd for 4-8 weeks. Maint: 20mg qd. Hypersecretory Conditions: Initial: 60mg qd, then adjust if needed. Divide dose if >80mg/day. Doses up to 120mg tid have been given. *H.pylori* Triple Therapy: 20mg + clarithromycin 500mg + amoxicillin 1g, all bid for 10 days. Give additional 18 days of omeprazole 20mg every morning if ulcer present initially. Dual Therapy: 40mg qd + clarithromycin 500mg tid for 14 days. Give additional 14 days of omeprazole 20mg every morning if ulcer present initially. Do not crush or chew. Take before eating. Can add contents of caps to applesauce if difficulty swallowing; swallow immediately without chewing.
*Pediatrics:* >2 yrs: GERD/Erosive Esophagitis: >20kg: 20mg qd. <20kg: 10mg qd. Do not crush or chew. Take before eating. Can add contents of caps to applesauce if difficulty swallowing; swallow immediately without chewing.

**HOW SUPPLIED:** Cap, Delayed Release: 10mg, 20mg, 40mg;

**WARNINGS/PRECAUTIONS:** Atrophic gastritis reported with long-term use. Symptomatic response does not preclude the presence of gastric malignancy.

**ADVERSE REACTIONS:** Headache, diarrhea, abdominal pain, asthenia, nausea, vomiting.

**INTERACTIONS:** May potentiate diazepam, warfarin, phenytoin and drugs metabolized by oxidation. May alter absorption of pH-dependent drugs (eg, ketoconazole, ampicillin esters, and iron salts). Monitor drugs metabolized by CYP450 (eg, cyclosporine, disulfiram, benzodiazepines). Increased levels with clarithromycin. Increases levels of clarithromycin.



**PREGNANCY:** Category C, not for use in nursing.

## PRILOSEC OTC

OTC

omeprazole magnesium (Procter & Gamble)

**THERAPEUTIC CLASS:** Proton pump inhibitor

**INDICATIONS:** Treatment of frequent heartburn (≥2 days per week).

**DOSAGE:** *Adults:* 20mg qd for 14 days. Take with water in the morning before food. May repeat q 4 months.

**HOW SUPPLIED:** Tab, Delayed Release: 20mg

**CONTRAINDICATIONS:** Trouble or pain swallowing food, vomiting with blood, or bloody or black stools.

**INTERACTIONS:** Caution with warfarin, diazepam, digoxin, antifungals, tacrolimus, and atazanavir.

**PREGNANCY:** Safety in pregnancy and nursing not known.

## PRIMACARE RX

minerals - folic acid - multiple vitamin (Ther-Rx)

**THERAPEUTIC CLASS:** Prenatal vitamin

**INDICATIONS:** Vitamin, mineral, and fatty acid supplementation for before, during, and after pregnancy.

**DOSAGE:** *Adults:* 1 cap qam and 1 tab qpm.

**HOW SUPPLIED:** Cap: (AM) Calcium 150mg-Linoleic Acid 25mg-Linolenic Acid 25mg-Omega-3 Fatty Acids 150mg-Vitamin D 170 IU-Vitamin E 30 IU; Tab: (PM) Biotin 0.035mg-Calcium 250mg-Chromium 0.045mg-Copper 1.3mg-Folic Acid 1mg-Iron 30mg-Molybdenum 0.05mg-Pantothenic Acid 7mg-Selenium 0.075mg-Vitamin $B_1$ 3mg-Vitamin $B_2$ 3.4mg-Vitamin $B_3$ 20mg-Vitamin $B_6$ 10mg-Vitamin $B_{12}$ 0.012mg-Vitamin C 100mg-Vitamin D 230 IU-Vitamin K 0.09mg-Zinc 11mg* *scored

**WARNINGS/PRECAUTIONS:** Accidental overdose of iron-containing products is a leading cause of fatal poisoning in children <6 yrs. Not for the treatment of pernicious anemia and other megaloblastic anemias where vitamin $B_{12}$ is deficient. Folic acid >0.1mg/day may obscure pernicious anemia.

**ADVERSE REACTIONS:** Allergic sensitization.

## PRIMACARE ONE RX

minerals - folic acid - multiple vitamin (Ther-Rx)

**THERAPEUTIC CLASS:** Prenatal vitamin

**INDICATIONS:** Vitamin, mineral, essential fatty acid supplementation throughout pregnancy, during the postnatal period for both lactating and non-lactating mothers, and throughout childbearing years. Also to improve nutritional status prior to conception.

**DOSAGE:** *Adults:* 1 cap qd.

**HOW SUPPLIED:** Cap: Omega-3 Fatty Acids 300mg-Linoleic Acid 30mg-Linolenic Acid 30mg-Folic Acid 1mg-Vitamin $B_6$ 25mg-Vitamin C 25mg-Vitamin $D_3$ 170 IU-Vitamin E 30 IU-Calcium 150mg-Iron 27mg.

**CONTRAINDICATIONS:** Known hypersensitivity to any of the ingredients.

**WARNINGS/PRECAUTIONS:** Folic acid in doses above 1mg daily may obscure pernicious anemia, in that hematologic remission can occur while neurological manifestations remain progressive.

**ADVERSE REACTIONS:** Allergic sensitization.

## PRIMAXIN I.M. RX

imipenem - cilastatin (Merck)

**THERAPEUTIC CLASS:** Thienamycin/dehydropeptidase I inhibitor

**INDICATIONS:** Treatment of lower respiratory tract (LRTI), skin and skin structure (SSSI), intra-abdominal, and gynecologic infections caused by susceptible strains of microorganisms. Not for severe or life-threatening infections.

**DOSAGE:** *Adults:* Dose according to imipenem. Mild to Moderate LRTI/SSSI/Gynecologic Infection: 500mg or 750mg IM q12h depending on severity. Intra-Abdominal Infection: 750mg IM q12h. Continue for at least 2 days after symptoms resolve. Elderly: Start at low end of dosing range. Continue for at least 2 days after symptoms resolve; do not treat >14 days. Max: 1500mg/day. Avoid if CrCl <20mL/min.
*Pediatrics:* >12 yrs: Dose according to imipenem. Mild to Moderate LRTI/SSSI/Gynecologic Infection: 500mg or 750mg IM q12h depending on severity. Intra-abdominal Infection: 750mg IM q12h. Continue for at least 2

P

days after symptoms resolve; do not treat >14 days. Max: 1500mg/day. Avoid if CrCl <20mL/min.

**HOW SUPPLIED:** Inj: (Imipenem-Cilastatin) 500mg-500mg

**CONTRAINDICATIONS:** Severe shock, heart block, hypersensitivity to local anesthetics of amide type (due to lidocaine diluent).

**WARNINGS/PRECAUTIONS:** Serious, fatal hypersensitivity reactions reported. Increased incidence of reactions with previous hypersensitivity to cephalosporins, penicillins, other β-lactams, and other allergens. Pseudomembranous colitis reported. Prolonged use may result in overgrowth of non-susceptible organisms. Avoid injection into blood vessel. Caution in elderly. CNS adverse events (eg, myoclonic activity, confusion, seizures) reported most commonly with CNS disorders and renal dysfunction; d/c if these occur.

**ADVERSE REACTIONS:** Injection site pain, nausea, diarrhea, fever, vomiting, rash, hypotension, seizures, dizziness, pruritus, urticaria, somnolence.

**INTERACTIONS:** Avoid probenecid. Do not mix or physically add with other antibiotics. May give concomitantly with other antibiotics.

**PREGNANCY:** Category C, caution in nursing.

## PRIMAXIN I.V. RX

imipenem - cilastatin (Merck)

**THERAPEUTIC CLASS:** Thienamycin/dehydropeptidase I inhibitor

**INDICATIONS:** Treatment of serious lower respiratory tract, urinary tract (UTI), intra-abdominal, gynecologic, skin and skin structure, bone and joint, septicemia, endocarditis, and polymicrobic infections caused by susceptible strains of microorganisms..

**DOSAGE:** *Adults:* >70kg and CrCl >70mL/min: Dose based on imipenem component. Uncomplicated UTI: 250mg q6h. Complicated UTI: 500mg q6h. Mild Infection: 250-500mg q6h. Moderate Infection: 500mg q6-8h or 1g q8h. Severe, Life Threatening Infection: 500mg-1g q6h or 1g q8h. Max dose: 50mg/kg/day or 4g/day, whichever is lower. Renal Impairment and/or <70kg: Refer to prescribing information. CrCl 6-20mL/min: 125-250mg q12h. CrCl <5mL/min: Administer hemodialysis within 48 hrs of dose.
*Pediatrics:* >3 months: Dose based on imipenem component. Non-CNS Infections: 15-25mg/kg q6h. Max: 2g/day if susceptible or 4g/day if moderately susceptible. May use up to 90mg/kg/day in older cystic fibrosis children. 4 weeks-3 months and ≥1500g: 25mg/kg q6h. 1-4 weeks and ≥1500g: 25mg/kg q8h. <1 week and ≥1500g: 25mg/kg q12h. Not recommended with CNS infection, and <30kg with impaired renal function.

**HOW SUPPLIED:** Inj: (Imipenem-Cilastatin) 250mg-250mg, 500mg-500mg

**WARNINGS/PRECAUTIONS:** Serious, fatal hypersensitivity reactions reported. Increased incidence of reactions with previous hypersensitivity to cephalosporins, penicillins, other β-lactams, and other allergens. Pseudomembranous colitis reported. Prolonged use may result in overgrowth of non-susceptible organisms. CNS adverse events (eg, myoclonic activity, confusion, seizures) reported most commonly with CNS disorders and renal dysfunction.

**ADVERSE REACTIONS:** Phlebitis/thrombophlebitis, nausea, diarrhea, vomiting, rash, fever, hypotension, seizures, dizziness, pruritus, urticaria, somnolence, hepatitis (including fulminant hepatitis), hepatic Failure.

**INTERACTIONS:** Seizures reported with ganciclovir; avoid concomitant use. Avoid probenecid. Do not mix or physically add to other antibiotics. May give concomitantly with other antibiotics.

**PREGNANCY:** Category C, caution in nursing.

## PRIMSOL
RX

trimethoprim HCl (FSC Laboratories)

**THERAPEUTIC CLASS:** Tetrahydrofolic acid inhibitor

**INDICATIONS:** Treatment of acute otitis media in pediatrics and urinary tract infection (UTI) in adults.

**DOSAGE:** *Adults:* UTI: Usual: 100mg q12h or 200mg q24h for 10 days. CrCl: 15-30mL/min: Give 50% of usual dose.
*Pediatrics:* Otitis Media: >6 months: 5mg/kg q12h for 10 days. CrCl: 15-30mL/min: Give 50% of usual dose.

**HOW SUPPLIED:** Sol: 50mg/5mL

**CONTRAINDICATIONS:** Megaloblastic anemia due to folate deficiency.

**WARNINGS/PRECAUTIONS:** May interfere with hematopoiesis. Serious blood disorders; monitor for sore throat, fever, pallor, and purpura. Caution with folate deficiency and renal/hepatic impairment, diarrhea, rash.

**ADVERSE REACTIONS:** Epigastric distress, nausea, vomiting, anemia, methemoglobinemia, hyperkalemia, hyponatremia, fever, elevation of serum transaminases and bilirubin, increases BUN and serum creatinine.

**INTERACTIONS:** May inhibit phenytoin metabolism.

**PREGNANCY:** Category C, caution in nursing.

## PRINIVIL
RX

lisinopril (Merck)

**ACE inhibitors can cause death/injury to developing fetus during 2nd and 3rd trimesters. Stop therapy if pregnancy detected.**

**THERAPEUTIC CLASS:** ACE inhibitor

**INDICATIONS:** Treatment of hypertension. Adjunct therapy in heart failure if inadequately controlled by diuretics and digitalis. Adjunct therapy in stable patients within 24 hrs of AMI to improve survival.

**DOSAGE:** *Adults:* HTN: If possible, discontinue diuretic 2-3 days prior to therapy. Initial: 10mg qd; 5mg qd with diuretic. Usual: 20-40mg qd. Resume diuretic if BP not controlled. Max: 80mg/day. CrCl 10-30mL/min: Initial: 5mg/day. Max: 40mg/day. CrCl <10mL/min: Initial: 2.5mg/day. Max: 40mg/day. Heart Failure: Initial: 5mg qd. Usual: 5-20mg qd. Hyponatremia or CrCl <30mL/min: Initial: 2.5mg qd. AMI: Initial: 5mg within 24 hrs, then 5mg after 24 hrs, then 10mg after 48 hrs, then daily. Use 2.5mg during 1st 3 days with low systolic BP. Maint: 10mg qd for 6 weeks, 2.5-5mg with hypotension. Discontinue with prolonged hypotension. Elderly: Caution with dose adjustment.

**HOW SUPPLIED:** Tab: 5mg*, 10mg, 20mg, 40mg *scored

**CONTRAINDICATIONS:** History of ACE inhibitor associated angioedema and hereditary or idiopathic angioedema.

**WARNINGS/PRECAUTIONS:** Intestinal/head/neck angioedema reported. D/C if angioedema, jaundice, or if marked LFT elevation occurs. Risk of hyperkalemia with DM, renal dysfunction. Persistent nonproductive cough reported. Monitor WBCs in renal and collagen vascular disease. Anaphylactoid reactions reported. Fetal/neonatal morbidity and death reported. Monitor for hypotension in high risk patients (eg, heart failure with systolic BP <100mmHg, surgery/anesthesia, hyponatremia, high dose diuretic therapy, severe volume and/or salt depletion). Caution with renal artery stenosis, CHF, renal dysfunction, or if obstruction to left ventricle outflow tract. Less effective on BP in blacks and more reports of angioedema than nonblacks. Caution in hypoglycemia and leukopenia/neutropenia. Patients should report any indication of infection which may be sign of leukopenia/neutropenia.

**ADVERSE REACTIONS:** Hypotension, diarrhea, headache, dizziness, cough, chest pain.

**INTERACTIONS:** May increase lithium levels. Hypotension risk with diuretics. May further decrease renal dysfunction with NSAIDs. Hyperkalemia with $K^+$-sparing diuretics, $K^+$-containing salt substitutes, or $K^+$ supplements. Nitroid reactions have been reported rarely in patients on therapy with injectable gold and concomitant ACE inhibitor therapy.

**PREGNANCY:** Category C (1st trimester) and D (2nd and 3rd trimesters), not for use in nursing.

## PRINZIDE RX

lisinopril - hydrochlorothiazide (Merck)

**ACE inhibitors can cause death/injury to developing fetus during 2nd and 3rd trimesters. Stop therapy if pregnancy detected.**

**THERAPEUTIC CLASS:** ACE inhibitor/thiazide diuretic

**INDICATIONS:** Treatment of hypertension. Not for initial therapy.

**DOSAGE:** *Adults:* Initial (if not controlled with lisinopril/HCTZ monotherapy): 10mg-12.5mg tab or 20mg-12.5mg tab daily. Titrate: May increase after 2-3 weeks. Initial (if controlled on 25mg HCTZ/day with hypokalemia): 10mg-12.5mg tab. Replacement Therapy: Substitute combination for titrated components.

**HOW SUPPLIED:** Tab: (Lisinopril-HCTZ) 10mg-12.5mg, 20mg-12.5mg, 20mg-25mg

**CONTRAINDICATIONS:** History of ACE inhibitor associated angioedema and hereditary or idiopathic angioedema. Anuria, sulfonamide hypersensitivity.

**WARNINGS/PRECAUTIONS:** D/C if angioedema, jaundice, or if marked LFT elevation occurs. Risk of hyperkalemia with DM, renal dysfunction. Persistent nonproductive cough reported. Monitor WBCs in renal and collagen vascular disease. Anaphylactoid reactions reported. Fetal/neonatal morbidity and death reported. Monitor for hypotension in high risk patients (eg, surgery/anesthesia, volume/salt depletion). Caution with CHF, renal or hepatic dysfunction, obstruction to left ventricle outflow tract, renal artery stenosis, elderly. More reports of angioedema in blacks than nonblacks. May exacerbate or activate SLE. Monitor electrolytes. Avoid if CrCl <30mL/min/1.73m$^2$. May increase cholesterol, TG. Hypercalcemia, hyperglycemia, hypomagnesemia, hyperuricemia may occur.

**ADVERSE REACTIONS:** Dizziness, cough, fatigue, orthostatic effects, diarrhea, nausea, muscle cramps, angioedema.

**INTERACTIONS:** Increase risk of hyperkalemia with $K^+$-sparing diuretics, $K^+$ supplements, or $K^+$-containing salt substitutes. Potentiates orthostatic hypotension with alcohol, barbiturates, and narcotics. Adjust antidiabetic drugs. Reduced absorption with cholestyramine, colestipol. Corticosteroids, ACTH deplete electrolytes. May decrease response to pressor amines. Potentiates other antihypertensives. May increase responsiveness to skeletal muscle relaxants. Risk of lithium toxicity. NSAIDs reduce effects and worsen renal dysfunction. Nitroid reactions have been reported rarely in patients on therapy with injectable gold and concomitant ACE inhibitor therapy. Patients on diuretics may experience an excessive reduction of blood pressure.

**PREGNANCY:** Category C (1st trimester) and D (2nd and 3rd trimesters), not for use in nursing.

## PROAIR HFA

RX

albuterol sulfate (Ivax)

**THERAPEUTIC CLASS:** $Beta_2$ agonist

**INDICATIONS:** Prevention and treatment of bronchospasm with reversible obstructive airway disease; prevention of exercise-induced bronchospasm (EIB) in patients ≥12 yrs.

**DOSAGE:** *Adults:* Bronchospasm or Asthmatic Symptoms: 2 inh q4-6h or 1 inh q4h. EIB: 2 inh 15-30 min before activity.
*Pediatrics:* ≥12 yrs: Bronchospasm or Asthmatic Symptoms: 2 inh q4-6h or 1 inh q4h. EIB: 2 inh 15-30 min before activity.

**HOW SUPPLIED:** MDI: 90mcg/inh [8.5g]

**WARNINGS/PRECAUTIONS:** Hypersensitivity reactions reported. Monitor for worsening asthma. Fatalities reported with excessive use. Caution with cardiovascular disorders, especially coronary insufficiency, arrhythmias and HTN. May need concomitant corticosteroids. Can produce paradoxical bronschospasm. Caution with DM, hyperthyroidism, and seizures. May cause transient hypokalemia.

**ADVERSE REACTIONS:** Pharyngitis, headache, rhinitis, dizziness, pain, tachycardia, tremor, nervousness.

**INTERACTIONS:** Avoid other sympathomimetic agents. Extreme caution with MAOIs and TCAs, and β-blockers. Monitor digoxin. May worsen ECG changes and/or hypokalemia with nonpotassium-sparing diuretics.

**PREGNANCY:** Category C, not for use in nursing.

## PROAMATINE

RX

midodrine HCl (Shire US)

> **Can cause marked elevation of supine BP. Clinical benefits of improving ability to carry out activities of daily living have not been verified.**

**THERAPEUTIC CLASS:** $Alpha_1$-agonist

**INDICATIONS:** Treatment of symptomatic orthostatic hypotension.

**DOSAGE:** *Adults:* Initial: 10mg tid; at 3-4 hr intervals, while awake. Max: 30mg/day. To avoid supine HTN during sleep, do not give <4 hrs before bedtime or after evening meal. Renal Dysfunction: Initial: 2.5mg tid.

**HOW SUPPLIED:** Tab: 2.5mg*, 5mg*, 10mg *scored

**CONTRAINDICATIONS:** Severe organic heart disease, acute renal disease, urinary retention, pheochromocytoma, thyrotoxicosis, persistent and excessive HTN.

**WARNINGS/PRECAUTIONS:** Risk of supine HTN; monitor for symptoms (eg, pounding in ears, headache, blurred vision), supine and standing BP; d/c if supine HTN persists. Caution with urinary retention, diabetes, renal or hepatic dysfunction. Decreased HR due to vagal reflex.

**ADVERSE REACTIONS:** Supine and sitting HTN, paresthesia, scalp pruritus, goosebumps, chills, urinary urge/retention/frequency.

**INTERACTIONS:** Monitor BP with vasoconstrictors (eg, phenylephrine, ephedrine, dihydroergotamine, pseudoephedrine). Fludrocortisone may potentiate supine HTN due to salt-retaining properties. OTC cold and diet products may potentiate pressor effects. Antagonized by a-blockers (eg, prazosin, terazosin, doxazosin). Metformin, cimetidine, ranitidine, procainamide, triamterene, flecainide, and quinidine may increase clearance. Caution with cardiac glycosides, psychopharmacologics, and β-blockers.

**PREGNANCY:** Category C, caution in nursing.

## PROBENECID
probenecid (Various)

RX

**THERAPEUTIC CLASS:** Uricosuric

**INDICATIONS:** Treatment of hyperuricemia associated with gout and gouty arthritis. Adjunct to penicillin, ampicillin, methicillin, oxacillin, cloxacillin, or nafcillin for elevation and prolongation of plasma levels.

**DOSAGE:** *Adults:* Gout: Initial: 250mg bid for 1 week. Titrate: May increase by 500mg every 4 weeks. Maint: 500mg bid. Max: 2g/day. May reduce by 500mg every 6 months if acute attack has been absent >6 months and serum urate levels are normal. Renal Impairment: Usual: 1g/day. Adjunct Antibiotic Therapy: 500mg qid. Elderly/Renal Impairment: Reduce dose. Decrease dose with gastric intolerance. May not be effective if CrCl <30mL/min.
*Pediatrics:* 2-14 yrs: Adjunct Antibiotic Therapy: Initial: 25mg/kg. Maint: 10mg/kg qid. >50kg: 500mg qid.

**HOW SUPPLIED:** Tab: 500mg

**CONTRAINDICATIONS:** Blood dyscrasias, uric acid kidney stones and children <2 yrs. Do not use in acute gout attack.

**WARNINGS/PRECAUTIONS:** Initiate therapy when acute gout attack subsides. Exacerbation of gout may occur; treat with colchicine. Use APAP if analgesic needed. Severe allergic reactions and anaphylaxis reported. D/C if hypersensitivity occurs. Caution with peptic ulcer. Monitor for glycosuria. Maintain liberal fluid intake and alkalization of urine.

**ADVERSE REACTIONS:** Headache, acute gouty arthritis, dizziness, hepatic necrosis, vomiting, nausea, anorexia, sore gums, nephrotic syndrome, uric acid stones, renal colic, costovertebral pain, urinary frequency, anaphylaxis, fever, urticaria, pruritus, blood dyscrasias, dermatitis, alopecia, flushing.

**INTERACTIONS:** Probenecid increases plasma levels of penicillin and other β-lactams; psychic disturbances reported. Avoid use with penicillin in the presence of renal impairment. Salicylates and pyrazinamide antagonize uricosuric effects. Increased plasma levels of methotrexate, sulfonamides, sulfonylureas, thiopental or ketamine-induced anesthesia, some NSAIDs (eg, indomethacin, naproxen), lorazepam, APAP, and rifampin. Possible false high plasma levels of theophylline.



**PREGNANCY:** Safety in pregnancy and nursing is not known.

## PROCANBID
procainamide HCl (King)

RX

**Positive ANA titer may develop with prolonged use.**

**THERAPEUTIC CLASS:** Class IA antiarrhythmic

**INDICATIONS:** Treatment of life-threatening ventricular arrhythmias.

**DOSAGE:** *Adults:* Initial: 25mg/kg q12h. >50 yrs or Renal/Hepatic/Cardiac Insufficiency: Reduce dose or increase intervals. Swallow tab whole.

**HOW SUPPLIED:** Tab, Extended Release: 500mg, 1000mg

**CONTRAINDICATIONS:** Complete heart block, 2nd-degree AV block, SLE, torsade de pointes.

**WARNINGS/PRECAUTIONS:** Monitor for QRS widening or QT prolongation. Should cardioconvert or digitalize before use with A-Fib/Flutter. Caution with AV conduction disturbances and 1st-degree heart block; reduce dose. Caution with myasthenia gravis; adjust dose of anticholinesterases. Caution in digitalis intoxication, pre-existing marrow failure, cytopenia, CHF, ischemic heart disease, cardiomyopathy. May induce lupoid syndrome. Reserve for life-threatening ventricular arrhythmias. Fatal blood dyscrasias reported; obtain CBC, WBC, differential, and platelets weekly for 1st 3 months, then periodically.

**ADVERSE REACTIONS:** GI disturbances, lupus-like symptoms, elevated LFTs, bitter taste, angioneurotic edema, flushing, psychosis, dizziness, depression, urticaria, pruritus, rash, agranulocytosis.

**INTERACTIONS:** Potentiated by amiodarone, cimetidine, ranitidine, trimethoprim. May require less than usual dose of neuromuscular blockers. Additive cardiac effects with other class 1A drugs (quinidine, disopyramide). Additive antivagal effects with anticholinergics. Alcohol decreases half-life.

**PREGNANCY:** Category C, not for use in nursing.

## PROCARDIA XL — RX

nifedipine (Pfizer)

**THERAPEUTIC CLASS:** Calcium channel blocker (dihydropyridine)

**INDICATIONS:** Management of vasospastic angina and chronic stable angina. Treatment of hypertension.

**DOSAGE:** *Adults:* Angina/HTN: Initial: 30-60mg qd. Titrate over 7-14 days. Max: 120mg/day. Caution if dose >90mg with angina.

**HOW SUPPLIED:** Tab, Extended Release: 30mg, 60mg, 90mg

**WARNINGS/PRECAUTIONS:** May cause hypotension; monitor BP initially or with titration. May exacerbate angina from β-blocker withdrawal. CHF risk, especially with aortic stenosis or β-blockers. Peripheral edema reported. May increase angina or MI with severe obstructive CAD. Caution in pre-existing severe GI narrowing.

**ADVERSE REACTIONS:** Dizziness, lightheadedness, giddiness, flushing, muscle cramps, headache, weakness, nausea, peripheral edema, nervousness/mood changes.

**INTERACTIONS:** β-Blockers may increase risk of CHF, severe hypotension, or angina exacerbation. Possible hypotension with fentanyl. Potentiates digoxin. Monitor quinidine, coumarin. Potentiated by cimetidine and grapefruit juice. Avoid grapefruit juice.

**PREGNANCY:** Category C, unknown use in nursing.



## PROCHLORPERAZINE — RX

prochlorperazine (Various)

**OTHER BRAND NAMES:** Compro (Paddock)

**THERAPEUTIC CLASS:** Phenothiazine derivative

**INDICATIONS:** Control of severe nausea and vomiting. Management of psychotic disorders (eg, schizophrenia). Short-term treatment of generalized non-psychotic anxiety.

**DOSAGE:** *Adults:* Nausea/Vomiting: (Tab) Usual: 5-10mg tid-qid. Max: 40mg/day. (IM) 5-10mg IM q3-4h prn. Max: 40mg/day. (IV) 2.5-10mg IV (not bolus). Max: 10mg single dose and 40mg/day. Nausea/Vomiting with Surgery: 5-10mg IM 1-2 hrs or 5-10mg IV 15-30 minutes before anesthesia, or during or after surgery; repeat once if needed. Non-Psychotic Anxiety: (Tab) 5mg tid-qid; Psychosis: Mild/Outpatient: 5-10mg PO tid-qid. Moderate-Severe/Hospitalized: Initial: 10mg PO tid-qid. May increase in small increments every 2-3 days. Severe: (PO) 100-150mg/day. (IM) 10-20mg, may repeat q2-4 hrs if needed. Switch to oral after obtain control or if needed, 10-20mg IM q4-6h. Elderly: use lower dosing range and titrate more gradually.
*Pediatrics:* Nausea/Vomiting: >2 yrs and >20lbs: (PO/PR) 20-29 lbs: Usual: 2.5mg qd-bid. Max: 7.5mg/day. 30-39 lbs: 2.5mg bid-tid. Max: 10mg/day. 40-85 lbs: 2.5mg tid or 5mg bid. Max: 15mg/day. (IM) 0.06mg/lb, usually single dose for control. Psychosis: (PO/PR) 2-12 yrs: Initial: 2.5mg bid-tid, up to 10mg/day on 1st day. Max: 2-5 yrs: 20mg/day. 6-12 yrs: 25mg/day. (IM) <12 yrs: 0.06mg/lb single dose. Switch to oral after obtain control.

**HOW SUPPLIED:** Inj: (prochlorperazine as edisylate) 5mg/mL; Sup: (prochlorperazine as edisylate) 2.5mg, (Compro) 25mg; Tab: (prochlorperazine as maleate) 5mg, 10mg

**CONTRAINDICATIONS:** Comatose states, concomitant large dose CNS depressants (alcohol, barbiturates, narcotics), pediatric surgery, pediatrics <2 yrs or <20 lbs.

**WARNINGS/PRECAUTIONS:** Secondary extrapyramidal symptoms can occur. Tardive dyskinesia, NMS may develop. Caution with activities requiring alertness. May mask symptoms of overdose of other drugs. May obscure diagnosis of intestinal obstruction, brain tumor, and Reye's syndrome. May interfere with thermoregulation. Caution with glaucoma, cardiac disorders. Caution in children with dehydration or acute illness and the elderly. Discontinue 48 hrs before myelography and may resume after 24 hrs post-procedure.

**ADVERSE REACTIONS:** Drowsiness, dizziness, amenorrhea, blurred vision, skin reactions, hypotension, NMS, cholestatic jaundice.

**INTERACTIONS:** Decreases oral anticoagulant effects. Potentiates αa-adrenergic blockade. Thiazide diuretics potentiate orthostatic hypotension. Increased levels of both drugs with propranolol. Anticonvulsants may need adjustment. Risk of encephalopathic syndrome with lithium. Antagonizes antihypertensive effects of guanethidine and related compounds.

**PREGNANCY:** Safety in pregnancy is not known; caution in nursing.

## PROCRIT RX

epoetin alfa (Ortho Biotech)

**Erythropoiesis-stimulating agents (ESAs) may increase risk for death and/or serious cardiovascular events when administered to a target Hgb >12g/dL. Use lowest dose that will gradually increase Hgb concentration to lowest level sufficient to avoid need for RBC transfusion. When ESAs are used preoperatively for reduction of allogenic RBC transfusions, a higher incidence of DVT was reported in patients not receiving prophylactic anticoagulation. Antithrombotic prophylaxis should be strongly considered when ESAs are used to reduce allogenic RBC transfusions.**



**THERAPEUTIC CLASS:** Erythropoiesis stimulator

**INDICATIONS:** Treatment of anemia of chronic renal failure (CRF), anemia related to zidovudine-treatment of HIV, chemotherapy-induced anemia in non-myeloid malignancies, and reduction of allogeneic blood transfusions in anemic patients (>10 to ≤13g/dL) scheduled for elective, noncardiac, nonvascular surgery.

**DOSAGE:** *Adults:* CRF: Initial: 50-100U/kg IV/SQ 3x/week. IV is preferred route in dialysis patients. Titrate: Reduce if Hgb approaches 12g/dL or if Hgb increases >1g/dL in any 2-week period. Increase when Hgb does not increase by 2g/dL after 8 weeks of therapy and Hgb is below target range (10-12g/dL). Maint: Individually titrate. Zidovudine-Treated HIV Patients: If serum erythropoietin levels ≤500mU/mL and zidovudine ≤4200mg/week give 100U/kg IV/SQ 3x/week for 8 weeks. Titrate: Increase by 50-100U/kg 3x/week after 8 weeks if necessary. Maint: If Hgb >13g/dL, discontinue until Hgb <12g/dL, then reduce dose by 25% when resume therapy. Max: 300U/kg 3x/week. Chemotherapy Induced Anemia: Initial: 150U/kg SQ 3x/week. Titrate: Reduce by 25% when Hgb approaches 12g/dL or Hgb increases >1g/dL in any 2-week period. If Hgb >13g/dL, withhold until Hgb <12g/dL then restart at 25% below previous dose. May increase to 300U/kg 3x/week if no response after 8 weeks of therapy. Max: 300U/kg 3x/week. Weekly Dosing: 40,000U SQ weekly. Titrate: If Hgb not increased by ≥1g/dL after 4 weeks, increase to 60,000U weekly. If Hgb >13g/dL, withhold until Hgb <12g/dL then restart with 25% dose reduction. Reduce dose by 25% if very rapid Hgb response (eg, increase >1g/dL in any 2-week period. Max: 60,000U weekly. Surgery: 300U/kg/day SQ for 10 days before surgery, on surgery day, and 4 days post-op or 600U/kg SQ once weekly on 21, 14, and 7 days before surgery and a 4th

dose on surgery day, with adequate iron supplement.
*Pediatrics:* CRF: Initial: 50U/kg 3x/week IV/SQ. Titrate: Reduce if Hgb approaches 12g/dL or if Hgb increases by >1g/dL in any 2-week period. Increase if Hgb does not increase by 2g/dL after 8 weeks of therapy and Hgb is below target range (10-12g/dL). Maint: Individually titrate.

**HOW SUPPLIED:** Inj: 2000U/mL, 3000U/mL, 4000U/mL, 10,000U/mL, 20,000U/mL, 40,000U/mL

**CONTRAINDICATIONS:** Uncontrolled HTN. Hypersensitivity to mammalian cell-derived products and albumin (human).

**WARNINGS/PRECAUTIONS:** Pure red cell aplasia and severe anemia (with or without other cytopenias) may occur. Caution with porphyria, HTN, or history of seizures. Evaluate iron stores before and during therapy; most patients need iron supplementation. Monitor Hgb, BP, iron levels, serum chemistry, and CBC. Menses may resume. Multidose formulation contains benzyl alcohol that has been associated with an increased incidence of neurological and other complications in premature infants which are sometimes fatal.

**ADVERSE REACTIONS:** HTN, headache, fatigue, arthralgias, nausea, vomiting, diarrhea, edema, rash, pyrexia, constipation, respiratory congestion, dyspnea, asthenia, skin reaction.

**INTERACTIONS:** Adjust anticoagulant dose in dialysis patients.

**PREGNANCY:** Category C, caution in nursing

## PROCTOCORT CREAM RX

hydrocortisone (Salix)

**THERAPEUTIC CLASS:** Corticosteroid

**INDICATIONS:** Corticosteroid responsive dermatoses.

**DOSAGE:** *Adults:* Apply bid-qid. May use occlusive dressings for psoriasis or recalcitrant conditions; discontinue dressings if infection develops.
*Pediatrics:* Apply bid-qid. May use occlusive dressings for psoriasis or recalcitrant conditions; discontinue dressings if infection develops.

**HOW SUPPLIED:** Cre: 1% [30g]

**WARNINGS/PRECAUTIONS:** May produce reversible HPA axis suppression, manifestations of Cushing's syndrome, hyperglycemia, and glucosuria. Caution when applied to large surface areas or under occlusive dressings. Use appropriate therapy with infections. Pediatrics may be more susceptible to systemic toxicity. Discontinue if irritation occurs. Avoid eyes.

**ADVERSE REACTIONS:** Burning, itching, irritation, dryness, folliculitis, hypertrichosis, acneiform eruptions, hypopigmentation, perioral dermatitis, allergic contact dermatitis, maceration skin, secondary infection, skin atrophy, striae, miliaria.

**PREGNANCY:** Category C, caution in nursing.

## PROCTOCORT SUPPOSITORY RX

hydrocortisone acetate (Salix)

**THERAPEUTIC CLASS:** Corticosteroid

**INDICATIONS:** For use in inflamed hemorrhoids and post irradiation (factitial) proctitis. Adjunct for chronic ulcerative colitis, cryptitis, other anorectum inflammation and pruritus ani.

**DOSAGE:** *Adults:* Nonspecific Proctitis: 1 sup rectally bid for 2 weeks. More Severe Cases: 1 sup rectally tid or 2 sup rectally bid. Factitial Proctitis: Use up to 6-8 weeks.

**HOW SUPPLIED:** Sup: 30mg [12s 24s]

**WARNINGS/PRECAUTIONS:** Discontinue if irritation develops. Discontinue if develop infection that does not respond to appropriate therapy. May stain fabric. Only use after adequate proctologic exam.

**ADVERSE REACTIONS:** Burning, itching, irritation, dryness, folliculitis, hypopigmentation, allergic contact dermatitis, secondary infection.

**PREGNANCY:** Category C, not for use in nursing.

## PROCTOFOAM-HC RX

pramoxine HCl - hydrocortisone acetate (Schwarz Pharma)

**THERAPEUTIC CLASS:** Corticosteroid/anesthetic

**INDICATIONS:** Corticosteroid responsive dermatoses of the anal region.

**DOSAGE:** *Adults:* Apply to anal/perianal area tid-qid.
*Pediatrics:* Apply to anal/perianal area tid-qid.

**HOW SUPPLIED:** Foam: (Hydrocortisone-Pramoxine) 1%-1% [10g]

**WARNINGS/PRECAUTIONS:** Discontinue if no improvement in 2-3 weeks. May produce reversible HPA axis suppression, manifestations of Cushing's syndrome, hyperglycemia, and glucosuria. Caution when applied to large surface areas or under occlusive dressings. Use appropriate therapy if infections develop; discontinue steroid if favorable response does not occur promptly. Discontinue if irritation develops. Pediatrics may be more susceptible to systemic toxicity. Avoid eyes.

**ADVERSE REACTIONS:** Burning, itching, irritation, dryness, folliculitis, hypertrichosis, acneiform eruptions, hypopigmentation, perioral dermatitis, allergic contact dermatitis, skin maceration, secondary infection, skin atrophy, striae, miliaria.

**PREGNANCY:** Category C, caution in nursing.

## PROFASI RX

chorionic gonadotropin (Serono)



**THERAPEUTIC CLASS:** Human chorionic gonadotropin

**INDICATIONS:** For prepubertal cryptorchidism not due to anatomic obstruction. For hypogonadotropic hypogonadism (secondary to a pituitary deficiency) in males. To induce ovulation (OI) and pregnancy in anovulatory, infertile women in whom anovulation is not due to primary ovarian failure and pretreated with human menotropins.

**DOSAGE:** *Adults:* Hypogonadism: 500-1000 U IM 3x/week (TIW) for 3 weeks, then twice weekly for 3 weeks; or 4000 U IM TIW for 6-9 months, then reduce to 2000 U TIW for 3 months. OI: 5000-10,000 U IM 1 day after last dose of menotropins.
Pediatrics: >4 yrs: Cryptorchidism: 4000 U IM TIW for 3 weeks; or 5000 U IM every 2nd day for 4 doses; or 15 doses of 500-1000 U over 6 weeks; or 500 U TIW for 4-6 weeks (if treatment fails, give 1000 U/injection starting 1 month later). Initiate therapy between 4-9 yrs. Hypogonadism: 500-1000 U IM TIW for 3 weeks, then twice weekly for 3 weeks; or 4000 U IM TIW for 6-9 months, then reduce to 2000 U TIW for 3 months.

**HOW SUPPLIED:** Inj: 10,000 U

**CONTRAINDICATIONS:** Precocious puberty, prostatic carcinoma or other androgen-dependent neoplasms, pregnancy.

**WARNINGS/PRECAUTIONS:** Potential ovarian hyperstimulation, enlargement or rupture of ovarian cysts, multiple births, and arterial thromboembolism with infertility treatment. D/C if precocious puberty occurs in cryptorchidism patients. Caution with cardiac or renal disease, epilepsy, migraine, asthma. Diluent contains benzyl alcohol. Not effective treatment for obesity.

**ADVERSE REACTIONS:** Headache, irritability, restlessness, depression, fatigue, edema, precocious puberty, gynecomastia, injection site pain, hypersensitivity reactions.

**PREGNANCY:** Category X, caution in nursing.

## PROGRAF RX

tacrolimus (Astellas)

**Increased susceptibility to infection and development of lymphoma.**

**THERAPEUTIC CLASS:** Macrolide immunosuppressant

**INDICATIONS:** Prophylaxis of organ rejection in allogenic liver, kidney, or heart transplants with concomitant adrenal corticosteroids. In heart transplant patients, azathioprine or mycophenolate mofetil co-administration is recommended.

**DOSAGE:** *Adults:* Initial (6h after transplantation): 0.03-0.05mg/kg/day (liver, kidney) or 0.01mg/kg/day (heart) IV infusion if cannot tolerate PO. Hepatic Transplant: 0.05-0.075mg/kg PO q12h with grapefruit juice; start 8-12 hrs after last IV dose. Kidney Transplant: 0.1mg/kg PO q12h, 24 hrs after transplant or until renal function recovered. Heart Transplant: 0.0375mg/kg PO q12h; start 8-12 hrs after last IV dose. Renal/Hepatic Impairment: Give lowest recommended dose. Severe Hepatic Impairment (Pugh >10): May require lower doses. Wait at least 48 hrs with post-op oliguria.
*Pediatrics:* Liver Transplant: Initial: 0.03-0.05mg/kg/day IV or 0.15-0.2mg/kg/day PO. Severe Hepatic Impairment (Pugh >10): May require lower doses.

**HOW SUPPLIED:** Cap: 0.5mg, 1mg, 5mg; Inj: 5mg/mL

**CONTRAINDICATIONS:** Hypersensitivity to HCO-60.

**WARNINGS/PRECAUTIONS:** Insulin-dependent post-transplant DM, HTN, myocardial hypertrophy, neurotoxicity, hyperkalemia, nephrotoxicity reported. Monitor drug levels frequently to prevent organ rejection and/or reduce potential toxicity. Monitor for anaphylaxis with infusion. Monitor levels closely with hepatic impairment.

**ADVERSE REACTIONS:** HTN, headache, insomnia, fever, pruritus, hyperglycemia, hyperkalemia, hypomagnesemia, diarrhea, nausea, vomiting, increased BUN, anorexia, constipation, tremor, rash, pleural effusion, gastroenteritis.

**INTERACTIONS:** CYP450 3A inducers (eg, carbamazepine, phenobarbital, phenytoin, rifabutin, rifampin, St. John's wort, etc.) may decrease plasma levels. Caution with other nephrotoxic drugs (eg. aminoglycosides, amphotericin B, cisplatin). May affect drugs metabolized by CYP450 3A. Avoid grapefruit juice. CYP450 3A inhibitors (eg, diltiazem, nicardipine, nifedipine, verapamil, azole antifungal, macrolides, cisapride, metoclopramide, etc) may increase plasma levels. Vaccination may be less effective. Avoid live vaccines, cyclosporine (when switching to tacrolimus, wait at least 24 hrs. after last cyclosporine dose), and $K^+$ sparing diuretics.

**PREGNANCY:** Category C, not for use in nursing.

## PROLASTIN RX

alpha1-proteinase inhibitor (human) (Talecris)

**THERAPEUTIC CLASS:** $Alpha_1$Proteinase Inhibitor

**INDICATIONS:** Chronic replacement therapy of individuals having congenital deficiency of $alpha_1$-proteinase inhibitor ($alpha_1$-antitrypsin deficiency) with clinically demonstrable panacinar emphysema.

**DOSAGE:** *Adults:* 60mg/kg IV once weekly.

**HOW SUPPLIED:** Inj: 500mg, 1000mg

P

**CONTRAINDICATIONS:** IgA deficiencies with known antibodies against IgA.

**WARNINGS/PRECAUTIONS:** May contain infectious agents (eg, viruses). May cause increase in plasma volume.

**ADVERSE REACTIONS:** Delayed fever, lightheadedness, dizziness, flu-like symptoms, allergic-like reactions, chills, dyspnea, rash, tachycardia.

**PREGNANCY:** Category C, caution in nursing.

## PROMETHAZINE — RX

promethazine HCl (Various)

**OTHER BRAND NAMES:** Phenergan (Wyeth) - Promethegan (G & W Labs)

**THERAPEUTIC CLASS:** Phenothiazine derivative

**INDICATIONS:** Allergic and vasomotor rhinitis, allergic conjunctivitis, blood or plasma allergic reactions, dermographism, urticaria, angioedema. Pre- and postoperative sedation. Adjunct in anaphylaxis, postoperative pain. Prevention and control of nausea, vomiting, and motion sickness.

**DOSAGE:** *Adults:* Allergy: 25mg qhs or 12.5mg ac and hs. Motion Sickness: Initial: 25mg 30-60 minutes before travel, then 25mg 8-12 hrs later if needed. Maint: 25mg bid. Prevention/Control of Nausea/Vomiting: 25mg initially, then 12.5-25mg q4-6h prn. Sedation: 25-50mg qhs. Preoperative: 50mg night before surgery, then 50mg preoperatively. Postoperative: 25-50mg.
*Pediatrics:* ≥2 yrs: Allergy: 25mg or 0.5mg/lb qhs or 6.25-12.5 tid. Motion Sickness: 12.5-25mg bid. Prevention/Control of Nausea/Vomiting: 25mg or 0.5mg/lb initially then 12.5-25mg or 0.5mg/lb q4-6h prn. Sedation: 12.5-25mg hs. Preoperative: 12.5-25mg night before surgery, then 0.5mg/lb preoperatively. Postoperative: 12.5-25mg.

**HOW SUPPLIED:** Sup: (Promethegan, Phenergan, Promethazine)12.5mg, 25mg, 50mg; Tab: (Phenergan, Promethazine)12.5mg*, 25mg*, 50mg *scored

**CONTRAINDICATIONS:** Treatment of lower respiratory tract symptoms (eg, asthma). Pediatric patients <2 yrs.

**WARNINGS/PRECAUTIONS:** Potential for fatal respiratory depression in pediatric patients <2 yrs. Caution in patients ≥2 yrs. Avoid with compromised respiratory function (eg, COPD, sleep apnea). Caution with bone marrow depression, narrow-angle glaucoma, stenosing peptic ulcer, bladder or pyloroduodenal obstruction, prostatic hypertrophy, CVD, hepatic dysfunction. Cholestatic jaundice reported. Alters HCG pregnancy tests. May lower seizure threshold, increase blood glucose, cause sun sensitivity. May impair mental/physical abilities.

**ADVERSE REACTIONS:** Drowsiness, sedation, blurred vision, dizziness, increased or decreased blood pressure, urticaria, dry mouth, nausea, vomiting.

**INTERACTIONS:** Additive sedative effects with CNS depressants (eg, alcohol, narcotic analgesics, sedatives, hypnotics, tranquilizers); reduce dose or eliminate these agents. Reduce barbiturate dose by one-half and analgesic depressant dose by one-quarter to one-half. Caution with drugs that alter seizure threshold (eg, narcotics, local anesthetics). Avoid sedatives and CNS depressants with sleep apnea.

**PREGNANCY:** Category C, not for use in nursing.



## PROMETHAZINE DM — RX

promethazine HCl - dextromethorphan hbr (Various)

**THERAPEUTIC CLASS:** Phenothiazine derivative/antitussive

**INDICATIONS:** For relief of coughs and upper respiratory symptoms associated with allergy or colds.

**DOSAGE:** *Adults:* 5mL q4-6h. Max: 30mL/24 hr.
*Pediatrics:* >12 yrs: 5mL q4-6h. Max: 30mL/24hr. 6-11 yrs: 2.5-5mL q4-6h. Max: 20mL/24hr. 2-5 yrs: 1.25-2.5mL q4-6h. Max: 10mL/24hr.

**HOW SUPPLIED:** Syrup: (Promethazine-Dextromethorphan) 6.25mg-15mg/5mL

**CONTRAINDICATIONS:** Treatment of lower respiratory tract symptoms (eg, asthma), concomitant MAOIs.

**WARNINGS/PRECAUTIONS:** May lower seizure threshold. Avoid with sleep apnea. Caution with narrow-angle glaucoma, stenosing peptic ulcer, atopic children, bladder or pyloroduodenal obstruction, cardiovascular disease, hepatic dysfunction. Cholestatic jaundice reported. Alters HCG pregnancy test reading. May increase blood glucose.

**ADVERSE REACTIONS:** Drowsiness, dizziness, sedation, GI disturbance, blurred vision, dry mouth, increased or decreased blood pressure, rash, nausea, vomiting.

**INTERACTIONS:** Hyperpyrexia, hypotension and death associated with MAOIs. Added sedative effects with alcohol, narcotic analgesics, sedatives, hypnotics, TCAs, and tranquilizers. Reduce barbiturate dose by one-half and narcotic analgesics by one-quarter to one-half.

**PREGNANCY:** Category C, caution in nursing.

## PROMETHAZINE VC — RX

promethazine HCl - phenylephrine HCl (Various)

**THERAPEUTIC CLASS:** Phenothiazine derivative/ sympathomimetic

**INDICATIONS:** For relief of upper respiratory symptoms (eg, nasal congestion) associated with allergy or colds.

**DOSAGE:** *Adults:* 5mL q4-6h. Max: 30mL/24 hr.
*Pediatrics:* >12 yrs: 5mL q4-6h. Max: 30mL/24 hr. 6-11 yrs: 2.5-5mL q4-6h. Max: 30mL/24 hr. 2-5 yrs: 1.25-2.5mL q4-6h.

**HOW SUPPLIED:** Syrup: (Promethazine-Phenylephrine) 6.25mg-5mg/5mL

**CONTRAINDICATIONS:** Treatment of lower respiratory tract symptoms (eg, asthma), HTN, peripheral vascular insufficiency, concomitant MAOIs.

**WARNINGS/PRECAUTIONS:** May lower seizure threshold. Avoid with sleep apnea. Caution with thyroid disease, diabetes, elderly, poor cerebral or coronary circulation, narrow-angle glaucoma, stenosing peptic ulcer, bladder or pyloroduodenal obstruction, cardiovascular disease, hepatic dysfunction. Cholestatic jaundice reported. Alters HCG pregnancy test reading. May increase blood glucose. Avoid prolonged exposure to sunlight.

**ADVERSE REACTIONS:** Drowsiness, dizziness, anxiety, tremor, sedation, blurred vision, dry mouth, increased or decreased blood pressure, rash, nausea, vomiting.

**INTERACTIONS:** Added sedative effects with alcohol, narcotic analgesics, sedatives, hypnotics, TCAs, tranquilizers. Reduce barbiturate dose by one-half and narcotic analgesics by one-quarter to one-half. Possible hypertensive crisis with MAOIs. Pressor response increased with TCAs. Excessive rise in BP with ergot alkaloids. Arrhythmias with other sympathomimetics. β-blockers block cardiostimulating effects. Reflex bradycardia blocked and pressor response enhanced with atropine. Pressor response decreased with β-blockers. Synergistic adrenergic response with amphetamines.

**PREGNANCY:** Category C, caution in nursing.

## PROMETHAZINE VC/CODEINE — CV

promethazine HCl - codeine phosphate - phenylephrine HCl (Various)

**THERAPEUTIC CLASS:** Phenothiazine derivative/antitussive/sympathomimetic

**INDICATIONS:** For relief of cough and upper respiratory symptoms (eg, nasal congestion) associated with allergy or colds.

**DOSAGE:** *Adults:* 5mL q4-6h. Max: 30mL/24hr.
*Pediatrics:* >12 yrs: 5mL q4-6h. Max: 30mL/24hr. 6-11 yrs: 2.5-5mL q4-6h. Max: 30mL/24hr. 2-5 yrs: 1.25-2.5mL q4-6h. Max: 18kg: 9mL/24hr. 16kg: 8mL/24hr. 14kg: 7mL/24hr. 12kg: 6mL/24hr.

**HOW SUPPLIED:** Syrup: (Promethazine-Codeine-Phenylephrine) 6.25mg-10mg-5mg/5mL

**CONTRAINDICATIONS:** Treatment of lower respiratory tract symptoms (eg, asthma), HTN, peripheral vascular insufficiency, concomitant MAOIs.

**WARNINGS/PRECAUTIONS:** May lower seizure threshold. Avoid with sleep apnea, asthma, acute febrile illness with productive cough, atopic children. Caution with acute abdominal conditions, convulsive disorders, significant renal dysfunction, fever, thyroid disease, diabetes, Addison's disease, ulcerative colitis, prostatic hypertrophy, recent GI or urinary tract surgery, elderly, debilitated, narrow-angle glaucoma, stenosing peptic ulcer, bladder or pyloroduodenal obstruction, cardiovascular disease, hepatic dysfunction. Cholestatic jaundice reported. Alters HCG pregnancy test reading. May increase blood glucose. Respiratory depressant effects may be exacerbated with head injury or increased intracranial pressure.

**ADVERSE REACTIONS:** Drowsiness, dizziness, sedation, tremor, anxiety, blurred vision, dry mouth, increased or decreased blood pressure, rash, nausea, vomiting, constipation, urinary retention.

**INTERACTIONS:** Added sedative effects with alcohol, narcotic analgesics, sedatives, hypnotics, TCAs, tranquilizers. Reduce barbiturate dose by one-half and narcotic analgesics by one-quarter to one-half. Possible hypertensive crisis with MAOIs. Pressor response increased with TCAs. Excessive rise in BP with ergot alkaloids. Arrhythmias with other sympathomimetics. β-blockers block cardiostimulating effects. Reflex bradycardia blocked and pressor response enhanced with atropine. Pressor response decreased with β-blockers. Synergistic adrenergic response with amphetamines.

**PREGNANCY:** Category C, caution in nursing.

## PROMETHAZINE W/CODEINE CV

promethazine HCl - codeine phosphate (Various)



**THERAPEUTIC CLASS:** Phenothiazine derivative/antitussive

**INDICATIONS:** For relief of coughs and upper respiratory symptoms associated with allergy or colds.

**DOSAGE:** *Adults:* 5mL q4-6h. Max: 30mL/24 hr.
*Pediatrics:* >12 yrs: 5mL q4-6h. Max: 30mL/24 hr. 6 to <12 yrs: 2.5-5mL q4-6h. Max: 30mL/24 hr. 2 to <6 yrs: 1.25-2.5mL q4-6h. Max: 2 to <6 yrs: 18kg: 9mL/24 hr. 16kg: 8mL/24 hr. 14kg: 7mL/24 hr. 12kg: 6mL/24 hr.

**HOW SUPPLIED:** Syrup: (Promethazine-Codeine) 6.25mg-10mg/5mL

**CONTRAINDICATIONS:** Treatment of lower respiratory tract symptoms (eg, asthma).

**WARNINGS/PRECAUTIONS:** Avoid prolonged sun exposure. May lower seizure threshold. Avoid with sleep apnea, asthma, acute febrile illness with productive cough, atopic children. Caution with acute abdominal conditions, convulsive disorders, significant renal dysfunction, fever, hypothyroidism, Addison's disease, ulcerative colitis, prostatic hypertrophy, recent GI or urinary tract surgery, elderly, debilitated, narrow-angle glaucoma, stenosing peptic ulcer, bladder or pyloroduodenal obstruction, cardiovascular disease, hepatic dysfunction. Cholestatic jaundice reported. Alters HCG pregnancy test reading. May increase blood glucose. Respiratory depressant effects may be exacerbated with head injury or increased intracranial pressure.

**ADVERSE REACTIONS:** Drowsiness, dizziness, sedation, blurred vision, dry mouth, increased or decreased blood pressure, rash, nausea, vomiting, constipation, urinary retention.

**INTERACTIONS:** Added sedative effects with alcohol, narcotic analgesics, sedatives, hypnotics, TCAs, and tranquilizers. Reduce barbiturate dose by one-half and narcotic analgesics by one-quarter to one-half. Possible adverse reactions with MAOIs.

**PREGNANCY:** Category C, caution in nursing.

## PROMETRIUM
progesterone (Solvay)

RX

**Progestins and estrogens should not be used for the prevention of cardiovascular disease. Increased risks of MI, stroke, invasive breast cancer, pulmonary emboli, DVT, and development of probable dementia in postmenopausal women.**

**THERAPEUTIC CLASS:** Progestogen

**INDICATIONS:** Prevention of endometrial hyperplasia in non-hysterectomized postmenopausal women receiving conjugated estrogens. For secondary amenorrhea.

**DOSAGE:** *Adults:* Prevention of Endometrial Hyperplasia: 200mg qpm for 12 days sequentially per 28 day cycle. Secondary Amenorrhea: 400mg qhs for 10 days.

**HOW SUPPLIED:** Cap: 100mg, 200mg

**CONTRAINDICATIONS:** Peanut allergy, undiagnosed abnormal genital bleeding, breast cancer, DVT, PE, thromboembolic disorders (stroke, myocardial infarction), liver dysfunction or disease, pregnancy.

**WARNINGS/PRECAUTIONS:** D/C if thrombotic disorders, papilledema, or retinal vascular lesions develop. D/C pending exam if sudden onset of proptosis, sudden partial or complete loss of vision, diplopia, or migraine. Include pap smear in pretreatment exam. Caution with depression, DM, and conditions aggravated by fluid retention (eg, epilepsy, migraine, asthma, cardiac/renal dysfunction).

**ADVERSE REACTIONS:** Dizziness, headache, breast pain, nausea, diarrhea, dizziness, abdominal pain and distension, emotional lability, upper respiratory infection.

**INTERACTIONS:** CYP3A4 inhibitors (eg, ketoconazole) may increase bioavailability of progesterone.

**PREGNANCY:** Category B, caution in nursing.

## PROPECIA
finasteride (Merck)

RX

**THERAPEUTIC CLASS:** Type II 5 alpha-reductase inhibitor

**INDICATIONS:** Treatment of male pattern hair loss (androgenetic alopecia). For men only.

**DOSAGE:** *Adults:* 1mg qd. Continue use to sustain benefit.

**HOW SUPPLIED:** Tab: 1mg [ProPak, 3 x 30 tabs]

**CONTRAINDICATIONS:** Pregnancy or women who may potentially become pregnant.

**WARNINGS/PRECAUTIONS:** Caution with hepatic dysfunction. Consider doubling PSA level results in men >41 yrs of age, without BPH, who are undergoing PSA test. Women who are pregnant or may become pregnant should not handle crushed or broken tablets; potential risk to a male fetus. Do not use in pediatrics or women.

**ADVERSE REACTIONS:** Decreased libido, erectile dysfunction, decreased volume of ejaculate, breast tenderness, hypersensitivity reactions.

**PREGNANCY:** Category X, not for use in nursing.

## PROPINE RX

dipivefrin HCl (Allergan)

**THERAPEUTIC CLASS:** Epinephrine (sympathomimetic) prodrug

**INDICATIONS:** Control of intraocular pressure in open-angle glaucoma.

**DOSAGE:** *Adults:* Usual: 1 drop q12h.

**HOW SUPPLIED:** Sol: 0.1% [5mL, 10mL, 15mL]

**CONTRAINDICATIONS:** Narrow-angle glaucoma.

**WARNINGS/PRECAUTIONS:** Macular edema may occur in aphakic patients.

**ADVERSE REACTIONS:** Tachycardia, arrhythmias, HTN, burning, stinging, follicular conjunctivitis, mydriasis, blurry vision, headache.

**PREGNANCY:** Category B, caution in nursing.

## PROPYLTHIOURACIL RX

propylthiouracil (Various)

**THERAPEUTIC CLASS:** Thiourea-derivative antithyroid agent

**INDICATIONS:** Treatment of hyperthyroidism.

**DOSAGE:** *Adults:* Initial: 300mg/day in 3 divided doses, q8h. Severe Hyperthyroidism/Very Large Goiters: Initial: 400mg/day in 3 divided doses; may give up to 600-900mg/day if needed. Maint: 100-150mg/day. *Pediatrics:* 6-10 yrs: Initial: 50-150mg/day. >10 yrs: Initial: 150-300mg/day. Maint: Determine by patient response.

**HOW SUPPLIED:** Tab: 50mg

**CONTRAINDICATIONS:** Nursing mothers.

**WARNINGS/PRECAUTIONS:** Discontinue with agranulocytosis, aplastic anemia, hepatitis, fever, or exfoliative dermatitis. Rare reports of severe hepatic reactions exist. Discontinue with significant hepatic abnormality, including transaminases >3X ULN. Caution with pregnancy, may cause fetal harm. Monitor PT and TFTs.

P

**ADVERSE REACTIONS:** Agranulocytosis, skin rash, urticaria, nausea, vomiting, epigastric distress, arthralgia, paresthesias, loss of taste, myalgia, headache, pruritus, drowsiness, neuritis, edema, vertigo, jaundice.

**INTERACTIONS:** May potentiate anticoagulant effects. Hyperthyroidism increases clearance of β-blockers; reduce β-blocker dose when patient becomes euthyroid. Increased digitalis glycoside levels when patient becomes euthyroid; reduce digitalis dose. Decreased theophylline clearance when patient becomes euthyroid; reduce theophylline dose. Caution with other drugs that cause agranulocytosis.

**PREGNANCY:** Category D, contraindicated in nursing.

## PROQUAD RX

mumps vaccine live - measles vaccine live - rubella vaccine live - varicella virus vaccine live (Merck)

**THERAPEUTIC CLASS:** Vaccine

**INDICATIONS:** Vaccination against measles, mumps, rubella, and varicella in children 12 months to 12 yrs of age.

**DOSAGE:** *Pediatrics:* 12 months-12 yrs: 0.5mL SQ. At least 1 month should elapse between dose of measles-containing vaccine and a dose of ProQuad. If for any reason a second dose of varicella-containing vaccine is required, at least 3 months should elapse between doses.

**HOW SUPPLIED:** Inj: 0.5mL

**CONTRAINDICATIONS:** Anaphylactic reactions to neomycin; hypsensitivity to gelatin; blood dyscrasias, leukemia, lymphomas, or other malignant neoplasms affecting the bone marrow or lymphatic system; immunosuppressive therapy; primary and acquired immunodeficiency states (e.g., AIDS/HIV); congenital or hereditary immunodeficiency; active untreated tuberculosis; active afebrile illness with fever >101.3°F; pregnant.

**WARNINGS/PRECAUTIONS:** Caution with egg allergy. May cause thrombocytopenia. Contains albumin, remote risk of viral infection transmission. Have epinephrine (1:1000) available.

**ADVERSE REACTIONS:** Injection Site: Pain/tenderness/soreness, erythema, swelling. Systemic: Fever, irritability, measles-like rash

**INTERACTIONS:** Do not give with immune globulin. Avoid use of salicylates for 6 weeks after vaccination. Avoid use of immunosuppressive doses of corticosteriods or other immunosuppressive drugs.

**PREGNANCY:** Category C, not for use in nursing.

## PROQUIN XR

RX

ciprofloxacin HCl (Esprit)

**THERAPEUTIC CLASS:** Fluoroquinolone

**INDICATIONS:** Treatment of uncomplicated urinary tract infections (acute cystitis) caused by *E.coli* and *K.pneumoniae*.

**DOSAGE:** *Adults:* 500mg qd with pm meal for 3 days. Administer at least 4 hrs before or 2 hrs after magnesium or aluminum containing antacids, sucralfate, Videx (didanosine) chewable/buffered tablets of pediatric powder, metal cations (eg, iron), multivitamins with zinc. Do not split, crush, or chew. Swallow tab whole.

**HOW SUPPLIED:** Tab, Extended-Release: 500mg

**WARNINGS/PRECAUTIONS:** Convulsions, increased intracranial pressure and toxic psychosis reported. Discontinue if dizziness, confusion, tremors, hallucinations, depression, or suicidal thoughts/acts. Caution with CNS disorders or if predisposed to seizures. Severe, fatal hypersensitivity reactions may occur. Pseudomembranous colitis; achilles, and other tendon ruptures reported. Discontinue at first sign of rash or if pain, inflammation, or ruptured tendon occurs. Maintain hydration; avoid alkaline urine. Avoid excessive sunlight and UV light. Not interchangeable with immediate-release or other extended-release oral formulations.

**ADVERSE REACTIONS:** Fungal infection, nasopharyngitis, headache, micturition urgency.

**INTERACTIONS:** Increases theophylline and caffeine levels and prolongs effects. Serious/fatal reactions have occurred with theophylline. Magnesium or aluminum containing antacids, sucralfate, Videx® (didanosine) chewable/buffered tablets or pediatric powder, and products containing calcium, iron, or zinc decrease serum and urine levels; administer at least 4 hrs before or 2 hrs after administration. Altered serum levels of phenytoin. Severe hypoglycemia with glyburide (rare). Potentiated by probenecid. Transient serum creatinine elevations with cyclosporine. Enhances oral anticoagulant effects. May increase risk of methotrexate toxic reactions due to inhibition of renal tubular transport. High dose quinolones shown to provoke convulsions with NSAIDs (not aspirin).

**PREGNANCY:** Category C, not for use in nursing.

## PROSCAR
RX

finasteride (Merck)

**THERAPEUTIC CLASS:** Type II 5 alpha-reductase inhibitor

**INDICATIONS:** Treatment of symptomatic benign prostatic hypertrophy (BPH) to improve symptoms, reduce the risk of acute urinary retention, and reduce the risk of the need for prostate surgery. To reduce the risk of symptomatic progression of BPH in combination with doxazosin.

**DOSAGE:** *Adults:* 5mg qd.

**HOW SUPPLIED:** Tab: 5mg

**CONTRAINDICATIONS:** Pregnancy.

**WARNINGS/PRECAUTIONS:** Not for use in pediatrics or women. Risk to male fetus in pregnancy. Pregnant women should not handle crushed or broken tablets. Rule out infection, prostate cancer, stricture disease, hypotonic bladder prior to initiating therapy. Caution with liver dysfunction. Decreases serum PSA levels by ~50% in patients with BPH, even with prostate cancer; adjust (double) PSA results to compare with normal values. Monitor for obstructive uropathy with large residual urinary volume and/or severely diminished urinary flow.

**ADVERSE REACTIONS:** Impotence, decreased libido, decreased ejaculate volume, hypersensitivity reactions (pruritus, urticaria, swelling of lips and face), testicular pain.

**PREGNANCY:** Category X, not for use in nursing.

## PROSED EC
RX

methenamine - benzoic acid - methylene blue - phenyl salicylate - atropine sulfate - hyoscyamine sulfate (Esprit)

**OTHER BRAND NAMES:** Prosed DS (Star)

**THERAPEUTIC CLASS:** Urinary tract analgesic

**INDICATIONS:** Relief of lower urinary tract discomfort due to hypermotility. Treatment of formaldehyde-susceptible cystitis, urethritis, trigonitis.

**DOSAGE:** *Adults:* 1 tab qid with plenty of fluid.
*Pediatrics:* >12 yrs: Individualize dose. Take with plenty of fluid.

**HOW SUPPLIED:** Tab, Enteric Coated: Atropine 0.06mg-Benzoic Acid 9mg-Hyoscyamine 0.06mg-Methenamine 81.6mg-Methylene Blue 10.8mg-Phenyl Salicylate 36.2mg

**CONTRAINDICATIONS:** Risk-benefit assessment in glaucoma, urinary bladder neck obstruction, pyloric or duodenal obstruction, cardiospasm.

**WARNINGS/PRECAUTIONS:** Discontinue if tachycardia, dizziness, or blurred vision occurs. Delay in gastric emptying time may obscure gastric ulcer therapy.

**ADVERSE REACTIONS:** Rapid pulse, flushing, blurred vision, dizziness, shortness of breath, difficult micturition, acute urinary retention, dry mouth, nausea, vomiting.

**INTERACTIONS:** May decrease absorption of other oral agents (dose 2 hrs after ketoconazole). Reduced effectiveness with urinary alkaliners, thiazide diuretics, antacids/antidiarrheals (space dosing by 1 hr). Antimuscarinic effects potentiated with other antimuscarinics, MAOIs. Caution with antimyasthenics. Increased risk of constipation with opioids. Increased risk of crystalluria with sulfonamides.

**PREGNANCY:** Category C, caution in nursing.

## PROSOM

estazolam (Abbott) **CIV**

**THERAPEUTIC CLASS:** Benzodiazepine

**INDICATIONS:** Short-term management of insomnia.

**DOSAGE:** *Adults:* Initial: 1mg qhs. May increase to 2mg qhs. Small/Debilitated/Elderly: Initial: 0.5mg qhs.

**HOW SUPPLIED:** Tab: 1mg*, 2mg* *scored

**CONTRAINDICATIONS:** Pregnancy.

**WARNINGS/PRECAUTIONS:** Avoid abrupt withdrawal after prolonged use. Caution with depression, elderly/debilitated, renal/hepatic impairment. May cause respiratory depression.

**ADVERSE REACTIONS:** Somnolence, hypokinesia, dizziness, abnormal coordination, constipation, dry mouth, amnesia, paradoxical reactions.

**INTERACTIONS:** Potentiated effects with anticonvulsants, antihistamines, alcohol, barbiturates, MAOIs, narcotics, phenothiazines, psychotropic medications, or other CNS depressants. Smoking may increase clearance.

**PREGNANCY:** Category X, not for use in nursing.

## PROSTIN E2

dinoprostone (Pharmacia & Upjohn) RX

**THERAPEUTIC CLASS:** Prostaglandin $E_2$

**INDICATIONS:** Termination of pregnancy between 12th to 20th week of gestation. Evacuation of uterine contents in the management of missed abortion or intrauterine fetal death up to 28 weeks gestation. Management of nonmetastatic gestational trophoblastic disease.

**DOSAGE:** *Adults:* Insert 1 sup high into vagina; remain in supine position for 10 minutes. Insert additional sups at 3-5 hr intervals until abortion occurs. Max: 2 days of continuous use.

**HOW SUPPLIED:** Sup: 20mg [$1^s$ $5^s$]

**CONTRAINDICATIONS:** Active pelvic inflammatory disease; active cardiac, pulmonary, renal, or hepatic disease.

**WARNINGS/PRECAUTIONS:** Adhere strictly to recommended dose. Use in facility able to provide intensive care and acute surgery. Not a feticidal agent. Can induce bone proliferation. If abortion fails, complete by other means. Caution with asthma, hypotension, HTN, cardiovascular disease, renal/hepatic disease, anemia, jaundice, diabetes, epilepsy, cervicitis, infected endocervical lesions, acute vaginitis, and compromised uteri. Transient pyrexia reported.

**ADVERSE REACTIONS:** Vomiting, diarrhea, nausea, temperature elevation, shivering, chills, transient BP decrease, headache.

**INTERACTIONS:** May augment activity of other oxytocic drugs; avoid concomitant use.

**PREGNANCY:** Category C, safety in nursing not known.

## PROSTIN VR PEDIATRIC

alprostadil (Pharmacia & Upjohn) RX

**Apnea occurs in about 10-12% of neonates, usually appearing during the 1st hr of drug infusion. Monitor respiratory status throughout treatment.**

**THERAPEUTIC CLASS:** Prostaglandin $E_1$

**INDICATIONS:** Palliative therapy to maintain patency of the ductus arteriosus until corrective surgery in neonates with congenital heart defects.

**DOSAGE:** Pediatrics: Initial: 0.05-0.1mcg/kg/min IV. Maint: 0.025-0.01mcg/kg/min IV. Max: 0.4mcg/kg/min.

**HOW SUPPLIED:** Inj: 0.5mg/mL

**WARNINGS/PRECAUTIONS:** May cause gastric outlet obstruction secondary to antral hyperplasia, monitor closely after 120 hrs of therapy. Limit infusion to minimum effective dose and time. May inhibit platelet aggregation; caution with bleeding tendencies. Cortical proliferation of long bones, localized and aneurysmal dilatations, vessel wall edema, intimal lacerations, decrease in medial muscularity and disruption of medial and internal lamina reported. Avoid in respiratory distress syndrome. Monitor arterial pressure intermittently; decrease rate of infusion with significant fall in pressure.

**ADVERSE REACTIONS:** Apnea, fever, seizures, bradycardia, flushing, diarrhea, hypotension, tachycardia.

**PREGNANCY:** Safety in pregnancy and nursing not known.

## PROTAMINE SULFATE RX

protamine sulfate (Various)

**THERAPEUTIC CLASS:** Heparin antagonist

**INDICATIONS:** Management of heparin overdose.

**DOSAGE:** *Adults:* Administer as slow IV infusion over 10 minutes, at doses not to exceed 50mg. Determine dose by blood coagulation studies. Each mg neutralizes about 90U heparin derived from lung tissue or 115U heparin derived from intestinal mucosa.

**HOW SUPPLIED:** Inj: 10mg/mL

**WARNINGS/PRECAUTIONS:** May cause allergic reactions with fish hypersensitivity. Rapid administration may cause severe hypotensive and anaphylactoid-like reactions. Caution in cardiac surgeries; hyperheparinemia or bleeding reported. Previous exposure to protamine/protamine-containing insulin may induce humoral immune response; severe hypersensitivity reaction, including life-threatening anaphylaxis reported. Increased risk of antiprotamine antibodies in infertile or vasectomized men.



**ADVERSE REACTIONS:** Hypotension, bradycardia, transitory flushing/feeling of warmth, lassitude, dyspnea, nausea, vomiting, back pain, anaphylaxis that causes severe respiratory distress, circulatory collapse, noncardiogenic pulmonary edema, acute pulmonary HTN.

**INTERACTIONS:** Incompatible with certain antibiotics, such as cephalosporins and penicillins.

**PREGNANCY:** Category C, caution in nursing.

## PROTONIX RX

pantoprazole sodium (Wyeth)

**OTHER BRAND NAMES:** Protonix IV (Wyeth)

**THERAPEUTIC CLASS:** Proton pump inhibitor

**INDICATIONS:** (Tab) Short-term treatment and maintenance of healing of erosive esophagitis associated with GERD. Long-term treatment of pathological hypersecretory conditions (eg, Zollinger-Ellison syndrome). (Inj) Short-term treatment of GERD with a history of erosive esophagitis as an alternative to oral therapy (not for initial treatment). Treatment of pathological hypersecretory (eg, Zollinger-Ellison Syndrome).

**DOSAGE:** *Adults:* (Tab) Erosive Esophagitis Treatment: 40mg qd for up to 8 weeks. May repeat for 8 weeks if needed. Maintenance: 40mg qd. Hypersecretory Conditions: Initial: 40mg bid. Adjust to patient's needs. Max: 240mg/day. (Inj) GERD: 40mg IV qd for 7-10 days. Pathological Hypersecretion: 80mg IV q12h. May adjust up to 80mg IV q8h based on acid output. Max: 240mg/day. Duration >6 days not studied. Do not split, crush or chew tabs.

**HOW SUPPLIED:** Inj: 40mg; Tab, Delayed Release: 20mg, 40mg

**WARNINGS/PRECAUTIONS:** Symptomatic response does not preclude the presence of gastric malignancy. Atrophic gastritis has been noted occasionally in gastric corpus biopsies from patients treated for long-term. False (+) urine screening test for THC reported. (Inj) Immediate hypersensitivity reactions reported (eg, thrombophlebitis, LFT elevation).

**ADVERSE REACTIONS:** (Inj) Abdominal pain, headache, constipation, dyspepsia, nausea. (Tab) Headache, flatulence, diarrhea, abdominal pain.

**INTERACTIONS:** May alter absorption of pH-dependent drugs (eg, ketoconazole, ampicillin esters, and iron salts).

**PREGNANCY:** Category B, not for use in nursing.

## PROTOPIC

tacrolimus (Astellas) — RX

**THERAPEUTIC CLASS:** Macrolide immunosuppressant

**INDICATIONS:** Short-term and intermittent long-term therapy of moderate to severe atopic dermatitis intolerant or unresponsive to conventional therapy.

**DOSAGE:** *Adults:* (0.03% or 0.1%) Apply thin layer bid. Rub in gently. Continue for 1 week after symptoms clear.
*Pediatrics:* >16 yrs: (0.03% or 0.1%) Apply thin layer bid. Rub in gently. Continue for 1 week after symptoms clear. 2-15 yrs: (0.03%) Apply thin layer bid. Rub in gently. Continue for 1 week after symptoms clear.

**HOW SUPPLIED:** Oint: 0.03%, 0.1% [30g, 60g, 100g]

**WARNINGS/PRECAUTIONS:** Do not use with occlusive dressings. Increased risk of varicella zoster, herpes simplex, or eczema herpeticum. Lymphadenopathy reported; monitor closely. Discontinue if unknown etiology of lymphadenopathy or presence of acute infectious mononucleosis. Avoid in Netherton's syndrome. Minimize or avoid exposure to natural or artificial sunlight. Long-term safety has not been established. Rare cases of malignancy (eg, skin and lymphoma) have been reported with topical calcineurin inhibitors; therefore, continuous long-term use should be avoided and application limited to areas of involvement. Not indicated for use in children <2 yrs. Only 0.03% ointment is indicated for use in children 2-15 yrs.

**ADVERSE REACTIONS:** Skin burning, pruritus, flu-like symptoms, allergic reaction, skin erythema, headache, skin infection, fever, herpes simplex, rhinitis.

**INTERACTIONS:** Caution with CYP3A4 inhibitors (eg, erythromycin, itraconazole, ketoconazole, fluconazole, calcium channel blockers, cimetidine) in widespread and/or erythrodermic disease. Increased risk for lymphomas in transplant patients receiving other immunosuppressive therapy.

**PREGNANCY:** Category C, not for use in nursing.

## PROVENTIL HFA

albuterol sulfate (Schering) — RX

**THERAPEUTIC CLASS:** $Beta_2$ agonist

**INDICATIONS:** Prevention and treatment of bronchospasm with reversible obstructive airway disease; prevention of exercise-induced bronchospasm (EIB) in patients ≥4 yrs old.

**DOSAGE:** *Adults:* Bronchospasm: 2 inh q4-6h or 1 inh q4h. EIB: 2 inh 15-30 min before activity.
*Pediatrics:* ≥4 yrs: Bronchospasm: 2 inh q4-6h or 1 inh q4h. EIB: 2 inh 15-30 min before activity.

**HOW SUPPLIED:** HFA: 90mcg/inh [6.7g]

**WARNINGS/PRECAUTIONS:** Hypersensitivity reactions reported. Monitor for worsening asthma. fatalities reported with excessive use. Caution with cardiovascular disorders, especially coronary insufficiency, arrhythmias and HTN. May need concomitant corticosteroids. Can produce paradoxical bronschospasm. Caution with DM, hyperthyroidism, and seizures. May cause transient hypokalemia.

**ADVERSE REACTIONS:** Tachycardia, tremor, dizziness, nausea/vomiting, palpitations, rihinitis, upper respiratory tract infection, fever, inhalation site and taste sensation, back pain, and nervousness.

**INTERACTIONS:** Avoid other sympathomimetic agents. Extreme caution wtih MAOIs and TCAs. Monitor digoxin. May worsen ECG changes and/or hypokalemia with nonpotassium-sparing diuretics. Antagonized by β-blockers.

**PREGNANCY:** Category C, not for use in nursing.

## PROVERA RX

medroxyprogesterone acetate (Pharmacia & Upjohn)

**THERAPEUTIC CLASS:** Progestogen

**INDICATIONS:** Secondary amenorrhea and for abnormal uterine bleeding due to hormonal imbalance in the absence of organic pathology, such as fibroids or uterine cancer. To reduce the incidence of endometrial hyperplasia in non-hysterectomized postmenopausal women receiving 0.625mg conjugated estrogen.

**DOSAGE:** *Adults:* Secondary Amenorrhea: 5-10mg qd for 5-10 days. Abnormal Uterine Bleeding: 5-10mg qd for 5-10 days beginning on day 16 or day 21 of cycle. Endometrial Hyperplasia: 5-10mg qd for 12-14 consecutive days per month beginning on day 1 or day 16 of cycle.

**HOW SUPPLIED:** Tab: 2.5mg*, 5mg*, 10mg* *scored

**CONTRAINDICATIONS:** Thrombophlebitis, thromboembolic disorders, cerebral apoplexy, liver dysfunction, malignancy of breast or genital organs, undiagnosed vaginal bleeding, missed abortion, pregnancy, as a diagnostic test for pregnancy.



**WARNINGS/PRECAUTIONS:** D/C if develop thrombotic disorders, papilledema, or retinal vascular lesions. D/C pending exam if sudden onset of proptosis, sudden partial or complete loss of vision, diplopia, or migraine. Include pap smear in pretreatment exam. Caution with depression, DM, and conditions aggravated by fluid retention (eg, epilepsy, migraine, asthma, cardiac, renal dysfunction).

**ADVERSE REACTIONS:** Breast tenderness, galactorrhea, urticaria, pruritus, edema, rash, thromboembolic phenomena, menstrual changes, edema, change in weight, cervical changes, cholestatic jaundice, depression, insomnia, nausea, somnolence.

**PREGNANCY:** Category X, caution in nursing.

## PROVIGIL CIV

modafinil (Cephalon)

**THERAPEUTIC CLASS:** Wakefulness-promoting agent

**INDICATIONS:** To improve wakefulness in patients with excessive daytime sleepiness associated with narcolepsy, obstructive sleep apnea/hypopnea syndrome (OSAHS), shiftwork sleep disorder (SWSD). As adjunct treatment for underlying obstruction in OSAHS.

**DOSAGE:** *Adults:* 200mg qd. Narcolepsy/OSAHS: Take in AM. SWSD: Take 1 hr prior to start of work shift. Hepatic Dysfunction: 100mg qd. Elderly: Consider dose reduction.

*Pediatrics:* ≥16 yrs: 200mg qd. Narcolepsy/OSAHS: Take in AM. SWSD: Take 1 hr prior to start of work shift. Hepatic Dysfunction: 100mg qd.

**HOW SUPPLIED:** Tab: 100mg, 200mg* *scored

**WARNINGS/PRECAUTIONS:** Avoid in history of left ventricular hypertrophy, ischemic ECG changes, chest pain, arrhythmia or other manifestations of mitral valve prolapse with CNS stimulants. Caution if recent MI, unstable angina, history of psychosis. Monitor hypertensive patients.

**ADVERSE REACTIONS:** Headache, infection, nausea, nervousness, anxiety, insomnia.

**INTERACTIONS:** Methylphenidate may delay absorption. May reduce efficacy of steroidal contraceptives up to 1 month after discontinuation. Caution with MAOIs. CYP3A4 inducers (eg, carbamazepine, phenobarbital, rifampin) may decrease levels. CYP3A4 inhibitors (eg, ketoconazole, itraconazole) may increase levels. May increase levels of drugs metabolized by CYP2C19 (eg, diazepam, propranolol, phenytoin) or CYP2C9 (eg, warfarin). Monitor for toxicity with phenytoin and PT with warfarin. May increase levels of clomipramine, desipramine. May decrease levels of drugs metabolized by CYP3A4 (eg, cyclosporine, steroidal contraceptives, theophylline). Avoid alcohol.

**PREGNANCY:** Category C, caution in nursing.

## PROZAC

fluoxetine HCl (Lilly)

RX

**Antidepressants increased the risk of suicidal thinking and behavior (suicidality) in short-term studies in children and adolescents with Major Depressive Disorder (MDD) and other psychiatric disorders. Fluoxetine is approved for use in pediatric patients with MDD and Obsessive Compulsive Disorder (OCD).**

**THERAPEUTIC CLASS:** Selective serotonin reuptake inhibitor

**INDICATIONS:** Treatment of MDD, OCD, bulimia nervosa, panic disorder with or without agoraphobia.

**DOSAGE:** *Adults:* MDD: Daily Dosing: Initial: 20mg qam; increase dose if no improvement after several weeks. Doses >20mg/day, give qam or bid (am and noon). Max: 80mg/day. OCD: Initial: 20mg/day. Maint: 20-60mg/day given qd-bid, am and noon. Max: 80mg/day. Bulimia Nervosa: 60mg qam. Max: 60mg/day. Panic Disorder: Initial: 10mg/day. May increase to 20mg/day after 1 week. May increase further after several weeks if no clinical improvement. Max: 60mg/day. Hepatic Impairment/Elderly: Use lower or less frequent dosage. *Pediatrics:* MDD: ≥8 yrs: Higher Weight Peds: Initial: 10 or 20mg/day. After 1 week at 10mg/day, may increase to 20mg/day. Lower Weight Peds: Initial: 10mg/day. Titrate: May increase to 20mg/day after several weeks if clinical improvement not observed. OCD: ≥7 yrs: Adolescents and Higher Weight Peds: Initial: 10mg/day. Titrate: Increase to 20mg/day after 2 weeks. Consider additional dose increases after several more weeks if clinical improvement not observed. Usual: 20-60mg/day. Lower Weight Peds: Initial: 10mg/day. Titrate: Consider additional dose increases after several weeks if clinical improvement not observed. Usual: 20-30mg/day. Max: 60mg/day.

**HOW SUPPLIED:** Cap: 10mg, 20mg, 40mg; Sol: 20mg/5mL [120mL]; Tab: 10mg* *scored

**CONTRAINDICATIONS:** During or within 14 days of MAOI therapy. Thioridazine within 5 weeks of discontinuation. Concomitant use of pimozide.

**WARNINGS/PRECAUTIONS:** D/C if unexplained allergic reaction occurs. Monitor for symptoms of mania/hypomania. Caution with diseases or conditions that could affect metabolism or hemodynamic responses, diabetes, history of seizures, suicidal tendencies. Altered platelet function, hyponatremia reported. Periodically monitor height and weight in pediatrics. Monitor for clinical worsening and/or suicidality, especially at initiation of therapy or dose changes. Avoid abrupt withdrawal. Monitor for discontinuation symptoms. Caution in third trimester of pregnancy due to risk of serious neonatal complications.

**ADVERSE REACTIONS:** Nausea, diarrhea, insomnia, anxiety, nervousness, dizziness, somnolence, tremor, decreased libido, sweating, anorexia, asthenia, dry mouth, dyspepsia, headache.

**INTERACTIONS:** See Contraindications. Antidiabetic drugs may need adjustment. May shift concentrations with plasma-bound drugs (eg, coumadin, digitoxin). May alter warfarin effects. May increase benzodiazepine, phenytoin, carbamazepine levels. Increased adverse effects with tryptophan. Caution with CNS drugs. Lithium levels may increase/decrease; monitor lithium levels. May potentiate drugs metabolized by CYP2D6, antipsychotics (eg, haloperidol, clozapine), other antidepressants. Avoid alcohol. Caution with drugs that interfere with hemostasis (eg, non-selective NSAIDs, aspirin, warfarin) due to increased risk of bleeding. Serotonin syndrome reported with use of an SSRI and a triptan; monitor closely.

**PREGNANCY:** Category C, not for use in nursing.

## PROZAC WEEKLY RX

fluoxetine HCl (Lilly)

**Antidepressants increased the risk of suicidal thinking and behavior (suicidality) in short-term studies in children and adolescents with Major Depressive Disorder (MDD) and other psychiatric disorders. Fluoxetine is approved for use in pediatric patients with MDD and obsessive compulsive disorder (OCD).**

**THERAPEUTIC CLASS:** Selective serotonin reuptake inhibitor

**INDICATIONS:** Treatment of MDD.

**DOSAGE:** *Adults:* One 90mg capsule every week starting 7 days after last daily dose of fluoxetine.

**HOW SUPPLIED:** Cap, Extended Release: 90mg

**CONTRAINDICATIONS:** During or within 14 days of MAOI therapy. Thioridazine within 5 weeks of discontinuation. Concomitant use of pimozide.

P

**WARNINGS/PRECAUTIONS:** Rash with systemic involvement and urticaria reported. Anxiety, nervousness, insomnia or activation of mania/hypomania reported. Weight loss and altered appetite; monitor weight changes. Caution with diseases or conditions that could affect metabolism or hemodynamic responses, diabetes, or history of seizures. May impair judgment, thinking or motor skills. Altered platelet function and hyponatremia reported. Monitor for clinical worsening and/or suicidality, especially at initiation of therapy or dose changes. Avoid abrupt withdrawal. Monitor for discontinuation symptoms. Caution in third trimester of pregnancy due to risk of neonatal complications.

**ADVERSE REACTIONS:** Nausea, diarrhea, insomnia, anxiety, nervousness, dizziness, somnolence, tremor, decreased libido, sweating, anorexia, asthenia, dry mouth, dyspepsia, headache.

**INTERACTIONS:** See Contraindications. Antidiabetic drugs may need adjustment. May shift concentrations with plasma-bound drugs (eg, coumadin, digitoxin). May alter warfarin effects. May increase benzodiazepine, phenytoin and carbamazepine levels. Increased adverse effects with tryptophan. Caution with CNS drugs. Lithium levels may increase/decrease; monitor lithium levels. May potentiate drugs metabolized by CYP2D6, antipsychotics (eg, haloperidol, clozapine) and other antidepressants. Avoid alcohol. Caution with drugs that interfere with hemostasis (eg, non-selective NSAIDs, aspirin, warfarin) due to increased risk of bleeding. Serotonin syndrome reported with use of an SSRI and a triptan; monitor closely.

**PREGNANCY:** Category C, not for use in nursing.

## PSORCON
RX

diflorasone diacetate (Dermik)

**OTHER BRAND NAMES:** Psorcon E (Dermik)

**THERAPEUTIC CLASS:** Corticosteroid

**INDICATIONS:** Corticosteroid responsive dermatoses.

**DOSAGE:** *Adults:* Apply qd-tid (Psorcon Oint/Psorcon E Cream) or qd-qid (Psorcon E Oint) or bid (Psorcon Cream) depending on the severity. May use occlusive dressings for psoriasis or recalcitrant conditions. D/C dressings if infection develops.

**HOW SUPPLIED:** Cre, Oint: 0.05% [15g, 30g, 60g]

**WARNINGS/PRECAUTIONS:** May produce reversible HPA axis suppression, manifestations of Cushing's syndrome, hyperglycemia, and glucosuria. Caution when applied to large surface areas or under occlusive dressings. Use appropriate antifungal or antibacterial agent with dermatological infections; d/c if infection does not clear. Pediatrics may be more susceptible to systemic toxicity. Avoid eyes. D/C if irritation occurs. Cre has an increased risk of producing adrenal suppression than Oint. Cre should not be used in treatment of rosacea or perioral dermatitis; avoid face, groin, or axillae.

**ADVERSE REACTIONS:** Burning, itching, irritation, dryness, folliculitis, hypertrichosis, acneiform eruptions, hypopigmentation, perioral dermatitis, allergic contact dermatitis, skin maceration, secondary infection, skin atrophy, striae, miliaria.

**PREGNANCY:** Category C, caution in nursing.

## PULMICORT
RX

budesonide (AstraZeneca LP)

**OTHER BRAND NAMES:** Pulmicort Respules (AstraZeneca LP) - Pulmicort Flexhaler (AstraZeneca LP)

**THERAPEUTIC CLASS:** Corticosteroid

**INDICATIONS:** (Respules) Treatment of asthma and as prophylactic therapy in children 12 months to 8 years of age. (Flexhaler) Maintenance treatment of asthma as prophylactic therapy in patients ≥6 years and to reduce or eliminate the need for oral systemic corticosteroidal therapy.

**DOSAGE:** *Adults:* (Flexhaler) Initial: 180-360mcg bid. Max: 720mcg bid. Individualize dose.
*Pediatrics:* (Flexhaler) >6 yrs: Initial: 180-360mcg bid. Max: 360mcg bid. Individualize dose. (Respules) 1-8 yrs: Previous Bronchodilator Only: Initial: 0.5mg qd or 0.25mg bid. Administer via jet nebulizer. Max: 0.5mg/day. Previous Inhaled Corticosteroid: 0.5mg qd or 0.25mg bid. Max: 1mg/day. Previous Oral Corticosteroid: 1mg qd or 0.5mg bid. Max: 1mg/day. Gradually reduce PO corticosteroid after 1 week of budesonide.

**HOW SUPPLIED:** Powder, Inhalation: (Flexhaler) 90mcg/dose, 180mcg/dose; Sus, Inhalation: (Respules) 0.25mg/2mL; 0.5mg/2mL [2mL, 30s]

**CONTRAINDICATIONS:** Primary treatment of status asthmaticus or other acute episodes of asthma where intensive measures are required.

**WARNINGS/PRECAUTIONS:** Deaths due to adrenal insufficiency have occurred with transfer from systemic corticosteroids to inhaled corticosteroids. Resume oral corticosteroids during stress or severe asthma attack. Transferring from oral to inhalation therapy may unmask allergic conditions (eg, rhinitis, conjunctivitis, arthritis, eosinophilic conditions, eczema). Observe for adrenal insufficiency, systemic corticosteroid withdrawal effects, and growth suppression (children). More susceptible to infections. Not for acute bronchospasm. D/C if bronchospasm occurs after dosing. Caution with TB of respiratory tract; untreated systemic fungal, bacterial, viral or parasitic infections; or ocular herpes simplex. *Candida* infection of mouth and pharynx reported.

**ADVERSE REACTIONS:** Nasopharyngitis, pharyngitis, headache, fever, sinusitis, pain, bronchospasm, bronchitis, respiratory infection, monoliasis.

**INTERACTIONS:** Oral ketoconazole increases plasma levels. CYP3A4 inhibitors (eg, itraconazole, clarithromycin, erythromycin) may inhibit metabolism and increase systemic exposure. (Respules) Slight decrease in clearance and increase in oral bioavailabilty with cimetidine.

**PREGNANCY:** (Respules) Category B, caution in nursing; (Flexhaler) Category B, not for use in nursing.

## PURINETHOL RX
mercaptopurine (Gate)

**THERAPEUTIC CLASS:** Purine analog

**INDICATIONS:** Remission induction and maintenance therapy of acute lymphatic leukemia (ALL).

**DOSAGE:** *Adults:* Induction: Initial: 2.5mg/kg/day. Calculate to nearest multiple of 25mg. Titrate: If no improvement after 4 weeks, increase to 5mg/kg/day. Discontinue with large rise or rapid fall in leukocytes or platelets. Resume when counts remain constant for 2-3 days or rises. Maint: 1.5-2.5mg/kg/day. Renal/Hepatic Impairment: Reduce dose.
*Pediatrics:* Induction: Initial: 2.5mg/kg qpm. Calculate to nearest multiple of 25mg. Titrate: If no improvement after 4 weeks, increase to 5mg/kg/day. Discontinue with large rise or rapid fall in leukocytes or platelets. Resume when counts remain constant for 2-3 days or rises. Maint: 1.5-2.5mg/kg/day. Renal/Hepatic Impairment: Reduce dose.

**HOW SUPPLIED:** Tab: 50mg* *scored

**CONTRAINDICATIONS:** Lack of definitive diagnosis of ALL. Prior resistance to mercaptopurine or thioguanine.

**WARNINGS/PRECAUTIONS:** Risk of dose-related bone marrow suppression. Monitor weekly platelet counts, Hgb, Hct, total WBC with differential; increase frequency during induction phase. Monitor closely for life-threatening infection or bleeding. Risk of hepatotoxicity, anorexia, diarrhea, jaundice, and ascites (especially with >2.5mg/kg dose). Perform LFTs weekly initially, then monthly; monitor more frequently with hepatotoxic drugs or pre-existing liver disease.



**ADVERSE REACTIONS:** Bone marrow toxicity, hepatotoxicity, hyperuricemia (reduce incidence by prehydration, urine alkalinization, prophylactic allopurinol), intestinal ulceration, rash, hyperpigmentation, alopecia, transient oligospermia.

**INTERACTIONS:** Reduce to 1/3-1/4 of usual dose with allopurinol to avoid toxicity. Reduce dose with myelosuppressants. Bone marrow suppression reported with trimethoprim-sulfamethoxazole. Cross-resistance with thioguanine.

**PREGNANCY:** Category D, not for use in nursing.

## PYRAZINAMIDE RX
pyrazinamide (Various)

**THERAPEUTIC CLASS:** Nicotinamide analogue

**INDICATIONS:** Adjunctive initial treatment of active tuberculosis (TB). For use after treatment failure with other primary drugs in active TB.

**DOSAGE:** *Adults:* Usual: 15-30mg/kg qd. Max: 3g/day. (CDC recommends Max: 2g/day). Alternate Regimen: 50-70mg/kg twice weekly. Dose based on lean body weight. Take initial 2 months of 6 month or longer regimen.
*Pediatrics:* Usual: 15-30mg/kg qd. Max: 3g/day. (CDC recommends Max: 2g/day). Alternate Regimen: 50-70mg/kg twice weekly. Dose based on lean body weight. Take initial 2 months of 6 month or longer regimen.

**HOW SUPPLIED:** Tab: 500mg* *scored

**CONTRAINDICATIONS:** Severe hepatic damage and active gout.

**WARNINGS/PRECAUTIONS:** Obtain baseline serum uric acid and LFTs before therapy. Caution with hepatic dysfunction or those at risk for drug-related hepatitis (eg, alcoholics) and DM. D/C if hyperuricemia with gouty arthritis or hepatocellular damage occurs. Inhibits renal excretion of urates.

**ADVERSE REACTIONS:** Gout, hepatotoxicity, nausea, vomiting, anorexia, arthralgia, myalgia, rash, urticaria, pruritus.

**PREGNANCY:** Category C, caution in nursing.

## PYRIDIUM RX

phenazopyridine HCl (Warner Chilcott)

**THERAPEUTIC CLASS:** Urinary tract analgesic

**INDICATIONS:** Symptomatic relief of urinary pain, burning, frequency and urgency associated with infection, trauma, and urinary procedures.

**DOSAGE:** *Adults:* 200mg tid pc. Concomitant Antibiotic for UTI: Do not exceed 2 days of pyridium therapy.

**HOW SUPPLIED:** Tab: 100mg, 200mg

**CONTRAINDICATIONS:** Renal insufficiency.

**WARNINGS/PRECAUTIONS:** Discontinue if skin or sclera develops a yellow color; may indicate impaired renal excretion. Caution in elderly, renal impairment. Produces orange to red urine; may stain fabric and contact lenses.

**ADVERSE REACTIONS:** Headache, rash, pruritus, GI distress, methemoglobinemia, hemolytic anemia, anaphylactoid-like reactions.

**PREGNANCY:** Category B, safety in nursing not known.

## PYRIDIUM PLUS RX

butabarbital - phenazopyridine HCl - hyoscyamine hydrobromide (Warner Chilcott)

**THERAPEUTIC CLASS:** Anticholinergic/barbiturate/analgesic

**INDICATIONS:** Symptomatic relief of urinary pain, burning, frequency and urgency associated with infection, trauma, and urinary procedures.

**DOSAGE:** *Adults:* 1 tab qid (pc and hs). Concomitant Antibiotic for UTI: Do not exceed 2 days of pyridium therapy.

**HOW SUPPLIED:** Tab: (Butabarbital-Hyoscyamine-Phenazopyridine) 15mg-0.3mg-150mg

**CONTRAINDICATIONS:** Renal or hepatic insufficiency, glaucoma, bladder neck obstruction, porphyria.

**WARNINGS/PRECAUTIONS:** Discontinue if skin or sclera develops a yellow color; may indicate impaired renal excretion. Caution in elderly, renal impairment. Produces orange to red urine; may stain fabric and contact lenses.

**ADVERSE REACTIONS:** Headache, rash, pruritus, GI distress, methemoglobinemia, hemolytic anemia, anaphylactoid-like reactions, dry mouth, dizziness, drowsiness, blurred vision.

**PREGNANCY:** Category C, safety in nursing not known.



## QUESTRAN RX

cholestyramine (Par)

**OTHER BRAND NAMES:** Questran Light (Par)

**THERAPEUTIC CLASS:** Bile acid sequestrant

**INDICATIONS:** Adjunct to reduce elevated cholesterol in primary hypercholesterolemia not responding to diet or to reduce LDL in hypertriglyceridemia. Relief of pruritus associated with partial biliary obstruction.

**DOSAGE:** *Adults:* Initial: 1 packet or scoopful qd or bid. Maint: 2-4 packets or scoopfuls/day, given bid. Titrate: Adjust at no less than 4 week intervals. Max: 6 packets/day or 6 scoopfuls/day. May also give as 1-6 doses/day. Mix with fluid or highly fluid food.
*Pediatrics:* Usual: 240mg/kg/day of anhydrous cholestyramine resin in 2-3 divided doses. Max: 8g/day.

**HOW SUPPLIED:** Powder: 4g/packet [60s, 378g], (Light) 4g/scoopful [60s, 268g]

**CONTRAINDICATIONS:** Complete biliary obstruction.

**WARNINGS/PRECAUTIONS:** May produce hyperchloremic acidosis with prolonged use. Caution in renal insufficiency, volume depletion. Chronic use may produce or worsen constipation. Avoid constipation with symptomatic CAD. May increase bleeding tendency due to vitamin K deficiency. Serum or red cell folate reduced with chronic use. Constipation may aggravate hemorrhoids. Light formulation contains phenylalanine. Measure cholesterol during 1st few months; periodically thereafter. Measure TG periodically.

**ADVERSE REACTIONS:** Constipation, heartburn, nausea, vomiting, abdominal pain, flatulence, diarrhea, anorexia, osteoporosis, rash, hyperchloremic acidosis (children), vitamin A and D deficiency, steatorrhea, hypoprothrombinemia (vitamin K deficiency).

**INTERACTIONS:** May interfere with absorption of fat-soluble vitamins (A, D, E, K), drugs that undergo enterohepatic circulation, and oral phosphate supplements. Take concomitant drugs 1hr before or 4-6 hrs after. Additive effects with HMG-CoA reductase inhibitors and nicotinic acid. Caution with spironolactone. May reduce or delay absorption of phenylbutazone, warfarin, thiazide diuretics, propranolol, tetracycline, penicillin G, phenobarbital, thyroid and thyroxine agents, estrogens, progestins, digitalis.

**PREGNANCY:** Category C, caution in nursing.

## QUINIDINE GLUCONATE INJECTION RX

quinidine gluconate (Various)

Q

**THERAPEUTIC CLASS:** Class IA antiarrhythmic/schizonticide antimalarial

**INDICATIONS:** Treatment of life-threatening Plasmodium flaciparum malaria. Conversion of atrial fibrillation/flutter (A-Fib/Flutter) to normal sinus rhythm. Treatment of ventricular arrhythmias.

**DOSAGE:** *Adults:* Malaria: LD: 15mg/kg base (24mg/kg gluconate) over 4 hrs. Maint: After 8 hrs, 7.5mg/kg (12mg/kg gluconate) IV q8h for 7 days. Alternate: Initial: 6.25mg/kg base (10mg/kg/min gluconate) IV over 1-2 hrs. Maint: 12.5mcg/kg/min base (20mcg/kg/min gluconate) for 72h. Switch to PO therapy when possible. A-Fib/Flutter and Ventricular Arrhythmia: 0.25mg/kg/minute. Max: 5-10mg/kg. Consider alternate therapy if conversion to sinus rhythm not achieved. Renal/Hepatic Impairment or CHF: Reduce dose. Elderly: Start at low end of dosing range.
*Pediatrics:* Malaria: LD: 15mg/kg base (24mg/kg gluconate) over 4 hrs. Maint: After 8 hrs, 7.5mg/kg (12mg/kg gluconate) IV q8h for 7 days. Alternate: Initial: 6.25mg/kg base (10mg/kg/min gluconate) IV over 1-2 hrs. Maint: 12.5mcg/kg/min base (20mcg/kg/min gluconate) for 72h. Switch to PO therapy when possible.

**HOW SUPPLIED:** Inj: 80mg/mL

**CONTRAINDICATIONS:** Cardiac rhythm dependent upon a junctional or idioventricular pacemaker (absent of functioning pacemaker), thrombocytopenic purpura with previous treatment, patients adversely affected by anticholinergics (eg, myasthenia gravis).

**WARNINGS/PRECAUTIONS:** Rapid infusion can cause peripheral vascular collapse and hypotension. May prolong QTc interval. Paradoxical increase in ventricular rate in A-Fib/Flutter. Caution in those at risk of complete AV block without implanted pacemakers, renal/hepatic dysfunction, elderly, and CHF. Physical/pharmacologic maneuvers to terminate paroxysmal supraventricular tachycardia may be ineffective. Exacerbated bradycardia in sick sinus syndrome.

**ADVERSE REACTIONS:** GI distress, lightheadedness, fatigue, palpitations, weakness, visual problems, nausea, vomiting, diarrhea, sleep disturbances, rash, headache, cinchonism, hepatotoxicity, autoimmune/inflammatory syndromes.

**INTERACTIONS:** Urine alkalinizers (eg, carbonic anhydrase inhibitors, sodium bicarbonate, thiazide diuretics) reduce renal elimination. CYP3A4 inducers (eg, phenobarbital, phenytoin, rifampin) may accelerate elimination. Verapamil, diltiazem decrease clearance. Caution with drugs metabolized by CYP2D6 (eg, mexiletine, phenothiazines, polycyclic antidepressants, codeine, hydrocodone) or by CYP3A4 (eg, nifedipine, felodipine, nicardipine, nimodipine). β-blockers may decrease clearance. May slow metabolism of nifedipine. Increases levels of digoxin, digitoxin, procainamide and haloperidol. Increased levels with ketoconazole, amiodarone, cimetidine. Potentiates warfarin, depolarizing and nondepolarizing neuromuscular blockers. Additive effects with anticholinergics, vasodilators, and negative inotropes. Antagonistic effects with cholinergics, vasoconstrictors, and positive inotropes.

**PREGNANCY:** Category C, not for use in nursing.

## QUINIDINE GLUCONATE ORAL — RX

quinidine gluconate (Various)

**THERAPEUTIC CLASS:** Class IA antiarrhythmic

**INDICATIONS:** Conversion of symptomatic atrial fibrillation/flutter (A-Fib/Flutter) to normal sinus rhythm, reduction of relapse frequency into A-Fib/Flutter, and suppression of ventricular arrhythmias.

**DOSAGE:** *Adults:* A-Fib/Flutter Conversion: Initial: 2 tabs q8h. Titrate: Increase cautiously if no effect after 3-4 doses. Alternate Regimen: 1 tab q8h for 2 days, then 2 tabs q12h for 2 days, then 2 tabs q8h up to 4 days. A-Fib/Flutter Relapse Reduction: 1 tab q8-12h. Titrate: Increase cautiously if needed. Ventricular Arrhythmia: Dosing regimens not adequately studied. Generally similar to A-Fib/Flutter. Renal/Hepatic Impairment or CHF: Reduce dose. May break tab in half. Do not chew or crush.

**HOW SUPPLIED:** Tab, Extended Release: 324mg

**CONTRAINDICATIONS:** Cardiac rhythm dependent upon a junctional or idioventricular pacemaker (absent of functioning pacemaker), thrombocytopenic purpura with previous treatment, myasthenia gravis.

**WARNINGS/PRECAUTIONS:** Increases risk of mortality, especially with structural heart disease. May prolong QTc interval. Paradoxical increase in ventricular rate in A-Fib/Flutter. Caution in those at risk of complete AV block without implanted pacemakers, renal/hepatic dysfunction, and CHF. Physical/pharmacologic maneuvers to terminate paroxysmal supraventricular tachycardia may be ineffective. Exacerbated bradycardia in sick sinus syndrome.

**ADVERSE REACTIONS:** Diarrhea, fever, rash, arrhythmia, abnormal ECG, nausea, vomiting, dizziness, headache.

**INTERACTIONS:** Urine alkalinizers (eg, carbonic anhydrase inhibitors, sodium bicarbonate, thiazide diuretics) reduce renal elimination. CYP3A4 inducers (eg, phenobarbital, phenytoin, rifampin) may accelerate elimination. Verapamil, diltiazem, β-blockers decrease clearance. Caution with drugs metabolized by CYP450 3A4 (eg, nifedipine, felodipine, nicardipine, nimodipine) and 2D6 (eg, mexiletine, phenothiazines, polycyclic antidepressants, codeine, hydrocodone). Increases levels of digoxin, digitoxin, procainamide and haloperidol. Increased levels with ketoconazole, amiodarone, cimetidine. Potentiates warfarin, depolarizing and nondepolarizing neuromuscular blockers. Additive effects with anticholinergics, vasodilators, and negative inotropics. Antagonistic effects with cholinergics, vasoconstrictors, and positive inotropes. Avoid grapefruit juice. Dietary salt may affect absorption.

**PREGNANCY:** Category C, not for use in nursing.

## QUINIDINE SULFATE — RX

quinidine sulfate (Various)

**THERAPEUTIC CLASS:** Class IA antiarrhythmic

**INDICATIONS:** Conversion of symptomatic atrial fibrillation/flutter (A-Fib/Flutter) to normal sinus rhythm, reduction of relapse frequency into A-Fib/Flutter, and suppression of ventricular arrhythmias.

**DOSAGE:** *Adults:* A-Fib/Flutter Conversion: Initial: 300mg q8-12h. Titrate: Increase cautiously if no result and levels are within therapeutic range. A-Fib/Flutter Relapse Reduction: 300mg q8-12h. Titrate: Increase cautiously if needed. Ventricular Arrhythmia: Dosing regimens not adequately studied. Monitor ECG for $QT_c$ prolongation.

**HOW SUPPLIED:** Tab, Extended Release: 300mg

**CONTRAINDICATIONS:** Cardiac rhythm dependent upon a junctional or idioventricular pacemaker (absent of functioning pacemaker), thrombocytopenic purpura with previous treatment, patients adversely affected by anticholinergics (eg, myasthenia gravis).

**WARNINGS/PRECAUTIONS:** Increases risk of mortality, especially with structural heart disease. May prolong QTc interval. Paradoxical increase in ventricular rate in A-Fib/Flutter. Adjust dose in renal/hepatic dysfunction, and CHF. Caution if at risk of complete AV-block in those without implanted pacemakers, or in elderly. Physical/pharmacologic maneuvers to terminate paroxysmal supraventricular tachycardia may be ineffective. Exacerbated bradycardia in sick sinus syndrome. Monitor blood counts, hepatic and renal function periodically with long-term therapy. D/C if bloody dyscrasia or hepatic/renal dysfunction occurs.

**ADVERSE REACTIONS:** Diarrhea, nausea, vomiting, esophagitis, lightheadedness, fatigue, palpitations, angina-like pain, weakness, rash, visual problems, cinchonism, hepatotoxicity, autoimmune/inflammatory syndromes.



**INTERACTIONS:** Urine alkalinizers (eg, carbonic anhydrase inhibitors, sodium bicarbonate, thiazide diuretics) reduce renal elimination. CYP3A4 inducers may accelerate elimination. Verapamil, diltiazem, β-blockers decrease clearance. Caution with drugs metabolized by CYP3A4 and 2D6. Increases levels of procainamide, haloperidol. Increased levels with ketoconazole, amiodarone, cimetidine. Potentiates warfarin, depolarizing and nondepolarizing neuromuscular blockers. Additive effects with anticholinergics, vasodilators, and negative inotropics. Avoid grapefruit juice. Dietary salt may affect absorption. Digoxin may need dose reduction.

**PREGNANCY:** Category C, not for use in nursing.

## QUININE SULFATE — RX

quinine sulfate (Various)

**THERAPEUTIC CLASS:** Cinchona alkaloid

**INDICATIONS:** For use in malaria.

**DOSAGE:** *Adults:* 1-3 tabs or caps tid for 6-12 days.

**HOW SUPPLIED:** Cap: 325mg; Tab: 260mg

**CONTRAINDICATIONS:** Pregnancy, glucose-6-phosphate dehydrogenase (G-6PD) deficiency, history of thrombocytopenic purpura associated with quinine sulfate, tinnitus, optic neuritis, and history of blackwater fever.

**WARNINGS/PRECAUTIONS:** May cause cinchonism (eg, headache, tinnitus, nausea, vision disturbance). Hemolysis reported with G-6PD deficiency; stop therapy if hemolysis appears. Discontinue if hypersensitivity occurs. Caution with atrial fibrillation.

**ADVERSE REACTIONS:** Headache, nausea, vomiting, epigastric pain, tinnitus, blurred vision, photophobia, hemolysis, thrombocytopenic purpura, diplopia, vertigo, restlessness, asthma symptoms, anginal symptoms.

**INTERACTIONS:** Decreased absorption with aluminum-containing antacids. May enhance the effect of warfarin and other oral anticoagulants. Potentiates neuromuscular blocking agents (eg, pancuronium, succinylcholine, tubocurarine). Increases digoxin and digitoxin plasma levels. Urinary alkalizers (eg, acetazolamide and sodium bicarbonate) may increase levels.

**PREGNANCY:** Category X, caution in nursing.

## QUIXIN

levofloxacin (Vistakon) RX

**THERAPEUTIC CLASS:** Fluoroquinolone

**INDICATIONS:** Treatment of bacterial conjunctivitis.

**DOSAGE:** *Adults:* Days 1-2: 1-2 drops q2h while awake, up to 8x/day. Days 3-7: 1-2 drops q4h while awake, up to qid.
Pediatrics: ≥1 yr: Days 1-2: 1-2 drops q2h while awake, up to 8x/day. Days 3-7: 1-2 drops q4h while awake, up to qid.

**HOW SUPPLIED:** Sol: 0.5% [5mL]

**WARNINGS/PRECAUTIONS:** Discontinue if hypersensitivity or superinfection occurs. Avoid contact lenses with conjunctivitis.

**ADVERSE REACTIONS:** Transient ocular burning, decreased vision, fever, foreign body sensation, headache, ocular pain, pharyngitis, photophobia.

**INTERACTIONS:** Systemic quinolone therapy may increase theophylline levels, interfere with caffeine metabolism, enhance warfarin effects, and elevate serum creatinine with cyclosporine.

**PREGNANCY:** Category C, caution in nursing.

## QVAR

beclomethasone dipropionate (Ivax) RX

Q

**THERAPEUTIC CLASS:** Corticosteroid

**INDICATIONS:** Maintenance treatment of asthma as prophylactic therapy in patients ≥5 tears; to reduce or eliminate the need for oral corticosteroidal therapy.

**DOSAGE:** *Adults:* Previous Bronchodilator Only: 40-80mcg bid. Max: 320mcg bid. Previous Inhaled Corticosteroid Therapy: 40-160mcg bid. Max: 320mcg bid. Maint With Oral Corticosteroids: May attempt gradual reduction of oral dose after 1 week on inhaled therapy.
*Pediatrics:* Adolescents: Previous Bronchodilator Only: 40-80mcg bid. Max: 320mcg bid. Previous Inhaled Corticosteroid Therapy: 40-160mcg bid. Max: 320mcg bid. 5-11 yrs: Previous Bronchodilator Only or Inhaled Corticosteroid Therapy: 40mcg bid. Max: 80mcg bid. >5 yrs: Maint With Oral Corticosteroids: May attempt gradual reduction of oral dose after 1 week on inhaled therapy.

**HOW SUPPLIED:** MDI: 40mcg/inh, 80mcg/inh [7.3g]

**CONTRAINDICATIONS:** Status asthmaticus, acute asthmatic attacks.

**WARNINGS/PRECAUTIONS:** Deaths due to adrenal insufficiency have occurred with transfer from systemic corticosteroids to inhaled corticosteroids. Resume oral corticosteroids during stress or severe asthma attack. Risk of adrenal insufficiency and withdrawal symptoms when replacing systemic corticosteroids. May unmask allergic conditions previously suppressed by systemic steroid therapy. Caution with TB, ocular herpes simplex, or untreated systemic bacterial, fungal, parasitic or viral infections. May suppress growth in children. Exposure to chickenpox or measles requires prophylaxis treatment. Not for rapid relief of bronchospasm.

**ADVERSE REACTIONS:** Headache, pharyngitis, upper respiratory tract infection, rhinitis, increased asthma symptoms, sinusitis.

**PREGNANCY:** Category C, not for use in nursing.

## RANEXA RX

ranolazine (CV Therapeutics)

**THERAPEUTIC CLASS:** Miscellaneous antianginal

**INDICATIONS:** Treatment of chronic angina. Because it prolongs the QT interval, use should be reserved for patients who have not achieved an adequate response with other antianginal drugs. For use in combination with amlodipine, β-blockers or nitrates. The effect on angina rate or exercise tolerance appeared to be smaller in women than men.

**DOSAGE:** *Adults:* Initial: 500mg bid. Max: 1000mg bid. Swallow whole; do not crush, break, or chew.

**HOW SUPPLIED:** Tab, Extended-Release: 500mg

**CONTRAINDICATIONS:** Pre-existing QT prolongation; hepatic impairment (Child-Pugh Classes A [mild], B [moderate], C [severe]); with QT prolonging drugs; with potent and moderately potent CYP3A inhibitors (including diltiazem).

**WARNINGS/PRECAUTIONS:** May prolong QTc interval in a dose-related manner; avoid with known QT prolongation (including congenital long QT syndrome, uncorrected hypokalemia), known history of ventricular tachycardia, hepatic dysfunction. Monitor BP with severe renal impairment.

**ADVERSE REACTIONS:** Dizziness, headache, constipation, nausea.

**INTERACTIONS:** See Contraindications. Increased levels with ketoconazole, diltiazem, verapamil, paroxetine. Avoid use with potent or moderately potent CYP3A inhibitors such as ketoconazole and other azole antifungals, diltiazem, verapamil, macrolide antibiotics, HIV protease inhibitors, grapefruit juice or grapefruit containing products. May increase levels of digoxin, simvastatin; consider dosage reduction of digoxin, simvastatin. Avoid with drugs that may prolong the QTc interval, such as Class Ia (eg, quinidine) and Class III (eg, dofetilide, sotalol) antiarrhythmics, and antipsychotics (eg, thioridazine, ziprasidone). May increase levels of drugs metabolized by CYP2D6 such as TCAs and some antipsychotics; consider dosage reduction of these drugs.



**PREGNANCY:** Category C, not for use in nursing.

## RAPAMUNE RX

sirolimus (Wyeth)

**Increased susceptibility to infection and development of lymphoma.**

**THERAPEUTIC CLASS:** Macrocyclic lactone immunosuppressant

**INDICATIONS:** Prophylaxis of organ rejection in renal transplant patients. Recommended to be used initially with cyclosporine and corticosteroids. In low-moderate risk patients, withdraw cyclosporine 2-4 months after transplantation and increase sirolimus dose to reach recommended blood levels.

**DOSAGE:** *Adults:* LD: 6mg. Maint: 2mg qd. Hepatic Impairment: Reduce maintenance dose by one-third.
*Pediatrics:* >13 yrs and <40kg: LD: $3mg/m^2$ Maint: $1mg/m^2$/day. Hepatic Impairment: Reduce maintenance dose by one-third. Take 4 hrs after cyclosporine.

**HOW SUPPLIED:** Sol: 1mg/mL [60mL]; Tab: 1mg, 2mg

**WARNINGS/PRECAUTIONS:** Increased cholesterol and triglycerides that may require treatment. Reduction in renal function due to long-term concomitant cyclosporine. Increased risk of lymphocele. Provide 1 year prophylaxis for *pneumocystis carinii* pneumonia and 3 months for cytomegalovirus after transplant. Limit exposure to sunlight and UV light. Not for use in liver or lung transplants. Interstitial lung disease reported. Increased susceptability to infection and the possible development of lymphoma and malignancy, especially of the skin, may result from immnosupression. Avoid in liver or lung transplant patients. Increased risk of angioedema, caution with concomitant use of angioedema-causing drugs, such as ACEI.

**ADVERSE REACTIONS:** Hypercholesterolemia, hyperlipemia, HTN, rash, acne, anemia, leukopenia, arthralgia, diarrhea, hypokalemia, thrombocytopenia, fever, abdominal pain, headache, constipation, creatinine increase, arthralgia, insomnia, dyspnea, upper respiratory infection, anaphylactic/anaphylactoid reactions, angioedema, hypersensitivity vasculitis.

**INTERACTIONS:** Increased levels with diltiazem. CYP3A4 inhibitors (eg, calcium channel blockers, antifungals, macrolide antibiotics) may increase levels of sirolimus, while CYP3A4 inducers (eg, anticonvulsants, rifabutin, St. John's wort) may decrease levels. Avoid live vaccines, grapefruit juice, rifampin, ketoconazole. Caution with other nephrotoxic drugs (eg, aminoglycosides, amphotericin B). Hepatic artery thrombosis reported with cyclosporine or tacrolimus, and increased death rate and graft loss with tacrolimus in liver transplant patients. Bronchial anastomotic dehiscence reported with immunosupressives in lung transplant patients. Cyclosporine is a substrate and inhibitor of CYP3A4 and P-gp. Caution with dosing. Monitor for rhabdomyolysis with cyclosporine and HMG Co-A reductase inhibitors/fibrates. Monitor renal function with cyclosporine. Grapefruit juice reduces CYP3A4 medicated drug metabolism, should not be administered with rapamune or used for dilution. Increased risk of deterioration of renal function, serum lipid abnormalities, and urinary tract infections with calcineurin inhibitors and corticosteriods.

**PREGNANCY:** Category C, not for use in nursing.

## RAPTIVA
efalizumab (Genentech)

RX

**THERAPEUTIC CLASS:** Monoclonal antibody/LFA-1 blocker

**INDICATIONS:** Chronic moderate to severe plaque psoriasis for candidates of systemic therapy or phototherapy.

**DOSAGE:** *Adults:* ≥18yrs: Initial: 0.7mg/kg SQ single dose. Maint: 1mg/kg SQ once weekly. Max: 200mg/dose.

**HOW SUPPLIED:** Inj: 125mg

**WARNINGS/PRECAUTIONS:** May increase risk of infection or reactivate latent, chronic infections. Avoid with clinically important infections. Serious infections may occur. Caution with chronic or history of recurrent infections or malignancies; d/c if serious infection or malignancy develops. Obtain baseline platelet counts and monitor periodically; d/c if thrombocytopenia develops. D/C if hemolytic anemia occurs.

**ADVERSE REACTIONS:** Headache, chills, fever, nausea, myalgia, flu syndrome, pain, back pain, acne, infections (may be serious), malignancies, thrombocytopenia, psoriasis worsening.

**INTERACTIONS:** Avoid other immunosuppressives, acellular, live and live-attenuated vaccines.

**PREGNANCY:** Category C, not for use in nursing.

## RAZADYNE ER

RX

galantamine hydrobromide (Ortho-McNeil)

**OTHER BRAND NAMES:** Razadyne (Ortho-McNeil)

**THERAPEUTIC CLASS:** Acetylcholinesterase Inhibitor

**INDICATIONS:** Treatment of mild to moderate dementia of the Alzheimer's type.

**DOSAGE:** *Adults:* (Sol, Tab) Initial: 4mg bid with am and pm meals. Titrate: Increase to 8mg bid after 4 weeks if tolerated, then increase to 12mg bid after 4 weeks if tolerated. Usual: 16-24mg/day. Max: 24mg/day. (Cap, ER) Initial: 8mg qd with am meal. Titrate: Increase to 16mg qd after 4 weeks, then increase to 24mg qd after 4 weeks if tolerated. Usual: 16-24mg/day. Max: 24mg/day. If therapy is interrupted, restart at lowest dose and increase to current dose. Moderate Renal/Hepatic Impairment (Child-Pugh: 7-9): Caution during dose titration. Max: 16mg/day. Avoid use with severe renal (CrCl <9mL/min) and severe hepatic impairment (Child-Pugh: 10-15).

**HOW SUPPLIED:** Sol: (Razadyne) 4mg/mL [100mL]; Tab: (Razadyne) 4mg, 8mg, 12mg. Cap, Extended-Release: (Razadyne ER) 8mg, 16mg, 24mg.

**WARNINGS/PRECAUTIONS:** Vagotonic effects; caution with supraventricular conduction disorder. May cause bradycardia and/or heart block. Caution with asthma or obstructive pulmonary disease. Monitor for active or occult GI bleeding and ulcers due to increased gastric acid secretion. Risk of generalized convulsions or bladder outflow obstruction. Ensure adequate fluid intake during treatment. Deaths reported with mild cognitive impairment.

**ADVERSE REACTIONS:** Nausea, vomiting, diarrhea, anorexia, weight loss, fatigue, dizziness, headache, depression, insomnia, abdominal pain, dyspepsia, UTI.

**INTERACTIONS:** Potential to interfere with anticholinergics. Synergistic effect with succinylcholine, other cholinesterase inhibitors, similar neuromuscular blockers or cholinergic agonists (eg, bethanechol). Increased levels with cimetidine, ketoconazole, and paroxetine. Caution with drugs that slow heart rate due to vagotonic effects. Monitor for GI bleed with NSAIDs.

**PREGNANCY:** Category B, not for use in nursing.

## REBETOL

RX

ribavirin (Schering)



**Not for monotherapy treatment of chronic hepatitis C. Primary toxicity is hemolytic anemia. Avoid with significant or unstable cardiac disease. Contraindicated in pregnancy and male partners of pregnant women. Use 2 forms of contraception during therapy and for 6 months after discontinuation.**

**THERAPEUTIC CLASS:** Nucleoside analogue

**INDICATIONS:** In combination with Intron A® for treatment of chronic hepatitis C in patients ≥3 yrs with compensated liver disease previously untreated with alpha interferon or in patients ≥18 yrs who relapsed after alpha interferon therapy. In combination with Peg-Intron® for treatment of chronic hepatitis C in patients ≥18 yrs with compensated liver disease previously untreated with interferon alpha.

**DOSAGE:** *Adults:* ≥18 yrs: With Intron A: <75kg: 400mg qam and 600mg qpm. >75kg: 600mg qam and 600mg qpm. Treat for 24-48 weeks interferon-naive; 24 weeks in relapse. With PEG-INTRON: 400mg bid, qam and qpm with food. Reduce to 600mg qd if Hgb <10g/dL with no cardiac history, or if Hgb decreases by >2g/dL during a 4 week-period with a cardiac history. D/C if Hgb <8.5g/L with no cardiac history or if Hgb <12g/dL after 4 weeks of dose reduction with a cardiac history. CrCl <50mL/min: Avoid use.
*Pediatrics:* ≥3 yrs: 15mg/kg/day in divided doses qam and qpm. Use sol if ≤25kg or cannot swallow caps. With Intron A: 25-36kg: 200mg bid, qam and

qpm. 37-49kg: 200mg qam and 400mg qpm. 50-61kg: 400mg bid, qam and qpm. >61kg: Dose as adult. Genotype 1: Treat for 48 weeks. Genotype 2/3: Treat for 24 weeks.

**HOW SUPPLIED:** Cap: 200mg; Sol: 40mg/mL [120mL]

**CONTRAINDICATIONS:** Pregnancy, male partners of pregnant women, hemoglobinopathies (eg, thalassemia major, sickle cell anemia). When used with Intron A or PEG-Intron, refer to the individual monograph.

**WARNINGS/PRECAUTIONS:** Severe depression, suicidal ideation, bone marrow suppression, autoimmune and infectious disorders, pulmonary dysfunction, pancreatitis, and DM reported. Assess for underlying cardiac disease (obtain EKG); fatal and nonfatal MI reported with anemia. Hemolytic anemia reported; monitor Hgb or Hct initially then at Week 2 and 4 (or more if needed) of therapy. Suspend therapy if symptoms of pancreatitis arise. Avoid if CrCl <50mL/min. Obtain negative pregnancy test prior to initiation then monthly, and for 6 months post-therapy.

**ADVERSE REACTIONS:** Hemolytic anemia, headache, fatigue, rigors, fever, nausea, anorexia, myalgia, arthralgia, insomnia, irritability, depression, dyspnea, alopecia.

**INTERACTIONS:** Dental and periodontal disorders reported with interferon or peginterferon combination therapy.

**PREGNANCY:** Category X, not for use in nursing.

## REBETRON

RX

ribavirin - interferon alfa-2b (Schering)

**Contraindicated in pregnancy and male partners of pregnant women. Use 2 forms of contraception during therapy and 6 months after discontinuation. May cause or aggravate fatal neuropsychiatric, autoimmune, ischemic, and infectious disorders. Monitor closely with periodic clinical and laboratory evaluations.**

**THERAPEUTIC CLASS:** Biological response modifier/nucleoside analogue

**INDICATIONS:** Treatment of chronic hepatitis C with compensated liver disease previously untreated with alfa interferon or in those relapsed after alpha interferon therapy.

**DOSAGE:** *Adults:* >18 yrs: Previously Untreated with Interferon: Treat for 24-48 weeks. Relapse After Interferon Treatment: Treat for 24 weeks. Usual: <75kg: Interferon 3MIU SQ three times weekly (TIW) with ribavirin 400mg PO qam and 600mg PO qpm. >75kg: Interferon 3MIU SQ TIW with ribavirin 600mg PO qam and 600mg PO qpm. Dose Reduction: If Hgb <10g/dL with no cardiac history, decrease ribavirin to 600mg PO qd. If >2g/dL decrease in Hgb during a 4-week period with a cardiac history, decrease interferon to 1.5MIU SQ TIW and ribavirin to 600mg PO qd. If WBC <1.5x$10^9$/L or neutrophils <0.75x$10^9$/L or platelets <50x$10^9$/L: Decrease interferon to 1.5MIU SQ TIW. Discontinue interferon and ribavirin if Hgb <8.5g/dL with no cardiac history, or Hgb <12g/dL after 4 weeks of dose reduction with a cardiac history, WBC <1x$10^9$/L, neutrophils <0.5x$10^9$/L, or platelets <25x$10^9$/L.

**HOW SUPPLIED:** Inj-Cap: (Interferon alpha-2b-Ribavirin) 3MIU/0.2mL-200mg, 3MIU/0.5mL-200mg

**CONTRAINDICATIONS:** Autoimmune hepatitis, pregnancy, male partners of pregnant women.

**WARNINGS/PRECAUTIONS:** Monitor CBC before therapy, at week 2 and 4, or more often if needed. Severe depression, suicidal ideation, hemolytic anemia, bone marrow suppression, sarcoidosis, pulmonary dysfunction, pancreatitis, and DM reported. Assess for underlying cardiac disease; fatal and nonfatal MI reported with anemia. Suspend or discontinue therapy if cardiovascular status deteriorates or if symptoms of pancreatitis develop. If pulmonary dysfunction develops, monitor closely and discontinue if needed. Avoid if CrCl <50mL/min. Caution with autoimmune disorders, psoriasis, organ transplants, decompensated hepatitis C, nonresponders to interferon, co-infection with hepatitis B virus or HIV infection. Perform visual exam before therapy in diabetic and hypertensive patients. Discontinue if resistant thyroid abnormalities occur. Maintain hydration. Avoid with significant or unstable cardiac disease and hemoglobinopathies (eg, thalassemia, sickle-cell anemia).

**ADVERSE REACTIONS:** Hemolytic anemia, headache, fatigue, rigors, flu-like symptoms, dizziness, nausea, dyspepsia, vomiting, anorexia, musculoskeletal pain, insomnia, irritability, depression, dyspnea, alopecia, rash, pruritus, elevated bilirubin and uric acid levels, thyroid abnormalities.

**INTERACTIONS:** Caution with myelosuppressives. Reduced absorption with antacids. Caution with coadministration of ribavirin with nucleoside analogues; may cause lactic acidosis. Only coadminister if benefit outweighs risks.

**PREGNANCY:** Category X, not for use in nursing.

## REBIF RX
interferon beta-1a (Pfizer/Serono)

**THERAPEUTIC CLASS:** Biological response modifier

**INDICATIONS:** Treatment of patients with relapsing forms of multiple sclerosis.

**DOSAGE:** *Adults:* Initial: 20% of prescribed dose SQ 3x/week (TIW); 4.4mcg for prescribed dose of 22mcg, 8.8mcg for prescribed dose of 44mcg. Titrate: Increase over a 4 week period to either 22mcg or 44mcg SQ TIW. Maint: 22mcg or 44mcg SQ TIW. Leukopenia/Elevated LFTs: Reduce dose by 20-50% until toxicity resolves. Administer dose at the same time everyday (late afternoon, evening) on the same 3 days/week at least 48 hrs apart.

**HOW SUPPLIED:** Inj: 22mcg/0.5mL, 44mcg/0.5mL; Titration Pack: 8.8mcg/0.2mL [6s] and 22mcg/0.5mL [6s]

**CONTRAINDICATIONS:** Hypersensitivity to human albumin.

**WARNINGS/PRECAUTIONS:** Caution with depression, alcohol abuse, active hepatic disease, increased serum SGPT (>2.5X ULN) , history of significant hepatic disease, seizure disorder. Consider discontinuing therapy if depression, jaundice/hepatic dysfunction develops. Reduce dose if serum SGPT >5X ULN. Contains albumin; risk of viral disease transmission. Monitor blood cell counts and LFTs at 1,3,6 months after initiation then periodically. Monitor thyroid function tests every 6 months in history of thyroid dysfunction.

**ADVERSE REACTIONS:** Psychiatric disorders, injection site disorders, influenza-like symptoms (eg, headache, fatigue, fever, rigors, chest pain), back pain, myalgia, abdominal pain, depression, elevation of liver enzymes, hematologic abnormalities.



**INTERACTIONS:** Monitor with myelosuppressive agents.

**PREGNANCY:** Category C, caution in nursing.

## RECLAST RX
zoledronic acid (Novartis)

**THERAPEUTIC CLASS:** Bisphosphonate

**INDICATIONS:** Treatment of Paget's disease.

**DOSAGE:** *Adults:* 5mg/100mL IV via vented infusion line. Infuse over ≥15 minutes at constant rate. Hydrate prior to administration.

**HOW SUPPLIED:** Inj: 5mg/100mL

**CONTRAINDICATIONS:** Hypocalcemia, pregnancy, lactation.

**WARNINGS/PRECAUTIONS:** Musculoskeletal pain and hypocalcemia may occur. Avoid during pregnancy. Monitor calcium and mineral levels; patient should receive calcium 1500mg/day and vitamin D 800 IU/day in divided doses. Not recommended in patient with severe renal impairment (CrCl <35mL/min). Osteonecrosis of the jaw reported with bisphosphonates.

**ADVERSE REACTIONS:** Influenza, hypocalcemia, headache, dizziness, lethargy, nausea, dyspnea, diarrhea, dyspepsia, arthralgia, myalgia, bone pain, pyrexia, fatigue, rigors.

**INTERACTIONS:** Caution with aminoglycosides and nephrotoxic drugs. Caution when used in combination with loop diuretics, may increase risk of hypocalcemia.

**PREGNANCY:** Category D, not for use in nursing.

## RECOMBIVAX HB — RX
hepatitis B (recombinant) (Merck)

**OTHER BRAND NAMES:** Recombivax HB Adult (Merck) - Recombivax HB Dialysis (Merck) - Recombivax HB Pediatric/Adolescent (Merck)

**THERAPEUTIC CLASS:** Vaccine

**INDICATIONS:** Vaccination against hepatitis B virus.

**DOSAGE:** *Adults:* Give IM into deltoid muscle. Give SQ if risk of hemorrhage. ≥20 yrs: 3-Dose Regimen: 10mcg at 0,1,6 months. Predialysis/Dialysis (Dialysis Formulation): 40mcg at 0,1,6, months; consider booster if anti-HBs level <10MIU/mL.
*Pediatrics:* Give IM into anterolateral thigh in infants/young children. Give SQ if risk of hemorrhage. 0-19 yrs: 3-Dose Regimen (Pediatric/Adolescent Formulation) 5mcg at 0,1,6 months. 11-15 yrs: 2-Dose Regimen (Adult Formulation): 10mcg 1st dose, 10mcg 4-6 months later. Infants Born to HBsAg Positive/Unknown Status Mothers: Give 3-dose regimen vaccine and 0.5mL HBIG in opposite anterolateral thigh.

**HOW SUPPLIED:** Inj: (Pediatric/Adolescent-Preservative Free) 5mcg/0.5mL, (Adult) 10mcg/mL, (Dialysis) 40mcg/mL

**CONTRAINDICATIONS:** Yeast hypersensitivity.

**WARNINGS/PRECAUTIONS:** Do not continue therapy if hypersensitivity occurs after injection. May not prevent hepatitis B with unrecognized infection. Caution with severely compromised cardiopulmonary status and those where febrile or systemic reaction is a significant risk. May delay use with serious active infection (eg, febrile illness). Have epinephrine available. Do not give intradermally or IV.

**ADVERSE REACTIONS:** Irritability, fever, diarrhea, fatigue/weakness, diminished appetite, rhinitis, injection site reactions.

**PREGNANCY:** Category C, caution in nursing.

## REFLUDAN — RX
lepirudin (Berlex)

**THERAPEUTIC CLASS:** Thrombin inhibitor

**INDICATIONS:** Anticoagulant for heparin-induced thrombocytopenia (HIT) and associated thromboembolic disease.

**DOSAGE:** *Adults:* LD: 0.4mg/kg (max 44mg) IV over 15-20 seconds. Initial: 0.15mg/kg/hr (max 16.5mg/hr) continuous infusion for 2-10 days. Adjust dose based on aPTT. If aPTT is above target range, stop infusion for 2 hrs and restart at 50% of previous rate. Check aPTT 4 hrs later. If aPTT is below target range, increase rate in steps of 20% and check aPTT 4 hrs later. Do not exceed 0.21mg/kg/hr. Renal Impairment: LD: 0.2mg/kg. Initial: CrCl 45-60 mL/min: 0.075mg/kg/hr. CrCl 30-44mL/min: 0.045mg/kg/hr. CrCl 15-29 mL/min: 0.0225mg/kg/hr. CrCl <15mL/min/Hemodialysis: Avoid or stop infusion. Concomitant Thrombolytic Therapy: LD: 0.2mg/kg. Initial: 0.1mg/kg/hr.

**HOW SUPPLIED:** Inj: 50mg

**WARNINGS/PRECAUTIONS:** Risk of bleeding. Weigh risks/benefits with recent puncture of large vessels or organ biopsy, anomaly of vessels or organs, recent CVA, stroke, intracerebral surgery or other neuraxial procedures, severe uncontrolled HTN, bacterial endocarditis, advanced renal impairment, hemorrhagic diathesis, recent major surgery or bleeding. Avoid with baseline aPTT >2.5. Monitor aPTT 4 hrs after initiate infusion and at least once daily. Liver injury may enhance anticoagulant effects. Antihirudin antibodies reported; may increase anticoagulant effects.

**ADVERSE REACTIONS:** Hemorrhagic events (eg, bleeding, anemia, hematoma, hematuria, epistaxis, hemothorax), fever, liver dysfunction, pneumonia, sepsis, allergic skin reactions, multiorgan failure.

**INTERACTIONS:** Thrombolytics increase risk of life-threatening intracranial bleeding or other bleeding complications and may enhance the effect on aPTT prolongation. Increased risk of bleeding with coumarin derivatives and other drugs that affect platelet function.

**PREGNANCY:** Category B, not for use in nursing.

## REFRESH CELLUVISC — OTC

carboxymethylcellulose sodium (Allergan)

**THERAPEUTIC CLASS:** Lubricant

**INDICATIONS:** Temporary relief of burning, irritation, and discomfort due to dryness of the eye or wind/sun exposure. As a protectant against further irritation.

**DOSAGE:** *Adults:* 1-2 drops in affected eye prn.

**HOW SUPPLIED:** Sol: 1% [0.4mL 30$^{s}$]

**WARNINGS/PRECAUTIONS:** Do not touch container tip to any surface to avoid contamination. Discontinue if eye pain or vision changes occur, if redness or irritation continues, or if condition worsens or persists >72 hrs. Do not reuse. Discard once opened.

**PREGNANCY:** Safety in pregnancy or nursing not known.

## REFRESH ENDURA — OTC

glycerin - polysorbate 80 (Allergan)

**THERAPEUTIC CLASS:** Lubricant

**INDICATIONS:** Temporary relief of burning, irritation, and discomfort due to dryness of the eye or wind/sun exposure. As a protectant against further irritation.

**DOSAGE:** *Adults:* 1-2 drops in affected eye prn.

**HOW SUPPLIED:** Sol: (Glycerin-Polysorbate 80) 1%-1% [0.3mL 20$^{s}$]

**WARNINGS/PRECAUTIONS:** Do not touch container tip to any surface to avoid contamination. Discontinue if eye pain or vision changes occur, if redness or irritation continues, or if condition worsens or persists >72 hrs. Do not reuse. Discard once opened.

**PREGNANCY:** Safety in pregnancy or nursing not known.

## REFRESH LIQUIGEL — OTC

carboxymethylcellulose sodium (Allergan)

**THERAPEUTIC CLASS:** Lubricant

**INDICATIONS:** Temporary relief of burning, irritation, and discomfort due to dryness of the eye or wind/sun exposure. As a protectant against further irritation.

**DOSAGE:** *Adults:* 1-2 drops in affected eye prn.

**HOW SUPPLIED:** Sol: 1% [15mL, 30mL]

**WARNINGS/PRECAUTIONS:** Do not touch container tip to any surface to avoid contamination. Discontinue if eye pain or vision changes occur, if redness or irritation continues, or if condition worsens or persists >72 hrs.

**PREGNANCY:** Safety in pregnancy or nursing not known.

## REFRESH PLUS — OTC

carboxymethylcellulose sodium (Allergan)

**THERAPEUTIC CLASS:** Lubricant

**INDICATIONS:** Temporary relief of burning, irritation, and discomfort due to dryness of the eye or wind/sun exposure and as a protectant against further irritation.

**DOSAGE:** *Adults:* 1-2 drops in affected eye prn.

**HOW SUPPLIED:** Sol: 0.5% [0.3mL 30s, 50s]

**WARNINGS/PRECAUTIONS:** Do not touch container tip to any surface to avoid contamination. Do not reuse, discard once opened. D/C if eye pain or vision changes occur, if redness or irritation continues, or if condition worsens or continues >72 hrs.

**PREGNANCY:** Safety in pregnancy or nursing not known.

## REFRESH TEARS — OTC

carboxymethylcellulose sodium (Allergan)

**THERAPEUTIC CLASS:** Lubricant

**INDICATIONS:** Temporary relief of burning, irritation, and discomfort due to dryness of the eye or wind/sun exposure and as a protectant against further irritation.

**DOSAGE:** *Adults:* 1-2 drops in affected eye prn.

**HOW SUPPLIED:** Sol: 0.5% [15mL, 30mL]

**WARNINGS/PRECAUTIONS:** Do not touch container tip to any surface to avoid contamination. D/C if eye pain or vision changes occur, if redness or irritation continues, or if condition worsens or continues >72 hrs.

**PREGNANCY:** Safety in pregnancy or nursing not known.

## REGRANEX — RX

becaplermin (Ortho-McNeil)



**THERAPEUTIC CLASS:** Platelet-derived growth factor (recombinant human)

**INDICATIONS:** Treatment of lower extremity diabetic neuropathic ulcers that extend into the subcutaneous tissue or beyond and have an adequate blood supply.

**DOSAGE:** *Adults:* Amount applied will vary depending on ulcer size. Measure the greatest length by the greatest width of the ulcer to determine amount of gel to apply. To calculate in inches: (For 15g or 7.5g tube) length x width x 0.6; (For 2g tube) length x width x 1.3. To calculate in centimeters: (For 15g or 7.5g tube) length x width/4; (For 2g tube) length x width/2. Adjust amount weekly or biweekly depending on the change in ulcer area. Squeeze gel onto clean measuring surface (eg, wax paper), then apply to ulcer with an application aid. Apply 1/16 of an inch thickness over entire ulcer area qd, then cover with moist saline dressing for 12 hrs. Remove dressing, rinse off residual gel with saline or water and cover again with moist saline dressing for 12 hrs and repeat. Reassess if ulcer does not decrease by 30% after 10 weeks or is not completely healed in 20 weeks.

*Pediatrics:* >16 yrs: Amount applied will vary depending on ulcer size. Measure the greatest length by the greatest width of the ulcer to determine amount of gel to apply. To calculate in inches: (For 15g or 7.5g tube) length x width x 0.6; (For 2g tube) length x width x 1.3. To calculate in centimeters: (For 15g or 7.5g tube) length x width/4; (For 2g tube) length x width/2. Adjust amount weekly or biweekly depending on the change in ulcer area. Squeeze gel onto clean measuring surface (eg, wax paper), then apply to ulcer with an application aid. Apply 1/16 of an inch thickness over entire ulcer area qd, then cover with moist saline dressing for 12 hrs. Remove dressing, rinse off residual gel with saline or water and cover again with moist saline dressing for 12 hrs and repeat. Reassess if ulcer does not decrease by 30% after 10 weeks or is not completely healed in 20 weeks.

**HOW SUPPLIED:** Gel: 0.01% [15g]

**CONTRAINDICATIONS:** Known neoplasm at application site.

**WARNINGS/PRECAUTIONS:** Do not use in wounds that close by primary intention.

**ADVERSE REACTIONS:** Erythematous rash.

**PREGNANCY:** Category C, caution in nursing.

## RELENZA — RX

zanamivir (GlaxoSmithKline)

**THERAPEUTIC CLASS:** Neuraminidase inhibitor

**INDICATIONS:** Treatment of uncomplicated acute illness due to influenza A and B virus in patients symptomatic for ≤2 days. Prophylaxis of influenza.

**DOSAGE:** *Adults:* Treatment: Usual: 2 inh (10mg) q12h for 5 days. Take 2 doses at least 2 hrs apart on 1st day. Prophylaxis: Household Setting: 2 inh (10mg) qd for 10 days. Community Setting: 2 inh (10mg) qd for 28 days. Administer at same time every day.
*Pediatrics:* Treatment: ≥7 yrs: Usual: 2 inh (10mg) q12h for 5 days. Take 2 doses at least 2 hrs apart on 1st day. Prophylaxis: ≥5 yrs: Household Setting: 2 inh (10mg) qd for 10 days. Community Setting: 2 inh (10mg) qd for 28 days. Administer at same time every day.

**HOW SUPPLIED:** Inh: 5mg/inh [20 blisters]

**WARNINGS/PRECAUTIONS:** Not recommended for use with underlying airways disease (eg, asthma, COPD). Serious cases of bronchospasm have been reported during treatment; d/c in any patient if bronchospasm or decline in respiratory function develops. D/C if allergic reaction occurs.

R

**ADVERSE REACTIONS:** Dizziness, headaches, diarrhea, nausea, sinusitis, bronchitis, cough, ear/nose/throat infections, nasal symptoms.

**INTERACTIONS:** Use inhaled bronchodilator before zanamivir.

**PREGNANCY:** Category C, caution in nursing

## RELPAX — RX

eletriptan hydrobromide (Pfizer)

**THERAPEUTIC CLASS:** 5-$HT_{1D,1B}$ agonist

**INDICATIONS:** Acute treatment of migraine with or without aura.

**DOSAGE:** *Adults:* >18 yrs: Initial: 20 or 40mg at onset of headache. If recurs after initial relief, may repeat after 2 hrs. Max: 40mg/dose or 80mg/day. Safety of treating >3 headaches/30 days not known. Severe Hepatic Impairment: Avoid use. Avoid within 72 hrs of potent CYP3A4 inhibitors.

**HOW SUPPLIED:** Tab: 20mg, 40mg

**CONTRAINDICATIONS:** Ischemic heart disease, coronary artery vasospasm (eg, Prinzmetal's angina) or other significant underlying cardiovascular disease, peripheral vascular disease, cerebrovascular syndromes, uncontrolled HTN, hemiplegic or basilar migraine, use within 24 hrs of other 5-$HT_1$ agonist or ergot-type agent (eg, dihydroergotamine, methysergide), severe hepatic impairment.

**WARNINGS/PRECAUTIONS:** Confirm diagnosis. Supervise 1st dose and monitor cardiac function in those at risk of CAD (eg, HTN, hypercholesterolemia, smoker, obesity, diabetes, CAD family history, postmenopausal women, males >40 yrs). Consider ECG during interval immediately following initial administration in patients with CAD risk factors. Monitor cardiac function in intermittent long-term users with CAD risk factors. Serious adverse cardiac events, increased BP, cerebrovascular events, vasospastic reactions reported. Caution in elderly. Possible long-term ophthalmic effects.

**ADVERSE REACTIONS:** Asthenia, chest tightness, dizziness, dry mouth, headache, nausea, paresthesia, somnolence, pain/pressure/heaviness in precordium/throat/jaw.

**INTERACTIONS:** Prolonged vasospastic reactions reported with ergot-containing drugs; avoid within 24 hours of each other. Avoid within 72 hrs of potent CYP3A4 inhibitors (eg, ketoconazole, itraconazole, nefazodone, troleandomycin, clarithromycin, ritonavir, nelfinavir). Avoid within 24 hours of other 5-$HT_1$ agonists. Propranolol, erythromycin, verapamil, fluconazole may increase levels.

**PREGNANCY:** Category C, caution in nursing.

## REMERON RX

mirtazapine (Organon)

**Antidepressants increased the risk of suicidal thinking and behavior (suicidality) in short-term studies in children and adolescents with Major Depressive Disorder (MDD) and other psychiatric disorders. Mirtazapine is not approved for use in pediatric patients.**

**OTHER BRAND NAMES:** Remeron SolTab (Organon)

**THERAPEUTIC CLASS:** Piperazino-azepine

**INDICATIONS:** Treatment of MDD.

**DOSAGE:** *Adults:* Initial: 15mg qhs. Titrate: May increase every 1-2 weeks. Max: 45mg/day. Disintegrating tabs disintegrate rapidly on tongue and can be swallowed with saliva; no water needed. Do not cut tabs in half.

**HOW SUPPLIED:** Tab: 15mg*, 30mg*, 45mg; Tab, Disintegrating: 15mg, 30mg, 45mg *scored

**WARNINGS/PRECAUTIONS:** Risk of agranulocytosis. D/C if sore throat, fever, or stomatitis, along with low WBC count, develop. May increase appetite, cholesterol, and triglycerides. Caution in history of seizures, mania/hypomania, hepatic or renal impairment, altered metabolic or hemodynamic conditions, elderly. Somnolence, dizziness reported. Close supervision with high risk suicide patients. May impair judgement, thinking, or motor skills.

**ADVERSE REACTIONS:** Somnolence, appetite increase, weight gain, dizziness, dry mouth, constipation, asthenia, flu syndrome, abnormal dreams.

**INTERACTIONS:** Alcohol and diazepam increase cognitive and motor skill impairment. Avoid MAOIs within 14 days of use.

**PREGNANCY:** Category C, caution in nursing.

## REMICADE RX

infliximab (Centocor)

**Reports of TB, invasive fungal infections, and other opportunistic infections. Evaluate for latent TB and treat if necessary prior to initiation of therapy.**

**THERAPEUTIC CLASS:** Monoclonal antibody/TNF-alpha receptor blocker

**INDICATIONS:** In combination with methotrexate (MTX), for reducing signs/symptoms, inhibiting structural damage progression and improving physical function in moderately to severely active rheumatoid arthritis (RA). For reducing signs/symptoms and inducing and maintaining clinical remission of moderately to severely active Crohn's disease, when response to conventional therapy is inadequate. For reducing the number of draining enterocutaneous and rectovaginal fistulas and maintaining fistula closure in fistulizing Crohn's disease. For reducing signs/symptoms in patients with active ankylosing spondylitis (AS). For reducing signs/symptoms of active arthritis, inhibiting structural damage progression, and improving physical function in patients with psoriatic arthritis. For reducing signs/symptoms, inducing and maintaining clinical remission and mucosal healing, and eliminating corticosteroid use in patients with moderately to severely active ulcerative colitis (UC) who have inadequate response to conventional therapy. Treatment of patients with chronic, severe plaque psoriasis who are candidates for systemic therapy and when other systemic therapies are medically less appropriate.

**DOSAGE:** *Adults*: RA (Combo with MTX): 3mg/kg as IV infusion; repeat at 2 and 6 weeks. Maint: 3mg/kg every 8 weeks. Incomplete Response: May increase to 10mg/kg or give every 4 weeks. Crohn's Disease/Fistulizing Crohn's Disease: Induction Regimen: 5mg/kg IV at 0, 2, and 6 weeks. Maint: 5mg/kg every 8 weeks. For patients who respond then lose their response, may increase to 10mg/kg. Consider discontinuing therapy if no response to by Week 14. Alkylosing Spondylitis: 5mg/kg as IV infusion; repeat at 2 and 6 weeks. Maint: 5mg/kg every 6 weeks. Psoriatic Arthritis: 5mg/kg as IV infusion; repeat at 2 and 6 weeks. Maint: 5mg/kg every 8 weeks. May be used with or without MTX. Ulcerative Colitis: 5mg/kg at 0, 2, and 6 weeks. Maint: 5mg/kg every 8 weeks. Plaque Psoriasis: 5mg/kg IV infusion; repeat at 2 and 6 weeks. Maint: 5mg/kg every 8 weeks.
*Pediatrics:* ≥6 yrs: Crohn's Disease: Induction Regimen: 5mg/kg IV at 0, 2, and 6 weeks. Maint: 5mg/kg every 8 weeks.

**HOW SUPPLIED:** Inj: 100mg

**CONTRAINDICATIONS:** Hypersensitivity to murine proteins. Moderate or severe CHF (NYHA Class III/IV) with doses >5mg/kg.

**WARNINGS/PRECAUTIONS:** Leukopenia, neutropenia, thrombocytopenia, and pancytopenia reported. Serious infections, including sepsis and pneumonia, reported. Avoid with active infection. Monitor for signs of infection during and after therapy; d/c if serious infection develops. Caution in patients who have resided in areas where histoplasmosis or coccidioidomycosis are endemic. Hypersensitivity reactions reported. Caution with optic neuritis, chronic and recurrent infections, CNS demyelinating disease (eg, MS) and seizure disorder. May result in autoantibody formation; d/c if lupus-like syndrome develops. Monitor closely and discontinue if new or worsening symptoms of heart failure appear. Lymphoma reported; caution with malignancies. Severe hepatic reactions, including acute liver failure, jaundice, hepatitis And cholestasis have been reported rarely. Caution in elderly.

**ADVERSE REACTIONS:** Nausea, infections, infusion reactions, headache, sinusitis, pharyngitis, coughing, abdominal pain, diarrhea, bronchitis, dyspepsia, fatigue, rhinitis, pain, arthralgia, hepatotoxicity.

**INTERACTIONS:** Do not give concurrently with live vaccines. May increase risk of serious infections and neutropenia with anakinra.

**PREGNANCY:** Category B, not for use in nursing.

## REMODULIN RX

treprostinil sodium (United Therapeutics)

**THERAPEUTIC CLASS:** Pulmonary and systemic vasodilator

**INDICATIONS:** Treatment of pulmonary arterial hypertension (PAH) in patients with NYHA Class II-IV symptoms to diminish symptoms associated with exercise.

**DOSAGE:** *Adults:* Initial: 1.25ng/kg/min SQ continuous infusion. Reduce rate to 0.625ng/kg/min if not tolerated. Titrate: Increase by no more than 1.25ng/kg/min per week for first 4 weeks, then no more than 2.5ng/kg/min per week thereafter, depending on clinical response.

**HOW SUPPLIED:** Inj: 1mg/mL, 2.5mg/mL, 5mg/mL, 10mg/mL [20mL]

**WARNINGS/PRECAUTIONS:** For SQ use only. Initiate therapy in adequate setting for monitoring and emergency care. Abrupt withdrawal or sudden large dose reduction may worsen PAH symptoms. Caution with hepatic or renal impairment.

**ADVERSE REACTIONS:** Infusion site pain/reactions, headache, diarrhea, nausea, rash, jaw pain, vasodilatation, dizziness, edema, pruritus, hypotension.

**INTERACTIONS:** Drugs that alter BP (eg, diuretics, antihypertensives, vasodilators) may potentiate BP reduction. Increased risk of bleeding with anticoagulants.

**PREGNANCY:** Category B, caution in nursing.

## RENAGEL RX

sevelamer HCl (Genzyme)

**THERAPEUTIC CLASS:** Phosphate binder

**INDICATIONS:** Reduction of serum phosphorus in end stage renal disease.

**DOSAGE:** *Adults:* Patients Not Taking a Phoshate Binder: Usual: 800-1600mg with each meal. Initial: Serum Phosphorus: >6 and <7.5mg/dL: 800mg tid. ≥7.5 and <9mg/dL: 1200mg-1600mg tid. ≥9mg/dL: 1600mg tid. Titration: Serum Phosphorus >6mg/dL: increase by 1 tab/cap per meal at 2 week intervals. 3.5-6mg/dL: Maintain dose. <3.5mg/dL: Decrease 1 tab/cap per meal at 2 week intervals. Swallow caps and tabs whole with meals. Switching from Calcium Acetate: Initial: based on calcium acetate dose.

**HOW SUPPLIED:** Tab: 400mg, 800mg

**CONTRAINDICATIONS:** Hypophosphatemia or bowel obstruction.

**WARNINGS/PRECAUTIONS:** Caution with dysphagia, swallowing disorders, severe GI motility or GI surgery. Monitor serum calcium, bicarbonate and chloride.

**ADVERSE REACTIONS:** Nausea, infection, thrombosis, cough increased, respiratory effects, constipation, diarrhea, flatulence, dyspepsia, vomiting.

**INTERACTIONS:** May bind other drugs; give drugs with narrow therapeutic index 1 hr before or 3 hrs after sevelamer. Caution with antiarrhythmic or anti-seizure medications. May decrease ciprofloxacin bioavailability by 50%.

**PREGNANCY:** Category C, unknown use in nursing.

## RENOVA RX

tretinoin (Ortho Neutrogena)

**THERAPEUTIC CLASS:** Retinoid

**INDICATIONS:** (0.05%) Adjunct to comprehensive skin care and sunlight avoidance programs, for mitigation of fine wrinkles, mottled hyperpigmentation, and tactile roughness of facial skin. (0.02%) Adjunct to comprehensive skin care and sunlight avoidance programs, for mitigation of fine facial wrinkles.

**DOSAGE:** *Adults:* (0.05%) 18-50 yrs: Wash face with mild soap, pat skin dry, and wait 20-30 minutes before use. Apply once daily in evening. Max: 48 weeks of therapy. (0.02%) 18-71 yrs: Wash face with mild soap, pat skin dry, and wait 20-30 minutes before use. Apply once daily in evening. Max: 52 weeks of therapy. May apply cosmetics 1 hr later. Use moisturizer every morning to prevent dryness.

**HOW SUPPLIED:** Cre: 0.02% [40g], 0.05% [40g, 60g]

**WARNINGS/PRECAUTIONS:** Avoid with sunburned skin, eczema, chronic skin conditions, and pregnancy. Larger amounts will not lead to better or faster results and may increase adverse effects. Avoid contact with eyes, mouth, paranasal creases, and mucous membranes. D/C if sensitivity, irritation, or systemic adverse reaction develops. Minimize sunlight exposure; avoid sunlamps. Wear protective clothing and use SPF >15. Causes photosensitivity. Extreme weather may increase skin irritation.

**ADVERSE REACTIONS:** Peeling, dry skin, burning, stinging, erythema, pruritus at the site of application.

**INTERACTIONS:** Caution with topical agents with strong drying effects, high concentration of alcohol, astringents, spices or lime, permanent wave solutions, electrolysis, hair depilatories, waxes or medicated or abrasive soaps, shampoos and cleansers. Increased phototoxicity with photosensitizers (eg, thiazides, tetracyclines, fluoroquinolones, phenothiazines, sulfonamides).

**PREGNANCY:** Category C, caution in nursing (0.05%), not for use in nursing (0.02%).

## REOPRO RX

abciximab (Lilly)

**THERAPEUTIC CLASS:** Glycoprotein IIb/IIIa inhibitor

**INDICATIONS:** Adjunct to percutaneous coronary intervention (PCI) for prevention of cardiac ischemic complications in patients undergoing PCI or with unstable angina unresponsive to conventional therapy when PCI is planned within 24 hrs.

**DOSAGE:** *Adults:* PCI: 0.25mg/kg IV bolus given 10-60 minutes before start PCI, followed by 0.125 mcg/kg/min IV infusion (Max: 10mcg/min) for 12 hrs. Angina: 0.25mg/kg IV bolus followed by 10mcg/min infusion for 18-24 hrs, concluding 1 hr after PCI.

R

**HOW SUPPLIED:** Inj: 2mg/mL

**CONTRAINDICATIONS:** Active internal bleeding, recent (within 6 weeks) significant GI or GU bleeding, CVA within 2 years, CVA with significant residual neurological deficit, bleeding diathesis, oral anticoagulants within 7 days (unless PT ≤1.2x control), thrombocytopenia, recent (within 6 weeks) major surgery or trauma, intracranial neoplasm, arteriovenous malformation, aneurysm, severe uncontrolled HTN, history of vasculitis, IV dextran use before PCI or during an intervention.

**WARNINGS/PRECAUTIONS:** Increased risk of bleeding. Monitor all potential bleeding sites (eg, catheter insertion sites, arterial and venous puncture sites, cutdown sites). Minimize vascular and other trauma. D/C if serious, uncontrollable bleeding, thrombocytopenia, or emergency surgery occurs. Anaphylaxis may occur. Antibody (HACA) formation may occur; risk of hypersensitivity, thrombocytopenia, decreased benefit with readministration. Monitor platelets, PT, APTT, ACT before infusion.

**ADVERSE REACTIONS:** Bleeding, thrombocytopenia, hypotension, bradycardia, nausea, vomiting, back/chest pain, headache.

**INTERACTIONS:** Caution with other drugs that affect hemostasis (eg, thrombolytics, heparin, oral anticoagulants, NSAIDs, dipyridamole, ticlopidine). Increased risk of bleeding with anticoagulants, thrombolytics, and antiplatelets. If have HACA titers, possible allergic reactions with monoclonal antibody agents.

**PREGNANCY:** Category C, caution in nursing.

## REPRONEX RX

menotropins (Ferring)

**THERAPEUTIC CLASS:** Follicle stimulating hormone/luteinizing hormone

**INDICATIONS:** With hCG, for multiple follicular development and ovulation in women who received pituitary suppression.

**DOSAGE:** *Adults:* Oligo-anovulation: Individualize dose. Initial: 150 IU SQ/IM qd for 5 days. Adjust subsequent dose to individual response at intervals no less than every 2 days and not exceeding 75-150 IU/adjustment. Max: 450 IU/day. Dosing >12 days is not recommended. If adequate response, give 5000-10,000 U hCG. May repeat course if inadequate response. Assisted Reproductive Technology: Initial: 225 IU SQ/IM. Adjust subsequent dose to individual response at intervals no less than every 2 days and not exceeding 75-150 IU/adjustment. Max: 450 IU/day. Dosing >12 days is not recommended. If adequate response, give 5000-10,000 U hCG.

**HOW SUPPLIED:** Inj: (FSH-LH) 75 IU-75 IU

**CONTRAINDICATIONS:** High FSH levels indicating primary ovarian failure, uncontrolled thyroid or adrenal dysfunction, organic intracranial lesions (eg, pituitary tumor), any cause of infertility other than anovulation (unless candidate for in vitro fertilization), abnormal bleeding of undetermined origin, ovarian cysts or enlargement not due to polycystic ovary syndrome, pregnancy.

**WARNINGS/PRECAUTIONS:** Exclude primary ovarian failure. Ovarian enlargement may occur; monitor ovarian response. Ovarian hyperstimulation syndrome (OHSS), hypersensitivity/anaphylactic reactions, multiple pregnancies, serious pulmonary and vascular complications reported. Avoid hCG if ovaries abnormally enlarged last day of therapy. Monitor follicular maturation by measuring estradiol levels and through ultrasonography.

**ADVERSE REACTIONS:** Pulmonary and vascular complications, OHSS, hemoperitoneum, adnexal torsion, ovarian enlargement, ovarian cysts, abdominal pain, GI symptoms, injection site reactions, rash.

**PREGNANCY:** Category X, caution in nursing.



## REQUIP RX

ropinirole HCl (GlaxoSmithKline)

**THERAPEUTIC CLASS:** Non-ergoline dopamine agonist

**INDICATIONS:** Treatment of symptoms of idiopathic Parkinson's disease. Treatment of moderate-to-severe primary Restless Legs Syndrome (RLS).

**DOSAGE:** *Adults:* Parkinson's: Initial: 0.25mg tid. Titrate: May increase weekly by 0.25mg tid (0.75mg/day) for 4 weeks. After week 4, may increase weekly by 1.5mg/day up to 9mg/day, then by 3mg/day weekly to 24mg/day. Max: 24mg/day. Withdrawal: Decrease dose to bid for 4 days, then qd for 3 days. RLS: Initial: 0.25mg qd, 1-3 hours before bedtime. Titrate: 0.5mg qd days 3-7, 1mg qd week 2, then increase by 0.5mg weekly. Max: 4mg.

**HOW SUPPLIED:** Tab: 0.25mg, 0.5mg, 1mg, 2mg, 3mg, 4mg, 5mg

**WARNINGS/PRECAUTIONS:** Falling asleep during activities of daily living reported; if significant, discontinue or warn patient to refrain from dangerous activities. Syncope, symptomatic hypotension, and hallucinations reported. Caution with severe renal or hepatic dysfunction. May cause or exacerbate pre-existing dyskinesia. Augmentation and rebound in RLS reported. Avoid abrupt withdrawal. Pathological gambling reported.

**ADVERSE REACTIONS:** Neuralgia, increased BUN, hallucinations, somnolence, vomiting, headache, sweating, asthenia, edema, fatigue, syncope, orthostatic symptoms.

**INTERACTIONS:** Adjust dose if CYP1A2 inhibitor or estrogen is stopped or started during treatment. Potentiated by ciprofloxacin. Decreased effects with dopamine antagonists (eg, phenothiazines, butyrophenones, thioxanthenes, metoclopramide). Drowsiness increased with sedatives. Caution with dopamine antagonists or alcohol.

**PREGNANCY:** Category C, not for use in nursing.

## RESCRIPTOR

RX

delavirdine mesylate (Pfizer)

**THERAPEUTIC CLASS:** Non-nucleoside reverse transcriptase inhibitor

**INDICATIONS:** Treatment of HIV-1 infection in combination with other antiretrovirals.

**DOSAGE:** *Adults:* Usual: 400mg tid. May disperse 100mg tab in ≥3 oz of water (200mg tab is not dispersible). Take with acidic beverage (eg, orange juice) if achlorhydria.
*Pediatrics:* >16yrs: Usual: 400mg tid. May disperse 100mg tab in at least 3 oz of water (200mg tab is not dispersible). Take with acidic beverage (eg, orange juice) if achlorhydria.

**HOW SUPPLIED:** Tab: 100mg, 200mg

**CONTRAINDICATIONS:** Contraindicated with drugs that are highly dependent on CYP3A for clearance (eg, astemizole, terfenadine, dihdroergotamine, egonovine, ergotamine, methylergonovine, cisapride, pimozide, alprazolam, midazolam, triazolam).

**WARNINGS/PRECAUTIONS:** Caution with hepatic dysfunction. D/C if severe rash develops. May cause immune reconstitution syndrome. May confer cross-resistance to other NNRTIs. May cause body fat redistribution/accumulation.

**ADVERSE REACTIONS:** Headache, fatigue, nausea, diarrhea, vomiting, increased ALT and AST, rash, maculopapular rash, pruritus, erythema, insomnia, upper respiratory infection.

**INTERACTIONS:** See Contraindications. Antacids decrease absorption; separate doses by 1 hr. $H_2$ antagonists reduce absorption; avoid chronic use. CYP3A inducers (eg, carbamazepine, phenobarbital, phenytoin, rifabutin, rifampin) may decrease plasma levels; avoid concomitant use. Increased plasma levels of drugs metabolized by CYP3A and 2C9 and amprenavir. Certain nonsedating antihistamines, sedative hypnotics, antiarrhythmics, calcium channel blockers, ergot agents, amphetamines, cisapride, and sildenafil (max of 25mg/48hrs of sildenafil) may result in potentially serious and/or life-threatening adverse events. Reduced effects of both delavirdine and didanosine; separate doses by 1 hr. Monitor LFTs with saquinavir. Increases indinavir plasma levels; reduce indinavir dose to 600mg tid.



**PREGNANCY:** Category C, not for use in nursing.

## RESERPINE

RX

reserpine (Various)

**THERAPEUTIC CLASS:** Rauwolfia alkaloid

**INDICATIONS:** Treatment of mild essential hypertension and adjunct treatment of severe hypertension. Relief of symptoms in agitated psychotic states.

**DOSAGE:** *Adults:* HTN: Initial: 0.5mg/day for 1-2 weeks. Maint: reduce to 0.1-0.25mg/day. Psychotic Disorders: Initial: 0.5mg/day. Range: 0.1-1mg/day.

**HOW SUPPLIED:** Tab: 0.1mg, 0.25mg

**CONTRAINDICATIONS:** Active or history of mental depression, active peptic ulcer, ulcerative colitis, current electroconvulsive therapy.

**WARNINGS/PRECAUTIONS:** Caution with renal insufficiency. May cause depression; discontinue at 1st sign. Caution with history of peptic ulcer, ulcerative colitis, or gallstones.

**ADVERSE REACTIONS:** GI effects, dry mouth, hypersecretion, arrhythmia, syncope, edema, dyspnea, muscle aches, dizziness, depression, nervousness, impotence, gynecomastia, rash.

**INTERACTIONS:** Avoid MAOIs or use extreme caution. Prolonged effect of direct-acting sympathomimetics (eg, epinephrine, isoproterenol). May inhibit effects of indirect-acting sympathomimetics (eg, ephedrine, tyramine). Risk of arrhythmia with quinidine or digoxin. Titrate carefully with other antihypertensives. Decreased effect with TCAs.

**PREGNANCY:** Category C, not for use in nursing.

## RESTASIS RX

cyclosporine (Allergan)

**THERAPEUTIC CLASS:** Topical immunomodulator

**INDICATIONS:** To increase tear production in patients with suppressed tear production due to ocular inflammation associated with keratoconjunctivitis sicca.

**DOSAGE:** *Adults:* 1 drop bid, q12h. Concomitant Artificial Tears: Space by 15 minutes.
*Pediatrics:* >16 yrs: 1 drop bid, q12h. Concomitant Artificial Tears: Space by 15 minutes.

**HOW SUPPLIED:** Emul: 0.05% [0.4mL 32[s]]

**CONTRAINDICATIONS:** Active ocular infections.

**WARNINGS/PRECAUTIONS:** Not studied in patients with a history of herpes keratitis. Not to be given while wearing contact lenses; lenses may be reinserted 15 minutes following administration.

**ADVERSE REACTIONS:** Ocular burning, conjunctival hyperemia, discharge, epiphora, eye pain, foreign body sensation, pruritus, stinging, visual disturbance (eg, blurring).

**PREGNANCY:** Category C, caution in nursing

R

## RESTORIL CIV

temazepam (Mallinckrodt)

**THERAPEUTIC CLASS:** Benzodiazepine

**INDICATIONS:** Short-term treatment of insomnia (7-10 days).

**DOSAGE:** *Adults:* Usual: 7.5-30mg qhs. Transient Insomnia: 7.5mg qhs. Elderly/Debilitated: Initial: 7.5mg qhs.

**HOW SUPPLIED:** Cap: 7.5mg, 15mg, 22.5mg, 30mg

**CONTRAINDICATIONS:** Pregnancy.

**WARNINGS/PRECAUTIONS:** Caution in elderly, debilitated, severely depressed, those with suicidal tendencies, hepatic/renal impairment, pulmonary insufficiency. Avoid abrupt discontinuation. If no improvement after 7-10 days, may indicate primary psychiatric and/or medical condition.

**ADVERSE REACTIONS:** Headache, dizziness, drowsiness, fatigue, nervousness, nausea, lethargy, hangover.

**INTERACTIONS:** Additive CNS depressant effects with alcohol and CNS depressants. May be synergistic with diphenhydramine.

**PREGNANCY:** Category X, caution in nursing.

## RETAVASE
RX

reteplase (PDL)

**THERAPEUTIC CLASS:** Thrombolytic agent

**INDICATIONS:** To improve ventricular function following acute myocardial infarction (AMI), reduce the incidence of congestive heart failure (CHF) and reduce the mortaility associated with AMI.

**DOSAGE:** *Adults:* 10 U IV over 2 minutes. Repeat in 30 minutes.

**HOW SUPPLIED:** Inj: 10.4 U

**CONTRAINDICATIONS:** Active internal bleeding, history of CVA, recent intracranial or intraspinal surgery or trauma, intracranial neoplasm, arteriovenous malformation, aneurysm, bleeding diathesis, severe uncontrolled HTN.

**WARNINGS/PRECAUTIONS:** Weigh benefits/risks with recent major surgery, previous puncture of noncompressible vessels, cerebrovascular disease, recent GI or GU bleeding, recent trauma, HTN, left heart thrombus, acute pericarditis, subacute bacterial endocarditis, hemostatic defects, severe hepatic or renal dysfunction, pregnancy, diabetic hemorrhagic retinopathy or other hemorrhagic ophthalmic conditions, septic thrombophlebitis or occluded AV cannula at a seriously infected site, elderly, any other bleeding condition that is difficult to manage. Cholesterol embolism and internal/superficial bleeding reported. Arrhythmias may occur with reperfusion. Avoid IM injection, noncompressible arterial puncture, and internal jugular or subclavian venous puncture.

**ADVERSE REACTIONS:** Bleeding, allergic reactions, dyspnea, hypotension.

**INTERACTIONS:** Increased risk of bleeding with heparin, vitamin K antagonists, and drugs that alter platelet function (eg, ASA, NSAIDs, dipyridamole, abciximab) before or after therapy. Weigh benefits/risks with oral anticoagulants.

**PREGNANCY:** Category C, caution in nursing.

## RETIN-A
RX

tretinoin (Ortho Neutrogena)

**OTHER BRAND NAMES:** Retin-A Micro (Ortho Neutrogena)

**THERAPEUTIC CLASS:** Retinoic acid derivative

R

**INDICATIONS:** Topical treatment of acne vulgaris.

**DOSAGE:** *Adults:* Cleanse area thoroughly, then apply qhs. May temporarily d/c or reduce dosing frequency if irritation occurs.
*Pediatrics:* >12 yrs: (Gel 0.04%, 0.1%) Cleanse area thoroughly, then apply qhs. May temporarily d/c or reduce dosing frequency if irritation occurs.

**HOW SUPPLIED:** (Retin-A) Cre: 0.025%, 0.05%, 0.1% [20g, 45g]; Gel: 0.01%, 0.025% [15g, 45g]; Sol: 0.05% [28mL]; (Retin-A Micro) Gel: 0.04%, 0.1% [20g, 45g]

**WARNINGS/PRECAUTIONS:** Avoid eyes, lips, paranasal creases, mucous membranes, and sunburned skin. Acne exacerbation during 1st weeks of therapy may occur. D/C if sensitivity or irritation occurs. Severe irritation with eczematous skin. Causes photosensitivity. Extreme weather (eg, cold, wind) may irritate skin.

**ADVERSE REACTIONS:** Local skin reactions (red, edematous, blistered, crusted), photosensitivity, temporary skin pigmentation changes.

**INTERACTIONS:** Caution with topical agents with strong drying effects, high concentration of alcohol, astringents, spices, or lime. Caution with sulfur, resorcinol, or salicylic acid, allow effects of these agents to subside before application of tretinoin.

**PREGNANCY:** Category C, caution in nursing.

## RETROVIR RX

zidovudine (GlaxoSmithKline)

**Associated with hematologic toxicity (eg, neutropenia, severe anemia), especially with advanced HIV disease. Prolonged use associated with symptomatic myopathy. Lactic acidosis and severe, possibly fatal hepatomegaly with steatosis reported.**

**THERAPEUTIC CLASS:** Nucleoside analogue

**INDICATIONS:** Treatment of HIV infection in combination with other antiretrovirals. Prevention of maternal-fetal HIV transmission.

**DOSAGE:** *Adults:* (Tab) 600mg/day in divided doses. (Inj) 1mg/kg IV over 1 hr 5-6 times/day. Prevention of Maternal-Fetal HIV Transmission: >14 weeks pregnancy: 100mg PO five times/day until start of labor. During labor and delivery: 2mg/kg IV over 1 hr followed by 1mg/kg/hr IV infusion until clamping of umbilical cord. End-Stage Renal Disease/Dialysis: 100mg PO q6-8h or 1mg/kg IV q6-8h. Significant Anemia/Neutropenia: May require dose interruption and adjunctive epoetin therapy. Less Severe Anemia/Neutropenia: Reduce daily dose.
*Pediatrics:* 6 weeks-12 yrs: 160mg/m$^2$ PO q8h. Max: 200mg PO q8h. Prevention of Maternal-Fetal HIV Transmission: Neonates: 2mg/kg PO q6h (or 1.5mg/kg IV over 30 min q6h) starting within 12 hrs after birth and continue through 6 weeks of age. End-Stage Renal Disease/Dialysis: 100mg PO q6-8h or 1mg/kg IV q6-8h. Significant Anemia/Neutropenia: May require dose interruption and adjunctive epoetin therapy. Pronounced Anemia: Reduce daily dose. Mild to Moderate Hepatic Impairment: Monitor for hematologic toxicity and reduce dose if needed.

**HOW SUPPLIED:** Cap: 100mg; Inj: 10mg/mL; Syrup: 50mg/5mL [240mL]; Tab: 300mg

**WARNINGS/PRECAUTIONS:** Adverse reactions increase with disease progression. Caution with compromised bone marrow or in elderly. Monitor for hematologic toxicity; reduce dose or stop therapy. Myopathy and myositis with pathological changes associated with prolonged use. Caution with obesity and liver disease; increased risk of lactic acidosis and hepatomegaly with steatosis. Increased risk of toxicity with prolonged exposure to nucleosides, in women, obesity, advanced HIV disease, severe hepatic impairment. Possible redistribution or accumuation of body fat. Hepatic decompensation has occurred in HIV/HCV co-infected patients receiving combination antiretroviral therapy for HIV and interferon alfa with or without ribavirin; monitor for treatment associated toxicities. Immune reconstitution syndrome has been reported with combination antiretroviral therapy.

**ADVERSE REACTIONS:** Headache, nausea, malaise, anorexia, vomiting, asthenia, constipation, anemia, neutropenia.

**INTERACTIONS:** Increased risk of hematologic toxicities with ganciclovir, interferon-alpha, bone marrow suppressives and cytotoxic drugs. Possible increased levels with phenytoin, atovaquone, fluconazole, methadone, probenecid, valproic acid. Possible decreased levels with nelfinavir, ritonavir, rifampin. Avoid with stavudine, ribavirin, doxorubicin, other combination products containing zidovudine. Prolonged exposure to antiretroviral nucleoside analogues increases risk of lactic acidosis and hepatomegaly with steatosis. May decrease phenytoin levels.

**PREGNANCY:** Category C, not for use in nursing.

## REVATIO RX

sildenafil citrate (Pfizer)

**THERAPEUTIC CLASS:** Phosphodiesterase type 5 inhibitor

**INDICATIONS:** Treatment of pulmonary arterial hypertension (WHO Group I) to improve exercise ability.

**DOSAGE:** *Adults:* 20mg tid 4-6 hours apart.

**HOW SUPPLIED:** Tab: 20mg

**CONTRAINDICATIONS:** Organic nitrates taken regularly and/or intermittently.

**WARNINGS/PRECAUTIONS:** Caution with MI, stroke, or life-threatening arrhythmia within last 6 months; with resting hypotension (BP<90/50), fluid depletion, severe left ventricular outflow obstruction, autonomic dysfunction, or HTN (BP>170/110); unstable angina due to cardiac failure or CAD; anatomical penile deformation; predisposition to priapism; and retinitis pigmentosa. Avoid in patients with veno-occlusive disease. Decrease in supine BP reported. If erection persists >4 hrs, seek immediate medical assistance; penile tissue damage and permanent loss of potency could result if priapism not treated immediately.

**ADVERSE REACTIONS:** Epistaxis, headache, flushing, dyspepsia, insomnia, erythema, dyspnea, rhinitis, diarrhea, myalgia, pyrexia, gastritis, sinusitis, paresthesia.

**INTERACTIONS:** See Contraindications. Reports of bleeding (epistaxis) with vitamin K antagonists. Increased levels with CYP3A4 inhibitors (eg, cimetidine, ketoconazole, itraconazole, erythromycin, saquinavir) and protease inhibitors (eg, ritonavir). CYP2C9 inhibitors may decrease sildenafil clearance. Decreased levels with CYP3A4 inducers (eg, bosentan; more potent inducers such as barbiturates, carbamazepine, phenytoin, efavirenz, nevirapine, rifampin, rifabutin). Co-administration with bosentan resulted in a decrease in AUC of sildenafil and increase in AUC of bosentan. Additional supine BP reduction with amlodipine reported. Simultaneous administration with alpha-blockers may lead to symptomatic hypotension.

**PREGNANCY:** Category B, caution in nursing.

## REV-EYES — RX

dapiprazole HCl (Bausch & Lomb)

**THERAPEUTIC CLASS:** Alpha adrenergic blocker

**INDICATIONS:** Treatment of iatrogenically induced mydriasis produced by adrenergic or parasympatholytic agents.

**DOSAGE:** *Adults:* Apply 2 drops to conjunctiva, repeat 5 minutes later. Administer after exam to reverse diagnostic mydriasis. Do not use more than once weekly.

**HOW SUPPLIED:** Sol: 0.5% [5mL]



**CONTRAINDICATIONS:** Anytime pupil constriction is undesirable (eg, acute iritis).

**WARNINGS/PRECAUTIONS:** For topical ophthalmic use only. Do not touch dropper tip to any surface to avoid contamination. May cause difficulty in dark adaptation and reduce vision field; caution in night driving or activities in poor illumination.

**ADVERSE REACTIONS:** Burning on instillation, ptosis, lid erythema/edema, chemosis, itching, punctate keratitis, corneal edema, browache, photophobia, headache.

**PREGNANCY:** Category B, caution in nursing.

## REVIA — RX

naltrexone HCl (Duramed)

**THERAPEUTIC CLASS:** Opioid antagonist

**INDICATIONS:** Treatment of alcohol dependence and to block effects of exogenously administered opioids.

**DOSAGE:** *Adults:* Alcoholism: 50mg qd up to 12 weeks. Opioid Dependence: Initial: 25mg qd. Maint: 50mg qd. Naloxone Challenge Test: 0.2mg IV, observe for 30 seconds, then 0.6mg IV, observe for 20 minutes; or 0.8mg SQ, observe for 20 minutes.

**HOW SUPPLIED:** Tab: 50mg

**CONTRAINDICATIONS:** Acute hepatitis, hepatic failure, patients failing naloxone challenge or opioid-dependent, concomitant opioid analgesics, acute opioid withdrawal, positive urine screen for opioids, phenanthrene sensitivity.

**WARNINGS/PRECAUTIONS:** Hepatotoxic with excessive doses; margin of separation between safe dose and hepatotoxic dose is 5-fold or less. Only treat patients opioid-free for 7-10 days. Attempting to overcome the opiate blockade is very dangerous. More sensitive to lower doses of opioids after naltrexone is discontinued. Safety in ultra rapid opiate detoxification is not known. Increased risk of suicide in substance abuse patients. Severe opioid withdrawal syndromes reported with accidental ingestion in opioid-dependent patients. Monitor closely during blockade reversal. Caution in renal or hepatic impairment. Perform naloxone challenge test if question of opioid dependence.

**ADVERSE REACTIONS:** Nausea, headache, dizziness, nervousness, fatigue, restlessness, insomnia, vomiting, anxiety, somnolence.

**INTERACTIONS:** Caution with other drugs. Do not use with disulfiram unless benefits outweigh risk of hepatotoxicity. Lethargy and somnolence reported with thioridazine. Antagonizes opioid-containing cough and cold, antidiarrheal, and analgesic agents.

**PREGNANCY:** Category C, caution in nursing.

## REVLIMID RX

lenalidomide (Celgene)

**Potential for human birth defects, hematological toxicity (neutropenia and thrombocytopenia), deep venous thrombosis (DVT) and pulmonary embolism (PE). Lenalidomide is an analogue of thalidomide. Thalidomide is a known human teratogen that causes severe life-threatening human birth defects. If taken during pregnancy, may cause birth defects or death to an unborn baby. Avoid pregnancy due to potential toxicity and to avoid fetal exposure. Only available under a special restricted distribution program called Revassist SM. Associated with significant neutropenia and thrombocytopenia in patients with del 5q MDS. CBC should be monitored weekly for the first 8 weeks of therapy and at least monthly thereafter. May require dose interruption and/or reduction and the use of blood product support and/or growth factors. Increased risk of DVT and PE in patients with multiple myeloma. Observe for signs and symptoms of thromboembolism.**

**THERAPEUTIC CLASS:** Thalidomide Analog

**INDICATIONS:** Transfusion-dependent anemia due to Low- or Intermediate-1-risk myelodysplastic syndromes associated with a deletion 5q cytogenetic abnormality with or without additional cytogenetic abnormalities. In combination with dexamethasone for the treatment of multiple myeloma in patients who have received at least one prior therapy.

**DOSAGE:** *Adults:* ≥18 yrs: Myelodysplastic Syndromes: 10mg daily with water. Multiple Myeloma: 25mg daily with water. Administer as single dose on Days 1-21 of repeated 28-day cycles. Do not break, chew, or open capsules. Adjust dose based on platelet and/or neutrophil counts.

**HOW SUPPLIED:** Cap: 5mg, 10mg, 15mg, 25mg

**CONTRAINDICATIONS:** Pregnancy.

**WARNINGS/PRECAUTIONS:** See Black Box Warning. Risk of adverse reactions may be greater in patients with impaired renal function.

**ADVERSE REACTIONS:** Thrombocytopenia, neutropenia, pruritus, rash, diarrhea, constipation, nausea, nasopharyngitis, fatigue, arthralgia, cough, pyrexia, peripheral edema, insomnia, asthenia.

**INTERACTIONS:** Co-administration increased digoxin $C_{max}$ by 14%; monitoring suggested.

**PREGNANCY:** Category X, not for use in nursing.

## REYATAZ RX
atazanavir sulfate (Bristol-Myers Squibb)

**THERAPEUTIC CLASS:** Protease inhibitor

**INDICATIONS:** Treatment of HIV-1 infection in combination with other antiretrovirals.

**DOSAGE:** *Adults:* Therapy-Naive: 400mg qd. Therapy-experienced: 300mg with ritonavir 100mg qd. Concomitant Efavirenz: Give atazanavir 300mg and ritonavir 100mg with efavirenz 600mg qd. Concomitant Buffered Didanosine: Give atazanavir 2 hrs before or 1 hr after didanosine. Concomitant Tenofovir: Give atazanavir 300mg with ritonavir 100mg and tenofovir 300mg. Moderate Hepatic Insufficiency (Child-Pugh Class B): 300mg qd. Take with food.

**HOW SUPPLIED:** Cap: 100mg, 150mg, 200mg, 300mg

**CONTRAINDICATIONS:** Concomitant administration with midazolam, triazolam, dihydroergotamine, ergotamine, ergonovine, methylergonovine, cisapride, pimozide.

**WARNINGS/PRECAUTIONS:** Prolongs PR interval; caution with pre-existing conduction system disease. New-onset DM, exacerbation of pre-existing DM, hyperglycemia, hyperbilirubinemia, increased bleeding with hemophilia Types A and B, Stevens-Johnson syndrome, erythema multiforme reported. Caution with hepatic impairment; avoid with severe hepatic insufficiency. Discontinue with severe rash. Possible redistribution/accumulation of body fat. Immune reconstitution syndrome reported with combination therapy. Nephrolithiasis reported.

**ADVERSE REACTIONS:** Headache, nausea, jaundice, abdominal pain, vomiting, diarrhea, rash, myalgia, peripheral neurologic symptoms.

**INTERACTIONS:** Avoid with rifampin, irinotecan, midazolam, triazolam, bepridil, ergot derivatives, cisapride, lovastatin, simvastatin, pimozide, indinavir, proton-pump inhibitors, St. John's wort. Avoid nevirapine, voriconazole, other protease inhibitors with atazanavir/ritonavir therapy. May increase levels of drugs metabolized by CYP3A or UGT1A1. CYP3A inducers may decrease levels. CYP3A inhibitors, voriconazole may increase levels. Decreased levels with buffered didanosine, tenofovir, efavirenz, antacids/buffered medications (give atazanavir 2 hrs before or 1 hr after), $H_2$-receptor antagonists (space dosing by 12 hrs). Increase levels of saquinavir, diltiazem (reduce dose by 50%), amiodarone, lidocaine (systemic), quinidine, warfarin, TCAs, rifabutin (reduce dose up to 75%), calcium channel blockers, oral contraceptives (use lowest possible dose), sildenafil/tadalafil/vardenafil (reduce dose), atorvastatin, cyclosporine, sirolimus, tacrolimus, clarithromycin (reduce dose by 50%; consider alternative therapy for infections other than *M.avium* complex). Increased levels with ritonavir (give atazanavir 300mg/day with ritonavir 100mg/day with food). Caution with high doses of ketoconazole, itrazonazole with atazanavir/ritonavir therapy. Atazanavir/ritonavir therapy may significantly increase plasma fluticasone propionate exposure resulting in significantly decreased serum cortisol concentrations.

**PREGNANCY:** Category B, not for use in nursing.

## RHINOCORT AQUA RX
budesonide (AstraZeneca LP)

**THERAPEUTIC CLASS:** Corticosteroid

**INDICATIONS:** Management of seasonal or perennial allergic rhinitis.

**DOSAGE:** *Adults*: 1 spray per nostril qd. Max: 4 sprays/nostril/day. *Pediatrics*: >6 yrs: 1 spray per nostril qd. Max: 6-12 yrs: 2 sprays/nostril/day. >12 yrs: 4 sprays/nostril/day.

**HOW SUPPLIED:** Spray: 32mcg/spray [8.6g]

**WARNINGS/PRECAUTIONS:** Risk of adrenal insufficiency and withdrawal symptoms when replacing systemic corticosteroids with a topical corticosteroids. Caution with active or quiescent TB, ocular herpes simplex, or untreated bacterial, fungal and systemic viral infections. Avoid with recent nasal trauma, surgery or septum ulcers. Risk for more severe/fatal course of infections (eg, chickenpox, measles) and for *Candida* infections of the nose and pharynx. Potential for growth velocity reduction in pediatrics.

**ADVERSE REACTIONS:** Nasal irritation, pharyngitis, cough, epistaxis.

**INTERACTIONS:** Oral ketoconazole and cimetidine increase plasma levels. CYP3A inhibitors (eg, itraconazole, clarithromycin, erythromycin) may decrease metabolism and increase systemic exposure. Concomitant systemic corticosteroids increases risk of hypercorticism and/or HPA axis suppression.

**PREGNANCY:** Category B, caution in nursing.

## RIDAURA — RX

auranofin (Prometheus)

**Risk of gold toxicity.**

**THERAPEUTIC CLASS:** Gold agent

**INDICATIONS:** Management of rheumatoid arthritis in patients with inadequate response to NSAIDs.

**DOSAGE:** *Adults:* Usual: 6mg qd or 3mg bid. If response not adequate after 6 months, increase to 3mg tid. If inadequate response with 9mg/day after 3 months, discontinue. Max: 9mg/day.

**HOW SUPPLIED:** Cap: 3mg

**CONTRAINDICATIONS:** History of gold induced disorders: anaphylactic reactions, necrotizing enterocolitis, pulmonary fibrosis, exfoliative dermatitis, bone marrow aplasia, or severe hematologic disorders.

**WARNINGS/PRECAUTIONS:** Gold toxicity manifests as a falling Hgb, leukopenia <4000 WBC/cu mm, granulocytes <1500/cu mm, decrease in platelets <150,000/cu mm, proteinuria, hematuria, pruritus, rash, stomatitis, or persistent diarrhea. Thrombocytopenia and proteinuria reported. Caution in renal/hepatic disease, inflammatory bowel disease, skin rash or a history of bone marrow depression. GI reactions, dermatitis, stomatitis, nephrotic syndrome, and blood dyscrasias reported.

**ADVERSE REACTIONS:** Diarrhea, nausea, constipation, anorexia, flatulence, dyspepsia, rash, conjunctivitis, anemia, proteinuria, hematuria, elevated liver enzymes.

**INTERACTIONS:** Increased phenytoin levels.

**PREGNANCY:** Category C, not for use in nursing.

## RIFADIN — RX

rifampin (Sanofi-Aventis)

**THERAPEUTIC CLASS:** Rifamycin derivative

**INDICATIONS:** Treatment of all forms of tuberculosis (TB). Treatment of asymptomatic carriers of *Neisseria meningitidis* to eliminate meningococci from the nasopharynx.

**DOSAGE:** *Adults:* TB: 10mg/kg PO/IV qd. Max: 600mg/day. Meningococcal Carriers: 600mg bid for 2 days. Take 1 hr before or 2 hrs after a meal with a full glass of water.
*Pediatrics:* TB: 10-20mg/kg PO/IV qd. Max: 600mg/day. Meningococcal Carriers: >1 month: 10mg/kg q12h for 2 days. Max: 600mg/dose. <1 month:

5mg/kg q12h for 2 days. Take 1 hr before or 2 hrs after a meal with a full glass of water.

**HOW SUPPLIED:** Cap: 150mg, 300mg; Inj: 600mg

**WARNINGS/PRECAUTIONS:** May produce liver dysfunction. May cause hyperbilirubinemia. Not for treatment of meningococcal disease. May produce reddish coloration of the urine, sweat, sputum, and tears. May permanently stain soft contact lenses.

**ADVERSE REACTIONS:** GI distress, thrombocytopenia, visual disturbances, menstrual disturbances, edema of face and extremities, elevated BUN and serum uric acid levels.

**INTERACTIONS:** May accelerate elimination of drugs metabolized by CYP450 (eg, anticonvulsants, antiarrhythmics, anticoagulants, azole antifungals, barbiturates, β-blockers, calcium channel blockers, chloramphenicol, clarithromycin, corticosteroids, cyclosporine, cardiac glycosides, clofibrate, oral or systemic contraceptives, dapsone, diazepam, doxycycline, fluoroquinolones, haloperidol, oral hypoglycemics, levothyroxine, methadone, narcotics, nortriptyline, progestins, quinine, tacrolimus, theophylline, TCAs, and zidovudine). Give antacids at least 1 hr before rifampin. Increased hepatotoxicity with halothane or isoniazid. Increased serum levels with probenecid and cotrimoxazole. Caution with other hepatotoxic agents. Concomitant ketoconazole decreases both drug serum levels. Decreased levels of enalapril, atovaquone. Increased levels with atovaquone.

**PREGNANCY:** Category C, not for use in nursing.

## RIFAMATE RX

rifampin - isoniazid (Sanofi-Aventis)

**Isoniazid associated with severe and sometimes fatal hepatitis. Monitor LFTs on a monthly basis.**

**THERAPEUTIC CLASS:** Isonicotinic acid hydrazide/rifamycin derivative

**INDICATIONS:** For pulmonary tuberculosis (TB). Not for initial therapy or prevention of TB.

**DOSAGE:** *Adults:* 2 caps qd. Take 1 hr before or 2 hrs after meals. Give with pyridoxine in the malnourished, those predisposed to neuropathy (eg, alcoholics, diabetics), and adolescents.

**HOW SUPPLIED:** Cap: (Isoniazid-Rifampin) 150mg-300mg



**CONTRAINDICATIONS:** Previous isoniazid-associated hepatic injury, severe adverse reactions to isoniazid (eg, drug fever, chills, and arthritis), acute liver disease.

**WARNINGS/PRECAUTIONS:** Monitor LFTs before therapy, periodically thereafter. Not for intermittent therapy. Urine, feces, saliva, sputum, sweat, and tears may be colored red-orange; may stain soft contact lenses permanently. Caution with chronic liver disease or severe renal dysfunction. Perform periodic ophthalmoscopic exams.

**ADVERSE REACTIONS:** Headache, drowsiness, fatigue, ataxia, dizziness, confusion, visual disturbances, weakness, GI effects, peripheral neuropathy, pyridoxine deficiency, anorexia, nausea, renal or hepatic insufficiency, blood dyscrasias.

**INTERACTIONS:** Anticoagulants may need dose increase. May decrease activity of methadone, oral hypoglycemics, digitoxin, quinidine, disopyramide, dapsone, and corticosteroids. Higher incidence of isoniazid hepatitis with daily alcohol ingestion. Risk of phenytoin toxicity. Caution with other hepatotoxic agents and phenytoin. May decrease effects of oral contraceptives; use alternative measures.

**PREGNANCY:** Safety in pregnancy not known, caution in nursing.

## RIFATER
RX

rifampin - isoniazid - pyrazinamide (Sanofi-Aventis)

**Isoniazid associated with severe and sometimes fatal hepatitis. Monitor LFTs on a monthly basis.**

**THERAPEUTIC CLASS:** Isonicotinic acid hydrazide/rifamycin derivative/nicotinamide analogue

**INDICATIONS:** For initial phase of pulmonary tuberculosis treatment.

**DOSAGE:** *Adults:* <44kg: 4 tabs single dose qd. 45-54kg: 5 tabs single dose. >55kg: 6 tabs single dose. Give pyridoxine in malnourished, if predisposed to neuropathy (eg, alcoholics, diabetics), and adolescents. Take 1 hr before or 2 hrs after meals with full glass of water. Treatment usually lasts 2 months. *Pediatrics:* >15 yrs: <44kg: 4 tabs single dose qd. 45-54kg: 5 tabs qd single dose. >55kg: 6 tabs qd single dose. Give pyridoxine in malnourished, if predisposed to neuropathy (eg, alcoholics, diabetics), and adolescents. Take 1 hr before or 2 hrs after meals with full glass of water. Treatment usually lasts 2 months.

**HOW SUPPLIED:** Tab: (Isoniazid-Pyrazinamide-Rifampin) 50mg-300mg-120mg

**CONTRAINDICATIONS:** Severe hepatic damage, adverse reactions to isoniazid (eg, drug fever, chills, arthritis), acute liver disease, acute gout.

**WARNINGS/PRECAUTIONS:** Liver dysfunction, hyperbilirubinemia, and hyperuricemia with acute gouty arthritis reported. Monitor LFTs (every 2-4 weeks), serum uric acid. Perform regular ophthalmologic exams. Caution with DM, severe renal dysfunction. May produce reddish coloration of urine, sweat, sputum, and tears. May permanently stain soft contact lenses.

**ADVERSE REACTIONS:** GI effects, cutaneous reactions, musculoskeletal pain, hepatitis, CNS and cardiorespiratory effects.

**INTERACTIONS:** Rifampin may accelerate metabolism of anticonvulsants (eg, phenytoin), antiarrhythmics (eg, disopyramide, mexiletine, quinidine, tocainide), anticoagulants, antifungals (eg, fluconazole, itraconazole, ketoconazole), barbiturates, β-blockers, calcium channel blockers (eg, diltiazem, nifedipine, verapamil), chloramphenicol, ciprofloxacin, corticosteroids, cyclosporine, cardiac glycosides, clofibrate, oral contraceptives, dapsone, diazepam, haloperidol, oral hypoglycemics (eg, sulfonylureas), methadone, narcotic analgesics, nortriptyline, progestins, theophylline. Antacids may reduce rifampin absorption. Avoid foods containing tyramine and histamine (eg, cheese, red wine, tuna). Anticoagulants may need dose increase. Higher incidence of isoniazid hepatitis with daily alcohol ingestion. Avoid halothane. INH inhibits certain CYP450 enzymes; monitor with anticonvulsants, benzodiazepines, haloperidol, ketoconazole, warfarin. Decreased levels with corticosteroids. Exaggerates CNS effects of meperidine, cycloserine, disulfiram. Excess catecholamine stimulation with L-dopa.

**PREGNANCY:** Category C, not for use in nursing.

## RILUTEK
RX

riluzole (Sanofi-Aventis)

**THERAPEUTIC CLASS:** Benzothiazole

**INDICATIONS:** Treatment of amyotrophic lateral sclerosis (ALS).

**DOSAGE:** *Adults:* 50mg q12h. Take 1 hr before or 2 hrs after meals.

**HOW SUPPLIED:** Tab: 50mg

**WARNINGS/PRECAUTIONS:** Caution in elderly, and hepatic or renal dysfunction. Perform baseline LFT's before therapy, every month during 1st 3 months, every 3 months, every 3 months for next 9 months, then periodically thereafter. Neutropenia reported; obtain WBC count with febrile illness.

**ADVERSE REACTIONS:** Asthenia, nausea, dizziness, decreased lung function, diarrhea, abdominal pain, pneumonia, vomiting, vertigo, paresthesia, anorexia, somnolence.

**INTERACTIONS:** Caution with potentially hepatotoxic drugs (eg, allopurinol, methyldopa, sulfinpyrazine). CYP1A2 inhibitors (eg, caffeine, phenacetin, theophylline, amitriptyline, quinolones) may decrease elimination. CYP1A2 inducers (eg, cigarette smoke, charcoal-broiled food, rifampicin, omeprazole) may increase elimination. Drugs metabolized by CYP1A2 (eg, theophylline, caffeine, tacrine) may interact with riluzole.

**PREGNANCY:** Category C, not for use in nursing.

## RIMSO-50 RX

dimethyl sulfoxide (Edwards)

**THERAPEUTIC CLASS:** Anti-inflammatory

**INDICATIONS:** Symptomatic relief of interstitial cystitis.

**DOSAGE:** *Adults:* Instill 50mL directly into bladder; allow to remain for 15 minutes. Repeat at 2 week intervals until symptomatic relief then increase intervals between treatments. Severe Cases/Very Sensitive Bladders: Initiate first few treatments under anesthesia.

**HOW SUPPLIED:** Sol: 50% [50mL]

**WARNINGS/PRECAUTIONS:** Hypersensitivity reactions may occur. Perform full eye exams prior to and periodically during treatment. Obtain LFTs, CBCs, renal function tests every 6 months. May be harmful with urinary tract malignancy due to DMSO-induced vasodilation.

**ADVERSE REACTIONS:** Garlic-like taste/breath/body odor, transient chemical cystitis, discomfort upon administration.

**PREGNANCY:** Category C, caution in nursing.

## RISPERDAL RX

risperidone (Janssen)

**Elderly patients with dementia-related psychosis treated with atypical antipsychotic drugs are at an increased risk of death; most appeared to be cardiovascular (eg, heart failure, sudden death) or infectious (eg, pneumonia) in nature. Risperidone is not approved for the treatment of patients with dementia-related psychosis.**



**OTHER BRAND NAMES:** Risperdal M-Tab (Janssen)

**THERAPEUTIC CLASS:** Benzisoxazole derivative

**INDICATIONS:** Treatment of schizophrenia. Short-term treatment of acute manic or mixed episodes associated with bipolar I disorder as monotherapy or with lithium or valproate. Treatment of irritability associated with autistic disorder in children and adolescents, including symptoms of aggression towards others, deliberate self-injuriousness, temper tantrums, and quickly changing moods.

**DOSAGE:** *Adults:* Schizophrenia: Initial: 1mg bid. Titrate: Increase by 1mg bid on the 2nd and 3rd day until target dose of 3mg bid by third day. Adjust further at intervals of at least 1 week. Usual: 4-8mg/day. Max: 16mg/day. Doses up to 8mg can be taken once daily. Bipolar Mania: Initial: 2-3mg qd. Titrate: Increase/Decrease by 1mg qd. Usual: 1-6mg/day. Max: 6mg/day. Elderly/Debilitated/Hypotension/Severe Renal or Hepatic Impairment: Initial: 0.5mg bid. Titrate: Increase by no more than 0.5mg bid. Increase at intervals of at least 1 week for dosages >1.5mg bid. Reassess periodically to determine maintenance treatment.

*Pediatrics:* 5-16 yrs: Irritability with Autistic Disorder: Initial: <20kg: 0.25mg/day; ≥20kg: 0.5mg/day. Titrate after at least 4 days: <20kg: Increase by 0.5mg/day; ≥20kg: 1mg/day. Maint: For minimum of 14 days. Inadequate Response: Increase at ≥2-wk intervals: <20kg: Increase by 0.25mg/day;

≥20kg: Increase by 0.5mg/day. Caution in patients <15kg. Max: <20kg: 1mg/day; ≥20kg: 2.5mg/day; >45kg: 3mg/day.

**HOW SUPPLIED:** Sol: 1mg/mL [30mL]; Tab: 0.25mg, 0.5mg, 1mg, 2mg, 3mg, 4mg; Tab, Disintegrating: (M-Tab) 0.5mg, 1mg, 2mg, 3mg, 4mg

**WARNINGS/PRECAUTIONS:** Neuroleptic malignant syndrome and/or tardive dyskinesia may occur. Monitor for hyperglycemia; perform fasting blood glucose testing if symptoms develop or with risk factors for DM. Cerebrovascular events (eg, stroke, TIA) reported in elderly with dementia-related psychosis. Not approved for the treatment of dementia-related psychosis. May induce orthostatic hypotension, elevate prolactin levels, have an antiemetic effect. Caution in elderly, renal/hepatic impairment, history of seizures, cardio- or cerebrovascular disease, suicidal tendencies, risk of aspiration pneumonia, conditions predisposing to hypotension (eg, hypovolemia, dehydration) or affecting metabolism or hemodynamic responses. May impair judgement, thinking, or motor skills; caution when operating hazardous machinery. May disrupt body temperature regulation; caution in patients exposed to temperature extremes. Re-evaluate periodically. Patients who receive antipsychotics are reported to have an increased sensitivity to antipsychotic medications.

**ADVERSE REACTIONS:** Insomnia, agitation, anxiety, somnolence, extrapyramidal symptoms, nausea, headache, dizziness, constipation, dyspepsia, rhinitis, diarrhea, akathisia, dystonia, parkinsonism.

**INTERACTIONS:** Caution with other CNS drugs or alcohol. May potentiate antihypertensives, antagonize levodopa and dopamine agonists, or increase valproate levels. Cimetidine and ranitidine may increase bioavailability. CYP3A4 inducers (eg, carbamazepine, phenytoin, rifampin, phenobarbital) may decrease levels. Clozapine, fluoxetine, and paroxetine may increase levels. Increased mortality with furosemide in elderly patients.

**PREGNANCY:** Category C, not for use in nursing.

## RISPERDAL CONSTA

RX

risperidone (Janssen)

**Elderly patients with dementia-related psychosis treated with atypical antipsychotic drugs are at an increased risk of death; most appeared to be cardiovascular (eg, heart failure, sudden death) or infectious (eg, pneumonia) in nature. Risperidone is not approved for the treatment of patients with dementia-related psychosis.**

**THERAPEUTIC CLASS:** Benzisoxazole derivative

**INDICATIONS:** Treatment of schizophrenia.

**DOSAGE:** *Adults*: 25mg IM every 2 weeks. Max: 50mg/dose. Give 1st injection with oral dosage form or other oral antipsychotic. Continue for 3 weeks, then d/c oral. Titrate: Increase at intervals of no more than every 4 weeks. Hepatic or Renal Impairment/Certain Drug Interactions/Poor Tolerability to Psychotropic Meds: Initial: 12.5mg.

**HOW SUPPLIED:** Inj: 12.5mg, 25mg, 37.5mg, 50mg

**WARNINGS/PRECAUTIONS:** Neuroleptic malignant syndrome and/or tardive dyskinesia may occur. Monitor for hyperglycemia; perform fasting blood glucose testing if symptoms develop or with risk factors for DM. Cerebrovascular events (eg, stroke, TIA) reported in elderly with dementia-related psychosis. Not approved for the treatment of dementia-related psychosis. May induce orthostatic hypotension, elevate prolactin levels, have an antiemetic effect. Caution in elderly, renal/hepatic impairment, history of seizures, cardio- or cerebrovascular disease, suicidal tendencies, risk of aspiration pneumonia, conditions predisposing to hypotension (eg, hypovolemia, dehydration) or affecting metabolism or hemodynamic responses. May impair judgement, thinking, or motor skills; caution when operating hazardous machinery. May disrupt body temperature regulation; caution in patients exposed to temperature extremes. Re-evaluate periodically. Patients who receive antipsychotics are reported to have an increased sensitivity to antipsychotic medications. Must inject into the gluteal muscle; avoid injection into blood vessel.

**ADVERSE REACTIONS:** Insomnia, somnolence, headache, dizziness, constipation, dyspepsia, rhinitis, diarrhea, akathisia, parkinsonism, hallucinations, somnolence, weight increase, dry mouth, fatigue.

**INTERACTIONS:** Caution with other CNS drugs or alcohol. May potentiate antihypertensives, antagonize levodopa and dopamine agonists, or increase valproate levels. Cimetidine and ranitidine may increase bioavailability. CYP3A4 inducers (eg, carbamazepine, phenytoin, rifampin, phenobarbital) may decrease levels. Clozapine, fluoxetine, and paroxetine may increase levels. Increased mortality with furosemide in elderly patients.

**PREGNANCY:** Category C, not for use in nursing.

## RITALIN

**CII**

methylphenidate HCl (Novartis)

**OTHER BRAND NAMES:** Ritalin LA (Novartis) - Ritalin SR (Novartis)

**THERAPEUTIC CLASS:** Sympathomimetic amine

**INDICATIONS:** (Cap, Extended-Release, Tab, Tab, Extended-Release) Treatment of attention deficit disorders. (Tab, Tab, Extended-Release) Treatment of narcolepsy.

**DOSAGE:** *Adults:* (Tab) 10-60mg/day given bid-tid 30-45 min ac. Take last dose before 6 pm if insomnia occurs. (Tab, Extended-Release) May use in place of immediate release (IR) when the 8 hr dose corresponds to the titrated 8 hr IR dose. Swallow whole; do not chew or crush.
*Pediatrics:* >6 yrs: (Tab) Initial: 5mg bid before breakfast and lunch. Titrate: Increase gradually by 5-10mg weekly. Max: 60mg/day. (Tab, Extended-Release) May use in place of immediate release (IR) when the 8 hr dose corresponds to the titrated 8 hr IR dose. Swallow whole; do not chew or crush. (Cap, ER) Initial: 10-20mg qam. Titrate: Adjust weekly by 10mg. Max: 60mg qam. Previous Methylphenidate Use: May use as qd in place of IR dosed bid or daily dose of methylphenidate-SR. Swallow whole or sprinkle over spoonful of applesauce. Do not crush, chew, or divide. Reduce dose or discontinue if paradoxical aggravation of symptoms occurs. Discontinue if no improvement after appropriate dose adjustment over 1 month.

**HOW SUPPLIED:** Cap, Extended-Release (Ritalin LA): 10mg, 20mg, 30mg, 40mg; Tab (Ritalin): 5mg, 10mg*, 20mg*; Tab, Extended-Release (Ritalin SR): 20mg *scored



**CONTRAINDICATIONS:** Marked anxiety, tension, and agitation; glaucoma; motor tics or family history or diagnosis of Tourette's syndrome; during or within 14 days of MAOI use.

**WARNINGS/PRECAUTIONS:** Monitor growth in children. Not for severe depression or fatigue. May exacerbate symptoms of behavior disturbance and thought disorder in psychotic children. Care should be taken in using stimulants to treat patients with comorbid bipolar disorder because of concern for possible induction of mixed/manic episode in such patients. Stimulants at usual doses can cause treatment emergent psychotic or manic symptoms (hallucinations, delusinal thinking, mania) in children and adolescents without prior history of psychotic illness. Aggressive behavior or hostility reported in clinical trials and the postmarketing experience of some medications indicated for the treatment of ADHD. May lower seizure threshold, especially with prior history of seizures or with prior EEG abnormalities; d/c if seizures occur. Caution with HTN and other underlying conditions that may be compromised such as heart failure, recent MI, or hyperthyroidism. Visual disturbances may occur (rare). Monitor CBC, differential, and platelets with prolonged use. Caution with emotionally-unstable patients or prior history of drug dependence or alcoholism; chronic use may lead to tolerance and psychological dependence. Monitor during withdrawal. Periodically d/c to assess condition. Avoid with known structural cardiac abnormalities or other serious cardiac problems.

**ADVERSE REACTIONS:** Nervousness, insomnia, hypersensitivity reactions, anorexia, nausea, dizziness, palpitations, headache, dyskinesia, drowsiness, BP and pulse changes, tachycardia, angina, arrhythmia, abdominal pain.

**INTERACTIONS:** See Contraindications. May decrease hypotensive effect of guanethidine. Caution with $a_2$-agonist (eg, clonidine) and pressor agents. Potentiates anticoagulants, anticonvulsants (eg, phenobarbital, diphenylhydantoin, primidone), phenylbutazone, TCAs (eg, imipramine, clomipramine, desipramine); monitor plasma drug levels or PT/INR. (Cap, Extended-Release) Antacids or acid suppressants may alter release characteristics of cap.

**PREGNANCY:** (Tab, ER) Safety in pregnancy and nursing not known. (Cap, ER) Category C, caution in nursing.

## RITUXAN RX

rituximab (Genentech/IDEC)

**Fatal infusion reactions reported and may manifest with hypoxia, pulmonary infiltrates, ARDS, MI, ventricular fibrillation, cardiogenic shock; discontinue if infusion reaction occurs. Acute renal failure reported in the setting of Tumor Lysis Syndrome (TLS) following treatment of non-Hodgkins Lymphoma. Severe mucocutaneous reactions reported. JC virus infection resulting in progressive multifocal leukoencephalopathy (PML) reported.**

**THERAPEUTIC CLASS:** Monoclonal antibody/CD20-blocker

**INDICATIONS:** Treatment of relapsed or refractory, low-grade or follicular, CD20 positive, B-Cell, non-Hodgkin's lymphoma (NHL). First-line treatment of follicular, CD-20 positive, B-cell NHL in combination with CVP chemotherapy. Treatment of low-grade, CD20 positive, B-Cell NHL in patients with stable disease or who achieve partial or complete response following first-line treatment with CVP chemotherapy. First-line treatment of diffuse large B-Cell, CD-20 positive, NHL in combination with CHOP or other anthracycline-based chemotherapy regimens. In combination with methotrexate to reduce signs and symptoms in adult patients with moderately- to severely-active rheumatoid arthritis (RA) who have had an inadequate response to one or more TNF-antagonist therapies.

**DOSAGE:** *Adults:* Give as infusion. Relapsed or Refractory, Low-Grade or Follicular, CD-20 Positive, B-Cell NHL: 375mg/$m^2$ IV once weekly for 4 or 8 doses. If progressive disease develops, re-treat with 375mg/$m^2$ IV once weekly for 4 doses. Previously Untreated, Follicular, CD20-Positive, B-Cell NHL: 375mg/$m^2$ IV on Day 1 of each CVP chemotherapy cycle for up to 8 doses. Previously Untreated, Low-Grade, CD20-Positive, B-Cell NHL: Following 6-8 cycles of CVP chemotherapy, 375mg/$m^2$ IV once weekly for 4 doses every 6 months for up to 16 doses. Diffuse Large B-Cell NHL: 375mg/$m^2$ IV given on Day 1 of each chemotherapy cycle for up to 8 infusions. RA: Give with methotrexate. Give two-1000mg IV infusions separated by 2 weeks. Administer methylprednisolone 100mg IV (or equivalent) 30 min prior to each infusion to reduce incidence and severity of infusion reactions. Do not administer as IV push or bolus.

**HOW SUPPLIED:** Inj: 10mg/mL

**WARNINGS/PRECAUTIONS:** Interrupt if severe infusion reaction develops; may resume at a 50% rate reduction when symptoms subside. Risk of TLS may increase with high numbers of circulating malignant cells or high tumor burden. HBV reactivation with fulminant hepatitis, hepatic failure, and death reported; d/c if viral hepatitis develops. Additional serious viral infections, either new, reactivated, or exacerbated have been reported. JC virus infection resulting in PML reported; d/c if PML develops. Hypersensitivity reactions may respond to infusion rate adjustment and medical management. D/C if serious arrhythmias occur. Caution with pre-existing cardiac conditions. Use with extreme caution in combination with cisplatin as renal failure may occur.

Severe renal toxicity reported; d/c if serum creatinine rises or oliguria occurs. D/C if mucocutaneous reactions develop. Monitor CBC and platelets regularly; more frequently with cytopenias. Abdominal pain, bowel obstruction and perforation reported.

**ADVERSE REACTIONS:** Arrhythmias, fever, chills, infection, PML, asthenia, nausea, lymphopenia, leukopenia, neutropenia, headache, abdominal pain, night sweats, rash, pruritus, pain.

**INTERACTIONS:** Renal toxicity reported with cisplatin. Vaccination with live virus vaccines not recommended. Observe closely for signs of infection if biologic agents and/or DMARDs are used concomitantly.

**PREGNANCY:** Category C, not for use in nursing.

## ROBAXIN — RX

methocarbamol (Schwarz)

**OTHER BRAND NAMES:** Robaxin-750 (Schwarz) - Robaxin Injection (Baxter)

**THERAPEUTIC CLASS:** Muscular analgesic (central-acting)

**INDICATIONS:** Adjunct for relief of acute, painful musculoskeletal conditions.

**DOSAGE:** *Adults:* (PO) Initial: (500mg tab) 1500mg qid for 2-3 days. Maint: 1000mg qid. Initial: (750mg tab) 1500mg qid for 2-3 days. Maint: 750mg q4h or 1500mg tid. Max: 6gm/d for 2-3 days; 8gm/d if severe. (Inj) Moderate Symptoms: 10mL IV/IM. IV Max Rate: 3mL undiluted drug/min. IM Max: 5mL into each gluteal region. Severe/Post-Op Condition: Max: 20-30mL/day up to 3 consecutive days. If feasible, continue with PO. Tetanus: 10-20mL up to 30mL. May repeat q6h until NG tube can be inserted. Continue with crushed tabs. Max: 24g/day PO.
*Pediatrics:* Tetanus: Initial: 15mg/kg. Repeat q6h prn. Administer through tubing or IV. Safety and effctiveness in pediatric patients have not been established except tetanus

**HOW SUPPLIED:** Inj: 100mg/mL; Tab: 500mg, 750mg

**CONTRAINDICATIONS:** (Inj) Renal pathology with injection due to propylene glycol content.

**WARNINGS/PRECAUTIONS:** May cause color interference in certain screening tests for 5-hydroxy-indoleacetic acid (5-HIAA) and vanillylmandelic acid (VMA). Caution in epilepsy with the injection. Injection rate should not exceed 3mL/min. Avoid extravasation with injection.

**ADVERSE REACTIONS:** Lightheadedness, dizziness, drowsiness, nausea, urticaria, pruritus, rash, conjunctivitis, nasal congestion, blurred vision, headache, fever, seizures, syncope, flushing.



**INTERACTIONS:** Additive adverse effects with alcohol and other CNS depressants. May inhibit effect of pyridostigmine; caution in patients with myasthemia gravis receiving anticholinergics.

**PREGNANCY:** Category C, caution in nursing.

## ROBINUL — RX

glycopyrrolate (Sciele)

**OTHER BRAND NAMES:** Robinul Forte (Sciele)

**THERAPEUTIC CLASS:** Anticholinergic

**INDICATIONS:** Adjunct treatment of peptic ulcer.

**DOSAGE:** *Adults:* Usual: (Tab) 1mg tid (am, pm and hs); may increase to 2mg qhs if needed. Maint: 1mg bid. (Forte) 2mg bid-tid. Max: 8mg/day.
*Pediatrics:* >12 yrs: Usual: (Tab) 1mg tid (am, pm & hs); may increase to 2mg qhs if needed. Maint: 1mg bid. (Forte) 2mg bid-tid. Max: 8mg/day.

**HOW SUPPLIED:** Tab: 1mg*, (Forte) 2mg* *scored

**CONTRAINDICATIONS:** Glaucoma, obstructive uropathy, GI tract obstruction, paralytic ileus, intestinal atony of elderly or debilitated, unstable cardiovascular status in acute hemorrhage, severe ulcerative colitis, toxic megacolon complicating ulcerative colitis, myasthenia gravis.

**WARNINGS/PRECAUTIONS:** May produce drowsiness and blurred vision; avoid operating machinery. Risk of heat prostration with high environmental temperature. Diarrhea may be early symptom of incomplete intestinal obstruction especially with ileostomy or colostomy. Caution in elderly, autonomic neuropathy, hepatic/renal disease, ulcerative colitis, hyperthyroidism, coronary heart disease, CHF, tachyarrhythmias, tachycardia, HTN, prostatic hypertrophy, hiatal hernia associated with reflux esophagitis.

**ADVERSE REACTIONS:** Blurred vision, dry mouth, urinary retention and hesitancy, increased ocular tension, tachycardia, decreased sweating, xerostomia, loss of taste, headache.

**PREGNANCY:** Safety in pregnancy is not known; not for use in nursing.

## ROBINUL INJECTION RX

glycopyrrolate (Baxter)

**THERAPEUTIC CLASS:** Anticholinergic

**INDICATIONS:** Preoperative antimuscarinic to reduce salivary tracheobronchial, and pharyngeal secretions; decrease gastric sections; and block cardiac vagal inhibitory reflexes during anesthesia induction and intubation. Intra-operatively to counteract drug-induced or vagal traction reflexes associated with arrhythmias. To protect against peripheral muscarinic effects of cholinergic agents. Adjunct therapy for treatment of peptic ulcer when rapid anticholinergic effect is desired or when oral medication is not tolerated.

**DOSAGE:** *Adults:* Preanesthesia: 0.002mg/lb IM 30-60 minutes before anesthesia induction or at the time of preanesthetic narcotic/sedative. Intraoperatively: 0.1mg IV, repeat prn every 2-3 minutes. Reverse Neuromuscular Blockade: 0.2mg IV for each 1mg neostigmine or 5mg pyridostigmine. Peptic Ulcer: 0.1mg IV/IM q4h, tid-qid. May use 0.2mg if needed.
*Pediatrics:* Preanesthesia: 1 month-12 yrs: 0.002mg/lb IM 30-60 minutes before anesthesia induction or at the time of preanesthetic narcotic/sedative. 1 month-2 yrs: May require up to 0.004mg/lb. Intraoperatively: 0.002mg/lb IV. Max: 0.1mg single dose. May repeat prn every 2-3 minutes. Reverse Neuromuscular Blockade: 0.2mg IV for each 1mg neostigmine or 5mg pyridostigmine. Peptic Ulcer: >12 yrs: 0.1mg IV/IM q4h, tid-qid. May use 0.2mg if needed.

**HOW SUPPLIED:** Inj: 0.2mg/mL

**CONTRAINDICATIONS:** Newborns (<1 month) due to benzyl alcohol content. For long treatment duration: Glaucoma, obstructive uropathy, obstructive disease of GI tract, paralytic ileus, intestinal atony of elderly or debilitated, unstable cardiovascular status in acute hemorrhage, severe ulcerative colitis, toxic megacolon complicating ulcerative colitis, myasthenia gravis.

**WARNINGS/PRECAUTIONS:** Caution with CAD, CHF, arrhythmias, HTN, hyperthyroidism, elderly, autonomic neuropathy, hepatic or renal disease, ulcerative colitis, or hiatal hernia. May produce drowsiness and blurred vision; caution when operating machinery. Risk of fever and heat stroke due to decreased sweating in high environmental temperature. Diarrhea may be early symptom of incomplete intestinal obstruction.

**ADVERSE REACTIONS:** Drowsiness, blurred vision, dry mouth, urinary retention and hesitancy, increased ocular tension, tachycardia, palpation, decreased sweating, loss of taste.

**INTERACTIONS:** Increased anticholinergic side effects with other anticholinergics, phenothiazines, antiparkinson drugs, TCAs. Increased severity of GI lesions with potassium chloride in a wax matrix.

**PREGNANCY:** Category B, caution in nursing.

## ROCALTROL

RX

calcitriol (Roche Labs)

**THERAPEUTIC CLASS:** Vitamin D analog

**INDICATIONS:** Predialysis: Management of secondary hyperparathyroidism and resultant metabolic bone disease with moderate to severe chronic renal failure (CrCl 15-55mL/min). Dialysis: Management of hypocalcemia and resultant metabolic bone disease. Hypoparathyroidism: Management of hypocalcemia and manifestations of postsurgical hypoparathyroidism, idiopathic hypoparathyroidism, and pseudohypoparathyroidism.

**DOSAGE:** *Adults:* Predialysis: Initial: 0.25mcg/day. Max: 0.5mcg/day. Hypoparathyroidism: Initial: 0.25mcg/day every am. Titrate: May increase at 2-4 week intervals to 0.5-2mcg/day. Elderly: Start at low end of dosing range. Dialysis: Initial: 0.25mcg/day. Titrate: May increase by 0.25mcg/day every 4-8 weeks to 0.5-1mcg/day. Monitor serum calcium levels twice weekly during titration. Normal to slightly reduced serum calcium, give 0.25mcg every other day. Discontinue with hypercalcemia; when calcium levels return to normal continue therapy and decrease dose by 0.25 mcg.
*Pediatrics:* Predialysis: >3 yrs: Initial: 0.25mcg/day. Max: 0.5mcg/day. <3yrs: Initial: 10-15ng/kg/day. Hypoparathyroidism: >6 yrs: Initial: 0.25mcg/day every am. Titrate: May increase at 2-4 week intervals to 0.5-2mcg/day. 1-5yrs: Initial: 0.25mcg/day every am. Titrate: May increase at 2-4 week intervals up to 0.75mcg/day. Monitor serum calcium levels twice weekly during titration. Discontinue with hypercalcemia; when calcium levels return to normal continue therapy and decrease dose by 0.25 mcg.

**HOW SUPPLIED:** Cap: 0.25mcg, 0.5mcg; Sol: 1mcg/mL [15mL]

**CONTRAINDICATIONS:** Hypercalcemia or vitamin D toxicity.

**WARNINGS/PRECAUTIONS:** Use non-aluminum phosphate binders and low phosphate diet to control serum phosphate. Chronic hypercalcemia can cause calcification of soft tissues. Monitor calcium levels twice a week initially. Avoid dehydration. Monitor serum creatinine. Maintain adequate calcium intake of at least 600mg/day. Caution in elderly. If treatment switched from ergocalciferol, may take several months for ergocalciferol level to decrease to baseline. May increase inorganic phosphate levels; ectopic calcification reported with renal failure. Monitor phosphorus, magnesium, alkaline phosphatase, and 24-hour urine periodically.

**ADVERSE REACTIONS:** Weakness, nausea, vomiting, dry mouth, constipation, muscle and bone pain, metallic taste, polyuria, polydipsia, weight loss, pancreatitis, photophobia, pruritus, decreased libido.



**INTERACTIONS:** Avoid vitamin D products and derivatives during therapy. Hypermagnesemia may occur with magnesium-containing antacids, especially in chronic renal dialysis. Caution with digoxin; hypercalcemia may precipitate arrhythmias. Reduced intestinal absorption with cholestyramine. May need to increase dose if given with phenytoin or phenobarbital. Caution with thiazides; risk of hypercalcemia. Ketoconazole may effect metabolism. Corticosteroids antagonize activity. Changes in diet or uncontrolled intake of calcium preparations can cause hypercalcemia. Adjust dose phosphate-binding agents.

**PREGNANCY:** Category C, not for use in nursing.

## ROCEPHIN

RX

ceftriaxone sodium (Roche Labs)

**THERAPEUTIC CLASS:** Cephalosporin (3rd generation)

**INDICATIONS:** Treatment of lower respiratory tract infections, skin and skin structure infections, bone and joint infections, intra-abdominal infections, acute otitis media, uncomplicated gonorrhea, pelvic inflammatory disease, UTI, septicemia, and meningitis. For surgical prophylaxis.

**DOSAGE:** *Adults:* Usual: 1-2g/day IV/IM given qd-bid. Max: 4g/day. Gonorrhea: 250mg IM single dose. Surgical Prophylaxis: 1g IV 1/2-2 hrs before surgery. *Pediatrics:* Skin Infections: 50-75mg/kg/day IV/IM given qd-bid. Max: 2g/day. Otitis Media: 50mg/kg (up to 1g) IM single dose. Serious Infections: 50-75mg/kg/day IM/IV given q12h. Max: 2g/day. Meningitis: Initial: 100mg/kg (up to 4g), then 100mg/kg/day given qd-bid for 7-14 days. Max: 4g/day.

**HOW SUPPLIED:** Inj: 250mg, 500mg, 1g, 2g, 10g

**WARNINGS/PRECAUTIONS:** Cross sensitivity to penicillins and other cephalosporins may occur. Pseudomembranous colitis reported. May result in overgrowth of nonsusceptible organisms. Altered PT, transient BUN, and serum creatinine elevations may occur. Do not exceed 2g/day and monitor blood levels with both hepatic and renal dysfunction. Caution with history of GI disease. D/C if develop gallbladder disease. May alter PT; monitor with impaired vitamin K synthesis or low vitamin K stores. Avoid in hyperbilirubinemic neonates, especially prematures.

**ADVERSE REACTIONS:** Injection site reactions, eosinophilia, thrombocytosis, diarrhea, SGOT and SGPT elevations.

**PREGNANCY:** Category B, caution in nursing.

## ROFERON-A RX

interferon alfa-2a, recombinant (Roche Labs)

**May cause or aggravate fatal or life-threatening neuropsychiatric, autoimmune, ischemic, and infectious disorders. Monitor closely with periodic clinical and laboratory evaluations. D/C with persistently severe or worsening signs or symptoms of these conditions.**

**THERAPEUTIC CLASS:** Biological response modifier

**INDICATIONS:** Treatment of chronic hepatitis C (HCV) and hairy cell leukemia. For chronic phase, Philadelphia chromosome positive chronic myelogenous leukemia (CML) in patients minimally pretreated.

**DOSAGE:** *Adults:* >18 yrs: HCV: 3MIU SQ 3x/week (TIW) for 48-52 weeks or 6MIU TIW for 12 weeks, then 3MIU TIW for 36 weeks. D/C if no response within 3 months. If intolerant to prescribed dose, temporarily reduce by 50%. May reinstate once adverse reactions resolve. Retreatment: 3MIU TIW or 6MIU TIW for 6-12 months. Hairy Cell Leukemia: Induction: 3MIU SQ qd for 16-24 weeks. Maint: 3MIU TIW. CML: 3MIU SQ qd for 3 days, 6MIU qd for 3 days, then to target dose of 9MIU qd. D/C or reduce dose or frequency of inj if severe adverse reactions occur.
*Pediatrics:* CML: 3MIU SQ qd for 3 days, 6MIU qd for 3 days, then to target dose of 9MIU qd. D/C or reduce dose or frequency of inj if severe adverse reactions occur.

**HOW SUPPLIED:** Inj: 3MIU/0.5mL, 6MIU/0.5mL, 9MIU/0.5mL

**CONTRAINDICATIONS:** Autoimmune hepatitis; hepatic decompensation (Child-Pugh class B & C) before or during treatment; neonates and infants (contains benzyl alcohol).

**WARNINGS/PRECAUTIONS:** Depression and suicidal behavior reported; extreme caution with history of depression. Cardiomyopathy reported; caution with cardiac disease or history of cardiac illness. Serious, acute hypersensitivity reactions reported. Transient liver abnormalities and/or GI hemorrhage reported. May suppress bone marrow function and result in severe cytopenias and anemia; caution with myelosuppression. May cause or aggravate hypothyroidism and hyperthyroidism. Hyperglycemia reported; monitor closely. May induce or aggravate dyspnea, pulmonary infiltrates, pneumonia, bronchiolitis obliterans, interstitial pneumonitis, and sarcoidosis; d/c with persistent or unexplained pulmonary infiltrates or pulmonary function impairment. Decrease/loss of vision and retinopathy reported; perform eye exam at baseline, if any ocular symptoms develop, and periodically with pre-existing disorder and d/c if new or worsening ophthalmologic disorders develop. Renal toxicities reported; monitor closely with impaired renal function and caution with CrCl <50mL/min. Development and exacerbation of autoimmune disease reported; monitor closely. Monitor CBC, platelets, and clinical chemistry tests before therapy and periodically thereafter. Severe infections reported; consider discontinuation. Pancreatitis reported; suspend if signs or symptoms observed; d/c if pancreatitis diagnosed.

**ADVERSE REACTIONS:** Depression, flu-like symptoms (fever, asthenia, fatigue, chills, myalgia), dizziness, headache, nausea, vomiting, diarrhea, rash, arthralgia, anorexia.

**INTERACTIONS:** May reduce theophylline clearance. Caution with agents that cause myelosuppression or are metabolized by CYP450. Synergistic myelosuppression with zidovudine. Anti-diabetic regimens may need adjustments. Use with interleukin-2 may increase risk of renal failure. May increase neurotoxic, hematotoxic or cardiotoxic effects of other drugs.

**PREGNANCY:** Category C, not for use in nursing.

## ROGAINE EXTRA STRENGTH — OTC

minoxidil (McNeill)

**THERAPEUTIC CLASS:** Vasodilator

**INDICATIONS:** To regrow hair on scalp.

**DOSAGE:** *Adults:* >18 yrs: Apply 1mL bid directly onto scalp in hair loss area.

**HOW SUPPLIED:** Sol: 5% [60mL]

**WARNINGS/PRECAUTIONS:** Avoid in women; may grow facial hair. Avoid if no family history of hair loss, sudden or patchy hair loss, or if scalp is inflamed, red, infected, irritated, or painful. Avoid eye contact. Not effective in hair loss due to medications, severe nutritional problems, low thyroid states, chemo, or conditions that cause scarring of the scalp. D/C if develop chest pain, rapid heartbeat, faintness/dizziness, sudden unexplained weight gain, swollen hands or feet, scalp irritation that continues or worsens.

**INTERACTIONS:** Avoid if using other medicines on the scalp.

**PREGNANCY:** Safety in pregnancy and nursing not known.

## ROGAINE FOR WOMEN — OTC

minoxidil (McNeill)

**THERAPEUTIC CLASS:** Vasodilator

**INDICATIONS:** To regrow hair on scalp.

**DOSAGE:** *Adults:* >18 yrs: Apply 1mL bid directly onto scalp in hair loss area.

**HOW SUPPLIED:** Sol: 2% [60mL]

**WARNINGS/PRECAUTIONS:** Avoid if scalp is red, inflamed, infected, irritated, painful to touch. Avoid eye contact. D/C if unwanted facial hair growth, chest pain, rapid heartbeat, faintness/dizziness, sudden unexplained weight gain, swollen hands or feet, or scalp irritation develops.

**ADVERSE REACTIONS:** Itching, skin irritation, unwanted facial hair growth.

**PREGNANCY:** Safety in pregnancy and nursing not known.



## ROMAZICON — RX

flumazenil (Roche Labs)

**THERAPEUTIC CLASS:** Benzodiazepine antagonist

**INDICATIONS:** Complete or partial reversal of sedative effects of benzodiazepines (BZDs) given with general anesthesia, or diagnostic and therapeutic procedures, and for the management of BZD overdose in adults. For reversal of BZD-induced conscious sedation in pediatrics (1-17 yrs old).

**DOSAGE:** *Adults:* Reversal of Conscious Sedation/General Anesthesia: Give IV over 15 seconds. Initial: 0.2mg. May repeat dose after 45 seconds and again at 60 second intervals up to a max of 4 additional times until reach desired level of consciousness. Max Total Dose: 1mg. In event of resedation, repeated doses may be given at 20-min intervals. Max: 1mg/dose (0.2mg/min) and 3mg/hr. BZD Overdose: Give IV over 30 seconds. Initial: 0.2mg. May repeat with 0.3mg after 30 seconds and then 0.5mg at 1-min intervals until reach desired level of consciousness. Max Total Dose: 3mg. In event of resedation, repeated doses may be given at 20-min intervals. Max: 1mg/dose (0.5mg/min); 3mg/hr. *Pediatrics*: >1yr: Give IV over 15 seconds. Initial: 0.01mg/kg (up to 0.2mg). May repeat dose after 45 seconds and again at 60-second intervals up to a max of 4 additional times until reach desired level of consciousness. Max Total Dose: 0.05mg/kg or 1mg, whichever is lower.

**HOW SUPPLIED:** Inj: 0.1mg/mL

**CONTRAINDICATIONS:** Patients given BZDs for life-threatening conditions (eg, control of intracranial pressure or status epilepticus), signs of serious cyclic antidepressant overdose.

**WARNINGS/PRECAUTIONS:** Caution in overdoses involving multiple drug combinations. Risk of seizures, especially with long-term BZD-induced sedation, cyclic antidepressant overdose, concurrent major sedative-hypnotic drug withdrawal, recent therapy with repeated doses of parenteral BZDs, myoclonic jerking or seizure prior to flumazenil administration. Monitor for resedation, respiratory depression, or other residual BZD effects (up to 2 hrs). Avoid use in the ICU; increased risk of unrecognized BZD dependence. Caution with head injury, alcoholism, and other drug dependencies. Does not reverse respiratory depression/hypoventilation or cardiac depression. May provoke panic attacks with history of panic disorder. Adjust subsequent doses in hepatic dysfunction. Not for use as treatment for BZD dependence or for management of protracted abstinence syndromes. May trigger dose-dependent withdrawal syndromes.

**ADVERSE REACTIONS:** Nausea, vomiting, dizziness, injection site pain, increased sweating, headache, abnormal or blurred vision, agitation.

**INTERACTIONS:** Avoid use until neuromuscular blockade effects are reversed. Toxic effects (eg, convulsions, cardiac dysrhythmias) may occur with mixed drug overdose (eg, cyclic antidepressants).

**PREGNANCY:** Category C, caution in nursing.

## RONDEC — RX

pseudoephedrine HCl - carbinoxamine maleate (Biovail)



**OTHER BRAND NAMES:** Rondec-TR (Biovail) - Rondec Oral Drops (Biovail)

**THERAPEUTIC CLASS:** Antihistamine/decongestant

**INDICATIONS:** (Drops) Seasonal/perennial allergic and vasomotor rhinitis. (Tab, Tab, Extended Release) Relief of upper respiratory symptoms associated with allergic rhinitis and the common cold.

**DOSAGE:** *Adults:* (Tab) 1 tab qid; (Tab, Extended Release) 1 tab bid. *Pediatrics:* (Sol) Give qid. 12-24 months: 1mL. 6-12 months: 3/4mL. 3-6 months: 1/2mL. 1-3 months: 1/4mL. (Tab) ≥6 yrs:1 tab qid. (Tab, Extended Release) ≥12 yrs: 1 tab bid.

**HOW SUPPLIED:** (Carbinoxamine-Pseudoephedrine) Sol: 1mg-15mg/mL [30mL]; Tab: 4mg-60mg; Tab, Extended Release: (Rondec TR) 8mg-120mg

**CONTRAINDICATIONS:** Severe HTN or CAD, MAOIs, narrow-angle glaucoma, urinary retention, peptic ulcer, during asthma attack.

**WARNINGS/PRECAUTIONS:** Caution in asthma, DM, HTN, heart disease, hyperthyroidism, increased IOP, prostatic hypertrophy, elderly. May cause excitability, especially in children.

**ADVERSE REACTIONS:** Sedation, dizziness, diplopia, vomiting, diarrhea, dry mouth, headache, nervousness, nausea, convulsions, CNS stimulation, cardiac arrhythmias, respiratory difficulty, increased HR or BP.

**INTERACTIONS:** May enhance effects of TCAs, benzodiazepines, barbiturates, alcohol, other CNS depressants. Increased sympathomimetic effects with MAOIs, beta blockers. May reduce antihypertensive effects of reserpine, veratrum alkaloids, methyldopa, mecamylamine.

**PREGNANCY:** Category C, safety in nursing not known.

## RONDEC SYRUP RX

pseudoephedrine HCl - brompheniramine maleate (Biovail)

**THERAPEUTIC CLASS:** Antihistamine/decongestant

**INDICATIONS:** Symptomatic relief of seasonal and perennial allergic rhinitis and vasomotor rhinitis.

**DOSAGE:** *Adults:* 5mL qid.
*Pediatrics:* ≥6 yrs: 5mL qid. 2-6 yrs: 2.5mL qid.

**HOW SUPPLIED:** (Brompheniramine-Pseudoephedrine) Syrup: 4mg-45mg/5mL

**CONTRAINDICATIONS:** Severe HTN or CAD, MAOIs, narrow-angle glaucoma, urinary retention, peptic ulcer, during asthma attack.

**WARNINGS/PRECAUTIONS:** Caution in asthma, DM, HTN, heart disease, hyperthyroidism, increased IOP, prostatic hypertrophy, elderly. May cause excitability, especially in children.

**ADVERSE REACTIONS:** Sedation, dizziness, diplopia, vomiting, diarrhea, dry mouth, headache, nervousness, nausea, convulsions, CNS stimulation, cardiac arrhythmias, respiratory difficulty, increased HR or BP.

**INTERACTIONS:** May enhance effects of TCAs, benzodiazepines, barbiturates, alcohol, other CNS depressants. Increased sympathomimetic effects with MAOIs, beta blockers. May reduce antihypertensive effects of reserpine, veratrum alkaloids, methyldopa, mecamylamine.

**PREGNANCY:** Category C, safety in nursing not known.

## RONDEC-DM DROPS RX



pseudoephedrine HCl - dextromethorphan hbr - carbinoxamine maleate (Biovail)

**THERAPEUTIC CLASS:** Antihistamine/decongestant/antitussive

**INDICATIONS:** Relief of coughs and upper respiratory symptoms associated with allergy or the common cold.

**DOSAGE:** *Pediatrics:* Give qid. 12-24 months: 1mL. 6-12 months: 3/4mL. 3-6 months: 1/2mL. 1-3 months: 1/4mL.

**HOW SUPPLIED:** (Carbinoxamine-Dextromethorphan-Pseudoephedrine) Sol: 1mg-4mg-15mg/mL [30mL]

**CONTRAINDICATIONS:** Severe HTN or CAD, during or within 2 weeks of MAOIs, narrow-angle glaucoma, urinary retention, peptic ulcer, during asthma attack.

**WARNINGS/PRECAUTIONS:** Caution with HTN, DM, heart disease, asthma, hyperthyroidism, increased IOP, prostatic hypertrophy and in atopic children, elderly, sedated, debilitated, or confined to supine positions. May cause excitability especially in children.

**ADVERSE REACTIONS:** Sedation, drowsiness, dizziness, diplopia, nausea, vomiting, diarrhea, dry mouth, headache, nervousness, convulsions, CNS stimulation, arrhythmias, increased HR or BP, tremors.

**INTERACTIONS:** Avoid during or within 2 weeks of MAOIs. May enhance effects of TCAs, barbiturates, alcohol, other CNS depressants. May reduce antihypertensive effects of reserpine, veratrum alkaloids, methyldopa, mecamylamine. Increased sympathomimetic effect with MAOIs, beta-blockers. Additive cough-suppressant effect with narcotic antitussives.

**PREGNANCY:** Category C, safety in nursing not known.

## RONDEC-DM SYRUP RX

pseudoephedrine HCl - dextromethorphan hbr - brompheniramine maleate (Biovail)

**OTHER BRAND NAMES:** Cardec DM (Alpharma) - Carbofed DM (Hi-Tech)

**THERAPEUTIC CLASS:** Antihistamine/decongestant/antitussive

**INDICATIONS:** Relief of coughs and upper respiratory symptoms, including nasal congestion, associated with allergy or the common cold.

**DOSAGE:** *Adults:* 5mL qid.
*Pediatrics:* >6 yrs: 5mL qid. 2-6 yrs: 2.5mL qid.

**HOW SUPPLIED:** Syrup: (Brompheniramine-Dextromethorphan-Pseudoephedrine) 4mg-15mg-45mg/5mL [120mL, 480mL]

**CONTRAINDICATIONS:** Severe HTN or CAD, narrow-angle glaucoma, urinary retention, peptic ulcer, acute asthma attack, with MAOI therapy.

**WARNINGS/PRECAUTIONS:** Caution with HTN, DM, ischemic heart disease, hyperthyroidism, BPH, asthma, and increased IOP. May produce CNS stimulation with convulsion, cardiovascular collapse and hypotension. Excitability reported especially in children. Do not exceed recommended doses. Caution in atopic children, elderly, sedated/debilitated, and patients confined to supine positions.

**ADVERSE REACTIONS:** Sedation, drowsiness, dizziness, diplopia, nausea, vomiting, diarrhea, dry mouth, headache, arrhythmias, increased heart rate, tremors, nervousness, insomnia, heartburn, dysuria, polyuria, increased BP.

**INTERACTIONS:** May enhance effects of TCAs, barbiturates, alcohol, other CNS depressants. May diminish antihypertensive effects of reserpine, veratrum alkaloids, methyldopa, mecamylamine. Increased sympathomimetic effect with beta-blockers and MAOIs. Additive cough-suppressant effect with narcotic antitussives. Do not use within 14 days of MAOI therapy.

**PREGNANCY:** Category C, caution in nursing.



## ROSAC RX

sulfur - sulfacetamide sodium (Stiefel)

**THERAPEUTIC CLASS:** Sulfonamide/sulfur combination

**INDICATIONS:** Topical control of acne vulgaris, acne rosacea and seborrheic dermatitis.

**DOSAGE:** *Adults*: Apply a thin film qd-tid.
*Pediatrics:* ≥12 yrs: Apply a thin film qd-tid.

**HOW SUPPLIED:** Cre: (Sulfacetamide-Sulfur) 10%-5% [45g]

**CONTRAINDICATIONS:** Kidney disease.

**WARNINGS/PRECAUTIONS:** Discontinue if irritation or hypersensitivity reaction occurs. Avoid contact with eyes. Caution if denuded or abraded skin. May cause reddening and scaling of epidermis.

**ADVERSE REACTIONS:** Local irritation.

**PREGNANCY:** Category C, caution in nursing.

## ROSULA RX
sulfur - sulfacetamide sodium (Doak)

**THERAPEUTIC CLASS:** Sulfonamide/sulfur combination

**INDICATIONS:** Topical treatment of acne vulgaris, acne rosacea, and seborrheic dermatitis.

**DOSAGE:** *Adults:* (Gel) Apply thin film qd-tid. (Cleanser) Wash for 10-20 seconds qd-bid.
*Pediatrics:* >12 yrs: (Gel) Apply thin film qd-tid. (Cleanser) Wash for 10-20 seconds qd-bid.

**HOW SUPPLIED:** (Sulfacetamide-Sulfur) Gel: 10%-5% [45mL]; Cleanser: 10%-5% [355mL]

**CONTRAINDICATIONS:** Kidney disease.

**WARNINGS/PRECAUTIONS:** Discontinue if irritation or hypersensitivity reaction occurs. Avoid contact with eyes, lips, and mucous membranes. Caution with denuded or abraded skin. Can cause reddening and scaling of epidermis.

**ADVERSE REACTIONS:** Local irritation.

**PREGNANCY:** Category C, caution in nursing.

## ROSULA NS RX
urea - sulfacetamide sodium (Doak)

**THERAPEUTIC CLASS:** Sulfonamide

**INDICATIONS:** Topical treatment of bacterial infections of the skin including *P.acne* and seborrheic dermatitis.

**DOSAGE:** *Adults:* Apply to affected area qd-bid.
*Pediatrics:* ≥12 yrs: Apply to affected area qd-bid.

**HOW SUPPLIED:** Swab: (Sulfacetamide-Urea) 10%-10% [30s]

**CONTRAINDICATIONS:** Kidney disease

**WARNINGS/PRECAUTIONS:** Discontinue if irritation or hypersensitivity reaction occurs. Avoid contact with eyes, lips, and mucous membranes. Caution with denuded or abraded skin. Cases of Stevens-Johnson syndrome and drug-induced systemic lupus erythematosus have been reported.

**ADVERSE REACTIONS:** Local hypersensitivity, instances of Stevens-Johnson syndrome.



**INTERACTIONS:** Incompatible with silver preparations.

**PREGNANCY:** Category C, caution in nursing.

## ROTATEQ RX
rotavirus vaccine, live (Merck)

**THERAPEUTIC CLASS:** Vaccine

**INDICATIONS:** Prevention of rotavirus gastroenteritis in infants and children caused by the serotypes G1, G2, G3, and G4 when administered as a 3-dose series to infants between the ages of 6-32 weeks. The first dose should be administered between 6-12 weeks of age.

**DOSAGE:** *Pediatrics:* Administer series of 3 doses orally starting at 6-12 weeks of age, with subsequent doses administered at 4-10 week intervals. Third dose should not be given after 32 weeks of age. Do not mix with any other vaccines or solutions. Do not reconstitute or dilute.

**HOW SUPPLIED:** Sus: 2mL

**WARNINGS/PRECAUTIONS:** Consider delaying use with febrile illness. Vaccination may not result in complete protection in all recipients. May increase risk of intussusception.

**ADVERSE REACTIONS:** Bronchiolitis, gastroenteritis, pneumonia, fever, UTI.

**INTERACTIONS:** Immunosuppressive therapies including irradiation, antimetabolites, alkylating agents, cytotoxic drugs, and corticosteroids (used in greater than physiologic doses) may reduce the immune response to vaccines.

**PREGNANCY:** Safety in pregnancy and nursing not known.

## ROWASA

mesalamine (Solvay) RX

**THERAPEUTIC CLASS:** Anti-inflammatory agent

**INDICATIONS:** Treatment of active mild to moderate distal ulcerative colitis, proctosigmoiditis or proctitis.

**DOSAGE:** *Adults:* Use 1 enema rectally qhs for 3-6 weeks. Retain for 8 hrs. Empty bowel prior to administration.

**HOW SUPPLIED:** Enema: 4g/60mL

**WARNINGS/PRECAUTIONS:** Discontinue if acute intolerance syndrome develops (eg, cramping, bloody diarrhea, abdominal pain, headache); consider sulfasalazine hypersensitivity. If rechallenge is considered, perform under careful observation. Caution with sulfasalazine hypersensitivity. Carefully monitor with renal dysfunction. Contains potassium metabisulfite; caution with sulfite sensitivity especially in asthmatics. Pancolitis, pericarditis (rare) reported.

**ADVERSE REACTIONS:** Abdominal problems, headache, flatulence, flu, fever, nausea, malaise/fatigue.

**PREGNANCY:** Category B, not for use in nursing.

## ROXANOL

morphine sulfate (Xanodyne) CII

**Highly concentrated, check dose carefully.**

**OTHER BRAND NAMES:** Roxanol-T (Xanodyne)

**THERAPEUTIC CLASS:** Opioid analgesic

**INDICATIONS:** Relief of severe acute and chronic pain.

**DOSAGE:** *Adults:* Usual: 10-30mg q4h. During first effective pain relief, dose should be maintained for at least 3 days before any dose reduction, if respiratory activity and other vital signs are adequate. Elderly/Very Ill/Respiratory Problems/Severe Renal and Hepatic Impairment: Lower doses may be required.

**HOW SUPPLIED:** Sol, Concentrate: 20mg/mL (Roxanol) [30mL, 120mL, 240mL], (Roxanol-T) [30mL, 120mL]

**CONTRAINDICATIONS:** Respiratory insufficiency or depression, severe CNS depression, attack of bronchial asthma, heart failure secondary to chronic lung disease, cardiac arrhythmias, increased intracranial or cerebrospinal pressure, head injuries, brain tumor, acute alcoholism, delirium tremens, convulsive disorders, after biliary tract surgery, suspected surgical abdomen, surgical anastomosis, concomitantly with MAOIs or within 14 days of such treatment.

**WARNINGS/PRECAUTIONS:** May cause tolerance, psychological, and physical dependence; withdrawal may occur on abrupt discontinuation. Caution with head injury, increased intracranial pressure, acute asthmatic attack, COPD, cor pulmonale, decreased respiratory reserve, pre-existing respiratory depression, hypoxia, hypercapnia, elderly, debilitated, severe hepatic/renal impairment, hypothyroidism, Addison's disease, prostatic hypertrophy, or urethral stricture. May cause orthostatic hypotension in ambulatory patients, severe hypotension with depleted blood volume. May obscure diagnosis/clinical course of acute abdominal conditions. May impair mental/physical abilities.

**ADVERSE REACTIONS:** Respiratory depression, lightheadedness, dizziness, sedation, nausea, vomiting, sweating, constipation.

**INTERACTIONS:** See Contraindications. Potentiated by alkalizing agents and antagonized by acidifying agents. Analgesic effect potentiated by chlorpromazine, methocarbamol. Enhanced depressant effects with other CNS depressants such as anesthetics, hypnotics, barbiturates, phenothiazines, chloral hydrate, glutethimide, sedatives, MAOIs (eg, procarbazine), antihistamines, β-blockers (eg, propranolol), alcohol, furazolidone, other narcotics, tranquilizers, and TCAs. May increase anticoagulant activity of coumarin and other anticoagulants.

**PREGNANCY:** Category C, caution in nursing.

## ROXICET — CII

acetaminophen - oxycodone HCl (Roxane)

**THERAPEUTIC CLASS:** Opioid analgesic

**INDICATIONS:** Relief of moderate-to-moderately severe pain.

**DOSAGE:** *Adults:* Usual: 5/325 tab/sol or 5/500 tab q6h prn. Titrate: May need to exceed usual dose based on individual response, pain severity and tolerance.

**HOW SUPPLIED:** (Oxycodone-APAP) Sol: 5mg-325mg/5mL [5mL, 10$^s$; 500mL]; Tab: 5mg-325mg, 5mg-500mg

**WARNINGS/PRECAUTIONS:** May cause drug dependence and tolerance; potential for abuse. Risk of respiratory depression. Capacity to elevate CSF pressure may be exaggerated with head injury, other intracranial lesions or a pre-existing increase in intracranial pressure. May obscure the diagnosis or clinical course with head injuries or with acute abdominal conditions. Caution with severe hepatic impairment, renal dysfunction, hypothyroidism, Addison's disease, prostatic hypertrophy, urethral stricture, the elderly or debilitated.

**ADVERSE REACTIONS:** Lightheadedness, dizziness, sedation, nausea, vomiting, euphoria, dysphoria, constipation, skin rash, pruritus.

**INTERACTIONS:** Additive CNS depression with narcotic analgesics, general anesthetics, phenothiazines, tranquilizers, sedatives-hypnotics, alcohol, and other CNS depressants; reduce dose of one or both agents.

**PREGNANCY:** Category C, caution in nursing.



## ROXICODONE — CII

oxycodone HCl (aaiPharma)

**THERAPEUTIC CLASS:** Opioid analgesic

**INDICATIONS:** Relief of moderate-to-moderately severe pain.

**DOSAGE:** *Adults:* Initial: Opioid Naive: 5mg to 15mg q4-6h prn. Titrate: Based on individual response. For chronic pain or severe chronic pain, use around the clock dosing schedule at lowest effective dose.

**HOW SUPPLIED:** Sol: 5mg/5mL [5mL, 40$^s$; 500mL], (Intensol) 20mg/mL [30mL]; Tab: 5mg*, 15mg*, 30mg* *scored

**WARNINGS/PRECAUTIONS:** Potential for physical dependence. May markedly exaggerate respiratory depressant effects in head injuries and increased intracranial pressure. May mask symptoms of acute abdominal conditions. Caution with history of drug abuse, the elderly, debilitated, hypothyroidism, Addison's disease, BPH, urethral stricture, severe hepatic and renal impairment.

**ADVERSE REACTIONS:** Dizziness, sedation, nausea, vomiting, euphoria, dysphoria, constipation, skin rash, pruritus, headache, insomnia, asthenia, somnolence.

**INTERACTIONS:** Additive CNS depression with narcotic analgesics, phenothiazines, tranquilizers, sedative-hypnotics, alcohol, and other CNS depressants; reduce dose. Mixed agonist/antagonist analgesics may reduce analgesic effect and/or cause withdrawal. May enhance effect of neuromuscular blockers. Avoid within 14 days of MAOIs.

**PREGNANCY:** Category B, not for use in nursing.

## ROZEREM RX
ramelteon (Takeda)

**THERAPEUTIC CLASS:** Melatonin receptor agonist

**INDICATIONS:** Treatment of insomnia characterized by difficulty with sleep onset.

**DOSAGE:** *Adults:* 8mg within 30 minutes of bedtime. Do not take with or after high fat meal.

**HOW SUPPLIED:** Tab: 8mg

**WARNINGS/PRECAUTIONS:** Sleep disturbances may be presenting manifestations of a physical and/or psychiatric disorder, initiate therapy only after careful evaluation. Do not use in severe hepatic impairment. A variety of abnormal thinking and behavior changes have been reported to occur in association with the use of hypnotics. In primarily depressed patients, worsening of depression, including suicidal ideation, has been reported in association with the use of hypnotics. May impair physical/mental abilities. Not recommended in patients with severe sleep apnea or severe COPD. Caution with alcohol. May affect reproductive hormones.

**ADVERSE REACTIONS:** Headache, somnolence, fatigue, dizziness, nausea, exacerbated insomnia, upper respiratory tract infection.

**INTERACTIONS:** Do not use with strong CYP1A2 inhibitors (fluvoxamine). Decreased efficacy with strong CYP inducers (rifampin). Caution with less strong CYP1A2 inhibitors, strong CYP3A4 inhibitors (ketoconazole), strong CYP2C9 inhibitors (fluconazole). Additive effect with alcohol.

**PREGNANCY:** Category C, not for use in nursing.

## RYNATAN RX
phenylephrine tannate - chlorpheniramine tannate (MedPointe)

**THERAPEUTIC CLASS:** Antihistamine/sympathomimetic

**INDICATIONS:** Symptomatic relief of coryza and nasal congestion with the common cold, sinusitis, allergic rhinitis, and other upper respiratory tract conditions.

**DOSAGE:** *Adults:* 1-2 tabs q12h.

**HOW SUPPLIED:** Tab: (Chlorpheniramine-Phenylephrine) 9mg-25mg

**CONTRAINDICATIONS:** Newborns, nursing mothers.

**WARNINGS/PRECAUTIONS:** Caution with HTN, cardiovascular disease, hyperthyroidism, DM, narrow angle glaucoma, prostatic hypertrophy, and elderly. May impair mental alertness. May cause mild stimulation or sedation in children.

**ADVERSE REACTIONS:** Drowsiness, sedation, dryness of mucous membranes, GI effects.

**INTERACTIONS:** Increased anticholinergic and sympathomimetic effects with MAOIs; avoid during or within 14 days of use. Additive CNS effects with alcohol or other CNS depressants (eg, sedative, hypnotics, tranquilizers).

**PREGNANCY:** Category C, not for use in nursing.

## RYNATAN PEDIATRIC RX
phenylephrine tannate - chlorpheniramine tannate (MedPointe)

**THERAPEUTIC CLASS:** Antihistamine/sympathomimetic

**INDICATIONS:** Symptomatic relief of coryza and nasal congestion with the common cold, sinusitis, allergic rhinitis, and other upper respiratory tract conditions.

**DOSAGE:** *Pediatrics:* >6 yrs: 5-10mL q12h. 2 to 6 yrs: 2.5-5mL q12h. <2 yrs: Titrate individually.

**HOW SUPPLIED:** Sus: (Chlorpheniramine-Phenylephrine) 4.5mg-5mg/5mL

**CONTRAINDICATIONS:** Newborns and nursing mothers.

**WARNINGS/PRECAUTIONS:** Caution with HTN, cardiovascular disease, hyperthyroidism, DM, narrow angle glaucoma, prostatic hypertrophy, and elderly. May impair mental alertness. Contains tartrazine.

**ADVERSE REACTIONS:** Drowsiness, sedation, dryness of mucous membranes, GI effects.

**INTERACTIONS:** Increased anticholinergic and sympathomimetic effects with MAOIs; avoid during or within 14 days of use. Additive CNS effects with alcohol or other CNS depressants (eg, sedative-hypnotics, tranquilizers).

**PREGNANCY:** Category C, not for use in nursing.

## RYNATUSS RX
ephedrine tannate - phenylephrine tannate - carbetapentane tannate - chlorpheniramine tannate (MedPointe)

**OTHER BRAND NAMES:** Rynatuss Pediatric (MedPointe)

**THERAPEUTIC CLASS:** Antitussive/antihistamine/bronchodilator/ sympathomimetic combination

**INDICATIONS:** Symptomatic relief of cough associated with respiratory tract conditions such as the common cold, bronchial asthma, acute and chronic bronchitis.

**DOSAGE:** *Adults:* 1-2 tabs q12h.
*Pediatrics:* >6 yrs: 5-10mL q12h. 2-6 yrs: 2.5-5mL q12h.

**HOW SUPPLIED:** (Carbetapentane-Chlorpheniramine-Ephedrine-Phenylephrine) Sus: (Rynatuss Pediatric) 30mg-4mg-5mg-5mg/5mL [240mL 480mL]; Tab: (Rynatuss) 60mg-5mg-10mg-10mg* *scored

R

**CONTRAINDICATIONS:** Newborns, nursing mothers.

**WARNINGS/PRECAUTIONS:** Caution with HTN, cardiovascular disease, hyperthyroidism, DM, narrow angle glaucoma, elderly or prostatic hypertrophy. Suspension contains FD&C Yellow No. 5 which may cause allergic-type reactions.

**ADVERSE REACTIONS:** Drowsiness, sedation, dryness of mucous membranes, GI effects.

**INTERACTIONS:** Avoid MAOI use within 14 days. Additive CNS effects with alcohol or other CNS depressants.

**PREGNANCY:** Category C, not for use in nursing.

## RYTHMOL RX
propafenone HCl (Reliant)

**THERAPEUTIC CLASS:** Class IC antiarrhythmic

**INDICATIONS:** To prolong the time to recurrence of paroxysmal atrial fibrillation/flutter (PAF) and paroxysmal supraventricular tachycardia (PSVT)

associated with disabling symptoms in patients without structural heart disease. Treatment of life-threatening documented ventricular arrhythmias.

**DOSAGE:** *Adults:* Initial: 150mg q8h. Titrate: May increase at minimum 3-4 day intervals to 225mg q8h, then to 300mg q8h if needed. Max: 900mg/day. Elderly/Marked Myocardial Damage: Increase more gradually during initial phase. Hepatic Dysfunction: Reduce dose by 20-30%.

**HOW SUPPLIED:** Tab: 150mg*, 225mg*, 300mg* *scored

**CONTRAINDICATIONS:** Uncontrolled CHF, cardiogenic shock, bradycardia, marked hypotension, bronchospastic disorders, electrolyte imbalance, and sinoatrial, atrioventricular (AV) and intraventricular disorders of impulse generation and/or conduction (eg, sick sinus node syndrome, AV block) in the absence of an artificial pacemaker.

**WARNINGS/PRECAUTIONS:** Avoid with non-life-threatening ventricular arrhythmias, bronchospastic disorders. May cause new or worsened arrhythmias. Caution with hepatic or renal dysfunction. Slows AV conduction and causes 1st-degree AV block. D/C if CHF worsens. Agranulocytosis, myasthenia gravis exacerbation, positive ANA titers reported. May alter pacing and sensing thresholds of artificial pacemakers.

**ADVERSE REACTIONS:** Taste disturbances, nausea, vomiting, dizziness, constipation, headache, fatigue, blurred vision, blood dyscrasias.

**INTERACTIONS:** Avoid quinidine. Local anesthetics may increase CNS side effects. Increases levels of cyclosporine, theophylline, desipramine, digoxin, β-blockers, warfarin. Cimetidine increases plasma levels. Decreased effects with rifampin.

**PREGNANCY:** Category C, not for use in nursing.

## RYTHMOL SR

propafenone HCl (Reliant)

RX

**THERAPEUTIC CLASS:** Class IC antiarrhythmic

**INDICATIONS:** To prolong the time to recurrence of symptomatic atrial fibrillation in patients without structural heart disease.

**DOSAGE:** *Adults:* Initial: 225mg q12h. Titrate: May increase at minimum 5 day intervals to 325mg q12h, then to 425mg q12h if needed. Hepatic Impairment/QRS Widening/2nd- or 3rd-degree AV Block: Reduce dose.

**HOW SUPPLIED:** Cap, Extended Release: 225mg, 325mg, 425mg

**CONTRAINDICATIONS:** CHF, cardiogenic shock, bradycardia, marked hypotension, bronchospastic disorders, electrolyte imbalance, and sinoatrial, atrioventricular (AV) and intraventricular disorders of impulse generation or conduction (eg, sick sinus node syndrome, AV block) unless paced.

**WARNINGS/PRECAUTIONS:** Avoid with non-life-threatening ventricular arrhythmias, bronchospastic disease, AV and intraventricular conduction defects unless paced. May cause new or worsened arrhythmias, provoke overt CHF. Caution with hepatic or renal dysfunction. 1st-degree AV block, agranulocytosis, myasthenia gravis exacerbation, positive ANA titers reported. May alter pacing and sensing thresholds of artificial pacemakers.

**ADVERSE REACTIONS:** Dizziness, chest pain, palpitations, taste disturbance, dyspnea, nausea, constipation, anxiety, fatigue, upper respiratory tract infection, influenza, 1st-degree heart block, vomiting.

**INTERACTIONS:** Avoid with drugs that prolong QT interval (eg, some phenothiazines, cisapride, bepridil, TCAs, oral macrolides, other antiarrhythmics), Class Ia and III antiarrhythmics (eg, quinidine, amiodarone). CYP2D6, CYP1A2, CYP3A4 inhibitors may increase levels. Local anesthetics may increase CNS side effects. Increases levels of cyclosporine, theophylline, desipramine, digoxin, β-blockers, warfarin. Cimetidine increases plasma levels. Decreased effects with rifampin.

**PREGNANCY:** Category C, caution in nursing.

## SAIZEN
somatropin (Serono)

RX

**THERAPEUTIC CLASS:** Human growth hormone

**INDICATIONS:** Long-term treatment of children with growth failure due to inadequate secretion of endogenous growth hormone. For replacement of endogenous growth hormone in adults who have growth hormone deficiency either alone, or associated with multiple hormone deficiencies, as a result of pituitary disease, hypothalamic disease, surgery, radiation therapy or trauma; or in patients who were growth hormone deficient during childhood as a result of congenital, genetic, acquired or idiopathic causes.

**DOSAGE:** *Adults:* Initial: ≤0.005mg/kg/day SQ. Titrate: May increase after 4 weeks to ≤0.01mg/kg/day depending on patient tolerance. Without Consideration of Body Weight: Initial: 0.2mg/day (0.15-0.3mg/day) SQ. Titrate: May increase by increments of 0.1-0.2mg/day every 1-2 months. Consider dose reduction in elderly.
*Pediatrics:* Individualize dose. Usual: 0.06mg/kg IM/SQ 3x/week. If epiphyses are fused, d/c therapy.

**HOW SUPPLIED:** Inj: 4mg, 5mg, 8.8mg

**CONTRAINDICATIONS:** Acute critical illness due to complications following open heart or abdominal surgery, accidental trauma or acute respiratory failure. Active proliferative or severe non-proliferative diabetic retinopathy. Active malignancy, or evidence of progression or recurrence of intracranial tumor. Prader-Willi syndrome when severely obese or have severe respiratory impairment, and in pediatric patients with closed epiphyses. Avoid reconstitution with bacteriostatic water if sensitive to benzyl alcohol.

**WARNINGS/PRECAUTIONS:** See Contraindications. Benzyl alcohol associated with toxicity in newborns; if sensitivity occurs, may reconstitute with SWFI. Insulin resistance reported; use caution with DM or family history of DM. Hypothyroidism may occur; bone maturation should be carefully followed. Increased incidence of slipped capital femoral epiphysis may develop with endocrine disorders; monitor for limping or hip/knee pain. Intracranial hypertension (IH) reported; d/c treatment if papilledema observed. Patients with Turner syndrome, chronic renal insufficiency or Prader-Willi syndrome may have increased risk for IH. If idiopathic IH confirmed, may restart therapy at lower dose after signs/symptoms resolve. Alternate injection sites to reduce development of tissue atrophy. Monitor for any malignant transformation of skin lesions.

**ADVERSE REACTIONS:** Arthalgia, headache, influenza-like symptoms, peripheral edema, back pain, myalgia, rhinitis, dizziness, upper respiratory tract infection, paraesthesia, hypoaesthesia, insomnia, nausea, generalized edema, depression.



**INTERACTIONS:** Diminished effects with concomitant glucocorticoid; adjust dose of accordingly. May alter clearance of CYP450 substrates (eg, corticosteroids, sex steroids, anticonvulsants, cyclosporine). May increase dose if taking oral estrogen replacement concomitantly. Adjust dose of insulin/oral antidiabetics when initiating therapy.

**PREGNANCY:** Category B, caution in nursing.

## SALAGEN
pilocarpine HCl (MGI Pharma)

RX

**THERAPEUTIC CLASS:** Cholinergic agonist

**INDICATIONS:** Treatment of dry mouth in Sjogren's syndrome, or from salivary gland hypofunction caused by radiotherapy for head and neck cancer.

**DOSAGE:** *Adults:* Cancer Patients: Initial: 5mg tid. Usual: 15-30mg/day for 12 weeks. Max: 10mg/dose. Sjogren's Syndrome: Usual: 5mg qid for 6 weeks.

**HOW SUPPLIED:** Tab: 5mg, 7.5mg

**CONTRAINDICATIONS:** Uncontrolled asthma, when miosis is undesirable (eg, acute iritis, narrow-angle glaucoma).

**WARNINGS/PRECAUTIONS:** Caution with significant cardiovascular disease, night driving, performing hazardous activities in reduced lighting, cholelithiasis, biliary tract disease, controlled asthma, chronic bronchitis, or COPD requiring pharmacotherapy. Monitor for toxicity and dehydration. May cause renal colic. Possible dose-related CNS effects

**ADVERSE REACTIONS:** Sweating, nausea, rhinitis, diarrhea, chills, flushing, urinary frequency, dizziness, asthenia, headache, dyspepsia, lacrimation, edema, amblyopia, vomiting, pharyngitis, HTN.

**INTERACTIONS:** Caution with β-adrenergic antagonists. May antagonize anticholinergic agents. Possible additive effects with parasympathomimetics.

**PREGNANCY:** Category C, not for use in nursing.

## SALFLEX RX
salsalate (Amarin)

**THERAPEUTIC CLASS:** Salicylate

**INDICATIONS:** Management of rheumatoid arthritis, osteoarthritis, and other rheumatic disorders.

**DOSAGE:** *Adults:* Usual: 1000mg tid or 1500mg bid.

**HOW SUPPLIED:** Tab: 500mg, 750mg* *scored

**WARNINGS/PRECAUTIONS:** Competes with thyroid hormone for binding to plasma proteins. Reye's syndrome may develop in viral infections (eg, chickenpox, influenza). Caution in chronic renal impairment and peptic ulcer. Bronchospasm reported with ASA-sensitivity. Monitor salicylic acid levels and urinary pH periodically with long-term therapy.

**ADVERSE REACTIONS:** Tinnitus, nausea, heartburn, rash, vertigo, hearing impairment.

**INTERACTIONS:** Avoid other salicylates. Antagonizes uricosuric agents. Decreased effects with agents that increase urinary pH. Potentiated by urinary acidifiers. Potential bleeding may occur with anticoagulants. Potentiates sulfonylureas. Competes for protein binding with methotrexate, corticosteroids, thyroxine, triiodothyronine, thiopental, sulfinpyrazone, phenytoin, naproxen, warfarin, and penicillin. Food slows absorption.

**PREGNANCY:** Category C, caution in nursing.

## SANCTURA RX
trospium chloride (Esprit)

S

**THERAPEUTIC CLASS:** Muscarinic antagonist

**INDICATIONS:** Overactive bladder with symptoms of urge urinary incontinence, urgency, and urinary frequency.

**DOSAGE:** *Adults:* 20mg bid. Take at least one hour before meals or on an empty stomach. CrCl <30mL/min: 20mg qhs. Elderly ≥75 yrs: May titrate to 20mg qd based upon tolerability.

**HOW SUPPLIED:** Tab: 20mg (14[s], 60[s])

**CONTRAINDICATIONS:** Active or risk of urinary retention, gastric retention, uncontrolled narrow-angle glaucoma.

**WARNINGS/PRECAUTIONS:** Caution with significant bladder outflow obstruction, GI obstructive disorders, ulcerative colitis, intestinal atony, myasthenia gravis, moderate or severe hepatic dysfunction. Reduce dose with severe renal insufficiency. Consider risks vs benefits with controlled narrow-angle glaucoma.

**ADVERSE REACTIONS:** Dry mouth, constipation, headache, rash.

**INTERACTIONS:** Increased adverse effects with other anticholinergics. May alter GI absorption of other drugs due to GI motility effects. Monitor closely with other drugs eliminated by active renal tubular secretion (eg, digoxin, procainamide, pancuronium, morphine, vancomycin, metformin, tenofovir).

**PREGNANCY:** Category C, caution in nursing.

## SANDIMMUNE

cyclosporine (Novartis)

RX

**Give with adrenal corticosteroids but not with other immunosuppressives. Increased susceptibility to infection and development of lymphoma. Sandimmune and Neoral are not bioequivalent. Monitor blood levels to avoid toxicity.**

**THERAPEUTIC CLASS:** Cyclic polypeptide immunosuppressant

**INDICATIONS:** Prophylaxis of organ rejection in kidney, liver, and heart allogeneic transplants with concomitant adrenal corticosteroids. Treatment of chronic rejection in patients previously treated with other immunosuppressives.

**DOSAGE:** *Adults:* Initial: PO: 15mg/kg single dose 4-12 hrs before transplant; continue same dose qd for 1-2 weeks. Usual: Taper by 5% per week until 5-10mg/kg/day. May mix oral solution with milk, chocolate milk, or orange juice. IV: 1/3 PO dose. Initial: 5-6mg/kg/day single dose; begin 4 to 12 hrs prior to transplantation. Maint: Continue single daily dose until PO forms are tolerated. Due to risk of anaphylaxis, only use injection if unable to take oral agents. *Pediatrics:* Initial: PO: 15mg/kg single dose 4-12 hrs before transplant; continue same dose qd for 1-2 weeks. Usual: Taper by 5% per week until 5-10mg/kg/day. May mix oral solution with milk, chocolate milk, or orange juice. IV: 1/3 PO dose. Initial: 5-6mg/kg/day single dose; begin 4 to 12 hrs prior to transplantation. Maint: Continue single daily dose until PO forms are tolerated. Due to risk of anaphylaxis, only use injection if unable to take oral agents.

**HOW SUPPLIED:** Cap: 25mg, 100mg; Inj: 50mg/mL; Sol: 100mg/mL [50mL]

**CONTRAINDICATIONS:** Hypersensitivity to Cremophor EL (polyoxyethylated castor oil).

**WARNINGS/PRECAUTIONS:** May cause hepatotoxicity and nephrotoxicity. Convulsions, elevated serum creatinine, and BUN levels reported. Thrombocytopenia and microangiopathic hemolytic anemia may develop. Monitor for hyperkalemia. Increases risk for development of lymphomas and other malignancies. Observe for 30 minutes after the start of infusion and frequently thereafter. Caution with malabsorption.



**ADVERSE REACTIONS:** Renal dysfunction, tremor, hirsutism, HTN, gum hyperplasia, HTN, glomerular capillary thrombosis, cramps, acne, convulsions, headache, diarrhea, hepatotoxity, abdominal discomfort, paresthesia, flushing.

**INTERACTIONS:** Ciprofloxacin, gentamicin, tobramycin, vancomycin, SMZ/TMP, amphotericin B, ketoconazole, melphalan, diclofenac, azapropazon, sulindac, naproxen, colchicine, cimetidine, ranitidine, tacrolimus, bezafirate, fenofibrate may potentiate renal dysfunction. Diltiazem, nicardipine, colchicine, fluconazole, itraconazole, ketoconazole, verapamil, azithromycin, clarithromycin, erythromycin, quinupristin/dalfopristin, allopurinol, amiodarone, bromocriptine, danazol, imatinib, metoclopramide, oral contraceptives, HIV protease inhibitors may increase levels. St. John's wort, grapefruit juice, carbamazepine, phenobarbital, phenytoin, rifampin, sulfinpyrazone, octreotide, orlistat, terbinafine, ticlopidine, and naficillin may decrease levels. Avoid with potassium-sparing diuretics. Caution with ACEIs, angiotensin II blockers, NSAIDs. Digitalis toxicity reported. Myotoxicity with statins, frequent gingival hyperplasia with nifedipine, and convulsions with high dose methylprednisolone reported. Increased levels of sirolimus; give 4 hrs after cyclosporine. Avoid live vaccines during therapy.

**PREGNANCY:** Category C, not for use in nursing.

## SANDOSTATIN RX

octreotide acetate (Novartis)

**THERAPEUTIC CLASS:** Somatostatin analog

**INDICATIONS:** To reduce blood levels of growth hormone and IGF-I in acromegaly inadequately responding to or cannot be treated with surgical resection, pituitary irradiation, and maximum dose bromocriptine mesylate. Symptomatic treatment of metastatic carcinoid tumors, where it suppresses or inhibits severe diarrhea and flushing episodes. Treatment of profuse watery diarrhea associated with VIP (Vasoactive Intestinal Peptide)-secreting tumors.

**DOSAGE:** *Adults:* Give SQ/IV. Acromegaly: Initial: 50mcg tid. Titrate: Adjust dose based on IGF-I levels every 2 weeks. Usual: 100mcg tid. Max: 500mcg tid. Reduce dose if no additional benefit with dose increase. Re-evaluate IGF-I or growth hormone levels every 6 months. Withdraw yearly for 4 weeks to assess disease activity after irradiation. Carcinoid Tumors: Initial: 100-600mcg/day given bid-qid (mean dose 300mcg/day) for 2 weeks. Max: 750mcg/day. VIPomas: Initial: 200-300mcg/day (range 150-750mcg) given bid-qid for 2 weeks. Max: 450mcg/day.

**HOW SUPPLIED:** Inj: 50mcg/mL, 100mcg/mL, 200mcg/mL, 500mcg/mL, 1000mcg/mL

**WARNINGS/PRECAUTIONS:** May inhibit gallbladder contractility and decrease bile secretions; increased risk of gallstones. May alter balance between insulin, glucagon, and growth hormone and lead to hypoglycemia or hyperglycemia. Hypothyroidism may result due to TSH suppression; monitor thyroid function at baseline and periodically. Cardiac conduction and other cardiovascular abnormalities may occur. Pancreatitis reported. Depressed vitamin $B_{12}$ levels and abnormal Schilling's test reported. May need dose adjustment in renal failure.

**ADVERSE REACTIONS:** Gallbladder and cardiac abnormalities, diarrhea, nausea, vomiting, abdominal distention, flatulence, constipation, headache, dizziness, hypo- and hyperglycemia, hyperthyroidism.

**INTERACTIONS:** May decrease cyclosporine effects. May need dose adjustments of insulin, oral hypoglycemics, β-blockers, calcium channel blockers, or agents that control fluid and electrolyte balance. Not compatible in TPN solutions. Increased availability of bromocriptine.

**PREGNANCY:** Category B, caution in nursing.

## SANDOSTATIN LAR RX

octreotide acetate (Novartis)



**THERAPEUTIC CLASS:** Somatostatin analog

**INDICATIONS:** Maintenance therapy of acromegaly. Long-term treatment of severe diarrhea and flushing associated with metastatic carcinoid tumors. Long-term treatment of profuse watery diarrhea associated with VIP (Vasoactive Intestinal Peptide)-secreting tumors. Use in patients who have responded to and tolerated Sandostatin Injection.

**DOSAGE:** *Adults:* Administer intragluteally. Acromegaly: Initial: 20mg IM every 4 weeks for 3 months. Titrate: If GH <2.5ng/mL, IGF-1 normal, and clinical symptoms controlled then maintain dose. If GH >2.5, IGF-1 elevated, and/or clinical symptoms uncontrolled then increase to 30mg every 4 weeks. If GH <1, IGF-1 normal, and clinical symptoms controlled then reduce to 10mg every 4 weeks. Max: 40mg every 4 weeks. Withdraw yearly for 8 weeks to assess disease activity after pituitary irradiation. Carcinoid Tumors/VIPomas: Initial: 20mg IM every 4 weeks for 2 months. Continue with Sandostatin® injection SQ for at least 2 weeks. Titrate: If symptoms not controlled, increase to 30mg every 4 weeks. If symptoms controlled at 20mg, reduce to 10mg. Max: 30mg every 4 weeks. For exacerbation of symptoms, give Sandostatin Injection SQ. for at least 2 weeks. Patients must be considered responders and tolerate the injection before switching to the depot. Renal Failure Requiring Dialysis: Reduce dose.

**HOW SUPPLIED:** Inj, Depot: 10mg, 20mg, 30mg

**WARNINGS/PRECAUTIONS:** May inhibit gallbladder contractility and decrease bile secretions; increased risk of gallstones. May alter balance between insulin, glucagon and growth hormone and lead to hypoglycemia or hyperglycemia. Hypothyroidism may result due to TSH suppression; monitor thyroid function at baseline and periodically. Cardiac conduction and other cardiovascular abnormalities may occur. Monitor zinc levels periodically with TPNs. Pancreatitis reported. Depressed vitamin $B_{12}$ levels and abnormal Schilling's test reported. May need dose adjustment in renal failure.

**ADVERSE REACTIONS:** Diarrhea, nausea, vomiting, abdominal discomfort, flatulence, constipation, hyperglycemia, injection site pain, upper respiratory infection, flu-like symptoms, fatigue, dizziness, headache, malaise, fever.

**INTERACTIONS:** May decrease cyclosporine levels. May need dose adjustments of insulin, oral hypoglycemics, β-blockers, calcium channel blockers, or agents that control fluid and electrolyte balance. May increase availability of bromocriptine. Caution with drugs that have a low therapeutic index and metabolized by CYP3A4 (eg, quinidine, terfenadine).

**PREGNANCY:** Category B, caution in nursing.

## SARAFEM

RX

fluoxetine HCl (Warner Chilcott/Lilly)

> **Antidepressants increased the risk of suicidal thinking and behavior (suicidality) in short-term studies in children and adolescents with Major Depressive Disorder (MDD) and other psychiatric disorders. Sarafem is not approved for use in pediatric patients.**

**THERAPEUTIC CLASS:** Selective serotonin reuptake inhibitor

**INDICATIONS:** Treatment of premenstrual dysphoric disorder.

**DOSAGE:** *Adults:* Continuous: Initial: 20mg qd. Maint: 20mg/day up to 6 months. Max: 60mg/day. Intermittent: Initial: 20mg qd; start 14 days before menses onset through 1st full day of menses. Maint: 20mg/day up to 3 months. Max: 60mg/day. Hepatic Impairment/Concurrent Disease/Concomitant Medications: Lower dose or less frequent dosing.

**HOW SUPPLIED:** Cap: 10mg, 20mg

**CONTRAINDICATIONS:** During or within 14 days of MAOI therapy. During or within 5 weeks of thioridazine use. Concurrent use with pimozide.



**WARNINGS/PRECAUTIONS:** Vasculitis reported. D/C if rash or allergic reaction develops. May impair thinking, judgment, or motor skills. May alter glycemic control. Changes in weight and appetite reported. Caution with cirrhosis.

**ADVERSE REACTIONS:** Chest pain, chills, hemorrhage, HTN, increased appetite, nausea, vomiting, anxiety, weight gain, agitation, amnesia, confusion, emotional lability, sleep disorder, taste perversion.

**INTERACTIONS:** See Contraindications. May increase benzodiazepine, thioridazine, TCAs, haloperidol, clozapine, phenytoin, and carbamazepine levels. Lithium levels may increase/decrease. Do not use with or within 14 days of MAOIs. May shift concentrations with plasma-bound drugs (eg, coumadin, digitoxin).

**PREGNANCY:** Category C, not for use in nursing.

## SCULPTRA RX
poly-l-lactic acid (Dermik)

**THERAPEUTIC CLASS:** Injectable implant

**INDICATIONS:** Restoration and/or correction of the signs of facial fat loss (lipoatrophy) in people with HIV.

**DOSAGE:** *Adults:* Reconstitute with 3-5mL of SWFI. Wait at least 2 hrs; agitate until uniform translucent suspension obtained. Inject into deep dermis or SC layer of skin using 26 G sterile needle. Limit to 0.1-0.2mL per injection; may require about 20 injections to cover target area. Use within 72 hrs of reconstitution.

**HOW SUPPLIED:** Inj: [3mL]

**WARNINGS/PRECAUTIONS:** Avoid with active skin inflammation or infection in/near target area. Injection procedure reactions reported. Should not be introduced into vasculature; may cause infarction or embolism. Use in deep dermis or SC layer; avoid superficial injections.

**ADVERSE REACTIONS:** Bruising, edema, discomfort, hematoma, inflammation, erythema, injection site SC papule.

**PREGNANCY:** Safety in pregnancy and nursing is not known.

## SEASONALE RX
levonorgestrel - ethinyl estradiol (Duramed)

**THERAPEUTIC CLASS:** Estrogen/progestogen combination

**INDICATIONS:** Prevention of pregnancy.

**DOSAGE:** Sunday start regimen. 1 tablet qd for 91 days, then repeat.

**HOW SUPPLIED:** (Ethinyl Estradiol-Levonorgestrel) Tab: 0.03mg/0.15mg

**CONTRAINDICATIONS:** Thrombophlebitis, DVT or thromboembolic disorders, pregnancy, cerebrovascular or CAD, valvular heart disease with complications, uncontrolled HTN, DM with vascular involvement, headaches with focal neurological symptoms, major surgery with prolonged immobilization, undiagnosed abnormal genital bleeding, cholestatic jaundice of pregnancy or jaundice with prior pill use, hepatic adenomas or carcinomas, active liver disease, breast cancer, endometrial carcinoma, or other estrogen-dependent neoplasia.

**WARNINGS/PRECAUTIONS:** Cigarette smoking increases risk of serious CV side effects. This risk increases with age (especially >35 yrs) and heavy smoking. Increased risk of MI, vascular disease, thromboembolism, stroke, HTN, and gallbladder disease. Retinal thrombosis, hepatic neoplasia, carcinoma of breast and reproductive organs reported. May cause glucose intolerance, fluid retention, breakthrough bleeding, and spotting. May increase BP, elevate LDL levels or cause other lipid changes. May cause or exacerbate migraine. May develop visual changes with contact lens. Increased risk of morbidity and mortality with certain inherited thrombophilias, HTN, hyperlipidemia, obesity, and diabetes. D/C if jaundice, significant depression, recurrent/persistent new headache patterns, or ophthalmic irregularities develop. Perform annual physical exam. Not for use before menarche or with uncontrolled HTN. May affect certain endocrine, LFTs, and blood components. Weigh benefit of fewer planned menses against inconvenience of increased intermenstrual bleeding or spotting.

**ADVERSE REACTIONS:** Nausea, vomiting, breakthrough bleeding, spotting, amenorrhea, migraine, depression, vaginal candidiasis, edema, weight changes.

**INTERACTIONS:** Reduced effects, increased breakthrough bleeding with rifampin, barbiturates, phenylbutazone, phenytoin, carbamazepine, felbamate, oxcarbazepine, griseofulvin, topiramate, St. John's wort, and possibly with ampicillin and tetracyclines. Atorvastatin, ascorbic acid, acetaminophen,

CYP3A4 inhibitors (eg, itraconazole, ketoconazole) may increase hormone levels. Protease inhibitors may increase or decrease levels. May increase levels of cyclosporine, prednisolone, theophylline. May decrease levels of acetaminophen. Increases clearance of temazepam, salicylic acid, morphine, clofibric acid.

**PREGNANCY:** Category X, not for use in nursing.

## SEASONIQUE

RX

levonorgestrel - ethinyl estradiol (Duramed)

**THERAPEUTIC CLASS:** Estrogen/progestogen combination

**INDICATIONS:** Prevention of pregnancy.

**DOSAGE:** *Adults*: 1 tablet qd for 91 days, then repeat. During first cycle of medication, start on 1st Sunday after onset of menstruation. Begin next and all subsequent 91-day courses without interruption on same day of week (Sunday) upon which first course began, following the same schedule.

**HOW SUPPLIED:** (Ethinyl Estradiol-Levonorgestrel) Tab: 0.03mg-0.15mg; (Ethinyl Estradiol) Tab: 0.01mg

**CONTRAINDICATIONS:** Thrombophlebitis, DVT or thromboembolic disorders, cerebrovascular or CAD, valvular heart disease with thrombogenic complications, uncontrolled HTN, DM with vascular involvement, headaches with focal neurological symptoms, major surgery with prolonged immobilization, breast cancer, endometrial cancer or other estrogen-dependent neoplasia, undiagnosed abnormal genital bleeding, cholestatic jaundice of pregnancy or jaundice with prior pill use, hepatic adenomas or carcinomas, active liver disease, or pregnancy.

**WARNINGS/PRECAUTIONS:** Cigarette smoking increases risk of serious CV side effects. This risk increases with age (especially >35 yrs) and heavy smoking. Increased risk of MI, vascular disease, thromboembolism, stroke, HTN, and gallbladder disease. Retinal thrombosis, hepatic neoplasia, carcinoma of breast and reproductive organs reported. May cause glucose intolerance, fluid retention, breakthrough bleeding, and spotting. May increase BP, elevate LDL levels or cause other lipid changes. May cause or exacerbate migraine. May develop visual changes with contact lens. Increased risk of morbidity and mortality with certain inherited thrombophilias, HTN, hyperlipidemia, obesity, and diabetes. D/C if jaundice, significant depression, recurrent/persistent new headache patterns, or ophthalmic irregularities develop. Perform annual physical exam. Not for use before menarche or with uncontrolled HTN. May affect certain endocrine, LFTs, and blood components. Weigh benefit of fewer planned menses against inconvenience of increased intermenstrual bleeding or spotting.



**ADVERSE REACTIONS:** Nausea, vomiting, breakthrough bleeding, spotting, amenorrhea, migraine, depression, vaginal candidiasis, edema, weight changes.

**INTERACTIONS:** Reduced effects, increased breakthrough bleeding, and menstrual irregularities with rifampin, barbiturates, phenylbutazone, phenytoin, carbamazepine, felbamate, oxcarbazepine, topiramate, hypericum perforatum, griseofulvin, ampicillin, and tetracyclines. Increased levels with atorvastatin, ascorbic acid, APAP, and CYP3A4 (eg, itraconazole, ketoconazole) inhibitors. Anti-HIV protease inhibitors may increase or decrease levels. May increase plasma levels of cyclosporine, prednisolone, and theophylline. May decrease levels of APAP. Increased clearance of temazepam, salicylic acid, morphine, and clofibric acid.

**PREGNANCY:** Category X, not for use in nursing.

## SECONAL SODIUM

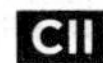


secobarbital sodium (Ranbaxy)

**THERAPEUTIC CLASS:** Barbiturate

**INDICATIONS:** Hypnotic, for the short-term treatment of insomnia (may lose effectiveness after 2 weeks); Preanesthetic.

**DOSAGE:** *Adults:* Hypnotic: 100mg hs; Preoperatively: 200-300mg, 1-2 hrs before surgery; Elderly/Debilitated/Renal or Hepatic Dysfunction: Reduce dose.
*Pediatrics:* Preoperatively: 2-6mg/kg. Max: 100mg.

**HOW SUPPLIED:** Cap: 100mg

**CONTRAINDICATIONS:** History of manifest or latent porphyria, marked impairment of liver function, or respiratory disease in which dyspnea or obstruction is evident.

**WARNINGS/PRECAUTIONS:** May be habit-forming; avoid abrupt cessation after prolonged use. Tolerance, psychological and physical dependence may occur with continued use. Use with caution, if at all, in patients who are mentally depressed, have suicidal tendencies, or have a history of drug abuse. In patients with hepatic damage, use with caution and initially reduce dose. Caution when administering to patients with acute or chronic pain. May impair mental and/or physical abilities. Avoid alcohol.

**ADVERSE REACTIONS:** Agitation, confusion, hyperkinesia, ataxia, CNS depression, somnolence, bradycardia, hypotension, nausea, vomiting, constipation, headache, hypersensitivity reactions, liver damage.

**INTERACTIONS:** May increase metabolism and decrease response to oral anticoagulants and enhance metabolism of exogenous corticosteroids. May interfere with absorption of griseofulvin, decreasing its blood level. May shorten half-life of doxycycline for up to 2 weeks after being discontinued. Variable effect on phenytoin and increased levels with sodium valproate and valproic acid; monitor blood levels and adjust dose appropriately. May cause additive depressant effects with other CNS depressants (eg, sedatives/hypnotics, antihistamines, tranquilizers, alcohol). Prolonged effects with MAOIs. May decrease effect of estradiol; alternative contraceptive methods should be suggested.

**PREGNANCY:** Category D, caution in nursing.

## SECTRAL

RX

acebutolol HCl (ESP Pharma)

**THERAPEUTIC CLASS:** Selective beta$_1$-blocker

**INDICATIONS:** Management of hypertension, ventricular arrhythmias.

**DOSAGE:** *Adults:* HTN: Initial: 400mg/day, given qd-bid. Usual: 200-800mg/day. Max: 1200mg/day. Ventricular Arrhythmia: Initial: 200mg bid. Maint: Increase gradually to 600-1200mg/day. Elderly: Lower daily doses. Max: 800mg/day. CrCl <50mL/min: Decrease daily dose by 50%. CrCl <25mL/min: Decrease daily dose by 75%.

**HOW SUPPLIED:** Cap: 200mg, 400mg

**CONTRAINDICATIONS:** Persistently severe bradycardia, 2nd- and 3rd-degree heart block, overt cardiac failure, cardiogenic shock.

**WARNINGS/PRECAUTIONS:** Withdrawal before surgery is controversial. Caution with bronchospastic disease, peripheral or mesenteric vascular disease, aortic or mitral valve disease, left ventricular dysfunction, heart failure controlled by digitalis and/or diuretics, hepatic or renal dysfunction. May mask hypoglycemia or hyperthyroidism symptoms. Avoid abrupt discontinuation. May develop antinuclear antibodies (ANA).

**ADVERSE REACTIONS:** Fatigue, dizziness, headache, constipation, diarrhea, dyspepsia, flatulence, nausea, dyspnea, urinary frequency, insomnia.

S

**INTERACTIONS:** Possible additive effects with catecholamine-depleting drugs. NSAIDs may reduce effects. Exaggerated hypertensive responses with alpha stimulants. May antagonize epinephrine. May potentiate insulin-induced hypoglycemia.

**PREGNANCY:** Category B, not for use in nursing.

## SELSUN RX — RX

selenium sulfide (Ross)

**THERAPEUTIC CLASS:** Antiseborrheic/antifungal

**INDICATIONS:** Treatment of tinea versicolor, seborrheic dermatitis of the scalp, and dandruff.

**DOSAGE:** *Adults:* Tinea Versicolor: Apply qd and lather with small amount of water. Rinse off after 10 minutes. Use for 7 days. Seborrheic Dermatitis/Dandruff: Massage into wet scalp, rinse off after 2-3 minutes and repeat. Usual: 2 applications/week for 2 weeks. Maint: Use weekly, every 2 weeks, or every 3-4 weeks.

**HOW SUPPLIED:** Lot: 2.5% [120mL]

**WARNINGS/PRECAUTIONS:** Avoid with inflammation, exudation, or broken skin. Avoid eyes, genital area, and skinfolds; may cause irritation. Not for treatment of tinea versicolor in pregnant women.

**ADVERSE REACTIONS:** Skin irritation, increased loss of hair, hair discoloration, oiliness or dryness of scalp.

**PREGNANCY:** Category C, safety in nursing is not known.

## SEMPREX-D — RX

acrivastine - pseudoephedrine HCl (Celltech)

**THERAPEUTIC CLASS:** Antihistamine/decongestant

**INDICATIONS:** Relief of symptoms associated with seasonal allergic rhinitis.

**DOSAGE:** *Adults:* 1 cap q4-6h, qid.
*Pediatrics:* >12 yrs: 1 cap q4-6h, qid.

**HOW SUPPLIED:** Cap: (Acrivastine-Pseudoephedrine) 8mg-60mg

**CONTRAINDICATIONS:** Severe HTN, CAD, MAOIs during or within 14 days of use. Hypersensitivity to alkylamine antihistamines.

**WARNINGS/PRECAUTIONS:** Not for use >14 days. Caution with HTN, DM, increased IOP, ischemic heart disease, hyperthyroidism, BPH, renal impairment, peptic ulcer, pyloroduodenal obstruction, and elderly. Sedation reported. Avoid with CrCl <48mL/min.



**ADVERSE REACTIONS:** Somnolence, headache, dry mouth, insomnia, dizziness, nervousness.

**INTERACTIONS:** MAOIs and β-agonists increase effects of sympathomimetics; avoid use during or within 14 days of MAOIs. Increased sedation with CNS depressants, alcohol.

**PREGNANCY:** Category B, caution in nursing.

## SENOKOT — OTC

senna (Purdue Products)

**THERAPEUTIC CLASS:** Stimulant laxative

**INDICATIONS:** To relieve functional constipation. Senokot-S also contains a stool softener.

**DOSAGE:** *Adults:* Take at bedtime. (Senokot/Senokot-S) 2 tabs qd. Max: 4 tabs bid. (SenokotXTRA) 1 tab qd. Max: 2 tabs bid. (Granules) 5mL qd. Max:

15mL bid. Granules may be eaten plain, mixed with liquids, or sprinkled on food.
*Pediatrics:* Take at bedtime. (Senokot/Senokot-S) >12 yrs: 2 tabs qd. Max: 4 tabs bid. 6-12 yrs: 1 tab qd. Max: 2 tabs bid. 2-6 yrs: 1/2 tab qd. Max: 1 tab bid. (SenokotXTRA) > 12 yrs: 1 tab qd. Max: 2 tabs bid. 6-12 yrs: 1/2 tab qd. Max: 1 tab bid. (Granules) ≥12 yrs: 1 tsp qd. Max: 2 tsp bid. 6-12 yrs: 1/2 tsp qd. Max: 1 tsp bid. 2-6 yrs: 1/4 tsp qd. Max: 1/2 tsp bid. Granules may be eaten plain, mixed with liquids, or sprinkled on food.

**HOW SUPPLIED:** Granules: 15mg/dose; Tab (Sennoside A and B): (Senokot) 8.6mg, (SenokotXTRA) 17mg; (Docusate Sodium-Sennoside A and B) (Senokot-S) 50mg-8.6mg

**WARNINGS/PRECAUTIONS:** Do not use with abdominal pain, nausea, or vomiting. Should not be used for longer than 1 week. Rectal bleeding or failure to have a bowel movement after use may indicate serious condition.

**INTERACTIONS:** Avoid mineral oil with Senokot-S.

**PREGNANCY:** Safety in pregnancy and nursing not known.

## SENSIPAR RX

cinacalcet HCl (Amgen)

**THERAPEUTIC CLASS:** Calcimimetic agent

**INDICATIONS:** Secondary hyperparathyroidism in patients with chronic kidney disease on dialysis. Hypercalcemia in parathyroid carcinoma.

**DOSAGE:** *Adults:* Take with food. Swallow whole. Secondary Hyperparathyroidism: Initial: 30mg qd. Titrate: Increase no more frequently than every 2-4 weeks through sequential doses of 60, 90, 120, and 180mg qd to target iPTH of 150-300pg/mL. Parathyroid Carcinoma: Initial: 30mg bid. Titrate: Increase every 2-4 weeks through sequential doses of 30mg bid, 60mg bid, 90mg bid, and 90mg tid-qid prn to normalize serum Ca levels. Adjust based on serum Ca levels (see labeling). May be used alone or in combination with vitamin D sterols and/or phosphate binders.

**HOW SUPPLIED:** Tab: 30mg, 60mg, 90mg

**WARNINGS/PRECAUTIONS:** Monitor closely for hypocalcemia, especially with history of seizure disorder. Do not initiate with serum Ca <8.4mg/dL. Measure serum Ca and phosphorus within 1 week and iPTH 1 to 4 weeks after initiation or dose adjustment. After maintenance dose reached, measure serum Ca and phosphorus monthly and iPTH every 1 to 3 months. Adynamic bone disease may develop with iPTH levels <100pg/mL; reduce dose or discontinue therapy if iPTH <150pg/mL. Caution with moderate/severe hepatic impairment.

**ADVERSE REACTIONS:** Nausea, vomiting, diarrhea, myalgia, dizziness, HTN, asthenia, anorexia, chest pain (non-cardiac), access infection.

**INTERACTIONS:** Drugs metabolized by CYP2D6 (eg, flecainide, vinblastine, thioridazine, most TCAs) may require dose adjustment. Increased amitriptyline, nortriptyline levels in CYP2D6 extensive metabolizers. Increased levels with strong CYP3A4 inhibitors (eg, ketoconazole, erythromycin, itraconazole); may require dose adjustments.

**PREGNANCY:** Category C, not for use in nursing.

## SENSORCAINE RX

bupivacaine HCl (Abraxis)

**OTHER BRAND NAMES:** Sensorcaine-MPF (Abraxis)

**THERAPEUTIC CLASS:** Local anesthetic

**INDICATIONS:** Production of local or regional anesthesia for surgery, oral surgery procedures, diagnostic and therapeutic procedures, and for obstetrical procedures. Only 0.25% and 0.5% are indicated for obstetrical anesthesia.

**DOSAGE:** *Adults:* Individualize dose. Dosage varies depending on procedure, area to be anesthetized, vascularity of tissues, number of neural segments to be blocked, depth and duration of anesthesia, degree of muscle relaxation required, and patient tolerance and physical condition. Single Dose Max: 175mg. May repeat once every 3 hrs. Total Daily Dose Max: 400mg. Epidural Anesthesia: 0.5% or 0.75% in 3-5mL increments. In obstetrics, use only 0.25% or 0.5%. Use 3-5mL increments of 0.5% solution not to exceed 50-100mg at any dosing interval. Repeat doses should be preceded by test dose containing epinephrine if not contraindicated. Young/Elderly/Debilitated/Cardiac or Liver Disease: Reduce dose.
*Pediatrics:* ≥12 yrs: Individualize dose. Dosage varies depending on procedure, area to be anesthetized, vascularity of tissues, number of neural segments to be blocked, depth and duration of anesthesia, degree of muscle relaxation required, and patient tolerance and physical condition. Single Dose Max: 175mg. May repeat once every 3 hrs. Total Daily Dose Max: 400mg. Epidural Anesthesia: 0.5% in 3-5mL increments. In obstetrics, use only 0.25% or 0.5%. Use 3-5mL increments of 0.5% solution not to exceed 50-100mg at any dosing interval. Repeat doses should be preceded by test dose containing epinephrine if not contraindicated.

**HOW SUPPLIED:** Inj: 0.25%, 0.5%; (MPF) 0.25%, 0.5%, 0.75%

**CONTRAINDICATIONS:** Obstetrical paracervical block anesthesia.

**WARNINGS/PRECAUTIONS:** The 0.75% strength is not recommended for obstetrical anesthesia. Acidosis, cardiac arrest, death reported from delay in toxicity management. Local anesthetic solutions containing antimicrobial preservatives should not be used for epidural or caudal anesthesia. Not recommended for IV regional anesthesia. Monitor cardiovascular and respiratory vital signs and state of consciousness after each injection. Caution with hepatic disease and impaired cardiovascular function. Monitor circulation and respiration with injections into head and neck area. Respiratory arrest following local anesthetic injection during retrobulbar blocks has been reported.

**ADVERSE REACTIONS:** Restlessness, anxiety, dizziness, tinnitus, blurred vision, tremors, convulsions, nausea, vomiting, chills, hypotension, bradycardia, ventricular arrhythmias, urticaria, pruritus, erythema, edema.

**INTERACTIONS:** Avoid use with any other local anesthetics.

**PREGNANCY:** Category C, not for use in nursing.

## SENSORCAINE WITH EPINEPHRINE RX

epinephrine - bupivacaine HCl (Abraxis)



**OTHER BRAND NAMES:** Sensorcaine-MPF w/Epinephrine (Abraxis)

**THERAPEUTIC CLASS:** Local anesthetic

**INDICATIONS:** Production of local or regional anesthesia for surgery, oral surgery procedures, diagnostic and therapeutic procedures, and for obstetrical procedures. Only 0.25% and 0.5% are indicated for obstetrical anesthesia.

**DOSAGE:** *Adults:* Individualize dose. Dosage varies depending on procedure, area to be anesthetized, vascularity of tissues, number of neural segments to be blocked, depth and duration of anesthesia, degree of muscle relaxation required, and patient tolerance and physical condition. Single Dose Max: 225mg. May repeat once every 3 hrs. Total Daily Dose Max: 400mg. Epidural Anesthesia: 0.5% or 0.75% in 3-5mL increments. In obstetrics, use only 0.25% or 0.5%. Use 3-5mL increments of 0.5% solution not to exceed 50-100mg at any dosing interval. Repeat doses should be preceded by test dose containing epinephrine if not contraindicated. Young/Elderly/Debilitated/Cardiac or Liver Disease: Reduce dose.
*Pediatrics:* ≥12 yrs: Individualize dose. Dosage varies depending on procedure, area to be anesthetized, vascularity of tissues, number of neural segments to be blocked, depth and duration of anesthesia, degree of muscle relaxation

required, and patient tolerance and physical condition. Single Dose Max: 225mg. May repeat once every 3 hrs. Total Daily Dose Max: 400mg. Epidural Anesthesia: 0.5% or 0.75% in 3-5mL increments. In obstetrics, use only 0.25% or 0.5%. Use 3-5mL increments of 0.5% solution not to exceed 50-100mg at any dosing interval. Repeat doses should be preceded by test dose containing epinephrine if not contraindicated.

**HOW SUPPLIED:** Inj: (Bupivacaine-Epinephrine) 0.25%/1:200,000, 0.5%/1:200,000; (MPF) 0.25%/1:200,000, 0.5%/1:200,000, 0.75%/1:200,000

**CONTRAINDICATIONS:** Obstetrical paracervical block anesthesia.

**WARNINGS/PRECAUTIONS:** The 0.75% strength is not recommended for obstetrical anesthesia. Acidosis, cardiac arrest, death reported from delay in toxicity management. Local anesthetic solutions containing antimicrobial preservatives should not be used for epidural or caudal anesthesia. Not recommended for IV regional anesthesia. Bupivacaine with epinephrine solutions contain sodium metabisulfite which may cause allergic-type reactions in susceptible people. Monitor cardiovascular and respiratory vital signs and state of consciousness after each injection. Caution when local anesthetic solutions containing a vasoconstrictor are used in areas of the body supplied by end arteries or having otherwise compromised blood supply; ischemic injury or necrosis may result with hypertensive vascular disease. Caution with hepatic disease and impaired cardiovascular function. Monitor circulation and respiration with injections into head and neck area. Respiratory arrest following local anesthetic injection during retrobulbar blocks has been reported.

**ADVERSE REACTIONS:** Restlessness, anxiety, dizziness, tinnitus, blurred vision, tremors, convulsions, nausea, vomiting, chills, hypotension, bradycardia, ventricular arrhythmias, urticaria, pruritus, erythema, edema.

**INTERACTIONS:** Avoid use with any other local anesthetics. Anesthetic solutions containing epinephrine or norepinephrine with MAOIs or TCAs may produce severe, prolonged HTN; avoid concurrent use or monitor closely if concurrent use is necessary. Concurrent administration of vasopressors and ergot-type oxytocic drugs may cause severe, persistent HTN or CVA. Phenothiazines and butyrophenones may reduce or reverse the pressor effect of epinephrine. Serious dose-related cardiac arrhythmias may occur with use during or following administration of potent inhalation anesthetics.

**PREGNANCY:** Category C, not for use in nursing.

## SEPTOCAINE

RX

epinephrine - articaine HCl (Septodont)

**THERAPEUTIC CLASS:** Anesthetic

**INDICATIONS:** For local, infiltrative, or conductive anesthesia in both simple and complex dental and periodontal procedures.

**DOSAGE:** *Adults:* Submucosal Infiltration: 0.5-2.5mL. Nerve Block: 0.5-3.4mL. Oral Surgery: 1-5.1mL. Max: 7mg/kg (0.175mL/kg) or 3.2mg/lb (0.0795mL/lb). *Pediatrics:* >4 yrs: Submucosal Infiltration/Nerve Block/Oral Surgery: up to 7mg/kg (0.175mL/kg) or 3.2mg/lb (0.0795mL/lb).

**HOW SUPPLIED:** Inj: (Articaine-Epinephrine) 4%-1:100,000/1.7mL, 4%-1:200,000/1.7ml.

**CONTRAINDICATIONS:** Hypersensitivity to sodium metabisulfite.

**WARNINGS/PRECAUTIONS:** Avoid intravascular injection; aspirate needle before use. Intravascular injection is associated with convulsions, followed by CNS or cardiorespiratory depression and coma progressing to respiratory arrest. Epinephrine can cause local tissue necrosis or systemic toxicity. Contains sodium metabisulfite which can cause allergic reactions. Exaggerated vasoconstrictive response may occur with peripheral vascular disease and hypertensive vascular disease. CNS or cardiovascular effects may occur with systemic absorption. Local anesthetics are capable of producing methemoglobinemia, with signs of cyanosis, fatigue, and weakness.

**ADVERSE REACTIONS:** Face edema, headache, infection, pain, gingivitis, swelling, paresthesia, trismus.

**INTERACTIONS:** MAOIs or TCAs may produce severe, prolonged HTN. Phenothiazines and butyrphenones may reduce or reverse pressor effect of epinephrine.

**PREGNANCY:** Category C, caution in nursing.

## SEPTRA — RX

trimethoprim - sulfamethoxazole (King)

**OTHER BRAND NAMES:** Septra DS (King) - Sulfatrim Pediatric (Alpharma)

**THERAPEUTIC CLASS:** Sulfonamide/tetrahydrofolic acid inhibitor

**INDICATIONS:** (Inj, Susp, Tab) Treatment of urinary tract infection (UTI), pneumocystitis carinii pneumonia (PCP) and enteritis caused by *Shigella*. (Susp, Tab). Treatment of acute exacerbation of chronic bronchitis (AECB), travelers' diarrhea, and acute otitis media.

**DOSAGE:** *Adults:* (Sus, Tab) UTI: 800mg-160mg PO q12h for 10-14 days. Shigellosis/Traveler's Diarrhea: 800mg-160mg PO q12h for 5 days. AECB: 800mg-160mg PO q12h for 14 days. PCP Treatment: 15-20mg/kg TMP and 75-100mg/kg SMX per 24 hrs given PO q6h for 14-21 days PCP Prophylaxis: 800mg-160mg PO qd. (Inj) Severe UTI: 8-10mg/kg TMP IV given in divided doses q6, 8 or 12h for up to 14 days. PCP Treatment: 15-20mg/kg TMP IV given in divided doses q6-8h for up to 14 days. Shigellosis: 8-10mg/kg TMP IV given in divided doses q6, 8 or 12h for 5 days. (Inj, Sus, Tab) Renal Impairment: CrCl 15-30mL/min: 50% usual dose. CrCl <15mL/min: Not recommended. *Pediatrics:* (Sus, Tab) >2 months: UTI/Otitis Media: 4mg/kg TMP and 20mg/kg SMX q12h for 10 days. Shigellosis/Traveler's Diarrhea: 4mg/kg TMP and 20mg/kg SMX q12h for 5 days. PCP Treatment: 15-20mg/kg TMP and 75-100mg/kg SMX/24 hrs given q6h for 14-21 days. PCP Prophylaxis: 150mg/m$^2$/day TMP and 750mg/m$^2$/day SMX PO given bid, on 3 consecutive days per week. Max: 320mg TMP and 1600mg SMX per day. (Inj) Severe UTI: 8-10mg/kg TMP IV given in divided doses q6, 8 or 12h for up to 14 days. PCP Treatment: 15-20mg/kg TMP IV given in divided doses q6-8h for up to 14 days. Shigellosis: 8-10mg/kg TMP IV given in divided doses q6, 8 or 12h for 5 days. (Inj, Sus, Tab) Renal Impairment: CrCl 15-30mL/min: 50% usual dose. CrCl <15mL/min: Not recommended.

**HOW SUPPLIED:** (Sulfamethoxazole [SMX]-Trimethoprim [TMP]) Inj: (Septra) 80mg-16mg/mL; Sus: (Sulfatrim Pediatric, Septra) 200mg-40mg/5mL [100mL, 473mL]; Tab: (Septra) 400mg-80mg*; Tab, DS: (Septra) 800mg-160mg* *scored

S

**CONTRAINDICATIONS:** Megaloblastic anemia due to folate deficiency, pregnancy at term, nursing, infants <2 months old.

**WARNINGS/PRECAUTIONS:** Fatal hypersensitivity reactions (eg, Stevens-Johnson syndrome, toxic epidermal necrolysis, fulminant hepatic necrosis, agranulocytosis, aplastic anemia) may occur. Pseudomembranous colitis, cough, SOB, and pulmonary infiltrates reported. Avoid with group A β-hemolytic streptococcal infections. Caution with hepatic/renal impairment, elderly, folate deficiency (eg, chronic alcoholics, anticonvulsants, malabsorption, malnutrition), bronchial asthma, and other allergies. In G6PD deficiency, hemolysis may occur. Increased incidence of adverse events in AIDS patients. Maintain adequate fluid intake.

**ADVERSE REACTIONS:** Anorexia, nausea, vomiting, rash, urticaria, cholestatic jaundice, agranulocytosis, anemia, hyperkalemia, renal failure, interstitial nephritis, hyponatremia, convulsions, arthralgia, myalgia, weakness.

**INTERACTIONS:** Increase risk of thrombocytopenia with purpura with diuretics (especially thiazides) in the elderly. Caution with warfarin; may prolong PT. Increased effects of phenytoin, methotrexate.

**PREGNANCY:** Category C, contraindicated in nursing.

## SEREVENT RX

salmeterol xinafoate (GlaxoSmithKline)

**Long-acting $\beta_2$-adrenergic agonists, such as salmeterol, may increase the risk of asthma-related deaths.**

**THERAPEUTIC CLASS:** $Beta_2$ agonist

**INDICATIONS:** Long-term maintenance treatment of asthma and COPD. Prevention of bronchospasm with reversible obstructive airway disease (including nocturnal asthma) when regular treatment with inhaled short-acting $\beta_2$-agonists is required. Prevention of exercise-induced bronchospasm (EIB).

**DOSAGE:** *Adults:* Asthma/COPD: 1 inh bid, am and pm (12 hrs apart). EIB Prevention: 1 inh 30 minutes before exercise (do not give preventive doses if already on bid dose).
*Pediatrics:* >4 yrs: Asthma: 1 inh bid, am and pm (12 hrs apart). EIB Prevention: 1 inh 30 minutes before exercise (do not give preventive doses if already on bid dose).

**HOW SUPPLIED:** Disk: 50mcg [28, 60 blisters]

**WARNINGS/PRECAUTIONS:** Avoid with significantly worsening or acutely deteriorating asthma. Not for acute treatment or substitute for oral/inhaled corticosteroids. Monitor for increasing use of inhaled $\beta_2$ agonists. QTc interval prolongation reported when exceeded recommended dose. D/C if paradoxical bronchospasm occurs. Immediate hypersensitivity and upper airway symptom reactions reported. Caution with cardiovascular disorder (eg, coronary insufficiency, arrhythmia, HTN), convulsive disorders, thyrotoxicosis, if usually unresponsive to sympathomimetic amines. May cause hypokalemia.

**ADVERSE REACTIONS:** Nasal/sinus congestion, pallor, rhinitis, headache, tracheitis/bronchitis, influenza, throat irritation.

**INTERACTIONS:** Caution with non-potassium-sparing diuretics. Extreme caution within 14 days of using MAOIs or TCAs. Avoid with β-blockers. Caution with >8 inhalations of short-acting $\beta_2$-agonists.

**PREGNANCY:** Category C, not for use in nursing.

## SEROMYCIN RX

cycloserine (Lilly)

**THERAPEUTIC CLASS:** Cell wall synthesis inhibitor

**INDICATIONS:** Adjunct treatment of active pulmonary and extrapulmonary tuberculosis (including renal disease) when primary agents (eg, streptomycin, isoniazid, rifampin, ethambutol) are inadequate. May be effective for treatment of acute urinary tract infection caused by *E.coli* and *Enterobacter* when conventional therapy failed.

**DOSAGE:** *Adults:* Initial: 250mg bid (q12h) for 2 weeks. Usual: 500mg-1g daily in divided doses; monitor by blood levels. Max: 1g/day.

**HOW SUPPLIED:** Cap: 250mg

**CONTRAINDICATIONS:** Epilepsy, depression, severe anxiety, psychosis, severe renal insufficiency, excessive concurrent alcohol use.

**WARNINGS/PRECAUTIONS:** D/C or reduce dose if allergic reaction or symptoms of CNS toxicity (eg, convulsions, somnolence, depression, confusion, headache, psychosis) occur. Increased risk of toxicity with blood levels >30mcg/mL. Narrow therapeutic index; caution in dosing. Increased risk of convulsions in chronic alcoholics. Monitor hematology, blood levels, renal and liver functions. Monitor cultures and susceptibility prior to therapy. Vitamin $B_{12}$ and/or folic acid deficiency, megaloblastic anemia and sideroblastic anemia; institute appropriate therapy.

**INTERACTIONS:** Contraindicated with excessive alcohol use. Increased neurotoxicity with ethionamide. Increased incidence of CNS effects with isoniazid.

**PREGNANCY:** Category C, not for use in nursing.

## SEROPHENE RX
clomiphene citrate (Serono)

**THERAPEUTIC CLASS:** Ovulatory stimulant

**INDICATIONS:** Treatment of ovulatory dysfunction in women desiring pregnancy.

**DOSAGE:** *Adults:* Initial: 50mg/day for 5 days. Start any time if no recent uterine bleeding. If progestin-induced bleeding is intended, or if spontaneous uterine bleeding occurs, start on the 5th day of the cycle. If ovulation does not occur, increase to 100mg qd for 5 days, 30 days after the 1st course. Max: 100mg qd for 5 days and 3 courses of therapy.

**HOW SUPPLIED:** Tab: 50mg

**CONTRAINDICATIONS:** Pregnancy, liver disease or history of liver dysfunction, abnormal uterine bleeding of undetermined origin, ovarian cysts or enlargement not due to polycystic ovarian syndrome, uncontrolled thyroid or adrenal dysfunction, organic intracranial lesion (eg, pituitary tumor).

**WARNINGS/PRECAUTIONS:** Increased incidence of visual symptoms with increasing total dose or therapy duration; d/c treatment and perform complete ophthalmological evaluation. Ovarian hyperstimulation syndrome reported; monitor for abdominal pain, nausea, vomiting, diarrhea, weight gain. Increased chance of multiple pregnancy. Perform pelvic exam before initiating therapy and before each course. Prolonged use may increase risk of borderline/invasive ovarian tumor.

**ADVERSE REACTIONS:** Ovarian enlargement, vasomotor flushes, nausea, vomiting, breast discomfort, abdominal-pelvic discomfort/distention/bloating, visual symptoms, headache, abnormal uterine bleeding.

**PREGNANCY:** Category X, caution in nursing.

## SEROQUEL RX
quetiapine fumarate (AstraZeneca LP)

**Elderly patients with dementia-related psychosis treated with atypical antipsychotic drugs are at an increased risk of death; most appeared to be cardiovascular (eg, heart failure, sudden death) or infectious (eg, pneumonia) in nature. Quetiapine is not approved for the treatment of patients with dementia-related psychosis. Antidepressants increased the risk of suicidal thinking and behavior (suicidality) in short-term studies in children and adolescents with Major Depressive Disorder (MDD) and other psychiatric disorders. Quetiapine is not approved for use in pediatric patients.**

**THERAPEUTIC CLASS:** Dibenzapine derivative

**INDICATIONS:** Treatment of schizophrenia. Treatment of acute manic episodes associated with bipolar I disorder, as monotherapy or adjunct therapy to lithium or divalproex. Treatment of depressive episodes associated with bipolar disorder.

**DOSAGE:** *Adults:* Bipolar Mania: Monotherapy/Adjunctive: Give bid. Initial: 100mg/day on Day 1. Titrate: Increase to 400mg/day on Day 4 in increments of up to 100mg/day in bid divided doses. Adjust doses up to 800mg/day by Day 6 in increments ≤200mg/day. Max: 800mg/day. Bipolar Depressive Episodes: Give once daily hs. Day 1: 50mg/day. Day 2: 100mg/day. Day 3: 200mg/day. Day 4: 300mg/day. Schizophrenia: Initial: 25mg bid. Titrate: Increase by 25-50mg bid-tid on the 2nd and 3rd day to 300-400mg/day given bid-tid by the 4th day. Adjust doses by 25-50mg bid at intervals of at least 2 days. Maint: Lowest effective dose. Max: 800mg/day. Hepatic Impairment: Initial: 25mg/day. Titrate: Increase by 25-50mg/day to effective dose. Elderly/Debilitated/Predisposition to Hypotension: Consider slower rate of dose titration and lower target dose.

**HOW SUPPLIED:** Tab: 25mg, 50mg, 100mg, 200mg, 300mg, 400mg

S

**WARNINGS/PRECAUTIONS:** NMS reported. May develop tardive dyskinesia. May induce orthostatic hypotension. Caution with cardiovascular disease, cerebrovascular disease, conditions which predispose to hypotension (eg, dehydration, hypovolemia), history of seizures. Monitor for cataracts at initiation, then every 6 months. Possible hypothyroidism. Hepatic enzyme, cholesterol and triglyceride elevations reported. May impair judgment, thinking and motor skills. Priapism reported. May disrupt body's ability to reduce core temperature. Caution in patients at risk for aspiration, elderly, debilitated. Depression may worsen in patients or suicidal thoughts and behaviors may also arise.

**ADVERSE REACTIONS:** Headache, dizziness, postural hypotension, dry mouth, dyspepsia, tachycardia, somnolence, constipation.

**INTERACTIONS:** Caution with other CNS drugs. Increased cognitive and motor effects of alcohol. May antagonize effects of levodopa and dopamine agonists. May enhance effects of antihypertensives. Phenytoin or other hepatic enzyme inducers (eg, carbamazepine, barbiturates, glucocorticoids) may reduce levels. Caution with inhibitors of CYP3A (eg, itraconazole, ketoconazole, fluconazole, erythromycin). Increased clearance with thioridazine. May reduce oral clearance of lorazepam.

**PREGNANCY:** Category C, not for use in nursing.

## SEROQUEL XR — RX

quetiapine fumarate (AstraZeneca)

**Elderly patients with dementia-related psychosis treated with atypical antipsychotic drugs are at an increased risk of death; most appeared to be cardiovascular (eg, heart failure, sudden death) or infectious (eg, pneumonia) in nature. Seroquel XR is not approved for the treatment of patients with dementia-related psychosis.**

**THERAPEUTIC CLASS:** Dibenzapine derivative

**INDICATIONS:** Treatment of schizophrenia

**DOSAGE:** *Adults:* Give qd, preferably in evening. Initial: 300mg/day. Titrate: To within range of 400-800mg/day depending on response and tolerance. Dose increases may be made at intervals as short as 1 day and in increments up to 300mg/day. Take without food or with light meal. Elderly/Hepatic Impairment: Start on Seroquel immediate-release 25mg/day; may increase in increments of 25-50 mg/day depending on response and tolerance. May switch to Seroquel XR when effective dose reached.

**HOW SUPPLIED:** Tab, Extended Release: 200mg, 300mg, 400mg

**WARNINGS/PRECAUTIONS:** Monitor DM patients regularly for hyperglycemia. NMS reported. May develop tardive dyskinesia. May induce orthostatic hypotension. Caution with cardiovascular or cerebrovascular disease, conditions which predispose to hypotension (eg, dehydration, hypovolemia and treatment with antihypertensives), history of seizures. Monitor for cataracts at initiation, then every 6 months. Possible hypothyroidism. Hepatic enzyme, cholesterol, and triglyceride elevations reported. May impair judgement, thinking, and motor skills. Priapism reported. May disrupt body's ability to reduce core temperature. Caution in patients at risk for aspiration, elderly, debilitated. Depression may worsen in patients or suicidal thoughts and behaviors may also arise.

**ADVERSE REACTIONS:** Dry mouth, constipation, dyspepsia, sedation, somnolence, dizziness, orthostatic hypotension.

**INTERACTIONS:** Caution with other CNS drugs. May ncrease cognitive and motor effects of alcohol. May antagonize effects of levodopa and dopamine agonists. May enhance effects of antihypertensives. Phenytoin or other hepatic enzyme inducers (eg, carbamazepine, barbiturates, glucocorticoids) may reduce levels. Caution with inhibitors of CYP3A (eg, itraconazole, ketoconazole, fluconazole, erythromycin). May reduce oral clearance of lorazepam.

**PREGNANCY:** Category C, not for use in nursing.

## SEROSTIM
RX

somatropin (Serono)

**THERAPEUTIC CLASS:** Human growth hormone

**INDICATIONS:** Treatment of AIDS wasting or cachexia.

**DOSAGE:** *Adults:* >55kg: 6mg SQ qhs. 45-55kg: 5mg SQ qhs. 35-44kg: 4mg SQ qhs. <35kg: 0.1mg/kg SQ qhs. Dose Reductions Due to Side Effects: Reduce total daily dose or number of doses/week. Rotate injection sites. Re-evaluate for infection if weight loss continues after 2 weeks of therapy.

**HOW SUPPLIED:** Inj: 4mg, 5mg, 6mg

**CONTRAINDICATIONS:** Acute critical illness due to complications after open heart or abdominal surgery, accidental trauma, acute respiratory failure.

**WARNINGS/PRECAUTIONS:** Monitor malnutrition, malabsorption and hypogonadism; may contribute to catabolism. Maintain nucleoside analogue therapy throughout treatment. Carpal tunnel syndrome reported. Perform periodic funduscopic exams.

**ADVERSE REACTIONS:** Fever, abdominal pain, diarrhea, neuropathy, nausea, vomiting, headache, fatigue, blood dyscrasias, lymphadenopathy, increased sweating, elevated LFTs, musculoskeletal discomfort, increased tissue turgor, albuminuria, insomnia, tachycardia, hyperglycemia.

**PREGNANCY:** Category B, caution in nursing.

## SILVADENE
RX

silver sulfadiazine (King)

**OTHER BRAND NAMES:** SSD (Basf)

**THERAPEUTIC CLASS:** Sulfonamide

**INDICATIONS:** Adjunct for prevention and treatment of wound sepsis in patients with 2nd- and 3rd-degree burns.

**DOSAGE:** *Adults:* Apply under sterile conditions qd-bid to thickness of approximately 1/16 inch. Re-apply if removed by patient activity. Continue until wound is healed.

**HOW SUPPLIED:** Cre: 1% [20g, 50g, 85g, 400g, 1000g]

**CONTRAINDICATIONS:** Late pregnancy, premature infants, newborns during 1st 2 months of life.

**WARNINGS/PRECAUTIONS:** Potential cross-sensitivity with other sulfonamides. Hemolysis may occur in G6PD deficient patients. Drug accumulation with hepatic and renal dysfunction. Monitor renal function and serum sulfa levels with extensive burns.



**ADVERSE REACTIONS:** Transient leukopenia, skin necrosis, erythema multiforme, skin discoloration, burning sensation, rash, interstitial nephritis, fungal superinfection, systemic sulfonamide reactions.

**INTERACTIONS:** May inactivate topical proteolytic enzymes. Leukopenia increased with cimetidine.

**PREGNANCY:** Category B, contraindicated in late pregnancy, and not for use in nursing.

## SIMULECT
RX

basiliximab (Novartis)

> **Manage patient in facility with adequate lab and supportive resources. Prescribing physician should be experienced with immunosuppressives and transplantation. Physician should have complete information requisite for patient follow-up.**

**THERAPEUTIC CLASS:** Monoclonal antibody/IL-2R alpha (CD25) blocker

**INDICATIONS:** Prophylaxis of acute organ rejection in renal transplantation.

**DOSAGE:** *Adults:* 20mg within 2 hrs prior to transplant, repeat 4 days after transplant. Withhold 2nd dose if graft loss or complications occur. *Pediatrics:* >35kg: 20mg within 2 hrs prior to transplant, repeat 4 days after transplant. <35kg: 10mg within 2 hrs prior to transplant, repeat 4 days after transplant. Withhold 2nd dose if graft loss or complications occur.

**HOW SUPPLIED:** Inj: 10mg, 20mg

**WARNINGS/PRECAUTIONS:** Only administer under qualified medical supervision. Increased risk of developing lymphoproliferative disorder and opportunistic infections. Anaphylaxis and other severe hypersensitivity reactions (eg, hypotension, cardiac failure, bronchospasm, respiratory failure, etc) reported and may necessitate discontinuation. Anti-idiotype antibodies may develop.

**ADVERSE REACTIONS:** GI effects, peripheral edema, fever, viral infection, hyperkalemia, hypokalemia, hyperglycemia, hypercholesterolemia, hypophosphatemia, hyperuricemia, UTI, dyspnea, upper respiratory infection, acne, HTN, headache, tremor, insomnia, anemia.

**PREGNANCY:** Category B, not for use in nursing.

## SINEMET CR

RX

levodopa - carbidopa (Bristol-Myers Squibb)

**OTHER BRAND NAMES:** Sinemet (Bristol-Myers Squibb)

**THERAPEUTIC CLASS:** Dopa-decarboxylase inhibitor/dopamine precursor

**INDICATIONS:** Treatment of symptoms of idiopathic Parkinson's disease, postencephalitic parkinsonism, and symptomatic parkinsonism.

**DOSAGE:** *Adults:* >18 yrs: Initial: (25mg-100mg tab) 1 tab tid. Titrate: Increase by 1 tab qd or every other day until 8 tabs/day. 10mg-100mg tab: Initial: 1 tab tid-qid. Titrate: Increase 1 tab qd or every other day until 2 tabs qid. 70-100mg/day carbidopa required. Max: 200mg/day carbidopa. (Tab, Extended-Release) No Prior Levodopa Use: Initial: 1 tab 50mg-200mg bid at intervals >6 hrs. Titrate: Increase or decrease dose or interval accordingly. Adjust dose every 3 days. Usual: 400-1600mg/day levodopa, given in 4-8 hr intervals while awake. Conversion to Extended-Release Tabs: See labeling.

**HOW SUPPLIED:** Tab: (Carbidopa-Levodopa) 10mg-100mg*, 25mg-100mg*, 25mg-250mg*; Tab, Extended Release: (Carbidopa-Levodopa) 25mg-100mg, 50mg-200mg* *scored

**CONTRAINDICATIONS:** MAOIs during or within 14 days of use, narrow-angle glaucoma, suspicious, undiagnosed skin lesions, history of melanoma.



**WARNINGS/PRECAUTIONS:** D/C levodopa 12 hrs before initiating therapy. Dyskinesias and mental disturbances may occur. Caution with severe cardiovascular or pulmonary disease, bronchial asthma, renal or hepatic disease, endocrine disease, chronic wide-angle glaucoma, peptic ulcer, and MI with residual arrhythmias. NMS reported during dose reduction or withdrawal. Dark color may appear in saliva, urine, or sweat. May cause false (+) ketonuria or false (-) glucosuria (glucose-oxidase method).

**ADVERSE REACTIONS:** Dyskinesias, nausea, cardiac irregularities, hypotension, dark saliva, GI bleeding, psychotic episodes, NMS, confusion, agitation, dizziness, somnolence, dream abnormalities.

**INTERACTIONS:** See Contraindications. Risk of postural hypotension with antihypertensives, selegiline. HTN and dyskinesia may occur with TCAs. Reduced effects with dopamine $D_2$ antagonists (eg, phenothiazines, butyrophenones, risperidone), isoniazid. Antagonized by phenytoin, papaverine, metoclopramide. Reduced bioavailability with iron salts, high-protein diets.

**PREGNANCY:** Category C, caution in nursing.

## SINGULAIR
montelukast sodium (Merck) RX

**THERAPEUTIC CLASS:** Leukotriene receptor antagonist

**INDICATIONS:** Prophylaxis and chronic treatment of asthma (≥12 months). Relief of symptoms of seasonal allergic rhinitis (≥2 yrs) and perennial allergic rhinitis (≥6 months). Prevention of exercise-induced bronchoconstriction (EIB) (≥15 yrs).

**DOSAGE:** *Adults:* Asthma: 10mg qpm. Allergic Rhinitis: 10mg qd. EIB: 10mg 2 hrs before exercise. Do not take additional dose within 24 hrs of previous dose. *Pediatrics:* Asthma: >15 yrs: 10mg qpm. 6-14 yrs: 5mg qpm. 2-5 yrs: 4mg qpm. 12-23 months: 4mg qpm. Seasonal/Perennial Allergic Rhinitis: >15 yrs: 10mg qd. 6-14 yrs: 5mg qd. 2-5 yrs: 4mg qd. Perennial Allergic Rhinitis: 6-23 months: 4mg qd. EIB: ≥15 yrs: 10mg 2 hrs before exercise. Do not take additional dose within 24 hrs of previous dose. Granules may be mixed with applesauce, carrots, rice or ice cream; give within 15 minutes of opening packet.

**HOW SUPPLIED:** Granules: 4mg/packet; Tab, Chewable: 4mg, 5mg; Tab: 10mg

**WARNINGS/PRECAUTIONS:** Not for treatment of acute asthma attacks. Do not abruptly substitute for inhaled or oral corticosteroids. Eosinophilic conditions reported (rare).

**ADVERSE REACTIONS:** (Adults, Pediatrics) Headache, cough. (Pediatrics) Pharyngitis, fever, flu, nausea, diarrhea, dyspepsia, rhinorrhea, upper respiratory infection.

**INTERACTIONS:** Monitor with potent CYP450 inducers (eg, phenobarbital, rifampin).

**PREGNANCY:** Category B, caution in nursing.

## SKELAXIN
metaxalone (King) RX

**THERAPEUTIC CLASS:** Muscular analgesic (central-acting)

**INDICATIONS:** Adjunct for acute, painful musculoskeletal conditions.

**DOSAGE:** *Adults:* 800mg tid-qid.
*Pediatrics:* >12 yrs: 800mg tid-qid.

**HOW SUPPLIED:** Tab: 800mg* *scored

**CONTRAINDICATIONS:** Tendency for drug-induced, hemolytic, and other anemias. Significant renal or hepatic impairment.

**WARNINGS/PRECAUTIONS:** Caution with pre-existing liver damage. Monitor hepatic function. False-positive Benedict's test reported.

S

**ADVERSE REACTIONS:** Nausea, vomiting, GI upset, drowsiness, dizziness, headache, nervousness, leukopenia, hemolytic anemia, jaundice.

**INTERACTIONS:** May enhance the effects of alcohol, barbiturates and other CNS depressants.

**PREGNANCY:** Not for use in pregnancy or nursing.

## SKELID
tiludronate disodium (Sanofi-Aventis) RX

**THERAPEUTIC CLASS:** Bisphosphonate

**INDICATIONS:** Treatment of Paget's disease when serum alkaline phosphatase is >2X ULN, or if symptomatic, or if at risk for future complications.

**DOSAGE:** *Adults:* 400mg qd for 3 months. After therapy, wait 3 months to assess response. Take with 6-8 oz of water. Take 2 hrs after food.

**HOW SUPPLIED:** Tab: 200mg

**WARNINGS/PRECAUTIONS:** May cause GI disorders (eg, dysphagia, esophagitis, esophageal or gastric ulcers). Maintain adequate Vitamin D and calcium intake. Avoid in severe renal failure. May cause osteonecrosis, primarily in the jaw and musculoskeletal pain.

**ADVERSE REACTIONS:** Pain, headache, dizziness, paresthesia, diarrhea, nausea, dyspepsia, vomiting, rhinitis, upper respiratory infection.

**INTERACTIONS:** Increased bioavailability with indomethacin; space dosing by 2 hrs. Decreased bioavailability with calcium supplements, ASA, and aluminum- or magnesium-containing antacids; space dosing by 2 hrs.

**PREGNANCY:** Category C, caution in nursing.

## SODIUM CHLORIDE IRRIGATION RX

sodium chloride (Baxter Healthcare Corporation)

**THERAPEUTIC CLASS:** Irrigation solution

**INDICATIONS:** For use as an arthroscopic irrigation fluid with endoscopic instruments during arthroscopic procedures requiring distention and irrigation of the knee, shoulder, elbow, or other bone joints.

**DOSAGE:** *Adults:* Irrigate as needed. May warm in overpouch to near body temperature in water bath or oven heated to not more than 45° C.

**HOW SUPPLIED:** Sol: 1000mL, 3000mL, 5000mL

**CONTRAINDICATIONS:** Not for injection by usual parenteral routes. An electrolyte solution should not be used for irrigation during electrosurgical procedures.

**WARNINGS/PRECAUTIONS:** Not for injection. Caution in CHF, severe renal insufficiency, and conditions where edema and sodium retention exists. Use opened containers promptly to reduce potential for bacterial contamination. Discard unused portion. Irrigation solutions must be regarded as systemic drugs since irrigating fluids can enter systemic ciruclation in large volumes.

**ADVERSE REACTIONS:** Infection, distension or disruption of tissues.

**INTERACTIONS:** Caution with corticosteroids or corticotropin; some of the fluid may be absorbed systemically.

**PREGNANCY:** Safety in pregnancy and nursing is not known.

## SOLAGE RX

mequinol - tretinoin (Galderma)

**THERAPEUTIC CLASS:** Retinoid

**INDICATIONS:** Solar lentigines.

**DOSAGE:** *Adults:* Apply to solar lentigines bid, morning and evening, at least 8 hrs apart. Avoid surrounding skin. Do not shower or bathe treated area for at least 6 hrs after application. Wait 30 minutes before applying cosmetics.

**HOW SUPPLIED:** Sol: (Mequinol-Tretinoin) 2%-0.01% [30mL]

**CONTRAINDICATIONS:** Women of childbearing potential and pregnancy.

**WARNINGS/PRECAUTIONS:** Caution with history/family history of vitiligo. Severe irritation with eczematous skin. Avoid/minimize exposure to sunlight/sunlamps or wear protective clothing. Avoid eyes, mouth, paranasal creases and mucous membranes. Discontinue if sensitivity, irritation, or systemic adverse reaction develops. Larger amounts will not lead to better or faster results and may increase adverse effects. Extreme weather may increase skin irritation. Caution when using with permanent wave solutions, electrolysis, hair depilatories or waxes.

**ADVERSE REACTIONS:** Erythema, burning/stinging/tingling, desquamation, pruritus, skin irritation, dry skin, hypopigmentation of treated lesions or surrounding skin.

**INTERACTIONS:** Avoid with photosensitizers (eg, thiazides, tetracyclines, fluoroquinolones, phenothiazines, sulfonamides); may cause augmented phototoxicity. Caution with other topicals products with a strong drying effect, high concentrations of alcohol, astringents, spices or lime, medicated soaps/shampoos.

**PREGNANCY:** Category X, caution in nursing.

## SOLAQUIN FORTE RX
hydroquinone (Valeant)

**THERAPEUTIC CLASS:** Depigmenting agent

**INDICATIONS:** For the gradual bleaching of hyperpigmented skin conditions (eg, chloasma, melasma, freckles, senile lentigines).

**DOSAGE:** *Adults:* Apply bid.
*Pediatrics:* >12 yrs: Apply bid.

**HOW SUPPLIED:** Cre: 4% [28.4g]; Gel: 4% [28.4g]

**WARNINGS/PRECAUTIONS:** Avoid sun exposure on bleached skin. Solaquin Forte contains sunscreen. May produce unwanted cosmetic effects if not used as directed. Test for skin sensitivity. Discontinue if no lightening effect after 2 months. Contains sodium metabisulfite, may cause serious allergic type reactions. Limit treatment to small areas of body at one time. Avoid contact with eyes.

**ADVERSE REACTIONS:** Cutaneous hypersensitivity (contact dermatitis).

**PREGNANCY:** Category C, caution in nursing.

## SOLARAZE RX
diclofenac sodium (Bioglan)

**THERAPEUTIC CLASS:** NSAID

**INDICATIONS:** Treatment of actinic keratoses.

**DOSAGE:** *Adults:* Apply generously to lesions bid for 60-90 days.

**HOW SUPPLIED:** Gel: 3% [50g,100g]

**CONTRAINDICATIONS:** Known hypersensitivity to benzyl alcohol, polyethylene glycol monomethyl ether 350, hyaluronate sodium.

**WARNINGS/PRECAUTIONS:** Anaphylactoid reactions may occur. Caution with ASA triad, GI ulceration or bleeding, severe renal/hepatic impairment. Do not apply to open skin wounds, infections, or exfoliative dermatitis. Avoid the eyes and sun/sunlamp exposure during therapy. Interrupt therapy if severe reactions occur.



**ADVERSE REACTIONS:** Contact dermatitis, dry skin, edema, exfoliation, pain, paresthesia, pruritis, rash.

**INTERACTIONS:** Minimize oral administration of NSAIDs. Safety of the concomitant use of sunscreens, cosmetics, or other topical medications is unknown.

**PREGNANCY:** Category B, not for use in nursing.

## SOLIRIS RX
eculizumab (Alexion)

**Increases the risk of meningococcal infections; vaccinate 2 weeks prior to receiving first dose.**

**THERAPEUTIC CLASS:** Monoclonal antibody/Protein C5 blocker

**INDICATIONS:** Treatment of paroxysmal nocturnal hemoglobinuria (PNH) to reduce hemolysis.

**DOSAGE:** *Adults:* Initial: 600mg every 7 days for first 4 weeks, then 900mg as 5th dose 7 days later, then 900mg every 14 days thereafter. Administer by IV infusion over 35 minutes.

**HOW SUPPLIED:** Inj: 10mg/mL

**CONTRAINDICATIONS:** Patients with unresolved serious *Neisseria meningitidis* infection and patients not vaccinated against it.

**WARNINGS/PRECAUTIONS:** Caution in patients with any systemic infection. After discontinuation, monitor for signs and symptoms of intravascular hemolysis and serum LDH levels.

**ADVERSE REACTIONS:** Meningococcal infections, headache, nasopharyngitis, back pain, nausea, fatigue, cough, herpes simplex infections, sinusitis, respiratory tract infection, constipation, myalgia, pain in extremities, influenza-like illness.

**PREGNANCY:** Category C, caution in nursing.

## SOLODYN

RX

minocycline HCl (Medicis)

**THERAPEUTIC CLASS:** Tetracycline derivative

**INDICATIONS:** Treatment of inflammatory lesions of non-nodular moderate to severe acne vulgaris in patients ≥12 yrs.

**DOSAGE:** *Adults:* 1mg/kg qd for 12 weeks. Reduce dose with renal impairment. *Pediatrics:* ≥12 yrs: 1mg/kg qd for 12 weeks. Reduce dose with renal impairment.

**HOW SUPPLIED:** Tab, Extended Release: 45mg, 90mg, 135mg.

**WARNINGS/PRECAUTIONS:** May cause fetal harm during pregnancy. Use during tooth development (last half of pregnancy, infancy, <8yrs) may cause permanent discoloration of the teeth or enamel hypoplasia; avoid use during this period. May decrease bone growth in premature infants. May cause pseudomembarnous colitis. Renal toxicity, hepatotoxicity, photosensitivity, increased BUN, superinfection, pseudotumor cerebri may occur. Caution in renal impairment; may lead to azotemia, hyperphosphatemia, and acidosis. Long-term use has been associated with lupus-like syndrome, autoimmune hepatitis And vasculitis. May cause serum sickness. May induce hyperpigmentation.

**ADVERSE REACTIONS:** Headache, fatigue, dizziness, pruritus, malaise, mood alteration.

**INTERACTIONS:** May require downward regulation of anticoagulant therapy. May interfere with bactericidal action of penicillin; avoid concurrent. May decrease efficacy of oral contraceptives. Impaired absorption with antacids containing aluminum, calcium or magnesium, and iron-containing preparations. Fatal renal toxicity with methoxyflurane reported.

**PREGNANCY:** Category D, not for use in nursing.

S

## SOLTAMOX

RX

tamoxifen citrate (Savient)

**For women with ductal carcinoma in situ (DCIS) and women at high risk for breast cancer. Fatal uterine malignancies (eg, endometrial adenocarcinoma, uterine sarcoma), stroke, and PE reported with use in risk reduction setting. Discuss benefits/risks of events with this patient population. Benefits of tamoxifen outweigh risks in women already diagnosed with breast cancer.**

**THERAPEUTIC CLASS:** Antiestrogen

**INDICATIONS:** Treatment of metastatic breast cancer in women and men. Treatment of node-positive and axillary node-negative breast cancer in women following mastectomy, axillary dissection and breast irradiation. To reduce risk of invasive breast cancer in women with DCIS. Reduction of breast cancer incidence in high risk women. Use for up to 5 yrs.

**DOSAGE:** *Adults:* Breast Cancer Treatment: 20-40mg qd. Divide dosages >20mg into AM and PM doses. Breast Cancer Risk Reduction/DCIS: 20mg qd for 5 yrs.

**HOW SUPPLIED:** Sol: 10mg/5mL

**CONTRAINDICATIONS:** Reduction in breast cancer incidence in high risk women and women with DCIS who require coumarin-type anticoagulant therapy or have a history of DVT, PE.

**WARNINGS/PRECAUTIONS:** Hypercalcemia reported in patients with bone metastases. Increased incidence of uterine malignancies (eg, endometrial cancer, uterine sarcoma) and endometrial changes including hyperplasia and polyps reported. Increased incidence of thromboembolic events (eg, DVT, PE). Malignant and non-malignant effects on the liver and ocular disturbances reported. Leukopenia, anemia, thrombocytopenia, neutropenia, pancytopenia reported. Promptly evaluate abnormal vaginal bleeding if receiving or previously received tamoxifen. Patients receiving or previously received tamoxifen should have annual gynecological exam. Do not become pregnant within 2 months of therapy. May cause fetal harm during pregnancy. Does not cause infertility even with menstrual irregularity.

**ADVERSE REACTIONS:** Hot flashes, increased bone and tumor pain, vaginal discharge, irregular menses; (men) loss of libido, impotence.

**INTERACTIONS:** Increases effects of coumarin-type anticoagulant; monitor PT. Increased risk of thromboembolic events with cytotoxic agents. Increased levels with bromocriptine. May decrease letrozole levels. Decreased levels with rifampin and aminoglutethimide. Decreased plasma levels of major metabolite, N-desmethyl tamoxifen with medroxyprogesterone.

**PREGNANCY:** Category D, not for use in nursing.

## SOLU-CORTEF RX

hydrocortisone sodium succinate (Pharmacia & Upjohn)

**THERAPEUTIC CLASS:** Corticosteroid

**INDICATIONS:** Steroid responsive disorders.

**DOSAGE:** *Adults:* Initial: 100-500mg IV/IM, depending on condition severity. May repeat dose at 2, 4, or 6 hrs based on clinical response. High dose therapy usually not >48-72 hrs; may use antacids prophylactically.
*Pediatrics:* Use lower adult doses. Determine dose by severity of condition and response. Dose should not be <25mg/day.

**HOW SUPPLIED:** Inj: 100mg, 250mg, 500mg, 1g

**CONTRAINDICATIONS:** Premature infants, systemic fungal infections.

**WARNINGS/PRECAUTIONS:** May need to increase dose before, during, and after stressful situations. May mask signs of infection or cause new infections. Prolonged use may produce glaucoma, optic nerve damage, secondary ocular infections. Increases BP, salt/water retention, potassium and calcium excretion. More severe/fatal course of infections reported with chickenpox, measles. Enhanced effect with hypothyroidism or cirrhosis. Caution with Strongyloides, latent TB, ocular herpes simplex, HTN, diverticulitis, fresh intestinal anastomoses, ulcerative colitis, osteoporosis, myasthenia gravis, renal insufficiency, peptic ulcer disease. Kaposi's sarcoma reported. Monitor for psychic disturbances. Acute myopathy with high doses. Avoid abrupt withdrawal. Monitor growth and development of children on prolonged therapy. Hypernatremia may occur with high dose therapy >48-72 hrs.

**ADVERSE REACTIONS:** Fluid and electrolyte disturbances, HTN, osteoporosis, muscle weakness, cushingoid state, menstrual irregularities, vertigo, headache, impaired wound healing, DM, ulcerative esophagitis, peptic ulcer, pancreatitis, increased sweating, increases intracranial pressure, carbohydrate intolerance, glaucoma, cataracts.

**INTERACTIONS:** Reduced efficacy and increased clearance with hepatic enzyme inducers (eg, phenobarbital, phenytoin, and rifampin). Increases clearance of chronic high dose ASA. Caution with ASA in hypoprothrombinemia. Effects on oral anticoagulants are variable; monitor PT/INR. Increased insulin and oral hypoglycemic requirements in DM. Avoid live vaccines with immunosuppressive doses. Possible decreased vaccine response with killed or inactivated vaccines with immunosuppressive doses. Decreased clearance with ketoconazole and troleandomycin.

**PREGNANCY:** Safety in pregnancy and nursing not known.

## SOLU-MEDROL RX

methylprednisolone sodium succinate (Pharmacia & Upjohn)

**THERAPEUTIC CLASS:** Glucocorticoid

**INDICATIONS:** Steroid responsive disorders.

**DOSAGE:** *Adults:* Usual: Initial: 10-40mg IV over several minutes. May repeat IV/IM dose at intervals based on clinical response. High Dose Therapy: 30mg/kg IV over at least 30 minutes, may repeat q4-6h for 48 hrs. High dose therapy usually not >48-72 hrs. Give antacids prophylactically. Multiple Sclerosis: (4mg methylprednisolone=5mg prednisolone): 200mg/day prednisolone for 1 week, then 80mg every other day for 1 month.
*Pediatrics:* Use lower adult doses. Determine dose by severity of condition and response. Dose should not be <0.5mg/kg q24h.

**HOW SUPPLIED:** Inj: 40mg, 125mg, 500mg, 1g, 2g

**CONTRAINDICATIONS:** Premature infants (due to benzyl alcohol diluent) and systemic fungal infections.

**WARNINGS/PRECAUTIONS:** May need to increase dose before, during, and after stressful situations. May mask signs of infection or cause new infections. Prolonged use may produce cataracts, glaucoma, secondary ocular infections. Increases BP, salt/water retention, calcium/potassium excretion. More severe/fatal course of infections reported with chickenpox, measles. Caution with latent TB, hypothyroidism, cirrhosis, ocular herpes simplex, HTN, diverticulitis, fresh intestinal anastomoses, ulcerative colitis, osteoporosis, myasthenia gravis, renal insufficiency, peptic ulcer disease. Kaposi's sarcoma reported. Growth and development of children on prolonged therapy should be monitored. Monitor for psychic disturbances. Avoid abrupt withdrawal. Reports of cardiac arrhythmias, circulatory collapse, cardiac arrest following rapid administration of large IV doses. Effectiveness not established for the treatment of sepsis syndrome and septic shock. Bradycardia reportedwith high doses.

**ADVERSE REACTIONS:** Fluid and electrolyte disturbances, HTN, osteoporosis, muscle weakness, cushingoid state, menstrual irregularities, insomnia, impaired wound healing, DM, ulcerative esophagitis, excessive sweating, increases intracranial pressure, carbohydrate intolerance, glaucoma, cataracts, nausea.

**INTERACTIONS:** Reduced efficacy with hepatic enzyme inducers (eg, phenobarbital, phenytoin, and rifampin). Increases clearance of chronic high dose ASA. Caution with ASA in hypoprothrombinemia. Effects on oral anticoagulants are variable; monitor PT/INR. Increased insulin and oral hypoglycemic requirements in DM. Avoid live vaccines with immunosuppressive doses. Possible decreased vaccine response with killed or inactivated vaccines with immunosuppressive doses. Mutual inhibition of metabolism with cyclosporine; convulsions reported. Decreased clearance with ketoconazole and troleandomycin.

**PREGNANCY:** Safety in pregnancy and nursing not known.

## SOMA
carisoprodol (MedPointe)

RX

**THERAPEUTIC CLASS:** Skeletal muscle relaxant (central-acting)

**INDICATIONS:** Adjunct for relief of discomfort associated with acute, painful musculoskeletal conditions.

**DOSAGE:** *Adults:* 350mg tid and hs.
*Pediatrics:* >12 yrs: 350mg tid and hs.

**HOW SUPPLIED:** Tab: 350mg

**CONTRAINDICATIONS:** Acute intermittent porphyria. Allergic or idiosyncratic reactions to meprobamate.

**WARNINGS/PRECAUTIONS:** May have sedative properties. Cases of drug abuse, dependence and withdrawal have been reported. Caution in addiction-prone patients. First-dose idiosyncratic reactions reported (rare). Occasionally within the period of teh fisrt to fourth dose, allergic reactions have occured. Rare reports of seizures in postmarketing surveillance. Caution with liver or renal dysfunction.

**ADVERSE REACTIONS:** Drowsiness, dizziness, nausea, vomiting, tachycardia, postural hypotension, idiosyncratic reactions.

**INTERACTIONS:** Additive effects with alcohol, other CNS depressants, and psychotropic drugs.

**PREGNANCY:** Safety in pregnancy and nursing not known.

## SOMA CMPD/CODEINE
aspirin - carisoprodol - codeine phosphate (MedPointe)

CIII

**THERAPEUTIC CLASS:** Central muscle relaxant/analgesic

**INDICATIONS:** Adjunct for pain, muscle spasm, and limited mobility associated with acute, painful musculoskeletal conditions.

**DOSAGE:** *Adults:* 1-2 tabs qid.
*Pediatrics:* >12 yrs: 1-2 tabs qid.

**HOW SUPPLIED:** Tab: (Carisoprodol-Codeine-Aspirin) 200mg-16mg-325mg

**CONTRAINDICATIONS:** Acute intermittent porphyria, bleeding disorders.

**WARNINGS/PRECAUTIONS:** First-dose idiosyncratic reactions reported (rare). Caution with liver or renal dysfunction, elderly, peptic ulcer, gastritis, addiction-prone patients and anticoagulant therapy. Contains sulfites.

**ADVERSE REACTIONS:** Drowsiness, dizziness, vertigo, ataxia, nausea, vomiting, gastritis, occult bleeding, constipation, diarrhea, miosis.



**INTERACTIONS:** Enhances methotrexate toxicity and hypoglycemia with oral antidiabetics. Corticosteroids and antacids decrease plasma levels. Increases GI bleeding risk with alcohol. Potentiated by urine acidifiers (eg, ammonium chloride). Antagonizes uricosuric effects of probenecid, sulfinpyrazone. Additive effects with alcohol, other CNS depressants, psychotropic drugs. Increases bleeding risk with anticoagulants.

**PREGNANCY:** Category C, not for use in nursing.

## SOMA COMPOUND
aspirin - carisoprodol (MedPointe)

RX

**THERAPEUTIC CLASS:** Central muscle relaxant/analgesic

**INDICATIONS:** Adjunct for pain, muscle spasm and limited mobility associated with acute, painful musculoskeletal conditions.

**DOSAGE:** *Adults:* 1-2 tabs qid.
*Pediatrics:* >12 yrs: 1-2 tabs qid.

**HOW SUPPLIED:** Tab: (Carisoprodol-ASA) 200mg-325mg

**CONTRAINDICATIONS:** Acute intermittent porphyria, bleeding disorders.

**WARNINGS/PRECAUTIONS:** First-dose idiosyncratic reactions reported (rare). Caution with liver or renal dysfunction, elderly, peptic ulcer, gastritis, addiction-prone patients and anticoagulant therapy.

**ADVERSE REACTIONS:** Drowsiness, dizziness, vertigo, ataxia, nausea, vomiting, gastritis, occult bleeding, constipation, diarrhea.

**INTERACTIONS:** Enhances methotrexate toxicity and hypoglycemia with oral antidiabetics. Corticosteroids and antacids decrease plasma levels. Increases GI bleeding risk with alcohol. Potentiated by urine acidifiers (eg, ammonium chloride). Antagonizes uricosuric effects of probenecid, sulfinpyrazone. Additive effects with alcohol, other CNS depressants, psychotropic drugs. Increases bleeding risk with anticoagulants.

**PREGNANCY:** Category C, not for use in nursing.

## SOMAVERT — RX

pegvisomant (Pharmacia & Upjohn)

**THERAPEUTIC CLASS:** Growth hormone receptor antagonist

**INDICATIONS:** Treatment of acromegaly in those who have had an inadequate response to surgery and/or radiation therapy, and/or other medical therapies, or for whom these therapies are not appropriate.

**DOSAGE:** *Adults:* LD: 40mg SQ. Maint: 10mg SQ qd. Titrate: Adjust dose by 5mg increments/decrements, based on IGF-I levels, every 4 to 6 weeks. Max: 30mg/day. LFTs >3X/<5X ULN (without symptoms of liver dysfunction): Monitor LFTs weekly. LFTs >5X ULN/Transaminase Elevations >3X ULN: Discontinue immediately and evaluate. Do not initiate if baseline LFTs >3X ULN until cause is determined.

**HOW SUPPLIED:** Inj: 10mg, 15mg, 20mg

**WARNINGS/PRECAUTIONS:** May expand and cause serious complications of tumors that secrete GH; monitor with periodic imaging scans of the sella turcica. May increase glucose tolerance and risk of hypoglycemia in diabetics. May result in functional GH deficiency. AST/ALT elevations reported; obtain baseline ALT, AST, TBIL, and ALP levels prior to initiation. Monitor LFTs monthly for first 6 months, quarterly for next 6 months, then biannually; monitor more frequently if elevations occur. Discontinue if liver injury is confirmed. Monitor IGF-I levels 4 to 6 weeks after initiation or dose adjustments; every 6 months after levels are normalized. Interferes with the measurement serum GH levels by commercially available GH assays; do not adjust dosage based on serum GH levels.

**ADVERSE REACTIONS:** Infection, abnormal LFTs, pain, injection site reactions, back pain, diarrhea, nausea, flu syndrome, chest pain, dizziness, paresthesia, HTN, sinusitis, peripheral edema.

**INTERACTIONS:** May need to reduce dosage of insulin and/or hypoglycemic agents. Concomitant opioids may increase dosage requirements of pegvisomant.

**PREGNANCY:** Category B; caution in nursing.

## SONATA — CIV

zaleplon (King)

**THERAPEUTIC CLASS:** Pyrazolopyrimidine (non-benzodiazepine)

**INDICATIONS:** Short-term treatment of insomnia.

**DOSAGE:** *Adults:* Insomnia: 10mg qhs. Low Weight Patients: Start with 5mg hs. Max: 20mg/day. Elderly/Debilitated/Concomitant Cimetidine: 5mg qhs. Max:

10mg/day. Mild to Moderate Hepatic Dysfunction: 5mg qhs. Take immediately prior to bedtime.

**HOW SUPPLIED:** Cap: 5mg, 10mg

**WARNINGS/PRECAUTIONS:** Monitor elderly/debilitated closely. Abnormal thinking and behavioral changes reported. Avoid abrupt withdrawal. Abuse potential exist. Caution in respiratory disorders, depression, conditions affecting metabolism or hemodynamic responses, and mild-to-moderate hepatic insufficiency. Not for use in severe hepatic impairment. May cause impaired coordination even the following day. Re-evaluate if no improvement of insomnia after 7-10 days of therapy. Contains tartrazine.

**ADVERSE REACTIONS:** Headache, asthenia, nausea, dizziness, amnesia, somnolence, eye pain, dysmenorrhea, abdominal pain.

**INTERACTIONS:** Potentiates CNS depression with psychotropics (eg, thioridazine, imipramine), anticonvulsants, antihistamines, alcohol and other CNS depressants. CYP3A4 inducers (eg, rifampin, phenytoin, carbamazepine and phenobarbital) decreases levels. Potentiated by cimetidine.

**PREGNANCY:** Category C, not for use in nursing.

## SORIATANE RX

acitretin (Stiefel)

**Avoid in pregnancy or becoming pregnant <3 yrs after discontinuation of therapy; use 2 reliable forms of contraception. Only use in females of reproductive potential with severe psoriasis unresponsive or contraindicated to other therapies, if receive warnings of therapy hazards and risk of contraception failure, if negative pregnancy test within 1 week before therapy, will begin therapy on the 2nd or 3rd day of next menstrual cycle, are capable of complying with contraceptive measures and are reliable. Repeat pregnancy testing and contraception counseling on a regular basis. It is not known whether residual acitretin in seminal fluid poses risk to fetus with male patients during or after therapy. Females should avoid ethanol during and 2 months after therapy.**

**THERAPEUTIC CLASS:** Retinoid

**INDICATIONS:** Treatment of severe psoriasis, including erythrodermic and generalized pustular types.

**DOSAGE:** *Adults:* Initial: 25-50mg single dose qd with main meal. Individualize dose based on intersubject variation in pharmacokinetics, clinical efficacy, and incidence of side effects. Maint: 25-50mg qd. Terminate therapy when lesions resolve. May treat relapses as outlined for initial therapy.

**HOW SUPPLIED:** Cap: 10mg, 25mg

**CONTRAINDICATIONS:** Pregnancy. See black box warnings.

**WARNINGS/PRECAUTIONS:** Risk of hepatotoxicity, pancreatitis, and pseudotumor cerebri. D/C if visual difficulties occur; decreased night vision and reduced tolerance to contact lenses reported. Bony abnormalities of the vertebral column, knees, and ankles reported. Increases TG and cholesterol and decreases HDL; perform lipid tests before therapy every 1-2 weeks until establish lipid response. Caution with severe hepatic/renal impairment. Transient worsening of psoriasis may occur initially. Do not donate blood during and for 3 yrs after therapy. Avoid sun lamps and excessive sun exposure. Depression and/or psychiatric symptoms (eg, aggressive feelings, thoughts of self-harm) reported.



**ADVERSE REACTIONS:** Ophthalmologic effects, cheilitis, rhinitis, dry mouth, epistaxis, alopecia, dry skin, rash, skin peeling, nail disorder, pruritus, paresthesia, paronychia, skin atrophy, sticky skin, xerophthalmia, arthralgia, rash.

**INTERACTIONS:** Caution with oral hypoglycemics. May increase risk of hepatotoxicity with methotrexate. Interferes with microdosed progestin"minipill" oral contraceptives. Females should avoid ethanol during and 2 months after therapy. Possible additive toxic effects with vitamin A doses that exceed minimum RDAs.

**PREGNANCY:** Category X, not for use in nursing.

## SPECTAZOLE RX
econazole nitrate (Ortho Neutrogena)

**THERAPEUTIC CLASS:** Azole antifungal

**INDICATIONS:** Treatment of tinea pedis, tinea cruris, and tinea corporis caused by *Trichophyton rubrum*, *Trichophyton mentagrophytes*, *Trichophyton tonsurans*, *Microsporum canis*, *Microsporum audouini*, *Microsporum gypseum*, and *Epidermophyton floccosum*. Treatment of cutaneous candidiasis and tinea versicolor.

**DOSAGE:** *Adults:* T.cruris/T.corporis/T.versicolor: Apply qd for 2 weeks. T.pedis: Apply qd for 4 weeks. Cutaneous Candidiasis: Apply bid for 2 weeks.

**HOW SUPPLIED:** Cre: 1% [15g, 30g, 85g]

**WARNINGS/PRECAUTIONS:** Avoid eyes.

**ADVERSE REACTIONS:** Burning, itching, stinging, erythema.

**PREGNANCY:** Category C, caution with nursing.

## SPECTRACEF RX
cefditoren pivoxil (Purdue Pharmaceutical)

**THERAPEUTIC CLASS:** Cephalosporin (3rd generation)

**INDICATIONS:** Treatment of acute bacterial exacerbations of chronic bronchitis (ABECB), pharyngitis/tonsillitis, community acquired pneumonia (CAP), and uncomplicated skin and skin-structure infections (SSSI).

**DOSAGE:** *Adults:* ABECB: 400mg bid for 10 days. Pharyngitis/Tonsillitis/SSSI: 200mg bid for 10 days. CAP: 400mg bid for 14 days. CrCl 30-49mL/min: 200mg bid. CrCl <30mL/min: 200mg qd. Take with meals.
*Pediatrics:* >12 yrs: ABECB: 400mg bid for 10 days. Pharyngitis/Tonsillitis/SSSI: 200mg bid for 10 days. CAP: 400mg bid for 14 days. CrCl 30-49mL/min: 200mg bid. CrCl <30mL/min: 200mg qd. Take with meals.

**HOW SUPPLIED:** Tab: 200mg

**CONTRAINDICATIONS:** Milk protein hypersensitivity, carnitine deficiency.

**WARNINGS/PRECAUTIONS:** Cross sensitivity to penicillins and other cephalosporins may occur. Pseudomembranous colitis reported. Not recommended for prolonged antibiotic therapy. Prolonged therapy may cause superinfection. May decrease PT.

**ADVERSE REACTIONS:** Diarrhea, nausea, vaginal moniliasis.

**INTERACTIONS:** Avoid antacids. H2 receptor antagonists may reduce absorption. Increased plasma levels with probenecid.

**PREGNANCY:** Category B, caution in nursing.



## SPIRIVA RX
tiotropium bromide (Boehringer Ingelheim/Pfizer)

**THERAPEUTIC CLASS:** Anticholinergic bronchodilator

**INDICATIONS:** Long-term maintenance treatment of bronchospasm associated with chronic obstructive pulmonary disease (COPD), including chronic bronchitis and emphysema.

**DOSAGE:** *Adults:* Inhale contents of one capsule (18mcg) qd, with HandiHaler device.

**HOW SUPPLIED:** Cap, Inhalation: 18mcg [5[s], 30[s]]

**CONTRAINDICATIONS:** Hypersensitivity to atropine or its derivatives (eg, ipratropium).

**WARNINGS/PRECAUTIONS:** Not for initial treatment of acute episodes. D/C if hypersensitivity (eg, angioedema) or paradoxical bronchospasm occurs. Caution with narrow-angle glaucoma, prostatic hyperplasia, bladder-neck obstruction. Monitor with moderate to severe renal impairment (CrCl ≤50mL/min).

**ADVERSE REACTIONS:** Dry mouth, arthritis, cough, flu-like symptoms, sinusitis, constipation, abdominal pain, UTI, moniliasis, rash, dizziness, dysphagia, hoarseness, intestinal obstruction-ileus paralytic, increased IOP, oral candidiasis, tachycardia, throat irritation.

**INTERACTIONS:** Avoid with other anticholinergics (eg, ipratropium).

**PREGNANCY:** Category C, caution in nursing.

## SPORANOX RX

itraconazole (Janssen/Ortho Biotech)

**Contraindicated with cisapride, pimozide, quinidine, or dofetilide. Serious cardiovascular events (eg, QT prolongation, torsade de pointes, ventricular tachycardia, cardiac arrest, and/or sudden death) reported with cisapride, pimozide, quinidine and other CYP3A4 inhibitors. Do not use caps for onychomycosis with ventricular dysfunction.**

**THERAPEUTIC CLASS:** Azole antifungal

**INDICATIONS:** (Cap) Onychomycosis of the toenail and fingernail in immunocompetent patients. Confirm diagnosis before therapy. (Cap, Inj) Treatment of blastomycosis and histoplasmosis. Treatment of aspergillosis if refractory to or intolerant to amphoteracin B. (Sol) Treatment of oropharyngeal and esophageal candidiasis. (Inj/Sol) Empiric therapy of febrile, neutropenic patients with suspected fungal infections (ETFN).

**DOSAGE:** *Adults:* (Cap) Take with full meal. If patient has achlorhydria or is also taking gastric acid suppressors give with a cola beverage. Toenail Onchomycosis: 200mg qd for 12 weeks. Fingernail Onchomycosis: 200mg bid for 1 week, then skip for 3 weeks, then 200mg bid for 1 week. Blastomycosis/Histoplasmosis: 200mg qd. May increase by 100mg increments if no improvement. Max: 400mg/day. Give bid if dose >200mg/day. Aspergillosis: 200-400mg/day. Life-Threatening Infections: LD: 200mg tid for 1st 3 days. Continue for at least 3 months. (IV) Give by IV infusion over 1 hour. Blastomycosis/Histoplasmosis/Aspergillosis: 200mg bid for 4 doses, then 200mg qd, up to 14 days. Continue with caps for at least 3 months. Treat for at least 3 months. ETFN/Life-Threatening Infections: 200mg IV bid for 4 doses, then 200mg qd for up to 14 days. Continue with solution 200mg PO bid, up to 28 days. (Sol) Oropharyngeal Candidiasis: 200mg/day for 1-2 weeks. Refractory to Fluconazole: 100mg bid (response in 2-4 weeks, may relapse shortly after discontinuation). Esophageal Candidiasis: 100-200mg/day for at least 3 weeks. Continue for 2 weeks after symptoms resolve. Take on empty stomach. Swish 10mL at a time for several seconds, then swallow.

S

**HOW SUPPLIED:** Cap: 100mg; Inj: 10mg/mL; Sol: 10mg/mL [150mL]

**CONTRAINDICATIONS:** (Cap, Inj, Sol) Concomitant cisapride, oral midazolam, pimozide, quinidine, dofetilide, triazolam, and HMG CoA-reductase inhibitors metabolized by CYP3A4 (eg, lovastatin, simvastatin). (Cap) Treatment of onychomycosis if pregnant or contemplating pregnancy, ventricular dysfunction (eg, CHF).

**WARNINGS/PRECAUTIONS:** Rare cases of hepatotoxicity reported. Monitor LFTs; discontinue if hepatic dysfunction develops. Avoid with liver disease. D/C if neuropathy or CHF occurs. Solution and capsules are not interchangeable. Consider alternative therapy if unresponsive in patients with cystic fibrosis. Avoid with ventricular dysfunction. Caution with ischemic/valvular disease, pulmonary disease, renal failure, other edematous disorders. Avoid injection if CrCl <30mL/min.

**ADVERSE REACTIONS:** Nausea, diarrhea, vomiting, abdominal pain, fever, cough, rash, increased sweating, headache, hypokalemia.

**INTERACTIONS:** See Contraindications. Increased levels with cisapride, pimozide, quinidine, dofetilide, oral midazolam, triazolam, HMG-CoA-reductase inhibitors; concurrent use is contraindicated. Increases levels of rifabutin, immunosuppressants, protease inhibitors, alfentanil, buspirone, methylprednisolone, trimetrexate, carbamazepine, HMG CoA-reductase inhibitors, digoxin, warfarin, busulfan, docetaxel, vinca alkaloids, astemizole, alprazolam, diazepam, oral midazolam, triazolam, dihydropyridine calcium channel blockers, verapamil, oral hypoglycemics. CYP3A4 inducers (eg, carbamazepine, phenobarbital, phenytoin, isoniazid, rifabutin, rifampin, nevirapine) decrease itraconazole levels. CYP3A4 inhibitors (eg, erythromycin, clarithromycin, indinavir, ritonavir) may increase itraconazole levels. Severe hypoglycemia with oral hypoglycemics. Additive negative inotropic effects with calcium channel blockers. Edema reported with dihydropyridine calcium channel blockers; adjust dose. Decreased absorption of capsules with antacids or gastric secretion suppressors.

**PREGNANCY:** Category C, not for use in nursing.

## SPRYCEL RX

dasatinib (Bristol-Myers Squibb)

**THERAPEUTIC CLASS:** Tyrosine kinase inhibitor

**INDICATIONS:** Treatment of chronic, accelerated, or myeloid or lymphoid blast phase chronic myeloid leukemia (CML) with resistance or intolerance to prior therapy including imatinib. Treament of Philadelphia chromosome-positive acute lymphoblastic leukemia (Ph+ ALL) with resistance or intolerance to prior therapy.

**DOSAGE:** *Adults*: 70mg bid. Swallow whole; do not crush. Dose Escalation: Chronic Phase CML: 90mg bid; Advanced Phase CML/Ph+ ALL: 100mg bid.

**HOW SUPPLIED:** Tab: 20mg, 50mg, 70mg

**WARNINGS/PRECAUTIONS:** Severe thrombocytopenia, neutropenia, and anemia reported; monitor CBC weekly for first 2 months, then monthly thereafter. Severe CNS hemorrhages including fatalities, gastrointestinal hemorrhage, and other hemorrhage cases reported; caution in patients on medications that inhibit platelet function or anticoagulants. Pleural and pericardial effusion reported. Severe ascities, generalized edema, severe pulmonary edema reported. QT prolongation reported; caution in patients at risk (eg, hypokalemia or hypomagnesemia, congenital long QT syndrome, concomitant anti-arrhythmics or other QT prolonging agents, cumulative high-dose anthracycline therapy); correct hypokalemia or hypomagnesemia prior to administration. Caution with hepatic impairment.

**ADVERSE REACTIONS:** Fluid retention events, diarrhea, nausea, abdominal pain, vomiting, bleeding events, pyrexia, pleural effusion, febrile neutropenia, gastrointestinal bleeding, pneumonia, thrombocytopenia, dyspnea, anemia, cardiac failure.

**INTERACTIONS:** Increased levels with CYP3A4 inhibitors (eg, ketoconazole, itraconazole, erythromycin, clarithromycin, ritonavir, atazanavir, indinavir, nefazodone, nelfinavir, saquinavir, telithromycin). Decreased levels with CYP3A4 inducers (eg, dexamethasone, phenytoin, carbamazepine, rifampicin, phenobarbital, St. John's wort). Avoid antacids; if necessary administer 2 hrs prior to or 2 hrs after dose. Concomitant use of $H_2$ blockers or PPIs is not recommended. Caution with CYP3A4 substrates with narrow therapeutic windows (eg, alfentanil, astemizole, terfenadine, cisapride, cyclosporine, fentanyl, pimozide, quinidine, sirolimus, tacrolimus, or ergot alkaloids such as ergotamine, dihydroergotamine).

**PREGNANCY:** Category D, not for use in nursing.

## SSKI
RX

potassium iodide (Upsher-Smith)

**THERAPEUTIC CLASS:** Expectorant

**INDICATIONS:** Symptomatic treatment of chronic pulmonary diseases complicated by tenacious mucus, including bronchial asthma, bronchitis and pulmonary emphysema.

**DOSAGE:** *Adults:* 0.3-0.6mL (300-600mg) tid-qid. Dilute in glassful of water, juice, or milk. Take with food or milk.

**HOW SUPPLIED:** Sol: 1g/mL [30mL]

**CONTRAINDICATIONS:** Iodide sensitivity.

**WARNINGS/PRECAUTIONS:** Caution with Addison's disease, cardiac disease, hyperthyroidism, myotonia congenita, tuberculosis, acute bronchitis, renal impairment. May cause fetal harm, abnormal thyroid function, and goiter in pregnant women. Prolonged use may lead to hypothyroidism or iodism; discontinue if iodism occurs. May alter thyroid function tests.

**ADVERSE REACTIONS:** Stomach upset/pain, diarrhea, nausea, vomiting, skin rash, salivary gland swelling/tenderness, thyroid adenoma, goiter, myxedema.

**INTERACTIONS:** May potentiate the hypothyroid and goitrogenic effects of lithium and other antithyroid drugs. Potassium-containing medications, potassium-sparing diuretics, and ACE inhibitors may cause hyperkalemia, cardiac arrhythmias, or cardiac arrest.

**PREGNANCY:** Category D, caution in nursing.

## STADOL NS
CIV

butorphanol tartrate (Bristol-Myers Squibb)

**THERAPEUTIC CLASS:** Opioid agonist-antagonist analgesic

**INDICATIONS:** Management of pain when the use of an opioid analgesic is appropriate.

**DOSAGE:** *Adults:* >18 yrs: Initial: 1 spray (1mg) in 1 nostril, may repeat after 60-90 minutes (after 90-120 minutes in elderly or renal/hepatic disease) and may repeat in 3-4 hrs after 2nd dose; or may use 1 spray in each nostril, may repeat after 3-4 hrs. Renal/Hepatic Disease: Increase dose interval to no less than 6 hrs.

**HOW SUPPLIED:** Nasal Spray: 10mg/mL [2.5mL]

**CONTRAINDICATIONS:** Hypersensitivity to benzethonium chloride.

S

**WARNINGS/PRECAUTIONS:** Not for use in narcotic-dependent patients. May result in physical dependence or tolerance. Avoid abrupt cessation. D/C if severe HTN occurs. Caution with hepatic or renal disease, acute MI, ventricular dysfunction, or coronary insufficiency. May impair ability to operate machinery. Increased respiratory depression with CNS disease or respiratory impairment. Severe risks with head injury.

**ADVERSE REACTIONS:** Somnolence, dizziness, nausea, vomiting, nasal congestion, insomnia.

**INTERACTIONS:** Increased CNS depression and respiratory depression with alcohol, barbiturates, tranquilizers, and antihistamines. May be potentiated by erythromycin, theophylline and other drugs that affect hepatic metabolism. Decreased absorption rate with nasal vasoconstrictors (eg, oxymetazoline). Diminished analgesic effect if administered shortly after sumatriptan nasal spray.

**PREGNANCY:** Category C, caution in nursing.

## STALEVO

RX

levodopa - carbidopa - entacapone (Novartis)

**THERAPEUTIC CLASS:** Dopa-decarboxylase inhibitor/dopamine precursor/COMT inhibitor

**INDICATIONS:** Treatment of idiopathic Parkinson's disease to substitute for equivalent doses of previously administered carbidopa/levodopa and entacapone or for those experiencing signs and symptoms of end-of-dose"wearing off" and are taking up to 600mg/day levodopa without experiencing dyskinesias.

**DOSAGE:** *Adults:* Currently Taking Carbidopa/Levodopa and Entacapone: May switch directly to corresponding strength of levodopa/carbidopa. Currently Taking Carbidopa/Levodopa but not Entacapone: First titrate individually with carbidopa/levodopa product and entacapone product then transfer to corresponding dose. Max: 8 tabs/day.

**HOW SUPPLIED:** Tab: (Carbidopa/Levodopa/Entacapone): Stalevo 50: 12.5mg/50mg/200mg; Stalevo 100: 25mg/100mg/200mg; Stalevo 150: 37.5mg/150mg/200mg

**CONTRAINDICATIONS:** MAOIs during or within 14 days of use, narrow-angle glaucoma, undiagnosed skin lesions, history of melanoma.

**WARNINGS/PRECAUTIONS:** Dyskinesia, mental disturbances, hypotension/syncope, hallucinations, rhabdomyolysis, hyperpyrexia, confusion, and fibrotic complications reported. Caution with biliary obstruction, severe cardiovascular or pulmonary disease, bronchial asthma, renal, hepatic or endocrine disease, chronic wide-angle glaucoma, history of MI with residual arrhythmias, peptic ulcer. Neuroleptic malignant syndrome reported with dose reductions or withdrawal. Avoid rapid withdrawal or abrupt dose reduction. May cause dark color to appear in saliva, urine, or sweat. May cause false (+) ketonuria, false (-) glucosuria (glucose-oxidase method), elevated LFTs, abnormal BUN, positive Coombs test. May depress prolactin secretion and increase growth hormone levels.

**ADVERSE REACTIONS:** Dyskinesia, hyperkinesia, hypokinesia, dizziness, nausea, diarrhea, abdominal pain, constipation, vomiting, urine discoloration, back pain, fatigue.

**INTERACTIONS:** See Contraindications. Increased HR, arrhythmias, and BP changes with drugs metabolized by COMT (eg, isoproterenol, epinephrine, norepinephrine, dopamine, dobutamine, alpha-methyldopa, apomorphine, isoetherine, bitolterol). Probenecid, cholestyramine, and some antibiotics (eg, erythromycin, rifampicin, ampicillin, chloramphenicol) may interfere with biliary excretion. Risk of postural hypotension with antihypertensives, selegiline. HTN and dyskinesia may occur with TCAs. Reduced effect with phenytoin, papaverine, metoclopramide, isoniazid, dopamine $D_2$ antagonists (eg, phenothiazines, butyrophenones, risperidone). Reduced bioavailability with iron salts. Caution with highly protein-bound drugs (eg, warfarin, salicylic acid, phenylbutazone, diazepam).

**PREGNANCY:** Category C, caution in nursing.

## STARLIX

RX

nateglinide (Novartis)

**THERAPEUTIC CLASS:** Meglitinide

**INDICATIONS:** Adjunt to diet and exercise, as monotherapy, to improve glycemic control in type 2 diabetics who have not been chronically treated with other antidiabetic agents. May be used in combination with metformin or a thiazolidinedione (TZD).

**DOSAGE:** *Adults:* Initial/Maint: 120mg tid before meals (with or without metformin or TZD). Take 1-30 minutes before meals. May use 60mg tid (with



S

or without metformin or TZD) in patients near goal $HbA_{1c}$. Skip dose if meal is skipped.

**HOW SUPPLIED:** Tab: 60mg, 120mg

**CONTRAINDICATIONS:** Type 1 diabetes, diabetic ketoacidosis.

**WARNINGS/PRECAUTIONS:** Caution in moderate to severe hepatic impairment. Transient loss of glucose control with trauma, surgery, fever, and infection; may need insulin therapy. Secondary failure may occur in prolonged therapy. Hypoglycemia risk in elderly, debilitated, malnourished, strenuous exercise, and with adrenal or pituitary insufficiency. Autonomic neuropathy may mask hypoglycemia.

**ADVERSE REACTIONS:** Upper respiratory infection, flu symptoms, dizziness, arthropathy, diarrhea, hypoglycemia, back pain, jaundice, cholestatic hepatitis, elevated liver enzymes.

**INTERACTIONS:** Potentiated hypoglycemia with alcohol, NSAIDs, salicylates, MAOIs, and non-selective β-blockers. Risk of hyperglycemia with thiazides, corticosteroids, thyroid products and sympathomimetics. May potentiate tolbutamide. Peak plasma levels reduced with liquid meals. β-blockers may mask hypoglycemic effects. Caution with highly protein-bound drugs.

**PREGNANCY:** Category C, not for use in nursing.

## STRATTERA RX
atomoxetine HCl (Lilly)

**Increased risk of suicidal ideation in short-term studies in children or adolescents with ADHD. Closely monitor for suicidality, clinical worsening, or unusual changes in behavior. Close observation/communication with prescriber by families and caregivers is advised.**

**THERAPEUTIC CLASS:** Selective norepinephrine reuptake inhibitor

**INDICATIONS:** Treatment of attention-deficit hyperactivity disorder (ADHD).

**DOSAGE:** *Adults:* Initial: 40mg/day given qam or evenly divided doses in the am and late afternoon/early evening. Titrate: Increase after minimum of 3 days to target dose of about 80mg/day. After 2-4 weeks, may increase to max of 100mg/day. Max: 100mg/day. Hepatic Insufficiency: Moderate (Child-Pugh Class B): Reduce initial and target doses to 50% of normal dose. Severe (Child-Pugh Class C): Reduce initial and target doses to 25% of normal dose. Concomitant CYP450 2D6 inhibitor (eg, paroxetine, fluoxetine, quinidine): Initial: 40mg/day. Titrate: Only increase to 80mg/day if symptoms fail to improve after 4 weeks.
*Pediatrics:* ≥6 yrs: ≤70kg: Initial: 0.5mg/kg/day given qam or evenly divided doses in the am and late afternoon or early evening. Titrate: Increase after minimum of 3 days to target dose of about 1.2mg/kg/day. Max: 1.4mg/kg/day or 100mg, whichever is less. >70kg: Initial: 40mg/day given qam or evenly divided doses in the am and late afternoon/early evening. Titrate: Increase after minimum of 3 days to target dose of about 80mg/day. After 2-4 weeks, may increase to max of 100mg/day. Max: 100mg/day. Hepatic Insufficiency: Moderate (Child-Pugh Class B): Reduce initial and target doses to 50% of the normal dose. Severe (Child-Pugh Class C): Reduce initial and target doses to 25% of normal dose. Concomitant CYP450 2D6 inhibitor (eg, paroxetine, fluoxetine, quinidine): ≥6 yrs: ≤70kg: Initial: 0.5mg/kg/day. Titrate: Only increase to 1.2mg/kg/day if symptoms fail to improve after 4 weeks. >70kg: Initial: 40mg/day. Titrate: Only increase to 80mg/day if symptoms fail to improve after 4 weeks.

**HOW SUPPLIED:** Cap: 10mg, 18mg, 25mg, 40mg, 60mg

**CONTRAINDICATIONS:** During or within 14 days of MAOI use; narrow angle glaucoma.

**WARNINGS/PRECAUTIONS:** Allergic reactions and orthostatic hypotension reported. Monitor growth. May increase BP and HR; caution with HTN, tachycardia, cardiovascular or cerebrovascular disease. May increase urinary retention and urinary hesitation. May cause severe liver injury in rare cases;

monitor liver enzymes and d/c with jaundice or liver injury. Reports of MI, stroke and sudden death in adults. Avoid with known structural cardiac abnormalities or other serious cardiac problems. Physical exam and evaluation of patient history is necessary. Stimulants at usual doses can cause treatment emergent psychotic or manic symptoms (eg, hallucinations, delusional thinking, mania) in children and adolescents without prior history of psychotic illness.

**ADVERSE REACTIONS:** (Adults) Dry mouth, headache, insomnia, nausea, decreased appetite, constipation, dysmenorrhea, ejaculation failure/disorder, urinary retention. (Pediatrics) Upper abdominal pain, headache, vomiting, decreased appetite, cough, irritability, dizziness, somnolence.

**INTERACTIONS:** See Contraindications. May potentiate the cardiovascular effects of albuterol or other $\beta_2$ agonists. Caution with pressor agents. Increased levels in extensive metabolizers with CYP2D6 inhibitors (eg, paroxetine, fluoxetine, quinidine); atomoxetine may need dose adjustment.

**PREGNANCY:** Category C, caution in nursing.

## STREPTASE RX

streptokinase (ZLB Behring)

**THERAPEUTIC CLASS:** Thrombolytic agent

**INDICATIONS:** For lysis of PE, DVT, and acute arterial thrombi and emboli. Alternative to surgical revision to clear totally or partially occluded arteriovenous (AV) cannulae. For lysis of intracoronary thrombi; ventricular function improvement; and reduction of mortality, CHF, and infarct size in AMI.

**DOSAGE:** *Adults:* AMI: IV: 1.5MIU within 60 minutes. Intracoronary: 20,000IU infusion bolus, then 2000IU/min for 60 minutes for total 140,000U. PE: LD: 250,000IU over 30 minutes. IV Infusion: 100,000IU/hr for 24 hrs (72 hrs if concurrent DVT). DVT: LD: 250,000IU over 30 minutes. IV Infusion: 100,000IU/hr for 72 hrs. Arterial Thrombosis or Embolism: LD: 250,000IU over 30 minutes. IV Infusion: 100,000IU/hr for 24-72 hrs. AV Cannulae Occlusion: Instill 250,000IU in 2mL of solution into occluded limb of cannula; clamp off cannula limb for 2 hrs. Aspirate contents after therapy, flush with saline, and reconnect cannula.

**HOW SUPPLIED:** Inj: 250,000IU, 750,000IU, 1.5MIU

**CONTRAINDICATIONS:** Active internal bleeding, recent CVA, recent intracranial or intraspinal surgery, intracranial neoplasm, severe uncontrolled HTN.

**WARNINGS/PRECAUTIONS:** Weigh benefits/risks with recent major surgery, previous puncture of noncompressible vessels, cerebrovascular disease, recent serious GI bleeding or trauma, HTN, left heart thrombus, subacute bacterial endocarditis, hemostatic defects, pregnancy, diabetic hemorrhagic retinopathy, septic thrombophlebitis or occluded AV cannula at a seriously infected site, >75 yrs, any other bleeding condition that is difficult to manage. Cholesterol embolism, non-cardiogenic pulmonary edema, hypotension, and bleeding reported. Arrhythmias may occur with reperfusion. Increased resistance due to antistreptokinase antibody.

**ADVERSE REACTIONS:** Bleeding, allergic reactions (eg, fever, shivering), respiratory depression.

**INTERACTIONS:** Antiplatelets and anticoagulants may cause bleeding problems.

**PREGNANCY:** Category C, safety not known in nursing.

## STREPTOMYCIN

RX

streptomycin sulfate (Various)

**Risk of severe neurotoxic reactions (eg, vestibular and cochlear disturbances) increased significantly with renal dysfunction or pre-renal azotemia. Optic nerve dysfunction, peripheral neuritis, arachnoiditis, and encephalopathy may occur. Monitor renal function; reduce dose with renal impairment and/or nitrogen retention. Do not exceed peak serum level of 20-25mcg/mL with kidney damage. Avoid other neurotoxic and/or nephrotoxic drugs (eg, neomycin, kanamycin, gentamicin, cephaloridine, paromomycin, viomycin, polymyxin B, colistin, tobramycin, cyclosporine). Respiratory paralysis can occur, especially if given soon after anesthesia or muscle relaxants. Reserve parenteral form when adequate lab and audiometric testing is available.**

**THERAPEUTIC CLASS:** Aminoglycoside

**INDICATIONS:** Treatment of moderate to severe infections such as mycobacterium tuberculosis (TB) and non-TB infections (eg, plague, tularemia, chancroid, granuloma inguinale, *H.influenzae* and *K.pneumoniae* infections, UTI, gram-negative bacillary bacteremia, endocardial infections).

**DOSAGE:** *Adults:* IM only. TB: 15mg/kg/day (Max: 1g), or 25-30mg/kg twice weekly (Max: 1.5g), or 25-30mg/kg three times weekly (Max: 1.5g). Do not exceed a total dose of 120g over the course of therapy unless no other therapeutic options exist. Elderly (>60 yrs): Reduce dose. Treat for minimum of 1 year if possible. Tularemia: 1-2g/day in divided doses for 7-14 days until afebrile for 5-7 days. Plague: 1g bid for minimum of 10 days. Streptococcal Endocarditis: With PCN, 1g bid for week 1, then 500mg bid for week 2. Elderly (>60 yrs): 500mg bid for 2 weeks. Enterococcal Endocarditis: With PCN, 1g bid for 2 weeks, then 500mg bid for 4 weeks. Renal Impairment: Reduce dose. Moderate/Severe Infections: 1-2g/day in divided doses q6-12h. Max: 2g/day. *Pediatrics:* IM only. TB: 20-40mg/kg/day (Max: 1g), or 25-30mg/kg twice weekly (Max: 1.5g), or 25-30mg/kg three times weekly (Max: 1.5g). Do not exceed a total dose of 120g over the course of therapy unless no other therapeutic options exist. Treat for minimum of 1 year if possible. Moderate/Severe Infections: 20-40mg/kg/day (8-20mg/lb/day) in divided doses q6-12h.

**HOW SUPPLIED:** Inj: 1g

**WARNINGS/PRECAUTIONS:** Vestibular and auditory dysfunction may occur. Contains sodium metabisulfite. Can cause fetal harm in pregnancy. Caution with dose selection in renal impairment. Alkalinize urine to minimize or prevent renal irritation with prolonged therapy. CNS depression (eg, stupor, flaccidity) reported in infants with higher than recommended doses. If syphilis is suspected when treating venereal infections, perform dark field exam before initiate treatment, and monthly serologic tests for at least 4 months. Overgrowth of nonsusceptible organisms may occur. Terminate therapy when toxic symptoms appear, when impending toxicity is feared, when organisms become resistant, or when full treatment effect has been obtained.



**ADVERSE REACTIONS:** Vestibular ototoxicity (nausea, vomiting, vertigo), paresthesia of face, rash, fever, urticaria, angioneurotic edema, eosinophilia.

**INTERACTIONS:** See Black Box Warning. Increased ototoxicity with ethacrynic acid, furosemide, mannitol and possibly other diuretics.

**PREGNANCY:** Category D, not for use in nursing.

## STRIANT

CIII

testosterone (Columbia Labs)

**THERAPEUTIC CLASS:** Androgen

**INDICATIONS:** Testosterone replacement therapy in males with primary or hypogonadotrophic hypogonadism.

**DOSAGE:** *Adults:* 30mg q12h to gum region, just above the incisor tooth on either side of mouth. Rotate sites with each application. Hold system in place for 30 seconds.

**HOW SUPPLIED:** Tab, Buccal: 30mg [6 blister packs, 10 buccal systems/blister]

**CONTRAINDICATIONS:** Women. Breast or prostate carcinoma in men.

**WARNINGS/PRECAUTIONS:** Caution in elderly; increased risk of prostatic hyperplasia/carcinoma. Risk of edema with pre-existing cardiac, renal, or hepatic disease; discontinue if edema occurs. May potentiate sleep apnea, especially with obesity or chronic lung diseases. Monitor Hgb, Hct, LFTs, PSA, cholesterol, lipids, serum testosterone.

**ADVERSE REACTIONS:** Gum/mouth irritation, bitter taste, gum pain/tenderness, headache, gynecomastia.

**INTERACTIONS:** May elevate oxyphenbutazone levels. May decrease blood glucose and, therefore, insulin requirements. Corticosteroids may enhance edema formation; caution with cardiac or hepatic disease.

**PREGNANCY:** Category X, not for use in nursing.

## STROMECTOL RX

ivermectin (Merck)

**THERAPEUTIC CLASS:** Avermectins derivative

**INDICATIONS:** Treatment of strongyloidiasis of the intestinal tract due to *Strongyloides stercoralis*, and onchocerciasis due to *Onchocerca volvulus*. Has no activity against adult *Onchocerca volvulus* parasites.

**DOSAGE:** *Adults:* Strongyloidiasis: 200mcg/kg single dose. Onchocerciasis: 150mcg/kg single dose. For mass distribution in international treatment programs, the usual dosing interval is 12 months. Usual dosing interval for retreatment for individual patients can be as short as 3 months. Take on empty stomach with water. To verify eradication of infection perform follow-up stool exams.
*Pediatrics:* >15kg: Strongyloidiasis: 200mcg/kg single dose. Onchocerciasis: 150mcg/kg single dose. For mass distribution in international treatment programs, the usual dosing interval is 12 months. Usual dosing interval for retreatment for individual patients can be as short as 3 months. Take on empty stomach with water. To verify eradication of infection perform follow-up stool exams.

**HOW SUPPLIED:** Tab: 3mg, 6mg* *scored

**WARNINGS/PRECAUTIONS:** May cause cutaneous and/or systemic reactions of varying severity (the Mazzotti reaction) and ophthalmological reactions. Patients with hyperreactive onchodermatitis (sowda) may be more likely to experience severe advisers reactions, especially edema and aggravation of onchodermatitis. Risk of serious or even fatal encephalopathy with onchocerciasis and *Loa loa* infection. Pretreatment assessment for loiasis and careful posttreatment follow-up should be performed in patients who were exposed to *Loa loa*-endemic areas of West or Central Africa.

**ADVERSE REACTIONS:** Diarrhea, nausea, dizziness, pruritis, decrease in leukocyte count, arthralgia/synovitis, axillary/cervical/inguinal lymph node enlargement, rash, fever, peipheral edema, tachycardia

**PREGNANCY:** Category C, caution in nursing.



## STROVITE FORTE RX

minerals - multiple vitamin (Everett)

**THERAPEUTIC CLASS:** Vitamin/mineral

**INDICATIONS:** For prophylactic or therapeutic nutritional supplementation in physiologically stressful conditions.

**DOSAGE:** *Adults:* 1 tab qd.

**HOW SUPPLIED:** Tab: Biotin 0.15mg-Calcium Pantothenate 25mg-Chromium 0.05mg-Copper 3mg-Folic Acid 1mg-Iron 10mg-Magnesium 50mg-Molybdenum 0.02mg-Niacin 100mg-Selenium 0.05mg-Vitamin A 4000 IU-Vitamin $B_1$ 20mg-Vitamin $B_2$ 20mg-Vitamin $B_6$ 25mg-Vitamin $B_{12}$ 0.05mg-Vitamin C 500mg-Vitamin D 400 IU-Vitamin E 60 IU-Zinc 15mg* *scored

**WARNINGS/PRECAUTIONS:** Accidental overdose of iron-containing products is a leading cause of fatal poisoning in children <6 yrs. Not for the treatment of pernicious anemia and other megaloblastic anemias where vitamin $B_{12}$ is deficient.

**ADVERSE REACTIONS:** GI intolerance, allergic and idiosyncratic reactions.

**INTERACTIONS:** Vitamin B6 may decrease efficacy of levodopa; avoid concomitant use.

## SUBLIMAZE

**CII**

fentanyl citrate (Akorn)

**THERAPEUTIC CLASS:** Opioid analgesic

**INDICATIONS:** For analgesic action of short duration during the anesthetic periods, premedication, induction and maintenance, and in the immediate postoperative period (recovery room) as the need arises. For use as a narcotic analgesic supplement in general or regional anesthesia. For administration with a neuroleptic as an anesthetic premedication, for the induction of anesthesia and as an adjunct in the maintenance of general and regional anesthesia. For use as an anesthetic agent with oxygen in selected high risk patients, such as those undergoing open heart surgery or certain complicated neurological or orthopedic procedures.

**DOSAGE:** *Adults:* ≥12 yrs: Individualize dose. Premedication: 50-100mcg IM 30-60 minutes prior to surgery. Adjunct to General Anesthesia: Low Dose: Total Dose: 2mcg/kg for minor surgery. Maint: 2mcg/kg. Moderate Dose: Total Dose: 2-20mcg/kg for major surgery. Maint: 2-20mcg/kg or 25-100mcg IM or IV if surgical stress or lightening of analgesia. High Dose: Total Dose: 20-50mcg/kg for open heart surgery, complicated neurosurgery, or orthopedic surgery. Maint: 20-50mcg/kg. Adjunct to Regional Anesthesia: 50-100mcg IM or slow IV over 1-2 minutes. Postoperative: 50-100mcg IM, repeat q 1-2 hrs as needed. General Anesthetic: 50-100mcg/kg with oxygen and a muscle relaxant, up to 150mcg/kg may be used.
*Pediatrics:* 2-12 yrs: Individualize dose. Induction/Maint: 2-3mcg/kg.

**HOW SUPPLIED:** Inj: 50mcg/mL

**WARNINGS/PRECAUTIONS:** Should only be administered by persons specifically trained in the use of IV anesthetics and management of the respiratory effects of potent opioids. An opioid antagonist, resuscitative and intubation equipment and oxygen should be readily available. Fluids and other countermeasures to manage hypotension should be available with tranquilizers. Initial dose reduction recommended with narcotic analgesia for recovery. May cause muscle rigidity particularly with muscles used for respiration. Adequate facilities should be available for postoperative monitoring and ventilation. Caution in respiratory depression susceptible patients (eg, comatose patients with head injury or brain tumor). Reduce dose for elderly and debilitated patients. Caution with obstructive pulmonary disease, decreased respiratory reserve, liver and kidney dysfunction, cardiac bradyarrhythmias. Monitor vital signs routinely.

**ADVERSE REACTIONS:** Respiratory depression, apnea, rigidity, bradycardia, HTN, hypotension, dizziness, blurred vision, nausea, emesis, diaphoresis, pruritus, urticaria, laryngospasms, anaphylaxis, euphoria, miosis, bradycardia, and bronchoconstriction.

**INTERACTIONS:** Severe and unpredictable potentiation by MAO inhibitors has been reported. Appropriate monitoring and availability of vasodilators and beta-blockers for the treatment of hypertension is indicated. Additive or potentiating effects with other CNS depressants (eg, barbiturates, tranquilizers, narcotics, general anesthetics). Reduce dose of other CNS depressants. Reports of cardiovascular depression with nitrous oxide. Alteration of respiration with certain forms of conduction anesthesia (eg, spinal anesthesia, some peridural anesthesia). Decreased pulmonary arterial pressure and hypotension with tranquilizers. Elevated blood pressure, with and without pre-existing hypertension, slower normalacy of EEG patterns with neuroleptics. Extreme caution with neuroleptics in the presense of risk factors for development of prolonged QT syndrome and torsade de pointes; ECG monitoring indicated.

**PREGNANCY:** Category C, caution with nursing.

## SUBOXONE

CIII

naloxone - buprenorphine (Reckitt Benckiser)

**OTHER BRAND NAMES:** Subutex (Reckitt Benckiser)

**THERAPEUTIC CLASS:** Partial opioid agonist/opioid antagonist

**INDICATIONS:** Opioid dependence.

**DOSAGE:** *Adults:* Give either agent SL as a single daily dose in the range of 12-16mg/day. Hold tabs under tongue until dissolved; swallowing tabs reduces bioavailability. Induction: Subutex: Give at least 4 hrs after last short-acting opioid (eg, heroin) use or preferably when early signs of opioid withdrawal appear. Maint: Suboxone: Range: 4mg-24mg/day. Target dose: 16mg/day. Titrate: Adjust by 2mg or 4mg to a level that maintains treatment and suppresses opioid withdrawal effects. Hepatic Impairment: Adjust dose and observe for precipitated opioid withdrawal. Concomitant CNS Depressants: Consider dose reduction.
*Pediatrics:* >16 yrs: Give either agent SL as a single daily dose in the range of 12-16mg/day. Hold tabs under tongue until dissolved; swallowing tabs reduces bioavailability. Induction: Subutex: Give at least 4 hrs after last short-acting opioid (eg, heroin) use or preferably when early signs of opioid withdrawal appear. Maint: Suboxone: Range: 4mg-24mg/day. Target dose: 16mg/day. Titrate: Adjust by 2mg or 4mg to a level that maintains treatment and suppresses opioid withdrawal effects. Hepatic Impairment: Adjust dose and observe for precipitated opioid withdrawal. Concomitant CNS Depressants: Consider dose reduction.

**HOW SUPPLIED:** Suboxone (Buprenorphine-Naloxone) Tab, SL: 2mg-0.5mg, 8mg-2mg. Subutex (Buprenorphine) Tab, SL: 2mg, 8mg

**WARNINGS/PRECAUTIONS:** Significant respiratory depression reported with buprenorphine; caution with compromised respiratory function. Naloxone may not be effective in reversing any respiratory depression produced by buprenorphine. Cytolytic hepatitis And hepatitis with jaundice reported. Obtain LFTs prior to initiation and periodically thereafter. Acute and chronic hypersensitivity reactions reported. May increase CSF pressure; caution with head injury, intracranial lesions. May cause miosis, changes in level of consciousness, and orthostatic hypotension. Caution with elderly, debilitated, myxedema, hypothyroidism, acute alcoholism, Addison's disease, CNS depression or coma, toxic psychoses, prostatic hypertrophy, urethral stricture, delirium tremens, kyphoscoliosis, biliary tract dysfunction or severe hepatic/renal/pulmonary impairment. Suboxone may cause opioid withdrawal symptoms. May obscure diagnosis of acute abdominal conditions. May produce dependence.

**ADVERSE REACTIONS:** Headache, infection, pain (general, abdomen, back), withdrawal syndrome, constipation, nausea, insomnia, sweating, asthenia, anxiety, depression, rhinitis.

**INTERACTIONS:** May need dose reduction with CYP3A4 inhibitors (eg, azole antifungals, macrolides and HIV protease inhibitors). General anesthetics, other narcotic analgesics, benzodiazepines, phenothiazines, other tranquilizers, sedative/hypnotics or other CNS depressants (including alcohol) may increase risk of CNS depression; consider dose reduction of one or both agents. Monitor closely with CYP3A4 inducers (eg, phenobarbital, carbamazepine, phenytoin, rifampicin).

**PREGNANCY:** Category C, not for use in nursing.

## SUDAFED — OTC
pseudoephedrine HCl (McNeil)

**THERAPEUTIC CLASS:** Decongestant

**INDICATIONS:** For the temporary relief of nasal congestion due to common cold, hay fever, or other upper respiratory allergies, and nasal congestion associated with sinusitus.

**DOSAGE:** *Adults:* Tab, ER: 120mg q12h or 240mg q24h. Max: 240mg/24h. *Pediatrics:*>12 yrs: Liquid/Tab/Tab, Chew: 60mg q4-6h. Max 240mg/24hrs. Tab, ER: 120mg q12h or 240mg q24h. Max: 240mg/24hrs. 6 to <12 yo: (Liquid/Tab/Tab, Chew) 30mg q4-6h. Max: 4 doses/24hrs. 2 to <6 yo: (Liquid/Tab/Tab, Chew) 15mg q4-6h. Max: 4 doses/24hrs.

**HOW SUPPLIED:** Liq: 15mg/5mL; Tab: 30mg, 60mg; Tab, Chewable: 15mg; Tab, Extended Release: 120mg, 240mg

**WARNINGS/PRECAUTIONS:** Do not exceed recommended dosage. If nervousness, dizziness, or sleeplessness occurs, discontinue use. Do not take this product if you have heart disease, high BP, thyroid disease, diabetes, or difficulty in urination due to prostate enlargement.

**INTERACTIONS:** Do not take with a MAOI or 14d after discontinuation.

**PREGNANCY:** Not rated in pregnancy or nursing.

## SUFENTA — CII
sufentanil citrate (Akorn)

**THERAPEUTIC CLASS:** Opioid analgesic

**INDICATIONS:** Analgesic adjunct in the maintenance of balanced general anesthesia in patients who are intubated and ventilated. Primary anesthetic agent of the induction and maintenance of anesthesia with 100% oxygen in patients undergoing major surgical procedures who are intubated or ventilated, such as cardiovascular surgery or neurosurgical procedures in the sitting position, to provide favorable myocardial and cerebral oxygen balance or when extended postoperative ventilation is anticipated. For epidural administrations an analgesic combined with low dose bupivacaine, usually 12.5mg per administration during labor and vaginal delivery.

**DOSAGE:** *Adults:* ≥12 yrs: Individualize dose. Premedication: Based on patients needs. Analgesic: Total Dose: 1-8mcg/kg. Maint: Incremental: 10-50mcg. Infusion: Based on induction dose not to exceed 1mcg/kg/hr. Anesthetic: Total Dose: 8-30mcg/kg. Maint: Incremental 0.5-10mcg/kg. Infusion: Based on induction dose not to exceed 30mcg/kg. Epidural: 10-15mcg with 10mL bupivacaine 0.125% with or without epinephrine. May repeat for a total of 3 doses in not less than 1 hour intervals.
*Pediatrics:* Individualize dose. 10-25mcg/kg with 100% oxygen. Maint: 25-50mcg supplemental doses.

**HOW SUPPLIED:** Inj: 50mcg/mL

**WARNINGS/PRECAUTIONS:** Should only be administered by persons specifically trained in the use of IV and epidural anesthetics and management of the respiratory effects of potent opioids. An opioid antagonist, resuscitative and intubation equipment and oxygen should be readily available. Prior to catheter insertion, the physician should be familiar with patient conditions (such as infection at the injection site, bleeding diathesis, anticoagulation therapy) which call for special evaluation of the benefit versus risk potential. May cause muscle rigidity of the neck and extremities. Adequate facilities should be available for postoperative monitoring and ventilation. Monitor vital signs routinely. Reduce dose for elderly and debilitated patients. Caution with pulmonary disease, decreased respiratory reserve, liver and kidney dysfunction, cardiac bradyarrhythmias. Reports of bradycardia responsive to atropine. May obscure clinical course of patients with head injuries.

**ADVERSE REACTIONS:** Respiratory depression, skeletal muscle rigidity, bradycardia, HTN, hypotension, chest wall rigidity, somnolence, pruritus, nausea, vomiting.

**INTERACTIONS:** Reports of cardiovascular depression with nitrous oxide. High doses of pancuronium may produce increase in heart rate. Reports of bradycardia and hypotension with other muscle relaxants. Greater incidence and degree of bradycardia and hypotension with chronic calcium channel blocker and beta-blocker therapy. Additive or potentiating effects with other CNS depressants (eg, barbiturates, tranquilizers, narcotics, general anesthetics). Reduce dose of either agent. Decrease in mean arterial pressure and systemic vascular resistance with benzodiazepines.

**PREGNANCY:** Category C, caution in nursing.

## SULAR — RX
nisoldipine (Sciele)

**THERAPEUTIC CLASS:** Calcium channel blocker (dihydropyridine)

**INDICATIONS:** Treatment of hypertension.

**DOSAGE:** *Adults:* Initial: 20mg qd. Titrate: Increase by 10mg weekly or longer. Maint: 20-40mg qd. Max: 60mg/day. Elderly (>65 yrs)/Hepatic Dysfunction: Initial: Do not exceed 10mg/day. Do not chew, divide, or crush tabs.

**HOW SUPPLIED:** Tab, Extended Release: 10mg, 20mg, 30mg, 40mg

**WARNINGS/PRECAUTIONS:** May increase angina or MI with severe obstructive CAD. May cause hypotension; monitor BP initially or with titration. Caution with heart failure or compromised ventricular function, especially with concomitant β-blockers. Caution with severe hepatic dysfunction or in elderly.

**ADVERSE REACTIONS:** Peripheral edema, headache, dizziness, pharyngitis, vasodilation, sinusitis, palpitations.

**INTERACTIONS:** Increased AUC and Cmax with cimetidine. Avoid phenytoin or CYP3A4 inducers. Decreased bioavailability with quinidine. High fat meals increase peak drug levels. Avoid high fat meals, grapefruit juice.

**PREGNANCY:** Category C, not for use in nursing.

## SULFACET-R — RX
sulfur - sulfacetamide sodium (Dermik)

S

**THERAPEUTIC CLASS:** Sulfonamide/sulfur combination

**INDICATIONS:** Topical treatment of acne vulgaris, acne rosacea, and seborrheic dermatitis.

**DOSAGE:** *Adults:* Shake well before use. Apply qd-tid. Expires after 4 months. *Pediatrics:* >12 yrs: Shake well before use. Apply qd-tid. Expires after 4 months.

**HOW SUPPLIED:** Lot: (Sulfacetamide-Sulfur) 10%-5% [25g]

**CONTRAINDICATIONS:** Kidney disease.

**WARNINGS/PRECAUTIONS:** D/C if irritation or hypersensitivity reaction occurs. Avoid eye contact. Contains sulfites. Caution with denuded or abraded skin. May cause reddening and scaling of epidermis.

**ADVERSE REACTIONS:** Local irritation.

**PREGNANCY:** Category C, caution in nursing.

## SULFAMYLON
RX

mafenide acetate (Mylan Bertek)

**THERAPEUTIC CLASS:** Sulfonamide

**INDICATIONS:** (Cre) Adjunct therapy for 2nd- and 3rd-degree burns. (Sol) Adjunct therapy for excised burn wounds.

**DOSAGE:** *Adults:* (Cre) Clean and debride wound, then apply qd-bid. Cream should cover wound at all times. Continue application until healing is progressing well or until site is ready for grafting. (Sol) Cover grafted area with mesh gauze and wet with solution using irrigation syringe/tubing q4h or prn to keep wet. If irrigation tube is not used, moisten gauze q6-8h or prn to keep wet. May use solution up to 5 days with same dressing.
*Pediatrics:* (Cre) Clean and debride wound, then apply qd-bid. Cream should cover wound at all times. Continue application until healing is progressing well or until site is ready for grafting. (Sol) 3 months-16 yrs: Cover grafted area with mesh gauze and wet with solution using irrigation syringe/tubing q4h or prn to keep wet. If irrigation tube is not used, moisten gauze q6-8h or prn to keep wet. May use solution up to 5 days with same dressing.

**HOW SUPPLIED:** Cre: 85mg/g [60g, 120g, 453.6g]; Sol: 50g/pkt [1[s], 5[s]]

**WARNINGS/PRECAUTIONS:** Fatal hemolytic anemia with DIC related to G6PD deficiency reported. Cream contains sodium metabisulfite. Monitor acid-base balance with pulmonary or renal dysfunction; risk of metabolic acidosis due to carbonic anhydrase inhibition. Fungal colonization may occur. D/C if hypersensitivity occurs, and for 24-48 hrs if acidosis occurs. Caution with acute renal failure.

**ADVERSE REACTIONS:** Facial edema, rash, burning sensation, pruritus, erythema, swelling, hyperventilation, tachypnea, acidosis.

**INTERACTIONS:** Possible cross sensitivity to other sulfonamides.

**PREGNANCY:** Category C, not for use in nursing.

## SULFOXYL LOTION REGULAR
RX

sulfur - benzoyl peroxide (Stiefel)

**OTHER BRAND NAMES:** Sulfoxyl Lotion Strong (Stiefel)

**THERAPEUTIC CLASS:** Antibacterial/keratolytic

**INDICATIONS:** Treatment of acne vulgaris.

**DOSAGE:** *Adults:* Apply qd for the first week, and bid thereafter. Shake well. Recommended to initiate Sulfoxyl Regular first, then Sulfoxyl Strong when patients demonstrate accommodation to Regular strength.



**HOW SUPPLIED:** Lot: (Benzoyl Peroxide-Sulfur) (Regular) 5%-2% [59mL]; (Strong) 10%-5% [59mL]

**WARNINGS/PRECAUTIONS:** Contact sensitization reactions may occur. For external use only; avoid eye contact or mucosal membranes. Avoid contact with hair, fabrics, or carpeting due to benzoyl peroxide's bleaching effect.

**ADVERSE REACTIONS:** Excessive erythema, peeling.

**PREGNANCY:** Category C, caution in nursing.

## SULINDAC
RX

sulindac (Various)

**NSAIDs may cause an increased risk of serious cardiovascular thrombotic events, MI, stroke and serious GI adverse events including bleeding, ulceration, and perforation of the stomach or intestines. Contraindicated for the treatment of peri-operative pain in the setting of coronary artery bypass graft (CABG) surgery.**

**OTHER BRAND NAMES:** Clinoril (Merck)

**THERAPEUTIC CLASS:** NSAID (indene derivative)

**INDICATIONS:** Acute or long-term use for osteoarthritis (OA), rheumatoid arthritis (RA), ankylosing spondylitis (AS), acute painful shoulder and acute gouty arthritis.

**DOSAGE:** *Adults:* OA/RA/AS: Initial: 150mg bid. Acute Painful Shoulder/Acute Gouty Arthritis: 200mg bid. Max: 400mg/day. Give with food.

**HOW SUPPLIED:** Tab: 150mg, 200mg* *scored

**CONTRAINDICATIONS:** ASA or other NSAID allergy that precipitates acute asthmatic attack, urticaria, or rhinitis. Treatment of peri-operative pain in the setting of CABG surgery.

**WARNINGS/PRECAUTIONS:** May lead to onset of new HTN or worsening of pre-existing HTN; monitor BP closely. Fluid retention and edema reported; caution with fluid retention or heart failure. Renal papillary necrosis and other renal injury reported after long-term use. Not recommended for use with advanced renal disease; if therapy must be initiated, monitor renal function. Anaphylactoid reactions may occur. May cause serious skin adverse events (eg, exfoliative dermatitis, Stevens-Johnson syndrome, and toxic epidermal necrolysis). Avoid in late pregnancy; may cause premature closure of ductus arteriosis. May cause elevations of LFTs; d/c if abnormal LFTs persist/worsen, liver disease develops, or systemic manifestations occur. Caution in elderly. Anemia may occur; monitor Hgb/Hct with long-term use. May inhibit platelet aggregation and prolong bleeding time; monitor with coagulation disorders. Caution with asthma and avoid with aspirin-sensitive asthma. Keep patients well-hydrated and caution with renal lithiasis. Pancreatitis reported; if pancreatitis suspected, d/c and do not restart. Adverse eye findings reported. Monitor closely with poor liver function and consider dose reduction.

**ADVERSE REACTIONS:** GI pain, dyspepsia, nausea, vomiting, diarrhea, constipation, rash, dizziness, headache, tinnitus, edema.

**INTERACTIONS:** Avoid DMSO, aspirin and other NSAIDs. May increase methotrexate and cyclosporine toxicities. Probenecid may increase plasma levels. Diflunisal may decrease plasma levels.

**PREGNANCY:** Category C, not for use in nursing.

## SUMYCIN — RX

tetracycline hydrochloride (Par)

**THERAPEUTIC CLASS:** *Streptomyces* derived bacteriostatic agent

**INDICATIONS:** Treatment of respiratory tract, urinary tract, and skin and skin structure infections, lymphogranuloma, psittacosis, trachoma, uncomplicated urethral/endocervical/rectal infection caused by *Chlamydia*, nongonococcal urethritis, chancroid, plague, cholera, brucellosis, and others. When PCN is contraindicated, treatment of uncomplicated gonorrhea, syphilis, listeriosis, anthrax, *Clostridium* species, and others. Adjunct therapy for amebicides and severe acne.

**DOSAGE:** *Adults:* Mild-Moderate: 250mg qid or 500mg bid. Severe: 500mg qid. Continue for 24-48 hrs after symptoms subside (minimum 10 days with Group A β-hemolytic streptococci). Severe Acne: Initial: 1g/day in divided doses. Maint: After improvement, 125-500mg/day. Brucellosis: 500mg qid for 3 weeks plus streptomycin 1g IM bid for 1 week, then qd for 1 week. Syphilis: 30-40g equally divided over 10-15 days. Gonorrhea: 500mg q6h for 7 days. *Chlamydia*: 500mg qid for at least 7 days. Renal Dysfunction: Reduce dose or extend dose interval.

*Pediatrics:* >8 yrs: Usual: 25-50mg/kg divided bid-qid. Continue for 24-48 hrs after symptoms subside (minimum 10 days with Group A β-hemolytic streptococci). Severe Acne: Initial: 1g/day in divided doses. Maint: After improvement, 125-500mg/day. Renal Dysfunction: Reduce dose or extend dose interval.

S

**HOW SUPPLIED:** Sus: 125mg/5mL; Tab: 250mg, 500mg

**WARNINGS/PRECAUTIONS:** May cause fetal harm with pregnancy, permanent tooth discoloration during tooth development (last half of pregnancy and children <8 yrs). May increase BUN. Photosensitivity, enamel hypoplasia reported. Superinfection with prolonged use. Suspension contains sodium metabisulfite. Bulging fontanels in infants and benign intracranial HTN in adults reported. Monitor renal/hepatic and hematopoietic function with long-term use. Caution with history of asthma, hay fever, urticaria, and allergy.

**ADVERSE REACTIONS:** GI effects, photosensitivity, increased BUN, hypersensitivity reactions, blood dyscrasias, dizziness, headache.

**INTERACTIONS:** May decrease PT; adjust anticoagulants. May interfere with bactericidal agents (eg, penicillin). May decrease effects of oral contraceptives. Take 1 hr before or 2 hrs after dairy products. Aluminum-, calcium-, iron- and magnesium-containing products impair absorption. Fatal renal toxicity reported with concurrent methoxyflurane.

**PREGNANCY:** Category D, not for use in nursing.

## SUPPRELIN LA — RX

histrelin acetate (Indevus)

**THERAPEUTIC CLASS:** Gonadotropin releasing hormone

**INDICATIONS:** Treatment of children with central precocious puberty.

**DOSAGE:** *Pediatrics:* ≥2 yrs: 50mg every 12 months. Inject SQ into inner aspect of upper arm. Remove after 12 months of therapy.

**HOW SUPPLIED:** Implant: 50mg

**CONTRAINDICATIONS:** Women who are or may become pregnant.

**WARNINGS/PRECAUTIONS:** Transient increase in estradiol in females and testosterone in both sexes with initial therapy. Proper surgical technique is critical during implant insertion and removal. Monitor LH, FSH, and estradiol or testosterone at 1 month post-implantation, then every 6 months. Assess height and bone age every 6-12 months.

**ADVERSE REACTIONS:** Implant site reactions, wound infection, dysmenorrhea, epistaxis, erythema, gynecomastia, headache, weight increase.

**PREGNANCY:** Category X, not for use in nursing.

## SUPRANE — RX

desflurane (Baxter Anesthesia)



**THERAPEUTIC CLASS:** Inhalation anesthetic

**INDICATIONS:** Induction and/or maintenance of anesthesia for inpatient and outpatient surgery in adults. Maintenance of anesthesia in infants and children after induction of anesthesia with other agents and tracheal intubation.

**DOSAGE:** *Adults:* Individualize dose. MAC Values: 70 yrs: 5.2 with oxygen 100% or 1.7 with nitrous oxide 60%. 45 yrs: 6 with oxygen 100% or 2.8 with nitrous oxide 60%. 25 yrs: 7.3 with oxygen 100% or 4 with nitrous oxide 60%. With Fentanyl or Midazolam: 31-65 yrs: No Fentanyl: 6.3. With 3mcg/kg Fentanyl: 3.1. With 6mcg/kg Fentanyl: 2.3. No Midazolam: 5.9. With Midazolam 25mcg/kg: 4.9. With Midazolam 50mcg/kg: 4.9. 18-30 yrs: No Fentanyl: 6.4. With Fentanyl 3mcg/kg: 3.5. With Fentanyl 6mcg/kg: 3. No Midazolam: 6.9. Pediatrics: Individualize dose. MAC Values: 7 yrs: 8.1 with oxygen 100%. 4 yrs: 8.6 with oxygen 100%. 3 yrs: 6.4 with nitrous oxide 60%. 2 yrs: 9.1 with oxygen 100%. 9 months: 10 with oxygen 100% or 7.5 with nitrous oxide 60%. 10 weeks: 9.4 with oxygen 100%. 2 weeks: 9.2 with oxygen 100%.

**HOW SUPPLIED:** Liq: [240mL]

**CONTRAINDICATIONS:** Known or suspected susceptibility to malignant hyperthermia.

**WARNINGS/PRECAUTIONS:** Not recommended for induction of general anesthesia via mask in infants or children. Produces dose-dependent decreases in BP. Concentrations >1 MAC may increase HR. Administer at 0.8 MAC or less, in conjunction with barbiturate induction and hyperventilation. Maintain normal hemodynamics with CAD. May cause sensitivity hepatitis in patients who have been sensitized by previous exposure to halogenated anesthetics. May trigger malignant hyperthermia. May produce a dose-dependent increase in CSF pressure when administered to patients with intracranial space occupying lesions. Not recommended for maintenence of anesthesia in non-intubated children.

**ADVERSE REACTIONS:** Coughing, breathholding, apnea, laryngospasm, oxyhemoglobin desaturation, increased secretions, bronchospasm, nausea, vomiting.

**INTERACTIONS:** Decreased MAC with benzodiazepines and opioids. May decrease the required dose of neuromuscular blocking agents.

**PREGNANCY:** Category B, caution in nursing.

## SUPRAX RX

cefixime (Lupin)

**THERAPEUTIC CLASS:** Cephalosporin (3rd generation)

**INDICATIONS:** Otitis media, pharyngitis, tonsillitis, acute bronchitis, acute exacerbation of chronic bronchitis, uncomplicated UTIs, and cervical/urethral gonorrhea caused by susceptible strains.

**DOSAGE:** *Adults:* Usual: 400mg qd. Gonorrhea: 400mg single dose. CrCl 21-60mL/min/Hemodialysis: Give 75% of standard dose. CrCl <20mL/min/CAPD: Give 50% of standard dose.
*Pediatrics:* >12 yrs or >50kg: (Tab/Sus) Usual: 400mg qd. ≥6 months: (Sus) 8mg/kg qd or 4mg/kg bid. Treat for at least 10 days with *S. pyogenes*. CrCl 21-60mL/min/Hemodialysis: Give 75% of standard dose. CrCl <20mL/min/CAPD: Give 50% of standard dose.

**HOW SUPPLIED:** Sus: 100mg/5mL [50mL, 75mL, 100mL]

**WARNINGS/PRECAUTIONS:** Caution with penicillin or other allergy, GI disease (eg, colitis). Anaphylactic/anaphylactoid reactions, pseudomembranous colitis reported. May cause false (+) direct Coombs, Benedict's, Fehling's solution, Clinitest.

**ADVERSE REACTIONS:** Diarrhea, abdominal pain, nausea, dyspepsia, flatulence, superinfection.

**INTERACTIONS:** May increase carbamazepine levels. Increased PT with anticoagulants (eg, warfarin).

**PREGNANCY:** Category B, not for use in nursing.



## SURMONTIL RX

trimipramine maleate (Odyssey)

**Antidepressants increased the risk of suicidal thinking and behavior (suicidality) in short-term studies in children and adolescents with Major Depressive Disorder (MDD) and other psychiatric disorders. Trimipramine is not approved for use in pediatric patients.**

**THERAPEUTIC CLASS:** Tricyclic antidepressant

**INDICATIONS:** Relief of symptoms of depression.

**DOSAGE:** *Adults:* Outpatient: Initial: 75mg/day in divided doses. Titrate: Increase to 150mg/day. Maint: 50-150mg/day. Max: 200mg/day. Hospitalized Patients: Initial: 100mg/day in divided doses. Titrate: Increase gradually to 200mg/day. If no improvement after 2-3 weeks, may increase up to 250-300mg/day. Elderly: Initial: 50mg/day. Titrate: Increase gradually to 100mg/day. Take at bedtime for at least 3 months.

*Pediatrics:* Adolescents: Initial: 50mg/day. Titrate: Increase gradually to 100mg/day. Take at bedtime for at least 3 months.

**HOW SUPPLIED:** Cap: 25mg, 50mg, 100mg

**CONTRAINDICATIONS:** Acute recovery period post-MI, within 14 days of MAOI therapy.

**WARNINGS/PRECAUTIONS:** Caution with cardiovascular disease, increased IOP, urinary retention, narrow-angle glaucoma, hyperthyroidism, seizure disorder, liver dysfunction. May impair ability to operate machinery. May alter glucose levels. May activate psychosis in schizophrenia. Manic or hypomanic episodes may occur. May increase hazards with electroshock therapy.

**ADVERSE REACTIONS:** Hypotension, HTN, arrhythmia, confusion, insomnia, incoordination, GI complaints, allergic reactions, gynecomastia, blood dyscrasias, dry mouth, blurred vision, urinary retention.

**INTERACTIONS:** Cimetidine inhibits elimination. Alcohol may exaggerate effects. May potentiate catecholamine or anticholinergic effects. Potentiated by CYP2D6 inhibitors (eg, quinidine) and substrates (eg, other antidepressants, phenothiazines, propafenone, fleccainide). Caution with SSRIs; wait 5 weeks after fluoxetine withdrawal before initiating therapy. Avoid MAOIs.

**PREGNANCY:** Category C, safety in nursing not known.

## SUSTIVA

RX

efavirenz (Bristol-Myers Squibb)

**THERAPEUTIC CLASS:** Non-nucleoside reverse transcriptase inhibitor

**INDICATIONS:** Treatment of HIV-1 infection in combination with other antiretrovirals.

**DOSAGE:** *Adults:* Initial: 600mg qd. Take on an empty stomach, preferably at bedtime.
*Pediatrics:* >3 yrs: 10 to <15kg: 200mg qd. 15 to <20kg: 250mg qd. 20 to <25kg: 300mg qd. 25 to <32.5kg: 350mg qd. 32.5 to <40kg: 400mg qd. >40kg: 600mg qd. Take on an empty stomach, preferably at bedtime.

**HOW SUPPLIED:** Cap: 50mg, 100mg, 200mg; Tab: 600mg

**CONTRAINDICATIONS:** Concomitant astemizole, bepridil, cisapride, midazolam, pimozide, triazolam, ergot derivatives, or standard doses of voriconazole.

**WARNINGS/PRECAUTIONS:** Not for monotherapy. Severe skin rash reported. Avoid pregnancy; use barrier contraception with other contraception methods and obtain (-) pregnancy test before therapy. Monitor LFTs with known or suspected hepatitis B or C. Monitor cholesterol and triglycerides. High fat meals may increase absorption. Possible redistribution or accumulation of body fat. Serious psychiatric adverse experiences and central nervous symptoms (dizziness, insomnia, impaired concentration, somnolence, abnormal dreams, hallucinations) have been reported.



**ADVERSE REACTIONS:** CNS symptoms (eg, dizziness, insomnia, impaired concentration, somnolence, abnormal dreams), psychiatric symptoms (eg, severe depression), rash, GI effects.

**INTERACTIONS:** Avoid astemizole, cisapride, midazolam, triazolam, voriconazole, St. John's wort, or ergot derivatives. St. John's wort decreases efavirenz to suboptimal levels; increases risk of resistance. Significantly decreased levels of voriconazole. CYP3A4 inducers (eg, phenobarbital, rifampin, rifabutin) may decrease plasma levels. Increased levels of ethinyl estradiol. Decreased levels of clarithromycin; consider alternative. Decreased levels of indinavir and rifabutin; adjust doses. Increased levels of ritonavir and efavirenz with concomitant use; monitor LFTs. Decreased levels of saquinavir, sertraline. May decrease methadone levels; monitor for signs of withdrawal. May affect warfarin levels. May decrease itraconazole, ketoconazole, amprenavir levels. Decreased levels of anticonvulsants (eg, phenytoin, phenobarbital, carbamazepine) and efavirenz; monitor anticonvulsant levels.

**PREGNANCY:** Category D, not for use in nursing.

## SUTENT RX
sunitinib malate (Pfizer)

**THERAPEUTIC CLASS:** Multikinase inhibitor

**INDICATIONS:** Treatment of gastrointestinal stromal tumor (GIST) after disease progression on or intolerance to imatinib mesylate. Treatment of advanced renal cell carcinoma (RCC).

**DOSAGE:** *Adults:* 50mg daily; 4 weeks on, 2 weeks off. Dose increase/reduction in 12.5mg increments is recommended based on individual safety and tolerability.

**HOW SUPPLIED:** Cap: 12.5mg, 25mg, 50mg

**WARNINGS/PRECAUTIONS:** Cases of decreased left ventricular ejection fraction (LVEF) reported. Patients with cardiac risk factors should be carefully monitored for signs and symptoms of CHF; baseline and periodic evaluation of LVEF should be considered. Discontinue if clinical manifestations of CHF occur. Prolongation of QT interval and torsade de pointes observed; consider monitoring ECG and electrolytes (magnesium, potassium). Cases of hemorrhagic events reported. Serious, sometimes fatal GI complications including GI perforation have occurred with intra-abdominal malignancies. Cases of HTN reported; monitor for HTN and treat as needed with standard antihypertensive therapy. Temporary suspension recommended if severe HTN occurs. Adrenal toxicity reported; monitor for adrenal insufficiency with stress, trauma, or severe infection. Myelosuppression, hypothyroidism, increases in serum lipase/amylase, and pancreatitis reported. Monitor CBCs, platelet count, thyroid function, and serum chemistries beginning each treatment cycle.

**ADVERSE REACTIONS:** Diarrhea, HTN, bleeding, mucositis, skin abnormalities, altered taste, electrolyte disturbances, peripheral neuropathy, seizures, periorbital edema, venous thromboembolic events, pancreatic and liver faliure.

**INTERACTIONS:** Concomitant CYP3A4 inhibitors (eg, ketoconazole) may increase plasma concentrations; dose reduction to 37.5mg daily is recommended with coadministration. CYP3A4 inducers (eg, rifampin) may decrease plasma concentrations; dose increase to 87.5mg daily should be considered with coadministration. Avoid concurrent St. Johnc‹s wort; may decrease plasma concentrations unpredictably.

**PREGNANCY:** Category D, not for use in nursing.

## SYMBICORT RX
formoterol - budesonide fumarate dihydrate (AstraZeneca)

**Long-acting beta2-adrenergic agonists (formoterol) may increase the risk of asthma-related death.**

**THERAPEUTIC CLASS:** Corticosteroid/beta$_2$ agonist

**INDICATIONS:** Long-term maintenance treatment of asthma in patients ≥12 yrs.

**DOSAGE:** *Adults:* CurrentMedium to High Doses Inhaled CS: 2 inh bid of 160/4.5. Current Low to Medium Doses Inhaled CS: 2 inh bid of 80/4.5. No Current Inhaled CS: 2 inh bid of 80/4.5 or 160/4.5 depending on asthma severity. Max: 640mcg/18mcg (2 inh bid of 160/4.5). Patients not responding to the starting dose after 1-2 weeks of therapy with 80/4.5, replace with 160/4.5 for better asthma control. Rinse mouth after use.
*Pediatrics:* ≥12 yrs: Current Medium to High Doses Inhaled CS: 2 inh bid of 160/4.5. Current Low to Medium Doses Inhaled CS: 2 inh bid of 80/4.5. No Current Inhaled CS: 2 inh bid of 80/4.5 or 160/4.5 depending on asthma severity. Max: 640mcg/18mcg (2 inh bid of 160/4.5). Patients not responding

to the starting dose after 1-2 weeks of therapy with 80/4.5, replace with 160/4.5 for better asthma control. Rinse mouth after use.

**HOW SUPPLIED:** MDI: (Budesonide-Formoterol) 80mcg-4.5mcg/inh, 160mcg-4.5mcg/inh [10.2g]

**CONTRAINDICATIONS:** Primary treatment of status asthmaticus or other acute asthma attacks.

**WARNINGS/PRECAUTIONS:** Do not use in patients with significantly worsening or acutely deteriorating asthma. Not for acute treatment of symptoms. Monitor for increasing use of inhaled, short-acting $beta_2$-agonists. Deaths due to adrenal insufficiency have occured with transfer from systemic corticosteroids to inhaled corticosteroids. Resume oral corticosteroids during stress or severe asthma attack. Transferring from oral to inhalation therapy may unmask allergic conditions (eg, rhinitis, conjunctivitis, eczema). Observe for adrenal insufficiency, systemic corticosteroid withdrawal effects, and growth suppression (children). More susceptible to infections. Not for acute bronchospasm. Do not use any additional inhaled long-acting $beta_2$-agonist for prevention of exercise induced bronchospasm or the maintenance treatment of asthma. D/C if paradoxical bronchospasm occurs. Immediate hypersensitivity and upper airway symptom reactions reported. Caution with cardiovascular disorder (eg, coronary insufficiency, arrythmia, HTN). QTc interval prolongation reported.

**ADVERSE REACTIONS:** Nasopharyngitis, headache, upper respiratory tract infections, sinusitis, back pain, nasal/sinus congestion, oral candidiasis, influenza, rhinitis, pharyngolaryngeal pain, vomiting.

**INTERACTIONS:** Oral ketoconazole increases plasma levels. CYP3A4 inhibitors (eg, itraconazole, clarithromycin, erythromycin) may inhibit metabolism and increase systemic exposure. Caution with non-potassium-sparing diuretics. Extreme caution within 14 days of using MAOIs or TCAs. Avoid with β-blockers.

**PREGNANCY:** Category C, caution in nursing.

## SYMBYAX RX

olanzapine - fluoxetine HCl (Lilly)

**Antidepressants increased the risk of suicidal thinking and behavior (suicidality) in short-term studies in children and adolescents with Major Depressive Disorder (MDD) and other psychiatric disorders. Fluoxetine is not approved for use in pediatric patients. Elderly patients with dementia-related psychosis treated with atypical antipsychotic drugs are at an increased risk of death; most appeared to be cardiovascular (eg, heart failure, sudden death) or infectious (eg, pneumonia) in nature. Symbyax is not approved for the treatment of patients with dementia-related psychosis.**



**THERAPEUTIC CLASS:** Thienobenzodiazepine/selective serotonin reuptake inhibitor

**INDICATIONS:** Treatment of depressive episodes associated with bipolar disorder.

**DOSAGE:** *Adults:* ≥18yrs: Initial: 6-25mg cap qd in evening. Titrate: Adjust dose based on efficacy and tolerability. Max: 18mg/75mg. Hypotension Risk/Hepatic Impairment/Slow Metabolizers: Initial: 3-25mg to 6-25mg qd in evening. Titrate: Increase cautiously. Re-evaluate periodically.

**HOW SUPPLIED:** Cap: (Olanzapine-Fluoxetine): 3-25mg, 6-25mg, 6-50mg, 12-25mg, 12-50mg

**CONTRAINDICATIONS:** During or within 14 days of MAOI use; during or within 5 weeks of discontinuation of thioridazine use; concomitant pimozide use.

**WARNINGS/PRECAUTIONS:** See Black Box Warning. Monitor for hyperglycemia, worsening of glucose control with DM, FBG levels with diabetes risk. Not for use with dementia-related psychosis. Risk of orthostatic hypotension, NMS, tardive dyskinesia, hyperprolactinemia, hyponatremia, seizures. Caution with cardio- or cerebrovascular disease, hypotension risk (eg, dehydration, hypovolemia), history of seizures or conditions that lower the seizure threshold, elderly (especially with dementia), hepatic impairment, risk of aspiration pneumonia, conditions that affect metabolism or hemodynamic responses, prostatic hypertrophy, narrow-angle glaucoma, history of paralytic ileus, suicidal tendencies. Discontinue if unexplained allergic reaction occurs. Elevated transaminases, bleeding episodes reported. Monitor for symptoms of mania/hypomania. May cause disruption of body temperature regulation. Serotonin syndrome reported; caution with MAOIs, other serotonergic drugs. Caution should be used when prescribing olanzapine and fluoxetine products concomitantly with symbyax.

**ADVERSE REACTIONS:** Asthenia, somnolence, weight gain, edema, increased appetite, peripheral edema, pharyngitis, abnormal thinking, tremor, erythema multiforme, fever, diarrhea, dry mouth, twitching, arthralgia.

**INTERACTIONS:** See Contraindications. Risk of orthostatic hypotension with antihypertensives, benzodiazepines, alcohol. May antagonize levodopa, dopamine agonists. Increased clearance with carbamazepine, omeprazole, rifampin, other inducers of CYP1A2 or glucuronyl transferase. Increase in clozapine, haloperidol, phenytoin levels. Caution with other CNS-drugs, sumatriptan, tryptophan, other highly protein bound drugs (eg, warfarin, digitoxin), hepatotoxic drugs, other olanzapine- or fluoxetine-containing products. Decreased clearance with fluvoxamine, fluoroquinolones, other CYP1A2 inhibitors. Monitor lithium levels. May increase TCA levels; may require reduction in TCA dose. Increased risk of bleeding with NSAIDs, aspirin, warfarin. Inhibits drugs metabolized by CYP2D6 (eg, flecainide, vinblastine, TCAs); initiate at lower end of dosage range.

**PREGNANCY:** Category C, not for use in nursing.

## SYMLIN

pramlintide acetate (Amylin)

RX

**Use with insulin. Risk of insulin-induced severe hypoglycemia, particularly with type 1 DM. Severe hypoglycemia usually occurs within 3 hours of injection. Serious injuries may occur if severe hypoglycemia occurs while operating a motor vehicle, heavy machinery, or other high-risk activities. Appropriate patient selection, careful patient instruction, and insulin dose adjustments are necessary to reduce this risk.**

**THERAPEUTIC CLASS:** Synthetic amylin analog

**INDICATIONS:** Adjunct treatment in patients with type 1 or type 2 DM who use mealtime insulin therapy and who have failed to achieve desired glucose control despite optimal insulin therapy. May be used with or without sulfonylurea and/or metformin in type 2 DM.

**DOSAGE:** *Adults:* Before initiating therapy reduce insulin dose by 50%. Monitor blood glucose frequently. Adjust insulin dose once target dose of pramlintide is maintained. Type 2 DM: Initial: 60mcg SQ immediately prior to meals. Titrate: 120mcg as tolerated. Type 1 DM: Initial: 15mcg SQ immediately prior to meals. Titrate: Increase by 15mcg increments to 30mcg or 60mcg as tolerated.

**HOW SUPPLIED:** Inj: 0.6mg/mL

**CONTRAINDICATIONS:** Confirmed diagnosis of gastroparesis; hypoglycemia unawareness.

**WARNINGS/PRECAUTIONS:** Do not mix with insulin; administer as separate injections.

**ADVERSE REACTIONS:** Nausea, headache, anorexia, vomiting, abdominal pain, fatigue, dizziness, coughing, pharyngitis.

**INTERACTIONS:** Do not administer with agents that alter gastrointestinal motility (eg, anticholinergic agents such as atropine), and agents that slow intestinal absorption of nutrients (eg, $\alpha$-glucosidase inhibitors). Administer analgesics and other oral agents that require rapid onset 1 hour before or 2 hours after injection.

**PREGNANCY:** Category C, caution in nursing.

## SYMMETREL

RX

amantadine HCl (Endo)

**THERAPEUTIC CLASS:** Dopamine agonist

**INDICATIONS:** Prophylaxis and treatment of uncomplicated influenza A infections. Treatment of parkinsonism and drug-induced extrapyramidal reactions.

**DOSAGE:** *Adults:* Influenza A Virus Prophylaxis/Treatment: 200mg qd or 100mg bid. Elderly: >65 yrs: 100mg qd. Parkinsonism: Initial: 100mg bid. Serious Associated Illness/Concomitant High Dose Antiparkinson Agent: Initial: 100mg qd. Titrate: May increase to 100mg bid after 1 to several weeks. Max: 400mg/day. Drug-Induced Extrapyramidal Reactions: 100mg bid. Titrate: May increase to 300mg/day in divided doses. CrCl 30-50mL/min: 200mg on Day 1, then 100mg qd. CrCl 15-29mL/min: 200mg on Day 1, then 100mg every other day. CrCl <15mL/min/Hemodialysis: 200mg every 7 days.
*Pediatrics:* Influenza A Virus Prophylaxis/Treatment: 9-12 yrs: 100mg bid. 1-9 yrs: 4.4-8.8mg/kg/day. Max: 150mg/day.

**HOW SUPPLIED:** Syrup: 50mg/5mL; Tab: 100mg

**WARNINGS/PRECAUTIONS:** Deaths reported from overdose. Suicide attempts, NMS reported. Caution with CHF, peripheral edema, orthostatic hypotension, renal or hepatic dysfunction, recurrent eczematoid rash, uncontrolled psychosis or severe psychoneurosis. Avoid in untreated angle closure glaucoma. Do not d/c abruptly in Parkinson's disease. May increase seizure activity.

**ADVERSE REACTIONS:** Nausea, dizziness, insomnia, depression, anxiety, hallucinations, confusion, anorexia, dry mouth, constipation, ataxia, livedo reticularis, peripheral edema, orthostatic hypotension, agranulocytosis.

**INTERACTIONS:** Caution with CNS stimulants. Anticholinergic agents may potentiate the anticholinergic side effects. Increased tremor in elderly Parkinson's patients with thioridazine. Increased plasma levels with trimethoprim-sulfamethoxazole, quinine, or quinidine. Avoid use of Attenuated Influenza Vaccine within 2 weeks before or 48 hours after.

**PREGNANCY:** Category C, not for use in nursing.

## SYNAGIS

RX

palivizumab (MedImmune)

**THERAPEUTIC CLASS:** Monoclonal antibody/RSV F-protein blocker



**INDICATIONS:** Prevention of serious lower respiratory tract disease caused by respiratory syncytial virus (RSV) in pediatrics at high risk of RSV.

**DOSAGE:** *Pediatrics:* 15mg/kg IM; give 1st dose before start of RSV season (November-April), then monthly throughout season. Give monthly also if develop RSV infection. Safety and efficacy established in infants with bronchopulmonary dysplasia (BPD) and infants with history of prematurity (<35 weeks gestational age).

**HOW SUPPLIED:** Inj: 50mg, 100mg

**WARNINGS/PRECAUTIONS:** Anaphylactoid reactions reported. Caution with thrombocytopenia or any coagulation disorder due to IM injection. Safety and efficacy not demonstrated for treatment of established RSV disease.

**ADVERSE REACTIONS:** Upper respiratory infection, otitis media, rash, pharyngitis, cough, bronchiolitis, pneumonia, bronchitis, asthma, croup, dyspnea, apnea, diarrhea, vomiting, nervousness, liver function abnormality, anemia.

**PREGNANCY:** Category C, safety in nursing not known.

## SYNALAR
RX

fluocinolone acetonide (Medicis)

**THERAPEUTIC CLASS:** Corticosteroid

**INDICATIONS:** Corticosteroid responsive dermatoses.

**DOSAGE:** *Adults:* Apply bid-qid. May use occlusive dressings for psoriasis or recalcitrant conditions; d/c dressings if infection develops.
*Pediatrics:* Apply bid-qid. May use occlusive dressings for psoriasis or recalcitrant conditions; d/c dressings if infection develops.

**HOW SUPPLIED:** Cre, Oint: 0.025% [15g, 60g]; Sol: 0.01% [20mL, 60mL]

**WARNINGS/PRECAUTIONS:** May produce reversible HPA axis suppression, manifestations of Cushing's syndrome, hyperglycemia, and glucosuria. Caution when applied to large surface areas or under occlusive dressings. Use appropriate antifungal or antibacterial agent with dermatological infections; d/c if infection does not clear. Peds may be more susceptible to systemic toxicity. Avoid eyes. D/C if irritation occurs.

**ADVERSE REACTIONS:** Burning, itching, irritation, dryness, folliculitis, hypertrichosis, acneiform eruptions, premolar dermatitis, hypopigmentation, allergic dermatitis, skin maceration, secondary infection, skin atrophy.

**PREGNANCY:** Category C, caution with nursing.

## SYNALGOS-DC
CIII

aspirin - caffeine - dihydrocodeine bitartrate (Women First)

**THERAPEUTIC CLASS:** Opioid analgesic

**INDICATIONS:** Relief of moderate to moderately severe pain.

**DOSAGE:** *Adults:* 2 caps q4h prn pain. Elderly: Start at low end of dosing range.
*Pediatrics:* >12 yrs: 2 caps q4h prn pain.

**HOW SUPPLIED:** Cap: (Dihydrocodeine-ASA-Caffeine) 16mg-356.4mg-30mg [Painpak, 12 caps]

**WARNINGS/PRECAUTIONS:** Caution in elderly, debilitated, and with peptic ulcer or coagulation abnormalities. May impair mental or physical abilities. Abuse potential.

**ADVERSE REACTIONS:** Lightheadedness, dizziness, drowsiness, sedation, nausea, vomiting, constipation, pruritus, skin reactions.

**INTERACTIONS:** Additive CNS depression with narcotic analgesics, general anesthetics, tranquilizers, sedative hypnotics, alcohol, and other CNS depressants. Enhanced effects of anticoagulants. Inhibits effects of uricosuric agents.

**PREGNANCY:** Safety in pregnancy and nursing is not known.



## SYNAREL
RX

nafarelin acetate (Searle)

**THERAPEUTIC CLASS:** Gonadotropin-releasing hormone analog

**INDICATIONS:** Management of endometriosis, including pain relief and reduction of lesions. Treatment of central precocious puberty (CPP) (gonadotropin-dependent precocious puberty) in children of both sexes.

**DOSAGE:** (Endometriosis) *Adults:* ≥18 yrs: 1 spray (200mcg) into one nostril qam and 1 spray into other nostril qpm. Initiate therapy between days 2-4 of menstrual cycle. Increase to 1 spray per nostril qam and qpm after 2 months (800mcg/day) if amenorrhea has not occurred. Treat for 6 months.
(CPP) *Pediatrics:* Usual: 2 sprays (400mcg) per nostril qam and qpm. Total Daily Dose: 1600mcg. Increase to 3 sprays into alternating nostrils tid

(1800mcg daily) if needed 30 seconds should elapse between sprays. Continue until resumption of puberty is desired.

**HOW SUPPLIED:** Spray: 200mcg/inh [8mL]

**CONTRAINDICATIONS:** Pregnancy, women who may become pregnant, nursing, undiagnosed abnormal vaginal bleeding.

**WARNINGS/PRECAUTIONS:** (Endometriosis) Ovarian cysts reported in adult women. Caution if risk factors for decreased bone mineral content present. Avoid sneezing during or after administration. Use nonhormonal methods of contraception. (CPP) Determine diagnosis before initiating therapy. Monitor regularly. Assess growth and bone age velocity within 3 to 6 months of initiation. Avoid sneezing during or after administration.

**ADVERSE REACTIONS:** (Endometriosis) Hot flashes, decreased libido, vaginal dryness, headache, emotional lability, myalgia, acne, nasal irritation, reduced breast size, insomnia, edema, seborrhea, weight gain, depression, hirsutism. (CPP) Acne, breast enlargement, vaginal bleeding, emotional lability, transient increase in pubic hair, rhinitis, body odor, seborrhea, white or brownish vaginal discharge.

**INTERACTIONS:** Avoid topical decongestants within 2 hrs after dosing.

**PREGNANCY:** Category X, not for use in nursing.

## SYNERA RX

lidocaine - tetracaine (Tapemark)

**THERAPEUTIC CLASS:** Acetamide local anesthetic

**INDICATIONS:** For use on intact skin to provide local dermal analgesia for superficial venous access and superficial dermatological procedures such as excision, electrodessication, and shave biopsy of skin lesions.

**DOSAGE:** *Adults:* Venipuncture or IV Cannulation: Apply to intact skin for 20-30 minutes prior to procedure. Superficial Dermatological Procedures: Apply to intact skin for 30 minutes prior to the procedure.
*Pediatrics:* ≥3 yrs: Venipuncture or IV Cannulation: Apply to intact skin for 20-30 minutes prior to procedure. Superficial Dermatological Procedure: Apply to intact skin for 30 minutes prior to the procedure.

**HOW SUPPLIED:** Patch: (Lidocaine-Tetracaine) 70mg-70mg

**CONTRAINDICATIONS:** PABA hypersensitivity.

**WARNINGS/PRECAUTIONS:** Serious adverse events may occur in children or pets if ingested. Caution in acutely ill or debillitated. Risk of allergic/anaphylactoid reactions (urticaria, angioedema, bronchospasm, shock). Increased risk of toxicity in severe hepatic disease. Avoid broken or inflamed skin, eye contact, larger area or longer duration than recommended.

S

**ADVERSE REACTIONS:** Erythema, blanching, edema, urticaria, angioedema, bronchospasm, shock.

**INTERACTIONS:** Additive toxic effect with concomitant Class I antiarrhythmics (eg, tocainide, mexiletine). Consider total amount absorbed from all formulations with other local anesthetics.

**PREGNANCY:** Category B, caution in nursing.

## SYNERCID RX

dalfopristin - quinupristin (King)

**THERAPEUTIC CLASS:** Streptogramin

**INDICATIONS:** Treatment of serious or life-threatening infections associated with vancomycin-resistant *Enterococcus faecium* (VREF) bacteremia and complicated skin and skin structure infections (SSSI) caused by *Staphylococcus aureus* (methicillin susceptible) or *Streptococcus pyogenes*.

**DOSAGE:** *Adults:* VREF: 7.5mg/kg IV q8h. Duration depends on site and severity of infection. Complicated SSSI: 7.5mg/kg IV q12h for at least 7 days. Hepatic Cirrhosis (Child Pugh A or B): May need dose reduction.
*Pediatrics:* >16 yrs: VREF: 7.5mg/kg IV q8h. Duration depends on site and severity of infection. Complicated SSSI: 7.5mg/kg IV q12h for at least 7 days. Hepatic Cirrhosis (Child Pugh A or B): May need dose reduction.

**HOW SUPPLIED:** Inj: (Dalfopristin-Quinupristin) 350mg-150mg per 500mg vial

**WARNINGS/PRECAUTIONS:** Pseudomembranous colitis reported. Flush vein with 5% dextrose after infusion to minimize venous irritation. Arthralgia, myalgia, and bilirubin elevation reported.

**ADVERSE REACTIONS:** Infusion site reactions (inflammation, pain, edema), nausea, diarrhea, rash.

**INTERACTIONS:** Significant inhibition of CYP3A4; caution with drugs metabolized by this system (eg, cyclosporin A, tacrolimus, midazolam, nifedipine, verapamil, diltiazem astemizole, terfenadine, delavirdine, nevirapine, indinavir, ritonavir, vinca alkaloids, docetaxel, paclitaxel, diazepam, HMG-CoA reductase inhibitors, methylprednisolone, carbamazepine, quinidine, lidocaine, disopyramide). Monitor cyclosporine levels. Avoid drugs metabolized by CYP3A4 that prolong QTc interval. May inhibit digoxin's gut metabolism.

**PREGNANCY:** Category B, caution in nursing.

## SYNTHROID RX

levothyroxine sodium (Abbott)

**THERAPEUTIC CLASS:** Thyroid replacement hormone

**INDICATIONS:** Hypothyroidism. As a pituitary TSH suppressant in the treatment and prevention of euthyroid goiters, including thyroid nodules, lymphocytic thyroiditis, and multinodular goiter. Adjunct to surgery and radioiodine therapy for thyrotropin-dependent well-differentiated thyroid cancer.

**DOSAGE:** *Adults:* Hypothyroidism: Usual: 1.7mcg/kg/day PO. Titrate: May increase by 12.5-25mcg every 6-8 weeks until euthyroid. >200mcg/day (seldom). Elderly/Cardiovascular Disease: Initial: 12.5-50mcg qd PO. Titrate: Increase by 12.5-25mcg every 3-6 weeks until euthyroid. Give 1/2 of oral dose for IV/IM, Pregnancy: May require increased doses. Subclinical Hypothyroidism: Lower doses required.
*Pediatrics:* Hypothyroidism: 0-3 months: 10-15mcg/kg/day. 3-6 months: 8-10mcg/kg/day. 6-12 months: 6-8mcg/kg/day. 1-5 yrs: 5-6mcg/kg/day. 6-12 yrs: 4-5mcg/kg/day. >12 yrs (growth/puberty complete): 2-3mcg/kg/day. Cardiac Risk: Lower starting dose. Infants with Serum $T_4$ <5mcg/dL: Initial: 50mcg/day. Chronic/Severe Hypothyroidism: Children: Initial: 25mcg/day. Titrate: Increase by 25mcg for 2 weeks then every 2-4 weeks until euthyroid. May crush tab and sprinkle over food (applesauce) or mix with 5-10mL water, formula (non-soy), or breast milk.

**HOW SUPPLIED:** Tab: 25mcg*, 50mcg*, 75mcg*, 88mcg*, 100mcg*, 112mcg*, 125mcg*, 137mcg*, 150mcg*, 175mcg*, 200mcg*, 300mcg* *scored

**CONTRAINDICATIONS:** Untreated thyrotoxicosis, uncorrected adrenal insufficiency.

**WARNINGS/PRECAUTIONS:** Do not use in the treatment of obesity; larger doses in euthyroid patients can cause serious or even life threatening toxicity. Caution with cardiovascular disorders, angina, CAD, HTN and the elderly. May aggravate DM, diabetes insipidus, or adrenal cortical insufficiency. Treatment of myxedema coma may require glucocorticoids. May lower seizure threshold.

**ADVERSE REACTIONS:** Craniosynostosis in infants, transient hair loss, pseudotumor cerebri in pediatrics (rare), hypersensitivity reactions, seizures (rare).

**INTERACTIONS:** Increased risk of coronary insufficiency with sympathomimetics and CAD. May potentiate oral anticoagulant effects; adjust dose and monitor PT/INR. Lithium blocks release of $T_4$ and $T_3$. Antidiabetic agents may need adjustment. Decreased absorption with cholestyramine resin, colestipol, ferrous sulfate, aluminum hydroxide, sodium polystyrene sulfonate, soybean flour (infant formula), sucralfate. Altered protein binding with clofibrate, estrogens, androgens/anabolic hormones, asparaginase, 5-FU, furosemide, glucocorticoids, meclofenamic acid, mefenamic acid, methadone, perphenazine, phenytoin, phenylbutazone, tamoxifen, salicylates. Altered thyroid hormone or TSH levels with aminoglutethimide, p-aminosalicyclic acid, amiodarone, androgens/anabolic hormones, complex anions (eg, thiocyanate, perchlorate, pertechnetate), antithyroid drugs, β-adrenergic blockers, carbamazepine, chloral hydrate, diazepam, dopamine/dopamine agonists, ethionamide, glucocorticoids, heparin, hepatic enzyme inducers, insulin, iodinated cholestographic agents, iodine-containing compounds, levodopa, lovastatin, lithium, 6-mercaptopurine, metoclopramide, mitotane, nitroprusside, phenobarbital, phenytoin, resorcinol, rifampin, somatostatin analogs, sulfonamides, sulfonylureas, thiazide diuretics. Adrenocorticoid clearance is decreased with hypothyroidism and increased with hyperthyroidism. May potentiate anticoagulants. Cytokines, amiodarone may induce hypo- or hyperthyroidism. Increased risk of arrhythmias with maprotiline. HTN and tachycardia reported with ketamine. Sympathomimetics may increase risk of coronary insufficiency with CAD. Adverse effects of both drugs with TCAs. Decreased clearance of theophylline with hypothyroidism. Impaired β-blocker effects. Decreased digitalis effects. Decreased uptake of iodine-containing radiolabeled ions. Altered levels of theophylline may occur. Use with somatrem/somatropin may accelerate epiphysea

**PREGNANCY:** Category A, caution in nursing.

## SYNVISC — RX

hylan g-f 20 (Wyeth)

**THERAPEUTIC CLASS:** Hylan polymer

**INDICATIONS:** Treatment of osteoarthritis (OA) knee pain inadequately responsive to conservative nonpharmacologic therapy and simple analgesics.

**DOSAGE:** *Adults:* Usual: Intra-articular injection once weekly (one week apart) for total of three injections.

**HOW SUPPLIED:** Inj: 8mg/mL

**CONTRAINDICATIONS:** Knee joint infections, hyaluronan hypersensitivity, skin diseases or infections in injection site area.

**WARNINGS/PRECAUTIONS:** Avoid with skin disinfectants containing quaternary ammonium salts; hyaluronan can precipitate in their presence. Do not inject extra-articularly or into synovial tissue and capsule. Intravascular injections may cause systemic adverse events. Caution with allergies to avian proteins, feathers, and egg products. Avoid with severely inflamed knee joints. Remove synovial fluid or effusion, if present, before injecting. Follow strict aseptic administration. Caution with lymphatic or venous stasis. Avoid strenuous activity or prolonged weight-bearing activities after injection. Packaging contains dry natural rubber latex.



**ADVERSE REACTIONS:** Injection site pain, knee swelling/effusion, rash, calf cramps, ankle edema, muscle pain.

**INTERACTIONS:** Do not inject anesthetics or other drugs into knee joint during therapy.

**PREGNANCY:** Safety in pregnancy and nursing not known.

## TACLONEX — RX

calcipotriene - betamethasone dipropionate (Warner Chilcott)

**THERAPEUTIC CLASS:** Vitamin $D_3$ analogue/corticosteroid

**INDICATIONS:** Topical treatment of psoriasis vulgaris for up to 4 weeks.

**DOSAGE:** *Adults:* ≥18yrs: Apply to affected area(s) qd for up to 4 weeks. Max: 100g/week. Treatment of >30% BSA not recommended. Do not apply to face, axillae, or groin.

**HOW SUPPLIED:** Oint: (Calcipotriene-Betamethasone) 0.005%-0.064% [15g, 30g, 60g]

**CONTRAINDICATIONS:** Known or suspected disorders of calcium metabolism; erythrodermic, exfoliative, and pustular psoriasis.

**WARNINGS/PRECAUTIONS:** Hypercalcemia reported; if elevation of serum calcium outside normal range occurs, discontinue treatment until normal calcium levels restored. May produce reversible hypothalamic-pituitary-adrenal axis suppression, manifestations of Cushing's syndrome, hyperglycemia, and glucosuria. Discontinue if irritation develops. Avoid in presence of pre-existing skin atrophy at treatment site.

**ADVERSE REACTIONS:** Pruritus, headache.

**PREGNANCY:** Category C, caution in nursing.

## TALACEN — CIV

acetaminophen - pentazocine HCl (Sanofi-Aventis)

**THERAPEUTIC CLASS:** Opioid agonist-antagonist analgesic

**INDICATIONS:** Relief of mild to moderate pain.

**DOSAGE:** *Adults:* 1 tab q4h prn. Max: 6 tabs/day.

**HOW SUPPLIED:** Tab: (Pentazocine-APAP) 25mg-650mg* *scored

**WARNINGS/PRECAUTIONS:** Contains sodium metabisulfite. Caution with head injury, increased intracranial pressure, acute CNS manifestations, MI, certain respiratory conditions, renal or hepatic dysfunction, and biliary surgery, seizure disorders and alcohol use. Potential for physical and psychological dependence.

**ADVERSE REACTIONS:** Nausea, vomiting, constipation, abdominal distress, anorexia, diarrhea, dizziness, lightheadedness, hallucinations, sedation, euphoria, headache, confusion, disorientation, sweating, tachycardia.

**INTERACTIONS:** Increased CNS depressant effects with alcohol. Withdrawal symptoms with narcotics.

**PREGNANCY:** Category C, caution in nursing.

## TALWIN NX — CIV

naloxone HCl - pentazocine HCl (Sanofi-Aventis)

**For oral use only. Severe, potentially lethal reactions may result from misuse by injection alone, or in combination with other agents.**

**THERAPEUTIC CLASS:** Opioid agonist-antagonist analgesic

**INDICATIONS:** Relief of moderate to severe pain.

**DOSAGE:** *Adults:* Usual: 1 tab q3-4h. May increase to 2 tabs q3-4h. Max: 12 tabs/day.
*Pediatrics:* >12 yrs: Usual: 1 tab q3-4h. May increase to 2 tabs q3-4h. Max: 12 tabs/day.

**HOW SUPPLIED:** Tab: (Pentazocine-Naloxone) 50mg-0.5mg* *scored

**WARNINGS/PRECAUTIONS:** Caution with elderly, drug dependence, head injury, increased intracranial pressure, certain respiratory conditions, acute CNS manifestations, renal or hepatic dysfunction, biliary surgery, and MI.

**ADVERSE REACTIONS:** Hypotension, tachycardia, hallucinations, dizziness, sedation, euphoria, sweating, nausea, vomiting, constipation, diarrhea, anorexia, facial edema, dermatitis, visual problems, chills, insomnia, urinary retention, paresthesia.

**INTERACTIONS:** Increased CNS depressant effects with alcohol. Withdrawal symptoms with narcotics.

**PREGNANCY:** Category C, caution in nursing.

## TAMBOCOR RX
flecainide acetate (Graceway)

**THERAPEUTIC CLASS:** Class IC antiarrhythmic

**INDICATIONS:** Prevention of paroxysmal supraventricular tachycardias (PSVT), paroxysmal atrial fibrillation/flutter (PAF) associated with disabling symptoms in patients without structural heart disease. Prevention of life-threatening ventricular arrhythmias (VT) .

**DOSAGE:** *Adults:* PSVT/PAF: Initial: 50mg q12h. Titrate: May increase by 50mg bid every 4 days. Max: 300mg/day. Sustained VT: Initial: 100mg q12h. Titrate: May increase by 50mg bid every 4 days. Max: 400mg/day. CrCl ≤35mL/min: Initial: 100mg qd or 50mg bid. Reduce dose by 50% with amiodarone. *Pediatrics:* <6 months: Initial: 50mg/m²/day given bid-tid. ≥6 months: Initial: 100mg/m²/day given bid-tid. Max: 200mg/m²/day. Reduce dose by 50% with amiodarone.

**HOW SUPPLIED:** Tab: 50mg, 100mg*, 150mg* *scored

**CONTRAINDICATIONS:** Right bundle branch block associated with left hemiblock (without a pacemaker), pre-existing 2nd- or 3rd-degree AV block, cardiogenic shock.

**WARNINGS/PRECAUTIONS:** Avoid with non-life-threatening ventricular arrhythmias. Increased mortality and non-cardiac arrests reported. Ventricular proarrhythmic effects may occur with atrial fibrillation/flutter. May cause or worsen CHF, arrhythmias. Slows cardiac conduction; dose related increases in PR, QRS, and QT intervals reported. Conduction changes may cause sinus pause, sinus arrest, bradycardia, 2nd- or 3rd-degree AV block. Extreme caution with sick sinus syndrome. May increase endocardial pacing thresholds and suppress ventricular escape with pacemakers. Correct hypokalemia or hyperkalemia before therapy. Monitor with significant hepatic impairment. Initiate treatment of sustained VT in the hospital.

**ADVERSE REACTIONS:** Arrhythmias, hepatic dysfunction, cardiac arrest, CHF, flushing, anxiety, vomiting, diarrhea, tinnitus.

**INTERACTIONS:** Additive negative inotropic effects with β-blockers (eg, propranolol). Potentiated by cimetidine, amiodarone, CYP2D6 inhibitors (eg, quinidine). Increases digoxin levels. Increased elimination with phenytoin, phenobarbital, carbamazepine. Diltiazem, nifedipine, verapamil, disopyramide not recommended.

**PREGNANCY:** Category C, safety in nursing unknown.



## TAMIFLU RX
oseltamivir phosphate (Roche Labs)

**THERAPEUTIC CLASS:** Neuraminidase inhibitor

**INDICATIONS:** Treatment of uncomplicated acute illness due to influenza in adults and children ≥1 yr who have been symptomatic for no more than 2 days. Prophylaxis of influenza in adults and children ≥1 yr.

**DOSAGE:** *Adults:* Prophylaxis: Begin within 2 days of exposure to infection. 75mg qd for at least 10 days, up to 6 weeks with community outbreak. CrCl 10-30mL/min: 75mg every other day. Treatment: Begin therapy within 2 days of symptom onset. 75mg bid for 5 days. CrCl 10-30mL/min: 75mg qd for 5 days. *Pediatrics:* Prophylaxis: ≥13 yr: Begin within 2 days of exposure to infection. 75mg qd for at least 10 days, up to 6 weeks with community outbreak. ≥1 yr: (Sus) ≤15kg: 30mg qd. >15-23kg: 45mg qd. >23-40kg: 60mg qd. >40kg: 75mg qd. Duration: 10 days. Treatment: ≥13 yrs: Begin therapy within 2 days of symptom onset. 75mg bid for 5 days. ≥1 yr: (Sus) ≤15kg: 30mg bid. >15-23kg: 45mg bid. >23-40kg: 60mg bid. >40kg: 75mg bid. Duration: 5 days.

**HOW SUPPLIED:** Cap: 75mg; Sus: 12mg/mL [25mL]

**WARNINGS/PRECAUTIONS:** Efficacy not known with chronic cardiac disease, respiratory disease, and immunocompromised. Not a substitute for influenza vaccine. Adjust dose with renal dysfunction. Postmarketing neuropsychiatric events (self-injury & delirium) reported.

**ADVERSE REACTIONS:** Nausea, vomiting, diarrhea, cough, headache, fatigue, toxic epidermal necrolysis, hepatitis, abnormal LFTs.

**INTERACTIONS:** Avoid admininstration of attenuated influenza vaccine within 2 weeks before or 48 hours after; may inhibit repliaction of live vaccine virus.

**PREGNANCY:** Category C, caution in nursing.

## TAMOXIFEN — RX

tamoxifen citrate (Various)

**For women with ductal carcinoma in situ (DCIS) and women at high risk for breast cancer; fatal uterine malignancies (eg, endometrial adenocarcinoma, uterine sarcoma), stroke, and PE reported with use in risk reduction setting. Discuss benefits/risks of events with this patient population. Benefits of tamoxifen outweigh risks in women already diagnosed with breast cancer.**

**THERAPEUTIC CLASS:** Antiestrogen

**INDICATIONS:** Treatment of metastatic breast cancer in women and men. Treatment of node-positive and axillary node-negative breast cancer in women following mastectomy, axillary dissection and breast irradiation. To reduce risk of invasive breast cancer in women with DCIS. Reduction of breast cancer incidence in high risk women. Use for up to 5 yrs.

**DOSAGE:** *Adults:* Breast Cancer Treatment: 20-40mg qd. Divide dosages >20mg into AM and PM doses. Breast Cancer Risk Reduction/DCIS: 20mg qd for 5 yrs.

**HOW SUPPLIED:** Tab: 10mg, 20mg

**CONTRAINDICATIONS:** Reduction in breast cancer incidence in high risk women and women wtih DCIS who require coumarin-type anticoagulant therapy or have a history of DVT, PE.

**WARNINGS/PRECAUTIONS:** Hypercalcemia reported in patients with bone metastases. Increased incidence of uterine malignancies (eg, endometrial cancer, uterine sarcoma) and endometrial changes including hyperplasia and polyps reported. Increased incidence of thromboembolic events (eg, DVT, PE). Malignant and non-malignant effects on the liver and ocular disturbances reported. Leukopenia, anemia, thrombocytopenia, neutropenia, pancytopenia reported. Promptly evaluate abnormal vaginal bleeding if receiving or previously received tamoxifen. Patients receiving or previously received tamoxifen should have annual gynecological exam. Do not become pregnant within 2 months of therapy. May cause fetal harm during pregnancy. Does not cause infertility even with menstrual irregularity.

**ADVERSE REACTIONS:** Hot flashes, increased bone and tumor pain, vaginal discharge, irregular menses; (men) loss of libido, impotence.

**INTERACTIONS:** Increases effects of coumarin-type anticoagulant; monitor PT. Increased risk of thromboembolic events with cytotoxic agents. Increased levels with bromocriptine. May decrease letrozole levels. Decreased levels with rifampin and aminoglutethimide. Decreased plasma levels of major metabolite, N-desmethyl tamoxifen with medroxyprogesterone.

**PREGNANCY:** Category D, not for use in nursing.

## TAPAZOLE
methimazole (King)

RX

**THERAPEUTIC CLASS:** Thyroid hormone synthesis inhibitor

**INDICATIONS:** Treatment of hyperthyroidism. To ameliorate hyperthyroidism prior to subtotal thyroidectomy or radioactive iodine therapy. Also indicated when thyroidectomy is contraindicated or not advisable.

**DOSAGE:** *Adults:* Initial: Mild Hyperthyroidism: 5mg q8h. Moderately Severe Hyperthyroidism: 30-40mg/day, in divided doses q8h. Severe Hyperthyroidism: 20mg q8h. Maint: 5-15mg/day.
*Pediatrics:* Initial: 0.4mg/kg/day, in divided doses q8h. Maint: 1/2 of initial dose.

**HOW SUPPLIED:** Tab: 5mg*, 10mg* *scored

**CONTRAINDICATIONS:** Nursing mothers.

**WARNINGS/PRECAUTIONS:** Can cause fetal harm. Agranulocytosis, leukopenia, thrombocytopenia, aplastic anemia may occur; monitor bone marrow function. Discontinue with agranulocytosis, aplastic anemia, or exfoliative dermatitis. Discontinue with liver abnormality (eg, hepatitis) including transaminases >3X ULN. Monitor thyroid function periodically. May cause hypoprothrombinemia and bleeding; monitor PT.

**ADVERSE REACTIONS:** Rash, urticaria, nausea, vomiting, arthralgia, paresthesia, myalgia, neuritis, vertigo, edema, altered taste, hair loss, lymphadenopathy, lupuslike syndrome, insulin autoimmune syndrome.

**INTERACTIONS:** May potentiate anticoagulants. β-blockers, digitalis, theophylline may need dose reduction when patient becomes euthyroid. Caution with other drugs that cause agranulocytosis.

**PREGNANCY:** Category D, contraindicated in nursing.

## TARCEVA
erlotinib (Genentech)

RX

**THERAPEUTIC CLASS:** Epidermal growth factor receptor tyrosine kinase inhibitor

**INDICATIONS:** Treatment of patients with locally advanced or metastatic non-small cell lung cancer (NSCLC) after failure of at least one prior chemotherapy regimen. First-line treatment of patients with locally advanced, unresectable or metastatic pancreatic cancer in combination with gemcitabine.

**DOSAGE:** *Adults:* NSCLC:150mg ≥1 hr before or 2 hrs after ingestion of food. Pancreatic Cancer: 100mg at least 1 hr before or 2 hrs after ingestion of food, in combination with gemcitabine. Continue until disease progression or unacceptable toxicity.

T

**HOW SUPPLIED:** Tab: 25mg, 100mg, 150mg

**WARNINGS/PRECAUTIONS:** Serious interstitial disease (ILD) including fatalities reported. Discontinue if ILD is diagnosed. Asymptomatic increases in liver transaminases observed. Dose reduction or interruption should be considered if changes in liver function are severe. Elevations in INR and infrequent reports of bleeding have been reported. Monitor closely with concomitant anticoagulants.

**ADVERSE REACTIONS:** Rash, diarrhea, anorexia, fatigue, dyspnea, cough, nausea, infection, vomiting, stomatitis, pruritus, dry skin, conjunctivitis, keratoconjunctivitis sicca, abdominal pain.

**INTERACTIONS:** Co-treatment with potent CYP3A4 inhibitor ketoconazole increases erlotinib AUC by 2/3. Caution should be used when administering or taking erlotinib with ketoconazole and other strong CYP3A4 inhibitors such as atazanavir, clarithromycin, indinavir, itraconazole, nefazodone, nelfinavir, ritonavir, saquinavir, telithromycin, troleandomycin, and voriconazole.

**PREGNANCY:** Category D, not for use in nursing.

## TARGRETIN CAPSULES

RX

bexarotene (Ligand)

**Retinoids are associated with birth defects. Avoid in pregnancy.**

**THERAPEUTIC CLASS:** Retinoid

**INDICATIONS:** Treatment of manifestations of cutaneous T-cell lymphoma in patients refractory to at least one prior systemic therapy.

**DOSAGE:** *Adults:* Initial: 300mg/m² qd with a meal. If toxicity occurs, adjust to 200mg/m²/day then to 100mg/m²/day, or temporarily suspend. Readjust upward if toxicity controlled. If no response after 8 weeks and 300mg/m² is tolerated, increase to 400mg/m²/day.

**HOW SUPPLIED:** Cap: 75mg

**CONTRAINDICATIONS:** Pregnancy.

**WARNINGS/PRECAUTIONS:** May induce lipid and LFT abnormalities, pancreatitis, hypothyroidism, leukopenia, cataracts. Perform fasting lipid levels before therapy, then weekly until lipid response to bexarotene (2-4 weeks), then at 8-week intervals. May need dose reduction or suspension if develop elevated triglycerides. Obtain baseline LFT; then monitor at 1, 2, and 4 weeks after initial therapy; then periodically if stable. Obtain WBC with differential at baseline, periodically thereafter. Minimize exposure to sunlight and artificial UV light. Great caution with hepatic dysfunction. Avoid if risk factors present for pancreatitis.

**ADVERSE REACTIONS:** Lipid abnormalities, anemia, nausea, headache, asthenia, infection, abdominal pain, chills, fever, flu syndrome, hypothyroidism, rash, dry skin, leukopenia, peripheral edema.

**INTERACTIONS:** Limit vitamin A intake to <1500 IU/day. CYP3A4 inhibitors (eg, ketoconazole, itraconazole, erythromycin, gemfibrozil, grapefruit juice) may increase levels and inducers (eg, rifampin, phenytoin, phenobarbital) may decrease levels. Avoid gemfibrozil. May increase metabolism of tamoxifen, hormonal contraceptives. May enhance hypoglycemia with insulin, sulfonylureas, or insulin sensitizers.

**PREGNANCY:** Category X, not for use in nursing.

## TARGRETIN GEL

RX

bexarotene (Ligand)

**THERAPEUTIC CLASS:** Retinoid

**INDICATIONS:** Topical treatment of cutaneous lesions associated with cutaneous T-cell lymphoma (CTCL) (Stage IA and IB) refractory to, intolerant to, or persistent after other therapies.

**DOSAGE:** *Adults:* Initial: Apply once every other day for 1 week. Titrate: Increase weekly to qd, then bid, then tid, and finally qid. Max: Apply qid. Allow to dry before covering with clothing. Reduce frequency if application site toxicity occurs. Discontinue temporarily if severe irritation occurs.

**HOW SUPPLIED:** Gel: 1% [60g]

**CONTRAINDICATIONS:** Pregnancy.

**WARNINGS/PRECAUTIONS:** Avoid normal skin, mucosal surfaces. Minimize exposure to sunlight and artificial UV light. Caution with retinoid hypersensitivity. Possible altered kinetics in renal dysfunction.

**ADVERSE REACTIONS:** Dermatitis, pruritus, rash, sweating, asthenia, skin disorder, pain, headache, edema, paresthesia, cough, pharyngitis.

**INTERACTIONS:** Avoid DEET-containing products (eg, insect repellents). Limit vitamin A intake to <1500 IU/day. Increased levels possible with ketoconazole, itraconazole, erythromycin, gemfibrozil, grapefruit juice.

**PREGNANCY:** Category X, not for use in nursing.

## TARKA

RX

trandolapril - verapamil HCl (Abbott)

**ACE inhibitors can cause death/injury to developing fetus during 2nd and 3rd trimesters. Stop therapy if pregnancy detected.**

**THERAPEUTIC CLASS:** ACE inhibitor/calcium channel blocker (nondihydropyridine)

**INDICATIONS:** Treatment of hypertension. Not for initial therapy.

**DOSAGE:** *Adults:* Replacement Therapy: 1 tab qd with food. Severe Hepatic Dysfunction: Give 30% of normal dose.

**HOW SUPPLIED:** Tab: (Trandolapril-Verapamil) 2mg-180mg, 1mg-240mg, 2mg-240mg, 4mg-240mg

**CONTRAINDICATIONS:** Severe ventricular dysfunction, hypotension, cardiogenic shock, sick sinus syndrome or 2nd- or 3rd-degree AV block (except with functioning ventricular pacemaker), A-Fib/Flutter with an accessory bypass tract, history of ACE inhibitor associated angioedema.

**WARNINGS/PRECAUTIONS:** Monitor for hypotension with surgery or anesthesia. Risk of hyperkalemia with renal insufficiency, DM. D/C if jaundice develops. Avoid with moderate to severe cardiac failure and ventricular dysfunction if taking a β-blocker. May cause angioedema, cough, fetal/neonatal morbidity, hypotension, AV block, anaphylactoid reactions, transient bradycardia, PR-interval prolongation. Monitor LFTs periodically. Give 30% of normal dose with severe hepatic dysfunction. Caution with CHF, hypertrophic cardiomyopathy, renal or hepatic dysfunction. Decrease dose in those with decreased neuromuscular transmission. Monitor WBC with collagen-vascular disease and/or renal disease.

**ADVERSE REACTIONS:** AV block, constipation, cough, dizziness, fatigue, headache, increased hepatic enzymes, chest pain, upper respiratory tract infection/congestion.

**INTERACTIONS:** May increase alcohol blood levels and prolong effects. Additive effects on HR, AV conduction, and contractility with β-blockers. Potentiates other antihypertensives. May increase digoxin, carbamazepine, theophylline, and cyclosporine levels. Avoid disopyramide within 48 hrs before or 24 hrs after verapamil. Additive negative inotropic effects and AV conduction prolongation with flecainide. Avoid quinidine with hypertrophic cardiomyopathy. Monitor lithium. Increased clearance with phenobarbital. Rifampin may reduce oral bioavailability. May potentiate neuromuscular blockers; both agents may need dose reduction. Risk of hyperkalemia with $K^+$-sparing diuretics, $K^+$ supplements. Caution with inhalation anesthetics.

**PREGNANCY:** Category C (1st trimester) and D (2nd and 3rd trimesters), not for use in nursing.



## TASMAR

RX

tolcapone (Valeant)

**Risk of fatal, acute fulminant liver failure. Withdraw if patients fail to show benefit within 3 weeks of initiation. Discontinue if develop hepatotoxicity, and do not consider retreatment. Perform LFTs before therapy, then every 2 weeks for 1st year, every 4 weeks for next 6 months, then every 8 weeks thereafter. Perform LFTs before increase dose to 200mg tid. Avoid with liver disease or if LFTs >2X ULN. Caution with severe dyskinesia or dystonia.**

**THERAPEUTIC CLASS:** COMT inhibitor

**INDICATIONS:** Adjunct to levodopa/carbidopa for the treatment of symptoms of idiopathic Parkinson's disease.

**DOSAGE:** *Adults:* Initial: 100mg tid. Use 200mg tid only if clinical benefit is justified. May need to decrease levodopa dose.

**HOW SUPPLIED:** Tab: 100mg, 200mg

**CONTRAINDICATIONS:** Liver disease, patients withdrawn from therapy due to drug-induced hepatocellular injury. History of non-traumatic rhabdomyolysis, hyperpyrexia or confusion related to medication.

**WARNINGS/PRECAUTIONS:** Hypotension/syncope, rhabdomyolysis, hallucinations, confusion, diarrhea, hematuria reported. Fibrotic complications can occur. Avoid with liver dysfunction. Caution with severe renal dysfunction. Closely monitor when discontinuing therapy.

**ADVERSE REACTIONS:** Dyskinesia, nausea, dystonia, excessive dreaming, anorexia, muscle cramps, orthostatic complaints, diarrhea, confusion, hallucination, vomiting, constipation, fatigue, increased sweating, xerostomia, urine discoloration, hepatotoxicity.

**INTERACTIONS:** Dobutamine, apomorphine and isoproterenol may need a dose reduction. Avoid non-selective MAOIs (eg, phenelzine, tranylcypromine). May increase risk of orthostatic hypotension and dyskinesia with levodopa. Caution with tolbutamide, desipramine, warfarin.

**PREGNANCY:** Category C, caution in nursing.

## TAVIST ALLERGY — OTC

clemastine fumarate (Novartis Consumer)

**THERAPEUTIC CLASS:** Antihistamine

**INDICATIONS:** Temporarily reduces symptoms of common cold, hay fever or other respiratory allergies.

**DOSAGE:** *Adults:* 1 tab q12h. Max: 2 tabs/24 hrs.
*Pediatrics:* >12 yrs: 1 tab q12h. Max: 2 tabs/24 hrs.

**HOW SUPPLIED:** Tab: 1.34mg* *scored

**WARNINGS/PRECAUTIONS:** May cause excitability in children. Caution with respiratory problems (eg, emphysema, chronic bronchitis), glaucoma, and enlarged prostate gland. May impair mental/physical abilities.

**ADVERSE REACTIONS:** Drowsiness, dizziness.

**INTERACTIONS:** Alcohol, sedatives, and tranquilizers may increase drowsiness.

**PREGNANCY:** Safety in pregnancy and nursing not known.

## TAXOL — RX

paclitaxel (Bristol-Myers Squibb)

> **Anaphylaxis, severe hypersensitivity reactions reported. Pretreat with corticosteroids, diphenhydramine, and $H_2$ antagonists. Do not rechallenge if severe hypersensitivity reaction occurs. Monitor CBC frequently.**

**THERAPEUTIC CLASS:** Antimicrotubule agent

**INDICATIONS:** First-line (with cisplatin) treatment of advanced ovarian carcinoma and non-small cell lung cancer. Subsequent treatment in advanced ovarian carcinoma. Treatment of breast cancer after failure with combination chemotherapy for metastatic disease or relapse within 6 months of adjuvant chemotherapy. Adjuvant treatment of node-positive breast cancer administered sequentially to doxorubicin-containing chemotherapy. Second-line treatment of AIDS-related Kaposi's sarcoma.

**DOSAGE:** *Adults:* IV: Ovarian Carcinoma: Previously Untreated: 175mg/m$^2$ over 3 hrs or 135mg/m$^2$ over 24 hrs every 3 weeks followed by cisplatin. Previous Treatment: 135mg/m$^2$ or 175mg/m$^2$ over 3 hrs every 3 weeks. Breast Cancer: 175mg/m$^2$ over 3 hrs every 3 weeks. Non-small Cell Lung Cancer: 135mg/m$^2$ over 24 hrs every 3 weeks followed by cisplatin. Kaposi's Sarcoma: 135mg/m$^2$ over 3 hrs every 3 weeks or 100mg/m$^2$ over 3 hrs every 2 weeks. Reduce dose of subsequent courses by 20% if neutrophils <500cells/mm$^3$ for >1 week or severe peripheral neuropathy occurs.

**HOW SUPPLIED:** Inj: 6mg/mL

**CONTRAINDICATIONS:** Hypersensitivity to drugs formulated in Cremophor® EL (eg, cyclosporine for injection concentrate, teniposide for injection concentrate), solid tumor patients with baseline neutrophils <1500 cells/mm³, AIDS-related Kaposi's sarcoma patients with baseline neutrophils <1000 cells/mm³.

**WARNINGS/PRECAUTIONS:** Severe conduction abnormalities, injection site reactions, peripheral neuropathy (more common in elderly) reported. Bone marrow suppression is dose dependent, dose limiting, and more common in elderly. Can cause fetal harm. Hypotension, bradycardia, and HTN may occur during administration. Toxicity enhanced with elevated liver enzymes. Contains dehydrated alcohol.

**ADVERSE REACTIONS:** Neutropenia, leukopenia, thrombocytopenia, anemia, infections, bleeding, bradycardia, hypotension, peripheral neuropathy, myalgia/arthralgia, nausea, vomiting, diarrhea, mucositis, alopecia.

**INTERACTIONS:** Increases doxorubicin levels. Caution with CYP450 2C8 and 3A4 substrates or inhibitors (eg, ritonavir, saquinavir, indinavir, nelfinavir). Myelosuppression more profound with cisplatin.

**PREGNANCY:** Category D, not for use in nursing.

## TAXOTERE RX

docetaxel (Sanofi-Aventis)

**Increased treatment-related mortality reported with hepatic dysfunction, high-dose therapy, and in non-small cell lung carcinoma previously treated with platinum-based chemotherapy with docetaxel 100mg/m². Avoid if neutrophils <1500cells/mm³, bilirubin >ULN, or SGOT/SGPT >1.5X ULN with alkaline phosphatase >2.5X ULN. Severe hypersensitivity reactions reported.**

**THERAPEUTIC CLASS:** Antimicrotubule agent

**INDICATIONS:** Treatment of locally advanced or metastatic breast cancer and non-small cell lung cancer (NSCLC) after failure of prior chemotherapy. In combination with doxorubicin and cyclophosphamide for the adjuvant treatment of operable, node-positive breast cancer. In combination with cisplatin for treatment of unresectable, locally advanced or metastatic NSCLC in those previously untreated with chemotherapy. Treatment of androgen independent (hormone refractory) metastatic prostate cancer in combination with prednisone. In combination with cisplatin and fluorouracil for the treatment of advanced gastric adenocarcinoma, including adenocarcinoma of the gastroesophageal junction, in patients who have not received prior chemotherapy for advanced disease. In combination with cisplatin and fluorouracil for the induction treatment of patients with inoperable locally advanced squamous cell carcinoma of the head and neck (SCCHN).

**DOSAGE:** *Adults:* Premedicate with oral corticosteroids. Adjust dose based on febrile neutropenia, neutrophil count, cutaneous reactions, peripheral neuropathy, neurosensory signs/symptoms, or GI toxicities (see package insert). Breast Cancer: 60-100mg/m² IV over 1 hr every 3 weeks. Adjuvant Treatment Operable Node-Positive Breast CA: 75mg/m² 1 hr after doxorubicin 50mg/m² and cyclophosphamide 500mg/m² every 3 weeks for 6 courses. NSCLC: 75mg/m² IV over 1 hr every 3 weeks. Prostate Cancer: 75mg/m² every 3 weeks over 1 hr with prednisone 5mg bid. Gastric Adenocarcinoma: Premedicate with antiemetics and appropriate hydration. 75mg/m² IV over 1 hr, followed by cisplatin 75mg/m² IV over 1-3 hrs (both on Day 1 only), followed by fluorouracil 750mg/m²/day IV over 24 hrs for 5 days, starting at end of cisplatin infusion. Repeat treatment every 3 weeks. SCCHN: 75mg/m² IV over 1 hr, followed by cisplatin 75mg/m² IV over 1 hr, on Day 1, followed by fluorouracil as a continuous IV infusion at 750mg/m²/day for five days administered every 3 weeks for 4 cycles.
*Pediatrics:* >16 yrs: Premedicate with oral corticosteroids. Adjust dose based on febrile neutropenia, neutrophil count, cutaneous reactions, peripheral neuropathy, neurosensory signs/symptoms, or GI toxicities (see package

insert). Breast Cancer: 60-100mg/m² IV over 1 hr every 3 weeks. Adjuvant Treatment Operable Node-Positive Breast CA: 75mg/m² 1 hr after doxorubicin 50mg/m² and cyclophosphamide 500mg/m² every 3 weeks for 6 courses. NSCLC: 75mg/m² IV over 1 hr every 3 weeks. Prostate Cancer: 75mg/m² every 3 weeks over 1 hr with prednisone 5mg bid. Gastric Adenocarcinoma: Premedicate with antiemetics and appropriate hydration. 75mg/m² IV over 1 hr, followed by cisplatin 75mg/m² IV over 1-3 hrs (both on Day 1 only), followed by fluorouracil 750mg/m²/day IV over 24 hrs for 5 days, starting at end of cisplatin infusion. Repeat treatment every 3 weeks. SCCHN: 75mg/m² IV over 1 hr, followed by cisplatin 75mg/m² IV over 1 hr, on Day 1, followed by fluorouracil as a continuous IV infusion at 750mg/m² per day for five days administered every 3 weeks for 4 cycles.

**HOW SUPPLIED:** Inj: 20mg/0.5mL

**CONTRAINDICATIONS:** Neutrophils <1500cells/mm³, hypersensitivity to polysorbate 80.

**WARNINGS/PRECAUTIONS:** Toxic deaths, febrile neutropenia, neutropenia, localized erythema of extremities with edema and desquamation, severe neurosensory symptoms, severe asthenia reported. Monitor for hypersensitivity reactions. Can cause fetal harm. Caution in elderly. Monitor CBC frequently; avoid subsequent cycles until neutrophils recover to >1500 cells/mm³ and platelets recover to >100,000cells/mm³.

**ADVERSE REACTIONS:** Arthralgia, myalgia, alopecia, stomatitis, nausea, vomiting, diarrhea, nail changes, cutaneous and neurosensory reactions, fluid retention, hypersensitivity reaction, leukopenia, thrombocytopenia, anemia, neutropenia, fever.

**INTERACTIONS:** Caution with agents that induce, inhibit, or are metabolized by CYP450 3A4 (eg, ketoconazole, erythromycin, terfenadine, astemizole, cyclosporine).

**PREGNANCY:** Category D, not for use in nursing.

## TAZICEF

ceftazidime (Hospira)

RX

**THERAPEUTIC CLASS:** Cephalosporin (3rd generation)

**INDICATIONS:** Treatment of lower respiratory tract (eg, pneumonia), skin and skin structure (SSSI), bone and joint, gynecologic, CNS (eg, meningitis), intra-abdominal, and urinary tract infections (UTI), and septicemia. For use in sepsis.

**DOSAGE:** *Adults:* Usual: 1g IM/IV q8-12h. Uncomplicated UTI: 250mg IM/IV q12h. Complicated UTI: 500mg IM/IV q8-12h. Bone and Joint Infection: 2g IV q12h. Uncomplicated Pneumonia/SSSI: 500mg-1g IM/IV q8h. Gynecological/Intra-Abdominal/Meningitis/Severe Life-Threatening Infection: 2g IV q8h. Lung Infection caused by Pseudomonas in Cystic Fibrosis (normal renal function): 30-50mg/kg IV q8h. Max: 6g/day. Renal Impairment: CrCl 31-50mL/min: 1g q12h. CrCl 16-30mL/min: 1g q24h. CrCl 6-15mL/min: 500mg q24h. CrCl <5mL/min: 500mg q48h. For severe infections (6g/day), increase renal impairment dose by 50% or increase dosing interval. Apply reduced dosage recommendations after initial 1g LD is given. Hemodialysis: Give 1g before and 1g after each hemodialysis. Intra-Peritoneal Dialysis/Continuous Ambulatory Peritoneal Dialysis: Give 1g followed by 500mg q24h, or add to fluid at 250mg/2L.
*Pediatrics:* Neonates (0-4 weeks): 30mg/kg IV q12h. 1 month-12 yrs: 30-50mg/kg IV q8h. Max: 6g/day. Higher doses for patients with cystic fibrosis or when treating meningitis. Renal impairment: CrCl 31-50mL/min: 1g q12h. CrCl 16-30mL/min: 1g q24h. CrCl 6-15mL/min: 500mg q24h. CrCl <5mL/min: 500mg q48h. For severe infections (6g/day), increase renal impairment dose by 50% or increase dosing interval. Apply reduced dosage recommendations after initial 1g LD is given. Hemodialysis: Give 1g before and 1g after each hemodialysis. Intra-Peritoneal Dialysis/Continuous Ambulatory Peritoneal Dialysis: Give 1g followed by 500mg q24h, or add to fluid at 250mg/2L.

**HOW SUPPLIED:** Inj: 1g, 2g, 6g

**WARNINGS/PRECAUTIONS:** Monitor renal function; potential for nephrotoxicity. May result in overgrowth of nonsusceptible organisms. Possible cross-sensitivity between penicillins, cephalosporins, and other beta-lactams. Pseudomembranous colitis reported. Elevated levels with renal insufficiency can lead to seizures, encephalopathy, asterixis, and neuromuscular excitability. Possible decrease in PT; caution with renal or hepatic impairment, poor nutritional state; monitor PT and give vitamin K if needed. Caution with colitis and other GI diseases. Distal necrosis can occur after inadvertent intra-arterial administration. Continue for 2 days after signs and symptoms of infection resolve, but may require longer therapy with complicated infections. Caution in elderly.

**ADVERSE REACTIONS:** Phlebitis and inflammation at injection site, pruritus, rash, fever, diarrhea, anaphylaxis.

**INTERACTIONS:** Nephrotoxicity reported with aminoglycosides or potent diuretics (eg, furosemide). Avoid with chloramphenicol; may decrease effect of beta-lactam antibiotics.

**PREGNANCY:** Category B, caution in nursing.

## TAZIDIME RX

ceftazidime (Lilly)

**THERAPEUTIC CLASS:** Cephalosporin (3rd generation)

**INDICATIONS:** Treatment of lower respiratory tract (eg, pneumonia), skin and skin structure (SSSI), bone and joint, gynecologic, CNS (eg, meningitis), intra-abdominal, and urinary tract infections (UTI), and septicemia. For use in sepsis.

**DOSAGE:** *Adults:* Usual: 1g IM/IV q8-12h. Uncomplicated UTI: 250mg IM/IV q12h. Complicated UTI: 500mg IM/IV q8-12h. Bone and Joint Infection: 2g IV q12h. Uncomplicated Pneumonia/Skin and Skin Structure Infection: 500mg-1g IM/IV q8h. Gynecological/Intra-Abdominal/Meningitis/Severe Life-Threatening Infection: 2g IV q8h. Lung Infection caused by Pseudomonas spp. in Cystic Fibrosis (normal renal function): 30-50mg/kg IV q8h. Max: 6g/day. Renal impairment: CrCl 31-50mL/min: 1g q12h. CrCl 16-30mL/min: 1g q24h. CrCl 6-15mL/min: 500mg q24h. CrCl <5mL/min: 500mg q48h. For severe infections (6g/day), increase renal impairment dose by 50% or increase dosing interval. Apply reduced dosage recommendations after initial 1g LD is given. Hemodialysis: Give 1g before then 1g after each hemodialysis. Intra-Peritoneal Dialysis/Continuous Ambulatory Peritoneal Dialysis: Give 1g followed by 500mg q24h, or add to fluid at 250mg/2L.
*Pediatrics:* Neonates (0-4 weeks): 30mg/kg IV q12h. 1 month-12 yrs: 30-50mg/kg IV q8h. Max: 6g/day. Higher doses for cystic fibrosis and meningitis. Renal Impairment: CrCl 31-50mL/min: 1g q12h. CrCl 16-30mL/min: 1g q24h. CrCl 6-15mL/min: 500mg q24h. CrCl <5mL/min: 500mg q48h. For severe infections (6g/day), increase renal impairment dose by 50% or increase dosing interval. Apply reduced dosage recommendations after initial 1g LD is given. Hemodialysis: Give 1g before then 1g after each hemodialysis. Intra-Peritoneal Dialysis/Continuous Ambulatory Peritoneal Dialysis: Give 1g followed by 500mg q24h, or add to fluid at 250mg/2L.

**HOW SUPPLIED:** Inj: 1g, 2g, 6g

**WARNINGS/PRECAUTIONS:** Monitor renal function; potential for nephrotoxicity. Prolonged use may result in overgrowth of nonsusceptible organisms. Possible cross-sensitivity between penicillins, cephalosporins, and other beta-lactam antibiotics. Pseudomembranous colitis reported. Elevated levels with renal insufficiency can lead to seizures, encephalopathy, asterixis and neuromuscular excitability. Possible decrease in PT; caution with renal or hepatic impairment, poor nutritional state; monitor PT and give vitamin K if needed. Caution with colitis and other GI diseases. Distal necrosis can occur after inadvertent intra-arterial administration. Continue therapy for 2 days after the signs and symptoms of infection have disappeared, but in complicated infections longer therapy may be required.

**ADVERSE REACTIONS:** Phlebitis and inflammation at injection site, pruritus, rash, fever, diarrhea.

**INTERACTIONS:** Nephrotoxicity reported with aminoglycosides or potent diuretics (eg, furosemide). Avoid with chloramphenicol; may decrease effect of beta-lactam antibiotics.

**PREGNANCY:** Category B, caution in nursing.

## TAZORAC — RX

tazarotene (Allergan)

**THERAPEUTIC CLASS:** Retinoic acid derivative

**INDICATIONS:** (Gel 0.05%, 0.1%) Stable plaque psoriasis of up to 20% body surface area involvement. (Cre 0.1%, Gel 0.1%) Acne vulgaris of mild to moderate severity. (Cre 0.05%, 0.1%) Treatment of plaque psoriasis.

**DOSAGE:** *Adults:* Cleanse and dry skin. Apply to skin qpm.
*Pediatrics:* >12 yrs: Cleanse and dry skin. Apply to acne or psoriatic lesions qpm.

**HOW SUPPLIED:** Cre: 0.05%, 0.1% [30g, 60g]; Gel: 0.05%, 0.1% [30g, 100g]

**CONTRAINDICATIONS:** Women who are or may become pregnant.

**WARNINGS/PRECAUTIONS:** Use adequate birth control measures. Avoid mouth, eyes, eyelids, sunlight exposure (including sunlamps), or eczematous skin. Stop therapy with pruritus, burning, skin redness, or peeling. Weather extremes (eg, wind, cold) may be irritating.

**ADVERSE REACTIONS:** Pruritus, burning/stinging, erythema, worsening of psoriasis, irritation, skin pain, desquamation, dry skin, rash, fissuring, localized edema, skin discoloration.

**INTERACTIONS:** Avoid topical agents that have a strong drying effect. Caution with photosensitizers (eg, thiazides, tetracyclines, fluoroquinolones, phenothiazines, sulfonamides).

**PREGNANCY:** Category X, caution in nursing.

## TEARS NATURALE FORTE — OTC

glycerin - dextran 70 - hydroxypropyl methylcellulose (Alcon)

**THERAPEUTIC CLASS:** Lubricant

**INDICATIONS:** Temporary relief of burning and irritation due to dryness of the eye and for use as a protectant against further irritation. Temporary relief of discomfort due to minor irritations of the eye or exposure to wind or sun.

**DOSAGE:** *Adults:* 1-2 drops in affected eye prn.

**HOW SUPPLIED:** Sol: (Dextran 70-Glycerin-Hydroxypropyl Methylcellulose) 0.1%-0.2%-0.3% [15mL, 30mL]

**WARNINGS/PRECAUTIONS:** Do not touch container tip to any surface to avoid contamination. Discontinue if eye pain or vision changes occur, if redness or irritation continues, or if condition worsens or persists >72 hrs.

**PREGNANCY:** Safety in pregnancy or nursing not known.

## TEARS NATURALE FREE — OTC

dextran 70 - hydroxypropyl methylcellulose (Alcon)

**THERAPEUTIC CLASS:** Lubricant

**INDICATIONS:** Temporary relief of burning and irritation due to dryness of the eye and for use as a protectant against further irritation. Temporary relief of discomfort due to minor irritations of the eye or exposure to wind or sun.

**DOSAGE:** *Adults:* 1-2 drops in affected eye prn.

**HOW SUPPLIED:** Sol: (Dextran 70-Hydroxypropyl Methylcellulose) 0.1%-0.3% [0.6mL 32s]

**WARNINGS/PRECAUTIONS:** Do not touch container tip to any surface to avoid contamination. D/C if eye pain or vision changes occur, if redness or irritation continues, or if condition worsens or persists >72 hrs.

**PREGNANCY:** Safety in pregnancy or nursing not known.

## TEGRETOL RX

carbamazepine (Novartis)

**Aplastic anemia and agranulocytosis reported. Obtain complete pretreatment hematological testing as a baseline. Discontinue if develop evidence of bone marrow depression.**

**OTHER BRAND NAMES:** Tegretol-XR (Novartis)

**THERAPEUTIC CLASS:** Carboxamide anticonvulsant

**INDICATIONS:** Treatment of partial seizures with complex symptomatology, general tonic-clonic seizures, and mixed seizure patterns of these or other partial or generalized seizures. Treatment of trigeminal or glossopharyngeal neuralgia pain.

**DOSAGE:** *Adults:* Epilepsy: Initial: (Immediate or Extended Release Tabs) 200mg bid or (Sus) 100mg qid. Titrate: (Immediate Release Tabs/Sus) Increase weekly by 200mg/day given tid-qid. (Extended Release Tabs) Increase weekly by 200mg/day given bid. Maint: 800-1200mg/day. Max: 1200mg/day. Trigeminal Neuralgia: Initial (Day 1): (Immediate or Extended Release Tabs) 100mg bid or (Sus) 50mg qid. Titrate: May increase by 100mg q12h (Tabs) or 50mg qid (Sus). Maint: 400-800mg/day. Max: 1200mg/day. Re-evaluate every 3 months. Swallow Extended Release Tabs whole; do not crush or chew.
*Pediatrics:* Epilepsy: >12 yrs: Initial: (Immediate or Extended Release Tabs) 200mg bid or (Sus) 100mg qid. Titrate: (Immediate Release Tabs/Sus) Increase weekly by 200mg/day given tid-qid. (Extended Release Tabs) Increase weekly by 200mg/day given bid. Max: 12-15 yrs: 1000mg/day. >15 yrs: 1200mg/day. 6-12 yrs: Initial: (Immediate or Extended Release Tabs) 100mg bid or (Sus) 50mg qid. Titrate: (Immediate Release Tabs/Sus) Increase weekly by 100mg/day given tid-qid. (Extended Release Tabs) Increase weekly by 100mg/day given bid. Maint: 400-800mg/day. Max: 1000mg/day. 6 months-6 yrs: Initial: (Immediate Release Tabs) 10-20mg/kg/day given bid-tid or (Sus) 10-20mg/kg/day given qid. Titrate: (Immediate Release Tabs/Sus) Increase weekly tid-qid. Max: 35mg/kg/day. Swallow Extended Release Tabs whole; do not crush or chew.

**HOW SUPPLIED:** Sus: 100mg/5mL; Tab: (Tegretol) 200mg*; Tab, Chewable: 100mg*; Tab, Extended Release: (Tegretol-XR) 100mg, 200mg, 400mg
*scored



**CONTRAINDICATIONS:** History of bone marrow depression, MAOI use within 14 days, hypersensitivity to TCAs.

**WARNINGS/PRECAUTIONS:** Lyell's syndrome and Stevens-Johnson syndrome, multi-organ hypersensitivity reactions reported. Caution with history of adverse hematologic reaction to any drug, increased IOP, the elderly, mixed seizure disorder with atypical absence seizure. Fetal harm with pregnancy. May activate latent psychosis. Caution with cardiac, hepatic, or renal damage. Perform eye exam and monitor LFTs and renal function at baseline and periodically. Suspension produces higher peak levels than the tablet.

**ADVERSE REACTIONS:** Dizziness, drowsiness, unsteadiness, nausea, vomiting, bone marrow depression, rash, urticaria, hypersensitivity reactions, photosensitivity reactions, CHF, edema, HTN, hypotension.

**INTERACTIONS:** Do not give suspension with other medicinal liquids or diluents. Metabolism is inhibited by CYP3A4 inhibitors (eg, cimetidine, macrolides) and induced by CYP3A4 inducers (eg, rifampin, phenytoin).

Decreases oral contraceptive effectiveness. Increases plasma levels of clomipramine, phenytoin and primidone. Decreases levels of APAP, alprazolam, clonazepam, clozapine, dicumarol, doxycycline, ethosuximide, haloperidol, lamotrigine, methsuximide, oral contraceptives, phensuximide, phenytoin, theophylline, tiagabine, topiramate, valproate, and warfarin. Increased risk of neurotoxic side effects with lithium. Avoid MAOIs.

**PREGNANCY:** Category D, not for use in nursing.

## TEKTURNA — RX

aliskiren (Novartis)

**Drugs that act directly on the renin-angiotensin system can cause injury/death to developing fetus during 2nd and 3rd trimesters of pregnancy. Stop therapy if pregnancy is detected.**

**THERAPEUTIC CLASS:** Renin inhibitor

**INDICATIONS:** Treatment of hypertension, alone or with other antihypertensives.

**DOSAGE:** *Adults:* Usual: 150mg qd. Titrate: May increase to 300mg/day if needed. Meals high in fat decrease absorption.

**HOW SUPPLIED:** Tab: 150mg, 300mg

**WARNINGS/PRECAUTIONS:** Caution with renal dysfunction (SrCr=1.7mg/dL (women) or 2mg/dL (men) and/or GFR <30mL/min), history of dialysis, nephortic syndrome, or renovascular hypertension. May increase serum potassium especially when used in combination with an ACE inhibitor in diabetic population. Angioedema of face, extremities, lips, tongue, glottis, and/or larynx reported; d/c and monitor until complete resolution of signs and symptoms. Hypotension rarely seen.

**ADVERSE REACTIONS:** Diarrhea, headache, nasopharyngitis, dizziness, fatigue, upper respiratory tract infection, back pain, cough.

**INTERACTIONS:** Co-administration with irbesartan or atorvastatin may increase $C_{max}$ up to 50% after multiple dosing. Co-administration of ketoconazole 200mg bid may result in an approximate 80% increase in plasma level. Co-administration with furosemide may reduce AUC and $C_{max}$ by 30% and 50%, respectively.

**PREGNANCY:** Categories C (first trimester) and D (second and third trimesters); not for use in nursing.

## TEMODAR — RX

temozolomide (Schering)

**THERAPEUTIC CLASS:** Alkylating agent (imidazotetrazine derivative)

**INDICATIONS:** Treatment of glioblastoma multiforme. Treatment of refractory anaplastic astrocytoma.

**DOSAGE:** *Adults:* Adjust according to nadir neutrophil and platelet counts of previous cycle and at time of initiating next cycle. Glioblastoma Multiforme: 75mg/m² qd for 42 days with focal radiotherapy. Maint: Cycle 1 (28 days): 150mg/m² qd for 5 days. Cycle 2-6 (28 days): If cycle 1 toxicity Grade≤2, ANC ≥1.5 x $10^9$/L and platelets ≥100 x $10^9$/L, increase to 200mg/m²/day for 5 consecutive days per 28-day cycle. Do not increase dose in subsequent cycles if dose not escalated at Cycle 2. Anaplastic Astrocytoma: Initial: 150mg/m² qd for 5 consecutive days per 28-day cycle. If ANC >1.5 x $10^9$/L and platelets >100 x $10^9$/L for both the nadir and day 29 (day 1 of next cycle), may increase to 200mg/m²/day for 5 consecutive days per 28-day cycle. Start next cycle when ANC >1.5 x $10^9$/L and platelets >100 x $10^9$/L . If ANC <1 x $10^9$/L or platelets <50 x $10^9$/L during any cycle, reduce next cycle by 50mg/m², but not <100mg/m². Swallow whole with water.

**HOW SUPPLIED:** Cap: 5mg, 20mg, 100mg, 140mg, 180mg, 250mg

T

**CONTRAINDICATIONS:** Hypersensitivity to DTIC (dacarbazine).

**WARNINGS/PRECAUTIONS:** Before therapy, must have ANC >1.5 x $10^9$/L and platelets >100 x $10^9$/L. Myelosuppression may occur; obtain CBC on day 22 (21 days after 1st dose) or within 48 hrs of that day, repeat weekly until ANC >1.5 x $10^9$/L and platelets >100 x $10^9$/L. Greater risk of myelosuppression in women and elderly. May cause fetal harm during pregnancy. Very rare cases of myelodysplastic syndrome and secondary malignancies, including myeloid leukemia have been observed. Do not open capsules. Caution in elderly, or severe renal/hepatic impairment.

**ADVERSE REACTIONS:** Headache, fatigue, myelosuppression (thrombocytopenia, neutropenia), nausea, vomiting, convulsions, hemiparesis, asthenia, fever, peripheral edema, constipation, dizziness, diarrhea.

**INTERACTIONS:** Valproic acid may decrease clearance.

**PREGNANCY:** Category D, not for use in nursing.

## TEMOVATE — RX

clobetasol propionate (GlaxoSmithKline)

**OTHER BRAND NAMES:** Temovate-E (GlaxoSmithKline) - Temovate Scalp (GlaxoSmithKline)

**THERAPEUTIC CLASS:** Corticosteroid

**INDICATIONS:** Corticosteroid responsive dermatoses. Temovate-E is also used to treat moderate to severe plaque-type psoriasis.

**DOSAGE:** *Adults:* Apply bid. Max: 50g/week or 50mL/week. Moderate-Severe Psoriasis: (Temovate-E) Apply bid for up to 4 weeks. May use on 5-10% of BSA. Max: 50g/week. Limit treatment to 2 consecutive weeks. Avoid with occlusive dressings.
*Pediatrics:* >12 yrs: Apply bid. Max: 50g/week or 50mL/week. Moderate-Severe Psoriasis: >16 yrs: (Temovate-E) Apply bid for up to 4 weeks. May use on 5-10% of BSA. Max: 50g/week. Limit treatment to 2 consecutive weeks. Avoid with occlusive dressings.

**HOW SUPPLIED:** (Temovate) Cre, Oint: 0.05% [15g, 30g, 45g, 60g]; Gel: 0.05% [15g, 30g, 60g]; Sol: 0.05% [25mL]; (Temovate-E) Cre: 0.05% [15g, 30g, 60g]; (Temovate Scalp) Sol: 0.05% [25mL, 50mL]

**CONTRAINDICATIONS:** (Scalp Sol) Primary scalp infections.

**WARNINGS/PRECAUTIONS:** Not for use on face, groin, or axillae, or for treatment of rosacea or perioral dermatitis. May produce reversible HPA axis suppression, manifestations of Cushing's syndrome, hyperglycemia, and glucosuria. Use appropriate antifungal or antibacterial agent with dermatological infections; d/c if infection does not clear. Peds may be more susceptible to systemic toxicity. Avoid eyes. D/C if irritation occurs.



**ADVERSE REACTIONS:** Burning, stinging, pruritus, skin atrophy, cracking/fissuring of the skin, erythema, folliculitis, numbness of fingers, telangiectasia, tingling (Sol), folliculitis (Sol).

**PREGNANCY:** Category C, caution in nursing.

## TENEX — RX

guanfacine HCl (Dr. Reddys)

**THERAPEUTIC CLASS:** $Alpha_2$-agonist

**INDICATIONS:** Treatment of hypertension.

**DOSAGE:** *Adults:* 1mg qhs. Titrate: May increase to 2mg qhs after 3-4 weeks. Max: 3mg/day.

**HOW SUPPLIED:** Tab: 1mg, 2mg

**WARNINGS/PRECAUTIONS:** Caution with severe coronary insufficiency, recent MI, cerebrovascular disease, chronic renal or hepatic failure. Avoid abrupt discontinuation. Dose-related drowsiness and sedation.

**ADVERSE REACTIONS:** Dry mouth, somnolence, asthenia, dizziness, constipation, impotence, headache.

**INTERACTIONS:** Additive sedation with other CNS depressants. Caution with CYP450 inducers (eg, phenobarbital, phenytoin) in renal dysfunction.

**PREGNANCY:** Category B, caution with nursing.

## TENORETIC RX

atenolol - chlorthalidone (AstraZeneca LP)

**THERAPEUTIC CLASS:** Selective $beta_1$-blocker/monosulfamyl diuretic

**INDICATIONS:** Treatment of hypertension. Not for initial therapy.

**DOSAGE:** *Adults:* Initial: 50mg-25mg tab qd. May increase to 100mg-25mg tab qd. CrCl 15-35mL/min: Max: 50mg atenolol/day. CrCl <15mL/min: Max: 50mg atenolol every other day.

**HOW SUPPLIED:** Tab: (Atenolol-Chlorthalidone) 50mg-25mg*, 100mg-25mg *scored

**CONTRAINDICATIONS:** Sinus bradycardia, >1st-degree heart block, cardiogenic shock, overt cardiac failure, anuria, sulfonamide hypersensitivity.

**WARNINGS/PRECAUTIONS:** Withdrawal before surgery is not recommended. Caution with bronchospastic disease, conduction abnormalities, left ventricular dysfunction, heart failure controlled by digitalis and/or diuretics, renal dysfunction. Can cause heart failure with prolonged use. May mask hypoglycemia or hyperthyroidism symptoms. Avoid abrupt discontinuation. Avoid with untreated pheochromocytoma. Possible fetal harm in pregnancy. May aggravate peripheral arterial circulatory disorders. Enhanced effects in postsympathectomy patient. Neonates born to mothers receiving atenolol may be at risk of hypoglycemia and bradycardia.

**ADVERSE REACTIONS:** Bradycardia, hypotension, dizziness, fatigue, nausea, depression, dyspnea, blood dyscrasias.

**INTERACTIONS:** Additive effects with catecholamine-depleting drugs (eg, reserpine), calcium channel blockers, and digitalis. Bradycardia, heart block, and left ventricular end diastolic pressure can rise with verapamil or diltiazem. Exacerbates rebound HTN with clonidine withdrawal. Prostaglandin synthase inhibitors (eg, indomethacin) may decrease hypotensive effects. Caution with anesthetic agents. May block epinephrine effects. May decrease arterial response to norepinephrine. Increases risk of lithium toxicity. Possible hypokalemia with corticosteroids or ACTH. May alter insulin requirements.

**PREGNANCY:** Category D, caution in nursing.

## TENORMIN RX

atenolol (AstraZeneca LP)



**THERAPEUTIC CLASS:** Selective $beta_1$-blocker

**INDICATIONS:** Management of hypertension. Long-term management of angina pectoris. To reduce cardiovascular mortality in hemodynamically stable patients with definite or suspected AMI.

**DOSAGE:** *Adults:* HTN: Initial: 50mg qd. Titrate: May increase after 1-2 weeks. Max: 100mg qd. Angina: Initial: 50mg qd. Titrate: May increase to 100mg after 1 week. Max: 200mg qd. AMI: Initial: 5mg IV over 5 minutes, repeat 10 minutes later. If tolerated, give 50mg PO 10 minutes after the last IV dose followed by another 50mg PO 12 hrs later. Maint: 100mg qd or 50mg bid for 6-9 days. Renal Impairment/Elderly: HTN: Initial: 25mg qd. HTN/Angina/AMI: Max: CrCl 15-35mL/min: 50mg/day. CrCl <15mL/min: 25mg/day. Hemodialysis: 25-50mg after each dialysis.

**HOW SUPPLIED:** Inj: 0.5mg/mL; Tab: 25mg, 50mg*, 100mg *scored

**CONTRAINDICATIONS:** Sinus bradycardia, >1st-degree heart block, cardiogenic shock, overt cardiac failure.

**WARNINGS/PRECAUTIONS:** Withdrawal before surgery is not recommended. Caution with bronchospastic disease, conduction abnormalities, left ventricular dysfunction, heart failure controlled by digitalis and/or diuretics, renal or hepatic dysfunction. Can cause heart failure with prolonged use, hyperuricemia, hypercalcemia, hypokalemia, hypophosphatemia. May mask hypoglycemia or hyperthyroidism symptoms. Avoid abrupt discontinuation. Avoid with untreated pheochromocytoma. Possible fetal harm in pregnancy. May aggravate peripheral arterial circulatory disorders. May manifest latent DM. Monitor for fluid or electrolyte imbalance. May develop antinuclear antibodies (ANA). Neonates born to mothers receiving atenolol may be at risk of hypoglycemia and bradycardia.

**ADVERSE REACTIONS:** Bradycardia, hypotension, dizziness, fatigue, nausea, depression, dyspnea.

**INTERACTIONS:** Additive effects with catecholamine-depleting drugs (eg, reserpine), calcium channel blockers, and digitalis. Bradycardia, heart block, and left ventricular end diastolic pressure can rise with verapamil or diltiazem. Exacerbates rebound HTN with clonidine withdrawal. Serious adverse reactions with IV atenolol and IV verapamil use. Prostaglandin synthase inhibitors (eg, indomethacin) may decrease hypotensive effects. Caution with drugs that depress the myocardium (eg, anesthesia). May block epinephrine effects.

**PREGNANCY:** Category D, caution in nursing.

## TENUATE CIV

diethylpropion HCl (Watson)

**OTHER BRAND NAMES:** Tenuate Dospan (Watson)

**THERAPEUTIC CLASS:** Sympathomimetic amine

**INDICATIONS:** Short term adjunct for exogenous obesity in patients with an initial BMI>30kg/m$^2$.

**DOSAGE:** *Adults:* (Tab)25mg tid 1 hour before meals, and mid-evening if needed for night hunger. (Tab, ER): 75mg at qd in mid-morning, swallowed whole.

*Pediatrics:* ≥16 yrs: (Tab) 25mg tid 1 hour before meals, and mid-evening if needed for night hunger. (Tab, ER): 75mg at qd in mid-morning, swallowed whole.

**HOW SUPPLIED:** Tab: (Tenuate) 25mg; Tab, Extended Release: (Tenuate Dospan) 75mg

**CONTRAINDICATIONS:** Advanced arteriosclerosis, hyperthyroidism, glaucoma, pulmonary HTN, severe HTN, within 14 days of MAOI use, agitated states, history of drug abuse, other concomitant anorectics.



**WARNINGS/PRECAUTIONS:** Possible risk of pulmonary hypertension and valvular heart disease. Caution in HTN, symptomatic cardiovascular disease. Avoid with heart murmur, valvular heart disease, severe HTN. May increase convulsions with epilepsy. Prolonged use may induce dependence with withdrawal symptoms. Discontinue if tolerance develops or if insignificant weight loss after 4 weeks of therapy.

**ADVERSE REACTIONS:** Palpitations, tachycardia, arrhythmias, blurred vision, dizziness, anxiety, insomnia, depression, urticaria, gynecomastia, nausea, vomiting, GI disturbances, bone marrow depression, impotence.

**INTERACTIONS:** MAOIs may cause hypertensive crisis. Avoid with other anorectic agents (prescription, OTC, herbal products) or if used within prior year. Phenothiazines may antagonize anorectic effects. Potential for arrhythmias with general anesthetics. May interfere with antihypertensives (eg, guanethidine, methyldopa). Adverse reactions with alcohol. Antidiabetic drug requirements may be altered. Valvular heart disease reported with fenfluramine or dexfenfluramine.

**PREGNANCY:** Category B, caution in nursing.

## TERAZOL 3 RX
terconazole (Ortho-McNeil)

**THERAPEUTIC CLASS:** Azole antifungal

**INDICATIONS:** Treatment of vulvovaginal candidiasis.

**DOSAGE:** *Adults:* 1 applicatorful or sup vaginally qhs for 3 nights.

**HOW SUPPLIED:** Cre: 0.8% [20g]; Sup: 80mg [3[s]]

**WARNINGS/PRECAUTIONS:** D/C if sensitization, irritation, fever, chills, or flu-like symptoms occur. Confirm diagnosis by KOH smears and/or cultures; reconfirm if no response. Do not use diaphragm with suppository.

**ADVERSE REACTIONS:** Sup: Localized burning, pruritus, genital pain, headache. Cre: Dysmenorrhea, headache, pruritus, burning, abdominal pain.

**PREGNANCY:** Category C, not for use in nursing.

## TERAZOL 7 RX
terconazole (Ortho-McNeil)

**THERAPEUTIC CLASS:** Azole antifungal

**INDICATIONS:** Treatment of vulvovaginal candidiasis.

**DOSAGE:** *Adults:* 1 applicatorful vaginally qhs for 7 nights.

**HOW SUPPLIED:** Cre: 0.4% [45g]

**WARNINGS/PRECAUTIONS:** D/C if sensitization, irritation, fever, chills, or flu-like symptoms occur. Confirm diagnosis by KOH smears and/or cultures; reconfirm if no response.

**ADVERSE REACTIONS:** Headache, body pain, burning, itching, irritation.

**PREGNANCY:** Category C, not for use in nursing.

## TERBUTALINE RX
terbutaline sulfate (Various)

**THERAPEUTIC CLASS:** $Beta_2$ agonist

**INDICATIONS:** Prevention and reversal of bronchospasm in asthma, and reversible bronchospasm in bronchitis and emphysema.

**DOSAGE:** *Adults:* (PO) Usual: 5mg tid. May reduce to 2.5mg tid. Max: 15mg/24hrs. (Inj) Usual: 0.25mg SQ into lateral deltoid area. May repeat within 15-30 minutes if no improvement. Max: 0.5mg/4hrs.
*Pediatrics:* (PO) 12-15 yrs: Usual: 2.5mg tid. Max: 7.5mg/24hrs. (Inj) >12 yrs: Usual: 0.25mg SQ into lateral deltoid area. May repeat within 15-30 minutes if no improvement. Max: 0.5mg/4hrs.

**HOW SUPPLIED:** Inj: 1mg/mL [1mL]; Tab: 2.5mg*, 5mg* *scored

**CONTRAINDICATIONS:** Hypersensitivity to sympathomimetic amines.

**WARNINGS/PRECAUTIONS:** Caution with ischemic heart disease, HTN, arrhythmias, hyperthyroidism, DM, seizures. Not approved for tocolysis. Hypersensitivity and exacerbation of bronchospasm reported. Monitor for transient hypokalemia.

**ADVERSE REACTIONS:** Nervousness, tremor, headache, somnolence, palpitations, dizziness, tachycardia, nausea.

**INTERACTIONS:** Avoid other sympathomimetic agents (except aerosol bronchodilators). Extreme caution with MAOIs and TCAs during or within 14

days of treatment. Decreased effects with β-blockers. Possible ECG changes and hypokalemia with loop or thiazide diuretics.

**PREGNANCY:** Category B, caution in nursing.

## TERRAMYCIN/POLYMYXIN B SULFATE RX

oxytetracycline HCl - polymyxin B sulfate (Pfizer)

**THERAPEUTIC CLASS:** Antibacterial combination

**INDICATIONS:** Treatment of superficial infections involving the conjuctiva and/or cornea.

**DOSAGE:** *Adults:* Apply 0.5 inch onto the lower eyelid bid-qid.

**HOW SUPPLIED:** Oint: (Oxytetracycline-Polymyxin B) 5mg/g [3.75g]

**WARNINGS/PRECAUTIONS:** D/C if superinfection occurs.

**ADVERSE REACTIONS:** Allergic or inflammatory reactions.

**PREGNANCY:** Safety in pregnancy and nursing not known.

## TESLAC CIII

testolactone (Bristol-Myers Squibb)

**THERAPEUTIC CLASS:** Non-steroidal aromatase inhibitor

**INDICATIONS:** Adjunctive therapy in the palliative treatment of advanced or disseminated breast cancer in postmenopausal women when hormonal therapy is indicated. May also be used in women diagnosed as having had disseminated breast carcinoma when premenopausal, in whom ovarian function has been subsequently terminated.

**DOSAGE:** *Adults:* 250mg qid. Continue for minimum of 3 months unless disease progresses.

**HOW SUPPLIED:** Tab: 50mg

**CONTRAINDICATIONS:** Treatment of breast cancer in men.

**WARNINGS/PRECAUTIONS:** Caution in elderly. Monitor calcium levels.

**ADVERSE REACTIONS:** Maculopapular erythema, increased BP, paresthesia, malaise, aches, peripheral edema, glossitis, anorexia, nausea, vomiting.

**INTERACTIONS:** May increase effects of anticoagulants; monitor/adjust anticoagulant dosage.

**PREGNANCY:** Category C, safety in nursing unknown.



## TESSALON RX

benzonatate (Forest)

**THERAPEUTIC CLASS:** Non-narcotic antitussive

**INDICATIONS:** Symptomatic relief of cough.

**DOSAGE:** *Adults:* Usual: 100-200mg tid as needed. Max: 600mg/day. *Pediatrics:* >10 yrs: Usual: 100-200mg tid as needed. Max: 600mg/day.

**HOW SUPPLIED:** Cap: 100mg, 200mg

**WARNINGS/PRECAUTIONS:** Severe hypersensitivity reactions; confusion and hallucinations reported in combination with other prescribed drugs. Swallow capsules without sucking/chewing to avoid local anesthesia adverse effects.

**ADVERSE REACTIONS:** Sedation, headache, dizziness, confusion, hallucinations, constipation, nausea, GI upset, pruritus.

**PREGNANCY:** Category C, caution in nursing.

## TESTIM

testosterone (Auxilium)

**THERAPEUTIC CLASS:** Androgen

**INDICATIONS:** Testosterone replacement in males with primary or hypogonadotropic hypogonadism.

**DOSAGE:** *Adults:* >18 yrs: Apply 5g qd, preferably in the am, to clean, dry, intact skin of shoulders and/or upper arms. Allow to dry prior to dressing. Titrate: May increase to 10g qd if response not achieved or serum concentration is below normal range. Do not apply to genitals or abdomen. To maintain serum testosterone levels, do not wash site of application for atleast 2 hrs.

**HOW SUPPLIED:** Gel: 1% [5g (50mg)/tube 30[s]]

**CONTRAINDICATIONS:** Breast or prostate carcinoma in men. Not for use by women. Pregnant and nursing women should avoid skin contact with application sites on men.

**WARNINGS/PRECAUTIONS:** Caution in elderly; increased risk of prostatic hypertrophy/carcinoma. Risk of edema with pre-existing cardiac, renal, or hepatic disease; discontinue if edema occurs, diuretic therapy may be required. Risk of gynecomastia. May potentiate sleep apnea especially with obesity or chronic lung diseases. Transfer of testosterone can occur with skin to skin contact. Risk of virilization of female partner. Advise patients to report persistent penis erections, changes in skin color, ankle swelling, unexplained nausea and vomitting, or breathing disturbances. Monitor serum testosterone, LFTs, Hgb, Hct, PSA, cholesterol, lipids. Prolonged use associated with serious hepatic effects (peliosis hepatitis, hepatic neoplasms, choleostatic hepatitis, jaundice).

**ADVERSE REACTIONS:** Application site reactions, benign prostatic hyperplasia, decreased DBP, increased BP, gynecomastia, headache, Hct/Hgb increases, hot flushes, insomnia, increased lacrimation, mood swings, smell disorder.

**INTERACTIONS:** May elevate oxyphenbutazone levels. May decrease blood glucose and insulin requirements. May increase clearance of propranolol. Corticosteroids may enhance edema; caution with cardiac or hepatic disease.

**PREGNANCY:** Category X, not for use in nursing.

## TESTRED

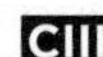

methyltestosterone (Valeant)

**THERAPEUTIC CLASS:** Androgen

**INDICATIONS:** Testosterone replacement therapy in males with primary hypogonadism or hypogonadotrophic hypogonadism. To stimulate puberty in males with delayed puberty. Secondary treatment of advancing inoperable metastatic (skeletal) breast cancer in females 1-5 yrs postmenopausal.

**DOSAGE:** *Adults:* Dose based on age, sex and diagnosis. Adjust dose according to clinical response and adverse events. Male Replacement Therapy: 10-50mg/day. Breast Carcinoma: 50-200mg/day.
*Pediatrics:* Dose based on age, sex and diagnosis. Adjust dose according to clinical response and adverse events. Delayed Puberty: Use lower range of 10-50mg/day for 4-6 months. Caution in children.

**HOW SUPPLIED:** Cap: 10mg

**CONTRAINDICATIONS:** Pregnancy. Males with breast or prostate carcinoma.

**WARNINGS/PRECAUTIONS:** D/C if hypercalcemia occurs in breast cancer; monitor calcium levels. Monitor for virilization in females. Risk of compromised stature in children; monitor bone growth every 6 months. Risk of hepatic damage with long-term use. D/C if jaundice, cholestatic hepatitis occurs. Risk of edema; caution with pre-existing cardiac, renal or hepatic disease. Caution

T

in the elderly; increased risk of prostatic hypertrophy and prostatic carcinoma. Should not be used for enhancement of athletic performance. Monitor LFTs, Hct, and Hgb periodically.

**ADVERSE REACTIONS:** Amenorrhea, virilization, menstrual irregularities, gynecomastia, excessive frequency/duration of penile erections, male pattern baldness, increased/decreased libido, oligospermia, hirsutism, acne, fluid and electrolyte disturbances, nausea, hypercholesterolemia, clotting factor suppression, polycythemia, altered LFTs, priapism, anxiety, depression.

**INTERACTIONS:** Potentiates oral anticoagulants and oxyphenbutazone. May decrease blood glucose and insulin requirements in diabetics.

**PREGNANCY:** Category X, not for use in nursing.

## TETANUS & DIPHTHERIA TOXOIDS ADSORBED — RX

tetanus toxoid - diphtheria toxoid (Sanofi Pasteur)

**THERAPEUTIC CLASS:** Toxoid combination

**INDICATIONS:** Active immunization against tetanus and diphtheria (Td).

**DOSAGE:** *Adults:* 0.5mL IM in the vastus lateralis or deltoid. Repeat 4-8 weeks later. Give 3rd dose 6-12 months after 2nd dose. Booster: 0.5mL IM every 10 yrs.
*Pediatrics:* >7 yrs: 0.5mL IM in the vastus lateralis or deltoid. Repeat 4-8 weeks later. Give 3rd dose 6-12 months after 2nd dose. Booster: 0.5mL IM every 10 yrs.

**HOW SUPPLIED:** Inj: 5LFU-2LFU/0.5mL

**CONTRAINDICATIONS:** Neurological or systemic allergic reaction to previous dose. Defer during febrile illness, acute infection, or an outbreak of poliomyelitis. Thimerosal hypersensitivity.

**WARNINGS/PRECAUTIONS:** Suboptimal response may occur in immunocompromised patients. Avoid booster more frequently than every 10 yrs especially with Arthus-type hypersensitivity reactions or temperature >39.4°C after a previous dose of tetanus toxoid. Caution with IM injection in thrombocytopenia or any coagulation disorder. Increased risk of local/systemic reactions to boosters doses. Have epinephrine available.

**ADVERSE REACTIONS:** Injection site reaction, fever, malaise, hypotension, nausea, arthralgia.

**INTERACTIONS:** Immunosuppressive therapy may reduce response to active immunization. Caution with anticoagulants.

**PREGNANCY:** Category C, safety in nursing not known.

## TETANUS TOXOID ADSORBED — RX

tetanus toxoid (Sanofi Pasteur)

**THERAPEUTIC CLASS:** Toxoid

**INDICATIONS:** Active immunization against tetanus.

**DOSAGE:** *Adults:* Primary Immunization: 0.5mL IM. Repeat 4-8 weeks later. Give 3rd dose 6-12 months after 2nd dose. Booster: 0.5mL IM every 10 yrs.
*Pediatrics:* <1 yr: 3 doses of 0.5mL IM 4 to 8 weeks apart, then 4th dose (0.5mL) 6 to 12 months after the 3rd dose. Last dose before 4 yrs. Give booster of 0.5mL at 4-6 yrs. No booster needed if last primary dose was given after 4 yrs. >1 yrs: Primary Immunization: 0.5mL IM. Repeat 4-8 weeks later. Give 3rd dose 6-12 months after 2nd dose. Booster: 0.5mL IM every 10 yrs.

**HOW SUPPLIED:** Inj: 5 LFU/0.5mL

**CONTRAINDICATIONS:** Neurological or systemic allergic reaction to previous dose. Defer during febrile illness, acute infection, or an outbreak of poliomyelitis. Thimerosal hypersensitivity.

**WARNINGS/PRECAUTIONS:** Suboptimal response may occur in immunocompromised patients. Avoid booster more frequently than every 10 yrs especially with Arthus-type hypersensitivity reactions or temperature >103°F after a previous dose of tetanus toxoid. Caution with IM injections in thrombocytopenia or any coagulation disorders. Have epinephrine injection available. Increased incidence of local/systemic reaction to booster doses.

**ADVERSE REACTIONS:** Local erythema, malaise, transient fever, pain, hypotension, nausea, arthralgia.

**INTERACTIONS:** Caution with anticoagulants. Immunosuppresive therapy (eg, radiation, corticosteroids, chemotherapy) may reduce antibody response to vaccine; defer routine vaccination. Separate syringes and sites should be used when Tetanus Immune Globulin (human) and vaccine are given concurrently.

**PREGNANCY:** Category C, safety in nursing not known.

## TEVETEN
eprosartan mesylate (Kos) RX

**Can cause death/injury to developing fetus during 2nd and 3rd trimesters. Stop therapy if pregnancy detected.**

**THERAPEUTIC CLASS:** Angiotensin II receptor antagonist

**INDICATIONS:** Treatment of hypertension, alone or with other antihypertensives.

**DOSAGE:** *Adults:* Initial: 600mg qd. Usual: 400-800mg/day, given qd-bid. Moderate to Severe Renal Impairment: Max: 600mg/day.

**HOW SUPPLIED:** Tab: 400mg*, 600mg *scored

**WARNINGS/PRECAUTIONS:** Can cause fetal injury/death. Correct volume or salt depletion before therapy. Changes in renal function may occur; caution with renal artery stenosis, severe CHF.

**ADVERSE REACTIONS:** Upper respiratory infection, rhinitis, pharyngitis, cough.

**INTERACTIONS:** Risk of hypotension with diuretics.

**PREGNANCY:** Category C (1st trimester) and D (2nd and 3rd trimesters), not for use in nursing.

## TEVETEN HCT
hydrochlorothiazide - eprosartan mesylate (Kos) RX

**Can cause death/injury to developing fetus during 2nd and 3rd trimesters. Stop therapy if pregnancy detected.**

**THERAPEUTIC CLASS:** Angiotensin II receptor antagonist/thiazide diuretic

**INDICATIONS:** Treatment of hypertension. Not for initial therapy.

**DOSAGE:** *Adults:* Usual (Not Volume Depleted): 600mg-12.5mg qd. Titrate: May increase to 600mg-25mg qd if needed. Renal Impairment: Max: 600mg/day (eprosartan).

**HOW SUPPLIED:** Tab: (Eprosartan-HCTZ) 600mg-12.5mg, 600mg-25mg

**CONTRAINDICATIONS:** Anuria, sulfonamide hypersensitivity.

**WARNINGS/PRECAUTIONS:** Hypersensitivity reactions reported. Fetal/neonatal morbidity and death reported. Monitor for hypotension in volume/salt depletion. Caution with CHF, renal or hepatic dysfunction. May exacerbate or activate SLE. Monitor electrolytes periodically. Hypercalcemia, hypomagnesemia, hyperuricemia, hyperglycemia may occur. Enhanced effects in post-sympathectomy patient.

**ADVERSE REACTIONS:** Dizziness, headache, back pain, fatigue, myalgia, upper respiratory tract infection, sinusitis, viral infection.

**INTERACTIONS:** Increased risk of hyperkalemia with potassium-sparing diuretics, potassium supplements, or potassium-containing salt substitutes. Potentiated orthostatic hypotension with alcohol, barbiturates, and narcotics. May need to adjust insulin and antidiabetic drugs. Impaired absorption with cholestyramine, colestipol. Corticosteroids and ACTH deplete electrolytes. May decrease response to pressor amines (eg, norepinephrine). Potentiated effect with other antihypertensives. May increase responsiveness to nondepolarizing skeletal muscle relaxants (eg, tubocurarine). Risk of lithium toxicity; avoid use. NSAIDs may decrease diuretic/antihypertensive effects.

**PREGNANCY:** Category C (1st trimester) and D (2nd and 3rd trimesters), not for use in nursing.

## TEV-TROPIN — RX

somatropin (Gate)

**THERAPEUTIC CLASS:** Human growth hormone

**INDICATIONS:** Long-term treatment of children who have growth failure due to an inadequate secretion of normal endogenous growth hormone.

**DOSAGE:** *Pediatrics:* 0.1mg/kg (0.3 IU/kg) SQ 3x week.

**HOW SUPPLIED:** Inj: 5mg

**CONTRAINDICATIONS:** Prader-Willi syndrome (PWS) with severe obesity or severe respiratory impairment. Growth failure due to PWS. Acute critical illness due to complications following open heart or abdominal surgery, multiple accidental traumas, acute respiratory failure; closed epiphyses; progression of an underlying intracranial lesion; active neoplasia, benzyl alcohol sensitivity.

**WARNINGS/PRECAUTIONS:** Reports of fatalities in pediatric patients with PWS. In PWS, evaluate for upper airway obstruction prior to initiation; monitor weight, for sleep apnea, signs of upper airway obstruction (eg, suspend therapy with onset of or increased snoring), respiratory infections (treat early and aggressively if occur). Monitor GHD secondary to intracranial lesion for progression/recurrence; glucose intolerance; hypothyroidism; intracranial hypertension (perform fundoscopic exam at start and periodically). Slipped capital femoral epiphysis may occur. Monitor for malignant transformation of any skin lesion. When injected SQ in the same site over a long period of time, may cause tissue atrophy; rotate injection site.

**ADVERSE REACTIONS:** Headaches, injection site reactions (pain, bruise), leukemia.

**INTERACTIONS:** Decreased effects with glucocorticoids.

**PREGNANCY:** Category C, caution with nursing.



## THALITONE — RX

chlorthalidone (King)

**THERAPEUTIC CLASS:** Monosulfamyl diuretic

**INDICATIONS:** Management of hypertension. Adjunct therapy in edema associated with CHF, hepatic cirrhosis, corticosteroid and estrogen therapy, renal dysfunction.

**DOSAGE:** *Adults:* HTN: Initial: 15mg qd. Titrate: May increase to 30mg qd, then to 45-50mg qd. Edema: Initial: 30-60mg/day or 60mg every other day, up to 90-120mg/day. Maint: May be lower than initial; adjust to patient. Take in the morning with food.

**HOW SUPPLIED:** Tab: 15mg

**CONTRAINDICATIONS:** Anuria, sulfonamide hypersensitivity.

**WARNINGS/PRECAUTIONS:** Caution in severe renal disease, liver dysfunction, allergy history, asthma. May exacerbate or activate SLE. Monitor for fluid and electrolyte imbalance. Hyperuricemia, hypomagnesemia, hypokalemia, hypercalcemia, hypophosphatemia, and hyperglycemia may occur. May manifest latent DM.

**ADVERSE REACTIONS:** Pancreatitis, jaundice, diarrhea, vomiting, constipation, nausea, blood dyscrasias, rash, photosensitivity, dizziness, headache, electrolyte disturbance, impotence.

**INTERACTIONS:** Potentiates action of other antihypertensive drugs. May increase responsiveness to tubocurarine. May decrease arterial effectiveness of norepinephrine. Antidiabetic agents may need adjustment. Risk of lithium toxicity. Orthostatic hypotension aggravated by alcohol, barbiturates, or narcotics.

**PREGNANCY:** Category B, not for use in nursing.

## THALOMID RX

thalidomide (Celgene)

**Severe, life-threatening human birth defects if taken during pregnancy. Women of childbearing potential should have a pregnancy test before starting therapy, then weekly for 1st month, and monthly thereafter. Males must use latex condoms in sexual intercourse with females of childbearing potential. Only prescribers and pharmacists registered with the** *S.T.E.P.S.®* distribution program can prescribe and dispense. The use of thalidomide in multiple myeloma results in an increased risk of venous thromboembolic events, such as deep vein thrombosis and pulmonary embolus.

**THERAPEUTIC CLASS:** Immunomodulatory agent

**INDICATIONS:** Acute treatment of the cutaneous manifestations of moderate to severe erythema nodosum leprosum (ENL). Maintenance therapy for prevention and suppression of the cutaneous manifestations of ENL recurrence. In combination with dexamethasone for the treatment of newly diagnosed multiple myeloma.

**DOSAGE:** *Adults:* Acute ENL: Initial: 100-300mg qhs with water at least 1 hr after evening meal. <50kg: Start therapy at lower end of dosing range. Severe Cutaneous ENL: Initial: 400mg qhs with water at least 1 hr after evening meal. Use with corticosteroids in moderate to severe neuritis with severe ENL. Taper steroid where neuritis is ameliorated. Duration of therapy is usually 2 weeks. Taper Dose: Decrease by 50mg every 2-4 weeks. Maintenance Therapy for Prevention/Suppression of ENL Recurrence: Use minimum dose to control reaction. Taper Dose: Every 3-6 months, attempt to decrease dose by 50mg every 2-4 weeks. Multiple Myeloma: 200mg qhs at least 1 hr after evening meal. Give with dexamethasone in 28 day treatment cycles.
*Pediatrics:* >12 yrs: Acute ENL: Initial: 100-300mg qhs with water at least 1 hr after evening meal. <50kg: Start therapy at lower end of dosing range. Severe Cutaneous ENL: Initial: 400mg qhs with water at least 1 hour after evening meal. Use with corticosteroids in moderate to severe neuritis with severe ENL. Taper steroid where neuritis is ameliorated. Duration of therapy is usually 2 weeks. Taper Dose: Decrease by 50mg every 2-4 weeks. Maintenance Therapy for Prevention/Suppression of ENL Recurrence: Use minimum dose to control reaction. Taper Dose: Every 3-6 months, attempt to decrease dose by 50mg every 2-4 weeks. Multiple Myeloma: 200mg qhs at least 1 hr after evening meal. Give with dexamethasone in 28 day treatment cycles.

**HOW SUPPLIED:** Cap: 50mg, 100mg, 200mg

**CONTRAINDICATIONS:** Women of childbearing potential unless alternative therapies are considered inappropriate and if precautions are taken to avoid pregnancy. Sexually mature males unless they comply with the *S.T.E.P.S.®* program and mandatory contraceptive measures.

**WARNINGS/PRECAUTIONS:** See Black Box Warning. If hypersensitivity reaction occurs such as rash, fever, or tachycardia, d/c drug. Stevens-Johnson syndrome and toxic epidermal necrolysis reported. May cause severe birth defects. Drowsiness and somnolence reported, caution when operating machinery. May cause neuropathy, monitor for symptoms. If symptoms of neuropathy arise, d/c immediately. Do not initiate if ANC <750/mm$^3$. Measure viral load of HIV patients after 1st and 3rd month of therapy and every 3 months thereafter.

**ADVERSE REACTIONS:** Drowsiness, somnolence, peripheral neuropathy, dizziness, orthostatic hypotension, neutropenia, increased HIV viral load, rash, constipation, hypocalcemia, thrombosis/embolism, dyspnea.

**INTERACTIONS:** Enhanced sedation with barbiturates, alcohol, chlorpromazine, and reserpine. Caution with drugs associated with peripheral neuropathy.

**PREGNANCY:** Category X, not for use in nursing.

## THEO-24 RX

theophylline (UCB Pharma)

**THERAPEUTIC CLASS:** Xanthine bronchodilator

**INDICATIONS:** Treatment of symptoms and reversible airflow obstruction associated with chronic asthma and other chronic lung diseases.

**DOSAGE:** *Adults:* Initial: 300-400mg/day. Titrate: After 3 days increase to 400-600mg/day if tolerated. May increase to >600mg/day if needed and tolerated after 3 more days. Renal/Liver Dysfunction/Elderly/CHF: Max: 400mg/day. May give in divided doses q12h in fast metabolizers. Swallow tab whole with full glass of water, do not crush. Dose should be titrated based on serum levels.
*Pediatrics:* 12-15 yrs: <45kg: Initial: 12-14mg/kg/day. Max: 300mg/day. Titrate: After 3 days increase to 16mg/kg/day. Max: 400mg/day. May increase to 20mg/kg/day if tolerated and needed after 3 more days. Max: 600mg/day. 12-15 yrs (>45kg): Follow adult dose schedule. Renal/Liver Dysfunction/CHF: Max: 16mg/kg/day or 400mg/day. May give in divided doses q12h in fast metabolizers. Swallow tab whole with full glass of water, do not crush. Dose should be titrated based on serum levels.

**HOW SUPPLIED:** Cap, Extended Release: 100mg, 200mg, 300mg, 400mg

**WARNINGS/PRECAUTIONS:** Extreme caution in peptic ulcer disease, seizure disorders and/or cardiac arrhythmias (except bradycardia). Caution in neonates, children <1 yr, and the elderly. Caution in pulmonary edema, CHF, fever >102°F for 24 hrs, cor-pulmonale, hypothyroidism, liver disease, reduced renal function, sepsis, shock, and HTN. If toxicity develops (eg, repetitive vomiting) monitor serum levels and adjust dosage.

**ADVERSE REACTIONS:** Diarrhea, nausea, vomiting, abdominal pain, nervousness, headache, insomnia, seizures, dizziness, tremor, tachycardia, arrhythmias, restlessness, tremor, transient diuresis.

**INTERACTIONS:** Potentiated by propranolol, allopurinol, erythromycin, cimetidine, interferon, ciprofloxacin, clarithromycin, disulfiram, enoxacin, methotrexate, beta adrenergic blockers, oral contraceptives, fluvoxamine, calcium channel blockers, corticosteroid, thyroid hormones, thiabendazole, ticlopidine, troleadomycin, carbamazepine, pentoxifylline, diuretics, tacrine, and isoniazid. Diminishes the effects of adenosine, diazepam, lithium, lorazepam, midazolam, and pancuronium. Synergistic CNS effects with ephedrine. Diminished effects with aminoglutethemide, phenytoin, phenobarbital, carbamazepine, rifampin, barbiturates, hydantoins, ketoconazole, diuretics sympathomimetics, and isoproterenol.

**PREGNANCY:** Category C, caution in nursing.

## THEOLAIR
RX

theophylline (Graceway)

**THERAPEUTIC CLASS:** Xanthine bronchodilator

**INDICATIONS:** Treatment of symptoms and reversible airflow obstruction associated with chronic asthma and other chronic lung diseases (eg, emphysema, chronic bronchitis).

**DOSAGE:** *Adults:* Initial: 300mg/day divided q6-8h. Titrate: if tolerated, after 3 days, increase to 400mg/day divided q6-8h. May increase to 600mg/day divided q6-8h if needed and tolerated after 3 more days.
*Pediatrics:* >1 yr and <45kg: Initial: 12-14mg/kg/day divided q4-6h. Max: 300mg/day. Titrate: If tolerated after 3 days, increase to 16mg/kg/day divided q6-8h. Max: 400mg/day. May increase to 20mg/kg/day divided q6-8h if tolerated and needed after 3 more days. Max: 600mg/day. >1 yr and >45kg: Follow adult dosage schedule.

**HOW SUPPLIED:** Tab: 125mg*, 250mg* *scored

**WARNINGS/PRECAUTIONS:** Extreme caution in peptic ulcer disease, seizure disorders and/or cardiac arrhythmias (except bradycardia). Caution in neonates, children <1 yr, and the elderly. Caution in pulmonary edema, CHF, fever >102°F for 24 hrs, cor-pulmonale, hyporthyroidism, liver disease, reduced renal function, sepsis, shock , and HTN. If toxicity develops (eg repetitive vomiting) monitor serum levels and adjust dosage.

**ADVERSE REACTIONS:** Nausea, vomiting, headache, insomnia, cardiac arrhythmias, intractable seizures, diarrhea, irritability, restlessness, fine skeletal muscle tremors, transient diuresis.

**INTERACTIONS:** Alcohol, propranolol, allopurinol, erythromycin, cimetidine, interferon, ciprofloxacin, clarithromycin, disulfiram, enoxacin, methotrexate, mexiletine, estrogen-containing oral contraceptives, propafenone, propranolol, verapamil, fluvoxamine, thiabendazole, ticlopidine, troleadomycin, pentoxifylline, and tacrine may increase levels. Diminishes the effects of adenosine, diazepam, lithium, flurazepam, lorazepam, midazolam, and pancuronium. Synergistic CNS effects with ephedrine. Aminoglutethemide, phenytoin, phenobarbital, carbamazepine, rifampin, barbiturates, hydantoins, moricizine, sulfinpyrazone and isoproterenol may decrease levels. Increased risk of ventricular arrhythmias with halothane. Ketamine may lower theophylline seizure threshold.

**PREGNANCY:** Category C, caution in nursing.

## THERACYS
RX

bcg live (Sanofi Pasteur)

**Contains live, attenuated mycobacteria. Potential risk for transmission; prepare, handle, and dispose of as a biohazard material. Nosocomial infections reported in immunosuppressed. Fatal reactions reported with intravesical BCG.**

**THERAPEUTIC CLASS:** Attenuated live BCG culture

**INDICATIONS:** Treatment and prophylaxis of carcinoma *in situ* of the bladder. Prophylaxis of primary or recurrent stage Ta and/or T1 papillary tumors following transurethral resection (TUR).

**DOSAGE:** *Adults:* Begin 7-14 days after biopsy or resection. Induction: 81mg intravesically weekly for 6 weeks. Maint: 81mg at 3, 6, 12, 18, and 24 months. Avoid fluids for 4 hrs before treatment. Empty badder before administration. Retain in bladder for 2 hrs, then void. During the 1st 15 minutes following instillation, patient should lie prone.

**HOW SUPPLIED:** Inj: 81mg

**CONTRAINDICATIONS:** Immunocompromised patients, congenital or acquired immune deficiency patients (eg, AIDS, cancer, immunosuppressives), concurrent febrile illness, UTI, gross hematuria, active TB. Wait 7-14 days after biopsy, TUR or traumatic catheterization.

**WARNINGS/PRECAUTIONS:** Not a vaccine for prevention of cancer. Risk of infectious complications; avoid with actively bleeding urinary mucosa; delay treatment for >1 week after TUR, biopsy, traumatic catheterization, or gross hematuria. Possible increased risk of severe local reactions with small bladder capacity. May cause tuberculin sensitivity. BCG infection of aneurysms and prosthetic devices (including arterial grafts, cardiac devices, and artificial joints) reported. Stopper of vial contains natural rubber latex which may cause allergic reactions. Evaluate for serious infectious complication if fever >101.3°F, or acute localized inflammation (eg, epididymitis, prostatitis, orchitis) persists >2-3 days. Febrile episodes with flu-like symptoms >72 hrs, fever >103°F, systemic manifestations increasing in intensity with repeated instillations, or persistent abnormal LFTs suggest systemic BCG infection and may require antituberculous therapy. D/C if fever persists or if acute febrile illness consistent with BCG infection occur. Administer >2 antimycobacterials while diagnostic evaluation is conducted. Sensitive to INH, rifampin, and ethambutol; not sensitive to pyrazinamide. Caution with groups at risk of HIV. Not recommended for stage TaG1 papillary tumors, unless judged to be at high risk of tumor recurrence. Persons with immunologic deficiency should not handle agent.

**ADVERSE REACTIONS:** Malaise, fever, chills, uveitis, conjunctivitis, iritis, keratitis, granulomatous choreoretinitis, arthritis, arthralgia, urinary symptoms, skin rash.

**INTERACTIONS:** Immunosuppressants, bone marrow depressants, and radiation may interfere with immune response; avoid concomitant use. Antimicrobials may interfere with efficacy. Avoid antituberculosis drugs (eg, INH) to prevent or treat the local, irritative toxicities of BCG Live.

**PREGNANCY:** Category C, not for use in nursing.

## THIOGUANINE RX

thioguanine (Various)

**THERAPEUTIC CLASS:** Purine analog

**INDICATIONS:** For remission induction, remission consolidation, and maintenance therapy of acute nonlymphocytic leukemias.

**DOSAGE:** *Adults:* Monotherapy: 2mg/kg/day. After 4 weeks, may increase to 3mg/kg/day if no improvement and leukocyte or platelet depression. Usual therapy is with other agents in combination.
*Pediatrics:* Monotherapy: 2mg/kg/day. After 4 weeks, may increase to 3mg/kg/day if no improvement and leukocyte or platelet depression. Usual therapy is with other agents in combination.

**HOW SUPPLIED:** Tab: 40mg* *scored

**CONTRAINDICATIONS:** Prior resistance to this drug.

**WARNINGS/PRECAUTIONS:** Dose-related bone marrow suppression. Increased sensitivity to myelosuppression with thiopurine methyltransferase (TPMT) deficiency. D/C temporarily at 1st sign of abnormally large fall in any formed elements of the blood. Withhold therapy with toxic hepatitis or biliary stasis. Monitor Hgb, Hct, platelets, WBCs, and differential frequently. Monitor LFTs weekly at start of therapy, monthly thereafter.

**ADVERSE REACTIONS:** Myelosuppression, hyperuricemia, hepatotoxicity, nausea, vomiting, anorexia, stomatitis.

**INTERACTIONS:** May be cross-resistant with mercaptopurine. Caution with TPMT inhibitors such as aminosalicylate derivatives (eg, olsalazine, mesalazine, sulfasalazine); increased sensitivity to myelosuppression. May need dose reduction with other drugs whose primary toxicity is myelosuppression. Esophageal varices reported with busulfan. Veno-occlusive liver disease reported with combination chemotherapy.

**PREGNANCY:** Category D, not for use in nursing.

## THIORIDAZINE

RX

thioridazine HCl (Various)

**Prolongation of QTc interval reported in a dose related manner. Associated with torsade de pointes and sudden death; reserve for patients who fail to respond to or cannot tolerate other antipsychotics.**

**THERAPEUTIC CLASS:** Piperidine phenothiazine

**INDICATIONS:** Management of schizophrenia in patients not responsive to or intolerant to other antipsychotics.

**DOSAGE:** *Adults:* Initial: 50-100mg tid. Titrate: Increase gradually. Usual: 200-800mg/day given bid-qid. Max: 800mg/day.
*Pediatrics:* Initial: 0.6mg/kg/day given in divided doses. Titrate: Increase gradually. Max: 3mg/kg/day.

**HOW SUPPLIED:** Tab: 10mg, 15mg, 25mg, 50mg, 100mg, 150mg, 200mg

**CONTRAINDICATIONS:** Severe CNS depression, comatose states, severe hypo- or hypertensive heart disease. Drugs that prolong QTc interval, congenital long QT syndrome, cardiac arrhythmias, drugs that inhibit CYP450 2D6 (eg, fluoxetine, paroxetine), patients with reduced activity of CYP450 2D6.

**WARNINGS/PRECAUTIONS:** Perform baseline ECG and measure baseline potassium level; monitor periodically thereafter. May develop tardive dyskinesia. NMS, seizures, leukopenia, agranulocytosis reported. Caution with activities requiring alertness. May elevate prolactin levels.

**ADVERSE REACTIONS:** Tardive dyskinesia, ECG changes, drowsiness, dry mouth, blurred vision, peripheral edema, galactorrhea, nausea, vomiting, gynecomastia, impotence, constipation, diarrhea.

**INTERACTIONS:** See Contraindications. May potentiate CNS depressants, alcohol, atropine, and phosphorus insecticides. Propranolol, fluvoxamine, pindolol increases thioridazine plasma levels; avoid concomitant use. Avoid CYP2D6 inhibitors (eg, fluoxetine, paroxetine); increased risk of arrhythmias.

**PREGNANCY:** Safety in pregnancy and nursing not known.

## THROMBIN-JMI

RX

thrombin (bovine origin) (King)

**THERAPEUTIC CLASS:** Topical Thrombin

**INDICATIONS:** An aid to hemostasis whenever oozing blood and minor bleeding from capillaries and small venules is accessible. In various types of surgery, may be used in conjuction with an Absorbable Gelatin Sponge, USP for hemostasis.

**DOSAGE:** *Adults:* Spray topically on surface of bleeding tissue. Reconstitute with sterile isotonic saline at a recommended concentration of 1,000-2,000 IU/mL. Profuse bleeding: Use 1,000 IU/mL. General use (eg, plastic surgery, dental extractions, skin grafting): 100 IU/mL. Intermediate strengths may be prepared by diluting in appropriate isotonic saline volume if needed. Oozing surfaces: Use dry form. May be used with FlowSeal™ NT.

**HOW SUPPLIED:** Powder: 5,000 IU, 20,000 IU; Kit: Powder: 20,000 IU [Spray; Syringe Spray]

**CONTRAINDICATIONS:** Sensitivity to material of bovine origin.

**WARNINGS/PRECAUTIONS:** The use of topical bovine thrombin preparations has occasionally been associated with abnormalities in hemostasis ranging from asymptomatic alterations in laboratory determinations, such as prothrombin time (PT) and partial thromboplastin time (PTT), to severe bleeding or thrombosis which rarely have been fatal. Consultation with an

T

expert is recommended if patient exhibits abnormal coagulation laboratory values, abnormal bleeding, or abnormal thrombosis. Should not be injected or allowed to enter large blood vessels. Extensive intravascular clotting and even death may result.

**ADVERSE REACTIONS:** Inhibitory antibodies which interfere with hemostasis may develop.

**PREGNANCY:** Category C, safety in nursing is not known

## THYROLAR RX

liotrix (Forest)

**THERAPEUTIC CLASS:** Thyroid replacement hormone

**INDICATIONS:** Hypothyroidism. As a pituitary TSH suppressant in the treatment or prevention of euthyroid goiters. Diagnostic agent in suppression tests to differentiate suspected hyperthyroidism or thyroid gland autonomy. Management of thyroid cancer.

**DOSAGE:** *Adults:* Hypothyroidism: Usual: 12.5mcg-50mcg to 25mcg-100mcg qd. Elderly/Coronary Artery Disease: Initial: 6.25mcg-25mcg qd. Chronic Myxedema: 3.1mcg-12.5mcg qd. Titrate: Increase by 3.1mcg-12.5mcg/d q 2-3 weeks. Reduce dose if angina occurs. Myxedema Coma: 400mcg IV levothyroxine sodium (100mcg/mL rapidly) followed by 100-200mcg/day IV. Switch to PO when stable. Thyroid Suppression: 1.56mg/kg/d levothyroxine ($T_4$) for 7-10 days.

*Pediatrics:* Hypothyroidism: >12 yrs: 18.75mcg-75mcg qd. 6-12 yrs: 12.5mcg-50mcg to 18.75mcg-75mcg qd. 1-5 yrs: 9.35mcg-37.5mcg to 12.5mcg-50mcg qd. 6-12 months: 6.25mcg-25mcg to 9.35mcg-37.5mcg qd. 0-6 months: 3.1mcg-12.5mcg to 6.25mcg-25mcg qd.

**HOW SUPPLIED:** (T3-T4) Tab: (1/4) 3.1mcg-12.5mcg, (1/2) 6.25mcg-25mcg, (1) 12.5mcg-50mcg, (2) 25mcg-100mcg, (3) 37.5mcg-150mcg

**CONTRAINDICATIONS:** Untreated thyrotoxicosis, uncorrected adrenal cortical insufficiency.

**WARNINGS/PRECAUTIONS:** Do not use in the treatment of obesity; larger doses in euthyroid patients can cause serious or even life threatening toxicity. Caution with angina pectoris and elderly; use lower doses. May aggravate diabetes mellitus or insipidus and adrenal cortical insufficiency. Excessive doses may cause craniosynostosis. Extreme caution with long standing myxedema especailly with cardiovascular impairment.

**INTERACTIONS:** May increase insulin or oral hypoglycemic requirements. Decreased absorption with cholestyramine and colestipol; space dosing by 4-5 hrs. Altered effect of oral anticoagulants; monitor PT/INR. Estrogens increase thyroxine-binding globulin; increase in thyroid dose may be needed. Serious or life-threatening side effects can occur with sympathomimetic amines. Androgens, corticosteroids, estrogens, iodine-containing preparations, and salicylates may interfere with thyroid lab tests.



**PREGNANCY:** Category A, caution in nursing.

## TIAZAC RX

diltiazem HCl (Forest)

**OTHER BRAND NAMES:** Taztia XT (Andrx)

**THERAPEUTIC CLASS:** Calcium channel blocker (nondihydropyridine)

**INDICATIONS:** Hypertension. Chronic stable angina.

**DOSAGE:** *Adults:* HTN: Initial: 120-240mg qd. Titrate: Adjust at 2 week intervals. Usual: 120-540mg qd. Max: 540mg qd. Angina: Initial: 120-180mg qd Titrate: Increase over 7-14 days. Max: 540mg qd.

**HOW SUPPLIED:** Cap, Extended Release: (Taztia XT, Tiazac) 120mg, 180mg, 240mg, 300mg, 360mg; (Tiazac) 420mg

**CONTRAINDICATIONS:** Sick sinus syndrome and 2nd- or 3rd-degree AV block (except with functioning pacemaker), severe hypotension (<90mm Hg systolic), acute MI, pulmonary congestion.

**WARNINGS/PRECAUTIONS:** Caution in renal, hepatic, or ventricular dysfunction. Monitor LFTs and renal function with prolonged use. D/C if persistent rash occurs. Symptomatic hypotension may occur. Acute hepatic injury reported.

**ADVERSE REACTIONS:** Headache, peripheral edema, vasodilation, dizziness, rash, dyspepsia.

**INTERACTIONS:** Increased levels of carbamazepine, midazolam, triazolam, lovastatin, and propranolol. Increased levels of diltiazem with cimetidine. Monitor digoxin, cyclosporine. Potentiates cardiac contractility, conductivity, and automaticity; and vascular dilation with anesthetics. Additive cardiac conduction effects with digitalis or β-blockers. Avoid rifampin and other CYP3A4 inducers. Potential additive effects with agents known to affect cardiac contractility and/or conduction.

**PREGNANCY:** Category C, not for use in nursing.

## TICE BCG

bcg live (Organon) RX

**Contains live, attenuated mycobacteria. Potential risk for transmission; prepare, handle, and dispose of as a biohazard material. Nosocomial infections reported. Fatal reactions reported with intravesical BCG.**

**THERAPEUTIC CLASS:** Attenuated live BCG culture

**INDICATIONS:** Treatment and prophylaxis of carcinoma *in situ* of the bladder. Prophylaxis of primary or recurrent stage Ta and/or T1 papillary tumors following transurethral resection (TUR). Not indicated for papillary tumors of stages higher than T1.

**DOSAGE:** *Adults:* Allow 7-14 days after biopsy before initiating therapy. Administer 1 vial (50mg) intravesically weekly for 6 weeks; may repeat schedule once if tumor remission not achieved. Then, continue monthly for 6-12 months. Retain in bladder for 2 hrs, then void. During bladder retention, reposition patient every 15 minutes to maximize bladder surface exposure.

**HOW SUPPLIED:** Inj: 50mg

**CONTRAINDICATIONS:** Immunocompromised patients, congenital or acquired immune deficiency patients (eg, AIDS, cancer, immunosuppressives), concurrent febrile illness, UTI, gross hematuria, active TB. Wait 7-14 days after biopsy, TUR or traumatic catheterization.

**WARNINGS/PRECAUTIONS:** Not a vaccine for prevention of cancer. Risk of infectious complications; avoid with actively bleeding urinary mucosa; delay treatment for >1 week after TUR, biopsy, traumatic catheterization, or gross hematuria. Possible increased risk of severe local reactions with small bladder capacity. May cause tuberculin sensitivity. Evaluate for serious infectious complication if fever >101.3°F, or acute localized inflammation (eg, epididymitis, prostatitis, orchitis) persists >2-3 days. Febrile episodes with flu-like symptoms >72 hrs, fever >103°F, systemic manifestations increasing in intensity with repeated instillations, or persistent abnormal LFTs suggest systemic BCG infection and may require antituberculous therapy. D/C if fever persists or if acute febrile illness consistent with BCG infection occur. Administer >2 antimycobacterials while diagnostic evaluation is conducted. Sensitive to INH, rifampin, and ethambutol; not sensitive to pyrazinamide. Caution with groups at risk of HIV. Not recommended for stage TaG1 papillary tumors, unless judged to be at high risk of tumor recurrence.

**ADVERSE REACTIONS:** Malaise, fever, chills, urinary symptoms, cramps/pain, rigors, nausea, vomiting, arthritis, myalgia.

**INTERACTIONS:** Immunosuppressants, bone marrow depressants, and radiation may interfere with immune response; avoid concomitant use.

Antimicrobials may interfere with efficacy; postpone BCG therapy. Avoid antituberculosis drugs (eg, INH) to prevent or treat the local, irritative toxicities of BCG Live.

**PREGNANCY:** Category C, not for use in nursing.

## TICLID RX
ticlopidine HCl (Roche Labs)

**Can cause life-threatening hematological adverse reactions, including neutropenia/agranulocytosis, thrombotic thrombocytopenic purpura (TTP), and aplastic anemia.**

**THERAPEUTIC CLASS:** Platelet aggregation inhibitor

**INDICATIONS:** To reduce risk of thrombotic stroke in stroke patients or those with stroke precursors who are ASA intolerant, allergic, or failed ASA therapy. Adjunct to ASA to reduce incidence of subacute stent thrombosis in patients undergoing successful coronary artery stent implantation.

**DOSAGE:** *Adults:* Take with food. Stroke: 250mg bid. Coronary Artery Stenting: 250mg bid with ASA up to 30 days after stent implant.

**HOW SUPPLIED:** Tab: 250mg

**CONTRAINDICATIONS:** Hematopoietic disorders (eg, neutropenia, thrombocytopenia), history of TTP or aplastic anemia, hemostatic disorders, active pathological bleeding, severe liver impairment.

**WARNINGS/PRECAUTIONS:** Monitor for hematologic toxicity before treatment, then every 2 weeks for 1st 3 months, and 2 weeks after discontinuation. Monitor more frequently if signs of hematological adverse reactions; d/c if neutrophils <1200/mm$^3$, aplastic anemia or TTP occurs. D/C 10-14 days before surgery. Caution in trauma, surgery, bleeding disorders. May need dose adjustment with renal or hepatic impairment. May elevate LFTs, TG, and cholesterol.

**ADVERSE REACTIONS:** Diarrhea, rash, nausea, GI pain, rash, dyspepsia, neutropenia.

**INTERACTIONS:** Adjust dose with drugs metabolized by CYP450 with low therapeutic ratios or with hepatic impairment. Potentiates ASA and NSAIDs effect on platelet aggregation. Antacids reduce plasma levels. Cimetidine reduces clearance. Decreases digoxin plasma levels. Significant decrease of theophylline plasma clearance. Caution with phenytoin, propranolol. Discontinue anticoagulants or fibrinolytics. Increased bioavailability with food.

**PREGNANCY:** Category B, not for use in nursing.

## TIGAN RX
trimethobenzamide HCl (King)

**THERAPEUTIC CLASS:** Emetic response modifier

**INDICATIONS:** Treatment of postoperative nausea and vomiting and for nausea associated with gastroenteritis.

**DOSAGE:** *Adults:* (Cap) 300mg tid-qid. (Inj) 200mg IM tid-qid.

**HOW SUPPLIED:** Cap: 300mg; Inj: 100mg/mL

**CONTRAINDICATIONS:** Injection in children.

**WARNINGS/PRECAUTIONS:** Caution in children; may cause EPS, which may be confused with CNS signs of undiagnosed primary disease (eg, Reye's syndrome) and may unfavorably alter the course of Reye's syndrome due to hepatotoxic potential. Caution with acute febrile illness, encephalitides, gastroenteritis, dehydration, electrolyte imbalance, and in elderly; CNS reactions reported. May produce drowsiness.

**ADVERSE REACTIONS:** Hypersensitivity reactions, parkinson-like symptoms, hypotension (inj), blood dyscrasias, blurred vision, coma, convulsions, mood depression, diarrhea, disorientation, dizziness, drowsiness, headache, jaundice, muscle cramps, opisthotonos.

**INTERACTIONS:** Caution with CNS agents (eg, phenothiazines, barbiturates, belladonna derivatives) in acute febrile illness, encephalitides, gastroenteritis, dehydration, and electrolyte imbalance. Adverse drug interactions reported with alcohol.

**PREGNANCY:** Safety in pregnancy and nursing not known.

## TIKOSYN
dofetilide (Pfizer) RX

**To minimize risk of arrhythmia, place patients initiated or reinitiated on therapy for minimum of 3 days in a facility that can provide CrCl, ECG monitoring, and cardiac resuscitation.**

**THERAPEUTIC CLASS:** Class III antiarrhythmic

**INDICATIONS:** Conversion to and maintenance of normal sinus rhythm in atrial fibrillation/flutter.

**DOSAGE:** *Adults:* CrCl: >60mL/min: 500mcg bid. CrCl 40-60mL/min: 250mcg bid. CrCl 20 to <40mL/min: 125mcg bid. Determine QTc interval 2-3 hrs after 1st dose and adjust dose if QTc >500msec or if >15% increase from baseline. QTc/Renal Dose Adjustment: Reduce 500mcg bid to 250mcg bid. Reduce 250mcg bid to 125mcg bid. Reduce 125mcg bid to 125mcg qd. Discontinue anytime after 2nd dose if QTc >500 milliseconds (550 msec with ventricular conduction abnormalities).

**HOW SUPPLIED:** Cap: 125mcg, 250mcg, 500mcg

**CONTRAINDICATIONS:** Long QT syndromes, baseline QT interval or QTc >440 msec (500 msec with ventricular conduction abnormalities), severe renal impairment (CrCl <20mL/min). Concomitant verapamil, cimetidine, trimethoprim, ketoconazole, and inhibitors of renal cation transport system (eg, megestrol, prochlorperazine).

**WARNINGS/PRECAUTIONS:** Can cause serious ventricular arrhythmia. Calculate CrCl before 1st dose; adjust dose based on CrCl. Caution in severe hepatic impairment. Maintain normal $K^+$ levels.

**ADVERSE REACTIONS:** Headache, chest pain, dizziness, arrhythmia, conduction disturbances, dyspnea, nausea, insomnia.

**INTERACTIONS:** Hypokalemia or hypomagnesemia may occur with $K^+$-depleting diuretics. CYP3A4 inhibitors (eg, macrolides, protease inhibitors, grapefruit juice, etc) may potentiate dofetilide. Avoid verapamil, cimetidine, trimethoprim, ketoconazole, and inhibitors of renal cationic secretion. Caution with drugs actively secreted by cationic secretion (eg, amiloride, triamterene, metformin). Not recommended with drugs that prolong the QT interval. Hold Class I and III antiarrhythmics for at least 3 half-lives before initiate dofetilide. Reduce amiodarone to <0.3mcg/mL or withdraw at least 3 months before initiate dofetilide.

**PREGNANCY:** Category C, not for use in nursing.

## TILADE
nedocromil sodium (King) RX

**THERAPEUTIC CLASS:** Pyranoquinoline anti-inflammatory agent

**INDICATIONS:** Maintenance therapy for mild to moderate asthma.

**DOSAGE:** *Adults:* 2 inh qid. May reduce to bid-tid once desired response is observed.
*Pediatrics:* >6 yrs: 2 inh qid. May reduce to bid-tid once desired response is observed.

**HOW SUPPLIED:** MDI: 1.75mg/inh [16.2g]

**WARNINGS/PRECAUTIONS:** Not for treatment of acute bronchospasm or status asthmaticus. Monitor when reducing systemic or inhaled steroid therapy. Stop therapy if bronchospasm occurs.

**ADVERSE REACTIONS:** Unpleasant taste, nausea, vomiting, dyspepsia, abdominal pain, pharyngitis, headache, cough, rhinitis.

**PREGNANCY:** Category B, caution with nursing

## TIMENTIN RX

ticarcillin disodium - clavulanate potassium (GlaxoSmithKline)

**THERAPEUTIC CLASS:** Broad-spectrum penicillin/beta-lactamase inhibitor

**INDICATIONS:** Treatment of lower respiratory tract, bone and joint, skin and skin structure, urinary tract (UTI), gynecologic, and intra-abdominal infections, and septicemia.

**DOSAGE:** *Adults:* >60kg: UTI/Systemic Infection: 3g-100mg (3.1g vial) IV q4-6h. Gynecologic Infections: Moderate: 200mg/kg/day ticarcillin IV given q6h. Severe: 300mg/kg/day ticarcillin IV given q4h. <60kg: Usual: 200-300mg/kg/day ticarcillin IV given q4-6h. UTI: 3g-200mg (3.2g vial) q8h. Renal Impairment (based on ticarcillin): CrCl 60-30mL/min: 2g IV q4h. CrCl 30-10mL/min: 2g IV q8h. CrCl <10mL/min: 2g IV q12h (2g IV q24h with hepatic dysfunction). Peritoneal Dialysis: 3.1g IV q12h. Hemodialysis: 2g IV q12h, and 3.1g after each dialysis. Apply reduced dosage after initial 3.1g LD is given. *Pediatrics:* >3 months: >60kg: Mild to Moderate: 3g-100mg (3.1g vial) IV q6h. Severe: 3g-100mg (3.1g vial) IV q4h. <60 kg: Mild to Moderate: 50mg/kg ticarcillin IV q6h. Severe: 50mg/kg ticarcillin IV q4h. Renal Impairment (based on ticarcillin): CrCl 60-30mL/min: 2g IV q4h. CrCl 30-10mL/min: 2g IV q8h. CrCl <10mL/min: 2g IV q12h (2g IV q24h with hepatic dysfunction). Peritoneal Dialysis: 3.1g IV q12h. Hemodialysis: 2g IV q12h, and 3.1g after each dialysis. Apply reduced dosage after initial 3.1g LD is given.

**HOW SUPPLIED:** Inj: (Ticarcillin-Clavulanate) 3g-100mg, 3g-100mg/100mL, 30g-1g

**WARNINGS/PRECAUTIONS:** Prolonged use may result in overgrowth of nonsusceptible organisms. Caution with penicillin, cephalosporin, and other allergen sensitivities. Pseudomembranous colitis reported. Risk of convulsions with high doses especially with renal impairment. Monitor renal, hepatic, hematopoietic functions, and serum K+ with prolonged therapy. Caution with fluid and electrolyte imbalance; hypokalemia reported. Clotting time, platelet aggregation, and PT abnormalities may occur especially with renal impairment; discontinue therapy. Continue therapy for at least 2 days after signs/symptoms disappear.Caution in elderly patient with impaired renal function.

**ADVERSE REACTIONS:** Hypersensitivity reactions, headache, giddiness, taste/smell disturbances, stomatitis, flatulence, nausea, vomiting, diarrhea, hematologic disturbances, hepatic/renal function tests abnormalities, local reactions.



**INTERACTIONS:** May inactivate aminoglycoside if mixed together in parenteral solution. Increased serum levels and prolonged half-life with probenecid.

**PREGNANCY:** Category B, caution in nursing.

## TIMOLOL GFS RX

timolol maleate (Falcon)

**THERAPEUTIC CLASS:** Nonselective beta-blocker

**INDICATIONS:** Treatment of elevated intraocular pressure in patients with open-angle glaucoma or ocular hypertension.

**DOSAGE:** *Adults:* Initial: 1 drop 0.25-0.5% qd. Evaluate IOP 4 weeks after starting treatment. Max: 1 drop 0.5% qd. Dose other ophthalmic drugs 10 minutes prior to gel forming drops.

**HOW SUPPLIED:** Sol, Gel Forming: 0.25%, 0.5% [2.5mL, 5mL]

**CONTRAINDICATIONS:** Bronchial asthma, history of bronchial asthma, severe COPD, sinus bradycardia, 2nd- or 3rd-degree AV block, overt cardiac failure, cardiogenic shock.

**WARNINGS/PRECAUTIONS:** May be absorbed systemically. Caution with cardiac failure, DM, and cerebrovascular insufficiency. May mask symptoms of hypoglycemia and hyperthyroidism. Avoid with COPD, bronchospastic disease. Not for use alone in angle-closure glaucoma. May potentiate muscle weakness. Discontinue if develop cardiac failure. Withdrawal before surgery is controversial.

**ADVERSE REACTIONS:** Ocular burning, ocular stinging, transient blurred vision.

**INTERACTIONS:** May potentiate systemic/ophthalmic β-blockers and catecholamine-depleting drugs (eg, reserpine). Oral/IV calcium antagonists can cause AV conduction disturbances, left ventricular failure, or hypotension. Digitalis can cause additive effects in prolonging AV conduction time. Quinidine may potentiate β-blockade. May antagonize epinephrine. Give other ophthalmic drugs 10 minutes before use.

**PREGNANCY:** Category C, not for use in nursing.

## TIMOLOL MALEATE

RX

timolol maleate (Various)

**THERAPEUTIC CLASS:** Nonselective beta-blocker

**INDICATIONS:** Treatment of hypertension. To reduce cardiovascular mortality and risk of reinfarction with previous MI. Migraine prophylaxis.

**DOSAGE:** *Adults:* HTN: Initial: 10mg bid. Maint: 20-40mg/day. Wait at least 7 days between dose increases. Max: 60mg/day given bid. MI: 10mg bid. Migraine: Initial: 10mg bid. Maint: 20mg qd. Max: 30mg/day in divided doses. May decrease to 10 mg qd. Discontinue if inadequate response after 6-8 weeks with max dose.

**HOW SUPPLIED:** Tab: 5mg, 10mg*, 20mg* *scored

**CONTRAINDICATIONS:** Active or history of bronchial asthma, severe COPD, sinus bradycardia, 2nd- and 3rd-degree AV block, overt cardiac failure, cardiogenic shock.

**WARNINGS/PRECAUTIONS:** Caution with well-compensated cardiac failure, DM, mild to moderate COPD, bronchospastic disease, dialysis, hepatic/renal impairment, or cerebrovascular insufficiency. Exacerbation of ischemic heart disease with abrupt cessation. May mask hyperthyroidism or hypoglycemia symptoms. Withdrawal before surgery is controversial. May potentiate weakness with myasthenia gravis. Can cause cardiac failure. Caution and consider monitoring renal function in elderly.

**ADVERSE REACTIONS:** Fatigue, headache, nausea, arrhythmia, pruritus, dizziness, dyspnea, asthenia, bradycardia, dizziness.

**INTERACTIONS:** Possible additive effects and hypotension and/or marked bradycardia with catecholamine-depleting drugs. NSAIDs may reduce antihypertensive effects. Quinidine may potentiate β-blockade. AV conduction time prolonged with digitalis and either diltiazem or verapamil. Hypotension, AV conduction disturbances, left ventricular failure reported with oral calcium antagonists. Caution with IV calcium antagonists, insulin, oral hypoglycemics. Avoid calcium antagonists with cardiac dysfunction. May exacerbate rebound HTN following clonidine withdrawal. May block effects of epinephrine.

**PREGNANCY:** Category C, not for use in nursing.

## TIMOPTIC
timolol maleate (Merck) RX

**OTHER BRAND NAMES:** Timoptic-XE (Merck) - Timoptic Ocudose (Preservative Free) (Merck)

**THERAPEUTIC CLASS:** Nonselective beta-blocker

**INDICATIONS:** Treatment of elevated IOP in patients with open-angle glaucoma or ocular hypertension.

**DOSAGE:** *Adults:* (Sol) Initial: 1 drop 0.25% bid. May increase to a max of 1 drop 0.5% bid. Maint: If adequate control, may attempt 1 drop 0.25-0.5% qd. (Sol, Gel Forming) Initial: 1 drop 0.25-0.5% qd. Max: 1 drop 0.5% qd. Dose other ophthalmic drugs 10 minutes prior to gel forming drops.

**HOW SUPPLIED:** Sol: (Timoptic) 0.25%, 0.5% [5mL, 10mL]; Sol: (Timoptic Ocudose) 0.25%, 0.5% [0.2mL 60s]; Sol, Gel Forming: (Timoptic-XE) 0.25%, 0.5% [5mL]

**CONTRAINDICATIONS:** Bronchial asthma, history of bronchial asthma, severe COPD, sinus bradycardia, 2nd- or 3rd-degree AV block, overt cardiac failure, cardiogenic shock.

**WARNINGS/PRECAUTIONS:** Severe cardiac and respiratory reactions reported. Caution with cardiac failure and cerebrovascular insufficiency; d/c if cardiac failure develops. May mask symptoms of hypoglycemia or hyperthyroidism; caution with DM or thyrotoxicosis. Avoid with COPD, bronchospastic disease. Not for use alone in angle-closure glaucoma. May potentiate muscle weakness. Withdrawal before surgery is controversial.

**ADVERSE REACTIONS:** Ocular: burning, stinging, blurred vision, pain, conjunctivitis, discharge, foreign body sensation, itching, tearing. Systemic: headache dizziness, upper respiratory infections.

**INTERACTIONS:** May potentiate systemic/ophthalmic β-blockers and catecholamine-depleting drugs (eg, reserpine). Oral/IV calcium antagonists may cause AV conduction disturbances, left ventricular failure, or hypotension. Digitalis may cause additive effects in prolonging AV conduction time. Potentiated systemic β-blockade reported with concomitant CYP2D6 inhibitors. Quinidine may potentiate systemic β-blockade. May antagonize epinephrine. May exacerbate rebound hypertension following clonidine withdrawal. Give other ophthalmic drugs 10 minutes before use.

**PREGNANCY:** Category C, not for use in nursing.

## TINDAMAX
tinidazole (Presutti) RX

**Avoid unnecessary use. Reserve only for indicated conditions.**

T

**THERAPEUTIC CLASS:** Antiprotozoal agent

**INDICATIONS:** Treatment of trichomoniasis caused by *Trichomonas vaginalis*, giardiasis caused by *Giardia duodenalis*, intestinal amebiasis and amebic liver abscess caused by *Entamoeba histolytica*, and bacterial vaginosis in non-pregnant women.

**DOSAGE:** *Adults:* Take with food. Trichomoniasis/Giardiasis: 2g single dose. Amebiasis: Intestinal: 2g qd for 3 days. Amebic Liver Abscess: 2g qd for 3-5 days. Hemodialysis: Give additional dose equivalent to one-half of recommended dose at the end of dialysis. For trichomoniasis, treat sexual partner with the same dose. Bacterial Vaginosis: 2g qd for 2 days or 1g qd for 5 days.
*Pediatrics:* >3 yrs: Take with food. Giardiasis: 50mg/kg single dose. Amebiasis: Intestinal: 50mg/kg qd for 3 days. Amebic Liver Abscess: 50mg/kg qd for 3-5 days. Max (for all): 2g/day. May crush tabs in cherry syrup.

**HOW SUPPLIED:** Tab: 250mg*, 500mg* *scored

**CONTRAINDICATIONS:** Treatment during 1st trimester of pregnancy.

**WARNINGS/PRECAUTIONS:** Seizures, peripheral neuropathy reported. Discontinue if abnormal neurological signs occur. Caution with hepatic impairment, blood dyscrasias, or CNS diseases.

**ADVERSE REACTIONS:** Metallic/bitter taste, nausea, anorexia.

**INTERACTIONS:** Avoid alcohol during and for 3 days after use and within 2 weeks of disulfiram. May potentiate oral anticoagulants. May reduce clearance of phenytoin (IV), fluorouracil. May increase levels of lithium, cyclosporine, tacrolimus, fluorouracil. Separate dosing with cholestyramine. Phenobarbital, rifampin, phenytoin, other hepatic enzyme inducers may decrease levels. Cimetidine, ketoconazole, other hepatic enzyme inhibitors may increase levels. Antagonized by oxytetracycline.

**PREGNANCY:** Category C, not for use in nursing.

## TIROSINT

levothyroxine sodium (IBSA) RX

**THERAPEUTIC CLASS:** Thyroid replacement hormone

**INDICATIONS:** Replacement or supplemental therapy in congenital or acquired hypothyroidism of any etiology, except transient hypothyroidism during the recovery phase of subacute thyroiditis, including primary, secondary, teritiary and subclinical hypothyroidism. Treatment or prevention of various euthyroid goiters including thyroid nodules, subacute or chronic lymphocytic throiditis (Hashimoto's thyroiditis) and multinodular goiter. Adjunct to surgery and radioiodine therapy in the management of thyrotropin-dependent well-differentiated thyroid cancer.

**DOSAGE:** *Adults:* Take in AM 1/2-1 hr before breakfast. Hypothyroidism: Usual: 1.7mcg/kg/day PO. Titrate: Adjust in 12.5-25mcg increments until patient is euthyroid. Elderly with Cardiac Disease: Initial: 12.5-25mcg qd PO. Titrate: May increase by 12.5-25mcg every 4-6 weeks until euthyroid. >50 yrs or <50 yrs with Underlying Cardiac Disease: Initial: 25-50mcg/day. Titrate: Gradual increments at 6-8 week intervals prn. Severe Hypothyroidism: Initial: 12.5-25mcg/day. Titrate: May increase by 25mcg/day every 2-4 weeks until TSH normalized. Pregnancy: May require increased doses. Subclinical Hypothyroidism: May require lower doses. Do not crush, cut or dissolve content in water.

*Pediatrics:* Take in AM 1/2-1hr before breakfast. Hypothyroidism: 0-3 months: 10-15mcg/kg/day. 3-6 months: 8-10mcg/kg/day. 6-12 months: 6-8mcg/kg/day. 6-12 yrs: 4-5mcg/kg/day. >12 yrs (growth/puberty incomplete): 2-3mcg/kg/day. >12 yrs (growth/puberty complete): 1.7mcg/kg/day. To minimize hyperactivity in older children give 1/4 of full replacement dose initially, then increase dose by same amount weekly until full replacement dose is achieved. Chronic/Severe Hypothyroidism: Initial: 25mcg/day. Titrate: Increase by 25mcg every 2-4 weeks until euthyroid. Do not crush, cut or dissolve content in water.

**HOW SUPPLIED:** Cap: 25mcg, 50mcg, 75mcg, 100mcg, 125mcg, 150mcg

**CONTRAINDICATIONS:** Untreated subclinical (suppressed serum TSH level with normal $T_3$ and $T_4$ levels) or overt thyrotoxicosis of any etiology, acute MI, uncorrected adrenal insufficiency or inability to swallow capsules.

**WARNINGS/PRECAUTIONS:** Do not use in treatment of obesity. Should not be used in treatment of male or female infertility unless condition is associated with hypothyroidism. Carefully titrate dose to avoid over/under treatment. Decreased bone mineral density with long term use. Caution with cardiovascular disease especially in elderly, adrenal insufficiency, non-toxic diffuse goiter or nodular thyroid disease and hypothalamic pituitary hormone deficiencies. Chronic autoimmune thyroiditis may occur in association with other autoimmune disorders; treat patients with concomitant adrenal insufficiency with replacement glucocorticoids before therapy. Infants with

T

congenital hypothyroidism may be at increased risk for other congenital abnormalities.

**ADVERSE REACTIONS:** Hyperthyroidism (increased appetite, weight loss, heat intolerance, hyperactivity, tremors, palpitations, tachycardia, diarrhea, vomiting, hair loss), pseudotumor cerebri, craniosynostosis and premature closure of the epiphyses in children.

**INTERACTIONS:** Dopamine/dopamine agonists, glucocorticoids and octreotide may result in transient reduction in TSH secretion. Aminoglutethimide, amiodarone, iodide (including iodine-containing radiographic contrast agents), lithium, methimazole, propylthiouracil, sulfonamides and tolbutamide may decrease thyroid hormone secretion. Amiodarone and iodide (including iodine-containing radiographic contrast agents) may increase thyroid hormone secretion. Antacids (eg, aluminum/magnesium), hydroxides (simethicone), bile acid sequestrants (cholestyramine, colestipol), calcium carbonate, cation exchange resins (kayexalate), ferrous sulfate and sucralfate may decrease T4 absorption. Clofibrate, estrogen-containing oral contraceptives, oral estrogens, heroin/methadone, 5-fluorouracil, mitotane and tamoxifen may increase serum TBG levels. Androgens/anabolic steroids, asparaginase, glucocorticoids and slow release nicotinic acid may decrease serum TBG levels. Furosemide (>80mg IV), heparin, hydantoins, NSAIDs (eg, fenamates, phenylbutazone) and salicylates (>2g/day) may cause protein-binding site displacement. Carbamazepine, hydantoins, phenobarbital and rifampin may increase hepatic metabolism. Amiodarone, β-adrenergic antagonists (eg, propranolol >160mg/day), glucocorticoids (eg, dexamethasone ≥4mg/day) and PTU may decrease T4 5'-deiodinase activity. Sympathomimetics may increase risk of coronary insufficiency with CAD. May potentate anticoagulants. Concurrent use of tri/tetracyclic antidepressants may increase effects of both agents; SSRIs (eg, sertraline) may result in increased levothyroxine requirements. May require higher doses of antidiabetic therapy. May decrease effect of digitalis glycosides. Cytokines (interferon-α, interleukin-2) may induce hypo/hyperthyroidism. Excessive use with somatrem or somatropin may accelerate epiphyseal closure. Concurrent use with ketamine may produce HTN and tachycardia. May decrease theophylline c

**PREGNANCY:** Category A, caution in nursing.

## TNKASE RX

tenecteplase (Genentech)

**THERAPEUTIC CLASS:** Thrombolytic agent

**INDICATIONS:** To reduce mortality with AMI.

**DOSAGE:** *Adults:* Administer as single IV bolus over 5 seconds. <60kg: 30mg. 60 to <70kg: 35mg. 70 to <80kg: 40mg. 80 to <90kg: 45mg. >90kg: 50mg. Max: 50mg/dose.



**HOW SUPPLIED:** Inj: 50mg

**CONTRAINDICATIONS:** Active internal bleeding, history of CVA, intracranial or intraspinal surgery or trauma within 2 months, intracranial neoplasm, arteriovenous malformation, aneurysm, bleeding diathesis, severe uncontrolled HTN .

**WARNINGS/PRECAUTIONS:** Weigh benefits/risks with recent major surgery, cerebrovascular disease, recent GI or GU bleeding, recent trauma, HTN, left heart thrombus, acute pericarditis, subacute bacterial endocarditis, hemostatic defects, severe hepatic dysfunction, pregnancy, diabetic hemorrhagic retinopathy or other hemorrhagic ophthalmic conditions, septic thrombophlebitis or occluded AV cannula at a seriously infected site, elderly, any other bleeding condition that is difficult to manage. Cholesterol embolism and internal/superficial bleeding reported. Arrhythmias may occur with reperfusion. Avoid IM injection, noncompressible arterial puncture, and internal jugular or subclavian venous puncture. Caution with readministration.

**ADVERSE REACTIONS:** Bleeding.

**INTERACTIONS:** Increased risk of bleeding with heparin, vitamin K antagonists, and drugs that alter platelet function (eg, ASA, NSAIDs, dipyridamole, GP IIb/IIIa inhibitors) before or after therapy. Weigh benefits/risks with oral anticoagulants, GP IIb/IIIa inhibitors.

**PREGNANCY:** Category C, caution in nursing.

## TOBI
tobramycin (Chiron) RX

**THERAPEUTIC CLASS:** Aminoglycoside

**INDICATIONS:** Management of cystic fibrosis patients with *P.aeruginosa.*

**DOSAGE:** *Adults:* Inhale via nebulizer 300mg q12h for 28 days, then stop for 28 days. Resume therapy for next 28 day on/28 day off cycle.
*Pediatrics:* >6 yrs: Inhale via nebulizer 300mg q12h for 28 days, then stop for 28 days. Resume therapy for next 28 day on/28 day off cycle.

**HOW SUPPLIED:** Sol: 60mg/mL (300mg/amp)

**WARNINGS/PRECAUTIONS:** Caution with muscular disorders (eg, myasthenia gravis, Parkinson's disease), and renal, auditory, vestibular, or neuromuscular dysfunction. May cause hearing loss, bronchospasm. Can cause fetal harm in pregnancy. D/C if nephrotoxicity occurs until serum level <2mcg/mL.

**ADVERSE REACTIONS:** Voice alteration, taste perversion, tinnitus.

**INTERACTIONS:** Avoid neurotoxic or ototoxic drugs. Hearing loss reported with previous or concomitant systemic aminoglycosides. Avoid ethacrynic acid, furosemide, urea, and mannitol.

**PREGNANCY:** Category D, not for use in nursing.

## TOBRADEX
tobramycin - dexamethasone (Alcon) RX

**THERAPEUTIC CLASS:** Aminoglycoside/corticosteroid

**INDICATIONS:** Ocular inflammation associated with infection or risk of infection.

**DOSAGE:** *Adults:* (Sus) 1-2 drops q4-6h. May increase to 1-2 drops q2h for first 24-48 hrs. (Oint) Apply 1/2 inch in conjunctival sac up to tid-qid. Max: 20mL or 8g for initial RX.
*Pediatrics:* >2 yrs: (Sus) 1-2 drops q4-6h. May increase to 1-2 drops q2h for first 24-48 hrs. (Oint) Apply 1/2 inch in conjunctival sac up to tid-qid. Max: 20mL or 8g for initial RX.

**HOW SUPPLIED:** Oint: (Tobramycin-Dexamethasone) 0.3-0.1% [3.5g]; Sus: 0.3-0.1% [2.5mL, 5mL, 10mL]

**CONTRAINDICATIONS:** Viral diseases of the cornea and conjunctiva including epithelial herpes simplex keratitis, vaccinia, and varicella. Mycobacterial infection and fungal diseases of the eye.

**WARNINGS/PRECAUTIONS:** Not for injection into the eye. Prolonged use may result in glaucoma, optic nerve damage, visual acuity and fields of vision defects, cataracts, secondary ocular infections (eg, fungal infections).

**ADVERSE REACTIONS:** Conjunctival erythema, hypersensitivity, lid itching and swelling, secondary infection.

**PREGNANCY:** Category C, caution in nursing.

# TOBRAMYCIN SULFATE RX

tobramycin sulfate (Various)

**Potential ototoxicity, nephrotoxicity, and neurotoxicity. Monitor peak and trough serum levels to avoid toxicity. Avoid prolonged serum levels >12mcg/mL. Rising trough levels (>2mcg/mL) may indicate tissue accumulation. Tissue accumulation, excessive peak levels, advanced age, and cumulative dose may contribute to ototoxicity and nephrotoxicity. Monitor urine, BUN, serum creatinine, and CrCl periodically. Obtain serial audiograms. D/C or adjust dose with renal, vestibular, or auditory dysfunction. Caution in premature and neonatal infants, advanced age, and dehydration. Avoid other neurotoxic or nephrotoxic agents, particularly other aminoglycosides, cephaloridine, viomycin, polymyxin B, colistin, cisplatin, and vancomycin. Avoid potent diuretics (eg, ethacrynic acid, furosemide). Risk of fetal harm during pregnancy.**

**THERAPEUTIC CLASS:** Aminoglycoside

**INDICATIONS:** Treatment of serious lower respiratory tract, CNS (eg, meningitis), intra-abdominal, bone, skin and skin structure, and complicated/recurrent urinary tract infections, and septicemia.

**DOSAGE:** *Adults:* IM/IV: Serious Infections: 3mg/kg/day given q8h. Life-Threatening Infections: Up to 5mg/kg/day given tid-qid. Reduce to 3mg/kg/day as soon as clinically indicated. Max: 5mg/kg/day unless serum levels monitored. Treat for 7-10 days; may need longer course in difficult and complicated infections. Severe Cystic Fibrosis: Initial: 10mg/kg/day given qid. Measure levels to determine subsequent doses. Renal Impairment: LD: 1mg/kg, followed by reduced doses given q8h or normal doses given at prolonged intervals based on either CrCl or serum creatinine. Do not use either method during dialysis. Obese Patients: Calculate dose based on estimated lean body weight plus 40% of the excess as the basic weight on which to figure mg/kg. ADD-Vantage vials are not for IM use.
*Pediatrics:* >1 week: IM/IV: 6-7.5mg/kg/day given tid-qid (eg, 2-2.5mg/kg q8h or 1.5-1.89mg/kg q6h). <1 week: Up to 2mg/kg q12h. Treat for 7-10 days; may need longer course in difficult and complicated infections. Severe Cystic Fibrosis: Initial: 10mg/kg/day given qid. Measure levels to determine subsequent doses. Renal Impairment: LD: 1mg/kg, followed by reduced doses given q8h or normal doses given at prolonged intervals based on either CrCl or serum creatinine. Do not use either method during dialysis. Obese Patients: Calculate dose based on estimated lean body weight plus 40% of the excess as the basic weight on which to figure mg/kg. ADD-Vantage vials are not for IM use.

**HOW SUPPLIED:** Inj: 10mg/mL, 40mg/mL, 1.2g

**CONTRAINDICATIONS:** History of serious toxic reactions to aminoglycosides.

**WARNINGS/PRECAUTIONS:** Increased risk of ototoxicity, nephrotoxicity, and neurotoxicity if treatment >10 days. Contains sodium bisulfite. D/C if allergic reaction occurs. Monitor serum calcium, magnesium, and sodium. For peak levels, measure about 30 minutes after IV infusion or 1 hr after IM injection. For trough levels, measure at 8 hrs or just before next dose. Prolonged or secondary apnea may occur with massive transfusions of citrated blood. Caution with muscular disorders (eg, myasthenia gravis, parkinsonism). Increased risk of neurotoxicity and nephrotoxicity after absorption from body surfaces with local irrigation or application. Not for intraocular and/or subconjunctival use. Overgrowth of nonsusceptible organisms may occur.

**ADVERSE REACTIONS:** Neurotoxicity (eg, dizziness, tinnitus, hearing loss, numbness, skin tingling, muscle twitching, convulsions), nephrotoxicity (eg, rising BUN/nonprotein nitrogen/serum creatinine, oliguria, cylindruria, increased proteinuria), blood dyscrasias, fever, rash, exfoliative dermatitis, urticaria, nausea, vomiting, diarrhea, headache, lethargy, injection site pain, confusion, disorientation, increased serum transaminases.

**INTERACTIONS:** Increased nephrotoxicity with cephalosporins. Do not premix with other drugs; administer separately. Possibility of prolonged or secondary apnea in anesthetized patients receiving neuromuscular blockers (eg, succinylcholine, tubocurarine, decamethonium). See Black Box Warning.

**PREGNANCY:** Category D, safety not known in nursing.

## TOBREX
tobramycin (Alcon) RX

**THERAPEUTIC CLASS:** Aminoglycoside

**INDICATIONS:** External infections of the eye and its adnexa.

**DOSAGE:** *Adults:* Mild to Moderate Infection: Apply half-inch ointment bid-tid or 1-2 drops q4h. Severe Infection: Apply half-inch ointment q3-4h or 2 drops hourly until improvement, reduce frequency prior to discontinuation.

**HOW SUPPLIED:** Oint: 0.3% [3.5g]; Sol: 0.3% [5mL]

**WARNINGS/PRECAUTIONS:** Ointment may retard corneal wound healing.

**ADVERSE REACTIONS:** Hypersensitivity, lid itching, swelling, conjunctival erythema, superinfection.

**INTERACTIONS:** Cross-sensitivity to other aminoglycoside antibiotics may occur.

**PREGNANCY:** Category B, not for use in nursing.

## TOFRANIL
imipramine HCl (Mallinckrodt) RX

**Antidepressants increased the risk of suicidal thinking and behavior (suicidality) in short-term studies in children and adolescents with Major Depressive Disorder (MDD) and other psychiatric disorders. Imipramine HCl is not approved for use in pediatric patients except for patients with nocturnal enuresis.**

**THERAPEUTIC CLASS:** Tricyclic antidepressant

**INDICATIONS:** Treatment of depression. Temporary adjunct in childhood enuresis in >6 years of age.

**DOSAGE:** *Adults:* Depression: Initial: (Inpatient) 100mg/day in divided doses. Titrate: Increase to 200mg/day; up to 250-300mg/day after 2 weeks if needed. (Outpatient) 75mg/day. Titrate: Increase to 150mg/day. Maint: 50-150mg/day. Max: 200mg/day. Elderly/Adolescents: Initial: 30-40mg/day. Max: 100mg/day.
*Pediatrics:* Depression: Adolescents: Initial: 30-40mg/day. Max: 100mg/day. Enuresis: ≥6 years old: Initial: 25mg/day 1 hour before bedtime. Titrate: 6-12 yrs: If inadequate response in 1 week, increase to 50mg before bedtime. ≥12 yrs: Increase to 75mg before bedtime after 1 week if needed. Max: 2.5mg/kg/day.

**HOW SUPPLIED:** Tab: 10mg, 25mg, 50mg

**CONTRAINDICATIONS:** Within 14 days of MAOI therapy, or during acute recovery period following MI.

**WARNINGS/PRECAUTIONS:** Caution with elderly, serious depression, cardiovascular disease, hyperthyroidism, urinary retention, narrow-angle glaucoma, increased IOP, seizure disorders, renal and hepatic impairment. May activate psychosis in schizophrenia; reduce dose. Limit electroshock therapy. May alter blood glucose levels. Photosensitivity reported. Discontinue prior to elective surgery, or with hypomanic or manic episodes. Discontinue with pathological neutrophil depression.

**ADVERSE REACTIONS:** Orthostatic hypotension, HTN, confusion, hallucinations, numbness, tremors, dry mouth, urticaria, nausea, vomiting, diarrhea, gynecomastia (male), breast enlargement (female), galactorrhea.

**INTERACTIONS:** See Contraindications. Increased levels with methylphenidate, CYP2D6 inhibitors (eg, quinidine, cimetidine, SSRIs) and enzyme substrates (eg, phenothiazines, other antidepressants, propafenone, flecainide). Wait 5 weeks after discontinuing SSRIs before initiating TCAs. Decreased levels with enzyme inducers (eg, barbiturates, phenytoin). Blocks effects of clonidine, guanethidine. Additive effects with anticholinergics, CNS depressants, alcohol. Caution with drugs that lower BP and thyroid drugs.

Paralytic ileus with anticholinergics. Avoid preparations that contain a sympathomimetic amine (eg, epinephrine, norepinephrine); may potentiate catecholamine effect.

**PREGNANCY:** Safety in pregnancy not known; not for use in nursing.

## TOFRANIL-PM

RX

imipramine pamoate (Mallinckrodt)

**Antidepressants increased the risk of suicidal thinking and behavior (suicidality) in short-term studies in children and adolescents with Major Depressive Disorder (MDD) and other psychiatric disorders. Imipramine is not approved for use in pediatric patients.**

**THERAPEUTIC CLASS:** Tricyclic antidepressant

**INDICATIONS:** Treatment of depression.

**DOSAGE:** *Adults:* (Inpatient) Initial: 100-150mg/day. Titrate: May increase to 200mg/day. After 2 weeks may increase up to 250-300mg/day if needed. (Outpatient) Initial: 75mg/day. Titrate: May increase to 150mg/day. Max: 200mg/day. (Inpatient/Outpatient) Maint: Following remission, maintain at lowest possible dose. Usual: 75-150mg/day. Elderly/Adolescents: Initiate with Tofranil 25-50mg/day. Switch to Tofranil-PM with doses ≥75mg. Max: 100mg/day.
*Pediatrics:* Adolescents: Initiate with Tofranil 25-50mg/day. Switch to Tofranil-PM with doses ≥75mg. Max: 100mg/day.

**HOW SUPPLIED:** Cap: 75mg, 100mg, 125mg, 150mg

**CONTRAINDICATIONS:** Within 14 days of MAOI therapy or during acute recovery period following MI.

**WARNINGS/PRECAUTIONS:** Caution with elderly, serious depression, cardiovascular disease, hyperthyroidism, urinary retention, narrow-angle glaucoma, increased IOP, seizure disorders, renal and hepatic impairment. May activate psychosis in schizophrenia; reduce dose. Limit electroshock therapy. May alter blood glucose levels. Photosensitivity reported. Discontinue prior to elective surgery, or with hypomanic or manic episodes. Discontinue with pathological neutrophil depression.

**ADVERSE REACTIONS:** Orthostatic hypotension, HTN, confusion, hallucinations, numbness, tremors, dry mouth, urticaria, nausea, vomiting, diarrhea, gynecomastia (male), breast enlargement (female), galactorrhea.

**INTERACTIONS:** See Contraindications. Increased levels with methylphenidate, CYP2D6 inhibitors (eg, quinidine, cimetidine, SSRIs) and enzyme substrates (eg, phenothiazines, other antidepressants, propafenone, flecainide). Wait 5 weeks after discontinuing SSRIs before initiating TCAs. Decreased levels with enzyme inducers (eg, barbiturates, phenytoin). Blocks effects of clonidine, guanethidine. Additive effects with anticholinergics, CNS depressants, alcohol. Caution with drugs that lower BP and thyroid drugs. Paralytic ileus with anticholinergics. Avoid preparations that contain a sympathomimetic amine (eg, epinephrine, norepinephrine); may potentiate catecholamine effect.



**PREGNANCY:** Safety in pregnancy not known; not for use in nursing.

## TOLMETIN

RX

tolmetin sodium (Various)

**NSAIDs may cause an increased risk of serious cardiovascular thrombotic events, MI, stroke, and serious GI adverse events including bleeding, ulceration and perforation of the stomach or intestines. Contraindicated for the treatment of peri-operative pain in the setting of coronary artery bypass graft (CABG) surgery.**

**OTHER BRAND NAMES:** Tolectin (Ortho-McNeil)

**THERAPEUTIC CLASS:** NSAID

**INDICATIONS:** Rheumatoid arthritis (RA). Osteoarthritis (OA). Juvenile rheumatoid arthritis (JRA). Fever. Relief of mild-to-moderate pain.

**DOSAGE:** *Adults:* OA/RA: Initial: 400mg tid. Usual: 200-600mg tid. Max: 1800mg/day. Take with antacids other than sodium bicarbonate if GI upset occurs.
*Pediatrics:* JRA: >2 yrs: Initial: 20mg/kg/day given tid-qid. Usual: 15-30mg/kg/day. Max: 30mg/kg/day. Take with antacids other than sodium bicarbonate if GI upset occurs.

**HOW SUPPLIED:** Cap: (DS) 400mg; Tab: 200mg*, 600mg *scored

**CONTRAINDICATIONS:** ASA or other NSAID allergy that precipitates asthma, rhinitis, urticaria, or allergic-type reactions. Treatment of peri-operative pain in the setting of CABG surgery.

**WARNINGS/PRECAUTIONS:** May cause adverse ocular events. Prolongs bleeding time. Risk of renal toxicity with heart failure, liver dysfunction, and elderly. Caution with compromised cardiac function, HTN, or other conditions predisposing to fluid retention. Borderline LFT elevations may occur. Decreased bioavailability with milk or food. Can cause serious skin adverse reactions such as exfoliative dermatitis, SJS, and TEN, which can be fatal. Avoid with aspirin-sensitive asthma and caution with preexisting asthma. Cannot be expected to substitute for corticosteroids or to treat corticosteroid insufficiency. Notable elevations of ALT or AST have been reported. Rare cases of severe hepatic reactions, including jaundice and fatal fulminant hepatitis, liver necrosis, and hepatic failure. Patients on long term treatment should have Hgb or Hct checked if exhibit signs or symptoms of anemia.

**ADVERSE REACTIONS:** Dyspepsia, GI distress, diarrhea, flatulence, vomiting, headache, asthenia, elevated blood pressure, dizziness, edema.

**INTERACTIONS:** Increased PT and bleeding with warfarin. May enhance methotrexate toxicity. May diminish the antihypertensive effect of ACEIs. Concomitant administration with aspirin is not recommended; potential for increased adverse effects. Can reduce the natriuretic effect of furosemide and thiazides. Can produce an elevation of plasma lithium levels and a reduction in renal lithium clearance.

**PREGNANCY:** Category C, not for use in nursing.

## TOPAMAX

topiramate (Ortho-McNeil) RX

**THERAPEUTIC CLASS:** Sulfamate-substituted monosaccharide antiepileptic

**INDICATIONS:** Monotherapy therapy in patients 10 yrs of age and older with partial onset or primary generalized tonic-clonic seizures. Adjunct therapy in patients 2-16 yrs of age and older with partial onset seizures, primary generalized tonic-clonic seizures, and seizures associated with Lennox-Gastaut syndrome. Migraine prophylaxis in adults.

**DOSAGE:** *Adults:* Seizures: Monotherapy: Initial: 25mg qam and qpm for one week. Titrate: Increase am and pm dose by 25mg every week until 200mg/day, then increase by 50mg every week until 400mg/day. Adjunct Therapy: ≥17 yrs: Initial: 25-50mg/day. Titrate: Increase by 25-50mg/week. Usual: Partial: 100-200mg bid. Tonic-Clonic: 200mg bid. Max: 1600mg/day. Migraine Prophylaxis: Titrate: Week 1: 25mg qpm. Week 2: 25mg bid. Week 3: 25mg qam and 50mg qpm. Week 4: 50mg bid. Usual: 50mg bid. Renal Dysfunction: 50% of usual dose. Swallow caps whole or sprinkle over food.
*Pediatrics:* Seizures: Monotherapy: ≥10 yrs: Initial: 25mg qam and qpm for one week. Titrate: Increase am and pm dose by 25mg every week until 200mg/day, then increase by 50mg every week until 400mg/day. Adjunct Therapy: 2-16 yrs: Initial: 1-3mg/kg nightly for 1 week. Titrate: Increase by 1-3mg/kg/day every 1-2 weeks. Usual: 2.5-4.5mg/kg bid. Swallow caps whole or sprinkle over food.

**HOW SUPPLIED:** Cap: 15mg, 25mg; Tab: 25mg, 50mg, 100mg, 200mg

**WARNINGS/PRECAUTIONS:** Hyperchloremic, non-anion gap, metabolic acidosis reported; obtain baseline and periodic serum bicarbonate levels. Withdraw gradually. Psychomotor slowing, difficulty with concentration, speech/language problems, paresthesia, acute myopia with secondary angle closure glaucoma, oligohidrosis, hyperthermia, and dose related depression or mood problems reported. May cause hyperammonemia and encephalopathy if used concomitantly with valproic acid. Risk of kidney stones; maintain adequate fluid intake. Caution with renal or hepatic dysfunction.

**ADVERSE REACTIONS:** Somnolence, fatigue, dizziness, ataxia, speech disorders, psychomotor slowing, abnormal vision, memory difficulty, paresthesia, diplopia, depression, anorexia, anxiety, mood problems, pancreatitis, hepatic failure.

**INTERACTIONS:** Phenytoin, carbamazepine, valproic acid decrease levels. Increases phenytoin, decreases valproic acid levels. May decrease AUC of digoxin. May potentiate CNS depression with alcohol, other CNS depressants. Increased risk of kidney stones with carbonic anhydrase inhibitors. May increase metformin levels; monitor diabetics regularly.

**PREGNANCY:** Category C, caution in nursing.

## TOPICORT RX
desoximetasone (Taro)

**OTHER BRAND NAMES:** Topicort LP (Taro)

**THERAPEUTIC CLASS:** Corticosteroid

**INDICATIONS:** Corticosteroid responsive dermatoses.

**DOSAGE:** *Adults:* Apply bid.
*Pediatrics:* (Cre, Gel) Apply bid. >10 yrs: (Oint) Apply bid.

**HOW SUPPLIED:** Cre: (LP) 0.05% [15g, 60g], 0.25% [15g, 60g]; Gel: 0.05% [15g, 60g]; Oint: 0.25% [15g, 60g]

**WARNINGS/PRECAUTIONS:** May produce reversible HPA axis suppression, manifestations of Cushing's syndrome, hyperglycemia, and glucosuria. Caution when applied to large surface areas or under occlusive dressings. Use appropriate antifungal or antibacterial agent with dermatological infections; d/c if infection does not clear. Peds may be more susceptible to systemic toxicity. Avoid eyes. D/C if irritation occurs.

**ADVERSE REACTIONS:** Burning, itching, irritation, dryness, folliculitis, hypertrichosis, acneiform eruptions, hypopigmentation, perioral dermatitis, allergic contact dermatitis, skin maceration, secondary infection, skin atrophy, striae, miliaria.

**PREGNANCY:** Category C, caution in nursing.



## TOPROL-XL RX
metoprolol succinate (AstraZeneca LP)

**THERAPEUTIC CLASS:** Selective beta$_1$-blocker

**INDICATIONS:** Treatment of hypertension, angina pectoris, and stable symptomatic (NYHA Class II or III) heart failure of ischemic, hypertensive or cardiomyopathic origin.

**DOSAGE:** *Adults:* HTN: Initial: 25-100mg qd. Titrate: May increase weekly. Max: 400mg/day. Angina: Initial: 100mg qd. Titrate: May increase weekly. Max: 400mg/day. Heart Failure: Initial: (NYHA Class II) 25mg qd for 2 weeks. Severe Heart Failure: 12.5mg qd for 2 weeks. Titrate: Double dose every 2 weeks as tolerated. Max: 200mg/day.

**HOW SUPPLIED:** Tab, Extended-Release: 25mg*, 50mg*, 100mg*, 200mg*
*scored

**CONTRAINDICATIONS:** Severe bradycardia, >1st-degree heart block, cardiogenic shock, sick sinus syndrome (unless a pacemaker is present), decompensated cardiac failure.

**WARNINGS/PRECAUTIONS:** Exacerbation of angina pectoris and MI reported following abrupt withdrawal; taper over 1-2 weeks. Caution with heart failure, bronchospastic disease, DM, hepatic dysfunction, hyperthyroidism, or peripheral vascular disease. May mask symptoms of hyperthyroidism and hypoglycemia. Withdrawal prior to surgery is controversial.

**ADVERSE REACTIONS:** Bradycardia, shortness of breath, fatigue, dizziness, depression, diarrhea, pruritus, rash, hepatitis, arthralgia.

**INTERACTIONS:** Additive effects with catecholamine-depleting drugs (eg, reserpine, MAOIs). CYP2D6 inhibitors (eg, quinidine, fluoxetine, paroxetine, propafenone) may increase levels. May exacerbate rebound hypertension following clonidine withdrawal. Caution when used with calcium channel blockers of the verapamil and diltiazem type. Concomitant use of digitalis glycosides and beta-blockers can increase the risk of bradycardia.

**PREGNANCY:** Category C, caution with nursing.

## TORISEL

RX

temsirolimus (Wyeth)

**THERAPEUTIC CLASS:** Kinase inhibitor

**INDICATIONS:** Treatment of advanced renal cell carcinoma.

**DOSAGE:** *Adults*: 25mg infused over 30-60 minutes once a week. Hold if ANC <1,000/mm³, platelet count <75,000/mm³, or NCI CTCAE grade 3 or greater adverse reactions. Restart by 5mg/week to a dose no lower than 15mg/week once toxicities have resolved to Grade 2 or less. Concomitant Strong CYP3A4 Inhibitors: Consider dose reduction to 12.5mg/week. If strong inhibitor is discontinued, allow wash out period of about 1 week before dose adjustment. Concomitant Strong CYP3A4 Inducers: Consider dose increase to 50mg/week. If strong inducer is discontinued, return to dose used prior to initiation of strong inducer.

**HOW SUPPLIED:** Inj: 25mg/mL

**WARNINGS/PRECAUTIONS:** Hypersensitivity reactions such as anaphylaxis, dyspnea, flushing, and chest pain have been observed. Give $H_1$ antihistamine before starting infusion. Hyperglycemia, glucose intolerance, and hyperlipemia may occur; monitor glucose and lipid profiles. Infections may result from immunosuppression. Monitor for interstitial lung disease (ILD); if ILD is suspected, d/c and consider use of corticosteroids and/or antibiotics. Bowel perforation may occur; monitor closely. Renal failure, sometimes fatal, reported; monitor renal function. May cause abnormal wound healing; caution during perioperative period. Caution with CNS tumors and/or anticoagulant therapy. Avoid live vaccines and close contact with those who have received live vaccines. Monitor CBC weekly and chemistry panel every 2 weeks.

**ADVERSE REACTIONS:** Rash, asthenia, mucositis, nausea, edema, anorexia, anemia, hyperlipemia, hyperglycemia, hypertriglyceridemia, lymphopenia, elevated alkaline phosphatase, AST, serum creatinine , leukopenia, hypophosphatemia, thrombocytopenia.

**INTERACTIONS:** Strong inducers of CYP3A4/5 (eg, dexamethasone, carbamazepine, phenytoin, phenobarbital, rifampacin) may decrease levels. Strong CYP3A4 inhibitors (eg, atazanavir, clarithromycin, indinavir, itraconazole, ketoconazole) may increase levels. If alternative treatment cannot be administered, dose adjustment should be considered. Concomitant use with sutinib may result in dose-limiting toxicity.

**PREGNANCY:** Category D, not for use in nursing.

## TOVALT ODT

**CIV**

zolpidem tartrate (Biovail)

**THERAPEUTIC CLASS:** Imidazopyridine

**INDICATIONS:** Short-term treatment of insomnia characterized by difficulties with sleep initiation.

**DOSAGE:** *Adult:* 10mg immediately before bedtime.
Elderly/Debilitated/Hepatic Insufficiency: Initial 5mg. Max: 10mg/24hrs. Do not chew, break or split tablet. Do not administer with or immediately after meals.

**HOW SUPPLIED:** Tab, Disintegrating: 5mg, 10mg

**WARNINGS/PRECAUTIONS:** Re-evaluate if insomnia fails to remit after 7-10 days of treatment. May impair mental/physical abilities, visual and auditory hallucinations; complex behavior such as sleep-driving reported. Amnesia, anxiety and other neuro-psychiatric symptoms may occur. Worsening of depression, including suicidal thinking, has been reported primarily in depressed patients. Severe anaphylactic and anaphylactoid reactions reported. Monitor elderly and debilitated patients for impaired motor performance. Caution with conditions that could affect metabolism or hemodynamic responses.

**ADVERSE REACTIONS:** Drowsiness, dizziness, headache, diarrhea, nausea, drugged feeling, lethargy, confusion, dependence.

**INTERACTIONS:** Increased effect with alcohol and other CNS depressants. Rifampin may decrease effects. Co-adminstration wtih imipramine or chlorpromazine may decrease alertness. Flumazenil reverses effect.

**PREGNANCY:** Category C, not for use in nursing

## TRACLEER

RX

bosentan (Actelion)

> **Potential liver injury; monitor LFTs before therapy, then monthly. Contraindicated in pregnancy; obtain monthly pregnancy tests. Prescribe through Tracleer Access Program.**

**THERAPEUTIC CLASS:** Endothelin receptor antagonist

**INDICATIONS:** Treatment of pulmonary arterial hypertension in patients with WHO Class III or IV symptoms, to improve exercise ability and decrease rate of clinical worsening.

**DOSAGE:** *Adults:* Initial: 62.5mg bid. Titrate/Maint: Increase to 125mg bid after 4 weeks. Low Weight (<40kg): Initial/Maint: 62.5mg bid. Adjust if Develop LFT Abnormality: >3 to <5X ULN: Reconfirm LFTs. Reduce dose or interrupt therapy. Monitor LFTs every 2 weeks. If LFTs return to pre-treatment levels, reintroduce or continue therapy. >5 to <8X ULN: Reconfirm LFTs. Stop treatment and monitor LFTs every 2 weeks. If LFTs return to pre-treatment values, may reintroduce therapy. >8X ULN: Stop treatment, do not reintroduce.
*Pediatrics:* >12 yrs: <40kg: Initial/Maint: 62.5mg bid.

**HOW SUPPLIED:** Tab: 62.5mg, 125mg

**CONTRAINDICATIONS:** Pregnancy, cyclosporine A, glyburide.

**WARNINGS/PRECAUTIONS:** May decrease Hgb and Hct; monitor 1 and 3 months after initiation, then every 3 months. Caution in elderly or mild hepatic impairment. Avoid with moderate to severe hepatic impairment, or LFTs >3X ULN. Discontinue gradually. Patients with severe chronic heart failure had an increased incidence of hospitalization for CHF associated with weight gain and increased leg edema during the first 4-8 weeks of treatment with tracleer. Should considered intervention with a diuretic, fluid management, or hospitalization for decompensating heart failure. If the signs of pulmonary edema occur when tracleer is administered the possibility of associated Pulmonary Veno-Occlusive Disease should be considered. Discontinue tracleer.

## TRANDATE

labetalol HCl (Prometheus)

RX

**THERAPEUTIC CLASS:** Nonselective beta-blocker/alpha$_1$ blocker

**INDICATIONS:** Management of hypertension.

**DOSAGE:** *Adults:* PO: Initial: 100mg bid. Titrate: May increase by 100mg bid every 2-3 days. Maint: 200-400mg bid. Severe HTN: 1200-2400mg/day given bid-tid. Titrate: Do not increase by more than 200mg bid. Elderly: Initial: 100mg bid. Titrate: May increase by 100mg bid. Maint: 100-200mg bid. IV: Repeated IV Injection: 20mg over 2 minutes. Slow IV Infusion: Titrate to response.

**HOW SUPPLIED:** Inj: 5mg/mL; Tab: 100mg*, 200mg*, 300mg* *scored

**CONTRAINDICATIONS:** Bronchial asthma, overt cardiac failure, greater than first degree heart block, cardiogenic shock, severe bradycardia, other conditions associated with hypotension, history of obstructive airway disease.

**WARNINGS/PRECAUTIONS:** (IV, PO) Caution with hepatic dysfunction. Do not withdraw abruptly, may exacerbate ischemic heart disease. Caution with latent cardiac insufficiency, may exacerbate cardiac failure, reduce sinus HR, and slow AV conduction. Avoid in overt CHF. Do not give with bronchospastic disease. Paradoxical HTN in pheochromocytoma was reported. Discontinue prior to surgery. Caution with DM, may mask symptoms of hypoglycemia. (IV) Caution when reducing severely elevated BP.

**ADVERSE REACTIONS:** Dizziness, fatigue, nausea, vomiting, dyspepsia, paresthesia, nasal stuffiness, ejaculation failure, impotence, edema, dyspnea, headache, vertigo, postural hypotension, increased sweating.

**INTERACTIONS:** Increased tremor with TCAs. Antagonizes effects of β-agonists (bronchodilators). Potentiated by cimetidine; may need to reduce dose. Synergistic effects with halothane. Synergistic antihypertensive effects blunts the reflex tachycardia with nitroglycerin. Caution with calcium antagonists. May need to adjust dose of antidiabetic drugs.

**PREGNANCY:** Category C, caution in nursing.

## TRANSDERM SCOP

scopolamine (Novartis Consumer)

RX

**THERAPEUTIC CLASS:** Anticholinergic agent

**INDICATIONS:** Prevention of nausea and vomiting associated with motion sickness or recovery from anesthesia and surgery.

**DOSAGE:** *Adults:* Motion Sickness: Apply 1 patch 4 hrs before travel. Replace after 3 days. Post-OP N/V: Apply 1 patch the evening before surgery or 1 hr prior to cesarean section. Keep in place for 24 hrs. Apply patch to a hairless area behind the ear. Do not cut patch in half.

**HOW SUPPLIED:** Patch: 0.33mg/24hr [4$^{s}$]

**CONTRAINDICATIONS:** Angle-closure (narrow angle) glaucoma, hypersensitivity to belladonna alkaloids.

**WARNINGS/PRECAUTIONS:** Monitor IOP with open-angle glaucoma. Not for use in children. Caution with pyloric obstruction, urinary bladder neck or intestinal obstruction, elderly. Increased CNS effects with liver or kidney dysfunction. May aggravate seizures or psychosis. Idiosyncratic reactions reported (rare). Remove patch before MRI.

**ADVERSE REACTIONS:** Dry mouth, drowsiness, blurred vision, dilation of pupils, dizziness, disorientation, confusion.

**INTERACTIONS:** Caution with anticholinergic drugs (eg, other belladonna alkaloids, antihistamines, TCAs, and muscle relaxants). Increased CNS effects with sedatives, tranquilizers, alcohol. May decrease absorption of oral medications due to delayed gastric emptying or decreased gastric motility.

**PREGNANCY:** Category C, caution in nursing.

# TRANXENE-SD

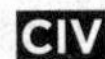

clorazepate dipotassium (Ovation)

**OTHER BRAND NAMES:** Tranxene T-Tab (Ovation) - Tranxene-SD Half Strength (Ovation)

**THERAPEUTIC CLASS:** Benzodiazepine

**INDICATIONS:** Management of anxiety disorders. Adjunct therapy for partial seizures. Symptomatic relief of acute alcohol withdrawal.

**DOSAGE:** *Adults:* Anxiety: Initial: (Tab) 15mg qhs. Usual: 30mg/day in divided doses. Max: 60mg/day. Elderly/Debilitated: Initial: 7.5-15mg/day. (Tab, Extended-Release) 22.5mg q24h, (may substitute for 7.5mg tid) or 11.25mg q24h (may substitute for 3.75mg tid). Do not use Extended-Release for initial therapy. Alcohol Withdrawal: Day 1: (Tab) 30mg, then 30-60mg/day. Day 2: 45-90mg/day. Day 3: 22.5-45mg/day. Day 4: 15-30mg. Give in divided doses. Reduce dose and continue with 7.5-15mg/day; discontinue when stable. Max: 90mg/day. Antiepileptic Adjunct: Initial: (Tab) 7.5mg tid. Titrate: Increase by no more than 7.5mg/week. Max: 90mg/day.
*Pediatrics:* >9 yrs: Anxiety: Initial: (Tab) 15mg qhs. Usual: 30mg/day in divided doses. Max: 60mg/day. (Tab, Extended-Release) 22.5mg q24h, (may substitute for 7.5mg tid) or 11.25mg q24h (may substitute for 3.75mg tid). Do not use Extended-Release for initial therapy. >12 yrs: Antiepileptic Adjunct: Initial: (Tab) 7.5mg tid. Titrate: Increase by no more than 7.5mg/week. Max: 90mg/day. 9-12 yrs: Initial: 7.5mg bid. Titrate: Increase by no more than 7.5mg/week. Max: 60mg/day.

**HOW SUPPLIED:** Tab: (Tranxene T-Tab) 3.75mg*, 7.5mg*, 15mg*; Tab, Extended Release: (Tranxene-SD) 22.5mg, (Tranxene-SD Half Strength) 11.25mg *scored

**CONTRAINDICATIONS:** Acute narrow-angle glaucoma.

**WARNINGS/PRECAUTIONS:** Avoid with depressive neuroses or psychotic reactions. Withdrawal symptoms with abrupt withdrawal; taper gradually. Caution with known drug dependency, renal/hepatic impairment. Suicidal tendencies reported; give lowest effective dose. Monitor LFTs and blood counts periodically with long-term therapy. Use lowest effective dose in elderly.

**ADVERSE REACTIONS:** Drowsiness, dizziness, GI complaints, nervousness, blurred vision, dry mouth, headache, mental confusion.

**INTERACTIONS:** Additive CNS depression with CNS depressants, alcohol. Potentiated by barbiturates, narcotics, phenothiazines, MAOIs, other antidepressants. Increased sedation with hypnotics.

**PREGNANCY:** Safety in pregnancy not known, not for use in nursing.

# TRASYLOL

RX

aprotinin (Bayer)

T

**May cause fatal anaphylactic or anaphylactoid reactions; increased risk if re-exposed to aprotinin-containing products. Weigh benefit against risks in primary CABG surgery if second exposure to aprotinin is required. Administer only in operative settings where cardiopulmonary bypass can be rapidly initiated.**

**THERAPEUTIC CLASS:** Broad spectrum protease inhibitor

**INDICATIONS:** Prophylactic use to reduce perioperative blood loss and the need for blood transfusion in patients undergoing cardiopulmonary bypass in the course of coronary artery bypass graft (CABG) surgery who are at an increased risk for blood loss and blood transfusion.

**DOSAGE:** *Adults:* IV: Administer through central line. Do not administer other drugs in the same line. Test Dose: 1mL 10 minutes before LD. Regimen A: LD:

200mL IV over 20-30 minutes. Pump Prime Dose: Add 200mL to recirculating priming fluid. Constant Infusion Dose: 50mL/hr. Regimen B: Give 1/2 doses of Regimen A.

**HOW SUPPLIED:** Inj: 10,000 KIU/mL

**CONTRAINDICATIONS:** Exposure to aprotinin within previous 12 months. Obtain full patient medical history as aprotinin may be a component in fibrant sealant products.

**WARNINGS/PRECAUTIONS:** D/C if hypersensitivity reactions occur. Take precautions with re-exposure to aprotinin: have emergency anaphylactic treatment available; give test dose and LD only when conditions for rapid cannulation present; delay aprotinin addition into pump prime solution until after LD safely given. Consider giving $H_1$ and $H_2$ blockers 15 minutes before test dose. Greater risk of hypersensitivity to aprotinin if history of allergic reactions to other agents. Administer test dose 10 minutes before LD. Administer LD in supine position over 20-30 minutes. Rapid IV administration may cause hypotension. May increase risk of renal dysfunction and possibly cause an increased need for dialysis in the perioperative period.

**ADVERSE REACTIONS:** Fever, infection, arrhythmia, hypotension, MI, CHF, pericarditis, peripheral edema, GI effects, confusion, insomnia, lung disorder, pleural effusion, atelectasis, dyspnea, pneumothorax, nausea, abnormal LFTs and renal function, urinary retention.

**INTERACTIONS:** May inhibit effects of fibrinolytic agents. May block acute hypotensive effect of captopril. Concomitant heparin may prolong activated clotting time. Caution with drugs that affect renal function (eg, aminoglycosides).

**PREGNANCY:** Category B, safety in nursing not known.

## TRAUMEEL

RX

botanical/mineral substances (Heel)

**THERAPEUTIC CLASS:** Homeopathic Complex

**INDICATIONS:** Treatment of symptoms associated with inflammatory, exudative, and degenerative processes due to acute trauma (eg, contusions, lacerations, fractures, sprains, post-op wounds), repetitive or overuse injuries (eg, tendonitis, bursitis, epicondylitis), and for minor aches and pains associated with such conditions. Treatment of minor aches and pains associated with backache, muscular aches, and minor pain from rheumatoid arthritis, osteoarthritis, gouty arthritis, and anklyosing spondylitis.

**DOSAGE:** *Adults:* 1 amp qd for acute disorders or 1-2 amps 1-3 times weekly. May administer IV, IM, SQ, or intradermally.
*Pediatrics:* >6 yrs: 1 amp qd for acute disorder or 1-2 amps 1-3 times weekly. 2-6 yrs: Half the adult dosage. May administer IV, IM, SQ, or intradermally.

**HOW SUPPLIED:** Inj: 2mL amps [$10^s$]

**WARNINGS/PRECAUTIONS:** Carefully re-evaluate if pain persists or worsens, if new symptoms occur, or if redness or swelling is present.

**ADVERSE REACTIONS:** Allergic reactions, anaphylactic reactions.

**PREGNANCY:** Category C, caution in nursing.

## TRAUMEEL TOPICAL

OTC

botanical/mineral substances (Heel)

**THERAPEUTIC CLASS:** Homeopathic Complex

**INDICATIONS:** Treatment of symptoms associated with inflammatory, exudative, and degenerative processes due to acute trauma (eg, contusions, lacerations, fractures, sprains, post-op wounds), repetitive or overuse injuries (eg, tendonitis, bursitis, epicondylitis), and for minor aches and pains associated with such conditions. Treatment of minor aches and pains associated with backache, muscular aches, and minor pain from rheumatoid arthritis, osteoarthritis, gouty arthritis, and anklyosing spondylitis.

**DOSAGE:** *Adults:* Individualize dose. Oint: Apply to affected area(s) morning and evening or more often if needed. Max: 5x/day. May also apply oint dressing. Gel: Apply to affected area(s) 1-2x/day or more often if needed. Max: 5x/day. May apply using mild compression and/or occlusive bandaging. *Pediatrics:* Individualize dose. Oint: Apply to affected area(s) morning and evening or more often if needed. Max: 5x/day. May also apply oint dressing. Gel: Apply to affected area(s) 1-2x/day or more often if needed. Max: 5x/day. May apply using mild compression and/or occlusive bandaging.

**HOW SUPPLIED:** Gel [50g, 250g]; Oint [50g, 100g]

**WARNINGS/PRECAUTIONS:** Avoid administration for pain for >10 days for adults or 5 days for children. Persistent or worsening pain, occurrence of new symptoms, or presence of redness or swelling may signify a serious condition. Avoid applying over larger areas. Only apply to unbroken skin. Ointment contains cetylstearyl alcohol which may cause local skin reactions (eg, contact dermatitis).

**ADVERSE REACTIONS:** Hypersensitivity reactions, local allergic reactions (cutaneous inflammation, redness, swelling, pruritus).

**PREGNANCY:** Safety in pregnancy not known, caution in nursing.

## TRAVATAN RX

travoprost (Alcon)

**OTHER BRAND NAMES:** Travatan Z (Alcon)

**THERAPEUTIC CLASS:** Prostaglandin analogue

**INDICATIONS:** Reduction of elevated IOP in open-angle glaucoma and ocular hypertension if intolerant to or unresponsive to other IOP therapies.

**DOSAGE:** *Adults:* 1 drop in affected eye(s) qd in the pm. Max: Once daily dosing.

**HOW SUPPLIED:** Sol: (Travatan) 0.004% [2.5mL]; (Travatan Z) 0.004% [2.5mL, 5mL]

**WARNINGS/PRECAUTIONS:** Contains benzalkonium chloride; remove contact lenses prior to administration, may reinsert after 15 minutes (Travatan). Avoid with active intraocular inflammation. Caution with history of intraocular inflammation (iritis/uveitis), aphakia, pseudophakia with torn posterior lens capsule, risk of macular edema. Increased ocular pigmentation (iris, eyelid, eyelashes) reported; may be permanent. Other eyelash changes reported. Not for the treatment of angle closure, inflammatory or neovascular glaucoma.

**ADVERSE REACTIONS:** Ocular hyperemia/pruritus/discomfort, foreign body sensation, decreased visual acuity, blepharitis, blurred vision, cataract, dry eye, photophobia, tearing.



**INTERACTIONS:** Space dosing of other ophthalmics by 5 minutes.

**PREGNANCY:** Category C, caution in nursing.

## TRAZODONE RX

trazodone HCl (Various)

**Antidepressants increased the risk of suicidal thinking and behavior (suicidality) in short-term studies in children and adolescents with Major Depressive Disorder (MDD) and other psychiatric disorders. Trazodone is not approved for use in pediatric patients.**

**THERAPEUTIC CLASS:** Triazolopyridine derivative

**INDICATIONS:** Treatment of depression.

**DOSAGE:** *Adults:* Initial: 150mg/day in divided doses pc. Titrate: May increase by 50mg/day every 3-4 days. Max: (Outpatient) 400mg/day, (Inpatient) 600mg/day.

**HOW SUPPLIED:** Tab: 50mg*, 100mg*, 150mg*, 300mg* *scored

**WARNINGS/PRECAUTIONS:** Avoid during initial recovery phase of MI. Caution in cardiac disease. Discontinue prior to elective surgery.

**ADVERSE REACTIONS:** Dry mouth, edema, constipation, blurred vision, fatigue, nervousness, drowsiness, dizziness, headache, insomnia, nausea, vomiting, musculoskeletal pain, hypotension, confusion, priaprism.

**INTERACTIONS:** Potent CYP3A4 inhibitors (eg, ritonavir, ketoconazole, indinavir, itraconazole, nefazodone) may increase levels. Carbamazepine decreases levels. Increases digoxin and phenytoin serum levels. Caution with antihypertensives and MAOIs. May enhance response to alcohol, barbiturates and other CNS depressants. May affect PT in patients on warfarin.

**PREGNANCY:** Category C, caution in nursing.

## TRECATOR

RX

ethionamide (Wyeth)

**THERAPEUTIC CLASS:** Peptide synthesis inhibitor

**INDICATIONS:** Treatment of active tuberculosis in patients with *M.tuberculosis* resistant to isoniazid or rifampin, or where there is intolerance to other drugs.

**DOSAGE:** *Adults:* 15-20mg/kg qd with food. May give in divided doses with poor GI tolerance. Max: 1g/day. Alternate Regimen: Initial: 250mg qd then titrate gradually to optimal doses as tolerated, or 250mg qd for 1-2 days, then 250mg bid for 1-2 days, then 1g/day in 3-4 divided doses. Continue therapy until bacteriological conversion has become permanent and maximal clinical improvement occurred.
*Pediatrics:* >12 yrs: 10-20 mg/kg/day in divided doses given bid or tid with food, or 15mg/kg/day as single dose. Continue therapy until bacteriological conversion has become permanent and maximal clinical improvement occurred.

**HOW SUPPLIED:** Tab: 250mg

**CONTRAINDICATIONS:** Severe hepatic impairment.

**WARNINGS/PRECAUTIONS:** Rapid development of resistance if used alone; should be used with at least 1 or 2 other drugs. Perform ophthalmologic exams before and periodically during therapy. Measure serum transaminases prior to initiation and monthly thereafter. Risk of hypoglycemia in diabetics; monitor blood glucose prior to initiation then periodically. Hypothroidism reported; monitor TFTs.

**ADVERSE REACTIONS:** Nausea, vomiting , diarrhea, abdominal pain, excessive salivation, metallic taste, stomatitis, anorexia, psychotic disturbances, drowsiness, dizziness, hypersensitivity reactions, increase in serum bilirubin, SGOT or SGPT.

**INTERACTIONS:** Discontinue all antituberculous medication with elevated serum transaminases until resolved; reintroduce sequentially to determine which drug is responsible. May raise isoniazid levels. May potentiate adverse effects of other antituberculous drugs. Convulsions reported with cycloserine. Risk of psychotic reactions with excessive ethanol ingestion. Give with pyridoxine.

**PREGNANCY:** Category C, not for use in nursing.

## TRELSTAR
RX

triptorelin pamoate (Watson)

**OTHER BRAND NAMES:** Trelstar LA (Watson) - Trelstar Depot (Watson)

**THERAPEUTIC CLASS:** Luteinizing hormone releasing hormone agonist

**INDICATIONS:** Palliative treatment of advanced prostate cancer.

**DOSAGE:** *Adults:* (Depot) 3.75mg IM every month or (LA) 11.25mg IM every 84 days.

**HOW SUPPLIED:** Inj: (Depot) 3.75mg, (LA) 11.25mg

**CONTRAINDICATIONS:** Pregnancy.

**WARNINGS/PRECAUTIONS:** Anaphylactic shock, angioedema, ureteral obstruction, spinal cord decompression reported. May worsen symptoms during 1st few weeks of treatment. Closely monitor patients with metastatic vertebral lesions and/or urinary tract obstruction during 1st few weeks of therapy. Monitor serum testosterone levels, PSA.

**ADVERSE REACTIONS:** Hot flushes, HTN, headache, skeletal pain, dysuria, leg edema, pain, impotence.

**INTERACTIONS:** Avoid hyperprolactinemic drugs.

**PREGNANCY:** Category X, not for use in nursing.

## TRENTAL
RX

pentoxifylline (Sanofi-Aventis)

**THERAPEUTIC CLASS:** Blood viscosity reducer

**INDICATIONS:** Treatment of intermittent claudication due to chronic occlusive arterial disease of the limbs.

**DOSAGE:** *Adults:* 400mg tid with meals for at least 8 weeks. Reduce to 400mg bid if digestive and GI side effects occur; discontinue if side effects persist.

**HOW SUPPLIED:** Tab, Extended Release: 400mg

**CONTRAINDICATIONS:** Recent cerebral and/or retinal hemorrhage, intolerance to methylxanthines (eg, caffeine, theophylline, theobromine).

**WARNINGS/PRECAUTIONS:** Monitor Hgb and Hct with risk factors complicated by hemorrhage (eg, recent surgery, peptic ulceration, cerebral/retinal bleeding).

**ADVERSE REACTIONS:** Bloating, dyspepsia, nausea, vomiting, dizziness, headache.

**INTERACTIONS:** Increase risk of bleeding with warfarin; monitor PT/INR more frequently. May increase in theophylline levels; risk of theophylline toxicity. May increase effect of antihypertensives.



**PREGNANCY:** Category C, not for use in nursing.

## TRIAVIL
RX

perphenazine - amitriptyline HCl (New River)

**Antidepressants increased the risk of suicidal thinking and behavior (suicidality) in short-term studies in children and adolescents with Major Depressive Disorder (MDD) and other psychiatric disorders.**

**THERAPEUTIC CLASS:** Piperazine phenothiazine/tricyclic antidepressant

**INDICATIONS:** Treatment of depression and anxiety.

**DOSAGE:** *Adults:* Initial: 25mg-2mg tab or 25mg-4mg tab tid-qid or 50mg-4mg bid. Maint: 25mg-2mg tab or 25mg-4mg tab bid-qid or 50mg-4mg bid. Max: 4 tabs/day of 50mg-4mg or 8 tabs/day any other strength. Severe Illness with Schizophrenia: Initial: 2 tabs of 25mg-4mg tid and hs prn. Elderly/Adolescents: Initial: 10mg-4mg tab tid-qid.

**HOW SUPPLIED:** Tab: (Amitriptyline-Perphenazine) 10mg-2mg, 25mg-2mg, 25mg-4mg

**CONTRAINDICATIONS:** CNS depression from drugs, bone marrow depression, MAOI use within 14 days, acute recovery phase following MI.

**WARNINGS/PRECAUTIONS:** Tardive dyskinesia may develop. NMS reported. May alter blood glucose levels. D/C before elective surgery. Caution with urinary retention, angle-closure glaucoma, increased IOP, hyperthyroidism, convulsive disorders, hepatic dysfunction and cardiovascular disorders. May increase prolactin levels. May obscure diagnosis of brain tumor or intestinal obstruction due to antiemetic effects. D/C if significant increase in body temperature develops. May impair mental/physical abilities.

**ADVERSE REACTIONS:** Sedation, hypotension, HTN, neurological impairment, dry mouth.

**INTERACTIONS:** See Contraindications. May block antihypertensive effects of guanethidine. May enhance response to alcohol, opiates, analgesics, atropine, and barbiturates. Delirium reported with disulfiram. Monitor closely with thyroid agents, anticholinergics and sympathomimetics. Anticonvulsants may need dose increase. Antagonizes epinephrine. Caution with SSRIs, ethchlorvynol. May need dose reduction with CYP2D6 inhibitors (eg, quinidine, cimetidine, propafenone, flecainide). May potentiate phosphorous insecticides. Reduced metabolism with cimetidine.

**PREGNANCY:** Not for use in pregnancy or nursing.

## TRIAZ

benzoyl peroxide (Medicis) RX

**THERAPEUTIC CLASS:** Antibacterial/keratolytic

**INDICATIONS:** Topical treatment of acne vulgaris.

**DOSAGE:** *Adults:* (Cleanser) Wash for 10-20 seconds qd-bid. (Gel) Apply qd-bid after washing with cleanser.

**HOW SUPPLIED:** Gel: 3%, 6%, 9% [42.5g]; Cleanser: 3%, 6%, 9% [170.3g, 340.2g]; Pads: 3%, 6%, 9% [30$^s$]

**WARNINGS/PRECAUTIONS:** External use only. Avoid contact with eyes, lips, and mucous membranes. Avoid sun exposure and use sunscreen. D/C if severe irritation develops.

**ADVERSE REACTIONS:** Dryness, contact dermatitis.

**PREGNANCY:** Category C, caution in nursing.

## TRICOR

fenofibrate (Abbott) RX

**THERAPEUTIC CLASS:** Fibric acid derivative

**INDICATIONS:** Adjunct to diet, for treatment of hypertriglyceridemia (Types IV and V) and to reduce elevated Total-C, LDL-C, Apo B, TG, and to increase HDL-C in primary hypercholesterolemia or mixed dyslipidemia (Types IIa and IIb).

**DOSAGE:** *Adults:* Hypercholesterolemia/Mixed Dyslipidemia: Initial: 145mg qd. Hypertriglyceridemia: Initial: 48-145mg/day. Titrate: Adjust if needed after repeat lipid levels at 4-8 week intervals. Max: 145mg/day. Renal Dysfunction/Elderly: Initial: 48mg/day. Take without regards to meals.

**HOW SUPPLIED:** Tab: 48mg, 145mg

**CONTRAINDICATIONS:** Pre-existing gallbladder disease, unexplained persistent hepatic function abnormality, hepatic or severe renal dysfunction (including primary biliary cirrhosis).

**WARNINGS/PRECAUTIONS:** Monitor LFTs regularly; discontinue if >3X ULN. May cause cholelithiasis; discontinue if gallstones found. D/C if myopathy or marked CPK elevation occurs. Decreased Hgb, Hct, WBCs, thrombocytopenia, and agranulocytosis reported; monitor CBC during first 12 months of therapy. Acute hypersensitivity reactions (rare) and pancreatitis reported. Monitor lipids periodically initially, discontinue if inadequate response after 2 months on 145mg/day. Minimize dose in severe renal impairment. Caution in elderly.

**ADVERSE REACTIONS:** Abdominal pain, back pain, headache, abnormal LFTs, respiratory disorder, increased creatinine phosphokinase.

**INTERACTIONS:** Potentiates coumarin anticoagulants; reduce anticoagulant dose and monitor PT/INR. Avoid HMG-CoA reductase inhibitors unless benefits outweigh risks. Bile acid sequestrants may impede absorption; take at least 1 hr before or 4-6 hrs after the resin. Evaluate benefits/risks with immunosuppressants (eg, cyclosporine) and other nephrotoxic agents.

**PREGNANCY:** Category C, not for use in nursing.

## TRIFLUOPERAZINE HCL RX

trifluoperazine HCl (Various)

**THERAPEUTIC CLASS:** Piperazine phenothiazine

**INDICATIONS:** Management of psychotic disorders (eg, schizophrenia) and for short-treatment of generalized non-psychotic anxiety (not as initial therapy).

**DOSAGE:** *Adults:* Psychotic Disorders: Initial: 2-5mg PO bid. Usual: 15-20mg/day. Max: 40mg/day or more if needed. Non-Psychotic Anxiety: 1-2mg bid. Max: 6mg/day or >12 weeks. Elderly: Lower dose and increase more gradually.

*Pediatrics:* Psychotic Disorders: 6-12 yrs: Initial: 1mg PO qd-bid. Titrate: Increase gradually until symptoms controlled. Usual: 15mg/day.

**HOW SUPPLIED:** Tab: 1mg, 2mg, 5mg, 10mg

**CONTRAINDICATIONS:** Comatose or greatly depressed states due to CNS depressants, bone marrow depression, blood dyscrasias, hepatic damage.

**WARNINGS/PRECAUTIONS:** May develop tardive dyskinesia, neuroleptic malignant syndrome. May elevate prolactin levels; caution with prolactin-dependent tumors. May mask drug toxicity and drug overdose due to antiemetic effects. May obscure diagnosis and treatment of intestinal obstruction, brain tumor, and Reye's syndrome. Risk of hypotension; avoid large doses and IV use with cardiovascular disease. Caution with glaucoma, angina, and elderly. May cause retinopathy; discontinue if retinal changes occur. Evaluate therapy periodically with prolonged use. May interfere with thermoregulatory mechanism; caution in extreme heat. Solution contains sodium bisulfite. Jaundice, hepatic damage reported. May cause false-positive PKU test.



**ADVERSE REACTIONS:** EPS, motor restlessness, dystonias, pseudo-parkinsonism, tardive dyskinesia, convulsions, dryness of mouth, headache, nausea, blood dycrasias.

**INTERACTIONS:** Additive CNS depression with other CNS depressants (eg, sedatives, narcotics, anesthetics, tranquilizers, alcohol). May decrease effects of guanethidine, oral anticoagulants. Propranolol may increase levels of both drugs. Thiazide diuretics may potentiate orthostatic hypotension. May lower seizure threshold; adjust anticonvulsants. May cause phenytoin toxicity. May potentiate a-adrenergic blockade. Risk of encephalopathic syndrome with lithium. Avoid with Amipaque®; discontinue 48 hrs before myelography, resume 24 hrs post procedure.

**PREGNANCY:** Safety in pregnancy not known. Not for use in nursing.

## TRIGLIDE
fenofibrate (Sciele)

RX

**THERAPEUTIC CLASS:** Fibric acid derivative

**INDICATIONS:** Adjunct to diet for treatment of hypertriglyceridemia (Types IV and V) and for the reduction of LDL-C, Total-C, TG, and Apo B in primary hypercholesterolemia or mixed dyslipidemia (Types IIa and IIb).

**DOSAGE:** *Adults:* Hypercholesterolemia/Mixed Hyperlipidemia: 160mg qd. Hypertriglyceridemia: Initial: 50-160mg/day. Titrate: Adjust if needed after repeat lipid levels at 4-8 week intervals. Max: 160mg/day. Renal Dysfunction/Elderly: Initial: 50mg/day. Take without regards to meals.

**HOW SUPPLIED:** Tab: 50mg, 160mg

**CONTRAINDICATIONS:** Severe renal dysfunction, hepatic dysfunction (including primary biliary cirrhosis and unexplained persistent liver function abnormality), pre-existing gallbladder disease.

**WARNINGS/PRECAUTIONS:** Monitor LFTs regularly; discontinue if >3X ULN. May cause cholelithiasis; discontinue if gallstones found. Discontinue if myopathy or marked CPK elevation occurs. Decreased Hgb, Hct, WBCs, thrombocytopenia, and agranulocytosis reported; monitor CBCs during first 12 months of therapy. Acute hypersensitivity reactions (rare) and pancreatitis reported. Monitor lipids periodically initially; discontinue if inadequate response after 2 months on 160mg/day. Minimize dose in severe renal impairment. Caution in elderly.

**ADVERSE REACTIONS:** Abdominal pain, back pain, headache, abnormal LFTs, respiratory disorder, increased creatinine phosphokinase/SGPT/SGOT.

**INTERACTIONS:** May potentiate coumarin anticoagulants; reduce anticoagulant dose and monitor PT/INR. Avoid HMG-CoA reductase inhibitors unless benefits outweigh risks. Bile acid sequestrants may impede absorption; take at least 1 hr before or 4-6 hrs after the resin. Evaluate benefits/risks with immunosuppressants (eg, cyclosporine) and other nephrotoxic agents; use lowest effective dose.

**PREGNANCY:** Category C, not for use in nursing.

## TRIHEXYPHENIDYL HCL
trihexyphenidyl HCl (Various)

RX

**THERAPEUTIC CLASS:** Anticholinergic/antispasmodic

**INDICATIONS:** Adjunct treatment for all forms of parkinsonism. To control extrapyramidal disorders caused by CNS drugs.

**DOSAGE:** *Adults:* Idiopathic Parkinsonism: 1mg on Day 1. Titrate: Increase by 2mg every 3-5 days. Usual: 6-10mg/day. Max: 15mg/day. Drug-Induced Parkinsonism: Initial: 1mg. If extrapyramidal manifestations not controlled in a few hrs, increase dose until achieve control. Usual: 5-15mg/day. Concomitant Levodopa: Trihexyphenidyl dose may need reduction. Usual: 3-6mg/day. Divide total daily dose into 3 doses. May divide doses >10mg/day into 4 doses. Take with meals and at bedtime.

**HOW SUPPLIED:** Sol: 2mg/5mL; Tab: 2mg, 5mg

**CONTRAINDICATIONS:** Narrow angle glaucoma.

**WARNINGS/PRECAUTIONS:** Monitor IOP. Caution with exposure in hot weather (esp. alcoholics), glaucoma, obstructive disease of GI or GU tract, prostatic hypertrophy, HTN, and cardiac, liver, or kidney disorders. Angle-closure glaucoma reported with long-term treatment. Neuroleptic Malignant Syndrome (NMS) reported with dose reduction or discontinuation. Avoid in tardive dyskinesia except in Parkinson's Disease. Use low initial dose with history of idiosyncrasy to other drugs or arteriosclerosis. Avoid abrupt withdrawal.

**ADVERSE REACTIONS:** Dry mouth, blurred vision, dizziness, nausea, nervousness, constipation, drowsiness, urinary hesitancy/retention, tachycardia, pupil dilation, increased intraocular tension, vomiting.

**INTERACTIONS:** Additive effects with cannabinoids, barbiturates, opiates, alcohol, and other CNS depressants. MAOIs and TCAs may intensify anticholinergic effects. Increased risk of tardive dyskinesia with neuroleptics. May need to reduce concomitant levodopa dose.

**PREGNANCY:** Safety in pregnancy not known, caution in nursing.

## TRILEPTAL RX

oxcarbazepine (Novartis)

**THERAPEUTIC CLASS:** Dibenzazepine

**INDICATIONS:** Monotherapy or adjunct therapy in adults and children 4-16 yrs with partial seizures.

**DOSAGE:** *Adults:* Monotherapy: Initial: 300mg bid. Titrate: Increase by 300mg/day every 3rd day. Maint: 1200mg/day. Adjunct Therapy: Initial: 300mg bid. Titrate: Increase weekly by a maximum of 600mg/day. Maint: 600mg bid. Conversion to Monotherapy: Initial: 300mg bid while reducing other AEDs. Titrate: Increase weekly by 600mg/day. Withdraw other AEDs over 3-6 weeks. Maint: 2400mg/day. Renal Impairment: CrCl <30mL/min: Initial: 300mg qd. Titrate: Increase gradually.
*Pediatrics:* 4-16yrs: Monotherapy: Initial: 4-5mg/kg bid. Titrate: Increase by 5mg/kg/day every 3rd day. Maint (mg/day): 20kg: Initial: 600mg. Max: 900mg. 25-30kg: Initial: 900mg. Max: 1200mg. 35-40kg: Initial: 900mg. Max: 1500mg. 45kg: Initial: 1200mg. Max: 1500mg. 50-55kg: Initial: 1200mg. Max: 1800mg. 60-65kg: Initial: 1200mg. Max: 2100mg. 70kg: Initial: 1500mg. Max: 2100mg. Adjunct Therapy: Initial: 4-5mg/kg bid. Max: 600mg/day. Titrate: Increase over 2 weeks. Maint (mg/day): 20-29kg: 900mg. 29.1-39kg: 1200mg. >39kg: 1800mg. Conversion to Monotherapy: Initial: 4-5mg/kg bid while reducing other AEDs. Titrate: Increase weekly by max of 10mg/kg/day to target dose. Withdraw other AEDs over 3-6 weeks. Renal Impairment: CrCl <30mL/min: Initial: 300mg qd. Titrate: Increase gradually.

**HOW SUPPLIED:** Sus: 300mg/5mL [250mL]; Tab: 150mg*, 300mg*, 600mg* *scored

**WARNINGS/PRECAUTIONS:** Risk of hyponatremia. Cross sensitivity with carbamazepine. Avoid abrupt withdrawal. Adjust dose in renal impairment. Reports of serious dermatologic reactions (eg, Stevens-Johnson syndrome, toxic epidermal necrolysis). CNS effects reported (eg, psychomotor slowing, concentration difficulty, speech or language problems, somnolence or fatigue, coordination abnormalities). Reports of multi-organ hypersensitivity reactions in close temporal association to initiation of therapy.

**ADVERSE REACTIONS:** Dizziness, somnolence, diplopia, nausea, vomiting, asthenia, nystagmus, ataxia, abnormal vision, tremor, abnormal gait, headache.

**INTERACTIONS:** Additive sedative effect with alcohol. Verapamil, carbamazepine, phenytoin, phenobarbital, valproic acid may decrease levels. Decreased plasma levels of felodipine and oral contraceptives. Increased plasma levels of phenytoin, phenobarbital.

**PREGNANCY:** Category C, not for use in nursing.

## TRI-LEVLEN RX

levonorgestrel - ethinyl estradiol (Berlex)

**THERAPEUTIC CLASS:** Estrogen/progestogen combination

**INDICATIONS:** Prevention of pregnancy.

**DOSAGE:** *Adults:* Start 1st Sunday after menses begin or 1st day of menses. *21-day:* 1 tab qd for 21 days, stop 7 days, then repeat. *28-day:* 1 tab qd for 28 days, then repeat.

**HOW SUPPLIED:** Tab: (Ethinyl Estradiol-Levonorgestrel) 0.03mg-0.05mg, 0.04mg-0.075mg, 0.03mg-0.125mg

**CONTRAINDICATIONS:** Thrombophlebitis, DVT or thromboembolic disorders, pregnancy, cerebrovascular or coronary artery disease, undiagnosed abnormal genital bleeding, cholestatic jaundice of pregnancy or jaundice with prior pill use, hepatic adenomas or carcinomas, breast cancer or other estrogen-dependent neoplasia.

**WARNINGS/PRECAUTIONS:** Cigarette smoking increases risk of serious cardiovascular side effects. This risk increases with age (especially >35 yrs) and heavy smoking. Increased risk of MI, vascular disease, thromboembolism, stroke and gallbladder disease. Retinal thrombosis, hepatic neoplasia, carcinoma of breast and reproductive organs reported. May cause glucose intolerance. May increase BP, elevate LDL levels or cause other lipid changes, fluid retention, breakthrough bleeding, and spotting. May cause or exacerbate migraine. May develop visual changes with contact lens. Increased risk of MI with HTN, hyperlipidemia, obesity, and diabetes. D/C if develop jaundice, significant depression or ophthalmic irregularities. Perform annual physical exam. Use before menarche is not indicated. May affect certain endocrine, LFTs and blood components.

**ADVERSE REACTIONS:** Nausea, vomiting, breakthrough bleeding, spotting, amenorrhea, migraine, depression, vaginal candidiasis, edema, weight changes.

**INTERACTIONS:** Reduced effects, increased breakthrough bleeding, and menstrual irregularities with rifampin, barbiturates, phenylbutazone, phenytoin, and possibly with griseofulvin, ampicillin, and tetracyclines. Increases or decreases levels of cyclosporine and theophylline.

**PREGNANCY:** Category X, not for use in nursing.

## TRILISATE RX

choline magnesium trisalicylate (Purdue Frederick)

**THERAPEUTIC CLASS:** Salicylate (non-acetylated)

**INDICATIONS:** Osteoarthritis, rheumatoid arthritis, acute painful shoulder, fever and mild-to-moderate pain.

**DOSAGE:** *Adults:* Initial: 1500mg bid. Max: 3g/d. Renal Dysfunction: Monitor salicylate level, adjust dose. Elderly: 750mg tid.
*Pediatrics:* >37kg: 2250mg/day given bid. 12-37kg: 50mg/kg/d given bid.

**HOW SUPPLIED:** Liq: 500mg/5mL [240mL]; Tab: 500mg*, 750mg*, 1000mg*
*scored

**WARNINGS/PRECAUTIONS:** Caution with renal or hepatic dysfunction, gastritis and peptic ulcer disease. Avoid with chickenpox, influenza or flu symptoms due to development of Reye syndrome in children and teenagers. Heavy alcohol use increases risk for adverse GI events.

**ADVERSE REACTIONS:** Tinnitus, nausea, vomiting, indigestion, heartburn, constipation, diarrhea, epigastric pain.

**INTERACTIONS:** Rise in urine pH (with chronic antacid use) increases salicylate clearance. Urine acidification decreases salicylate clearance. May potentiate anticoagulants, sulfonylureas, insulin, methotrexate, phenytoin, valproic acid and carbonic anhydrase inhibitors. Corticosteroids decrease salicylate levels. Salicylates may decrease effects of uricosuric agents.

**PREGNANCY:** Category C, caution with nursing.

## TRI-LUMA RX

tretinoin - hydroquinone - fluocinolone acetonide (Galderma)

**THERAPEUTIC CLASS:** Corticosteroid/depigmenting agent/keratolytic

**INDICATIONS:** Short-term treatment of moderate to severe melasma of the face.

**DOSAGE:** *Adults:* Gently wash face and neck with mild cleanser. Apply thin film to hyperpigmented areas of melasma including 0.5 inch of normal skin surrounding lesion, at least 30 minutes before bedtime.

**HOW SUPPLIED:** Cre: (Fluocinolone-Hydroquinone-Tretinoin) 0.01%-4%-0.05% [30g]

**WARNINGS/PRECAUTIONS:** Contains sodium metabisulfite. Discontinue if ochronosis, sensitivity, or irritation occurs. Cutaneous hypersensitivity reported. May produce reversible HPA axis suppression, manifestations of Cushing's syndrome, hyperglycemia, and glucosuria. Avoid eyes, nose, angles of mouth, occlusive dressings, or sunlight/UV exposure. Extreme weather (eg, cold, wind) may irritate skin.

**ADVERSE REACTIONS:** Erythema, desquamation, burning, dryness, pruritus, acne, paresthesia, telangiectasia.

**INTERACTIONS:** Avoid medicated/abrasive soaps or cleansers, soaps/cosmetics with drying effects, products with high concentration of alcohol/astringent, and other irritants or keratolytic agents. Caution with other photosensitizers. Use non-hormonal birth control.

**PREGNANCY:** Category C, caution in nursing.

## TRI-NORINYL RX

norethindrone - ethinyl estradiol (Watson)

**THERAPEUTIC CLASS:** Estrogen/progestogen combination

**INDICATIONS:** Prevention of pregnancy.

**DOSAGE:** *Adults:* Start 1st Sunday after menses begins or the 1st day of menses. *28-day:* 1 tab qd for 28 days, then repeat.

**HOW SUPPLIED:** Tab: (Ethinyl Estradiol-Norethindrone) 0.035mg-0.5mg, 0.035mg-1mg

**CONTRAINDICATIONS:** Thrombophlebitis, DVT or thromboembolic disorders, pregnancy, cerebrovascular or coronary artery disease, undiagnosed abnormal genital bleeding, cholestatic jaundice of pregnancy or jaundice with prior pill use, hepatic adenomas or carcinomas, breast cancer or other estrogen-dependent neoplasia.

**WARNINGS/PRECAUTIONS:** Cigarette smoking increases risk of serious cardiovascular side effects. This risk increases with age (especially >35 yrs) and heavy smoking. Increased risk of MI, vascular disease, thromboembolism, stroke and gallbladder disease. Retinal thrombosis, hepatic neoplasia, carcinoma of breast and reproductive organs reported. May cause glucose intolerance. May increase BP, elevate LDL levels or cause other lipid changes, fluid retention, breakthrough bleeding, and spotting. May cause or exacerbate migraine. May develop visual changes with contact lens. Increased risk of MI with HTN, hyperlipidemia, obesity, and diabetes. Discontinue if develop jaundice, significant depression or ophthalmic irregularities. Perform annual physical exam. Use before menarche is not indicated. May affect certain endocrine, LFTs and blood components.

**ADVERSE REACTIONS:** Nausea, vomiting, breakthrough bleeding, spotting, amenorrhea, migraine, depression, vaginal candidiasis, edema, weight changes.

**INTERACTIONS:** Reduced effects, increased breakthrough bleeding, and menstrual irregularities with rifampin, barbiturates, phenylbutazone, phenytoin, and possibly with griseofulvin, ampicillin, and tetracyclines.

**PREGNANCY:** Category X, not for use in nursing.

## TRIPEDIA

RX

tetanus toxoid - diphtheria toxoid - pertussis vaccine, acellular
(Sanofi Pasteur)

**THERAPEUTIC CLASS:** Vaccine/toxoid combination

**INDICATIONS:** Active immunization against diphtheria, tetanus, and pertussis in pediatrics 6 weeks to 7 yrs of age (prior to 7th birthday). Combined with ActHIB for active immunization in pediatrics 15-18 months previously immunized against diphtheria, tetanus, and pertussis with 3 doses of whole-cell pertussis DTP or acellular pertussis vaccine and 3 or fewer doses of ActHIB® within 1st year of life for prevention of *H. influenzae* type b, diphtheria, tetanus, and pertussis.

**DOSAGE:** *Pediatrics:* <7 yrs: Primary Series: 3 doses of 0.5mL IM at 4-8 week intervals. 1st dose usually at 2 months, but can give at 6 weeks up to 7th birthday. Booster: 4th dose (0.5mL IM) at 15-20 months, at least 6 months after 3rd dose, 5th dose at 4-6 yrs; prior to school entry. May give to complete the 4th or 5th dose of primary series of 3 doses of whole-cell pertussis DTP (4th dose at 15-20 months and 5th dose before school if 4th dose not given on or before 4th birthday). May combine with ActHIB® for 4th dose at 15-18 months.

**HOW SUPPLIED:** Inj: (Diphtheria-Pertussis-Tetanus) 6.7LFU-46.8mcg-5LFU/0.5mL

**CONTRAINDICATIONS:** Hypersensitivity to thimersal and gelatin, immediate anaphylactic reaction associated with previous dose, encephalopathy not due to an identifiable cause within 7 days of prior pertussis immunization. Defer during poliomyelitis outbreak or acute febrile illness.

**WARNINGS/PRECAUTIONS:** Caution if within 48 hrs of previous whole-cell DTP or acellular DTP vaccine, fever >105°F not due to another identifiable cause, collapse or shock-like state, or inconsolable crying lasting >3 hrs occurs, or if convulsions occur within 3 days. For high seizure risk, give APAP at time of vaccination and q4-6h for 24 hrs. Caution with neurologic or CNS disorders. Avoid with coagulation disorders. Have epinephrine available. Suboptimal response may occur in immunocompromised patients.

**ADVERSE REACTIONS:** Local erythema and swelling, irritability, drowsiness, anorexia, fever.

**INTERACTIONS:** Avoid with anticoagulants. Immunosuppressive therapy (eg, irradiation, antimetabolites, alkylating agents, cytotoxic drugs, corticosteroids) may decrease response. Do not combine through reconstitution with any vaccine for infants <15 months.

**PREGNANCY:** Category C, safety in nursing not known.

## TRIPHASIL

RX

levonorgestrel - ethinyl estradiol (Wyeth)

T

**OTHER BRAND NAMES:** Enpresse (Barr)

**THERAPEUTIC CLASS:** Estrogen/progestogen combination

**INDICATIONS:** Prevention of pregnancy.

**DOSAGE:** *Adults:* Start 1st Sunday after menses begins or the 1st day of menses. *21-day:* 1 tab qd for 21 days, stop 7 days, then repeat. *28-day:* 1 tab qd for 28 days, then repeat.

**HOW SUPPLIED:** Tab: (Ethinyl Estradiol-Levonorgestrel) 0.03mg-0.05mg, 0.04mg-0.075mg, 0.03mg-0.125mg

**CONTRAINDICATIONS:** Thrombophlebitis, DVT or thromboembolic disorders, pregnancy, cerebrovascular or coronary artery disease, undiagnosed abnormal genital bleeding, cholestatic jaundice of pregnancy or jaundice with prior pill use, hepatic adenomas or carcinomas, breast cancer or other estrogen-dependent neoplasia, thrombogenic valvulopathies, thrombogenic rhythm disorders, diabetes with vascular involvement, uncontrolled HTN, endometrium carcinoma, active liver disease if liver function has not returned to normal.

**WARNINGS/PRECAUTIONS:** Cigarette smoking increases risk of serious cardiovascular side effects. This risk increases with age (especially >35 yrs) and heavy smoking. Increased risk of MI, vascular disease, thromboembolism, stroke and gallbladder disease. Retinal thrombosis, hepatic neoplasia, carcinoma of breast and reproductive organs reported. May cause glucose intolerance. May increase BP, elevate LDL levels or cause other lipid changes, fluid retention, breakthrough bleeding, and spotting. May cause or exacerbate migraine. May develop visual changes with contact lens. Diarrhea and vomiting may decrease hormone absorption. Increased risk of MI with HTN, hyperlipidemia, obesity, and diabetes. Discontinue if develop jaundice, significant depression or ophthalmic irregularities. Perform annual physical exam. Use before menarche is not indicated. May affect certain endocrine, LFTs and blood components.

**ADVERSE REACTIONS:** Nausea, vomiting, breakthrough bleeding, spotting, amenorrhea, migraine, depression, vaginal candidiasis, edema, weight changes.

**INTERACTIONS:** Reduced effects, increased breakthrough bleeding, and menstrual irregularities with rifampin, rifabutin, barbiturates, phenylbutazone, phenytoin, griseofulvin, topiramate, some protease inhibitors, modafinil, ampicillin, other penicillins, tetracyclines and possibly with St. John's wort. Troleadomycin may increase risk of intrahepatic cholestasis. Increased levels with ascorbic acid, APAP, CYP3A4 inhibitors (eg, indinavir, fluconazole, troleandomycin), and atorvastatin. May alter levels of cyclosporine, theophylline, and corticosteroids.

**PREGNANCY:** Category X, not for use in nursing.

## TRISENOX RX

arsenic trioxide (Cell Therapeutics)

**Acute promyelocytic leukemia (APL) differentiation syndrome reported. Can cause QT interval prolongation and complete AV block. Perform ECG and assess serum electrolytes and creatinine before therapy.**

**THERAPEUTIC CLASS:** DNA fragmentation agent

**INDICATIONS:** For induction of remission and consolidation of APL refractory to or relapsed from retinoid and anthracycline chemotherapy, and has t(15;17) translocation or PML/RAR-alpha gene expression.

T

**DOSAGE:** *Adults:* Induction: 0.15mg/kg IV qd until bone marrow remission. Max: 60 doses. Consolidation: 0.15mg/kg IV qd for 25 doses over 5 weeks. Begin 3-6 weeks after complete induction therapy.
*Pediatrics:* >5 yrs: Induction: 0.15mg/kg IV qd until bone marrow remission. Max: 60 doses. Consolidation: 0.15mg/kg IV qd for 25 doses over 5 weeks. Begin 3-6 weeks after complete induction therapy.

**HOW SUPPLIED:** Inj: 1mg/mL

**WARNINGS/PRECAUTIONS:** Hyperleukocytosis, QT interval prolongation, torsade de pointes, and complete AV block reported. Caution with renal failure. Monitor electrolyte, hematologic, and coagulation profiles at least twice weekly, and more frequently in unstable patients during induction. Obtain ECG weekly, and more frequently for unstable patients.

**ADVERSE REACTIONS:** Fatigue, pyrexia, edema, chest pain, injection site pain, nausea, vomiting, abdominal pain, constipation, hypokalemia, hypomagnesemia, hyperglycemia, increased ALT, headache, insomnia, dyspnea.

**INTERACTIONS:** Caution with agents that prolong the QT interval (eg, certain antiarrhythmics, thioridazine) or lead to electrolyte abnormalities (eg, diuretics, amphotericin B).

**PREGNANCY:** Category D, not for use in nursing.

## TRIVORA RX
levonorgestrel - ethinyl estradiol (Watson)

**OTHER BRAND NAMES:** Enpresse (Barr)

**THERAPEUTIC CLASS:** Estrogen/progestogen combination

**INDICATIONS:** Prevention of pregnancy.

**DOSAGE:** *Adults:* Start 1st Sunday after menses begin or the 1st day of menses. *28-day:* 1 tab qd for 28 days, then repeat.

**HOW SUPPLIED:** Tab: (Ethinyl Estradiol-Levonorgestrel) 0.03mg-0.05mg, 0.04mg-0.075mg, 0.03mg-0.125mg

**CONTRAINDICATIONS:** Thrombophlebitis, deep vein thrombophlebitis, thromboembolic disorders, pregnancy, cerebrovascular or coronary artery disease, undiagnosed abnormal genital bleeding, cholestatic jaundice of pregnancy or jaundice with prior pill use, hepatic carcinoma, benign liver tumor, breast cancer, endometrial cancer, or other estrogen-dependent neoplasia.

**WARNINGS/PRECAUTIONS:** Cigarette smoking increases risk of serious cardiovascular side effects. This risk increases with age (especially >35 yrs) and heavy smoking. Increased risk of MI, vascular disease, thromboembolism, stroke, and gallbladder disease. Retinal thrombosis, hepatic neoplasia reported. May cause glucose intolerance. May increase BP, elevate LDL levels or cause other lipid changes, fluid retention, breakthrough bleeding, and spotting. May cause or exacerbate migraine. May develop visual changes with contact lens. Morbidity and mortality risk increased with HTN, hyperlipidemia, obesity, and diabetes. Discontinue if develop jaundice, significant depression or ophthalmic irregularities. Perform annual physical exam. Use before menarche is not indicated. May affect certain endocrine, LFTs, and blood components.

**ADVERSE REACTIONS:** Nausea, vomiting, breakthrough bleeding, spotting, amenorrhea, migraine, depression, vaginal candidiasis, edema, weight changes.

**INTERACTIONS:** Reduced effects, increased breakthrough bleeding, and menstrual irregularities with rifampin, barbiturates, phenylbutazone, phenytoin, and possibly with griseofulvin, ampicillin, and tetracyclines.

**PREGNANCY:** Category X, not for use in nursing.

## TRIZIVIR RX
lamivudine - zidovudine - abacavir sulfate (GlaxoSmithKline)

**Fatal hypersensitivity reactions reported; discontinue if hypersensitivy reaction suspected and do not restart. Hematologic toxicities, lactic acidosis, and severe hepatomegaly with steatosis (including fatal cases) reported. Severe exacerbations of hepatitis B in patients co-infected with HIV upon discontinuation; monitor hepatic function.**

**THERAPEUTIC CLASS:** Nucleoside analog combination

**INDICATIONS:** Treatment of HIV-1 infection alone or in combination with other antiretrovirals.

**DOSAGE:** *Adults:* >40kg and CrCl >50mL/min: 1 tab bid.
*Pediatrics:* Adolescents: >40kg and CrCl >50mL/min: 1 tab bid.

**HOW SUPPLIED:** Tab: (Abacavir-Lamivudine-Zidovudine) 300mg-150mg-300mg

**WARNINGS/PRECAUTIONS:** Hypersensitivity; discontinue if suspected and register patients by calling 1-800-270-0425. Caution with bone marrow compromise. Prolonged use associated with myopathy and myositis with pathological changes. Avoid with mild to moderate hepatic impairment or liver cirrhosis. Recurrent hepatitis upon discontinuation of lamivudine reported in hepatitis B patients. Lamivudine-resistant hepatitis B virus reported.

**ADVERSE REACTIONS:** Nausea, vomiting, diarrhea, loss of appetite, insomnia, fever, chills, fatigue.

**INTERACTIONS:** Ethanol decreases elimination. Ganciclovir, interferon alpha, and other bone marrow suppressants or cytotoxic agents may increase hematologic toxicity. Antagonistic effects with stavudine. Increased lamivudine exposure with trimethoprim 160mg/sulfamethoxazole 800mg. Avoid zalcitabine. Hepatic decompensation reported in patients on combination antiretroviral therapy for HIV and interferon alfa with or without ribavarin; monitor closely for treatment-associated toxicities.

**PREGNANCY:** Category C, not for use in nursing.

## TROBICIN RX

spectinomycin HCl (Pharmacia & Upjohn)

**THERAPEUTIC CLASS:** Aminocyclitol

**INDICATIONS:** Treatment of acute gonorrheal urethritis and proctitis in men and acute gonorrheal cervicitis in women due to *Neisseria gonorrhoeae*. Treatment of men and women recently exposed to gonorrhea.

**DOSAGE:** *Adults:* Administer 2g (5mL) IM into upper outer quandrant of gluteal muscle. Use 4g (10mL) for treatment in geographic areas with prevalent antibiotic resistance. Divide dose between 2 gluteal sites.

**HOW SUPPLIED:** Inj: 2g

**WARNINGS/PRECAUTIONS:** Contains benzyl alcohol. May mask or delay symptoms of incubating syphilis. Perform serologic test for syphilis at time of diagnosis and after 3 months. Caution in atopic individuals. Monitor for resistance by *N.gonorrhoeae*.

**ADVERSE REACTIONS:** Injection site soreness, urticaria, dizziness, nausea, chills, fever, insomnia

**PREGNANCY:** Category B, caution in nursing.

## TRUSOPT RX

dorzolamide HCl (Merck)

T

**THERAPEUTIC CLASS:** Carbonic anhydrase inhibitor

**INDICATIONS:** Treatment of open-angle glaucoma and ocular hypertension.

**DOSAGE:** *Adults:* 1 drop tid. Space dosing other ophthalmic drugs by 10 minutes.
*Pediatrics:* 1 drop tid. Space dosing other ophthalmic drugs by 10 minutes.

**HOW SUPPLIED:** Sol: 2% [5mL, 10mL]

**WARNINGS/PRECAUTIONS:** Systemically absorbed. Avoid with sulfonamide allergy or severe renal impairment. Caution with hepatic impairment. Not studied in acute angle-closure glaucoma. Local ocular adverse effects (conjunctivitis, lid reactions) reported with chronic use. Bacterial keratitis reported with contaminated containers.

**ADVERSE REACTIONS:** Ocular burning, stinging, discomfort, superficial punctate keratitis, bitter taste, blurred vision, eye redness, tearing, dryness, photophobia, ocular allergic reactions, lid reactions, conjunctivitis.

**INTERACTIONS:** Caution with high-dose salicylates. Acid-base disturbances with oral carbonic anhydrase inhibitors. Avoid oral carbonic anhydrase inhibitors due to additive effects. Wait 10 minutes before using another ophthalmic drug.

**PREGNANCY:** Category C, not for use in nursing.

## TRUVADA

RX

emtricitabine - tenofovir disoproxil fumarate (Gilead)

**Lactic acidosis and severe hepatomegaly with steatosis, including fatal cases, reported with nucleoside analogs alone or with concomitant antiretrovirals. Severe acute exacerbations of hepatitis B reported in patients coinfected with HBV and HIV upon discontinuation of emtricitabine or tenofovir disoproxil fumarate (DF).**

**THERAPEUTIC CLASS:** Nucleoside analog combination

**INDICATIONS:** Treatment of HIV-1 infection in combination with other antiretrovirals.

**DOSAGE:** *Adults:* ≥18 years: CrCl ≥50mL/min: 1 tab qd. CrCl 30-49mL/min: 1 tab q48h.

**HOW SUPPLIED:** Tab: (Emtricitabine-Tenofovir Disoproxil Fumarate) 200mg-300mg

**WARNINGS/PRECAUTIONS:** Obesity and prolonged nucleosides exposure may be risk factors for lactic acidosis and severe hepatomegaly with steatosis. Avoid in patients with CrCl <30mL/min or patients requiring hemodialysis. Tenofovir DF may cause renal impairment. Monitor serum creatinine and phosphorous in patients at risk or with a history of renal dysfunction and those receiving concomitant nephrotoxic agents. May decrease in bone mineral density; monitor bone density in patients with history of pathologic bone fracture or at risk for osteopenia. Possible redistribution/accumulation of body fat. Hepatic function should be monitored closely for at least several months in patients who are coinfected with HIV and HBV and d/c Viread.

**ADVERSE REACTIONS:** Dizziness, diarrhea, nausea, vomiting, headache, asthenia, abdominal pain, depression, flatulence, rash, paresthesia, dyspepsia, insomnia, neuropathy, increased cough, rhinitis.

**INTERACTIONS:** May increase levels of didanosine; use caution when coadministering, monitor for didanosine-associated adverse effects, and d/c if these adverse effects develop. Atazanavir and lopinavir/ritonavir may increase tenofovir DF-concentrations; monitor for emtricitabine/tenofovir DF associated adverse effects. Atazanavir without ritonavir should not be coadministered with emtricitabine/tenofovir DF. Drugs that reduce renal function or compete for active tubular secretion may increase serum levels of emtricitabine, tenofovir DF, and/or other renally eliminated drugs (eg, adefovir, dipivoxil, cidofovir, acyclovir, valacyclovir, ganciclovir, valganciclovir). Avoid coadministration with other drugs containing lamivudine. Avoid with concurrent or recent use of nephrotoxic agents. Do not coadminister with Atripla, Emtriva or Viread.

**PREGNANCY:** Category B, not for use in nursing.



## TUCKS OINTMENT

OTC

mineral oil - zinc oxide - pramoxine HCl (McNeil)

**THERAPEUTIC CLASS:** Anesthetic agent

**INDICATIONS:** Temporary relief of pain, soreness, burning, and itching associated with hemorrhoids and anorectal disorders.

**DOSAGE:** *Adults:* Cleanse area with soap and water, then rinse and dry. Apply externally to affected area. Max: 5 times/day for 7 days. To use dispensing cap, attach it to tube, lubricate well, then gently insert part way into anal canal. Squeeze tube to deliver medication.
*Pediatrics:* >12 yrs: Cleanse area with soap and water, then rinse and dry. Apply externally to affected area. Max: 5 times/day for 7 days. To use dispensing cap,

attach it to tube, lubricate well, then gently insert part way into anal canal. Squeeze tube to deliver medication.

**HOW SUPPLIED:** Oint: (Mineral Oil-Pramoxine-Zinc Oxide) 46.6%-1%-12.5%

**WARNINGS/PRECAUTIONS:** Allergic reactions may develop. D/C if redness, irritation, swelling, pain, or other symptoms develop or increase. Do not administer into rectum by using fingers or any mechanical device or applicator.

**PREGNANCY:** Safety in pregnancy and nursing not known.

## TUCKS SUPPOSITORIES OTC

starch (McNeil)

**THERAPEUTIC CLASS:** Anesthetic agent

**INDICATIONS:** To give temporary relief from itching, burning, and discomfort associated with hemorrhoids and other anorectal disorders.

**DOSAGE:** *Adults:* Cleanse area with soap and water, then rinse and dry. Insert 1 sup rectally. Max: 6 times/day for 7 days.
*Pediatrics:* >12 yrs: Cleanse area with soap and water, then rinse and dry. Insert 1 sup rectally. Max: 6 times/day for 7 days.

**HOW SUPPLIED:** Sup: 51%

**PREGNANCY:** Safety in pregnancy and nursing not known.

## TUSSEND CIII

pseudoephedrine HCl - hydrocodone bitartrate - chlorpheniramine maleate (King)

**THERAPEUTIC CLASS:** Cough suppressant

**INDICATIONS:** Relief of cough and congestion of the respiratory tract. Relief of hay fever symptoms.

**DOSAGE:** *Adults:* 1 tab or 10mL q4-6h. Max: 4 doses/24 hrs.
*Pediatrics:* >12 yrs: 1 tab or 10mL q4-6h. Max: 4 doses/24 hrs. 6-12 yrs: 1/2 tab or 5mL q4-6h. Max: 4 doses/24 hrs.

**HOW SUPPLIED:** (Hydrocodone-Chlorpheniramine-Pseudophedrine) Syrup: 2.5mg-2mg-30mg/5mL; Tab: 5mg-4mg-60mg

**CONTRAINDICATIONS:** Severe CAD, MAOI therapy, narrow-angle glaucoma, urinary retention, peptic ulcer, during an asthma attack, nursing mothers and infants. Hypersensitivity to other sympathomimetic amines.

**WARNINGS/PRECAUTIONS:** Caution with HTN, ischemic heart disease, DM, asthma, increased IOP, elderly/debilitated, severe impairment of hepatic or renal function, hyperthyroidism, or prostatic hypertrophy. Caution with head injury, intracranial lesions or pre-existing increase in intracranial pressure. May obscure the diagnosis/clinical course with acute abdominal conditions. May impair the mental and physical abilities.

**ADVERSE REACTIONS:** Lightheadedness, dizziness, sedation, nausea, vomiting, constipation, urethral spasm, urinary retention.

**INTERACTIONS:** Narcotics, antipsychotics, antianxiety agents, alcohol, and other CNS depressants may potentiate CNS depression. Increased effect of antidepressant or hydrocodone with MAOIs or TCAs. Anticholinergics may produce paralytic ileus. Digitalis glycosides may increase risk of cardiac arrhythmias. Decreased hypotensive effects of guanethidine, mecamylamine, methyldopa, reserpine, and veratrum alkaloids. TCAs may antagonize the effects of pseudoephedrine. Risk of hypertensive crises with pseudoephedrine and MAOIs, indomethacin, or with β-adrenergic blockers and methyldopa.

**PREGNANCY:** Category C, not for use in nursing.

## TUSSEND EXPECTORANT CIII

guaifenesin - pseudoephedrine HCl - hydrocodone bitartrate (King)

**THERAPEUTIC CLASS:** Cough suppressant/expectorant/decongestant

**INDICATIONS:** For exhausting, nonproductive cough accompanying respiratory tract congestion associated with the common cold, influenza, sinusitis and bronchitis.

**DOSAGE:** *Adults:* 10mL q4-6h. Max: 10mL qid prn. May take with meals.
*Pediatrics:* 6-12 yrs: 5mL q4-6h. Max: 5mL qid prn. May take with meals.

**HOW SUPPLIED:** Sol: (Hydrocodone-Guaifenesin-Pseudophedrine) 2.5mg-100mg-30mg/5mL

**CONTRAINDICATIONS:** Severe HTN, severe CAD, MAOI therapy and nursing women. Hypersensitivity to sympathomimetics and phenanthrene derivatives.

**WARNINGS/PRECAUTIONS:** Caution with severe respiratory impairment , HTN, DM, ischemic heart disease, hyperthyroidism, increased IOP, prostatic hypertrophy, and in elderly or debilitated patients. May impair mental and physical abilities. May produce drug dependence of the morphine type.

**ADVERSE REACTIONS:** GI upset, nausea, drowsiness, constipation, tachycardia, palpitations, headache, dizziness.

**INTERACTIONS:** Hydrocodone may potentiate effects of narcotics, general anesthetics, tranquilizers, sedatives and hypnotics, alcohol, and other CNS depressants. Increased effect of antidepressant or hydrocodone with MAOIs or TCAs. Decreased hypotensive effects of mecamylamine, methyldopa, reserpine, and veratrum alkaloids. MAOIs and β-adrenergic blockers potentiate the sympathomimetic effect of pseudoephedrine.

**PREGNANCY:** Category C, not for use in nursing.

## TUSSI-12 RX

carbetapentane tannate - chlorpheniramine tannate (Wallace)

**THERAPEUTIC CLASS:** Antitussive/antihistamine

**INDICATIONS:** Symptomatic relief of cough.

**DOSAGE:** *Adults:* 1-2 tabs q12h.
*Pediatrics:* >6 yrs: 5-10mL q12h. 2-6 yrs: 2.5-5mL q12h.

**HOW SUPPLIED:** (Carbetapentane-Chlorpheniramine) Sus: 30mg-4mg/5mL [118mL]; Tab: 60mg-5mg* *scored

**CONTRAINDICATIONS:** Newborns, nursing mothers.

**WARNINGS/PRECAUTIONS:** Caution with HTN, cardiovascular disease, hyperthyroidism, DM, elderly, narrow angle glaucoma, or prostatic hypertrophy. Excitation in children may occur. Suspension contains tartrazine.

**ADVERSE REACTIONS:** Drowsiness, sedation, dryness of mucous membranes, GI effects.

**INTERACTIONS:** Avoid with or within 14 days of discontinuation of MAOIs. Additive CNS effects with alcohol, CNS depressants.

**PREGNANCY:** Category C, not for use in nursing.

## TUSSIONEX PENNKINETIC CIII

hydrocodone polistirex - chlorpheniramine polistirex (UCB)

**THERAPEUTIC CLASS:** Opioid antitussive/antihistamine

**INDICATIONS:** Relief of cough and upper respiratory symptoms associated with allergy and cold.

**DOSAGE:** *Adults:* 5mL q12h. Max: 10mL/24 hrs.
*Pediatrics:* >12 yrs: 5mL q12h. Max: 10mL/24 hrs. 6-12 yrs: 2.5mL q12h. Max: 5mL/24 hrs.

T

**HOW SUPPLIED:** Sus: (Hydrocodone-Chlorpheniramine) 10mg-8mg/5mL

**WARNINGS/PRECAUTIONS:** May produce dose-related respiratory depression. Caution with pulmonary disease, post-surgery, head injury, intracranial lesions or pre-existing increase in intracranial pressure, narrow angle glaucoma, asthma, BPH, elderly, debilitated, impaired hepatic/renal functions, hypothyroidosis, Addison's disease or urethral stricture. May mask acute abdominal conditions and the clinical course of head injuries. May cause obstructive bowel disease. Consider risk/benefit ratio in pediatrics especially in croup. Impairment of mental and physical performance.

**ADVERSE REACTIONS:** Sedation, drowsiness, lethargy, anxiety, dysphoria, euphoria, dizziness, psychotic dependence, rash, pruritus, nausea, vomiting, ureteral spasm, urinary retention, respiratory depression, dryness of the pharynx, tightness of the chest.

**INTERACTIONS:** Additive CNS depression with narcotics, antipsychotics, antianxiety agents, and alcohol. Increased effect of antidepressant or hydrocodone with MAOIs or TCAs. Concurrent anticholinergics may cause paralytic ileus.

**PREGNANCY:** Category C, not for use in nursing.

## TUSSI-ORGANIDIN DM NR — RX

guaifenesin - dextromethorphan hydrobromide (MedPointe)

**OTHER BRAND NAMES:** Gani-Tuss-DM NR (Cypress) - Tussi-Organidin DM S NR (MedPointe)

**THERAPEUTIC CLASS:** Antitussive/expectorant

**INDICATIONS:** Temporary relief of cough due to minor throat and bronchial irritation.

**DOSAGE:** *Adults:* 10mL q4h. Max: 60mL/24hrs.
*Pediatrics:* >12 yrs: 10mL q4h. Max: 60mL/24hrs. 6 to <12 yrs: 5mL q4h. Max: 30mL/24hrs. 2 to <6 yrs: 2.5mL q4h. Max: 15mL/24hrs. 6 months to <2 yrs: 0.6-1.25mL q4h or 2.5mL q6-8h. Max: 7.5mL/24hrs.

**HOW SUPPLIED:** Liq: (Dextromethorphan-Guaifenesin) 10mg/5mL-100mg/5mL

**CONTRAINDICATIONS:** MAOIs.

**ADVERSE REACTIONS:** Drowsiness, GI disturbance.

**INTERACTIONS:** Avoid MAOIs use during or within 2 weeks of discontinuation. Additive CNS depression with alcohol, antihistamines, psychotropics, or other CNS depressants.

**PREGNANCY:** Category C, not for use in nursing.

## TWINJECT — RX

epinephrine (Verus)

**THERAPEUTIC CLASS:** Sympathomimetic catecholamine

**INDICATIONS:** Emergency treatment of severe allergic reactions (type 1) including anaphylaxis to insect stings or bites, allergens, foods, drugs, diagnostic testing substances, as well as idiopathic or exercise-induced anaphylaxis.

**DOSAGE:** *Adults:* Administer SQ or IM into thigh. 15-30kg: (Twinject 0.15mg) 0.15mg. May repeat if needed. ≥30kg: (Twinject 0.3mg) 0.3mg. May repeat if needed.
*Pediatrics:* Administer SQ or IM into thigh. 15-30kg: (Twinject 0.15mg) 0.15mg. May repeat if needed. ≥30kg: (Twinject 0.3mg) 0.3mg. May repeat if needed.

**HOW SUPPLIED:** Inj: (Twinject 0.15mg, Twinject 0.3mg) 1mg/mL

**WARNINGS/PRECAUTIONS:** Inject into anterolateral aspect of thigh; avoid injecting into hands, feet, or buttock. Avoid IV use. Contains sodium bisulfite.

Caution with cardiac arrhythmias, coronary artery or organic heart disease, or hypertension. May precipitate/aggravate angina pectoris or produce ventricular arrhythmias with coronary insufficiency or ischemic heart disease. Light sensitive; store in tube provided.

**ADVERSE REACTIONS:** Anxiety, apprehensiveness, restlessness, tremor, weakness, dizziness, sweating, palpitations, pallor, nausea, vomiting, headache, respiratory difficulties, hypertension.

**INTERACTIONS:** Monitor for cardiac arrhythmias with cardiac glycosides or diuretics. Effects may be potentiated by TCAs, MAOIs, levothyroxine, and certain antihistamines (notably chlorpheniramine, tripelennamine, diphenhydramine). Cardiostimulating and bronchodilating ffects antagonized by beta-adrenergic blockers (eg, propranolol). Vasoconstricting and hypertensive effects antagonized by alpha-adrenergic blockers (eg, phentolamine). Ergot alkaloids and phenothiazines may reverse pressor effects.

**PREGNANCY:** Category C, safety in nursing not known.

## TWINRIX — RX

hepatitis B (recombinant) - hepatitis A vaccine (inactivated)
(GlaxoSmithKline)

**THERAPEUTIC CLASS:** Vaccine

**INDICATIONS:** Active immunization against hepatitis A virus and hepatitis B virus in patients >18yrs of age.

**DOSAGE:** *Adults:* ≥18 yrs: 3-Dose Schedule: 1mL IM in deltoid region at 0, 1, and 6 months. Alternatively, 4-Dose Schedule: 1 ml IM in deltoid region on Days 0, 7 and 21-30 followed by booster dose at 12 months.

**HOW SUPPLIED:** Inj: (Hepatitis A-Hepatitis B) 720 ELISA U-20mcg/mL

**CONTRAINDICATIONS:** Hypersensitivity to monovalent hepatitis A or B vaccines.

**WARNINGS/PRECAUTIONS:** Anaphylaxis reported (rare). Hepatitis A and B have long incubation periods, so vaccine may be ineffective with unrecognized hepatitis. May not prevent disease if protective antibody titers are not achieved. Delay vaccine with moderate to severe acute illness. Caution with thrombocytopenia or bleeding disorders. Suboptimal response may occur in immunocompromised patients. Have epinephrine (1:1000) available.

**ADVERSE REACTIONS:** Injection site reactions (soreness, redness, swelling, induration), respiratory infection, headache, fatigue, diarrhea, nausea, fever.

**INTERACTIONS:** Caution with anticoagulants. Immunosuppressive therapy may reduce response.

**PREGNANCY:** Category C, caution in nursing.



## TYGACIL — RX

tigecycline (Wyeth)

**THERAPEUTIC CLASS:** Glycylcycline

**INDICATIONS:** Treatment of complicated skin and skin structure infections (cSSSI) caused by *Escherichia coli*, *Enterococcus faecalis* (vancomycin-susceptible isolates only), *Staphylococcus aureus* (methicillin-susceptible and resistant isolates), *Streptococcus agalactiae*, *Streptococcus anginosus* grp. (includes *S.anginosus*, *S.intermedius*, and *S.constellatus*), *Streptococcus pyogenes*, and *Bacteroides fragilis*. Treatment of complicated intra-abdominal infections (cIAI) caused by *Citrobacter freundii*, *Enterobacter cloacae*, *Escherichia coli*, *Klebsiella oxytoca*, *Klebsiella pneumoniae*, *Enterococcus faecalis* (vancomycin-susceptible isolates only), *Staphylococcus aureus* (methicillin-susceptible isolates only), *Streptococcus anginosus* grp. (includes

*S.anginosus*, *S.intermedius*, and *S.constellatus*), *Bacteroides fragilis*, *Bacteroides thetaiotaomicron*, *Bacteroides uniformis*, *Bacteroides vulgatus*, *Clostridium perfringens*, and *Peptostreptococcus micros*.

**DOSAGE:** *Adults:* 100mg IV over 30-60 minutes then 50mg q12hrs over 30-60 minutes for 5-14 days. Severe hepatic impairment (Child-Pugh C): 100mg IV over 30-60 minutes then 25mg q12hrs.

**HOW SUPPLIED:** Inj: 50mg/5mL

**WARNINGS/PRECAUTIONS:** Structurally similar to tetracyclines and may have similar adverse effects: photosensitivity, pseudotumor, cerebri, pancreatitis, and anti-anabolic action (may lead to increased BUN, azotemia, acidosis, and hypophosphatemia). Caution in patients with known hypersensitivity to tetracyclines. May cause fetal harm, and permanent tooth discoloration (yellow-gray-brown) when administered during tooth development (last half of pregnancy to 8 years). Monitor for pseudomembranous colitis. Caution when used for cIAI secondary to clinical apparent intestinal perforations.

**ADVERSE REACTIONS:** Nausea, vomiting, diarrhea, abdominal pain, infection, fever, headache, HTN, thrombocythemia, anemia, hypoproteinemia, increased lactic dehydrogenase, increased SGOT, increased SGPT.

**INTERACTIONS:** Decreased effectiveness of oral contraceptives. Monitor PT with warfarin.

**PREGNANCY:** Category D, caution in nursing.

## TYKERB RX

lapatinib (GlaxoSmithKline)

**THERAPEUTIC CLASS:** Kinase inhibitor

**INDICATIONS:** Treatment of patients with advanced or metastatic breast cancer, in combination with capecitabine, whose tumors overexpress HER2 and recieved prior therapy including an anthracycline, a taxane, and trastuzumab.

**DOSAGE:** *Adults:* Usual: 1250mg qd on Days 1-21 continuously with capecitabine 2000mg/m$^2$/day (administered orally in 2 doses 12 hrs apart) on Days 1-14 in a repeating 21 day cycle. Give at least 1 hr before or after a meal (however, give capecitabine with food).

**HOW SUPPLIED:** Tab: 250mg

**WARNINGS/PRECAUTIONS:** Decreased left ventricular ejection fraction reported; confirm normal LVEF prior to therapy and evaluate during treatment. Reduce dose in patients with severe hepatic impairment. Severe diarrhea reported; manage with anti-diarrheals, replace electrolytes. Prolongs the QT interval in some patients; consider ECG and electrolyte monitoring. Fetal harm may occur if administered to pregnant women; women should not become pregnant during therapy.

**ADVERSE REACTIONS:** Diarrhea, nausea, vomiting, stomatitis, dyspepsia, palmar-plantar erythrodysesthesia, rash, dry skin, mucosal inflammation, pain in extremity, back pain, dyspnea, insomnia.

**INTERACTIONS:** May increase exposure to concominant drugs metabolized by CYP3A4 or CYP2C8. Avoid coadministration with strong CYP3A4 inhibitors and inducers; if unavoidable, consider dose reduction with concomitant CYP3A4 inhibitors, and gradual dose increase with concomitant CYP3A4 inducers. Levels may increase if given with a P-glycoprotein inhibitor.

**PREGNANCY:** Category D, not for use in nursing.

## TYLENOL OTC

acetaminophen (McNeil Consumer)

**OTHER BRAND NAMES:** Tylenol 8 Hour (McNeil Consumer) - Tylenol Junior (McNeil Consumer) - Tylenol Infant's (McNeil Consumer) - Tylenol Children's (McNeil Consumer) - Tylenol Arthritis Pain (McNeil Consumer) - Tylenol Extra Strength (McNeil Consumer) - Tylenol Regular Strength (McNeil Consumer)

**THERAPEUTIC CLASS:** Analgesic

**INDICATIONS:** Temporary relief of minor aches and pains. Temporary reduction of fever.

**DOSAGE:** *Adults:* ≥12 yrs: (Regular Strength) 650mg q4-6h prn. Max: 3900mg/day. (Extra Strength Tabs, Caplets, or Geltabs) 1000mg q4-6h prn. Max: 4000mg/day. (Arthritis Pain, 8 Hour) 2 caplets or geltabs q8h with water. Max: 6 caplets or geltabs/day.

*Pediatrics:* Max: 5 doses/day. 0-3 mths (6-11 lbs): 40mg q4h prn. 4-11 mths (12-17 lbs): 80mg q4h prn. 12-23 mths (18-23 lbs): 120mg q4h prn. 2-3 yrs (24-35 lbs): 160mg q4h prn. 4-5 yrs (36-47 lbs): 240mg q4h prn. 6-8 yrs (48-59 lbs): 320mg q4h prn. 9-10 yrs (60-71 lbs): 400mg q4h prn. 11 yrs (72-95 lbs): 480mg q4h prn. 12 yrs (≥96 lbs): 640mg q4h prn. Older Children: Regular Strength: 6-11 yrs: 325mg q4-6h prn. Max: 1625mg/day.

**HOW SUPPLIED:** Caplets: (Arthritis Pain, 8 Hour) 650mg; Drops: (Infants') 80mg/0.8mL; Geltabs: (Arthritis Pain, 8 Hour) 650mg; Sol: (Extra Strength) 500mg/15mL; Sus: (Children's) 160mg/5mL; Tab: (Regular Strength) 325mg; (Extra Strength Tabs, EZ Tabs, GoTabs, Caplets, Cool Caplet, Geltabs, Rapid Release Gels) 500mg; Tab, Chewable: (Children's) 80mg, (Junior) 160mg

**WARNINGS/PRECAUTIONS:** May cause liver damage.

**INTERACTIONS:** Increased risk of hepatotoxicity with excessive alcohol use (≥3 drinks/day).

**PREGNANCY:** Safety in pregnancy or nursing not known.

## TYLENOL WITH CODEINE CIII

acetaminophen - codeine phosphate (Ortho-McNeil)

**THERAPEUTIC CLASS:** Opioid analgesic

**INDICATIONS:** Relief of mild to moderately severe pain.

**DOSAGE:** *Adults:* (Tab) Usual: 15-60mg codeine/dose and 300-1000mg APAP/dose up to q4h prn. Max: 60mg codeine/dose, 360mg codeine/day and 4g APAP/day. (Elixir): 15mL q4h prn.

*Pediatrics:* (Elixir): Usual: 7-12 yrs: 10mL tid-qid. 3-6 yrs: 5mL tid-qid.

**HOW SUPPLIED:** (Codeine-APAP) Elixir: (CV) 12-120mg/5mL; Tab: (#3, CIII) 30-300mg, (#4, CIII) 60-300mg

**WARNINGS/PRECAUTIONS:** Respiratory depressant effects may be exacerbated with head injury or increased intracranial pressure. May obscure head injuries, acute abdominal conditions. Caution in the elderly, debilitated, severe hepatic or renal dysfunction, hypothyroidism, Addison's disease, prostatic hypertrophy or urethral stricture. Potential for physical dependence, tolerance. Tabs contain sulfites.

**ADVERSE REACTIONS:** Lightheadedness, dizziness, sedation, shortness of breath, nausea, vomiting, allergic reactions, euphoria, dysphoria, constipation, abdominal pain, pruritus.

**INTERACTIONS:** Additive CNS depression with narcotic analgesics, antipsychotics, antianxiety agents, alcohol, other CNS depressants. Anticholinergics may produce paralytic ileus.

**PREGNANCY:** Category C, caution in nursing.

## TYLOX

CII

acetaminophen - oxycodone HCl (Ortho-McNeil)

**OTHER BRAND NAMES:** Roxilox (Roxane)

**THERAPEUTIC CLASS:** Opioid analgesic

**INDICATIONS:** Moderate to moderately severe pain.

**DOSAGE:** *Adults:* Usual: 1 cap q6h prn.

**HOW SUPPLIED:** Cap: (Oxycodone-APAP) 5mg-500mg

**WARNINGS/PRECAUTIONS:** Contains sulfites. Monitor with head injury; may increase respiratory depressant effects, increase cerebrospinal fluid, obscure acute abdominal conditions. Caution in elderly, debilitated, severe hepatic or renal dysfunction, hypothyroidism, Addison's disease, prostatic hypertrophy, or urethral stricture. Potential for physical dependence, tolerance. Inappropriate for intractable/severe pain.

**ADVERSE REACTIONS:** Dizziness, sedation, nausea, vomiting, euphoria, dysphoria, constipation, abdominal pain, pruritus.

**INTERACTIONS:** Additive CNS depression with alcohol, narcotic analgesics, general anesthetics, phenothiazines, antipsychotics, antianxiety agents, other CNS depressants. May produce paralytic ileus with anticholinergics.

**PREGNANCY:** Category C, caution in nursing.

## TYSABRI

RX

natalizumab (Biogen Idec/Elan)

**Increases the risk of progressive multifocal leukoencephalopathy (PML), an opportunistic viral infection of the brain that usually leads to death or severe disabilty. Because of PML, natalizumab must be administered only to patients who are enrolled in and met all the conditions of the special restricted distribution program. Monitor patients for any new signs or symptoms that may be suggestive of PML. Dosing should be withheld immediately at the first sign or symptom suggestive of PML.**

**THERAPEUTIC CLASS:** Monoclonal antibody/VCAM-1 blocker

**INDICATIONS:** Treatment of patients with relapsing forms of multiple sclerosis (MS) to delay the accumulation of physical disability and reduce the frequency of clinical exacerbations.

**DOSAGE:** *Adults:* 300mg IV infusion every 4 weeks.

**HOW SUPPLIED:** Inj: 300mg/15mL

**CONTRAINDICATIONS:** Progressive multifocal leukoencephalopathy (PML).

**WARNINGS/PRECAUTIONS:** Possible hypersensitivity reactions, including anaphylaxis. Increased risk of infections. Concurrent use with antineoplastic, immunosuppressive, or immunomodulating agents may further increase the risk of infections. Induces increases in circulating lymphocytes, monocytes, eosinophils, basophils, and nucleated red blood cells.

**ADVERSE REACTIONS:** Headache, fatigue, UTI, depression, lower respiratory tract infection, arthralgia, abdominal discomfort, rash, gastroenteritis, vaginitis, allergic reaction, urinary urgency/frequency, irregular menstruation/dysmenorrhea, dermatitis, abnormal liver function test.

**INTERACTIONS:** Reduced clearance of natalizumab with concomitant interferon beta-1a.

**PREGNANCY:** Category C, caution in nursing.

## TYZEKA RX

telbivudine (Novartis)

**Lactic acidosis and severe hepatomegaly with steatosis reported. Discontinuation may result in severe acute exacerbations of hepatitis; monitor hepatic function closely for at least several months following discontinuation of therapy.**

**THERAPEUTIC CLASS:** Nucleoside analogue

**INDICATIONS:** Treatment of chronic hepatitis B.

**DOSAGE:** *Adults:* CrCl ≥50mL/min: 600mg qd. CrCl 30-49mL/min: 600mg every 48 hrs. CrCl <30mL/min (not requiring dialysis): 600mg every 72 hrs. ESRD: 600mg every 96 hrs.
*Pediatrics:* ≥16 yrs: CrCl ≥50mL/min: 600mg qd. CrCl 30-49mL/min: 600mg every 48 hrs. CrCl <30mL/min (not requiring dialysis): 600mg every 72 hrs. ESRD: 600mg every 96 hrs.

**HOW SUPPLIED:** Tab: 600mg

**WARNINGS/PRECAUTIONS:** Myopathy reported; interrupt therapy if myopathy suspected and d/c if myopathy diagnosed. Monitor renal function.

**ADVERSE REACTIONS:** Upper respiratory tract infection, fatigue, malaise, abdominal pain, nasopharyngitis, headache, elevated blood CPK, cough, nausea, vomiting, influenza, flu-like symptoms, diarrhea, loose stools, pharyngolaryngeal pain.

**INTERACTIONS:** Drugs that alter renal function may alter plasma concentrations of telbivudine.

**PREGNANCY:** Category B, not for use in nursing.

## ULTANE RX

sevoflurane (Abbott)

**THERAPEUTIC CLASS:** Inhalation anesthetic

**INDICATIONS:** For induction and maintenance of general anesthesia in adult and pediatric patients for inpatient and outpatient surgery.

**DOSAGE:** *Adults:* Individualize dose. MAC Values: 80 yrs: 1.4% sevoflurane in oxygen or 0.7% sevoflurane in 65% nitrous oxide/35% oxygen. 60 yrs: 1.7% sevoflurane in oxygen or 0.9% sevoflurane in 65% nitrous oxide/35% oxygen. 40 yrs: 2.1% sevoflurane in oxygen or 1.1% sevoflurane in 65% nitrous oxide/35% oxygen. 25 yrs: 2.6% sevoflurane in oxygen or 1.4% sevoflurane in 65% nitrous oxide/35% oxygen.
*Pediatrics:* Individualize dose. MAC Values: 3-12 yrs: 2.5% sevoflurane in oxygen. 6 months-<3 yrs: 2.8% sevoflurane in oxygen or 2% sevoflurane in 65% nitrous oxide/35% oxygen. 1-<6 months: 3% sevoflurane in oxygen. 0-1 month: 3.3% sevoflurane in oxygen.

**HOW SUPPLIED:** Liq: [250mL]

**CONTRAINDICATIONS:** Susceptibility to malignant hyperthermia.

**WARNINGS/PRECAUTIONS:** Potential for renal injury. May be associated with glycosuria and proteinuria. May cause malignant hyperthermia. May cause perioperative hyperkalemia resulting in cardiac arrhythmias. May decrease BP. Rare cases of seizures have been reported. Transient changes in postoperative LFTs and very rare cases of post-operative hepatic dysfunction or hepatitis reported. Concomitant use of desiccated $CO_2$ absorbents (eg, potassium hydroxide) are not recommended, may result in rare cases of extreme heat, smoke, and/or spontaneous fire in anesthesia breathing circuit; replace $CO_2$ absorbent routinely.

**ADVERSE REACTIONS:** Bradycardia, hypotension, agitation, laryngospasm, airway obstruction, breathholding, cough, tachycardia, shivering, somnolence, dizziness, increased salivation, nausea, vomiting.

**INTERACTIONS:** Decreased anesthetic requirement with nitrous oxide. May increase both the intensity and duration of neuromuscular blockade induced by nondepolarizing muscle relaxants.

**PREGNANCY:** Category B, caution in nursing.

## ULTIVA CII

remifentanil HCl (Abbott)

**THERAPEUTIC CLASS:** Opioid analgesic

**INDICATIONS:** As an analgesic agent for use during the induction and maintenance of general anesthesia. For continuation as an analgesic into the immediate postoperative period in adults under the direct supervision of an anesthesia practitioner in a postoperative anesthesia care unit or intensive care setting. As an analgesic component of monitored anesthesia care in adults.

**DOSAGE:** *Adults:* Continuous IV Infusion: Induction: 0.5-1mcg/kg/min. Maint: 0.4mcg/kg with nitrous oxide 66%; 0.25mcg/kg with isoflurane (0.4-1.25 MAC); 0.25 with propofol (100-200mcg/kg/min). Post-Op Continuation: 0.1mcg/kg/min. CABG: Induction/Maint/Continuation: 1mcg/kg/min. Elderly (>65 yrs): Use 50% of adult dose. Titrate carefully.
*Pediatrics:* Anesthesia Maint: Continuous IV Infusion: 1-12 yrs: 0.25mcg/kg/min with halothane (0.3-1.5 MAC), sevoflurane (0.3-1.5 MAC, or isoflurane (0.4-1.5 MAC). Range: 0.05-1.3mcg/kg/min. Birth-2 months: 0.4mcg/kg/min. Range: 0.4-1mcg/kg/min.

**HOW SUPPLIED:** Inj: 1mg, 2mg, 5mg

**CONTRAINDICATIONS:** Epidural or intrathecal administration, hypersensitivity to fentanyl analogs.

**WARNINGS/PRECAUTIONS:** Administer only with infusion device. IV bolus administration should be used only during the maintenance of general anesthesia. Interruption of infusion will result in rapid offset of effect. Use associated with apnea and respiratory depression. Not for use in diagnostic or therapeutic procedures outside the monitored anesthesia care setting. Resuscitative and intubation equipment, oxygen, and opioid antagonist must be readily available. May cause skeletal muscle rigidity and is related to the dose and speed of administration. Do not administer into the same IV tubing with blood due to potential inactivation by nonspecific esterases in blood products. Continuously monitor vital signs and oxygenation. Bradycardia, hypotension, intraoperative awareness reported. Not recommended as sole agent for induction of anesthesia.

**ADVERSE REACTIONS:** Nausea, vomiting, hypotension, muscle rigidity, bradycardia, shivering, fever, dizziness, visual disturbances, respiratory depression, apnea.

**INTERACTIONS:** Synergism with thiopental, propafol, isoflurane, midazolam; reduce doses of these drugs by up to 75%.

**PREGNANCY:** Category C, caution in nursing.



## ULTRACET RX

acetaminophen - tramadol HCl (Ortho-McNeil)

**THERAPEUTIC CLASS:** Central acting analgesic

**INDICATIONS:** Short-term management of acute pain.

**DOSAGE:** *Adults:* 2 tabs q4-6h prn for 5 days or less. Max: 8 tabs/24hrs. CrCl <30mL/min: Max: 2 tabs q12h.

**HOW SUPPLIED:** Tab: (Tramadol-APAP) 37.5mg-325mg

**CONTRAINDICATIONS:** Acute alcohol intoxication, hypnotics, narcotics, centrally-acting analgesics, opioids or psychotropics.

**WARNINGS/PRECAUTIONS:** Seizures and anaphylactic reactions reported. May complicate acute abdominal conditions. Caution with risk of respiratory depression, increased intracranial pressure, or head injury. Avoid abrupt withdrawal. Caution in elderly. Avoid use in opioid-dependent patients and with hepatic impairment.

**ADVERSE REACTIONS:** Constipation, diarrhea, nausea, somnolence, anorexia, increased sweating, dizziness.

**INTERACTIONS:** Caution and reduce dose with CNS depressants (eg, alcohol, opioids, anesthetics, phenothiazines, tranquilizers, sedatives, hypnotics). May need dose adjustment with carbamazepine. Possible digoxin toxicity and altered warfarin effects. Caution with quinidine. CYP2D6 inhibitors (eg, fluoxetine, paroxetine, amitriptyline) may potentiate tramadol. May potentiate seizure risk with MAOIs, SSRIs, naloxone (with overdose), TCAs, tricyclics (eg, cyclobenzaprine, promethazine), neuroleptics, opioids and drugs that lower seizure threshold. Avoid other APAP containing products and alcohol.

**PREGNANCY:** Category C, not for use in nursing.

## ULTRAM — RX

tramadol HCl (Ortho-McNeil)

**OTHER BRAND NAMES:** Ultram ER (Ortho-McNeil)

**THERAPEUTIC CLASS:** Central acting analgesic

**INDICATIONS:** Management of moderate to moderately severe pain.

**DOSAGE:** *Adults:* >17 yrs: (Tab) Initial: 25mg qam. Titrate: Increase by 25mg every 3 days to 25mg qid, then increase by 50mg every 3 days to 50mg qid. Usual: 50-100mg q4-6h as needed. Max: 400mg/day. Elderly: Start at low end of dosing range. >75 yrs: Max: 300mg/day. CrCl <30mL/min: Dose q12h. Max: 200mg/day. Cirrhosis: 50mg q12h. Concomitant carbamazepine (up to 800mg/day): May need 2x recommended dose of tramadol. ≥18 yrs: (Tab, ER) Initial: 100mg qd. Titrate: Increase by 100mg increments every 5 days. Max: 300mg/day. Avoid in CrCl <30mL/min and severe hepatic impairment (Child-Pugh Class C).

**HOW SUPPLIED:** Tab: 50mg* *scored; Tab, Extended-Release: 100mg, 200mg, 300mg

**CONTRAINDICATIONS:** Acute alcohol intoxication, hypnotics, narcotics, centrally-acting analgesics, opioids or psychotropics.

**WARNINGS/PRECAUTIONS:** Seizures and anaphylactoid reactions reported. Do not use in opioid-dependent patients. Caution if at risk for respiratory depression, or with increased ICP or head trauma. May complicate acute abdominal conditions. Do not d/c abruptly. Adjust dose with renal or hepatic impairment.

**ADVERSE REACTIONS:** Dizziness, nausea, constipation, headache, somnolence, vomiting, nervousness, sweating, asthenia, dyspepsia, dry mouth, diarrhea, CNS stimulation, pruritus.

**INTERACTIONS:** Caution and reduce dose with CNS depressants (eg, alcohol, opioids, anesthetics, phenothiazines, tranquilizers, sedatives, hypnotics). May need dose adjustment with carbamazepine. Possible digoxin toxicity and altered warfarin effects. Caution with quinidine. CYP2D6 inhibitors (eg, fluoxetine, paroxetine, amitriptyline) may potentiate tramadol. May potentiate seizure risk with MAOIs, SSRIs, naloxone (with overdose), TCAs, tricyclics (eg, cyclobenzaprine, promethazine), neuroleptics, opioids and drugs that lower seizure threshold.

**PREGNANCY:** Category C, not for use in nursing.

## ULTRAVATE RX

halobetasol propionate (Westwood-Squibb)

**THERAPEUTIC CLASS:** Corticosteroid

**INDICATIONS:** Corticosteroid responsive dermatoses.

**DOSAGE:** *Adults:* Apply qd-bid. Rub in gently. Limit treatment to 2 weeks. Max: 50g/week.
*Pediatrics:* >12 yrs: Apply qd-bid. Rub in gently. Limit treatment to 2 weeks. Max: 50g/week.

**HOW SUPPLIED:** Cre, Oint: 0.05% [15g, 50g]

**WARNINGS/PRECAUTIONS:** Avoid face, groin, or axillae. Not for treatment of rosacea or perioral dermatitis. May produce reversible HPA axis suppression, manifestations of Cushing's syndrome, hyperglycemia, and glucosuria. Caution when applied to large surface areas or under occlusive dressings. Use appropriate antifungal or antibacterial agent with dermatological infections; discontinue if infection does not clear. Pediatrics may be more susceptible to systemic toxicity. Avoid eyes. Discontinue if irritation occurs. Reassess if no improvement after 2 weeks.

**ADVERSE REACTIONS:** Stinging, burning, itching, irritation, dryness, folliculitis, hypertrichosis, acneiform eruptions, hypopigmentation, perioral dermatitis, allergic contact dermatitis, skin maceration, secondary infection, skin atrophy, striae, miliaria.

**PREGNANCY:** Category C, caution in nursing.

## UNASYN RX

sulbactam sodium - ampicillin sodium (Pfizer)

**THERAPEUTIC CLASS:** Semisynthetic penicillin/beta lactamase inhibitor

**INDICATIONS:** Treatment of skin and skin structure (SSSI), intra-abdominal, and gynecological infections caused by susceptible microorganisms.

**DOSAGE:** *Adults:* 1.5-3g (ampicillin¢lbactam) IM/IV q6h. Max: 4g/day sulbactam. Renal Impairment: CrCl >30mL/min: 1.5-3g q6-8h. CrCl 15-29mL/min: 1.5-3g q12h. CrCl 5-14mL/min: 1.5-3g q24h.
*Pediatrics:* >1 yr: SSSI: 1.5-3g (ampicillin¢lbactam) IM/IV q6h. Max: 4g/day sulbactam.

**HOW SUPPLIED:** Inj: (Ampicillin-Sulbactam) 1g-0.5g, 2g-1g, 10g-5g

**WARNINGS/PRECAUTIONS:** Serious, fatal hypersensitivity reactions reported. Pseudomembranous colitis reported. Increased risk of skin rash with mononucleosis, use alternate agent.

**ADVERSE REACTIONS:** Injection site pain, thrombophlebitis, diarrhea, rash, nausea, vomiting, malaise, headache, chest pain, flatulence, dysuria, edema, erythema, chills, epistaxis.



**INTERACTIONS:** Probenecid increases and prolongs blood levels. Increased incidence of rash with allopurinol. Do not reconstitute with aminoglycosides; may inactivate aminoglycosides.

**PREGNANCY:** Category B, caution in nursing.

## UNIPHYL RX

theophylline (Purdue Pharmaceutical)

**THERAPEUTIC CLASS:** Xanthine bronchodilator

**INDICATIONS:** Treatment of the symptoms and reversible airflow obstruction associated with chronic asthma and other chronic lung disease (eg, emphysema, chronic bronchitis).

**DOSAGE:** *Adults:* Initial: 300-400mg qd for 3 days with meals. Titrate: Increase to 400-600mg qd. After 3 days and if needed/tolerated, increase dose according to blood levels. Tab may be split in half; do not chew or crush. Renal Dysfunction/Elderly (>60 yrs): Max: 400mg/day. Conversion from Immediate-Release Theophylline: Give same daily dose as once daily. *Pediatrics:* 12-15 yrs: (<45kg): Initial: 12-14mg/kg/day up to 300mg qd for 3 days with meals. Titrate: Increase to 16mg/kg/day up to 400mg qd. After 3 days if needed/tolerated increase to 20mg/kg/day up to 600mg qd. (>45kg): Follow adult dose schedule. Tab may be split in half; do not chew or crush. Conversion from Immediate-Release Theophylline: >12 yrs: Give same daily dose as once daily. Renal Dysfunction: Max: 400mg qd.

**HOW SUPPLIED:** Tab, Extended Release: 400mg*, 600mg* *scored

**WARNINGS/PRECAUTIONS:** Extreme caution in peptic ulcer disease, seizure disorders and/or cardiac arrhythmias (except bradycardia). Caution in neonates, children <1 yr, and the elderly. Caution in pulmonary edema, CHF, fever >102°F for 24 hrs, cor-pulmonale, hypothyroidism, liver disease, reduced renal function, sepsis, shock, and HTN. If toxicity develops (eg, repetitive vomiting) monitor serum levels and adjust dosage.

**ADVERSE REACTIONS:** Vomiting, headache, insomnia, diarrhea, restlessness, tremors, hematemesis, hypokalemia, hyperglycemia, tachycardia, hypotension/shock, nervousness, disorientation, arrhythmias, seizures.

**INTERACTIONS:** Diminished effects with charcoal broiled food, phenytoin, carbamazepine, phenobarbital, hydantoins, rifampin, ritonavir, aminoglutethimide, barbiturates, ketoconazole, sulfinpyrazone, INH, loop diuretics, sympathomimetics, high protein/low carbohydrate diet, St. John's wort. Potentiated by propranolol, allopurinol, erythromycin, troleandomycin, ciprofloxacin, quinolone antibiotics, oral contraceptives, calcium channel blockers, corticosteroids, disulfiram, ephedrine, influenza virus vaccine, interferon, macrolides, mexiletine, thiabendazole, thyroid hormones, carbamazepine, loop diuretics

**PREGNANCY:** Category C, caution in nursing.

## UNIRETIC RX

hydrochlorothiazide - moexipril HCl (Schwarz)

**ACE inhibitors can cause death/injury to developing fetus during 2nd and 3rd trimesters. Stop therapy if pregnancy detected.**

**THERAPEUTIC CLASS:** ACE inhibitor/thiazide diuretic

**INDICATIONS:** Treatment of hypertension. Not for initial therapy.

**DOSAGE:** *Adults:* Initial (if not controlled on moexipril/HCTZ monotherapy): Switch to 7.5mg-12.5mg tab, 15mg-12.5mg tab, or 15mg-25mg tab qd. Titrate: May increase after 2-3 weeks. Initial (if controlled on 25mg HCTZ/day with hypokalemia): 3.75mg-6.25mg (1/2 of 7.5mg-12.5mg tab). If excessive Reduction with 7.5mg-12.5mg tab, may switch to 3.75mg-6.25mg. Replacement Therapy: Substitute combination for titrated components. Take 1 hr before meals.

U

**HOW SUPPLIED:** Tab: (Moexipril-HCTZ) 7.5mg-12.5mg*, 15mg-12.5mg*, 15mg-25mg* *scored

**CONTRAINDICATIONS:** History of ACE inhibitor-associated angioedema, anuria, sulfonamide hypersensitivity.

**WARNINGS/PRECAUTIONS:** Discontinue if angioedema, jaundice, or if marked LFT elevation occurs. Intestinal angioedema reported. Risk of hyperkalemia with DM, renal dysfunction. Persistent nonproductive cough reported. Monitor WBCs in renal and collagen vascular disease. Anaphylactoid reactions reported. Fetal/neonatal morbidity and death reported. Monitor for hypotension in high risk patients (eg, surgery/anesthesia, volume/salt depletion). Caution in elderly, CHF, renal or hepatic dysfunction. More reports of angioedema in blacks than nonblacks. May exacerbate or activate SLE.

Monitor electrolytes. Avoid if CrCl <40mL/min/1.73m$^2$. May increase cholesterol, TG. Hypercalcemia, hypomagnesemia, hyperuricemia may occur.

**ADVERSE REACTIONS:** Cough, dizziness, fatigue.

**INTERACTIONS:** Increase risk of hyperkalemia with $K^+$-sparing diuretics, $K^+$ supplements, or $K^+$-containing salt substitutes. Potentiates orthostatic hypotension with alcohol, barbiturates, and narcotics. Adjust antidiabetic drugs. Reduced absorption with cholestyramine, colestipol. Corticosteroids, ACTH deplete electrolytes. May decrease response to pressor amines. Potentiates other antihypertensives. May increase responsiveness to skeletal muscle relaxants. Risk of lithium toxicity. NSAIDs reduce effects. Increased absorption of HCTZ with guanabenz and propantheline.

**PREGNANCY:** Category C (1st trimester) and D (2nd and 3rd trimesters), not for use in nursing.

## UNISOM — OTC
doxylamine succinate (Chattem)

**THERAPEUTIC CLASS:** Antihistamine

**INDICATIONS:** As a sleep aid 30 minutes before retiring.

**DOSAGE:** *Adult:* 1 tab 30 minutes prior to going to bed. Max: 1 tab qhs.
*Pediatrics:* >12 yrs: 1 tab 30 minutes prior to going to bed. Max: 1 tab qhs.

**HOW SUPPLIED:** Tab: 25mg

**CONTRAINDICATIONS:** Pregnancy, nursing, asthma, glaucoma, prostate enlargement.

**WARNINGS/PRECAUTIONS:** Caution in emphysema, chronic bronchitis, glaucoma, and difficulty in urination due to BPH. Caution with alcohol. Re-evaluate therapy if sleeplessness persists >2 weeks.

**ADVERSE REACTIONS:** Anticholinergic effects.

**PREGNANCY:** Not for use in pregnancy or nursing.

## UNITHROID — RX
levothyroxine sodium (Lannett)

**THERAPEUTIC CLASS:** Thyroid replacement hormone

**INDICATIONS:** Hypothyroidism. As a pituitary TSH suppressant in the treatment and prevention of euthyroid goiters, including thyroid nodules, lymphocytic thyroiditis, and multinodular goiter. Adjunct to surgery and radioiodine therapy for thyrotropin-dependent well-differentiated thyroid cancer.

**DOSAGE:** *Adults:* Take in the AM at least 1/2-1 hr before food. Hypothyroid: Usual: 1.7mcg/kg/day. >200mcg/day (seldom). >50 yrs/<50 yrs with Cardiac Disease: Initial: 25-50mcg/day. Titrate: Increase by 12.5-25mcg/day every 6-8 weeks until euthyroid. Elderly with Cardiac Disease: Initial: 12.5-25mcg/day. Titrate: Increase by 12.5-25mcg/day every 4-6 weeks until euthyroid. Severe Hypothyroidism: Initial: 12.5-25mcg/day. Titrate: Increase by 25mcg/day every 2-4 weeks until euthyroid. Pregnancy: May increase dose requirements. Subclinical Hypothyroidism: Lower doses required.
*Pediatrics:* Take in the AM at least 1/2-1 hr before food. Hypothyroidism: 0-3 months: 10-15mcg/kg/day. 3-6 months: 8-10mcg/kg/day. 6-12 months: 6-8mcg/kg/day. 1-5 yrs: 5-6mcg/kg/day. 6-12 yrs: 4-5mcg/kg/day. >12 yrs: 2-3mcg/kg/day. Growth/Puberty Complete: 1.7mcg/kg/day. Cardiac Risk: Initial: Use lower dose. Titrate: Increase dose every 4-6 weeks until euthyroid. Infants with Serum $T_4$ <5mcg/dL: Initial: 50mcg/day. Chronic/Severe Hypothyroidism: Children: Initial: 25mcg/day. Titrate: Increase by 25mcg/day every 2-4 weeks until desired effect. Minimize Hyperactivity in Older Children: Initial: Give 1/4 of full replacement dose. Titrate: Increase by same amount weekly until full dose achieved. May crush tab and mix with 5-10mL water.

**HOW SUPPLIED:** Tab: 25mcg*, 50mcg*, 75mcg*, 88mcg*, 100mcg*, 112mcg*, 125mcg*, 150mcg*, 175mcg*, 200mcg*, 300mcg* *scored

**CONTRAINDICATIONS:** Untreated thyrotoxicosis, acute MI, uncorrected adrenal insufficiency.

**WARNINGS/PRECAUTIONS:** Do not use in the treatment of obesity; larger doses in euthyroid patients can cause serious or even life threatening toxicity. Caution with cardiovascular disease, CAD, adrenal insufficiency, autonomous thyroid tissue, hypothalamic/pituitary hormone deficiencies, and the elderly with risk of occult cardiac disease. Carefully titrate dose to avoid over or under treatment. Decreased bone mineral density with long term use. With adrenal insufficiency supplement with glucocorticoids before therapy.

**INTERACTIONS:** Sympathomimetics may increase risk of coronary insufficiency with CAD. Upward dose adjustments needed for insulin and oral hypoglycemic agents. Decreased absorption with soybean flour (infant formula), cotton seed meal, walnuts, and fiber. May potentiate oral anticoagulant effects; adjust dose and monitor PT/INR. May decrease levels and effects of digitalis glycosides. Cholestyramine, colestipol, ferrous sulfate, aluminum hydroxide, sodium polystyrene, soybean flour, sucralfate may decrease absorption. Reduced TSH secretion with dopamine/dopamine agonists, glucocorticoids, octreotide. Decreased thyroid hormone secretion with aminoglutethimide, amiodarone, iodine (including iodine-containing radiographic contrast agents), lithium, methimazole, PTU, sulfonamides, tolbutamide. Increased thyroid hormone secretion with amiodarone, iodide (including iodine-containing radiographic contrast agents). Decreased $T_4$ absorption with antacids (aluminum & magnesium hydroxides), simethicone, bile acid sequestrants (cholestyramine, colestipol), calcium carbonate, cation exchange resins (eg, Kayexalate), ferrous sulfate, sucralfate. Increased serum TBG concentration with clofibrate, estrogens, heroin/methadone, 5-FU, mitotane, tamoxifen. Decreased serum TBG concentration with androgens/anabolic steroids, asparaginase, glucocorticoids, nicotinic acid (slow-release). Protein-binding site displacement with furosemide, heparin, hydantoins, NSAIDs, salicylates. Increased hepatic metabolism with carbamazepine, hydantoins, phenobarbital, rifampin. Decreased conversion of $T_4$ to $T_3$ levels with amiodarone, β-adrenergic antagonists (propranolol >160mg/day), glucocorticoids (dexamethasone >4mg/day), PTU. Additive effects of both agents with antidepressants. Interferon-(alpha) may cause development of antithyroid microsomal antibodies causing transient hypothyroidism, hyperthyroidism, or both. Interl

**PREGNANCY:** Category A, caution in nursing.

## UNIVASC

RX

moexipril HCl (Schwarz)

**ACE inhibitors can cause death/injury to developing fetus during 2nd and 3rd trimesters. Stop therapy if pregnancy detected.**

**THERAPEUTIC CLASS:** ACE inhibitor

**INDICATIONS:** Treatment of hypertension.

**DOSAGE:** *Adults:* If possible, discontinue diuretic 2-3 days prior to therapy. Take 1 hr before meals. Initial: 7.5mg qd, 3.75mg with concomitant diuretic therapy. Maint: 7.5-30mg/day given qd-bid. Resume diuretic if BP not controlled. Max: 60mg/day. CrCl <40mL/min: Initial: 3.75mg qd. Max: 15mg/day.

**HOW SUPPLIED:** Tab: 7.5mg*, 15mg* *scored

**CONTRAINDICATIONS:** History of ACE inhibitor associated angioedema.

**WARNINGS/PRECAUTIONS:** Discontinue if angioedema, jaundice, or if marked LFT elevation occurs. Intestinal angioedema reported. Risk of hyperkalemia with DM, renal dysfunction. Persistent nonproductive cough reported. Monitor WBCs in renal and collagen vascular disease. Anaphylactoid reactions reported. Fetal/neonatal morbidity and death reported. Monitor for hypotension in high risk patients (heart failure, surgery/anesthesia, prolonged diuretic therapy, volume and/or salt depletion, etc). Caution with CHF, renal dysfunction, and renal artery stenosis. Less effective on BP in blacks and more reports of angioedema than nonblacks.

**ADVERSE REACTIONS:** Cough, dizziness, diarrhea, flu syndrome, fatigue, pharyngitis, flushing, rash, myalgia.

**INTERACTIONS:** May increase lithium levels. Hypotension risk with diuretics. Increased risk of hyperkalemia with $K^+$-sparing diuretics, $K^+$-containing salt substitutes or $K^+$ supplements.

**PREGNANCY:** Category C (1st trimester) and D (2nd and 3rd trimesters), not for use in nursing.

## URECHOLINE

RX

bethanechol chloride (Merck/Odyssey)

**THERAPEUTIC CLASS:** Cholinergic agent

**INDICATIONS:** Treatment of acute postoperative and postpartum nonobstructive urinary retention and for neurogenic atony of the urinary bladder with retention

**DOSAGE:** *Adults:* Initial: 5-10mg. Titrate: May repeat every hr until satisfactory response or 50mg given. Usual: 10-50mg tid-qid. Max: 200mg/day.

**HOW SUPPLIED:** Tab: 5mg*, 10mg*, 25mg*, 50mg* *scored

**CONTRAINDICATIONS:** GI or bladder wall strength or integrity is in question or with mechanical obstruction, if increased muscular activity of GI tract or urinary bladder may be harmful, bladder neck obstruction, spastic GI disturbances, acute inflammatory lesions of GI tract, peritonitis, marked vagotonia, hyperthyroidism, peptic ulcer, bronchial asthma, bradycardia, hypotension, vasomotor instability, CAD, epilepsy, parkinsonism.

**WARNINGS/PRECAUTIONS:** If sphincter fails to relax, urine may be forced up ureter into kidney pelvis; may increase risk of reflux infection.

**ADVERSE REACTIONS:** Malaise, abdominal cramps/discomfort, nausea, belching, diarrhea, salivation, urinary urgency, headache, fall in BP with reflex tachycardia, vasomotor response, flushing, sweating, bronchial constriction, lacrimation.

**INTERACTIONS:** Caution with ganglionic blockers; a critical fall in BP may occur.

**PREGNANCY:** Category C, not for use in nursing.

## URIMAX

RX

methenamine - methylene blue - phenyl salicylate - sodium biphosphate - hyoscyamine sulfate (Xanodyne)



**THERAPEUTIC CLASS:** anticholinergic/antibacterial/antiseptic/analgesic/Acidifier

**INDICATIONS:** Treatment of symptoms of irritative voiding. For relief of local symptoms that accompany lower urinary tract infections (eg, inflammation, hypermotility, pain). For relief of urinary tract symptoms caused by diagnostic procedures.

**DOSAGE:** *Adults:* 1 tab qid with plenty of fluid.
*Pediatrics:* >6 yrs: Individualize dose. Take with plenty of fluid.

**HOW SUPPLIED:** Tab, Extended Release: (Hyoscyamine-Methenamine-Methylene Blue-Phenyl Salicylate-Sodium Biphosphate) 0.12mg-81.6mg-10.8mg-36.2mg-40.8mg

**CONTRAINDICATIONS:** Consider risk-benefit with the following: cardiac disease, GI tract obstructive disease, glaucoma, myasthenia gravis, obstructive uropathy.

**WARNINGS/PRECAUTIONS:** Discontinue if rapid pulse, dizziness, or blurred vision occurs. Intolerance may occur if intolerant to belladonna alkaloids or salicylates. Delay in gastric emptying could complicate management of gastric ulcers. Infants and children are especially susceptible to toxic effect of belladonna alkaloids. Caution in elderly. Urine and feces may become blue to blue-green due to methylene blue.

**ADVERSE REACTIONS:** Rapid pulse, flushing, blurred vision, dizziness, shortness of breath, difficult micturition, acute urinary retention, dry mouth, nausea, vomiting.

**INTERACTIONS:** May decrease absorption of urinary alkalizers, thiazide diuretics, antimuscarinics, antacids/antidiarrheals. Space dosing by 1 hr with antimyasthenics, MAOIs, opioids, sulfonamides. Space dosing by 2 hrs with ketoconazole. Thiazide diuretics may decrease effectiveness of methenamine. Intensified antimuscarinic effects of hyoscyamine with antimuscarinics. Antacids/antidiarrheals may reduce absorption of hyoscyamine and may reduce effectiveness of methenamine.

**PREGNANCY:** Category C, caution in nursing.

## URISED RX

methenamine - benzoic acid - methylene blue - phenyl salicylate - atropine sulfate - hyoscyamine sulfate (PolyMedica)

**THERAPEUTIC CLASS:** anticholinergic/antiseptic/antibacterial/analgesic

**INDICATIONS:** Relief of lower urinary tract discomfort due to hypermotility. Treatment of formaldehyde-susceptible cystitis, urethritis, trigonitis.

**DOSAGE:** *Adults:* Usual: 2 tabs qid with plenty of fluid.
*Pediatrics:* >6 yrs: Individualize dose. Take with plenty of fluid.

**HOW SUPPLIED:** Tab: Atropine 0.03mg-Benzoic Acid 4.5mg-Hyoscyamine 0.03mg-Methenamine 40.8mg-Methylene Blue 5.4mg-Phenyl Salicylate 18.1mg

**CONTRAINDICATIONS:** Glaucoma, pyloric or duodenal obstruction, urinary bladder neck obstruction, or cardiospasm.

**WARNINGS/PRECAUTIONS:** Caution with cardiovascular disorders. May precipitate acute urinary retention in prostatic hypertrophy.

**ADVERSE REACTIONS:** Rash, dry mouth, flushing, difficult micturition, rapid pulse, dizziness, blurred vision, urine/feces discoloration.

**INTERACTIONS:** Avoid alkalinizing agents/foods. Sulfonamides may precipitate in the urine; avoid concomitant use.

**PREGNANCY:** Category C, caution in nursing.

## URISPAS RX

flavoxate HCl (Ortho-McNeil)

**THERAPEUTIC CLASS:** Smooth muscle antispasmodic

**INDICATIONS:** Relief of dysuria, urgency, nocturia, suprapubic pain, frequency and incontinence.

**DOSAGE:** *Adults:* 100-200mg tid-qid. Reduce dose with improvement.
*Pediatrics:* >12 yrs: 100-200mg tid-qid. Reduce dose with improvement.

**HOW SUPPLIED:** Tab: 100mg

**CONTRAINDICATIONS:** Pyloric or duodenal obstruction, obstructive intestinal lesions or ileus, achalasia, GI hemorrhage, and obstructive uropathies of the lower urinary tract.

**WARNINGS/PRECAUTIONS:** Caution with glaucoma and while operating machinery where alertness is required. Drowsiness, blurred vision may occur.

**ADVERSE REACTIONS:** Drowsiness, dry mouth, nausea, vomiting, tachycardia, leukopenia, vertigo, nervousness, confusion, fatigue, headache, hyperpyrexia, constipation, urticaria, blurred vision.

**PREGNANCY:** Category B, caution in nursing.

## URO KP NEUTRAL RX

sodium phosphate - disodium phosphate - dipotassium phosphate
(Esprit)

**THERAPEUTIC CLASS:** Phosphate supplement

**INDICATIONS:** Prevention of recurrent calcium oxalate stones; increases urinary phosphate and pyrophosphate.

**DOSAGE:** *Adults:* 1-2 tab qid with a full glass of water.

**HOW SUPPLIED:** Tab: (Phosphorous-Potassium-Sodium) 258mg-49.4mg-262.4mg

**CONTRAINDICATIONS:** Infected phosphate stones. Severe renal impairment (<30% of normal). Hyperphosphatemia.

**WARNINGS/PRECAUTIONS:** Caution with potassium and/or sodium adjustments. May experience laxative effect during first few days of therapy; reduce daily dose or discontinue if severe. Caution with cardiac disease (eg, digitalized patients), severe adrenal insufficiency (eg, Addison's disease), acute dehydration, severe renal insufficiency/impairment or chronic renal disease, extensive tissue breakdown (eg, severe burns), myotonia congenita, cardiac failure, liver cirrhosis or severe hepatic disease, peripheral or pulmonary edema, hypernatremia, HTN, toxemia of pregnancy, hypoparathyroidism, acute pancreatitis. High serum phosphate may increase incidence of extraskeletal calcification. May be beneficial in rickets; use with caution. Monitor renal function and serum electrolytes.

**ADVERSE REACTIONS:** Diarrhea, nausea, stomach pain, vomiting, bone and joint pain.

**INTERACTIONS:** Antacids containing aluminum, magnesium or calcium may prevent absorption. Hypernatremia with concurrent diazoxide, guanethidine, hydralazine, methyldopa, rauwolfia alkaloids, mineralocorticoids. Calcium products and/or vitamin D may antagonize effects in hypercalcemia treatment. Hyperkalemia with concurrent potassium sparing diuretics or potassium-containing products.

**PREGNANCY:** Category C, caution in nursing.

## UROCIT-K RX

potassium citrate (Mission)

U

**THERAPEUTIC CLASS:** Urinary tract alkalinizer

**INDICATIONS:** Management of renal tubular acidosis (RTA) with calcium stones, hypocitraturic calcium oxalate nephrolithiasis of any etiology, and uric acid lithiasis with or without calcium stones.

**DOSAGE:** *Adults:* Initial: Severe Hypocitraturia (urinary citrate <150mg/day): 20mEq tid or 15mEq qid. Mild-Moderate Hypocitraturia (urinary citrate >150mg/day): 10mEq tid. Max: 100mEq/day. Measure urinary pH and 24-hr urinary citrate after 1st dose before titration.

**HOW SUPPLIED:** Tab, Extended Release: 5mEq, 10mEq

**CONTRAINDICATIONS:** Hyperkalemia, conditions with predisposition to hyperkalemia (eg, chronic renal failure, uncontrolled DM, acute dehydration, strenuous exercise, adrenal insufficiency, extensive tissue breakdown, K+-

sparing agents), delayed gastric emptying, esophageal compression, intestinal obstruction or stricture, anticholinergics, UTI, renal insufficiency, and PUD.

**WARNINGS/PRECAUTIONS:** Avoid with impaired mechanisms for excreting $K^+$ (eg, chronic renal failure, severe myocardial damage, or heart failure). Do not crush, chew, or suck tablet. GI mucosal lesions reported; d/c with severe vomiting, abdominal pain, or GI bleeding. Monitor serum electrolytes, serum creatinine and CBC every 4 months. D/C with hyperkalemia, urinary citrate and/or pH, increased serum creatinine, or decreased Hct or Hgb. Limit salt intake.

**ADVERSE REACTIONS:** Abdominal discomfort, vomiting, diarrhea, nausea.

**INTERACTIONS:** Avoid $K^+$-sparing diuretics. Increased GI irritation with drugs that slow GI transit time (eg, anticholinergics).

**PREGNANCY:** Category C, caution in nursing.

## UROGESIC BLUE RX

methenamine - methylene blue - phenyl salicylate - sodium biphosphate - hyoscyamine sulfate **(Edwards)**

**THERAPEUTIC CLASS:**
anticholinergic/antibacterial/antiseptic/analgesic/Acidifier

**INDICATIONS:** Treatment of symptoms of irritative voiding. Relief of lower urinary tract discomfort.

**DOSAGE:** *Adults:* 1 tab qid with plenty of fluid.
*Pediatrics:* >6 yrs: Individualize dose. Take with plenty of fluid.

**HOW SUPPLIED:** Tab: Hyoscyamine 0.12mg-Methenamine 81.6mg-Methylene Blue 10.8mg-Phenyl Salicylate 36.2mg-Sodium Biphosphate 40.8mg

**CONTRAINDICATIONS:** Consider risk-benefit with: cardiac disease, GI tract obstructive disease, glaucoma, myasthenia gravis, obstructive uropathy.

**WARNINGS/PRECAUTIONS:** Discontinue if rapid pulse, dizziness, or blurred vision occurs. Delay in gastric emptying may obscure gastric ulcer therapy. Caution in elderly.

**ADVERSE REACTIONS:** Rapid pulse, flushing, blurred vision, dizziness, shortness of breath, difficult micturition, acute urinary retention, dry mouth, nausea, vomiting, urine/feces discoloration.

**INTERACTIONS:** May decrease absorption of other oral agents (dose 2 hrs after ketoconazole). Reduced effectiveness with urinary alkaliners, thiazide diuretics, antacids/antidiarrheals (space dosing by 1 hr). Antimuscarinic effects potentiated with other antimuscarinics, MAOIs. Caution with antimyasthenics. Increased risk of constipation with opioids. Sulfonamides may precipitate in the urine.

**PREGNANCY:** Category C, safety in nursing not known.

## UROXATRAL RX

alfuzosin HCl **(Sanofi-Aventis)**



**THERAPEUTIC CLASS:** Alpha$_1$-blocker

**INDICATIONS:** Treatment of signs and symptoms of benign prostatic hyperplasia.

**DOSAGE:** *Adults:* 10mg qd, taken immediately after the same meal each day.

**HOW SUPPLIED:** Tab, Extended-Release: 10mg

**CONTRAINDICATIONS:** Moderate or severe hepatic insufficiency. Concomitant potent CYP3A4 inhibitors (eg, ketoconazole, itraconazole, ritonavir).

**WARNINGS/PRECAUTIONS:** Monitor for postural hypotension, syncope. Rule out prostate cancer. Discontinue with new or worsening angina. Caution with severe renal insufficiency. Caution in patients with congenital or aquired QT prolongation.

**ADVERSE REACTIONS:** Dizziness, upper respiratory tract infection, headache, fatigue, urticaria, angioedema, pruritis, rhinitis, tachycardia, chest pain, priapism, diarrhea, flushing, edema, angina pectoris.

**INTERACTIONS:** Increased levels with potent CYP3A4 inhibitors (eg, ketoconazole, itraconazole, ritonavir); concomitant use is contraindicated. Avoid use with other alpha-blockers. Increased levels with cimetidine, diltiazem, atenolol. Possibility of significant hypotension with other antihypertensives.

**PREGNANCY:** Category B, not for use in nursing.

## URSO

ursodiol (Axcan Scandipharm) RX

**OTHER BRAND NAMES:** Urso 250 (Axcan Scandipharm) - Urso Forte (Axcan Scandipharm)

**THERAPEUTIC CLASS:** Bile acid

**INDICATIONS:** Treatment of primary biliary cirrhosis.

**DOSAGE:** *Adults:* Usual: 13-15mg/kg/day given bid-qid with food.

**HOW SUPPLIED:** Tab: (Urso 250) 250mg, (Urso Forte) 500mg

**WARNINGS/PRECAUTIONS:** Administer appropriate specific treatment with variceal bleeding, hepatic encephalopathy, ascites, or when in need of urgent liver transplant.

**ADVERSE REACTIONS:** Diarrhea, leukopenia, peptic ulcer, hyperglycemia, skin rash, increased creatinine.

**INTERACTIONS:** Decreased absorption with bile acid sequestering agents (eg, cholestyramine, colestipol), aluminum-based antacids. Estrogens, oral contraceptives, clofibrate and perhaps other cholesterol-lowering agents may counteract effectiveness.

**PREGNANCY:** Category B, caution in nursing.

## VAGIFEM

estradiol (Novo Nordisk) RX

**Estrogens increase the risk of endometrial cancer.**

**THERAPEUTIC CLASS:** Estrogen

**INDICATIONS:** Treatment of atrophic vaginitis.

**DOSAGE:** *Adults:* Initial: Insert 1 tab vaginally qd for 2 weeks. Maint: Insert 1 tab twice weekly. Attempt to discontinue or taper at 3-6 month intervals.

**HOW SUPPLIED:** Tab, Vaginal: 25mcg

V

**CONTRAINDICATIONS:** Breast carcinoma or other estrogen dependent neoplasia, abnormal genital bleeding, pregnancy, porphyria, thrombophlebitis, thromboembolic disorders. History of thrombophlebitis, thrombosis, or thromboembolic disorders associated with estrogen use.

**WARNINGS/PRECAUTIONS:** Risk of gallbladder disease, thromboembolism, thrombotic disease. Elevated BP and hepatic adenomas reported. Monitor for hypercalcemia in breast cancer and bone metastases. Caution in asthma, epilepsy, migraine, cardiac or renal dysfunction due to fluid retention. Excessive uterine bleeding and mastodynia reported. Caution in liver dysfunction, metabolic bone disease associated with hypercalcemia, diabetes. May cause hypercoagulability and hyperlipoproteinemia. Caution in young patients.

**ADVERSE REACTIONS:** Vaginal spotting, vaginal discharge, allergic reactions, headache, abdominal pain, respiratory infection, genital moniliasis, back pain, rash.

**PREGNANCY:** Category X, caution in nursing.

## VAGISTAT-1 OTC

tioconazole (Novartis)

**THERAPEUTIC CLASS:** Azole antifungal

**INDICATIONS:** Treatment of recurrent vaginal yeast infections.

**DOSAGE:** *Adults:* Insert applicatorful intravaginally hs single dose. *Pediatrics:* >12 yrs: Insert applicatorful intravaginally hs single dose.

**HOW SUPPLIED:** Oint: 6.5% [4.6g]

**WARNINGS/PRECAUTIONS:** Do not use if abdominal pain, fever (>100°F), chills, nausea, vomiting, diarrhea, or foul smelling discharge. Do not use with tampons. Do not rely on condoms or diaphragm to prevent STDs or pregnancy until 3 days after last use.

**PREGNANCY:** Not for use in pregnancy, safety in nursing not known.

## VALCYTE RX

valganciclovir HCl (Roche Labs)

> **Granulocytopenia, anemia, and thrombocytopenia reported. Carcinogenic, teratogenic, and may cause aspermatogenesis based on animal studies.**

**THERAPEUTIC CLASS:** Synthetic guanine derivative nucleoside analogue

**INDICATIONS:** Treatment of cytomegalovirus (CMV) retinitis in AIDS patients. Prevention of CMV disease in kidney, heart, and kidney-pancreas transplant patients at high risk (Donor CMV seropositive/Recipient CMV seronegative).

**DOSAGE:** *Adults:* Treatment of CMV retinitis: Initial: 900mg bid for 21 days. Maint: 900mg qd. Prevention of CMV disease: 900mg qd starting within 10 days of transplantation until 100 days posttransplantation. CrCl 40-59mL/min: Initial: 450mg bid. Maint: 450mg qd. CrCl 25-39mL/min: Initial: 450mg qd. Maint: 450mg every other day. CrCl 10-21mL/min: Initial: 450mg every other day. Maint: 450mg twice weekly. CrCl <10mL/min: Not recommended. Take with food.

**HOW SUPPLIED:** Tab: 450mg

**CONTRAINDICATIONS:** Hypersensitivity to ganciclovir.

**WARNINGS/PRECAUTIONS:** Avoid if the neutrophils <500cells/mcL. Severe leukopenia, neutropenia, anemia, thrombocytopenia, pancytopenia, bone marrow depression, and aplastic anemia observed. Adjust dose in renal impairment. Do not substitute with ganciclovir caps.

**ADVERSE REACTIONS:** Diarrhea, nausea, vomiting, graft rejection, abdominal pain, pyrexia, headache, neutropenia, anemia, insomnia, peripheral neuropathy, convulsions, dizziness, ataxia, confusion.

**INTERACTIONS:** Greater risk for neutropenia and anemia with zidovudine. Monitor for toxicity with probenecid. Increased levels of metabolites of both drugs with mycophenolate mofetil. Increased risk of didanosine toxicity. Caution with myelosuppressive drugs or irradiation.

**PREGNANCY:** Category C, not for use in nursing.

## VALIUM

CIV

diazepam (Roche Labs)

**THERAPEUTIC CLASS:** Benzodiazepine

**INDICATIONS:** Management of anxiety disorders and short-term relief of anxiety symptoms. Symptomatic relief of acute alcohol withdrawal. Adjunct therapy in skeletal muscle spasm and convulsive disorders.

**DOSAGE:** *Adults:* Anxiety: 2-10mg bid-qid. Alcohol Withdrawal: 10mg tid-qid for 24 hours. Maint: 5mg tid-qid prn. Skeletal Muscle Spasm: 2-10mg tid-qid: Seizure Disorders: 2-10mg bid-qid. Elderly/Debilitated: 2-2.5mg qd-bid initially; may increase gradually as needed and tolerated.
*Pediatrics:* >6 months: 1-2.5mg tid-qid initially; may increase gradually as needed and tolerated.

**HOW SUPPLIED:** Tab: 2mg*, 5mg*, 10mg* *scored

**CONTRAINDICATIONS:** Acute narrow angle glaucoma, untreated open angle glaucoma, patients <6 months.

**WARNINGS/PRECAUTIONS:** Monitor blood counts and LFTs in long-term use. Neutropenia and jaundice reported. Increase in grand mal seizures reported. Avoid abrupt withdrawal. Caution with kidney or hepatic dysfunction.

**ADVERSE REACTIONS:** Drowsiness, fatigue, ataxia, paradoxical reactions, minor EEG changes.

**INTERACTIONS:** Phenothiazines, narcotics, barbiturates, MAOIs, and other antidepressants may potentiate effects. Delayed clearance with cimetidine. Avoid alcohol and other CNS-depressants. Risk of seizure with flumazenil.

**PREGNANCY:** Not for use during pregnancy, safety in nursing not known.

## VALTREX

RX

valacyclovir HCl (GlaxoSmithKline)

**THERAPEUTIC CLASS:** Nucleoside analogue

**INDICATIONS:** Treatment of herpes zoster (shingles) and herpes labialis (cold sores). Treatment or suppression of genital herpes in immunocompetent patients and for the suppression of recurrent genital herpes in HIV-infected patients.

**DOSAGE:** *Adults:* Herpes Zoster: 1g q8h for 7 days. Start within 48-72 hrs after onset of rash. CrCl 30-49mL/min: 1g q12h. CrCl 10-29mL/min: 1g q24h. CrCl <10mL/min: 500mg q24h. Genital Herpes: Initial: 1g q12h for 10 days. Start within 48-72 hrs after onset of symptoms. CrCl 10-29mL/min: 1g q24h. CrCl <10mL/min: 500mg q24h. Recurrent Episodes: Treatment: 500mg bid for 3 days. Start within 24 hrs after onset of symptoms. CrCl <29mL/min: 500mg q24h. Suppressive Therapy with Normal Immune Function:1g q24h. CrCl <29mL/min: 500mg q24h. Alternative: (<9 episodes/yr) 500mg q24h. CrCl <29mL/min: 500mg q48h. Suppressive Therapy with HIV and CD4 >100cells/mm³: 500mg q12h. CrCl <29mL/min: 500mg q24h. Herpes Labialis: 2g q12h for 1 day. Start at earliest symptom of cold sore. CrCl 30-49mL/min: 1g q12h. 10-29mL/min: 500mg q12h. <10mL/min: 500mg single dose. Administer therapy for 1 day. Initiate at earliest symptoms of a cold sore.
*Pediatrics:* Post-Pubertal: Herpes Zoster: 1g q8h for 7 days. Start within 48-72 hrs after onset of rash. CrCl 30-49mL/min: 1g q12h. CrCl 10-29mL/min: 1g q24h. CrCl <10mL/min: 500mg q24h. Genital Herpes: Initial: 1g q12h for 10 days. Start within 48-72 hrs after onset of symptoms. CrCl 10-29mL/min: 1g q24h. CrCl <10mL/min: 500mg q24h. Recurrent Episodes: Treatment: 500mg bid for 3 days. Start within 24 hrs after onset of symptoms. CrCl <29mL/min: 500mg q24h. Suppressive Therapy with Normal Immune Function:1g q24h. CrCl <29mL/min: 500mg q24h. Alternative: (<9 episodes/yr ) 500mg q24h. CrCl <29mL/min: 500mg q48h. Suppressive Therapy with HIV and CD4 >100cells/mm³: 500mg q12h. CrCl <29mL/min: 500mg q24h. Herpes Labialis: 2g q12h for 1 day. Start at earliest symptom of cold sore. CrCl 30-49mL/min: 1g

q12h. 10-29mL/min: 500mg q12h. <10mL/min: 500mg single dose. Administer therapy for 1 day. Initiate at earliest symptoms of a cold sore.

**HOW SUPPLIED:** Tab: 500mg, 1g

**CONTRAINDICATIONS:** Acyclovir hypersensitivity.

**WARNINGS/PRECAUTIONS:** Thrombotic thrombocytopenic purpura/hemolytic uremic syndrome reported with advanced HIV disease, allogenic bone marrow or renal transplants. Reduce dose with renal dysfunction. Possible renal and CNS toxicity in elderly.

**ADVERSE REACTIONS:** Nausea, headache, vomiting, dizziness, abdominal pain.

**INTERACTIONS:** Renal and CNS toxicity with nephrotoxic drugs.

**PREGNANCY:** Category B, caution in nursing.

## VANAMIDE RX

urea (Dermik)

**THERAPEUTIC CLASS:** Debriding/Healing Agent

**INDICATIONS:** Debridement and promotion of normal healing of surface lesions, particularly where healing is retarded by local infection, necrotic tissue, fibrinous or purulent debris, or eschar.

**DOSAGE:** *Adults*: Apply until absorbed. May cover with adhesive bandage or gauze. Keep dry and occlusive for 3-7 days.

**HOW SUPPLIED:** Cre: 40% [85g, 199g]

**WARNINGS/PRECAUTIONS:** Avoid contact with eyes. Discontinue if redness or irritation occurs.

**ADVERSE REACTIONS:** Transient stinging, burning, itching, irritation.

**PREGNANCY:** Safety in pregnancy or nursing not known.

## VANCOCIN RX

vancomycin HCl (Baxter)

**THERAPEUTIC CLASS:** Tricyclic glycopeptide antibiotic

**INDICATIONS:** Treatment of severe infections caused by susceptible strains of methicillin-resistant staphylococci. Indicated for penicillin-allergic patients, those who cannot receive or have failed to respond to other drugs, and for vancomycin-susceptible organisms that are resistant to other antimicrobials.

**DOSAGE:** *Adults:* Usual: 500mg IV q6h or 1g IV q12h. Mild to Moderate Renal Impairment: Initial: 15mg/kg/day. Maint: 1.9mg/kg/d. Administer 10mg/minute or over at least 60 minutes, whichever is longer. Renal Dysfunction: Initial: 15mg/kg. Dose is about 15x the GFR in mL/min (refer to table in labeling). Elderly: Require greater dose reduction. Functionally Anephric: Initial: 15mg/kg, then 1.9mg/kg/24hrs. Marked Renal Dysfunction: 250-1000mg every several days. Anuria: 1000mg every 7-10 days.
*Pediatrics:* Usual: 10mg/kg IV q6h. Infants/Neonates: Initial: 15mg/kg, then 10mg/kg q12h for neonates in the 1st week of life and q8h thereafter until 1 month of age. Administer over at least 60 minutes. Renal Dysfunction: Initial: 15mg/kg. Dose is about 15x the GFR in mL/min (refer to table in labeling). Premature Infants: Require greater dose reduction.

**HOW SUPPLIED:** Inj: 500mg/100mL, 1g/200mL

**CONTRAINDICATIONS:** Known allergy to corn or corn products because the solution contains dextrose.

**WARNINGS/PRECAUTIONS:** Only for colitis treatment; not systemically absorbed. Rapid bolus may cause hypotension, cardiac arrest (rare). Administer in a dilute solution over at least 60 minutes. Ototoxicity, pseudomembranous colitis reported. Adjust dose in renal dysfunction. Prolonged use may result in the overgrowth of nonsusceptible organisms.

Monitor renal and auditory function. Reversible neutropenia reported; monitor leukocyte count periodically. Intrathecal safety has not been assessed.

**ADVERSE REACTIONS:** Infusion-related events, hypotension, wheezing, pruritus, pain, chest and head muscle spasm, dyspnea, urticaria,"Red Man Syndrome," nephrotoxicity, pseudomembranous colitis, ototoxicity, neutropenia, phlebitis.

**INTERACTIONS:** Infusion-related events (eg, erythema, flushing, anaphylactoid reactions) increases with anesthetic agents. Carefully monitor with other neurotoxic or nephrotoxic drugs (eg, amphotericin B, aminoglycosides, bacitracin, polymyxin B, colistin, or cisplatin).

**PREGNANCY:** Category C, not for use in nursing.

## VANCOCIN ORAL — RX

vancomycin HCl (Viro Pharma)

**THERAPEUTIC CLASS:** Tricyclic glycopeptide antibiotic

**INDICATIONS:** Staphylococcal enterocolitis and antibiotic-associated pseudomembranous colitis caused by *C. difficile.*

**DOSAGE:** *Adults:* 500mg-2g/day given tid-qid for 7-10 days.
*Pediatrics:* 40mg/kg/day given tid-qid for 7-10 days. Max: 2g/day.

**HOW SUPPLIED:** Cap: 125mg, 250mg

**WARNINGS/PRECAUTIONS:** Not effective for other types of infection. Caution with inflammatory disorders of intestinal mucosa, renal impairment; increased risk of systemic absorption. Ototoxicity reported. Monitor auditory function.

**ADVERSE REACTIONS:** Nephrotoxicity, ototoxicity, reversible neutropenia, anaphylactoid reactions (hypotension, wheezing,"Red Man Syndrome," pruritus), superinfection.

**INTERACTIONS:** Monitor renal function with aminoglycosides.

**PREGNANCY:** Category B (Caps) or C (Susp), not for use in nursing.

## VANIQA — RX

eflornithine HCl (SkinMedica)

**THERAPEUTIC CLASS:** Ornithine decarboxylase inhibitor

**INDICATIONS:** Reduction of unwanted facial hair in women. Usage is limited to the face and areas under the chin.

**DOSAGE:** *Adults:* Apply to affected areas bid, at least 8 hrs apart. Rub in thoroughly. May wash area after 4 hrs. May apply 5 minutes after other hair removal techniques. May apply sunscreen or cosmetics after cream dries.
*Pediatrics:* >12 yrs: Apply to affected areas bid, at least 8 hrs apart. Rub in thoroughly. May wash area after 4 hrs. May apply 5 minutes after other hair removal techniques. May apply sunscreen or cosmetics after cream dries.



**HOW SUPPLIED:** Cre: 13.9% [30g]

**WARNINGS/PRECAUTIONS:** Discontinue if hypersensitivity or continued irritation occurs. Transient stinging/burning with abraded/broken skin. Condition may return to pretreatment levels 8 weeks after discontinuation.

**ADVERSE REACTIONS:** Acne, stinging/tingling skin, burning/dry skin, pseudofolliculitis barbae, alopecia.

**PREGNANCY:** Category C, caution in nursing.

## VANOS RX
fluocinonide (Medicis)

**THERAPEUTIC CLASS:** Corticosteroid

**INDICATIONS:** Corticosteroid responsive dermatoses.

**DOSAGE:** *Adults:* Apply thin layer to affected area qd-bid. Max: 60g/week. Do not exceed 2 weeks.
*Pediatrics:* ≥12 yrs: Appy thin layer to affected area qd-bid. Max: 60g/week. Do not exceed 2 weeks.

**HOW SUPPLIED:** Cre: 0.1% [30g, 60g]

**WARNINGS/PRECAUTIONS:** May produce reversible HPA axis suppression, manifestations of Cushing's syndrome, hyperglycemia, and glucosuria. Caution when applied to large surface areas or under occlusive dressings. Use appropriate antifungal or antibacterial agent with dermatological infections. Discontinue if infection does not clear or if irritation develops. Do not use for more than 2 weeks at a time.

**ADVERSE REACTIONS:** Headache, application site burning, nasopharyngitis, nasal congestion, unspecified application site reaction.

**PREGNANCY:** Category C, not for use in nursing.

## VANTAS RX
histrelin acetate (Valera)

**THERAPEUTIC CLASS:** Luteinizing hormone releasing hormone agonist

**INDICATIONS:** Palliative treatment of advanced prostate cancer.

**DOSAGE:** *Adults:* 50mg every 12 months. Inject SQ into inner aspect of the upper arm. Refrain from wetting the inserted arm for 24 hours. Refrain from heavy lifting or strenuous exercise of the inserted arm for 7 days after implant insertion. Must remove after 12 months of therapy.

**HOW SUPPLIED:** Implant: 50mg

**CONTRAINDICATIONS:** Women and pediatric patients.

**WARNINGS/PRECAUTIONS:** Transient increase in serum testosterone and worsening of symptoms of prostate cancer with initial therapy. Urethral obstruction and spinal cord compression reported. Anaphylactic reactions may occur.

**ADVERSE REACTIONS:** Hot flashes, fatigue, implant site reaction, testicular atrophy, renal impairment, gynecomastia, constipation, erectile dysfunction.

**PREGNANCY:** Category X, not for use in nursing.

## VANTIN RX
cefpodoxime proxetil (Pharmacia & Upjohn)

**THERAPEUTIC CLASS:** Cephalosporin (3rd generation)

**INDICATIONS:** Acute otitis media, pharyngitis/tonsillitis, community acquired pneumonia (CAP), acute bacterial exacerbation of chronic bronchitis (ABECB), acute uncomplicated urethral and cervical gonorrhea, acute uncomplicated ano-rectal infections in women, uncomplicated skin and skin structure infections (SSSI), acute maxillary sinusitis, uncomplicated urinary tract infections (UTI).

**DOSAGE:** *Adults:* Take tabs with food. Pharyngitis/Tonsillitis: 100mg q12h for 5-10 days. CAP: 200mg q12h for 14 days. ABECB: 200mg q12h for 10 days. Uncomplicated Gonorrhea (men and women)/Rectal Gonococcal Infections (women): 200mg single dose. SSSI: 400mg q12h for 7-14 days. Sinusitis: 200mg q12h for 10 days. UTI: 100mg q12h for 7 days. CrCl <30mL/min: Increase interval to q24h. Hemodialysis: Dose 3 times weekly after dialysis.

*Pediatrics:* >12 yrs: Take tabs with food. Pharyngitis/Tonsillitis: 100mg q12h for 5-10 days. CAP: 200mg q12h for 14 days. ABECB: 200mg q12h for 10 days. Uncomplicated Gonorrhea (men and women)/Rectal Gonococcal Infections (women): 200mg single dose. SSSI: 400mg q12h for 7-14 days. Sinusitis: 200mg q12h for 10 days. UTI: 100mg q12h for 7 days. 2 months-11 yrs: Otitis Media: 5mg/kg q12h for 5 days. Max: 200mg/dose. Pharyngitis/Tonsillitis: 5mg/kg q12h for 5-10 days. Max: 100mg/dose. Sinusitis: 5mg/kg q12h for 10 days. Max: 200mg/dose. CrCl <30mL/min: Increase interval to q24h. Hemodialysis: Dose 3 times weekly after dialysis.

**HOW SUPPLIED:** Sus: 50mg/5mL [50mL, 100mL], 100mg/5mL [50mL, 75mL, 100mL]; Tab: 100mg, 200mg

**WARNINGS/PRECAUTIONS:** Cross sensitivity to penicillins and other cephalosporins may occur. Pseudomembranous colitis reported. Positive direct Coombs' tests reported. Caution with renal dysfunction.

**ADVERSE REACTIONS:** Diarrhea, nausea, vaginal fungal infections, vulvovaginal infections, abdominal pain, headache, superinfection.

**INTERACTIONS:** Decreased plasma levels and absorption with antacids and $H_2$ blockers. Delayed peak plasma levels with anticholinergics. Probenecid inhibits renal excretion. Closely monitor renal function with nephrotoxic agents.

**PREGNANCY:** Category B, not for use in nursing.

## VAPRISOL

RX

conivaptan HCl (Astellas)

**THERAPEUTIC CLASS:** Arginine vasopressin antagonist

**INDICATIONS:** Treatment of euvolemic hyponatremia in hospitalized patients.

**DOSAGE:** *Adults:* IV use only. Use large veins and change infusion site every 24 hrs. Loading Dose: 20mg IV over 30 min. Follow with 20mg continuous IV over 24 hrs. Following initial day of treatment, administer for an additional 1-3 days in a continuous infusion of 20mg/day. Titrate: May increase to 40mg/day if needed. Total duration of infusion should not exceed 4 days

**HOW SUPPLIED:** Inj: 5mg/mL

**CONTRAINDICATIONS:** Hypovolemic hyponatremia. Concurrent potent CYP3A4 inhibitors (eg, ketoconazole, itraconazole, clarithromycin, ritonavir, and indinavir).

**WARNINGS/PRECAUTIONS:** Safety in CHF not established. Monitor sodium concentration and neurologic status during administration; discontinue if rapid rise in serum sodium. Caution with hepatic or renal impairment. Rotate infusion site every 24 hrs.

**ADVERSE REACTIONS:** Infusion site reactions, erythema/pain/phlebitis at infusion site, anemia, constipation, diarrhea, dry mouth, nausea, vomiting, peripheral edema, pyrexia, thirst, hypokalemia, headache, polyuria, cardiac failure, atrial dyrthythmias, and sepsis.

**INTERACTIONS:** See Contraindications. CYP3A4 inhibitors may increase levels. May increase levels of drugs primarily metabolized by CYP3A4 and digoxin.



**PREGNANCY:** Category C, caution in nursing.

## VAQTA

RX

hepatitis A vaccine (inactivated) (Merck)

**THERAPEUTIC CLASS:** Vaccine

**INDICATIONS:** Active immunization against hepatitis A virus in persons 12 months of age and older. Give primary immunization at least 2 weeks before expected exposure.

**DOSAGE:** *Adults:* ≥19 yrs: 1mL (50 U) IM followed by a booster of 1mL (50 U) 6-18 months later.
*Pediatrics:* 1-18 yrs: 0.5mL (25 U) IM followed by a booster of 0.5mL (25 U) 6-18 months later.

**HOW SUPPLIED:** Inj: 25 U/0.5mL, 50 U/mL

**WARNINGS/PRECAUTIONS:** Have epinephrine (1:1000) available. May not prevent hepatitis A with unrecognized infection. Caution with bleeding disorders. Defer use with acute infection or febrile illness. Suboptimal response may occur in immunocompromised patients.

**ADVERSE REACTIONS:** Injection-site pain, tenderness, erythema, swelling, warmth, fever.

**INTERACTIONS:** Immunosuppressive therapy may reduce response to active immunization.

**PREGNANCY:** Category C, caution in nursing.

## VASERETIC RX

hydrochlorothiazide - enalapril maleate (Merck)

**ACE inhibitors can cause death/injury to developing fetus during 2nd and 3rd trimesters. Stop therapy if pregnancy detected.**

**THERAPEUTIC CLASS:** ACE inhibitor/thiazide diuretic

**INDICATIONS:** Treatment of hypertension. Not for initial therapy.

**DOSAGE:** *Adults:* Initial (if not controlled with enalapril/HCTZ monotherapy): 5mg-12.5mg tab or 10mg-25mg tab qd. Titrate: May increase after 2-3 weeks. Max: 20mg enalapril/50mg HCTZ per day. Replacement Therapy: Substitute combination for titrated components.

**HOW SUPPLIED:** Tab: (Enalapril-HCTZ) 5mg-12.5mg, 10mg-25mg

**CONTRAINDICATIONS:** History of ACE inhibitor associated angioedema and hereditary or idiopathic angioedema. Anuria, sulfonamide hypersensitivity.

**WARNINGS/PRECAUTIONS:** D/C if angioedema, jaundice, or if marked LFT elevation occurs. Risk of hyperkalemia with DM, renal dysfunction. Persistent nonproductive cough reported. Monitor WBCs in renal and collagen vascular disease. Anaphylactoid reactions reported. Fetal/neonatal morbidity and death reported. Monitor for hypotension in high risk patients (surgery/anesthesia, hyponatremia, severe volume/salt depletion, etc). Caution with CHF, renal or hepatic dysfunction, obstruction to left ventricle outflow tract, elderly, renal artery stenosis. More reports of angioedema in blacks than nonblacks. May exacerbate or activate SLE. Monitor serum electrolytes. Avoid if CrCl <30mL/min/1.73m$^2$. May increase cholesterol, TG, uric acid levels, and blood glucose.

**ADVERSE REACTIONS:** Dizziness, cough, fatigue, orthostatic effects, diarrhea, nausea, muscle cramps, asthenia, impotence.

**INTERACTIONS:** Increase risk of hyperkalemia with $K^+$-sparing diuretics, $K^+$ supplements, or $K^+$-containing salt substitutes. Potentiates orthostatic hypotension with alcohol, barbiturates, and narcotics. Adjust insulin and antidiabetic drugs. Impaired absorption with cholestyramine, colestipol. Corticosteroids and ACTH deplete electrolytes. May decrease response to pressor amines. Potentiates other antihypertensives. May increase responsiveness to skeletal muscle relaxants. Risk of lithium toxicity. NSAIDs may reduce antihypertensive effect and worsen renal dysfunction.

**PREGNANCY:** Category C (1st trimester) and D (2nd and 3rd trimesters), not for use in nursing.

## VASOCON-A OTC

naphazoline HCl - antazoline phosphate (Novartis Ophthalmics)

**THERAPEUTIC CLASS:** Antihistamine/decongestant

**INDICATIONS:** Temporary relief of minor allergic symptoms of the eye, including itching and redness due to pollen and animal hair.

**DOSAGE:** *Adults:* 1-2 drops prn. Max: 4 doses/day.
*Pediatrics:* >6 yrs: 1-2 drops prn. Max: 4 doses/day.

**HOW SUPPLIED:** Sol: (Antazoline-Naphazoline) 0.5%-0.05% [15mL]

**WARNINGS/PRECAUTIONS:** Do not use if solution changes color or becomes cloudy. D/C if develop eye pain, vision changes, redness or irritaton continues, or if condition worsens or persists >72hrs. Supervision required with heart disease, HTN, or narrow angle glaucoma.

**PREGNANCY:** Safety in pregnancy and nursing not known.

## VASOTEC RX

enalapril maleate (Merck)

**ACE inhibitors can cause death/injury to developing fetus during 2nd and 3rd trimesters. Stop therapy if pregnancy detected.**

**THERAPEUTIC CLASS:** ACE inhibitor

**INDICATIONS:** Treatment of hypertension. Treatment of symptomatic CHF usually in combination with diuretics and digitalis. To decrease overt heart failure development and hospitalization in stable asymptomatic left ventricular dysfunction.

**DOSAGE:** *Adults:* HTN: If possible, discontinue diuretic 2-3 days prior to therapy. Initial: 5mg qd, 2.5mg qd with concomitant diuretic. Usual: 10-40mg/day given qd or bid. Resume diuretic if BP not controlled. CrCl <30mL/min: Initial: 2.5mg/day. Dialysis: 2.5mg/day on dialysis days. Heart Failure: Initial: 2.5mg/day. Usual: 2.5-20mg given bid. Max: 40mg/day. Left Ventricular Dysfunction: Initial: 2.5mg bid. Titrate: Increase to 20mg/day. Hyponatremia or SrCr 1.6mg/dL with Heart Failure: Initial: 2.5mg qd. Titrate: Increase to 2.5mg bid, then 5mg bid. Max: 40mg/day.
*Pediatrics:* HTN: 1 month-16 yrs: Initial: 0.08mg/kg (up to 5mg) qd. Titrate: Adjust according to response. Max: 0.58mg/kg/dose (or 40mg/dose). Avoid if GFR <30mL/min/1.73m$^2$. (To prepare 200mL of 1mg/mL sus: Add 50mL of BicitraB to polyethylene terephthalate bottle with ten 20mg tabs and shake for at least 2 minutes. Let stand for 60 minutes, then shake again for 1 minute. Add 150mL of Ora-Sweet SFC` and shake, then refrigerate. Can store up to 30 days.)

**HOW SUPPLIED:** Tab: 2.5mg*, 5mg*, 10mg, 20mg *scored

**CONTRAINDICATIONS:** History of ACE inhibitor associated angioedema and hereditary or idiopathic angioedema.

**WARNINGS/PRECAUTIONS:** D/C if angioedema, jaundice, or if marked LFT elevation occurs. Risk of hyperkalemia with DM, renal dysfunction. Persistent nonproductive cough reported. Monitor WBCs in renal or collagen vascular disease. Anaphylactoid reactions reported. Fetal/neonatal morbidity and death reported. Monitor for hypotension in high risk patients (heart failure, surgery/anesthesia, hyponatremia, high dose diuretic therapy, severe volume and/or salt depletion, etc). Caution with CHF, obstruction to left ventricle outflow tract, renal dysfunction, and renal artery stenosis. Less effective on BP in blacks and more reports of angioedema than nonblacks.

**ADVERSE REACTIONS:** Fatigue, orthostatic effects, asthenia, diarrhea, nausea, headache, dizziness, cough, rash, hypotension, vomiting.

**INTERACTIONS:** May increase lithium levels. Hypotension risk with diuretics. May further decrease renal dysfunction with NSAIDs. Increase risk of hyperkalemia with $K^+$-sparing diuretics, $K^+$-containing salt substitutes or $K^+$

supplements. Augmented effect by antihypertensives that cause renin release (eg, thiazides). NSAIDs may diminish antihypertensive effect.

**PREGNANCY:** Category C (1st trimester) and D (2nd and 3rd trimesters), not for use in nursing.

## VASOTEC I.V.

enalaprilat (Merck)

RX

**ACE inhibitors can cause death/injury to developing fetus during 2nd and 3rd trimesters. Stop therapy if pregnancy detected.**

**THERAPEUTIC CLASS:** ACE inhibitor

**INDICATIONS:** Treatment of hypertension when oral therapy is not practical.

**DOSAGE:** *Adults:* Administer IV over 5 minutes. Usual: 1.25mg q6h for no longer than 48 hrs. Max: 20mg/day. Concomitant Diuretic/CrCl <30mL/min: Initial: 0.625mg, may repeat after 1 hr. Maint: 1.25mg q6h. Risk of Excessive Hypotension: Initial: 0.625mg over 5 minutes to 1 hr. PO/IV Conversion: Give 5mg/day PO for 1.25mg IV q6h and 2.5mg/day PO for 0.625mg q6h IV.

**HOW SUPPLIED:** Inj: 1.25mg/mL

**CONTRAINDICATIONS:** History of ACE inhibitor associated angioedema and hereditary or idiopathic angioedema.

**WARNINGS/PRECAUTIONS:** D/C if angioedema, jaundice, or if marked LFT elevation occurs. Risk of hyperkalemia with DM, renal dysfunction. Persistent nonproductive cough reported. Monitor WBCs in renal or collagen vascular disease. Anaphylactoid reactions reported. Fetal/neonatal morbidity and death reported. Monitor for hypotension in high risk patients (heart failure, surgery/anesthesia, hyponatremia, high dose diuretic therapy, severe volume and/or salt depletion, etc). Caution with CHF, obstruction to left ventricle outflow tract, renal dysfunction, and renal artery stenosis. Less effective on BP in blacks and more reports of angioedema than nonblacks.

**ADVERSE REACTIONS:** Hypotension, headache, angioedema, myocardial infarction, fatigue, dizziness, fever, rash, constipation, cough.

**INTERACTIONS:** May increase lithium levels. Hypotension risk with diuretics. May further decrease renal dysfunction with NSAIDs. Increase risk of hyperkalemia with $K^+$-sparing diuretics, $K^+$-containing salt substitutes or $K^+$ supplements. Augmented effect by antihypertensives that cause renin release (eg, thiazides). NSAIDs may diminish antihypertensive effect.

**PREGNANCY:** Category C (1st trimester) and D (2nd and 3rd trimesters), not for use in nursing.

## VECTIBIX

panitumumab (Amgen)

RX

**Dermatologic toxicities and severe infusion reactions reported.**

**THERAPEUTIC CLASS:** Monoclonal antibody/EGFR-blocker

**INDICATIONS:** Treatment of EGFR-expressing, metastatic colorectal carcinoma with disease progression on or following fluoropyrimidine-, oxaliplatin-, and irinotecan-containing chemotherapy regimens.

**DOSAGE:** *Adults:* 6mg/kg IV infusion over 60 min every 14 days. Infuse doses >1000mg over 90 min. Reduce infusion rate by 50% with mild or moderate (Grade 1 or 2) infusion reaction for duration of that infusion. Immediately and permanently d/c infusion with severe (Grade 3 or 4) infusion reactions. Withhold for dermatologic toxicities that are ≥ Grade 3 or considered intolerable. If toxicity does not improve to ≤ Grade 2 within 1 month, permanently d/c. If dermatologic toxicity improves to ≤ Grade 2 and symptoms improve after withholding no more than 2 doses, treatment may be

V

resumed at 50% of original dose. If toxicities recur, permanently d/c. If toxicities do not recur, subsequent doses may be increased by increments of 25% of original dose until recommended dose of 6mg/kg is reached.

**HOW SUPPLIED:** Inj: 20mg/mL

**WARNINGS/PRECAUTIONS:** Toxicity involving GI mucosa, eye, and nail reported. Pulmonary fibrosis reported. Diarrhea may occur; incidence and severity may increase when used in combination with irinotecan. Use with leucovorin not recommended. Hypomagnesemia and hypocalcemia reported; monitor electrolytes during and for 8 weeks following therapy. Sunlight may exacerbate any skin reactions that may occur; use sunscreen and/or hats and limit sun exposure during therapy. Detection of EGFR protein expression is necessary for selection of appropriate patients.

**ADVERSE REACTIONS:** Rash, hypomagnesemia, paronychia, fatigue, abdominal pain, nausea, diarrhea, constipation, vomiting, erythema, acneiform dermatitis, pruritus, skin exfoliation, skin fissures, cough.

**PREGNANCY:** Category C, not for use in nursing.

## VECURONIUM RX

vecuronium bromide (Various)

**Administer by adequately trained individuals familiar with actions, characteristics, and hazards.**

**THERAPEUTIC CLASS:** Skeletal muscle relaxant (nondepolarizing)

**INDICATIONS:** Adjunct to general anesthesia, to facilitate endotracheal intubation, and to provide skeletal muscle relaxation during surgery or mechanical ventilation.

**DOSAGE:** *Adults:* Individualize dose. Initial: 0.08-0.1mg/kg IV bolus. Maint: 0.01-0.015mg/kg IV within 25-40 minutes of initial dose. Administer subsequent doses at 12-15 minute intervals under balanced anesthesia and slightly longer with inhalation agents. Max: 0.15-0.28mg/kg. Prior Succinylcholine: Reduce dose to 0.04-0.06mg/kg with inhalation anesthesia and 0.05-0.06mg/kg with balanced anesthesia. Continuous Infusion: Initial: 1mcg/kg/min administered 20-40 minutes after intubating dose of 80-100mcg/kg. Administer infusion after evidence of recovery from bolus. Adjust infusion rate to maintain 90% suppression of twitch response. Maint: 0.8-1.2mcg/kg/min. Concurrent Steady-State Enflurane/Isoflurane: Reduce rate 25-60%, 45-60 minutes after intubating dose.
*Pediatrics:* 10-17 yrs: Individualize dose. Initial: 0.08-0.1mg/kg IV bolus. Maint: 0.01-0.015mg/kg IV within 25-40 minutes of initial dose. Administer subsequent dose at 12-15 minute intervals under balanced anesthesia and slightly longer with inhalation agents. Max: 0.15-0.28mg/kg. Prior Succinylcholine: Reduce dose to 0.04-0.06mg/kg with inhalation anesthesia and 0.05-0.06mg/kg with balanced anesthesia. Continuous Infusion: Initial: 1mcg/kg/min administered 20-40 minutes after intubating dose of 80-100mcg/kg. Administer infusion after evidence of recovery from bolus. Adjust infusion rate to maintain 90% suppression of twitch response. Maint: 0.8-1.2mcg/kg/min. Concurrent Steady-State Enflurane/Isoflurane: Reduce rate 25-60%, 45-60 minutes after intubating dose. 1-10 yrs: May require a slightly higher initial dose and may also require supplementation slightly more often than adults.



**HOW SUPPLIED:** Inj: 10mg, 20mg

**WARNINGS/PRECAUTIONS:** May have profound effect in myasthenia gravis or myasthenic (Eaton Lambert) syndrome; use small test dose and monitor closely. Prolongation of neuromuscular blockade may occur in anephric patients; consider lower initial dose. Conditions associated with slower circulation time in cardiovascular disease, old age, and edematous states may delay onset time; dosage should not be increased. Prolonged recovery time reported with cirrhosis or cholestasis. In ICU, long-term use may be associated with prolonged paralysis and/or skeletal muscle weakness. Monitor neuromuscular transmission of ICU patients continuously with a nerve stimulator. Severe obesity and neuromuscular disease may pose airway or ventilatory problems. Electrolyte imbalances may alter neuromuscular blockade.

**ADVERSE REACTIONS:** Skeletal muscle weakness and paralysis.

**INTERACTIONS:** Enhanced neuromuscular blocking action with pancuronium, d-tubocurarine, metocurine, gallamine, enflurane, isoflurane, halothane, aminoglycosides, tetracyclines, bacitracin, polymyxin B, colistin, sodium colistimethate, and magnesium salts. Possible synergistic or antagonistic effects with other muscle relaxants. Prior administration of succinylcholine may enhance neuromuscular blocking effect.

**PREGNANCY:** Category C, safety in nursing not known.

## VELCADE RX

bortezomib (Millennium)

**THERAPEUTIC CLASS:** Proteasome inhibitor

**INDICATIONS:** Treatment of multiple myeloma and mantle cell lymphoma in patients who have received at least 1 prior therapy.

**DOSAGE:** *Adults:* Initial 1.3mg/m$^2$/dose IV bolus twice weekly for 2 weeks (days 1,4,8, and 11) followed by a 10-day rest period (days 12-21). At least 72 hrs should elapse between consecutive doses. Grade 3 Non-Hematological/Grade 4 Hematological Toxicities (excluding neuropathy): Withhold therapy until symptoms of toxcitiy resolve. Reinitiate at 25% reduced dose. Peripheral Neuropathy: Grade 1 with pain or Grade 2 (interfering with function but not activities of daily living): Reduce dose to 1mg/m$^2$. Grade 2 with pain or Grade 3 (interfering with activities of daily living): Withhold dose until toxicity resolves. Reinitiate at 0.7mg/m$^2$ once weekly. Grade 4 (permanent sensory loss interfering with funtion): Discontinue therapy.

**HOW SUPPLIED:** Inj: 3.5mg

**CONTRAINDICATIONS:** Hypersensitivity to boron or mannitol.

**WARNINGS/PRECAUTIONS:** Avoid pregnancy. May cause or worsen peripheral neuropathy along with reports of severe sensory and motor peripheral neuropathy. Thrombocytopenia and neutropenia reported; monitor CBC and platelets frequently. May cause orthostatic/postural hypotension; caution with history of syncope or dehydration. May cause an acute development or exacerbation of CHF and/or a new onset of decreased left ventricular ejection fraction. There have been rare reports of acute diffuse infiltrative pulmonary disease of unknown etiology such as pneumonitis, interstitial pneumonia, lung infiltration and Acute Respiratory Distress Syndrome. May cause nausea, diarrhea, constipation, and vomiting; use of antiemetic and antidiarrheal medications may be necessary. Rare reports of Reversible Posterior Leukoencephalopathy Syndrome have been reported. May cause tumor lysis syndrome. Hepatic impairment may decrease clearance. Closely monitor if CrCl <13mL/min or on hemodialysis. Patients on oral antidiabetic agents may require close monitoring of blood glucose levels. Monitor CBC frequently.

**ADVERSE REACTIONS:** Asthenic disorders, psychiatric disorders, nausea, diarrhea, decreased appetite, anorexia, constipation, thrombocytopenia, peripheral neuropathy, pyrexia, vomiting, anemia, headache, cough, dyspnea, reactivation of herpes infection, blurred vision, rash, hypotension.

**INTERACTIONS:** Caution with concomitant use of medications associated with peripheral neuropathy (eg, amiodarone, antivirals, isoniazid, nitrofurantoin, statins) or hypotension. Oral antidiabetic agents may require dosage adjustment. Caution with CYP3A4 inducers and inhibitors; may alter levels.

**PREGNANCY:** Category D, not for use in nursing.

## VENOFER

RX

iron sucrose (American Regent)

**THERAPEUTIC CLASS:** Iron supplement

**INDICATIONS:** Treatment of iron deficiency anemia in the following patients: non-dialysis dependent chronic kidney disease (NDD-CKD) patients receiving and not receiving erythropoietin; hemodialysis dependent chronic kidney disease (HDD-CKD) patients receiving an erythropoietin; peritoneal dialysis dependent chronic kidney disease (PDD-CKD) patients receiving an erythropoietin.

**DOSAGE:** *Adults:* HDD-CKD: 100mg IV injection over 2-5 minutes or 100mg infusion over at least 15 minutes per consecutive hemodialysis session for a total cumulative dose of 1000mg. NDD-CKD: 1000mg over a 14 day period as a 200mg slow IV injection undiluted over 2-5 minutes on 5 different occasions within the 14 day period.

**HOW SUPPLIED:** Inj: 20mg/mL

**CONTRAINDICATIONS:** Iron overload, anemia not caused by iron deficiency.

**WARNINGS/PRECAUTIONS:** Fatal hypersensitivity reactions characterized by anaphylactic shock, collapse, hypotension, and dyspnea reported. Caution with administration; hypotension may occur. Monitor hematologic and hematinic parameters periodically.

**ADVERSE REACTIONS:** Headache, fever, pain, asthenia, malaise, hypotension, chest pain, HTN, hypervolemia, nausea, vomiting, elevated LFTs, dizziness, cramps, musculoskeletal pain, dyspnea, cough, pruritus, application site reaction.

**INTERACTIONS:** Avoid oral iron preparations.

**PREGNANCY:** Category B, caution in nursing.

## VENTAVIS

RX

iloprost (CoTherix)

**THERAPEUTIC CLASS:** Systemic and pulmonary arterial vasulcar bed dilator

**INDICATIONS:** Treatment of pulmonary arterial hypertension (WHO Group I) in patients with NYHA Class III or IV symptoms.

**DOSAGE:** *Adults:* Initial: 2.5mcg via Prodose AAD System. Maint: 5mcg. Max: 45mcg/day. Should be taken 6 to 9 times per day.

**HOW SUPPLIED:** Sol, Inhalation: 20mcg/2mL

**WARNINGS/PRECAUTIONS:** Risk of syncope and hypotension. If signs of pulmonary edema occur when inhaled iloprost is administered, the treamtent should be immediately stopped. Avoid oral ingestion and contact with skin or eyes. Administration only via I-neb® AAD or Prodose® AAD System.

**ADVERSE REACTIONS:** Vasodilation, increased cough, headache, trismus, insomnia, nausea, hypotension, vomiting, flu syndrome, back pain, syncope, palpitations, muscle cramps, inreased GGT, increased alk phos.

**INTERACTIONS:** Iloprost has the potential to increase the hypotensive effect of vasodilators and antihypertensive agents. Increased risk of bleeding with anticoagulants.

**PREGNANCY:** Category C, not recommended in nursing.

## VENTOLIN HFA
RX

albuterol sulfate (GlaxoSmithKline)

**THERAPEUTIC CLASS:** $Beta_2$ agonist

**INDICATIONS:** Prevention and treatment of bronchospasm with reversible obstructive airway disease. Prevention of Exercise-Induced Bronchospasm (EIB).

**DOSAGE:** *Adults:* Bronchospasm: 2 inh q4-6h or 1 inh q4h. EIB: 2 inh 15-30 minutes before activity.
*Pediatrics:* ≥4 yrs: Bronchospasm: 2 inh q4-6h or 1 inh q4h. EIB: 2 inh 15-30 minutes before activity.

**HOW SUPPLIED:** MDI: 90mcg/inh [18g]

**WARNINGS/PRECAUTIONS:** D/C if paradoxical bronchospasm or cardiovascular events occur. Avoid excessive use. Caution with coronary insufficiency, arrhythmias, HTN, DM, hyperthyroidism, seizures, sensitivity to sympathomimetics. Hypersensitivity reactions may occur. May cause transient hypokalemia.

**ADVERSE REACTIONS:** Throat irritation, viral respiratory infections, upper respiratory inflammation, cough, musculoskeletal pain.

**INTERACTIONS:** Avoid other short-acting sympathomimetic bronchodilators; caution with oral sympathomimetics. Extreme caution with MAOIs, TCAs during or within 2 weeks of discontinuation. May cause severe bronchospasm with β-blockers. Decreases digoxin levels. ECG changes and/or hypokalemia with nonpotassium-sparing diuretics.

**PREGNANCY:** Category C, not for use in nursing.

## VEPESID
RX

etoposide (Bristol-Myers Squibb)

**Severe myelosuppression with bleeding or infection may occur.**

**THERAPEUTIC CLASS:** Podophyllotoxin derivative

**INDICATIONS:** (Inj) Adjunct therapy for management of refractory testicular tumors. (Cap, Inj) First line combination therapy for management of small cell lung cancer (SCLC).

**DOSAGE:** *Adults:* (Inj) Testicular Cancer: Range: 50-100mg/m$^2$/day IV on days 1-5 to 100mg/m$^2$/day IV on days 1, 3, and 5. SCLC: Range: 35mg/m$^2$/day IV for 4 days to 50mg/m$^2$/day for 5 days. After adequate recovery from toxicity, repeat course for either therapy at 3-4 week intervals. CrCl 15-50mL/min: 75% of dose. (PO) SCLC: Two times the IV dose and round to nearest 50mg.

**HOW SUPPLIED:** Cap: 50mg; Inj: 20mg/mL

**WARNINGS/PRECAUTIONS:** Observe for myelosuppression during and after therapy. Risk of anaphylactic reaction manifested by chills, fever, tachycardia, bronchospasm, dyspnea, and hypotension. Increased risk of toxicity with a low serum albumin. Perform CBC before each dose, during, and after therapy. May cause fetal harm in pregnancy.

**ADVERSE REACTIONS:** Myelosuppression, nausea, vomiting, anaphylactic-like reactions, hypotension (after rapid IV use), alopecia, anorexia.

**INTERACTIONS:** High dose oral cyclosporine reduces clearance.

**PREGNANCY:** Category D, not for use in nursing.

## VERAMYST

RX

fluticasone furoate (GlaxoSmithKline)

**THERAPEUTIC CLASS:** Corticosteroid

**INDICATIONS:** Treatment of the symptoms of seasonal and perennial allergic rhinitis in patients ≥2 yrs.

**DOSAGE:** *Adults:* Initial: 2 sprays per nostril qd. Maint: 1 spray per nostril qd. *Pediatrics:* ≥12 yrs: Initial: 2 sprays per nostril qd. Maint: 1 spray per nostril qd. 2-11 yrs: Initial: 1 spray per nostril qd. Titrate: If inadequate response, may increase to 2 sprays per nostril.

**HOW SUPPLIED:** Spray: 27.5mcg/spray [10g]

**WARNINGS/PRECAUTIONS:** Excessive use may cause hypercorticism and adrenal suppression. Risk of adrenal insufficiency and withdrawal symptoms when replacing systemic corticosteroids with topical corticosteroids. Caution with active or quiescent TB, ocular herpes simplex, or untreated bacterial, fungal, and systemic viral infections. Risk for more severe/fatal course of infections (eg, chickenpox, measles); avoid exposure in patients who have not had disease or have not been properly immunized. Epistaxis and nasal ulcerations may occur. Candida infection of nose reported. Avoid with recent nasal trauma, ulcers, or surgery. May result in glaucoma and cataracts. Potential for growth velocity reduction in pediatrics.

**ADVERSE REACTIONS:** Headache, epistaxis, nasopharyngitis, pyrexia, pharynolaryngeal pain, cough, nasal ulceration, back pain.

**INTERACTIONS:** Ketoconazole or other potent CYP3A4 inhibitors may increase serum fluticasone levels; co-administer with caution. Increased levels with ritonavir; avoid use.

**PREGNANCY:** Category C, caution in nursing.

## VERDESO

RX

desonide (Stiefel)

**THERAPEUTIC CLASS:** Corticosteroid

**INDICATIONS:** Mild-to-moderate atopic dermatitis.

**DOSAGE:** *Adults:* Apply thin layer to affected area bid. Max Duration: 4 consecutive weeks. Not to dispense directly on face; use hands to gently massage. Avoid occlusive dressings.
*Pediatrics:* ≥3 months: Apply thin layer to affected area bid. Max Duration: 4 consecutive weeks. Not to dispense directly on face; use hands to gently massage. Avoid occlusive dressings.

**HOW SUPPLIED:** Foam: 0.05% [50g, 100g]

**WARNINGS/PRECAUTIONS:** May produce reversible HPA axis suppression, manifestations of Cushing's syndrome, hyperglycemia, and glucosuria. Discontinue if irritation occurs. Caution when applied to large surface areas. Pediatrics may be more susceptible to systemic toxicity. Use an appropriate antifungal or antibacterial with concomitatnt skin infections; discontinue if infection does not clear.



**ADVERSE REACTIONS:** Application site burning, upper respiratory tract infection, cough.

**PREGNANCY:** Category C, caution in nursing.

## VERELAN

RX

verapamil HCl (Schwarz)

**THERAPEUTIC CLASS:** Calcium channel blocker (nondihydropyridine)

**INDICATIONS:** Management of hypertension.

**DOSAGE:** *Adults:* Usual: 240mg qam. Titrate: May increase by 120mg qam. Max: 480mg qam. Elderly/Small People: Initial: 120mg qam. Titrate: May increase to 180mg qam, then 240mg qam, then 360mg qam, then 480mg qam. May sprinkle on applesauce; do not crush or chew.

**HOW SUPPLIED:** Cap, Extended Release: 120mg, 180mg, 240mg, 360mg

**CONTRAINDICATIONS:** Severe ventricular dysfunction, hypotension, cardiogenic shock, sick sinus syndrome or 2nd- or 3rd-degree AV block (except with functioning ventricular pacemaker), A-Fib/Flutter with an accessory bypass tract.

**WARNINGS/PRECAUTIONS:** Avoid with moderate to severe cardiac failure, and ventricular dysfunction if taking a β-blocker. May cause hypotension, AV block, transient bradycardia, PR interval prolongation. Monitor LFTs periodically; hepatocellular injury reported. Give 30% of normal dose with severe hepatic dysfunction. Caution with hypertrophic cardiomyopathy, renal or hepatic dysfunction. Decrease dose in those with decreased neuromuscular transmission

**ADVERSE REACTIONS:** Constipation, dizziness, nausea, hypotension, headache, peripheral edema, infection, flu syndrome, fatigue, bradycardia, AV block.

**INTERACTIONS:** Additive negative effects on HR, AV conduction, and contractility with β-blockers. Potentiates other antihypertensives. May increase digoxin, carbamazepine, theophylline, cyclosporine, and alcohol levels. Avoid disopyramide within 48 hrs before or 24 hrs after verapamil. Additive negative inotropic effects and AV conduction prolongation with flecainide. Avoid quinidine with hypertrophic cardiomyopathy. Monitor lithium levels. Increased clearance with phenobarbital. Rifampin may reduce oral bioavailability. May potentiate neuromuscular blockers; both agents may need dose reduction. Caution with inhalation anesthetics. Increased bleeding time with ASA. Increased efficacy of doxorubicin. Reduced absorption with COPP and VAC cytotoxic drug regimens. May decrease clearance of paclitaxel. CYP3A4 inhibitors (eg, erythromycin, ritonavir) or grapefruit juice may increase levels. CYP3A4 inducers (eg, rifampin) may may lower levels.

**PREGNANCY:** Category C, not for use in nursing.

## VERELAN PM

verapamil HCl (Schwarz) RX

**THERAPEUTIC CLASS:** Calcium channel blocker (nondihydropyridine)

**INDICATIONS:** Management of hypertension.

**DOSAGE:** *Adults:* Usual: 200mg qhs. Titrate: May increase to 300mg qhs, then 400mg qhs. Renal or Hepatic Dysfunction/Elderly/Small People: Initial: 100mg qhs. Max: 400mg qhs. May sprinkle on applesauce; do not crush or chew.

**HOW SUPPLIED:** Cap, Extended Release: 100mg, 200mg, 300mg

**CONTRAINDICATIONS:** Severe ventricular dysfunction, hypotension, cardiogenic shock, sick sinus syndrome or 2nd- or 3rd-degree AV block (except with functioning ventricular pacemaker), A-Fib/Flutter with an accessory bypass tract.

**WARNINGS/PRECAUTIONS:** Avoid with moderate to severe cardiac failure, and ventricular dysfunction if taking a β-blocker. May cause hypotension, AV block, transient bradycardia, PR interval prolongation. Monitor LFTs periodically; hepatocellular injury reported. Give 30% of normal dose with severe hepatic dysfunction. Caution with hypertrophic cardiomyopathy, renal or hepatic dysfunction. Decrease dose in those with decreased neuromuscular transmission.

**ADVERSE REACTIONS:** Constipation, dizziness, nausea, hypotension, headache, peripheral edema, infection, flu syndrome, fatigue, bradycardia, AV block.

**INTERACTIONS:** Additive negative effects on HR, AV conduction, and contractility with β-blockers. Potentiates other antihypertensives. May increase digoxin, carbamazepine, theophylline, cyclosporine, and alcohol levels. Avoid disopyramide within 48 hrs before or 24 hrs after verapamil. Additive negative inotropic effects and AV conduction prolongation with flecainide. Avoid quinidine with hypertrophic cardiomyopathy. Monitor lithium levels. Increased clearance with phenobarbital. Rifampin may reduce oral bioavailability. May potentiate neuromuscular blockers; both agents may need dose reduction. Caution with inhalation anesthetics. Increased bleeding time with ASA. Increased efficacy of doxorubicin. Reduced absorption with COPP and VAC cytotoxic drug regimens. May decrease clearance of paclitaxel. CYP3A4 inhibitors (eg, erythromycin, ritonavir) or grapefruit juice may increase levels. CYP3A4 inducers (eg, rifampin) may decrease levels.

**PREGNANCY:** Category C, not for use in nursing.

## VERSED INJECTION CIV

midazolam HCl (Roche Labs)

**Associated with respiratory depression and respiratory arrest especially when used for sedation in noncritical care settings. Do not administer by rapid injection to neonates. Continuous monitoring required.**

**THERAPEUTIC CLASS:** Benzodiazepine

**INDICATIONS:** For sedation, anxiolysis, and amnesia induction pre-op, prior to or during diagnostic, therapeutic, or endoscopic procedures, either alone or in combination with other CNS depressants. For induction of general anesthesia. For sedation of intubated and ventilated patients.

**DOSAGE:** *Adults:* IV: Sedation/Anxiolysis/Amnesia Induction: <60 yrs: Initial: 1-2.5mg IV over 2 min. Max: 5mg. Titrate: In small increments at 2 min intervals if needed. Concomitant Narcotics/Other CNS Depressants: Reduce by 30%. >60 yrs/Debilitated/Chronically Ill: Initial: 1-1.5mg IV over 2 min. Max: 3.5mg. Titrate: In small increments at 2 min intervals if needed. Concomitant Narcotics/Other CNS Depressants. Reduce by 50%. Maint: 25% of sedation dose by slow titration. IM: Preoperative Sedation/Anxiolysis/Amnesia: <60 yrs: 0.07-0.08mg/kg IM up to 1 hr before surgery. >60 yrs/Debilitated: 1-3mg IM. Anesthesia Induction: Unpremedicated: <55 yrs: Initially: 0.3-0.35mg/kg IV over 20-30 seconds. May give additional doses of 25% of initial dose to complete induction. >55 yrs: Initial: 0.3mg/kg IV. Debilitated: Initial: 0.15-0.25mg/kg IV. Premedicated: <55 yrs: Initial: 0.25mg/kg IV over 20-30 seconds. >55 yrs: Initial: 0.2mg/kg IV. Debilitated: 0.15mg/kg IV. Maintenance Sedation: LD: 0.01-0.05mg/kg IV. May repeat dose at 10-15 min intervals until adequate sedation. Maint: 0.02-0.1mg/kg/hr. Titrate to desired level of sedation using 25-50% adjustments. Infusion rate should be decreased 10-25% every few hrs to find minimum effective infusion rate.

*Pediatrics:* Sedation/Anxiolysis/Amnesia Induction: IV: <6 months: Limited information; titrate with small increments and monitor. 6 months-5 yrs: Initial: 0.05-0.1mg/kg IV over 2-3 min, up to 0.6mg/kg if needed. Max: 6mg. 6-12 yrs: Initial: 0.025-0.05mg/kg IV over 2-3 min, up to 0.4mg/kg if needed. Max: 10mg. 12-16 yrs: 1-2.5mg IV over 2 min. Titrate: In small increments at 2 min intervals if needed. Max: 10mg. IM: 0.1-0.15mg/kg IM, up to 0.5mg/kg if needed. Max: 10mg. Sedation: LD: 0.05-0.2mg/kg IV infusion over 2-3 min. Maint: 0.06-0.12mg/kg/hr IV infusion. May adjust dose by 25%. Sedation in Critical Care: Neonatal Dose: <32 weeks: Initial: 0.03mg/kg/hr IV infusion. >32 weeks: Initial: 0.06mg/kg/hr IV infusion. Adjust to lowest effective dose.

**HOW SUPPLIED:** Inj: 1mg/mL, 5mg/mL

**CONTRAINDICATIONS:** Acute narrow-angle glaucoma, untreated open-angle glaucoma, intrathecal or epidural use.

**WARNINGS/PRECAUTIONS:** Agitation, involuntary movements, hyperactivity, and combativeness reported. Caution with CHF, chronic renal failure, pulmonary disease, uncompensated acute illnesses (eg, severe fluid or electrolyte disturbances), elderly or debilitated. Avoid use with shock or coma, or in acute alcohol intoxication with depression of vital signs. Contains benzyl alcohol.

**ADVERSE REACTIONS:** Decreased tidal volume and/or respiratory rate, BP/HR variations, apnea, hypotension, pain and local reactions at injection site, hiccoughs, nausea, vomiting, desaturation.

**INTERACTIONS:** Prolonged sedation with CYP450 3A4 inhibitors (eg, erythromycin, diltiazem, verapamil, ketoconazole, itraconazole, saquinavir, cimetidine). Increased sedative effects with morphine, meperidine, fentanyl, secobarbital, droperidol or other CNS depressants. Avoid use with acute alcohol intoxication. Decreases concentration of halothane and thiopental required for anesthesia. May cause severe hypotension with concomitant use of fentanyl in neonates.

**PREGNANCY:** Category D, caution in nursing.

## VERSED SYRUP

CIV

midazolam HCl (Roche Labs)

**Associated with respiratory depression and respiratory arrest especially when used for sedation in noncritical care settings. Reports of airway obstruction, desaturation, hypoxia, and apnea especially with other CNS depressants. Continuous monitoring required.**

**THERAPEUTIC CLASS:** Benzodiazepine

**INDICATIONS:** Use in pediatric patients for sedation, anxiolysis and amnesia prior to diagnostic procedures or before induction of anesthesia.

**DOSAGE:** *Pediatrics:* 0.25-1mg/kg single dose. Max: 20mg.

**HOW SUPPLIED:** Syrup: 2mg/mL [118mL]

**CONTRAINDICATIONS:** Acute narrow-angle glaucoma.

**WARNINGS/PRECAUTIONS:** Monitor for respiratory adverse events and paradoxical reactions.

**ADVERSE REACTIONS:** Emesis, nausea, agitation, hypoxia, laryngospasm, bradycardia, prolonged sedation, rash.

**INTERACTIONS:** Decreased levels with CYP3A4 inducers (eg, rifampin, carbamazepine, phenytoin). Increased levels with CYP3A4 inhibitors (eg, azole antimycotics, protease inhibitors, calcium channel blockers, macrolide antibiotics, cimetidine). Increased sedative and respiratory effects with narcotics, propofol, ketamine, nitrous oxide, droperidol, barbiturates, alcohol and other CNS depressants. Caution with anesthetics.

**PREGNANCY:** Category D, caution in nursing.

## VESANOID

RX

tretinoin (Roche Labs)

**Administer under strict supervision of experienced physician and institution. Risk of retinoic acid-APL syndrome and leukocytosis. High risk of teratogenic effects.**

**THERAPEUTIC CLASS:** Retinoid

**INDICATIONS:** Induction of remission in acute promyelocytic leukemia (APL) in those resistant to anthracycline therapy or those where anthracycline-based therapy is contraindicated.

**DOSAGE:** *Adults:* 45mg/m$^2$/day in 2 divided doses. D/C 30 days after achieving complete remission or after 90 days of therapy, whichever occurs 1st.
*Pediatrics:* 45mg/m$^2$/day in 2 divided doses. D/C 30 days after achieving complete remission or after 90 days of therapy, whichever occurs 1st.

**HOW SUPPLIED:** Cap: 10mg

**CONTRAINDICATIONS:** Sensitivity to parabens.

**WARNINGS/PRECAUTIONS:** May cause abortion or fetal abnormalities. Females should use contraception during and 1 month after therapy. Confirm APL diagnosis. Pseudotumor cerebri reported, especially in pediatrics. Reversible hypercholesterolemia, hypertriglyceridemia reported. Elevated LFTs reported; d/c if >5x ULN. Monitor for signs of respiratory compromise or leukocytosis. Check hematologic profile, coagulation profile, LFTs, and cholesterol frequently.

**ADVERSE REACTIONS:** Malaise, shivering, hemorrhage, infections, peripheral edema, pain, chest discomfort, edema, disseminated intravascular coagulation, weight change, injection site reactions, dyspnea, pleural effusion, respiratory insufficiency, pneumonia.

**INTERACTIONS:** Possible interactions with drugs that affect CYP450 system. Aggravated symptoms of hypervitaminosis A with vitamin A. Cases of fatal thrombotic complications with antifibrinolytic agents (eg, tranexamic acid, aminocaproic acid).

**PREGNANCY:** Category D, not for use in nursing.

## VESICARE — RX

solifenacin succinate (Yamanouchi)

**THERAPEUTIC CLASS:** Muscarinic receptor antagonist

**INDICATIONS:** Treatment of overactive bladder with symptoms of urge urinary incontinence, urgency, and urinary frequency.

**DOSAGE:** *Adults:* Usual: 5mg qd. Max: 10mg qd. Renal Impairment (CrCl< 30mL/min)/ Moderate Hepatic Impairment (Child-Pugh B)/ Potent CYP3A4 Inhibitors: Max: 5mg qd. Do not use in severe hepatic impairment (Child-Pugh C).

**HOW SUPPLIED:** Tab: 5mg, 10mg

**CONTRAINDICATIONS:** Urinary retention, gastric retention, uncontrolled narrow-angle glaucoma.

**WARNINGS/PRECAUTIONS:** Caution with bladder outflow obstruction, decreased gastrointestinal motility, and narrow-angle glaucoma. Caution with renal and hepatic impairment.

**ADVERSE REACTIONS:** Dry mouth, constipation, nausea, dyspepsia, UTI, blurred vision.

**INTERACTIONS:** Do not exceed 5mg daily dose when administered with therapeutic doses of ketoconazole or other potent CYP3A4 inhibitors.

**PREGNANCY:** Category C, not for use in nursing.

## VEXOL — RX

rimexolone (Alcon)

**THERAPEUTIC CLASS:** Corticosteroid

**INDICATIONS:** Management of postoperative inflammation. Treatment of anterior uveitis.



**DOSAGE:** *Adults:* Postoperative Inflammation: 1-2 drops qid beginning 24 hrs postoperative; continue for 2 weeks thereafter. Anterior Uveitis: 1-2 drops every hourr while awake for 1st week, then 1 drop q2h while awake in 2nd week, then taper dose until resolved.

**HOW SUPPLIED:** Sus: 1% [5mL, 10mL]

**CONTRAINDICATIONS:** Viral diseases of the cornea and conjunctiva including epithelial herpes simplex keratitis, vaccinia, and varicella. Mycobacterial infection and fungal diseases of the eye. Acute purulent untreated infections.

**WARNINGS/PRECAUTIONS:** Not for injection into the eye. Prolonged use may result in ocular HTN/glaucoma, optic nerve damage, visual acuity and vision field defects, cataracts, secondary ocular infections (eg, fungal infections). Monitor IOP after 10 days of therapy. Re-evaluate if no response after 2 days.

**ADVERSE REACTIONS:** Elevated IOP, secondary ocular infections, blurred vision, ocular pain, discharge, hyperemia, pruritus, foreign body sensation, discomfort.

**PREGNANCY:** Category C, not for use in nursing.

## VFEND RX

voriconazole (Pfizer)

**THERAPEUTIC CLASS:** Triazole antifungal

**INDICATIONS:** Treatment of invasive aspergillosis, esophageal candidiasis. Treatment of serious fungal infections caused by *Scedosporium apiospermum* and *Fusarium* spp. including *Fusarium solani* in patientsintolerant of, or refractory to, other therapy. Treatment of candidemia in non-neutropenic patients and the following *Candida* infections: disseminated infections in skin and infections in abdomen, kidney, bladder wall, and wounds.

**DOSAGE:** *Adults:* Invasive Aspergillosis/Infections Due to *Fusarium* spp. and *Scedosporium apiospermum*: (Inj) LD: 6mg/kg IV q12h x 1st 24 hrs. Maint: 4mg/kg IV q12h; may reduce to 3mg/kg if unable to tolerate. Switch to PO when appropriate. (PO) Maint: ≥40kg: 200mg q12h. <40kg: 100mg q12h. Esophageal Candidiasis: (PO) ≥40kg: 200mg q12h. <40kg: 100mg q12h. Treat for minimum of 14 days and at least 7 days following resolution of symptoms. Candidemia Non-Neutropenic Patients/Deep Tissue *Candida* Infections: (Inj) LD: 6mg/kg IV q12h x 1st 24 hrs. (Inj) Maint: 3-4mg/kg IV q12h. (PO) Maint: ≥40kg: 200mg q12h. <40kg: 100mg q12h. Treat for at least 14 days following resolution of symptoms or following last positive culture, whichever is longer. For PO maint dosing, if inadequate response may increase from 200mg q12h to 300mg q12h for ≥40kg or from 100mg q12h to 150mg q12h for <40kg. If unable to tolerate higher PO maint doses, may reduce by 50mg steps from 300mg q12h to minimum of 200mg q12h for ≥40kg or from 150mg q12h to minimum of 100mg q12h for <40kg. Concomitant Phenytoin: Maint: IV: 5mg/kg q12h. PO: ≥40kg: 400mg q12h. <40kg: 200mg q12h. Concomitant Efavirenz: Maint: 400mg q12h and efavirenz 300mg q24h. Mild to Moderate Hepatic Cirrhosis: Maint: Use 1/2 of maint dose. CrCl <50mL/min: Use PO. Take PO 1 hr before or 1 hr after a meal. Base duration on severity of underlying disease, recovery from immunosuppression, and clinical response.

**HOW SUPPLIED:** Inj: 200mg; Sus: 40mg/mL; Tab: 50mg, 200mg

**CONTRAINDICATIONS:** Concomitant CYP3A4 substrates (terfenadine, astemizole, cisapride, pimozide, quinidine), sirolimus, rifampin, carbamazepine, long-acting barbiturates, high-dose ritonavir (400mg q12h), standard doses of efavirenz (adjusted dose may be adminstered), rifabutin, ergot alkaloids.

**WARNINGS/PRECAUTIONS:** Monitor visual function with treatment >28 days. Hepatic reactions (clinical hepatitis, cholestasis, fulminant hepatic failure) reported; monitor LFTs at initiation and during therapy. Discontinue if liver dysfunction occurs. Tabs contain lactose; avoid with galactose intolerance, Lapp lactase deficiency, or glucose-galactose malabsorption. Anaphylactoid-type reactions reported with infusion. Avoid strong, direct sunlight. Monitor renal function. May prolong QT interval; caution with proarrhythmic conditions. Correct electrolyte disturbances before starting therapy. If rash develops, monitor closely and consider discontinuation of voriconazole.

**ADVERSE REACTIONS:** Visual disturbances, fever, chills, rash, headache, nausea, vomiting, sepsis, peripheral edema, abdominal pain, respiratory disorder, increased LFTs and alkaline phosphatase.

**INTERACTIONS:** See Contraindications. Avoid with low-dose ritonavir (100mg q12h). May increase levels of CYP3A4 inhibitors; monitor for adverse events and toxicity with HIV protease inhibitors, NNRTIs, benzodiazepines, HMG Co-A reductase inhibitors, dihydropyridine calcium channel blockers, and vinca alkaloids. May increase levels of CYP2C9 inhibitors; monitor phenytoin, warfarin, hypoglycemics, tacrolimus (reduce tacrolimus to 1/3 of initial dose), and cyclosporine (reduce cyclosporine to 1/2 of initial dose). Omeprazole is CYP2C19/3A4 inhibitor; reduce omeprazole by 1/2 if voriconazole ≥40mg. Proton pump inhibitors that are CYP2C19 substrates may increase levels. Phenytoin may decrease levels. Oral contraceptives containing ethinyl estradiol and norethindrone may increase levels. May increase levels of oral contraceptives containing ethinyl estradiol and norethindrone. May increase levels of methadone; may prolong QT interval; dose reduction may be needed. Do not infuse into same line or cannula with other drug infusions or parenteral nutrition. Do not infuse simultaneously with blood products or electrolyte supplements.

**PREGNANCY:** Category D, not for use in nursing.

## VIADUR — RX

leuprolide acetate (Bayer)

**THERAPEUTIC CLASS:** Synthetic gonadotropin releasing hormone analog

**INDICATIONS:** Palliative treatment of advanced prostate cancer.

**DOSAGE:** *Adults:* Insert 1 implant SQ in upper arm every 12 months.

**HOW SUPPLIED:** Implant: 65mg

**CONTRAINDICATIONS:** Women, pregnancy, pediatrics.

**WARNINGS/PRECAUTIONS:** Transient worsening of symptoms may occur during 1st few weeks of therapy. Closely monitor patients with metastatic vertebral lesions and/or urinary tract obstruction during 1st few weeks of therapy. Monitor serum testosterone, PSA. Ureteral obstruction and spinal cord decompression reported.

**ADVERSE REACTIONS:** Headache, asthenia, hot flashes, extremity pain, diarrhea, ecchymosis, anemia, peripheral edema, depression, sweating, gynecomastia, nocturia, urinary frequency, testis atrophy, breast pain, impotence.

**PREGNANCY:** Category X, safety in nursing not known.

## VIAGRA — RX

sildenafil citrate (Pfizer)

**THERAPEUTIC CLASS:** Phosphodiesterase type 5 inhibitor

**INDICATIONS:** Treatment of erectile dysfunction.

**DOSAGE:** *Adults:* Usual: 50mg 1 hr (range 0.5-4 hrs) prior to sexual activity at frequency of up to once daily. Titrate: May decrease to 25mg qd or increase to 100mg qd. Max: 100mg qd. Elderly/Hepatic Impairment/CrCl <30mL/min/Concomitant CYP450 3A4 Inhibitors (eg, ketoconazole, itraconazole, erythromycin, saquinavir): Initial: 25mg qd. Concomitant Ritonavir: Max: 25mg q48h. Concomitant alpha-blocker: Avoid doses >25mg sildenafil within 4 hours of an alpha-blocker.

**HOW SUPPLIED:** Tab: 25mg, 50mg, 100mg

**CONTRAINDICATIONS:** Organic nitrates taken regularly and/or intermittently.

**WARNINGS/PRECAUTIONS:** Caution with MI, stroke or life-threatening arrhythmia within last 6 months; with resting hypotension (BP<90/50) or HTN (BP>170/110); unstable angina due to cardiac failure or CAD; anatomical penile deformation; predisposition to priapism; and retinitis pigmentosa. Avoid in men where sexual activity is inadvisable due to underlying CV status. Decrease in supine BP reported. Rare reports of non-arteritic anterior ischemic optic neuropathy (NAION) with PDE5 inhibitors. Caution when PDE5 inhibitors are given concomitantly with alpha-blockers. PDE5 inhibitors and alpha-adrenergic blocking agents are both vasodilators with BP-lowering effects; additive effect on BP may be anticipated.

**ADVERSE REACTIONS:** Headache, flushing, dyspepsia, nasal congestion, UTI, abnormal vision (eg, color tinge, increased light sensitivity, blurred vision), diarrhea, cardiovascular events.

**INTERACTIONS:** Increased levels with CYP3A4 inhibitors (eg, cimetidine, ketoconazole, itraconazole, erythromycin, saquinavir) and protease inhibitors (eg, ritonavir). CYP2C9 inhibitors may decrease sildenafil clearance. CYP3A4 inducers (eg, rifampin) may decrease levels. Potentiates hypotensive effects of nitrates. Additional supine BP reduction with amlodipine reported. Simultaneous administration with alpha-blockers may lead to symptomatic hypotension; sildenafil dose should not exceed 25mg and should not be taken within 4 hrs of taking an alpha-blocker. Avoid with other ED treatments.

**PREGNANCY:** Category B, not for use in nursing.

## VIBRAMYCIN

RX

doxycycline hyclate (Pfizer)

**OTHER BRAND NAMES:** Vibra-Tabs (Pfizer)

**THERAPEUTIC CLASS:** Tetracycline derivative

**INDICATIONS:** Treatment of susceptible infections including respiratory, urinary, skin and skin structure, lymphogranuloma, psittacosis, trachoma, uncomplicated urethral/endocervical/rectal, nongonococcal urethritis, rickettsiae, chancroid, plague, cholera, brucellosis, anthrax. When penicillin is contraindicated, treatment of uncomplicated gonorrhea, syphilis, listeriosis, *Clostridium* species, and others. Adjunct therapy for amebiasis and severe acne. Prophylaxis of malaria.

**DOSAGE:** *Adults:* Usual: 100mg q12h on day 1, then 100mg qd or 50mg q12h. Severe Infection: 100mg q12h. Treat for 10 days with strep infection. Uncomplicated Gonococcal Infection (Except Anorectal in Men): 100mg bid for 7 days or 300mg followed by 300mg in 1 hour. Uncomplicated Urethral/Endocervical/Rectal Infection and Nongonococcal Urethritis: 100mg bid for 7 days. Syphilis: 100mg bid for 2 weeks. Syphilis for >1 yr: 100mg bid for 4 weeks. Acute Epididymo-orchitis: 100mg bid for at least 10 days. Inhalation Anthrax (Post-Exposure): 100mg bid for 60 days. Malaria Prophylaxis: 100mg qd. Begin 1-2 days before travel and continue for 4 weeks after leaving malarious area.
*Pediatrics:* >8 yrs: <100 lbs: 1mg/lb bid on day 1, then 1mg/lb qd or 0.5mg/lb bid. Severe Infections: Maint: 2mg/lb. >100lbs: Usual: 100mg q12h on day 1, then 100mg qd or 50mg q12h. Severe Infection: 100mg q12h. Treat for 10 days with strep infection. Inhalation Anthrax (Post-Exposure): <100lbs: 1mg/lb bid for 60 days. >100lbs: 100mg bid for 60 days. Malaria Prophylaxis: 2mg/kg qd. Max: 100mg/day. Begin 1-2 days before travel and continue for 4 weeks after leaving malarious area.

**HOW SUPPLIED:** Cap: (Doxycycline Hyclate) 50mg, 100mg; Syr: (Doxycycline Calcium) 50mg/5mL; Sus: (Doxycycline Monohydrate) 25mg/5mL [60mL]; Tab: (Vibra-Tabs) 100mg

**WARNINGS/PRECAUTIONS:** May cause fetal harm with pregnancy. Permanent tooth discoloration during tooth development (last half of pregnancy and children <8 yrs) reported. May increase BUN. Photosensitivity, enamel hypoplasia reported. Superinfection with prolonged use. Syrup contains sodium metabisulfite. Bulging fontanels in infants and benign intracranial HTN in adults reported. Monitor renal/hepatic and hematopoietic function with long-term use. Take adequate fluids with caps or tabs to reduce esophageal irritation. Take with food or milk if GI irritation occurs.

**ADVERSE REACTIONS:** GI effects, photosensitivity, increased BUN, hypersensitivity reactions, blood dyscrasias.

**INTERACTIONS:** May decrease PT, adjust anticoagulants. May interfere with bactericidal agents (eg, penicillin). May decrease effects of oral contraceptives. Aluminum-, calcium-, iron- and magnesium-containing products and bismuth subsalicylate impair absorption. Decreased half-life with barbiturates, carbamazepine, and phenytoin. Fatal renal toxicity with methoxyflurane.

**PREGNANCY:** Category D, not for use in nursing.

## VIBRAMYCIN IV

RX

doxycycline hyclate (Pfizer)

**THERAPEUTIC CLASS:** Tetracycline derivative

**INDICATIONS:** Treatment of rickettsiae, *Mycoplasma pneumoniae*, psittacosis, ornithosis, lymphogranuloma venereum, granuloma inguinale, relapsing fever, chancroid, *Pasteurella pestis, Pasturella tularensis, Bartonella bacilliformis, Bacteroides* species, *Vibrio comma, Vibrio fetus, Brucella* species, *E.coli, Enterobacter aerogenes, Shigella* species, *Mima* species, *Herellea* species, *Haemophilus influenzae, Klebsiella* species, *Streptococcus* species, *Diplococcus pneumoniae, Staphylococcus aureus*, anthrax, and trachoma. When PCN is contraindicated; treatment of *Neisseria gonorrhoeae, N.meningitidis*, syphilis, yaws, *Listeria monocytogenes, Clostridium* species, *Fusobacterium fusiforme* and *Actinomyces* species. Adjunct therapy for amebiasis.

**DOSAGE:** *Adults:* Usual: 200mg IV divided qd-bid on Day 1 then 100-200mg/day IV depending on severity, with 200mg administered in 1 or 2 infusions. Primary/Secondary Syphilis: 300mg/day IV for at least 10 days. Inhalational Anthrax (Post-Exposure): 100mg IV bid. Institute oral therapy as soon as possible and continue therapy for a total of 60 days.
*Pediatrics:* >8 yrs: >100 lbs: Usual: 200mg IV divided qd-bid on Day 1 then 100-200mg/day IV depending on severity, with 200mg administered in 1 or 2 infusions. <100 lbs: 2mg/lb IV divided qd-bid on Day 1 then 1-2mg/lb/day IV divided qd-bid depending on severity. Inhalational Anthrax (Post-Exposure): <100 lbs: 1 mg/lb IV bid. Institute oral therapy as soon as possible and continue therapy for a total of 60 days.

**HOW SUPPLIED:** Inj: 100mg, 200mg

**WARNINGS/PRECAUTIONS:** May cause fetal harm during pregnancy. Permanent tooth discoloration during tooth development (last half of pregnancy and children <8 yrs) reported; avoid use in this age group except for anthrax treatment. Decreased bone growth in premature infants reported. May increase BUN. Photosensitivity, enamel hypoplasia reported. Superinfection with prolonged use. Monitor hematopoietic, renal and hepatic values periodically with long term therapy. Bulging fontanels in infants and benign intracranial HTN in adults reported.

**ADVERSE REACTIONS:** GI effects, increased BUN, rash, hypersensitivity reactions, hemolytic anemia, thrombocytopenia.

**INTERACTIONS:** May decrease PT; adjust anticoagulants. Avoid use with bactericidal agents (eg, penicillin).

**PREGNANCY:** Safety in pregnancy not known; not for use in nursing.

## VICODIN

CIII

V

acetaminophen - hydrocodone bitartrate (Abbott)

**OTHER BRAND NAMES:** Vicodin ES (Abbott) - Vicodin HP (Abbott)

**THERAPEUTIC CLASS:** Opioid analgesic

**INDICATIONS:** Relief of moderate to moderately severe pain.

**DOSAGE:** *Adults:* Usual: Vicodin: 1-2 tabs q4-6h prn. Max: 8 tabs/day. Vicodin HP: 1 tab q4-6h prn. Max: 6 tabs/day. Vicodin ES: 1 tab q4-6h prn. Max: 5 tabs/day.

**HOW SUPPLIED:** (Hydrocodone-APAP) Tab: Vicodin: 5mg-500mg*; Vicodin HP: 10mg-660mg*; Vicodin ES: 7.5mg-750mg* *scored

**WARNINGS/PRECAUTIONS:** Caution in elderly, debilitated, severe hepatic or renal dysfunction, hypothyroidism, Addison's disease, prostatic hypertrophy, urethral stricture, pulmonary disease and postoperative use. May obscure acute abdominal conditions or head injuries. May produce dose-related respiratory depression. Monitor for tolerance. Suppresses cough reflex.

**ADVERSE REACTIONS:** Lightheadedness, dizziness, sedation, nausea, vomiting, constipation, rash, respiratory depression.

**INTERACTIONS:** Additive CNS depression with other narcotic analgesics, antihistamines, antipsychotics, antianxiety agents, alcohol and other CNS depressants. Increased effect of antidepressant or hydrocodone with MAOIs or TCAs.

**PREGNANCY:** Category C, not for use in nursing.

## VICON FORTE — RX

minerals - multiple vitamin (UCB Pharma)

**OTHER BRAND NAMES:** Vitacon Forte (Amide)

**THERAPEUTIC CLASS:** Vitamin/Mineral Combination

**INDICATIONS:** Treatment or prevention of vitamin And mineral deficiencies.

**DOSAGE:** *Adults:* 1 cap qd.

**HOW SUPPLIED:** Cap: Ascorbic Acid 150mg-Calcium Pantothenate 10mg-Folic Acid 1mg-Magnesium 70mg-Manganese 4mg-Niacinamide 25mg-Pyridoxine 2mg-Riboflavin 5mg-Thiamine 10mg-Vitamin A 8000 IU-Vitamin $B_{12}$ 10mcg-Vitamin E 50 IU-Zinc 80mg

**WARNINGS/PRECAUTIONS:** Folic acid may obscure signs of pernicious anemia.

**PREGNANCY:** Safety in pregnancy and nursing not known.

## VICOPROFEN — CIII

ibuprofen - hydrocodone bitartrate (Abbott)

**OTHER BRAND NAMES:** Reprexain (Watson)

**THERAPEUTIC CLASS:** Opioid analgesic

**INDICATIONS:** Short-term (generally <10 days) management of acute pain.

**DOSAGE:** *Adults:* Usual: 1 tab q4-6h prn. Max: 5 tabs/day. Elderly: Use lowest dose or longest interval.
*Pediatrics:* >16 yrs: Usual: 1 tab q4-6h prn. Max: 5 tabs/day.

**HOW SUPPLIED:** (Hydrocodone-Ibuprofen) Tab: (Vicoprofen) 7.5mg-200mg; (Reprexain) 5mg-200mg* *scored

**CONTRAINDICATIONS:** ASA or other NSAID allergy that precipitates asthma, urticaria, or other allergic reaction.

**WARNINGS/PRECAUTIONS:** May produce dose-related respiratory depression. May obscure acute abdominal conditions or head injuries. Avoid with ASA triad, late pregnancy, advanced renal disease, ASA-sensitive asthma. Caution in elderly, debilitated, dehydration, renal disease, intrinsic coagulation defects, severe hepatic dysfunction, asthma, hypothyroidism, Addison's disease, prostatic hypertrophy, urethral stricture, heart failure, HTN, ulcer disease, pulmonary disease, postoperative use. May be habit-forming. Suppresses cough reflex. Risk of GI ulceration, bleeding, perforation. Anemia, fluid retention, edema, severe hepatic reactions reported. Possible risk of aseptic meningitis, especially in SLE patients. Increased risk of serious cardiovascular thrombotic events, MI and stroke. Fluid retention and edema observed. Skin reactions (eg, exfoliative dermatitis, TEN, SJS) can occur.

**ADVERSE REACTIONS:** Headache, somnolence, dizziness, constipation, dyspepsia, nausea, vomiting, infection, edema, nervousness, anxiety, pruritus, diarrhea, asthenia, abdominal pain, insomnia, dry mouth, sweating.

**INTERACTIONS:** Additive CNS depression with other narcotics, antihistamines, antipsychotics, antianxiety agents, alcohol, CNS depressants. Increased effect of antidepressant or hydrocodone with MAOIs or TCAs. May produce paralytic ileus with anticholinergics. May decrease effects of furosemide and thiazide diuretics, ACE-inhibitors. Avoid ASA. Risk of serious GI bleeding with warfarin. May enhance methotrexate toxicity. Monitor for lithium toxicity.

**PREGNANCY:** Category C, not for use in nursing.

## VIDAZA RX

azacitidine (Pharmion)

**THERAPEUTIC CLASS:** Pyrimidine nucleoside analog

**INDICATIONS:** Treatment of myelodysplastic syndrome subtypes: refractory anemia or refractory anemia with ringed sideroblasts (if accompanied by neutropenia or thrombocytopenia or requiring transfusions), refractory anemia with excess blasts, refractory anemia with excess blasts in transformation, and chronic myelomonocytic leukemia.

**DOSAGE:** *Adults:* Initial: 75mg/m² SQ or IV (administer over 10-40 minutes) daily for 7 days. Repeat cycle every 4 weeks. May increase to 100mg/m² after 2 cycles if no beneficial effect and no toxicity. Treat ≥4 cycles. Adjust dose based on hematology lab values, renal function, and serum electrolytes.

**HOW SUPPLIED:** Inj: 100mg

**CONTRAINDICATIONS:** Advanced malignant hepatic tumors.

**WARNINGS/PRECAUTIONS:** May cause fetal harm. Avoid pregnancy in women of childbearing potential. Neutropenia and thrombocytopenia may occur; monitor CBC periodically (at minimum, before each cycle). May cause hepatotoxicity; caution with liver disease. Renal abnormalities reported; reduce dose or hold for unexplained reductions in serum bicarbonate <20mEq/L or elevations of BUN or serum creatinine occur. Monitor for toxicity with renal impairment.

**ADVERSE REACTIONS:** (SQ) Nausea, anemia, thrombocytopenia, vomiting, pyrexia, leukopenia, diarrhea, fatigue, injection site erythema, constipation, neutropenia, ecchymosis, cough, dyspnea, weakness; (IV) Petechiae, rigors, weakness, hypokalemia.

**PREGNANCY:** Category D, not for use in nursing.

## VIDEX RX

didanosine (Bristol-Myers Squibb)

**Fatal/nonfatal pancreatitis, lactic acidosis, and severe hepatomegaly with steatosis reported. Suspend therapy if suspect pancreatitis and discontinue if pancreatitis confirmed. Fatal lactic acidosis reported in pregnant women receiving concomitant stavudine.**

**OTHER BRAND NAMES:** Videx EC (Bristol-Myers Squibb)

V

**THERAPEUTIC CLASS:** Nucleoside analogue

**INDICATIONS:** Treatment of HIV-1 infection in combination with other antiretrovirals (use Videx EC when management requires once daily dosing or alternative didanosine formulation).

**DOSAGE:** *Adults:* >60kg: (Cap) 400mg qd; (Sol) 200mg bid or 400mg qd. <60kg: (Cap) 250mg qd; (Sol) 125mg bid or 250mg qd. CrCl 30-59mL/min: >60kg: (Cap) 200mg qd; (Sol) 200mg qd or 100mg qd. <60kg: (Cap) 125mg qd; (Sol) 150mg qd or 75mg bid. CrCl 10-29mL/min: >60kg: (Cap) 125mg qd; (Sol) 150mg qd. <60kg: (Cap) 125mg qd; (Sol) 100mg qd. CrCl <10mL/min: >60kg: (Cap) 125mg qd; (Sol) 100mg qd. <60kg: (Sol) 75mg qd. Concomitant Viread: CrCl ≥60mL/min :≥60kg: 250mg qd; <60kg: 200mg qd. Take on empty stomach at least 30 minutes before or 2 hrs after meals. Swallow caps

whole.
*Pediatrics:* 2 weeks-8 months: (Sol) 100mg/m² bid. >8 months: 120mg/m² bid.

**HOW SUPPLIED:** Sol: 2g, 4g [120mL, 240mL]; Cap, Delayed Release: (Videx EC) 125mg, 200mg, 250mg, 400mg

**WARNINGS/PRECAUTIONS:** Risk of toxicity with CrCl <60mL/min; reduce dose. Retinal changes and optic neuritis reported; perform periodic retinal exams. Peripheral neuropathy reported. Caution with hepatic dysfunction. May cause asymptomatic hyperuricemia. Twice daily dosing is preferred over once daily dosing. Chewable tabs contain phenylalanine. Caution with sodium restricted diets; buffered powder solution contains 1380mg sodium. Monitor for lactic acidosis in pregnancy if used with stavudine. Possible redistribution or accumulation of fat. Immune reconstitution syndrome has been reported in patients treated with combination antiretroviral therapy. Fatal and non-fatal pancreatitis reported; increased risk in combination with stavudine, with or without hydroxyurea.

**ADVERSE REACTIONS:** Pancreatitis, lactic acidosis, hepatomegaly, visual changes, diarrhea, neuropathy, abdominal pain, headache, nausea, vomiting, rash, elevated LFTs.

**INTERACTIONS:** Extreme caution with drugs that may cause pancreatitis. Increase risk of peripheral neuropathy with neurotoxic agents (eg, stavudine). Aluminum- and magnesium-containing antacids may potentiate adverse events. Space dose by 2 hrs of drugs whose absorption can be affected by stomach acidity (eg, ketoconazole, itraconazole). Increased serum levels with oral ganciclovir. Space dose by 2 hrs after or 6 hrs before ciprofloxacin. Avoid allopurinol. Decreased serum levels with methadone. Caution with tenofovir or ribavirin; monitor closely for didanosine-related toxicities and suspend therapy if signs of pancreatitis, symptomatic hyperlactatemia, or lactic acidosis develop.

**PREGNANCY:** Category B, not for use in nursing.

## VIGAMOX — RX
moxifloxacin HCl (Alcon)

**THERAPEUTIC CLASS:** Fluoroquinolone

**INDICATIONS:** Treatment of bacterial conjunctivitis.

**DOSAGE:** *Adults:* 1 drop tid for 7 days.
*Pediatrics:* ≥1 yr: 1 drop tid for 7 days.

**HOW SUPPLIED:** Sol: 0.5% [3mL]

**WARNINGS/PRECAUTIONS:** Not for injection. Do not inject subconjunctivally or into the anterior chamber of the eye. Superinfection may result with prolonged use. Fatal hypersensitivity reactions reported after first dose of systemic quinolone therapy. Avoid contact lenses when symptoms are present.

**ADVERSE REACTIONS:** Conjunctivitis, decreased visual acuity, dry eye, keratitis, ocular discomfort/hyperemia, ocular pain/pruritus, subconjunctival hemorrhage, tearing.

**PREGNANCY:** Category C, caution in nursing.



## VINBLASTINE — RX
vinblastine sulfate (Various)

**For IV use only; fatal if given intrathecally. Considerable irritation if leakage occurs into surrounding tissue. If this occurs, discontinue and restart in another vein. Heat and hyaluronidase minimize discomfort and cellulitis.**

**THERAPEUTIC CLASS:** Vinca alkaloid

**INDICATIONS:** Palliative treatment of generalized Hodgkin's disease (Stages III and IV), lymphocytic lymphoma, histiocytic lymphoma, advanced mycosis fungoides, advanced testis carcinoma, Kaposi's sarcoma, Letterer-Siwe disease, and resistant choriocarcinoma and unresponsive breast carcinoma.

**DOSAGE:** *Adults:* Dose at intervals of <7 days. 1st Dose: 3.7mg/m$^2$. 2nd Dose: 5.5mg/m$^2$. 3rd Dose: 7.4mg/m$^2$. 4th Dose: 9.25mg/m$^2$. 5th Dose: 11.1mg/m$^2$. Max: 18.5mg/m$^2$. Do not increase dose after that dose which reduces WBC to 3000 cells/mm$^3$. Maint: Use dose of 1 increment smaller than this dose at weekly intervals. Reduce to 50% dose if direct serum bilirubin >3mg/100mL. Only dose if WBC >4000cells/mm$^3$.
*Pediatrics:* Dose at intervals of <7 days. 1st Dose: 2.5mg/m$^2$. 2nd Dose: 3.75mg/m$^2$. 3rd Dose: 5mg/m$^2$. 4th Dose: 6.25mg/m$^2$. 5th Dose: 7.5mg/m$^2$. Max: 12.5mg/m$^2$. Do not increase dose after that dose which reduces WBC to 3000 cells/mm$^3$. Maint: Use dose of 1 increment smaller than this dose at weekly intervals. Reduce to 50% dose if direct serum bilirubin >3mg/100mL. Only dose if WBC >4000cells/mm$^3$.

**HOW SUPPLIED:** Inj: 1mg/mL, 10mg

**CONTRAINDICATIONS:** Significant granulocytopenia (unless result of disease being treated), bacterial infections.

**WARNINGS/PRECAUTIONS:** Avoid pregnancy. Acute shortness of breath, severe bronchospasm, aspermia, stomatitis, neurologic toxicity reported. Increased toxicity with hepatic insufficiency. Monitor for infection with WBC <2000cells/mm$^3$. Avoid with malignant-cell infiltration of bone marrow, or in older persons with cachexia or ulcerated skin. Small daily amounts for long periods is not advised. Avoid eye contamination. Monitor WBCs. May cause fetal harm during pregnancy.

**ADVERSE REACTIONS:** Leukopenia (granulocytopenia), anemia, thrombocytopenia, alopecia, constipation, anorexia, nausea, vomiting, abdominal pain, diarrhea, HTN, paresthesis.

**INTERACTIONS:** May increase phenytoin metabolism/elimination, or decrease phenytoin absorption. Caution with CYP3A inhibitors (eg, erythromycin, doxorubicin, etoposide), or with hepatic dysfunction; may cause earlier onset and/or an increased severity of side effects. Increased risk of acute shortness of breath and severe bronchospasm with mitomycin-C.

**PREGNANCY:** Category D, not for use in nursing.

## VINCRISTINE SULFATE RX

vincristine sulfate (Various)

**For IV use only; fatal if given intrathecally. Considerable irritation if leakage occurs into surrounding tissue. If this occurs, discontinue and restart in another vein. Heat and hyaluronidase minimize discomfort and cellulitis.**

**THERAPEUTIC CLASS:** Vincaleukoblastine mitotic inhibitor

**INDICATIONS:** Treatment of acute leukemia. As adjunct therapy in Hodgkin's disease, non-Hodgkin's malignant lymphomas, rhabdomyosarcoma, neuroblastoma and Wilm's tumor.

**DOSAGE:** *Adults:* Usual: 1.4mg/m$^2$ IV once a week. If billirubin >3mg/100mL reduce dose by 50%. If given together with L-asparaginase, give 12-24 hrs before the enzyme.
*Pediatrics:* Usual: 1.5-2mg/m$^2$ IV once a week. <10kg: 0.05mg/kg once a week.

**HOW SUPPLIED:** Inj: 1mg/mL

**CONTRAINDICATIONS:** Demyelinating form of Charcot-Marie-Tooth syndrome.

**WARNINGS/PRECAUTIONS:** Reports of acute uric acid nephropathy. Does not pass BBB; if CNS leukemia diagnosed, additional agents may be needed. Caution in pre-existing neuromuscular disease. Acute SOB and severe bronchospasm reported; caution with pulmonary dysfunction. May cause fetal harm during pregnancy.

**ADVERSE REACTIONS:** Anaphylaxis, alopecia, leukopenia, neuritic pain, constipation, paresthesia, difficulty in walking, loss of deep-tendon reflexes, muscle wasting, rash, edema, abdominal cramps, weight loss, polyuria, dysuria, urinary retention, HTN, hypotension, motor difficulties, ataxia, paralysis, dehydration, azotemia, anemia, thrombocytopenia.

**INTERACTIONS:** May increase phenytoin metabolism/elimination, or decrease phenytoin absorption. Caution with CYP3A inhibitors (eg, itraconazole), or with hepatic dysfunction; may cause earlier onset and/or an increased severity of neuromuscular side effects. Avoid use with radiation therapy through parts that include the liver. Increased risk of neurological side effects with neurotoxic potential. Risk of acute SOB and severe bronchospasm with mitomycin C.

**PREGNANCY:** Category D, not for use in nursing.

## VIOKASE — RX

lipase - amylase - protease (Axcan Scandipharm)

**THERAPEUTIC CLASS:** Pancreatic enzyme supplement

**INDICATIONS:** Treatment of pancreatic exocrine insufficiency (eg, cystic fibrosis, chronic pancreatitis, pancreatectomy, and pancreatic ductal obstruction).

**DOSAGE:** *Adults:* (Powder) Cystic Fibrosis: 0.7g (1/2 tsp) with meals. (Tab) Cystic Fibrosis/Pancreatitis: 8,000-32,000 U Lipase with meals. Pancreatectomy/Pancreatic Duct Obstruction: 8,000-16,000 U Lipase q2h. *Pediatrics:* (Powder) Cystic Fibrosis: 0.7g (1/2 tsp) with meals. (Tab) Cystic Fibrosis/Pancreatitis: 8,000-32,000 U Lipase with meals. Pancreatectomy/Pancreatic Duct Obstruction: 8,000-16,000 U Lipase q2h.

**HOW SUPPLIED:** (Amylase-Lipase-Protease) Powder: 70,000 U-16,800 U-70,000 U/0.7g [240g]; Tab: (Viokase 8) 30,000 U-8,000 U-30,000 U; (Viokase 16) 60,000 U-16,000 U-60,000 U

**CONTRAINDICATIONS:** Pork protein hypersensitivity.

**WARNINGS/PRECAUTIONS:** May have allergic reactions if previously sensitized to trypsin, pancreatin or pancrelipase. Irritating to oral mucosa if held in mouth. Inhalation of powder can cause an asthma attack. High doses can cause hyperuricemia and hyperuricosuria.

**ADVERSE REACTIONS:** Irritation to nasal mucosa and respiratory tract with inhaled powder.

**PREGNANCY:** Category C, caution in nursing.

## VIRA-A — RX

vidarabine (King)

**THERAPEUTIC CLASS:** Purine nucleoside antiviral

**INDICATIONS:** Treatment of acute keratoconjunctivitis and recurrent epithelial keratitis due to HSV1 and HSV2. Effective in superficial keratitis due to HSV unresponsive to or intolerant to idoxuridine.

**DOSAGE:** *Adults:* Apply 1/2 inch 5 times daily at 3-hr intervals. Discontinue, if no improvement after 7 days or incomplete re-epithelialization by 21 days. Continue for 7 more days at a reduced dose (eg, bid) after re-epithelialization. *Pediatrics:* >2 yrs: Apply 1/2 inch 5 times daily at 3 hr intervals. Discontinue, if no improvement after 7 days or incomplete re-epithelialization by 21 days. Continue for 7 more days at a reduced dose (eg, bid) after re-epithelialization.

**HOW SUPPLIED:** Oint: 3% [3.5g]

**WARNINGS/PRECAUTIONS:** May produce temporary visual haze. Establish diagnosis of keratoconjunctivitis due to HSV before starting therapy. Not for RNA virus, adenoviral ocular infection, bacterial, fungal or chlamydial infections.

**ADVERSE REACTIONS:** Lacrimation, foreign body sensation, conjunctival injection, burning, irritation, superficial punctate keratitis, pain, photophobia, punctal occlusion.

**PREGNANCY:** Category C, not for use in nursing.

## VIRACEPT RX
nelfinavir mesylate (Pfizer)

**THERAPEUTIC CLASS:** Protease inhibitor

**INDICATIONS:** Treatment of HIV infection in combination with other antiretrovirals.

**DOSAGE:** *Adults:* 1250mg bid or 750mg tid. Concomitant rifabutin: Reduce rifabutin dose by one-half and nelfinavir 1250mg bid is preferred dose. Take with a meal or light snack. May crush or dissolve whole tab in water or mix in food and consume immediately. May store mixture under refrigeration up to 6 hrs.
*Pediatrics:* 2-13 yrs: 20-30mg/kg tid. Take with a meal or light snack. May mix powder with non-acidic liquid (eg, water, milk, formula, etc.); consume immediately. May store up to 6 hrs under refrigeration.

**HOW SUPPLIED:** Sus: (powder) 50mg/g [144g]; Tab: 250mg, 625mg

**CONTRAINDICATIONS:** Concomitant pimozide, triazolam, midazolam, ergot derivatives, amiodarone or quinidine.

**WARNINGS/PRECAUTIONS:** Powder contains phenylalanine. New-onset DM, exacerbation of DM and hyperglycemia reported. Register pregnant patients (800-258-4263). Caution with hepatic dysfunction. Increased bleeding reported. Possible redistribution or accumulation of fat.

**ADVERSE REACTIONS:** Diarrhea, nausea, flatulence, rash, redistribution of body fat, jaundice, hypersensitivity reactions, bilirubinemia, hyperglycemia, metabolic acidosis.

**INTERACTIONS:** See Contraindications. Avoid pimozide, triazolam, midazolam, ergot derivatives, amiodarone or quinidine; potential for life-threatening adverse events. Avoid rifampin. Avoid lovastatin or simvastatin; caution with other HMG-CoA reductase inhibitors. May increase sildenafil levels and adverse effects. Avoid St. John's wort; may decrease levels of nelfinavir. May increase levels of drugs metabolized by CYP450 3A (eg, dihydropyridine calcium channel blockers, immunosuppressants, etc). Use alternative or additional contraception with oral contraceptives. May increase levels of cyclosporine, tacrolimus, sirolimus, atorvastatin, cerivastatin, fluticasone, azithromycin. Carbamazepine, phenobarbital may decrease levels of nelfinavir. May decrease levels of phenytoin, methadone. Give didanosine 1 hr before or 2 hrs after nelfinavir. Omeprazole decreases levels of nelfinavir; concomitant use with proton pump inhibitors may lead to loss of virologic response and development of resistance.

**PREGNANCY:** Category B, not for use in nursing.

## VIRAMUNE RX
nevirapine (Boehringer Ingelheim)



**Severe, life-threatening, in some cases fatal, hepatotoxicity and skin reactions (eg, Stevens-Johnson syndrome, toxic epidermal necrolysis, hypersensitivity) reported. Women, including pregnant women, and/or patients with higher CD4 counts are at higher risk of hepatotoxicity. Permanently discontinue following severe hepatitic, skin or hypersensitivity reactions.**

**THERAPEUTIC CLASS:** Non-nucleoside reverse transcriptase inhibitor

**INDICATIONS:** Treatment of HIV-1 infection in combination with other antiretrovirals.

**DOSAGE:** *Adults:* 200mg qd for 14 days (lead-in period), then 200mg bid. Do not increase dose if rash occurs, until it resolves. Retitrate if interrupt >7 days.

*Pediatrics:* 2 months-8 yrs: 4mg/kg qd for 14 days, then 7mg/kg bid. Max: 400mg/day. >8 yrs: 4mg/kg qd for 14 days, then 4mg/kg bid. Max: 400mg/day. Do not increase dose if rash occurs, until it resolves. Retitrate if interrupt >7 days.

**HOW SUPPLIED:** Sus: 50mg/5mL [240mL]; Tab: 200mg* *scored

**WARNINGS/PRECAUTIONS:** Avoid with severe hepatic impairment. Caution with moderate impairment and dialysis. Perform laboratory tests (eg, LFTs) at baseline and during first 18 weeks of therapy. Possible redistribution or accumulation of body fat.

**ADVERSE REACTIONS:** Headache, fever, severe rash, GI effects, fatigue, thrombocytopenia, fatigue, hepatotoxicity, granulocytopenia (pediatrics).

**INTERACTIONS:** Avoid use of prednisone for prevention of therapy-associated rash. Decreased levels of clarithromycin; consider alternative. Decreased levels of efavirenz, indinavir, nelfinavir, saquinavir. May decrease effectiveness of oral contraceptives and other hormonal contraceptives; use alternate or additional method of contraception. Increased levels with fluconazole. Avoid with ketoconazole, St. John's wort, rifampin. Decreased levels of lopinavir; adjust lopinavir/ritonavir doses. May decrease levels of methadone; monitor for signs of withdrawal. Increased levels of rifabutin. Possible decreased levels with antiarrhythmics (eg, amiodarone, disopyramide, lidocaine), anticonvulsants (eg, carbamazepine, clonazepam, ethosuximide), itraconazole, calcium channel blockers (eg, diltiazem, nifedipine, verapamil), cyclophosphamide, ergotamine, immunosuppressants (eg, cyclosporine, tacrolimus, sirolimus), cisapride, fentanyl. Monitor with warfarin.

**PREGNANCY:** Category C, not for use in nursing.

## VIRAZOLE

RX

ribavirin (Valeant)

**Sudden deterioration of respiratory function associated with initiation in infants. Monitor respiratory function carefully. Not for use in adults. Use with mechanical ventilator assistance with staff familiar with mode of administration and specific type of ventilator.**

**THERAPEUTIC CLASS:** Nucleoside analogue

**INDICATIONS:** Treatment of hospitalized infants and young children with severe lower respiratory tract infections due to respiratory syncytial virus.

**DOSAGE:** *Pediatrics:* Continuous aerosol administration of 20mg/mL in the drug reservoir of the SPAG-2 unit for 12-18 hrs/day for 3-7 days.

**HOW SUPPLIED:** Sol, Inhalation: 6g

**CONTRAINDICATIONS:** Women who are or may become pregnant during exposure to drug.

**WARNINGS/PRECAUTIONS:** Monitor respiratory function and fluid status according to SPAG-2 manual. Accumulation of drug precipitate can result in mechanical ventilator dysfunction and associated increased pulmonary pressures.

**ADVERSE REACTIONS:** Worsening of respiratory status, bronchospasm, pulmonary edema, hypoventilation, cyanosis, dyspnea, bacterial pneumonia, pneumothorax, apnea, atelectasis, ventilator dependence, cardiac arrest, hypotension, bradycardia.

**INTERACTIONS:** Digoxin toxicity reported.

**PREGNANCY:** Category X, safety in nursing not known.

## VIREAD
tenofovir disoproxil fumarate (Gilead) RX

**Lactic acidosis and severe hepatomegaly with steatosis, including fatal cases, reported with nucleoside analogs alone or with concomitant antiretrovirals.**

**THERAPEUTIC CLASS:** Nucleotide analog reverse transcriptase inhibitor

**INDICATIONS:** Treatment of HIV-1 infection in combination with other antiretrovirals.

**DOSAGE:** *Adults:* 300mg qd without regard to food.

**HOW SUPPLIED:** Tab: 300mg

**WARNINGS/PRECAUTIONS:** Obesity and prolonged nucleoside exposure may be risk factors for lactic acidosis and severe hepatomegaly with steatosis. Caution if risk factors for hepatic disease present or with hepatic insufficiency. Monitor hepatic function with both clinical and laboratory follow-up for at least several months in patients who are coinfected with HIV and HBV and d/c Viread. All patients should have creatinine clearance calculated prior to and during therapy. Dose adjust and monitor renal function when creatinine clearance <50 mL/min. May cause renal impairment. Monitor serum creatinine and phosphorous in patients at risk or with a history of renal dysfunction and those receiving concomitant nephrotoxic agents. Bone monitoring should be considered for HIV patients at risk for osteopenia. Cases of osteomalacia have been reported. Possible fat redistribution and accumulation of body fat.

**ADVERSE REACTIONS:** Nausea, diarrhea, vomiting, flatulence, asthenia, headache, abdominal pain, anorexia.

**INTERACTIONS:** Increases levels of didanosine; use caution when co-administering, monitor for didanosine-associated adverse effects (suppression of CD4 cell counts), and discontinue if these adverse events develop. Renally eliminated drugs (eg, cidofovir, acyclovir, valacyclovir, ganciclovir, valganciclovir) may increase levels of itself or tenofovir. Indinavir, lopinavir/ritonavir, and drugs that decrease renal function may increase tenofovir plasma levels. May decrease lamivudine, indinavir, lopinavir, and ritonavir plasma levels. Avoid with concurrent or recent use of nephrotoxic agents.

**PREGNANCY:** Category B, not for use in nursing.

## VIROPTIC
trifluridine (King) RX

**THERAPEUTIC CLASS:** Fluorinated pyrimidine nucleoside antiviral

**INDICATIONS:** Treatment of primary keratoconjunctivitis and recurrent epithelial keratitis due to herpes simplex virus, types 1 and 2.

**DOSAGE:** *Adults:* 1 drop q2h while awake until re-epithelialization. Max: 9 drops/day. Following Re-epithelialization: 1 drop q4h while awake for 7 days; minimum of 5 drops/day. If no improvement after 7 days or if complete re-epithelialization has not occurred after 14 days, consider other therapy. Avoid using >21 days.

*Pediatrics:* >6 yrs: 1 drop q2h while awake until re-epithelialization. Max: 9 drops/day. Following Re-epithelialization: 1 drop q4h while awake for 7 days; minimum of 5 drops/day. If no improvement after 7 days or if complete re-epithelialization has not occurred after 14 days, consider other therapy. Avoid using >21 days.

**HOW SUPPLIED:** Sol: 1% [7.5mL]

**WARNINGS/PRECAUTIONS:** Only use with a clinical diagnosis of herpetic keratitis. May cause transient, mild local irritation of the conjunctiva and cornea when instilled.

**ADVERSE REACTIONS:** Burning, stinging, palpebral edema, superficial punctate keratopathy, epithelial keratopathy, hypersensitivity reaction, stromal edema, irritation, keratitis sicca, hyperemia, increased IOP.

**PREGNANCY:** Category C, caution in nursing.

## VISICOL
sodium phosphate (InKine) RX

**THERAPEUTIC CLASS:** Bowel cleanser

**INDICATIONS:** Bowel cleanser for colonoscopy.

**DOSAGE:** *Adults:* Drink only clear liquids 12 hrs before dose. Evening Before Exam: 3 tabs with 8 oz clear liquids every 15 min for a total of 20 tabs (last dose is 2 tabs). Repeat on the day of exam 3-5 hrs before procedure. May retreat after 7 days.

**HOW SUPPLIED:** Tab: (Sodium Phosphate Monobasic Monohydrate-Sodium Phosphate Dibasic Anhydrous) 1.102g-0.398g* *scored

**CONTRAINDICATIONS:** Patients with biopsy-proven acute phosphate nephropathy.

**WARNINGS/PRECAUTIONS:** Fatalities reported from electrolyte imbalances and arrhythmias if administered with other sodium phosphate-containing products. May induce QT prolongation, colonic mucosal aphthous ulcerations and exacerbate IBS. Caution with severe renal insufficiency (creatinine clearance less than 30 mL/minute), CHF, ascites, unstable angina, acute bowel obstruction, bowel perforation, toxic megacolon, gastric retention, ileus, pseudo-obstruction of the bowel, severe chronic constipation, acute colitis, gastric bypass, stapling surgery, or hypomotility syndrome. Correct electrolyte disturbance before use. Caution within 3 months of acute MI or cardiac surgery. Do not use additional enema or laxative. Reports of generalized tonic-clonic seizures and/or loss of consciousness in patients with no prior history of seizures.

**ADVERSE REACTIONS:** Nausea, vomiting, abdominal bloating, dizziness, headache, abdominal pain.

**INTERACTIONS:** May reduce absorption of other drugs. Caution with sodium phosphate-containing products, agents that prolong QT interval or affect electrolyte levels.

**PREGNANCY:** Category C, safety in nursing not known.

## VISINE A.C.
zinc sulfate - tetrahydrozoline HCl (McNeil) OTC

**THERAPEUTIC CLASS:** Decongestant/astringent

**INDICATIONS:** Temporary relief of discomfort and redness of the eyes due to minor eye irritations.

**DOSAGE:** *Adults:* 1-2 drops in affected eye up to qid.
*Pediatrics:* >6 yrs: 1-2 drops in affected eye up to qid.

**HOW SUPPLIED:** Sol: (Tetrahydrozoline-Zinc) 0.05%-0.25% [15mL, 30mL]

**WARNINGS/PRECAUTIONS:** May temporarily enlarge pupils. Overuse may cause more redness. Remove contact lenses before use. Do not touch container tip to any surface to avoid contamination. D/C if eye pain or vision changes occur, if redness or irritation continues, or if condition worsens or continues >72 hrs. Supervision required with glaucoma.

**ADVERSE REACTIONS:** Brief tingling sensation.

**PREGNANCY:** Safety in pregnancy and nursing not known.

## VISINE ADVANCED RELIEF OTC

povidone - dextran 70 - polyethylene glycol 400 - tetrahydrozoline HCl (McNeil)

**THERAPEUTIC CLASS:** Decongestant/lubricant

**INDICATIONS:** Relief of eye redness due to minor eye irritations. Use as a protectant against further irritation or to relieve eye dryness.

**DOSAGE:** *Adults:* 1-2 drops in affected eye up to qid.
*Pediatrics:* >6 yrs: 1-2 drops in affected eye up to qid.

**HOW SUPPLIED:** Sol: (Dextran 70-Polyethylene Glycol 400-Povidone, Tetrahydrozoline) 0.05%-0.1%-1%-1%-0.05% [15mL, 30mL]

**WARNINGS/PRECAUTIONS:** May temporarily enlarge pupils. Overuse may cause more redness. Remove contact lenses before use. Do not touch container tip to any surface to avoid contamination. D/C if eye pain or vision changes occur, if redness or irritation continues, or if condition worsens or continues >72 hrs. Supervision required with glaucoma.

**PREGNANCY:** Safety in pregnancy and nursing not known.

## VISINE FOR CONTACTS OTC

glycerin - hydroxypropyl methylcellulose (McNeil)

**THERAPEUTIC CLASS:** Lubricant

**INDICATIONS:** To moisten daily wear soft lenses while on the eyes during the day. To moisten extended wear soft lenses upon awakening, prior to retiring at night, and as needed during the day.

**DOSAGE:** *Adults:* Use prn throughout the day. Minor Irritation/Discomfort/Blurring With Lenses: Instill 1-2 drops on eye and blink 2-3 times. If discomfort continues; remove lenses.
*Pediatrics:* Use prn throughout the day. Minor Irritation/Discomfort/Blurring With Lenses: Instill 1-2 drops on eye and blink 2-3 times. If discomfort continues; remove lenses.

**HOW SUPPLIED:** Sol: [15mL, 30mL]

**WARNINGS/PRECAUTIONS:** Eye problems including corneal ulcers can occur; remove contacts if eye discomfort, excessive tearing, vision changes or eye redness occur. Do not touch container tip to any surface to avoid contamination.

**ADVERSE REACTIONS:** Eye irritation, excessive tearing, unusual eye secretions, eye redness, reduced visual acuity, blurred vision, photophobia, dry eyes.

**PREGNANCY:** Safety in pregnancy and nursing not known.

## VISINE L.R. OTC

oxymetazoline HCl (McNeil)

**THERAPEUTIC CLASS:** Decongestant



**INDICATIONS:** Relief of eye redness due to minor eye irritations.

**DOSAGE:** *Adults:* 1-2 drops in affected eye q6h prn.
*Pediatrics:* >6 yrs: 1-2 drops in affected eye q6h prn.

**HOW SUPPLIED:** Sol: 0.025% [15mL, 30mL]

**WARNINGS/PRECAUTIONS:** Overuse may cause more redness. Remove contact lenses before use. Do not touch container tip to any surface to avoid contamination. D/C if eye pain or vision changes occur, if redness or irritation continues, or if condition worsens or continues >72 hrs. Supervision required with glaucoma.

**PREGNANCY:** Safety in pregnancy and nursing not known.

## VISINE ORIGINAL

OTC

tetrahydrozoline HCl (McNeil)

**THERAPEUTIC CLASS:** Decongestant

**INDICATIONS:** Relief of eye redness due to minor eye irritations.

**DOSAGE:** *Adults:* 1-2 drops in affected eye up to qid.
*Pediatrics:* >6 yrs: 1-2 drops in affected eye up to qid.

**HOW SUPPLIED:** Sol: 0.05% [15mL, 30mL]

**WARNINGS/PRECAUTIONS:** May temporarily enlarge pupils. Overuse may cause more redness. Remove contact lenses before use. Do not touch container tip to any surface to avoid contamination. D/C if eye pain or vision changes occur, if redness or irritation continues, or if condition worsens or continues >72 hrs. Supervision required with glaucoma.

**PREGNANCY:** Safety in pregnancy and nursing not known.

## VISINE TEARS

OTC

glycerin - polyethylene glycol 400 - hydroxypropyl methylcellulose (McNeil)

**THERAPEUTIC CLASS:** Lubricant

**INDICATIONS:** Temporary relief of burning and irritation due to dryness of the eye and protection against further irritation.

**DOSAGE:** *Adults:* 1-2 drops prn.
*Pediatrics:* >6 yrs: 1-2 drops prn.

**HOW SUPPLIED:** Sol: (Glycerin-Hydroxypropyl Methylcellulose-Polyethylene Glycol 400) 0.2%-0.2%-1% [15mL, 30mL]

**WARNINGS/PRECAUTIONS:** Remove contact lenses before use. Do not touch container tip to any surface to avoid contamination. D/C if eye pain or vision changes occur, if redness or irritation continues, or if condition worsens or continues >72 hrs.

**PREGNANCY:** Safety in pregnancy and nursing not known.

## VISINE-A

OTC

naphazoline HCl - pheniramine maleate (McNeil)

**THERAPEUTIC CLASS:** Decongestant/antihistamine

**INDICATIONS:** Temporary relief of itchy, red eyes due to pollen, ragweed, grass, animal hair, and dander.

**DOSAGE:** *Adults:* 1-2 drops in affected eye up to qid.
*Pediatrics:* >6 yrs: 1-2 drops in affected eye up to qid.

**HOW SUPPLIED:** Sol: (Naphazoline-Pheniramine) 0.025%-0.3% [15mL]

**WARNINGS/PRECAUTIONS:** May temporarily enlarge pupils. Overuse may cause more redness. Remove contact lenses before use. Do not touch container tip to any surface to avoid contamination. D/C if eye pain or vision changes occur, if redness or irritation continues, or if condition worsens or continues >72 hrs. Supervision required with glaucoma.

**ADVERSE REACTIONS:** Brief tingling sensation.

**PREGNANCY:** Safety in pregnancy and nursing not known.

# VISTIDE

RX

cidofovir (Gilead)

**Renal impairment is a major toxicity; prehydrate with IV normal saline (NS) and administer probenecid with each dose. Monitor serum creatinine (SCr) and urine protein within 48 hrs prior to each dose. Modify dose with renal function changes. Contraindicated with nephrotoxic agents. Neutropenia reported; monitor neutrophils. Carcinogenic, teratogenic, and hypospermatic in animal studies.**

**THERAPEUTIC CLASS:** Viral DNA synthesis inhibitor

**INDICATIONS:** Treatment of cytomegalovirus (CMV) retinitis in AIDS patients.

**DOSAGE:** *Adults:* IV: Induction: 5mg/kg once weekly for 2 weeks. Maint: 5mg/kg once every 2 weeks. Reduce maint from 5mg/kg to 3mg/kg for an increase in SCr of 0.3-0.4mg/dL above baseline. D/C with increase in SCr >0.5mg/dL above baseline or >3+ proteinuria. Administer probenecid 2g PO 3 hrs before cidofovir, then 1g at 2 hrs and 8 hrs after completion of cidofovir infusion. Administer at least 1L 0.9% NS immediately before infusion. If tolerated, give 2nd liter at start of or immediately after infusion.

**HOW SUPPLIED:** Inj: 75mg/mL

**CONTRAINDICATIONS:** SCr >1.5mg/dL, CrCl <55mL/min, or urine protein >100mg/dL ( >2+ proteinuria) with therapy initiation. Nephrotoxic agents (discontinue at least 7 days before therapy), severe hypersensitivity to probenecid or other sulfa-containing agents, direct intraocular use.

**WARNINGS/PRECAUTIONS:** Dose-dependent nephrotoxicity. Monitor IOP, visual acuity, ocular symptoms, uveitis/iritis, and renal function periodically. Monitor WBC with differential before each dose. Avoid during pregnancy. Adequate contraception for both sexes during and following treatment is advised. May cause male infertility. Potentially carcinogenic. .

**ADVERSE REACTIONS:** Nausea, vomiting, neutropenia, proteinuria, decreased IOP/ocular hypotony, anterior uveitis/iritis, metabolic acidosis, nephrotoxicity, pneumonia, dyspnea, infection, fever, creatinine >2mg/dL, decreased sodium bicarbonate.

**INTERACTIONS:** Avoid nephrotoxic agents (aminoglyosides, amphotericin B, foscarnet, IV pentamidine, vancomycin, and NSAIDs); discontinue nephrotoxic agents at least 7 days before therapy. Temporarily discontinue zidovudine or decrease zidovudine by 50% with probenecid.

**PREGNANCY:** Category C, not for use in nursing.

# VISUDYNE

RX

verteporfin (Novartis Ophthalmics)

**THERAPEUTIC CLASS:** Photosensitizing agent

**INDICATIONS:** Treatment of age-related macular degeneration with subfoveal choroidal neovascularization.

**DOSAGE:** *Adults:* 6mg/m$^2$ IV over 10 minutes at 3mL/min. Photoactivation with laser light therapy with nonthermal diode laser 15 minutes after start IV infusion. Re-evaluate every 3 months and repeat if choroidal neovascular leakage is detected on fluorescein angiography.

**HOW SUPPLIED:** Inj: 15mg

**CONTRAINDICATIONS:** Porphyria.

**WARNINGS/PRECAUTIONS:** Avoid direct sunlight or bright indoor light for 5 days. Avoid extravasation. If extravasation occurs, protect area from direct light until swelling and discoloration fade. Protect from intense light if surgery within 48 hrs after therapy. Do not retreat if severe vision decrease of 4 lines or more occurs within 1 week after therapy. Only use compatible lasers. Caution with moderate to severe hepatic dysfunction. Reduced effects with increasing age.

**ADVERSE REACTIONS:** Headache, injection site reactions, visual disturbances, asthenia, HTN, eczema, constipation, nausea, anemia, arthralgia, vertigo, pharyngitis.

**INTERACTIONS:** Calcium channel blockers, polymyxin B, and radiation therapy may enhance rate of uptake by vascular endothelium. Increased photosensitivity with tetracyclines, sulfonamides, phenothiazines, sulfonylureas, thiazide diuretics, and griseofulvin. Decreased effects with dimethyl sulfoxide, β-carotene, ethanol, formate, mannitol, and drugs that decrease clotting, vasoconstriction, or platelet aggregation (eg, thromboxane $A_2$inhibitors).

**PREGNANCY:** Pregnancy C, caution in nursing.

## VITAFOL-PN RX

minerals - folic acid - multiple vitamin (Everett)

**THERAPEUTIC CLASS:** Prenatal vitamin

**INDICATIONS:** Vitamin and mineral supplementation for before, during, and after pregnancy.

**DOSAGE:** *Adults:* 1 tab qd.

**HOW SUPPLIED:** Tab: Calcium 125mg-Folic Acid 1mg-Iron 65mg-Magnesium 25mg-Niacin 15mg-Vitamin A 1700 IU-Vitamin $B_1$ 1.6mg-Vitamin $B_2$ 1.8mg-Vitamin $B_6$ 2.5mg-Vitamin $B_{12}$ 0.005mg-Vitamin C 60mg-Vitamin D 400 IU-Vitamin E 30 IU-Zinc 15mg

**CONTRAINDICATIONS:** Untreated and uncomplicated pernicious anemia, hemachromatosis, pyridoxine responsive anemia, liver cirrhosis, cobalt sensitivity, iron storage disease or the potential for this disease due to chronic hemolytic anemia.

**WARNINGS/PRECAUTIONS:** Accidental overdose of iron-containing products is a leading cause of fatal poisoning in children <6 yrs. Folic acid may partially correct hematological damage due to vitamin $B_{12}$ deficiency of pernicious anemia, while neurological damage progresses. Prolonged use of iron salts may cause iron storage disease.

**ADVERSE REACTIONS:** GI disturbances, allergic sensitization, black tarry stools.

## VITAPLEX RX

multiple vitamin (Amide)

**THERAPEUTIC CLASS:** Vitamin Supplement

**INDICATIONS:** For nutritional supplementation in conditions requiring water-soluble vitamins.

**DOSAGE:** *Adults:* 1 tab qd.

**HOW SUPPLIED:** Tab: Folic Acid 0.5mg-Niacin 100mg-Pantothenic Acid 18mg-Vitamin $B_1$ 15mg-Vitamin $B_2$ 15mg-Vitamin $B_6$ 4mg-Vitamin $B_{12}$ 5mcg-Vitamin C 500mg

**WARNINGS/PRECAUTIONS:** Not for treatment of pernicious anemia or other megoblastic anemias, or severe specific deficiencies.

**ADVERSE REACTIONS:** Allergic and idiosyncratic reactions.

**INTERACTIONS:** May decrease efficacy of levodopa.

## VITAPLEX PLUS

RX

minerals - multiple vitamin (Amide)

**THERAPEUTIC CLASS:** Vitamin/Mineral Supplements

**INDICATIONS:** For prophylactic or therapeutic nutritional supplementation in physiologically stressful conditions.

**DOSAGE:** *Adults:* 1 tab qd.

**HOW SUPPLIED:** Tab: Biotin 0.15mg-Chromium 0.1mg-Copper 3mg-Folic Acid 0.8mg-Iron 27mg-Magnesium 50mg-Manganese 5mg-Niacin 100mg-Pantothenic Acid 25mg-Vitamin A 5000IU-Vitamin $B_1$ 20mg-Vitamin $B_2$ 20mg-Vitamin $B_6$ 25mg-Vitamin $B_{12}$ 50mcg-Vitamin C 500mg-Vitamin E 30IU-Zinc 22.5mg

**WARNINGS/PRECAUTIONS:** Not for treatment of pernicious anemia or other megoblastic anemias, or severe specific deficiencies.

**ADVERSE REACTIONS:** Allergic and idiosyncratic reactions, GI intolerance.

**INTERACTIONS:** May decrease efficacy of levodopa.

## VITRASERT

RX

ganciclovir (Bausch & Lomb)

**THERAPEUTIC CLASS:** Nucleoside analogue antiviral

**INDICATIONS:** Treatment of cytomegalovirus (CMV) retinitis in AIDS patients.

**DOSAGE:** *Adults:* Each implant releases 4.5mg over 5-8 months. Remove and replace when there is evidence of progression of retinitis.
*Pediatrics:* >9 yrs: Each implant releases 4.5mg over 5-8 months. Remove and replace when there is evidence of progression of retinitis.

**HOW SUPPLIED:** Implant: 4.5mg

**CONTRAINDICATIONS:** Hypersensitivity to acyclovir, patients with contraindication for intraocular surgery (eg, external infection, severe thrombocytopenia).

**WARNINGS/PRECAUTIONS:** For intravitreal implantation only. Monitor for extraocular CMV disease. Implant does not treat systemic CMV. Complications from surgery include vitreous loss or hemorrhage, cataract formation, retinal detachment, uveitis, endophthalmitis, decrease in visual acuity. Immediate decrease in visual acuity will last 2-4 weeks postop. Maintain sterility of the surgical field, implant. Handle implant by suture tab to avoid damage to polymer coating. Handling and disposal of the implant should follow guidelines for antineoplastics.

**ADVERSE REACTIONS:** Visual acuity loss, vitreous hemorrhage, retinal detachments, cataract formation/lens opacities, macular abnormalities, IOP spikes, optic disk/nerve changes, uveitis, hyphemas.

**PREGNANCY:** Category C, not for use in nursing.



## VIVACTIL

RX

protriptyline HCl (Odyssey)

**Antidepressants increased the risk of suicidal thinking and behavior (suicidality) in short-term studies in children and adolescents with Major Depressive Disorder (MDD) and other psychiatric disorders. Protriptyline is not approved for use in pediatric patients.**

**THERAPEUTIC CLASS:** Tricyclic antidepressant

**INDICATIONS:** Treatment of symptoms of depression in those under close medical supervision.

**DOSAGE:** *Adults:* Usual: 15-40mg/day taken tid-qid. Titrate: May increase to 60mg/day. Max: 60mg/day. Elderly: Initial: 5mg tid. Titrate: Increase gradually if needed. Monitor cardiovascular system with doses >20mg/day. *Pediatrics:* Adolescents: Initial: 5mg tid. Titrate: Increase gradually if needed.

**HOW SUPPLIED:** Tab: 5mg, 10mg

**CONTRAINDICATIONS:** Within 14 days of MAOI therapy, cisapride, acute recovery period following MI.

**WARNINGS/PRECAUTIONS:** Caution with history of seizures, urinary retention, increased IOP, cardiovascular disorders, hyperthyroidism, elderly. May aggravate psychotic symptoms in schizophrenia, manic symptoms in manic-depressive psychosis, and anxiety/agitation in overactive/agitated patients. D/C several days before elective surgery.

**ADVERSE REACTIONS:** Tachycardia, hypotension, confusion, anxiety, insomnia, nightmares, seizures, EPS, dizziness, headache, anticholinergic effects, rash, photosensitivity, blood dyscrasias, GI effects, impotence, decreased libido, flushing.

**INTERACTIONS:** Risk of hyperpyrexia with anticholinergics and neuroleptics. Reduced hepatic metabolism with cimetidine. Enhanced seizure risk with tramadol. Enhanced response to alcohol, barbiturates, other CNS depressants. Use with CYP2D6 enzyme inhibitors (eg, quinidine, cimetidine, other antidepressants, phenothiazines, propafenone, flecainide, SSRIs) require lower doses for either TCA or other drug. Hyperpyretic crises, severe convulsions, and deaths reported with MAOIs. May block antihypertensive effect of guanethidine, or similarly acting compounds.

**PREGNANCY:** Safety in pregnancy and nursing not known.

## VIVELLE RX

estradiol (Novartis)

**Estrogens increase risk of endometrial cancer in postmenopausal women. Estrogens, with or without progestins, should not be used for the prevention of cardiovascular disease. Increased risks of MI, stroke, invasive breast cancer, PE, and DVT in postmenopausal women (50-79 yrs of age) reported. Increased risk of developing probable dementia in postmenopausal women ≥65 yrs of age reported.**

**OTHER BRAND NAMES:** Vivelle-Dot (Novartis)

**THERAPEUTIC CLASS:** Estrogen

**INDICATIONS:** Treatment of moderate to severe vasomotor symptoms and/or vulvar/vaginal atrophy associated with menopause. Treatment of hypoestrogenism due to hypogonadism, castration, or primary ovarian failure. Prevention of postmenopausal osteoporosis.

**DOSAGE:** *Adults:* Vasomotor Symptoms/Vulvar/Vaginal Atrophy: Initial: 0.0375mg/day twice weekly. Titrate: Adjust after at least 1 month. Discontinue or taper at 3-6 month intervals. Wait 1 week after withdrawal of oral therapy before initiating therapy. Osteoporosis Prevention: Minimum Effective Dose: 0.025mg/day twice weekly. Apply to clean, dry area of the trunk; avoid breasts and waistline. Rotate sites; allow 1 week between same site. Without intact uterus, may give continuously; with intact uterus, may give cyclically (3 weeks on, 1 week off) with a progestin.

**HOW SUPPLIED:** Patch: 0.025mg/day, 0.0375mg/day, 0.05mg/day, 0.075mg/day, 0.1mg/day [(Vivelle-Dot) $8^{s}$, $24^{s}$ (Vivelle) $8^{s}$, $48^{s}$]

**CONTRAINDICATIONS:** Pregnancy, undiagnosed abnormal genital bleeding, breast cancer, estrogen dependent neoplasia, DVT/PE, active or recent (eg, within past year) arterial thromboembolic disease (eg, stroke, MI), liver dysfunction or disease.

**WARNINGS/PRECAUTIONS:** May increase risk of cardiovascular events (eg, MI, stroke), venous thrombosis, and PE; d/c immediately if any of these events occur or are suspected. May increase risk of breast/endometrial cancer and gallbladder disease. May lead to severe hypercalcemia with breast cancer and bone metastases; monitor and d/c if hypercalcemia occurs. Retinal vascular thrombosis reported; monitor and d/c if papilledema or retinal vascular lesions occur. Consider addition of a progestin if no hysterectomy. May elevate BP; monitor at regular intervals. May cause elevations of plasma triglycerides with pre-existing hypertriglyceridemia. Caution with history of cholestatic jaundice associated with past estrogen use or with pregnancy; d/c with recurrence. May lead to increased thyroid-binding globulin levels; monitor thyroid function. May cause fluid retention; caution with cardiac/renal dysfunction. Caution with severe hypocalcemia. May increase risk of ovarian cancer. May exacerbate endometriosis, asthma, DM, epilepsy, migraine, porphyria, SLE, and hepatic hemangiomas; use with caution.

**ADVERSE REACTIONS:** Altered vaginal bleeding, vaginal candidiasis, breast tenderness/enlargement, nausea, vomiting, melasma, headache, weight changes, edema, altered libido.

**INTERACTIONS:** CYP3A4 inducers (eg, St. John's wort, phenobarbital, carbamazepine, rifampin) may decrease levels which may decrease therapeutic effects and/or change uterine bleeding profile. CYP3A4 inhibitors (eg, erythromycin, clarithromycin, ketoconazole, itraconazole, ritonavir, grapefruit juice) may increase levels which may result in side effects.

**PREGNANCY:** Contraindicated in pregnancy, caution in nursing.

## VIVITROL RX

naltrexone (Cephalon)

**THERAPEUTIC CLASS:** Opioid antagonist

**INDICATIONS:** Treatment of alcohol dependence.

**DOSAGE:** *Adults:* Administer 380mg IM gluteal injection every 4 weeks or once a month using alternating buttocks.

**HOW SUPPLIED:** Inj, Extended Release: 380mg

**CONTRAINDICATIONS:** Concomitant opioid analgesics, physiologic opioid dependence, acute opiate withdrawal, positive urine screen for opioids.

**WARNINGS/PRECAUTIONS:** Hepatotoxic with excessive doses; margin of separation between safe dose and hepatotoxic dose is 5-fold or less. May cause eosinophilic pneumonia. Only treat patients opioid-free for 7-10 days. Perform naloxone challenge test if risk of precipitating withdrawal. Attempting to overcome the opiate blockade using opioids is very dangerous. More sensitive to lower doses of opioids after naltrexone is discontinued. In an emergency situation, suggested plan for pain management is regional analgesia, conscious sedation with a benzodiazepine, or use of non-opioid analgesics or general anesthesia. Monitor for development of depression or suicidal thinking. Caution in renal or hepatic impairment. Administration will not eliminate or diminish alcohol withdrawal symptoms.

**ADVERSE REACTIONS:** Nausea, vomiting, diarrhea, abdominal pain, upper respiratory tract infection, pharyngitis, insomnia, anxiety, depression, injection site reactions, arthralgia, muscle cramps, dizziness, syncope, appetite disorder.

**INTERACTIONS:** See Contraindications.

**PREGNANCY:** Category C, not for use in nursing.



## VOLTAREN OPHTHALMIC RX

diclofenac sodium (Novartis Ophthalmics)

**THERAPEUTIC CLASS:** NSAID

**INDICATIONS:** Treatment of postoperative inflammation following cataract surgery. Temporary relief of pain and photophobia in corneal refractive surgery.

**DOSAGE:** *Adults:* Cataract Surgery: 1 drop qid, start 24 hrs after surgery and continue for 2 weeks. Corneal Refractive Surgery: 1-2 drops within 1 hr prior to, and within 15 minutes after surgery. Continue qid for up to 3 days.

**HOW SUPPLIED:** Sol: 0.1% [2.5mL, 5mL]

**WARNINGS/PRECAUTIONS:** May delay wound healing. Caution with bleeding tendencies. Monitor for 1 yr after use in corneal refractive procedures. May increase bleeding of ocular tissues.

**ADVERSE REACTIONS:** Transient burning/stinging, keratitis, elevated IOP, lacrimation, abnormal vision, conjunctivitis, eyelid swelling, discharge, iritis, itching.

**INTERACTIONS:** Caution with agents that prolong bleeding time (eg, NSAIDs). Potential for cross-sensitivity to acetylsalicylic acid, phenylacetic acid derivatives, and other NSAIDs.

**PREGNANCY:** Category C, safety in nursing not known.

## VOLTAREN-XR — RX

diclofenac sodium (Novartis)

**NSAIDs may cause an increased risk of serious cardiovascular thrombotic events, MI, stroke and serious GI adverse events including bleeding, ulceration, and perforation of the stomach or intestines. Contraindicated for the treatment of peri-operative pain in the setting of coronary artery bypass graft (CABG) surgery.**

**OTHER BRAND NAMES:** Voltaren (Novartis)

**THERAPEUTIC CLASS:** NSAID (benzeneacetic acid derivative)

**INDICATIONS:** (Voltaren) Relief of signs and symptoms of osteoarthritis (OA), rheumatoid arthritis (RA), and ankylosing spondylitis (AS). (Voltaren-XR) Relief of signs and symtpoms of OA and RA.

**DOSAGE:** *Adults:* Voltaren: OA: 50mg bid-tid or 75mg bid. Max: 150mg/day. RA: 50mg tid-qid or 75mg bid. Max: 200mg/day. AS: 25mg qid and 25mg qhs prn. Max: 125mg/day. Voltaren-XR: OA: 100mg qd. RA: 100mg qd-bid.

**HOW SUPPLIED:** Tab, Delayed Release: (Voltaren) 25mg, 50mg, 75mg; Tab, Extended Release: (Voltaren-XR) 100mg

**CONTRAINDICATIONS:** ASA or other NSAID allergy that precipitates asthma, urticaria, or allergic-type reactions. Treatment of peri-operative pain in the setting of CABG surgery.

**WARNINGS/PRECAUTIONS:** May lead to onset of new HTN or worsening of pre-existing HTN; monitor BP closely. Fluid retention and edema reported; caution with fluid retention or heart failure. Caution with considerable dehydration. Renal papillary necrosis and other renal injury reported after long-term use. Not recommended for use with advanced renal disease; if therapy must be initiated, monitor renal function. Anaphylactoid reactions may occur. May cause serious skin adverse events (eg, exfoliative dermatitis, Stevens-Johnson syndrome, and toxic epidermal necrolysis). Avoid in late pregnancy; may cause premature closure of ductus arteriosis. May cause elevations of LFTs; d/c if liver disease develops or systemic manifestations occur. Caution in elderly. Anemia may occur; with long-term use, monitor Hgb/Hct if signs or symptoms of anemia develop. May inhibit platelet aggregation and prolong bleeding time; monitor with coagulation disorders. Caution with asthma and avoid with aspirin-sensitive asthma.

**ADVERSE REACTIONS:** Fluid retention, dizziness, rash, nausea, abdominal cramps, LFT abnormalities, constipation, diarrhea, heartburn, tinnitus, GI ulceration, flatulence.

**INTERACTIONS:** Avoid with other diclofenac products. Increased adverse effects with ASA; avoid use. May enhance methotrexate toxicity; caution when co-administering. May increase nephrotoxicity of cyclosporine; caution when co-administering. May diminish antihypertensive effect of ACE-inhibitors. May reduce natriuretic effect of furosemide and thiazides; monitor for renal failure. May increase lithium levels; monitor for toxicity. Synergistic effects on GI bleeding with warfarin.

**PREGNANCY:** Category C, not for use in nursing.

## VoSoL HC
RX

acetic acid - hydrocortisone (Wallace)

**OTHER BRAND NAMES:** Acetasol HC (Alpharma)

**THERAPEUTIC CLASS:** Antibacterial/corticosteroid combination

**INDICATIONS:** Treatment of superficial infections of the external auditory canal complicated by inflammation.

**DOSAGE:** *Adults:* Remove cerumen and debris. Insert cotton wick into ear canal; saturate cotton before or after insertion. Add 3-5 drops q4-6h to keep moist. Remove after 24 hrs; continue with 5 drops tid-qid as long as indicated.
*Pediatrics:* >3 yrs: Remove cerumen and debris. Insert cotton wick into ear canal; saturate cotton before or after insertion. Add 3-4 drops q4-6h to keep moist. Remove after 24 hrs; continue with 3-4 drops tid-qid as long as indicated.

**HOW SUPPLIED:** Sol: (Acetic Acid-Hydrocortisone) 2%-1% [10mL]

**CONTRAINDICATIONS:** Herpes simplex, vaccinia, varicella, perforated tympanic membrane.

**WARNINGS/PRECAUTIONS:** Discontinue promptly if sensitization occurs.

**ADVERSE REACTIONS:** Transient stinging, burning.

**PREGNANCY:** Safety in pregnancy and nursing not known.

## VoSpire ER
RX

albuterol sulfate (Odyssey)

**THERAPEUTIC CLASS:** Beta$_2$ agonist

**INDICATIONS:** Treatment of bronchospasm in reversible obstructive airway disease.

**DOSAGE:** *Adults:* Usual: 4-8mg q12h. Low Body Weight: Initial: 4mg q12h. Titrate: May increase to 8mg q12h. Max: 32mg/day in divided doses. Swallow whole with liquids; do not chew or crush.
*Pediatrics:* >12 yrs: Usual: 4-8mg q12h. Low Body Weight: Initial: 4mg q12h. Titrate: May increase to 8mg q12h. Max: 32mg/day in divided doses. 6-12 yrs: Usual: 4mg q12h. Max: 24mg/day in divided doses. Swallow whole with liquids; do not chew or crush.

**HOW SUPPLIED:** Tab, Extended Release: 4mg, 8mg

**WARNINGS/PRECAUTIONS:** Hypersensitivity reactions reported. Caution with cardiovascular disorders, especially coronary insufficiency, arrhythmias and HTN. Increased doses may signify need for concomitant corticosteroids. Can produce paradoxical bronchospasm. Caution with DM, hyperthyroidism, seizures. May produce transient hypokalemia. Erythema multiforme and Stevens-Johnson (rare) reported in children.

**ADVERSE REACTIONS:** Tremor, headache, nervousness, tachycardia, palpitations, nausea, vomiting, muscle cramps.

**INTERACTIONS:** Avoid oral sympathomimetic agents. Extreme caution within 14 days of MAOI or TCA therapy. Monitor digoxin. May worsen ECG changes and/or hypokalemia with nonpotassium-sparing diuretics. Antagonized by β-blockers.

**PREGNANCY:** Category C, not for use in nursing.

## Vumon
RX

teniposide (Bristol-Myers Squibb)

**Cytotoxic. Severe myelosuppression, with resulting infection or bleeding, and/or hypersensitivity reactions may occur.**

**THERAPEUTIC CLASS:** Type II topoisomerase inhibitor

**INDICATIONS:** With other anticancer agents, for induction therapy of refractory childhood acute lymphoblastic leukemia.

**DOSAGE:** *Pediatrics:* 165mg/m² with cytarabine 300mg/m² IV twice weekly for 8-9 doses; or 250mg/m² with vincristine 1.5mg/m² IV weekly for 4-8 weeks and prednisone 40mg/m² PO for 28 days.

**HOW SUPPLIED:** Inj: 10mg/mL

**CONTRAINDICATIONS:** Hypersensitivity to Cremophor EL (polyoxyethylated castor oil).

**WARNINGS/PRECAUTIONS:** Monitor CBC, hepatic and renal function before and during therapy. Avoid rapid IV infusion. May cause fetal harm. Dose-limiting bone marrow suppression. D/C if significant hypotension occurs. Hypersensitivity (HS) reactions manifested by chills, fever, urticaria, tachycardia, bronchospasm, dyspnea, HTN, and hypotension may occur. If re-treating patient with earlier HS reaction, pretreat with corticosteroid and antihistamine. Continuously observe for at least 60 minutes after starting infusion and frequently thereafter. Use gloves when handling or preparing solution. Reduce dose or d/c if severe reactions occur.

**ADVERSE REACTIONS:** Myelosuppression, leukopenia, neutropenia, thrombocytopenia, anemia, mucositis, diarrhea, nausea, vomiting, infection, alopecia, bleeding, hypersensitivity reactions, rash, fever.

**INTERACTIONS:** Risk of CNS depression with antiemetics and high dose teniposide. Tolbutamide, sodium salicylate, and sulfamethizole displace protein-bound teniposide; may potentiate toxicity. Increased plasma clearance of methotrexate.

**PREGNANCY:** Category D, not for use in nursing.

## VYTONE RX

iodoquinol - hydrocortisone **(Dermik)**

**THERAPEUTIC CLASS:** Corticosteroid/Anti-infective

**INDICATIONS:** "Possibly" Effective: Contact or atopic dermatitis, impetiginized eczema, nummular eczema, endogenous chronic infectious dermatitis, stasis dermatitis, pyoderma, nuchal eczema and chronic eczematoid otitis externa, acne urticata, localized or disseminated neurodermatitis, lichen simplex chronicus, anogenital pruritus (vulvae, scroti, ani), folliculitis, bacterial dermatoses, mycotic dermatoses such as tinea (capitis, cruris, corporis, pedis), monliasis, intertrigo.

**DOSAGE:** *Adults:* Apply to affected area(s) tid-qid.
*Pediatrics:* >12 yrs: Apply tid-qid.

**HOW SUPPLIED:** Cre: (Hydrocortisone-Iodoquinol) 1%-1% [30g]

**WARNINGS/PRECAUTIONS:** For external use only. Avoid eyes. Discontinue if irritation develops. May stain skin, hair, or fabrics. Risk of systemic absorption with treatment of extensive areas or use of occlusive dressings. Increased risk of systemic absorption in children. Iodoquinol may interfere with thyroid tests. False-positive phenylketonuria test reported.

**ADVERSE REACTIONS:** Burning, itching, irritation, dryness, folliculitis, hypertrichosis, acneiform eruptions, hypopigmentation, perioral dermatitis, allergic dermatitis, skin maceration, secondary infection, skin atrophy, striae, miliaria.

**PREGNANCY:** Category C, caution in nursing.

## VYTORIN

RX

ezetimibe - simvastatin (Merck/Schering-Plough)

**THERAPEUTIC CLASS:** Cholesterol absorption inhibitor/HMG-CoA reductase inhibitor

**INDICATIONS:** When treatment with both components is appropriate, used as an adjunct to diet for the reduction of elevated total-C, LDL-C, Apo B, TG, non-HDL-C, and to increase HDL-C in primary hypercholesterolemia (heterozygous familial and non-familial) or mixed hyperlipidemia. For the reduction of elevated total-C, LDL-C in homozygous familial hypercholesterolemia as an adjunct to other lipid-lowering treatments or if such treatments are unavailable.

**DOSAGE:** *Adults:*Take once daily in the evening. Initial: 10mg/20mg qd. Less aggressive LDL-C reductions: Initial: 10mg/10mg qd. LDL-C reduction >55%: Initial: 10mg/40mg qd. Titrate: Adjust at ≥2 weeks. Homozygous Familial Hypercholesterolemia: 10mg/40mg or 10mg/80mg qd. Severe Renal Insufficiency: Avoid unless tolerant of ≥5mg of simvastatin; monitor closely. Concomitant Bile Acid Sequestrant: Take either ≥2 hours before or ≥4 hours after bile acid sequestrant. Concomitant Cyclosporine: Avoid unless tolerant of ≥5mg of simvastatin. Max: 10mg/10mg/day. Concomitant Amiodarone/Verapamil: Max: 10mg/20mg/day.

**HOW SUPPLIED:** Tab: (ezetimibe-simvastatin) 10mg/10mg, 10mg/20mg, 10mg/40mg, 10mg/80mg

**CONTRAINDICATIONS:** Active liver disease, unexplained persistent elevations in serum transaminases, pregnancy, lactation.

**WARNINGS/PRECAUTIONS:** Rhabdomyolysis (rare), myopathy reported. Discontinue therapy if myopathy is suspected or diagnosed, if AST or ALT ≥3X ULN persist, a few days prior to major surgery or when any major medical or surgical condition supervenes. Monitor LFTs prior to therapy and thereafter when clinically indicated. With 10mg/80mg dose, monitor LFTs prior to titration, 3 months after titration and periodically thereafter for the first year. Caution with heavy alcohol use, severe renal insufficiency, or history of hepatic disease. Avoid use in moderate or severe hepatic insufficiency.

**ADVERSE REACTIONS:** Headache, upper respiratory tract infection, myalgia, CK and transaminase elevations, urticaria, arthralgia.

**INTERACTIONS:** Avoid use with concomitant itraconazole, ketoconazole, erythromycin, clarithromycin, telithromycin, HIV protease inhibitors, nefazodone, grapefruit juice (>1 quart/day); increased risk of myopathy/rhabdomyolysis. Max 10/10mg daily with gemfibrozil, cyclosporin, danazol. Max 10/20mg daily with amiodarone, verapamil. Caution with other fibrates, ≥1g/day of niacin. Incremental LDL-C reductions with concomitant cholestyramine. Monitor digoxin, warfarin.

**PREGNANCY:** Category X, not for use in nursing.

## VYVANSE

CII

lisdexamfetamine dimesylate (Shire)

V

**High abuse potential; prolonged periods of administration may lead to dependence. Misuse of amphetamine may cause sudden death and serious cadiovascular events.**

**THERAPEUTIC CLASS:** Sympathomimetic Amine

**INDICATIONS:** Treatment of attention deficit hyperactivity disorder (ADHD) in children 6 to 12 yrs old.

**DOSAGE:** *Pediatrics:* 6-12 yrs: Usual: 30mg qam. Titrate: If needed, increase at increments of 20mg/day at weekly intervals. Max: 70mg/day. Swallow caps or dissolve contents in glass of water; do not store once dissolved. Re-evaluate in long-term use.

**HOW SUPPLIED:** Cap: 30mg, 50mg, 70mg

**CONTRAINDICATIONS:** Advanced arteriosclerosis, symptomatic cardiovscular disease, moderate to severe HTN, hyperthyroidism, glaucoma, agitated states, history of drug abuse, during or within 14 days of MAOI use.

**WARNINGS/PRECAUTIONS:** May exacerbate symptoms of behavior disturbance and thought disorder in psychotic patients. Caution with comorbid bipolar disorder; concern for possible induction of mixed/manic episode. Aggressive behavior or hostility reported. Monitor growth in children. Stimulants may lower the convulsive threshold; d/c in the presence of seizures. Difficulties with accommodation and blurring of vision reported. May exacerbate Tourette's syndrome and phonic or motor tics. Caution with HTN, heart failure, MI, or ventricular arrhythnmia; monitor BP and HR. Avoid use with structural cardiac abnormalities, cardiomyopathy, serious heart rhythm abnormalities, or other serious cardiac problems; sudden death reported. Treatment emergent psychotic or manic symptoms may occur (eg, hallucinations, delusional thinking, or mania, without prior history of psychotic illness); d/c treatment if needed.

**ADVERSE REACTIONS:** Decreased appetite, insomnia, upper abdominal pain, headache, weight loss, irritability, vomiting, nausea, dry mouth, dizziness, affect lability, rash.

**INTERACTIONS:** GI acidifying agents (eg, guanethidine, reserpine, glutamic acid, etc.) and urinary acidifying agents (eg, ammonium chloride, etc) decrease efficacy. MAOIs may cause hypertensive crisis. Potentiated effects of both agents with TCAs. May delay absorption of phenytoin, ethosuximide, phenobarbital. Potentiates meperidine, norepinephrine, phenobarbital, phenytoin. Antagonized by haloperidol, chlorpromazine, lithium. Inhibits adrenergic blockers, antihistamines, antihypertensives (veratrum alkaloids), methanamine therapy. Methenamine increases urinary excretion. Potentiated by propoxyphene overdose; fatal convulsions may occur.

**PREGNANCY:** Pregnancy C, not for use in nursing.

## WART-OFF OTC
salicylic acid (McNeil)

**THERAPEUTIC CLASS:** Keratolytic Agent

**INDICATIONS:** Removal of common warts and plantar warts on the bottom of the foot.

**DOSAGE:** Wash and dry affected area. Apply 1 drop to cover each wart, may repeat qd or bid (until wart is removed) up to 12 weeks.

**HOW SUPPLIED:** Sol: 17% [13.5mL]

**WARNINGS/PRECAUTIONS:** Do not use if diabetic or have poor blood circulation. Do not use on irritated skin, area that is infected or reddened, moles, birthmarks, warts with hair, genital warts, or warts on the face or mucous membranes. Avoid inhaling vapors and eye contact. Flammable product.

**PREGNANCY:** Not known, unknown use in nursing.

## WELCHOL RX
colesevelam HCl (Sankyo)

**THERAPEUTIC CLASS:** Bile acid sequestrant

**INDICATIONS:** As monotherapy or with an HMG-CoA reductase inhibitor as adjunct therapy to reduce elevated LDL cholesterol in primary hypercholesterolemia (Type IIa).

**DOSAGE:** *Adults:* 3 tabs bid or 6 tabs qd. Max: 7 tabs/day. Take with liquids and a meal.

**HOW SUPPLIED:** Tab: 625mg

**CONTRAINDICATIONS:** Bowel obstruction.

**WARNINGS/PRECAUTIONS:** Exclude secondary causes of hypercholesterolemia and perform a lipid profile. Monitor cholesterol and TG based on NCEP guidelines. Caution if TG levels >300mg/dL, dysphagia,. swallowing disorders, GI motility disorders, major GI tract surgery, and those susceptible to vitamin K or fat soluble vitamin deficiencies.

**ADVERSE REACTIONS:** Asthenia, constipation, dyspepsia, pharyngitis, myalgia.

**INTERACTIONS:** Decreases levels of sustained-release verapamil.

**PREGNANCY:** Category B, safety not known for nursing.

## WELLBUTRIN SR

RX

bupropion HCl (GlaxoSmithKline)

**Antidepressants increased the risk of suicidal thinking and behavior (suicidality) in short-term studies in children and adolescents with Major Depressive Disorder (MDD) and other psychiatric disorders. Bupropion is not approved for use in pediatric patients.**

**OTHER BRAND NAMES:** Wellbutrin (GlaxoSmithKline)

**THERAPEUTIC CLASS:** Aminoketone

**INDICATIONS:** Treatment of MDD.

**DOSAGE:** *Adults:* >18 yrs: (Tab, Extended-Release) Initial: 150mg qd, may increase to 150mg bid after 3 days. Usual: 150mg bid. Max: 200mg bid. Separate doses by at least 8 hrs. Severe Hepatic Cirrhosis: 100mg/day or 150mg every other day. Mild-Moderate Hepatic Cirrhosis/Renal Impairment: Reduce frequency and/or dose. (Tab) Initial: 100mg bid, may increase to 100mg tid after 3 days. Usual: 100mg tid. Max: 450mg/day, given in divided doses of not more than 150mg each. Severe Hepatic Cirrhosis: Max: 75mg qd.

**HOW SUPPLIED:** Tab: 75mg, 100mg; Tab, Extended-Release: 100mg, 150mg, 200mg

**CONTRAINDICATIONS:** Seizure disorder, bulimia or anorexia nervosa, within 14 days of MAOIs, other forms of bupropion, abrupt discontinuation of alcohol or sedatives.

**WARNINGS/PRECAUTIONS:** Dose-related risk of seizures. D/C and do not restart if seizure occurs. Extreme caution with history of seizure, cranial trauma, severe hepatic cirrhosis. Agitation, insomnia, psychosis, confusion and other neuropsychiatric signs reported. Caution with bipolar disorder, recent MI, unstable heart disease, renal impairment. Altered appetite/weight, allergic reactions, HTN reported. Monitor for clinical worsening and/or suicidality, especially at initiation of therapy or dose changes.

**ADVERSE REACTIONS:** Headache, dry mouth, nausea, insomnia, dizziness, pharyngitis, infection, abdominal pain, constipation, diarrhea, tinnitus, agitation, anxiety, rash, anorexia.

**INTERACTIONS:** See Contraindications. Extreme caution with drugs that lower seizure threshold (eg, antidepressants, antipsychotics, theophylline, systemic steroids). Increased seizure risk with opioid, cocaine, or stimulant addiction, OTC stimulants or anorectics, oral hypoglycemics, insulin, excessive use or abrupt discontinuation of alcohol or sedatives. Caution with levodopa, amantadine, and drugs that are metabolized by CYP2D6 (eg, SSRIs, TCAs, antipsychotics, beta-blockers, type 1C antiarrhythmics); use low initial dose and gradually titrate. Avoid other bupropion-containing drugs. Monitor HTN with transdermal nicotine. Caution with CYP2B6 substrates or inhibitors (eg, orphenadrine, cyclophosphamide, thiotepa). Carbamazepine, phenytoin, cimetidine, and phenobarbital may induce metabolism of bupropion. Minimize or avoid alcohol.



**PREGNANCY:** Category C, not for use in nursing.

## WELLBUTRIN XL

RX

bupropion HCl (GlaxoSmithKline)

**Antidepressants increased the risk of suicidal thinking and behavior (suicidality) in short-term studies in children and adolescents with Major Depressive Disorder (MDD) and other psychiatric disorders. Bupropion is not approved for use in pediatric patients.**

**THERAPEUTIC CLASS:** Aminoketone

**INDICATIONS:** Treatment of MDD and prevention of seasonal major depressive episodes in patients diagnosed with seasonal affective disorder (SAD).

**DOSAGE:** *Adults:* ≥18 yrs: Give in AM. Swallow whole. MDD: Initial: 150mg qd. May increase to 300mg qd on Day 4. Usual: 300mg qd. Max: 450mg qd. SAD: Start in autumn; stop in early spring. Initial: 150mg qd. May increase to 300mg after 1 week. Usual/Max: 300mg qd. Taper dose for 2 weeks prior to discontinuation. Mild-Moderate Hepatic Cirrhosis/Renal Impairment: Reduce frequency and/or dose. Severe Hepatic Cirrhosis: Max: 150mg every other day.

**HOW SUPPLIED:** Tab, Extended Release: 150mg, 300mg

**CONTRAINDICATIONS:** Seizure disorder, bulimia or anorexia nervosa, within 14 days of MAOIs, other forms of bupropion, abrupt discontinuation of alcohol or sedatives.

**WARNINGS/PRECAUTIONS:** Dose-related risk of seizures. Discontinue and do not restart if seizure occurs. Extreme caution with history of seizure, cranial trauma, severe hepatic cirrhosis. Agitation, insomnia, psychosis, confusion and other neuropsychiatric signs reported. Caution with bipolar disorder, recent MI, unstable heart disease, renal impairment. Altered appetite/weight, allergic reactions, HTN reported. Monitor for clinical worsening and/or suicidality, especially at initiation of therapy or dose changes.

**ADVERSE REACTIONS:** Headache, dry mouth, nausea, insomnia, dizziness, pharyngitis, abdominal pain, agitation, diarrhea, palpitations, myalgia, anxiety, tinnitus, constipation, sweating, rash.

**INTERACTIONS:** See Contraindications. Extreme caution with drugs that lower seizure threshold (eg, antidepressants, antipsychotics, theophylline, systemic steroids). Increased seizure risk with opioid, cocaine, or stimulant addiction, OTC stimulants or anorectics, oral hypoglycemics, insulin, excessive use or abrupt discontinuation of alcohol or sedatives. Caution with levodopa, amantadine, and drugs that are metabolized by CYP2D6 (eg, SSRIs, TCAs, antipsychotics, beta-blockers, type 1C antiarrhythmics); use low initial dose and gradually titrate. Monitor HTN with transdermal nicotine. Caution with CYP2B6 substrates or inhibitors (eg, orphenadrine, cyclophosphamide, thiotepa). Carbamazepine, phenytoin, cimetidine, and phenobarbital may induce metabolism of bupropion. Minimize or avoid alcohol.

**PREGNANCY:** Category C, not for use in nursing.

## WESTCORT

RX

hydrocortisone valerate (Westwood-Squibb)

**THERAPEUTIC CLASS:** Corticosteroid

**INDICATIONS:** Corticosteroid responsive dermatoses.

**DOSAGE:** *Adults:* Apply bid-tid. May use occlusive dressings for psoriasis or recalcitrant conditions; discontinue dressings if infection develops. *Pediatrics:* Apply bid-tid. May use occlusive dressings for psoriasis or recalcitrant conditions; discontinue dressings if infection develops.

**HOW SUPPLIED:** Cre, Oint: 0.2% [15g, 45g, 60g]

**WARNINGS/PRECAUTIONS:** May produce reversible HPA axis suppression, manifestations of Cushing's syndrome, hyperglycemia, and glucosuria. Caution when applied to large surface areas or under occlusive dressings. Use appropriate antifungal or antibacterial agent with dermatological infections;

discontinue if infection does not clear. Pediatrics may be more susceptible to systemic toxicity. Avoid eyes. Discontinue if irritation occurs.

**ADVERSE REACTIONS:** Burning, itching, dryness, irritation, folliculitis, hypertrichosis, acneiform eruptions, hypopigmentation, allergic contact dermatitis, skin maceration, secondary infection, skin atrophy, striae, miliaria.

**PREGNANCY:** Category C, caution in nursing.

## WIGRAINE RX

caffeine - ergotamine tartrate (Organon)

**THERAPEUTIC CLASS:** Alpha adrenergic antagonist/vasoconstrictor

**INDICATIONS:** To abort or prevent vascular headaches (eg, migraine, migraine variants, histamine cephalalgia).

**DOSAGE:** *Adults:* 2 tabs at start of headache, then 1 tab every 30 minutes prn. Max: 6 tabs/headache or 10 tabs/week.

**HOW SUPPLIED:** Tab: (Ergotamine-Caffeine) 1mg-100mg

**CONTRAINDICATIONS:** Pregnancy, peripheral vascular disease, CAD, HTN, hepatic or renal dysfunction, sepsis.

**WARNINGS/PRECAUTIONS:** Risk of ergotism.

**ADVERSE REACTIONS:** Precordial distress/pain, muscle pains, numbness/tingling in fingers/toes, tachycardia, bradycardia, vomiting, nausea, leg weakness, diarrhea, edema, itching.

**PREGNANCY:** Category X, not for use in nursing.

## WINRHO SDF RX

rho (d) immune globulin (Baxter)

**THERAPEUTIC CLASS:** Immuneglobulin

**INDICATIONS:** Treatment of non-splenectomized, $Rh_o$(D) positive children with chronic or acute immune thrombocytopenic purpura (ITP), adults with chronic ITP, or children and adults with ITP secondary to HIV infection. To prevent Rh immunization in $Rh_o$ (D) negative mothers who had not been previously sensitized to $Rh_o$ (D) factor. To suppress Rh isoimmunization in non-sensitized, $Rh_o$(D) negative women within 72 hours after spontaneous or induced abortions, amniocentesis, chorionic villus sampling, ruptured tubal pregnancy, abdominal trauma or transplacental hemorrhage or in the normal course of pregnancy, unless fetus or father is known to be $Rh_o$(D) negative. To suppress Rh isoimmunization in $Rh_o$(D) negative female children and adults transfused with $Rh_o$(D) positive blood products.

**DOSAGE:** *Adults:* ITP: Initial: 50mcg/kg IV as a single dose or in 2 divided doses on separate days. Hgb <10g/dL: 25-40mcg/kg. Subsequent/Maint: 25-60mcg/kg. Hgb 8-10g/dL: 25-40mcg/kg. Hgb >10g/dL: 50-60mcg/kg. Hgb <8g/dL: Use caution. Rh Suppression: Pregnancy: Give as IM or IV. 28 Weeks Gestation: 300mcg. If early in pregnancy, give at 12 week intervals. Postpartum: With Rh Positive Baby: 120mcg at birth, but no later than 72 hours after. Rh Status of Baby Unknown at 72 Hours: Administer to mother at 72 hours after birth. May give up to 28 days after birth. Abortion/Amniocentesis or Other Manipulation After 34 Weeks Gestation: 120mcg dose within 72 hours. Amniocentesis Before 34 Weeks Gestation/Post Chorionic Villus Sampling: 300mcg dose immediately after procedure. Repeat every 12 weeks. Threatened Abortion: 300mcg as soon as possible. Transfusion: Exposure to $Rh_o$(D) Positive Blood: 9mcg/mL blood given as 600mcg q8h IV or 12mcg/mL blood given as 1200mcg q12h IM. Exposure to $Rh_o$(D) Positive RBCs: 18mcg/mL cells given as 600mcg q8h IV or 24mcg/mL cells given as 1200mcg q12h IM.

*Pediatrics:* ITP: Initial: 50mcg/kg IV as a single dose or in 2 divided doses on separate days. Hgb <10g/dL: 25-40mcg/kg. Subsequent/Maint: 25-60mcg/kg.

Hgb 8-10g/dL: 25-40mcg/kg. Hgb >10g/dL: 50-60mcg/kg. Hgb <8g/dL: Use caution. Transfusion: Exposure to $Rh_o$(D) Positive Blood: 9mcg/mL blood given as 600mcg q8h IV or 12mcg/mL blood given as 1200mcg q12h IM. Exposure to $Rh_o$(D) Positive RBCs: 18mcg/mL cells given as 600mcg q8h IV or 24mcg/mL cells given as 1200mcg q12h IM.

**HOW SUPPLIED:** Inj: 120mcg (600 IU), 300mcg (1500 IU), 1000mcg (5000 IU)

**CONTRAINDICATIONS:** When used to prevent Rh alloimmunization, should not be adminstered to $Rh_o$(D) positive individuals including babies; $Rh_o$(D) negative women who are Rh immunized as evidenced by standard manual Rh antibody screening test; individuals with a history of anaphylactic or other severe systemic reaction to immune globulins. When used to treat patients with ITP, should not be administered to $Rh_o$(D) negative individuals; splenectomized individuals; individuals with known hypersensitivity to plasma products.

**WARNINGS/PRECAUTIONS:** May transmit disease. Avoid use in $Rh_o$(D) negative, $Rh_o$(D) negative who are Rh immunized, or spelenectomized patients. Not for replacement therapy for immuneglobulin deficiency syndromes. Caution with IgA deficiency; anaphylactic reactions may occur. (ITP): Monitor for intravascular hemolysis, clinically compromising anemia, renal insufficiency. If transfused, use $Rh_o$(D) negative RBCs. Caution if platelets from $Rh_o$(D) positive donors are transfused.

**ADVERSE REACTIONS:** Headache, chills, fever, decreased Hgb, back pain, intravascular hemolysis.

**INTERACTIONS:** May interfere with response to live vaccines; delay immunization for 3 months.

**PREGNANCY:** Category C, safety in nursing not known.

## XALATAN RX

latanoprost (Pharmacia & Upjohn)

**THERAPEUTIC CLASS:** Prostaglandin analogue

**INDICATIONS:** Reduction of elevated IOP in open-angle glaucoma or ocular hypertension.

**DOSAGE:** *Adults:* Usual: 1 drop qd in the pm. Max: Once daily dosing. Space dosing with other ophthalmic drugs by 5 minutes.

**HOW SUPPLIED:** Sol: 0.005% [2.5mL, 2.5mL x 3]

**CONTRAINDICATIONS:** Hypersensitivity to benzalkonium chloride.

**WARNINGS/PRECAUTIONS:** Changes to pigmented tissues, growth of eyelashes, and macular edema reported. May change eye color. Caution with history of intraocular inflammation, aphakic patients, pseudophakic patients with a torn posterior lens capsule, patients at risk of macular edema. Avoid with active intraocular inflammation. Do not administer with contact lenses.

**ADVERSE REACTIONS:** Eyelash changes (increased length, thickness, pigmentation, number of lashes), eyelid skin darkening, intraocular inflammation, iris pigmentation changes, macular edema.

**INTERACTIONS:** Administer at least 5 minutes apart from other topical ophthalmic agents.

**PREGNANCY:** Category C, caution in nursing.

## XANAX CIV

alprazolam (Pharmacia & Upjohn)



**THERAPEUTIC CLASS:** Benzodiazepine

**INDICATIONS:** Anxiety disorders and short-term relief of anxiety symptoms. Panic disorder with or without agoraphobia.

**DOSAGE:** *Adults:* Anxiety: Initial: 0.25-0.5mg tid. Titrate: May increase every 3-4 days. Max: 4mg/day. Elderly/Advanced Liver Disease/Debilitated: Initial: 0.25mg bid-tid. Titrate: Increase gradually as tolerated. Panic Disorder: Initial: 0.5mg tid. Titrate: Increase by no more than 1mg/day every 3-4 days; slower titration if >4mg/day. Usual: 1-10mg/day. Decrease dose slowly (no more than 0.5mg every 3 days).

**HOW SUPPLIED:** Tab: 0.25mg*, 0.5mg*, 1mg*, 2mg* *scored

**CONTRAINDICATIONS:** Acute narrow angle glaucoma, untreated open angle glaucoma, concomitant ketoconazole or itraconazole.

**WARNINGS/PRECAUTIONS:** Risk of dependence. Withdrawal symptoms, including seizures, reported with dose reduction or abrupt discontinuation; avoid abrupt withdrawal. Caution with impaired renal, hepatic, or pulmonary function, severe depression, obesity, elderly, and debilitated. May cause fetal harm. Hypomania/mania reported with depression. Weak uricosuric effect. Periodically reassess usefulness.

**ADVERSE REACTIONS:** Drowsiness, light-headedness, depression, headache, confusion, insomnia, dry mouth, constipation, diarrhea, nausea/vomiting, tachycardia/palpitations, blurred vision, nasal congestion.

**INTERACTIONS:** See Contraindications. Increases plasma levels of imipramine, desipramine. Additive CNS depressant effects with psychotropics, anticonvulsants, antihistamines, ethanol. Potentiated by fluoxetine, fluvoxamine, nefazodone, cimetidine, oral contraceptives. Propoxyphene decreases plasma levels. Caution with diltiazem, isoniazid, macrolides, grapefruit juice, sertraline, paroxetine, ergotamine, cyclosporine, amiodarone, nicardipine, nifedipine and other CYP3A inhibitors. Avoid azole antifungals.

**PREGNANCY:** Category D, not for use in nursing.

## XANAX XR

**CIV**

alprazolam (Pharmacia & Upjohn)

**THERAPEUTIC CLASS:** Benzodiazepine

**INDICATIONS:** Panic disorder with or without agoraphobia.

**DOSAGE:** *Adults:* >18 yrs: Initial: 0.5-1mg qd, preferably in the am. Titrate: Increase by no more than 1mg/day every 3-4 days. Maint: 1-10mg/day. Usual: 3-6mg/day. Decrease dose slowly (no more than 0.5mg every 3 days). Elderly/Advanced Liver Disease/Debilitated: Initial: 0.5mg qd.

**HOW SUPPLIED:** Tab, Extended Release: 0.5mg, 1mg, 2mg, 3mg

**CONTRAINDICATIONS:** Acute narrow angle glaucoma, untreated open angle glaucoma, concomitant ketoconazole or itraconazole.

**WARNINGS/PRECAUTIONS:** Risk of dependence. Withdrawal symptoms, including seizures, reported with dose reduction or abrupt discontinuation; avoid abrupt withdrawal. Caution with impaired renal, hepatic, or pulmonary function, severe depression, obesity, elderly, and debilitated. May cause fetal harm. Hypomania/mania reported with depression. Weak uricosuric effect. Periodically reassess usefulness.

**ADVERSE REACTIONS:** Sedation, somnolence, memory impairment, dysarthria, abnormal coordination, fatigue, depression, constipation, mental impairment, ataxia, dry mouth, decreased libido, increased/decreased appetite.

**INTERACTIONS:** See Contraindications. Increases plasma levels of imipramine, desipramine. Additive CNS depressant effects with psychotropics, anticonvulsants, antihistamines, ethanol. Potentiated by fluoxetine, fluvoxamine, nefazodone, cimetidine, oral contraceptives. Decreased levels with CYP3A inducers (eg, carbamazepine) or propoxyphene. Caution with diltiazem, isoniazid, macrolides, grapefruit juice, sertraline, paroxetine, ergotamine, cyclosporine, amiodarone, nicardipine, nifedipine and other CYP3A inhibitors. Avoid azole antifungals.

**PREGNANCY:** Category D, not for use in nursing.

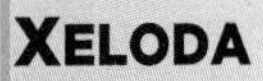

## XELODA
capecitabine (Roche Labs)

RX

**Altered coagulation parameters and/or bleeding, including death, reported with coumarin-derivative anticoagulants (eg, warfarin). Monitor PT/INR frequently to adjust anticoagulant dose.**

**THERAPEUTIC CLASS:** Fluoropyrimidine carbamate

**INDICATIONS:** First-line treatment of metastatic colorectal carcinoma when fluoropyrimidine therapy alone is preferred. Adjuvant treatment in patients with Dukes' C colon cancer who have undergone complete resection of the primary tumor when treatment with fluoropyrimidine therapy alone is preferred. Treatment of metastatic breast cancer in combination with docetaxel after failure of prior anthracycline-containing chemotherapy. Treatment of metastatic breast cancer in patients resistant to paclitaxel and anthracycline-containing chemotherapy or resistant to paclitaxel and for whom further anthracycline therapy is not indicated.

**DOSAGE:** *Adults:* Take with water within 30 minutes after meals. Usual/Concomitantly w/ docetoxel: 1250mg/m² bid for 2 weeks, then 1 week off. Give as 3-week cycles. For adjuvant treatment of Dukes' C colon cancer give as 3-week cycles for a total of 8 cycles (24 weeks). CrCl 30-50mL/min: Reduce to 75% of starting dose. Interrupt and/or reduce dose if toxicity occurs. Readjust according to adverse effects (see labeling for details).

**HOW SUPPLIED:** Tab: 150mg, 500mg

**CONTRAINDICATIONS:** Hypersensitivity to 5-FU, dihydropyrimidine dehydrogenase (DPD) deficiency, severe renal impairment (CrCl <30mL/min).

**WARNINGS/PRECAUTIONS:** Reduce dose with moderate renal dysfunction. Carefully monitor for adverse events with mild to moderate renal dysfunction. Carefully monitor with severe diarrhea fluid/electrolyte balance; may need dose adjustment. Patients >80 yrs may experience increased grade 3 and 4 adverse events (see full prescribing info). Possible fetal harm with pregnancy. Monitor for hand-and-foot syndrome. Cardiotoxicity reported; more common with history of CAD. Carefully monitor with mild to moderate hepatic dysfunction due to hepatic metastases. Hyperbilirubinemia, neutropenia, thrombocytopenia, and decrease in hemoglobin reported.

**ADVERSE REACTIONS:** Diarrhea, hand and foot syndrome, pyrexia, anemia, nausea, fatigue, vomiting, dermatitis, neutropenia, thrombocytopenia, stomatitis, anorexia, hyperbilirubinemia, abdominal pain, paresthesia.

**INTERACTIONS:** May increase phenytoin levels; reduce phenytoin dose. Leucovorin may increase levels and toxicity of 5-FU. Altered coagulation parameters and/or bleeding reported with anticoagulants (eg, coumarin, phenprocoumon); monitor PT/INR frequently. Caution with CYP2C9 substrates. Aluminum and/or magnesium antacids may increase levels.

**PREGNANCY:** Category D, not for use in nursing.

## XENICAL
orlistat (Roche Labs)

RX

**THERAPEUTIC CLASS:** Lipase inhibitor

**INDICATIONS:** For weight loss and weight maintenance and to reduce the risk of weight regain after weight loss in obese patients with an initial BMI ≥30kg/m² or ≥27kg/m² in the presence of other risk factors.

**DOSAGE:** *Adults:* 120mg tid with each main meal containing fat. Take during or up to 1 hr after meals. Use with reduced calorie diet with about 30% of calories from fat. Omit dose if meal is missed or contains no fat. Separate multivitamin (containing fat-soluble vitamins) by at least 2 hrs.
*Pediatrics:≥12 yrs:* 120mg tid with each main meal containing fat. Take during or up to 1 hr after meals. Use with reduced calorie diet with about 30% of

calories from fat. Omit dose if meal is missed or contains no fat. Separate multivitamin (containing fat-soluble vitamins) by at least 2 hrs.

**HOW SUPPLIED:** Cap: 120mg

**CONTRAINDICATIONS:** Chronic malabsorption syndrome, cholestasis.

**WARNINGS/PRECAUTIONS:** Exclude organic causes of obesity. Caution with history of hyperoxaluria or calcium oxalate nephrolithiasis. Gastrointestinal effects may increase with a diet high in fat (>30%). Weight loss may improve metabolic control; monitor dosage of antidiabetic agents. Increased risk of cholelithiasis due to substantial weight loss.

**ADVERSE REACTIONS:** Oily spotting, flatus with discharge, fecal urgency, fatty/oily stool, oily evacuation, increased defecation, fecal incontinence.

**INTERACTIONS:** Monitor warfarin and cyclosporine (separate cyclosporine dose by 2 hrs). May decrease absorption of fat soluble vitamins and beta carotene; supplement with fat-soluble multivitamin.

**PREGNANCY:** Category B, not for use in nursing.

## XIBROM

bromfenac (Ista) RX

**THERAPEUTIC CLASS:** NSAID

**INDICATIONS:** Treatment of postoperative inflammation after cataract extraction.

**DOSAGE:** *Adults:* 1 drop bid in affected eye(s), start 24 hours post-op and continue for 2 weeks.

**HOW SUPPLIED:** Sol: 0.09% [5mL]

**WARNINGS/PRECAUTIONS:** Contains sodium sulfite, may cause allergic-type reactions including anaphylactic symptoms and life-threatening or less severe asthmatic episodes. Potential cross-sensitivity to acetylsalicylic acid, phenylacetic acid derivatives, and other NSAIDs. May cause increased bleeding of ocular tissues; slow or delay healing; keratitis. Continued use may lead to sight-threatening epithelial breakdown, corneal thinning, corneal erosion, corneal ulceration, corneal perforation; discontinue use if this occurs. Caution in complicated ocular surgeries, corneal denervation, corneal epithelial defects, DM, ocular surface diseases (eg, dry eye syndrome), RA, repeat ocular surgeries within a short period of time, bleeding tendencies, or receiving other medication which may prolong bleeding time.

**ADVERSE REACTIONS:** Abnormal sensation in eye, conjunctival hyperemia, eye irritation (burning/stinging), eye pain, eye pruritus, eye redness, headache, iritis.

**INTERACTIONS:** Concomitant use of topical NSAIDs and topical steroids may increase potential for healing problems. Caution with other medications which may prolong bleeding time.

**PREGNANCY:** Category C, caution in nursing.

## XIFAXAN

rifaximin (Salix) RX

**THERAPEUTIC CLASS:** Semi-synthetic rifampin analog

**INDICATIONS:** Traveler's diarrhea caused by noninvasive strains of *E.coli*

**DOSAGE:** *Adults:* 1 tab tid for 3 days.
*Pediatrics:* ≥12 yrs: 1 tab tid for 3 days.

**HOW SUPPLIED:** Tab: 200mg

**WARNINGS/PRECAUTIONS:** Avoid in diarrhea complicated by fever or blood in the stool or diarrhea due to pathogens other than *E.coli*. Discontinue if diarrhea symptoms worsen or persist >24-48 hrs; consider alternative antibiotic therapy. Pseudomembranous colitis reported.

**ADVERSE REACTIONS:** Flatulence, headache, abdominal pain, rectal tenesmus, defecation urgency, nausea, constipation, pyrexia.

**PREGNANCY:** Category C; not for use in nursing.

## XIGRIS RX
drotrecogin alfa (Lilly)

**THERAPEUTIC CLASS:** Activated protein C

**INDICATIONS:** For reduction of mortality in severe sepsis (associated with acute organ dysfunction) in patients at a high risk of death.

**DOSAGE:** *Adults:* 24mcg/kg/hr IV for 96 hrs.

**HOW SUPPLIED:** Inj: 5mg, 20mg

**CONTRAINDICATIONS:** Active internal bleeding, hemorrhagic stroke within 3 months, intracranial or intraspinal surgery or severe head trauma within 2 months, trauma with an increased risk of life-threatening bleeding, epidural catheter, intracranial neoplasm or mass lesion, evidence of cerebral herniation.

**WARNINGS/PRECAUTIONS:** Increased risk of bleed with platelets <30,000 x $10^6$/L (even if platelets increased by transfusions), PT-INR >3, GI bleed within 6 weeks, ischemic stroke within 3 months, intracranial arteriovenous malformation or aneurysm, known bleeding diathesis, chronic severe hepatic disease, or condition where bleeding is a significant hazard or difficult to manage due to location. If bleeding occurs, stop infusion. Discontinue 2 hrs before invasive surgical procedures or procedures with risk of bleeding. Patients with single organ dysfunction and recent surgery may not be at high risk of death irrespective of APACHE II score and therefore may not be among the indicated population; use in these patients only after careful consideration.

**ADVERSE REACTIONS:** Bleeding.

**INTERACTIONS:** Caution with drugs that affect hemostasis; increased risk of bleed with therapeutic heparin, thrombolytic therapy within 3 days, and oral anticoagulants, ASA >650mg, platelet inhibitors or glycoprotein IIb/IIIa inhibitors within 7 days.

**PREGNANCY:** Category C, not for use in nursing.

## XOLAIR RX
omalizumab (Genentech)

**THERAPEUTIC CLASS:** Monoclonal antibody/IgE-blocker

**INDICATIONS:** Moderate-severe persistent asthma in those who have a positive skin test or *in vitro* reactivity to a perennial aeroallergen and whose symptoms are inadequately controlled with inhaled corticosteroids.

**DOSAGE:** *Adults:* 150-375mg SQ every 2 or 4 weeks based on body weight and pretreatment serum total IgE level. Max: 150mg/site. 30-90kg & IgE >30-100 IU/mL: 150mg q4 weeks; >90-150kg & IgE >30-100 IU/mL OR 30-90kg & IgE >100-200 IU/mL OR 30-60kg & IgE >200-300 IU/mL: 300mg q4 weeks; >90-150kg & IgE >100-200 IU/mL OR >60-90kg & IgE >200-300 IU/mL OR 30-70kg & IgE >300-400 IU/mL: 225mg q2 weeks; >90-150kg & IgE >200-300 IU/mL OR >70-90kg & IgE >300-400 IU/mL OR 30-70kg & IgE >400-500 IU/mL OR 30-60kg & IgE >500-600 IU/mL: 300mg q2 weeks; >70-90kg & IgE >400-500 IU/mL OR >60-70kg & IgE >500-600 IU/mL OR 30-60kg & IgE >600-700 IU/mL: 375mg q2 weeks.
*Pediatrics:* ≥12 yrs: 150-375mg SQ every 2 or 4 weeks based on body weight and pretreatment serum total IgE level. Max injection = 150mg/site. 30-90kg & IgE >30-100 IU/mL: 150mg q4 weeks; >90-150kg & IgE >30-100 IU/mL OR 30-90kg & IgE >100-200 IU/mL OR 30-60kg & IgE >200-300 IU/mL: 300mg q4 weeks; >90-150kg & IgE >100-200 IU/mL OR >60-90kg & IgE >200-300 IU/mL OR 30-70kg & IgE >300-400 IU/mL: 225mg q2 weeks; >90-150kg and IgE >200-300 IU/mL OR >70-90kg & IgE >300-400 IU/mL OR 30-70kg & IgE

>400-500 IU/mL OR 30-60kg & IgE >500-600 IU/mL: 300mg q2 weeks; >70-90kg & IgE >400-500 IU/mL OR >60-70kg & IgE >500-600 IU/mL OR 30-60kg & IgE >600-700 IU/mL: 375mg q2 weeks.

**HOW SUPPLIED:** Inj.: 150mg [5mL]

**WARNINGS/PRECAUTIONS:** Malignant neoplasms reported. Serious life-threatening anaphylaxis reported usually within 2 hrs of dose; monitor closely. Not for use in treatment of acute bronchospasm or status asthmaticus. Systemic or inhaled corticosteroids should not be abruptly discontinued when initiating therapy. Malignant neoplasms and anaphylaxis reported. Not for use in treatment of acute bronchospasm or status asthmaticus. Systemic or inhaled corticosteroids should not be abruptly discontinued when initiating therapy.

**ADVERSE REACTIONS:** Injection site reactions, viral infections, upper respiratory infection, sinusitis, headache, pharyngitis, pain, arthralgia, leg pain.

**PREGNANCY:** Category B, caution in nursing.

## XOPENEX RX

levalbuterol HCl (Sepracor)

**THERAPEUTIC CLASS:** $Beta_2$ agonist

**INDICATIONS:** Prevention and treatment of bronchospasm with reversible obstructive airway disease.

**DOSAGE:** *Adults:* Initial: 0.63mg tid, q6-8h. Severe Asthma: 1.25mg tid, q6-8h. Administer by nebulizer.
*Pediatrics:* >12 yrs: Initial: 0.63mg tid, q6-8h. Severe Asthma: 1.25mg tid, q6-8h. 6-11 yrs: 0.31mg tid. Max: 0.63mg tid. Administer by nebulizer.

**HOW SUPPLIED:** Sol: 0.31mg/3mL, 0.63mg/3mL, 1.25mg/3mL [3mL, $24^s$]

**WARNINGS/PRECAUTIONS:** Hypersensitivity reactions reported. Discontinue immediately if paradoxical bronchospasm occurs. May produce ECG changes; caution with cardiovascular disorders, coronary insufficiency, arrhythmias, and HTN. Caution with convulsive disorders, hyperthyroidism, and diabetes. May produce transient hypokalemia.

**ADVERSE REACTIONS:** Tachycardia, migraine, dyspepsia, leg cramps, nervousness, dizziness, tremor, rhinitis, increased cough, chest pain, HTN, hypotention, diarrhea, dry mouth, anxiety, insomnia, paresthesia, wheezing.

**INTERACTIONS:** Avoid other sympathomimetic agents. Extreme caution with MAOIs and TCAs. Monitor digoxin. ECG changes and/or hypokalemia with nonpotassium-sparing diuretics. Antagonized by β-blockers.

**PREGNANCY:** Category C, not for use in nursing.

## XOPENEX HFA RX

levalbuterol tartrate (Sepracor)

**THERAPEUTIC CLASS:** $Beta_2$ agonist

**INDICATIONS:** Prevention and treatment of bronchospasm with reversible obstructive airway disease.

**DOSAGE:** *Adults:* 2 inh (90mcg) q4-6hrs or 1 inh (45mcg) q4hrs may be sufficient.
*Pediatrics:* ≥4 yrs: 2 inh (90mcg) q4-6hrs or 1 inh (45mcg) q4hrs may be sufficient.



**HOW SUPPLIED:** MDI: 45mcg/inh [15g]

**WARNINGS/PRECAUTIONS:** Discontinue immediately if paradoxical bronchospasm occurs. May produce ECG changes; caution with cardiovascular disorders, coronary insufficiency, arrhythmias, and HTN. Caution with convulsive disorders, hyperthyroidism, and diabetes. May produce transient hypokalemia.

**ADVERSE REACTIONS:** Asthma, pharyngitis, rhinitis, pain, vomiting.

**INTERACTIONS:** Avoid other sympathomimetic agents. Extreme caution with MAOIs and TCAs. Monitor digoxin. ECG changes and/or hypokalemia with nonpotassium-sparing diuretics. Antagonized by β-blockers.

**PREGNANCY:** Category C, not for use in nursing.

## Xylocaine Injection

RX

lidocaine HCl (Abraxis)

**OTHER BRAND NAMES:** Xylocaine-MPF (Abraxis)

**THERAPEUTIC CLASS:** Local anesthetic

**INDICATIONS:** For production of local or regional anesthesia by infiltration techniques such as percutaneous injection and IV regional anesthesia by peripheral nerve block techniques such as brachial plexus and intercostal and by central neural techniques such as lumbar and caudal epidural blocks.

**DOSAGE:** *Adults:* Dosage varies depending on procedure, depth and duration of anesthesia, degree of muscular relaxation, and patient physical condition. Max: 4.5mg/kg or total dose of 300mg. Epidural/Caudal Anesthesia: Max: Intervals not less than 90 minutes. Paracervical Block: Max: 200mg/90 minutes. Regional Anesthesia: IV: Max: 4mg/kg. Children/Elderly/Debilitated/Cardiac or Liver Disease: Reduce dose. *Pediatrics:* >3 yrs: Max: 1.5-2mg/lb. Regional Anesthesia: IV: Max: 3mg/kg.

**HOW SUPPLIED:** Inj: 0.5%, 1%, 2%; (MPF) 0.5%, 1%, 1.5%, 2%

**WARNINGS/PRECAUTIONS:** Acidosis, cardiac arrest, death reported from delay in toxicity management. Local anesthetic solutions containing antimicrobial preservatives should not be used for epidural or spinal anesthesia. Use lowest effective dose. During epidural anesthesia, administer initial test dose and monitor for CNS and cardiovascular toxicity as well as for signs of unintended intrathecal administration. Reduce dose with debilitated, elderly, acutely ill, and children. Extreme caution when using lumbar and caudal epidural anesthesia with existing neurological disease, spinal deformities, septicemia, and severe HTN. Monitor cardiovascular and respiratory vital signs and state of consciousness after each injection. Caution with hepatic disease, cardiovascular disorders. Monitor circulation and respiration with injections into head and neck area.

**ADVERSE REACTIONS:** Lightheadedness, nervousness, euphoria, confusion, dizziness, drowsiness, tinnitus, blurred vision, vomiting, heat/cold sensations, twitching, tremors, convulsions, respiratory depression, bradycardia, hypotension, urticaria, edema, anaphylactoid reactions.

**PREGNANCY:** Category B, caution in nursing.

## Xylocaine Jelly

RX

lidocaine HCl (Abraxis)

**THERAPEUTIC CLASS:** Acetamide local anesthetic

**INDICATIONS:** Prevention and control of pain in procedures involving the male and female urethra. Topical treatment of painful urethritis. Anesthetic lubricant for endotracheal intubation.

**DOSAGE:** *Adults:* Max: 600mg/12 hrs. Surface Anesthesia of Male Urethra: Instill about 15mL (300mg). Instill an additional dose of not more than 15mL if needed. Prior to Sounding or Cystoscopy: A total dose of 30mL (600mg) is usually required. Prior to Catheterization: 5-10mL usually adequate. Surface Anesthesia of Female Urethra: Instill 3-5mL. Elderly/Debilitated: Reduce dose. *Pediatrics:* Determine dose by age and weight. Max: 4.5mg/kg.

**HOW SUPPLIED:** Jelly: 2% [Tube: 5mL, 30mL; Syringe: 10mL, 20mL]

**WARNINGS/PRECAUTIONS:** Avoid excessive dosage or frequent administration; may result in serious adverse effects requiring resuscitative measures. Caution with heart block and severe shock. Extreme caution if mucosa traumatized or sepsis is present in the area of application; risk of rapid systemic absorption.

**ADVERSE REACTIONS:** Lightheadedness, nervousness, confusion, euphoria, dizziness, drowsiness, blurred vision, tremors, convulsions, respiratory depression, bradycardia, hypotension, urticaria, edema, anaphylactoid reactions.

**PREGNANCY:** Category B, caution in nursing.

## XYLOCAINE VISCOUS — RX

lidocaine HCl (Abraxis)

**THERAPEUTIC CLASS:** Acetamide local anesthetic

**INDICATIONS:** Topical anesthesia of irritated or inflamed mucous membranes of the mouth and pharynx. To reduce gagging during X-ray or dental procedures.

**DOSAGE:** *Adults:* Irritated/Inflamed Mucous Membranes: Usual: 15mL undiluted. (Mouth) Swish and spit out. (Pharynx) Gargle and may swallow. Do not administer in <3 hr intervals. Max: 8 doses/24hr; (Single Dose) 4.5mg/kg or total of 300mg.
*Pediatrics:* >3 yrs: Max: Determine by age and weight. Infants <3 yrs: Apply 1.25mL with cotton-tipped applicator to immediate area. Do not administer in <3 hour intervals. Max: 8 doses/24hr.

**HOW SUPPLIED:** Sol: 2% [100mL, 450mL]

**WARNINGS/PRECAUTIONS:** Reduce dose in elderly, debilitated, acutely ill and children. Caution with heart block and severe shock. Excessive dosage or too frequent administration may result in high plasma levels and serious adverse effects requiring resuscitative measures. Extreme caution if mucosa traumatized; risk of rapid systemic absorption. Overdose reported in pediatrics due to inappropriate dosing.

**ADVERSE REACTIONS:** Lightheadedness, nervousness, confusion, euphoria, dizziness, drowsiness, blurred vision, tremors, convulsions, respiratory depression, bradycardia, hypotension, urticaria, edema, anaphylactoid reactions.

**PREGNANCY:** Category B, caution in nursing.

## XYLOCAINE WITH EPINEPHRINE — RX

epinephrine - lidocaine HCl (Abraxis)

**OTHER BRAND NAMES:** Xylocaine-MPF with Epinephrine (Abraxis)

**THERAPEUTIC CLASS:** Local anesthetic

**INDICATIONS:** For production of local or regional anesthesia by infiltration techniques such as percutaneous injection and IV regional anesthesia by peripheral nerve block techniques such as brachial plexus and intercostal and by central neural techniques such as lumbar and caudal epidural blocks.

**DOSAGE:** *Adults:* Dosage varies depending on procedure, depth and duration of anesthesia, degree of muscular relaxation, and patient physical condition. Max: 7mg/kg or total dose of 500mg. Epidural/Caudal Anesthesia: Max: Intervals not less than 90 minutes. Paracervical Block: Max: 200mg/90 minutes. Regional Anesthesia: IV: Max: 4mg/kg.
Children/Elderly/Debilitated/Cardiac or Liver Disease: Reduce dose.
*Pediatrics:* >3 yrs: Max: 1.5-2mg/lb. Regional Anesthesia: IV: Max: 3mg/kg.

**HOW SUPPLIED:** Inj: (Lidocaine-Epinephrine) 0.5%/1:200,000, 1%/1:100,000, 2%/1:100,000; (MPF) 1%/1:200,000, 1.5%/1:200,000, 2%/1:200,000

**WARNINGS/PRECAUTIONS:** Acidosis, cardiac arrest, death reported from delay in toxicity management. Local anesthetic solutions containing antimicrobial preservatives should not be used for epidural or spinal anesthesia. Xylocaine with epinephrine solutions contain sodium metabisulfite which may cause allergic-type reactions in susceptible people. Use lowest effective dose. During epidural anesthesia, administer initial test dose and monitor for CNS and cardiovascular toxicity as well as for signs of unintended intrathecal administration. Reduce dose with debilitated, elderly, acutely ill, and children. Extreme caution when using lumbar and caudal epidural anesthesia with existing neurological disease, spinal deformities, septicemia, and severe HTN. Caution when local anesthetic injections containing a vasoconstrictor are used in areas of the body supplied by end arteries or having otherwise compromised blood supply; ischemic injury or necrosis may result with peripheral or hypertensive vascular disease due to exaggerated vasoconstrictor response. Monitor cardiovascular and respiratory vital signs and state of consciousness after each injection. Caution with hepatic disease, cardiovascular disorders. Monitor circulation and respiration with injections into head and neck area.

**ADVERSE REACTIONS:** Lightheadedness, nervousness, euphoria, confusion, dizziness, drowsiness, tinnitus, blurred vision, vomiting, heat/cold sensations, twitching, tremors, convulsions, respiratory depression, bradycardia, hypotension, urticaria, edema, anaphylactoid reactions.

**INTERACTIONS:** Anesthetic solutions containing epinephrine or norepinephrine with MAOIs or TCAs may produce severe, prolonged HTN; avoid concurrent use or monitor closely if concurrent use is essential. Phenothiazines and butyrophenones may reduce or reverse pressor effect of epinephrine; avoid concurrent use or monitor closely if concurrent use is essential. Vasopressors, ergot-type oxytocic drugs may cause severe, persistent HTN or CVA.

**PREGNANCY:** Category B, caution in nursing.

## XYREM

**CIII**

sodium oxybate (Orphan Medical)

**Sodium oxybate is GHB (gamma hydroxybutyrate), a known drug of abuse. Do not use with alcohol or other CNS depressants. Associated with confusion, depression, and other neuropsychiatric events. Available only through the Xyrem Success Program, call 1-866-XYREM88.**

**THERAPEUTIC CLASS:** CNS Depressant

**INDICATIONS:** Treatment of excessive daytime sleepiness and cataplexy in patients with narcolepsy.

**DOSAGE:** *Adults:* Initial: 2.25g qhs, then take 2.25g 2.5-4 hrs later. Titrate: Increase by 0.75g/dose every 1-2 weeks. Range: 6-9g/night. Max: 9g/night. Hepatic Insufficiency: Initial: Decrease by 50%. Titrate dose increments to effect. Take 1st dose at bedtime while in bed and the 2nd dose while sitting in bed. Dilute each dose with 2 ounces of water.

*Pediatrics:* ≥16 yrs: Initial: 2.25g qhs, then take 2.25g 2.5-4 hrs later. Titrate: Increase by 0.75g/dose every 1-2 weeks. Range: 6-9g/night. Max: 9g/night. Hepatic Insufficiency: Initial: Decrease by 50%. Titrate dose increments to effect. Take 1st dose at bedtime while in bed and the 2nd dose while sitting in bed. Dilute each dose with 2 ounces of water.

**HOW SUPPLIED:** Sol: 500mg/mL [180mL]

**CONTRAINDICATIONS:** Sedative hypnotic agents, succinic semialdehyde dehydrogenase deficiency.

**WARNINGS/PRECAUTIONS:** Rapid onset of CNS depressant effects; ingest only at bedtime and while in bed. Avoid engaging in activities requiring mental alertness for 6 hrs after ingestion. Daily sodium intake ranges from 0.5g (with 3g dose) to 1.6g (with 9g dose); caution in heart failure, HTN, or renal impairment. Caution with compromised respiratory function, hepatic insufficiency, history of depressive illness or suicide attempts, elderly. Evaluate patients who develop through disorders or behavior abnormalities. Sleepwalking reported. Rule out worsening sleep apnea or nocturnal seizures if incontinence develops.

**ADVERSE REACTIONS:** Headache, nausea, dizziness, pain, somnolence, pharyngitis, infection, flu syndrome, diarrhea, urinary incontinence, vomiting, rhinitis, asthenia, sinusitis, nervousness, back pain, confusion, sleepwalking, depression, dyspepsia, abdominal pain, abnormal dreams, insomnia.

**INTERACTIONS:** Avoid alcohol, sedative hypnotics, or other CNS depressants. Food decreases bioavailability.

**PREGNANCY:** Category B, caution in nursing.

## XYZAL RX
levocetirizine dihydrochloride (UCB)

**THERAPEUTIC CLASS:** $H_1$ antagonist

**INDICATIONS:** Seasonal and perennial allergic rhinitis. Chronic idiopathic urticaria.

**DOSAGE:** *Adults:* 5mg qd in evening. Adjust dose with decreased renal function.
*Pediatrics:* ≥12 yrs: 5mg qd in evening. Adjust dose with decreased renal function. 6-11 yrs:2.5mg (1/2 tab) qd in evening.

**HOW SUPPLIED:** Tab: 5mg* *scored

**CONTRAINDICATIONS:** End stage renal disease (CrCl <10mL/min) or hemodialysis. Pediatrics 6-11 yrs with renal impairment.

**WARNINGS/PRECAUTIONS:** May impair mental/physical abilities.

**ADVERSE REACTIONS:** Somnolence, fatigue, dry mouth, headache, pharyngitis, abdominal pain, cough, epistaxis.

**INTERACTIONS:** Avoid alcohol and CNS depressants. Possible decreased clearance with large doses of theophylline.

**PREGNANCY:** Category B, not for use in nursing.

## YASMIN RX
drospirenone - ethinyl estradiol (Berlex)

**THERAPEUTIC CLASS:** Estrogen/progestogen combination

**INDICATIONS:** Prevention of pregnancy.

**DOSAGE:** *Adults:* Start 1st Sunday after menses begins or the 1st day of menses. 1 tab qd for 28 days, then repeat.

**HOW SUPPLIED:** Tab: (Ethinyl Estradiol-Drospirenone) 0.03mg-3mg

**CONTRAINDICATIONS:** Renal or adrenal insufficiency, hepatic dysfunction, thrombophlebitis, thromboembolic disorders, history of deep vein thrombophlebitis, cerebrovascular or CAD, breast carcinoma, endometrial carcinoma, estrogen-dependent neoplasia, undiagnosed abnormal genital bleeding, cholestatic jaundice of pregnancy or jaundice with prior pill use, liver tumor, active liver disease, pregnancy, heavy smoking (>15 cigarettes daily) and >35 yrs.

**WARNINGS/PRECAUTIONS:** Cigarette smoking increases risk of serious CV side effects. This risk increases with age (especially >35 yrs) and heavy smoking. Increased risk of MI, thromboembolism, thrombotic disease, cerebrovascular events, and gallbladder disease. Monitor $K^+$ levels during first cycle with conditions predisposing to hyperkalemia. Retinal thrombosis, hepatic neoplasia, carcinoma of breast and reproductive organs reported. May cause glucose intolerance. May increase BP, elevate LDL levels or cause other lipid changes, fluid retention, breakthrough bleeding and spotting. May cause or exacerbate migraine. May develop visual changes with contact lens. Increased risk of MI with HTN, hyperlipidemia, obesity and DM. Discontinue if develop jaundice, significant depression or ophthalmic irregularities. Use before menarche is not indicated.

**ADVERSE REACTIONS:** Nausea, vomiting, breakthrough bleeding, spotting, amenorrhea, migraine, depression, vaginal candidiasis, edema, weight changes.

**INTERACTIONS:** Reduced effects, increased breakthrough bleeding, and menstrual irregularities with rifampin, phenobarbital, phenytoin, carbamazepine, possibly with griseofulvin, ampicillin, tetracycline, St. John's wort, and phenylbutazone. Increased levels with atorvastatin, ascorbic acid and APAP. Risk of hyperkalemia with ACE inhibitors, angiotensin-II receptor antagonists, potassium-sparing diuretics, heparin, aldosterone antagonists, and NSAIDs; monitor $K^+$ levels during 1st cycle. Increased levels of cyclosporine, prednisolone, and theophylline. May decrease APAP levels and increase clearance of temazepam, salicylic acid, morphine, and clofibric acid.

**PREGNANCY:** Category X, not for use in nursing.

## YAZ

RX

drospirenone - ethinyl estradiol (Berlex)

**THERAPEUTIC CLASS:** Estrogen/progestogen combination

**INDICATIONS:** Prevention of pregnancy. Treatment of symptoms of premenstrual dysphoric disorder (PMDD). Treatment of moderate acne vulgaris in women 14 yrs and older.

**DOSAGE:** *Adults:* 1 tab qd for 28 days (24 active plus 4 inert pills), then repeat. Start 1st Sunday after menses begin or 1st day of menses.
*Pediatrics:* ≥14 yrs: Acne: 1 tab qd for 28 days (24 active plus 4 inert pills), then repeat. Start 1st Sunday after menses begin or 1st day of menses.

**HOW SUPPLIED:** Tab: (Ethinyl Estradiol-Drospirenone) 0.02mg-3mg

**CONTRAINDICATIONS:** Renal or adrenal insufficiency, hepatic dysfunction, thrombophlebitis, thromboembolic disorders, history of deep vein thrombophlebitis, valvular heart disease with thrombogenic complications, severe HTN, DM with vascular involvement, HA with focal neurological symptoms, major surgery with prolonged immobilization, cerebrovascular or CAD, breast carcinoma, endometrial carcinoma, estrogen-dependent neoplasia, undiagnosed abnormal genital bleeding, cholestatic jaundice of pregnancy or jaundice with prior pill use, liver tumor, active liver disease, pregnancy, heavy smoking (>15 cigarettes daily) and >35 yrs.

**WARNINGS/PRECAUTIONS:** Cigarette smoking increases risk of serious CV side effects. Risk increases with age (especially >35 yrs) and with heavy smoking. Increased risk of MI, thromboembolism, thrombotic disease, cerebrovascular events, and gallbladder disease. Monitor $K^+$ levels during first cycle with conditions predisposing to hyperkalemia. Retinal thrombosis, hepatic neoplasia, carcinoma of breast and reproductive organs reported. May cause glucose intolerance. May increase BP, elevate LDL levels or cause other lipid changes, fluid retention, breakthrough bleeding and spotting. May cause or exacerbate migraine. May develop visual changes with contact lens. Increased risk of MI with HTN, hyperlipidemia, obesity and DM. D/C if jaundice, significant depression or ophthalmic irregularities develop. Use before menarche is not indicated.

**ADVERSE REACTIONS:** Nausea, vomiting, breakthrough bleeding, spotting, amenorrhea, migraine, mental depression, vaginal candidiasis, edema, weight changes, depression decrease in serum folate levels, aggravation of varicose veins, uritcaria, angioedema, severe reactions with respiratory and circulatory symptoms, dysmenorrhea.

**INTERACTIONS:** Reduced effects, increased breakthrough bleeding, and menstrual irregularities with rifampin, phenobarbital, phenytoin, carbamazepine, possibly with griseofulvin, ampicillin, tetracycline, St. John's wort, and phenylbutazone. Increased levels with atorvastatin, ascorbic acid and APAP. Risk of hyperkalemia with ACE inhibitors, angiotensin-II receptor antagonists, potassium-sparing diuretics, heparin, aldosterone antagonists, and NSAIDs; monitor $K^+$ levels during 1st cycle. Increased levels of cyclosporine, prednisolone, and theophylline. May decrease APAP levels and increase clearance of temazepam, salicylic acid, morphine, and clofibric acid.

**PREGNANCY:** Category X, not for use in nursing.

## YF-VAX

RX

yellow fever vaccine (Sanofi Pasteur)

**THERAPEUTIC CLASS:** Vaccine

**INDICATIONS:** Active immunization of persons ≥9 months living or traveling to endemic areas or for international travel when required or laboratory personnel who might be exposed to virulent yellow fever virus.

**DOSAGE:** *Adults:* Primary Vaccination: 0.5mL (4.74 $log_{10}$ PFU) SQ. Booster: 0.5mL (4.74 $log_{10}$ PFU) every 10 yrs. Desensitization: 0.05mL of 1:10 dilution, then 0.05mL of full strength, then 0.10mL of full strength, then 0.15mL of full strength, then 0.20mL of full strength SQ at 15-20 minute intervals. *Pediatrics:* ≥9 months: Primary Vaccination: 0.5mL (4.74 $log_{10}$ PFU) SQ. Booster: 0.5mL (4.74 $log_{10}$ PFU) every 10 years. Desensitization: 0.05mL of 1:10 dilution, then 0.05mL of full strength, then 0.10mL of full strength, then 0.15mL of full strength, then 0.20mL of full strength SQ at 15-20 minute intervals.

**HOW SUPPLIED:** Inj: 4.74 $log_{10}$ PFU/0.5mL

**CONTRAINDICATIONS:** Hypersensitivity to eggs or egg products. Immunosuppressed patients due to illness (eg, HIV infection, leukemia, lymphoma, thymoma, generalized malignancy) or drug therapy (eg, corticosteriods, alkylating drugs, or antimetabolites) or radiation.

**WARNINGS/PRECAUTIONS:** Epinephrine (1:1000) should be immediately available. Vaccine-associated viscerotropic disease (rare) and vaccine-associated neurotropic disease (rare).

**ADVERSE REACTIONS:** Systemic: Headache, myalgia, low-grade fevers. Local: Edema, hypersensitivity, pain or mass at injection site.

**INTERACTIONS:** Prednisone and other corticosteroids may decrease immunogenicity and increase risk of adverse events.

**PREGNANCY:** Category C, not for use in nursing.

## YOCON

RX

yohimbine HCl (Glenwood)

**THERAPEUTIC CLASS:** $Alpha_2$ receptor blocker

**INDICATIONS:** As a sympatholytic and mydriatic for erectile dysfunction.

**DOSAGE:** *Adults:* Usual: 5.4mg tid. Decrease to 2.7mg (1/2 tab) if side effects occur, then increase to 5.4mg tid gradually. Max: 10 weeks of therapy.

**HOW SUPPLIED:** Tab: 5.4mg

**CONTRAINDICATIONS:** Renal disease.

**WARNINGS/PRECAUTIONS:** Not for use in females, especially in pregnancy. Not for use in pediatrics, geriatrics, or cardio-renal patients with gastric or duodenal ulcer history. Do not use in psychiatric patients.

**ADVERSE REACTIONS:** Anti-diuresis, increased blood pressure and heart rate, increased motor activity, irritability, tremor, sweating, nausea, vomiting, dizziness, headache, skin flushing.

**INTERACTIONS:** Avoid with antidepressants or other mood-modifying drugs.

**PREGNANCY:** Safety in pregnancy and nursing is not known.

## ZADITOR OTC
ketotifen fumarate (Novartis Ophthalmics)

**THERAPEUTIC CLASS:** $H_1$ antagonist and mast cell stabilizer

**INDICATIONS:** Temporary prevention of itching of the eye due to allergic conjunctivitis.

**DOSAGE:** *Adults:* 1 drop q8-12h.
*Pediatrics:* >3 yrs: 1 drop q8-12h.

**HOW SUPPLIED:** Sol: 0.025% [5mL]

**WARNINGS/PRECAUTIONS:** Not for contact lens irritation. Do not wear a contact lens if eye is red. If eyes are not red, wait 10 minutes after instillation before inserting contacts. Soft contact lens can absorb benzalkonium chloride.

**ADVERSE REACTIONS:** Rhinitis, allergic reactions, burning, stinging, conjunctivitis, dry eye, eye pain, eyelid disorder, itching, keratitis, lacrimation disorder, mydriasis, photophobia, headache, rash.

**PREGNANCY:** Category C, caution in nursing.

## ZANAFLEX RX
tizanidine HCl (Acorda)

**THERAPEUTIC CLASS:** Centrally acting $alpha_2$-adrenergic agonist

**INDICATIONS:** Short-term treatment of spasticity.

**DOSAGE:** *Adults:* Initial: 4mg single dose q6-8h. Titrate: Increase by 2-4mg. Usual: 8mg single dose q6-8h. Max: 3 doses/24h or 36mg/day.

**HOW SUPPLIED:** Cap: 2mg, 4mg, 6mg; Tab: 2mg*, 4mg* *scored

**CONTRAINDICATIONS:** Concomitant use with fluvoxamine, ciprofloxacin or potent inhibitors of CYP1A2.

**WARNINGS/PRECAUTIONS:** May prolong QT interval. May cause liver damage; monitor baseline LFTs and at 1, 3, and 6 months. Retinal degeneration and corneal opacities reported. Caution with renal impairment or elderly. May cause hypotension, caution with antihypertensives; avoid ciprofloxacin and fluvoxamine. Use with extreme cautions in patients with hepatic impairment. May cause sedation and hallucinations. Avoid concomitant use with oral contraceptives. When discontinuing, taper dose to avoid withdrawal and rebound hypertension, tachycardia, and hypertonia.

**ADVERSE REACTIONS:** Dry mouth, somnolence, asthenia, dizziness, UTI, urinary frequency, flu-like syndrome, rhinitis.

**INTERACTIONS:** See Contraindications. Potentiated depressant effect with alcohol. Potentiated by oral contraceptives. Avoid alpha-adrenergic agonists. Avoid with CYP1A2 inhibitors.

**PREGNANCY:** Category C, caution in nursing.

## ZANOSAR RX
streptozocin (Sicor)

**Associated with dose-related renal toxicity, nausea, vomiting, liver dysfunction, diarrhea, and hematological changes.**

**THERAPEUTIC CLASS:** Alkylating Agent

**INDICATIONS:** Treatment of metastatic islet cell carcinoma of the pancreas.

**DOSAGE:** *Adults:* Daily Schedule: $500mg/m^2$ IV daily for 5 days every 6 weeks until maximum benefit or treatment-limiting toxicity occurs. Weekly Schedule: $1g/m^2$ IV at 1 week intervals for 1st two doses. Titrate: May increase dose for subsequent courses if response not achieved. Max: $1.5g/m^2$/dose. Significant Renal Toxicity: Reduce dose or discontinue.

**HOW SUPPLIED:** Inj: 1gm

**WARNINGS/PRECAUTIONS:** Monitor renal function before and after each course of therapy. Obtain urinalysis, BUN, SCr, electrolytes, and CrCl prior to, at least weekly during, and 4 weeks after drug is given. May cause extravasation. Monitor CBCs and LFTs at least weekly. Caution in elderly. May impair mental/physical activities.

**ADVERSE REACTIONS:** Nausea, vomiting, diarrhea, hepatic and renal toxicity, glucose tolerance abnormality.

**INTERACTIONS:** Additive toxicity with other cytotoxic drugs. Avoid other potential nephrotoxins. May prolong doxorubicin half-life and lead to severe bone marrow suppression; consider reducing doxorubicin dose.

**PREGNANCY:** Category D, not for use in nursing.

## ZANTAC

RX

ranitidine HCl (GlaxoSmithKline)

**THERAPEUTIC CLASS:** $H_2$ blocker

**INDICATIONS:** (PO) Short-term treatment of active duodenal (DU) and benign gastric ulcers (GU). Maintenance therapy for duodenal and gastric ulcers. Treatment of pathological hypersecretory conditions (eg, Zollinger-Ellison) and GERD. Treatment and maintenance of erosive esophagitis. (Inj) Hospitalized patients with pathological hypersecretory conditions or intractable duodenal ulcer. Short term alternate to oral therapy.

**DOSAGE:** *Adults:* (PO) DU/GU: 150mg bid or (DU) 300mg after evening meal or qhs. Maint: 150mg qhs. GERD: 150mg bid. Erosive Esophagitis: 150mg qid. Maint: 150mg bid. Hypersecretory Conditions: 150mg bid. May give up to 6g/day with severe disease. (Inj) Usual: 50mg IV/IM q6-8 hrs or 6.25mg/hr continuous IV. Max: 400mg/day. Zollinger-Ellison: Initial: 1mg/kg/hr. Titrate: May increase after 4 hrs by 0.5mg/kg/hr increments. Max: 2.5mg/kg/hr or 220mg/hr. CrCl <50mL/min: 50mg IV q18-24 hrs or 150mg PO q24h. Give more frequent (q12h) if necessary. Hemodialysis: Give dose at end of treatment. Dissolve each 150mg effervescent tab in 6-8oz of water before administration.
*Pediatrics:* 1 month-16 yrs: (PO) DU/GU: 2-4mg/kg bid. Max: 300mg/day. Maint: 2-4mg/kg qd. Max: 150mg/day. GERD/Erosive Esophagitis: 2.5-5mg/kg bid. (Inj) DU: 2-4mg/kg/day IV given q6-8 hrs. Max: 50mg q6-8 hrs. CrCl <50mL/min: 50mg IV q18-24 hrs or 150mg PO q24h. Give more frequent (q12h) if necessary. Hemodialysis: Give dose at end of treatment. Dissolve each 25mg effervescent tab in 5mL of water before administration.

**HOW SUPPLIED:** Inj: 1mg/mL, 25mg/mL; Syrup: 15mg/mL; Tab: 150mg, 300mg; Tab, Effervescent: 25mg, 150mg

**WARNINGS/PRECAUTIONS:** Do not exceed recommended infusion rates; bradycardia reported with rapid infusion. Caution with liver and renal dysfunction. Monitor SGPT if on IV therapy for >5 days at dose >100mg qid. Avoid use with history of acute porphyria. Symptomatic response does not preclude the presence of gastric malignancy. May cause false (+) urine protein test. Granules and effervescent tablets contain phenylalanine.

**ADVERSE REACTIONS:** Headache, constipation, diarrhea, nausea, abdominal discomfort, vomiting, hepatitis, blood dyscrasias, rash, injection site reactions (IV/IM).

**INTERACTIONS:** Increases plasma levels of triazolam. Monitor anticoagulants.

**PREGNANCY:** Category B, caution with nursing.

## ZANTAC OTC

OTC

ranitidine HCl (McNeil)

**OTHER BRAND NAMES:** Zantac 75 (McNeil) - Zantac 150 (McNeil)

**THERAPEUTIC CLASS:** $H_2$ blocker

**INDICATIONS:** For prevention and relief of heartburn associated with acid indigestion and sour stomach brought on by certain foods and beverages.

**DOSAGE:** *Adults:* Treatment/Relief of Heartburn: 75-150mg with water. Heartburn Prevention: 75-150mg 30-60 minutes before eating food or drinking beverages that cause heartburn. Max: 150mg/24 hrs.
*Pediatrics:* >12 yrs: Treatment/Relief of Heartburn: 75-150mg with water. Heartburn Prevention: 75-150mg 30-60 minutes before eating food or drinking beverages that cause heartburn. Max: 150mg/24 hrs.

**HOW SUPPLIED:** Tab: 75mg, 150mg

**CONTRAINDICATIONS:** Trouble or pain swallowing food, vomiting with blood, or bloody or black stools.

**WARNINGS/PRECAUTIONS:** Trouble swallowing or persistent abdominal pain may indicate a more serious condition.

**INTERACTIONS:** Avoid other acid reducers.

**PREGNANCY:** Safety in pregnancy and nursing not known.

## ZARONTIN

RX

ethosuximide (Parke-Davis)

**THERAPEUTIC CLASS:** Succinimide

**INDICATIONS:** Control of absence (petit mal) epilepsy.

**DOSAGE:** *Adults:* 500mg qd. Titrate: May increase daily dose by 250mg every 4-7 days. Max: 1.5g/day.
*Pediatrics:* Initial: 3-6 yrs: 250mg qd. >6 yrs: 500mg qd. Titrate: May increase daily dose by 250mg every 4-7 days. Usual: 20mg/kg/day. Max: 1.5g/day.

**HOW SUPPLIED:** Cap: 250mg; Syrup: 250mg/5mL

**WARNINGS/PRECAUTIONS:** Extreme caution in liver and renal dysfunction. Monitor blood counts, liver and renal function periodically. SLE, blood dyscrasias reported. Adjust dose slowly and avoid abrupt withdrawal. May increase grand mal seizures in mixed types of epilepsy when used alone. Caution with mental/physical activities.

**ADVERSE REACTIONS:** Anorexia, nausea, vomiting, abdominal pain, blood dyscrasias, drowsiness, headache, urticaria, SLE, myopia.

**INTERACTIONS:** May increase phenytoin levels. Valproic acid may alter levels.

**PREGNANCY:** Safety in pregnancy and nursing not known.

## ZAROXOLYN

RX

metolazone (Celltech)

**Do not interchange rapid and complete bioavailability metolazone formulations for other slow and incomplete bioavailability metolazone formulations; they are not therapeutically equivalent.**

**THERAPEUTIC CLASS:** Quinazoline diuretic

**INDICATIONS:** Treatment of hypertension and of salt and water retention in edema accompanying CHF or renal disease.

**DOSAGE:** *Adults:* Edema: 5-20mg qd. HTN: 2.5-5mg qd. Elderly: Start at low end of dosing range.

**HOW SUPPLIED:** Tab: 2.5mg, 5mg, 10mg

**CONTRAINDICATIONS:** Anuria, hepatic coma or precoma.

**WARNINGS/PRECAUTIONS:** Risk of hypokalemia, orthostatic hypotension, hypercalcemia, hyperuricemia, azotemia and rapid onset hyponatremia. Cross-allergy with sulfonamide-derived drugs, thiazides, or quinethazone. Sensitivity reactions may occur with 1st dose. Monitor electrolytes. May cause hyperglycemia and glycosuria in diabetics. Caution in elderly or severe renal impairment. May exacerbate or activate SLE.

**ADVERSE REACTIONS:** Chest pain/discomfort, orthostatic hypotension, syncope, neuropathy, necrotizing angiitis, hepatitis, jaundice, pancreatitis, blood dyscrasias, joint pain.

**INTERACTIONS:** Furosemide and other loop diuretics prolong fluid and electrolyte loss. Adjust dose of other antihypertensives. Potentiates hypotensive effects of alcohol, barbiturates, and narcotics. Lithium, digitalis toxicity. Corticosteroids and ACTH increase hypokalemia and salt and water retention. Enhanced neuromuscular blocking effects of curariform drugs. Salicylates and NSAIDs decrease effects. Decreased arterial response to norepinephrine. Decrease in methenamine efficacy. Adjust anticoagulants, antidiabetics.

**PREGNANCY:** Category B, not for use in nursing.

## ZEBETA

RX

bisoprolol fumarate (Duramed)

**THERAPEUTIC CLASS:** Selective $beta_1$-blocker

**INDICATIONS:** Management of hypertension.

**DOSAGE:** *Adults:* Initial: 2.5-5mg qd. Max: 20mg/day. Hepatic Dysfunction or CrCl <40mL/min: Initial: 2.5mg qd; caution with dose titration.

**HOW SUPPLIED:** Tab: 5mg*, 10mg *scored

**CONTRAINDICATIONS:** Cardiogenic shock, overt cardiac failure, 2nd- or 3rd-degree AV block, marked sinus bradycardia.

**WARNINGS/PRECAUTIONS:** Avoid abrupt withdrawal. May mask hypoglycemia or hyperthyroidism symptoms. Caution with compensated cardiac failure, DM, bronchospastic disease, hepatic/renal impairment, or peripheral vascular disease. May precipitate cardiac failure.

**ADVERSE REACTIONS:** Diarrhea, upper respiratory infection, fatigue.

**INTERACTIONS:** May block epinephrine effects. Caution with clonidine withdrawal. Excessive reduction of sympathetic activity with catecholamine-depleting drugs. Avoid other β-blockers. Caution with calcium channel blockers (eg, verapamil, diltiazem), antiarrhythmics (eg, disopyramide), and anesthetics that depress myocardial function. Rifampin increases clearance. Antidiabetic agents may need adjustment.

**PREGNANCY:** Category C, caution in nursing.

## ZEGERID

RX

omeprazole - sodium bicarbonate (Santarus)

**THERAPEUTIC CLASS:** Proton pump inhibitor

**INDICATIONS:** (Cap, Powder) Short-term treatment of erosive esophagitis diagnosed by endoscopy, active duodenal ulcer, and active benign gastric ulcer. Treatment of heartburn and other symptoms associated with GERD. Maintain healing of erosive espophagitis. (Powder, 40mg-1680mg) Reduction of risk of upper GI bleeding in critically ill patients.

**DOSAGE:** *Adults:* Cap/Powder: Duodenal Ulcer: 20mg qd for 4-8 weeks. Gastric Ulcer: 40mg qd for 4-8 weeks. GERD: 20mg qd for up to 4 weeks without esophageal lesions and for 4-8 weeks with erosive esophagitis. Maintenance of Healing Erosive Esophagitis: 20mg qd. Powder (40mg-1680mg): Risk Reduction of Upper GI Bleeding in Critically Ill Patients: Initial: 40mg, followed by 40mg after 6-8 hrs. Maint: 40mg qd for 14 days. Take 1 hr before a meal. Add packet contents to 2 tablespoons of water; do not use other liquids or foods. Stir powder well and drink immediately. Swallow caps whole with water.

**HOW SUPPLIED:** (Omeprazole-Sodium Bicarbonate) Cap: 20mg-1100mg, 40mg-1100mg; Powder: 20mg-1680mg/packet [30s], 40mg-1680mg/packet [30s].

**WARNINGS/PRECAUTIONS:** Atrophic gastritis reported with long-term use. Symptomatic response does not preclude the presence of gastric malignancy. Due to sodium bicarbonate content, avoid with metabolic alkalosis, hypocalcemia and use caution with a sodium-restricted diet, Bartter's syndrome, hypocalcemia, respiratory alkalosis. Long-term use of bicarbonate with calcium or milk may cause milk-alkali syndrome.

**ADVERSE REACTIONS:** Abdominal pain, headache, nausea, vomiting.

**INTERACTIONS:** May prolong elimination of diazepam, warfarin, phenytoin, and drugs metabolized by oxidation. May alter absorption of pH-dependent drugs (eg, ketoconazole, ampicillin esters, and iron salts). Monitor when given with drugs metabolized by CYP450 (eg, cyclosporine, disulfiram, benzodiazepines). Clarithromycin may increase levels. May increase levels of tacrolimus, clarithromycin. May reduce levels of atazanavir.

**PREGNANCY:** Category C, not for use in nursing.

## ZELAPAR — RX

selegiline HCl (Valeant)

**THERAPEUTIC CLASS:** Monoamine oxidase inhibitor (Type B)

**INDICATIONS:** Adjunct in the management of Parkinson's disease in patients exhibiting a deteriorated response to levodopa/carbidopa therapy.

**DOSAGE:** *Adults:* 1.25mg every AM without liquid for 6 weeks. Titrate: After 6 weeks, may increase to 2.5mg if desired benefit not achieved. Max: 2.5mg/day.

**HOW SUPPLIED:** Tab, Orally Disintigrating: 1.25mg

**CONTRAINDICATIONS:** Concomitant meperidine, tramadol, methadone, propoxyphene dextromethorphan, and other MAOIs.

**WARNINGS/PRECAUTIONS:** Do not exceed 2.5mg/day; risk of non-selective MAO inhibition. Greater risk of orthostatic hypotension and dizziness in geriatric patients. Decrease levodopa/carbidopa to prevent exacerbation of levodopa side effects. Perform periodic dermatologic screening. May increase frequency of mild oropharyngeal abnormality. Caution with renal or hepatic impairment. Neuroleptic malignant syndrome reported in association with rapid dose reduction, withdrawal of, or changes in antiparkinsonian therapy.

**ADVERSE REACTIONS:** Nausea, dizziness, pain, headache, insomnia, rhinitis, skin disorders, dyskinesia, backache, dyspepsia, stomatitis, constipation, hallucinations, pharyngitis, rash.

**INTERACTIONS:** See Contraindications. Serious, sometimes fatal, reactions have been precipitated with meperidine, tramadol, methadone, and propoxyphene; avoid concomitant use. Episodes of psychosis or bizarre behavior reported with dextromethorphan; avoid concomitant use. Severe toxicity reported with SSRIs or TCAs; avoid concurrent use and allow 2 weeks between discontinuation of selegiline and initiation of TCAs or SSRIs. Allow 5 weeks for fluoxetine due to a longer half-life. Caution with sympathomimetics and CYP3A4 inducers (eg, phenytoin, carbamazepine, nafcillin, phenobarbital, and rifampin).

**PREGNANCY:** Category C, not for use in nursing.

## ZEMAIRA

RX

alpha1-proteinase inhibitor (human) (ZLB Behring)

**THERAPEUTIC CLASS:** Alpha$_1$-Proteinase Inhibitor

**INDICATIONS:** Chronic augmentation and maintenance therapy in individuals with alpha$_1$-proteinase inhibitor (A$_1$-PI) deficiency and clinical evidence of emphysema.

**DOSAGE:** *Adults:* 60mg/kg IV once weekly.

**HOW SUPPLIED:** Inj: 1000mg

**CONTRAINDICATIONS:** IgA deficiencies with known antibodies against IgA.

**WARNINGS/PRECAUTIONS:** May contain infectious agents (eg, viruses). Infusion rates and clinical status should be monitored closely during infusion. May cause increase in plasma volume.

**ADVERSE REACTIONS:** Asthenia, injection site pain, dizziness, headache, paresthesia, pruritus.

**PREGNANCY:** Category C, caution in nursing.

## ZEMPLAR

RX

paricalcitol (Abbott)

**THERAPEUTIC CLASS:** Vitamin D analog

**INDICATIONS:** Prevention and treatment of secondary hyperparathyroidism associated with Stage 3 and 4 chronic kidney disease.

**DOSAGE:** *Adults:* Initial: Baseline iPTH Level ≤500pg/mL: 1mcg qd or 2mcg tiw. Baseline iPTH Level >500pg/mL: 2mcg qd or 4mcg tiw. May need dose adjustment based on iPTH level relative to baseline (see labeling).

**HOW SUPPLIED:** Cap: 1mcg, 2mcg, 4mcg

**CONTRAINDICATIONS:** Vitamin D toxicity, hypercalcemia.

**WARNINGS/PRECAUTIONS:** May cause over suppression of PTH, hypercalcemia, hypercalciuria, hyperphosphatemia, and adynamic bone disease. Overdose may cause progressive hypercalcemia.

**ADVERSE REACTIONS:** Pain, allergic reactions, headache, infection, hypotension, HTN, diarrhea, nausea, vomiting, constipation, edema, arthritis, dizziness, vertigo, rhinitis, rash.

**INTERACTIONS:** Digitalis toxicity potentiated by hypercalcemia. Caution with strong CYP 3A inhibitors (ketoconazole, atazanavir, clarithromycin, indinavir, itraconazole, nefazodone, nelfinavir, ritonavir, saquinavir, telithromycin, voriconazole). Drugs that may impair intestinal absorption of fat-soluble vitamins (cholestyramine) may intefere with absorption.

**PREGNANCY:** Category C, not for use in nursing.

## ZEMPLAR IV

RX

paricalcitol (Abbott)

**THERAPEUTIC CLASS:** Vitamin D analog

**INDICATIONS:** Prevention and treatment of secondary hyperparathyroidism associated with chronic renal failure.

**DOSAGE:** *Adults:* Initial: 0.04-0.1mcg/kg bolus no more frequently than every other day during dialysis. Max: 0.24mcg/kg (16.8mcg). Titrate: May increase by 2-4mcg at 2-4 week intervals. Monitor serum Ca and phosphorus more frequently during dose adjustments. Reduce or interrupt dose if elevated Ca level or Ca x P product >75, may reinitiate at lower dose once normalized. May need dose decrease as PTH levels decrease (see labeling).
*Pediatrics:* ≥5 yrs: (Inj) Initial: 0.04-0.1mcg/kg bolus no more frequently than every other day during dialysis. Max: 0.24mcg/kg (16.8mcg). Titrate: May

increase by 2-4mcg at 2-4 week intervals. Monitor serum Ca and phosphorus more frequently during dose adjustments. Reduce or interrupt dose if elevated Ca level or Ca x P product >75, may reinitiate at lower dose once normalized. May need dose decrease as PTH levels decrease (see labeling).

**HOW SUPPLIED:** Inj: 2mcg/mL, 5mcg/mL

**CONTRAINDICATIONS:** Vitamin D toxicity, hypercalcemia.

**WARNINGS/PRECAUTIONS:** Overdose may cause progressive hypercalcemia. Should supplement wiht calcium and restrict phosphorus. May need phosphate-binding compounds to control serum phosphorus levels.

**ADVERSE REACTIONS:** Nausea, vomiting, edema, chills, flu, GI bleeding, lightheadness, pneumonia, pain, allergic reaction, headache, HTN, diarrhea, arthritis, rash.

**INTERACTIONS:** Digitalis toxicity potentiated by hypercalcemia. Avoid excessive use of aluminum containing compounds.

**PREGNANCY:** Category C, caution in nursing.

## ZEMURON RX

rocuronium bromide (Organon USA)

**THERAPEUTIC CLASS:** Skeletal muscle relaxant (nondepolarizing)

**INDICATIONS:** Adjunct to general anesthesia to facilitate both rapid sequence and routine tracheal intubation, and to provide skeletal muscle relaxation during surgery or mechanical ventilation

**DOSAGE:** *Adults:* Individualize dose. Rapid Sequence Intubation: 0.6-1.2mg/kg; Tracheal Intubation: Initial: 0.6mg/kg. Maint: 0.1, 0.15, or 0.2mg/kg. Continous Infusion: Initial: 10-12mcg/kg/min. Range: 4-16mcg/kg/min. *Pediatrics:* 3 months-14 yrs: Individualize dose. Initial: 0.6mg/kg.

**HOW SUPPLIED:** Inj: 10mg/mL

**WARNINGS/PRECAUTIONS:** Employ peripheral nerve stimulator to monitor drug response. May have profound effects with myasthenia gravis or myasthenic (Eaton-Lambert) syndrome; use small test dose and monitor closely. Do not mix with alkaline solutions (eg, barbiturate solutions) in the same syringe or administer simultaneously during IV infusion through the same needle. Anaphylactic reactions reported. Tolerance may develop during chronic administration. Not recommended for rapid sequence induction in Cesarean section. Caution with clinically significant hepatic disease. Conditions associated with slower circulation time (eg, cardiovascular disease or advanced age) may delay onset time. Electrolyte imbalances may enhance neuromuscular blockade.

**ADVERSE REACTIONS:** Arrhythmia, abnormal ECG, tachycardia, nausea, vomiting, asthma, hiccup, rash, injection site edema, pruritus.

**INTERACTIONS:** Use of inhalation anesthetics has been shown to enhance the activity of other neuromuscular blocking agents. Resistance observed with chronic anticonvulsant therapy. Certain antibiotics (eg, aminoglycosides, vancomycin; tetracyclines, bacitracin, polymyxins, colistin, and sodium colistimethate) may cause prolongation of neuromuscular block. Quinidine injection during recovery from use of other muscle relaxants suggests that recurrent paralysis may occur. Magnesium salts may enhance neuromuscular blockade.

**PREGNANCY:** Category C, safety in nursing not known.

## ZENAPAX RX

daclizumab (Roche Labs)

**THERAPEUTIC CLASS:** Immunosuppressive agent

**INDICATIONS:** For prophylaxis of acute organ rejection in renal transplants, in combination with cyclosporine and corticosteroids.

**DOSAGE:** *Adults:* 1mg/kg IV over 15 minutes for 5 doses. Administer 1st dose no more than 24 hrs prior to transplant and remaining 4 doses at 14-day intervals.
*Pediatrics:* >11 months: 1mg/kg IV over 15 minutes for 5 doses. Administer 1st dose no more than 24 hrs prior to transplant and remaining 4 doses at 14-day intervals.

**HOW SUPPLIED:** Inj: 25mg/5mL

**WARNINGS/PRECAUTIONS:** Increased risk of lymphoproliferative disorder and opportunistic infections. Anaphylactic reactions reported. Caution in elderly. Re-administration after initial course of therapy has not been studied in humans.

**ADVERSE REACTIONS:** Constipation, nausea, vomiting, diarrhea, abdominal pain, pyrosis, dyspepsia, abdominal distention, epigastric pain.

**PREGNANCY:** Category C, not for use in nursing.

## ZERIT

RX

stavudine (Bristol-Myers Squibb)

**Lactic acidosis and severe, fatal hepatomegaly reported. Fatal and non-fatal pancreatitis reported with didanosine.**

**THERAPEUTIC CLASS:** Synthetic thymidine nucleoside analogue

**INDICATIONS:** Treatment of HIV-1 infection in combination with other antiretrovirals.

**DOSAGE:** *Adults:* >60kg: 40mg q12h. <60kg: 30mg q12h. Interrupt therapy if develop peripheral neuropathy, resume at 1/2 dose when neuropathy resolves. D/C permanently if neuropathy recurs after resumption. Suspend therapy if lactic acidosis or hepatotoxicity occurs. CrCl 26-50mL/min: >60kg: 20mg q12h. <60kg: 15mg q12h. CrCl 10-25mL/min: >60kg: 20mg q24h. <60kg: 15mg q24h.
*Pediatrics:* >60kg: 40mg q12h. 30-59 kg: 30mg q12h. >14 days and <30kg: 1mg/kg q12h. Birth-13 days: 0.5mg/kg q12h. Interrupt therapy if develop peripheral neuropathy, resume with 1/2 dose when neuropathy resolves. D/C permanently if neuropathy recurs after resumption. Suspend therapy if lactic acidosis or hepatotoxicity occurs. Renal Impairment: Reduce dose and/or increase interval.

**HOW SUPPLIED:** Cap: 15mg, 20mg, 30mg, 40mg; Sus: 1mg/mL [200mL]

**WARNINGS/PRECAUTIONS:** Obesity and prolonged nucleoside exposure may increase risk to lactic acidosis and hepatomegaly. Caution with risk factors for hepatic disease. Peripheral neuropathy reported. Monitor for lactic acidosis in pregnancy if used with didanosine. D/C if motor weakness develops.

**ADVERSE REACTIONS:** Peripheral neuropathy, rash, elevated LFTs and amylase, headache, diarrhea, nausea, vomiting.

**INTERACTIONS:** Avoid zidovudine. Increased risk of neuropathy with neurotoxic drugs (eg, didanosine). Increased risk of hepatotoxicity with didanosine and hydroxyurea. Motor weakness reported with other antiretrovirals.

**PREGNANCY:** Category C, not for use in nursing.

## ZESTORETIC

RX

lisinopril - hydrochlorothiazide (AstraZeneca LP)

**ACE inhibitors can cause death/injury to developing fetus during 2nd and 3rd trimesters. Stop therapy if pregnancy detected.**

**THERAPEUTIC CLASS:** ACE inhibitor/thiazide diuretic

**INDICATIONS:** Treatment of hypertension. Not for initial therapy.

**DOSAGE:** *Adults:* Initial (if not controlled with lisinopril/HCTZ monotherapy): 10mg-12.5mg tab or 20mg-12.5mg tab daily. Titrate: May increase after 2-3 weeks. Initial (if controlled on 25mg HCTZ/day with hypokalemia): 10mg-12.5mg tab. Replacement Therapy: Substitute combination for titrated components.

**HOW SUPPLIED:** Tab: (Lisinopril-HCTZ) 10mg-12.5mg, 20mg-12.5mg, 20mg-25mg

**CONTRAINDICATIONS:** History of ACE inhibitor associated angioedema, hereditary or idiopathic angioedema, anuria, sulfonamide hypersensitivity.

**WARNINGS/PRECAUTIONS:** D/C if angioedema, jaundice, or marked LFT elevation occur. Risk of hyperkalemia with DM, renal dysfunction. Persistent nonproductive cough reported. Monitor WBCs in renal and collagen vascular disease. Anaphylactoid reactions reported. Fetal/neonatal morbidity and death reported. Monitor for hypotension in high risk patients (eg, surgery/anesthesia, volume/salt depletion). Caution with CHF, renal or hepatic dysfunction. More reports of angioedema in blacks than nonblacks. May exacerbate or activate SLE. Monitor electrolytes. Avoid if CrCl <30mL/min/1.7m$^2$. May increase cholesterol, TG. Hypercalcemia, hypomagnesemia, hyperuricemia may occur. Caution with left ventricle outflow obstruction.

**ADVERSE REACTIONS:** Dizziness, headache, cough, fatigue, orthostatic effects, diarrhea, nausea, muscle cramps, angioedema.

**INTERACTIONS:** Increase risk of hyperkalemia with $K^+$-sparing diuretics, $K^+$ supplements, or $K^+$-containing salt substitutes. Potentiates orthostatic hypotension with alcohol, barbiturates, and narcotics. Adjust antidiabetic drugs. Reduced absorption with cholestyramine, colestipol. Corticosteroids, ACTH deplete electrolytes. May decrease response to pressor amines. Potentiates other antihypertensives. May increase responsiveness to skeletal muscle relaxants. Risk of lithium toxicity. NSAIDs reduce effects and worsen renal dysfunction.

**PREGNANCY:** Category C (1st trimester) and D (2nd and 3rd trimesters), not for use in nursing.

## ZESTRIL

RX

lisinopril (AstraZeneca LP)

**ACE inhibitors can cause death/injury to developing fetus during 2nd and 3rd trimesters. Stop therapy if pregnancy detected.**

**THERAPEUTIC CLASS:** ACE inhibitor

**INDICATIONS:** Treatment of hypertension. Adjunct therapy in heart failure if inadequately controlled by diuretics and digitalis. Adjunct therapy in stable patients within 24 hrs of AMI to improve survival.

**DOSAGE:** *Adults:* HTN: If possible, d/c diuretic 2-3 days prior to therapy. Initial: 10mg qd, 5mg qd with diuretic. Usual: 20-40mg qd. Resume diuretic if BP not controlled. Max: 80mg/day. CrCl 10-30mL/min: Initial: 5mg/day. Max: 40mg/day. CrCl <10mL/min: Initial: 2.5mg/day. Max: 40mg/day. Heart Failure: Initial: 5mg qd. Usual: 5-40mg qd. May increase by 10mg every 2 weeks. Max: 40mg/day. Hyponatremia or CrCl <30mL/min: Initial: 2.5mg qd. AMI: Initial: 5mg within 24 hrs, then 5mg after 24 hrs, then 10mg after 48 hrs, then 10mg qd. Use 2.5mg during 1st 3 days with low systolic BP. Maint: 10mg qd for 6 weeks, 2.5-5mg with hypotension. D/C with prolonged hypotension. Elderly: Caution with dose adjustment.

**HOW SUPPLIED:** Tab: 2.5mg, 5mg*, 10mg, 20mg, 30mg, 40mg *scored

**CONTRAINDICATIONS:** History of ACE inhibitor associated angioedema.

**WARNINGS/PRECAUTIONS:** D/C if angioedema, jaundice, or marked LFT elevation occur. Risk of hyperkalemia with DM, renal dysfunction. Persistent nonproductive cough reported. Monitor WBCs in renal and collagen vascular disease. Anaphylactoid reactions reported. Fetal/neonatal morbidity and death reported. Monitor for hypotension in high risk patients (heart failure with systolic BP <100 mmHg, surgery/anesthesia, hyponatremia, high dose diuretic therapy, severe volume and/or salt depletion, etc.). Caution with CHF, renal dysfunction, and renal artery stenosis. Less effective on BP in blacks and more reports of angioedema than non-blacks.

**ADVERSE REACTIONS:** Hypotension, diarrhea, headache, dizziness, hyperkalemia, increase creatinine and non-protein nitrogen, syncope, chest pain.

**INTERACTIONS:** May increase lithium levels. Hypotension risk with diuretics. Increase risk of hyperkalemia with $K^+$-sparing diuretics, $K^+$-containing salt substitutes or $K^+$ supplements. Indomethacin may reduce effects.

**PREGNANCY:** Category C (1st trimester) and D (2nd and 3rd trimesters), not for use in nursing.

## ZETACET — RX

sulfur - sulfacetamide sodium (Stiefel)

**THERAPEUTIC CLASS:** Sulfonamide/sulfur combination

**INDICATIONS:** Topical treatment of acne vulgaris, acne rosacea, and seborrheic dermatitis.

**DOSAGE:** *Adults:* Apply a thin layer qd-tid. Shake well before use. *Pediatrics:* >12 yrs: Apply a thin layer qd-tid. Shake well before use.

**HOW SUPPLIED:** Lot: (Sulfacetamide-Sulfur) 10%-5% [25g]

**CONTRAINDICATIONS:** Kidney disease.

**WARNINGS/PRECAUTIONS:** Caution with denuded or abraded skin. Caution in patients prone to hypersensitivity to topical sulfonamides. Discontinue if irritation occurs. For external use only; avoid eye contact. Can cause reddening and scaling of epidermis.

**ADVERSE REACTIONS:** Local irritation.

**PREGNANCY:** Category C, caution in nursing.

## ZETIA — RX

ezetimibe (Merck/Schering-Plough)

**THERAPEUTIC CLASS:** Cholesterol absorption inhibitor

**INDICATIONS:** Adjunct to diet, as monotherapy or with concomitant HMG-CoA reductase inhibitors, to reduce total-C, LDL-C, and Apo B levels in primary (heterozygous familial and nonfamilial) hypercholesterolemia. Adjunct to diet, with concomitant fenofibrate, to reduce elevated total-C, LDL-C, Apo B, and non-HDL-C in mixed hyperlipidemia. Adjunct to other lipid-lowering treatments or if such treatments are unavailable, with concomitant atorvastatin or simvastatin, to reduce total-C and LDL-C in homozygous familial hypercholesterolemia. Adjunct to diet, to reduce sitosterol and campesterol levels in homozygous familial sitosterolemia.

**DOSAGE:** *Adults:* 10mg qd. May give with HMG-CoA reductase inhibitor (with primary hypercholesterolemia) or fenofibrate (with mixed hyperlipidemia) for incremental effect. Concomitant Bile Sequestrant: Give either ≥2 hrs before or ≥4 hrs after bile acid sequestrant.

**HOW SUPPLIED:** Tab: 10mg

**CONTRAINDICATIONS:** When used with a statin, refer to the HMG-CoA reductase inhibitor monographs.

**WARNINGS/PRECAUTIONS:** Monitor LFTs with concurrent statin therapy. Not recommended with moderate or severe hepatic insufficiency.

**ADVERSE REACTIONS:** Back pain, arthralgia, diarrhea, sinusitis, abdominal pain, myalgia.

**INTERACTIONS:** Incremental LDL-C reduction may be reduced with concomitant cholestyramine. Fibrates may increase cholesterol excretion into the bile; concurrent use is not recommended. Increased levels with fenofibrate and gemfibrozil. Monitor cyclosporine levels with concomitant use of cyclosporine. Monitor INR when administered with warfarin.

**PREGNANCY:** Category C, contraindicated in nursing.

## ZEVALIN RX

ibritumomab tiuxetan (Biogen Idec)

**Discontinue if severe infusion reactions occurs. Severe and prolonged cytopenias reported; avoid if >25% lymphoma marrow involvement and/or impaired bone marrow reserve. Severe, some fatal, cutaneous and mucocutaneous reactions reported. Do not exceed the maximum dose. Avoid patients with altered biodistribution.**

**THERAPEUTIC CLASS:** Monoclonal antibody

**INDICATIONS:** Treatment of relapsed or refractory low grade, follicular, or transformed B-cell non-Hodgkin's lymphoma, including rituximab refractory follicular non-Hodgkin's lymphoma.

**DOSAGE:** *Adults:* Day 1: Rituximab 250mg/m$^2$ IV single infusion. Within 4 hrs, give 5mCi of In-111 ibritumomab IV. Assess biodistribution by conducting 1st image at 2-24 hrs, 2nd image at 48-72 hrs, and optional 3rd image at 90-120 hrs. If biodistribution acceptable, Day 7-9: Rituximab 250mg/m$^2$ IV. Within 4 hrs, give Y-90 Ibritumomab 0.4mCi/kg (or 0.3mCi/kg if platelets 100,000-149,000 cells/mm$^3$). Max: Y-90 ibritumomab 32mCi.

**HOW SUPPLIED:** Inj: 3.2mg/2mL

**CONTRAINDICATIONS:** Type I hypersensitivity or anaphylactic reactions to murine proteins or to any component of this product including rituximab, yttrium chloride, and indium chloride.

**WARNINGS/PRECAUTIONS:** Use with rituximab, Contains albumin; remote risk of transmission of viral disease and CJD. Single course treatment only. Minimize radiation exposure during and after radiolabeling. Monitor CBC and platelets weekly until levels recover. Increased risk of hypersensitivity reactions with HAMA from prior murine protein use. Caution with transfusion. Secondary leukemia and mylodysplastic syndrome reproted.

**ADVERSE REACTIONS:** Neutropenia, thrombocytopenia, anemia, nausea, vomiting, diarrhea, increased cough, dyspnea, arthralgia, anorexia, anxiety, ecchymosis.

**INTERACTIONS:** Increased risk of bleeding and hemorrhage with drugs that interfere with platelet function or coagulation; monitor for thrombocytopenia more frequently. Safety of immunization with live viral vaccines not studied.

**PREGNANCY:** Category D, not for use in nursing.

## ZIAC RX

hydrochlorothiazide - bisoprolol fumarate (Duramed)

**THERAPEUTIC CLASS:** Selective beta$_1$-blocker/thiazide diuretic

**INDICATIONS:** Management of hypertension.

**DOSAGE:** *Adults:* Initial: 2.5mg-6.25mg tab qd. Maint: May increase every 14 days. Max: 20mg bisoprolol-12.5mg HCTZ/day. Renal/Hepatic Dysfunction: Caution in dosing/titrating.

**HOW SUPPLIED:** Tab: (Bisoprolol-HCTZ) 2.5mg-6.25mg, 5mg-6.25mg, 10mg-6.25mg

**CONTRAINDICATIONS:** Cardiogenic shock, overt cardiac failure, 2nd- or 3rd-degree AV block, marked sinus bradycardia, anuria, sulfonamide hypersensitivity.

**WARNINGS/PRECAUTIONS:** Caution with compensated cardiac failure, DM, bronchospastic disease, hepatic/renal impairment, or peripheral vascular disease. Avoid abrupt withdrawal. Photosensitivity reactions, hypokalemia, hypercalcemia, hypophosphatemia reported. May activate/exacerbate SLE. Enhanced effects in post-sympathectomy patients. May mask hyperthyroidism or hypoglycemia symptoms. Monitor for fluid/electrolyte imbalance. May precipitate hyperuricemia, acute gout, cardiac failure.

**ADVERSE REACTIONS:** Cough, diarrhea, myalgia, headache, dizziness, fatigue, upper respiratory infection.

**INTERACTIONS:** Alcohol, barbiturates, or narcotics may potentiate orthostatic hypotension. Adjust dose of antidiabetic drugs. Potentiates other antihypertensives. Avoid other β-blockers. Impaired absorption with cholestyramine, colestipol. Corticosteroids, ACTH intensify electrolyte depletion. May decrease response to pressor amines. May increase response to nondepolarizing muscle relaxants. Risk of lithium toxicity. NSAIDs may reduce effects. May block epinephrine effects. Excessive reduction of sympathetic activity with catecholamine-depleting drugs. Caution with clonidine withdrawal. Increased clearance with rifampin. Caution with calcium channel blockers, myocardial depressants, anesthesia, and antiarrhythmics.

**PREGNANCY:** Category C, not for use in nursing.

## ZIAGEN RX

abacavir sulfate (GlaxoSmithKline)

**Fatal hypersensitivity reactions, lactic acidosis, severe hepatomegaly with steatosis, including fatal cases reported. Discontinue if hypersensitivity reaction is suspected and do not restart.**

**THERAPEUTIC CLASS:** Synthetic carbocyclic nucleoside analogue

**INDICATIONS:** Treatment of HIV-1 infection in combination with other antiretrovirals.

**DOSAGE:** *Adults:* >16 yrs:300mg bid or 600mg qd.
*Pediatrics:* 3 months-16 yrs: 8mg/kg bid. Max: 300mg bid.

**HOW SUPPLIED:** Sol: 20mg/mL [240mL]; Tab: 300mg

**WARNINGS/PRECAUTIONS:** Register abacavir hypersensitive patients at 800-270-0425. Caution with liver disease; lactic acidosis and severe hepatomegaly with steatosis, including fatal cases, have been reported. Not for monotherapy when antiretroviral regimens are changed. Immune reconstitution syndrome reported. Should not be coadministered with Epzicom or Trizivir.

**ADVERSE REACTIONS:** Hypersensitivity reactions (eg, fever, rash, fatigue, GI symptoms), nausea, vomiting, diarrhea, loss of appetite, insomnia, chills, headache, fatigue.

**INTERACTIONS:** Decreased elimination with ethanol.

**PREGNANCY:** Category C, not for use in nursing.

## ZIANA RX

tretinoin - clindamycin phosphate (Medicis)

**THERAPEUTIC CLASS:** Lincosamide derivative/retinoid

**INDICATIONS:** Topical treatment of acne vulgaris.

**DOSAGE:** *Adults:* Apply pea-sized amount to entire face qd at bedtime. Avoid eyes, mouth, angles of nose, or mucous membranes. Not for oral, ophthalmic, or intravaginal use.
*Pediatrics:* ≥12 yrs: Apply pea-sized amount to entire face qd at bedtime.

Avoid eyes, mouth, angles of nose, or mucous membranes. Not for oral, ophthalmic, or intravaginal use.

**HOW SUPPLIED:** Gel: (Clindamycin-Tretinoin) 1.2%-0.025% [2g, 30g, 60g]

**CONTRAINDICATIONS:** Regional enteritis, ulcerative colitis, or history of antibiotic-associated colitis.

**WARNINGS/PRECAUTIONS:** May cause severe colitis; d/c if significant diarrhea occurs. Avoid exposure to sunlight and sunlamps; wear sunscreen daily.

**ADVERSE REACTIONS:** Nasopharyngitis, erythema, scaling, itching, burning.

**INTERACTIONS:** Caution with concomitant topical medications, medicated/abrasive soaps and cleansers, soaps/cosmetics with strong drying effect, products with high concentrations of alcohol, astringents, spices, or lime. Avoid with erythromycin-containing products. Caution with neuromuscular blocking agents.

**PREGNANCY:** Category C, not for use in nursing.

## ZINECARD — RX

dexrazoxane (Pharmacia & Upjohn)

**THERAPEUTIC CLASS:** EDTA derivative

**INDICATIONS:** To reduce the incidence and severity of cardiomyopathy associated with doxorubicin in women with metastatic breast cancer who received a cumulative doxorubicin dose of 300mg/m² and who will continue doxorubicin therapy.

**DOSAGE:** *Adults:* IV: 10:1 ratio of dexrazoxaneDO,xorubicin (eg, 500mg/m² dexrazoxane:50mg/m² doxorubicin). Hepatic Impairment: Reduce dose proportionally. Give by slow IV push or rapid IV infusion. Give doxorubicin within 30 minutes after start of infusion.

**HOW SUPPLIED:** Inj: 250mg, 500mg

**CONTRAINDICATIONS:** Chemotherapy regimens not containing an anthracycline.

**WARNINGS/PRECAUTIONS:** Not for use with initiation of doxorubicin therapy. Monitor cardiac function. May cause secondary malignancies. Obtain frequent CBCs. Caution with moderate or severe renal insufficiency; reduce dose by 50% if CrCl <40mL/min.

**ADVERSE REACTIONS:** Alopecia, nausea, vomiting, fatigue, malaise, anorexia, stomatitis, fever, infection, diarrhea, pain on injection, sepsis, neurotoxicity, streaking/erythema.

**INTERACTIONS:** Avoid use during the initiation of FAC (fluorouracil, doxorubicin, cyclophosphamide) therapy. Additive myelosuppression with other chemotherapies.

**PREGNANCY:** Category C, not for use in nursing.

## ZITHROMAX — RX

azithromycin (Pfizer)

**THERAPEUTIC CLASS:** Macrolide antibiotic

**INDICATIONS:** (PO) Treatment of acute bacterial exacerbations of COPD, acute bacterial sinusitis (ABS), community acquired pneumonia (CAP), pharyngitis/tonsillitis, uncomplicated skin and skin structure, urethritis/cervicitis, genital ulcer disease (men), acute otitis media, prevention of disseminated *Mycobacterium avium* complex (MAC) disease in advanced HIV infection. (IV) Treatment of CAP and pelvic inflammatory disease (PID).

**DOSAGE:** *Adults:* (PO) COPD/CAP/Pharyngitis/Tonsillitis (second line therapy)/SSSI: >16 yrs: 500mg on day 1, then 250mg qd on days 2-5. COPD:

500mg qd for 3 days. ABS: 500mg qd for 3 days. Genital Ulcer Disease and Non-Gonococcal Urethritis/Cervicitis: 1g single dose. Urethritis/Cervicitis due to *N.gonorrhea:* 2g single dose. MAC Prophylaxis: 1200mg once weekly. MAC Treatment: 600mg qd with ethambutol 15mg/kg/day. (IV) >16 yrs: CAP: 500mg qd for at least 2 days, then 500mg PO to complete 7-10 day course. PID: 500mg qd for 1-2 days, then 250mg PO to complete 7 day course. *Pediatrics:* (Sus) Otitis Media: >6 months: 30mg/kg single dose; 10mg/kg qd for 3 days; or 10mg/kg qd on day 1, then 5mg/kg qd on days 2-5. ABS: ≥6 months: 10mg/kg qd for 3 days. CAP: >6 months: 10mg/kg qd on day 1, then 5mg/kg qd on days 2-5. (Sus, Tab) Pharyngitis/Tonsillitis: >2 yrs: 12mg/kg qd for 5 days. 1g sus not for pediatric use.

**HOW SUPPLIED:** Inj: 500mg; Sus: 100mg/5mL [15mL], 200mg/5mL [15mL, 22.5mL, 30mL], 1g/pkt [3s 10s]; Tab: 250mg [Z-PAK, 6 tabs], 500mg [TRI-PAK, 3 tabs], 600mg

**WARNINGS/PRECAUTIONS:** D/C if allergic reaction occurs. Oral therapy is only for community acquired pneumonia of mild severity. Hypersensitivity reactions may recur after initial successful symptomatic treatment. Monitor for pseudomembranous colitis. Caution with renal/hepatic dysfunction. 1g sus not for pediatric use.

**ADVERSE REACTIONS:** Diarrhea/loose stools, nausea, abdominal pain.

**INTERACTIONS:** Monitor theophylline, terfenadine, cyclosporine, hexobarbital, phenytoin, warfarin. May increase digoxin, carbamazepine levels. Potentiates triazolam. Aluminum- and magnesium-containing antacids reduce oral levels. Acute ergot toxicity may occur with ergotamine or dihydroergotamine. Monitor for azithromycin side effects (eg, liver enzyme abnormalities, hearing impairment) with nelfinavir.

**PREGNANCY:** Category B, caution in nursing.

## ZMAX
azithromycin (Pfizer) RX

**THERAPEUTIC CLASS:** Macrolide Antibiotics

**INDICATIONS:** Treatment of mild to moderate acute bacterial sinusitis due to *Haemophilus influenzae, Moraxella catarrhalis*, or *Streptococcus pneumoniae*. Treatment of community-acquired pneumonia due to *Chlamydophila pneumoniae, Haemophilus influenzae, Mycoplasma pneumoniae*, or *Streptococcus pneumoniae* in patients appropriate for oral therapy.

**DOSAGE:** *Adults:* 2g single dose. Take on an empty stomach (1 hour before or 2 hours after a meal).

**HOW SUPPLIED:** Suspension, Extended-Release: 2g

**CONTRAINDICATIONS:** Hypersensitivity to macrolide or ketolide antibiotics.

**WARNINGS/PRECAUTIONS:** Rare reports of angioedema, anaphylaxis, and dermatologic reactions including Stevens-Johnson syndrome and toxic epidermal necrolysis. Discontinue if allergic reaction occurs. Hypersensitivity reactions may recur after initial successful symptomatic treatment. Monitor for pseudomembranous colitis. Caution with renal/hepatic dysfunction and patients with increased risk for prolonged cardiac repolarization.

**ADVERSE REACTIONS:** Diarrhea/loose stools, nausea, abdominal pain, headache, vomiting.

**INTERACTIONS:** Monitor for azithromycin side effects (eg, liver enzyme abnormalities, hearing impairment) with nelfinavir. Monitor cyclosporine, hexobarbital, phenytoin, warfarin concentrations. May increase digoxin levels. Acute ergot toxicity may occur with ergotamine or dihydroergotamine.

**PREGNANCY:** Category B, caution in nursing.

## ZOCOR
simvastatin (Merck)

RX

**THERAPEUTIC CLASS:** HMG-CoA reductase inhibitor

**INDICATIONS:** May initiate with diet in patients with, or at high risk for, coronary heart disease (CHD). In high risk patients with CHD, diabetes, peripheral vessel disease, history of stroke or other cerebrovascular disease to reduce risk of total mortality by reducing CHD deaths, risk of non-fatal MI and stroke, need for revascularization procedures. To reduce elevated total-C, LDL-C, Apo B, TG, and increase HDL-C in primary hypercholesterolemia (heterozygous familial and nonfamilial) and mixed dyslipidemia (Types IIa and IIb). To treat hypertriglyceridemia (Type IV) and primary dysbetalipoproteinemia (Type III). To reduce total-C, LDL-C in homozygous familial hypercholesterolemia as adjunct to other lipid-lowering agents or if such treatments are unavailable. To reduce total-C, LDL-C, Apo B in adolescents 10-17 yrs old, at least 1yr post-menarche, with heterozygous familial hypercholesterolemia. To reduce elevated LDL-C, TG in Type IIb hyperlipidemia.

**DOSAGE:** *Adults:* Initial: 20-40mg qpm. Usual: 5-80mg/day. Titrate: Adjust at ≥4-week intervals. High Risk for CHD Events: Initial: 40mg/day. Homozygous Familial Hypercholesterolemia: 40mg qpm or 80mg/day given as 20mg bid plus 40mg qpm. Concomitant Cyclosporine: Initial: 5mg/day. Max: 10mg/day. Concomitant Gemfibrozil (try to avoid): Max: 10mg/day. Concomitant Amiodarone/Verapamil: Max: 20mg/day. Severe Renal Insufficiency: 5mg/day; monitor closely.
*Pediatrics:* Heterozygous Familial Hypercholesterolemia: 10-17 yrs (at least 1yr postmenarchal): Initial: 10mg qpm. Usual: 10-40mg/day. Titrate: Adjust at ≥4-week intervals. Max: 40mg/day.

**HOW SUPPLIED:** Tab: 5mg, 10mg, 20mg, 40mg, 80mg

**CONTRAINDICATIONS:** Active liver disease, unexplained persistent elevations of serum transaminases, pregnancy, nursing mothers.

**WARNINGS/PRECAUTIONS:** Caution with heavy alcohol use, severe renal insufficiency or history of hepatic disease. Monitor LFT's prior to therapy, periodically thereafter for 1st year, or until 1 year after last dose elevation (additional test at 3 months for 80mg dose). D/C if AST or ALT ≥3X ULN persist, if myopathy is suspected or diagnosed, a few days prior to major surgery. Rhabomyolysis (rare), myopathy reported.

**ADVERSE REACTIONS:** Abdominal pain, headache, CK and transaminase elevations.

**INTERACTIONS:** Avoid use with concomitant itraconazole, ketoconazole, erythromycin, clarithromycin, telithromycin, HIV protease inhibitors, nefazodone, grapefruit juice (>1 quart/day); increased risk of myopathy/rhabdomyolysis. Max 10mg/day with gemfibrozil, cyclosporin, danazol. Max 20mg/day with amiodarone, verapamil. Caution with other fibrates, ≥1g/day of niacin. Monitor digoxin, warfarin.

**PREGNANCY:** Category X, not for use in nursing.

## ZODERM
benzoyl peroxide (Doak)

RX

**THERAPEUTIC CLASS:** Antibacterial/keratolytic

**INDICATIONS:** Acne vulgaris.

**DOSAGE:** *Adults*: (Cleanser) Wash and rinse affected area qd-bid. (Cre, Gel) Apply to cleansed area qd-bid.

**HOW SUPPLIED:** Cleanser: 4.5%, 6.5%, 8.5% [400mL]; Cre, Gel: 4.5%, 6.5%, 8.5% [125mL]

**WARNINGS/PRECAUTIONS:** Avoid eyes, mouth, mucous membranes, sun exposure. Discontinue if severe irritation occurs. May bleach fabrics or hair.

**ADVERSE REACTIONS:** Allergic contact dermatitis, dryness.

**PREGNANCY:** Category C, caution in nursing.

## ZOFRAN

RX

ondansetron (GlaxoSmithKline)

**THERAPEUTIC CLASS:** 5-$HT_3$ antagonist

**INDICATIONS:** (Inj) Prevention of nausea and vomiting associated with initial and repeat courses of emetogenic cancer chemotherapy, including high-dose cisplatin. Prevention of postoperative nausea and/or vomiting. (Sol/Tab) Prevention of nausea and vomiting associated with: highly emetogenic cancer chemotherapy, including cisplatin ≥50mg/$m^2$; initial and repeat courses of moderately emetogenic cancer chemotherapy; and radiotherapy in patients receiving either total body irradiation, single high-dose fraction to the abdomen, or daily fractions to the abdomen. Prevention of postoperative nausea and/or vomiting.

**DOSAGE:** *Adults:* Prevention of Chemotherapy-Induced Nausea/Vomiting: (Inj) 32mg single dose or three 0.15mg/kg doses, 1st dose 30 minutes before chemotherapy, then 4 and 8 hours after the 1st dose. Prevention of Nausea/Vomiting Associated With Highly Emetogenic Cancer Chemotherapy: (Tab) 24mg single dose tab 30 minutes before chemotherapy. Prevention of Nausea/Vomiting Associated With Moderately Emetogenic Cancer Chemotherapy: (Sol/Tab) 8mg bid, 1st dose 30 minutes before chemotherapy, then 8 hrs later, then bid for 1-2 days after chemotherapy. Prevention of Post-Op Nausea/Vomiting: (Inj) 4mg IM/IV immediately before anesthesia or post-op after surgery if nausea or vomiting occurs. (Sol/Tab) 16mg 1 hr before anesthesia. Prevention of Nausea/Vomiting Associated with Radiation Therapy: (Sol/Tab) Usual: 8mg tid. Total Body Irradiation: 8mg 1-2 hrs before therapy daily. Single High-Dose Therapy To Abdomen: 8mg 1-2 hrs before therapy then q8h after 1st dose for 1-2 days after completion of therapy. Daily Fractionated Therapy To Abdomen: 8mg 1-2 hrs before therapy then q8h after 1st dose. Severe Hepatic Dysfunction (Child-Pugh[2] ≥10): Max: 8mg/day IV single dose infused over 15 minutes, start 30 minutes before chemotherapy or 8mg/day PO.

*Pediatrics:* Prevention of Chemotherapy-Induced Nausea/Vomiting: (Inj) 6 months-18 yrs: Three 0.15mg/kg doses, 1st dose 30 minutes before chemotherapy, then 4 and 8 hrs after the 1st dose. (Sol/Tab) Prevention of Nausea/Vomiting Associated With Moderately Emetogenic Cancer Chemotherapy: >12 yrs: 8mg bid, 1st dose 30 minutes before chemotherapy, then 8mg 8 hrs later, then bid for 1-2 days. 4-11 yrs: 4mg tid, 1st dose 30 minutes before chemotherapy, then 4 and 8 hrs after 1st dose, then tid for 1-2 days. Prevention of Post-Op Nausea/Vomiting: (Inj) >12 yrs: 4mg IM/IV immediately before anesthesia or post-op after surgery if nausea or vomiting occurs. 1 month-12 yrs: <40kg: 0.1mg/kg single dose. >40kg: 4mg single dose. Severe Hepatic Dysfunction: Max: 8mg/day IV single dose infused over 15 minutes, start 30 minutes before chemotherapy or 8mg/day PO.

**HOW SUPPLIED:** Inj: 2mg/mL, 32mg/50mL; Sol: 4mg/5mL [50mL]; Tab: 4mg, 8mg, 24mg; Tab, Disintegrating: 4mg, 8mg

**WARNINGS/PRECAUTIONS:** Hypersensitivity reactions have been reported in those hypersensitive to other 5-$HT_3$ receptor antagonists. Transient ECG changes including QT interval prolongation have been reported with IV administration. May mask a progressive ileus or gastric distension. Orally disintegrating tablets contain phenylalanine; caution in phenylketonurics.

**ADVERSE REACTIONS:** Headache, diarrhea, dizziness, drowsiness, malaise/fatigue, constipation, LFT abnormalities.

**INTERACTIONS:** Ondansetron is metabolized by CYP450 enzymes; inducers or inhibitors of these enzymes may change the clearance and half-life of ondansetron.

**PREGNANCY:** Category B, caution in nursing.

## ZOLADEX 1-MONTH RX
goserelin acetate (AstraZeneca LP)

**THERAPEUTIC CLASS:** Synthetic gonadotropin releasing hormone analog

**INDICATIONS:** Palliative treatment of advanced prostate cancer and advanced breast cancer in pre-and perimenopausal women. Adjunct to and during radiotherapy and in combination with flutamide for management of locally confined Stage T2b-T4 (Stage B2-C) prostate cancer. Management of endometriosis, including pain relief and reduction of endometriotic lesions. Use as an endometrial thinning agent prior to ablation for dysfunctional uterine bleeding.

**DOSAGE:** *Adults:* Inject SQ into anterior abdominal wall below navel line. Advanced Prostate/Breast Cancers: 3.6mg every 28 days. Stage B2-C Prostate Cancer: 3.6mg starting 8 weeks before radiotherapy then 10.8mg formulation 28 days after 1st injection or 3.6mg at 28 day intervals for 4 doses (2 before and 2 during radiotherapy). Endometriosis: 3.6mg every 28 days for up to 6 months. Endometrial Thinning: 3.6mg then surgery 4 weeks later, or 3.6mg for 2 doses (4 weeks apart) followed by surgery 2-4 weeks after 2nd dose.

**HOW SUPPLIED:** Implant: 3.6mg

**CONTRAINDICATIONS:** Pregnancy, nursing.

**WARNINGS/PRECAUTIONS:** Exclude pregnancy before initiating therapy. Premenopausal women should use nonhormonal contraception during and 12 weeks post-therapy. Worsening of symptoms of prostate and breast cancer with initial therapy. Ureteral obstruction and spinal cord compression reported with prostate cancer. Temporary increases in bone pain may occur. Ovarian cysts reported. Hypercalcemia reported in prostate and breast cancer patients with bone metastases. May increase cervical resistance. Hypersensitivity, antibody formation and acute anaphylactic reactions may occur.

**ADVERSE REACTIONS:** (Males) hot flashes, sexual dysfunction, decreased erections, lower urinary tract symptoms, lethargy, pain (worsened in the first 30 days), edema, upper respiratory infection, rash, sweating, diarrhea, nausea. (Females, Endometriosis Treatment) Hot flashes, vaginitis, emotional lability, decreased libido, sweating, depression, headache, acne, breast atrophy. (Breast Cancer Treatment) hot flashes. tumor flare, nausea, edema, malaise/fatigue/lethargy, vomiting.

**INTERACTIONS:** Ovarian hyperstimulation syndrome reported when used concomitantly with other gonadotropins.

**PREGNANCY:** Category X (endometriosis and endometrial thinning), Category D (breast cancer), not for use in nursing.

## ZOLADEX 3-MONTH RX
goserelin acetate (AstraZeneca LP)

**THERAPEUTIC CLASS:** Synthetic gonadotropin releasing hormone analog

**INDICATIONS:** Palliative treatment of advanced prostate cancer. Adjunct to radiotherapy and flutamide for management of locally confined Stage T2b-T4 (Stage B2-C) prostate cancer.

**DOSAGE:** *Adults:* Inject SQ into anterior abdominal wall below navel line. Advanced Prostate Cancer: 10.8mg every 12 weeks. Stage B2-C Prostate Cancer: 3.6mg depot formulation 8 weeks before radiotherapy then 10.8mg 28 days after 1st injection.

**HOW SUPPLIED:** Implant: 10.8mg

**CONTRAINDICATIONS:** Pregnancy, 10.8mg implant is not indicated in women.

**WARNINGS/PRECAUTIONS:** Worsening of symptoms of prostate cancer with initial therapy. Ureteral obstruction and spinal cord compression reported. Temporary increase in bone pain may occur. Hypersensitivity, antibody formation and acute anaphylactic reactions may occur.

**ADVERSE REACTIONS:** Hot flashes, sexual dysfunction, decreased erections, osteoporosis, pain, asthenia, gynecomastia.

**PREGNANCY:** Category X, not for use in nursing.

## ZOLINZA
vorinostat (Merck) RX

**THERAPEUTIC CLASS:** Histone deacetylase inhibitor

**INDICATIONS:** Treatment of cutaneous manifestations in patients with cutaneous T-cell lymphoma who have progressive, persistent, or recurrent disease on or following two systemic therapies.

**DOSAGE:** *Adults:* 400mg PO qd with food. Intolerant to Therapy: May reduce dose to 300mg PO qd with food. If necessary, may further reduce dose to 300mg PO qd with food for 5 consecutive days each week.

**HOW SUPPLIED:** Cap: 100mg

**WARNINGS/PRECAUTIONS:** Pulmonary embolism and DVT reported; monitor for signs and symptoms. Dose-related thrombocytopenia and anemia may occur; consider dose modification or discontinuation. GI disturbances reported. Hyperglycemia observed; monitor glucose levels. QTc prolongation reported; monitor electrolytes and ECGs at baseline and periodically during treatment. Monitor CBC and chemistry tests every 2 weeks during the first 2 months of therapy and monthly thereafter.

**ADVERSE REACTIONS:** Diarrhea, fatigue, nausea, thrombocytopenia, anorexia, dysgeusia, decreased weight, muscle spasms, alopecia, dry mouth, increased SrCr, chills, vomiting, constipation, dizziness.

**INTERACTIONS:** Prolongation of PT and INR observed with coumarin-derivative anticoagulants; monitor closely. Severe thrombocytopenia and GI bleeding reported with concomitant use of other histone deacetylase inhibitors (eg, valproic acid); monitor platelet count every 2 weeks for the first two months of therapy.

**PREGNANCY:** Category D, not for use in nursing.

## ZOLOFT
sertraline HCl (Pfizer) RX

**Antidepressants increased the risk of suicidal thinking and behavior (suicidality) in short-term studies in children and adolescents with Major Depressive Disorder (MDD) and other psychiatric disorders. Sertraline HCl is not approved for use in pediatric patients except for patients with obsessive compulsive disorder (OCD).**

**THERAPEUTIC CLASS:** Selective serotonin reuptake inhibitor

**INDICATIONS:** Treatment of MDD, social anxiety disorder (SAD), OCD, panic disorder with or without agoraphobia, premenstrual dysphoric disorder (PMDD) and posttraumatic stress disorder (PTSD).

**DOSAGE:** *Adults:* MDD/OCD: 50mg qd. Titrate: Adjust dose at 1 week intervals. Max: 200mg/day. Panic Disorder/PTSD/SAD: Initial: 25mg qd. Titrate: Increase to 50mg qd after 1 week. Adjust dose at 1 week intervals. Max: 200mg/day. PMDD: Initial: 50mg qd continuous or limited to luteal phase of cycle. Titrate: Increase 50mg/cycle if needed up to 150mg/day for continuous or 100mg/day for luteal phase dosing. If 100mg/day is established for luteal phase dosing, a 50mg/day titration step for 3 days should take place at the beginning of each luteal phase dosing period. Hepatic Impairment: Use lower or less frequent doses. Dilute solution with 4oz of water, ginger ale, lemon/lime soda, lemonade or orange juice. Take immediately after mixing.
*Pediatrics:* OCD: Initial: 6-12 yrs: 25mg qd. 13-17 yrs: 50mg qd. Titrate: Adjust dose at 1 week intervals. Max: 200mg/day. Hepatic Impairment: Use lower or less frequent doses. Dilute solution with 4oz of water, ginger ale, lemon/lime soda, lemonade or orange juice. Take immediately after mixing.

**HOW SUPPLIED:** Sol: 20mg/mL [60mL]; Tab: 25mg*, 50mg*, 100mg* *scored

**CONTRAINDICATIONS:** Concomitant use with MAOIs or pimozide. Concomitant disulfiram with solution.

**WARNINGS/PRECAUTIONS:** Activation of mania/hypomania reported. Monitor weight loss. Caution with conditions that could affect metabolism or hemodynamic responses, seizure disorder. Dose adjust with liver dysfunction. Altered platelet function and hyponatremia reported. Weak uricosuric effects reported. Caution with latex sensitivity; solution dropper dispenser contains rubber. Monitor for clinical worsening and/or suicidality, especially at initiation of therapy or dose changes. Avoid abrupt withdrawal. Monitor for discontinuation symptoms.

**ADVERSE REACTIONS:** Ejaculation failure, dry mouth, increased sweating, somnolence, tremor, anorexia, dizziness, headache, vomiting, diarrhea, dyspepsia, nausea, agitation, insomnia, nervousness, abnormal vision.

**INTERACTIONS:** See Contraindications. Increased levels with cimetidine. Avoid with alcohol, pimozide or MAOIs. Decreases clearance of tolbutamide. Rare reports of weakness, hyperreflexia, incoordination with an SSRI and sumatriptan. May potentiate drugs metabolized by CYP2D6 (eg, TCAs, Type 1C antiarrhythmics). Caution with CNS drugs (eg, diazepam). Monitor lithium. Caution with TCAs; may need dose adjustment. May shift concentrations with plasma protein-bound drugs (eg, warfarin, digitoxin). Monitor PT with warfarin. Caution with OTC products. May induce metabolism of cisapride. Caution with drugs that interfere with hemostasis (eg, non-selective NSAIDs, aspirin, warfarin) due to increased risk of bleeding.

**PREGNANCY:** Category C, caution in nursing.

## ZOMETA RX

zoledronic acid (Novartis)

**THERAPEUTIC CLASS:** Bisphosphonate

**INDICATIONS:** Treatment of hypercalcemia of malignancy. Treatment of multiple myeloma and bone metastases from solid tumors, in conjunction with antineoplastic therapy.

**DOSAGE:** *Adults:* Hypercalcemia of Malignancy: Max: 4mg IV over no less than 15 minutes. Retreatment (if necessary): Wait at least 7 days from initial dose. Multiple Myeloma/Bone Metastases: 4mg IV over 15 minutes every 3-4 weeks. CrCl 50-60mL/min: 3.5mg; CrCl 40-49mL/min: 3.3mg; CrCl 30-39mL/min: 3.0mg. Measure serum creatinine prior to each dose. Withhold dose with renal deterioration; resume when serum creatinine returns to within 10% of baseline. Take with oral calcium 500mg/day and Vitamin D 400 IU/day.

**HOW SUPPLIED:** Inj: 4mg/5mL

**WARNINGS/PRECAUTIONS:** Caution with hepatic insufficiency, aspirin-sensitive asthma, and the elderly. Risk of renal toxicity/failure. In severe renal impairment, avoid with bone metastases and use caution with hypercalcemia of malignancy. Rehydrate before use with hypercalcemia of malignancy. Monitor serum creatinine before each dose, and serum calcium, electrolytes, phosphate, magnesium, and Hct/Hgb regularly. May cause fetal harm during pregnancy. Osteonecrosis of the jaw reported in cancer patients treated with bisphosphonates; avoid invasive dental procedures during therapy.

**ADVERSE REACTIONS:** Fever, chills, bone pain, arthralgia, myalgia, nausea, vomiting, diarrhea, constipation, injection site reactions, conjunctivitis, hypomagnesemia, abnormal serum creatinine, hypophosphatemia, hypocalcemia.

**INTERACTIONS:** Additive effect/risk of hypocalcemia with aminoglycosides and loop diuretics. Caution with other nephrotoxic drugs. Increased risk of renal dysfunction with thalidomide in multiple myeloma patients.

**PREGNANCY:** Category D, not for use in nursing.

## ZOMIG

RX

zolmitriptan (AstraZeneca LP)

**OTHER BRAND NAMES:** Zomig-ZMT (AstraZeneca LP) - Zomig Nasal Spray (AstraZeneca LP)

**THERAPEUTIC CLASS:** 5-$HT_{1D,1B}$ agonist

**INDICATIONS:** Acute treatment of migraine attacks with or without aura.

**DOSAGE:** *Adults:* >18 yrs: (Spray) 5mg single dose; may repeat once after 2 hours. Max: 10mg/24 hrs. Safety of treating >4 headaches/30 days unknown. (Tab) Initial: 2.5mg or lower (2.5mg tab may be broken in 1/2), may repeat after 2 hrs. Max: 10mg/24 hrs. Safety of treating >3 headaches in 30 days is unknown. (ZMT) Dissolve on tongue without water. Hepatic Impairment: Use low dose and monitor blood pressure.

**HOW SUPPLIED:** Nasal Spray: 5mg [0.1mL 6$^{s}$]; Tab: 2.5mg*; 5mg; Tab, Disintegrating: (ZMT) 2.5mg, 5mg *scored

**CONTRAINDICATIONS:** Ischemic heart disease, coronary artery vasospasm (eg, Prinzmetal's angina), uncontrolled HTN, other significant cardiovascular disease, hemiplegic or basilar migraine, MAOI use during or within 14 days, other 5-$HT_1$ agonist or ergot-type agent use within 24 hrs.

**WARNINGS/PRECAUTIONS:** Confirm diagnosis. Supervise 1st dose and monitor cardiac function in those at risk of CAD (eg, HTN, hypercholesterolemia, smoker, obesity, diabetes, CAD family history, postmenopausal women, males >40 yrs). Serious adverse cardiac events, cerebrovascular events, vasospastic reactions reported with 5-$HT_1$ agonists. Disintegrating tabs contain phenylalanine. Caution with hepatic dysfunction. Reconsider diagnosis before 2nd dose.

**ADVERSE REACTIONS:** Paresthesia, asthenia, warm/cold sensation, neck/throat/jaw pain, dry mouth, nausea, dizziness, somnolence, unusual taste (nasal spray).

**INTERACTIONS:** Ergot-agents may prolong vasospastic reactions. Avoid MAOIs, during or within 14 days of therapy. SSRIs may cause weakness, hyperreflexia, and incoordination. Half-life and AUC doubled with cimetidine. Avoid 5-$HT_{1B/1D}$ agonists within 24 hrs.

**PREGNANCY:** Category C, caution in nursing.

## ZONALON

RX

doxepin HCl (Bioglan)

**THERAPEUTIC CLASS:** $H_1/H_2$ receptor blocker

**INDICATIONS:** Short-term management of moderate pruritus in atopic dermatitis, and lichen simplex chronicus.

**DOSAGE:** *Adults:* Apply qid up to 8 days. Wait at least 3-4 hrs between applications. Avoid occlusive dressings.

**HOW SUPPLIED:** Cre: 5% [30g, 45g]

**CONTRAINDICATIONS:** Untreated narrow angle glaucoma, urinary retention.

**WARNINGS/PRECAUTIONS:** Significant drowsiness reported when applied to >10% of BSA; may need to reduce amount or area covered, or number of applications. Avoid eyes.

**ADVERSE REACTIONS:** Drowsiness, dry mouth, dry lips, thirst, headache, fatigue, dizziness, emotional changes, taste changes.

**INTERACTIONS:** Discontinue MAOIs at least 2 weeks before therapy. Alcohol may potentiate sedation. Caution with drugs metabolized by CYP2D6 (eg, other antidepressants, phenothiazines, carbamazepine, flecainide, encainide, propafenone, quinidine). Poor metabolizers may have increased plasma levels. Possible serum level fluctuations with cimetidine. Hypoglycemia reported when oral doxepin was added to tolazamide therapy.

**PREGNANCY:** Category B, not for use in nursing.

## ZONEGRAN RX

zonisamide (Eisai)

**THERAPEUTIC CLASS:** Sulfonamide anticonvulsant

**INDICATIONS:** Adjunctive therapy in the treatment of partial seizures.

**DOSAGE:** *Adults:* Initial: 100mg qd for 2 weeks. Titrate: Increase to 200mg/day for 2 weeks, then increase to 300mg/day, then to 400mg/day at 2 week intervals. Max: 400mg/day.
*Pediatrics:* >16 yrs: Initial: 100mg qd for 2 weeks. Titrate: Increase to 200mg/day for 2 weeks, then increase to 300mg/day, then to 400mg/day at 2 week intervals. Max: 400mg/day.

**HOW SUPPLIED:** Cap: 25mg, 50mg, 100mg

**CONTRAINDICATIONS:** Sulfonamide hypersensitivity.

**WARNINGS/PRECAUTIONS:** Sulfonamide hypersensitivity reactions (eg, Stevens-Johnson syndrome, toxic epidermal necrolysis, fulminant hepatic necrosis, blood dyscrasias), cognitive/neuropsychiatric effects, kidney stones, sudden death reported. Discontinue with unexplained rash. Increased risk of oligohydrosis and hyperthermia in pediatrics; monitor for decreased sweating and increased body temperature. Advise females to use contraceptives to prevent pregnancy. Caution with renal/hepatic impairment. Avoid abrupt withdrawal.

**ADVERSE REACTIONS:** Somnolence, anorexia, dizziness, tremor, convulsion, dry mouth, incoordination, amblyopia, tinnitus, GI effects, flu syndrome, ataxia, nystagmus, pruritus.

**INTERACTIONS:** Enzyme inducers increase metabolism and clearance. Caution with drugs that predispose patients to heat-related disorders (eg, carbonic anhydrase inhibitors, anticholinergic drugs).

**PREGNANCY:** Category C, not for use in nursing.

## ZORBTIVE RX

somatropin (Serono)

**THERAPEUTIC CLASS:** Human Growth Hormone

**INDICATIONS:** Treatment of Short Bowel Syndrome in patients recieving specialized nutritional support.

**DOSAGE:** *Adults:* 0.1mg/kg qd SC for 4 weeks. Max: 8mg qd. Rotate injection site.

**HOW SUPPLIED:** Inj: 8.8mg

**CONTRAINDICATIONS:** Acute critical illness due to complications folowing open heart or abdominal surgery, multiple accidental trauma, or acute respiratory failure; active neoplasia (either newly diagnosed or recurrent); benzyl alcohol sensitivity.

**WARNINGS/PRECAUTIONS:** Associated with acute pancreatitis. New onset impaired glucose intolerance, new onset type 2 DM, exacerbation of pre-existing DM, ketoacidosis, diabetic coma reported; closely monitor with risk factors for glucose intolerance. Perform funduscopic evaluations periodically. Increased tissue turgor, musculoskeletal discomfort, and carpal tunnel syndrome may occur.

**ADVERSE REACTIONS:** Peripheral/facial edema, chest/back pain, fever, flu-like disorder, malaise, flatulence, abdominal pain, nausea, vomiting, viral infection, dizziness, headache, rash.

**PREGNANCY:** Category B, caution in nursing.

## ZOSTAVAX
zoster vaccine live (Merck) RX

**THERAPEUTIC CLASS:** Vaccine

**INDICATIONS:** Prevention of herpes zoster in individuals ≥60.

**DOSAGE:** *Adults*: ≥60 yrs: Inject SQ immediately after reconstitution with supplied diluent.

**HOW SUPPLIED:** Inj: 19,400 PFU/0.65mL

**CONTRAINDICATIONS:** Anaphylactic/anaphylactoid reactions to gelatin or neomycin. Primary or acquired immunodeficiency states (eg, leukemia); lymphomas or other malignant neoplasms affecting the bone marrow or lymphatic system; AIDS or other clinical manifestations HIV infections. Immunosuppressive therapy, including high-dose corticosteroids. Active untreated tuberculosis. Pregnancy.

**WARNINGS/PRECAUTIONS:** More extensive vaccine-associated rash or disseminated disease with immunosuppression. Anaphlactic/anaphylactoid reaction may occur. Deferral of vaccination should be considered in acute illness.

**ADVERSE REACTIONS:** Erythema, pain, tenderness, swelling, pruritus.

**INTERACTIONS:** See Contraindications.

**PREGNANCY:** Category C, caution in nursing.

## ZOSYN
tazobactam - piperacillin sodium (Wyeth) RX

**THERAPEUTIC CLASS:** Broad-spectrum penicillin/beta lactamase inhibitor

**INDICATIONS:** Treatment of appendicitis, peritonitis, uncomplicated/complicated skin and skin structure infections, postpartum endometritis, pelvic inflammatory disease, moderate severity of community acquired pneumonia, and moderate to severe nosocomial pneumonia.

**DOSAGE:** *Adults:* Usual: 3.375g q6h for 7-10 days. Nosocomial Pneumonia: 4.5g q6h for 7-14 days plus aminoglycoside. CrCl 20-40mL/min: 2.25g q6h. CrCl <20mL/min: 2.25g q8h. Hemodialysis: Max: 2.25g q12h. Give 1 additional 0.75g dose after each dialysis period.

**HOW SUPPLIED:** Inj: (Piperacillin-Tazobactam) 40mg-5mg/mL, 60mg-7.5mg/mL, 2g-0.25g, 3g-0.375g, 4g-0.5g, 4g-0.5g/100mL, 36g-4.5g

**CONTRAINDICATIONS:** History of allergic reactions to cephalosporins.

**WARNINGS/PRECAUTIONS:** Serious, fatal hypersensitivity reactions may occur with penicillin allergy. Pseudomembranous colitis reported. D/C if bleeding manifestations occur. May experience neuromuscular excitability or convulsions with higher doses. Contains 2.35mEq/g Na; caution with restricted salt intake. Increased incidence of rash and fever in cystic fibrosis. Monitor electrolyte periodically with low $K^+$ reserves.

**ADVERSE REACTIONS:** Rash, pruritus, diarrhea, nausea, vomiting, phlebitis, injection site reaction, pain, inflammation.

**INTERACTIONS:** May inactivate aminoglycosides. Probenecid prolongs half-life. Monitor coagulation parameters with heparin, oral anticoagulants, or drugs that affect blood coagulation system or thrombocyte function. May prolong neuromuscular blockade of vecuronium.

**PREGNANCY:** Category B, caution in nursing.

## ZOVIRAX
RX

acyclovir (GlaxoSmithKline)

**THERAPEUTIC CLASS:** Nucleoside analogue

**INDICATIONS:** Acute treatment of herpes zoster (shingles). Treatment of initial and recurrent episodes of genital herpes. Treatment of chickenpox (varicella).

**DOSAGE:** *Adults:* Herpes Zoster: 800mg q4h, 5x/day for 7-10 days. Start within 72 hrs after onset of rash. Genital Herpes: Initial: 200mg q4h, 5x/day for 10 days. Chronic Therapy: 400mg bid or 200mg 3-5x/day up to 12 months, then re-evaluate. Intermittent Therapy: 200mg q4h, 5x/day for 5 days. Start with 1st sign/symptom of recurrence. Chickenpox: 800mg qid for 5 days. CrCl 10-25mL/min: For a dose of 800mg q4h, give 800mg q8h. CrCl 0-10mL/min: For a dose of 200mg q4h, give 200mg q12h. For a dose of 400mg q12h, give 200mg q12h. For a dose of 800mg q4h, give 800mg q12h. Elderly: Reduce dose.
*Pediatrics:* >2 yrs: <40kg: Chickenpox: 20mg/kg qid for 5 days. >40kg: 800mg qid for 5 days.

**HOW SUPPLIED:** Cap: 200mg; Sus: 200mg/5mL; Tab: 400mg, 800mg

**CONTRAINDICATIONS:** Hypersensitivity to valacyclovir.

**WARNINGS/PRECAUTIONS:** Adust dose in renal impairment, elderly. Renal failure and death reported. Thrombotic thrombocytopenic purpura/hemolytic uremic syndrome in immunocompromised patients reported.

**ADVERSE REACTIONS:** Nausea, vomiting, diarrhea, headache, malaise, renal dysfunction.

**INTERACTIONS:** Probenecid increased levels of IV formulation. Caution with potentially nephrotoxic agents.

**PREGNANCY:** Category B, caution in nursing.

## ZOVIRAX CREAM
RX

acyclovir (Biovail)

**THERAPEUTIC CLASS:** Nucleoside analogue antiviral

**INDICATIONS:** Treatment of recurrent herpes labialis (cold sores).

**DOSAGE:** *Adults:* Apply5x/day for 4 days. Initiate with 1st sign/symptom.
*Pediatrics:* ≥12 yrs: Apply 5x/day for 4 days. Initiate with 1st sign/symptom.

**HOW SUPPLIED:** Cre: 5% [2g]

**WARNINGS/PRECAUTIONS:** Cutaneous use only; not for use in the eye, mouth or nose.

**ADVERSE REACTIONS:** Dry lips, desquamation, dryness of skin, cracked lips, burning skin, pruritus, flakiness of skin, stinging on skin.

**PREGNANCY:** Category B, caution in nursing.

## ZOVIRAX OINTMENT
RX

acyclovir (Biovail)

**THERAPEUTIC CLASS:** Nucleoside analogue antiviral

**INDICATIONS:** Management of initial genital herpes and in limited non life-threatening mucocutaneous herpes simplex infections in immunocompromised patients.

**DOSAGE:** *Adults:* Apply to all lesions q3h, 6x/day for 7 days. Apply with finger cot or rubber glove to prevent autoinoculation and transmission. Initiate with 1st sign/symptom.

**HOW SUPPLIED:** Oint: 5% [15g]

**WARNINGS/PRECAUTIONS:** Not for use for the prevention of recurrent HSV infections. Cutaneous use only; avoid eyes.

**ADVERSE REACTIONS:** Pain with application, transient burning and stinging, pruritus.

**PREGNANCY:** Category B, caution in nursing.

## ZYBAN
bupropion HCl (GlaxoSmithKline) RX

**Antidepressants increased the risk of suicidal thinking and behavior (suicidality) in short-term studies in children and adolescents with Major Depressive Disorder (MDD) and other psychiatric disorders. Bupropion is not approved for use in pediatric patients.**

**THERAPEUTIC CLASS:** Aminoketone

**INDICATIONS:** Aid to smoking cessation treatment.

**DOSAGE:** *Adults:* ≥18 yrs: Initial: 150mg qd for 3 days. Usual: 150mg bid; separate dose intervals by at least 8 hrs. Max: 300mg/day. Initiate treatment while patient is still smoking. Patients should set a"target quit date" within the first 2 weeks. Treat for 7 to 12 weeks; d/c at 7 weeks if no progress seen. Renal/Hepatic Dysfunction: Reduce dose. Severe Hepatic Cirrhosis: 150mg every other day.

**HOW SUPPLIED:** Tab, Extended Release: 150mg

**CONTRAINDICATIONS:** Seizure disorder, bulimia or anorexia nervosa, within 14 days of MAOIs, other forms of bupropion, abrupt discontinuation of alcohol or sedatives.

**WARNINGS/PRECAUTIONS:** Dose-related risk of seizures. D/C and do not restart if seizure occurs. Extreme caution with history of seizure, cranial trauma, severe hepatic cirrhosis. Caution with recent MI, unstable heart disease, renal impairment. Agitation, insomnia, psychosis, confusion and other neuropsychiatric phenomena reported. Allergic reactions, HTN reported. May precipitate manic episodes in bipolar disorder.

**ADVERSE REACTIONS:** Anxiety, dizziness, anorexia, myalgia, pruritus, dry mouth, insomnia, nausea, constipation, tremor, dream abnormality, rash, confusion.

**INTERACTIONS:** Extreme caution with drugs that lower seizure threshold (eg, antidepressants, antipsychotics, theophylline, systemic steroids). Increased seizure risk with opioid, cocaine, or stimulant addiction, OTC stimulants or anorectics, oral hypoglycemics or insulin, excessive use or abrupt discontinuation of alcohol or sedatives. Caution with levodopa, amantadine, and drugs that are metabolized by CYP2D6 (eg, SSRIs, TCAs, antipsychotics, β-blockers, type 1C antiarrhythmics); use low initial dose and gradually titrate. Avoid other bupropion-containing drugs and MAOIs. Monitor HTN with transdermal nicotine. Caution with CYP2B6 substrates or inhibitors (eg, orphenadrine, cyclophosphamide). Carbamazepine, phenytoin, cimetidine, and phenobarbital may induce metabolism of bupropion. Minimize or avoid alcohol.

**PREGNANCY:** Pregnancy B, not for use in nursing.

## ZYDONE
acetaminophen - hydrocodone bitartrate (Endo) CIII

**THERAPEUTIC CLASS:** Opioid analgesic

**INDICATIONS:** Relief of moderate to moderately severe pain.

**DOSAGE:** *Adults:* (5/400): 1-2 tabs q4-6h prn. Max: 8 tabs/day. (7.5/400, 10/400): 1 tab q4-6h prn. Max: 6 tabs/day.

**HOW SUPPLIED:** Tab: (Hydrocodone-APAP) 5mg-400mg, 7.5mg-400mg, 10mg-400mg

**WARNINGS/PRECAUTIONS:** May produce dose-related respiratory depression. May obscure diagnosis of acute abdominal conditions or head injuries. Caution in elderly, debilitated, severe hepatic or renal dysfunction, hypothyroidism, Addison's disease, prostatic hypertrophy, urethral stricture, pulmonary disease and postoperative use. May be habit-forming. Suppresses cough reflex.

**ADVERSE REACTIONS:** Lightheadedness, dizziness, sedation, nausea, vomiting.

**INTERACTIONS:** Additive CNS depression with opioids, antihistamines, antipsychotics, antianxiety agents, or other CNS depressants (including alcohol). Increased effect of antidepressant or hydrocodone with MAOIs or TCAs.

**PREGNANCY:** Category C, not for use in nursing.

## ZYFLO CR — RX

zileuton (Critical Therapeutics)

**OTHER BRAND NAMES:** Zyflo (Critical Therapeutics)

**THERAPEUTIC CLASS:** Leukotriene inhibitor

**INDICATIONS:** Prophylaxis and chronic treatment of asthma.

**DOSAGE:** *Adults:* 600mg qid, with meals and at bedtime. (Tab, Extended-Release) 1200mg bid within 1 hr after am and pm meals. Max: 2400mg/day. *Pediatrics:* >12 yrs: 600mg qid, with meals and at bedtime. (Tab, Extended-Release) 1200mg bid within 1 hr after am and pm meals. Max: 2400mg/day.

**HOW SUPPLIED:** Tab, Extended-Release: 600mg; Tab: 600mg* *scored

**CONTRAINDICATIONS:** Active liver disease or transaminase elevations (>3X ULN).

**WARNINGS/PRECAUTIONS:** Not for treatment of acute attacks. Evaluate liver function prior to therapy and periodically thereafter. D/C if signs of liver disease occur.

**ADVERSE REACTIONS:** (Zyflo, Zyflo CR) Headache, ALT elevation, dyspepsia, pain, nausea, asthenia, myalgia. (Zyflo CR) Sinusitis, pharyngolaryngeal pain.

**INTERACTIONS:** Monitor drugs metabolized by CYP450 3A4. Increases theophylline levels; reduce theophylline by 50% and monitor levels. Potentiates warfarin, propranolol. (Zyflo) Potentiates terfenadine.

**PREGNANCY:** Category C, not for use in nursing.

## ZYLET — RX

tobramycin - loteprednol etabonate (Bausch & Lomb)

**THERAPEUTIC CLASS:** Aminoglycoside/corticosteriod

**INDICATIONS:** Treatment of steroid-responsive inflammatory ocular conditions for which a corticosteroid is indicated and where superficial bacterial ocular infection or a risk of bacterial ocular infection exists.

**DOSAGE:** *Adults:* Initial: 1-2 drops q4-6h. May increase to 1-2 drops q1-2h for first 24-48 hours. Max: 20mL for initial Rx.

**HOW SUPPLIED:** Sus: 2.5mL, 5mL, 10mL

**CONTRAINDICATIONS:** Viral diseases of the cornea and conjunctiva including epithelial herpes simplex keratitis (dendritic keratitis), vaccinia, and varicella, and also in mycobacterial infection of the eye and fungal diseases of ocular structures.

**WARNINGS/PRECAUTIONS:** Not for injection into the eye. Prolonged use may result in glaucoma, optic nerve damage, visual acuity and fields of vision defects, cataracts, secondary ocular infections. May exacerbate the severity of many viral infections of the eye (including herpes simplex). May delay healing and increase incidence of bleb formation after cataract surgery.

**ADVERSE REACTIONS:** Injection and superficial punctate keratitis, increased IOP, burning, stinging, headache, secondary infection, vision disorders, discharge, itching, lacrimation disorder, photophobia, corneal deposits, ocular discomfort, eyelid disorder.

**PREGNANCY:** Category C, caution in nursing.

## ZYLOPRIM RX

allopurinol (Prometheus)

**THERAPEUTIC CLASS:** Xanthine oxidase inhibitor

**INDICATIONS:** Management of symptoms of primary and secondary gout. Management of hyperuricosuria and hyperuricemia due to chemotherapy. Management of recurrent calcium oxalate calculi in those with hyperuricosuria (uric acid excretion >800mg/day in males and >750mg/day in females).

**DOSAGE:** *Adults:* Gout: Initial: 100mg/day. Titrate: Increase by 100mg/week until serum uric acid level is <6mg/dL. Mild Gout: Usual: 200-300mg/day. Moderately Severe Gout: Usual: 400-600mg/day. Max: 800mg/day. Recurrent Calcium Oxalate Stones: Usual: 200-300mg/day. Prevention of Uric Acid Nephropathy with Chemotherapy: Usual: 600-800mg/day for 2-3 days with high fluid intake. CrCl 10-20mL/min: 200mg/day. CrCl <10mL/min: Max: 100mg/day. CrCl <3mL/min: Also increase dosing intervals. Take after meals. Divide dose if >300mg.
*Pediatrics:* Hyperuricemia with Malignancies: 6-10 yrs: 300mg/day. <6 yrs: 150mg/day. Evaluate response after 48 hrs. Take after meals.

**HOW SUPPLIED:** Tab: 100mg*, 300mg* *scored

**WARNINGS/PRECAUTIONS:** Discontinue if skin rash occurs. Severe hypersensitivity reactions, hepatotoxicity, and bone marrow depression reported. Monitor LFTs during early stages of therapy with liver disease. Caution with activities that require alertness. Caution with renal impairment. Renal failure reported with hyperuricemia secondary to neoplastic diseases. Fluid intake should yield >2 liters of urinary output/day. Maintain neutral or slightly alkaline urine. Acute gout attacks increase during early stages of therapy; give colchicine.

**ADVERSE REACTIONS:** Acute gout attacks, rash, diarrhea, SGOT/SGPT increase, alkaline phosphatase increase, nausea.

**INTERACTIONS:** Increased toxicity with thiazide diuretics or renal impairment; monitor renal function. Reduce mercaptopurine or azathioprine to 1/3 or 1/4 of usual dose. Potentiates dicumarol, chlorpropamide and cyclosporine. Decreased effects with uricosurics. Increased skin rash with ampicillin, amoxicillin. Enhanced bone marrow suppression with cytotoxic agents (eg, cyclophosphamide). Caution with sulfinpyrazone.

**PREGNANCY:** Category C, caution in nursing.

## ZYMAR RX

gatifloxacin (Allergan)

**THERAPEUTIC CLASS:** Fluoroquinolone

**INDICATIONS:** Treatment of bacterial conjunctivitis.

**DOSAGE:** *Adults:* 1 drop q2h while awake, up to 8x/day for 2 days; then 1 drop up to qid while awake for 5 days.
*Pediatrics:* ≥1 yr: 1 drop q2h while awake, up to 8x/day for 2 days; then 1 drop up to qid while awake for 5 days.

**HOW SUPPLIED:** Sol: 0.3% [5mL]

**WARNINGS/PRECAUTIONS:** Not for injection. Do not inject subconjunctivally or into the anterior chamber of the eye. Superinfection may result with prolonged use. Fatal hypersensitivity reactions reported after 1st dose of systemic quinolone therapy. Avoid contact lenses when symptoms are present.

**ADVERSE REACTIONS:** Conjunctival irritation, increased lacrimation, keratitis, papillary conjunctivitis, chemosis, conjunctival hemorrhage, dry eye, eye discharge/irritation/pain, red eye, eyelid edema, headache, reduced visual acuity, taste disturbance.

**INTERACTIONS:** Systemic quinolone therapy may increase theophylline levels, interfere with caffeine metabolism, enhance warfarin effects, and elevate serum creatinine with cyclosporine.

**PREGNANCY:** Category C, caution in nursing.

## ZYMASE RX

lipase - amylase - protease (Organon)

**THERAPEUTIC CLASS:** Pancreatic enzyme supplement

**INDICATIONS:** Treatment of conditions with pancreatic enzyme deficiency with resultant inadequate fat digestion (eg, chronic pancreatitis, pancreatectomy, cystic fibrosis, steatorrhea).

**DOSAGE:** *Adults:* 1-2 caps with each meal or snack. Contents of cap may be mixed with liquids or soft foods that do not require chewing.
*Pediatrics:* 1-2 caps with each meal or snack. Contents of cap may be mixed with liquids or soft foods that do not require chewing.

**HOW SUPPLIED:** Cap, Delayed Release: (Amylase-Lipase-Protease) 24,000U-12,000U-24,000U

**CONTRAINDICATIONS:** Pork protein hypersensitivity.

**WARNINGS/PRECAUTIONS:** Do not chew or crush contents of capsules. High doses can cause hyperuricemia and hyperuricosuria.

**PREGNANCY:** Safety in pregnancy and nursing not known.

## ZYPREXA RX

olanzapine (Lilly)

**Elderly patients with dementia-related psychosis treated with atypical antipsychotic drugs are at an increased risk of death; most appeared to be cardiovascular (eg, heart failure, sudden death) or infectious (eg, pneumonia) in nature. Olanzapine is not approved for the treatment of patients with dementia-related psychosis.**

**OTHER BRAND NAMES:** Zyprexa Zydis (Lilly) - Zyprexa IntraMuscular (Lilly)

**THERAPEUTIC CLASS:** Thienobenzodiazepine

**INDICATIONS:** (Tab) Treatment of schizophrenia. Treatment of acute mixed or manic episodes in Bipolar I Disorder. Short-term treatment of acute manic episodes associated with Bipolar I Disorder in combination with lithium or valproate. (Inj) Agitation associated with schizophrenia, bipolar I mania.

**DOSAGE:** *Adults:* (Tab) Schizophrenia: Initial/Usual: 5-10mg qd. Titrate: Adjust by 5mg daily at weekly intervals. Max: 20mg/day. Bipolar Mania: Initial: 10-15mg qd. Titrate: Increase by 5mg daily. Max: 20mg/day. With Lithium or Valproate: Initial/Usual: 10mg qd. Max: 20mg/day. Debilitated/Hypotension Risk/Slow metabolizers/Sensitivity to olanzapine effects: Initial: 5mg qd. Titrate: Increase cautiously. (IM) Agitation: Initial: 10mg IM. Usual: 2.5-10mg IM. Max: 3 doses of 10mg q 2-4h. Elderly: 5mg IM. Debilitated/Hypotension Risk/Sensitivity to olanzapine effects: 2.5mg IM. May initiate PO therapy when clinically appropriate.

**HOW SUPPLIED:** Inj: 10mg; Tab: 2.5mg, 5mg, 7.5mg, 10mg, 15mg, 20mg; Tab, Disintegrating: (Zydis) 5mg, 10mg, 15mg, 20mg

**WARNINGS/PRECAUTIONS:** Monitor for hyperglycemia, worsening of glucose control with DM, FBG levels with diabetes risk. Risk of NMS, tardive dyskinesia, orthostatic hypotension, seizures. Caution in hepatic impairment, prostatic hypertrophy, narrow-angle glaucoma, history of paralytic ileus, elderly patients with dementia or Parkinson's disease, cardio- or cerebrovascular disease, hypotension risk (eg, hypovolemia, dehydration), risk for aspiration pneumonia, suicidal tendencies. Elevated transaminases, hyperprolactinemia reported. May cause disruption of body temperature regulation. Re-evaluate periodically.

**ADVERSE REACTIONS:** Postural hypotension, constipation, dry mouth, weight gain, somnolence, dizziness, personality disorder, akathisia, asthenia, dyspepsia, tremor, increased appetite, ecchymosis, rhinitis, joint pain

**INTERACTIONS:** May potentiate antihypertensives. Decreased levels with activated charcoal. Increased clearance with carbamazepine. Increased levels with fluvoxamine; lower olanzapine dose. Caution with other CNS drugs, alcohol. May antagonize levodopa, dopamine agonists. Inducers of CYP1A2 or glucuronyl transferase (eg, omeprazole, rifampin) may increase clearance. Inhibitors of CYP1A2 may decrease clearance.

**PREGNANCY:** Category C, not for use in nursing.

## ZYRTEC

RX

cetirizine HCl (Pfizer)

**THERAPEUTIC CLASS:** $H_1$ antagonist

**INDICATIONS:** Seasonal or perennial allergic rhinitis. Chronic idiopathic urticaria.

**DOSAGE:** *Adults:* 5-10mg qd. Hepatic Impairment/Hemodialysis/CrCl <31mL/min: 5mg qd.
*Pediatrics:* >12 yrs: 5-10mg qd. 6-11 yrs: 5-10mg qd. 2-5 yrs: 2.5mg qd. Max: 5mg qd or 2.5mg q12h. Perennial Allergic Rhinitis/Urticaria: 6 months-23 months: 2.5mg qd. 12 months-23 months: May increase to max 5mg/day given as 2.5mL q12h. Hepatic Impairment/Hemodialysis/CrCl <31mL/min: >12 yrs: 5mg qd. 6-11 yrs: Use lower the recommended dose. <6 yrs: Not recommended.

**HOW SUPPLIED:** Syrup: 1mg/mL [120mL, 480mL]; Tab: 5mg, 10mg; Tab, Chewable: 5mg, 10mg

**CONTRAINDICATIONS:** Hydroxyzine hypersensitivity.

**WARNINGS/PRECAUTIONS:** Adjust dose with hepatic or renal impairment. May impair mental/physical abilities.

**ADVERSE REACTIONS:** Somnolence, fatigue, dry mouth, headache, pharyngitis, abdominal pain, cough, epistaxis, diarrhea, bronchospasm.

**INTERACTIONS:** Avoid alcohol and CNS depressants. Possible decreased clearance with large doses of theophylline.

**PREGNANCY:** Category B, not for use in nursing.

## ZYRTEC-D

RX

cetirizine HCl - pseudoephedrine HCl (Pfizer)

**THERAPEUTIC CLASS:** Antihistamine/decongestant

**INDICATIONS:** Relief of nasal and non-nasal symptoms associated with seasonal or perennial allergic rhinitis.

**DOSAGE:** *Adults:* 1 tab bid. Hepatic Impairment/Renal Dysfunction (CrCl <31mL/min): 1 tab qd. Swallow tabs whole.
*Pediatrics:* >12 yrs: 1 tab bid. Hepatic Impairment/Renal Dysfunction (CrCl <31mL/min): 1 tab qd. Swallow tabs whole.

**HOW SUPPLIED:** Tab, Extended Release: (Cetirizine-Pseudoephedrine) 5mg-120mg

**CONTRAINDICATIONS:** Narrow angle glaucoma, urinary retention, MAOIs during or within 14 days of use, severe HTN, severe CAD, hypersensitivity to adrenergics.

**WARNINGS/PRECAUTIONS:** Caution with HTN, DM, ischemic heart disease, increased IOP, hyperthyroidism, renal impairment, or prostatic hypertrophy. May produce CNS stimulation with convulsions or cardiovascular collapse.

**ADVERSE REACTIONS:** Insomnia, dry mouth, fatigue, somnolence.

**INTERACTIONS:** Avoid MAOIs during or within 14 days of use.

**PREGNANCY:** Category C, not for use in nursing.

## ZYVOX

RX

linezolid (Pfizer)

**THERAPEUTIC CLASS:** Oxazolidinone class antibacterial

**INDICATIONS:** Vancomycin resistant *Enterococcus faecium* (VRE) infections, nosocomial pneumonia caused by *Staphylococcus aureus* (methicillin-susceptible and -resistant strains) or *Streptococcus pneumoniae* (including multi-drug resistant strains [MDRSP]), complicated skin and skin structure infections (SSSI) including diabetic foot infections without concomitant osteomyelitis caused by *Staphylococcus aureus* (methicillin-susceptible and -resistant strains), *Streptococcus pyogenes*, or *Streptococcus agalactiae*, uncomplicated SSSI caused by *Staphylococcus aureus* (methicillin-susceptible only) or *Streptococcus pyogenes*, community-acquired pneumonia (CAP) caused by *Streptococcus pneumoniae* (MDRSP), including concurrent bacteremia, or *Staphylococcus aureus* (methicillin-susceptible strains only).

**DOSAGE:** *Adults:* Complicated SSSI/CAP/Nosocomial Pneumonia: 600mg IV/PO q12h for 10-14 days. VRE: 600mg IV/PO q12h for 14-28 days. Uncomplicated SSSI: 400mg PO q12h for 10-14 days.
*Pediatrics:* Complicated SSSI/CAP/Nosocomial Pneumonia: Treat for 10-14 days. ≥12 yrs: 600mg IV/PO q12h. Birth-11yrs: 10mg/kg IV/PO q8h. VRE: Treat for 14-28 days: >12 yrs: 600mg IV/PO q12h; Birth-11 yrs: 10mg/kg IV/PO q8h. Uncomplicated SSSI: Treat for 10-14 days: >12 yrs: 600mg PO q12h; 5-11 yrs: 10mg/kg PO q12h; <5 yrs: 10mg/kg PO q8h. Neonates <7 days should be initiated with dosing regimen of 10mg/kg q12h; may increase to 10mg/kg q8h if sub-optimal response. All neonatal patients should receive 10mg/kg q8h by 7 days of life.

**HOW SUPPLIED:** Inj: 2mg/mL [100mL, 200mL, 300mL]; Sus: 100mg/5mL; Tab: 400mg, 600mg

**WARNINGS/PRECAUTIONS:** Myelosuppression including anemia, thrombocytopenia, pancytopenia, and leukopenia reported; monitor CBC weekly. Superinfection and pseudomembranous colitis may occur. May permit overgrowth of clostridia. Oral suspension contains phenylalanine. Peripheral and optic neuropathy have been reported; monitor visual function if on for extended periods (=3 months). Lactic acidosis reported.

**ADVERSE REACTIONS:** Diarrhea, headache, nausea, vomiting.

**INTERACTIONS:** Potential interaction with adrenergic and serotonergic agents. May enhance pressor response to sympathomimetics, vasopressors, and dopaminergic agents; caution with dopamine, epinephrine, pseudoephedrine, and phenylpropanolamine. Serotonin syndrome may occur with SSRIs and other antidepressants. Avoid large quantities of tyramine-containing foods or beverages.

**PREGNANCY:** Category C, caution in nursing.

# Appendix: Reference Tables

# ABBREVIATIONS, ACRONYMS AND SYMBOLS

| ABBREVIATIONS | DESCRIPTIONS |
|---|---|
| - (eg, 6-8) | to (eg, 6 to 8) |
| / | per |
| < | less than |
| > | greater than |
| ≤ | less than or equal to |
| ≥ | greater than or equal to |
| 5-FU | 5-fluorouracil |
| 5-HT | 5-hydroxytriptamine (serotonin) |
| ABECB | acute bacterial exacerbation of chronic bronchitis |
| aa | of each |
| ACTH | adrenocorticotrophic hormone |
| ad | right ear |
| ADHD | attention-deficit/hyperactivity disorder |
| A-fib | atrial fibrillation |
| A-flutter | atrial flutter |
| AIDS | acquired immunodeficiency syndrome |
| ALT | alanine transaminase (SGPT) |
| am | morning |
| AMI | acute myocardial infarction |
| ANA | antinuclear antibodies |
| ANC | absolute neutrophil count |
| APAP | acetaminophen |
| as | left ear |
| ASA | aspirin |
| AST | aspartate transaminase (SGOT) |
| au | each ear |
| AUC | area under the curve |
| AV | atrioventricular |
| bid | twice daily |
| BMI | body mass index |
| BP | blood pressure |
| BPH | benign prostatic hypertrophy |
| BSA | body surface area |
| BUN | blood urea nitrogen |
| CABG | coronary artery bypass graft |
| CAD | coronary artery disease |
| Cap | capsule |
| CAP | community-acquired pneumonia |
| CBC | complete blood count |
| CF | cystic fibrosis |
| CHF | congestive heart failure |
| cm | centimeter |
| CMV | cytomegalovirus |
| $C_{max}$ | maximum (peak) concentration |
| CNS | central nervous system |
| COPD | chronic obstructive pulmonary disease |
| CrCl | creatinine clearance |
| CRF | chronic renal failure |
| CSF | cerebrospinal fluid |
| CVA | cerebrovascular accident |
| CVD | cardiovascular disease |

*(Continued)*

| ABBREVIATIONS | DESCRIPTIONS |
|---|---|
| CYP450 | cytochrome P450 |
| d/c | discontinue |
| DM | diabetes mellitus |
| DVT | deep vein thrombosis |
| ECG | electrocardiogram |
| EEG | electroencephalogram |
| eg | for example |
| EPS | extrapyramidal symptom |
| ESRD | end-stage renal disease |
| g | gram |
| GABA | gamma-aminobutyric acid |
| GAD | general anxiety disorder |
| GERD | gastroesophageal reflux disease |
| GFR | glomerular filtration rate |
| GI | gastrointestinal |
| GVHD | graft versus host disease |
| HCG | human chorionic gonadotropin |
| Hct | hematocrit |
| HCTZ | hydrochlorothiazide |
| HDL | high density lipoprotein |
| Hgb | hemoglobin |
| HIV | human immunodeficiency virus |
| HMG-CoA | 3-hydroxy-3-methylglutaryl-coenzyme A |
| HR | heart rate |
| hr or hrs | hour or hours |
| hs | bedtime |
| HSV | herpes simplex virus |
| HTN | hypertension |
| IBD | inflammatory bowel disease |
| IBS | irritable bowel syndrome |
| ICH | intracranial hemorrhage |
| IM | intramuscular |
| INH | isoniazid |
| Inj | injection |
| IOP | intraocular pressure |
| IU | international unit |
| IV | intravenous/intravenously |
| $K^+$ | potassium |
| kg | kilogram |
| KIU | kallikrein inhibitor unit |
| L | liter |
| lbs | pounds |
| LD | loading dose |
| LDL | low density lipoprotein |
| LFT | liver function test |
| Lot | lotion |
| Loz | lozenge |
| LVH | left ventricular hypertrophy |
| M | molar |
| MAC | mycobacterium avium complex |
| Maint | maintenance |
| MAOI | monoamine oxidase inhibitor |
| Max | maximum |
| mcg | microgram |

*(Continued)*

| ABBREVIATIONS | DESCRIPTIONS |
|---|---|
| mEq | milli-equivalent |
| mg | milligram |
| MI | myocardial infarction |
| min | minute (usually as mL/min) |
| mL | milliliter |
| mm | millimeter |
| mM | millimolar |
| MRI | magnetic resonance imaging |
| MS | multiple sclerosis |
| msec | millisecond |
| MTX | methotrexate |
| $Na^+$ | sodium |
| NaCl | sodium chloride |
| NG | nasogastric |
| NKA | no known allergies |
| NMS | neuroleptic malignant syndrome |
| npo | nothing by mouth |
| NSAID | nonsteroidal anti-inflammatory drug |
| NV | nausea and vomiting |
| OA | osteoarthritis |
| OCD | obsessive-compulsive disorder |
| od | right eye |
| Oint | ointment |
| os | left eye |
| ou | each eye |
| PAT | paroxysmal atrial tachycardia |
| pc | after meals |
| PD | Parkinson's disease |
| PID | pelvic inflammatory disease |
| pm | evening |
| po | orally |
| PONV | postoperative nausea and vomiting |
| pr | rectally |
| prn | as needed |
| PSA | prostate-specific antigen |
| PSVT | paroxysmal supraventricular tachycardia |
| pya | prior to admission |
| PT/INR | prothrombin time/international normalized ratio |
| PTSD | post-traumatic stress disorder |
| PTT | partial thromboplastin time |
| PTU | propylthiouracil |
| PUD | peptic ulcer disease |
| PVD | peripheral vascular disease |
| q4h, q6h, q8h… | every four hours, every six hours, every eight hours… |
| qd | once daily |
| qh | every hour |
| qid | four times daily |
| qod | every other day |
| qs | a sufficient quantity |
| qs ad | a sufficient quantity up to |
| RA | rheumatoid arthritis |
| RBC | red blood cells |

(Continued)

| ABBREVIATIONS | DESCRIPTIONS |
|---|---|
| RDIs | reference daily intakes |
| RDS | respiratory distress syndrome |
| REM | rapid eye movement |
| SAH | subarachnoid hemorrhage |
| SBP | systolic blood pressure |
| SGOT | serum glutamic-oxaloacetic transaminase (AST) |
| SGPT | serum glutamic-pyruvic transaminase (ALT) |
| SIADH | syndrome of inappropriate antidiuretic hormone secretion |
| SLE | systemic lupus erythematosus |
| SOB | shortness of breath |
| Sol | solution |
| SQ | subcutaneous |
| SrCr | serum creatinine |
| SSRI | selective serotonin reuptake inhibitor |
| SSSI | skin and skin structure infection |
| STD | sexually transmitted disease |
| Sup | suppository |
| Sus | suspension |
| SVT | supraventricular tachycardia |
| $t_{1/2}$ | half-life |
| Tab | tablet |
| Tab, SL | sublingual tablet |
| TB | tuberculosis |
| TBG | thyroxine binding globulin |
| tbl | tablespoon |
| TCA | tricyclic antidepressant |
| TD | tardive dyskinesia |
| TFT | thyroid function test |
| TG | triglyceride |
| tid | three times daily |
| $T_{max}$ | time to maximum concentration |
| TNF | tumor necrosis factor |
| TPN | total parenteral nutrition |
| TSH | thyroid stimulating hormone |
| tsp | teaspoonful |
| TTP | thrombotic thrombocytopenic purpura |
| U | unit |
| ud | as directed |
| ULN | upper limit of normal |
| URI | upper respiratory infection |
| UTI | urinary tract infection |
| UV | ultraviolet |
| WBC | white blood cell count |
| Vd | volume of distribution |
| VTE | venous thromboembolism |
| X | times (eg, >2X ULN) |
| yr or yrs | year or years |

# CALCULATIONS AND FORMULAS

## WEIGHTS AND MEASURES

| | |
|---|---|
| **METRIC MEASURES** | |
| 1 kilogram (kg) | 1000 g |
| 1 gram (g) | 1000 mg |
| 1 milligram (mg) | 0.001 g |
| 1 microgram (mcg or µg) | 0.001 mg; 1 x $10^{-6}$ g |
| 1 liter (L) | 1000 mL |
| 1 milliliter (mL) | 0.001 L; 1 cc (cubic centimeter) |
| **APOTHECARY MEASURES (AP)** | |
| 1 scruple | 20 grains (gr) |
| 1 drachm | 3 scruples; 60 gr |
| 1 ounce (oz) | 8 drachms; 24 scruples; 480 gr |
| 1 pound (lb) | 12 oz; 96 drachms; 288 scruples; 5760 gr |
| **U.S. FLUID MEASURES** | |
| 1 fluidrachm | 60 minim |
| 1 fluidounce | 8 fluidrachm; 480 minim |
| 1 pint (pt) | 16 fl oz; 7680 minim |
| 1 quart (qt) | 2 pt; 32 fl oz |
| 1 gallon (gal) | 4 qt; 128 fl oz |
| **AVOIRDUPOIS WEIGHT (AV)** | |
| 1 ounce | 437.5 gr |
| 1 pound | 16 oz |
| **CONVERSION FACTORS** | |
| 1 gram | 15.4 gr |
| 1 grain | 64.8 mg |
| 1 ounce (Av) | 28.35 g; 437.5 gr |
| 1 ounce (Ap) | 31.1 g; 480 gr |
| 1 pound (Av) | 453.6 g; 2.68 lb (Ap); 2.20 lb (Av) |
| 1 fluidounce | 29.57 mL |
| 1 fluidrachm | 3.697 mL |
| 1 minim | 0.06 mL |
| **COMMON MEASURES** | |
| 1 teaspoonful | 5 mL; 1/6 fl oz |
| 1 tablespoonful | 15 mL; 1/2 fl oz |
| 1 wineglassful | 60 mL; 2 fl oz |
| 1 teacupful | 120 mL; 4 fl oz |
| 1 gallon | 3800 mL; 128 fl oz |
| 1 quart | 960 mL; 32 fl oz |
| 1 pint | 480 mL; 16 fl oz (exactly 473.2 mL) |
| 8 fluid ounces | 240 mL |
| 4 fluid ounces | 120 mL |
| 2.2 lb | 1 kg |

## DOSE EQUIVALENTS

| WEIGHT (METRIC) | WEIGHT (APOTHECARY) |
|---|---|
| 30 g | 1 ounce |
| 15 g | 4 drams |
| 10 g | 2 1/2 drams |
| 7.5 g | 2 drams |
| 6 g | 90 grains |
| 5 g | 75 grains |
| 4 g | 60 grains; 1 dram |
| 3 g | 45 grains |
| 2 g | 30 grains; 1/2 dram |
| 1.5 g | 22 grains |
| 1 g | 15 grains |
| 750 mg | 12 grains |
| 600 mg | 10 grains |
| 500 mg | 7 1/2 grains |
| 400 mg | 6 grains |
| 300 mg | 5 grains |
| 250 mg | 4 grains |

*(Continued)*

## DOSE EQUIVALENTS *(Continued)*

| WEIGHT (METRIC) | WEIGHT (APOTHECARY) |
|---|---|
| 200 mg | 3 grains |
| 150 mg | 2 1/2 grains |
| 125 mg | 2 grains |
| 100 mg | 1 1/2 grains |
| 75 mg | 1 1/4 grains |
| 60 mg | 1 grain |
| 50 mg | 3/4 grain |
| 40 mg | 2/3 grain |
| 30 mg | 1/2 grain |
| 25 mg | 3/8 grain |
| 20 mg | 1/3 grain |
| 15 mg | 1/4 grain |
| 12 mg | 1/5 grain |
| 10 mg | 1/6 grain |
| 8 mg | 1/8 grain |
| 6 mg | 1/10 grain |
| 5 mg | 1/12 grain |
| 4 mg | 1/15 grain |
| 3 mg | 1/20 grain |
| 2 mg | 1/30 grain |
| 1.5 mg | 1/40 grain |
| 1.2 mg | 1/50 grain |
| 1 mg | 1/60 grain |
| **LIQUID MEASURES (METRIC)** | **LIQUID MEASURES (APOTHECARY)** |
| 1000 mL | 1 quart |
| 750 mL | 1 1/2 pints |
| 500 mL | 1 pint |
| 230 mL | 8 fluid ounces |
| 200 mL | 7 fluid ounces |
| 100 mL | 3 1/2 fluid ounces |
| 50 mL | 1 3/4 fluid ounces |
| 30 mL | 1 fluid ounces |
| 15 mL | 4 fluid drams |
| 10 mL | 2 1/2 fluid drams |
| 8 mL | 2 fluid drams |
| 5 mL | 1 1/4 fluid drams |
| 4 mL | 1 fluid dram |
| 3 mL | 45 minims |
| 2 mL | 30 minims |
| 1 mL | 15 minims |
| 0.75 mL | 12 minims |
| 0.6 mL | 10 minims |
| 0.5 mL | 8 minims |
| 0.3 mL | 5 minims |
| 0.25 mL | 4 minims |
| 0.2 mL | 3 minims |
| 0.1 mL | 1 1/2 minims |
| 0.06 mL | 1 minim |
| 0.05 mL | 3/4 minim |
| 0.03 mL | 1/2 minim |

## MILLIEQUIVALENT (mEq) AND MILLIMOLE (mmol)

**CALCULATIONS**

$$\text{moles} = \frac{\text{weight of a substance (grams)}}{\text{molecular weight of that substance (grams)}} \quad \textbf{OR} \quad = \frac{\text{equivalent}}{\text{valence of ion}}$$

$$\text{millimoles} = \frac{\text{weight of a substance (milligrams)}}{\text{molecular weight of that substance (milligrams)}} \quad \textbf{OR} \quad = \frac{\text{milliequivalents}}{\text{valence of ion}} \quad \textbf{OR} \quad = \text{moles} \times 1000$$

equivalents = moles x valence of ion

milliequivalents = millimoles x valence of ion **OR** = equivalents x 1000

*(Continued)*

## CONVERSIONS

| | |
|---|---|
| mg/100mL to mEq/L | mEq/L = $\frac{(mg/100mL) \times 10 \times valence}{atomic\ weight}$ |
| mEq/L to mg/100mL | mg/100mL = $\frac{(mEq/L) \times atomic\ weight}{10 \times valence}$ |
| mEq/L to volume percent of a gas | volume % = $\frac{(mEq/L) \times 22.4}{10}$ |

# ACID-BASE ASSESSMENT

## DEFINITIONS

| | |
|---|---|
| $PIO_2$ | Oxygen partial pressure of inspired gas (mmHg); 150 mmHg in room air at sea level |
| $FiO_2$ | Fractional pressure of oxygen in inspired gas (0.21 in room air) |
| $PAO_2$ | Alveolar oxygen partial pressure |
| $PACO_2$ | Alveolar carbon dioxide partial pressure |
| $PaO_2$ | Arterial oxygen partial pressure |
| $PaCO_2$ | Arterial carbon dioxide partial pressure |
| R | Respiratory exchange quotient (typically 0.8, increases with high carbohydrate diet, decreases with high fat diet) |

## HENDERSON-HASSELBALCH EQUATION

$pH = 6.1 + \log [HCO_3^- / (0.03)(pCO_2)]$

## ALVEOLAR GAS EQUATION

$PIO_2 = FiO_2 \times$ (total atmospheric pressure - vapor pressure of $H_2O$ at 37°C)
$= FiO_2 \times (760\ mmHg - 47\ mmHg)$

$PaO_2 = PIO_2 - PaCO_2/R$

## ALVEOLAR/ARTERIAL OXYGEN GRADIENT

$PAO_2 - PaO_2$

# ACID-BASE DISORDERS

| Disorder | pH | $HCO_3^-$ | $PCO_2$ | Compensation |
|---|---|---|---|---|
| Metabolic acidosis | < 7.35 | Primary decrease | Compensatory decrease | 1.2-mmHg decrease in $PCO_2$ for every 1-mmol/L decrease in $HCO_3^-$ **or** $PCO_2 = (1.5 \times HCO_3^-) + 8 (\pm 2)$ **or** $PCO_2 = HCO_3^- + 15$ **or** $PCO_2$ = last 2 digits of pH x 100 |
| Metabolic alkalosis | > 7.45 | Primary increase | Compensatory increase | 0.6-0.75 mmHg increase in $PCO_2$ for every 1-mmol/L increase in $HCO_3^-$. $PCO_2$ should not rise above 60 mm Hg in compensation. |
| Respiratory acidosis | < 7.35 | Compensatory increase | Primary increase | ***Acute:*** 1-2 mmol decrease in $HCO_3^-$. for every 10-mmHg decrease in $PCO_2$. ***Chronic:*** 3-4 mmol increase in $HCO_3^-$. for every 10-mmHg increase in $PCO_2$. |
| Respiratory alkalosis | > 7.45 | Compensatory decrease | Primary decrease | ***Acute:*** 1-2 mmol increase in $HCO_3^-$. for every 10-mmHg increase in $PCO_2$. ***Chronic:*** 4-5 mmol decrease in $HCO_3^-$. for every 10-mmHg decrease in $PCO_2$. |

## ACID-BASE EQUATION

$H^+$ (in mEq/L) = $(24 \times PaCO_2)$ divided by $HCO_3^-$

*(Continued)*

# OTHER CALCULATIONS

## ANION GAP

Anion gap = $Na^+$ - ($Cl^-$ + $HCO_3^-$ measured)

## AA GRADIENT

Aa gradient [(713) ($FiO_2$ - ($PaCO_2$ divided by 0.8))] - $PaO_2$

## OSMOLALITY

**Definition:**
Osmolality is a measure of the total number of particles in a solution.

U.S. units (sodium as mEq/L, BUN (blood urea nitrogen) and glucose as (mg/dL)
Plasma osmolality (mOsm/kg) = 2([$Na^+$] + [$K^+$]) + ([BUN]/2.8) + ([glucose]/18)

SI units (all variables in mmol/L):
Plasma osmolality (mOsm/kg) = 2[$Na^+$] + [urea] + [glucose]
Normal range plasma omolality: 280 - 303 mOsm/kg

**Corrected Sodium**
Corrected Na+ = measured $Na^+$ + [1.5 x (glucose - 150 divided by 100)]*
*Do not correct for glucose <150.

**Total Serum Calcium Corrected for Albumin Level**
[(Normal albumin - patient's albumin) x 0.8] + patient's measured total calcium

**Water Deficit**
Water deficit = 0.6 x body weight [1 - (140 divided by $Na^+$)]*
*Body weight is estimated weight in kg; $Na^+$ is serum or plasma sodium.

**Bicarbonate Deficit**
$HCO_3^-$ deficit = [0.4 x weight (kg)] x ($HCO_3^-$ desired - $HCO_3^-$ measured)

## CHILD-PUGH SCORE

The Child-Pugh classification used to assess the prognosis of chronic liver disease, mainly cirrhosis. Child-Pugh is also used to determine the required strength of treatment and the necessity of liver transplantation.

Score:
The score employs five clinical measures of liver disease. Each measure is scored 1-3, with 3 indicating most severe derangement.

| Measure | 1 point | 2 points | 3 points | Units |
|---|---|---|---|---|
| Bilirubin (total)* | <34 (<2) | 34-50 (2-3) | >50 (>3) | mol/L (mg/dL) |
| Serum albumin | >3 | 528-35 | <28 | mg/L |
| INR* | <1.7 | 1.71-2.20 | > 2.20 | no unit |
| Ascites | None | Suppressed with medication | Refractory | no unit |
| Hepatic encephalopathy | None | Grade I-II (or suppressed with medication) | Grade III-IV (or refractory) | no unit |

* In primary sclerosing cholangitis and primary biliary cirrhosis, the bilirubin references are changed to reflect the fact that these diseases feature high conjugated bilirubin levels. The upper limit for 1 point is 68 mol/L (4 mg/dL) and the upper limit for 2 points is 170 mol/L (10 mg/dL).

** Some older reference works substitute PT prolongation for INR.

Interpretation:
Chronic liver disease is classified into Child-Pugh class A to C, employing the added score from above.

| Points | Class | One year survival | Two year survival |
|---|---|---|---|
| 5-6 | A | 100% | 85% |
| 7-9 | B | 81% | 57% |
| 10-15 | C | 45% | 35% |

## CREATININE CLEARANCE

Clinically, creatinine clearance is a useful measure for estimating the glomerular filtration rate (GFR) of the kidneys.

| Factors | Abbreviations |
|---|---|
| Creatinine clearance | $Cl_{Cr}$ |
| Plasma creatinine concentration | $P_{Cr}$ |
| Serum creatinine concentration | $S_{Cr}$ |
| Urine creatinine concentration | $U_{Cr}$ |
| Urine flow rate | V |
| Plasma creatinine concentration | $P_{Cr}$ |

*(Continued)*

## CREATININE CLEARANCE *(Continued)*

**Calculations:**

$$Cl_{Cr} = \frac{U_{Cr} \times V}{P_{Cr}}$$

**Example:**

Patient with $P_{Cr}$ 1 mg/dL, $U_{Cr}$ 60 mg/dL, and V of 0.5 dL/hr.

$$Cl_{Cr} = \frac{60 \text{ mg/dL} \times 0.5 \text{ dL/hr}}{1 \text{ mg/dL}} = 30 \text{ dL/hr}$$

**Cockcroft-Gault formula:** Estimates creatinine clearance (mL/min).

**Male:**

$$Cl_{Cr} = \frac{(140 - \text{age}) \times \text{mass (kg)}}{72 \times S_{Cr} \text{ (mg/dL)}}$$

**Example:**

Male patient, 67 years of age, weight 75 kg, and $S_{Cr}$ 1 mg/dL.

$$Cl_{Cr} = \frac{(140 - 67) \times 75}{72 \times 1} = 76 \text{ mL/min}$$

**Female:**

$$Cl_{Cr} = \frac{(140 - \text{age}) \times \text{mass (kg)}}{72 \times S_{Cr} \text{ (mg/dL)}} \times 0.85 \text{ if female}$$

**Example:**

Female patient, 67 years of age, weight 75 kg, and $S_{Cr}$ 1 mg/dL.

$$Cl_{Cr} = \frac{(140 - 67) \times 75}{72 \times 1} \times 0.85 = 64.6 \text{ mL/min}$$

Note: Using actual body weight (ABW) in obese patients can significantly overestimate creatinine clearance. Adjusted ideal body weight (IBW) can provide more approximate estimate. Adjusted IBW = IBW + 0.4 (ABW - IBW).

## BASAL ENERGY EXPENDITURE (BEE)

Basal energy expenditure: the amount of energy required to maintain the body's normal metabolic activity (ie, respiration, maintenance of body temperature, etc).

H = height (cm), W = weight (kg), A = age (years)

**Male:**

BEE = 66.67 + 13.75W + 5H - 6.76A

**Female:**

BEE = 665.1 + 9.56W +1.85H -4.68A

## BODY MASS INDEX (BMI)

$$BMI = \frac{\text{weight (kg)}}{[\text{height (m)}]^2}$$

## BODY SURFACE AREA (BSA)

$$BSA\ (m^2) = \sqrt{\frac{\text{height (in)} \times \text{weight (lb)}}{3131}}$$

**OR**

$$BSA\ (m^2) = \sqrt{\frac{\text{height (cm)} \times \text{weight (kg)}}{3600}}$$

## IDEAL BODY WEIGHT (IBW)

Adults (18 years and older; IBW is in kg):

IBW (male) = 50 + (2.3 x height [inches] over 5 feet)
IBW (female) = 45.5 + (2.3 x height [inches] over 5 feet)

Children (IBW is in kg; height is in cm):

1-18 years of age:

$$IBW = \frac{(\text{height}^2 \times 1.65)}{100}$$

5 feet and taller:

IBW (male) = 39 + (2.27 x height [inches] over 5 feet)
IBW (female) = 42.2 + (2.27 x height [inches] over 5 feet)

*(Continued)*

## POUNDS/KILOGRAM CONVERSION

| 1 pound = 0.45359 kilogram | | | | 1 kilogram = 2.2 pounds | | | |
|---|---|---|---|---|---|---|---|
| lb | kg | lb | kg | lb | kg | lb | kg |
| 1 | 0.45 | 105 | 47.63 | 210 | 95.25 | 315 | 142.88 |
| 5 | 2.27 | 110 | 49.89 | 215 | 97.52 | 320 | 145.15 |
| 10 | 4.54 | 115 | 52.16 | 220 | 99.79 | 325 | 147.42 |
| 15 | 6.80 | 120 | 54.43 | 225 | 102.06 | 330 | 149.68 |
| 20 | 9.07 | 125 | 56.70 | 230 | 104.33 | 335 | 151.95 |
| 25 | 11.34 | 130 | 58.97 | 235 | 106.59 | 340 | 154.22 |
| 30 | 13.61 | 135 | 61.23 | 240 | 108.86 | 345 | 156.49 |
| 35 | 15.88 | 140 | 63.50 | 245 | 111.13 | 350 | 158.76 |
| 40 | 18.14 | 145 | 65.77 | 250 | 113.40 | 355 | 161.02 |
| 45 | 20.41 | 150 | 68.04 | 255 | 115.67 | 360 | 163.29 |
| 50 | 22.68 | 155 | 70.31 | 260 | 117.93 | 365 | 165.56 |
| 55 | 24.95 | 160 | 72.57 | 265 | 120.20 | 370 | 167.83 |
| 60 | 27.22 | 165 | 74.84 | 270 | 122.47 | 375 | 170.10 |
| 65 | 29.48 | 170 | 77.11 | 275 | 124.74 | 380 | 172.36 |
| 70 | 31.75 | 175 | 79.38 | 280 | 127.01 | 385 | 174.63 |
| 75 | 34.02 | 180 | 81.65 | 285 | 129.27 | 390 | 176.90 |
| 80 | 36.29 | 185 | 83.91 | 290 | 131.54 | 395 | 179.17 |
| 85 | 38.56 | 190 | 86.18 | 295 | 133.81 | 400 | 181.44 |
| 90 | 40.82 | 195 | 88.45 | 300 | 136.08 | 405 | 183.70 |
| 95 | 43.09 | 200 | 90.72 | 305 | 138.34 | 405 | 183.70 |
| 100 | 45.36 | 205 | 92.99 | 310 | 140.61 | 415 | 188.24 |

## TEMPERATURE CONVERSION

| Fahrenheit to Celsius = (°F - 32) x 5/9 = °C | | | | Celsius to Fahrenheit = (°C x 9/5) + 32 = °F | | | |
|---|---|---|---|---|---|---|---|
| °F | °C | °F | °C | °C | °F | °C | °F |
| 0.0 | -17.8 | 92.0 | 33.3 | 0.0 | 32.0 | 49.0 | 120.2 |
| 5.0 | -15.0 | 93.0 | 33.9 | 5.0 | 41.0 | 50.0 | 122.0 |
| 10.0 | -12.2 | 94.0 | 34.4 | 10.0 | 50.0 | 51.0 | 123.8 |
| 15.0 | -9.4 | 95.0 | 35.0 | 15.0 | 59.0 | 85.0 | 185.0 |
| 20.0 | -6.7 | 96.0 | 35.6 | 20.0 | 68.0 | 52.0 | 125.6 |
| 25.0 | -3.9 | 97.0 | 36.1 | 25.0 | 77.0 | 53.0 | 127.4 |
| 30.0 | -1.1 | 98.0 | 36.7 | 30.0 | 86.0 | 54.0 | 129.2 |
| 35.0 | 1.7 | 98.6 | 37.0 | 35.0 | 95.0 | 55.0 | 131.0 |
| 40.0 | 4.4 | 99.0 | 37.2 | 36.0 | 96.8 | 56.0 | 132.8 |
| 45.0 | 7.2 | 100.0 | 37.8 | 37.0 | 98.6 | 57.0 | 134.6 |
| 50.0 | 10.0 | 101.0 | 38.3 | 38.0 | 100.4 | 58.0 | 136.4 |
| 55.0 | 12.8 | 102.0 | 38.9 | 39.0 | 102.2 | 59.0 | 138.2 |
| 60.0 | 15.6 | 103.0 | 39.4 | 40.0 | 104.0 | 60.0 | 140.0 |
| 65.0 | 18.3 | 104.0 | 40.0 | 41.0 | 105.8 | 65.0 | 149.0 |
| 70.0 | 21.1 | 105.0 | 40.6 | 42.0 | 107.6 | 70.0 | 158.0 |
| 75.0 | 23.9 | 106.0 | 41.1 | 43.0 | 109.4 | 75.0 | 167.0 |
| 80.0 | 26.7 | 107.0 | 41.7 | 44.0 | 111.2 | 80.0 | 176.0 |
| 85.0 | 29.4 | 108.0 | 42.2 | 45.0 | 113.0 | 90.0 | 194.0 |
| 90.0 | 32.2 | 109.0 | 42.8 | 46.0 | 114.8 | 95.0 | 203.0 |
| 91.0 | 32.8 | 110.0 | 43.3 | 47.0 | 116.6 | 100.0 | 212.0 |
| | | | | 48.0 | 118.4 | 105.0 | 221.0 |

*(Continued)*

## PEDIATRIC DOSAGE ESTIMATION FORMULAS

The following formulas can be used to estimate the approximate pediatric dosage of a medication. These formulas are based on the adult dose and either the child's age or weight. These formulas should be used with caution as the response to any drug is not always directly proportional to the age or weight of the child relative to the usual adult dose. Dosage will also vary based on the formula used. Care should be taken when using any of these methods to calculate the child's dosage. Some products have FDA approved pediatric indications and dosages, always refer to full prescribing information first before calculating a pediatric dosage.

### BASED ON WEIGHT

**Augsberger's Rule:**

$$\frac{[(1.5 \times \text{weight [kg]}) + 10]}{100} \times \text{adult dose} = \text{approximate child's dose}$$

**Example:** If the child's weight is 15 kg (33 lb) and the adult dose is 50 mg then the child's dose is 16.25 mg.

$$\frac{[(1.5 \times 15\text{ kg}) + 10]}{100} \times 50\text{ mg} = 0.325 \times 50\text{ mg} = 16.25\text{ mg}$$

**Clark's Rule:**

(weight [lb]/150) x adult dose = approximate child's dose

**Example:** If the child's weight is 15 kg (33 lb) and the adult dose is 50 mg then the child's dose is 11 mg.

(33/150) x 50 mg = 0.22 x 50 mg = 11 mg

### Based on Age

**Augsberger's Rule:**

$$\frac{[(4 \times \text{age [years]}) + 20]}{100} \times \text{adult dose} = \text{approximate child's dose}$$

**Example:** If the child's age is 8 years and the adult dose is 50 mg then the child's dose is 26 mg.
[(4 x 8) + 20)/100] x 50 mg = 0.52 X 50 mg = 26 mg

**Dilling's Rule:**

(age [years]/20) x adult dose = approximate child's dose

**Example:** If the child's age is 8 years and the adult dose is 50 mg then the child's dose is 20 mg.
(8/20) x 50 mg = 0.40 x 50 mg = 20 mg

**Cowling's Rule:**

$$\frac{[\text{age at next birthday (years)}]}{24} \times \text{adult dose} = \text{approximate child's dose}$$

**Example:** If the child is going to turn 8 years old in few months and the adult dose is 50 mg then the child's dose is 16.7 mg. (8/24) x 50 mg = 0.33 x 50 mg = 16.7 mg

**Younge's Rule:**

$$\frac{[\text{age (years)}]}{\text{age} + 12} \times \text{adult dose} = \text{approximate child's dose}$$

**Example:** If the child's age is 8 years and the adult dose is 50 mg then the child's dose is 20 mg.
[8/(8+12)] x 50 mg = 0.4 x 50 mg = 20 mg

**Fried's Rule** (younger than 1 year):

$$\frac{[\text{age (months)}]}{150} \times \text{adult dose} = \text{approximate infant's dose}$$

**Example:** If the child's age is 10 months and the adult dose is 50 mg then the child's dose is 3.33 mg.
(10/150) x 50 mg = 0.067 x 50 mg = 3.33 mg

# Drug Information Centers

## ALABAMA

### BIRMINGHAM

**Drug Information Service**
**University of Alabama**
**UAB Hospital Pharmacy**

Drug Information-JT1720
619 S. 19th St.
Birmingham, AL 35249-6860
Mon.-Fri. 8 AM-5 PM
205-934-2162
www.health.uab.edu/pharmacy

**Global Drug**
**Information Service**
**Samford University**
**McWhorter School**
**of Pharmacy**

800 Lakeshore Dr.
Birmingham, AL 35229-7027
Mon.-Wed. 8 AM-9 PM
Thurs.-Fri. 8 AM-4:30 PM
205-726-2519 or 2891
www.samford.edu/schools/pharmacy/dic/index.html

### HUNTSVILLE

**Huntsville Hospital Drug Information Center**

101 Sivley Rd.
Huntsville, AL 35801
Mon.-Fri. 7 AM-3:30 PM
256-265-8284

## ARIZONA

### TUCSON

**Arizona Poison and Drug**
**Information Center**
**Arizona Health**
**Sciences Center**
**University Medical Center**

1501 N. Campbell Ave.
Room 1156
Tucson, AZ 85724
7 days/week, 24 hours
520-626-6016
800-222-1222 **(Emergency)**
www.pharmacy.arizona.edu

## ARKANSAS

### LITTLE ROCK

**Arkansas Drug Information Center**

4301 W. Markham St.
Slot 522-2
Little Rock, AR 72205
Mon.-Fri. 8:30 AM-5 PM
501-686-5072
(Little Rock area only - **for healthcare professionals only)**
800-228-1233
(AR only - **for healthcare professionals only)**

## CALIFORNIA

### LOS ANGELES

**Los Angeles Regional**
**Drug Information Center**
**LAC & USC Medical Center**

1200 N. State St.
Trailer 25
Los Angeles, CA 90033
Mon.-Fri. 8 AM-4 PM
Closed 12 PM to 1 PM
323-226-7741

### SAN DIEGO

**Drug Information Service**
**University of California**
**San Diego Medical Center**

200 West Arbor Dr.
MC 8925
San Diego, CA 92103-8925
Mon.-Fri. 9 AM-5 PM
619-543-6971
**(for healthcare professionals only)**

### SAN FRANCISCO

**Drug Information Analysis Service**
**University of California,**
**San Francisco**

533 Parnassus Ave.
Room U12
San Francisco, CA 94143-0622
Mon.-Fri. 8:30 AM-4:30 PM
415-502-9540
**(for healthcare professionals only)**

### STANFORD

**Drug Information Center**
**University of California**
**Stanford Hospital and Clinics**

300 Pasteur Dr.
Room H-0301
Stanford, CA 94305
Mon.-Fri. 8 AM-4 PM
650-723-6422

## COLORADO

### DENVER

**Rocky Mountain Poison**
**and Drug Center**

990 Bannock St.
(Physical address)
777 Bannock St.
(Mailing address)
Denver, CO 80264
303-739-1123
800-222-1222 **(Emergency)**
www.rmpdc.org

## CONNECTICUT

### FARMINGTON

**Drug Information Service**
**University of Connecticut Health Center**

263 Farmington Ave.
Farmington, CT 06030
Mon.-Fri. 7:30 AM-4 PM
860-679-2783

### HARTFORD

**Drug Information Center Hartford Hospital**

P.O. Box 5037
80 Seymour St.
Hartford, CT 06102
Mon.-Fri. 8:30 AM-5 PM
860-545-2221
860-545-2961(After 5 PM)
www.hartfordhospital.org

### NEW HAVEN

**Drug Information Center**
**Yale-New Haven Hospital**

20 York St.
New Haven, CT 06540-3202
Mon.-Fri. 8:30 AM-5 PM
203-688-2248
www.ynhh.org

## DISTRICT OF COLUMBIA

**Drug Information Service**
**Howard University Hospital**

Room BB06
2041 Georgia Ave. NW
Washington, DC 20060
Mon.-Fri. 8:30 AM-4 PM
202-865-1325
800-222-1222 **(Emergency)**
www.huhosp.org/patientpublic/pharmacy.htm

## FLORIDA

### FT. LAUDERDALE

**Nova Southeastern University**
**College of Pharmacy**
**Drug Information Center**

3200 S. University Dr.
Ft. Lauderdale, FL 33328
Mon.-Fri. 9 AM-5 PM
954-262-3103
http://pharmacy.nova.edu

### GAINESVILLE

**Drug Information & Pharmacy Resource Center Shands Hospital at University of Florida**

P.O. Box 100316
Gainesville, FL 32610-0316
Mon.-Fri. 9 AM-5 PM
352-265-0408
**(for healthcare professionals only)**
http://shands.org/professional/drugs

### JACKSONVILLE

**Drug Information Service Shands Jacksonville**

655 W. 8th St.
Jacksonville, FL 32209
Mon.-Fri. 8:30 AM-5 PM
904-244-4185
**(for healthcare professionals only)**
904-244-4700
(for consumers, Mon.-Fri. 9:30 AM-4 PM)

### ORLANDO

**Orlando Regional Drug Information Service Orlando Regional Healthcare System**

1414 Kuhl Ave., MP 192
Orlando, FL 32806
Mon.-Fri. 8 AM-4 PM
321-841-8717

### TALLAHASSEE

**Drug Information Education Center Florida Agricultural and Mechanical University College of Pharmacy and Pharmaceutical Sciences**

Tallahassee, FL 32307
Mon.-Fri. 9 AM-5 PM
850-488-5239

### WEST PALM BEACH

**Drug Information Center Nova Southeastern University, West Palm Beach**

3970 RCA Blvd., Suite 7006A
Palm Beach Gardens, FL 33410
Mon.-Fri. 9 AM-5 PM
561-622-0658
**(for healthcare professionals only)**

## GEORGIA

### ATLANTA

**Emory University Hospital Dept. of Pharmaceutical Services-Drug Information**

1364 Clifton Rd. NE
Atlanta, GA 30322
Mon.-Fri. 8 AM-1 PM
404-712-4644
**(for healthcare professionals only)**

**Drug Information Service Northside Hospital**

1000 Johnson Ferry Rd. NE
Atlanta, GA 30342
Mon.-Fri. 9 AM-5 PM
404-851-8676 (GA only)

### AUGUSTA

**Drug Information Center Medical College of Georgia Hospital and Clinic**

BI2101
1120 15th St.
Augusta, GA 30912
Mon.-Fri. 8:30 AM-5 PM
706-721-2887

### COLUMBUS

**Columbus Regional Drug Information Center**

710 Center St.
Columbus, GA 31902
Mon.-Fri. 8 AM-5 PM
706-571-1934
**(for healthcare professionals only)**

## IDAHO

### POCATELLO

**Drug Information Center Idaho State University School of Pharmacy**

970 S. 5th St.
Campus Box 8092
Pocatello, ID 83209
Mon.-Thur. 8:30 AM-5 PM
Fri. 8:30 AM-3 PM
208-282-4689
800-334-7139 (ID only)
http://pharmacy.isu.edu

## ILLINOIS

### CHICAGO

**Drug Information Center Northwestern Memorial Hospital**

Feinberg Pavilion, LC 700
251 E. Huron St.
Chicago, IL 60611
Mon.-Fri. 8:30 AM-5 PM
312-926-7573

**Drug Information Services University of Chicago Hospitals**

5841 S. Maryland Ave.
MC 0010
Chicago, IL 60637-1470
Mon.-Fri. 9 AM-5 PM
773-702-1388

**Drug Information Center University of Illinois at Chicago**

833 S. Wood St.
MC 886
Chicago, IL 60612-7231
Mon.-Fri. 8 AM-4 PM
312-996-5332
**(for healthcare professionals only)**
312-996-3682
(for consumers, Mon.-Fri. 9 AM-12 PM)
www.uic.edu/pharmacy/services/di/index.html

### HARVEY

**Drug Information Center Ingalls Memorial Hospital**

1 Ingalls Dr.
Harvey, IL 60426
Mon.-Fri. 8 AM-4:30 PM
708-333-2300

### HINES

**Drug Information Service Hines Veterans Administration Hospital**

2100 S. 5th Ave.
Pharmacy Services
MC119
P.O. Box 5000
Hines, IL 60141-5000
Mon.-Fri. 8 AM-4:30 PM
708-202-8387, ext. 23780

### PARK RIDGE

**Drug Information Center Advocate Lutheran General Hospital**

1775 Dempster St.
Park Ridge, IL 60068
Mon.-Fri. 7:30 AM-4 PM
847-723-8128
**(for healthcare professionals only)**

## INDIANA

### INDIANAPOLIS

**Drug Information Center**
**St. Vincent Hospital**
**and Health Services**

2001 W. 86th St.
Indianapolis, IN 46260
Mon.-Fri. 8 AM-4 PM
317-338-3200
**(for healthcare professionals only)**

**Drug Information Service**
**Clarian Health Partners**

Pharmacy Department I-65 at 21st St.
Room CG04
Indianapolis, IN 46202
Mon.-Fri. 8 AM-4:30 PM
317-962-1750

### MUNCIE

**Drug Information Center**
**Ball Memorial Hospital**

2401 University Ave.
Muncie, IN 47303
Mon.-Fri. 8 AM-4:30 PM
765-747-3035

## IOWA

### DES MOINES

**Regional Drug Information Center**
**Mercy Medical Center-Des Moines**

1111 Sixth Ave.
Des Moines, IA 50314
Mon.-Fri. 8 AM-4:30 PM
(regional service; in-house service answered 7 days/week, 24 hours)
515-247-3286

### IOWA CITY

**Drug Information Center**
**University of Iowa**
**Hospitals and Clinics**

200 Hawkins Dr.
Iowa City, IA 52242
Mon.-Fri. 8 AM-4:30 PM
319-356-2600

## KANSAS

### KANSAS CITY

**Drug Information Center**
**University of Kansas**
**Medical Center**

3901 Rainbow Blvd.
Kansas City, KS 66160
Mon.-Fri. 8:30 AM-4:30 PM
913-588-2328
**(for healthcare professionals only)**

## KENTUCKY

### LEXINGTON

**University of Kentucky**
**Central Pharmacy**
**Chandler Medical Center**

800 Rose St., C-114
Lexington, KY 40536-0293
7 days/week, 24 hours
859-323-5642

## LOUISIANA

### MONROE

**Louisiana Drug and Poison**
**Information Center**
**University of Louisiana at Monroe**
**College of Pharmacy**

Sugar Hall
Monroe, LA 71209-6430
Mon.-Fri. 8 AM-4:30 PM
318-342-1710

### NEW ORLEANS

**Xavier University Drug Information Center Tulane University Hospital and Clinic**

1440 Canal St.
Suite 808
New Orleans, LA 70112
Mon.-Fri. 9 AM-5 PM
504-588-5670

## MARYLAND

### ANDREWS AFB

**Drug Information Services**

79 MDSS/SGQP
1050 W. Perimeter Rd.
Suite D1-119
Andrews AFB, MD 20762-6660
Mon.-Fri. 7:30 AM-5 PM
240-857-4565

### BALTIMORE

**Drug Information Service**
**Johns Hopkins Hospital**

600 N. Wolfe St.
Carnegie 180
Baltimore, MD 21287-6180
Mon.-Fri. 8:30 AM-5 PM
410-955-6348

**Drug Information Service**
**University of Maryland**
**School of Pharmacy**

Pharmacy Hall Room 760
20 North Pine St.
Baltimore, MD 21201
Mon.-Fri. 8:30 AM-5 PM
410-706-7568
**(for consumers only)**
410-706-0898
**(for healthcare professionals only)**
www.pharmacy.umaryland.edu/umdi

### EASTON

**Drug Information**
**Pharmacy Dept.**
**Memorial Hospital**

219 S. Washington St.
Easton, MD 21601
7 days/week, 7 AM-5:30 PM
410-822-1000, ext. 5645

## MASSACHUSETTS

### BOSTON

**Drug Information Services**
**Brigham and Women's Hospital**

75 Francis St.
Boston, MA 02115
Mon.-Fri. 7 AM-3 PM
617-732-7166

### WORCESTER

**Drug Information Pharmacy**
**UMass Memorial**
**Medical Center**
**Healthcare Hospital**

55 Lake Ave. North
Worcester, MA 01655
Mon.-Fri. 8:30 AM-5 PM
508-856-3456
508-856-2775 (24-hour)

## MICHIGAN

### ANN ARBOR

**Drug Information Service Dept. of Pharmacy Services**
**University of Michigan**
**Health System**

1500 East Medical Center Dr.
UH B2D301
Box 0008
Ann Arbor, MI 48109-0008
Mon.-Fri. 8 AM-5 PM
734-936-8200

### DETROIT

**Drug Information Center**
**Department of Pharmacy Services**
**Detroit Receiving Hospital and**
**University Health Center**

4201 St. Antoine Blvd.
Detroit, MI 48201
Mon.-Fri. 9 AM-5 PM
313-745-4556
www.dmcpharmacy.org

### LANSING

**Drug Information Services**
**Sparrow Hospital**

1215 East Michigan Ave.
Lansing, MI 48912
7 days/week, 24 hours
517-364-2444

### *PONTIAC*

**Drug Information Center**
**St. Joseph Mercy Oakland**

44405 Woodward Ave.
Pontiac, MI 48341
Mon.-Fri. 8 AM-4:30 PM
248-858-3055

### *ROYAL OAK*

**Drug Information Services**
**William Beaumont Hospital**

3601 West 13 Mile Rd.
Royal Oak, MI 48073-6769
Mon.-Fri. 8 AM-4:30 PM
248-898-4077

### *SOUTHFIELD*

**Drug Information Service**
**Providence Hospital**

16001 West 9 Mile Rd.
Southfield, MI 48075
Mon.-Fri. 8 AM-4 PM
248-849-3125

## MISSISSIPPI

### *JACKSON*

**Drug Information Center**
**University of Mississippi**
**Medical Center**

2500 N. State St.
Jackson, MS 39216
Mon.-Fri. 8 AM-4:30 PM
601-984-2060

## MISSOURI

### *KANSAS CITY*

**University of**
**Missouri-Kansas City**
**Drug Information Center**

2411 Holmes St., MG-200
Kansas City, MO 64108
Mon.-Fri. 9 AM-4 PM
816-235-5490
http://druginfo.umkc.edu/

### *SPRINGFIELD*

**Drug Information Center**
**St. John's Hospital**

1235 E. Cherokee St.
Springfield, MO 65804
Mon.-Fri. 8 AM-4:30 PM
417-820-3488

### *ST. JOSEPH*

**Regional Medical Center Pharmacy**

5325 Faraon St.
St. Joseph, MO 64506
7 days/week, 24 hours
816-271-6141

## MONTANA

### *MISSOULA*

**Drug Information Service**
**University of Montana School of Pharmacy and Allied Health Sciences**

32 Campus Dr.
1522 Skaggs Bldg.
Missoula, MT 59812-1522
Mon.-Fri. 8 AM-5 PM
406-243-5254
800-501-5491
www.umt.edu/druginfo

## NEBRASKA

### *OMAHA*

**Drug Informatics Service**
**School of Pharmacy**
**Creighton University**

2500 California Plaza
Health Science Library
Room 204
Omaha, NE 68178
Mon.-Fri. 8:30 AM-4:30 PM
402-280-5101
http://druginfo.creighton.edu

## NEW JERSEY

### *NEWARK*

**New Jersey Poison Information and Education System**

65 Bergen St.
Newark, NJ 07107
Mon.-Fri. 8 AM- 5 PM
973-972-9280
800-222-1222 **(Emergency)**
www.njpies.org

### *NEW BRUNSWICK*

**Drug Information Service**
**Robert Wood Johnson**
**University Hospital**

Pharmacy Department
1 Robert Wood Johnson Pl.
New Brunswick, NJ 08901
Mon.-Fri. 8:30 AM-4:30 PM
732-937-8842

## NEW MEXICO

### *ALBUQUERQUE*

**New Mexico Poison Center**
**University of New Mexico**
**Health Sciences Center**

MSC09 5080
1 University of New Mexico
Albuquerque, NM 87131
7 days/week, 24 hours
505-272-4261
800-222-1222 **(Emergency)**
http://hsc.unm.edu/pharmacy/poison

## NEW YORK

### *BROOKLYN*

**International Drug**
**Information Center**
**Long Island University**
**Arnold & Marie Schwartz College of Pharmacy & Health Sciences**

75 DeKalb Ave.
RM-HS509
Brooklyn, NY 11201
Mon.-Fri. 9 AM-5 PM
718-488-1064
www.liu.edu

### *NEW HYDE PARK*

**Drug Information Center**
**St. John's University at Long Island Jewish Medical Center**

270-05 76th Ave.
New Hyde Park, NY 11040
Mon.-Fri. 8 AM-3 PM
718-470-DRUG (3784)

### *NEW YORK CITY*

**Drug Information Center**
**Memorial Sloan-Kettering Cancer Center**

1275 York Ave.
RM S-702
New York, NY 10021
Mon.-Fri. 9 AM-5 PM
212-639-7552

**Drug Information Center**
**Mount Sinai Medical Center**

1 Gustave Levy Pl.
New York, NY 10029
Mon.-Fri. 9 AM-5 PM
212-241-6619
**(for in-house healthcare professionals only)**

**Drug Information Service**
**New York Presbyterian Hospital**

Room K04
525 E. 68th St.
New York, NY 10021
Mon.-Fri. 9 AM-5 PM
212-746-0741

### *ROCHESTER*

**Finger Lakes Poison and Drug Information Center University of Rochester**

601 Elmwood Ave.
Rochester, NY 14642
Mon.-Fri. 8 AM-5 PM
585-275-3718

*ROCKVILLE CENTER*

**Drug Information Center**
**Mercy Medical Center**

1000 North Village Ave.
Rockville Center, NY 11571-9024
Mon.-Fri. 8 AM-4 PM
516-705-1053

## NORTH CAROLINA

*BUIES CREEK*

**Drug Information Center School of Pharmacy Campbell University**

P.O. Box 1090
Buies Creek, NC 27506
Mon.-Fri. 8:30 AM-4:30 PM
910-893-1200, ext. 2701
800-760-9697 (Toll free)
ext. 2701
800-327-5467 (NC only)

*CHAPEL HILL*

**University of North Carolina Hospitals Drug Information Center Dept. of Pharmacy**

101 Manning Dr.
Chapel Hill, NC 27514
Mon.-Fri. 8 AM-4:30 PM
919-966-2373

*DURHAM*

**Drug Information Center Duke University Health Systems**

DUMC Box 3089
Durham, NC 27710
Mon.-Fri. 8 AM-5 PM
919-684-5125

*GREENVILLE*

**Eastern Carolina Drug Information Center Pitt County Memorial Hospital Dept. of Pharmacy Service**

P.O. Box 6028
2100 Stantonsburg Rd.
Greenville, NC 27835
Mon.-Fri. 8 AM-5 PM
252-847-4257

*WINSTON-SALEM*

**Drug Information Service Center**
**Wake-Forest University**
**Baptist Medical Center**

Medical Center Blvd.
Winston-Salem, NC 27157
Mon.-Fri. 8 AM-5 PM
336-716-2037
**(for healthcare professionals only)**

## OHIO

*ADA*

**Drug Information Center**
**Raabe College of Pharmacy**
**Ohio Northern University**

Ada, OH 45810
Mon.-Thurs. 8:30 AM-5 PM,
7-10 PM
Fri. 8:30 AM- 4 PM;
Sun. 2 PM-10 PM
419-772-2307
www.onu.edu/pharmacy/druginfo

*CINCINNATI*

**Drug and Poison Information Center**
**Children's Hospital**
**Medical Center**

3333 Burnet Ave. VP-3
Cincinnati, OH 45229
Mon.-Fri. 9 AM-5 PM
513-636-5054
(Administration)
513-636-5111
(7 days/week, 24 hours)

*CLEVELAND*

**Drug Information Service**
**Cleveland Clinic Foundation**

9500 Euclid Ave.
Cleveland, OH 44195
Mon.-Fri. 8:30 AM-4:30 PM
216-444-6456
**(for healthcare professionals only)**

*COLUMBUS*

**Drug Information Center**
**Ohio State University Hospital**
**Dept. of Pharmacy**

Doan Hall 368
410 W. 10th Ave.
Columbus, OH 43210-1228
7 days/week, 24 hours
614-293-8679
**(for in-house healthcare professionals only)**

**Drug Information Center**
**Riverside Methodist Hospital**

3535 Olentangy River Road
Columbus, OH 43214
7 days/week, 24 hours
614-566-5425

*TOLEDO*

**Drug Information Services**
**St. Vincent Mercy Medical Center**

2213 Cherry St.
Toledo, Ohio 43608-2691
Mon.-Fri. 7 AM-5 PM
419-251-4227
www.rx.medctr.ohio-state.edu

## OKLAHOMA

*OKLAHOMA CITY*

**Drug Information Service**
**Integris Health**

3300 Northwest Expressway
Oklahoma City, OK 73112
Mon.-Fri. 8 AM-4:30 PM
405-949-3660

**Drug Information Center**
**OU Medical Center**
**Presbyterian Tower**

700 NE 13th St.
Oklahoma City, OK 73104
Mon.-Fri. 8 AM-4:30 PM
405-271-6226
Fax: 405-271-6281

*TULSA*

**Drug Information Center**
**Saint Francis Hospital**

6161 S. Yale Ave.
Tulsa, OK 74136
Mon.-Fri. 8 AM-4:30 PM
918-494-6339
**(for healthcare professionals only)**

## PENNSYLVANIA

*PHILADELPHIA*

**Drug Information Center**
**Temple University Hospital**
**Dept. of Pharmacy**

3401 N. Broad St.
Philadelphia, PA 19140
Mon.-Fri. 8 AM-4:30 PM
215-707-4644

**Drug Information Service**
**Tenet Health System**
**Hahnemann University Hospital**
**Department of Pharmacy**

MS 451
Broad and Vine Streets
Philadelphia, PA 19102
Mon.-Fri. 8 AM-4 PM
215-762-DRUG (3784)
**(for healthcare professionals only)**

**Drug Information Service**
**Dept. of Pharmacy**
**Thomas Jefferson**
**University Hospital**

111 S. 11th St.
Philadelphia, PA 19107-5089
Mon.-Fri. 8 AM-5 PM
215-955-8877

**University of Pennsylvania Health System Drug Information Service Hospital of the University of Pennsylvania Department of Pharmacy**

3400 Spruce St.
Philadelphia, PA 19104
Mon.-Fri. 8:30 AM-4 PM
215-662-2903

### PITTSBURGH

**Pharmaceutical Information CenterMylan School of Pharmacy Duquesne University**

431 Mellon Hall
Pittsburgh, PA 15282
Mon.-Fri. 8 AM-4 PM
412-396-4600

**Drug Information Center University of Pittsburgh**

302 Scaife Hall
200 Lothrop St.
Pittsburgh, PA 15213
Mon.-Fri. 8:30 AM-4:30 PM
412-647-3784
**(for healthcare professionals only)**

### UPLAND

**Drug Information Center Crozer-Chester Medical Center Dept. of Pharmacy**

1 Medical Center Blvd.
Upland, PA 19013
Mon.-Fri. 8 AM-4:30 PM
610-447-2851
**(for in-house healthcare professionals only)**

## PUERTO RICO

### PONCE

**Centro Informacion Medicamentos Escuela de Medicina de Ponce**

P.O. Box 7004
Ponce, PR 00732-7004
Mon.-Fri. 8 AM-4:30 PM
787-840-2575

### SAN JUAN

**Centro de Informacion de Medicamentos-CIM Escuela de Farmacia-RCM**

P.O. Box 365067
San Juan, PR 00936-5067
Mon.-Fri. 8 AM-5:30 PM
787-758-2525, ext. 1516

## SOUTH CAROLINA

### CHARLESTON

**Drug Information Service Medical University of South Carolina**

150 Ashley Ave.
Rutledge Tower Annex
Room 604
P.O. Box 250584
Charleston, SC 29425-0810
Mon.-Fri. 9 AM-5:30 PM
843-792-3896
800-922-5250

### COLUMBIA

**Drug Information Service University of South Carolina College of Pharmacy**

Columbia, SC 29208
Mon.-Fri. 8 AM-5 PM
803-777-7804
www.pharm.sc.edu

### SPARTANBURG

**Drug Information Center Spartanburg Regional Healthcare System**

101 E. Wood St.
Spartanburg, SC 29303
Mon.-Fri. 8 AM-4:30 PM
864-560-6910

## TENNESSEE

### KNOXVILLE

**Drug Information Center University of Tennessee Medical Center at Knoxville**

1924 Alcoa Highway
Knoxville, TN 37920-6999
Mon.-Fri. 8 AM-4:30 PM
865-544-9124

### MEMPHIS

**South East Regional Drug Information Center VA Medical Center**

1030 Jefferson Ave.
Memphis, TN 38104
Mon.-Fri. 6:30 AM-4 PM
901-523-8990, ext. 6720

**Drug Information Center University of Tennessee**

875 Monroe Ave.
Suite 116
Memphis, TN 38163
Mon.-Fri. 8 AM-5 PM
901-448-5556

## TEXAS

### AMARILLO

**Drug Information Center Texas Tech Health Sciences Center School of Pharmacy**

1300 Coulter Rd.
Amarillo, TX 79106
Mon.-Fri. 8 AM-5 PM
806-356-4008

### GALVESTON

**Drug Information Center University of Texas Medical Branch**

301 University Blvd.
Galveston, TX 77555-0701
Mon.-Fri. 8 AM-5 PM
409-772-2734

### HOUSTON

**Drug Information Center Ben Taub General Hospital Texas Southern University/HCHD**

1504 Taub Loop
Houston, TX 77030
Mon.-Fri. 8:30 AM-5 PM
713-873-3710

### LACKLAND A.F.B.

**Drug Information Center Dept. of Pharmacy Wilford Hall Medical Center**

2200 Bergquist Dr.
Suite 1
Lackland A.F.B., TX 78236
7 days/week, 24 hours
210-292-5414

### LUBBOCK

**Drug Information and Consultation Service Covenant Medical Center**

3615 19th St.
Lubbock, TX 79410
Mon.-Fri. 8 AM-5 PM
806-725-0408

### SAN ANTONIO

**Drug Information Service University of Texas Health Science Center at San Antonio Department of Pharmacology**

7703 Floyd Curl Drive
San Antonio, TX 78229-3900
Mon.-Fri. 8 AM-4 PM
210-567-4280

### TEMPLE

**Drug Information Center Scott and White Memorial Hospital**

2401 S. 31st St.
Temple, TX 76508
Mon.-Fri. 8 AM-5 PM
254-724-4636

## UTAH

### SALT LAKE CITY

**Drug Information Service University of Utah Hospital**

421 Wakara Way
Suite 204
Salt Lake City, UT 84108
Mon.-Fri. 7 AM-5 PM
801-581-2073

## VIRGINIA

### *HAMPTON*

**Drug Information Center**
**Hampton University School of Pharmacy**

Hampton Harbors Annex
Hampton, VA 23668
Mon.-Fri. 9 AM-4 PM
757-728-6693

## WEST VIRGINIA

### *MORGANTOWN*

**West Virginia Center for Drug and Health Information**
**West Virginia University**
**Robert C. Byrd Health Sciences Center**

1124 HSN, P.O. Box 9520
Morgantown, WV 26506
Mon.-Fri. 8:30 AM-5 PM
304-293-6640
800-352-2501 **(WV only)**
www.hsc.wvu.edu/SOP

## WYOMING

### *LARAMIE*

**Drug Information Center**
**University of Wyoming**

P.O. Box 3375
Laramie, WY 82071
Mon.-Fri. 8:30 AM-4:30 PM
307-766-6988

# POISON CONTROL CENTERS

The American Association of Poison Control Centers (AAPCC) uses a single, nationwide emergency number to automatically link callers with their regional poison center. This toll-free number, **800-222-1222**, also works for **teletype lines (TTY)** for the hearing-impaired and **telecommunication devices (TTD)** for individuals who are deaf. However, a few local poison centers and the ASPCA/Animal Poison Control Center are not part of this nationwide system and continue to use separate numbers.

Most of the centers listed below are certified by the AAPCC. Certified centers are marked by an asterisk after the name. Each has to meet certain criteria. It must, for example, serve a large geographic area; it must be open 24 hours a day and provide direct-dial or toll-free access; it must be supervised by a medical director; and it must have registered pharmacists or nurses available to answer questions from the public.

Within each state, centers are listed alphabetically by city. Some state poison centers also list their original emergency numbers (including TTY/TDD) that only work within that state. For these listings, callers may use either the state number or the nationwide 800 number.

## ALABAMA

### BIRMINGHAM

**Regional Poison Control Center, The Children's Hospital of Alabama (*)**

1600 7th Ave. South
Birmingham, AL 35233-1711
Business: 205-939-9201
**Emergency:** 800-222-1222
www.chsys.org

### TUSCALOOSA

**Alabama Poison Center (*)**

2503 Phoenix Dr.
Tuscaloosa, AL 35405
Business: 205-345-0600
**Emergency:** 800-222-1222
800-462-0800 (AL)
www.alapoisoncenter.org

## ALASKA

### JUNEAU

**Alaska Poison Control System**

Section of Community
Health and EMS
410 Willoughby Ave., Room 103
Box 110616
Juneau, AK 99811-0616
Business: 907-465-3027
**Emergency:** 800-222-1222
www.chems.alaska.gov

### (PORTLAND, OR)

**Oregon Poison Center (*)**
**Oregon Health Sciences University**

3181 SW Sam Jackson Park Rd.
CB550
Portland, OR 97239
Business: 503-494-8311
**Emergency:** 800-222-1222
www.oregonpoison.com

## ARIZONA

### PHOENIX

**Banner Poison Control Center (*)**
**Banner Good Samaritan Medical Center**

901 E. Willetta St.
Room 2701
Phoenix, AZ 85006
Business: 602-495-4884
**Emergency:** 800-222-1222
www.bannerpoisoncontrol.com

### TUCSON

**Arizona Poison and Drug Information Center (*)**
**Arizona Health Sciences Center**

1501 N. Campbell Ave.
Room 1156
Tucson, AZ 85724
Business: 520-626-7899
**Emergency:** 800-222-1222

## ARKANSAS

### LITTLE ROCK

**Arkansas Poison and Drug Information Center**
**College of Pharmacy - UAMS**

4301 West Markham St.
Mail Slot 522-2
Little Rock, AR 72205-7122
Business: 501-686-5540
**Emergency:** 800-222-1222
800-376-4766 (AR)
TDD/TTY: 800-641-3805

## ASPCA/Animal Poison Control Center

1717 South Philo Rd.
Suite 36
Urbana, IL 61802
Business: 217-337-5030
**Emergency:** 888-426-4435
800-548-2423
www.napcc.aspca.org

## CALIFORNIA

### FRESNO/MADERA

**California Poison Control System-Fresno/Madera Div.(*)**
**Children's Hospital of Central California**

9300 Valley Children's Place MB 15
Madera, CA 93638-8762
Business: 559-622-2300
**Emergency:** 800-222-1222
800-876-4766 (CA)
TDD/TTY: 800-972-3323
www.calpoison.org

### SACRAMENTO

**California Poison Control System-Sacramento Div.(*)**
**UC Davis Medical Center**

Room HSF 1024
2315 Stockton Blvd.
Sacramento, CA 95817
Business: 916-227-1400
**Emergency:** 800-222-1222
800-876-4766 (CA)
TDD/TTY: 800-972-3323
www.calpoison.org

### SAN DIEGO

**California Poison Control System-San Diego Div. (*)**
**UC San Diego Medical Center**

200 West Arbor Dr.
San Diego, CA 92103-8925
Business: 858-715-6300
**Emergency:** 800-222-1222
800-876-4766 (CA)
TDD/TTY: 800-972-3323
www.calpoison.org

### SAN FRANCISCO

**California Poison Control System-San Francisco Div.(*)**
**San Francisco General Hospital**
**University of California San Francisco**

Box 1369
San Francisco, CA 94143-1369
Business: 415-502-6000
**Emergency:** 800-222-1222
800-876-4766 (CA)
TDD/TTY: 800-972-3323
www.calpoison.org

## COLORADO

### DENVER

**Rocky Mountain Poison and Drug Center (*)**

777 Bannock St.
Mail Code 0180
Denver, CO 80204-4507
Business: 303-739-1100
**Emergency:** 800-222-1222
TDD/TTY: 303-739-1127 (CO)
www.RMPDC.org

## CONNECTICUT

### FARMINGTON

**Connecticut Regional Poison Control Center (*) University of Connecticut Health Center**

263 Farmington Ave.
Farmington, CT 06030-5365
Business: 860-679-4540
**Emergency:** 800-222-1222
TDD/TTY: 866-218-5372
http://poisoncontrol.uchc.edu

## DELAWARE

### (PHILADELPHIA, PA)

**The Poison Control Center (*) Children's Hospital of Philadelphia**

34th St. & Civic Center Blvd.
Philadelphia, PA 19104-4303
Business: 215-590-2003
**Emergency:** 800-222-1222
800-722-7112 (DE)
TDD/TTY: 215-590-8789
www.poisoncontrol.chop.edu

## DISTRICT OF COLUMBIA

### WASHINGTON, DC

**National Capital Poison Center (*)**

3201 New Mexico Ave., NW
Suite 310
Washington, DC 20016
Business: 202-362-3867
**Emergency:** 800-222-1222
www.poison.org

## FLORIDA

### JACKSONVILLE

**Florida Poison Information Center-Jacksonville (*) SHANDS Hospital**

655 West 8th St.
Jacksonville, FL 32209
Business: 904-244-4465
**Emergency:** 800-222-1222
http://fpicjax.org

### MIAMI

**Florida Poison Information Center-Miami (*) University of Miami–Department of Pediatrics**

P.O. Box 016960 (R-131)
Miami, FL 33101
Business: 305-585-5250
**Emergency:** 800-222-1222
www.miami.edu/poison-center

### TAMPA

**Florida Poison Information Center-Tampa (*) Tampa General Hospital**

P.O. Box 1289
Tampa, FL 33601-1289
Business: 813-844-7044
**Emergency:** 800-222-1222
www.poisoncentertampa.org

## GEORGIA

### ATLANTA

**Georgia Poison Center (*) Hughes Spalding Children's Hospital, Grady Health System**

80 Jesse Hill Jr. Dr., SE
P.O. Box 26066
Atlanta, GA 30303-3050
Business: 404-616-9237
**Emergency:** 800-222-1222
404-616-9000 (Atlanta)
TDD: 404-616-9287
www.georgiapoisoncenter.org

## Hawaii

### (DENVER, CO)

**Rocky Mountain Poison and Drug Center (*)**

777 Bannock St.
Mail Code 0180
Denver, CO 80204-4507
Business: 303-739-1100
**Emergency:** 800-222-1222
www.RMPDC.org

## IDAHO

### (DENVER, CO)

**Rocky Mountain Poison and Drug Center (*)**

777 Bannock St.
Mail Code 0180
Denver, CO 80204-4507
Business: 303-739-1100
**Emergency:** 800-222-1222
www.RMPDC.org

## ILLINOIS

### CHICAGO

**Illinois Poison Center (*)**

222 South Riverside Plaza
Suite 1900
Chicago, IL 60606
Business: 312-906-6136
**Emergency:** 800-222-1222
TDD/TTY: 312-906-6185
www.illinoispoisoncenter.org

## INDIANA

### INDIANAPOLIS

**Indiana Poison Control Center (*) Clarian Health Partners Methodist Hospital**

I-65 at 21st St.
Indianapolis, IN 46206-1367
Business: 317-962-2335
**Emergency:** 800-222-1222
800-382-9097
317-962-2323 (Indianapolis)
TTY: 317-962-2336
www.clarian.org/poisoncontrol

## IOWA

### SIOUX CITY

**Iowa Statewide Poison Control Center Iowa Health System and the University of Iowa Hospitals and Clinics**

401 Douglas St., Suite 402
Sioux City, IA 51101
Business: 712-279-3710
**Emergency:** 800-222-1222
712-277-2222 (IA)
www.iowapoison.org

## KANSAS

### KANSAS CITY

**Mid-America Poison Control Center University of Kansas Medical Center**

3901 Rainbow Blvd.
Room B-400
Kansas City, KS 66160-7231
Business 913-588-6638
**Emergency:** 800-222-1222
800-332-6633 (KS)
TDD: 913-588-6639
www.kumc.edu/poison

## KENTUCKY

### LOUISVILLE

**Kentucky Regional Poison Center (*)**

P.O. Box 35070
Louisville, KY 40232-5070
Business: 502-629-7264
**Emergency:** 800-222-1222
502-589-8222 (Louisville)
www.krpc.com

## LOUISIANA

### MONROE

**Louisiana Drug and Poison Information Center (*)**
**University of Louisiana at Monroe**

700 University Ave.
Monroe, LA 71209-6430
Business: 318-342-3648
**Emergency:** 800-222-1222
www.lapcc.org

## MAINE

### PORTLAND

**Northern New England Poison Center**

Maine Medical Center
22 Bramhall St.
Portland, ME 04102
Business: 207-662-7220
**Emergency:** 800-222-1222
207-871-2879 (ME)
TDD/TTY: 877-299-4447 (ME)
207-871-2879 (ME)
www.nnepc.org

## MARYLAND

### BALTIMORE

**Maryland Poison Center (*)**
**University of Maryland at Baltimore School of Pharmacy**

20 North Pine St., PH 772
Baltimore, MD 21201
Business: 410-706-7604
**Emergency:** 800-222-1222
TDD: 410-706-1858
www.mdpoison.com

### (WASHINGTON, DC)

**National Capital Poison Center (*)**

3201 New Mexico Ave., NW
Suite 310
Washington, DC 20016
Business: 202-362-3867
**Emergency:** 800-222-1222
TDD/TTY: 202-362-8563 (MD)
www.poison.org

## MASSACHUSETTS

### BOSTON

**Regional Center for Poison Control and Prevention (*)**
**(Serving Massachusetts and Rhode Island)**

300 Longwood Ave.
Boston, MA 02115
Business: 617-355-6609
**Emergency:** 800-222-1222
TDD/TTY: 888-244-5313
www.maripoisoncenter.com

## MICHIGAN

### DETROIT

**Regional Poison Control Center (*)**
**Children's Hospital of Michigan**

4160 John R. Harper
Professional Office Bldg.
Suite 616
Detroit, MI 48201
Business: 313-745-5335
**Emergency:** 800-222-1222
TDD/TTY: 800-356-3232
www.mitoxic.org/pcc

### GRAND RAPIDS

**DeVos Children's Hospital Regional Poison Center (*)**

100 Michigan St., NE
Grand Rapids, MI 49503
Business: 616-391-3690
**Emergency:** 800-222-1222
http://poisoncenter.devoschildrens.org

## MINNESOTA

### MINNEAPOLIS

**Minnesota Poison Control System (*)**
**Hennepin County Medical Center**

701 Park Ave.
Mail Code RL
Minneapolis, MN 55415
Business: 612-873-3144
**Emergency:** 800-222-1222
www.mnpoison.org

## MISSISSIPPI

### JACKSON

**Mississippi Regional Poison Control Center, University of Mississippi Medical Center**

2500 North State St.
Jackson, MS 39216
Business: 601-984-1680
**Emergency:** 800-222-1222

## MISSOURI

### ST. LOUIS

**Missouri Regional Poison Center (*) Cardinal Glennon Children's Hospital**

7980 Clayton Rd.
Suite 200
St. Louis, MO 63117
Business: 314-772-5200
**Emergency:** 800-222-1222
TDD/TTY: 314-612-5705
www.cardinalglennon.com

## MONTANA

### (DENVER, CO)

**Rocky Mountain Poison and Drug Center (*)**

777 Bannock St.
Mail Code 0180
Denver, CO 80204-4507
Business: 303-739-1100
**Emergency:** 800-222-1222
TDD/TTY: 303-739-1127
www.RMPDC.org

## NEBRASKA

### OMAHA

**The Poison Center (*)**
**Children's Hospital**

8401 W. Dodge St., Suite 115
Omaha, NE 68114
Business: 402-955-5555
**Emergency:** 800-222-1222
www.nebraskapoison.com

## NEVADA

### (DENVER, CO)

**Rocky Mountain Poison and Drug Center (*)**

777 Bannock St.
Mail Code 0180
Denver, CO 80204-4507
Business: 303-739-1100
**Emergency:** 800-222-1222
www.RMPDC.org

### (PORTLAND, OR)

**Oregon Poison Center (*)**
**Oregon Health Sciences University**

3181 SW Sam Jackson Park Rd.
Portland, OR 97201
Business: 503-494-8600
**Emergency:** 800-222-1222
www.oregonpoison.com

## NEW HAMPSHIRE

### *(PORTLAND, ME)*

**Northern New England Poison Center**

Maine Medical Center
22 Bramhall St.
Portland, ME 04102
Business: 207-662-7220
**Emergency:** 800-222-1222
www.nnepc.org

## NEW JERSEY

### *NEWARK*

**New Jersey Poison Information and Education System (*) UMDNJ**

65 Bergen St.
Newark, NJ 07101
Business: 973-972-9280
**Emergency:** 800-222-1222
TDD/TTY: 973-926-8008
www.njpies.org

## NEW MEXICO

### *ALBUQUERQUE*

**New Mexico Poison and Drug Information Center (*)**

MSC09-5080
1 University of New Mexico
Albuquerque, NM 87131-0001
Business: 505-272-4261
**Emergency:** 800-222-1222
http://HSC.UNM.edu/pharmacy/poison

## NEW YORK

### *BUFFALO*

**Western New York Regional Poison Control Center (*) Children's Hospital of Buffalo**

219 Bryant St.
Buffalo, NY 14222
Business: 716-878-7654
**Emergency:** 800-222-1222
www.fingerlakespoison.org

### *MINEOLA*

**Long Island Regional Poison and Drug Information Center (*) Winthrop University Hospital**

259 First St.
Mineola, NY 11501
Business: 516-663-2650
**Emergency:** 800-222-1222
TDD: 516-747-3323 (Nassau)
516-924-8811 (Suffolk)
www.lirpdic.org

### *NEW YORK CITY*

**New York City Poison Control Center (*) NYC Dept. of Health**

455 First Ave., Room 123
New York, NY 10016
Business: 212-447-8152
**Emergency:** 800-222-1222
(English) 212-340-4494
212-POISONS
(212-764-7667)
**Emergency:** 212-venenos
(Spanish) (212-836-3667)
TDD: 212-689-9014

### *ROCHESTER*

**Finger Lakes Regional Poison and Drug Information Center (*) University of Rochester Medical Center**

601 Elmwood Ave.
Box 321
Rochester, NY 14642
Business: 585-273-4155
**Emergency:** 800-222-1222
TTY: 585-273-3854

### *SYRACUSE*

**Central New York Poison Center (*) SUNY Upstate Medical University**

750 East Adams St.
Syracuse, NY 13210
Business: 315-464-7078
**Emergency:** 800-222-1222
www.cnypoison.org

## NORTH CAROLINA

### *CHARLOTTE*

**Carolinas Poison Center (*) Carolinas Medical Center**

P.O. Box 32861
Charlotte, NC 28232
Business: 704-512-3795
**Emergency:** 800-222-1222
TDD: 800-735-8262
TTY: 800-735-2962
www.ncpoisoncenter.org

## NORTH DAKOTA

### *(MINNEAPOLIS, MN)*

**Minnesota Poison Control System (*) Hennepin County Medical Center**

701 Park Ave.
Mail Code 820
Minneapolis, MN 55415
Business: 612-873-3144
**Emergency:** 800-222-1222
www.ndpoison.org

## OHIO

### *CINCINNATI*

**Cincinnati Drug and Poison Information Center (*) Regional Poison Control System**

3333 Burnet Ave.
Vernon Place, 3rd Floor
Cincinnati, OH 45229
Business: 513-636-5111
**Emergency:** 800-222-1222
TDD/TTY: 800-253-7955
www.cincinnatichildrens.org/dpic

### *CLEVELAND*

**Greater Cleveland Poison Control Center**

11100 Euclid Ave.
MP 6007
Cleveland, OH 44106-6007
Business: 216-844-1573
**Emergency:** 800-222-1222
216-231-4455 (OH)

### *COLUMBUS*

**Central Ohio Poison Center (*)**

700 Children's Dr.
Room L032
Columbus, OH 43205-2696
Business: 614-722-2635
**Emergency:** 800-222-1222
TTY: 614-228-2272
www.bepoisonsmart.com

## OKLAHOMA

### *OKLAHOMA CITY*

**Oklahoma Poison Control Center (*) Children's Hospital at OU Medical Center**

940 Northeast 13th St.
Room 3510
Oklahoma City, OK 73104
Business: 405-271-5062
**Emergency:** 800-222-1222
www.oklahomapoison.org

## OREGON

### *PORTLAND*

**Oregon Poison Center (*) Oregon Health Sciences University**

3181 S.W. Sam Jackson Park Rd., CB550
Portland, OR 97239
Business: 503-494-8968
**Emergency:** 800-222-1222
www.oregonpoison.com

## PENNSYLVANIA

### PHILADELPHIA

**The Poison Control Center (*)**
**Children's Hospital of Philadelphia**

34th Street & Civic Center Blvd.
Philadelphia, PA 19104-4399
Business: 215-590-2003
**Emergency:** 800-222-1222
215-386-2100 (PA)
TDD/TTY: 215-590-8789
www.poisoncontrol.chop.edu

### PITTSBURGH

**Pittsburgh Poison Center (*)**
**Children's Hospital of Pittsburgh**

3705 Fifth Ave.
Pittsburgh, PA 15213
Business: 412-390-3300
**Emergency:** 800-222-1222
412-681-6669
www.chp.edu/clinical/03a_poison.php

## PUERTO RICO

### SANTURCE

**San Jorge Children's Hospital Poison Center**

268 San Jorge St.
Santurce, PR 00912
Business: 787-726-5660
**Emergency:** 800-222-1222
TTY: 787-641-1934
www.poisoncenter.net

## RHODE ISLAND

### (BOSTON, MA)

**Regional Center for Poison Control and Prevention (*)**
**(Serving Massachusetts and Rhode Island)**

300 Longwood Ave.
Boston, MA 02115
Business: 617-355-6609
**Emergency:** 800-222-1222
TDD/TTY: 888-244-5313
www.maripoisoncenter.com

## SOUTH CAROLINA

### COLUMBIA

**Palmetto Poison Center (*)**
**College of Pharmacy**
**University of South Carolina**

Columbia, SC 29208
Business: 803-777-7909
Drug Info: 803-777-7805
**Emergency:** 800-222-1222
800-922-1117 (SC)
http://poison.sc.edu

## SOUTH DAKOTA

### (MINNEAPOLIS, MN)

**Hennepin Regional Poison Center (*)**
**Hennepin County Medical Center**

701 Park Ave.
Minneapolis, MN 55415
Business: 612-873-3144
**Emergency:** 800-222-1222
www.mnpoison.org

### SIOUX FALLS

**Provides education only—Does not manage exposure cases.**

**Sioux Valley Poison Control Center (*)**

1305 W. 18th St.
Box 5039
Sioux Falls, SD 57117-5039
Business: 605-328-6670
www.sdpoison.org

## TENNESSEE

### NASHVILLE

**Tennessee Poison Center (*)**

1161 21st Ave. South
501 Oxford House
Nashville, TN 37232-4632
Business: 615-936-0760
**Emergency:** 800-222-1222
www.poisonlifeline.org

## TEXAS

### AMARILLO

**Texas Panhandle Poison Center (*)**
**Northwest Texas Hospital**

1501 S. Coulter Dr.
Amarillo, TX 79106
Business: 806-354-1630
**Emergency:** 800-222-1222
www.poisoncontrol.org

### DALLAS

**North Texas Poison Center (*)**
**Texas Poison Center Network**
**Parkland Health and Hospital System**

5201 Harry Hines Blvd.
Dallas, TX 75235
Business: 214-589-0911
**Emergency:** 800-222-1222
www.poisoncontrol.org

### EL PASO

**West Texas Regional Poison Center (*)**
**Thomason Hospital**

4815 Alameda Ave.
El Paso, TX 79905
Business 915-534-3800
**Emergency:** 800-222-1222
www.poisoncontrol.org

### GALVESTON

**Southeast Texas Poison Center (*)**
**The University of Texas Medical Branch**

3.112 Trauma Bldg.
301 University Ave.
Galveston, TX 77555-1175
Business: 409-766-4403
**Emergency:** 800-222-1222
www.poisoncontrol.org

### SAN ANTONIO

**South Texas Poison Center (*)**
**The University of Texas Health Science Center–San Antonio**

7703 Floyd Curl Dr., MC 7849
San Antonio, TX 78229-3900
Business: 210-567-5762
**Emergency:** 800-222-1222
www.poisoncontrol.org

### TEMPLE

**Central Texas Poison Center (*)**
**Scott & White Memorial Hospital**

2401 South 31st St.
Temple, TX 76508
Business: 254-724-7401
**Emergency:** 800-222-1222
www.poisoncontrol.org

## UTAH

### SALT LAKE CITY

**Utah Poison Control Center (*)**

585 Komas Dr.
Suite 200
Salt Lake City, UT 84108
Business: 801-587-0600
**Emergency:** 800-222-1222
801-587-0600 (UT)
http://uuhsc.utah.edu/poison

## VERMONT

### (PORTLAND, ME)

**Northern New England Poison Center**

Maine Medical Center
22 Bramhall St.
Portland, ME 04102
Business: 207-662-7220
**Emergency:** 800-222-1222
www.nnepc.org

## VIRGINIA

### CHARLOTTESVILLE

**Blue Ridge Poison Center (*)**
**University of Virginia Health System**

P.O. Box 800774
Charlottesville, VA 22908-0774
Business: 434-924-0347
**Emergency:** 800-222-1222
www.healthsystem.virginia.edu.brpc

### RICHMOND

**Virginia Poison Center (*)**
**Virginia Commonwealth University**

P.O. Box 980522
Richmond, VA 23298-0522
Business: 804-828-4780
**Emergency:** 800-222-1222
804-828-9123
www.vcu.edu/mcved/vpc

## WASHINGTON

### SEATTLE

**Washington Poison Center (*)**

155 NE 100th St.
Suite 400
Seattle, WA 98125-8011
Business: 206-517-2350
**Emergency:** 800-222-1222
206-526-2121 (WA)
TDD: 800-572-0638 (WA)
www.wapc.org

## WEST VIRGINIA

### CHARLESTON

**West Virginia Poison Center (*)**

3110 MacCorkle Ave. SE
Charleston, WV 25304
Business: 304-347-1212
**Emergency:** 800-222-1222
www.wvpoisoncenter.org

## WISCONSIN

### MILWAUKEE

**Children's Hospital of Wisconsin**
**Statewide Poison Center**

9000 W. Wisconsin Ave.
P.O. Box 1997, Mail Station 677A
Milwaukee, WI 53226
Business: 414-266-2952
**Emergency:** 800-222-1222
TDD/TTY: 414-266-2542
www.chw.org

## Wyoming

### (OMAHA, NE)

**The Poison Center (*)**
**Children's Hospital**

8401 W. Dodge St., Suite 115
Omaha, NE 68114
Business: 402-955-5555
**Emergency:** 800-222-1222
www.nebraskapoison.com

# Antipyretic Products

| BRAND | INGREDIENT/STRENGTH | DOSE |
|---|---|---|
| **ACETAMINOPHEN** | | |
| Anacin Aspirin Free tablets | Acetaminophen 500mg | **Adults & Peds: ≥12 yrs:** 2 tabs q6h. **Max:** 8 tabs q24h. |
| Feverall Childrens' suppositories | Acetaminophen 120mg | **Peds: 3-6 yrs:** 1-2 supp. q4-6h. **Max:** 6 supp q24h. |
| Feverall Infants' suppositories | Acetaminophen 80mg | **Peds: 3-11 months:** 1 supp q6h. **12-36 months:** 1 supp q4h. **Max:** 6 supp q24h. |
| Feverall Jr. Strength suppositories | Acetaminophen 325mg | **Peds: 6-12 yrs:** 1 supp q4-6h. **Max:** 6 supp q24h. |
| Tylenol 8 Hour caplets | Acetaminophen 650mg | **Adults & Peds: ≥12 yrs:** 2 tabs q8h prn. **Max:** 6 tabs q24h. |
| Tylenol 8 Hour geltabs | Acetaminophen 650mg | **Adults & Peds: ≥12 yrs:** 2 tabs q8h prn. **Max:** 6 tabs q24h. |
| Tylenol Arthritis caplets | Acetaminophen 650mg | **Adults:** 2 tabs q8h prn. **Max:** 6 tabs q24h. |
| Tylenol Arthritis geltabs | Acetaminophen 650mg | **Adults:** 2 tabs q8h prn. **Max:** 6 tabs q24h. |
| Tylenol Children's Meltaways tablets | Acetaminophen 80mg | **Peds: 2-3 yrs (24-35 lbs):** 2 tabs. **4-5 yrs (36-47 lbs):** 3 tabs. **6-8 yrs (48-59 lbs)**: 4 tabs. **9-10 yrs (60-71 lbs):** 5 tabs. **11 yrs (72-95 lbs):** 6 tabs. May repeat q4h. **Max:** 5 doses q24h. |
| Tylenol Children's suspension | Acetaminophen 160mg/5mL | **Peds: 2-3 yrs (24-35 lbs):** 1 tsp (5mL). **4-5 yrs (36-47 lbs):** 1.5 tsp (7.5mL). **6-8 yrs (48-59 lbs):** 2 tsp (10mL). **9-10 yrs (60-71 lbs):** 2.5 tsp (12.5mL). **11 yrs (72-95 lbs):** 3 tsp (15mL). May repeat q4h. **Max:** 5 doses q24h. |
| Tylenol Extra Strength caplets | Acetaminophen 500mg | **Adults & Peds: ≥12 yrs:** 2 tabs q4-6h prn. **Max:** 8 tabs q24h. |
| Tylenol Extra Strength Cool caplets | Acetaminophen 500mg | **Adults & Peds: ≥12 yrs:** 2 tabs q4-6h prn. **Max:** 8 tabs q24h. |
| Tylenol Extra Strength gelcaps | Acetaminophen 500mg | **Adults & Peds: ≥ 12 yrs:** 2 caps q4-6h prn. **Max:** 8 caps q24h. |
| Tylenol Extra Strength Geltabs | Acetaminophen 500mg | **Adults & Peds: ≥12 yrs:** 2 tabs q4-6h prn. **Max:** 8 tabs q24h. |
| Tylenol Extra Strength liquid | Acetaminophen 1000mg/30mL | **Adults & Peds: ≥12 yrs:** 2 tbl (30mL) q4-6h prn. **Max:** 8 tbl (120mL) q24h. |
| Tylenol Extra Strength tablets | Acetaminophen 500mg | **Adults & Peds: ≥12 yrs:** 2 tabs q4-6h prn. **Max:** 8 tabs q24h. |
| Tylenol Infants' suspension | Acetaminophen 80mg/0.8mL | **Peds: 2-3 yrs (24-35 lbs):** 1.6 mL q4h prn. **Max:** 5 doses (8mL) q24h. |
| Tylenol Junior Meltaways tablets | Acetaminophen 160mg | **Peds: 6-8 yrs (48-59 lbs):** 2 tabs. **9-10 yrs (60-71 lbs):** 2.5 tabs. **11 yrs (72-95 lbs):** 3 tabs. **12 yrs (≥96 lbs):** 4 tabs. May repeat q4h. **Max:** 5 doses q24h. |
| Tylenol Regular Strength tablets | Acetaminophen 325mg | **Adults & Peds: ≥12 yrs:** 2 tabs q4-6h prn. **Max:** 12 tabs q24h. **Peds: 6-11 yrs:** 1 tab q4-6h. **Max:** 5 tabs q24h. |

*(Continued)*

| BRAND | INGREDIENT/STRENGTH | DOSE |
|---|---|---|
| **NONSTEROIDAL ANTI-INFLAMMATORY DRUGS (NSAIDs)** | | |
| Advil Children's Chewables tablets | Ibuprofen 50mg | **Peds: 2-3 yr (24-35 lb):** 2 tabs q6-8h. **4-5 yr (36-47 lb):** 3 tabs q6-8h. **6-8 yr (45-89 lb):** 4 tabs q6-8h. **9-10 yr (60-71 lb):** 5 tabs q6-8h. **11 yr (72-95 lb):** 6 tabs q6-8h. **Max:** 4 doses q24h |
| Advil Children's suspension | Ibuprofen 100mg/5mL | **Peds: 2-3 yrs (24-35 lbs):** 1 tsp (5mL). **4-5 yrs (36-47 lbs):** 1.5 tsp (7.5mL). **6-8 yrs (48-59 lbs):** 2 tsp (10mL). **9-10 yrs (60-71 lbs):** 2.5 tsp (12.5mL). **11 yrs (72-95 lbs):** 3 tsp (15mL). May repeat q6-8h. **Max:** 4 doses q24h. |
| Advil gelcaps | Ibuprofen 200mg | **Adults & Peds: ≥12 yrs:** 1-2 caps q4-6h. **Max:** 6 caps q24h. |
| Advil Infants' drops | Ibuprofen 50mg/1.25mL | **Peds: 6-11 months (12-17 lbs):** 1.25mL. **12-23 months (18-23 lbs):** 1.875mL. May repeat q6-8h. **Max:** 4 doses q24h. |
| Advil Junior Strength tablets | Ibuprofen 100mg | **Peds: 6-10 yrs (48-71 lbs):** 2 tabs. **11 yrs (72-95 lbs):** 3 tabs. May repeat q6-8h. **Max:** 4 doses q24h. |
| Advil liqui-gels | Ibuprofen 200mg | **Adults & Peds: ≥12 yrs:** 1-2 caps q4-6h. **Max:** 6 caps q24h. |
| Advil tablets | Ibuprofen 200mg | **Adults & Peds: ≥12 yrs:** 1-2 tabs q4-6h. **Max:** 6 tabs q24h. |
| Aleve caplets | Naproxen Sodium 220mg | **Adults: ≥65 yrs:** 1 tab q12h. **Max:** 2 tabs q24h. **Adults & Peds: ≥12 yrs:** 1 tab q8-12h. **Max:** 3 tabs q24h. |
| Aleve gelcaps | Naproxen Sodium 220mg | **Adults: ≥65 yrs:** 1 cap q12h. **Max:** 2 caps q24h. **Adults & Peds: ≥12 yrs:** 1 cap q8-12h. **Max:** 3 caps q24h. |
| Aleve tablets | Naproxen Sodium 220mg | **Adults: ≥65 yrs:** 1 tab q12h. **Max:** 2 tabs q24h. **Adults & Peds: ≥12 yrs:** 1 tab q8-12h. **Max:** 3 tabs q24h. |
| Motrin Children's suspension | Ibuprofen 100mg/5mL | **Peds: 2-3 yrs (24-35 lbs):** 1 tsp (5mL). **4-5 yrs (36-47 lbs):** 1.5 tsp (7.5mL). **6-8 yrs (48-59 lbs):** 2 tsp (10mL). **9-10 yrs (60-71 lbs):** 2.5 tsp (12.5mL). **11 yrs (72-95 lbs):** 3 tsp (15mL). May repeat q6-8h. **Max:** 4 doses q24h. |
| Motrin IB caplets | Ibuprofen 200mg | **Adults & Peds: ≥12 yrs:** 1-2 tabs q4-6h. **Max:** 6 tabs q24h. |
| Motrin IB tablets | Ibuprofen 200mg | **Adults & Peds: ≥12 yrs:** 1-2 tabs q4-6h. **Max:** 6 tabs q24h. |
| Motrin Infants' drops | Ibuprofen 50mg/1.25mL | **Peds: 6-11 months (12-17 lbs):** 1.25mL. **12-23 months (18-23 lbs):** 1.875mL. May repeat q6-8h. **Max:** 4 doses q24h. |
| Motrin Junior Strength chewable tablets | Ibuprofen 100mg | **Peds: 6-8 yrs (48-59 lbs):** 2 tabs. **9-10 yrs (60-71 lbs):** 2.5 tabs. **11 yrs (72-95 lbs):** 3 tabs. May repeat q6-8h. **Max:** 4 doses q24h. |
| Nuprin caplets | Ibuprofen 200mg | **Adults & Peds: ≥12 yrs:** 1-2 tabs q4-6h. **Max:** 6 tabs q24h. |
| Nuprin tablets | Ibuprofen 200mg | **Adults & Peds: ≥12 yrs:** 1-2 tabs q4-6h. **Max:** 6 tabs q24h. |

*(Continued)*

| BRAND | INGREDIENT/STRENGTH | DOSE |
|---|---|---|
| **SALICYLATES** | | |
| Anacin 81 tablets | Aspirin 81mg | **Adults & Peds: ≥12 yrs:** 4-8 tabs q4h. **Max:** 48 tabs q24h. |
| Aspergum chewable tablets | Aspirin 227mg | **Adults & Peds: ≥12 yrs:** 2 tabs q4h. **Max:** 16 tabs q24h. |
| Bayer Aspirin Extra Strength caplets | Aspirin 500mg | **Adults & Peds: ≥12 yrs:** 1-2 tabs q4-6h. **Max:** 8 tabs q24h. |
| Genuine Bayer Aspirin coated caplets | Aspirin 325mg | **Adults & Peds: ≥12 yrs:** 1-2 tabs q4h or 3 tabs q6h. **Max:** 12 tabs q24h. |
| Bayer Aspirin safety coated caplets | Aspirin 325mg | **Adults & Peds: ≥12 yrs:** 1-2 tabs q4h or 3 tabs q6h. **Max:** 12 tabs q24h. |
| Bayer Children's Aspirin chewable tablets | Aspirin 81mg | **Adults & Peds: ≥12 yrs:** 4-8 tabs q4h. **Max:** 48 tabs q24h. |
| Bayer Low Dose Aspirin tablets | Aspirin 81mg | **Adults & Peds: ≥12 yrs:** 4-8 tabs q4h. **Max:** 48 tabs q24h. |
| Ecotrin Adult Low Strength tablets | Aspirin 81mg | **Adults:** 4-8 tabs q4h. **Max:** 48 tabs q24h. |
| Ecotrin Enteric Low Strength tablets | Aspirin 81mg | **Adults:** 4-8 tabs q4h. **Max:** 48 tabs q24h. |
| Ecotrin Enteric Regular Strength tablets | Aspirin 325mg | **Adults & Peds: ≥12 yrs:** 1-2 tabs q4h. **Max:** 12 tabs q24h. |
| Ecotrin Maximum Strength tablets | Aspirin 500mg | **Adults & Peds: ≥12 yrs:** 2 tabs q6h. **Max:** 8 tabs q24h. |
| Ecotrin Regular Strength tablets | Aspirin 325mg | **Adults & Peds: ≥12 yrs:** 1-2 tabs q4h. **Max:** 12 tabs q24h. |
| Halfprin 162mg tablets | Aspirin 162mg | **Adults & Peds: ≥12 yrs:** 2-4 tabs q4h. **Max:** 24 tabs q24h. |
| Halfprin 81mg tablets | Aspirin 81mg | **Adults & Peds: ≥12 yrs:** 4-8 tabs q4h. **Max:** 48 tabs q24h. |
| St. Joseph Adult Low Strength chewable tablets | Aspirin 81mg | **Adults & Peds: ≥12 yrs:** 4-8 tabs q4h. **Max:** 48 tabs q24h. |
| St. Joseph Adult Low Strength tablets | Aspirin 81mg | **Adults & Peds: ≥12 yrs:** 4-8 tabs q4h. **Max:** 48 tabs q24h. |
| **SALICYLATES, BUFFERED** | | |
| Bayer Extra Strength Plus caplets | Aspirin Buffered with Calcium Carbonate 500mg | **Adults & Peds: ≥12 yrs:** 1-2 tabs q4-6h. **Max:** 8 tabs q24h. |
| Bufferin Extra Strength tablets | Aspirin Bufferred with Calcium Carbonate/ Magnesium Oxide/Magnesium Carbonate 500mg | **Adults & Peds: ≥12 yrs:** 2 tabs q6h. **Max:** 8 tabs q24h. |
| Bufferin tablets | Aspirin Bufferred with Calcium Carbonate/ Magnesium Oxide/Magnesium Carbonate 325mg | **Adults & Peds: ≥12 yrs:** 2 tabs q4h. **Max:** 12 tabs q24h. |

# HEADACHE/MIGRAINE PRODUCTS

| BRAND | INGREDIENT/STRENGTH | DOSE |
|---|---|---|
| **ACETAMINOPHEN** | | |
| Anacin Aspirin Free tablets | Acetaminophen 500mg | **Adults & Peds: ≥12 yrs:** 2 tabs q6h. **Max:** 8 tabs q24h. |
| Tylenol 8 Hour caplets | Acetaminophen 650mg | **Adults & Peds: ≥12 yrs:** 2 tabs q8h prn. **Max:** 6 tabs q24h. |
| Tylenol 8 Hour geltabs | Acetaminophen 650mg | **Adults & Peds: ≥12 yrs:** 2 tabs q8h prn. **Max:** 6 tabs q24h. |
| Tylenol Arthritis caplets | Acetaminophen 650mg | **Adults:** 2 tabs q8h prn. **Max:** 6 tabs q24h. |
| Tylenol Arthritis geltabs | Acetaminophen 650mg | **Adults:** 2 tabs q8h prn. **Max:** 6 tabs q24h. |
| Tylenol Children's Meltaway tablets | Acetaminophen 80mg | **Peds: 2-3 yrs (24-35 lbs):** 2 tabs **4-5 yrs (36-47 lbs):** 3 tabs. **6-8 yrs (48-59 lbs):** 4 tabs. **9-10 yrs (60-71 lbs):** 5 tabs. **11 yrs (72-95 lbs):** 6 tabs. May repeat q4h. **Max:** 5 doses q24h. |
| Tylenol Children's suspension | Acetaminophen 160mg/5mL | **Peds: 2-3 yrs (24-35 lbs):** 1 tsp (5mL). **4-5 yrs (36-47 lbs):** 1.5 tsp (7.5mL). **6-8 yrs (48-59 lbs):** 2 tsp (10mL). **9-10 yrs (60-71 lbs):** 2.5 tsp (12.5mL). **11 yrs (72-95 lbs):** 3 tsp (15mL). May repeat q4h. **Max:** 5 doses q24h. |
| Tylenol Extra Strength caplets | Acetaminophen 500mg | **Adults & Peds: ≥12 yrs:** 2 tabs q4-6h prn. **Max:** 8 tabs q24h. |
| Tylenol Extra Strength Cool caplets | Acetaminophen 500mg | **Adults & Peds: ≥12 yrs:** 2 tabs q4-6h prn. **Max:** 8 tabs q24h. |
| Tylenol Extra Strength gelcaps | Acetaminophen 500mg | **Adults & Peds: ≥ 12 yrs:** 2 caps q4-6h prn. **Max:** 8 caps q24h. |
| Tylenol Extra Strength liquid | Acetaminophen 1000mg/30mL | **Adults & Peds: ≥12 yrs:** 2 tbl (30mL) q4-6h prn. **Max:** 8 tbl (120mL) q24h. |
| Tylenol Extra Strength tablets | Acetaminophen 500mg | **Adults & Peds: ≥12 yrs:** 2 tabs q4-6h prn. **Max:** 8 tabs q24h. |
| Tylenol Infants' suspension | Acetaminophen 80mg/0.8mL | **Peds: 2-3 yrs (24-35 lbs):** 1.6 mL q4h prn. **Max:** 5 doses (8mL) q24h. |
| Tylenol Junior Meltaways tablets | Acetaminophen 160mg | **Peds: 6-8 yrs (48-59 lbs):** 2 tabs. **9-10 yrs (60-71 lbs):** 2.5 tabs. **11 yrs (72-95 lbs):** 3 tabs. **12 yrs (≥96 lbs):** 4 tabs. May repeat q4h. **Max:** 5 doses q24h. |
| Tylenol Regular Strength tablets | Acetaminophen 325mg | **Adults & Peds: ≥12 yrs:** 2 tabs q4-6h prn. **Max:** 12 tabs q24h. **Peds: 6-11 yrs:** 1 tab q4-6h. **Max:** 5 tabs q24h. |
| **ACETAMINOPHEN COMBINATIONS** | | |
| Excedrin Extra Strength caplets | Acetaminophen/Aspirin/Caffeine 250mg-250mg-65mg | **Adults & Peds: ≥12 yrs:** 2 tabs q6h. **Max:** 8 tabs q24h. |
| Excedrin Extra Strength geltabs | Acetaminophen/Aspirin/Caffeine 250mg-250mg-65mg | **Adults & Peds: ≥12 yrs:** 2 tabs q6h. **Max:** 8 tabs q24h. |
| Excedrin Extra Strength tablets | Acetaminophen/Aspirin/Caffeine 250mg-250mg-65mg | **Adults & Peds: ≥12 yrs:** 2 tabs q6h. **Max:** 8 tabs q24h. |
| Excedrin Migraine caplets | Acetaminophen/Aspirin/Caffeine 250mg-250mg-65mg | **Adults:** 2 tabs prn. **Max:** 2 tabs q24h. |
| Excedrin Migraine geltabs | Acetaminophen/Aspirin/Caffeine 250mg-250mg-65mg | **Adults:** 2 tabs prn. **Max:** 2 tabs q24h. |
| Excedrin Migraine tablets | Acetaminophen/Aspirin/Caffeine 250mg-250mg-65mg | **Adults:** 2 tabs prn. **Max:** 2 tabs q24h. |

*(Continued)*

| BRAND | INGREDIENT/STRENGTH | DOSE |
|---|---|---|
| **ACETAMINOPHEN COMBINATIONS** *(Continued)* | | |
| Excedrin Sinus Headache caplets | Acetaminophen/Phenylephrine HCl 325mg-5mg | **Adults & Peds: ≥12 yrs:** 2 tabs q4h. **Max:** 12 tabs q24h. |
| Excedrin Sinus Headache tablets | Acetaminophen/Phenylephrine HCl 325mg-5mg | **Adults & Peds: ≥12 yrs:** 2 tabs q4h. **Max:** 12 tabs q24h. |
| Excedrin Tension Headache caplets | Acetaminophen/Caffeine 500mg-65mg | **Adults & Peds: ≥12 yrs:** 2 tabs q6h. **Max:** 8 tabs q24h. |
| Excedrin Tension Headache geltabs | Acetaminophen/Caffeine 500mg-65mg | **Adults & Peds: ≥12 yrs:** 2 tabs q6h. **Max:** 8 tabs q24h. |
| Excedrin Tension Headache tablets | Acetaminophen/Caffeine 500mg-65mg | **Adults & Peds: ≥12 yrs:** 2 tabs q6h. **Max:** 8 tabs q24h. |
| Goody's Extra Strength Headache Powders | Acetaminophen/Aspirin/Caffeine 260mg-520mg-32.5mg | **Adults & Peds: ≥12 yrs:** 1 powder q4-6h. **Max:** 4 powders q24h. |
| Tylenol Sinus Congestion & Pain Daytime gelcaps | Acetaminophen/Phenylephrine HCl 325mg/5mg | **Adults & Peds: ≥12 yrs:** 2 caps q4h. **Max:** 12 caps q24h. |
| Tylenol Sinus Congestion & Pain Daytime coolburst caplets | Acetaminophen/Phenylephrine HCl 325mg/5mg | **Adults & Peds: ≥12 yrs:** 2 caps q4h. **Max:** 12 caps q24h. |
| Vanquish caplets | Acetaminophen/Aspirin/Caffeine 194mg-227mg-33mg | **Adults & Peds: ≥12 yrs:** 2 tabs q6h. **Max:** 8 tabs q24h. |
| **ACETAMINOPHEN/SLEEP AID** | | |
| Excedrin PM caplets | Acetaminophen/Diphenhydramine 500mg-38mg | **Adults & Peds: ≥12 yrs:** 2 tabs qhs. |
| Excedrin PM geltabs | Acetaminophen/Diphenhydramine citrate 500mg-38 mg | **Adults & Peds: ≥12 yrs:** 2 tabs qhs. |
| Excedrin PM tablets | Acetaminophen/Diphenhydramine citrate 500mg-38 mg | **Adults & Peds: ≥12 yrs:** 2 tabs qhs. |
| Goody's PM Powder | Acetaminophen/Diphenhydramine 1000mg-76mg/dose | **Adults & Peds: ≥12 yrs:** 1 packet (2 powders) qhs. |
| Tylenol PM caplets | Acetaminophen/Diphenhydramine 500mg-25mg | **Adults & Peds: ≥12 yrs:** 2 tabs qhs. |
| Tylenol PM gelcaps | Acetaminophen/Diphenhydramine 500mg-25mg | **Adults & Peds: ≥12 yrs:** 2 caps qhs. |
| Tylenol PM geltabs | Acetaminophen/Diphenhydramine 500mg-25mg | **Adults & Peds: ≥12 yrs:** 2 tabs qhs. |
| Tylenol Sinus Night Time caplets | Acetaminophen/Pseudoephedrine HCl/ Doxylamine Succinate 500mg-30mg-6.25mg | **Adults & Peds: ≥12 yrs:** 2 tbl (30mL) qhs. **Max:** 8 tbl (120mL) q24h. |
| **NONSTEROIDAL ANTI-INFLAMMATORY DRUGS (NSAIDs)** | | |
| Advil caplets | Ibuprofen 200mg | **Adults & Peds: ≥12 yrs:** 1-2 tabs q4-6h. **Max:** 6 tabs q24h. |
| Advil Children's Chewables tablets | Ibuprofen 50mg | **Peds: 2-3 yr (24-35 lbs):** 2 tabs q6-8h. **4-5 yr (36-47 lbs):** 3 tabs q6-8h. **6-8 yr (45-89 lbs):** 4 tabs q6-8h. **9-10 yr (60-71 lbs):** 5 tabs q6-8h. **11 yr (72-95 lbs):** 6 tabs q6-8h. **Max:** 4 doses q24h |
| Advil Children's suspension | Ibuprofen 100mg/5mL | **Peds: 2-3 yrs (24-35 lbs):** 1 tsp (5mL). **4-5 yrs (36-47 lbs):** 1.5 tsp (7.5mL). **6-8 yrs (48-59 lbs):** 2 tsp (10mL). **9-10 yrs (60-71 lbs):** 2.5 tsp (12.5mL). **11 yrs (72-95 lbs):** 3 tsp (15mL). May repeat q6-8h. **Max:** 4 doses q24h. |
| Advil gelcaps | Ibuprofen 200mg | **Adults & Peds: ≥12 yrs:** 1-2 caps q4-6h. **Max:** 6 caps q24h. |
| Advil Infants' drops | Ibuprofen 50mg/1.25mL | **Peds: 6-11 months (12-17 lbs):** 1.25mL. **12-23 months (18-23 lbs):** 1.875mL. May repeat q6-8h. **Max:** 4 doses q24h. |
| Advil Junior Strength tablets | Ibuprofen 100mg | **Peds: 6-10 yrs (48-71 lbs):** 2 tabs. **11 yrs (72-95 lbs):** 3 tabs. May repeat q6-8h. **Max:** 4 doses q24h. |

*(Continued)*

| BRAND | INGREDIENT/STRENGTH | DOSE |
|---|---|---|
| **NONSTEROIDAL ANTI-INFLAMMATORY DRUGS (NSAIDs)** *(Continued)* | | |
| Advil liqui-gels | Ibuprofen 200mg | **Adults & Peds: ≥12 yrs:** 1-2 caps q4-6h. **Max:** 6 caps q24h. |
| Advil Migraine capsules | Ibuprofen 200mg | **Adults:** 2 caps prn. **Max:** 2 caps q24h. |
| Advil tablets | Ibuprofen 200mg | **Adults & Peds: ≥12 yrs:** 1-2 tabs q4-6h. **Max:** 6 tabs q24h. |
| Aleve caplets | Naproxen Sodium 220mg | **Adults: ≥65 yrs:** 1 tab q12h. **Max:** 2 tabs q24h. **Adults & Peds: ≥12 yrs:** 1 tab q8-12h. **Max:** 3 tabs q24h. |
| Aleve gelcaps | Naproxen Sodium 220mg | **Adults: ≥65 yrs:** 1 cap q12h. **Max:** 2 caps q24h. **Adults & Peds: ≥12 yrs:** 1 cap q8-12h. **Max:** 3 caps q24h. |
| Aleve tablets | Naproxen Sodium 220mg | **Adults: ≥65 yrs:** 1 tab q12h. **Max:** 2 tabs q24h. **Adults & Peds: ≥12 yrs:** 1 tab q8-12h. **Max:** 3 tabs q24h. |
| Motrin Children's suspension | Ibuprofen 100mg/5mL | **Peds: 2-3 yrs (24-35 lbs):** 1 tsp (5mL). **4-5 yrs (36-47 lbs):** 1.5 tsp (7.5mL). **6-8 yrs (48-59 lbs):** 2 tsp (10mL). **9-10 yrs (60-71 lbs):** 2.5 tsp (12.5mL). **11 yrs (72-95 lbs):** 3 tsp (15mL). May repeat q6-8h. **Max:** 4 doses q24h. |
| Motrin IB caplets | Ibuprofen 200mg | **Adults & Peds: ≥12 yrs:** 1-2 tabs q4-6h. **Max:** 6 tabs q24h. |
| Motrin IB tablets | Ibuprofen 200mg | **Adults & Peds: ≥12 yrs:** 1-2 tabs q4-6h. **Max:** 6 tabs q24h. |
| Motrin Infants' Drops | Ibuprofen 50mg/1.25mL | **Peds: 6-11 months (12-17 lbs):** 1.25mL. **12-23 months (18-23 lbs):** 1.875mL. May repeat q6-8h. **Max:** 4 doses q24h. |
| Motrin Junior Strength chewable tablets | Ibuprofen 100mg | **Peds: 6-8 yrs (48-59 lbs):** 2 tabs. **9-10 yrs (60-71 lbs):** 2.5 tabs. **11 yrs (72-95 lbs):** 3 tabs. May repeat q6-8h. **Max:** 4 doses q24h. |
| Nuprin caplets | Ibuprofen 200mg | **Adults & Peds: ≥12 yrs:** 1-2 tabs q4-6h. **Max:** 6 tabs q24h. |
| Nuprin tablets | Ibuprofen 200mg | **Adults & Peds: ≥12 yrs:** 1-2 tabs q4-6h. **Max:** 6 tabs q24h. |
| **NSAID COMBINATIONS** | | |
| Aleve Sinus & Headache caplets | Naproxen Sodium/Pseudoephedrine HCl 220 mg-120 mg | **Adults & Peds: ≥12 yrs:** 1 tab q12h. **Max:** 2 tabs q24h. |
| Nuprin Cold and Sinus caplets | Ibuprofen/Pseudoephedrine HCl 200mg-30 mg | **Adults & Peds: ≥12 yrs:** 1-2 tabs q4-6h. **Max:** 6 tabs q24h. |
| **SALICYLATES** | | |
| Anacin 81 tablets | Aspirin 81mg | **Adults & Peds: ≥12 yrs:** 4-8 tabs q4h. **Max:** 48 tabs q24h. |
| Aspergum chewable tablets | Aspirin 227mg | **Adults & Peds: ≥12 yrs:** 2 tabs q4h. **Max:** 16 tabs q24h. |
| Bayer Aspirin Extra Strength caplets | Aspirin 500mg | **Adults & Peds: ≥12 yrs:** 1-2 tabs q4-6h. **Max:** 8 tabs q24h. |
| Genuine Bayer Aspirin safety coated tablets | Aspirin 325mg | **Adults & Peds: ≥12 yrs:** 1-2 tabs q4h or 3 tabs q6h. **Max:** 12 tabs q24h. |
| Bayer Aspirin safety coated caplets | Aspirin 325mg | **Adults & Peds: ≥12 yrs:** 1-2 tabs q4h or 3 tabs q6h. **Max:** 12 tabs q24h. |
| Bayer Children's Aspirin chewable tablets | Aspirin 81mg | **Adults & Peds: ≥12 yrs:** 4-8 tabs q4h. **Max:** 48 tabs q24h. |
| Bayer Low Dose Aspirin tablets | Aspirin 81mg | **Adults & Peds: ≥12 yrs:** 4-8 tabs q4h. **Max:** 48 tabs q24h. |

*(Continued)*

| BRAND | INGREDIENT/STRENGTH | DOSE |
|---|---|---|
| **SALICYLATES** *(Continued)* | | |
| Doan's Extra Strength caplets | Magnesium Salicylate Tetrahydrate 580mg | **Adults & Peds: ≥12 yrs:** 2 tabs q6h. **Max:** 8 tabs q24h. |
| Ecotrin Adult Low Strength tablets | Aspirin 81mg | **Adults:** 4-8 tabs q4h. **Max:** 48 tabs q24h. |
| Ecotrin Enteric Low Strength tablets | Aspirin 81mg | **Adults:** 4-8 tabs q4h. **Max:** 48 tabs q24h. |
| Ecotrin Enteric Regular Strength tablets | Aspirin 325mg | **Adults & Peds: ≥12 yrs:** 1-2 tabs q4h. **Max:** 12 tabs q24h. |
| Ecotrin Maximum Strength tablets | Aspirin 500mg | **Adults & Peds: ≥12 yrs:** 2 tabs q6h. **Max:** 8 tabs q24h. |
| Ecotrin Regular Strength tablets | Aspirin 325mg | **Adults & Peds: ≥12 yrs:** 1-2 tabs q4h. **Max:** 12 tabs q24h. |
| Halfprin 162mg tablets | Aspirin 162mg | **Adults & Peds: ≥12 yrs:** 2-4 tabs q4h. **Max:** 24 tabs q24h. |
| Halfprin 81mg tablets | Aspirin 81mg | **Adults & Peds: ≥12 yrs:** 4-8 tabs q4h. **Max:** 48 tabs q24h. |
| St. Joseph Adult Low Strength chewable tablets | Aspirin 81mg | **Adults & Peds: ≥12 yrs:** 4-8 tabs q4h. **Max:** 48 tabs q24h. |
| St. Joseph Adult Low Strength tablets | Aspirin 81mg | **Adults & Peds: ≥12 yrs:** 4-8 tabs q4h. **Max:** 48 tabs q24h. |
| **SALICYLATES, BUFFERED** | | |
| Ascriptin Maximum Strength tablets | Aspirin Buffered with Maalox/Calcium Carbonate 500mg | **Adults & Peds: ≥12 yrs:** 2 tabs q4h. **Max:** 8 tabs q24h. |
| Ascriptin Regular Strength tablets | Aspirin Buffered with Maalox/Calcium Carbonate 325mg | **Adults & Peds: ≥12 yrs:** 2 tabs q4h. **Max:** 12 tabs q24h. |
| Bayer Extra Strength Plus caplets | Aspirin Buffered with Calcium Carbonate 500mg | **Adults & Peds: ≥12 yrs:** 1-2 tabs q4-6h. **Max:** 8 tabs q24h. |
| Bufferin Extra Strength tablets | Aspirin Bufferred with Calcium Carbonate/Magnesium Oxide/Magnesium Carbonate 500mg | **Adults & Peds: ≥12 yrs:** 2 tabs q6h. **Max:** 8 tabs q24h. |
| Bufferin tablets | Aspirin Bufferred with Calcium Carbonate/Magnesium Oxide/Magnesium Carbonate 325mg | **Adults & Peds: ≥12 yrs:** 2 tabs q4h. **Max:** 12 tabs q24h. |
| **SALICYLATE COMBINATIONS** | | |
| Alka-Seltzer effervescent tablets | Aspirin/Citric Acid/Sodium Bicarbonate 325mg-1000mg-1916mg | **Adults & Peds: ≥12 yrs:** 2 tabs q4h. **Max:** 8 tabs q24h. |
| Alka-Seltzer Extra Strength effervescent tablets | Aspirin/Citric Acid/Sodium Bicarbonate 500mg-1000mg-1985mg | **Adults & Peds: ≥12 yrs:** 2 tabs q6h. **Max:** 7 tabs q24h. |
| Alka-Seltzer Morning Relief effervescent tablets | Aspirin/Caffeine 500mg-65mg | **Adults & Peds: ≥12 yrs:** 2 tabs q6h. **Max:** 8 tabs q24h. |
| Anacin Pain Reliever caplets | Aspirin/Caffeine 400mg-32mg | **Adults & Peds: ≥12 yrs:** 2 tabs q6h. **Max:** 8 tabs q24h. |
| Anacin Extra Strength tablets | Aspirin/Caffeine 500mg-32mg | **Adults & Peds: ≥12 yrs:** 2 tabs q6h. **Max:** 8 tabs q24h. |
| Anacin tablets | Aspirin/Caffeine 400mg-32mg | **Adults & Peds: ≥12 yrs:** 2 tabs q6h. **Max:** 8 tabs q24h. |
| Bayer Back & Body Pain caplets | Aspirin/Caffeine 500mg-32.5mg | **Adults & Peds: ≥12 yrs:** 2 tabs q6h. **Max:** 8 tabs q24h. |
| BC Arthritis Strength powders | Aspirin/Caffeine/Salicylamide 742mg-38mg-222mg | **Adults & Peds: ≥12 yrs:** 1 powder q3-4h. **Max:** 4 powders q24h. |
| BC Original powders | Aspirin/Caffeine/Salicylamide 650mg-33.3mg-195mg | **Adults & Peds: ≥12 yrs:** 1 powder q3-4h. |
| **SALICYLATE/SLEEP AID** | | |
| Alka-Seltzer PM Pain Reliever & Sleep Aid effervescent tablets | Aspirin/Diphenhydramine Citrate 325mg-38 mg | **Adults & Peds: ≥12 yrs:** 2 tabs qpm. |
| Bayer PM Relief caplets | Aspirin/Diphenhydramine 500mg-38.3mg | **Adults & Peds: ≥12 yrs:** 2 tabs qhs. |
| Doan's Extra Strength PM caplets | Magnesium Salicylate Tetrahydrate/Diphenhydramine 580mg-25mg | **Adults & Peds: ≥12 yrs:** 2 tabs qhs. |

# INSOMNIA PRODUCTS

| BRAND | INGREDIENT/STRENGTH | DOSE |
|---|---|---|
| **DIPHENHYDRAMINE** | | |
| Nytol Quickcaps caplets | Diphenhydramine 25mg | **Adults & Peds: ≥12 yrs:** 2 tabs qpm. |
| Nytol Quickgels Maximum Strength | Diphenhydramine 50mg | **Adults & Peds: ≥12 yrs:** 1 tab qpm. |
| Simply Sleep Nighttime Sleep Aid caplets | Diphenhydramine 25mg | **Adults & Peds: ≥12 yrs:** 2 tabs qpm. |
| Simply Sleep Nighttime Sleep Aid mini caplets | Diphenhydramine 25mg | **Adults & Peds: ≥12 yrs:** 2 tabs qpm. |
| Sominex tablets | Diphenhydramine 25mg | **Adults & Peds: ≥12 yrs:** 2 tabs qpm. |
| Sominex Maximum Strength caplets | Diphenhydramine 50mg | **Adults & Peds: ≥12 yrs:** 1 tab qpm. |
| Unisom Sleepgels | Diphenhydramine 50mg | **Adults & Peds: ≥12 yrs:** 1 tab qpm. |
| **DIPHENHYDRAMINE COMBINATION** | | |
| Alka-Seltzer PM | Aspirin/Diphenhydramine Citrate 325mg-38mg | **Adults & Peds: ≥12 yrs:** 2 tabs qpm. |
| Bayer PM Relief caplets | Aspirin/Diphenhydramine 500mg-38.3mg | **Adults & Peds: ≥12 yrs:** 2 tabs qhs. |
| Doan's Extra Strength PM caplets | Magnesium Salicylate Tetrahydrate/ Diphenhydramine 580mg-25mg | **Adults & Peds: ≥12 yrs:** 2 tabs qhs. |
| Excedrin PM caplets | Acetaminophen/Diphenhydramine 500mg-38mg | **Adults & Peds: ≥12 yrs:** 2 tabs qhs. |
| Excedrin PM geltabs | Acetaminophen/Diphenhydramine 500mg-38mg | **Adults & Peds: ≥12 yrs:** 2 tabs qhs. |
| Excedrin PM tablets | Acetaminophen/Diphenhydramine 500mg-38mg | **Adults & Peds: ≥12 yrs:** 2 tabs qhs. |
| Goody's PM Powders | Acetaminophen/Diphenhydramine 1000mg-76mg/dose | **Adults & Peds: ≥12 yrs:** 1 packet (2 powders) qhs. |
| Tylenol PM caplets | Acetaminophen/Diphenhydramine 500mg-25mg | **Adults & Peds: ≥12 yrs:** 2 tabs qhs. |
| Tylenol PM gelcaps | Acetaminophen/Diphenhydramine 500mg-25mg | **Adults & Peds: ≥12 yrs:** 2 caps qhs. |
| Tylenol PM geltabs | Acetaminophen/Diphenhydramine 500mg-25mg | **Adults & Peds: ≥12 yrs:** 2 tabs qhs. |
| Tylenol PM liquid | Acetaminophen/Diphenhydramine 1000g-50mg/30mL | **Adults & Peds: ≥12 yrs:** 2 tbl (30mL) qhs. **Max:** 8 tbl (120mL) q24h. |
| **DOXYLAMINE** | | |
| Unisom Sleeptabs | Doxylamine Succinate 25mg | **Adults & Peds: ≥12 yrs:** 1 tab 30 min before hs. |

# SMOKING CESSATION PRODUCTS

| BRAND | INGREDIENT/STRENGTH | DOSE |
|---|---|---|
| Commit Stop Smoking 2mg lozenges | Nicotine Polacrilex 2mg | **Adults:** If smoking first cigarettte >30 minutes after waking up use 2mg lozenge. **Weeks 1 to 6:** 1 lozenge q1-2h. **Weeks 7 to 9:** 1 lozenge q2-4h. **Weeks 10 to 12:** 1 lozenge q4-8h. **Max:** 5 lozenges/6 hours; 20 lozenges/day. Stop using at the end of 12 weeks. |
| Commit Stop Smoking 4mg lozenges | Nicotine Polacrilex 4mg | **Adults:** If smoking first cigarettte within 30 minutes after waking up use 4mg lozenge. **Weeks 1 to 6:** 1 lozenge q1-2h. **Weeks 7 to 9:** 1 lozenge q2-4h. **Weeks 10 to 12:** 1 lozenge q4-8h. **Max:** 5 lozenges/6 hours; 20 lozenges/day. Stop using at the end of 12 weeks. |
| NicoDerm CQ Step 1 clear patch | Nicotine 21mg | **Adults:** If smoking >10 cigarettes/day. **Step 1-Weeks 1 to 6:** Apply one 21mg patch/day. **Step 2-Weeks 7 to 8:** Apply one 14mg patch/day. **Step 3-Weeks 9 to 10:** Apply one 7mg patch/day. |
| NicoDerm CQ Step 2 clear patch | Nicotine 14mg | **Adults:** If smoking <10 cigarettes/day. **Step 2-Weeks 1 to 6:** Apply one 14mg patch/day. **Step 3-Weeks 7 to 8:** Apply one 7mg patch/day. |
| NicoDerm CQ Step 3 clear patch | Nicotine 7mg | **Adults:** Apply 1 patch qd Weeks 9 to 10 if smoking >10 cigarettes/day or Weeks 7 to 8 if smoking ≤10 cigarettes/day. |
| Nicorette 2mg, Original/Mint/Orange gum | Nicotine Polacrilex 2mg | **Adults:** If smoking <25 cigarettes/day use 2mg gum. **Weeks 1 to 6:** 1 piece q1-2h. **Weeks 7 to 9:** 1 piece q2-4h. **Weeks 10 to 12:** 1 piece q4-8h. **Max:** 24 pieces/day. |
| Nicorette 4mg, Original/Mint/Orange gum | Nicotine Polacrilex 4mg | **Adults:** If smoking ≥25 cigarettes/day use 4mg gum. **Weeks 1 to 6:** 1 piece q1-2h. **Weeks 7 to 9:** 1 piece q2-4h. **Weeks 10 to 12:** 1 piece q4-8h. **Max:** 24 pieces/day. |
| Habitrol Nicotine Transdermal System Patch Step 1 | Nicotine 21mg/24hr | **Adults:** If smoking >10 cigarettes/day. **Step 1-Weeks 1 to 4:** Apply one 21mg patch/day. **Step 2-Weeks 5 to 6:** Apply one 14mg patch/day. **Step 3-Weeks 7 to 8:** Apply one 7mg patch/day. |
| Habitrol Nicotine Transdermal System Patch Step 2 | Nicotine 14mg/24hr | **Adults:** If smoking >10 cigarettes/day. **Step 1-Weeks 1 to 4:** Apply one 21mg patch/day. **Step 2-Weeks 5 to 6:** Apply one 14mg patch/day. **Step 3-Weeks 7 to 8:** Apply one 7mg patch/day. |
| Habitrol Nicotine Transdermal System Patch Step 3 | Nicotine 7mg/24hr | **Adults:** If smoking >10 cigarettes/day. **Step 1-Weeks 1 to 4:** Apply one 21mg patch/day. **Step 2-Weeks 5 to 6:** Apply one 14mg patch/day. **Step 3-Weeks 7 to 8:** Apply one 7mg patch/day. |

# Weight Management Products

| BRAND | INGREDIENT/STRENGTH | DOSE |
|---|---|---|
| 1-EZ Diet Appetite Suppressant capsules | Chromium (as Chromium Picolinate), Citrimax *(Garcinia cambogial)* (Fruit) (standardized to 50% Hydrocycitric Acid), Advantra Z and Zhi Shi *(Citrus aurantium)* (Fruit) (standardized to 6% Synephrines), Jujube Extract *(Zyzyphus jujube)* (Fruit), Bitter Melon Extract *(Momordica charantia)* (Fruit), Kola Nut *(Coca acuminate)* (Seed), Green Tea *(Camellia sinensis)* (Leaf) (Standardized to 70% Polyphenols), Gugulipids *(Commiphora mukul)* (Gum Resin) (standardized to 2.5% Guggulsterones),Gelatin, Magnesium Stearate, Silicon Dioxide | **Adults:** Take 2 caps with meals bid. |
| 1-EZ Diet Fat & Carb Blocker capsules | Chromium (as Chromium Picolinate), Chitosan, White Kidney Bean, Oat Bran, Gelatin, Magnesium Stearate, Silicon Dioxide | **Adults:** Take 2 caps with meals bid. |
| Applied Nutrition Diet System 6 capsules | Vitamin C, Vitamin E, Thiamin (B1), Riboflavin (B2), Niacin (B3),Vitamin B12, Pantothenic Acid, Selenium, Chromium, *Garcinia cambogia* Extract, Kola Nut Extract, L-Carnitine, L-Tyrosine, Green Tea Extract, Choline, Inositol, Cayenne Powder, Ginger Root Powder, Spirulina, Bioperine Complex, Proprietary Xendrol Blend | **Adults:** Take 2 caps with meals bid. |
| Applied Nutrition Diet System 6, Carbo Binding Diet Program caplets | Calcium Carbonate, Microcrystalline Cellulose, Stearic Acid, Croscarmellose Sodium, Magnesium Stearate, Silicon Dioxide, Hydroxypropyl Methylcellulose, Polyethylene Glycol | **Adults:** Take 2 caps with meals bid. |
| Applied Nutrition Green Tea Fat Burner | Chromium (From Chromium Picolinate), Green Tea Extract (Leaf, 50% EGCG, 2% Caffeine), Natural Caffeine, Xenedrol Blend (Bitter Orange Extract) (Fruit, 30% Synephrine), Betaine HCl, Bladderwrack Powder (Root, Stem and Leaf), Cayenne Powder (Fruit), Eleuthero Powder (Root), Ginger Powder, Gotu Kola Powder (Aerial), Licorice Powder (Root), Yerba Maté Powder (Leaf), Soybean Oil, Gelatin, Water, Glycerin, Sorbitol, Beeswax, Lecithin, Sodium, Copper, Chlorophyllin, Titanium Dioxide | **Adults:** Take 2 caps with meals bid. |
| Applied Nutrition Hoodia Diet capsules | Green Tea Extract (Leaf, 20% Caffeine), *Hoodia gordonii* (Aerial, 20:1), Natural Caffeine, Garcinia Extract (Fruit, 50% Hydroxycitric Acid), Choline (as Choline Bitartrate), Inositol, L-Methionine, Soybean Oil, Gelatin, Glycerin, Purified Water, Lecithin, Beeswax, Sodium Copper Chlorophyllin, Titanium Dioxide | **Adults:** Take 2 caps with meals bid. |
| Applied Nutrition Natural Fat Burner capsules | Vitamin C (as Ascorbic Acid with Bioflavinoids), Vitamin E (as Dl-Alpha Tocopheryl Acetate), Niacin (as Niacinamide), Vitamin B6 (as Pyridoxine Hydrochloride), Folic Acid, Vitamin B12 (as Cyanocobalamin), Green Tea Extract (leaf, 50% EGCG, 2% Caffeine), Cinnamon extract, Natural Caffeine, Red Leaf Lettuce, Cranberry Extract, Noni Extract, Blueberry Extract, Pomegranate Extract, Apple Cider Vinegar, Soybean Oil, Gelatin, Purified Water, Lecithin, Beeswax, Glycerin, Silicon Dioxide, Annatto, Titanium Dioxide, St. John's wort, Turmeric | **Adults:** Take 2 caps with meals bid. |
| Applied Nutrition The New Grapefruit Diet capsules | Vitamin B6 (as Pyridoxine HCl), Iodine, Kelp, Chromium (as Chromium Picolinate), Soy Lecithin, Grapefruit Powder Extract, Cider Vinegar Powder, Bioperine Black Pepper Extract (Fruit), Gelatin, Silica, Magnesium Stearate | **Adults:** Take 2 caps with meals bid. |
| Aqua-Ban Maximum Strength Diuretic tablets | Pamabrom, Carnauba Wax, Croscarmellose Sodium, Hypromellose, Lactose, Magnesium Stearate, Microcrystalline Cellulose, Polyethylene Glycol, Polysorbate 80, Starch, Titanium Dioxide | **Adults:** Take 1 tab with meals qid. **Max:** 4 tabs q24h. |

*(Continued)*

| BRAND | INGREDIENT/STRENGTH | DOSE |
|---|---|---|
| Atkins Essential Oils Vita-Nutrient Supplement Formula softgels | Flaxseed Oil, Borage Seed Oil, Fish Oil, Oleic Acid, Linoleic Acid, Gamma Linolenic Acid, Eicosapentaenoic Acid (EPA), Docoshexaenoic Acid (DHA), Vitamin E (d-Alpha Tocopherol) | **Adults:** Take 1-2 caps with meals qd. |
| BioMD Nutraceuticals Metabolism T3 capsules | Calcium Phosphate, Gum Guggle Extract, L-Tyrosine, *Garcinia cambogia*, Dipotassium Phosphate, Sodium Phosphate, Disodium Phosphate, Phosphatidyl Choline | **Adults:** Take 2 caps with meal tid. |
| Biotest Hot-Rox capsules | A7-E Super-Thermogenic Gel (lauroyl macrogol-32 glycerides, p-merthylcarboylethylphenol 3, 17-dihydroxydelta 5-etiocholane-7-one diethyl-carbonate, Carbolin 19 [forskolin 1, 9-carbonate] piperine, yohibine HCl) Biotest GBX (guarana-berry extract containing theophylline and caffeine) Gelatin, Cellulose, Magnesium Stearate, Titanium Dioxide | **Adults:** Take 1-2 caps with bid. **Max:** 4 caps q24h. |
| Bodyonics Pinnacle Estrolean Fat Burner Supreme capsules | Apple Extract, Pomegranate Extract, Sea Vegetable Extract, Lipase Protease, Amylase, Guarana Extract, Green Tea Extract, Yerba Maté Extract (Standardized for 66.6mg Caffeine), Ginger Root Extract *(Zingiber officinale)* Black Pepper Extract *(Piper nigrum)* Licorice *(Glycyrrhiza glabra)*, *Citrus Aurantum* (Bitter Orange) (standardized for 4% synephrine, *Rhodiola* rosea Extract (standardized for 3% Rosavins), *Rhododendron caucasicum* Extract (standardized for 3% Taxifolian), Chromium Polynicotinate, L-Carnitine Tartrate, Garcinia Cambogia Extract, Grapefruit Extract, Cinnamon Twig Bar, Dong Quai Extract, Barberry Extract, Chaste Berry Extract | **Adults:** Take 2 caps with meal qam. |
| Bodyonics Pinnacle SugarEase capsules | Banabalean leaves, Promolin Fenugreek Extract Seeds, Dang Shen, Bai Zhu, Fu Ling, Gan Cao, Sheng Jiang, Da Zao, Yerba Maté Extract, Cocoa extract, tyramine, Citrus Naringinean, Natural Caffeine | **Adults:** Take 1 cap with meal tid. |
| Carb Cutter Original Formula tablets | Vitamin C (as Ascorbic Acid), Chromium (as Chromium Dinicotinate Glycinate), Absorptive Vegetable Fiber, Banaba Leaf Extract *(Lagerstroemia speciosa)*, Gymnema Sylvestre Leaf and Gymnema Sylvestre Leaf Extract (25% Gymnemic Acids), Fenugreek Seed Extract, Super Hydroxycitric Extract of *Garcinia cambogia* Fruit], Vanadium (as BMOV), Guarana Seed Extract (Supplying 60mg Caffeine), Korean Ginseng Root Extract (5% Ginsenosides), Eleuthero Root Extract (0.8% Eleutherosides), Green Tea Leaf Extract (36% Total Polyphenols), Dicalcium Phosphate, Microcrystalline Cellulose, Croscarmellose Sodium, Stearic Acid, Magnesium Stearate, Silica, Pharmaceutical Glaze | **Adults:** Take 1-2 tabs with meals bid. |
| Carb Cutter Phase 2 Starch Neutralizer tablets | Phase 2 Starch Neutralizer *(Phaseolus vulgaris)* (from White Kidney Bean Extract), *Gymnema Sylvestre* Leaf, Fenugreek Seed, *Garcina cambogia* Fruit Extract 50.0%, Hydroxycitric Acid, Vanadium (as Vanadyl Sulfate) Dicalcium Phosphate, Microcrystalline Cellulose, Croscarmellose Sodium, Stearic Acid, Magnesium Stearate, Silica, Pharmaceutical Glaze | **Adults:** Take 1-2 tabs with meals bid. |
| Chroma Slim Apple Cider Vinegar caplets | Apple Cider Vinegar Complex, Grapefruit Powder, Premium Herbal Blend, Soy Lecithin, Vitamin B6, Chromium Microcrystalline Cellulose, Maltodextrin, Dicalcium Phosphate, Crospovidone, Modified Food Starch, Hydroxypropyl Methylcellulose, Calcium Silicate, Silica, Magnesium Stearate, PEG | **Adults:** Take 2 caps with meals bid. |

*(Continued)*

| BRAND | INGREDIENT/STRENGTH | DOSE |
|---|---|---|
| Chroma Slim Chitosan-C with Chromium Picolinate capsules | Dicalcium Phosphate, Calcium Carbonate, Microcrystalline Cellulose, Croscarmellose Sodium, Stearic Acid, Sodium Lauryl Sulfate, Magnesium Stearate, Silica, Hydroxypropyl Methylcellulose, Hydroxypropylcellulose, PEG, Natural Peppermint Flavor, Carnuba Wax | **Adults:** Take 2 caps with meals bid. |
| Chroma Slim Ultra with Biotrol | Cellulose, Dicalcium Phosphate, Silica, Croscarmellose Sodium, Magnesium Stearate, Hydroxypropyl Methylcellulose, Stearic Acid, Maltodextrin, PEG | **Adults:** Take 3 caps before breakfast and 3 caps before dinner. |
| CortiLess Anti-Stress Weight Loss Supplement capsules | Vitamin C, Calcium, Chromium, Magnolia Bark Extract, Theanine, Green Tea Leaf Extract, Cocoa Bean Extract (contains Theobromine), Banaba Leaf (contains Corosolic Acid), Anadyl Sulfate (derived from Vanadium), Gelatin, Cellulose, Magnesium Stearate, Silica | **Adults:** Take 1 cap with meals bid. **Max:** 6 caps q24h. |
| Cortislim Cortisol Control Weight Loss Formula capsules | Vitamin C, Calcium, Chromium, Cortiplex Blend (Magnolia Bark Extract, Beta-Sitosterol, Theanine), Leptiplex Blend (Green Tea Extract, Bitter Orange Peel Extract), Insutrol Blend (Banaba Leaf Extract, Vanadium), Microcrystalline Cellulose, Gelatin, Magnesium Stearate, Water, Silicon Dioxide | **Adults:** Take 2 caps with meals bid-tid. **Max:** 6 caps q24h. |
| CSE Naturally hGH chewable tablets | Homeopathic Recombinant Human Growth Hormone (HrhGH) 6C+100C+200C (Anti-Aging) | **Adults:** Chew 1 tab with meals tid. |
| Dexatrim Decaf Green Tea Formula caplets | Chromium, Green Tea Leaf Standardized Extract with Epigallocatechin Gallate (EGCG) and Caffeine, Asian (Panax) Ginseng Root, Theobromine, Microcrystalline Cellulose, Dicalcium Phosphate, Croscarmellose Sodium, Stearic Acid, Pharmaceutical Glaze, Carnauba Wax | **Adults:** Take 1 cap with meals tid. |
| Dexatrim Max Maximum Weight Loss Power, Ephedra Free caplets | Thiamin (B1), Riboflavin (B2), Niacin (B3), Vitamin B6, Vitamin B12, Pantothenic Acid, Chromium, Green Tea Leaf Extract, Asian Ginseng Standardized Extract | **Adults:** Take 1-2 tabs qd. |
| Dexatrim Natural Extra Energy Formula caplets | Calcium, Chromium, Green Tea Leaf Standardized Extract with Epigallocatechin Gallate (EGCG) and Caffeine, Asian (Panax), Ginseng Root, Microcrystalline Cellulose, Croscarmellose Sodium, Stearic Acid, Hypromellose, Silica, Magnesium Stearate | **Adults:** Take 1cap with meals tid. |
| Dexatrim Natural Green Tea Formula caplets | Calcium, Chromium, Green Tea Leaf Standardized Extract, Asian (Panax), Ginseng Root, Microcrystalline Cellulose, Croscarmellose Sodium, Stearic Acid, Silica, Magnesium Stearate, Hypromellose, Hydroxypropyl Cellulose, PEG 400, Titanium Dioxide, Riboflavin, Caramel (245-8) | **Adults:** Take 1 cap with meal tid. |
| Dexatrim Max Evening Appetite Control caplets | L-Theanine (from Green Tea Leaf), 5-HTP (natural 5-hydroxytryptophan), Chamomile Flower, English Lavender Flower, Lemon Balm Leaf, Orange Blossom. | **Adults:** Take 2 caps 30 minutes before evening meal. **Max:** 6 caps q24h. |
| Diet Lean Weight Loss Multivitamin tablets | Vitamin A, Vitamin C, Vitamin D, Vitamin E, Vitamin K, Thiamin (B1), Riboflavin (B2), Niacin (B3), Vitamin B6, Folate, Folic Acid, Folacin, Vitamin B12, Pantothenic Acid, Calcium, Iron, Magnesium, Zinc, Selenium, Copper, Manganese, Chromium, EGCG | **Adults:** Take 1 tab with meal qd. |
| Diurex Long Acting Water capsules | Caffeine Anhydrous, Acetaminophen, Potassium Salicylate, Non-Parilell Seeds, Magnesium Oxide, Titanium Dioxide | **Adults:** Take 1 cap qam after breakfast. |
| EAS CLA capsules | Green Tea *(Camellia sinensis)* Leaf, Total Polyphenols, Catechins, Epigallocatechin Gallates (EGCG), Gelatin, Microcellulose, Magnesium Stearate, Silica. | **Adults:** Take 2 caps with meals tid. |

*(Continued)*

| BRAND | INGREDIENT/STRENGTH | DOSE |
|---|---|---|
| EAS Lean DynamX, Orange Cream powder (EAS) | Green Tea *(Camellia sinensis)* Leaf: Total Polyphenols, Catechins, Epigallocatechin Gallates (EGCG), Gelatin, Microcellulose, Magnesium Stearate, Silica | **Adults:** Mix 1 tsp with 8oz of water bid-tid. |
| EAS Thermo DynamX capsules | Calcium, Chromium, Conjugated Linoleic Acid, Calcium B-Hydroxy B-Methylbutyrate, Maté, L-Carnitine, L-Tartrate | **Adults:** Take 2-3 caps bid before meals. |
| Estrin-D capsules | Vitamin B6, Magnesium, Estrin-D Blend | **Adults:** Take 2 caps with meals qd. **Max:** 6 caps q24h. |
| Health and Nutrition Systems Eat Less Dietary Supplement capsules | Galactomannan, Kola Nut Extract, Cellulose, Green Tea Leaf Extract, Glucomannan, Cinnamon Twig Extract, Galangal Rhizome Extract, Apple Pectin, Citrus Pectin | **Adults:** Take 1-2 caps with meals bid. |
| Hydroxycut Advanced Weight Loss Formula, Ephedra Free capsules | Hydroxycitrate, Polynictinate, *Garcinia cambogia, Gymnema sylvestre* leaf extract, Soy Photolipids, *Rhodiola rosea* extract, *Withania somnifera* extract, Hydroxytea, Green Tea Extract, Caffeine Anhydrous, Hydroxypropy Cellulose, Microcrystalline Cellulose, Polyvinylpyrrolidone, Croscarmellose Sodium (Sodium Chloride, Sodium Glycolate), Vegetable Stearine, Magnesium Stearate, Coating (Polyvinyl Aclohol, Titanium Dioxide, Polyethylene Glycol, Talc), Silica, Acesulfame-Potassium, Maltodextrin, Propylene Oxide | **Adults:** Take 3 caps with meals tid. **Max:** 4 caps q24h. |
| Hydroxycut Caffeine-Free Weight Loss Formula, capsules | Hydroxycitrate, Polynictinate, *Garcinia cambogia, Gymnema sylvestre* leaf extract, Glucomannan, Alpha Lipoic Acid, Willow Bark extract, L-Carnitine, Caffeine-Free Green Tea Leaf Extract, Microcrystalline Cellulose, Hydroxypropyl Cellulose, Polyvinylpyrrolidone, Croscarmellose Sodium (Sodium Chloride, Sodium Glycolate), Vegetable Stearine, Magnesium Stearate, Coating (Polyvinyl Alcohol, Titanium Dioxide, Polyethylene Glycol, Talc, Silica, Acesulfame Potassium, Maltodextrin, Propylene Oxide) | **Adults:** Take 2 caps with meals tid. **Max:** 6 caps q24h. |
| Hydroxycut Fat Loss Support Formula, Caffeine-Free capsules | Hydroxycitrate, Polynictinate, *Garcinia cambogia, Gymnema sylvestre* leaf extract, Glucomannan, Alpha Lipoic Acid, Willow Bark Extract, L-Carnitine, Hydroxy Tea, Epigallocatechin Gallate (EGCG), Caffeine, Guarana Extract, Gelatin, Magnesium Stearate, Silica, Cellulose | **Adults:** Take 3 caps with meals tid. **Max:** 9 caps q24h. |
| Isatori Lean System 7 Triple Action Fat-Loss Formula with 7-Keto capsules | Yerba Maté, Guarana extract, *Citrus aurantium* Fruit Extract, *Forslean coleus forskohilli* extract, 7-Keto, Dandelion Leaf and Root Powder, Bioperine, Gelatin, Rice Flour, Magnesium Stearate, Titanium Dioxide | **Adults:** Take 3 caps with meals bid. **Max:** 6 caps q24h. |
| Metab-O-Fx Ephedra Free caplets | Guarana Seed, Yerba Maté Leaf, Kola Nut Seed, Bitter Orange Extract, Green Tea Extract, Cocoa Nut, Black Tea Extract, Korean Ginseng Root, *Rhodiola rosea* Extract, Dicalcium Phosphate, Cellulose, Croscarmellose, Silica, Vegetable Stearic Acid, Acacia gum, Vegetable Magnesium Stearate, Cellulose Coating | **Adults:** Take 1 tab with meal bid-tid. **Max:** 3 tabs q24h. |
| Metabolife Ephedra Free Dietary Supplement tablets | Calcium (as Hydroxycitrate and Dicalcium Phosphate), Chromium (as Chromium Picolinate), Sodium, Potassium, and a Proprietary Blend of the Following: Green Tea Extract (Leaf) (standardized for EGCG and total Catechins), Super Citrimax *Garcinia cambogia* Extract (Fruit) (standardized for Hydroxycitric Acid), Guarana Extract (Seed) (standardized for Caffeine), Yerba Maté extract (leaf) (standardized for Caffeine). Maltodextrin, Modified Cellulose, Caffeine, Dicalcium Phosophate, Stearic Acid, Sodium Bicarbonate, Dextrin, Silica, Citric Acid, Sodium Copper Chlorophyllin, Dextrose, Lecithin, Sodium Carboxymethylcellulose, Sodium Citrate | **Adults:** Take 2 tabs with meals tid. |

*(Continued)*

| BRAND | INGREDIENT/STRENGTH | DOSE |
|---|---|---|
| Metabolife Metabolife Ultra caplets | Thiamin, Riboflavin, Vitamin B6, Pantothenic Acid, Calcium, Magnesium, Potassium, Modified Cellulose, Maltodextrin, Caffeine, Dicalcium Phosphate, Stearic Acid, Dextrin, Dextrose, Lecithin, Sodium Carboxymethylcellulose, Magnesium Stearate, Sodium Citrate, Caffeine, Synephrine | **Adults:** Take 2-3 caps with meals bid-tid. **Max:** 6 caps q24h. |
| Metabolife Ultra Caffeine Free caplets | Thiamin (B1), Riboflavin (B2), Niacin (B3), Vitamin B6, Pantothenic acid, Calcium, Chromium, Potassium, Modified Cellulose, Maltodextrin, Stearic Acid, Silica, Dextrin, Titanium Dioxide, Polyethylene Glycol, Lecithin, Dextrose, Sodium Carboxymethylcellulose, Sodium Citrate | **Adults:** Take 2 tabs with meals tid. **Max:** 6 tabs q24h. |
| Metabolife Ultra Weight Management caplets | Green Tea Extract, L-Tyrosine, Cayenne, Caffeine, Maltodextrin, Cellulose, Croscarmellose Sodium, Stearic Acid, Sodium Bicarbonate, Silica, Citric Acid, Glycerin | **Adults:** Take 2 tabs with meals tid. **Max:** 6 tabs q24h. |
| MHP TakeOff, Hi-Energy Fat Burner capsules | *Citrus aurantium* Extract, Guarana Seed Extract and Green Tea Leaf Extract, L-Tyrosine, Triple-Ginseng Concentrate, Adrenal Support Blend, *Ginkgo biloba* Leaf Extract, Dicalcium Phosphate, Microcrystalline Cellulose, Croscarmellose Sodium, Stearic Acid, Magnesium Stearate, Silica and Film Coat (Hydroxypropyl Methylcellulose, Hydroxypropyl Cellulose, Polyethylene Glycol, Propylene Glycol, Titanium Dioxide, and Sodium Citrate). Triple-Ginseng Concentrate: Panax Ginseng Root Extract, American Ginseng Root Extract and Siberian Ginseng Root Extract. Adrenal Support Blend: Licorice Root Extract, Astragalus Root Extract and Schizandra Berry Extract. | **Adults:** Take 1-2 caps with meal prn. |
| MHP Thyro-Slim A.M./P.M. tablets | Selenium, Copper, Chromium, Guarana Seed Extract, Green Tea Leaf, *Garcinia cambogia* Fruit extract, Bitter Orange Fruit Extract, Citrus aurantium, Thyrogenic T-3 Complex: Guggulipid, Dicalcium Phosphate, Microcrystalline Cellulose, Hydroxypropyl Methylcellulose, Methylcellulose, Stearic Acid, Vegetable Stearin, Silica, Magnesium Stearate, Hydroxypropyl Cellulose, Polyethylene Glycol, Croscarmellose Sodium | **Adults:** Take 2 tabs with meals bid. |
| Natrol Carb Intercept with Phase 2 Starch Neutralizer capsules | White Kidney Bean Extract, Silica, Magnesium Stearate, Gelatin | **Adults:** Take 2 caps with meals tid. |
| Natrol Chitosan 500mg capsules | Chitosan, Magnesium Stearate, Silica, Gelatin | **Adults:** Take 3 caps with meals qd. **Max:** 6 caps q24h. |
| Natrol CitriMax Balance tablets | Vitamin B6, Magnesium, Chromium, Vanadium, Hydroxycitric Acid (HCA) Extract, Green Tea Extract, *Gymnerna sylvestre* Extract, Bitter Orange Extract, Cellulose, Stearic Acid, Cellulose Gum, Silica, Magnesium Stearate, Methylcellulose, Glycerine | **Adults:** Take 2 tabs with meals tid. |
| Natrol Green Tea 500mg capsules | Green Tea Extract, Polyphenols, Catechins, Caffeine, Gelatin, Magnesium Stearate, Rice Powder, Silica | **Adults:** Take 1 cap with meals qd. |
| Natural Balance Fat Magnet capsules | Chitosan, Psyllium Husk, Malic Acid, Vegetarian Lipase, Aloe Vera, Gelatin, Microcrystalline Cellulose, Stearic Acid, Magnesium Stearate | **Adults:** Take 2 caps with meals bid. |
| Nature Made High Potency Chromium Picolinate, 200mcg tablets | Dibasic Calcium Phosphate, Cellulose, Magnesium Stearate, Chromium Picolinate, Croscarmellose Sodium | **Adults:** Take 1 tab with meals qd. |
| Nature's Bounty Super Green Tea Diet capsules | Green Tea *(Camellia sinensis)* (Leaf); Caffeine; Guarana *(Paullinia cupana)* (Seed); Ginger *(Zingiber officinale)* (Root); Bladderwrack Extract *(Fucus vesiculosus)* (Whole Plant); Uva Ursi *(Arctistaohylos uva-ursi)* (Leaf); Vitamin B-6 (as Pyridoxine Hydrochloride); Chromium (as Chromium Polynicotinate) | **Adults:** Take 1 cap with meals bid. |

*(Continued)*

| BRAND | INGREDIENT/STRENGTH | DOSE |
|---|---|---|
| Nature's Bounty Xtreme Lean Zn-3 Ephedra Free capsules | Yerba Maté, *Ilex paraguatensis,* Guarana, *Paulinia cupana,* Damiana, *Turnera aphrodisiacal, Schizonepeta, Nepeta tenuifolia,* Green Tea Extract, *Camellia sinensis,* White Pepper, *Piper nigrum,* Tibet-seng, *Rhodiola crenulata,* Panax Ginseng, Maca Root, *Lepidium meyenii,* Cocoa Nut *(Theobroma cacao),* Kola Nut *(Cola acuminate),* Thea Sinensis Complex | **Adults:** Take 1 cap with meals tid. |
| Nunaturals LevelRight for Blood Sugar Management capsules | *Gymenema sylvestre* Extract, Fenugreek Extract, Bitter Melon Extract, Siberian Ginseng Extract, Alpha Lipoic Acid, Cinnamon Bark Extract, Banaba Leaf Extract, Biotin, Chromium Polynicotinate, Chromium Picolinate, Vanadium | **Adults:** Take 1 cap with meals tid. |
| One-A-Day Weight Smart Dietary Supplement tablets | Vitamin A, C, D, E, K; Thiamin (B1); Riboflavin (B2); Niacin (B3); Vitamin B6, B12; Folic Acid; Calcium; Iron; Magnesium; Zinc; Selenium; Copper Calcium Carbonate, Cellulose, Magnesium Oxide, Green Tea Extract, Ascorbic Acid, Ferrous Fumarate, Acacia, dl-Alpha Tocopherol Acetate, Niacinamide, Croscarmellose Sodium, Zinc Oxide, Dextrin, d-Calcium Pantothenate, Dicalcium Phosphate, Caffeine Powder, Silicon Dioxide, Hypromellose, Magnesium Stearate, Titanium Dioxide, Gelatin, Corn Starch, Crospovidone, Glucose, Manganese Sulfate, Calcium Silicate, Cupric Sulfate, Polyethylene Glycol, Pyridoxine, Hydrochloride, Riboflavin, Dextrose, Lecithin, Beta Carotene, Chromium Chloride, Resin, Sodium Selenate, Phytonadione, Tricalcium Phosphate, Cholecalciferol, Cyanocobalamin | **Adults:** Take 1 tab with meals qd. |
| PatentLean Effective and Trusted Fat and Weight Loss Supplement | 3-Acetyl-7-Oxo-Dehydroepiandrosterone, Magnesium Stearate, Maltodextrin, Gelatin, Titanium Dioxide | **Adults:** Take 1 cap with meals bid. **Max:** 2 caps q24h. |
| Prolab BCAA Plus capsules | Vitamin C, Vitamin B6, L-Leucine, L-Isoleucine, L-Valine | **Adults:** Take 6 caps after workout. |
| Prolab Enhanced CLA softgels | CLA (Conjugated Linoleic Acid), Flax Seed Oil, Alpha Linoleic Acid, Linoleic Acid | **Adults:** Take 3 caps with meals qd. |
| Relora Anti-Anxiety & Stress Relief, 250mg capsules | Relora (a patent-pending plant extract from *Magnolia officinalis* and Philodendron) | **Adults:** Take 1 cap with meals tid. |
| Slim Form patch | Marine Algae *(Fucus vesiculosus),* Mannitol, Chlorides, Potassium, Sodium, Magnesium, Amino Acids, Calcium, Glucose, Phosphate, Fucose | **Adults:** Apply patch as directed. |
| Stacker 2 Ephedra Free capsules | Proprietary Blend: Kola Nut (Seed), Yerba Maté (Fruit), *Cassia mimosoides* Extract (Leaf/Stem/Pod) White Willow Bark; Caffeine (Anhydrous); Tri-Gugg Lyptoid Complex: Green Tea (Leaf), Guggulsterone (Whole Plant), Gymnema (Leaf) | **Adults:** Use as directed. **Max:** 3 caps tid. |
| Tetrazene ES-50 Ultra High-Energy Weight Loss Catalyst capsules | Vitamin B6 (as Pyridoxine HCl); Biotin; Tetrazene Proprietary Blend: GKM-90 (Super-Class) Konjac Glucomannan), Glutamine, Olive Leaf Extract. ES-50 Thermogenic Complex: L-Tyrosine, Camellia Sinensis (Green Tea Leaf Extract, Standardized for EGCG and Caffeine), Pharmaceutical Grade Caffeine, Vinpocetine. | **Adults:** Take 2 caps with meals tid. **Max:** 6 caps q24h. |
| Tetrazene KGM-90 Rapid Weight Loss Catalyst capsules | Vitamin B6; Biotin; Propietary Blend as Follows: KGM-90 (SuperClass Pharmaceutical Grade Glucomannan) Glutamine, Olive Leaf Extract | **Adults:** Take 2 caps with meals tid. **Max:** 6 caps q24h. |
| Thermogenics Plus Stimulant-Free capsules | Proprietary Blend (Phosphosterine): Calcium Phosphate, *Commiphora phytosterol* extract, *Garcinia cambogia,* L-Tyrosine, Dipotassium Phosphate, Sodium Phosphate, Disodium Phosphate, Phosphatidyl Choline, *Scutellaria* (Root), *Bupleurum* (Root), *Epimedium* (Herb) | **Adults:** Take 2 caps tid. |

*(Continued)*

| BRAND | INGREDIENT/STRENGTH | DOSE |
|---|---|---|
| ThyroStart with Thydrazine, Thyroid Support capsules | Vitamin A (as Beta-Carotene), Vitamin C (Ascorbic Acid), Vitamin E (d-Alpha Tocopheryl Acetate), Thiamin (B1), Riboflavin (B2), Vitamin B6, Pyridoxine HCl, Folate, Folic Acid, Folacin, Vitamin B12, Cyanocobalamin, Biotin, Pantothenic Acid, Magnesium Amino Acid Chelate, Zinc Amino Acid, Proprietary Blend (Thydrazine) | **Adults:** Take 2 caps with meals tid. |
| Twinlab GTF Chromium, 200mcg tablets | Calicum from Dicalcium Phosphate Dehydrate; Chromium from Chromium Yeast; Brewers Yeast, Cellulose, Stearic Acid, Croscarmellose Sodium, Magnesium Stearate, Silica | **Adults:** Take 1 tab qd. |
| Twinlab Mega L-Carnitine 500mg tablets | Cellulose, Calcium Phosphate, Vegetable Oil (Palm Olein, Soy, Coconut and High Oleic Sunflower Oils), Povidone, Croscarmellose Sodium, Silica, Magnesium Stearate, Polyethylene Glycol, Water; L-Carnitine from L-Carnipure, L-Carnitine, L-Tartrate | **Adults:** Take 1-4 tabs with meals qd. |
| Twinlab Metabolift, Ephedra Free Formula capsules | Guarana Seed Extract, Citrus Aurantium Fruit Extract, Proprietary Thermogenic and Metabolic Blend, St. John's wort Extract, L-Phenylalanine, Green Tea Leaf Extract, Quercetin Dihydrate, Citrus Bioflavonoid Complex, Ginger Root, Cayenne Fruit | **Adults:** Take 2 caps with meals tid. **Max:** 6 caps q24h. |
| Ultra Diet Pep tablets | Vitamin B12 (Cyanocobalamin), Vitamin B6 (as Pyridoxine HCl), Pantothenic Acid (as d-Calcium Pantothenate), DynaChrome Chromium (as Arginate/Cheildamate), Potassium (as Potassium Chloride), Proprietary Blend Siberian Ginseng (Root) Guarana (standardized Seed Extract), Green Tea (standardized Seed Extract), Dandelion (Leaf); Ginger (Root), Passion Flower (Aerial Portion Extract), Kelp (Leaf) | **Adults:** Take 1 ab with meals bid. |
| Xenadrine EFX capsules | Tyroplex (Proprietary Blend of L-Tyrosine and Acetyl-L-Tyrosine), Green Tea Extract (standardized for Epigallocatechin Gallate, Caffeine and Polyphenols), Seropo (Proprietary Cocoa Extract standardized for PEA [Phenylethylamine], Tyramine and Theobromine), Yerba Maté (standardized for Caffeine and Methylxanthines), dl-Methionine, Ginger Root (standardized for Gingerols), Isotherm (proprietary blend of 3, 3', 4', 5-7 Pentahydroxyflavone and 3, 3', 4', 7-Tetrahydroxyflavone), DMAE (2-Dimethylaminoethanol), Grape Seed Extract (standardized for Catechins). | **Adults:** Take 2 caps with meals bid. **Max:** 4 caps q24h. |
| Xenadrine NRG 8 Hour Power tablets | Calcium Phosphate, Cellulose, Sorbitol, Gamma Cyclodextrin, Cephalins (Phosphatidyl Ethanolamine and Serine), Xanthan Gum, Inulin, Magnesium Stearate. Natural Protective Coating Utilized. Proprietary Thermoxanthin Blend: Methylxanthine Complex Proprietary Blend (Providing Total Methylxanthines, Including Caffeine, Theobromine and Theophylline), Yerba Maté Leaf *(Ilex Paraguariensis)*, Guarana Seed *(Paullinia cupana)*, Cocoa Seed *(Theobroma cacao)*, Green Tea Leaf *(Camellia sinensis)*, Green Coffee Bean Extract *(Coffee arabica)*, Naturally Infused Caffeine, Amino Acid Complex Proprietary Blend: L-Tyrosine, L-Theanine. | **Adults:** Take 3 tabs qd. **Max:** 12 caps q24h. |

*(Continued)*

| BRAND | INGREDIENT/STRENGTH | DOSE |
|---|---|---|
| XtremeLean Advanced Formula, Ephedra Free capsules | Vitamin C (as Ascorbic Acid), Vitamin B-6 (as Pyridoxine Hydrochloride), Pantothenic Acid (as d-Calcium Pantothenate), Magnesium (as Magnesium Oxide), Proprietary XtremeLean, Thermo Complex (Yerba Maté Extract [Leaf]) (standardized for Methylxanthines [Caffeine]), Green Tea Extract *(Camellia sinensis)* (Leaf) (standardized for Epigallocatechin Gallate, Caffeine, Polyphenols), Metabromine Cocoa Extract (standardized for Theobromine, Caffeine), Bitter Orange Extract *(Citrus aurantium)* (Fruit) (standardized for Synepherine, N-Methyltyramine, Hordenine, Octopamine, Tyramine), Tyrosine Complex (L-Tyrosine, Acetyl L-Tyrosine), L-Methionine, Ginger Extract *(Zingiber officinale)* (Root), Grape Seed Extract (Seed); Flavone Complex (Proprietary Blend of: 3, 3', 4', 5-7- Pentahydroxyflavone, 3, 3', 4', 7 Tetrahydroxyflavone), DMAE (Dimethylaminoethanol), Gelatin, Vegetable Magnesium Stearate, Silica | **Adults:** Take 2 caps with meals bid. |
| Zantrex 3, Ephedrine Free | Rice Flour, Zantrex-3 Proprietary Blend Containing: Yerba Maté (Leaf), Caffeine, Guarana (Seed), Damiana (Leaf, Stem), Green Tea (Leaf), Kola Nut, *Schizonepeta* (Spica), *Piper nigrum* (Fruit), Tibetan Ginseng (Root), Panax Ginseng (Root), Maca Root, Cocoa Nut, Thea Sinensis Complex (Leaf). | **Adults:** Take 2 caps with meals qd. **Max:** 6 cap q24h. |

# ACNE PRODUCTS

| BRAND | INGREDIENT/STRENGTH | DOSE |
|---|---|---|
| **BENZOYL PEROXIDE** | | |
| Clean & Clear Continuous Control Acne Cleanser | Benzoyl Peroxide 10% | **Adults & Peds:** Use bid. |
| Clean & Clear Persa-Gel 10, Maximum Strength | Benzoyl Peroxide 10% | **Adults & Peds:** Use qd-tid. |
| Clearasil Daily Acne Control cream | Benzoyl Peroxide 10% | **Adults & Peds:** Use qd-tid. |
| Clearasil Maximum Strength Acne Treatment vanishing cream | Benzoyl Peroxide 10% | **Adults & Peds:** Use qd-tid. |
| Clearasil Total Control Acne Crisis Clear Up | Benzoyl Peroxide 10% | **Adults & Peds:** Use qd-tid. |
| Clearasil Ultra Acne Treatment tinted cream | Benzoyl Peroxide 10% | **Adults & Peds:** Use tid. |
| Clearasil Ultra Acne Treatment vanishing cream | Benzoyl Peroxide 10% | **Adults & Peds:** Use tid. |
| Neutrogena Clear Pore Cleanser Mask | Benzoyl Peroxide 3.5% | **Adults & Peds:** Use biw-tiw. |
| Neutrogena On-the-Spot Acne Treatment vanishing cream | Benzoyl Peroxide 2.5% | **Adults & Peds:** Apply qd initially, then bid-tid. |
| Oxy 10 Balance Oil-Free Maximum Strength Acne Wash | Benzoyl Peroxide 10% | **Adults & Peds:** Use bid-tid. |
| Oxy Balance Acne Treatment for Sensitive Skin vanishing cream | Benzoyl Peroxide 5% | **Adults & Peds:** Use qd-tid. |
| Oxy Balance Maximum Acne Treatment tinted lotion | Benzoyl Peroxide 10% | **Adults & Peds:** Use qd-tid. |
| Oxy Spot Treatment | Benzoyl Peroxide 10% | **Adults & Peds:** Use qd-tid. |
| PanOxyl Aqua Gel Maximum Strength gel | Benzoyl Peroxide 10% | **Adults & Peds:** Apply qd initially, then bid-tid. |
| PanOxyl Bar 10% Maximum Strength | Benzoyl Peroxide 10% | **Adults & Peds:** Apply qd initially, then bid-tid. |
| PanOxyl Bar 5% | Benzoyl Peroxide 5% | **Adults & Peds:** Use qd initially, then bid-tid. |
| ZAPZYT Maximum Strength Acne Treatment gel | Benzoyl Peroxide 10% | **Adults & Peds:** Use qd-tid. |
| ZAPZYT Treatment Bar | Benzoyl Peroxide 10% | **Adults & Peds:** Use qd-tid. |
| **SALICYLIC ACID** | | |
| Aveeno Clear Complexion Cleansing Bar | Salicylic Acid 0.5% | **Adults & Peds:** Use daily. |
| Aveeno Clear Complexion Foaming Cleanser | Salicylic Acid 0.5% | **Adults & Peds:** Use daily. |
| Aveeno Correcting Treatment, Clear Complexion | Salicylic Acid 1% | **Adults & Peds:** Use qd-tid. |
| Biore Blemish Fighting Cleansing Cloths | Salicylic Acid 0.5% | **Adults & Peds:** Use qd-tid. |
| Biore Blemish Fighting Ice Cleanser | Salicylic Acid 2% | **Adults & Peds:** Use qd. |
| Bye Bye Blemish Acne Lemon Scrub | Salicylic Acid 1% | **Adults & Peds:** Use qd-tid. |
| Bye Bye Blemish Anti-Acne Moisturizer | Salicylic Acid 0.5% | **Adults & Peds:** Use qd-tid. |
| Bye Bye Blemish Anti-Acne Serum | Salicylic Acid 1% | **Adults & Peds:** Use qd-tid. |
| Bye Bye Blemish Drying Lotion | Salicylic Acid 2% | **Adults & Peds:** Use pm. |

*(Continued)*

| BRAND | INGREDIENT/STRENGTH | DOSE |
|---|---|---|
| **SALICYLIC ACID** *(Continued)* | | |
| Bye Bye Blemish Purifying Acne Mask | Salicylic Acid 0.5% | **Adults & Peds:** Use qd. |
| Clean & Clear Advantage Acne Cleanser | Salicylic Acid 2% | **Adults & Peds:** Use qd. |
| Clean & Clear Advantage Acne Spot Treatment | Salicylic Acid 2% | **Adults & Peds:** Use qd. |
| Clean & Clear Advantage Daily Cleansing Pads | Salicylic Acid 2% | **Adults & Peds:** Use qd. |
| Clean & Clear Blackhead Clearing Astringent | Salicylic Acid 1% | **Adults & Peds:** Use qd. |
| Clean & Clear Blackhead Clearing Daily Cleansing Pads | Salicylic Acid 1% | **Adults & Peds:** Use qd. |
| Clean & Clear Blackhead Clearing Scrub | Salicylic Acid 2% | **Adults & Peds:** Use qd. |
| Clean & Clear Clear Advantage Daily Acne Clearing lotion | Salicylic Acid 1% | **Adults & Peds:** Use qd. |
| Clean & Clear Continuous Control Acne Wash, Oil Free | Salicylic Acid 2% | **Adults & Peds:** Use qd. |
| Clean & Clear Facial Cleansing Bar, Blackhead Clearing | Salicylic Acid 0.5% | **Adults & Peds:** Use qd. |
| Clean & Clear Oil-Free Dual Action Moisturizer lotion | Salicylic Acid 0.5% | **Adults & Peds:** Use qd-tid. |
| Clearasil 3 in 1 Acne Defense Cleanser | Salicylic Acid 2% | **Adults & Peds:** Use qd-tid. |
| Clearasil Acne Fighting Cleansing Wipes | Salicylic Acid 2% | **Adults & Peds:** Use qd. |
| Clearasil Acne Fighting Facial Moisturizer | Salicylic Acid 2% | **Adults & Peds:** Use qd-tid. |
| Clearasil Acne Fighting Foaming Cleanser | Salicylic Acid 2% | **Adults & Peds:** Use qd-tid. |
| Clearasil Blackhead Clearing Pads with Targeted Action | Salicylic Acid 2% | **Adults & Peds:** Use qd-tid. |
| Clearasil Blackhead Clearing Scrub | Salicylic Acid 2% | **Adults & Peds:** Use qd. |
| Clearasil Daily Acne Control Pore Cleansing Pads | Salicylic Acid 2% | **Adults & Peds:** Use qd. |
| Clearasil Daily Blackhead Control Astringent | Salicylic Acid 1% | **Adults & Peds:** Use qd. |
| Clearasil Daily Oil Control Cream Cleanser | Salicylic Acid 1% | **Adults & Peds:** Use qd. |
| Clearasil Icewash, Acne Gel Cleanser | Salicylic Acid 2% | **Adults & Peds:** Use qd. |
| Clearasil Maximum Strength Pore Cleansing Pads | Salicylic Acid 2% | **Adults & Peds:** Use qd-tid. |
| Clearasil Oil Control Acne Wash | Salicylic Acid 2% | **Adults & Peds:** Use qd. |
| Clearasil Overnight Acne Defense Gel | Salicylic Acid 2% | **Adults & Peds:** Use qd-tid. |
| Clearasil Total Control Daily Skin Perfecting Treatment | Salicylic Acid 0.5% | **Adults & Peds:** Use qd. |
| Clearasil Total Control Deep Pore Cream Cleanser | Salicylic Acid 2% | **Adults & Peds:** Use qd. |
| Clearasil Ultra Acne Clearing Scrub | Salicylic Acid 2% | **Adults & Peds:** Use qd. |
| Clearasil Ultra Deep Pore Cleansing Pads | Salicylic Acid 2% | **Adults & Peds:** Use qd-tid. |
| L'Oreal Pure Zone Pore Unclogging Scrub Cleanser | Salicylic Acid 1% | **Adults & Peds:** Use bid. |
| L'Oreal Pure Zone Skin Clearing Foaming Cleanser | Salicylic Acid 2% | **Adults & Peds:** Use bid. |

*(Continued)*

| BRAND | INGREDIENT/STRENGTH | DOSE |
|---|---|---|
| **SALICYLIC ACID** *(Continued)* | | |
| Neutrogena Clear Pore Treatment - Night Time | Salicylic Acid 2% | **Adults & Peds:** Use qd. |
| Neutrogena Advanced Solutions Acne Mark Fading Peel with CelluZyme | Salicylic Acid 2% | **Adults & Peds:** Use qw-tiw. |
| Neutrogena Blackhead Eliminating Astringent | Salicylic Acid 0.5% | **Adults & Peds:** Use qd. |
| Neutrogena Blackhead Eliminating Daily Scrub | Salicylic Acid 2% | **Adults & Peds:** Use prn. |
| Neutrogena Blackhead Eliminating Treatment Mask | Salicylic Acid 0.5% | **Adults & Peds:** Use biw-tiw. |
| Neutrogena Body Clear Body Scrub | Salicylic Acid 2% | **Adults & Peds:** Use qd. |
| Neutrogena Body Clear Body Wash | Salicylic Acid 2% | **Adults & Peds:** Use qd. |
| Neutrogena Clear Pore Oil-Controlling Astringent | Salicylic Acid 2% | **Adults & Peds:** Use qd-tid. |
| Neutrogena Maximum Strength Oil Controlling Pads | Salicylic Acid 2% | **Adults & Peds:** Use qd-tid. |
| Neutrogena Multi-Vitamin Acne Treatment | Salicylic Acid 1.5% | **Adults & Peds:** Use prn. |
| Neutrogena Oil Free Acne Stress Control Power Clear scrub | Salicylic Acid 2% | **Adults & Peds:** Use qd. |
| Neutrogena Oil Free Acne Stress Control Power Foam wash | Salicylic Acid 2% | **Adults & Peds:** Use qd. |
| Neutrogena Acne Stress Control 3-in-1 Hydrating Acne Treatment | Salicylic Acid 2% | **Adults & Peds:** Use qd. |
| Neutrogena Oil Free Acne Wash Cleansing Cloths | Salicylic Acid 2% | **Adults & Peds:** Use qd. |
| Neutrogena Oil Free Acne Wash Cream Cleanser | Salicylic Acid 2% | **Adults & Peds:** Use qd. |
| Neutrogena Rapid Clear Acne Defense Lotion | Salicylic Acid 2% | **Adults & Peds:** Use qd-tid. |
| Neutrogena Rapid Clear Acne Eliminating Gel | Salicylic Acid 2% | **Adults & Peds:** Use qd-tid. |
| Neutrogena Skin Clearing Face Wash | Salicylic Acid 1.5% | **Adults & Peds:** Use bid. |
| Neutrogena Skin Clearing Moisturizer | Salicylic Acid 2% | **Adults & Peds:** Use prn. |
| Noxzema Continuous Clean Clarifying Toner | Salicylic Acid 2% | **Adults & Peds:** Use qd-tid. |
| Noxzema Continuous Clean Deep Foaming Cleanser | Salicylic Acid 2% | **Adults & Peds:** Use qd. |
| Noxzema Continuous Clean Microbead Cleanser | Salicylic Acid 2% | **Adults & Peds:** Use qd. |
| Noxzema Triple Clean Pads | Salicylic Acid 2% | **Adults & Peds:** Use qd-tid. |
| Olay Daily Facials Clarity Daily Scrub | Salicylic Acid 2% | **Adults & Peds:** Apply qd. |
| Olay Daily Facials Clarity, Purifying Toner | Salicylic Acid 2% | **Adults & Peds:** Apply qd-tid. |
| Olay Daily Facials Night Cleansing Cloths | Salicylic Acid 2% | **Adults & Peds:** Apply qd-tid. |
| Olay Daily Facials Self-Foaming Discs | Salicylic Acid 2% | **Adults & Peds:** Apply qd-tid. |
| Oxy Balance Daily Cleansing Pads, Sensitive Skin | Salicylic Acid 0.5% | **Adults & Peds:** Use qd-tid. |
| Oxy Balance Deep Pore Cleansing Pads, Gentle | Salicylic Acid 0.5% | **Adults & Peds:** Use qd-tid. |

*(Continued)*

| BRAND | INGREDIENT/STRENGTH | DOSE |
|---|---|---|
| **SALICYLIC ACID** *(Continued)* | | |
| Oxy Deep Pore Acne Medicated Cleansing Pads, Maximum Strength | Salicylic Acid 2% | **Adults & Peds:** Use qd-tid. |
| Oxy Body Wash | Salicylic Acid 2% | **Adults & Peds:** Use qd. |
| Phisoderm Anti-Blemish Gel Facial Wash | Salicylic Acid 2% | **Adults & Peds:** Use qd. |
| St. Ives Medicated Apricot Scrub | Salicylic Acid 2% | **Adults & Peds:** Use qd. |
| Stridex Facewipes to Go with Acne Medication | Salicylic Acid 0.5% | **Adults & Peds:** Use qd-tid. |
| Stridex Triple Action Acne Pads Maximum Strength, Alcohol Free | Salicylic Acid 2% | **Adults & Peds:** Use qd-tid. |
| Stridex Triple Action Acne Pads with Salicylic Acid, Super Scrub | Salicylic Acid 0.5% | **Adults & Peds:** Use qd-tid. |
| Stridex Triple Action Medicated Acne Pads, Sensitive Skin | Salicylic Acid 0.5% | **Adults & Peds:** Use qd-tid. |
| ZAPZYT Acne Wash Treatment For Face & Body | Salicylic Acid 2% | **Adults & Peds:** Use bid. |
| ZAPZYT Acne Wash with Soothing Aloe & Chamomile | Salicylic Acid 2% | **Adults & Peds:** Use qd-tid. |
| ZAPZYT Pore Treatment Gel | Salicylic Acid 2% | **Adults & Peds:** Use qd-tid. |

# ANTIFUNGAL PRODUCTS

| BRAND | INGREDIENT/STRENGTH | DOSE |
|---|---|---|
| **BUTENAFINE** | | |
| Lotrimin Ultra Antifungal cream | Butenafine HCl 1% | **Adults & Peds ≥12 yrs:** Use bid. |
| **CLOTRIMAZOLE** | | |
| Clearly Confident Triple Action Fungus Treatment | Clortrimazole 1% | **Adults:** Apply to affected area qd. |
| FungiCure Anti-Fungal Liquid Spray | Clotrimazole 1% | **Adults & Peds:** Use bid. |
| Lotrimin AF Antifungal Athlete's Foot cream | Clotrimazole 1% | **Adults & Peds≥2 yrs:** Use bid. |
| Lotrimin AF Antifungal Athlete's Foot topical solution | Clotrimazole 1% | **Adults & Peds≥2 yrs:** Use bid. |
| Lotrimin AF For Her Antifungal cream | Clotrimazole 1% | **Adults & Peds≥2 yrs:** Use bid. |
| Swabplus Foot Care Athlete's Foot Relief Swabs | Clotrimazole 1% | **Adults & Peds:** Use bid. |
| **MICONAZOLE** | | |
| Desenex Antifungal liquid spray | Miconazole Nitrate 2% | **Adults:** Apply to affected area bid. |
| Desenex Antifungal powder | Miconazole Nitrate 2% | **Adults:** Apply to affected area bid. |
| Desenex Antifungal spray powder | Miconazole Nitrate 2% | **Adults:** Apply to affected area bid. |
| DiabetAid Antifungal Foot Bath tablets | Miconazole Nitrate 2% | **Adults & Peds ≥2yrs:** Use prn. |
| Diabet-X Antifungal Skin Treatment cream | Miconazole Nitrate 2% | **Adults & Peds ≥2yrs:** Use prn. |
| Lotrimin AF Antifungal Aerosol liquid spray | Miconazole Nitrate 2% | **Adults & Peds ≥2yrs:** Use prn. |
| Lotrimin AF Antifungal Jock Itch aerosol powder spray | Miconazole Nitrate 2% | **Adults & Peds ≥2yrs:** Use prn. |
| Lotrimin AF Antifungal powder | Miconazole Nitrate 2% | **Adults & Peds ≥2yrs:** Use prn. |
| Micatin Antifungal liquid spray | Miconazole Nitrate 2% | **Adults & Peds ≥12yrs:** Use prn. |
| Micatin Antifungal Spray Powder | Miconazole Nitrate 2% | **Adults & Peds ≥12yrs:** Use prn. |
| Micatin Athlete's Foot cream | Miconazole Nitrate 2% | **Adults:** Apply to affected area bid. **Max:** 2 weeks. |
| Micatin Athlete's Foot spray liquid | Miconazole Nitrate 2% | **Adults:** Apply to affected area bid. **Max:** 2 weeks. |
| Micatin Athlete's Foot spray powder | Miconazole Nitrate 2% | **Adults:** Apply to affected area bid. **Max:** 2 weeks. |
| Micatin Jock Itch Spray powder | Miconazole Nitrate 2% | **Adults:** Apply to affected area bid. **Max:** 2 weeks. |
| Micatin Jock Itch Antifungal cream | Miconazole Nitrate 2% | **Adults:** Apply to affected area bid. **Max:** 2 weeks. |
| Neosporin AF Antifungal cream | Miconazole Nitrate 2% | **Adults & Peds ≥12yrs:** Use bid. |
| Neosporin AF Athlete's Foot Spray liquid | Miconazole Nitrate 2% | **Adults & Peds ≥12yrs:** Use bid. |
| Neosporin AF Athlete's Foot Spray powder | Miconazole Nitrate 2% | **Adults & Peds ≥12yrs:** Use bid. |
| Neosporin AF Jock Itch Antifungal cream | Miconazole Nitrate 2% | **Adults & Peds ≥12yrs:** Use qd. **Max: 2 weeks** |
| Zeasorb Super Absorbent Antifungal powder | Miconazole Nitrate 2% | **Adults & Peds:** Use bid. |

*(Continued)*

| BRAND | INGREDIENT/STRENGTH | DOSE |
|---|---|---|
| **TERBINAFINE** | | |
| Lamisil AT Antifungal cream | Terbinafine HCl 1% | **Adults & Peds ≥12yrs:** Use bid. |
| Lamisil AT Antifungal Spray Pump | Terbinafine HCl 1% | **Adults & Peds ≥12yrs:** Use bid. |
| Lamisil AT Athlete's Foot cream | Terbinafine HCl 1% | **Adults & Peds ≥12yrs:** Use bid. |
| Lamisil AT Athlete's Foot gel | Terbinafine HCl 1% | **Adults & Peds ≥12yrs:** Use bid. |
| Lamisil AT Athlete's Foot Spray Pump | Terbinafine HCl 1% | **Adults & Peds ≥12yrs:** Use bid. |
| Lamisil AT for Women cream | Terbinafine HCl 1% | **Adults & Peds ≥12yrs:** Use bid. |
| Lamisil AT Jock Itch cream | Terbinafine HCl 1% | **Adults & Peds ≥12yrs:** Use bid. |
| Lamisil AT Jock Itch Spray Pump | Terbinafine HCl 1% | **Adults & Peds ≥12yrs:** Use bid. |
| **TOLNAFTATE** | | |
| Aftate Antifungal Liquid Spray for Athlete's Foot | Tolnaftate 1% | **Adults:** Apply to affected area qd-bid. |
| FungiCure Anti-Fungal Gel | Tolnaftate 1% | **Adults & Peds:** Use bid. |
| Gold Bond Antifungal Foot Swabs | Tolnaftate 1% | **Adults & Peds:** Use bid. |
| Miracle of Aloe Miracle Anti-Fungal | Tolnaftate 1% | **Adults & Peds ≥12yrs:** Use bid. |
| Swabplus Foot Care Fungus Relief Swabs | Tolnaftate 1% | **Adults & Peds:** Use bid. |
| Tinactin Antifungal Aerosol Deodorant Powder Spray | Tolnaftate 1% | **Adults & Peds:** Use bid. |
| Tinactin Antifungal Aerosol liquid spray | Tolnaftate 1% | **Adults & Peds:** Use bid. |
| Tinactin Antifungal Aerosol powder spray | Tolnaftate 1% | **Adults & Peds:** Use bid. |
| Tinactin Antifungal cream | Tolnaftate 1% | **Adults & Peds:** Use bid. |
| Tinactin Antifungal Foot powder | Tolnaftate 1% | **Adults & Peds:** Use bid. |
| Tinactin Antifungal Jock Itch powder spray | Tolnaftate 1% | **Adults & Peds:** Use bid. |
| **UNDECYLENIC ACID** | | |
| Fungi Nail Anti-fungal Solution | Undecylenic Acid 25% | **Adults & Peds:** Use bid. |
| FungiCure Anti-fungal Liquid | Undecylenic Acid 10% | **Adults & Peds:** Use bid. |
| Tineacide Antifungal cream | Undecylenic Acid 10% | **Adults & Peds ≥12yrs:** Use bid. |

# ANTISEBORRHEAL PRODUCTS

| BRAND | INGREDIENT/STRENGTH | DOSE |
|---|---|---|
| **COAL TAR** | | |
| DHS Tar Dermatological Hair & Scalp Shampoo | Coal Tar 0.5% | **Adults & Peds:** Use biw. |
| DHS Tar Shampoo | Coal Tar 0.5% | **Adults & Peds:** Use at least biw. |
| Neutrogena T/Gel Shampoo Orignial Formula | Coal Tar 0.5% | **Adults & Peds:** Use at least biw. |
| Neutrogena T/Gel Stubborn Itch Shampoo | Coal Tar 0.5% | **Adults & Peds:** Use at least biw. |
| Polytar shampoo | Coal Tar 0.5% | **Adults & Peds:** Use at least biw. |
| Polytar soap | Coal Tar 0.5% | **Adults & Peds:** Apply to affected area prn. |
| Psoriasin Liquid dab-on | Coal Tar 0.66% | **Adults:** Apply to affected area qd-qid. |
| Ionil-T Shampoo | Coal Tar 1% | **Adults & Peds:** Use at least biw. |
| Neutrogena T/Gel Shampoo Extra Strength | Coal Tar 1% | **Adults & Peds:** Use at least biw. |
| Psoriasin gel | Coal Tar 1.25% | **Adults:** Apply to affected area qd-qid. |
| Ionil-T Plus Shampoo | Coal Tar 2% | **Adults & Peds:** Use at least biw. |
| MG217 Ointment | Coal Tar 2% | **Adults & Peds:** Apply to affected area qd-qid. |
| Denorex Therapeutic Protection 2-in-1 shampoo | Coal Tar 2.5% | **Adults & Peds:** Use at least biw. |
| Denorex Therapeutic Protection shampoo | Coal Tar 2.5% | **Adults & Peds:** Use at least biw. |
| MG217 Tar Shampoo | Coal Tar 3% | **Adults & Peds:** Use at least biw. |
| Ionil T Therapeutic Coal Tar Shampoo | Coal Tar 5% | **Adults & Peds:** Use biw. |
| **CORTICOSTEROIDS** | | |
| Aveeno Anti-Itch Cream 1% | Hydrocortisone 1% | **Adults & Peds: ≥2 yrs:** Apply to affected area tid-qid. |
| Cortaid Advanced 12-Hour Anti-Itch Cream | Hydrocortisone 1% | **Adults & Peds: ≥2 yrs:** Apply to affected area tid-qid. |
| Cortaid Intensive Therapy Cooling Spray | Hydrocortisone 1% | **Adults & Peds: ≥2 yrs:** Apply to affected area tid-qid. |
| Cortaid Intensive Therapy Moisturizing Cream | Hydrocortisone 1% | **Adults & Peds: ≥2 yrs:** Apply to affected area tid-qid. |
| Cortaid Maximum Strength Cream | Hydrocortisone 1% | **Adults & Peds: ≥2 yrs:** Apply to affected area tid-qid. |
| Cortaid Maximum Strength Ointment | Hydrocortisone 1% | **Adults & Peds: ≥2 yrs:** Apply to affected area tid-qid. |
| Cortizone-10 Cream | Hydrocortisone 1% | **Adults & Peds: ≥2 yrs:** Apply to affected area tid-qid. |
| Cortizone-10 Maximum Strength Anti-Itch Ointment | Hydrocortisone 1% | **Adults & Peds: ≥2 yrs:** Apply to affected area tid-qid. |
| Cortizone-10 Ointment | Hydrocortisone 1% | **Adults & Peds: ≥2 yrs:** Apply to affected area tid-qid. |
| Cortizone-10 Plus Maximum Strength Cream | Hydrocortisone 1% | **Adults & Peds: ≥2 yrs:** Apply to affected area tid-qid. |
| Cortizone-10 Quick Shot Spray | Hydrocortisone 1% | **Adults & Peds: ≥2 yrs:** Apply to affected area tid-qid. |

*(Continued)*

| BRAND | INGREDIENT/STRENGTH | DOSE |
|---|---|---|
| **PYRITHIONE ZINC** | | |
| Denorex Dandruff Shampoo, Daily Protection | Pyrithione Zinc 2% | **Adults & Peds:** Use biw. |
| Garnier Fructis Fortifying Shampoo, Anti-Dandruff | Pyrithione Zinc 1% | **Adults & Peds:** Use biw. |
| Head & Shoulders Dandruff Conditioner, Dry Scalp Care | Pyrithione Zinc 0.5% | **Adults & Peds:** Use biw. |
| Head & Shoulders Dandruff Conditioner, Extra Fullness | Pyrithione Zinc 0.5% | **Adults & Peds:** Use biw. |
| Head & Shoulders Dandruff Shampoo Plus Conditioner, Smooth & Silky | Pyrithione Zinc 1% | **Adults & Peds:** Use biw. |
| Head & Shoulders Dandruff Shampoo, Citrus Breeze | Pyrithione Zinc 1% | **Adults & Peds:** Use biw. |
| Head & Shoulders Dandruff Shampoo, Classic Clean | Pyrithione Zinc 1% | **Adults & Peds:** Use biw. |
| Head & Shoulders Dandruff Shampoo, Dry Scalp Care | Pyrithione Zinc 1% | **Adults & Peds:** Use biw. |
| Head & Shoulders Dandruff Shampoo, Extra Volume | Pyrithione Zinc 1% | **Adults & Peds:** Use biw. |
| Head & Shoulders Dandruff Shampoo, Ocean Lift | Pyrithione Zinc 1% | **Adults & Peds:** Use biw. |
| Head & Shoulders Dandruff Shampoo, Refresh | Pyrithione Zinc 1% | **Adults & Peds:** Use biw. |
| Head & Shoulders Dandruff Shampoo, Restoring Shine | Pyrithione Zinc 1% | **Adults & Peds:** Use biw. |
| Head & Shoulders Dandruff Shampoo, Sensitive Care | Pyrithione Zinc 1% | **Adults & Peds:** Use biw. |
| Head & Shoulders Dandruff Shampoo, Smooth & Silky | Pyrithione Zinc 1% | **Adults & Peds:** Use biw. |
| L'Oreal VIVE for Men Shampoo, Thickening Anti-Dandruff | Pyrithione Zinc 1% | **Adults & Peds:** Use biw. |
| Neutrogena T-Gel Daily Control Dandruff Shampoo | Pyrithione Zinc 1% | **Adults & Peds:** Use biw. |
| Pantene Pro-V Shampoo + Conditioner, Anti-Dandruff | Pyrithione Zinc 1% | **Adults & Peds:** Use biw. |
| Pert Plus Shampoo Plus Conditioner, Dandruff Control | Pyrithione Zinc 1% | **Adults & Peds:** Use biw. |
| Selsun Blue Dandruff Conditioner | Pyrithione Zinc 0.75% | **Adults & Peds:** Use biw. |
| Suave for Men 2 in 1 Shampoo/Conditioner, Dandruff | Pyrithione Zinc 0.5% | **Adults & Peds:** Use biw. |
| **SALICYLIC ACID** | | |
| Neutrogena T/Gel Conditioner | Salicylic Acid 2% | **Adults & Peds:** Use at least biw. |
| Psoriasin Therapeutic Body Wash With Aloe | Salicylic Acid 3% | **Adults & Peds:** Use biw. |
| Psoriasin Therapeutic Shampoo With Panthenol | Salicylic Acid 3% | **Adults & Peds:** Use biw. |
| Neutrogena T/Sal Shampoo, Scalp Build-up Control | Salicylic Acid 3% | **Adults & Peds:** Use biw. |
| Scalpicin Anti-Itch Liquid Scalp Treatment (Combe) | Salicylic Acid 3% | **Adults:** Apply to affected area qd-qid. |
| **SALICYLIC ACID/SULFUR/COAL TAR** | | |
| Sebex-T Tar Shampoo | Salicylic acid/sulfur/coal tar 2%-2%-5% | **Adults & Peds:** Use qw to biw. |
| Sebutone | Salicylic acid/sulfur/coal tar 2%-2%-1.5% | **Adults & Peds:** Use qw to biw. |

*(Continued)*

| BRAND | INGREDIENT/STRENGTH | DOSE |
|---|---|---|
| **SELENIUM SULFIDE** | | |
| Head & Shoulders Dandruff Shampoo, Intensive Treatment | Selenium Sulfide 1% | **Adults & Peds:** Use biw. |
| Selsun Blue Dandruff Shampoo, Medicated Treatment | Selenium Sulfide 1% | **Adults & Peds:** Use biw. |
| Selsun Blue Dandruff Shampoo | Selenium Sulfide 1% | **Adults & Peds:** Use biw. |
| Plus Conditioner | Selenium Sulfide 1% | **Adults & Peds:** Use biw. |
| Selsun Blue Dandruff Shampoo, | Selenium Sulfide 1% | **Adults & Peds:** Use biw. |
| Balanced Treatment | Selenium Sulfide 1% | **Adults & Peds:** Use biw. |
| Selsun Blue Dandruff Shampoo, Moisturizing Treatment | Selenium Sulfide 1% | **Adults & Peds:** Use biw. |
| **SULFUR/SALICYLIC ACID** | | |
| Sebulex Medicated Dandruff Shampoo | Sulfur/Salicylic Acid 2%-2% | **Adults & Peds:** Use qd. |

# CONTACT DERMATITIS PRODUCTS

| BRAND | INGREDIENT/STRENGTH | DOSE |
|---|---|---|
| **ANTIHISTAMINE** | | |
| Benadryl Extra Strength Gel Pump | Diphenhydramine HCl 2% | **Adults & Peds ≥12 yrs:** Apply to affected area tid-qid. |
| **ANTIHISTAMINE COMBINATION** | | |
| Benadryl Extra Strength Cream | Diphenhydramine HCl/Zinc Acetate 2%-0.1% | **Adults & Peds ≥12 yrs:** Apply to affected area tid-qid. |
| Benadryl Extra Strength Spray | Diphenhydramine HCl/Zinc Acetate 2%-0.1% | **Adults & Peds ≥12 yrs:** Apply to affected area tid-qid. |
| Benadryl Itch Relief Spray | Diphenhydramine HCl/Zinc Acetate 2%-0.1% | **Adults & Peds ≥2 yrs:** Apply to affected area tid-qid. |
| Benadryl Itch Relief Stick | Diphenhydramine HCl/Zinc Acetate 2%-0.1% | **Adults & Peds ≥2 yrs:** Apply to affected area tid-qid. |
| Benadryl Original Cream | Diphenhydramine HCl/Zinc Acetate 1%-0.1% | **Adults & Peds ≥2 yrs:** Apply to affected area tid-qid. |
| CalaGel Anti-Itch Gel | Diphenhydramine HCl/Zinc Acetate/Benzenthonium Chloride 2%-0.215%-15% | **Adults & Peds ≥2 yrs:** Apply to affected area tid-qid. |
| Ivarest Anti-Itch Cream | Diphenhydramine HCl/Calamine 2%-14% | **Adults & Peds ≥2 yrs:** Apply to affected area tid-qid. |
| **ASTRINGENT** | | |
| Domeboro Powder Packets | Aluminum Acetate/Aluminum Sulfate 938mg-1191mg | **Adults & Peds:** Dissolve 1-2 packets and apply to affected area for 15-30 min tid. |
| Ivy-Dry Super Lotion Extra Strength | Zinc Acetate/Benzyl Alcohol 2%-10% | **Adults & Peds: ≥ 6 yrs:** Apply to affected area qd-tid. |
| **ASTRINGENT COMBINATION** | | |
| Aveeno Anti-Itch Cream | Calamine/Pramoxine HCl 3%-1% | **Adults & Peds ≥2 yrs:** Apply to affected area tid-qid. |
| Aveeno Anti-Itch Lotion | Calamine/Pramoxine HCl/ Camphor 3%-1%-0.47% | **Adults & Peds ≥2 yrs:** Apply to affected area tid-qid. |
| Caladryl Clear Lotion | Zinc Acetate/Pramoxine HCl 0.1%-1% | **Adults & Peds ≥2 yrs:** Apply to affected area tid-qid. |
| Caladryl Lotion | Calamine/Pramoxine HCl 8%-1% | **Adults & Peds ≥2 yrs:** Apply to affected area tid-qid. |
| Calamine lotion (generic) | Calamine/Zinc Oxide 6.971%-6.971% | **Adults & Peds:** Apply to affected area prn. |
| **CLEANSER** | | |
| Ivy-Dry Scrub | Polyethylene, sodium lauryl sulfoacetate, cetearyl alcohol, nonoxynol-9, camellia sinensis oil, phenoxyethanol, methylparaben, propylparaben, triethanolamine, carbomer, erythorbic acid, aloe barbadensis extract, tocopheryl acetate extract, tetrasodium EDTA | **Adults & Peds:** Wash affected area prn. |
| IvyStat! Gel/Exfoliant | Hydrocortisone 1% (gel); Cocamidopropyl-sultaine, PEG-4 laurate, cocamide DEA, polyethylene beads, sodium chloride, benzethonium chloride (cleanser) | **Adults & Peds:** Apply to affected area tid-qid. |
| **CORTICOSTEROID** | | |
| Aveeno Anti-Itch Cream 1% | Hydrocortisone 1% | **Adults & Peds ≥2 yrs:** Apply to affected area tid-qid. |
| Cortaid Advanced 12-Hour Anti-Itch Cream | Hydrocortisone 1% | **Adults & Peds ≥2 yrs:** Apply to affected area tid-qid. |
| Cortaid Intensive Therapy Cooling Spray | Hydrocortisone 1% | **Adults & Peds ≥2 yrs:** Apply to affected area tid-qid. |
| Cortaid Intensive Therapy Moisturizing Cream | Hydrocortisone 1% | **Adults & Peds ≥2 yrs:** Apply to affected area tid-qid. |
| Cortaid Maximum Strength Cream | Hydrocortisone 1% | **Adults & Peds ≥2 yrs:** Apply to affected area tid-qid. |

*(Continued)*

| BRAND | INGREDIENT/STRENGTH | DOSE |
|---|---|---|
| Cortaid Maximum Strength Ointment | Hydrocortisone 1% | **Adults & Peds ≥2 yrs:** Apply to affected area tid-qid. |
| Cortizone-10 Cream | Hydrocortisone 1% | **Adults & Peds ≥2 yrs:** Apply to affected area tid-qid. |
| Cortizone-10 Maximum Strength Anti-Itch Ointment | Hydrocortisone 1% | **Adults & Peds ≥2 yrs:** Apply to affected area tid-qid. |
| Cortizone-10 Ointment | Hydrocortisone 1% | **Adults & Peds ≥2 yrs:** Apply to affected area tid-qid. |
| Cortizone-10 Plus Maximum Strength Cream | Hydrocortisone 1% | **Adults & Peds ≥2 yrs:** Apply to affected area tid-qid. |
| Cortizone-10 Quick Shot Spray | Hydrocortisone 1% | **Adults & Peds ≥2 yrs:** Apply to affected area tid-qid. |
| Dermarest Eczema Lotion | Hydrocortisone 1% | **Adults & Peds ≥2 yrs:** Apply to affected area tid-qid. |
| **COUNTERIRRITANT** | | |
| Gold Bond First Aid Quick Spray | Menthol/Benzethonium Chloride 1%-0.13% | **Adults & Peds ≥2 yrs:** Apply to affected area tid-qid. |
| Gold Bond Medicated Maximum Strength Anti-Itch Cream | Menthol/Pramoxine HCl 1%-1% | **Adults & Peds ≥2 yrs:** Apply to affected area tid-qid. |
| Ivy Block Lotion | Bentoquatam 5% | **Adults & Peds ≥2 yrs:** Apply q4h for continued protection. |
| **LOCAL ANESTHETIC** | | |
| Solarcaine Aloe Extra Burn Relief Gel | Lidocaine HCl 0.5% | **Adults & Peds ≥2 yrs:** Apply to affected area tid-qid. |
| Solarcaine Aloe Extra Spray | Lidocaine HCl 0.5% | **Adults & Peds ≥2 yrs:** Apply to affected area tid-qid. |
| Solarcaine First Aid Medicated Spray | Benzocaine/Triclosan 20%-0.13% | **Adults & Peds ≥2 yrs:** Apply to affected area qd-tid. |
| **LOCAL ANESTHETIC COMBINATION** | | |
| Bactine First Aid Liquid | Lidocaine HCl/Benzalkonium Chloride 2.5%-0.13% | **Adults & Peds ≥2 yrs:** Apply to affected area qd-tid. |
| Bactine Pain Relieving Cleansing Spray | Lidocaine HCl/Benzalkonium Chloride 2.5%-0.13% | **Adults & Peds ≥2 yrs:** Apply to affected area qd-tid. |
| Lanacane Maximum Strength Cream | Benzocaine/Benzethonium Chloride 20%-0.2% | **Adults & Peds ≥2 yrs:** Apply to affected area qd-tid. |
| Lanacane Maximum Strength Spray | Benzocaine/Benzethonium Chloride/Ethanol 20%-0.2%-36% | **Adults & Peds ≥2 yrs:** Apply to affected area qd-tid. |
| Lanacane Original Formula Cream | Benzocaine/Benzethonium Chloride 6%-0.2% | **Adults & Peds ≥2 yrs:** Apply to affected area qd-tid. |
| **SKIN PROTECTANT** | | |
| Aveeno Skin Relief Moisturizing Cream | Dimethicone 2.5% | **Adults & Peds:** Apply to affected area prn. |
| **SKIN PROTECTANT COMBINATION** | | |
| Aveeno Itch Relief Lotion | Dimethicone/Menthol 2.5%-0.1% | **Adults & Peds ≥2 yrs:** Apply to affected area tid-qid. |
| Gold Bond Extra Strength Medicated Body Lotion | Dimethicone/Menthol 5%-0.5% | **Adults & Peds:** Apply to affected area prn. |
| Gold Bond Medicated Body Lotion | Dimethicone/Menthol 5%-0.15% | **Adults & Peds:** Apply to affected area prn. |
| Gold Bond Medicated Extra Strength Powder | Zinc Oxide/Menthol 5%-0.8% | **Adults & Peds ≥2 yrs:** Apply to affected area tid-qid. |
| Vaseline Intensive Care Lotion Advanced Healing | Dimethicone 1%-White Petrolatum | **Adults & Peds:** Apply to affected area prn. |

# DANDRUFF PRODUCTS

| BRAND | INGREDIENT/STRENGTH | DOSE |
|---|---|---|
| **COAL TAR** | | |
| Denorex Dandruff Shampoo + Conditioner, Therapeutic | Coal Tar 2.5% | **Adults & Peds:** Use biw. |
| DHS Tar Dermatological Hair & Scalp Shampoo | Coal Tar 0.5% | **Adults & Peds:** Use biw. |
| Ionil T Therapeutic Coal Tar Shampoo | Coal Tar 2.5% | **Adults & Peds:** Use biw. |
| Neutrogena T-Gel Original Shampoo | Coal Tar 0.5% | **Adults & Peds:** Use biw. |
| Neutrogena T-Gel Shampoo, Extra Strength | Coal Tar 1% | **Adults & Peds:** Use biw. |
| Neutrogena T-Gel Shampoo, Stubborn Itch Control | Coal Tar 0.5% | **Adults & Peds:** Use biw. |
| **KETOCONAZOLE** | | |
| Nizoral Anti-Dandruff Shampoo | Ketoconazole 1% | **Adults & Peds ≥12:** Use q3-4d prn. |
| **PYRITHIONE ZINC** | | |
| Denorex Dandruff Shampoo, Daily Protection | Pyrithione Zinc 2% | **Adults & Peds:** Use biw. |
| Garnier Fructis Fortifying Shampoo, Anti-Dandruff | Pyrithione Zinc 1% | **Adults & Peds:** Use biw. |
| Head & Shoulders Dandruff Conditioner, Dry Scalp Care | Pyrithione Zinc 0.5% | **Adults & Peds:** Use biw. |
| Head & Shoulders Dandruff Conditioner, Extra Fullness | Pyrithione Zinc 0.5% | **Adults & Peds:** Use biw. |
| Head & Shoulders Dandruff Shampoo Plus Conditioner, Smooth & Silky | Pyrithione Zinc 1% | **Adults & Peds:** Use biw. |
| Head & Shoulders Dandruff Shampoo, Citrus Breeze | Pyrithione Zinc 1% | **Adults & Peds:** Use biw. |
| Head & Shoulders Dandruff Shampoo, Classic Clean | Pyrithione Zinc 1% | **Adults & Peds:** Use biw. |
| Head & Shoulders Dandruff Shampoo, Dry Scalp Care | Pyrithione Zinc 1% | **Adults & Peds:** Use biw. |
| Head & Shoulders Dandruff Shampoo, Extra Volume | Pyrithione Zinc 1% | **Adults & Peds:** Use biw. |
| Head & Shoulders Dandruff Shampoo, Ocean Lift | Pyrithione Zinc 1% | **Adults & Peds:** Use biw. |
| Head & Shoulders Dandruff Shampoo, Refresh | Pyrithione Zinc 1% | **Adults & Peds:** Use biw. |
| Head & Shoulders Dandruff Shampoo, Restoring Shine | Pyrithione Zinc 1% | **Adults & Peds:** Use biw. |
| Head & Shoulders Dandruff Shampoo, Sensitive Care | Pyrithione Zinc 1% | **Adults & Peds:** Use biw. |
| Head & Shoulders Dandruff Shampoo, Smooth & Silky | Pyrithione Zinc 1% | **Adults & Peds:** Use biw. |
| L'Oreal VIVE for Men Shampoo, Thickening Anti-Dandruff | Pyrithione Zinc 1% | **Adults & Peds:** Use biw. |
| Neutrogena T-Gel Daily Control Dandruff Shampoo | Pyrithione Zinc 1% | **Adults & Peds:** Use biw. |
| Pantene Pro-V Shampoo + Conditioner, Anti-Dandruff | Pyrithione Zinc 1% | **Adults & Peds:** Use biw. |
| Pert Plus Shampoo Plus Conditioner, Dandruff Control | Pyrithione Zinc 1% | **Adults & Peds:** Use biw. |
| Selsun Blue Dandruff Conditioner | Pyrithione Zinc 0.75% | **Adults & Peds:** Use biw. |
| Suave for Men 2 in 1 Shampoo/ Conditioner, Dandruff | Pyrithione Zinc 0.5% | **Adults & Peds:** Use biw. |

*(Continued)*

| BRAND | INGREDIENT/STRENGTH | DOSE |
|---|---|---|
| **SALICYLIC ACID** | | |
| Denorex Dandruff Shampoo, Extra Strength | Salicylic Acid 3% | **Adults & Peds:** Use biw. |
| Neutrogena T/Sal Shampoo, Scalp Build-up Control | Salicylic Acid 3% | **Adults & Peds:** Use biw. |
| Scalpicin Anti-Itch Liquid Scalp Treatment | Salicylic Acid 3% | **Adults & Peds:** Apply to affected area qd-qid. |
| **SELENIUM SULFIDE** | | |
| Head & Shoulders Dandruff Shampoo, Intensive Treatment | Selenium Sulfide 1% | **Adults & Peds:** Use biw. |
| Selsun Blue Dandruff Shampoo, Medicated Treatment | Selenium Sulfide 1% | **Adults & Peds:** Use biw. |
| Selsun Blue Dandruff Shampoo Plus Conditioner | Selenium Sulfide 1% | **Adults & Peds:** Use biw. |
| Selsun Blue Dandruff Shampoo, Balanced Treatment | Selenium Sulfide 1% | **Adults & Peds:** Use biw. |
| Selsun Blue Dandruff Shampoo, Moisturizing Treatment | Selenium Sulfide 1% | **Adults & Peds:** Use biw. |
| **SULFUR/SALICYLIC ACID** | | |
| Sebulex Medicated Dandruff Shampoo | Sulfur/Salicylic Acid 2%-2% | **Adults & Peds ≥12yrs:** Use qd. |

# Diaper Rash Products

| BRAND | INGREDIENT/STRENGTH | DOSE |
|---|---|---|
| **WHITE PETROLATUM** | | |
| Balmex Extra Protective Clear Ointment | White Petrolatum 51% | **Peds:** Apply prn. |
| Vaseline Baby, Baby Fresh Scent | White Petrolatum (strength n/a) | **Peds:** Apply prn. |
| Vaseline Petroleum Jelly | White Petrolatum (strength n/a) | **Peds:** Apply prn. |
| **ZINC OXIDE** | | |
| Aveeno Baby Soothing Relief Diaper Rash Cream | Zinc Oxide 13% | **Peds:** Apply prn. |
| Balmex Diaper Rash Ointment with Aloe & Vitamin E | Zinc Oxide 11.3% | **Peds:** Apply prn. |
| Boudreaux's Butt Paste, Diaper Rash Ointment | Zinc Oxide 16% | **Peds:** Apply prn. |
| California Baby Diaper Rash Cream | Zinc Oxide 12% | **Peds:** Apply prn. |
| Canus Li'l Goat's Milk Ointment | Zinc Oxide 40% | **Peds:** Apply prn. |
| Desitin Diaper Rash Ointment, Creamy, Fresh Scent | Zinc Oxide 10% | **Peds:** Apply prn. |
| Desitin Diaper Rash Ointment, Hypoallergenic | Zinc Oxide 40% | **Peds:** Apply prn. |
| Huggies Diaper Rash Cream | Zinc Oxide 10% | **Peds:** Apply prn. |
| Johnson's Baby Diaper Rash Cream with Zinc Oxide | Zinc Oxide 13% | **Peds:** Apply prn. |
| Mustela Bebe Vitamin Barrier Cream | Zinc Oxide 10% | **Peds:** Apply prn. |
| Mustela Dermo-Pediatrics, Stelactiv Diaper Rash | Zinc Oxide 10% | **Peds:** Apply prn. |
| **COMBINATION PRODUCTS** | | |
| A+D Original Ointment, Diaper Rash and All-Purpose Skincare Formula | Petrolatum/Lanolin 53.4%-15.5% | **Peds:** Apply prn. |
| A+D Zinc Oxide Diaper Rash Cream with Aloe | Dimethicone/Zinc Oxide 1%-10% | **Peds:** Apply prn. |

# Dry Skin Products

| BRAND | INGREDIENTS | DOSE |
|---|---|---|
| AmLactin Moisturizing Cream | Lactic acid, ammonium hydroxide, light mineral oil, glyceryl stearate, PEG-100 stearate, glycerin, propylene glycol, magnesium aluminum silicate, laureth 4, polyoxyl 40 stearate, cetyl alcohol, methylcellulose, methyl and propylparabens | **Adults & Peds:** Apply to affected area bid. |
| AmLactin Moisturizing Lotion | Lactic acid, ammonium hydroxide, light mineral oil, glyceryl stearate, PEG-100 stearate, glycerin, propylene glycol, magnesium aluminum silicate, laureth 4, polyoxyl 40 stearate, cetyl alcohol, methylcellulose, methyl and propylparabens | **Adults & Peds:** Apply to affected area bid. |
| AmLactin XL Moisturizing Lotion Ultraplex Formulation | Ammonium lactate, potassium lactate, sodium lactate, emulsifyin wax, light mineral oil, white petrolatum, glycerin, propylene glycol, stearic acid, xanthum gum, methyl and propylparabens | **Adults & Peds:** Apply to affected area bid. |
| Aquaphor Baby Healing Ointment | Petrolatum, mineral oil, cerein, lanolin alcohol | **Adults & Peds:** Apply to affected area prn. |
| Aquaphor Original Ointment | Petrolatum, mineral oil, cerein, lanolin alcohol | **Adults & Peds:** Apply to affected area prn. |
| Aveeno Baby Essential Moisture Bath | Deionized water, cocamidopropyl betaine, decyl glucoside, PEG 80 sorbitan laurate, disodium lauroamphodiacetate, lauryl methyl gluceth 10 hydroxypropyl dimonium chloride, DI PPG 2 myreth-10 adipate, avena sativa kernel extract (oat), hydrolized oats, hydrolized milk protein, hydroxylated milk glycerides, hydrolized soy protein, PEG 25 soy sterol, coco glucoside, glycerol oleate, PEG 150 distearate, glycol distearate, acrylates/c10-30 alkyl acrylate crosspolymer, glycerin, tetrasodium EDTA, laureth-4, polyquaternium 10, PEG 14m, quaternium 15, sodium hydroxide, citric acid, fragrance | **Adults & Peds:** Apply to affected area prn. |
| Aveeno Baby Moisture Soothing Relief Cream | Glycerin, petrolatum, mineral oil, cetyl alcohol, dimethicone, avena sativa kernel flour, carbomer, sodium hydroxide, ceteareth-6, hydrolyzed milk protein, hydrolyzed oats, hydrolyzed soy protein, PEG-25 soya sterol, tetrasodium EDTA, methylparaben, citric acid, sodium citrate, benzalkonium chloride, benzaldehyde, butylene glycol, butylparaben, ethylparaben, ethyl alcohol, isobutylparaben, phenoxyethanol, propylparaben, stearyl alcohol | **Adults & Peds:** Apply to affected area prn. |
| Aveeno Bath Moisturizing Packets | Colloidal oatmeal 43% | **Adults & Peds:** Bathe in 1 packet for 15-20 min qd-bid. |
| Aveeno Daily Baby Lotion | Dimethicone 1.2% | **Peds:** Apply prn. |
| Aveeno Daily Moisturizer, Ultra-Calming SPF 15 | Avobenzone/octinoxate/octisalate 3%-7.5%-2.% | **Adults:** Use qd. |
| Aveeno Daily Moisturizing Lotion | Dimethicone 1.25% | **Adults:** Use prn. |
| Aveeno Intense Relief Hand Cream | Glycerin, distearyldimonium chloride, petrolatum, isopropyl palmitate, cetyl alcohol, aluminum starch octenylsuccinate, dimethicone, avena sativa kernel flour, benzyl alcohol, sodium chloride | **Adults & Peds:** Apply to affected area prn. |
| Aveeno Moisturizing Bar for Dry Skin | Oat flour, cetearyl alcohol, stearic acid, sodium cocoyl isethionate, water, disodium lauryl sulfosuccinate, glycerin, hydrogenated vegetable oil, titanium dioxide, citric acid, sodium trideceth sulfate, hydrogenated castor oil | **Adults & Peds:** Wash face daily. |
| Aveeno Moisturizing Lotion, Skin Relief | Dimethicone 1.25% | **Adult & Peds:** ≥2 yrs: Use daily. |

*(Continued)*

| BRAND | INGREDIENTS | DOSE |
|---|---|---|
| Aveeno Positively Radiant Moisturizing Lotion | Glycerin, emulsifying wax, ethylhexyl isononanoate, glycine soja (soybean) seed extract, propylene glycol isoceteth-3 acetate, dimethicone, polyacrylamide, cyclomethicone, stearic acid, phenoxyethanol, c13-14 isoparaffin, dimethicone copolyol, benzyl alcohol, titanium dioxide, fragrance, iodopropynyl butylcarbamate, glyceryl laurate, laureth-7, methylparaben, silica, mica, polymethyl-methacrylate, cetearyl alcohol, tetrasodium EDTA, butylparaben, ethylparaben, isobutylparaben, propylparaben, DMDM hydantoin, panthenyl ethyl ether, tocopheryl acetate, panthenol, BHT, citric acid | **Adults:** Apply daily. |
| Aveeno Positively Radiant Daily Moisturizer SPF 15 | Avobenzone/octinoxate/octisalate arachidyl alcohol, arachidyl glucoside, behenyl alcohol, benzalkonium chloride, benzyl alcohol, BHT, bisphenylpropyl dimethicone, butylparaben, c12-15 alkyl benzoate, c13-14 isoparaffin, cetearyl alcohol, cetearyl glucoside, dimethicone, disodium EDTA, ethylene/acrylic acid copolymer, ethylparaben, fragrance, glycerin, glycine soja (soybean) seed extract, iodopropyl butylcarbamate, isobutylparaben, laureth-7, methylparaben, mica, panthenol, phenoxyethanol, polyacrylamide, polymethyl methacrylate, propylparaben, silica, steareth 2, steareth 21, titanium dioxide, water, sodium hydroxide, citric acid | **Adults:** Use daily. |
| Aveeno Positively Radiant Daily Cleansing Pads | Cocamidopropyl betaine, decyl glucoside, glycerin, disodium lauroamphodiacetate, PEG-16 soy sterol, polysorbate 20, PPG-2 hydroxyethyl cocamide, phenoxyethanol, tetrasodium EDTA, butylene glycol, sodium coco PG-dimonium chloride phosphate, sodium citrate, glycine soja (soybean) protein, citric acid, PEG-14m, methylparaben, butylparaben, ethylparaben, isobutylparaben, propylparaben, fragrance | **Adults:** Use daily. |
| Aveeno Positively Smooth Facial Moisturizer | C12-15 alkyl benzoate, cetearyl alcohol, bis-phenylpropyl dimethicone, glycine, soja seed extract, butylene glycol, arachidyl alcohol, glycine soja protein, dimethicone, glycerin, panthenol, polyacrylamide, phenoxyethanol, cetearyl glucoside, behenyl alcohol, benzyl alcohol, C13-14 isoparaffin, DMDM hydantoin, arachidyl glucoside, disodium EDTA, methylparaben, laureth 7, BHT, ethylparaben, butylparaben, propylparaben, isobutylparaben, fragrance, iodopropynyl butylcarbamate | **Adults:** Use prn. |
| Aveeno Positively Smooth Moisturizing Lotion | Glycerin, emulsifying wax, isononanoate, gylcine soja seed extract, propylene glycol isoceteth-3 acetate, dimethicone, cyclomethicone, polyacrylamide, stearic acid, panthenyl ethyl ether, tocopheryl acetate, panthenol, phenoxyethanol, C13-14 isoparaffin, dimethicone copolyol, benzyl alcohol, DMDM hydantoin, glyceryl laurate, laureth 7, methylparaben, cetearyl alcohol, tetrasodium EDTA, butylparaben, ethylparaben, BHT, propylparaben, isobutylparaben, fragrance, iodopropyl butylcarbamate | **Adults:** Use prn. |
| Aveeno Positively Smooth Moisturizing Pads | Cocamidopropyl betaine, decyl glucoside, glycerin, disodium lauroamphodiacetate, PEG-16 soy sterol, polysorbate 20, PPG-2 hydroxyethyl cocamide, phenoxyethanol, tetrasodium EDTA, butylene glycol, sodium coco PG-dimonium chloride phosphate, sodium citrate, glycine soja protein, citric acid, PEG-14M, methylparaben, butylparaben, ethylparaben, isobutylparaben, propylparaben, fragrance | **Adults:** Use daily. |
| Aveeno Radiant Skin Daily Moisturizer with SPF 15 | Octinoxate (octyl methoxycinnamate)/avobenzone 3%/octisalate (octyl salicylate) 7.5%-3%-2% | **Adults:** Use prn. |
| Aveeno Skin Relief Body Wash, Fragrance Free | Glycerin, cocamidopropyl betaine, sodium laureth sulfate, decyl glucoside, oat flour, glycol stearate, sodium lauroampho-PG-acetate phosphate, guar hydroxypropyltrimonium chloride, hydroxypropyltrimonium hydrolyzed wheat protein, PEG 20 glycerides, hydroxypropyltrimonium hydrolyzed wheat starch, PEG 150 pentaerythrityl tetrastearate, PEG 120 methyl glucose trioleate, tetrasodium EDTA, PEG-6 caprylic/capric glyceride, quaternium 15, coriandum sativum extract, elettaria cardamomum seed extract, conmiphora myhrrha extract | **Adults:** Use prn. |

*(Continued)*

| BRAND | INGREDIENTS | DOSE |
|---|---|---|
| Carmol-10 Lotion | Urea 10% | **Adults & Peds:** Apply to affected area qd-bid. |
| Carmol-20 Cream | Urea 20% | **Adults & Peds:** Apply to affected area qd-bid. |
| Cetaphil Daily Facial Moisturizer SPF 15 | Avobenzone 3%, octocrylene 10%, diisopropyl adipate, cyclomethicone, glyceryl stearate, PEG-100 stearate, glycerin, polymethyl methacrylate, phenoxyethanol, benzyl alcohol, acrylates/C10-30 alkyl acrylate crosspolymer, tocopheryl acetate, carbomer 940, disodium EDTA, triethanolamine | **Adults & Peds:** Apply to affected area prn. |
| Cetaphil Moisturizing Cream | Glyceryl polymethacrylate, propylene glycol, petrolatum, dicaprylyl ether, PEG-5 glyceryl stearate, glycerin, dimethicone, dimethiconol, cetyl alcohol, sweet almond oil, acrylates/C10-30 alkylacrylate crosspolymer, tocopheryl acetate, phenoxyethanol, benzyl alcohol, disodium EDTA, sodium hydroxide, lactic acid | **Adults & Peds:** Apply to affected area prn. |
| Cetaphil Moisturizing Lotion | Glycerin, hydrogenated polyisobutene, cetearyl alcohol, ceteareth-20, macadamia nut oil, dimethicone, tocopheryl acetate, stearoxytrimethylsilane, stearyl alcohol, panthenol, farnesol, benzyl alcohol, phenoxyethanol, acrylates/C10-30 alkyl acrylate crosspolymer, sodium hydroxide, citric acid | **Adults & Peds:** Apply to affected area prn. |
| Cetaphil Therapeutic Hand Cream | Glycerin, cetearyl alcohol, oleth-2, PEG-2 stearate, butyrospermum parkii, ethylhexyl methoxycinnamate, dimethicone, stearyl alcohol, glyceryl stearate, PEG-100 stearate, methylparaben, tocopherol, arginine PCA, chlorhexidine digluconate | **Adults & Peds:** Apply to affected area prn. |
| Corn Huskers Lotion | Glycerin, SD alcohol 40, sodium calcium aginate, oleyl sarcosine, methylparaben, guar gum, triethanolamine, calcium sulfate, calcium chloride, fumaric acid, boric acid | **Adults & Peds:** Apply to affected area prn. |
| Eucerin Creme Original | Petrolatum, mineral oil, ceresin, lanolin alcohol, methylchloroisothiazolinone, methylisothiazolinone | **Adults & Peds:** Apply to affected area prn. |
| Eucerin Dry Skin Therapy Calming Crème | Glycerin, cetyl palmitate, mineral oil, caprylic/capric triglyceride, octyldodecanol, cetyl alcohol, glycerly stearate, colloidal oatmeal, dimethicone, PEG-40 stearate, phenoxyethanol, DMDM hydantoin | **Adults:** Apply to affected area prn. |
| Eucerin Dry Skin Therapy Plus Intensive Repair Lotion | Mineral oil, PEG-7 hydrogenated castor oil, isohexadecane, sodium lactate, urea, glycerin, isopropyl palmitate, panthenol, microcrystalline wax, magnesium sulfate, lanolin alcohol, bisabolol, methylchloroisothiazolinone, methylisothiazolinone | **Adults:** Apply to affected area prn. |
| Eucerin Gentle Hydrating Cleanser | Sodium laureth sulfate, cocamidopropyl betaine, disodium cocoamphodiacetate, glycol distearate, PEG-7 glyceryl cocoate, PEG-5 lanolate, cocamide MEA, laureth 10, citric acid, PEG-120 methyl glucose dioleate, lanolin alcohol, imidazolidinyl urea | **Adults:** Use on affected area qd. |
| Eucerin Hand Creme Extensive Repair | Glycerin, urea, glyceryl stearate, stearyl alcohol, dicaprylyl ether, sodium lactate, dimethicone, PEG-40 stearate, cyclopentasiloxane, cyclohexasiloxane, aluminum starch octenylsuccinate, lactic aid, xanthan gum, phenoxyethanol, methylparaben, propylparaben | **Adults & Peds:** Apply to affected area qd. |
| Eucerin Lotion Daily Replenishing | Sunflower seed oil, petrolatum, glycerin, glyceryl stearate SE, octyldodecanol, caprylic/capric triglyceride, stearic acid, dimethicone, cetearyl alcohol, lanolin alcohol, panthenol, tocopheryl acetate, cholesterol, carbomer, disodium EDTA, sodium hydroxide, phenoxyethanol, methylparaben, ethylparaben, propylparaben, butylparaben, BHT | **Adults & Peds:** Apply to affected area qd. |
| Eucerin Lotion Original | Mineral oil, isopropyl myristate, PEG-40 sorbitan peroleate, glyceryl lanolate, sorbitol, propylene glycol, cetyl palmitate, magnesium sulfate, aluminum stearate, lanolin alcohol, BHT, methylchloroisothiazolinone, methylisothiazolinone | **Adults & Peds:** Apply to affected area prn. |
| Eucerin Lotion Plus Intensive Repair | Mineral oil, PEG-7 hydrogenated castor oil, isohexadecane, sodium lactate, urea, glycerin, isopropyl palmitate, panthenol, microcrystalline wax, magnesium sulfate, lanolin alcohol, bisabolol, methylchloroisothiazolinone, methylisothiazolinone | **Adults & Peds:** Apply to affected area prn. |

*(Continued)*

| BRAND | INGREDIENTS | DOSE |
|---|---|---|
| Eucerin Redness Relief Daily Perfecting Lotion | Octinoxate, octisalate, titanium dioxide, glycerin, dimethicone, olyglyceryl-3 methylglucose distearate, butyrospermum parkii, lauroyl lysine, squalane, alcohol Denat., sorbitan stearate, phenoxyethanol, butylene glycol, magnesium aluminum silicate, glycyrrhiza inflata root extract xanthan gum, methylparaben, propylparaben, ethylparaben, iodopropynyl butylcarbamate, trimethoxycaprylylsilane, chromium oxide greens, chromium hydroxide green, ultramarines | **Adults & Peds:** Apply to affected area prn. |
| Eucerin Redness Relief Soothing Cleanser | Glycerin, sodium laureth sulfate, carbomer, phenoxyethanol, PEG-40 hydrogenated castor oil, sodium methyl cocoyl taurate, PEG-7 glyceryl cocoate, decyl glucoside, glycyrrhiza inflata root extract, xanthan gum, sodium hydroxide, methylparaben, butylparaben, ethylparaben, isobutylparaben, propylparaben, benzophenone-4 | **Adults & Peds:** Apply to affected area qam and qpm. |
| Eucerin Redness Relief Soothing Moisture Lotion | Octinoxate, octisalate, titanium dioxide, water, glycerin, dimethicone, polyglyceryl-3 methyl glucose distearate, butyrospermum parkii (shea butter), squalane, alcohol denat., dicaprylyl carbonate, sorbitan stearate, lauroyl lysine, glycyrrhiza inflata root extract, phenoxyethanol, 1,2-hexanediol, magnesium aluminum silicate, xanthan gum, trimethoxycaprylylsilane, methylparaben, propylparaben, ethylparaben | **Adults & Peds:** Apply to affected area qam and qpm. |
| Eucerin Redness Relief Soothing Night Creme | Glycerin, panthenol, caprylic/capric triglyceride, dicaprylyl carbonate, octyldodecanol, C12-15 alkyl benzoate, dimethicone, squalane, tapioca starch, cetearyl alcohol, glyceryl stearate citrate, myristyl myristate, butylene glycol, benzyl alcohol, glycyrrhiza inflata root extract, carbomer, phenoxyethanol, ammonium acryloydimethyltaurate/VP copolymer, sodium hydroxide, methylparaben, propylparaben, iodopropynyl butylcarbamate | **Adults & Peds:** Apply to affected area qpm. |
| Gold Bond Ultimate Healing Skin Therapy Lotion | Glycerin, dimethicone, petrolatum, jojoba esters, cetyl alcohol, aloe barbadensis leaf juice, stearyl alcohol, distearyldimonium chloride, cetearyl alcohol, steareth-21, steareth-2, propylene glycol, chamomilla recutita flower extract, polysorbate 60, stearamidopropyl PG-dimonium chloride phosphate, methyl gluceth 20, tocopheryl acetate, magnesium ascorbyl phosphate, hydrolyzed collagen, hydrolyzed elastin, retinyl palmitate, hydrolyzed jojoba esters, glyceryl stearate, dipotassium EDTA, fragrance, triethanolamine, diazolidinyl urea, methylparaben, propylparaben | **Adults & Peds:** Apply to affected area prn. |
| Gold Bond Ultimate Healing Skin Therapy Powder | Corn starch, sodium bicarbonate, silica, fragrance, ascrobyl palmitate, aloe barbadensis leaf extract, lavandula angustifolia extract, chamomilla recutita flower extract, rosmarinus officinalis leaf extract, acacia farnesiana extract, tocopheryl acetate, retinyl palmitate, polyoxymethylene urea, isopropyl myristate, benzethonium chloride | **Adults & Peds:** Apply to affected area prn. |
| Keri Moisture Therapy Advance Extra Dry Skin Lotion | Glycerin, stearic acid, hydrogenated polyisobutene, petrolatum, cetyl alcohol, aloe barbadensis gel, tocopheryl acetate, cyclopentasiloxane, dimethicone copolyol, glyceryl stearate, PEG-100 stearate, dimethicone, carbomer, methylparaben, PEG-5 soya sterol, magnesium aluminum silicate, propylparaben, phenoxyethanol, disodium EDTA, diazolidinyl urea, sodium hydroxide | **Adults & Peds:** Apply to affected area prn. |
| Keri Moisture Therapy Lotion, Sensitive Skin | Glycerin, stearic acid, hydrogenated polyisobutene, petrolatum, cetyl alcohol, aloe barbadensis gel, tocopheryl acetate, cyclopentasiloxane, dimethicone copolyol, glyceryl stearate, PEG-100 Stearate, dimethicone, carborner, methylparaben, PEG-5 soya sterol, magnesium aluminum silicate, propylparaben, phenoxyethanol, disodium EDTA, diazolidinyl urea, sodium hydroxide | **Adults:** Apply to skin prn. |
| Keri Original Formula Lotion | Mineral oil, propylene glycol, PEG-40 stearate, glyceryl stearate/PEG-100 stearate, PEG-4 dilaurate, laureth-4, lanolin oil, methylparaben, carbomer, propylparaben, fragrance, triethanolamine, dioctyl sodium sulfosuccinate, quaternium-15 | **Adults & Peds:** Apply to affected area prn. |

*(Continued)*

| BRAND | INGREDIENTS | DOSE |
|---|---|---|
| Keri Shea Butter Moisture Therapy Lotion | Mineral oil, glycerin, butyrospermum parkii, PEG-40 stearate, glyceryl stearate, PEG-100 stearate, PEG-4 dilaurate, laureth 4, aloe barbadensis leaf juice, helianthus annuus seed oil, tocopheryl Acetate, carbomer, methylparaben, propylparaben, DMDM hydantoin, iodopropynyl butylcarbamate, sodium hydroxide, sodium EDTA | **Adults & Peds:** Apply to affected area prn. |
| Lac-Hydrin Five Lotion | Lactic acid, ammonium hydroxide, glycerin, petrolatum, squalane, steareth-2, POE-21-stearyl ether, propylene glycol dioctanoate, cetyl alcohol, dimethicone, methylchloroisothiazoline, methylisothiazolinone | **Adults & Peds:** Apply to affected area bid. |
| Lubriderm Advanced Therapy Lotion | Cetyl alcohol, glycerin, mineral oil, cyclomethicone, propylene glycol dicaprylate/dicaprate, PEG-40 stearate, isopropyl isostearate, emulsifying wax, lecithin, carbomer, diazolidinyl urea, titanium dioxide, sodium benzoate, BHT, PPG-3 myristyl ether citrate, disodium EDTA, retinyl palmitate, tocopheryl acetate, sodium pyruvate, fragrance, sodium hydroxide, xanthan gum, iodopropynyl butylcarbamate | **Adults & Peds:** Apply to affected area prn. |
| Lubriderm Daily Moisture Fragrance Free Lotion | Mineral oil, petrolatum, sorbitol solution, stearic acid, lanolin, lanolin alcohol, cetyl alcohol, glyceryl stearate/ PEG-100 stearate, triethanolamine, dimethicone, propylene glycol, microcrystalline wax, PPG-3 myristyl ether citrate, disodium EDTA, methylparaben, ethylparaben, propylparaben, xanthan gum, butylparaben, methyldibromo glutaronitrile | **Adults & Peds:** Apply to affected area prn. |
| Lubriderm Daily Moisture Lotion | Mineral oil, petrolatum, sorbitol solution, stearic acid, lanolin, lanolin alcohol, cetyl alcohol, glyceryl stearate/ PEG-100 stearate, triethanolamine, Dimethicone, Propylene Glycol, microcrystalline wax, PPG-3 myristyl ether citrate, disodium EDTA, methylparaben, ethylparaben, propylparaben, xanthan gum, butylparaben, methyldibromo glutaronitrile | **Adults & Peds:** Apply to affected area prn. |
| Lubriderm Sensitive Skin Lotion | Butylene glycol, mineral oil, petrolatum, glycerin, cetyl alcohol, propylene glycol dicaprylate/dicaprate, PEG-40 stearate, C11-13 isoparaffin, glyceryl stearate, PPG-3 myristyl ether citrate, emulsifying wax, dimethicone, DMDM hydantoin, methylparaben, carbomer 940, ethylparaben, propylparaben, titanium dioxide, disodium EDTA, sodium hydroxide, butylparaben, xanthan gum | **Adults & Peds:** Apply to affected area prn. |
| Lubriderm Daily UV Moisturizer Lotion, SPF 15 | Octyl methoxycinnamate/octyl salicylate/oxybenzone 7.5%-4%-3% | **Adults & Peds: >6 mo:** Apply to skin prn. |
| Lubriderm Lotion, Skin Therapy, Fresh Scent | Mineral oil, petrolatum, sorbitol solution, stearic acid, lanolin, lanolin alcohol, cetyl alcohol, glyceryl stearate, PEG-100 stearate, triethanolamine, dimethicone, propylene glycol, tri (PPG-3 myristyl ether) citrate, disodium EDTA, methylparaben, ethylparaben, propylparaben, fragrance, xanthan gum, butylparaben, methyldibromo glutaronitrile | **Adults:** Apply to skin prn. |
| Lubriderm Skin Nourishing Moisturizing Lotion with Premium Oat Extract | Caprylic/capric triglycerides, glycerin, glyceryl stearate se, petrolatum, camellia oleifera seed oil, castor oil, cocoa butter, cetyl alcohol, wax, brassica alba seed extract, oat kernel extract, cassia angustifolia seed polysaccharide, glyceryl stearate, PEG 100 stearate, diazolidinyl urea, xanthan gum, disodium EDTA, fragrance, iodopropynyl butylcarbamate, soybean oil | **Adults:** Apply to skin prn. |
| Lubriderm Skin Nourishing Moisturizing Lotion with Shea and Cocoa Butters | Glycerin, cetyl alcohol, glyceryl stearate SE, petrolatum, emulsifying wax, caprylic/capric triglyceride, castor oil, octyldodecanol, shea butter, cocoa butter, dimethicone, tocopheryl acetate, diazolidinyl urea, xanthan gum, disodium EDTA, fragrance, iodopropynyl butylcarbamate | **Adults:** Apply to skin prn. |
| Lubriderm Skin Nourishing Moisturizing Lotion with Sea Kelp Extract | Glycerin, glyceryl, stearate SE, cetyl alcohol, emulsifying wax, petrolatum, caprylic/caprictriglyceride, castor oil, octyldodecanol, dimethicone, diazolidinyl urea, propylene glycol, xanthan gum, disodium EDTA, fragrance, giant kelp leaf extract, iodopropynyl butylcarbamate | **Adults:** Apply to skin prn. |
| Neutrogena Body Moisturizer Cream | Glycerin, emulsifying wax, octyl isononanoate, dimethicone, propylene glycol isoceteth-3 acetate, cyclomethicone, stearic acid, aloe extract, matricaria extract, tocopheryl acetate, dimethicone copolyol, acrylates/C10-30 alkyl acrylate crosspolymer, cetearyl alcohol, sodium cetearyl sulfate, sodium sulfate, hydrogenated lanolin, glyceryl laurate, tetrasodium EDTA, triethanolamine, BHT, geranium, dipropylene glycol, propylene glycol, methylparaben, ethylparaben, propylparaben, diazolidinyl urea, benzalkonium chloride | **Adults & Peds:** Apply to affected area prn. |

*(Continued)*

| BRAND | INGREDIENTS | DOSE |
|---|---|---|
| Neutrogena Comforting Butter Body Cream | Glycerin, distearyldimonium chloride, petrolatum, isopropyl palmitate, cetyl alcohol, dimethicone, panthenol, butyrospermum parkii, cocoa (theobroma cacao) seed butter, mango (mangifera indica) seed butter, benzyl alcohol, BHT, sodium chloride, yellow 5, yellow 6, fragrance | **Adults & Peds:** Apply to affected area prn. |
| Neutrogena Comforting Butter Hand Cream | Glycerin, distearyldimonium chloride, petrolatum, isopropyl palmitate, cetyl alcohol, dimethicone, panthenol, butyrospermum parkii, cocoa (theobroma cacao) seed butter, mango (mangifera indica) seed butter, benzyl alcohol, phytantriol, BHT, sodium chloride, yellow 5, yellow 6, fragrance | **Adults & Peds:** Apply to affected area prn. |
| Neutrogena Fragrance-Free Body Moisturizer Cream | Glycerin, emulsifying wax, octyl isononanoate, dimethicone, propylene glycol isoceteth-3 acetate, cyclomethicone, stearic acid, aloe extract, matricaria extract, tocopheryl acetate, dimethicone copolyol, acrylates/C10-30 alkyl acrylate crosspolymer, cetearyl alcohol, sodium cetearyl sulfate, sodium sulfate, hydrogenated lanolin, glyceryl laurate, tetrasodium EDTA, triethanolamine, BHT, geranium, dipropylene glycol, propylene glycol, methylparaben, ethylparaben, propylparaben, diazolidinyl urea, benzalkonium chloride | **Adults & Peds:** Apply to affected area prn. |
| Neutrogena Moisture for Sensitive Skin | Glycerin, octyl palmitate, dimethicone, petrolatum, cyclomethicone, soy sterol, isopropyl isostearate, cetyl alcohol, PEG-10 soya sterol, glyceryl stearate, PEG-100 stearate, C12-15 alkyl benzoate, tetrasodium EDTA, sodium hydroxide, diazolidinyl urea, ethylparaben, methylparaben, propylparaben | **Adults & Peds:** Apply to affected area prn. |
| Neutrogena Norwegian Formula Body/Hand Cream | Glycerin, cetearyl alcohol, stearic acid, sodium cetearyl sulfate, methylparaben, propylparaben, dilauryl thiodipropionate, sodium sulfate | **Adults & Peds:** Apply to affected area qd. |
| Neutrogena Summer Glow Moisturizer | Avobenzone, octisalate, oxybenzone, glycerin, dimethicone, dihydroxy acetone, silica, diethylhexyl 2,6 naphthalate, c12-15 alkyl benzoate, potassium cetyl phosphate, hydroxypropyl starch phosphate, glyceryl stearate, PEG 100 stearate, hydrogenated palm glycerides, cetyl alcohol, BHT, magnesium aluminum silicate, chlorphenesin, tetrasodium EDTA, citric acid, sodium citrate, phenoxyethanol, methylparaben | **Adults & Peds:** Apply to affected area qd. |
| Nivea Body Age Defying Moisturizer | Glycerin, mineral oil, caprylic/capric triglycerides, cetyl alcohol, dimethicone, glyceryl stearate, cyclopentasiloxane, cyclohexasiloxane, PEG 40 stearate, creatine, 1-methylhydantoin-2-imide, ubiquinone, fragrance, carbomer, sodium hydroxide, phenoxyethanol, methylparaben, propylparaben | **Adults:** Apply to damp skin prn. |
| Nivea Body Creamy Conditioning Oil, Very Dry, Flaky Skin | Mineral oil, isopropyl myristate, PEG-40 sorbitan peroleate, glyceryl lanolate, sorbitol, propylene glycol, cetyl palmitate, magnesium sulfate, aluminum stearate, lanolin alcohol, fragrance, BHT, methylchloroisothiazolinone, methylisothiazolinone | **Adults:** Apply to damp skin prn. |
| Nivea Body Original Lotion, Dry Skin | Mineral oil, glycerin, isopropyl palmitate, glyceryl stearate SE, cetearyl alcohol, tocopheryl acetate, isopropyl myristate, simethicone, fragrance, carbomer, hydroxypropyl methylcellulose, sodium hydroxide, methylchloroisothiazolinone, methylisothiazolinone | **Adults:** Apply to damp skin prn. |
| Nivea Body Original Skin Oil, Extremely Dry, Chapped Skin | Mineral oil, triple purified water, lanolin, petrolatum, glyceryl lanolate, lanolin alcohol, fragrance, sodium borate, methylchloroisothiazolinone, methylisothiazolinone | **Adults:** Apply to affected area prn. |
| Nivea Body Sheer Moisture Lotion, Normal to Dry Skin | Mineral oil, caprylic/capric triglycerides, SD alcohol 40B, glycerin, glyceryl stearate citrate, cetearyl alcohol, dimethicone, tocopheryl acetate, panthenol, lanolin alcohol, fragrance, carbomer, sodium hydroxide, methylchloroisothiazolinone, methylisothiazolinone | **Adults:** Apply to damp skin prn. |
| Nivea Smooth Sensation Daily Lotion, Dry Skin | Glycerin, mineral oil, caprylic/capric triglycerides, cetyl alcohol, dimethicone, glyceryl stearate, cyclopentasiloxane, cyclohexasiloxane, PEG 40 stearate, ginkgo biloba leaf extract, tocopheryl acetate, butyrospermum parkii (shea butter), phenoxyethanol, fragrance, carbomer, sodium hydroxide, EDTA, methylparaben, propylparaben | **Adults:** Apply to damp skin prn. |

*(Continued)*

| BRAND | INGREDIENTS | DOSE |
|---|---|---|
| Nivea Creme | Mineral oil, petrolatum, glycerin, isohexadecane, microcrystalline wax, lanolin alcohol, paraffin, panthenol, magnesium sulfate, decyl oleate, octyldodecanol, aluminum stearate, methylchloroisothiazolinone, methylisothiazolinone, citric acid, magnesium stearate | **Adults & Peds:** Apply to affected area prn. |
| Nivea Extra-Enriched Lotion | Mineral oil, isohexadecane, PEG-40 sorbitan peroleate, polyglyceryl-3 diisostearate, glycerin, petrolatum, isopropyl palmitate, cetyl palmitate, tocopheryl acetate (vitamin E), glyceryl lanolate, lanolin alcohol, magnesium sulfate, aluminum stearate, phenoxyethanol, methyldibromo glutaronitrile | **Adults & Peds:** Apply to damp skin after shower or bath. |
| Pacquin Hand & Body Cream | Glycerin, stearic acid, potassium stearate, sodium stearate, cetyl alcohol, fragrance, diisopropyl sebacate, carbomer 940, methylparaben, propylparaben | **Adults & Peds:** Apply to affected area qd. |
| Pacquin Plus Hand & Body Cream | Glycerin, stearic acid, potassium stearate, carbomer, cetyl alcohol, cetyl esters wax, diisopropyl sebacate, lanolin, myristyl lactate, sodium stearate, methyl- and propylparabens | **Adults & Peds:** Apply to affected area qd. |
| Vaseline Dual Action Petroleum Jelly Cream | Petrolatum, glycerin, potassium lactate, stearic acid, butylene glycol, glycol stearate, PEG-100 stearate, caprylic/capric triglyceride, lactic acid, dimethicone, helianthus annuus seed pil or glycine Soya (soybean) oil, glyceryl stearate, tocopheryl acetate, tocopheryl acetate, fragrance, cetyl alcohol, xanthan gum, glycine soja sterols, ethylhexyl methoxyethylcellulose, stearamide AMP, lecithin, methylparaben, DMDM hydantoin, disodium EDTA | **Adults & Peds:** Apply to affected area prn. |
| Vaseline Intensive Care Advanced Healing Fragrance Free | White petrolatum, glycerin, stearic acid, glycol stearate, helianthus annuus seed oil, glycine soja sterol, lecithin, tocopheryl acetate, retinyl palmitate, urea, collagen amino scids, sodium stearoyl lactate, mineral water, sodium PCA, potassium lactate, lactic acid, cetyl alcohol, glyceryl stearate, magnesium aluminum silicate, carbomer, stearamide AMP, ethylene brassylate, trolamine, corn oil, disodium EDTA, methylparaben, DMDM hydantoin, BHT, titanium dioxide | **Adults & Peds:** Apply to affected area prn. |
| Vaseline Intensive Care Cocoa Butter Deep Conditioning Lotion | Petrolatum, glycerin, stearic acid, isopropyl palmitate, glycol stearate, dimethicone, theobroma cacao seed butter (cocoa), butyrospermum parkii (shea butter), helianthus annuus seed oil or glycine soja oil (sunflower, soybean), glycine soja sterol (soybean), tocopheryl acetate (vitamin E acetate), retinyl palmitate (vitamin A palmitate), sodium stearoyl-2-lactylate, collagen amino acids, urea, glyceryl stearate, cetyl alcohol, magnesium aluminum silicate, carbomer, lecithin, mineral water, sodium pca, potassium lactate, lactic acid, fragrance, stearamide amp, triethanolamine, methylparaben, DMDM hydantoin, disodium EDTA, caramel, titanium dioxide | **Adults & Peds:** Apply to affected area prn. |
| Vaseline Intensive Care Firming & Radiance Age-Defying Lotion | Octinoxate 1.25% | **Adults & Peds:** Apply to affected area prn. |
| Vaseline Intensive Care Healthy Body Complexion Nourishing Body Lotion | Glycerin, dimethicone, potassium lactate, stearic acid, sodium hydroxypropyl starch phosphate, mineral oil, glycol stearate, lactic acid, glycine soja sterol, lecithin, petrolatum, tocopheryl acetate, retinyl palmitate, helianthus annuus seed acid, sodium PCA, sodium stearoyl lactate, urea, collagen amino acids, mineral water, glyceryl stearate, cetyl alcohol, magnesium aluminum silicate, fragrance, stearamide AMP, ethylhexyl methoxycinnamate, corn oil, methylparaben, DMDM hydantoin, disodium EDTA, xanthan gum, BHT | **Adults & Peds:** Apply to affected area prn. |
| Vaseline Intensive Care Healthy Hand & Nail Lotion | Potassium lactate, sodium hydroxypropyl starch phosphate, glycerin, stearic acid, mineral oil, dimethicone, lactic acid, glycol stearate, PEG 100 stearate, keratin, glycine soja sterol, lecithin, tocopheryl acetate, retinyl palmitate, healianthus annuus seed oil, sodium PCA, sodium stearoyl lactate, urea, collagen amino acids, ethylhexyl methoxycinnamate, petrolatum, mineral water, cetyl alcohol, stearamide AMP, cyclomethicone, magnesium aluminum silicate, glyceryl stearate, fragrance, xanthan gum, corn oil, BHT, disodium EDTA, methylparaben, DMDM hydantoin | **Adults & Peds:** Apply to affected area prn. |

*(Continued)*

| BRAND | INGREDIENTS | DOSE |
|---|---|---|
| Vaseline Intensive Care Lotion Aloe and Naturals | Glycerin, stearic acid, aloe barbadensis leaf juice glycol stearate, helianthus annuus, seed oil, glycine soja sterols, lecithin, panthenol, tocopheryl acetate, retinyl palmitate, sucumis sativus extract, urea, collagen amino acids, sodium stearoyl lactate, mineral water, sodium PCA, potassium lactate, lactic acid, petrolatum, dimethicone, glyceryl stearate, cetyl alcohol, methyl palmitate, magnesium aluminum silicate, eucalyptus globulus oil, lavandula angustifolia oil, citrus aurantium dulcis oil, carbomer, stearamide AMP, triethanolamine, corn oil, butylene glycol, methylparaben, DMDM hydantoin, disodium EDTA, BHT, titanium dioxide | **Adults & Peds:** Apply to affected area prn. |
| Vaseline Intensive Care Lotion Total Moisture | Glycerin, stearic acid, glycol stearate, petrolatum, helianthus annuus seed oil, glycine soja sterols, lecithin, tocopheryl acetate, retinyl palmitate, urea, collagen amino acids, sodium stearoyl lactylate, mineral water, sodium PCA, potassium lactate, lactic acid, dimethicone, avena sativa kernel flour, keratin, glyceryl stearate, cetyl alcohol, magnesium aluminum silicate, fragrance, carbomer, stearamide AMP, triethanolamine, corn oil, methylparaben, DMDM hydantoin, iodopropynyl butylcarbamate, disodium EDTA, BHT, propylene glycol, titanium dioxide | **Adults & Peds:** Apply to affected area prn. |
| Vaseline Intensive Care Lotion Total Moisture | Glycerin, stearic acid, glycol stearate, petrolatum, helianthus annuus seed oil, glycine soja sterols, lecithin, tocopheryl acetate, retinyl palmitate, urea, collagen amino acids, sodium stearoyl lactylate, mineral water, sodium PCA, potassium lactate, lactic acid, dimethicone, avena sativa kernel flour, keratin, glyceryl stearate, cetyl alcohol, magnesium aluminum silicate, fragrance, carbomer, stearamide AMP, triethanolamine, corn oil, methylparaben, DMDM hydantoin, iodopropynyl butylcarbamate, disodium EDTA, BHT, propylene glycol, titanium dioxide | **Adults & Peds:** Apply to affected area prn. |
| Vaseline Intensive Care Nightly Renewal Light Body Lotion | Glycerin, isopropyl myristate, dimethicone, cyclopentasiloxane, stearic acid, tapioca starch, glycol stearate, helianthus annuus seed oil, glycine soja oil, glycine soja sterol (soybean), vitis vinefera seed extract, lavendula angustifolia extract, lecithin, tocopheryl acetate, retinyl palmitate, urea, collagen amino acids, sodium PCA, potassium lactate, lactic acid, cetyl alcohol, glyceryl stearate, magnesium aluminum silicate, carbomer, methyl methacrylate crosspolymer, fragrance | **Adults & Peds:** Apply to affected area prn. |
| Vaseline Intensive Rescue Moisture Locking Lotion | Glycerin, petrolatum, stearic acid, glycol stearate, dimethicone, isopropyl isostearate, tapioca starch, cetyl alcohol, glyceryl stearate, magnesium aluminum silicate, carbomer, ethylene brassylate, triethanolamine, disodium EDTA, phenoxyethanol, methylparaben, propylparaben, titanium dioxide | **Adults & Peds:** Apply to affected area prn. |
| Vaseline Jelly | White petrolatum | **Adults & Peds:** Apply to affected area prn. |
| Vaseline Petroleum Jelly Cream Deep Moisture | White petrolatum 10% | **Adults & Peds:** Apply to affected area prn. |
| Vaseline Soothing Moisture, Moisturizing Cream w/ Cocoa Butter | Petrolatum, caprylic/capric triglyceride, stearic acid, glycerin, sodium hydroxypropyl starch phosphate, glycol stearate, PEG-100 stearate, cocoa butter, cyclomethicone, glyceryl stearate, cetyl alcohol, tocopheryl acetate, acrylates/C10-30 alkyl acrylate crosspolymer, fragrance, stearamide AMP, potassium hydroxide, DMDM hydantoin, disodium EDTA, iodopropyl butylcarbamate, titanium dioxide | **Adults & Peds:** Apply to affected area prn. |

# Psoriasis Products

| BRAND | INGREDIENT/ STRENGTH | DOSE |
|---|---|---|
| **COAL TAR** | | |
| Denorex Psoriasis Overnight Treatment cream | Coal Tar (strength n/a) | **Adults & Peds:** Apply to affected area qhs prn. |
| Denorex Therapeutic Protection 2-in-1 shampoo | Coal Tar 2.5% | **Adults & Peds:** Use at least biw. |
| Denorex Therapeutic Protection shampoo | Coal Tar 2.5% | **Adults & Peds:** Use at least biw. |
| DHS tar Shampoo | Coal Tar 0.5% | **Adults & Peds:** Use at least biw. |
| Ionil-T Plus Shampoo | Coal Tar 2% | **Adults & Peds:** Use at least biw. |
| Ionil-T Shampoo | Coal Tar 1% | **Adults & Peds:** Use at least biw. |
| MG217 Ointment | Coal Tar 2% | **Adults & Peds:** Apply to affected area qd-qid. |
| MG217 tar Shampoo | Coal Tar 3% | **Adults & Peds:** Use at least biw. |
| Neutrogena T/Gel Shampoo Extra Strength | Coal Tar 1% | **Adults & Peds:** Use at least biw. |
| Neutrogena T/Gel Shampoo Orignial Formula | Coal Tar 0.5% | **Adults & Peds:** Use at least biw. |
| Neutrogena T/Gel Stubborn Itch Shampoo | Coal Tar 0.5% | **Adults & Peds:** Use at least biw. |
| Polytar shampoo | Coal Tar 0.5% | **Adults & Peds:** Use at least biw. |
| Polytar soap | Coal Tar 0.5% | **Adults & Peds:** Apply to affected area prn. |
| Psoriasin Multi-Symptom Psoriasis Relief Gel | Coal Tar 1.25% | **Adults & Peds:** Apply to affected area qd-qid. |
| Psoriasin Multi-Symptom Psoriasis Relief Ointment | Coal Tar 2% | **Adults & Peds:** Apply to affected area qd-qid. |
| **CORTICOSTEROIDS** | | |
| Aveeno Anti-Itch Cream 1% | Hydrocortisone 1% | **Adults & Peds: >2 yrs:** Apply to affected area tid-qid. |
| Cortaid Advanced 12-Hour Anti-Itch Cream | Hydrocortisone 1% | **Adults & Peds: >2 yrs:** Apply to affected area tid-qid. |
| Cortaid Intensive Therapy Cooling Spray | Hydrocortisone 1% | **Adults & Peds: >2 yrs:** Apply to affected area tid-qid. |
| Cortaid Intensive Therapy Moisturizing Cream | Hydrocortisone 1% | **Adults & Peds: >2 yrs:** Apply to affected area tid-qid. |
| Cortaid Maximum Strength Cream | Hydrocortisone 1% | **Adults & Peds: >2 yrs:** Apply to affected area tid-qid. |
| Cortaid Maximum Strength Ointment | Hydrocortisone 1% | **Adults & Peds: >2 yrs:** Apply to affected area tid-qid. |
| Cortizone-10 Cream | Hydrocortisone 1% | **Adults & Peds: >2 yrs:** Apply to affected area tid-qid. |
| Cortizone-10 Maximum Strength Anti-Itch Ointment | Hydrocortisone 1% | **Adults & Peds: >2 yrs:** Apply to affected area tid-qid. |
| Cortizone-10 Ointment | Hydrocortisone 1% | **Adults & Peds: >2 yrs:** Apply to affected area tid-qid. |
| Cortizone-10 Plus Maximum Strength Cream | Hydrocortisone 1% | **Adults & Peds: >2 yrs:** Apply to affected area tid-qid. |
| Cortizone-10 Quick Shot Spray | Hydrocortisone 1% | **Adults & Peds: >2 yrs:** Apply to affected area tid-qid. |
| **SALICYLIC ACID** | | |
| Denorex Psoriasis Daytime Treatment cream | Salicylic Acid 3% | **Adults & Peds:** Apply to affected area qd-qid. |
| Dermarest Psoriasis Medicated Foam Shampoo | Salicylic Acid 3% | **Adults & Peds:** Apply to affected are at least biw. |
| Dermarest Psoriasis Medicated Moisturizer | Salicylic Acid 2% | **Adults & Peds:** Apply to affected area qd-qid. |

*(Continued)*

| BRAND NAME | INGREDIENT/STRENGTH | DOSE |
|---|---|---|
| **SALICYLIC ACID** *(Continued)* | | |
| Dermarest Psoriasis Medicated Scalp Treatment | Salicylic Acid 3% | **Adults & Peds:** Apply to affected area qd-qid. |
| Dermarest Psoriasis Medicated Scalp Treatment mousse | Salicylic Acid 3% | **Adults & Peds:** Apply to affected area qd-qid. |
| Dermarest Psoriasis Medicated Shampoo/Conditioner | Salicylic Acid 3% | **Adults & Peds:** Apply to affected area at least biw. |
| Dermarest Psoriasis Skin Treatment | Salicylic Acid 3% | **Adults & Peds:** Apply to affected area qd-qid. |
| Neutrogena T/Gel Conditioner | Salicylic Acid 2% | **Adults & Peds:** Use at least biw. |
| Psoriasin Therapeutic Body Wash With Aloe | Salicylic Acid 3% | **Adults & Peds:** Use biw. |
| Psoriasin Therapeutic Shampoo With Panthenol | Salicylic Acid 3% | **Adults & Peds:** Use biw. |

# Wound Care Products

| BRAND | INGREDIENT/STRENGTH | DOSE |
|---|---|---|
| **NEOMYCIN/POLYMYXIN B/BACITRACIN COMBINATIONS** | | |
| Bacitracin ointment | Bacitracin<br>500 U | **Adults & Peds:** Apply to affected area qd-tid. |
| Bactine Pain Relieving Protective Antibiotic | Neomycin/polymyxin B/bacitracin/pramoxine<br>3.5mg-10,000 U- 500 U- 1% | **Adults & Peds:** Apply to affected area qd-tid. |
| Neosporin ointment | Neomycin/polymyxin B/bacitracin<br>3.5mg-5,000 U-400 U | **Adults & Peds:** Apply to affected area qd-tid. |
| Neosporin Plus Pain Relief cream | Neomycin/polymyxin B/pramoxine<br>3.5mg-10,000 U-10mg | **Adults & Peds:** Apply to affected area qd-tid. |
| Neosporin Plus Pain Relief ointment | Neomycin/polymyxin B/bacitracin/pramoxine<br>3.5mg-10,000 U-500 U-10mg | **Adults & Peds:** Apply to affected area qd-tid. |
| Neosporin To Go ointment | Neomycin/polymyxin B/bacitracin<br>3.5mg-5,000 U-400 U | **Adults & Peds:** Apply to affected area qd-tid. |
| Polysporin ointment | Polymyxin B/bacitracin<br>10,000 U-500 U | **Adults & Peds:** Apply to affected area qd-tid. |
| **BENZALKONIUM CHLORIDE COMBINATIONS** | | |
| Bactine First Aid Liquid | Lidocaine HCl/benzalkonium chloride<br>2.5%-0.13% | **Adults & Peds: ≥2 yrs:** Apply to affected area qd-tid. |
| Bactine Pain Relieving Cleansing Spray | Lidocaine HCl/benzalkonium chloride<br>2.5%-0.13% | **Adults & Peds: ≥2 yrs:** Apply to affected area qd-tid. |
| Bactine Pain Relieving Cleansing Wipes | Benzalkonium chloride/pramoxine HCl<br>0.13%-1.0% | **Adults & Peds: ≥2 yrs:** Use 1 wipe qd-tid. |
| Band-Aid Antiseptic Foam, One-Step Cleansing and Infection Protection | Benzalkonim chloride 0.13% | **Adults & Peds: ≥3 yrs:** Use tid. |
| **BENZETHONIUM CHLORIDE COMBINATIONS** | | |
| Gold Bond First Aid Quick Spray | Menthol/benzethonium chloride 1%-0.13% | **Adults & Peds: ≥2 yrs:** Apply to affected area tid-qid. |
| Lanacane Maximum Strength Cream | Benzocaine/benzethonium chloride 20%-0.1% | **Adults & Peds: ≥2 yrs:** Apply to affected area tid-qid. |
| **CHLORHEXIDINE GLUCONATE** | | |
| Hibiclens | Chlorhexidine gluconate 4% | **Adults & Peds:** Apply sparingly to affected area prn. |
| **IODINE** | | |
| Betadine Skin Cleanser | Povidone-iodine 7.5% | **Adults & Peds:** Apply to affected area for 3 minutes and rinse. Repeat bid-tid. |
| Betadine solution | Povidone-iodine 10% | **Adults & Peds:** Apply to affected area qd-tid. |
| Betadine spray | Povidone-iodine 10% | **Adults & Peds:** Apply to affected area qd-tid. |
| Betadine Surgical Scrub | Povidone-iodine 7.5% | **Adults & Peds:** Apply to affected area for 5 minutes. |
| Betadine swab | Povidone-iodine 10% | **Adults & Peds:** Apply to affected area qd-tid. |
| **MISCELLANEOUS** | | |
| Aquaphor Healing Ointment | Petrolatum, mineral oil, ceresin, lanolin, alcohol, panthenol, glycerin, bisabolol | **Adults & Peds:** Apply to affected area prn. |
| Curad Spray Bandage | Ethyl acetate, pentane, methylacrylate, menthol, carbon dioxide | **Adults & Peds:** Apply to affected area prn. |
| Proxacol Hydrogen Peroxide | Hydrogen peroxide 3% | **Adults:** Apply to affected area qd-tid. |
| Wound Wash Sterile Saline spray | Sterile sodium chloride solution 0.9% | **Adults & Peds:** Apply to affected area prn. |

# ANTACID AND HEARTBURN PRODUCTS

| BRAND | INGREDIENT/STRENGTH | DOSE |
|---|---|---|
| **ANTACID** | | |
| Alka-Mints chewable tablets | Calcium Carbonate 850mg | **Adults & Peds: ≥12 yrs:** 1-2 tabs q2h. **Max:** 9 tabs q24h. |
| Alka-Seltzer Gold tablets | Citric Acid/Potassium Bicarbonate/ Sodium Bicarbonate 1000mg-344mg-1050mg | **Adults: ≥60 yrs:** 2 tabs q4h prn. **Max:** 6 tabs q24h. **Adults & Peds: ≥12 yrs:** 2 tabs q4h prn. **Max:** 8 tabs q24h. **Peds: ≤12 yrs:** 1 tab q4h prn. **Max:** 4 tabs q24h. |
| Alka-Seltzer Heartburn Relief tablets | Citric Acid/Sodium Bicarbonate 1000mg-1940mg | **Adults: ≥60 yrs:** 2 tabs q4h prn. **Max:** 4 tabs q24h. **Adults & Peds: ≥12 yrs:** 2 tabs q4h prn. **Max:** 8 tabs q24h. |
| Alka-Seltzer tablets, Extra-Strength | Aspirin/Sodium Bicarbonate/Citric Acid 500mg-1985mg-1000mg | **Adults: ≥60 yrs:** 2 tabs q6h prn. **Max:** 3 tabs q24h. **Adults & Peds: ≥12 yrs:** 2 tabs q6h prn. **Max:** 7 tabs q24h. |
| Brioschi powder | Sodium Bicarbonate/Tartaric Acid 2.69g-2.43g/dose | **Adults & Peds: ≥12 yrs:** 1 capful (6g) dissolved in 4-6 oz water q1h. **Max:** 6 doses q24h. |
| Dulcolax Milk of Magnesia liquid | Magnesium Hydroxide 400mg/5mL | **Adults & Peds: ≥12 yrs:** 1-3 tsp (5-15mL) qd-qid. |
| Gaviscon Extra Strength liquid | Aluminum Hydroxide/Magnesium Carbonate 254mg-237.5mg/5mL | **Adults:** 2-4 tsp (10-20mL) qid. |
| Gaviscon Extra Strength tablets | Aluminum Hydroxide/Magnesium Carbonate 160mg-105mg | **Adults:** 2-4 tabs qid. |
| Gaviscon Original chewable tablets | Aluminum Hydroxide/Magnesium Trisilicate 80mg-20mg | **Adults:** 2-4 tabs qid. |
| Gaviscon Regular Strength liquid | Aluminum Hydroxide/Magnesium Carbonate 95mg-358mg/5mL | **Adults:** 2-4 tsp (10-20mL) qid. |
| Gaviscon Acid Breakthrough, chewable tablets | Calcium Carbonate 500mg | **Adults:** 2 tabs prn. |
| Maalox Quick Dissolve Regular Strength chewable tablets | Calcium Carbonate 600mg | **Adults:** 1-2 tabs prn. **Max:** 12 tabs q24h. |
| Mylanta, Children's | Calcium Carbonate 400 mg | **Peds: 6-11 yrs (48-95 lbs):** Take 2 tab prn. **Peds: 2-5 yrs (24-47 lbs):** Take 1 tab prn |
| Mylanta gelcaps | Calcium Carbonate/Magnesium Hydroxide 550mg-125mg | **Adults:** 2-4 caps prn. **Max:** 12 caps q24h. |
| Mylanta Supreme Antacid liquid | Calcium Carbonate/Magnesium Hydroxide 400mg-135mg/5mL | **Adults:** 2-4 tsp (10-20mL) qid. **Max:** 18 tsp (90mL) q24h. |
| Mylanta Ultra chewable tablets | Calcium Carbonate/Magnesium Hydroxide 700mg-300mg | **Adults:** 2-4 tabs qid. **Max:** 10 tabs q24h. |
| Pepto-Bismol Children's Chewable tablets | Calcium Carbonate 400 mg | **Peds: 2-5 yrs (24-47 lbs):** Take 1 tab q24h. **Peds: 6-11 yrs (48-95 lbs):** Take 2 tab q24h. |
| Phillips Milk of Magnesia liquid | Magnesium Hydroxide 400mg/5mL | **Adults & Peds: ≥12 yrs:** 30-60mL qd. **Peds: 6-11 yrs:** 15-30mL qd. **2-5 yrs:** 5-15mL qd. |
| Rolaids Extra Strength Softchews | Calcium Carbonate 1177mg | **Adults:** 2-3 chews q1h prn. **Max:** 6 chews q24h. |
| Rolaids Extra Strength tablets | Calcium Carbonate/Magnesium Hydroxide 675mg-135mg | **Adults:** 2-4 tabs q1h prn. **Max:** 10 tabs q24h. |
| Rolaids tablets | Calcium Carbonate/Magnesium Hydroxide 550mg-110mg | **Adults:** 2-4 tabs q1h prn. **Max:** 12 tabs q24h. |
| Titralac chewable tablets | Calcium Carbonate 420mg | **Adults:** 2 tabs q2-3h prn. **Max:** 19 tabs q24h. |

*(Continued)*

| BRAND | INGREDIENT/STRENGTH | DOSE |
|---|---|---|
| **ANTACID** *(Continued)* | | |
| Tums chewable tablets | Calcium Carbonate 500mg | **Adults:** 2-4 tabs q1h prn. **Max:** 15 tabs q24h. |
| Tums E-X chewable tablets | Calcium Carbonate 750mg | **Adults:** 2-4 tabs prn. **Max:** 10 tabs q24h. |
| Tums Lasting Effects chewable tablets | Calcium Carbonate 500mg | **Adults:** 2 tabs prn. **Max:** 15 tabs q24h. |
| Tums Smooth Dissolve tablets | Calcium Carbonate 750mg | **Adults:** 2-4 tabs prn. **Max:** 10 tabs q24h. |
| Tums Ultra Maximum Strength chewable tablets | Calcium Carbonate 1000mg | **Adults:** 2-3 tabs prn. **Max:** 7 tabs q24h. |
| **ANTACID/ANTIFLATULENT** | | |
| Gas-X with Maalox capsules | Calcium Carbonate/Simethicone 250mg-62.5mg | **Adults:** 2-4 caps prn. **Max:** 8 caps q24h. |
| Gas-X Extra Strength with Maalox capsules | Calcium Carbonate/Simethicone 500mg-125mg | **Adults:** 1-2 caps prn. **Max:** 4 caps q24h. |
| Gelusil chewable tablets | Aluminum Hydroxide/Magnesium Hydroxide/Simethicone 200mg-200mg-20mg | **Adults:** 2-4 tabs qid. |
| Maalox Max liquid | Aluminum Hydroxide/Magnesium Hydroxide/Simethicone 400mg-400mg-40mg/5mL | **Adults & Peds: ≥12 yrs:** 2-4 tsp (10-20mL) qid. **Max:** 12 tsp (60mL) q24h. |
| Maalox Max Quick Dissolve Maximum Strength tablets | Calcium Carbonate/Simethicone 1000mg-60mg | **Adults:** 1-2 tabs prn. **Max:** 8 tabs q24h. |
| Maalox Regular Strength liquid | Aluminum Hydroxide/Magnesium Hydroxide/Simethicone 200mg-200mg-20mg/5mL | **Adults & Peds: ≥12 yrs:** 2-4 tsp (10-20mL) qid. **Max:** 16 tsp (80mL) q24h. |
| Mylanta Maximum Strength liquid | Aluminum Hydroxide/Magnesium Hydroxide/Simethicone 400mg-400mg-40mg/5mL | **Adults & Peds: ≥12 yrs:** 2-4 tsp (10-20mL) qid. **Max:** 12 tsp (60mL) q24h. |
| Mylanta Regular Strength liquid | Aluminum Hydroxide/Magnesium Hydroxide/Simethicone 200mg-200mg-20mg/5mL | **Adults & Peds: ≥12 yrs:** 2-4 tsp (10-20mL) qid. **Max:** 12 tsp (60mL) q24h. |
| Rolaids Multi-Sympton chewable tablets | Calcium Carbonate/Magnesium Hydroxide/Simethicone 675mg-135mg-60mg | **Adults:** 2 tabs qid prn. **Max:** 8 tabs q24h. |
| Titralac Plus chewable tablets | Calcium Carbonate/Simethicone 420mg-21mg | **Adults:** 2 tabs q2-3h prn. **Max:** 19 tabs q24h. |
| **BISMUTH SUBSALICYLATE** | | |
| Maalox Total Stomach Relief Maximum Strength liquid | Bismuth Subsalicylate 525mg/15mL | **Adults & Peds: ≥12 yrs:** 2 tbl (30mL) q1/2-1h. **Max:** 8 tbl (120mL) q24h. |
| Pepto Bismol chewable tablets | Bismuth Subsalicylate 262mg | **Adults & Peds: ≥12 yrs:** 2 tabs q1/2-1h. **Max:** 8 doses q24h. |
| Pepto Bismol caplets | Bismuth Subsalicylate 262mg | **Adults & Peds: ≥12 yrs:** 2 tabs q1/2-1h. **Max:** 8 doses q24h. |
| Pepto Bismol liquid | Bismuth Subsalicylate 262mg/15mL | **Adults & Peds: ≥12 yrs:** 2 tbl (30mL) q1/2-1h. **Max:** 8 doses (240mL) q24h. |
| Pepto Bismol Maximum Strengtth liquid | Bismuth Subsalicylate 525mg/15mL | **Adults & Peds: ≥12 yrs:** 2 tbl (30mL) q1h. **Peds: 9-12 yrs:** 1 tbl (15mL) q1h. **6-9 yrs:** 2 tsp (10mL) q1h. **3-6 yrs:** 1 tsp (5mL). **Max:** of 8 doses (240mL) q24h. |
| **$H_2$-RECEPTOR ANTAGONIST** | | |
| Pepcid AC chewable tablets | Famotidine 10mg | **Adults & Peds: ≥12 yrs:** 1 tab qd. **Max:** 2 tabs q24h. |

*(Continued)*

| BRAND | INGREDIENT/STRENGTH | DOSE |
|---|---|---|
| **$H_2$-RECEPTOR ANTAGONIST** *(Continued)* | | |
| Pepcid AC gelcaps | Famotidine 10mg | **Adults & Peds: ≥12 yrs:** 1 tab qd. **Max:** 2 tabs q24h. |
| Pepcid AC Maximum Strength tablets | Famotidine 20mg | **Adults & Peds: ≥12 yrs:** 1 tab qd. **Max:** 2 tabs q24h. |
| Pepcid AC tablets | Famotidine 10mg | **Adults & Peds: ≥12 yrs:** 1 tab qd. **Max:** 2 tabs q24h. |
| Tagamet HB tablets | Cimetidine 200mg | **Adults & Peds: ≥12 yrs:** 1 tab qd. **Max:** 2 tabs q24h. |
| Zantac 150 tablets | Ranitidine 150mg | **Adults & Peds: ≥12 yrs:** 1 tab qd. **Max:** 2 tabs q24h. |
| Zantac 75 tablets | Ranitidine 75mg | **Adults & Peds: ≥12 yrs:** 1 tab qd. **Max:** 2 tabs q24h. |
| **$H_2$-RECEPTOR ANTAGONIST/ANTACID** | | |
| Pepcid Complete chewable tablets | Famotidine/Calcium Carbonate/ Magnesium Hydroxide 10mg-800mg-165mg | **Adults & Peds: ≥12 yrs:** 1 tab qd. **Max:** 2 tabs q24h. |
| **PROTON PUMP INHIBITOR** | | |
| Prilosec OTC tablets | Omeprazole 20mg | **Adults:** 1 tab qd x 14 days. May repeat 14 day course q 4 months. |

# ANTIDIARRHEAL PRODUCTS

| BRAND | INGREDIENT/STRENGTH | DOSE |
|---|---|---|
| **ABSORBENT AGENTS** | | |
| Equalactin chewable tablets | Calcium Polycarbophil 625mg | **Adults: ≥12 yrs:** 2 tabs q30min prn. **Max:** 6 doses q24h. **Peds: 6-12 yrs:** 1 tab q30min. **Max:** 6 doses q24h. **3-6 yrs:** 1 tab q30min. **Max:** 3 doses q24h. |
| Fibercon caplets | Calcium Polycarbophil 625mg | **Adults: ≥12 yrs:** 2 tabs q30min prn. **Max:** 6 doses q24h. **Peds: 6-12 yrs:** 1 tab q30min. **Max:** 6 doses q24h. **3-6 yrs:** 1 tab q30min. **Max:** 3 doses q24h. |
| Fiber-Lax tablets | Calcium Polycarbophil 625mg | **Adults: ≥12 yrs:** 2 tabs q30min prn. **Max:** 6 doses q24h. **Peds: 6-12 yrs:** 1 tab q30min. **Max:** 6 doses q24h. **3-6 yrs:** 1 tab q30min. **Max:** 3 doses q24h. |
| Kapectolin | Kaolin/Pectin 90g-2g/30mL | **Adults:** 60-120mL after each loose bowel movement. **Peds: ≥12 yrs:** 45-60mL after each loose bowel movement. **6-12 yrs:** 30-60mL after each loose bowel movement. **3-6 yrs:** 15-30mL after each loose bowel movement. |
| Konsyl Fiber tablets | Calcium Polycarbophil 625mg | **Adults: ≥12 yrs:** 2 tabs q30min prn. **Max:** 6 doses q24h. **Peds: 6-12 yrs:** 1 tab q30min. **Max:** 6 doses q24h. **3-6 yrs:** 1 tab q30min. **Max:** 3 doses q24h. |
| Phillip's Fibercaps | Calcium Polycarbophil 625mg | **Adults: ≥12 yrs:** 2 tabs q30min prn. **Max:** 6 doses q24h. **Peds: 6-12 yrs:** 1 tab q30min. **Max:** 6 doses q24h. **3-6 yrs:** 1 tab q30min. **Max:** 3 doses q24h. |
| **ANTIPERISTALTIC AGENTS** | | |
| Imodium A-D caplet | Loperamide HCl 2mg | **Adults: ≥12 yrs:** 2 caplets after first loose stool; 1 caplet after each subsequent loose stool. **Max:** 4 caplets q24h. **Peds: 9-11 yrs (60-95lbs):** 1 caplet after first loose stool; ½ caplet after each subsequent loose stool. **Max:** 3 caplets q24h. **6-8 yrs (48-59 lbs):** 1 caplet after first loose stool; ½ caplet after each subsequent loose stool. **Max:** 2 caplets q24h. |
| Imodium A-D E-Z Chews | Loperamide HCl 2mg | **Adults: ≥12 yrs:** 2 caplets after first loose stool; 1 caplet after each subsequent loose stool. **Max:** 4 caplets q24h. **Peds: 9-11 yrs (60-95 lbs):** 1 caplet after first loose stool; ½ caplet after each subsequent loose stool. **Max:** 3 caplets q24h. **6-8 yrs (48-59 lbs):** 1 caplet after first loose stool; 1/2 caplet after each subsequent loose stool. **Max:** 2 caplets q24h. |
| Imodium A-D liquid | Loperamide HCl 1mg/7.5mL | **Adults: ≥12 yrs:** 30mL (6 tsp) after first loose stool; 15mL (3 tsp) after each subsequent loose stool. **Max:** 60mL (12 tsp) q24h. **Peds: 9-11 yrs (60-95 lbs):** 15mL (3 tsp) after first loose stool; 7.5mL (1½ tsp) after each subsequent loose stool. **Max:** 45mL (9 tsp) q24h. **6-8 yrs (48-59 lbs):**15 mL (3 tsp) after first loose stool; 7.5mL (1½ tsp) after each subsequent loose stool. **Max:** 30mL (6 tsp) q24h. |

*(Continued)*

| BRAND | INGREDIENT/STRENGTH | DOSE |
|---|---|---|
| **ANTIPERISTALTIC/ANTIFLATULENT AGENTS** | | |
| Imodium Advanced caplet | Loperamide HCl/Simethicone 2mg-125mg | **Adults: ≥12 yrs:** 2 caplets after first loose stool; 1 caplet after each subsequent loose stool. **Max:** 4 caplets q24h. **Peds: 9-11 yrs (60-95 lbs):** 1 caplet after first loose stool; 1/2 caplet after each subsequent loose stool. **Max:** 3 caplets q24h. **6-8 yrs (48-59 lbs):** 1 caplet after first loose stool; ½ caplet after each subsequent loose stool. **Max:** 2 caplets q24h. |
| Imodium Advanced chewable tablet | Loperamide HCl/Simethicone 2mg-125mg | **Adults: ≥12 yrs:** 2 caplets after first loose stool; 1 caplet after each subsequent loose stool. **Max:** 4 caplets q24h. **Peds: 9-11 yrs (60-95 lbs):** 1 caplet after first loose stool; ½ caplet after each subsequent loose stool. **Max:** 3 caplets q24h. **6-8 yrs (48-59lbs):** 1 caplet after first loose stool; ½ caplet after each subsequent loose stool. **Max:** 2 caplets q24h. |
| **BISMUTH SUBSALICYLATE** | | |
| Kaopectate caplet | Bismuth Subsalicylate 262mg | **Adults & Peds: ≥12 yrs:** 2 caplets q½-1h. **Max:** 8 doses q24h. |
| Kaopectate Extra Strength liquid | Bismuth Subsalicylate 525mg/15mL | **Adults: ≥12 yrs:** 2 tbl (30mL). **Peds: 9-12 yrs:** 1 tbl (15mL) q1h prn. **6-9 yrs:** 2 tsp (10mL) q1h prn. **3-6 yrs:** 1 tsp (5mL) q1h prn. **Max:** 8 doses q24h. |
| Kaopectate liquid | Bismuth Subsalicylate 262mg/15mL | **Adults: ≥12 yrs:** 2 tbl (30mL). **Peds: 9-12 yrs:** 1 tbl (15mL) q1h prn. **6-9 yrs:** 2 tsp (10mL) q1h prn. **3-6 yrs:** 1 tsp (5mL) q1h prn. **Max:** 8 doses q24h. |
| Pepto Bismol chewable tablets | Bismuth Subsalicylate 262mg | **Adults & Peds: ≥12 yrs:** 2 tabs q½-1h. **Max:** 8 doses q24h. |
| Pepto Bismol caplets | Bismuth Subsalicylate 262mg | **Adults & Peds: ≥12 yrs:** 2 tabs q½-1h. **Max:** 8 doses q24h. |
| Pepto Bismol liquid | Bismuth Subsalicylate 262mg/15mL | **Adults & Peds: ≥12 yrs:** 2 tbl (30mL) q½-1h. **Max:** 8 doses q24h. |
| Pepto Bismol Maximum Strength | Bismuth Subsalicylate 525mg/15mL | **Adults: ≥12 yrs:** 2 tbl (30mL). **Peds: 9-12 yrs:** 1 tbl (15mL) q1h prn. **6-9 yrs:** 2 tsp (10mL) q1h prn. **3-6 yrs:** 1 tsp (5mL) q1h prn. **Max:** 8 doses q24h. |

# ANTIFLATULANT PRODUCTS

| BRAND | INGREDIENT/STRENGTH | DOSE |
|---|---|---|
| **ALPHA-GALACTOSIDASE** | | |
| Beano Food Enzyme Dietary Supplement drops | Alpha-Galactosidase Enzyme 150 GalU | **Adults:** Add 5 drops before meals. |
| Beano Food Enzyme Dietary Supplement tablets | Alpha-Galactosidase Enzyme 150 GalU | **Adults:** Take 3 tabs before meals. |
| **ANTACID/ANTIFLATULENCE** | | |
| Gas-X with Maalox capsules | Calcium Carbonate/Simethicone 250mg-62.5mg | **Adults:** 2-4 caps prn. **Max:** 8 caps q24h. |
| Gas-X Extra Strength with Maalox capsules | Calcium Carbonate/Simethicone 500mg-125mg | **Adults:** 1-2 caps prn. **Max:** 4 caps q24h. |
| Gelusil chewable tablets | Aluminum Hydroxide/Magnesium Hydroxide/Simethicone 200mg-200mg-20mg | **Adults:** 2-4 tabs qid. |
| Maalox Max liquid | Aluminum Hydroxide/Magnesium Hydroxide/Simethicone 400mg-400mg-40mg/5mL | **Adults & Peds: ≥12 yrs:** 2-4 tsp (10-20mL) qid. **Max:** 12 tsp (60mL) q24h. |
| Maalox Max Quick Dissolve Maximum Strength tablets | Calcium Carbonate/Simethicone 1000mg-60mg | **Adults:** 1-2 tabs prn. **Max:** 8 tabs q24h. |
| Maalox Regular Strength liquid | Aluminum Hydroxide/Magnesium Hydroxide/Simethicone 200mg-200mg-20mg/5mL | **Adults & Peds: ≥12 yrs:** 2-4 tsp (10-20mL) qid. **Max:** 16 tsp (80mL) q24h. |
| Mylanta Maximum Strength liquid | Aluminum Hydroxide/Magnesium Hydroxide/Simethicone 400mg-400mg-40mg/5mL | **Adults & Peds: ≥12 yrs:** 2-4 tsp (10-20mL) qid. **Max:** 12 tsp (60mL) q24h. |
| Mylanta Regular Strength liquid | Aluminum Hydroxide/Magnesium Hydroxide/Simethicone 200mg-200mg-20mg/5mL | **Adults & Peds: ≥12 yrs:** 2-4 tsp (10-20mL) qid. **Max:** 24 tsp (120mL) q24h. |
| Rolaids Antacid & Antigas Soft Chews | Calcium Carbonate/Simethicone 1177mg-80mg | **Adults:** 2-3 chews hourly prn. |
| Titralac Plus chewable tablets | Calcium Carbonate/Simethicone 420mg-21mg | **Adults:** 2 tabs q2-3h prn. **Max:** 19 tabs q24h. |
| **SIMETHICONE** | | |
| GasAid Maximum Strength Anti-Gas softgels | Simethicone 125mg | **Adults:** Take 1-2 caps prn and qhs. **Max:** 4 caps q24h. |
| Gas-X Infant Drops | Simethicone 20mg/0.3mL | **Peds: ≥2 yrs (≥24 lbs):** 0.6mL prn. **Peds: <2 yrs (<24 lbs):** 0.3mL prn. **Max:** 6 doses q24h. |
| Gas-X Thin Strips | Simethicone 62.5mg | **Adults:** Allow 2-4 strips to dissolve prn. **Max:** 8 strips q24h. |
| Gas-X Antigas Chewable tablets | Simethicone 80mg | **Adults:** Take 1-2 caps prn and qhs. **Max:** 6 caps q24h. |
| Gas-X Extra Strength Antigas softgels | Simethicone 125mg | **Adults:** Take 1-2 caps prn and qhs. **Max:** 4 caps q24h. |
| Gas-X Maximum Strength Antigas softgels | Simethicone 166mg | **Adults:** Take 1-2 caps prn and qhs. **Max:** 3 caps q24h. |
| Little Tummys Gas Relief drops | Simethicone 20mg/0.3mL | **Peds: ≥2 yrs (≥24 lbs):** 0.6mL prn. **Peds: <2 yrs (<24 lbs):** 0.3mL prn. **Max:** 12 doses q24h. |
| Mylanta Gas Maximum Strength Chewable tablets | Simethicone 125mg | **Adults:** Chew 1-2 tab prn and qhs. |
| Mylanta Gas Regular Strength Chewable tablets | Simethicone 80mg | **Adults:** Chew 1-2 tab prn and qhs. |
| Mylicon Infant's Gas Relief drops | Simethicone 20mg/0.3mL | **Peds: ≥2 yrs (≥24 lbs):** 0.6mL prn. **Peds: <2 yrs (<24 lbs):** 0.3mL prn. **Max:** 12 doses q24h. |

# HEMORRHOIDAL PRODUCTS

| BRAND | INGREDIENT/STRENGTH | DOSE |
|---|---|---|
| **ANESTHETICS/ANESTHETIC COMBINATIONS** | | |
| Tucks Hemorrhoidal Ointment | Pramoxine HCl/Zinc Oxide/Mineral Oil 1%-12.5% - 46.6% | **Adults: ≥12 yrs:** Apply to affected area prn. **Max:** 5 times q24h. |
| Fleet Pain Relief Pre-Moistened Anorectal Pads | Pramoxine HCl/Glycerin 1%-12% | **Adults & Peds: ≥12 yrs:** Apply to affected area prn. **Max:** 5 times q24h. |
| Hemorid Maximum Strength Hemorrhoidal Creme with Aloe | Petrolatum/Mineral Oil/ Pramoxine HCl/Phenylephrine HCl 30%-20%-1%-0.25% | **Adults & Peds: ≥12 yrs:** Apply to affected area qid. |
| Nupercainal ointment | Dibucaine 1% | **Adults & Peds: ≥12 yrs:** Apply to affected area tid-qid. |
| Preparation H Hemorrhoidal Cream, Maximum Strength Pain Relief | Glycerin/Phenylephrine HCl/ Pramoxine HCl/White Petrolatum 14.4%-0.25%-1%-15% | **Adults & Peds: ≥12 yrs:** Apply to affected area tid-qid. |
| Tronolane Anesthetic Hemorrhoid Cream | Pramoxine HCl/Zinc Oxide 1%-5% | **Adults:** Apply to affected area prn. **Max:** 5 times q24h. |
| **BULK-FORMING LAXATIVES** | | |
| Citrucel caplets | Methylcellulose 500mg | **Adults: ≥12 yrs:** 2-4 tabs qd. **Max:** 12 tabs q24h. **Peds: 6-12 yrs:** 1 tabs qd. **Max:** 6 tabs q24h. |
| Citrucel powder | Methylcellulose 2g/tbl | **Adults: ≥12 yrs:** 1 tbl (11.5g) qd-tid. **Peds: 6-12 yrs:** 1/2 tbl (5.75g) qd. |
| Equalactin chewable tablet | Calcium Polycarbophil 625mg | **Adults & Peds: ≥12 yrs:** 2 tabs qd. **Max:** 8 tabs qd. |
| Fibercon caplets | Calcium Polycarbophil 625mg | **Adults & Peds: ≥12 yrs:** 2 tabs qd. **Max:** 8 tabs qd. |
| Fiber-Lax tablets | Calcium Polycarbophil 625mg | **Adults & Peds: ≥12 yrs:** 2 tabs qd. **Max:** 8 tabs qd. |
| Konsyl Easy Mix powder | Psyllium 6g/tsp | **Adults & Peds: ≥12 yrs:** 1 tsp qd-tid. **Max:** 1/2 tsp qd-tid. |
| Konsyl Fiber tablets | Calcium Polycarbophil 625mg | **Adults & Peds: ≥12 yrs:** 2 tabs qd. **Max:** 8 tabs qd. |
| Konsyl Orange powder | Psyllium 3.4g | **Adults & Peds: ≥12 yrs:** 1 tsp qd-tid. **Max:** 1/2 tsp qd-tid. |
| Konsyl Original powder | Psyllium 6g/tsp | **Adults ≥12 yrs:** 1 tsp qd-tid. **Peds: 6-12 yrs:** 1/2 tsp qd-tid. |
| Konsyl-D powder | Psyllium 3.4g/tsp | **Adults ≥12 yrs:** 1 tsp qd-tid. **Peds: 6-12 yrs:** 1/2 tsp qd-tid. |
| Metamucil capsules | Psyllium 0.52g | **Adults & Peds: ≥12 yrs:** 5 caps qd-tid. |
| Metamucil Original Texture powder | Psyllium 3.4g/tbs | **Adults ≥12 yrs:** 1 tbs qd-tid. **Peds: 6-12 yrs:** 1/2 tsp qd-tid. |
| Metamucil Smooth Texture powder | Psyllium 3.4g/tbs | **Adults ≥12 yrs:** 1 tbs qd-tid. **Peds: 6-12 yrs:** 1/2 tsp qd-tid. |
| Metamucil wafers | Psyllium 3.4g/dose | **Adults ≥12 yrs:** 2 wafers qd-tid. **Peds: 6-12 yrs:** 1 wafer qd-tid. |
| **HYDROCORTISONE** | | |
| Tucks Anti-Itch Ointment | Hydrocortisone Acetate 1.12% | **Adults & Peds: ≥12 yrs:** Apply to affected area ud. |
| Cortizone 10 External Anal Itch Relief Cream with Aloe | Hydrocortisone 1% | **Adults & Peds: ≥12 yrs:** Apply to affected area tid-qid. |
| Preparation H Anti-Itch Cream | Hydrocortisone 1.0% | **Adults & Peds: ≥12 yrs:** Apply to affected area tid-qid. |

*(Continued)*

| BRAND | INGREDIENT/STRENGTH | DOSE |
|---|---|---|
| **STOOL SOFTENER** | | |
| Colace capsules | Docusate Sodium 100mg | **Adults: ≥12 yrs:** 1-3 caps qd.<br>**Peds: 2-12 yrs:** 1 cap qd. |
| Colace capsules | Docusate Sodium 50mg | **Adults: ≥12 yrs:** 1-6 caps qd.<br>**Peds: 2-12 yrs:** 1-3 cap qd. |
| Colace liquid | Docusate Sodium 10mg/mL | **Adults: ≥12 yrs:** 5-15mL qd-bid.<br>**Peds: 2-12 yrs:** 5-15mL qd. |
| Colace syrup | Docusate Sodium 60mg/15mL | **Adults: ≥12 yrs:** 15-90mL qd.<br>**Peds: 2-12 yrs:** 5-37.5mL qd. |
| Correctol Stool Softener Laxative soft-gels | Docusate Sodium 100mg | **Adults: ≥12 yrs:** Take 1-3 cap qd.<br>**Peds: 6-12 yrs:** Take 1 cap qd. |
| Docusol Constipation Relief, Mini Enemas | Docusate Sodium 283mg | **Adults: ≥12 yrs:** Take 1-3 units qd.<br>**Peds: 6-12 yrs:** Take 1 unit qd. |
| Dulcolax Stool Softener capsules | Docusate Sodium 100mg | **Adults: ≥12 yrs:** 1-3 caps qd.<br>**Peds: 6-12 yrs:** 1 cap qd. |
| Ex-Lax Stool Softener tablets | Docusate Sodium 100mg | **Adults: ≥12 yrs:** 1-3 caps qd.<br>**Peds: 2-12 yrs:** 1 cap qd. |
| Kaopectate Liqui-Gels | Docusate Calcium 240mg | **Adults & Peds: ≥12 yrs:** 1 cap qd until normal bowel movement. |
| Phillips Stool Softener capsules | Docusate Sodium 100mg | **Adults: ≥12 yrs:** 1-3 caps qd.<br>**Peds: 2-12 yrs:** 1 cap qd. |
| **WITCH HAZEL/WITCH HAZEL COMBINATIONS** | | |
| Hemspray Hemorrhoid Relief Spray | Witch Hazel/Glycerin/ Phenylephrine HCl/Camphor 50%-20%-0.25%-0.15% | **Adults & Peds: ≥12 yrs:** Apply to affected area prn.<br>**Max:** 5 times q24h. |
| Hemspray Hemorrhoid Relief Swabs | Witch Hazel/Glycerin/ Phenylephrine HCl/Camphor 50%-20%-0.25%-0.15% | **Adults & Peds: ≥12 yrs:** Apply to affected area prn.<br>**Max:** 5 times q24h. |
| Preparation H Hemorrhoidal Cooling Gel | Phenylephrine HCl/Witch Hazel 0.25%-50.0% | **Adults & Peds: ≥12 yrs:** Apply to affected area qid. |
| Preparation H Medicated Wipes | Witch Hazel 50% | **Adults & Peds: ≥12 yrs:** Apply to affected area prn.<br>**Max:** 6 times q24h. |
| T.N. Dickinson's Witch Hazel Hemorrhoidal Pads | Witch Hazel 50% | **Adults & Peds: ≥12 yrs:** Apply to affected area prn.<br>**Max:** 6 times q24h. |
| Tucks Hemorrhoidal Pads with Witch Hazel | Witch Hazel 50% | **Adults & Peds: ≥12 yrs:** Apply to affected area prn.<br>**Max:** 6 times q24h. |
| Tucks Hemorrhoidal Towelettes with Witch Hazel | Witch Hazel 50% | **Adults & Peds: ≥12 yrs:** Apply to affected area prn.<br>**Max:** 6 times q24h. |
| **MISCELLANEOUS** | | |
| Preparation H Hemorrhoidal Ointment | Mineral Oil/Petrolatum/ Phenylephrine HCl/Shark Liver Oil 14%-71.9%-0.25%-3.0% | **Adults & Peds: ≥12 yrs:** Apply to affected area qid. |
| Preparation H Hemorrhoidal Suppositories | Cocoa Butter/Phenylephrine HCl/ Shark Liver Oil 85.5%-0.25%-3.0% | **Adults & Peds: ≥12 yrs:** Insert 1 supp qid. |
| Rectal Medicone Suppositories | Phenylephrine HCl 0.25% | **Adults & Peds: ≥12 yrs:** Insert 1 supp tid-qid. |
| Tronolane Suppositories | Hard Fat/Phenylephrine HCl 88.7%-0.25% | **Adults & Peds: ≥12 yrs:** Insert 1 supp tid-qid. |
| Tucks Topical Starch Hemorrhoidal Suppositories | Topical Starch 51% | **Adults & Peds: ≥12 yrs:** Insert 1 supp prn.<br>**Max:** 6 times q24h. |

# LAXATIVE PRODUCTS

| BRAND | INGREDIENT/STRENGTH | DOSE |
|---|---|---|
| **BULK-FORMING** | | |
| Citrucel caplets | Methylcellulose 500mg | **Adults: ≥12 yrs:** 2-4 tabs qd. **Max:** 12 tabs q24h. **Peds: 6-12 yrs:** 1 tabs qd. **Max:** 6 tabs q24h. |
| Citrucel powder | Methylcellulose 2g/tbl | **Adults: ≥12 yrs:** 1 tbl (11.5g) qd tid. **Peds: 6-12 yrs:** 1/2 tbl (5.75g) qd. |
| Equalactin chewable tablet | Calcium Polycarbophil 625mg | **Adults & Peds: ≥12 yrs:** 2 tabs qd. **Max:** 8 tabs qd. |
| Fibercon caplets | Calcium Polycarbophil 625mg | **Adults & Peds: ≥12 yrs:** 2 tabs qd. **Max:** 8 tabs qd. |
| Fiber-Lax tablets | Calcium Polycarbophil 625mg | **Adults & Peds: ≥12 yrs:** 2 tabs qd. **Max:** 8 tabs qd. |
| Konsyl Easy Mix powder | Psyllium 6g/tsp | **Adults: ≥12 yrs:** 1 tsp qd-tid. **Peds: 6-12 yrs:** 1/2 tsp qd-tid. |
| Konsyl Fiber tablets | Calcium Polycarbophil 625mg | **Adults & Peds: ≥12 yrs:** 2 tabs qd. **Max:** 8 tabs qd. |
| Konsyl Orange powder | Psyllium 3.4g | **Adults: ≥12 yrs:** 1 tsp qd-tid. **Peds: 6-12 yrs:** 1/2 tsp qd-tid. |
| Konsyl Original powder | Psyllium 6g/tsp | **Adults: ≥12 yrs:** 1 tsp qd-tid. **Peds: 6-12 yrs:** 1/2 tsp qd-tid. |
| Konsyl-D powder | Psyllium 3.4g/tsp | **Adults: ≥12 yrs:** 1 tsp qd-tid. **Peds: 6-12 yrs:** 1/2 tsp qd-tid. |
| Metamucil capsules | Psyllium 0.52g | **Adults & Peds: ≥12 yrs:** 5 caps qd-tid. |
| Metamucil Original Texture powder | Psyllium 3.4g/tbs | **Adults: ≥12 yrs:** 1 tbs qd-tid. **Peds: 6-12 yrs:** 1/2 tsp qd-tid. |
| Metamucil Smooth Texture powder | Psyllium 3.4g/tbs | **Adults: ≥12 yrs:** 1 tbs qd-tid. **Peds: 6-12 yrs:** 1/2 tsp qd-tid. |
| Metamucil wafers | Psyllium 3.4 g/dose | **Adults: ≥12 yrs:** 2 wafers qd-tid. **Peds: 6-12 yrs:** 1 wafer qd-tid. |
| **HYPEROSMOTICS** | | |
| Fleet Children's Babylax suppositories | Glycerin 2.3g | **Peds: 2-5 yrs:** 1 supp. qd. |
| Fleet Glycerin suppositories | Glycerin 2g | **Adults & Peds: ≥6 yrs:** 1 supp qd. |
| Fleet Liquid Glycerin suppositories | Glycerin 5.6g | **Adults & Peds: ≥6 yrs:** 1 supp qd. |
| Fleet Mineral Oil Enema | Mineral Oil 133mL | **Adults: ≥12 yrs:** 1 bottle (133mL). **Peds: 2-12 yrs:** 1/2 bottle (66.5mL) |
| **HYPEROSMOTIC COMBINATION** | | |
| Fleet Pain Relief Pre-Moistened Anorectal Pads | Glycerin/Pramoxine HCl 12%-1% | **Adults & Peds: ≥12 yrs:** Apply to affected area five times daily. |
| **SALINES** | | |
| Ex-Lax Milk of Magnesia liquid | Magnesium Hydroxide 400mg/5mL | **Adults & Peds: ≥12 yrs:** Take 2-4 tbs hs. **Peds: 6-11 yrs:** 1-2 tbs hs. **2-5 yrs:** 1-3 tbs hs. |
| Fleet Children's Enema | Monobasic Sodium Phosphate/Dibasic Sodium Phosphate 9.5g-3.5g/66mL | **Peds: 5-11 yrs:** 1 bottle (66mL). **2-5 yrs:** 1/2 bottle (33mL). |
| Fleet Enema | Monobasic Sodium Phosphate/Dibasic Sodium Phosphate 19g-7g/133mL | **Adults & Peds: ≥12 yrs:** 1 bottle (133mL). |
| Fleet Phospho-Soda | Monobasic Sodium Phosphate/Dibasic Sodium Phosphate 2.4g-0.9g/5mL | **Adults: ≥12 yrs:** 4-9 tsp qd. **Peds: 10-11 yrs:** 2-4 tsp qd. **5-9 yrs:** 1-2 tsp qd. |
| Magnesium Citrate solution | Magnesium Citrate 1.75gm/30mL | **Adults: ≥12 yrs:** 300mL. **Peds: 6-12 yrs:** 90-210mL. **2-6 yrs:** 60-90mL. |

*(Continued)*

| BRAND | INGREDIENT/STRENGTH | DOSE |
|---|---|---|
| **SALINES** *(Continued)* | | |
| Phillips Antacid/Laxative chewable tablets | Magnesium Hydroxide 311mg | **Adults: ≥ 12 yrs:** 6-8 tabs qd. **Peds: 6-11 yrs:** 3-4 tabs qd. **2-5 yrs:** 1-2 tabs qd. |
| Phillips Soft Chews, Laxative | Magnesium/Sodium 500mg-10 mg | **Adults & Peds: ≥12 yrs:** Take 2-4 tab qd. **Max:** 4 tab q24h. |
| Phillips Cramp-free Laxative caplets | Magnesium 500 mg | **Adults & Peds: ≥12 yrs:** Take 2-4 tab qd. **Max:** 4 tab q24h. |
| Phillips Milk of Magnesia Concentrated liquid | Magnesium Hydroxide 800mg/5mL | **Adults: ≥12 yrs:** 15-30mL qd. **Peds: 6-11 yrs:** 7.5-15mL qd. **2-5 yrs:** 2.5-7.5mL qd. |
| Phillips Milk of Magnesia liquid | Magnesium Hydroxide 400mg/5mL | **Adults: ≥12 yrs:** 30-60mL qd. **Peds: 6-11 yrs:** 15-30mL qd. **2-5 yrs:** 5-15mL qd. |
| **SALINE COMBINATION** | | |
| Phillips M-O liquid | Magnesium Hydroxide/Mineral Oil 300mg-1.25mL/5mL | **Adults: ≥12 yrs:** 30-60mL qd. **Peds: 6-11 yrs:** 5-15mL qd. |
| **STIMULANTS** | | |
| Alophen Enteric Coated Stimulant Laxative pills | Bisacodyl 5mg | **Adults: ≥12 yrs:** Take 1-3 tab qd. **Peds: 6-12 yrs:** Take 1 tab qd. |
| Carter's Laxative, Sodium Free pills | Bisacodyl 5mg | **Adults: ≥12 yrs:** Take 1-3 tab (usually 2 tab) qd. **Peds: 6-12 yrs:** Take 1 tab qd. |
| Castor Oil | Castor Oil | **Adults: ≥12 yrs:** 15-60mL. **Peds: 2-12 yrs:** 5-15mL. |
| Correctol Stimulant Laxative Tablets For Women | Bisacodyl 5mg | **Adults: ≥12 yrs:** Take 1-3 tab qd. **Peds: 6-12 yrs:** Take 1 tab qd. |
| Doxidan capsules | Bisacodyl 5mg | **Adults: ≥12 yrs:** 1-3 caps (usually 2) qd. **Peds: 6-12 yrs:** 1 cap qd. |
| Dulcolax Overnight Relief Laxative tablets | Bisacodyl 5mg | **Adults: ≥12 yrs:** 1-3 tabs (usually 2) qd. **Peds: 6-12 yo:** 1 tab qd. |
| Dulcolax suppository | Bisacodyl 10mg | **Adults: ≥12 yrs:** 1 supp qd. **Peds: 6-12 yrs:** 1/2 supp qd. |
| Dulcolax tablets | Bisacodyl 5mg | **Adults: ≥12 yrs:** 1-3 tabs (usually 2) qd. **Peds: 6-12 yrs:** 1 tab qd. |
| Ex-Lax Maximum Strength tablets | Sennosides 25mg | **Adults: ≥12 yrs:** 2 tabs qd-bid. **Peds: 6-12 yrs:** 1 tab qd-bid. |
| Ex-Lax tablets | Sennosides 15mg | **Adults: ≥12 yrs:** 2 tabs qd-bid. **Peds: 6-12 yrs:** 1 tab qd-bid. |
| Ex-Lax Ultra Stimulant Laxative tablets | Bisacodyl 5mg | **Adults: ≥12 yrs:** 1-3 tabs qd. **Peds: 6-12 yrs:** 1 tab qd. |
| Fleet Bisacodyl suppositories | Bisacodyl 10mg | **Adults: ≥12 yrs:** 1 supp. qd. **Peds: 6-12 yrs:** 1/2 supp. qd. |
| Fleet Stimulant Laxative tablets | Bisacodyl 5mg | **Adults: ≥12 yrs:** 1-3 tabs (usually 2) qd. **Peds: 6-12 yrs:** 1 tab qd. |
| Nature's Remedy caplets | Aloe/Cascara Sagrada 100mg-150mg | **Adults: ≥12 yrs:** 2 tabs qd-bid. **Max:** 4 tabs bid. **Peds: 6-12 yrs:** 1 tab qd-bid. **Max:** 2 tab bid. **2-6 yrs:** 1/2 tab qd-bid. **Max:** 1 tab bid. |
| Perdiem Overnight Relief tablets | Sennosides 15mg | **Adults: ≥12 yrs:** 2 tabs qd-bid. **Peds: 6-12 yrs:** 1 tab qd-bid. |
| Senokot tablets | Sennosides 8.6mg | **Adults: ≥12 yrs:** 2 tabs qd. **Max:** 4 tabs bid. **Peds: 6-12 yrs:** 1 tab qd. **Max:** 2 tabs bid. **2-6 yrs:** 1/2 tab qd. **Max:** 1 tab bid. |
| **STIMULANT COMBINATIONS** | | |
| Perdiem powder | Senna/Psyllium 0.74g-3.25g/6g | **Adults: ≥12 yrs:** 1-2 tsp qd-bid. **Peds:** 6-12 yo: 1 tsp qd-bid. |

*(Continued)*

| BRAND | INGREDIENT/STRENGTH | DOSE |
|---|---|---|
| **STIMULANT COMBINATIONS** *(Continued)* | | |
| Peri-Colace tablets | Sennosides/Docusate 8.6mg-50mg | **Adults: ≥12 yrs:** 2-4 tabs qd. **Peds: 6-12 yrs:** 1-2 tabs qd. **2-6 yrs:** 1 tab qd. |
| SennaPrompt capsules | Sennosides/Psyllium 500mg/9mg | **Adults & Peds: ≥12 yrs:** 5 caps qd-bid. |
| Senokot S tablets | Sennosides/Docusate 8.6mg-50mg | **Adults: ≥12 yrs:** 2 tabs qd. **Max:** 4 tabs bid. **Peds: 6-12 yrs:** 1 tab qd. **Max:** 2 tabs bid. **2-6 yrs:** 1/2 tab qd. **Max:** 1 tab bid. |
| **SURFACTANTS (STOOL SOFTENERS)** | | |
| Colace capsules | Docusate Sodium 100mg | **Adults: ≥12 yrs:** 1-3 caps qd. **Peds: 2-12 yrs:** 1 cap qd. |
| Colace capsules | Docusate Sodium 50mg | **Adults: ≥12 yrs:** 1-6 caps qd. **Peds: 2-12 yrs:** 1-3 caps qd. |
| Colace Glycerin suppositories | Glycerin 2.1g; 1.2g | **Adults: ≥6 yrs:** 2.1g supp qd. **Peds: 2-6 yrs:** 1.2g supp qd. |
| Colace liquid | Docusate Sodium 10mg/mL | **Adults: ≥12 yrs:** 5-15mL qd-bid. **Peds: 2-12 yrs:** 5-15mL qd. |
| Colace syrup | Docusate Sodium 60mg/15mL | **Adults: ≥12 yrs:** 15-90mL qd. **Peds: 2-12 yrs:** 5-37.5mL qd. |
| Correctol Stool Softener Laxative soft-gels | Docusate Sodium 100mg | **Adults: ≥12 yrs:** Take 1-3 cap qd. **Peds: 6-12 yrs:** Take 1 cap qd |
| Docusol Constipation Relief, mini enemas | Docusate Sodium 283mg | **Adults: ≥12 yrs:** Take 1-3 units qd. **Peds: 6-12 yrs:** Take 1 unit qd |
| Dulcolax Stool Softener capsules | Docusate Sodium 100mg | **Adults: ≥12 yrs:** 1-3 caps qd. **Peds: 2-12 yrs:** 1 cap qd. |
| Ex-Lax Stool Softener tablets | Docusate Sodium 100mg | **Adults: ≥12 yrs:** 1-3 caps qd. **Peds: 2-12 yrs:** 1 cap qd. |
| Fleet Sof-Lax tablets | Docusate Sodium 100mg | **Adults: ≥12 yrs:** 1-3 caps qd. **Peds: 2-12 yrs:** 1 cap qd. |
| Kaopectate Liqui-Gels | Docusate Calcium 240mg | **Adults & Peds: ≥12 yrs:** 1 cap qd until normal bowel movement. |
| Phillips Stool Softener capsules | Docusate Sodium 100mg | **Adults: ≥12 yrs:** 1-3 caps qd. **Peds: 2-12 yrs:** 1 cap qd. |

# ARTIFICIAL TEAR PRODUCTS

| BRAND | INGREDIENT/STRENGTH | DOSE |
|---|---|---|
| Akwa Tears Lubricant Eye Drops Hypotonic | Polyvinyl Alcohol/Benzalkonium Chloride 1.4%-0.005% | **Adults:** Instill 1-2 drops to affected eye prn. |
| Akwa Tears Lubricant Ophthalmic Ointment | White Petrolatum/Mineral Oil/ Lanolin 83%-15%-21% | **Adults:** Place 1/4 in oint inside eyelid qd. |
| All Clear AR Maximum Redness Relief Lubricant Eye Drops | Hydroxypropyl Methylcellulose/ Naphazoline HCl/Benzalkonium Chloride | **Adults:** Instill 1-2 drops to affected eye qid. |
| All Clear Redness & Irritation Relief drops | Polyethylene Glycol 300/Naphazoline HCl/ Benzalkonium Chloride | **Adults:** Instill 1-2 drops to affected eye qid. |
| Allergan Lacri-Lube S.O.P. Lubricant Eye Ointment | Mineral Oil/White Petrolatum 42.5%-56.8% | **Adults:** Place 1/4 in oint inside eyelid qd. |
| Allergan Refresh Celluvisc Lubricant Eye Drops | Carboxymethylcellulose Sodium 1% | **Adults:** Instill 1-2 drops to affected eye prn. |
| Allergan Refresh Endura Lubricant Eye Drops | Glycerin/Polysorbate 80. 1%-1% | **Adults:** Instill 1-2 drops to affected eye prn. |
| Allergan Refresh Liquigel Lubricant Eye Drops | Carboxymethylcellulose Sodium 1% | **Adults:** Instill 1-2 drops to affected eye prn. |
| Allergan Refresh Lubricant Eye Drops | Polyvinyl Alcohol/Povidone 1.4%-0.6% | **Adults:** Instill 1-2 drops to affected eye prn. |
| Allergan Refresh Plus Lubricant Eye Drops | Carboxymethylcellulose Sodium 0.5% | **Adults:** Instill 1-2 drops to affected eye prn. |
| Allergan Refresh PM Lubricant Eye Ointment | White Petrolatum/Mineral Oil 57.3%-42.5% | **Adults:** Place 1/4 in oint inside eyelid. |
| Allergan Refresh Tears Lubricant Eye Drops | Carboxymethylcellulose Sodium 0.5% | **Adults:** Instill 1-2 drops to affected eye prn. |
| AMO Blink Contacts Lubricant Eye Drops | Purified water, sodium hyaluronate, sodium chloride, potassium chloride, calcium chloride, magnesium chloride, boric acid | **Adults:** Instill 1-2 drops to affected eye prn. |
| Bausch & Lomb Eye Wash | Boric acid, purified water, sodium borate, sodium chloride | **Adults:** Flush affected eye prn. |
| Bion Tears Lubricant Eye Drops | Dextran 70/Hydroxypropyl Methylcellulose 2910 0.01%-0.3% | **Adults:** Instil 1-2 drops to affected eye prn. |
| CIBA Vision Rewetting Drops | Purified Water, Sodium Chloride, Borate Buffer, Ciba E.A. (carbamide), EDTA (2%), Poloxamer 407, Sorbic Acid (.15%) | **Adults:** Instill 1-2 drops to affected eye prn. |
| Clear Eyes Eye Drops for Dry Eyes | Carboxymethylcellulose Sodium/ Glycerine 1.0%-0.25% | **Adults:** Instill 1-2 drops to affected eye prn. |
| Clear Eyes Eye Drops for Dry Eyes, Plus Removes Redness | Hypromellose/ Glycerine/Naphazoline HCl 0.8%-0.25%-0.012% | **Adults:** Instill 1-2 drops to affected eye prn. |
| Clerz 2 Lubricating and Rewetting Drops | Purified water, sodium chloride, potassium chloride, sodium borate, edetate disodium, hydroxyethylcellulose, boric acid, sorbic acid and poloxamer 407 | **Adults:** Instil 1-2 drops to affected eye 6 times daily. **Max:** 12 drops q24h. |
| GenTeal Mild Dry Eyes drops | Hypromellose 0.2% | **Adults:** Instill 1-2 drops to affected eye prn. |
| GenTeal Moderate Dry Eyes drops | Hypromellose 0.3% | **Adults:** Instill 1-2 drops to affected eye prn. |
| GenTeal PF Dry Eye drops | Hypromellose 0.3% | **Adults:** Instill 1-2 drops to affected eye prn. |
| Moisture Eyes Lubricant Eye Drops | Propylene Glycol 1.0% | **Adults:** Instill 1-2 drops to affected eye prn. |
| Moisture Eyes PM Preservative Free Lubricant Eye Ointment | White Petrolatum/Mineral Oil 80%-20% | **Adults:** Place 1/4 in oint inside eyelid as directed. |
| Murine Plus Tears Plus Eye Drops | Polyvinyl Alcohol/Povidone/ Tetrahydrozoline HCl 0.5%-0.6%-0.05% | **Adults:** Instill 1-2 drops to affected eye qid. |
| Murine Tears Lubricant Eye Drops | Polyvinyl Alcohol/Povidone 0.5%-0.6% | **Adults:** Instill 1-2 drops to affected eye prn. |

*(Continued)*

| BRAND | INGREDIENT/STRENGTH | DOSE |
|---|---|---|
| Muro 128 Sterile Ophthalmic 5% Solution | Sodium Chloride 5% | **Adults:** Instill 1-2 drops to affected eye q3-4h. |
| Muro 128 Sterile Ophthalmic 2% Solution | Sodium Chloride 2% | **Adults:** Instill 1-2 drops to affected eye q3-4h. |
| Optics Laboratory Minidrops Eye Therapy | Polyvinylpyrrolidone/ Polyvinyl Alcohol 6mg-14mg | **Adults:** Instill 1-2 drops to affected eye prn. |
| Rohto V For Eyes Lubricant/Redness Reliever Eye Drops | Naphazoline HCl/ Polysorbate 80 0.012%-0.2% | **Adults:** Instill 1-2 drops to affected eye qid. |
| Rohto Zi For Eyes Lubricant Eye Drops | Povidone 1.8% | **Adults:** Instill 1-2 drops to affected eye prn. |
| Systane Lubricant Eye Drops | Polyethylene Glycol 400/ Propylene Glycol 0.4%-0.3% | **Adults:** Instill 1-2 drops to affected eye prn. |
| Tears Naturale Forte Lubricant Eye Drops | Dextran 70 0.1%, Glycerin 0.2%, Hydroxypropyl Methylcellulose 0.3% | **Adults:** Instill 1-2 drops to affected eye prn. |
| Tears Naturale Free Lubricant Eye Drops | Dextran 70/Hydroxypropyl Methylcellulose 2910 0.1%-0.3% | **Adults:** Instill 1-2 drops to affected eye prn. |
| Tears Naturale II Polyquad Lubricant Eye Drops | Dextran 70/Hydroxypropyl Methylcellulose 2910 0.1%-0.3% | **Adults:** Instill 1-2 drops to affected eye prn. |
| Tears Naturale P.M. Lubricant Eye Ointment | White Petrolatum/Mineral Oil | **Adults:** Place 1/4 in oint inside eyelid qd. |
| TheraTears Liquid Gel Lubricant Eye Gel | Sodium Carboxymethylcellulose 1% | **Adults:** Instill 1-2 drops to affected eye prn. |
| TheraTears Lubricant Eye Drops | Sodium Carboxymethylcellulose 0.25% | **Adults:** Instil 1-2 drops to affected eye prn. |
| Visine Pure Tears Lubricant Eye Drops | Glycerin/Hypromellose/Polyethylene Glycol 400 0.2%-0.2%-1% | **Adults:** Instill 1-2 drops to affected eye prn. |
| Viva-Drops Lubricant Eye Drops | Polysorbate 80 | **Adults:** Instill 1-2 drops to affected eye prn. |

# OPHTHALMIC DECONGESTANT/ANTIHISTAMINE PRODUCTS

| BRAND | INGREDIENT/STRENGTH | DOSE |
|---|---|---|
| **NAPHAZOLINE** | | |
| Clear Eyes drops | Naphazoline HCl/Glycerin 0.012%-0.2% | **Adults:** Instill 1-2 drops to affected eye qid. |
| Clear Eyes ACR Seasonal Relief | Naphazoline HCl/Glycerin/Zinc Sulfate 0.012%-0.2%-0.25% | **Adults:** Instill 1-2 drops to affected eye qid. |
| All Clear AR Maximum Redness Relief Lubricant drops | Naphazoline HCl/Hydroxypropyl Methylcellulose/Benzalkonium Chloride 0.03%-0.5%-0.01% | **Adults:** Instill 1-2 drops to affected eye qid. |
| Clear Eyes for Dry Eyes Plus Removes Redness Drops | Naphazoline HCl/Hypromellose/ Glycerine 0.012%-0.8%-0.25% | **Adults:** Instill 1-2 drops to affected eye prn. |
| Naphcon-A Allergy Relief drops | Naphazoline HCl/Pheniramine Maleate 0.025%-0.3% | **Adults:** Apply 1-2 drops to affected eye qid. |
| Visine-A Allergy Relief drops | Naphazoline HCl/ Pheniramine Maleate 0.025%-0.3% | **Adults & Peds: ≥6 yrs:** Instill 1-2 drops to affected eye qid. |
| Advanced Eye Relief Opcon-A Allergy Relief drops | Naphazoline HCl/ Pheniramine Maleate 0.03%-0.32% | **Adults & Peds: ≥6 yrs:** Instill 1-2 drops to affected eye qid. |
| All Clear Redness & Irritation Relief drops | Naphazoline HCl/Polyethylene Glycol 300/ Benzalkonium Chloride 0.012%-0.2%-0.01% | **Adults:** Instill 1-2 drops to affected eye qid. |
| Rohto V Cool Redness Relief drops | Naphazoline HCl/ Polysorbate 80 0.012%-0.2% | **Adults:** Instill 1-2 drops to affected eye qid. |
| **OXYMETAZOLINE** | | |
| Visine L.R. Redness Reliever drops | Oxymetazoline HCl 0.025% | **Adults & Peds: ≥6 yrs:** Instill 1-2 drops to affected eye prn. |
| **PHENYLEPHRINE** | | |
| Allergan Relief Redness Reliever & Lubricant Eye Drops | Phenylephrine HCl/ Polyvinyl Alcohol 0.12%-1.4% | **Adults:** Instill 1-2 drops to affected eye qid. |
| **TETRAHYDROZOLINE** | | |
| Visine Original drops | Tetrahydrozoline HCl 0.05% | **Adults:** Instill 1-2 drops to affected eye qid. |
| Visine Advanced Redness Reliever drops | Tetrahydrozoline HCl/Polyethylene Glycol 400/ Povidone/Dextran 70 0.05%-1%-1%-0.1% | **Adults:** Instill 1-2 drops to affected eye qid. |
| Murine Tears Plus Eye Drops | Tetrahydrozoline HCl/Polyvinyl Alcohol/ Povidone 0.05%-0.5%-0.6% | **Adults:** Instill 1-2 drops to affected eye qid. |
| Visine A.C. Astringent Redness Reliever drops | Tetrahydrozoline HCl/ Zinc Sulfate 0.05%-0.25% | **Adults:** Instill 1-2 drops to affected eye qid. |

# ALLERGIC RHINITIS PRODUCTS

| BRAND | INGREDIENT/STRENGTH | DOSE |
|---|---|---|
| **ANTIHISTAMINE** | | |
| Alavert 24-Hour Allergy tablets | Loratadine 10mg | **Adults & Peds: ≥6 yrs:** 1 tab qd. **Max:** 1 tab q24h. |
| Benadryl Allergy capsules | Diphenhydramine HCl 25mg | **Adults: ≥12 yrs:** 1-2 caps q4-6h. **Peds:** 6-12 **yrs:** 1 cap q4-6h. **Max:** 6 doses q24h. |
| Benadryl Allergy chewable tablets | Diphenhydramine HCl 12.5mg | **Adults: ≥12 yrs:** 2-4 tabs q4-6h. **Peds:** 6-12 **yrs:** 1-2 tabs q4-6h. **Max:** 6 doses q24h. |
| Benadryl Allergy liquid | Diphenhydramine HCl 12.5mg/5mL | **Adults: ≥12 yrs:** 2-4 tsp (10-20mL) q4-6h. **Peds: 6-12 yrs:** 1-2 tsp (5-10mL) q4-6h. **Max:** 6 doses q24h. |
| Benadryl Allergy Ultratab | Diphenhydramine HCl 25mg | **Adults: ≥12 yrs:** 1-2 tabs q4-6h. **Peds:** 6-12 **yrs:** 1 tab q4-6h. **Max:** 6 doses q24h. |
| Benadryl Children's Allergy fastmelt tablets | Diphenhydramine Citrate HCl 19mg | **Adults: ≥12 yrs:** 2-4 tabs q4-6h. **Peds:** 6-12 tant **Max:** 6 doses q24h. |
| Chlor-Trimeton 4-Hour Allergy tablets | Chlorpheniramine Maleate 4mg | **Adults: ≥12 yrs:** 1 tab q4-6h. **Max:** 6 tabs q24h. **Peds: 6-12 yrs:** 1/2 tab q4-6h. **Max:** 3 tabs q24h. |
| Claritin 24 Hour Allergy tablets | Loratadine 10mg | **Adults & Peds: ≥6 yrs:** 1 tab qd. **Max:** 1 tab q24h. |
| Claritin Children's syrup | Loratadine 5mg/5mL | **Adults: ≥6 yrs:** 2 tsp qd. **Max:** 2 tsp q24h. **Peds: 2-6 yrs:** 1 tsp qd. **Max:** 1 tsp q24h. |
| Claritin RediTabs | Loratadine 10mg | **Adults & Peds: ≥6 yrs:** 1 tab qd. **Max:** 1 tab q24h. |
| Dimetapp ND Children's Allergy liquid | Loratadine 5mg/5mL | **Adults: ≥6 yrs:** 2 tsp qd. **Max:** 2 tsp q24h. **Peds: 2-6 yrs:** 1 tsp qd. **Max:** 1 tsp q24h. |
| Dimetapp ND Children's Allergy tablets | Loratadine 10mg | **Adults & Peds: ≥6 yrs:** 1 tab qd. **Max:** 1 tab q24h. |
| Tavist Allergy tablets | Clemastine Fumarate 1.34mg | **Adults & Peds: ≥12 yrs:** 1 tab q12h. **Max:** 2 tabs q24h. |
| Tavist ND 24-Hour Allergy tablets | Loratadine 10mg | **Adults & Peds: ≥6 yrs:** 1 tab qd. **Max:** 1 tab q24h. |
| Triaminic Allerchews | Loratadine 10mg | **Adults & Peds: ≥6 yrs:** 1 tab qd. **Max:** 1 tab q24h. |
| **ANTIHISTAMINE COMBINATIONS** | | |
| Advil Allergy Sinus caplets | Chlorpheniramine Maleate/ Ibuprofen/Pseudoephedrine HCl 2mg-200mg-30mg | **Adults & Peds: ≥12 yrs:** 1 tab q4-6h. **Max:** 6 tabs q24h. |
| Alavert D-12 Hour Allergy tablets | Loratadine/Pseudoephedrine Sulfate 5mg-120mg | **Adults & Peds: ≥12 yrs:** 1 tab q12h. **Max:** 2 tabs q24h. |
| Benadryl Allergy & Sinus Headache caplets | Diphenhydramine HCl/ Acetaminophen/Phenylephrine HCl/ 12.5mg-325mg-5mg | **Adults & Peds: ≥12 yrs:** 2 caps q4h. **Max:** 12 caps q24h. |
| Benadryl Severe Allergy & Sinus Headache caplets | Diphenhydramine HCl/ Acetaminophen/Phenylephrine HCl 25mg-325mg-5mg | **Adults & Peds: ≥12 yrs:** 2 tabs q4h. **Max:** 12 tabs q24h. |
| Benadryl-D Allergy & Sinus Liquid | Diphenhydramine HCl/ Pseudoephedrine HCl 12.5mg-30mg/5mL | **Adults & Peds: ≥12 yrs:** 2 tsp q4-6h. **Peds: 6-12 yrs:** 1 tsp q4-6h. **Max:** 4 doses q24h. |
| Benadryl-D Allergy & Sinus tablets | Diphenhydramine HCl/ Phenylephrine HCl 25mg-10mg | **Adults & Peds: ≥12 yrs:** 1 tab q4h. **Max:** 6 tabs q24h. |

*(Continued)*

| BRAND | INGREDIENT/STRENGTH | DOSE |
|---|---|---|
| **ANTIHISTAMINE COMBINATIONS** *(Continued)* | | |
| Claritin-D 12 Hour Allergy & Congestion tablets | Loratadine/Pseudoephedrine Sulfate 5mg-120mg | **Adults & Peds: ≥12 yrs:** 1 tab q12h. **Max:** 2 tabs q24h. |
| Claritin-D 24 Hour Allergy & Congestion tablets | Loratadine/Pseudoephedrine Sulfate 10mg-240mg | **Adults & Peds: ≥12 yrs:** 1 tab q12h. **Max:** 1 tabs q24h. |
| Drixoral Allergy Sinus sustained-action tablets | Dexbrompheniramine Maleate/Acetaminophen/ Pseudoephedrine HCl 3mg-500mg-60mg | **Adults & Peds: ≥12 yrs:** 2 tabs q12h. **Max:** 4 tabs q24h. |
| Sinutab Sinus caplets | Acetaminophen/Phenylephrine HCl 325mg-5mg | **Adults & Peds: ≥12 yrs:** 2 tabs q4h. **Max:** 12 tabs q24h. |
| Sudafed PE Sinus & Allergy tablets | Chlorpheniramine Maleate/Phenylephrine HCl 4mg-10mg | **Adults: ≥12 yrs:** 1 tab q4h. **Peds: 6-12 yrs:** 1/2 tab q4h. **Max:** 6 doses q24h. |
| Tylenol Allergy Complete Multi-Symptom Cool Burst caplets | Chlorpheniramine Maleate/ Acetaminophen/Phenylephrine HCl 2mg-325mg-5mg | **Adults & Peds: ≥12 yrs:** 2 tabs q4h. **Max:** 12 tabs q24h. |
| Tylenol Allergy Complete Nighttime Cool Burst caplets | Diphenhydramine HCl/ Acetaminophen/Phenylephrine HCl 25mg-325mg-5mg | **Adults & Peds: ≥12 yrs:** 2 tabs q4h. **Max:** 12 tabs q24h. |
| Tylenol Allergy Complete caplets | Chlorpheniramine Maleate/ Acetaminophen/Pseudoephedrine HCl 2mg-500mg-30mg | **Adults & Peds: ≥12 yrs:** 2 tabs q4-6h. **Max:** 8 tabs q24h. |
| Tylenol Allergy Complete Night Time caplets | Diphenhydramine HCl/ Acetaminophen/Pseudoephedrine HCl 25mg-500mg-30mg | **Adults & Peds: ≥12 yrs:** 2 tabs q4-6h. **Max:** 8 tabs q24h. |
| Tylenol Severe Allergy caplets | Diphenhydramine HCl/ Acetaminophen 12.5mg-500mg | **Adults & Peds: ≥12 yrs:** 2 tabs q4-6h. **Max:** 8 tabs q24h. |
| **TOPICAL NASAL DECONGESTANTS** | | |
| 4-Way Fast Acting Nasal Decongestant Spray | Phenylephrine HCl 1% | **Adults & Peds: ≥12 yrs:** Instill 2-3 sprays per nostril q4h. |
| 4-Way Nasal Decongestant Spray, 12 Hour | Phenylephrine HCl 1% | **Adults & Peds: ≥12 yrs:** Instill 2-3 sprays per nostril q4h. |
| 4-Way No Drip Nasal Decongestant Spray | Phenylephrine HCl 1% | **Adults & Peds: ≥12 yrs:** Instill 2-3 sprays per nostril q4h. |
| Afrin Extra Moisturizing Nasal Spray | Oxymetazoline HCl 0.05% | **Adults & Peds: ≥6 yrs:** Instill 2-3 sprays per nostril q10-12h. |
| Afrin No Drip Nasal Spray | Oxymetazoline HCl 0.05% | **Adults & Peds: ≥6 yrs:** Instill 2-3 sprays per nostril q10-12h. |
| Afrin No Drip Sinus Nasal Spray | Oxymetazoline HCl 0.05% | **Adults & Peds: ≥6 yrs:** Instill 2-3 sprays per nostril q10-12h. |
| Afrin Original Nasal Spray | Oxymetazoline HCl 0.05% | **Adults & Peds: ≥6 yrs:** Instill 2-3 sprays per nostril q10-12h. |
| Afrin Original Pumpmist Nasal Spray | Oxymetazoline HCl 0.05% | **Adults & Peds: ≥6 yrs:** Instill 2-3 sprays per nostril q10-12h. |
| Afrin Severe Congestion Nasal Spray | Oxymetazoline HCl 0.05% | **Adults & Peds: ≥6 yrs:** Instill 2-3 sprays per nostril q10-12h. |
| Afrin Sinus Nasal Spray | Oxymetazoline HCl 0.05% | **Adults & Peds: ≥6 yrs:** Instill 2-3 sprays per nostril q10-12h. |
| Benzedrex Inhaler | Propylhexedrine 250mg | **Adults & Peds: ≥6 yrs:** Inhale 2 sprays per nostril q2h |
| Neo-Synephrine 12 Hour Extra Moisturizing Nasal Spray | Oxymetazoline HCl 0.05% | **Adults & Peds: ≥6 yrs:** Instill 2-3 sprays per nostril q10-12h. |
| Neo-Synephrine 12 Hour Nasal Decongestant Spray | Oxymetazoline HCl 0.05% | **Adults & Peds: ≥6 yrs:** Instill 2-3 sprays per nostril q10-12h. |
| Neo-Synephrine Extra Strength Nasal Decongestant Drops | Phenylephrine HCl 1% | **Adults & Peds: ≥12 yrs:** Instill 2-3 drops per nostril q4h. |

*(Continued)*

| BRAND | INGREDIENT/STRENGTH | DOSE |
|---|---|---|
| **TOPICAL NASAL DECONGESTANTS** *(Continued)* | | |
| Neo-Synephrine Extra Strength Nasal Spray | Phenylephrine HCl 1% | **Adults & Peds: ≥6 yrs:** Instill 2-3 sprays per nostril q4h. |
| Neo-Synephrine Mild Formula Nasal Spray | Phenylephrine HCl 0.25% | **Adults & Peds: ≥6 yrs:** Instill 2-3 sprays per nostril q4h. |
| Neo-Synephrine Regular Strength Nasal Decongestant Spray | Phenylephrine HCl 0.5% | **Adults & Peds: ≥12 yrs:** Instill 2-3 sprays per nostril q4h. |
| Nostrilla 12 Hour Nasal Decongestant | Oxymetazoline HCl 0.05% | **Adults & Peds: ≥6 yrs:** Instill 2-3 sprays per nostril q10-12h. |
| Vicks Sinex 12 Hour Ultra Fine Mist For Sinus Relief | Oxymetazoline HCl 0.05% | **Adults & Peds: ≥12 yrs:** Instill 2-3 sprays per nostril q10-12h. |
| Vicks Sinex Long Acting Nasal Spray For Sinus Relief | Oxymetazoline HCl 0.05% | **Adults & Peds: ≥12 yrs:** Instill 2-3 sprays per nostril q10-12h. |
| Vicks Sinex Nasal Spray For Sinus Relief | Phenylephrine HCl 0.5% | **Adults & Peds: ≥12 yrs:** Instill 2-3 sprays per nostril q4h. |
| **TOPICAL NASAL MOISTURIZERS** | | |
| 4-Way Saline Moisturizing Mist | Water, Boric Acid, Glycerin, Sodium Chloride, Sodium Borate, Eucalyptol, Menthol, Polysorbate 80, Benzalkonium Chloride | **Adults & Peds: ≥2 yrs:** Instill 2-3 sprays per nostril prn. |
| Ayr Baby's Saline Nose Spray, Drops | Sodium Chloride 0.65% | **Peds:** Instill 2 to 6 drops in each nostril. |
| Ayr Saline Nasal Gel | Aloe Vera Gel, Carbomer, Diazolidinyl Urea, Dimethicone Copolyol, FD&C Blue 1, Geranium Oil, Glycerin, Glyceryl Polymethacrylate, Methyl Gluceth 10, Methylparaben, Poloxamer 184, Propylene Glycol, Propylparaben, Sodium Chloride, Tocopherol Acetate, Triethanolamine, Xanthan Gum, Water | **Adults & Peds: ≥12 yrs:** Apply to nostril prn. |
| Ayr Saline Nasal Gel, No-Drip Sinus Spray | Water, Sodium Carbomethyl Starch, Propylene Glycol, Glycerin, Aloe Barbadensis Leaf Juice (Aloe Vera Gel), Sodium Chloride, Cetyl Pyridinium Chloride, Citric Acid, Disodium EDTA, Glycine Soja (Soybean Oil), Tocopheryl Acetate, Benzyl Alcohol, Benzalkonium Chloride, Geranium Maculatum Oil | **Adults & Peds: ≥12 yrs:** Use prn as directed. |
| Ayr Saline Nasal Mist | Sodium Chloride 0.65% | **Adults & Peds: ≥12 yrs:** Instill 2 sprays per nostril prn. |
| ENTSOL Mist, Buffered Hypertonic Nasal Irrigation Mist | Purified Water, Sodium Chloride, Sodium Phosphate Dibasic Edetate Disodium, Potassium Phosphate Monobasic, Benzalkonium Chloride | **Adults & Peds: ≥12 yrs:** Instill 1-2 sprays per nostril prn. |
| ENTSOL Single Use, Pre-Filled Nasal Wash Squeeze Bottle | Purified Water, Sodium Chloride, Sodium Phosphate Dibasic, Potassium Phosphate Monobasic | **Adults & Peds: ≥12 yrs:** Use as directed. |
| ENTSOL Spray, Buffered Hypertonic Saline Nasal Spray | Purified Water, Sodium Chloride Phosphate Dibasic, Potassium Phosphate Monobasic | **Adults & Peds: ≥12 yrs:** Instill 1 spray per nostril bid, 6 times daily |
| Little Noses Saline Spray/Drops, Non-Medicated | Sodium Chloride 0.65% | **Peds:** 2-6 drops per nostril as directed. |
| Ocean Premium Saline Nasal Spray | Sodium Chloride 0.65%, Phenylcarbinol, Benzalkonium Chloride | **Adults & Peds: ≥6 yrs:** Instill 2 sprays per nostril prn. |
| Simply Saline Sterile Saline Nasal Mist | Sodium Chloride 0.9% | **Adults & Peds: ≥12 yrs:** Use prn as directed. |

*(Continued)*

| BRAND | INGREDIENT/STRENGTH | DOSE |
|---|---|---|
| **TOPICAL NASAL MOISTURIZERS** *(Continued)* | | |
| SinoFresh Moisturizing Nasal & Sinus Spray | Cetylpyridinium Chloride 0.05% | **Adults & Peds: ≥12 yrs:** Instill 1-3 sprays per nostril qd. |
| Zicam Nasal Moisturizer | Purified Water, High Purity Sodium Chloride, Aloe Vera | **Adults & Peds: ≥12 yrs:** Use as directed. |
| **MISCELLANEOUS** | | |
| NasalCrom Allergy Prevention Nasal Spray | Cromolyn Sodium 5.2mg | **Adults & Peds: ≥6 yrs:** Instill 1 spray per nostril q4-6h. |
| NasalCrom Nasal Allergy Symptom Controller, Nasal Spray | Cromolyn Sodium 5.2mg | **Adults & Peds: ≥2 yrs:** Instill 1 spray per nostril q4-6h. |
| Similasan Hay Fever Relief, Non-Drowsy Formula, Nasal Spray | Cardiospermum HPUS 6X, Galphimia Glauca HPUS 6X, Luffa Operculata HPUS 6X, Sabadilla HPUS 6x | **Adults & Peds: ≥12 yrs:** Use as directed. |
| Zicam Allergy Relief, Homeopathic Nasal Solution, Pump | Luffa Operculata 4x, 12x, 30x, Galphimia Glauca 12x, 30x, Histaminum Hydrochloricum 12x, 30x, 200x, Sulphur 12x, 30x, 200x | **Adults & Peds: ≥6 yrs:** Instill 2-3 sprays per nostril q4h. |

# Is it a Cold, the Flu, or an Allergy?

| | COLD | FLU | AIRBORNE ALLERGY |
|---|---|---|---|
| **SYMPTOMS** | | | |
| Chest discomfort | Mild to moderate | Common; can become severe | Sometimes |
| Cough | Common (hacking cough) | Sometimes | Sometimes |
| Duration | 3-14 days | Days to weeks | Weeks (eg, 6 weeks for ragweed or grass pollen seasons) |
| Extreme exhaustion | Never | Early and prominent | Never |
| Fatigue, weakness | Sometimes | Can last up to 2-3 weeks | Sometimes |
| Fever | Rare | Characteristic, high (100-102 °F); lasts 3-4 days | Never |
| General aches, pains | Slight | Usual; often severe | Never |
| Headache | Rare | Prominent | Sometimes |
| Itchy eyes | Rare or never | Rare or never | Common |
| Runny nose | Common | | Common |
| Sneezing | Usual | Sometimes | Usual |
| Sore throat | Common | Sometimes | Sometimes |
| Stuffy nose | Common | Sometimes | Common |
| **TREATMENT** | | | |
| | Antihistamines | Amantadine | Antihistamines |
| | Decongestants | Rimantadine | Nasal steroids |
| | Nonsteroidal antiflammatories | Oseltamivir | Decongestants |
| | Temporary symptom relief | Zanamavir | |
| **PREVENTION** | | | |
| | Wash your hands often; avoid close contact with anyone with a cold | Annual vaccination<br>Amantadine<br>Rimantadine<br>Oseltamivir | Avoid allergens such as pollen, house flies, dust mites, mold pet dander, cockroaches |
| **COMPLICATIONS** | | | |
| | Sinus infection | Bronchitis | Sinus infections |
| | Middle ear infection | Pneumonia | Asthma |
| | Asthma | Can be life-threatening | |

Adapted from the National Institute of Allergy and Infectious Diseases, September 2005.

# Cough-Cold-Flu Products

| BRAND NAME | ANALGESIC | ANTIHISTAMINE | DECONGESTANT | COUGH SUPPRESSANT | EXPECTORANT | DOSE |
|---|---|---|---|---|---|---|
| **ANTIHISTAMINE + DECONGESTANT** | | | | | | |
| Actifed Cold & Allergy tablets | | Chlorpheniramine Maleate 4mg | Phenylephrine HCl 10mg | | | **Adults: ≥12 yrs:** 1 tabs q4-6h. **Max:** 4 tabs q24h. **Peds: 6-12 yrs:** 1/2 tab q4-6h. **Max:** 2 tabs q24h. |
| Benadryl Children's Allergy & Cold Fastmelt tablets | | Diphenhydramine HCl 19mg | Pseudoephedrine HCl 30mg | | | **Adults: ≥12 yrs:** 2 tabs q4h. **Max:** 8 tabs q24h. **Peds: 6-12 yrs:** 1 tab q4h. **Max:** 4 tabs q24h. |
| Benadryl-D Allergy/Sinus Tablets | | Diphenhydramine HCl 25mg | Phenylephrine HCl 10mg | | | **Adults & Peds: ≥12 yrs:** 1 tab q4h. **Max:** 6 tab q24h. |
| Children's Benadryl-D Allergy & Sinus Liquid | | Diphenhydramine HCl 12.5mg/5mL | Pseudophedrine HCl 30mg/5mL | | | **Adults: ≥12 yrs:** 2 tsp (10mL) q4-6h. **Peds: 6-12 yrs:** 1 tsp (5mL) q4-6h. **Max:** 4 doses q24h. |
| Children's Benadryl Allergy & Cold Fastmelt Tablets | | Diphenhydramine HCl 19mg | Pseudoephedrine HCl 30mg | | | **Adult & Peds ≥12 yrs:** 2 tabs q4h. **Max:** 8 tabs q24h. **Peds: 6-12 yrs:** 1 tab q4hr. **Max:** 6 doses q24h. |
| Dimetapp Children's Cold & Allergy elixir | | Brompheniramine Maleate 1mg/5mL | Phenylephrine HCl 2.5mg/5mL | | | **Adults: ≥12 yrs:** 4 tsp (20mL) q4h. **Peds: 6-12 yrs:** 2 tsp (10mL) q4h. **Max:** 6 doses q24h. |
| Triaminic Cold & Allergy liquid | | Chlorpheniramine Maleate 1mg/5mL | Phenylephrine HCl 2.5mg/5mL | | | **Adults: ≥12 yrs:** 1 tsp (5mL) q4h. **Max:** 6 doses q24h. **Peds: 6-12 yrs:** 2 tsp (10mL). |
| Triaminic Nighttime Cough & Cold liquid | | Diphenhydramine HCl 6.25mg/5mL | Phenylephrine HCl 2.5mg/5mL | | | **Adults: ≥12 yrs:** 1 tsp (5mL) q4h. **Max:** 6 doses q24h. **Peds: 6-12 yrs:** 2 tsp (10mL). |
| **ANTIHISTAMINE + DECONGESTANT + ANALGESIC** | | | | | | |
| Actifed Cold & Sinus caplets | Acetaminophen 500mg | Chlorpheniramine Maleate 2mg | Pseudoephedrine HCl 30mg | | | **Adults & Peds: ≥12 yrs:** 2 tabs q6h. **Max:** 8 tabs q24h. |
| Advil Multi-Symptom Cold caplets | Ibuprofen 200mg | Chlorpheniramine Maleate 2mg | Pseudoephedrine HCl 30mg | | | **Adults & Peds: ≥12 yrs:** 1 tab q4-6h. **Max:** 6 tabs q24h. |
| Alka-Seltzer Plus Cold effervescent tablets | Acetaminophen 250mg | Chlorpheniramine Maleate 2mg | Phenylephrine HCl 5mg | | | **Adults & Peds: ≥12 yrs:** 2 tabs q4h. **Max:** 8 tabs q24h. |

| BRAND NAME | ANALGESIC | ANTIHISTAMINE | DECONGESTANT | COUGH SUPPRESSANT | EXPECTORANT | DOSE |
|---|---|---|---|---|---|---|
| Benadryl Allergy & Cold caplets | Acetaminophen 500mg | Diphenhydramine HCl 12.5mg | Phenylephrine HCl 5mg | | | **Adults & Peds: ≥12 yrs:** 2 cap q4h. **Max:** 12 q24h. **Peds: 6-12 yrs:** 1 cap q4h. **Max:** 5 tabs q24h. |
| Benadryl Allergy & Sinus Headache caplets | Acetaminophen 325mg | Diphenhydramine HCl 12.5mg | Phenylephrine HCl 5mg | | | **Adults & Peds: ≥12 yrs:** 2 tab q4h. **Max:** 12 tab q24h. **Peds: 6-12 yrs:** 1 cap q4h. **Max:** 5 tabs q24h. |
| Benadryl Severe Allergy & Sinus Headache caplets | Acetaminophen 325mg | Diphenhydramine HCl 25mg | Phenylephrine HCl 5mg | | | **Adults & Peds: ≥12 yrs:** 2 caps q4h. **Max:** 12 caps q24h. |
| Comtrex Acute Head Cold caplets | Acetaminophen 500mg | Brompheniramine Maleate 2mg | Pseudoephedrine HCl 30mg | | | **Adults & Peds: ≥12 yrs:** 2 tabs q6h. **Max:** 8 tabs q24h. |
| Comtrex Flu Therapy Nightime liquid | Acetaminophen 1000mg/30mL | Chlorpheniramine Maleate 4mg/30mL | Pseudoephedrine HCl 60mg/30mL | | | **Adults & Peds: ≥12 yrs:** 2 tbl (30mL) q6h. **Max:** 8 tbl (240mL) q24h. |
| Comtrex Flu Therapy Day & Night tablets | Acetaminophen 500mg | Chlorpheniramine Maleate 2mg | Pseudoephedrine HCl 30mg | | | **Adults & Peds: ≥12 yrs:** 2 tabs q6h. **Max:** 4 daytime tabs q24h. |
| Comtrex Nighttime Acute Head Cold liquid | Acetaminophen 1000mg/30mL | Brompheniramine Maleate 4mg/30mL | Pseudoephedrine HCl 60mg/30mL | | | **Adults & Peds: ≥12 yrs:** 2 tbl (30mL) q6h. **Max:** 8 tbl (240mL) q24h. |
| Contac Cold & Flu Maximum Strength caplets | Acetaminophen 500mg | Chlorpheniramine Maleate 2mg | Phenylephrine HCl 5mg | | | **Adults & Peds: ≥12 yrs:** 2 caps q4-6h **Max:** 8 caps q24h. |
| Dristan Cold Multi-Symptom tablets | Acetaminophen 325mg | Chlorpheniramine Maleate 2mg | Phenylephrine HCl 5mg | | | **Adults & Peds: ≥12 yrs:** 2 tabs q4h. **Max:** 12 caps q24h. |
| Robitussin Cold & Congestion tablets | Acetaminophen 325mg | Chlorpheniramine Maleate 2mg | Phenylephrine HCl 5mg | | | **Adults & Peds: ≥12 yrs:** 2 tabs q4h. **Max:** 12 caps q24h. |
| Sudafed Sinus PE Nighttime Cold caplets | Acetaminophen 325mg | Diphenhydramine HCl 25mg | Phenylephrine HCl 5mg | | | **Adults & Peds: ≥12 yrs:** 2 tabs q4h. **Max:** 12 tabs q24h. |
| Sudafed PE Severe Cold caplets | Acetaminophen 325mg | Diphenhydramine HCl 12.5mg | Phenylephrine HCl 5mg | | | **Adults & Peds: ≥12 yrs:** 2 tabs q4h. **Max:** 12 tabs q24h. **Peds: 6-12 yrs:** 1 tab q4h. **Max:** 5 tabs q24h. |
| Theraflu Cold & Sore Throat Hot Liquid | Acetaminophen 325mg/packet | Pheniramine Maleate 20mg/packet | Phenylephrine HCl 10mg/packet | | | **Adults & Peds: ≥12 yrs:** 1 packet q4h. **Max:** 6 packets q24h. |
| Theraflu Nighttime Severe Cold Hot Liquid | Acetaminophen 650mg/packet | Pheniramine Maleate 20mg/packet | Phenylephrine HCl 10mg/packet | | | **Adults & Peds: ≥12 yrs:** 1 packet q4h. **Max:** 6 packets q24h. |

*(Continued)*

| BRAND NAME | ANALGESIC | ANTIHISTAMINE | DECONGESTANT | COUGH SUPPRESSANT | EXPECTORANT | DOSE |
|---|---|---|---|---|---|---|
| **ANTIHISTAMINE + DECONGESTANT + ANALGESIC** *(Continued)* | | | | | | |
| Theraflu Flu & Sore Throat Liquid | Acetaminophen 650mg/packet | Pheniramine Maleate 20mg/packet | Phenylephrine HCl 10mg/packet | | | **Adults & Peds: ≥12 yrs:** 1 packet q4h. **Max:** 6 packets q24h. |
| Tylenol Children's Plus Cold liquid | Acetaminophen 160mg/5mL | Chlorpheniramine Maleate 1mg/5mL | Phenylephrine HCl 2.5mg/5mL | | | **Peds: 6-11 yrs (48-95 lbs):** 2 tsp (10mL) q4h. **Max:** 5 doses q24h. |
| Tylenol Children's Plus Cold & Allergy liquid | Acetaminophen 160mg/5mL | Diphenhydramine HCl 12.5mg/5mL | Phenylephrine HCl 2.5mg/5mL | | | **Peds: 6-11 yrs (48-95 lbs):** 2 tsp (10mL) q4-6h. **Max:** 4 doses q24h. |
| Tylenol Children's Plus Cold Nighttime suspension | Acetaminophen 160mg/5mL | Chlorpheniramine Maleate 1mg/5mL | Pseudoephedrine HCl 15mg/5mL | | | **Peds: 6-12 yrs (48-95 lbs):** 2 tsp (10mL) q4-6h. **Max:** 8 tsp (40mL) q24h. |
| Tylenol Flu Nighttime gelcaps | Acetaminophen 500mg | Diphenhydramine HCl 25mg | Pseudoephedrine HCl 30mg | | | **Adults & Peds: ≥12 yrs:** 2 caps q6h. **Max:** 8 caps q24h. |
| Tylenol Sinus Congestion & Pain Nighttime caplets | Acetaminophen 325mg | Chlorpheniramine Maleate 2mg | Phenylephrine HCl 5mg | | | **Adults & Peds: ≥12 yrs:** 2 caps q4h. **Max:** 12 caps q24h. |
| Tylenol Sinus Nighttime caplets | Acetaminophen 500mg | Doxylamine Succinate 6.25mg | Pseudoephedrine HCl 30mg | | | **Adults & Peds: ≥12 yrs:** 2 tabs q4-6h. **Max:** 8 tabs q24h. |
| **COUGH SUPPRESSANT** | | | | | | |
| Delsym 12 Hour Cough Relief liquid | | | | Dextromethorphan Polistrex 30mg/5mL | | **Adults: ≥12 yrs:** 2 tsp (10mL) q12h. **Peds: 6-12 yrs:** 1 tsp (5mL) q12h. 2-6 yrs: 1/2 tsp (2.5mL) q12h. **Max:** 4 doses q24h. |
| PediaCare Long-Acting Cough liquid | | | | Dextromethorphan HBr 7.5mg/5mL | | **Peds: 6-12 yrs:** 2 tsp q6-8h. 2-6 yrs: 1 tsp q6-8h. **Max:** 4 doses q24h. |
| Robitussin Cough Long-Acting liquid | | | | Dextromethorphan HBr 15mg/5mL | | **Adults & Peds: ≥12 yrs:** 2 tsp (10mL) q6-8h. **Max:** 8 tsp (40mL) q24h. |
| Robitussin CoughGels liqui-gels | | | | Dextromethorphan HBr 15mg | | **Adults & Peds: ≥12 yrs:** 2 caps q6-8h. **Max:** 8 caps q24h. |
| Robitussin Pediatric Cough liquid | | | | Dextromethorphan HBr 7.5mg/5mL | | **Adults: ≥12 yrs (≥96 lbs):** 4 tsp (20mL) q6-8h. **Peds: 6-12 yrs (48-95 lbs):** 2 tsp (10mL) q6-8h. 2-6yrs: 1 tsp (5mL) q6-8h. **Max:** 4 doses q24h. |

| BRAND NAME | ANALGESIC | ANTIHISTAMINE | DECONGESTANT | COUGH SUPPRESSANT | EXPECTORANT | DOSE |
|---|---|---|---|---|---|---|
| Simply Cough liquid | | | | Dextromethorphan HBr 5mg/5mL | | **Peds: 6-12 yrs (48-95 lbs):** 2 tsp (10mL) q4h. **2-6 yrs (24-47 lbs):** 1 tsp (5mL) q4h. **Max:** 4 doses q24h. |
| Theraflu Long Acting Cough thin strips | | | | Dextromethorphan 11mg/strip | | **Adults & Peds: ≥12 yrs:** 2 strips q6-8h. **Max:** 8 strips q24h. |
| Triaminic Long Acting Cough thin strips | | | | Dextromethorphan 5.5mg/strip | | **Peds: 6-12 yrs:** 2 strips q6-8h. **Max:** 8 strips q24h. |
| Vicks DayQuil Cough liquid | | | | Dextromethorphan HBr 15mg/15mL | | **Adults & Peds: ≥12 yrs:** 2 tbl (30mL) q6-8h. **Peds: 6-12 yrs:** 1 tbl (15mL) q6-8h. **Max:** 4 doses q24h. |
| Vicks 44 liquid | | | | Dextromethorphan HBr 30mg/15mL | | **Adults & Peds: ≥12 yrs:** 1 tbl (15mL) q6-8h. **Peds: 6-12 yrs:** 1.5 tsp (7.5mL) q6-8h. **Max:** 4 doses q24h. |
| Vicks BabyRub | | | | Eucalyptus, petrolatum, fragrance, aloe extract, eucalyptus oil, lavender oil, rosemary oil | | **Peds: ≥3 mth:** Apply q8h. |
| Vicks Cough Drops Cherry Flavor | | | | Menthol 1.7mg | | **Adults & Peds: ≥5 yrs:** 3 drops q1-2h. |
| Vicks Cough Drops Original Flavor | | | | Menthol 3.3mg | | **Adults & Peds: ≥5 yrs:** 2 drops q1-2h. |
| Vicks VapoRub | | | | Camphor 5.2% Menthol 2.8%, Eucalyptus 1.2% | | **Adults & Peds: ≥2 yrs:** Apply q8h. |
| Vicks VapoRub cream | | | | Camphor 4.8% Menthol 2.6%, Eucalyptus 1.2% | | **Adults & Peds: ≥2 yrs:** Apply q8h. |
| Vicks VapoSteam | | | | Camphor 6.2% | | **Adults & Peds: ≥2 yrs:** 1 tbl/quart q8h. |
| **COUGH SUPPRESSANT + ANTIHISTAMINE** | | | | | | |
| Coricidin HBP Cough & Cold tablets | | Chlorpheniramine Maleate 4mg | | Dextromethorphan HBr 30mg | | **Adults & Peds: ≥12 yrs:** 1 tabs q6h. **Max:** 4 tabs q24h. |
| Dimetapp Long-Acting Cold Plus Cough elixir | | Chlorpheniramine Maleate 1mg/5mL | | Dextromethorphan HBr 7.5mg/5mL | | **Peds: ≥12 yrs:** 4 tsp (20mL) q6h. **6-12 yrs:** 2 tsp (10 mL) q6h. **Max:** 4 doses q24h. |

*(Continued)*

| BRAND NAME | ANALGESIC | ANTIHISTAMINE | DECONGESTANT | COUGH SUPPRESSANT | EXPECTORANT | DOSE |
|---|---|---|---|---|---|---|
| **COUGH SUPPRESSANT + ANTIHISTAMINE** *(Continued)* | | | | | | |
| Robitussin Cough & Cold Long-Acting liquid | | Chlorpheniramine Maleate 2mg/5mL | | Dextromethorphan HBr 15mg/5mL | | **Adults:** **≥12 yrs:** 2 tsp (10mL) q6h. **Max:** 4 doses q24h. |
| Triaminic Softchews Cough & Runny Nose | | Chlorpheniramine Maleate 1mg | | Dextromethorphan HBr 5mg | | **Adults & Peds:** **≥12 yrs:** 1 tabs q4-6h. Max: 6 tabs q24h. |
| Vicks Children's NyQuil liquid | | Chlorpheniramine Maleate 2mg/15mL | | Dextromethorphan HBr 15mg/15mL | | **Adults:** **≥12 yrs:** 2 tbl (30mL) q6h. **Peds:** **6-11 yrs:** 1 tbl (15mL) q6h. **Max:** 4 doses q24h. |
| Vicks NyQuil Cough liquid | | Doxylamine Succinate 6.25mg/15mL | | Dextromethorphan HBr 15mg/15mL | | **Adults & Peds:** **≥12 yrs:** 2 tbl (30mL) q6h. **Max:** 8 tbl (120mL) q24h. |
| **COUGH SUPPRESSANT + ANTIHISTAMINE + ANALGESIC** | | | | | | |
| Alka-Seltzer Plus Flu effervescent tablets | Aspirin 500mg | Chlorpheniramine Maleate 2mg | | Dextromethorphan HBr 15mg | | **Adults & Peds:** **≥12 yrs:** 2 tabs q6h. **Max:** 8 tabs q24h. |
| Alka-Seltzer Plus Nighttime Liquid Gels | Acetaminophen 325mg | Doxylamine Succinate 6.25mg | | Dextromethorphan HBr 15mg | | **Adults & Peds:** **≥12 yrs:** 2 tabs q6h. **Max:** 12 tabs q24h. |
| Coricidin HBP Maximum Strength Flu tablets | Acetaminophen 500mg | Chlorpheniramine Maleate 2mg | | Dextromethorphan HBr 15mg | | **Adults & Peds:** **≥12 yrs:** 2 tabs q6h. **Max:** 8 tabs q24h. |
| Triaminic Flu Cough & Fever liquid | Acetaminophen 160mg/5mL | Chlorpheniramine Maleate 1mg/5mL | | Dextromethorphan HBr 7.5mg/5mL | | **Adults & Peds:** **≥12 yrs:** 1 tsp (5mL) q6h. **Max:** 4 doses (20mL) q24h. |
| Tylenol Nighttime Cough & Sore Throat Cool Burst liquid | Acetaminophen 1000mg/30mL | Doxylamine 12.5mg/30mL | | Dextromethorphan HBr 30mg/30mL | | **Adults & Peds:** **≥12 yrs:** 2 tbl (30mL) q6h. **Max:** 8 tbl (120mL) q24h. |
| Vicks 44M liquid | Acetaminophen 162.5mg/5mL | Chlorpheniramine Maleate 1mg/5mL | | Dextromethorphan HBr 7.5mg/5mL | | **Adults & Peds:** **≥12 yrs:** 4 tsp (20mL) q6h. **Max:** 16 tsp (80mL) q24h. |
| Vicks NyQuil liquicaps | Acetaminophen 325mg | Doxylamine Succinate 6.25mg | | Dextromethorphan HBr 15mg | | **Adults & Peds:** **≥12 yrs:** 2 caps q6h. **Max:** 8 caps q24h. |
| Vicks NyQuil liquid | Acetaminophen 500mg/15mL | Doxylamine Succinate 6.25mg/15mL | | Dextromethorphan HBr 15mg/15mL | | **Adults & Peds:** **≥12 yrs:** 2 tbl (30mL) q6h. **Max:** 8 tbl (120mL) q24h. |
| **COUGH SUPPRESSANT + ANTIHISTAMINES + ANALGESIC + DECONGESTANT** | | | | | | |
| Alka-Seltzer Plus Cough & Cold Liquid Gels | Acetaminophen 325mg | Chlorpheniramine Maleate 2mg | Phenylephrine HCl 5mg | Dextromethorphan HBr 10mg | | **Adults & Peds:** **≥12 yrs:** 2 tabs q4h. **Max:** 12 tabs q24h. |
| Alka-Seltzer Plus Nighttime effervescent tablets | Acetaminophen 250mg | Doxlamine Succinate 6.25mg | Phenylephrine HCl 5mg | Dextromethorphan HBr 10mg | | **Adults & Peds:** **≥12 yrs:** 2 tabs q4h. **Max:** 8 tabs q24h. |

| BRAND NAME | ANALGESIC | ANTIHISTAMINE | DECONGESTANT | COUGH SUPPRESSANT | EXPECTORANT | DOSE |
|---|---|---|---|---|---|---|
| Alka-Seltzer Plus Cough & Cold effervescent tablets | Acetaminophen 250mg | Chlorpheniramine Maleate 2mg | Phenylephrine HCl 5mg | Dextromethorphan HBr 10mg | | **Adults & Peds: ≥12 yrs:** 2 tabs q4h. **Max:** 8 tabs q24h. |
| Alka-Seltzer Plus Cough & Cold liquid | Acetaminophen 162.5mg/5mL | Chlorpheniramine Maleate 1mg/5mL | Phenylephrine HCl 2.5mg/5mLmg | Dextromethorphan HBr 5mg/5mL | | **Adults & Peds: ≥12 yrs:** 4 tsp q4h. **Max:** 24 tsp q24h. |
| Comtrex Cold & Cough Nighttime caplets | Acetaminophen 500mg | Chlorpheniramine Maleate 2mg | Pseudoephedrine HCl 30mg | Dextromethorphan HBr 15mg | | **Adults & Peds: ≥12 yrs:** 2 tabs q6h. **Max:** 8 tabs q24h. |
| Comtrex Nighttime Cold & Cough liquid | Acetaminophen 1000mg/30mL | Chlorpheniramine Maleate 4mg/30mL | Pseudoephedrine HCl 60mg/30mL | Dextromethorphan HBr 30mg/30mL | | **Adults & Peds: ≥12 yrs:** 2 tbl (30mL) q6h. **Max:** 8 tbl (240mL) q24h. |
| Dimetapp Children's Nighttime Flu liquid | Acetaminophen 160mg/5mL | Chlorpheniramine Maleate 1mg/5mL | Phenylephrine HCl 2.5mg/5mL | Dextromethorphan HBr 5mg/5mL | | **Adults: ≥12 yrs:** 4 tsp (20mL) q4h. **Peds: 6-12 yrs:** 2 tsp (10mL) q4h. **Max:** 5 doses q24h. |
| Robitussin Cold Cough & Flu liquid | Acetaminophen 160mg/5mL | Chlorpheniramine Maleate 1mg/5mL | Phenylephrine HCl 2.5mg/5mL | Dextromethorphan HBr 5mg/5mL | | **Adults: ≥12 yrs:** 4 tsp (20mL) q4h. **Peds: 6-12 yrs:** 2 tsp (10mL) q4h. **Max:** 5 doses q24h. |
| Tylenol Children's Plus Flu liquid | Acetaminophen 160mg/5mL | Chlorpheniramine Maleate 1mg/5mL | Phenylephrine HCl 2.5mg/5mL | Dextromethorphan HBr 7.5mg/5mL | | **Peds: 6-11 yrs (48-95 lbs):** 2 tsp (10mL) q6-8h. **Max:** 4 doses q24h. |
| Tylenol Cold & Flu Severe Nighttime Cool Burst liquid | Acetaminophen 1000mg/30mL | Doxylamine 12.5mg/30mL | Pseudoephedrine HCl 60mg/30mL | Dextromethorphan HBr 30mg/30mL | | **Adults & Peds: ≥12 yrs:** 2 tbl (30mL) q6h. **Max:** 8 tbl (120mL) q24h. |
| Tylenol Cold Head Congestion Nighttime caplets | Acetaminophen 325mg | Chlorpheniramine Maleate 2mg | Phenylephedrine HCl 5mg | Dextromethorphan HBr 10mg | | **Adults & Peds: ≥12 yrs:** 2 caps q4h. **Max:** 12 caps q24h. |
| Tylenol Cold Multi-Symptom Nighttime caplets | Acetaminophen 325mg | Chlorpheniramine Maleate 2mg | Phenylephedrine HCl 5mg | Dextromethorphan HBr 10mg | | **Adults & Peds: ≥12 yrs:** 2 caps q4h. **Max:** 12 caps q24h. |
| Tylenol Cold Multi-Symptom Nighttime liquid | Acetaminophen 325mg/15mL | Doxylamine 6.25mg/30mL | Phenylephedrine HCl 5mg/15mL | Dextromethorphan HBr 10mg/15mL | | **Adults & Peds: ≥12 yrs:** 2 tbl (30mL) q4h. **Max:** 12 tbl (180mL) q24h. |
| Tylenol Cold Nighttime Cool Burst caplets | Acetaminophen 325mg | Chlorpheniramine Maleate 2mg | Pseudoephedrine HCl 30mg | Dextromethorphan HBr 15mg | | **Adults & Peds: ≥12 yrs:** 2 tabs q6h. **Max:** 8 tabs q24h. |
| **COUGH SUPPRESSANT + ANTIHISTAMINE + DECONGESTANT** | | | | | | |
| Dimetapp DM Children's Cold & Cough elixir | | Brompheniramine Maleate 1mg/5mL | Phenylephrine HCl 2.5mg/5mL | Dextromethorphan HBr 5mg/5mL | | **Adults: ≥12 yrs:** 4 tsp (20mL) q4h. **Peds: 6-12 yrs:** 2 tsp (10mL) q4h. **Max:** 6 doses q24h. |
| Robitussin Allergy & Cough liquid | | Chlorpheniramine Maleate 2mg/5mL | Phenylephrine HCl 5mg/5mL | Dextromethorphan HBr 10mg/5mL | | **Adults: ≥12 yrs:** 2 tsp (10mL) q4h. **Peds: 6-12 yrs:** 1 tsp (5mL) q4h. **Max:** 6 doses q24h. |

*(Continued)*

| BRAND NAME | ANALGESIC | ANTIHISTAMINE | DECONGESTANT | COUGH SUPPRESSANT | EXPECTORANT | DOSE |
|---|---|---|---|---|---|---|
| **COUGH SUPPRESSANT + ANTIHISTAMINE + DECONGESTANT** *(Continued)* | | | | | | |
| Robitussin Pediatric Cough & Cold Nighttime liquid | | Chlorpheniramine Maleate 1mg/5mL | Phenylephrine HCl 2.5mg/5mL | Dextromethorphan HBr 5mg/5mL | | **Adults & Peds: ≥12 yrs** (≥ 96 lbs): 4 tsp (20mL) q4h. **Peds: 6-12 yrs (48-95 lbs):** 2 tsp (10mL) q4h. |
| Robitussin Cough & Cold Nighttime liquid | | Chlorpheniramine Maleate 1mg/5mL | Phenylephrine HCl 2.5mg/5mL | Dextromethorphan HBr 5mg/5mL | | **Adults: ≥12 yrs:** 4 tsp (20mL) q4h. **Peds: 6-12 yrs:** 2 tsp (10mL) q4h. **Max:** 6 doses q24h. |
| Theraflu Cold & Cough Hot Liquid | | Pheniramine Maleate 20mg/packet | Phenylephrine HCl 10mg/packet | Dextromethorphan HBr 20mg/packet | | **Adults & Peds: ≥12 yrs:** 1 packet q4h. **Max:** 6 packets q24h. |
| **COUGH SUPPRESSANT + DECONGESTANT** | | | | | | |
| PediaCare Children's Multi-Symptom Cold Liquid | | | Phenylephrine HCl 2.5mg/5mL | Dextromethorphan HBr 5mg/5mL | | **Peds: 6-12 yrs:** 2 tsp (10mL) q4h. 2-6 yrs: 1 tsp (5mL) q4h. **Max:** 6 doses q24h. |
| PediaCare Decongestant & Cough Infants' drops | | | Phenylephrine HCl 1.25mg/0.8mL | Dextromethorphan HBr 2.5mg/0.8mL | | **Peds: 2-3 yrs:** 1.6mL q4h. **Max:** 6 doses q24h. |
| Vicks 44D Cough & Congestion Relief liquid | | | Phenylephrine HCl 10mg/15mL | Dextromethorphan HBr 30mg/15mL | | **Adults: ≥12 yrs:** 1 tbl (15mL) q4h. **Peds: 6-12 yrs:** 1.5 tsp (7.5mL) q4h. **Max:** 6 doses q24h. |
| **COUGH SUPPRESSANT + DECONGESTANT + ANALGESIC** | | | | | | |
| Alka-Seltzer Plus Day Cold liquid gels | Acetaminophen 325mg | | Phenylephrine HCl 5mg | Dextromethorphan HBr 10mg | | **Adults & Peds: ≥12 yrs:** 2 tabs q4h. **Max:** 12 tabs q24h. |
| Alka-Seltzer Plus Day & Night liquid gels | Acetaminophen 325mg | | Phenylephrine HCl 5mg | Dextromethorphan HBr 10mg | | **Adults & Peds: ≥12 yrs:** 2 tabs q4h. **Max:** 12 tabs q24h. |
| Alka-Seltzer Plus Day & Night effervescent tablets | Acetaminophen 250mg | | Phenylephrine HCl 5mg | Dextromethorphan HBr 10mg | | **Adults & Peds: ≥12 yrs:** 2 tabs q4h. **Max:** 8 tabs q24h. |
| Alka-Seltzer Plus Day Cold Liquid | Acetaminophen 162.5mg/5mL | | Phenylephrine HCl 2.5mg/5mL | Dextromethorphan HBr 5mg/5mL | | **Adults & Peds: ≥12 yrs:** 4 tsps q4h. **Max:** 6 doses q24h. |
| Sudafed PE Cold & Cough caplets | Acetaminophen 325mg | | Phenylephrine HCl 5mg | Dextromethorphan HBr 10mg | | **Adults & Peds: ≥12 yrs:** 2 caps q4h. **Max:** 12 tabs q24h. |
| Theraflu Daytime Severe Cold caplets | Acetaminophen 325mg | | Phenylephrine HCl 5mg | Dextromethorphan HBr 5mg | | **Adults & Peds: ≥12 yrs:** 2 tabs q6h. **Max:** 8 tabs q24h. |

| BRAND NAME | ANALGESIC | ANTIHISTAMINE | DECONGESTANT | COUGH SUPPRESSANT | EXPECTORANT | DOSE |
|---|---|---|---|---|---|---|
| Tylenol Cold & Flu Severe Daytime Cool Burst liquid | Acetaminophen 1000mg/30mL | | Pseudoephedrine HCl 60mg/30mL | Dextromethorphan HBr 30mg/30mL | | **Adults & Peds: ≥12 yrs:** 2 tbl (30mL) q6h. **Max:** 8 tbl (120mL) q24h. |
| Tylenol Cold Daytime Cool Burst caplets | Acetaminophen 325mg | | Pseudoephedrine HCl 30mg | Dextromethorphan HBr 15mg | | **Adults & Peds: ≥12 yrs:** 2 tabs q6h. **Max:** 8 tabs q24h. |
| Tylenol Cold Head Congestion Daytime capsules | Acetaminophen 325mg | | Phenylepheprine HCl 5mg | Dextromethorphan HBr 10mg | | **Adults & Peds: ≥12 yrs:** 2 caps q4h. **Max:** 12 caps q24h. |
| Tylenol Cold Head Congestion Day/Night pack | Acetaminophen 325mg | | Phenylephedrine HCl 5mg | Dextromethorphan HBr 10mg | | **Adults & Peds: ≥12 yrs:** 2 caps q4h. **Max:** 12 caps q24h. |
| Tylenol Cold Multi-Symptom Daytime capsules | Acetaminophen 325mg | | Phenylephrine HCl 5mg | Dextromethorphan HBr 10mg | | **Adults & Peds: ≥12 yrs:** 2 caps q4h. **Max:** 12 caps q24h. |
| Tylenol Cold Multi-Symptom Day/Night pack | Acetaminophen 325mg | | Phenylephrine HCl 5mg | Dextromethorphan HBr 10mg | | **Adults & Peds: ≥12 yrs:** 2 caps q4h. **Max:** 12 caps q24h. |
| Tylenol Plus Cold & Cough Infants' drops | Acetaminophen 80mg/0.8mL | | Phenylephrine HCl 1.25mg/0.8mL | Dextromethorphan HBr 2.5mg/0.8mL | | **Peds: 2-3 yrs (24-35 lbs):** 1.6mL q4h. **Max:** 5 doses q24h. |
| Tylenol Flu Daytime gelcaps | Acetaminophen 500mg | | Pseudoephedrine HCl 30mg | Dextromethorphan HBr 15mg | | **Adults & Peds: ≥12 yrs:** 2 caps q6h. **Max:** 8 caps q24h. |
| Vicks DayQuil liquicaps | Acetaminophen 325mg | | Phenylephrine HCl 30mg | Dextromethorphan HBr 10mg | | **Adults & Peds: ≥12 yrs:** 2 caps q4. **Max:** 6 caps q24h. |
| Vicks DayQuil liquid | Acetaminophen 325mg/15mL | | Phenylephrine HCl 5mg/15mL | Dextromethorphan HBr 10mg/15mL | | **Adults & Peds: ≥12 yrs:** 2 tbl (30mL) q4h. **Max:** 12 tbl (120mL) q24h. |
| **COUGH SUPPRESSANT + DECONGESTANT + EXPECTORANT** | | | | | | |
| Robitussin CF liquid | | | Phenylephrine HCl 5mg/5mL | Dextromethorphan HBr 10mg/5mL | Guaifenesin 100mg/5mL | **Adults: ≥12 yrs:** 2 tsp (10mL) q4h. **Peds: 6-12 yrs:** 1 tsp (5mL) q4h. **2-6 yrs:** 1/2 tsp (2.5mL) q4h. **Max:** 6 doses q24h. |
| **COUGH SUPPRESSANT + DECONGESTANT + EXPECTORANT + ANALGESIC** | | | | | | |
| Comtrex Chest Cold capsules | Acetaminophen 250mg | | Pseudoephedrine HCl 30mg | Dextromethorphan HBr 10mg | Guaifenesin 100mg | **Adults & Peds: ≥12 yrs:** 2 caps q4h. **Max:** 12 caps q24h. |
| Tylenol Cold Multi-Symptom Severe liquid | Acetaminophen 325mg/15mL | | Phenylephrine HCl 5mg/15ml | Dextromethorphan HBr 10mg/15mL | Guaifenesin 200mg/15mL | **Adults & Peds: ≥12 yrs:** 2 tbs q4h. **Max:** 12 tbs q24h. |
| Tylenol Cold Multi-Symptom Severe caplets | Acetaminophen 325mg | | Phenylephrine HCl 5mg | Dextromethorphan HBr 10mg | Guaifenesin 200mg | **Adults & Peds: ≥12 yrs:** 2 tabs q4h. **Max:** 12 tabs q24h. |

*(Continued)*

| BRAND NAME | ANALGESIC | ANTIHISTAMINE | DECONGESTANT | COUGH SUPPRESSANT | EXPECTORANT | DOSE |
|---|---|---|---|---|---|---|
| **COUGH SUPPRESSANT + DECONGESTANT + EXPECTORANT & ANALGESIC** *(Continued)* | | | | | | |
| Tylenol Severe Head Congestion caplets | Acetaminophen 325mg | | Phenylephrine HCl 5mg | Dextromethorphan HBr 10mg | Guaifenesin 200mg | **Adults & Peds: ≥12 yrs:** 2 tabs q4h. **Max:** 12 tabs q24h. |
| **COUGH SUPPRESSANT & EXPECTORANT** | | | | | | |
| Coricidin HBP Chest Congestion & Cough softgels | | | | Dextromethorphan HBr 10mg | Guaifenesin 200mg | **Adults & Peds: ≥12 yrs:** 1-2 caps q4h. **Max:** 12 caps q24h. |
| Mucinex DM extended-release tablets | | | | Dextromethorphan HBr 30mg | Guaifenesin 600mg | **Adults & Peds: ≥12 yrs:** 1-2 tabs q12h. **Max:** 4 tabs q24h. |
| Robitussin Cough & Congestion liquid | | | | Dextromethorphan HBr 10mg/5mL | Guaifenesin 200mg/5mL | **Adults: ≥12 yrs:** 2 tsp (10mL) q4h.<br>**Peds: 6-12 yrs:** 1 tsp (5mL) q4h.<br>**2-6 yrs:** 1/2 tsp (2.5mL) q4h.<br>**Max:** 6 doses q24h. |
| Robitussin DM Infant Drops | | | | Dextromethorphan HBr 5mg/2.5mL | Guaifenesin 100mg/2.5mL | **Peds 2-6 yrs (24-47lbs):** 2.5mL q4h.<br>**Max:** 6 doses q24h. |
| Robitussin DM liquid | | | | Dextromethorphan HBr 10mg/5mL | Guaifenesin 100mg/5mL | **Adults: ≥12 yrs:** 2 tsp (10mL) q4h.<br>**Peds: 6-12 yrs:** 1 tsp (5mL) q4h.<br>**2-6 yrs:** 1/2 tsp (2.5mL) q4h.<br>**Max:** 6 doses q24h. |
| Robitussin Sugar Free Cough liquid | | | | Dextromethorphan HBr 10mg/5mL | Guaifenesin 100mg/5mL | **Adults: ≥12 yrs:** 2 tsp (10mL) q4h.<br>**Peds: 6-12 yrs:** 1 tsp (5mL) q4h.<br>**2-6 yrs:** 1/2 tsp (2.5mL) q4h.<br>**Max:** 6 doses q24h. |
| Vicks 44E liquid | | | | Dextromethorphan HBr 20mg/15mL | Guaifenesin 200mg/15mL | **Adults: ≥12 yrs:** 1 tbl (15mL) q4h.<br>**Peds: 6-12 yrs:** 1.5 tsp (7.5mL) q4h.<br>**Max:** 6 doses q24h. |
| Vicks 44E Pediatric liquid | | | | Dextromethorphan HBr 10mg/15mL | Guaifenesin 100mg/15mL | **Adults: ≥12 yrs:** 2 tbl (30mL) q4h.<br>**Peds: 6-12 yrs:** 1 tbl (15mL) q4h.<br>**2-5 yrs:** 0.5 tbl (7.5mL) q4h.<br>**Max:** 6 doses q24h. |
| **DECONGESTANT** | | | | | | |
| Contac-D Cold Decongestant tablets | | | Phenylephrine HCl 10mg | | | **Adults & Peds: ≥12 yrs:** 1 tabs q4h. **Max:** 6 tabs q24h. |

| BRAND NAME | ANALGESIC | ANTIHISTAMINE | DECONGESTANT | COUGH SUPPRESSANT | EXPECTORANT | DOSE |
|---|---|---|---|---|---|---|
| Dimetapp Children's Cold & Allergy Chewable tablets | | | Phenylephrine HCl 1.25mg | | | **Peds: 6-12 yrs:** 2 tabs q4h. **Max:** 6 tabs q24h. |
| Dimetapp Toddler's Drops Decongestant | | | Phenylephrine HCl 1.25mg/0.8mL | | | **Peds: 2-6 yrs:** 1.6mL q4h. **Max:** 6 doses q24h. |
| PediaCare Decongestant Infants' drops | | | Phenylephrine HCl 1.25mg/0.8mL | | | **Peds: 2-3 yrs:** 1.6mL q4h. **Max:** 6 doses q24h. |
| PediaCare Children's Decongestant liquid | | | Phenylephrine HCl 2.5mg/5mL | | | **Peds: 6-12 yrs:** 2 tsp (10mL) q4h. **2-6 yrs:** 1 tsp (5mL) q4h. **Max:** 6 doses q24h. |
| Sudafed 12 Hour tablets | | | Pseudoephedrine HCl 120mg | | | **Adults & Peds: ≥12 yrs:** 1 tab q12h. **Max:** 2 tabs q24h. |
| Sudafed 24 Hour tablets | | | Pseudoephedrine HCl 240mg | | | **Adults & Peds: ≥12 yrs:** 1 tab q24h. **Max:** 1 tab q24h. |
| Sudafed Children's liquid | | | Pseudoephedrine HCl 15mg/5mL | | | **Adults: ≥12 yrs:** 4 tsp (20mL) q4-6h. **Peds: 6-12 yrs:** 2 tsp (10mL) q4-6h. **2-6 yrs:** 1 tsp (5mL) q4-6h. **Max:** 4 doses q24h. |
| Sudafed PE tablets | | | Phenylephrine HCl 10mg | | | **Adults & Peds: ≥12 yrs:** 1 tab q4h. **Max:** 6 tabs q24h. |
| Sudafed PE Quick Dissolve Strips | | | Phenylephrine HCl 10mg | | | **Adults & Peds: ≥12 yrs:** 1 film q4h. **Max:** 6 films q24h. |
| Sudafed tablets | | | Pseudoephedrine HCl 30mg | | | **Adults: ≥12 yrs:** 2 tabs q4-6h. **Peds: 6-12 yrs:** 1 tab q4-6h. **Max:** 4 doses q24h. |
| Vicks Sinex 12-hour nasal spray | | | Oxymetazoline HCl 0.05% | | | **Adults & Peds: ≥6 yrs:** 2-3 sprays q10-12h. **Max:** 2 doses q24h. |
| Vicks Sinex Nasal Spray | | | Phenylephrine HCl 0.5% | | | **Adults & Peds: ≥12 yrs:** 2-3 sprays q4h. **Max:** 18 sprays q24h. |
| Vicks Sinex UltraFine Mist | | | Phenylephrine HCl 0.5% | | | **Adults & Peds: ≥12 yrs:** 2-3 sprays q4h. **Max:** 18 sprays q24h. |
| Vicks Sinex 12 Hour UltraFine Mist | | | Oxymetazoline HCl 0.05% | | | **Adults & Peds: ≥6 yrs:** 2-3 sprays q10-12h. **Max:** 2 doses q24h |

*(Continued)*

| BRAND NAME | ANALGESIC | ANTIHISTAMINE | DECONGESTANT | COUGH SUPPRESSANT | EXPECTORANT | DOSE |
|---|---|---|---|---|---|---|
| **DECONGESTANT** *(Continued)* | | | | | | |
| Vicks Vapor Inhaler | | | Levmetamfetamine 50mg | | | **Adults: ≥12 yrs:** 2 inhalations q2h. **Max:** 24 inhalations q24h **Peds: 6-12 yrs:** 1 inhalation q2h. **Max:** 12 inhalations q24h. |
| **DECONGESTANT + ANALGESIC** | | | | | | |
| Advil Children's Cold liquid | Ibuprofen 100mg | | Pseudoephedrine HCl 15mg | | | **Peds: 6-11 yrs (48-95 lbs):** 2 tsp (10mL) q6h. **2-5 yrs (24-47 lbs):** 1 tsp (5mL) q6h. **Max:** 4 doses q24h |
| Advil Cold & Sinus caplets/liqui-gels | Ibuprofen 200mg | | Pseudoephedrine HCl 30mg | | | **Adults & Peds: ≥12 yrs:** 1-2 caps q4-6h. **Max:** 6 caps q24h. |
| Alka-Seltzer Plus Cold & Sinus tablets | Acetaminophen 250mg | | Phenylephrine HCl 5mg | | | **Adults & Peds: ≥12 yrs:** 2 tabs q4h. **Max:** 8 tab q24h. |
| Alka-Seltzer Plus Cold & Sinus Effervescent tablets | Acetaminophen 250mg | | Phenylephrine HCl 5mg | | | **Adults & Peds: ≥12 yrs:** 2 tabs q4h. **Max:** 8 tab q24h. |
| Contac Cold & Flu Day & Night caplets | Acetaminophen 500mg | | Phenylephrine HCl 5mg | | | **Adults & Peds: ≥12 yrs:** 2 caps q4-6h. **Max:** 8 tab q24h. |
| Contac Cold & Flu Maximum Strength caplets | Acetaminophen 500mg | | Phenylephrine HCl 5mg | | | **Adults & Peds: ≥12 yrs:** 2 caps q4-6h. **Max:** 8 tab q24h. |
| Motrin Children's Cold suspension | Ibuprofen 100mg/5mL | | Pseudoephedrine HCl 15mg/5mL | | | **Peds: 6-12 yrs (48-95 lbs):** 2 tsp (10mL) q6h. **2-6 yrs (24-47 lbs):** 1 tsp (5mL) q6h. **Max:** 4 doses q24h. |
| Sinutab Sinus tablets | Acetaminophen 500mg | | Phenylephrine HCl 5mg | | | **Adults & Peds: ≥12 yrs:** 2 tabs q6h. **Max:** 8 tabs q24h. |
| Sudafed PE Sinus Headache caplets | Acetaminophen 325mg | | Phenylephrine HCl 5mg | | | **Adults & Peds: ≥12 yrs:** 2 caps q4h. **Max:** 12 caps q24h. |
| Theraflu Daytime Severe Cold Hot liquid | Acetaminophen 650mg | | Phenylephrine HCl 10mg | | | **Adults & Peds: ≥12 yrs:** 1 packet q4h. **Max:** 6 packets q24h. |
| Tylenol Sinus Congestion & Pain Daytime gelcaps | Acetaminophen 325mg | | Phenylephrine HCl 5mg | | | **Adults & Peds: ≥12 yrs:** 2 caps q4h. **Max:** 12 caps q24h. |
| Tylenol Sinus Congestion & Pain Day/Night pack | Acetaminophen 325mg | | Phenylephrine HCl 5mg | | | **Adults & Peds: ≥12 yrs:** 2 caps q4h. **Max:** 12 caps q24h. |

| BRAND NAME | ANALGESIC | ANTIHISTAMINE | DECONGESTANT | COUGH SUPPRESSANT | EXPECTORANT | DOSE |
|---|---|---|---|---|---|---|
| Vicks DayQuil Sinus liquicaps | Acetaminophen 325mg | | Phenylephrine HCl 5mg | | | **Adults & Peds: ≥12 yrs:** 2 caps q4h. **Max:** 6 caps q24h. |
| **DECONGESTANT + EXPECTORANT** | | | | | | |
| Robitussin PE Head & Chest liquid | | | Phenylephrine HCl 5mg/5mL | | Guaifenesin 100mg/5mL | **Adults: ≥12 yrs:** 2 tsp (10mL) q4h. **Peds: 6-12 yrs:** 1 tsp (5mL) q4h. **Max:** 6 doses q24h. |
| Sinutab Non-Drying liquid caps | | | Pseudoephedrine HCl 30mg | | Guaifenesin 200mg | **Adults & Peds: ≥12 yrs:** 2 cap q4h. **Max:** 12 q24h |
| Sudafed Non-Drying Sinus liquid caps | | | Phenylephrine HCl 5mg | | Guaifenesin 200mg | **Adults & Peds: ≥12 yrs:** 2 caps q4h. **Max:** 8 caps q24h. |
| Triaminic Chest & Nasal liquid | | | Phenylephrine HCl 2.5mg/5mL | | Guaifenesin 50mg/5mL | **Adults & Peds: ≥12 yrs:** 1 tsp q 4h. **Max:** 6 doses q24h. **Peds: 6-12 yrs:** 2 tsp (10mL). **2-6 yrs:** 1 tsp (5mL). |
| **DECONGESTANT + EXPECTORANT + ANALGESIC** | | | | | | |
| Tylenol Sinus Congestion & Severe pain caplets | Acetaminophen 325 mg | | Phenylephrine HCl 5mg | | Guaifenesin 200mg | **Adults & Peds: ≥12 yrs:** 2 caps q4h. **Max:** 12 caps q24h. |
| **EXPECTORANT** | | | | | | |
| Mucinex extended-release tablets | | | | | Guaifenesin 600mg | **Adults & Peds: ≥12 yrs:** 1-2 tabs q12h. **Max:** 4 tabs q24h. |
| Robitussin liquid | | | | | Guaifenesin 100mg/5mL | **Adults: ≥12 yrs:** 2-4 tsp (10-20mL) q4h. **Peds: 6-12 yrs:** 1-2 tsp (5-10mL) q4h. **2-6 yrs:** 1/2-1 tsp (2.5-5mL) q4h. **Max:** 6 doses q24h. |

# NASAL DECONGESTANT/MOISTURIZING PRODUCTS

| BRAND | INGREDIENT/STRENGTH | DOSE |
|---|---|---|
| **PSEUDOEPHEDRINE** | | |
| Dimetapp Decongestant Toddler's drops | Phenylephrine HCl 1.25mg/0.8mL | **Peds: 2-6 yrs:** 1.6mL q4h. **Max:** 6 doses/day. |
| Sudafed 12 Hour tablets | Pseudoephedrine HCl 120mg | **Adults & Peds: ≥12 yrs:** 1 tab q12h. **Max:** 2 tabs/day. |
| Sudafed 24 Hour tablets | Pseudoephedrine HCl 240mg | **Adults & Peds: ≥12 yrs:** 1 tab q24h. **Max:** 1 tab/day. |
| Sudafed Children's Nasal Decongestant chewable tablets | Pseudoephedrine HCl 15mg | **Peds: 6-12 yrs:** 2 tabs q4-6h. **Max:** 4 doses/day. |
| Sudafed Children's Nasal Decongestant liquid | Pseudoephedrine HCl 15mg | **Adults: ≥12 yrs:** 4 tsp q4-6h. **Peds: 6-12 yrs:** 2 tsp q4-6h. **2-6 yrs:** 1 tsp q4-6h. **Max:** 4 doses/day. |
| Sudafed Nasal Decongestant tablets | Pseudoephedrine HCl 30mg | **Adults: ≥12 yrs:** 2 tabs q4-6h. **Peds: 6-12 yrs:** 1 tab q4-6h. **Max:** 4 doses/day. |
| **TOPICAL NASAL DECONGESTANTS** | | |
| 4-Way Fast Acting Nasal Decongestant spray | Phenylephrine HCl 1% | **Adults & Peds: ≥12 yrs:** Instill 2-3 sprays per nostril q4h. |
| 4-Way Nasal Decongestant spray, 12 Hour | Phenylephrine HCl 1% | **Adults & Peds: ≥12 yrs:** Instill 2-3 sprays per nostril q4h. |
| 4-Way No Drip Nasal Decongestant spray | Phenylephrine HCl 1% | **Adults & Peds: ≥12 yrs:** Instill 2-3 sprays per nostril q4h. |
| Afrin Extra Moisturizing Nasal spray | Oxymetazoline HCl 0.05% | **Adults & Peds: ≥6 yrs:** Instill 2-3 sprays per nostril q10-12h. |
| Afrin No Drip Nasal Spray | Oxymetazoline HCl 0.05% | **Adults & Peds: ≥6 yrs:** Instill 2-3 sprays per nostril q10-12h. |
| Afrin No Drip Sinus Nasal spray | Oxymetazoline HCl 0.05% | **Adults & Peds: ≥6 yrs:** Instill 2-3 sprays per nostril q10-12h. |
| Afrin Original Nasal spray | Oxymetazoline HCl 0.05% | **Adults & Peds: ≥6 yrs:** Instill 2-3 sprays per nostril q10-12h. |
| Afrin Original Pumpmist Nasal spray | Oxymetazoline HCl 0.05% | **Adults & Peds: ≥6 yrs:** Instill 2-3 sprays per nostril q10-12h. |
| Afrin Severe Congestion Nasal spray | Oxymetazoline HCl 0.05% | **Adults & Peds: ≥6 yrs:** Instill 2-3 sprays per nostril q10-12h. |
| Afrin Sinus Nasal spray | Oxymetazoline HCl 0.05% | **Adults & Peds: ≥6 yrs:** Instill 2-3 sprays per nostril q10-12h. |
| Benzedrex Inhaler | Propylhexedrine 250 mg | **Adults & Peds: ≥6 yrs:** Inhale 2 sprays per nostril q2h. |
| Neo-Synephrine 12 Hour Extra Moisturizing Nasal spray | Oxymetazoline HCl 0.05% | **Adults & Peds: ≥6 yrs:** Instill 2-3 sprays per nostril q10-12h. |
| Neo-Synephrine 12 Hour Nasal Decongestant spray | Oxymetazoline HCl 0.05% | **Adults & Peds: ≥6 yrs:** Instill 2-3 sprays per nostril q10-12h. |
| Neo-Synephrine Extra Strength Nasal Decongestant Drops | Phenylephrine HCl 1% | **Adults & Peds: ≥12 yrs:** Instill 2-3 drops per nostril q4h. |
| Neo-Synephrine Extra Strength Nasal spray | Phenylephrine HCl 1% | **Adults & Peds: ≥6 yrs:** Instill 2-3 sprays per nostril q4h. |
| Neo-Synephrine Mild Formula Nasal spray | Phenylephrine HCl 0.25% | **Adults & Peds: ≥6 yrs:** Instill 2-3 sprays per nostril q4h. |
| Neo-Synephrine Regular Strength Nasal Decongestant spray | Phenylephrine HCl 0.5% | **Adults & Peds: ≥12 yrs:** Instill 2-3 sprays per nostril q4h. |
| Nostrilla 12 Hour Nasal Decongestant | Oxymetazoline HCl 0.05% | **Adults & Peds: ≥6 yrs:** Instill 2-3 sprays per nostril q10-12h. |
| Vicks Sinex 12 Hour Ultra Fine Mist For Sinus Relief | Oxymetazoline HCl 0.05% | **Adults & Peds: ≥12 yrs:** Instill 2-3 sprays per nostril q10-12h. |
| Vicks Sinex Long Acting Nasal Spray For Sinus Relief | Oxymetazoline HCl 0.05% | **Adults & Peds: ≥12 yrs:** Instill 2-3 sprays per nostril q10-12h. |
| Vicks Sinex Nasal Spray For Sinus Relief | Phenylephrine HCl 0.5% | **Adults & Peds: ≥12 yrs:** Instill 2-3 sprays per nostril q4h. |

*(Continued)*

| BRAND | INGREDIENT/STRENGTH | DOSE |
|---|---|---|
| **TOPICAL NASAL MOISTURIZERS** | | |
| 4-Way Saline Moisturizing Mist | Water, Boric Acid, Glycerin, Sodium Chloride, Sodium Borate, Eucalyptol, Menthol, Polysorbate 80, Benzalkonium Chloride | **Adults & Peds: ≥2 yrs:** Instill 2-3 sprays per nostril prn. |
| Ayr Baby's Saline Nose Spray, Drops | Sodium Chloride 0.65% | **Peds:** Instill 2 to 6 drops in each nostril. |
| Ayr Saline Nasal Gel | Aloe Vera Gel, Carbomer, Diazolidinyl Urea, Dimethicone Copolyol, FD&C Blue 1, Geranium Oil, Glycerin, Glyceryl Polymethacrylate, Methyl Gluceth 10, Methylparaben, Poloxamer 184, Propylene Glycol, Propylparaben, Sodium Chloride, Tocopherol Acetate, Triethanolamine, Xanthan Gum, Water | **Adults & Peds: ≥12 yrs:** Apply to nostril prn. |
| Ayr Saline Nasal Gel, No-Drip Sinus Spray | Water, Sodium Carbomethyl Starch, Propylene Glycol, Glycerin, Aloe Barbadensis Leaf Juice (Aloe Vera Gel), Sodium Chloride, Cetyl Pyridinium Chloride, Citric Acid, Disodium EDTA, Glycine Soja (Soybean Oil), Tocopheryl Acetate, Benzyl Alcohol, Benzalkonium Chloride, Geranium Maculatum Oil | **Adults & Peds: ≥12 yrs:** Use prn as directed. |
| Ayr Saline Nasal Mist | Sodium Chloride 0.65% | **Adults & Peds: ≥12 yrs:** Instill 2 sprays per nostril prn. |
| ENTSOL Mist, Buffered Hypertonic Nasal Irrigation Mist | Purified Water, Sodium Chloride, Sodium Phosphate Dibasic Edetate Disodium, Potassium Phosphate Monobasic, Benzalkonium Chloride | **Adults & Peds: ≥12 yrs:** Instill 1-2 sprays per nostril prn. |
| ENTSOL Single Use, Pre-Filled Nasal Wash Squeeze Bottle | Purified Water, Sodium Chloride, Sodium Phosphate Dibasic, Potassium Phosphate Monobasic | **Adults & Peds: ≥12 yrs:** Use as directed. |
| ENTSOL Spray, Buffered Hypertonic Saline Nasal Spray | Purified Water, Sodium Chloride Phosphate Dibasic, Potassium Phosphate Monobasic | **Adults & Peds: ≥12 yrs:** Instill 1 spray per nostril bid, 6 times daily |
| Little Noses Saline Spray/Drops, Non-Medicated | Sodium Chloride 0.65% | **Peds:** 2-6 drops per nostril as directed. |
| Ocean Premium Saline Nasal Spray | Sodium Chloride 0.65%, Phenylcarbinol, Benzalkonium Chloride | **Adults & Peds: ≥6 yrs:** Instill 2 sprays per nostril prn. |
| Simply Saline Sterile Saline Nasal Mist | Sodium Chloride 0.9% | **Adults & Peds: ≥12 yrs:** Use prn as directed. |
| SinoFresh Moisturizing Nasal & Sinus spray | Cetylpyridinium Chloride 0.05% | **Adults & Peds: ≥12 yrs:** Instill 1-3 sprays per nostril qd. |
| Zicam Nasal Moisturizer | Purified Water, High Purity Sodium Chloride, Aloe Vera | **Adults & Peds: ≥12 yrs:** Use as directed. |

# ANALGESIC PRODUCTS

| BRAND | INGREDIENT/STRENGTH | DOSE |
|---|---|---|
| **ACETAMINOPHEN** | | |
| Anacin Aspirin Free tablets | Acetaminophen 500mg | **Adults & Peds: ≥12 yrs:** 2 tabs q6h. **Max:** 8 tabs q24h. |
| Feverall Childrens' suppositories | Acetaminophen 120mg | **Peds: 3-6 yrs:** 1-2 supp. q4-6h. max 6 supp. q24h. |
| Feverall Infants' suppositories | Acetaminophen 80mg | **Peds: 3-11 months:** 1 supp. q6h. **12-36 months:** 1 supp. q4h. **Max:** 6 supp. q24h. |
| Feverall Jr. Strength suppositories | Acetaminophen 325mg | **Peds: 6-12 yrs:** 1 supp. q4-6h. **Max:** 6 supp. q24h. |
| Tylenol 8 Hour caplets | Acetaminophen 650mg | **Adults & Peds: ≥12 yrs:** 2 tabs q8h prn. **Max:** 6 tabs q24h. |
| Tylenol 8 Hour geltabs | Acetaminophen 650mg | **Adults & Peds: ≥12 yrs:** 2 tabs q8h prn. **Max:** 6 tabs q24h. |
| Tylenol Arthritis caplets | Acetaminophen 650mg | **Adults:** 2 tabs q8h prn. **Max:** 6 tabs q24h. |
| Tylenol Arthritis geltabs | Acetaminophen 650mg | **Adults:** 2 tabs q8h prn. **Max:** 6 tabs q24h. |
| Tylenol Children's Meltaways tablets | Acetaminophen 80mg | **Peds: 2-3 yrs (24-35 lbs):** 2 tabs **4-5 yrs (36-47 lbs):** 3 tabs. **6-8 yrs (48-59 lbs)**: 4 tabs. **9-10 yrs (60-71 lbs):** 5 tabs. **11 yrs (72-95 lbs):** 6 tabs. May repeat q4h. **Max:** 5 doses q24h. |
| Tylenol Children's suspension | Acetaminophen 160mg/5mL | **Peds: 2-3 yrs (24-35 lbs):** 1 tsp (5mL). **4-5 yrs (36-47 lbs):** 1.5 tsp (7.5mL). **6-8 yrs (48-59 lbs):** 2 tsp (10mL). **9-10 yrs (60-71 lbs):** 2.5 tsp (12.5mL). **11 yrs (72-95 lbs):** 3 tsp (15mL). May repeat q4h. **Max:** 5 doses q24h. |
| Tylenol Extra Strength caplets | Acetaminophen 500mg | **Adults & Peds: ≥12 yrs:** 2 tabs q4-6h prn. **Max:** 8 tabs q24h. |
| Tylenol Extra Strength Cool caplets | Acetaminophen 500mg | **Adults & Peds: ≥12 yrs:** 2 tabs q4-6h prn. **Max:** 8 tabs q24h. |
| Tylenol Extra Strength gelcaps | Acetaminophen 500mg | **Adults & Peds: ≥ 12 yrs:** 2 caps q4-6h prn. **Max:** 8 caps q24h. |
| Tylenol Rapid Blast liquid | Acetaminophen 500mg/15mL | **Adults & Peds: ≥12 yrs:** 2 tbl (30mL) q4-6h prn. **Max:** 8 tbl (120mL) q24h. |
| Tylenol Extra Strength EZ tablets | Acetaminophen 500mg | **Adults & Peds: ≥12 yrs:** 2 tabs q4-6h prn. **Max:** 8 tabs q24h. |
| Tylenol Extra Strength Go tablets | Acetaminophen 500mg | **Adults & Peds: ≥12 yrs:** 2 tabs q4-6h prn. **Max:** 8 tabs q24h. |
| Tylenol Infants' suspension | Acetaminophen 80mg/0.8mL | **Peds: 2-3 yrs (24-35 lbs):** 1.6 mL q4h prn. **Max:** 5 doses (8mL) q24h. |
| Tylenol Junior Meltaways tablets | Acetaminophen 160mg | **Peds: 6-8 yrs (48-59 lbs):** 2 tabs. **9-10 yrs (60-71 lbs):** 2.5 tabs. **11 yrs (72-95 lbs):** 3 tabs. **12 yrs (≥96 lbs):** 4 tabs. May repeat q4h. **Max:** 5 doses q24h. |
| Tylenol Regular Strength tablets | Acetaminophen 325mg | **Adults & Peds: ≥12 yrs:** 2 tabs q4-6h prn. **Max:** 12 tabs q24h. **Peds: 6-11 yrs:** 1 tab q4-6h. **Max:** 5 tabs q24h. |
| **ACETAMINOPHEN COMBINATIONS** | | |
| Anacin Advanced Headache tablets | Acetaminophen/Aspirin/Caffeine 250mg-65mg | **Adults & Peds: ≥12 yrs:** 2 tabs q6h. Max: 8 tabs q24h. |

*(Continued)*

| BRAND | INGREDIENT/STRENGTH | DOSE |
|---|---|---|
| **ACETAMINOPHEN COMBINATIONS** *(Continued)* | | |
| Excedrin Back & Body caplets | Acetaminophen/Aspirin Buffered 250mg-250mg | **Adults & Peds:** ≥**12 yrs:** 2 tabs q6h **Max:** 8 tabs q24h. |
| Excedrin Extra Strength caplets | Acetaminophen/Aspirin/Caffeine 250mg-250mg-65mg | **Adults & Peds:** ≥**12 yrs:** 2 tabs q6h. **Max:** 8 tabs q24h. |
| Excedrin Extra Strength geltabs | Acetaminophen/Aspirin/Caffeine 250mg-250mg-65mg | **Adults & Peds:** ≥**12 yrs:** 2 tabs q6h. **Max:** 8 tabs q24h. |
| Excedrin Extra Strength tablets | Acetaminophen/Aspirin/Caffeine 250mg-250mg-65mg | **Adults & Peds:** ≥**12 yrs:** 2 tabs q6h. **Max:** 8 tabs q24h. |
| Excedrin Migraine caplets | Acetaminophen/Aspirin/Caffeine 250mg-250mg-65mg | **Adults:** 2 tabs prn. **Max:** 2 tabs q24h. |
| Excedrin Migraine geltabs | Acetaminophen/Aspirin/Caffeine 250mg-250mg-65mg | **Adults:** 2 tabs prn. **Max:** 2 tabs q24h. |
| Excedrin Migraine tablets | Acetaminophen/Aspirin/Caffeine 250mg-250mg-65mg | **Adults:** 2 tabs prn. **Max:** 2 tabs q24h. |
| Excedrin Quicktabs tablets | Acetaminophen/Caffeine 500mg-65mg | **Adults & Peds:** ≥**12 yrs:** 2 tabs q6h. **Max:** 8 tabs q24h. |
| Excedrin Sinus Headache caplets | Acetaminophen/Phenylephrine HCl 325mg-5mg | **Adults & Peds:** ≥**12 yrs:** 2 tabs q4h. **Max:** 12 tabs q24h. |
| Excedrin Sinus Headache tablets | Acetaminophen/Phenylephrine HCl 325mg-5mg | **Adults & Peds:** ≥**12 yrs:** 2 tabs q4h. **Max:** 12 tabs q24h. |
| Excedrin Tension Headache caplets | Acetaminophen/Caffeine 500mg-65mg | **Adults & Peds:** ≥**12 yrs:** 2 tabs q6h. **Max:** 8 tabs q24h. |
| Excedrin Tension Headache geltabs | Acetaminophen/Caffeine 500mg-65mg | **Adults & Peds:** ≥**12 yrs:** 2 tabs q6h. **Max:** 8 tabs q24h. |
| Excedrin Tension Headache tablets | Acetaminophen/Caffeine 500mg-65mg | **Adults & Peds:** ≥**12 yrs:** 2 tabs q6h. **Max:** 8 tabs q24h. |
| Goody's Extra Strength Headache Powders | Acetaminophen/Aspirin/Caffeine 260mg-520mg-32.5mg | **Adults & Peds:** ≥**12 yrs:** 1 powder q4-6h. **Max:** 4 powders q24h. |
| Midol Menstrual Headache caplets | Acetaminophen/Caffeine 500mg-65g | **Adults & Peds:** ≥**12 yrs:** 2 tabs q6h. **Max:** 8 tabs q24h. |
| Midol Menstrual Complete caplets | Acetaminophen/Caffeine/Pyrilamine Maleate 500mg-60mg-15mg | **Adults & Peds:** ≥**12 yrs:** 2 tabs q6h. **Max:** 8 tabs q24h. |
| Midol Menstrual Complete caplets | Acetaminophen/Caffeine/Pyrilamine Maleate 500mg-60mg-15mg | **Adults & Peds:** ≥**12 yrs:** 2 tabs q6h. **Max:** 8 tabs q24h. |
| Midol PMS caplets | Acetaminophen/Pamabrom/Pyrilamine 500mg-25mg-15mg | **Adults & Peds:** ≥**12 yrs:** 2 tabs q6h. **Max:** 8 tabs q24h. |
| Midol Teen caplets | Acetaminophen/Pamabrom 500mg-25mg | **Adults & Peds:** ≥**12 yrs:** 2 tabs q6h. **Max:** 8 tabs q24h. |
| Pamprin Multi-Symptom caplets | Acetaminophen/Pamabrom/Pyrilamine 500mg-25mg-15mg | **Adults & Peds:** ≥**12 yrs:** 2 tabs q4-6h. **Max:** 8 tabs q24h. |
| Premsyn PMS caplets | Acetaminophen/Pamabrom/Pyrilamine 500mg-25mg-15mg | **Adults & Peds:** ≥**12 yrs:** 2 tabs q4-6h. **Max:** 8 tabs q24h. |
| Tylenol Women's caplets | Acetaminophen/Pamabrom 500mg-25mg | **Adults & Peds:** ≥**12 yrs:** 2 tabs q4-6h. **Max:** 8 tabs q24h. |
| Vanquish caplets | Acetaminophen/Aspirin/Caffeine 194mg-227mg-33mg | **Adults & Peds:** ≥**12 yrs:** 2 tabs q6h. **Max:** 8 tabs q24h. |
| **ACETAMINOPHEN/SLEEP AIDS** | | |
| Excedrin PM caplets | Acetaminophen/Diphenhydramine 500mg-38mg | **Adults & Peds:** ≥**12 yrs:** 2 tabs qhs. |
| Excedrin PM geltabs | Acetaminophen/Diphenhydramine citrate 500mg-38 mg | **Adults & Peds:** ≥**12 yrs:** 2 tabs qhs. |
| Excedrin PM tablets | Acetaminophen/Diphenhydramine citrate 500mg-38 mg | **Adults & Peds:** ≥**12 yrs:** 2 tabs qhs. |
| Goody's PM Powder | Acetaminophen/Diphenhydramine 1000mg-76mg/dose | **Adults & Peds:** ≥**12 yrs:** 1 packet (2 powders) qhs. |
| Tylenol PM caplets | Acetaminophen/Diphenhydramine 500mg-25mg | **Adults & Peds:** ≥**12 yrs:** 2 tabs qhs. |
| Tylenol PM gelcaps | Acetaminophen/Diphenhydramine 500mg-25mg | **Adults & Peds:** ≥**12 yrs:** 2 caps qhs. |

*(Continued)*

| BRAND | INGREDIENT/STRENGTH | DOSE |
|---|---|---|
| **ACETAMINOPHEN/SLEEP AIDS** *(Continued)* | | |
| Tylenol PM geltabs | Acetaminophen/Diphenhydramine 500mg-25mg | **Adults & Peds: ≥12 yrs:** 2 tabs qhs. |
| Tylenol PM liquid | Acetaminophen/Diphenhydramine 1000g-50mg/30 mL | **Adults & Peds: ≥12 yrs:** 2 tbl (30mL) qhs. **Max:** 8 tbl (120mL) q24h. |
| **NSAIDs** | | |
| Advil caplets | Ibuprofen 200mg | **Adults & Peds: ≥12 yrs:** 1-2 tabs q4-6h. **Max:** 6 tabs q24h. |
| Advil Children's Chewables tablets | Ibuprofen 50mg | **Peds: 2-3 yr (24-35 lb):** 2 tabs q6-8h. **4-5 yr (36-47 lb):** 3 tabs q6-8h. **6-8 yr (45-89 lb):** 4 tabs q6-8h. **9-10 yr (60-71 lb):** 5 tabs q6-8h. **11 yr (72-95 lb):** 6 tabs q6-8h. **Max:** 4 doses q24h |
| Advil Children's suspension | Ibuprofen 100mg/5mL | **Peds: 2-3 yrs (24-35 lbs):** 1 tsp (5mL). **4-5 yrs (36-47 lbs):** 1.5 tsp (7.5mL). **6-8 yrs (48-59 lbs):** 2 tsp (10mL). **9-10 yrs (60-71 lbs):** 2.5 tsp (12.5mL). **11 yrs (72-95 lbs):** 3 tsp (15mL). May repeat q6-8h. **Max:** 4 doses q24h. |
| Advil gelcaps | Ibuprofen 200mg | **Adults & Peds: ≥12 yrs:** 1-2 caps q4-6h. **Max:** 6 caps q24h. |
| Advil Infants' Drops | Ibuprofen 50mg/1.25mL | **Peds: 6-11 months (12-17 lbs):** 1.25mL. **12-23 months (18-23 lbs):** 1.875mL. May repeat q6-8h. **Max:** 4 doses q24h. |
| Advil Junior Strength tablets | Ibuprofen 100mg | **Peds: 6-10 yrs (48-71 lbs):** 2 tabs. **11 yrs (72-95 lbs):** 3 tabs. May repeat q6-8h. **Max:** 4 doses q24h. |
| Advil Junior Strength Chewable tablets | Ibuprofen 100mg | **Peds: 6-10 yrs (48-71 lbs):** 2 tabs. **11 yrs (72-95 lbs):** 3 tabs. May repeat q6-8h. **Max:** 4 doses q24h. |
| Advil liqui-gels | Ibuprofen 200mg | **Adults & Peds: ≥12 yrs:** 1-2 caps q4-6h. **Max:** 6 caps q24h. |
| Advil Migraine capsules | Ibuprofen 200mg | **Adults:** 2 caps prn. **Max:** 2 caps q24h. |
| Advil tablets | Ibuprofen 200mg | **Adults & Peds: ≥12 yrs:** 1-2 tabs q4-6h. **Max:** 6 tabs q24h. |
| Aleve caplets | Naproxen Sodium 220mg | **Adults: ≥65 yrs:** 1 tab q12h. **Max:** 2 tabs q24h. **Adults & Peds: ≥12 yrs:** 1 tab q8-12h. **Max:** 3 tabs q24h. |
| Aleve gelcaps | Naproxen Sodium 220mg | **Adults: ≥65 yrs:** 1 cap q12h. **Max:** 2 caps q24h. **Adults & Peds: ≥12 yrs:** 1 cap q8-12h. **Max:** 3 caps q24h. |
| Aleve tablets | Naproxen Sodium 220mg | **Adults: ≥65 yrs:** 1 tab q12h. **Max:** 2 tabs q24h. **Adults & Peds: ≥12 yrs:** 1 tab q8-12h. **Max:** 3 tabs q24h. |
| Midol Cramps and Body Aches tablets | Ibuprofen 200mg | **Adults & Peds: ≥12 yrs:** 1-2 tabs q4-6h. **Max:** 6 tabs q24h. |
| Midol Extended Relief caplets | Naproxen Sodium 220mg | **Adults & Peds: ≥12 yrs:** 1 tabs q8-12h. **Max:** 3 tabs q24h. |
| Motrin Children's suspension | Ibuprofen 100mg/5mL | **Peds: 2-3 yrs (24-35 lbs):** 1 tsp (5mL). **4-5 yrs (36-47 lbs):** 1.5 tsp (7.5mL). **6-8 yrs (48-59 lbs):** 2 tsp (10mL). **9-10 yrs (60-71 lbs):** 2.5 tsp (12.5mL). **11 yrs (72-95 lbs):** 3 tsp (15mL). May repeat q6-8h. **Max:** 4 doses q24h. |

*(Continued)*

| BRAND | INGREDIENT/STRENGTH | DOSE |
|---|---|---|
| **NSAIDs** *(Continued)* | | |
| Motrin IB caplets | Ibuprofen 200mg | **Adults & Peds: ≥12 yrs:** 1-2 tabs q4-6h. **Max:** 6 tabs q24h. |
| Motrin IB gelcaps | Ibuprofen 200mg | **Adults & Peds: ≥12 yrs:** 1-2 tabs q4-6h. **Max:** 6 tabs q24h. |
| Motrin IB tablets | Ibuprofen 200mg | **Adults & Peds: ≥12 yrs:** 1-2 tabs q4-6h. **Max:** 6 tabs q24h. |
| Motrin Infants' Drops | Ibuprofen 50mg/1.25mL | **Peds: 6-11 months (12-17 lbs):** 1.25mL. **12-23 months (18-23 lbs):** 1.875mL. May repeat q6-8h. **Max:** 4 doses q24h. |
| Motrin Junior Strength chewable tablets | Ibuprofen 100mg | **Peds: 6-8 yrs (48-59 lbs):** 2 tabs. **9-10 yrs (60-71 lbs):** 2.5 tabs. **11 yrs (72-95 lbs):** 3 tabs. May repeat q6-8h. **Max:** 4 doses q24h. |
| Nuprin caplets | Ibuprofen 200mg | **Adults & Peds: ≥12 yrs:** 1-2 tabs q4-6h. **Max:** 6 tabs q24h. |
| Nuprin tablets | Ibuprofen 200mg | **Adults & Peds: ≥12 yrs:** 1-2 tabs q4-6h. **Max:** 6 tabs q24h. |
| **SALICYLATES** | | |
| Anacin 81 tablets | Aspirin 81mg | **Adults & Peds: ≥12 yrs:** 4-8 tabs q4h. **Max:** 48 tabs q24h. |
| Aspergum chewable tablets | Aspirin 227mg | **Adults & Peds: ≥12 yrs:** 2 tabs q4h. **Max:** 16 tabs q24h. |
| Bayer Aspirin Extra Strength caplets | Aspirin 500mg | **Adults & Peds: ≥12 yrs:** 1-2 tabs q4-6h. **Max:** 8 tabs q24h. |
| Bayer Aspirin safety coated caplets | Aspirin 325mg | **Adults & Peds: ≥12 yrs:** 1-2 tabs q4h or 3 tabs q6h. **Max:** 12 tabs q24h. |
| Bayer Children's Aspirin chewable tablets | Aspirin 81mg | **Adults & Peds: ≥12 yrs:** 4-8 tabs q4h. **Max:** 48 tabs q24h. |
| Bayer Low Dose Aspirin tablets | Aspirin 81mg | **Adults & Peds: ≥12 yrs:** 4-8 tabs q4h. **Max:** 48 tabs q24h. |
| Bayer Sugar Free Low Dose Aspirin tablets | Aspirin 81mg | **Adults & Peds: ≥12 yrs:** 4-8 tabs q4h. **Max:** 48 tabs q24h. |
| Bayer Genuine Aspirin tablets | Aspirin 325mg | **Adults & Peds: ≥12 yrs:** 1-2 tabs q4h or 3 tabs q6h. **Max:** 12 tabs q24h. |
| Bayer Extra-Strength Plus caplets | Aspirin 500mg | **Adults & Peds: ≥12 yrs:** 2 tabs q6h. **Max:** 8 tabs q24h. |
| Doan's Regular Strength caplets | Magnesium Salicylate Tetrahydrate 377mg | **Adults & Peds: ≥12 yrs:** 2 tabs q4h. **Max:** 12 tabs q24h. |
| Ecotrin Adult Low Strength tablets | Aspirin 81mg | **Adults:** 4-8 tabs q4h. **Max:** 48 tabs q24h. |
| Ecotrin Enteric Low Strength tablets | Aspirin 81mg | **Adults:** 4-8 tabs q4h. **Max:** 48 tabs q24h. |
| Ecotrin Enteric Regular Strength tablets | Aspirin 325mg | **Adults & Peds: ≥12 yrs:** 1-2 tabs q4h. **Max:** 12 tabs q24h. |
| Ecotrin Maximum Strength tablets | Aspirin 500mg | **Adults & Peds: ≥12 yrs:** 2 tabs q6h. **Max:** 8 tabs q24h. |
| Ecotrin Regular Strength tablets | Aspirin 325mg | **Adults & Peds: ≥12 yrs:** 1-2 tabs q4h. **Max:** 12 tabs q24h. |
| Halfprin 162mg tablets | Aspirin 162mg | **Adults & Peds: ≥12 yrs:** 2-4 tabs q4h. **Max:** 24 tabs q24h. |
| Halfprin 81mg tablets | Aspirin 81mg | **Adults & Peds: ≥12 yrs:** 4-8 tabs q4h. **Max:** 48 tabs q24h. |
| St. Joseph Adult Low Strength chewable tablets | Aspirin 81mg | **Adults & Peds: ≥12 yrs:** 4-8 tabs q4h. **Max:** 48 tabs q24h. |
| St. Joseph Adult Low Strength tablets | Aspirin 81mg | **Adults & Peds: ≥12 yrs:** 4-8 tabs q4h. **Max:** 48 tabs q24h. |

*(Continued)*

| BRAND | INGREDIENT/STRENGTH | DOSE |
|---|---|---|
| **SALICYLATES, BUFFERED** | | |
| Ascriptin Maximum Strength tablets | Aspirin Buffered with Maalox/Calcium Carbonate 500mg | **Adults & Peds: ≥12 yrs:** 2 tabs q4h. **Max:** 8 tabs q24h. |
| Ascriptin Regular Strength tablets | Aspirin Buffered with Maalox/Calcium Carbonate 325mg | **Adults & Peds: ≥12 yrs:** 2 tabs q4h. **Max:** 12 tabs q24h. |
| Bayer Extra Strength Plus caplets | Aspirin Buffered with Calcium Carbonate 500mg | **Adults & Peds: ≥12 yrs:** 1-2 tabs q4-6h. **Max:** 8 tabs q24h. |
| Bufferin Extra Strength tablets | Aspirin Bufferred with Calcium Carbonate/Magnesium Oxide/Magnesium Carbonate 500mg | **Adults & Peds: ≥12 yrs:** 2 tabs q6h. **Max:** 8 tabs q24h. |
| Bufferin tablets | Aspirin Bufferred with Calcium Carbonate/Magnesium Oxide/Magnesium Carbonate 325mg | **Adults & Peds: ≥12 yrs:** 2 tabs q4h. **Max:** 12 tabs q24h. |
| **SALICYLATE COMBINATIONS** | | |
| Alka-Seltzer effervescent tablets | Aspirin/Citric Acid/Sodium Bicarbonate 325mg-1000mg-1916mg | **Adults & Peds: ≥12 yrs:** 2 tabs q4h. **Max:** 8 tabs q24h. |
| Alka-Seltzer Extra Strength effervescent tablets | Aspirin/Citric Acid/Sodium Bicarbonate 500mg-1000mg-1985mg | **Adults & Peds: ≥12 yrs:** 2 tabs q6h. **Max:** 7 tabs q24h. |
| Alka-Seltzer Morning Relief effervescent tablets | Aspirin/Caffeine 500mg-65mg | **Adults & Peds: ≥12 yrs:** 2 tabs q6h. **Max:** 8 tabs q24h. |
| Anacin Pain Reliever caplets | Aspirin/Caffeine 400mg-32mg | **Adults & Peds: ≥12 yrs:** 2 tabs q6h. **Max:** 8 tabs q24h. |
| Anacin Extra Strength tablets | Aspirin/Caffeine 500mg-32mg | **Adults & Peds: ≥12 yrs:** 2 tabs q6h. **Max:** 8 tabs q24h. |
| Anacin tablets | Aspirin/Caffeine 400mg-32mg | **Adults & Peds: ≥12 yrs:** 2 tabs q6h. **Max:** 8 tabs q24h. |
| Bayer Back & Body Pain caplets | Aspirin/Caffeine 500mg-32.5mg | **Adults & Peds: ≥12 yrs:** 2 tabs q6h. **Max:** 8 tabs q24h. |
| BC Arthritis Strength powders | Aspirin/Caffeine/Salicylamide 742mg-38mg-222mg | **Adults & Peds: ≥12 yrs:** 1 powder q3-4h. **Max:** 4 powders q24h. |
| BC Original powders | Aspirin/Caffeine/Salicylamide 650mg-33.3mg-195mg | **Adults & Peds: ≥12 yrs:** 1 powder q3-4h. |
| **SALICYLATE/SLEEP AID** | | |
| Alka-Seltzer PM Pain Reliever & Sleep Aid, effervescent tablets | Aspirin/Diphenhydramine Citrate 325mg-38 mg | **Adults & Peds: ≥12 yrs:** 2 tabs qpm. |
| Bayer PM Relief caplets | Aspirin/Diphenhydramine 500mg-38.3mg | **Adults & Peds: ≥12 yrs:** 2 tabs qhs. |
| Doan's Extra Strength PM caplets | Magnesium Salicylate Tetrahydrate/Diphenhydramine 580mg-25mg | **Adults & Peds: ≥12 yrs:** 2 tabs 2 tabs qhs. |

# CANKER AND COLD SORE PRODUCTS

| BRAND | INGREDIENT/STRENGTH | DOSE |
|---|---|---|
| Abreva Cold Sore/Fever Blister Treatment | Docosanol 10% | **Adults & Peds: ≥12 yrs:** Use 5 times a day till healed. |
| Anbesol Cold Sore Therapy Ointment | Allantoin/Benzocaine/Camphor/ White Petrolatum 1%-20%-3%-64.9% | **Adults & Peds: ≥2 yrs:** Apply to affected area tid-qid. |
| Anbesol Jr. Gel | Benzocaine 10% | **Adults & Peds: ≥2 yrs:** Apply to affected area qid. |
| Anbesol Maximum Strength Gel | Benzocaine 20% | **Adults & Peds: ≥2 yrs:** Apply to affected area qid. |
| Anbesol Regular Strength Gel | Benzocaine 10% | **Adults & Peds: ≥2 yrs:** Apply to affected area qid. |
| Anbesol Regular Strength Liquid | Benzocaine 10% | **Adults & Peds: ≥2 yrs:** Apply to affected area qid. |
| Campho-Phenique Cold Sore for Scab Relief Cream | Pramoxine HCl/White Petrolatum 1%-30% | **Adults & Peds: ≥2 yrs:** Apply to affected area tid-qid. |
| Campho-Phenique Cold Sore Gel | Camphor/Phenol 10.8%-4.7% | **Adults & Peds: ≥2 yrs:** Apply to affected area qd-tid |
| Carmex Cold Sore Reliever and Lip Moisturizer | Menthol/Camphor/Phenol 0.4%-1.7%-0.4% | **Adults & Peds: ≥12 yrs:** Apply to affected area prn. |
| ChapStick Cold Sore Therapy | Allantoin/Benzocaine/Camphor/White Petrolatum 1%-20%-3%-64.9% | **Adults & Peds: ≥2 yrs:** Apply to affected area tid-qid. |
| Chloraseptic Mouth Pain Spray | Phenol 1.4% | **Peds: ≥2 yrs:** Apply to affected area prn. |
| Herpecin-L Lip Balm Stick, SPF 30 | Dimethicone/Methyl Anthranilate/ Octyl Methoxycinnamate/Octyl Salicylate/ Oxybenzone 1%-5%-7.5%-5%- 6% | **Adults & Peds: ≥12 yrs:** Apply prn. |
| Kank-A Soft Brush Mouth Pain Gel | Benzocaine 20% | **Adults & Peds: ≥2 yrs:** Apply to affected area qid. |
| Kanka-A Mouth Pain Liquid | Benzocaine 20% | **Adults & Peds: ≥2 yrs:** Apply to affected area qid. |
| Novitra Cold Sore Maximum Strength Cream | Zincum Oxydatum 2X HPUS | **Adults & Peds: ≥2 yrs:** Apply to affected area q2-3h, 6 to 8 times daily. |
| Orabase Maximum Strength Oral Pain Reliever | Benzocaine 20% | **Adults & Peds: ≥2 yrs:** Apply to affected area qid. |
| Orabase Soothe-N-Seal, Liquid Protectant for Canker Sore Pain Relief | Formulated 2-Octyl Cyanoacrylate | **Adults:** Apply prn. |
| Orajel Canker Sore Ultra Gel | Benzocaine/Menthol 15%-2% | **Adults & Peds: ≥2 yrs:** Apply to affected area qid. |
| Orajel Maximum Strength Gel Oral Pain Reliever | Benzocaine 20% | **Adults & Peds: ≥2 yrs:** Apply to affected area qid. |
| Orajel Mouth Sore Gel | Benzocaine/Benzalkonium Chloride/Zinc | **Adults & Peds: ≥2 yrs:** Chloride 20%-0.02%-0.1% Apply to affected area qid. |
| Orajel Mouth Sore Swabs | Benzocaine 20% | **Adults & Peds: ≥2 yrs:** Apply to affected area qid. |
| Releev 1-Day Cold Sore Treatment | Benzalkonium Chloride 0.13% | **Adults & Peds: ≥2 yrs:** Apply to clean dry affected area tid-qid. |
| Swabplus Mouth Sore Relief Swabs | Benzocaine 20% | **Adults & Peds: ≥2 yrs:** Apply to affected area qid. |
| Tanac Liquid | Benzalkonium Chloride/Benzocaine 0.12%-10% | **Adults & Peds: ≥2 yrs:** Apply to affected area tid-qid. |
| Zilactin Cold Sore Gel | Benzyl Alcohol 10% | **Adults & Peds: ≥2 yrs:** Apply to affected area qid. |

# ACE INHIBITORS

| DRUG | PEEK PLASMA LEVEL | FOOD EFFECT ON AMOUNT ABSORBED | HYPERTENSION DOSING* | HEART FAILURE DOSING | RENAL DOSE ADJUSTMENT |
|---|---|---|---|---|---|
| Benazepril | 1-2 hrs (fasting); 2-4 hrs (non-fasting**) | None | Initial: 10mg qd.<br>Usual: 20-40mg/day given qd-bid.<br>Max: 80mg/day. | Not FDA approved. | CrCl<30mL/min/1.73$m^2$:<br>Initial: 5mg qd.<br>Max: 40mg/day. |
| Captopril | 1 hr | Reduced*** | Initial: 25mg bid-tid.<br>Usual: 25-150mg bid-tid.<br>Max: 450mg/day. | Initial: 25mg tid.<br>Usual: 50-100mg tid.<br>Max: 450mg/day. | Significant Renal Dysfunction: Lower initial dose and titrate slowly. |
| Enalapril | 3-4 hrs** | None | Initial: 5mg qd.<br>Usual: 10-40mg/day given qd-bid.<br>Max: 40mg/day.† | Initial: 2.5mg qd.<br>Usual: 2.5-20mg given bid.<br>Max: 40mg/day. | HTN: CrCl ≤30mL/min:<br>Initial: 2.5mg/day.<br>Max: 40mg/day.<br>Dialysis: 2.5mg/day on dialysis day.<br>HF: SCr 1.6mg/dL:<br>Initial: 2.5mg qd.<br>Max: 40mg/day. |
| Fosinopril | 3 hrs** | None | Initial: 10mg qd.<br>Usual: 20-40mg/day.<br>Max: 80mg/day. | Initial: 10mg qd.<br>Usual: 20-40mg qd.<br>Max: 40mg/day. | HTN: No dosage adjustment needed.<br>HF: Moderate to severe renal failure/vigorous diuresis: 5mg qd. |
| Lisinopril | 7 hrs | None | Initial: 10mg qd.<br>Usual: 20-40mg qd.<br>Max: 80mg/day. | (Prinivil)<br>Initial: 5mg qd.<br>Usual: 5-20mg qd.<br>(Zestril)<br>Initial: 5mg qd.<br>Usual: 5-40mg qd.<br>Max: 40mg/day. | HTN: CrCl 10-30mL/min:<br>Initial: 5mg qd.<br>Max: 40mg/day.<br>CrCl <10mL/min:<br>Initial: 2.5mg qd.<br>Max: 40mg/day.<br>HF: CrCl ≤30mL/min:<br>Initial: 2.5mg qd. |
| Moexipril | 1-1.5 hrs** | Reduced*** | Initial: 7.5mg qd.<br>Usual: 7.5-30mg/day given qd-bid.<br>Max: 60mg/day. | Not FDA approved. | CrCl ≤40mL/min/1.73$m^2$:<br>Initial: 3.75mg qd.<br>Max: 15mg/day. |
| Perindopril | 3-7 hrs** | None | Initial: 4mg qd.<br>Usual: 4-8mg/day given qd-bid.<br>Max: 16mg/day. | Not FDA approved. | CrCl >30mL/min:<br>Initial: 2mg qd.<br>Max: 8mg/day. |
| Quinapril | 2 hrs** | Reduced (after high fat meals) | Initial: 10-20mg qd.<br>Usual: 20-80mg/day given qd-bid. | Initial: 5mg bid.<br>Usual: 10-20mg bid. | CrCl 30-60mL/min:<br>Initial: 5mg/day.<br>CrCl 10-30mL/min:<br>Initial: 2.5mg/day. |
| Ramipril | 2-4 hrs** | None | Initial: 2.5mg qd.<br>Usual: 2.5-20mg/day given qd-bid. | Post MI:<br>Initial: 2.5mg bid; 1.25mg bid if hypotensive.<br>Titrate to 5mg bid. | HTN:<br>Initial: 1.25mg qd.<br>Max: 5mg/day.<br>Post MI:<br>Initial: 1.25mg/day.<br>Max: 2.5mg/bid. |
| Trandolapril | 4-10 hrs** | None | Initial: 1mg qd in non-black patients. 2mg qd in black patients.<br>Usual: 2-4mg/day.<br>Max: 8mg/day. | Post MI:<br>Initial: 1mg qd.<br>Titrate to 4mg qd if tolerated. | CrCl <30mL/min:<br>Initial: 0.5mg qd. |

* Reduce dose with concomitant diuretic.
** Peak effect of active metabolite.
*** Administer 1 hour before meals (captopril) or on an empty stomach (moexipril).
† Refer to monograph for pediatric dosing.

# ARBs* and Combinations

| DRUG | BRAND | USUAL HTN† DOSAGE RANGE (mg/day) | HOW SUPPLIED‡ |
|---|---|---|---|
| **ANGIOTENSIN II RECEPTOR BLOCKERS** | | | |
| Candesartan | Atacand | 8–32 | **Tab:** 4mg, 8mg, 16mg, 32mg |
| Eprosartan | Teveten | 400–800 | **Tab:** 400mg, 600mg |
| Irbesartan | Avapro | 150–300 | **Tab:** 75mg, 150mg, 300mg |
| Losartan | Cozaar | 25–100 | **Tab:** 25mg, 50mg, 100mg |
| Olmesartan | Benicar | 20–40 | **Tab:** 5mg, 20mg, 40mg |
| Telmisartan | Micardis | 20–80 | **Tab:** 20mg, 40mg, 80mg |
| Valsartan | Diovan | 80–320 | **Tab:** 40mg, 80mg, 160mg, 320mg |
| **COMBINATIONS** | | | |
| Candesartan-Hydrochlorothiazide | Atacand HCT | *See individual listing. Monotherapy recommended first.* | **Tab:** 16mg-12.5mg, 32mg-12.5mg |
| Eprosartan-Hydrochlorothiazide | Teveten HCT | | **Tab:** 600mg-12.5mg, 600mg-25mg |
| Irbesartan-Hydrochlorothiazide | Avalide | | **Tab:** 150mg-12.5mg, 300mg-12.5mg, 300mg-25mg |
| Losartan-Hydrochlorothiazide | Hyzaar | | **Tab:** 50mg-12.5mg, 100mg-25mg, 100mg-12.5mg |
| Olmesartan-Hydrochlorothiazide | Benicar HCT | | **Tab:** 20mg-12.5mg, 40mg-12.5mg, 40mg-25mg |
| Telmisartan-Hydrochlorothiazide | Micardis HCT | | **Tab:** 40mg-12.5mg, 80mg-12.5mg, 80mg-25mg |
| Valsartan-Hydrochlorothiazide | Diovan HCT | | **Tab:** 80mg-12.5mg, 160mg-12.5mg, 160mg-25mg, 320mg-12.5mg, 320mg-25mg |

*ARBs: Angiotensin II Receptor Blockers.

†HTN: Hypertension.

‡Adopted from the Seventh Report of the Joint National Committee on Prevention, Detection, Evaluation, and Treatment of High Blood Pressure (JNC 7) http://www.nhlbi.nih.gov/guidelines/hypertension/jnc7full.htm

# CALCIUM CHANNEL BLOCKERS

| DRUG | BRAND | HOW SUPPLIED | HYPERTENSION DOSING* | ANGINA DOSING* |
|---|---|---|---|---|
| **DIHYDROPYRIDINES** | | | | |
| **Amlodipine besylate** | Norvasc | Tab: 2.5mg, 5mg, 10mg | Initial: 5mg qd.<br>Max: 10mg qd. | Initial/Usual:<br>10mg qd. |
| **Felodipine** | Plendil | Tab, ER: 2.5mg, 5mg, 10mg | Initial: 5mg qd.<br>Usual: 2.5-10mg qd. | Not FDA approved |
| **Isradipine** | DynaCirc | Cap: 2.5mg, 5mg | Initial: 2.5mg bid.<br>Max: 20mg/day. | Not FDA approved |
| | DynaCirc CR | Tab, CR: 5mg, 10mg | Initial: 5mg qd.<br>Max: 20mg/day. | Not FDA approved |
| **Nicardipine HCl** | Cardene | Cap: 20mg, 30mg | Initial: 20mg tid.<br>Usual: 20-40mg tid. | Initial: 20mg tid.<br>Usual: 20-40mg tid. |
| | Cardene SR | Cap, ER: 30mg, 45mg, 60mg | Initial: 30mg bid.<br>Usual: 30-60mg bid. | Not FDA approved |
| **Nifedipine** | Adalat CC | Tab, ER: 30mg, 60mg, 90mg | Initial: 30mg qd.<br>Usual: 30-60mg qd.<br>Max: 90mg/day. | Not FDA approved |
| | Procardia | Cap: 10mg, 20mg | Not FDA approved | Initial: 10mg tid.<br>Usual: 10-20mg tid.<br>Max: 180mg/day. |
| | Procardia XL | Tab, ER: 30mg, 60mg, 90mg | Initial: 30-60mg qd.<br>Max: 120mg/day. | Initial: 30-60mg qd.<br>Max: 90-120mg/day. |
| **Nisoldipine** | Sular | Tab, ER: 10mg, 20mg, 30mg, 40mg | Initial: 20mg qd.<br>Usual: 20-40mg qd.<br>Max: 60mg/day. | Not FDA approved |
| **NON-DIHYDROPYRIDINES** | | | | |
| **Diltiazem HCl** | Cardizem | Tab: 30mg, 60mg, 90mg, 120mg | Not FDA approved | Initial: 30mg qid.<br>Usual: 180-360mg/day. |
| | Cardizem CD, Cartia XT | Cap, ER: 120mg, 180mg, 240mg, 300mg, (Cardizem CD) 360mg | Initial: 180-240mg qd.<br>Usual: 240-360mg qd.<br>Max: 480mg qd. | Initial: 120-180mg qd.<br>Max: 480mg/day. |
| | Cardizem LA | Tab, ER: 120mg, 180mg, 240mg, 300mg, 360mg, 420mg | Initial: 180-240mg qd.<br>Max: 540mg/day. | Not FDA approved |
| | Dilacor XR, Diltia XT | Cap, ER: 120mg, 180mg, 240mg | Initial: 180-240mg qd.<br>Usual: 180-480mg qd.<br>Max: 540mg qd. | Initial: 120mg qd.<br>Max: 480mg/day. |
| | Tiazac | Cap, ER: 120mg, 180mg, 240mg, 300mg, 360mg, 420mg | Initial: 120-240mg qd.<br>Usual: 120-540mg qd.<br>Max: 540mg qd. | Initial: 120-180mg qd.<br>Max: 540mg qd. |
| **Verapamil HCl** | Calan** | Tab: 40mg, 80mg, 120mg | Initial: 80mg tid.<br>Usual: 360-480mg/day. | Usual: 80-120mg tid. |
| | Calan SR, Isoptin SR | Tab, ER: 120mg, 180mg, 240mg | Initial: 180mg qam.<br>Max: 480mg/day. | Not FDA approved |
| | Covera HS | Tab, ER: 180mg, 240mg | Initial: 180mg qhs.<br>Max: 480mg qhs. | Initial: 180mg qhs.<br>Max: 480mg qhs. |
| | Verelan | Cap, ER: 120mg, 180mg, 240mg, 360mg | Usual: 240mg qam.<br>Max: 480mg qam. | Not FDA approved |
| | Verelan PM | Cap, ER: 100mg, 200mg, 300mg | Usual: 200mg qhs.<br>Max: 400mg qhs. | Not FDA approved |

* NOTE: Adult dosing shown is for monotherapy. Dosage needs to be adjusted by titration to individual patient needs. Dosages may need to be reduced in the elderly, or with renal/hepatic impairment. When used in combination with other antihypertensives the dosage of the calcium channel blocker or the concomitant antihypertensives may need to be adjusted due to possible additive effect. Monitor patient closely. For more detailed information refer to the individual monograph listings in the Cardiovascular section or the drug's labeling.

** For additional indications refer to the monograph listings or the drug's FDA-approved labeling.

# CHOLESTEROL-LOWERING AGENTS

| BRAND (GENERIC) | HOW SUPPLIED (MG)* | USUAL DOSAGE RANGE** | T-CHOL (% DECREASE) | LDL (% DECREASE) | HDL (% DECREASE) | TG (% DECREASE) |
|---|---|---|---|---|---|---|
| **HMG-CoA REDUCTASE INHIBITORS (STATINS)** | | | | | | |
| Lipitor (Atrovastatin) | Tabs: 10, 20, 40 80 | 10-80mg/day | 29 to 45 | 39 to 60 | 5 to 9 | 19 to 37 |
| Lescol (Fluvastatin) | Tabs: 20, 40 | 20-80mg/day | 17 to 27 | 22 to 36 | 3 to 6 | 12 to 18 |
| Lescol XL (Fluvastatin) | Tabs, ER: 80 | 20-80mg/day | 17 to 27 | 22 to 36 | 3 to 6 | 12 to 18 |
| Altoprev (Lovastatin) | Tab, ER: 20, 40, 80 | 20-60mg/day | 17 to 29 | 24 to 40 | 6.6 to 9.5 | 10 to 19 |
| Mevacor (Lovastatin) | Tabs: 10, 20, 40 | 10-80mg/day given qd or bid | 17 to 29 | 24 to 40 | 6.6 to 9.5 | 10 to 19 |
| Pravachol (Pravastatin) | Tabs: 10, 20, 40, 80 | 10-80mg/day | 16 to 27 | 22 to 37 | 2 to 12 | 11 to 24 |
| Crestor (Rosuvastatin) | Tabs: 5, 10, 20, 40 | 5-40mg/day | 33 to 46 | 45 to 63 | 8 to 14 | 10 to 35 |
| Zocor (Simvastatin) | Tabs: 5, 10, 20, 40, 80 | 5-80mg/day | 19 to 36 | 26 to 47 | 8 to 16 | 12 to 33 |
| **FIBRATES** | | | | | | |
| Tricor (Fenofibrate) | Tab: 48, 148 | 48-145mg/day | 18.7 | 20.6 | 11 | 28.9 |
| Lofibra (Fenofibrate) | Tabs: 54, 160 | 54-160mg/day | 18.7 | 20.6 | 11 | 28.9 |
| Antara (Fenofibrate) | Caps: 43, 87, 130 | 43-130mg/day | 18.7 | 20.6 | 11 | 28.9 |
| Triglide (Fenofibrate) | Tabs: 50, 160 | 50-160mg/day | 18.7 | 20.6 | 11 | 28.9 |
| Lopid (Gemfibrozil) | Tab: 600 | 1200mg/day in divided doses | n/a | 4.1 | 12.6 | Not specified-but decrease |
| **BILE-ACID SEQUESTRANTS** | | | | | | |
| Questran, Questran Light (Cholestyramine) | Can: 268, 378 | 2-4 packets or scoopfuls daily (8-16 g) divided into two doses | 7.2 | 10.4 | n/a | n/a |
| WelChol (Colesevelam HCl) | Tabs: 625 | 3750mg/day given qd for bid Increase | 7 to 10 | 15 to 18 | 3 | 9 to 10 |
| **CHOLESTROL ABSORPTION INHIBITOR** | | | | | | |
| Zetia (Ezetimibe) | Tab: 10 | 10mg qd | 13 | 18 | 1 | 8 |
| **NICOTINIC ACID DERIVATIVE** | | | | | | |
| Nispan (Niacin, Extended Release) | Tabs, ER: 500, 750, 1000 | 1-2g hs | 3 to 10 | 5 to 14 | 18 to 22 | 13 to 28 |
| **COMBINATIONS** | | | | | | |
| Caduet (Amlodipine/ Atorvastatin) | Tabs: 2.5/10, 2.5/20, 2.5/40, 5/10, 5/20, 5/40, 5/80, 10/10, 10/ 20, 10/40, 10/80 | 10/20mg to 10/80mg | n/a | n/a | n/a | n/a |
| Vytorin (Ezetimibe/ Simvastatin) | Tabs: 10/10, 10/20, 10/40, 10/80 | 10/10 to 10/80mg/day | 31 to 43 | 45 to 60 | 6 to 8 | 23 to 31 |
| Advicor (Niacin ER/ Lovastatin) | Tabs: 500/20, 750/20, 1000/20, 1000/40 | 500/20mg to 2000mg/40mg | Not specified | 30 to 42 | 20 to 30 | 32 to 44 |

* Unless otherwise indicated

** NOTE: Dosage shown is for adults and may need to be adjusted to individual patient needs. For pediatric dosing and additional information please refer to the individual monograph listing or the drug's FDA-approved labeling. According to NCEP-ATP III guidelines, lipid-altering agents should be used in addition to a diet restricted in saturated fat and cholesterol only when the response to diet and other nonpharmacological measures has been inadequate.

Abbreviation: ER: Extended-Release

# LIPID MANAGEMENT

| DRUG | BRAND | HOW SUPPLIED (mg)* | USUAL DOSAGE RANGE** | COMMENTS |
|---|---|---|---|---|
| **HMG-CoA REDUCTASE INHIBITORS (STATINS)**** | | | | |
| Atorvastatin | Lipitor | Tab: 10, 20, 40, 80 | 10-80mg/day | CI: Active liver disease, unexplained persistent elevations of serum transaminases, pregnancy, nursing mothers.<br>Generally LFTs should be monitored prior to therapy, at 12 weeks, with dose elevations, and periodically thereafter.<br>Increased risk of myopathy with concomitant use of cyclosporine, fibrates, erythromycin, niacin, or azole antifungals.<br>Use with fibrates and niacin should generally be avoided. |
| Fluvastatin | Lescol | Cap: 20, 40 | 20-80mg/day | |
| | Lescol XL | Tab, ER: 80 | | |
| Lovastatin | Altoprev | Tab, ER: 10, 20, 40, 60 | 10-60mg/day | |
| | Mevacor | Tab: 10, 20, 40 | 10-80mg/day given qd or bid | |
| Pravastatin | Pravachol | Tab: 10, 20, 40, 80 | 10-80mg/day | |
| Rosuvastatin | Crestor | Tab: 5, 10, 20, 40 | 5-40mg/day | |
| Simvastatin | Zocor | Tab: 5, 10, 20, 40, 80 | 5-80mg/day | |
| **FIBRATES** | | | | |
| Fenofibrate | Tricor<br><br>Lofibra | Tab: 48, 145<br><br>Cap: 67,134, 200<br>Tab: 54, 160 | 48-145mg/day<br><br>67-200mg/day<br>54-160mg/day | Use with statins should generally be avoided.<br>CI: Pre-existing gallbladder disease, hepatic or severe renal dysfunction. |
| Gemfibrozil | Lopid | Tab: 600 | 1200mg/day in divided doses | |
| **BILE-ACID SEQUESTRANTS** | | | | |
| Cholestyramine | Questran<br>Questran Light | 4g/pkt or scoop | 8-16g/day, given bid | CI: Complete biliary obstruction. Mix with fluid or highly fluid food.<br>(Light): Contains phenylalanine. |
| Colesevelam HCl | WelChol | Tab: 625 | 3750mg/day given qd or bid | CI: Bowel obstruction.<br>Take with liquids and a meal. |
| **CHOLESTEROL ABSORPTION INHIBITOR** | | | | |
| Ezetimibe | Zetia | Tab: 10 | 10mg qd | Not recommended with moderate or severe hepatic insufficiency or with concurrent use of fibrates. |
| **NICOTINIC ACID DERIVATIVE** | | | | |
| Niacin, extended-release | Niaspan | Tab, ER: 500, 750, 1000 | 1-2g qhs | CI: Hepatic dysfunction, active peptic ulcer disease, arterial bleeding. May pretreat with ASA or NSAIDs 30 minutes before to reduce flushing. |
| **COMBINATIONS** | | | | |
| Amlodipine/ Atorvastatin | Caduet | Tab: (Amlodipine/ Atorvastatin): 2.5/10, 2.5/20, 2.5/40, 5/10, 5/20, 5/40, 5/80, 10/10, 10/20, 10/40, 10/80 | 5mg/20mg to 10mg/80mg | See Statins. |
| Ezetimbe/ Simvastatin | Vytorin | Tab: (Ezetimbe/ Simvastatin): 10/10, 10/20, 10/40, 10/80 | 10/10 to 10/80mg/day | See Statins. Avoid use in moderate to severe hepatic insufficiency. |
| Niacin/ Lovastatin | Advicor | Tab: (Niacin, ER/Lovastatin) 500/20, 750/20, 1000/20 | 500mg/20mg to 2000mg/40mg | See Statins and Niacin. Do not substitute for equivalent dose of immediate-release niacin. |

* Unless otherwise indicated.

** **NOTE:** Dosages shown are for adults and may need to be adjusted to individual patient needs. For pediatric dosing and additional information please refer to the individual monograph listings or the drug's FDA-approved labeling. According to NCEP-ATP III guidelines, lipid-altering agents should be used in addition to a diet restricted in saturated fat and cholesterol only when the response to diet and other nonpharmacological measures has been inadequate.

Abbreviations: CI: Contraindications, ER: Extended-Release.

# ACNE MANAGEMENT: SYSTEMIC THERAPIES

| DRUG (BRAND) | HOW SUPPLIED | DOSAGE | SIDE EFFECTS |
|---|---|---|---|
| **ANTIBIOTICS** | | | |
| **Doxycycline hyclate** (Doryx, Vibramycin) | Cap: 75mg, 100mg | 100mg q12h on 1st day, followed by 100mg qd. | Anorexia, nausea, vomiting, diarrhea, dysphagia, enterocolitis, rash, exfoliative dermatitis, renal toxicity, hypersensitivity reactions, blood dyscrasias |
| **Doxycycline monohydrate** (Minodox) | Cap: 50mg, 100mg | 100mg q12h or 50mg q6h for 1 day, then 100mg/day. | GI effects, photosensitivity, rash, monohydrate, blood dyscrasias, hypersensitivity reactions |
| **Minocycline hydrochloride** (Dynacin, Minocin) | Cap: 50mg, 75mg, 100mg; Tab: 50mg, 75mg, 100mg | 200mg initially, then 100mg q12h; alternative is 100-200mg initially, then 50mg qid. | Anorexia, nausea, vomiting, diarrhea, dysphagia, enterocolitis, pancreatitis, increased LFTs, hepatitis, liver failure, renal toxicity, rash, exfoliative, dermatitis, Stevens-Johnson syndrome, skin and mucous, membrane, pigmentation, blood, dyscrasias, headache, tooth discoloration |
| **Minocycline hydrochloride** (Solodyn) | Tab, Extended-Release: 45mg, 90mg, 135mg. | 1mg/kg qd for 12 weeks. | Headache, fatigue, dizziness, pruritus, malaise, mood alteration |
| **Tetracycline hydrochloride** (Sumycin) | Sus: 125mg/5mL; Tab: 250mg, 500mg | Mild-Moderate: 250mg qid or 500mg bid. Severe: 500mg qid. Severe Acne: Initial: 1g/day in divided doses. Maint: After improvement, 125-500mg/day | GI effects, photosensitivity, increased BUN, hypersensitivity reactions, blood dyscrasias, dizziness, headache |
| **RETINOID** | | | |
| **Isotretinoin** (Accutane) | Cap: 10mg, 20mg, 40mg | 0.5-1mg/kg/day given bid for 15-20 weeks. | Cheilitis, dry skin and mucous membranes, conjunctivitis, blood dyscrasias, epistaxis, decreased HDL, elevated cholesterol and TG, elevated blood sugar, arthralgias, back pain, hearing/vision impairment, rash, photosensitivity reactions, psychiatric disorders |
| **VITAMIN/MINERAL** | | | |
| **Nicotinamide/ Folic acid/Zinc** (Nicomide) | Tab: (Nicotinamide-Folic acid-Zinc) 750mg-500mcg-25mg | 1 tab qd-bid. | Nausea, vomiting, transient LFT elevations, allergic sensitization |

**Source:**

FDA-Approved Product Labeling.

# ACNE MANAGEMENT: TOPICAL THERAPIES

| DRUG (BRAND) | HOW SUPPLIED | DOSAGE | SIDE EFFECTS |
|---|---|---|---|
| **ANTIBACTERIAL/KERATOLYTIC AGENTS & COMBINATIONS** | | | |
| **Benzoyl peroxide** (Benzac AC, Benzagel, Triaz) | Benzac AC: (Gel) 5%, 10% [60g], (Wash) 10% [60g]; Benzagel: (Gel) 5%, 10% [42.5g], (Wash) 10% [60g]; Triaz: (Gel) 3%, 6%, 9% [42.5g], (Cleanser) 3%, 6%, 9% [170.3g, 240.2g], (Pads) 3%, 6%, 9% [30g] | (Benzac) Apply qd-bid. (Benzagel) Apply wash qd-bid; apply gel qd initially or qhs for light skin. (Triaz) Apply gel/ wash qd-bid. | Erythema, peeling, contact dermatitis, dryness |
| **Benzoyl peroxide/ Sulfur** (Sulfoxyl Lotion Regular/Strong) | Lot: (Regular): 10%-2% [59mL]; (Strong): 10%-5% [59mL] | Apply initially once daily for the first week then twice daily, as tolerated. | Erythema, peeling, contact, dermatitis, dryness, irritation, itching, redness |
| **Clindamycin/ Benzoyl peroxide** (Benzaclin, Duac) | Benzaclin: (Gel) 1%-5% [25g, 50g]; Duac: (Gel) 1%-5% [45g] | (Benzaclin) Apply qd. (Duac) Apply once in the evening. | Dry skin, erythema, peeling, and burning |
| **Benzoyl peroxide/ Erythromycin** (Benzamycin) | Gel: 5%-3% [46.6g, 60s] | Apply bid. | Dryness, urticaria, skin irritation, skin discoloration, oiliness |
| **Benzoyl peroxide** (Brevoxyl, Zoderm) | Brevoxyl: (Gel) 4%, 8% [42.5g, 90g], (Lot, Cleanser) 4%, 8% [297g], (Lot, Creamy Wash) 4%, 8% [170g]; Zoderm: (Cleanser) 4.5%, 6.5%, 8.5% [400mL], (Cre/Gel) 4.5%, 6.5%, 8.5% [125mL] | (Brevoxyl) Apply gel qd-bid; apply lotion qd for first week then bid as tolerated. (Zoderm) Apply qd-bid. | Erythema, peeling, contact dermatitis, dryness |
| **ANTIBIOTICS & COMBINATIONS** | | | |
| **Clindamycin** (Cleocin T, Clindagel, Clindets, Evoclin Foam) | Cleocin T: (Gel) 1% [30g, 60g], (Lot) 1% [60mL], (Sol) 1% [30mL, 60mL], (Swab, Pledgets) 1% [60s]; Clindagel: 1% [40, 75mL]; Clindets: (Swab) 1% [69]; Evoclin: (Foam) 1% [50g, 100g] | (Cleocin T) Apply bid. (Clindagel) Apply qd. (Clindets) Apply bid. (Evoclin Foam) Apply qd. | Local irritation, stains clothing |
| **Clindamycin/ Tretinoin** (Ziana) | Gel: 1.2%-0.025% [2g, 30g, 60g] | Apply qd at bedtime. | Nasopharyngitis, erythema, scaling, itching, burning |
| **Dapsone** (Aczone) | Gel: 5% [30g] | Apply bid. | Erythema, dryness, oiliness/peeling, nasopharyngitis, headache |
| **Erythromycin** (A/T/S, Emgel, Erycette, Erygel) | A/T/S: (Gel) 2% [30g], (Sol) 2% [60mL]; Emgel: (Gel) 2% [27g, 50g]; Erycette: (Swab) 2% [60g]; Erycette: (Swab) 2% [60g]; Erygel: 2% [30g, 60g] | (A/T/S) Apply gel qd-bid; apply solution bid. (Emgel) Apply bid. (Erycette) Apply bid. (Erygel) Apply qd-bid. | Local irritation, stains clothing |
| **Gentamicin** (Garamycin Topical) | Cre, Oint: 0.1% [15g] | Apply tid-qid. | Irritation (erythema and pruritus) |
| **Sulfacetamide** (Klaron) | Lot: 10% [118mL] | Apply bid. | Itching, redness, irritation |
| **Sulfacetamide/ Sulfur** (Plexion TS, Sulfacet-R, Zetacet) | Plexion TS: (Lot) 10%-5% [30g]; Sulfacet-R/Zetacet: (Lot) 10%-5% [25g] | Apply qd-tid. | Itching, redness, irritation |
| **Sulfacetamide/ Sulfur** (Plexion SCT, Rosac) | Plexion SCT: (Cre) 10%-5% [120g]; Rosac: (Cre) 10%-5% [45g] | Apply qd-tid. | Local irritation |
| **Sulfacetamide/ Sulfur** (Clenia, Plexion, Rosula) | Clenia: (Cleanser) 10%-5% [170g, 340g], Cre: 10%-5% [28g]; Plexion: (Cleanser) 10%-5% [170.3g, 340.2g]; Rosula: (Cleanser) 10%-5% [355mL], Gel 10%-5% [45mL] | Apply cream qd initially then titrate to bid-tid prn. (Plexion) Apply qd-bid. (Rosula) Apply cleanser qd-bid; apply gel qd-tid. | Local irritation |

*(Continued)*

| **DRUG** (BRAND) | **HOW SUPPLIED** | **DOSAGE** | **SIDE EFFECTS** |
|---|---|---|---|
| **ANTIBIOTICS & COMBINATIONS** *(Continued)* | | | |
| **Sulfacetamide/ Urea** (Rosula NS Dicarboxylic Acids) | (Swab) 10%-10% [30$^{s}$] | Apply qd-bid. | Local hypersensitivity, instances of Stevens-Johnson syndrome |
| **Azelaic acid** (Azelex, Finevin) | (Cre) 20% [30g, 50g] | Apply bid. | Dryness, scaling, erythema, burning, irritation, pruritus; rarely, hypopigmentation |
| **Azelaic acid** (Finacea, Retinoids) | (Gel) 15% [30g] | Apply bid. | Burning, stinging, tingling, pruritus, scaling, dry skin |
| **Adapalene** (Differin) | (Cre, Gel) 0.1% [45g]; (Pledglets) 0.1% [60$^{s}$]; (Sol) 0.1% [30mL] | Apply hs. | Erythema, scaling, dryness, pruritus, burning, sunburn, acne flares |
| **Tazarotene** (Tazorac) | (Cre) 0.05%, 0.1% [30g, 60g]; (Gel) 0.05%, 0.1% [30g, 100g] | Apply hs. | Pruritus, burning/stinging, erythema, irritation, skin pain, desquamation, dry skin, rash |
| **Tretinoin** (Avita, Retin-A) | (Cre) 0.025%, 0.05%, 0.1% [20g, 45g]; (Gel) 0.01%, 0.025% [15g, 45g]; (Sol) 0.05% [28mL] | Apply hs. | Local skin reactions (red, edematous, blistered, crusted), photosensitivity, temporary skin pigmentation changes |
| **Tretinoin microsphere** (Retin-A-Micro) | (Gel) 0.04%, 0.1% [20g, 45g] | Apply hs. | |

**Source:**
FDA-Approved Product Labeling.

# Psoriasis Management: Systemic Therapies

| **DRUG** (BRAND) | **HOW SUPPLIED** | **DOSAGE** | **SIDE EFFECTS** |
|---|---|---|---|
| **ANTIMETABOLITE** | | | |
| **Methotrexate** | Inj: 20mg, 1g, 25mg/mL; Tab: 2.5mg, 5mg, 7.5mg, 10mg, 15 mg | Initial: 10-25mg weekly until response or use divided oral dose schedule, 2.5mg at 12-hr intervals for 3 doses. Titrate: Increase gradually until optimal response. Maint: Reduce to lowest effective dose. Max: 30mg/wk. | Ulcerative stomatitis, leukopenia, nausea, abdominal distress, malaise, fatigue, chills, fever, dizziness, decreased resistance to infection |
| **IMMUNOSUPPRESSIVES** | | | |
| **Alefacept** (Amevive) | Inj: (IV) 7.5mg, (IM) 15mg | 7.5mg IV bolus or 15mg IM once wkly for 12 wks. May repeat cycle 12 wks after first cycle complete. Adjust dose, D/C, based on CD4+ T-lymphocyte counts. | Lymphopenia, injection-site reactions, influenza-like symptoms, pruritus |
| **Cyclosporin** (Neoral) | Cap: 25mg, 100mg; Sol: 100mg/mL [50mL] | Initial: 1.25mg/kg bid for 4 wks. Titrate: May increase by 0.5mg/kg/day every 2 weeks. Max: 4mg/kg/day. | Infection, renal dysfunction, HTN, malignancy risk w/certain psoriasis therapies |
| **MONOCLONAL ANTIBODIES** | | | |
| **Efalizumab** (Raptiva) | Inj: 125mg | Initial dose: 0.7mg/kg SQ x 1. Maint: 1mg/kg SQ per wk. Max: 200mg/dose. | Influenza-like symptoms, URI, acne, psoriasis exacerbation, thrombocytopenia |
| **Infliximab** (Remicade) | Inj: 100mg | 5mg/kg IV infusion; repeat at 2 and 6 weeks. Maint: 5mg/kg every 8 weeks. | Infusion reactions, URI, pruritus, headache, sore throat; potential risk of reactivating TB |
| **PSORALENS** | | | |
| **Methoxsalen*** (8-Mop, Oxsoralen-Ultra) | Cap: 10mg | Take with food or milk. Initial: <30kg: 10mg. 30-50kg: 20mg. 51-65kg: 30mg. 66-80kg: 40mg. 81-90kg: 50mg. 91-115kg: 60mg. >115kg: 70mg. Take 2 hrs before UVA exposure. Titrate: May increase by 10mg after 15th treatment under certain conditions. Max: Do not treat more often than qod. | Nausea, nervousness, insomnia, depression, pruritus, erythema |
| **RETINOID** | | | |
| **Acitretin** (Soriatane) | Cap: 10mg, 25mg | Initial: 25-50mg qd w/food. Individualize dose based on intersubject variation in pharmacokinetics, clinical efficacy, and incidence of side effects. Maint: 25-50mg qd. Terminate therapy when lesions resolve. May treat relapses. | Ophthalmologic effects, cheilitis, rhinitis, dry mouth, epistaxis, alopecia, dry skin, rash, skin peeling, nail disorder, pruritus, paresthesia, paronychia, skin atrophy, sticky skin, xerophthalmia, arthralgia, rash. |
| **TNF-BLOCKING AGENT** | | | |
| **Etanercept** (Enbrel) | Inj: 25mg [vial], 50mg/mL [syringe] | Initial: 50mg SQ twice weekly given 3 or 4 days apart for 3 months. May begin with 25-50mg/wk. Maint: 50mg/wk. | Injection site reactions, infections, headache |

* Oxsoralen-Ultra and 8-MOP are not interchangeable due to significantly greater bioavailability and earlier photosensitization onset time of Oxsoralen-Ultra.

**References:**

1. FDA-Approved Product Labeling.
2. Luba KM, Stulberg DL. Chronic plaque psoriasis. *Am Fam Physician.* 2006 Feb 15;73(4):636-44. Review.

# PSORIASIS MANAGEMENT: TOPICAL THERAPIES

| DRUG (BRAND) | HOW SUPPLIED | DOSAGE | SIDE EFFECTS |
|---|---|---|---|
| **TOPICAL IMMUNOSUPPRESSANT** | | | |
| **Pimecrolimus** (Elidel) | Cre: 1% [30g, 60g, 100g] | Apply bid. | Burning, headache, nasopharyngitis, pyrexia |
| **TOPICAL STEROIDS** | | | |
| **Clobetasol** (Temovate, Clobex, Embeline E, Olux) | (Temovate) Cre, Oint: 0.05% [15g, 30g, 45g, 60g]; Gel: 0.05% [15g, 30g, 60g]; Sol: 0.05% [25mL]; (Clobex) Lot: 0.05% [30mL, 59mL]; Shampoo: 0.05% [118mL]; Spray: 0.05% [2oz]; (Embeline E) Cre: 0.05% [15g, 30g, 60g]; (Olux) Foam: 0.05% [50g, 100g] | Apply bid. | Hypopigmentation, striae, skin atrophy, tachyphylaxis |
| **Fluocinolone** (Synalar) | Cre, Oint: 0.025% [15g, 60g]; Sol: 0.01% [20mL, 60mL] | Apply bid-qid. | Dryness, folliculitis, acne, skin atrophy, burning, itching, irritation |
| **Fluocinolone** (Lidex, Vanos) | (Lidex) Cre, Gel, Oint: 0.05% [15g, 30g, 60g]; Sol: 0.05% [60mL]; (Vanos) Cre: 0.1% [30mg, 60mg] | (Lidex) Apply bid-tid. (Vanos) Apply qd-bid. | Burning, itching, irritation, dryness, folliculitis, acne, hypopigmentation, skin atrophy |
| **Halcinonide** | (Halog) Cre, Oint: 0.1% [15g, 30g, (Halog, Halog-E) 60g, 240g]; Sol: 0.1% [20mL, 60mL]; (Halog-E) Cre: 0.1% in a hydrophilic vanishing cream [30g, 60g] | (Cre, Oint, Sol) Apply bid-tid. (Cre, hydrophilic base) Apply qd-tid. | Burning, itching, irritation, dryness, folliculitis, hypopigmentation, contact dermatitis, skin maceration |
| **Hydrocortisone** (Hytone, Locoid, Pandel, Westcor) | (Hytone 1%) Lot: 1% [30mL, 120mL]; (Locoid) Cre, Oint: 0.1% [15g, 45g]; Sol: 0.1% [20mL, 60mL]; (Pandel) Cre: 0.1% [15g, 45g, 80g]; (Westcort) Cre, Oint: 0.2% [15g, 45g, 60g] | (Hytone 1%, Locoid) Apply tid-qid. (Pandel) Apply qd-bid. (Westcort) Apply bid-tid. | Burning, stinging, moderate paresthesia, itching, dryness, folliculitis, hypopigmentation, skin atrophy |
| **Hydrocortisone/ Pramoxine** (Epifoam, Novacort, Pramosone) | (Epifoam) Foam: (Hydrocortisone-Pramoxine) 1%-1% [10g]; (Novacort) Gel: 2%-1% [29g]; (Pramosone) Cre: 1%-1%, 1%-2.5% Lot: 1%-1% [60mL, 120mL, 240mL], 1%-2.5% [60mL, 120mL]; Oint: 1%-1%, 1%-2.5% [30g] | Apply tid-qid. | Burning, itching, irritation, dryness, folliculitis, hypopigmentation, maceration, skin atrophy |
| **Mometasone** (Elocon) | Cre, Oint: 0.1% [15g, 45g]; Lot: 0.1% [30mL, 60mL] | Apply qd. | Burning, pruritus, skin atrophy, rosacea, acneiform reaction, tingling, stinging, furunculosis, folliculitis |
| **Triamcinolone** (Kenalog) | (Kenalog) Cre: 0.1% [15g, 60g, 80g], 0.5% [20g]; Lot: 0.025%, 0.1% [60mL]; Oint: 0.1% [15g, 60g]; Spray: 0.147mg/g [63g] | (Kenalog) Cre, Lot, Oint: Apply 0.025% bid-qid. Apply 0.1% or 0.5% bid-tid. Spray: Apply tid-qid. | Burning, itching, irritation, dryness, folliculitis, hypopigmentation, allergic contact dermatitis |
| **TOPICAL RETINOID** | | | |
| **Tazarotene** (Tazorac) | Cre: 0.05%, 0.1% [30g, 60g]; Gel: 0.05%, 0.1% [30g, 100g] | Apply hs. | Pruritus, erythema, irritation, dry skin, rash, skin discoloration |
| **VITAMIN D DERIVATIVES & COMBINATIONS** | | | |
| **Calcipotriene** (Dovonex, Dovonex Scalp) | (Dovonex) Cre, Oint: 0.005% [60g, 120g]; (Dovonex Scalp) Sol: 0.005% [60mL] | (Dovonex) Apply bid. (Dovonex Scalp) Apply bid. | Skin irritation, pruritus, burning, hypercalcemia |
| **Calcipotriene/ betamethasone** (Taclonex) | Oint: (Calcipotriene-Betamethasone) 0.005%-0.064% [15g, 30g, 60g] | Apply qd. | Pruritus, headache |

*(Continued)*

| **DRUG** (BRAND) | **HOW SUPPLIED** | **DOSAGE** | **SIDE EFFECTS** |
|---|---|---|---|
| **MISCELLANEOUS AGENTS** | | | |
| **Anthralin** (Anthra-Derm) | Cre: 1% [50g] | Apply qd-bid. | Skin irritation, erythema, staining (skin and clothing), odor |
| **Coal Tar** (Zetar) | Sol 10%: 2% [3.8oz] | Apply hs. | Skin irritation, folliculitis, odor, staining of clothing |
| **Urea** (Carmol 40) | Cre: 40% [28.35g, 85g, 198.6g]; Gel: 40% [15mL]; Lot: 40% [236.6 mL] | Apply bid. | Transient stinging, burning, itching, irritation |

**References:**

1. FDA-Approved Drug Labeling.
2. Luba KM, Stulberg DL. Chronic plaque psoriasis. *Am Fam Physician.* 2006 Feb 15;73(4):636-44. Review.

# Topical Corticosteroids

| STEROID | DOSAGE FORM(S) | STRENGTH (%) | POTENCY | FREQUENCY |
|---|---|---|---|---|
| Alclometasone Dipropionate (Aclovate) | Cre, Oint | 0.05 | Low | bid/tid |
| Augmented Betamethasone Dipropionate | Oint | 0.05 | Very High | qd/bid |
| (Diprolene, Diprolene AF) | Cre, Lot | 0.05 | High | qd/bid |
| Betamethasone Dipropionate | Cre, Lot, Oint | 0.05 | High | qd/bid |
| Betamethasone Valerate (Beta-Val) | Cre, Lot | 0.1 | Medium | qd/tid |
| (Luxiq) | Foam, Lot | 0.12, 0.1 | Medium | bid |
| Clobetasol Propionate (Clobex, Cormax, Olux,Temovate, Temovate-E) | Cre, Foam (Olux), Gel, Lotion (Clobex), Oint, Shampoo (Clobex), Sol | 0.05 | Very High | bid<br>qd (shampoo) |
| Clocortolone Pivalate (Cloderm) | Cre | 0.1 | Low | tid |
| Desonide (DesOwen, Verdeso) | Cre, Foam, Lot, Oint | 0.05 | Low | bid/tid |
| Desoximetasone | Cre | 0.05 | Medium | bid |
| (Topicort, Topicort LP) | Cre, Oint | 0.25 | High | bid |
| | Gel | 0.05 | High | bid |
| Diflorasone Diacetate | Cre, Oint (Maxiflor) | 0.05 | High | qd/tid |
| (Maxiflor, Psorcon) | Oint (Psorcon) | 0.05 | Very High | qd/qid |
| Fluocinolone Acetonide | Cre, Oint | 0.025 | Medium | bid/qid |
| (Capex, Derma-Smoothe/FS, Synalar) | Sol | 0.01 | Medium | bid/qid |
| | Oil (Derma-Smoothe/FS) | 0.01 | Medium | qd/tid |
| | Shampoo (Capex) | 0.01 | Medium | qd |
| Fluocinonide | Cre, Gel, Oint, Sol | 0.05 | High | bid/qid |
| (Lidex, Lidex-E, Vanos) | Cre | 0.1 | Very High | qd/bid |
| Flurandrenolide | Cre, Oint | 0.025 | Medium | bid/tid |
| (Cordran, Cordran SP) | Cre, Lot, Oint | 0.05 | Medium | bid/tid |
| | Tape | 4mcg/cm$^2$ | Medium | qd/bid |
| Fluticasone Propionate | Cre, Lot | 0.05 | Medium | qd/bid |
| (Cutivate) | Oint | 0.005 | Medium | bid |
| Halcinonide (Halog, Halog-E) | Cre, Oint, Sol | 0.1 | High | qd/tid |
| Halobetasol Propionate (Ultravate) | Cre, Oint | 0.05 | Very High | qd/bid |
| Hydrocortisone | Cre, Lot, Oint | 0.5 | Low | tid/qid |
| (Ala-Cort, Ala-Scalp, Anusol HC, Cetacort, | Cre, Lot, Oint, Sol | 1 | Low | tid/qid |
| Hi-Cort, Hytone, Nutracort, Stie-Cort, | Lot | 2 | Low | tid/qid |
| Synacort, Texacort) | Cre, Lot, Oint, Sol | 2.5 | Low | tid/qid |
| Hydrocortisone Butyrate (Locoid, Locoid Lipo Cream) | Cre, Lot, Oint, Sol | 0.1 | Medium | bid/tid |
| Hydrocortisone Probutate (Pandel) | Cre | 0.1 | Medium | qd/bid |
| Hydrocortisone Valerate (Westcort) | Cre, Oint | 0.2 | Medium | bid/tid |
| Mometasone Furoate (Elocon) | Cre, Lot, Oint | 0.1 | Medium | qd |
| Prednicarbate (Dermatop) | Cre, Oint | 0.1 | Medium | bid |
| Triamcinolone Acetonide | Cre, Lot, Oint | 0.025 | Medium | bid/qid |
| (Kenalog, Triderm) | Cre, Lot, Oint | 0.1 | Medium | bid/tid |
| | Cre, Oint | 0.5 | High | bid/tid |
| | Spray | 0.147 | Medium | tid/qid |

# INSULIN FORMULATIONS

| TYPE OF INSULIN | BRAND | ONSET* (hrs) | PEAK* (hrs) | DURATION* (hrs) | COMMON PITFALLS** |
|---|---|---|---|---|---|
| **Rapid-acting** | | | | | |
| Insulin Glulisine | Apidra | – | 0.5 to 1.7 | 1 to 3 | See individual comments. |
| Human Insulin Inhalation Powder | Exubera | 10-20 min | 0.5 to 1.5 | 6 | See individual comments. |
| Insulin Lispro | Humalog | <0.25 | 0.5 to 1.5 | 3 to 5 | Hypoglycemia occurs if lag time is too long or the patient exercises within 1 hr of dose; with high-fat meals, the dose should be adjusted downward. |
| Insulin Aspart | Novolog | <0.25 | 0.5 to 1 | 3 to 5 | |
| **Short-acting** | | | | | Lag time is not used appropriately; the insulin should be given 20 to 30 minutes before the patient eats. |
| Regular Insulin | Humulin R† | 0.5 to 1 | 2 to 4 | 4 to 12 | |
| | Novolin R | 0.5 to 1 | 2 to 5 | 8 | |
| **Intermediate-acting** | | | | | In many patients, breakfast injection does not last the evening until the evening meal; administration with the evening meal does not meet insulin needs on awakening. |
| NPH (Isophane) | Humulin N<br>Novolin R | 1 to 3 | 6 to 12 | 18 to 24 | |
| **Long-acting** | | | | | |
| Insulin glargine | Lantus | 1 | Flat | 24 | Administer once daily at the same time every day. |
| Insulin detemir | Levemir | – | 6 to 8 | 24 | See individual comments. |
| **Combinations** | | | | | |
| Isophane insulin suspension (70%)/regular insulin (30%) | Humulin 70/30<br>Novolin 70/30 | 0.5 to 1 | 4 to 6 | 24 | See individual comments. |
| Isophane insulin suspension (50%)/regular insulin (50%) | Humulin 50/50 | 0.5 to 1 | 3 to 5 | 24 | See individual comments. |
| Insulin lispro protamine (75%)/insulin lispro (25%) | Humalog Mix 75/25 | ≤0.25 | 0.5 to 4 | 24 | See individual comments. |
| Insulin aspart protamine (70%)/ insulin aspart (30%) | Novolog Mix 70/30 | ≤0.25 | 1 to 4 | 24 | See individual comments. |

*Approximate parameters following SC injection of an average patient dose; insulin concentration: 100U/mL. (Not applicable for inhalation insulin.)

**Source: Hirsch, IB. Type 1 Diabetes Mellitus and the Use of Flexible Insulin Regimens. *Am Fam Physician.* November 1999;60(8):2343-2352,2355-2356.

†Also available 500 U/mL for insulin resistant patients (rapid onset; up to 24 hour duration).

# ORAL ANTIDIABETIC AGENTS

| DRUG | HOW SUPPLIED | INITIAL* & (MAX) DOSE | USUAL DOSE RANGE* |
|---|---|---|---|
| **BIGUANIDES** | | | |
| **Metformin HCl** | | | |
| Fortamet | Tab, ER: 500mg, 1000mg | 1000mg qd (2500mg/day). | 500-2500mg qd. |
| Glucophage | Tab: 500mg, 850mg, 1000mg | 500mg bid or 850mg qd (2550mg/day). | 1-2g daily in divided doses. |
| Glucophage XR | Tab, ER: 500mg | 500mg qd (2000mg/day). | 500mg-2g qd. |
| **DIPEPTIDYL PEPTIDASE-4 INHIBITOR** | | | |
| **Sitagliptin**<br>Januvia | Tab: 25mg, 50mg, 100mg | 100mg qd. | 100mg qd. |
| **GLUCOSIDASE INHIBITORS** | | | |
| **Acarbose**<br>(Precose) | Tab: 25mg, 50mg, 100mg | 25mg tid (300mg/day). | 25-100mg tid. |
| **Miglitol**<br>(Glyset) | Tab: 25mg, 50mg, 100mg | 25mg tid (300mg/day). | 50-100mg tid. |
| **MEGLITINIDES** | | | |
| **Nateglinide**<br>Starlix | Tab: 60mg, 120mg | 120mg tid (360mg/day). | 120mg tid. |
| **Repaglinide**<br>Prandin | Tab: 0.5mg, 1mg, 2mg (16mg/day). | 0.5-2mg with each meal | 0.5-4mg with each meal. |
| **SULFONYLUREAS** | | | |
| **Glimepiride**<br>Amaryl | Tab: 1mg, 2mg, 4mg | 1-2mg qd (8mg/day). | 1-4mg qd. |
| **Glipizide**<br>Glucotrol | Tab: 5mg, 10mg | 5mg qd (40mg/day). | 5-40mg qd or divided if >15mg/day. |
| Glucotrol XL | Tab, ER: 2.5mg, 5mg, 10mg | 5mg qd (20mg/day). | 5-10mg qd. |
| **Glyburide**<br>Diabeta, Micronase | Tab: 1.25mg, 2.5mg, 5mg | 2.5-5mg qd (20mg/day). | 1.25-20mg qd or divided doses. |
| **Glynase**<br>PresTab | Tab: 1.5mg, 3mg, 6mg | 1.5-3mg qd (12mg/day). | 0.75-12mg qd divided doses. |
| **THIAZOLIDINEDIONES** | | | |
| **Pioglitazone HCl**<br>Actos | Tab: 15mg, 30mg, 45mg | 15-30mg qd (45mg/day). | 15-30mg qd. |
| **Rosiglitazone maleate**<br>Avandia | Tab: 2mg, 4mg, 8mg | 2mg bid or 4mg qd (8mg/day). | 4mg bid or 8mg qd. |
| **COMBINATIONS** | | | |
| **Glipizide/ Metformin HCl**<br>Metaglip | Tab: 2.5mg/250mg, 2.5mg/500mg, 5mg/500mg | 2.5mg/250mg qd or 2.5mg/500mg bid | 1-2 tab qd-bid. (10mg/1g qd or 20mg/2g divided doses). |
| **Glyburide/ Metformin HCl**<br>Glucovance | Tab: 1.25mg/250mg, 2.5mg/500mg, 5mg/500mg | 1.25mg/250mg qd or bid (20mg/2g/day). | 1-2 tabs bid. |
| **Pioglitazone/ Glimepiride**<br>Duetact | Tab: 30mg/2mg, 30mg/4mg (once daily at any strength). | 30mg/2mg qd or 30mg/4mg qd | 1 tab am. |

*(Continued)*

| DRUG | HOW SUPPLIED | INITIAL* & (MAX) DOSE | USUAL DOSE RANGE* |
|---|---|---|---|
| **COMBINATIONS** *(Continued)* | | | |
| **Pioglitazone/ Metformin HCl** Actoplus Met | Tab: 15mg/500mg, 15mg/850mg | 15mg/500mg or 15mg/850mg qd-bid (45mg/2250mg/day). | 1 tab qd-bid. |
| **Rosiglitazone/ Glimepiride** Avandaryl | Tab: 4mg/1mg, 4mg/2mg, 4mg/4mg | 4mg/1mg or 4mg/2mg qd (8mg/4mg qd). | 1 tab am. |
| **Rosiglitazone/ Metformin HCl** Avandamet | Tab: 1mg/500mg, 2mg/500mg, 4mg/500mg, 2mg/1g, 4mg/1g | 2mg/500mg qd-bid. (8mg/2g/day). | 1-2 tabs bid. |
| **Sitagliptin/ Metformin** Janumet | Tab: 50mg/500mg, 50mg/1000mg bid (100mg/2g qd). | 50mg/500mg or 50mg/1000mg | 1 tab bid. |

*NOTE: Usual dose ranges are derived from the drug's FDA-approved labeling. There is no fixed dosage regimen for the management of diabetes mellitus with any hypoglycemic agent. The initial and maintenance dosing should be conservative, depending on the patient's individual needs, especially in elderly, debilitated or malnourished patients, and with impaired renal or hepatic function. Management of type 2 diabetes should include blood glucose and HbA1c monitoring, nutritional counseling, exercise, and weight reduction as needed. For more detailed information refer to the individual monograph listings or the drug's FDA-approved labeling.

# $H_2$ ANTAGONISTS AND PPIs COMPARISON

| DRUG | HOW SUPPLIED | INDICATIONS: Heartburn | PUD | GERD | Zollinger-Ellison | H.pylori | NSAID† Induced | Upper GI‡ Bleeding |
|---|---|---|---|---|---|---|---|---|
| **$H_2$ ANTAGONISTS** | | | | | | | | |
| **CIMETIDINE** | | | | | | | | |
| Tagamet | Inj: 150mg/mL, 300mg/50mL; Sol: 300mg/5mL Tab: 200mg, 300mg, 400mg, 800mg | | X | X | X | | | X |
| Tagamet HB* | Tab: 200mg | X | | | | | | |
| **FAMOTIDINE** | | | | | | | | |
| Pepcid | Inj: 0.4mg/mL, 10mg/mL Sus: 40mg/5mL Tab: 20mg, 40mg Tab, Disintegrating: 20mg, 40mg | | X | X | X | | | |
| Pepcid AC* | Cap: 10mg Tab: 10mg, 20mg Tab, Chewable: 10mg | X | | | | | | |
| Pepcid Complete* | Tab, Chewable: (Famotidine-Calcium Carbonate-Magnesium Hydroxide) 10mg-800mg-165mg | X | | | | | | |
| **NIZATIDINE** | | | | | | | | |
| Axid | Cap: 150mg, 300mg Sol: 15mg/mL | | X | X | | | | |
| **RANITIDINE** | | | | | | | | |
| Zantac | Inj: 1mg/mL, 25mg/mL Syrup: 15mg/mL Tab: 150mg, 300mg Tab, Effervescent: 25mg, 150mg | | X | X | X | | | |
| Zantac OTC* | Tab: 75mg, 150mg | X | | | | | | |
| **PROTON PUMP INHIBITORS** | | | | | | | | |
| **ESOMEPRAZOLE** | | | | | | | | |
| Nexium | Cap, Delayed-Release: 20mg, 40mg Inj: 20mg, 40mg | | | X | X | X | X | |
| **LANSOPRAZOLE** | | | | | | | | |
| Prevacid | Cap, Delayed-Release: 15mg, 30mg; Inj: 30mg Sus: 15mg/packet, 30mg/packet Tab, Disintegrating: 15mg, 30mg | | X | X | X | X | X | |
| Prevpac | Cap: (Amoxicillin) 500mg Tab: (Clarithromycin) 500mg Cap, Delayed-Release: (Lansoprazole) 30mg | | | | | X | | |
| Prevacid NapraPAC | Cap, Delayed-Release: (Naproxen Lansoprazole): 500mg-15mg | | | | | | X | |
| **OMEPRAZOLE** | | | | | | | | |
| Prilosec | Cap, Delayed-Release: 10mg, 20mg, 40mg | | X | X | X | X | | |
| Prilosec OTC* | Tab: 20mg | X | | | | | | |
| Zegerid | (Omeprazole-Sodium Bicarbonate) Cap: 20mg-1100mg, 40mg-1100mg; Pow: 20mg-1680mg/packet, 40mg-1680mg/packet | | X | X | | | | X |
| **PANTOPRAZOLE** | | | | | | | | |
| Protonix | Inj: 40mg Tab, Delayed-Release: 20mg, 40mg | | | X | X | | | |
| **RABEPRAZOLE** | | | | | | | | |
| Aciphex | Tab, Delayed-Release: 20mg | | X | X | X | X | | |

*OTC. †Prevention of NSAID-induced gastric ulcers. ‡Prevention of upper GI bleeding in critically ill patients.

# ANTIBIOTIC SENSITIVITY - AMINOGLYCOSIDES*

| ORGANISMS | Amikacin | Gentamicin | Streptomycin | Tobramycin | |
|---|---|---|---|---|---|
| **ANAEROBES** | | | | | |
| *Actinomyces* | | | | | |
| *Bacillus anthracis* | | | | | |
| *Bacteroides fragilis* | | | | | |
| *Clostridium difficile* | | | | | |
| *Clostridium species* | | | | | |
| **GRAM-NEGATIVE AEROBES** | | | | | |
| *Acinetobacter baumannii* | ++ | + | | ++ | |
| *Aeromonas hydrophila* | ++ | ++ | | ++ | |
| *Bartonella henselae* | | ++ | | | |
| *Bordetella species* | | | | | |
| *Burkholderia cepacia* | | | | | |
| *Campylobacter jejuni* | | + | | | |
| *Citrobacter species* | ++ | +++ | | +++ | |
| *Coxiella burnetti* | | | | | |
| *Enterobacter species* | +++ | +++ | | +++ | |
| *Escherichia coli* | + | ++ | | ++ | |

+++ = excellent activity (1st line recommendation). ++ = good activity (2nd line recommendation). + = moderate activity (acceptable in vitro data suggesting some isolates may be sensitive).
Blank = no or insufficient activity, or unknown.
†† 2nd line against *S. typhi.* † Penicillin sensitive; MIC ≤1.0 mcg/mL. §§ Penicillin resistant; MIC ≥2.0 mcg/mL.
*These are generalizations. There are major differences among countries, areas, and hospitals depending on antibiotic usage patterns.

| ORGANISMS | Amikacin | Gentamicin | Streptomycin | Tobramycin | |
|---|---|---|---|---|---|
| **GRAM-NEGATIVE AEROBES** *(Continued)* | | | | | |
| *Francisella tularensis* | | +++ | +++ | + | |
| *Haemophilus influenzae* | + | + | | + | |
| *Klebsiella species* | ++ | ++ | | ++ | |
| *Legionella species* | | | | | |
| *Moraxella catarrhalis* | + | + | | + | |
| *Morganella morganii* | ++ | ++ | | ++ | |
| *Neisseria gonorrhoeae* | | | | | |
| *Neisseria meningitidis* | | | | | |
| *Pasturella multocida* | | | | | |
| *Proteus mirabilis* | ++ | +++ | | ++ | |
| *Proteus vulgaris* | ++ | +++ | | ++ | |
| *Providencia stuartii* | ++ | ++ | | ++ | |
| *Pseudomonas aeruginosa* | +++ | +++ | | +++ | |
| *Rickettsia species* | | | | | |
| *Salmonella species* | | | | | |
| *Serratia species* | ++ | ++ | | ++ | |
| *Shigella species* | + | + | | + | |
| *Stenotrophomonas maltophilia* | | | | | |

+++ = excellent activity (1st line recommendation). ++ = good activity (2nd line recommendation). + = moderate activity (acceptable in vitro data suggesting some isolates may be sensitive).
Blank = no or insufficient activity, or unknown.
†† 2nd line against *S. typhi.* † Penicillin sensitive; MIC ≤1.0 mcg/mL. §§ Penicillin resistant; MIC ≥2.0 mcg/mL.
*These are generalizations. There are major differences among countries, areas, and hospitals depending on antibiotic usage patterns.

**AMINOGLYCOSIDES (CONTINUED)**

| ORGANISMS | Amikacin | Gentamicin | Streptomycin | Tobramycin | |
|---|---|---|---|---|---|
| **GRAM-NEGATIVE AEROBES** *(Continued)* | | | | | |
| *Vibrio vulnificus* | | | | | |
| *Yersinia enterocolitica* | ++ | ++ | | ++ | |
| *Yersinia pestis* | | ++ | +++ | + | |
| **GRAM-POSITIVE AEROBES** | | | | | |
| *Enterococcus faecalis* | | ++ | ++ | | |
| *Enterococcus faecium* | | + | + | | |
| *Enterococcus faecium (VRE)* | | + | + | | |
| *Listeria monocytogenes* | + | + | | + | |
| *Nocardia* | ++ | | | | |
| *Staphylococcus aureus (MSSA)* | | | | | |
| *Staphylococcus aureus (MRSA)* | | | | | |
| *Staphylococcus epidermidis* | | + | | | |
| *Staphylococcus epidermidis (MRSE)* | | + | | | |
| *Streptococcus pneumoniae†* | | | | | |
| *Streptococcus pneumoniae§§* | | | | | |

+++ = excellent activity (1st line recommendation). ++ = good activity (2nd line recommendation). + = moderate activity (acceptable in vitro data suggesting some isolates may be sensitive).
Blank = no or insufficient activity, or unknown.
†† 2nd line against *S. typhi.* † Penicillin sensitive; MIC ≤1.0 mcg/mL. §§ Penicillin resistant; MIC ≥2.0 mcg/mL.
*These are generalizations. There are major differences among countries, areas, and hospitals depending on antibiotic usage patterns.

| ORGANISMS | Amikacin | Gentamicin | Streptomycin | Tobramycin | |
|---|---|---|---|---|---|
| **GRAM-POSITIVE AEROBES** *(Continued)* | | | | | |
| *Streptococcus (Group A,B,C,F,G)* | | | | | |
| *Streptococcus species* | | + | | | |
| **MISCELLANEOUS** | | | | | |
| *Chlamydia pneumoniae* | | | | | |
| *Chlamydia trachomatis* | | | | | |
| *Ehrlichia/Anaplasma species* | | | | | |
| **MYCOBACTERIA** | | | | | |
| *Mycobacterium avium (MAI) (non-HIV)* | ++ | | + | | |
| *Mycoplasma pneumoniae* | | | | | |
| **SPIROCHETES** | | | | | |
| *Leptospira interrogans* | | | | | |
| *Treponema pallidum (syphilis)* | | | | | |

+++ = excellent activity (1st line recommendation). ++ = good activity (2nd line recommendation). + = moderate activity (acceptable in vitro data suggesting some isolates may be sensitive).
Blank = no or insufficient activity, or unknown.
†† 2nd line against *S. typhi.* † Penicillin sensitive; MIC ≤1.0 mcg/mL. §§ Penicillin resistant; MIC ≥2.0 mcg/mL.
*These are generalizations. There are major differences among countries, areas, and hospitals depending on antibiotic usage patterns.

# ANTIBIOTIC SENSITIVITY – CARBAPENEMS/MONOBACTAMS*

| ORGANISMS | Aztreonam | Ertapenem | Imipenem/Cilastatin | Meropenem | |
|---|---|---|---|---|---|
| **ANAEROBES** | | | | | |
| *Actinomyces* | | | ++ | ++ | |
| *Bacillus anthracis* | | | | | |
| *Bacteroides fragilis* | | +++ | +++ | +++ | |
| *Clostridium difficile* | | | | | |
| *Clostridium species* | | ++ | ++ | ++ | |
| **GRAM-NEGATIVE AEROBES** | | | | | |
| *Acinetobacter baumannii* | + | | +++ | +++ | |
| *Aeromonas hydrophila* | ++ | + | ++ | ++ | |
| *Bartonella henselae* | | | | | |
| *Bordetella species* | | + | + | + | |
| *Burkholderia cepacia* | | + | + | ++ | |
| *Campylobacter jejuni* | | + | + | + | |
| *Citrobacter species* | ++ | +++ | +++ | +++ | |
| *Coxiella burnetti* | | | | | |
| *Enterobacter species* | ++ | ++ | +++ | +++ | |
| *Escherichia coli* | ++ | ++ | ++ | ++ | |

+++ = excellent activity (1st line recommendation). ++ = good activity (2nd line recommendation). + = moderate activity (acceptable in vitro data suggesting some isolates may be sensitive).
Blank = no or insufficient activity, or unknown.
†† 2nd line against *S. typhi.* † Penicillin sensitive; MIC ≤1.0 mcg/mL. §§ Penicillin resistant; MIC ≥2.0 mcg/mL.
*These are generalizations. There are major differences among countries, areas, and hospitals depending on antibiotic usage patterns.

| ORGANISMS | Aztreonam | Ertapenem | Imipenem/Cilastatin | Meropenem | |
|---|---|---|---|---|---|
| **GRAM-NEGATIVE AEROBES** *(Continued)* | | | | | |
| *Francisella tularensis* | | | | | |
| *Haemophilus influenzae* | ++ | ++ | ++ | ++ | |
| *Klebsiella species* | ++ | ++ | ++ | ++ | |
| *Legionella species* | | | | | |
| *Moraxella catarrhalis* | ++ | ++ | ++ | ++ | |
| *Morganella morganii* | ++ | ++ | ++ | ++ | |
| *Neisseria gonorrhoeae* | + | | + | + | |
| *Neisseria meningitidis* | ++ | | ++ | ++ | |
| *Pasturella multocida* | | | ++ | ++ | |
| *Proteus mirabilis* | ++ | ++ | ++ | ++ | |
| *Proteus vulgaris* | ++ | ++ | ++ | ++ | |
| *Providencia stuartii* | ++ | ++ | ++ | ++ | |
| *Pseudomonas aeruginosa* | +++ | | +++ | +++ | |
| *Rickettsia species* | | | | | |
| *Salmonella species* | ++ | ++ | ++ | ++ | |
| *Serratia species* | ++ | ++ | ++ | ++ | |
| *Shigella species* | ++ | ++ | ++ | ++ | |
| *Stenotrophomonas maltophilia* | | | | | |

+++ = excellent activity (1st line recommendation). ++ = good activity (2nd line recommendation). + = moderate activity (acceptable in vitro data suggesting some isolates may be sensitive).
Blank = no or insufficient activity, or unknown.
†† 2nd line against *S. typhi.* † Penicillin sensitive; MIC ≤1.0 mcg/mL. §§ Penicillin resistant; MIC ≥2.0 mcg/mL.
*These are generalizations. There are major differences among countries, areas, and hospitals depending on antibiotic usage patterns.

**CARBAPENEMS/MONOBACTAMS (CONTINUED)**

| ORGANISMS | Aztreonam | Ertapenem | Imipenem/Cilastatin | Meropenem | |
|---|---|---|---|---|---|
| **GRAM-NEGATIVE AEROBES** *(Continued)* | | | | | |
| *Vibrio vulnificus* | | | | | |
| *Yersinia enterocolitica* | ++ | | | | |
| *Yersinia pestis* | | | | | |
| **GRAM-POSITIVE AEROBES** | | | | | |
| *Enterococcus faecalis* | | + | ++ | + | |
| *Enterococcus faecium* | | | + | | |
| *Enterococcus faecium (VRE)* | | | | | |
| *Listeria monocytogenes* | | | + | + | |
| *Nocardia* | | | ++ | | |
| *Staphylococcus aureus (MSSA)* | | ++ | ++ | ++ | |
| *Staphylococcus aureus (MRSA)* | | | | | |
| *Staphylococcus epidermidis* | | ++ | ++ | ++ | |
| *Staphylococcus epidermidis (MRSE)* | | | | | |
| *Streptococcus pneumoniae†* | | ++ | ++ | ++ | |
| *Streptococcus pneumoniae§§* | | ++ | ++ | ++ | |

+++ = excellent activity (1st line recommendation). ++ = good activity (2nd line recommendation). + = moderate activity (acceptable in vitro data suggesting some isolates may be sensitive).
Blank = no or insufficient activity, or unknown.
†† 2nd line against *S. typhi.* † Penicillin sensitive; MIC ≤1.0 mcg/mL. §§ Penicillin resistant; MIC ≥2.0 mcg/mL.
*These are generalizations. There are major differences among countries, areas, and hospitals depending on antibiotic usage patterns.

| ORGANISMS | Aztreonam | Ertapenem | Imipenem/Cilastatin | Meropenem | |
|---|---|---|---|---|---|
| **GRAM-POSITIVE AEROBES** *(Continued)* | | | | | |
| *Streptococcus (Group A,B,C,F,G)* | | ++ | ++ | ++ | |
| *Streptococcus species* | | ++ | ++ | ++ | |
| **MISCELLANEOUS** | | | | | |
| *Chlamydia pneumoniae* | | | | | |
| *Chlamydia trachomatis* | | | | | |
| *Ehrlichia/Anaplasma species* | | | | | |
| **MYCOBACTERIA** | | | | | |
| *Mycobacterium avium (MAI) (non-HIV)* | | | | | |
| *Mycoplasma pneumoniae* | | | | | |
| **SPIROCHETES** | | | | | |
| *Leptospira interrogans* | | | | | |
| *Treponema pallidum (syphilis)* | | | | | |

+++ = excellent activity (1st line recommendation). ++ = good activity (2nd line recommendation). + = moderate activity (acceptable in vitro data suggesting some isolates may be sensitive).
Blank = no or insufficient activity, or unknown.
†† 2nd line against *S. typhi.* † Penicillin sensitive; MIC ≤1.0 mcg/mL. §§ Penicillin resistant; MIC ≥2.0 mcg/mL.
*These are generalizations. There are major differences among countries, areas, and hospitals depending on antibiotic usage patterns.

# ANTIBIOTIC SENSITIVITY – CEPHALOSPORINS*

| ORGANISMS | Cefaclor | Cefadroxil | Cefazolin | Cefdinir | Cefepime | Cefixime | Cefotaxime | Cefoxitin | Cefpodoxime Proxetil | Cefprozil | Ceftazidime | Ceftibuten | Ceftizoxime | Ceftriaxone | Cefuroxime Axetil | Cephalexin |
|---|---|---|---|---|---|---|---|---|---|---|---|---|---|---|---|---|
| **ANAEROBES** | | | | | | | | | | | | | | | | |
| *Actinomyces* | | | | | | | + | | | | | | + | ++ | | |
| *Bacillus anthracis* | | | | | | | | | | | | | | | | |
| *Bacteroides fragilis* | | | | | | | | ++ | | | | | + | | | |
| *Clostridium difficile* | | | | | | | | | | | | | | | | |
| *Clostridium species* | + | | + | | + | | + | ++ | | + | + | | + | + | + | |
| **GRAM-NEGATIVE AEROBES** | | | | | | | | | | | | | | | | |
| *Acinetobacter baumannii* | | | | | ++ | | + | | | | ++ | | + | + | | |
| *Aeromonas hydrophila* | | | | | ++ | ++ | ++ | + | | | ++ | | ++ | ++ | + | |
| *Bartonella henselae* | | | | | | | | | | | | | | | | |
| *Bordetella species* | | | | | | | | | | | | | | | | |
| *Burkholderia cepacia* | | | | | + | | | | | | ++ | | + | | | |
| *Campylobacter jejuni* | | | | | + | | + | | | | | | | + | | |
| *Citrobacter species* | | | | | +++ | | ++ | | | | ++ | | ++ | ++ | + | |
| *Coxiella burnetti* | | | | | | | | | | | | | | | | |
| *Enterobacter species* | | | | | +++ | | + | | | | ++ | | ++ | ++ | | |
| *Escherichia coli* | ++ | +++ | +++ | ++ | ++ | ++ | +++ | ++ | ++ | +++ | ++ | ++ | ++ | +++ | ++ | +++ |

+++ = excellent activity (1st line recommendation). ++ = good activity (2nd line recommendation). + = moderate activity (acceptable in vitro data suggesting some isolates may be sensitive).
Blank = no or insufficient activity, or unknown.
†† 2nd line against *S. typhi.* † Penicillin sensitive; MIC ≤1.0 mcg/mL. §§ Penicillin resistant; MIC ≥2.0 mcg/mL.
*These are generalizations. There are major differences among countries, areas, and hospitals depending on antibiotic usage patterns.

| ORGANISMS | Cefaclor | Cefadroxil | Cefazolin | Cefdinir | Cefepime | Cefixime | Cefotaxime | Cefoxitin | Cefpodoxime Proxetil | Cefprozil | Ceftazidime | Ceftibuten | Ceftizoxime | Ceftriaxone | Cefuroxime Axetil | Cephalexin |
|---|---|---|---|---|---|---|---|---|---|---|---|---|---|---|---|---|
| **GRAM-NEGATIVE AEROBES** *(Continued)* | | | | | | | | | | | | | | | | |
| *Francisella tularensis* | | | | | | | | | | | | | | | | |
| *Haemophilus influenzae* | ++ | | | +++ | ++ | ++ | +++ | ++ | +++ | ++ | ++ | ++ | +++ | +++ | ++ | |
| *Klebsiella species* | + | ++ | ++ | ++ | ++ | ++ | +++ | ++ | ++ | ++ | ++ | ++ | +++ | +++ | ++ | ++ |
| *Legionella species* | | | | | | | | | | | | | | | | |
| *Moraxella catarrhalis* | +++ | + | + | +++ | ++ | ++ | +++ | + | +++ | +++ | + | +++ | +++ | +++ | +++ | + |
| *Morganella morganii* | | | | | ++ | | +++ | + | | | ++ | ++ | +++ | +++ | + | |
| *Neisseria gonorrhoeae* | + | | | | ++ | +++ | ++ | ++ | ++ | + | + | ++ | ++ | +++ | ++ | |
| *Neisseria meningitidis* | | | | | ++ | + | ++ | + | | | + | | ++ | ++ | ++ | |
| *Pasturella multocida* | | | + | ++ | ++ | ++ | ++ | | ++ | | ++ | ++ | ++ | ++ | ++ | + |
| *Proteus mirabilis* | ++ | ++ | ++ | +++ | ++ | ++ | +++ | ++ | +++ | +++ | ++ | +++ | +++ | +++ | +++ | ++ |
| *Proteus vulgaris* | | | | | ++ | ++ | +++ | + | + | | ++ | + | +++ | +++ | ++ | |
| *Providencia stuartii* | | | | | +++ | | +++ | + | + | | +++ | + | +++ | +++ | + | |
| *Pseudomonas aeruginosa* | | | | | +++ | | | | | | +++ | | | | | |
| *Rickettsia species* | | | | | | | | | | | | | | | | |
| *Salmonella species* | | | | | | | +++†† | | | | | | | +++ | | |
| *Serratia species* | | | | + | +++ | + | +++ | + | + | | ++ | | +++ | +++ | | |

+++ = excellent activity (1st line recommendation). ++ = good activity (2nd line recommendation). + = moderate activity (acceptable in vitro data suggesting some isolates may be sensitive).
Blank = no or insufficient activity, or unknown.
†† 2nd line against *S. typhi.* † Penicillin sensitive; MIC ≤1.0 mcg/mL. §§ Penicillin resistant; MIC ≥2.0 mcg/mL.
*These are generalizations. There are major differences among countries, areas, and hospitals depending on antibiotic usage patterns.

**CEPHALOSPORINS (CONTINUED)**

| ORGANISMS | Cefaclor | Cefadroxil | Cefazolin | Cefdinir | Cefepime | Cefixime | Cefotaxime | Cefoxitin | Cefpodoxime Proxetil | Cefprozil | Ceftazidime | Ceftibuten | Ceftizoxime | Ceftriaxone | Cefuroxime Axetil | Cephalexin |
|---|---|---|---|---|---|---|---|---|---|---|---|---|---|---|---|---|
| **GRAM-NEGATIVE AEROBES** *(Continued)* | | | | | | | | | | | | | | | | |
| *Shigella species* | | | | + | ++ | | ++ | + | ++ | + | ++ | + | ++ | ++ | ++ | |
| *Stenotrophomonas maltophilia* | | | | | | | | | | | + | | | | | |
| *Vibrio vulnificus* | | | | | | | ++ | | | | +++ | | | | | |
| *Yersinia enterocolitica* | | | | ++ | ++ | ++ | ++ | + | ++ | | ++ | ++ | ++ | ++ | + | |
| *Yersinia pestis* | | | | | | | + | | | | | | | + | | |
| **GRAM-POSITIVE AEROBES** | | | | | | | | | | | | | | | | |
| *Enterococcus faecalis* | | | | | | | | | | | | | | | | |
| *Enterococcus faecium* | | | | | | | | | | | | | | | | |
| *Enterococcus faecium (VRE)* | | | | | | | | | | | | | | | | |
| *Listeria monocytogenes* | | | | | | | | | | | | | | | | |
| *Nocardia* | | | | | | | ++ | | | | | | | ++ | + | |
| *Staphylococcus aureus (MSSA)* | + | +++ | +++ | ++ | ++ | | ++ | + | ++ | + | + | + | ++ | ++ | ++ | ++ |
| *Staphylococcus aureus (MRSA)* | | | | | | | | | | | | | | | | |

+++ = excellent activity (1st line recommendation). ++ = good activity (2nd line recommendation). + = moderate activity (acceptable in vitro data suggesting some isolates may be sensitive).

Blank = no or insufficient activity, or unknown.

†† 2nd line against *S. typhi.* † Penicillin sensitive; MIC ≤1.0 mcg/mL. §§ Penicillin resistant; MIC ≥2.0 mcg/mL.

*These are generalizations. There are major differences among countries, areas, and hospitals depending on antibiotic usage patterns.

| ORGANISMS | Cefaclor | Cefadroxil | Cefazolin | Cefdinir | Cefepime | Cefixime | Cefotaxime | Cefoxitin | Cefpodoxime Proxetil | Cefprozil | Ceftazidime | Ceftibuten | Ceftizoxime | Ceftriaxone | Cefuroxime Axetil | Cephalexin |
|---|---|---|---|---|---|---|---|---|---|---|---|---|---|---|---|---|
| **GRAM-POSITIVE AEROBES** *(Continued)* | | | | | | | | | | | | | | | | |
| *Staphylococcus epidermidis* | + | ++ | ++ | | + | | + | + | + | ++ | | | + | + | ++ | ++ |
| *Staphylococcus epidermidis (MRSE)* | | | | | | | | | | | | | | | | |
| *Streptococcus pneumoniae†* | ++ | ++ | ++ | ++ | ++ | ++ | ++ | + | ++ | ++ | + | + | ++ | ++ | ++ | ++ |
| *Streptococcus pneumoniae§§* | | | | | + | | +++ | | + | | | | ++ | +++ | | |
| *Streptococcus (Group A,B,C,F,G)* | ++ | ++ | ++ | ++ | ++ | ++ | ++ | + | ++ | ++ | + | + | ++ | ++ | ++ | ++ |
| *Streptococcus species* | ++ | ++ | ++ | ++ | ++ | ++ | ++ | + | ++ | ++ | + | + | + | ++ | ++ | ++ |
| **MISCELLANEOUS** | | | | | | | | | | | | | | | | |
| *Chlamydia pneumoniae* | | | | | | | | | | | | | | | | |
| *Chlamydia trachomatis* | | | | | | | | | | | | | | | | |
| *Ehrlichia/Anaplasma species* | | | | | | | | | | | | | | | | |
| **MYCOBACTERIA** | | | | | | | | | | | | | | | | |
| *Mycobacterium avium (MAI) (non-HIV)* | | | | | | | | | | | | | | | | |

+++ = excellent activity (1st line recommendation). ++ = good activity (2nd line recommendation). + = moderate activity (acceptable in vitro data suggesting some isolates may be sensitive).

Blank = no or insufficient activity, or unknown.

†† 2nd line against *S. typhi.* † Penicillin sensitive; MIC ≤1.0 mcg/mL. §§ Penicillin resistant; MIC ≥2.0 mcg/mL.

*These are generalizations. There are major differences among countries, areas, and hospitals depending on antibiotic usage patterns.

**CEPHALOSPORINS (CONTINUED)**

| ORGANISMS | Cefaclor | Cefadroxil | Cefazolin | Cefdinir | Cefepime | Cefixime | Cefotaxime | Cefoxitin | Cefpodoxime Proxetil | Cefprozil | Ceftazidime | Ceftibuten | Ceftizoxime | Ceftriaxone | Cefuroxime axetil | Cephalexin |
|---|---|---|---|---|---|---|---|---|---|---|---|---|---|---|---|---|
| **MYCOBACTERIA** *(Continued)* | | | | | | | | | | | | | | | | |
| *Mycoplasma pneumoniae* | | | | | | | | | | | | | | | | |
| **SPIROCHETES** | | | | | | | | | | | | | | | | |
| *Leptospira interrogans* | | | | | | | | | | | | | | ++ | | |
| *Treponema pallidum (syphilis)* | | | | | | | ++ | | | | | | + | ++ | | |

+++ = excellent activity (1st line recommendation). ++ = good activity (2nd line recommendation). + = moderate activity (acceptable in vitro data suggesting some isolates may be sensitive).
Blank = no or insufficient activity, or unknown.
†† 2nd line against *S. typhi.* † Penicillin sensitive; MIC ≤1.0 mcg/mL. §§ Penicillin resistant; MIC ≥2.0 mcg/mL.
*These are generalizations. There are major differences among countries, areas, and hospitals depending on antibiotic usage patterns.

# ANTIBIOTIC SENSITIVITY - FLUOROQUINOLONES*

| ORGANISMS | Ciprofloxacin | Gemifloxacin | Levofloxacin | Moxifloxacin | Norfloxacin | Ofloxacin |
|---|---|---|---|---|---|---|
| **ANAEROBES** | | | | | | |
| *Actinomyces* | | | | + | | |
| *Bacillus anthracis* | +++ | | ++ | ++ | | ++ |
| *Bacteroides fragilis* | | | | + | | |
| *Clostridium difficile* | | | | | | |
| *Clostridium species* | | | | + | | |
| **GRAM-NEGATIVE AEROBES** | | | | | | |
| *Acinetobacter baumannii* | ++ | | ++ | + | | + |
| *Aeromonas hydrophila* | +++ | | +++ | +++ | + | +++ |
| *Bartonella henselae* | + | | | | | |
| *Bordetella species* | + | | + | + | | |
| *Burkholderia cepacia* | ++ | | + | + | | |
| *Campylobacter jejuni* | +++ | | ++ | +++ | ++ | ++ |
| *Citrobacter species* | ++ | | ++ | + | + | + |
| *Coxiella burnetti* | ++ | | ++ | | | ++ |
| *Enterobacter species* | ++ | | ++ | ++ | ++ | ++ |
| *Escherichia coli* | ++ | | ++ | ++ | +++ | ++ |

+++ = excellent activity (1st line recommendation). ++ = good activity (2nd line recommendation). + = moderate activity (acceptable in vitro data suggesting some isolates may be sensitive).
Blank = no or insufficient activity, or unknown.
†† 2nd line against *S. typhi.* † Penicillin sensitive; MIC ≤1.0 mcg/mL. §§ Penicillin resistant; MIC ≥2.0 mcg/mL.
*These are generalizations. There are major differences among countries, areas, and hospitals depending on antibiotic usage patterns.

**FLUOROQUINOLONES (CONTINUED)**

| ORGANISMS | Ciprofloxacin | Gemifloxacin | Levofloxacin | Moxifloxacin | Norfloxacin | Ofloxacin |
|---|---|---|---|---|---|---|
| **GRAM-NEGATIVE AEROBES** *(Continued)* | | | | | | |
| *Francisella tularensis* | ++ | | | | | |
| *Haemophilus influenzae* | ++ | ++ | ++ | ++ | | ++ |
| *Klebsiella species* | ++ | + | ++ | ++ | ++ | ++ |
| *Legionella species* | +++ | ++ | +++ | +++ | | +++ |
| *Moraxella catarrhalis* | ++ | ++ | ++ | ++ | | ++ |
| *Morganella morganii* | ++ | | ++ | + | ++ | + |
| *Neisseria gonorrhoeae* | +++ | | +++ | ++ | + | +++ |
| *Neisseria meningitidis* | ++ | | ++ | ++ | | ++ |
| *Pasturella multocida* | ++ | | + | | | + |
| *Proteus mirabilis* | ++ | | ++ | ++ | +++ | ++ |
| *Proteus vulgaris* | ++ | | ++ | ++ | +++ | ++ |
| *Providencia stuartii* | ++ | | ++ | + | ++ | + |
| *Pseudomonas aeruginosa* | +++ | | +++ | ++ | ++ | ++ |
| *Rickettsia species* | ++ | | ++ | + | | ++ |
| *Salmonella species* | +++ | ++†† | +++ | +++ | +++ | +++ |
| *Serratia species* | +++ | | +++ | ++ | ++ | ++ |
| *Shigella species* | +++ | | +++ | +++ | +++ | +++ |
| *Stenotrophomonas maltophilia* | + | | + | ++ | + | + |

+++ = excellent activity (1st line recommendation). ++ = good activity (2nd line recommendation). + = moderate activity (acceptable in vitro data suggesting some isolates may be sensitive).

Blank = no or insufficient activity, or unknown.

†† 2nd line against *S. typhi.* † Penicillin sensitive; MIC ≤1.0 mcg/mL. §§ Penicillin resistant; MIC ≥2.0 mcg/mL.

*These are generalizations. There are major differences among countries, areas, and hospitals depending on antibiotic usage patterns.

| ORGANISMS | Ciprofloxacin | Gemifloxacin | Levofloxacin | Moxifloxacin | Norfloxacin | Ofloxacin | |
|---|---|---|---|---|---|---|---|
| **GRAM-NEGATIVE AEROBES** *(Continued)* | | | | | | | |
| *Vibrio vulnificus* | + | | + | + | | | |
| *Yersinia enterocolitica* | ++ | | ++ | ++ | ++ | ++ | |
| *Yersinia pestis* | + | | + | | | | |
| **GRAM-POSITIVE AEROBES** | | | | | | | |
| *Enterococcus faecalis* | + | | ++ | ++ | + | + | |
| *Enterococcus faecium* | + | | + | + | | + | |
| *Enterococcus faecium (VRE)* | | | | | | | |
| *Listeria monocytogenes* | | | | | | | |
| *Nocardia* | | | | | | | |
| *Staphylococcus aureus (MSSA)* | + | ++ | ++ | ++ | + | + | |
| *Staphylococcus aureus (MRSA)* | | | + | + | | | |
| *Staphylococcus epidermidis* | + | | + | + | + | + | |
| *Staphylococcus epidermidis (MRSE)* | + | | + | + | | + | |
| *Streptococcus pneumoniae†* | + | ++ | ++ | ++ | | + | |
| *Streptococcus pneumoniae§§* | + | +++ | +++ | +++ | | + | |

+++ = excellent activity (1st line recommendation). ++ = good activity (2nd line recommendation). + = moderate activity (acceptable in vitro data suggesting some isolates may be sensitive).
Blank = no or insufficient activity, or unknown.
†† 2nd line against *S. typhi.* † Penicillin sensitive; MIC ≤1.0 mcg/mL. §§ Penicillin resistant; MIC ≥2.0 mcg/mL.
*These are generalizations. There are major differences among countries, areas, and hospitals depending on antibiotic usage patterns.

**FLUOROQUINOLONES (CONTINUED)**

| ORGANISMS | Ciprofloxacin | Gemifloxacin | Levofloxacin | Moxifloxacin | Norfloxacin | Ofloxacin | |
|---|---|---|---|---|---|---|---|
| **GRAM-POSITIVE AEROBES** *(Continued)* | | | | | | | |
| *Streptococcus (Group A,B,C,F,G)* | + | + | + | + | | + | |
| *Streptococcus species* | + | ++ | ++ | ++ | + | + | |
| **MISCELLANEOUS** | | | | | | | |
| *Chlamydia pneumoniae* | ++ | ++ | ++ | ++ | | ++ | |
| *Chlamydia trachomatis* | | | ++ | ++ | | ++ | |
| *Ehrlichia/Anaplasma species* | + | | + | | | + | |
| **MYCOBACTERIA** | | | | | | | |
| *Mycobacterium avium (MAI) (non-HIV)* | ++ | | ++ | ++ | | ++ | |
| *Mycoplasma pneumoniae* | ++ | ++ | ++ | ++ | | ++ | |
| **SPIROCHETES** | | | | | | | |
| *Leptospira interrogans* | | | | | | | |
| *Treponema pallidum (syphilis)* | | | | | | | |

+++ = excellent activity (1st line recommendation). ++ = good activity (2nd line recommendation). + = moderate activity (acceptable in vitro data suggesting some isolates may be sensitive).
Blank = no or insufficient activity, or unknown.
†† 2nd line against *S. typhi.* † Penicillin sensitive; MIC ≤1.0 mcg/mL. §§ Penicillin resistant; MIC ≥2.0 mcg/mL.
*These are generalizations. There are major differences among countries, areas, and hospitals depending on antibiotic usage patterns.

# ANTIBIOTIC SENSITIVITY - MACROLIDES & CLINDAMYCIN*

| ORGANISMS | Azithromycin | Clarithromycin | Clindamycin | Erythromycin | Telithromycin | |
|---|---|---|---|---|---|---|
| **ANAEROBES** | | | | | | |
| *Actinomyces* | ++ | ++ | ++ | ++ | | |
| *Bacillus anthracis* | | + | ++ | + | | |
| *Bacteroides fragilis* | | | ++ | | | |
| *Clostridium difficile* | | | ++ | | | |
| *Clostridium species* | | | | | | |
| **GRAM-NEGATIVE AEROBES** | | | | | | |
| *Acinetobacter baumannii* | | | | | | |
| *Aeromonas hydrophila* | | | | | | |
| *Bartonella henselae* | +++ | +++ | | +++ | | |
| *Bordetella species* | +++ | +++ | | +++ | ++ | |
| *Burkholderia cepacia* | | | | | | |
| *Campylobacter jejuni* | +++ | +++ | ++ | +++ | | |
| *Citrobacter species* | | | | | | |
| *Coxiella burnetti* | | | | + | | |
| *Enterobacter species* | | | | | | |
| *Escherichia coli* | | | | | | |

+++ = excellent activity (1st line recommendation). ++ = good activity (2nd line recommendation). + = moderate activity (acceptable in vitro data suggesting some isolates may be sensitive).

Blank = no or insufficient activity, or unknown.

†† 2nd line against *S. typhi.* † Penicillin sensitive; MIC ≤1.0 mcg/mL. §§ Penicillin resistant; MIC ≥2.0 mcg/mL.

*These are generalizations. There are major differences among countries, areas, and hospitals depending on antibiotic usage patterns.

**MACROLIDES & CLINDAMYCIN (CONTINUED)**

| ORGANISMS | Azithromycin | Clarithromycin | Clindamycin | Erythromycin | Telithromycin |
|---|---|---|---|---|---|
| **GRAM-NEGATIVE AEROBES** *(Continued)* | | | | | |
| *Francisella tularensis* | | | | | |
| *Haemophilus influenzae* | ++ | ++ | | + | ++ |
| *Klebsiella species* | | | | | |
| *Legionella species* | +++ | +++ | | ++ | ++ |
| *Moraxella catarrhalis* | +++ | +++ | | ++ | ++ |
| *Morganella morganii* | | | | | |
| *Neisseria gonorrhoeae* | ++ | | | + | |
| *Neisseria meningitidis* | | | | | |
| *Pasturella multocida* | + | | | | |
| *Proteus mirabilis* | | | | | |
| *Proteus vulgaris* | | | | | |
| *Providencia stuartii* | | | | | |
| *Pseudomonas aeruginosa* | | | | | |
| *Rickettsia species* | | | | + | + |
| *Salmonella species* | ++ | | | | |
| *Serratia species* | | | | | |
| *Shigella species* | + | | | | |
| *Stenotrophomonas maltophilia* | | | | | |

+++ = excellent activity (1st line recommendation). ++ = good activity (2nd line recommendation). + = moderate activity (acceptable in vitro data suggesting some isolates may be sensitive).

Blank = no or insufficient activity, or unknown.

†† 2nd line against *S. typhi*. † Penicillin sensitive; MIC ≤1.0 mcg/mL. §§ Penicillin resistant; MIC ≥2.0 mcg/mL.

*These are generalizations. There are major differences among countries, areas, and hospitals depending on antibiotic usage patterns.

| ORGANISMS | Azithromycin | Clarithromycin | Clindamycin | Erythromycin | Telithromycin | |
|---|---|---|---|---|---|---|
| **GRAM-NEGATIVE AEROBES** *(Continued)* | | | | | | |
| *Vibrio vulnificus* | | | | | | |
| *Yersinia enterocolitica* | | | | | | |
| *Yersinia pestis* | | | | | | |
| **GRAM-POSITIVE AEROBES** | | | | | | |
| *Enterococcus faecalis* | | | | | | |
| *Enterococcus faecium* | | | | | | |
| *Enterococcus faecium (VRE)* | | | | | | |
| *Listeria monocytogenes* | | | | ++ | | |
| *Nocardia* | ++ | ++ | ++ | + | ++ | |
| *Staphylococcus aureus (MSSA)* | | | ++ | | | |
| *Staphylococcus aureus (MRSA)* | + | + | ++ | + | | |
| *Staphylococcus epidermidis* | + | + | ++ | + | | |
| *Staphylococcus epidermidis (MRSE)* | ++ | ++ | ++ | ++ | ++ | |
| *Streptococcus pneumoniae†* | | | ++ | | +++ | |
| *Streptococcus pneumoniae§§* | ++ | ++ | ++ | ++ | ++ | |

+++ = excellent activity (1st line recommendation). ++ = good activity (2nd line recommendation). + = moderate activity (acceptable in vitro data suggesting some isolates may be sensitive).
Blank = no or insufficient activity, or unknown.
†† 2nd line against *S. typhi.* † Penicillin sensitive; MIC ≤1.0 mcg/mL. §§ Penicillin resistant; MIC ≥2.0 mcg/mL.
*These are generalizations. There are major differences among countries, areas, and hospitals depending on antibiotic usage patterns.

**MACROLIDES & CLINDAMYCIN (CONTINUED)**

| ORGANISMS | Azithromycin | Clarithromycin | Clindamycin | Erythromycin | Telithromycin | |
|---|---|---|---|---|---|---|
| **GRAM-POSITIVE AEROBES** *(Continued)* | | | | | | |
| *Streptococcus (Group A,B,C,F,G)* | ++ | ++ | ++ | ++ | | |
| *Streptococcus species* | | | | | | |
| **MISCELLANEOUS** | | | | | | |
| *Chlamydia pneumoniae* | +++ | +++ | | +++ | ++ | |
| *Chlamydia trachomatis* | +++ | ++ | ++ | ++ | | |
| *Ehrlichia/Anaplasma species* | ++ | +++ | | | | |
| **MYCOBACTERIA** | | | | | | |
| *Mycobacterium avium (MAI) (non-HIV)* | +++ | +++ | | +++ | ++ | |
| *Mycoplasma pneumoniae* | | | | ++ | | |
| **SPIROCHETES** | | | | | | |
| *Leptospira interrogans* | + | | | + | | |
| *Treponema pallidum (syphilis)* | | | | | | |

+++ = excellent activity (1st line recommendation). ++ = good activity (2nd line recommendation). + = moderate activity (acceptable in vitro data suggesting some isolates may be sensitive).
Blank = no or insufficient activity, or unknown.
†† 2nd line against *S. typhi.* † Penicillin sensitive; MIC ≤1.0 mcg/mL. §§ Penicillin resistant; MIC ≥2.0 mcg/mL.
*These are generalizations. There are major differences among countries, areas, and hospitals depending on antibiotic usage patterns.

# ANTIBIOTIC SENSITIVITY - PENICILLINS*

| ORGANISMS | Amoxicillin | Amoxicillin + Clavulanate | Ampicillin | Ampicillin + Sulbactam | Dicloxacillin | Nafcillin/ Oxacillin | Penicillin | Piperacillin | Piperacillin + Tazobactam | Ticarcillin + Clavulanic Acid |
|---|---|---|---|---|---|---|---|---|---|---|
| **ANAEROBES** | | | | | | | | | | |
| *Actinomyces* | +++ | ++ | +++ | ++ | | | +++ | | | |
| *Bacillus anthracis* | ++ | + | ++ | + | | | ++ | | | |
| *Bacteroides fragilis* | | +++ | | +++ | | | | + | +++ | +++ |
| *Clostridium difficile* | | | | | | | | | | |
| *Clostridium species* | ++ | ++ | ++ | ++ | | | +++ | ++ | ++ | ++ |
| **GRAM-NEGATIVE AEROBES** | | | | | | | | | | |
| *Acinetobacter baumannii* | | | | ++ | | | | + | ++ | ++ |
| *Aeromonas hydrophila* | | | | | | | | + | + | + |
| *Bartonella henselae* | | | | | | | | | | |
| *Bordetella species* | | | | | | | | | | |
| *Burkholderia cepacia* | | | | | | | | | + | + |
| *Campylobacter jejuni* | ++ | + | | | | | | | | + |
| *Citrobacter species* | | | | | | | | ++ | ++ | ++ |
| *Coxiella burnetti* | | | | | | | | | | |
| *Enterobacter species* | | | | | | | | ++ | ++ | ++ |
| *Escherichia coli* | +++ | ++ | +++ | ++ | | | | ++ | ++ | ++ |

+++ = excellent activity (1st line recommendation). ++ = good activity (2nd line recommendation). + = moderate activity (acceptable in vitro data suggesting some isolates may be sensitive).
Blank = no or insufficient activity, or unknown.
†† 2nd line against *S. typhi.* † Penicillin sensitive; MIC ≤1.0 mcg/mL. §§ Penicillin resistant; MIC ≥2.0 mcg/mL.
*These are generalizations. There are major differences among countries, areas, and hospitals depending on antibiotic usage patterns.

**PENICILLINS (CONTINUED)**

| ORGANISMS | Amoxicillin | Amoxicillin + Clavulanate | Ampicillin | Ampicillin + Sulbactam | Dicloxacillin | Nafcillin/ Oxacillin | Penicillin | Piperacillin | Piperacillin + Tazobactam | Ticarcillin + Clavulanic Acid |
|---|---|---|---|---|---|---|---|---|---|---|
| **GRAM-NEGATIVE AEROBES** *(Continued)* | | | | | | | | | | |
| *Francisella tularensis* | | | | | | | | | | |
| *Haemophilus influenzae* | + | +++ | + | ++ | | | | | ++ | ++ |
| *Klebsiella species* | | ++ | | ++ | | | | ++ | ++ | ++ |
| *Legionella species* | | | | | | | | | | |
| *Moraxella catarrhalis* | | +++ | | ++ | | | | | ++ | ++ |
| *Morganella morganii* | | | | | | | | ++ | ++ | ++ |
| *Neisseria gonorrhoeae* | | ++ | | ++ | | | | | ++ | ++ |
| *Neisseria meningitidis* | + | ++ | ++ | ++ | | | +++ | ++ | | |
| *Pasturella multocida* | ++ | +++ | ++ | ++ | | | +++ | ++ | ++ | ++ |
| *Proteus mirabilis* | +++ | ++ | +++ | ++ | | | | ++ | ++ | ++ |
| *Proteus vulgaris* | | | | | | | | ++ | ++ | ++ |
| *Providencia stuartii* | | | | | | | | ++ | ++ | ++ |
| *Pseudomonas aeruginosa* | | | | | | | | +++ | +++ | ++ |
| *Rickettsia species* | | | | | | | | | | |
| *Salmonella species* | + | ++ | + | ++ | | | | ++ | ++ | ++ |
| *Serratia species* | | | | | | | | ++ | ++ | ++ |
| *Shigella species* | ++ | ++ | ++ | + | | | | + | + | + |

+++ = excellent activity (1st line recommendation). ++ = good activity (2nd line recommendation). + = moderate activity (acceptable in vitro data suggesting some isolates may be sensitive).
Blank = no or insufficient activity, or unknown.
†† 2nd line against *S. typhi.* † Penicillin sensitive; MIC ≤1.0 mcg/mL. §§ Penicillin resistant; MIC ≥2.0 mcg/mL.
*These are generalizations. There are major differences among countries, areas, and hospitals depending on antibiotic usage patterns.

| ORGANISMS | Amoxicillin | Amoxicillin + Clavulanate | Ampicillin | Ampicillin + Sulbactam | Dicloxacillin | Nafcillin/ Oxacillin | Penicillin | Piperacillin | Piperacillin + Tazobactam | Ticarcillin + Clavulanic Acid |
|---|---|---|---|---|---|---|---|---|---|---|
| **GRAM-NEGATIVE AEROBES** *(Continued)* | | | | | | | | | | |
| *Stenotrophomonas maltophilia* | | | | | | | | + | + | ++ |
| *Vibrio vulnificus* | | | | ++ | | | | | ++ | |
| *Yersinia enterocolitica* | | + | | ++ | | | | ++ | ++ | ++ |
| *Yersinia pestis* | + | | + | | | | | | | |
| **GRAM-POSITIVE AEROBES** | | | | | | | | | | |
| *Enterococcus faecalis* | +++ | ++ | +++ | ++ | | | +++ | ++ | ++ | |
| *Enterococcus faecium* | + | + | + | + | | | + | + | + | |
| *Enterococcus faecium (VRE)* | | | | | | | | | | |
| *Listeria monocytogenes* | +++ | ++ | +++ | ++ | | | ++ | ++ | ++ | ++ |
| *Nocardia* | + | ++ | + | ++ | | | | | | |
| *Staphylococcus aureus (MSSA)* | | ++ | | ++ | +++ | +++ | | | ++ | ++ |
| *Staphylococcus aureus (MRSA)* | | | | | | | | | | |
| *Staphylococcus epidermidis* | | ++ | | ++ | +++ | +++ | | | ++ | ++ |
| *Staphylococcus epidermidis (MRSE)* | | | | | | | | | | |
| *Streptococcus pneumoniae†* | +++ | ++ | ++ | ++ | + | + | +++ | ++ | ++ | ++ |
| *Streptococcus pneumoniae§§* | ++ | ++ | ++ | ++ | | | ++ | + | + | + |

+++ = excellent activity (1st line recommendation). ++ = good activity (2nd line recommendation). + = moderate activity (acceptable in vitro data suggesting some isolates may be sensitive).
Blank = no or insufficient activity, or unknown.
†† 2nd line against *S. typhi.* † Penicillin sensitive; MIC ≤1.0 mcg/mL. §§ Penicillin resistant; MIC ≥2.0 mcg/mL.
*These are generalizations. There are major differences among countries, areas, and hospitals depending on antibiotic usage patterns.

**PENICILLINS (CONTINUED)**

| ORGANISMS | Amoxicillin | Amoxicillin + Clavulanate | Ampicillin | Ampicillin + Sulbactam | Dicloxacillin | Nafcillin/ Oxacillin | Penicillin | Piperacillin | Piperacillin + Tazobactam | Ticarcillin + Clavulanic Acid |
|---|---|---|---|---|---|---|---|---|---|---|
| **GRAM-POSITIVE AEROBES** *(Continued)* | | | | | | | | | | |
| *Streptococcus (Group A,B,C,F,G)* | +++ | + | +++ | + | + | + | +++ | + | + | + |
| *Streptococcus species* | +++ | + | ++ | + | + | + | +++ | ++ | + | + |
| **MISCELLANEOUS** | | | | | | | | | | |
| *Chlamydia pneumoniae* | | | | | | | | | | |
| *Chlamydia trachomatis* | | | | | | | | | | |
| *Ehrlichia/Anaplasma species* | | | | | | | | | | |
| **MYCOBACTERIA** | | | | | | | | | | |
| *Mycobacterium avium (MAI) (non-HIV)* | | | | | | | | | | |
| *Mycoplasma pneumoniae* | | | | | | | | | | |
| **SPIROCHETES** | | | | | | | | | | |
| *Leptospira interrogans* | ++ | | +++ | | | | +++ | | | |
| *Treponema pallidum (syphilis)* | ++ | | ++ | | | | +++ | | | |

+++ = excellent activity (1st line recommendation). ++ = good activity (2nd line recommendation). + = moderate activity (acceptable in vitro data suggesting some isolates may be sensitive).

Blank = no or insufficient activity, or unknown.

†† 2nd line against *S. typhi.* † Penicillin sensitive; MIC ≤1.0 mcg/mL. §§ Penicillin resistant; MIC ≥2.0 mcg/mL.

*These are generalizations. There are major differences among countries, areas, and hospitals depending on antibiotic usage patterns.

## ANTIBIOTIC SENSITIVITY – SULFONAMIDES*

| ORGANISMS | Trimethoprim + Sulfamethoxazole |
|---|---|
| **ANAEROBES** | |
| *Actinomyces* | |
| *Bacillus anthracis* | |
| *Bacteroides fragilis* | |
| *Clostridium difficile* | |
| *Clostridium species* | |
| **GRAM-NEGATIVE AEROBES** | |
| *Acinetobacter baumannii* | + |
| *Aeromonas hydrophila* | ++ |
| *Bartonella henselae* | |
| *Bordetella species* | ++ |
| *Burkholderia cepacia* | +++ |
| *Campylobacter jejuni* | |
| *Citrobacter species* | ++ |
| *Coxiella burnetti* | |
| *Enterobacter species* | ++ |

## ANTIBIOTIC SENSITIVITY – TETRACYCLINES*

| ORGANISMS | Doxycycline | Minocycline | Tetracycline | |
|---|---|---|---|---|
| **ANAEROBES** | | | | |
| *Actinomyces* | ++ | ++ | ++ | |
| *Bacillus anthracis* | ++ | | ++ | |
| *Bacteroides fragilis* | + | | + | |
| *Clostridium difficile* | | | | |
| *Clostridium species* | + | | + | |
| **GRAM-NEGATIVE AEROBES** | | | | |
| *Acinetobacter baumannii* | ++ | ++ | ++ | |
| *Aeromonas hydrophila* | ++ | ++ | ++ | |
| *Bartonella henselae* | +++ | ++ | ++ | |
| *Bordetella species* | + | | + | |
| *Burkholderia cepacia* | | ++ | | |
| *Campylobacter jejuni* | ++ | ++ | ++ | |
| *Citrobacter species* | | | | |
| *Coxiella burnetti* | +++ | +++ | +++ | |
| *Enterobacter species* | | | | |

+++ = excellent activity (1st line recommendation). ++ = good activity (2nd line recommendation). + = moderate activity (acceptable in vitro data suggesting some isolates may be sensitive).
Blank = no or insufficient activity, or unknown.
†† 2nd line against *S. typhi.* † Penicillin sensitive; MIC $\leq$1.0 mcg/mL. §§ Penicillin resistant; MIC $\geq$2.0 mcg/mL.
*These are generalizations. There are major differences among countries, areas, and hospitals depending on antibiotic usage patterns.

**SULFONAMIDES (CONTINUED)**

| ORGANISMS | Trimethoprim + Sulfamethoxazole |
|---|---|
| **GRAM-NEGATIVE AEROBES** *(Continued)* | |
| *Escherichia coli* | +++ |
| *Francisella tularensis* | |
| *Haemophilus influenzae* | +++ |
| *Klebsiella species* | +++** |
| *Legionella species* | ++ |
| *Moraxella catarrhalis* | +++ |
| *Morganella morganii* | |
| *Neisseria gonorrhoeae* | |
| *Neisseria meningitidis* | |
| *Pasturella multocida* | ++ |
| *Proteus mirabilis* | ++ |
| *Proteus vulgaris* | ++ |
| *Providencia stuartii* | ++ |
| *Pseudomonas aeruginosa* | |
| *Rickettsia species* | |
| *Salmonella species* | ++ |
| *Serratia species* | + |

**TETRACYCLINES (CONTINUED)**

| ORGANISMS | Doxycycline | Minocycline | Tetracycline | |
|---|---|---|---|---|
| **GRAM-NEGATIVE AEROBES** *(Continued)* | | | | |
| *Escherichia coli* | + | + | + | |
| *Francisella tularensis* | ++ | ++ | ++ | |
| *Haemophilus influenzae* | ++ | ++ | ++ | |
| *Klebsiella species* | + | + | | |
| *Legionella species* | ++ | ++ | ++ | |
| *Moraxella catarrhalis* | ++ | ++ | ++ | |
| *Morganella morganii* | ++ | ++ | ++ | |
| *Neisseria gonorrhoeae* | + | + | + | |
| *Neisseria meningitidis* | + | + | + | |
| *Pasturella multocida* | ++ | | ++ | |
| *Proteus mirabilis* | + | + | + | |
| *Proteus vulgaris* | + | + | + | |
| *Providencia stuartii* | | | | |
| *Pseudomonas aeruginosa* | | | | |
| *Rickettsia species* | +++ | +++ | +++ | |
| *Salmonella species* | + | + | + | |
| *Serratia species* | | | | |

+++ = excellent activity (1st line recommendation). ++ = good activity (2nd line recommendation). + = moderate activity (acceptable in vitro data suggesting some isolates may be sensitive).
Blank = no or insufficient activity, or unknown.
†† 2nd line against *S. typhi*. † Penicillin sensitive; MIC ≤1.0 mcg/mL. §§ Penicillin resistant; MIC ≥2.0 mcg/mL.
*These are generalizations. There are major differences among countries, areas, and hospitals depending on antibiotic usage patterns.

| ORGANISMS | Trimethoprim + Sulfamethoxazole |
|---|---|
| **GRAM-NEGATIVE AEROBES** *(Continued)* | |
| *Shigella species* | ++ |
| *Stenotrophomonas maltophilia* | +++ |
| *Vibrio vulnificus* | |
| *Yersinia enterocolitica* | +++ |
| *Yersinia pestis* | + |
| **GRAM-POSITIVE AEROBES** | |
| *Enterococcus faecalis* | |
| *Enterococcus faecium* | |
| *Enterococcus faecium (VRE)* | |
| *Listeria monocytogenes* | ++ |
| *Nocardia* | +++ |
| *Staphylococcus aureus (MSSA)* | ++ |
| *Staphylococcus aureus (MRSA)* | ++ |
| *Staphylococcus epidermidis* | ++ |
| *Staphylococcus epidermidis (MRSE)* | ++ |
| *Streptococcus pneumoniae†* | ++ |

| ORGANISMS | Doxycycline | Minocycline | Tetracycline | |
|---|---|---|---|---|
| **GRAM-NEGATIVE AEROBES** *(Continued)* | | | | |
| *Shigella species* | + | + | + | |
| *Stenotrophomonas maltophilia* | | + | | |
| *Vibrio vulnificus* | +++ | +++ | +++ | |
| *Yersinia enterocolitica* | | | | |
| *Yersinia pestis* | ++ | ++ | ++ | |
| **GRAM-POSITIVE AEROBES** | | | | |
| *Enterococcus faecalis* | + | + | + | |
| *Enterococcus faecium* | | | | |
| *Enterococcus faecium (VRE)* | + | + | + | |
| *Listeria monocytogenes* | + | + | + | |
| *Nocardia* | ++ | ++ | + | |
| *Staphylococcus aureus (MSSA)* | ++ | ++ | + | |
| *Staphylococcus aureus (MRSA)* | ++ | ++ | + | |
| *Staphylococcus epidermidis* | ++ | ++ | + | |
| *Staphylococcus epidermidis (MRSE)* | ++ | ++ | ++ | |
| *Streptococcus pneumoniae†* | ++ | ++ | ++ | |

+++ = excellent activity (1st line recommendation). ++ = good activity (2nd line recommendation). + = moderate activity (acceptable in vitro data suggesting some isolates may be sensitive).
Blank = no or insufficient activity, or unknown.
†† 2nd line against *S. typhi.* † Penicillin sensitive; MIC ≤1.0 mcg/mL. §§ Penicillin resistant; MIC ≥2.0 mcg/mL.
*These are generalizations. There are major differences among countries, areas, and hospitals depending on antibiotic usage patterns.

**SULFONAMIDES (CONTINUED)**

| ORGANISMS | Trimethoprim + Sulfamethoxazole |
|---|---|
| **GRAM-POSITIVE AEROBES** *(Continued)* | |
| *Streptococcus pneumoniae§§* | |
| *Streptococcus (Group A,B,C,F,G)* | ++ |
| *Streptococcus species* | ++ |
| **MISCELLANEOUS** | |
| *Chlamydia pneumoniae* | |
| *Chlamydia trachomatis* | + |
| *Ehrlichia/Anaplasma species* | |
| **MYCOBACTERIA** | |
| *Mycobacterium avium (MAI) (non-HIV)* | |
| *Mycoplasma pneumoniae* | |
| **SPIROCHETES** | |
| *Leptospira interrogans* | |
| *Treponema pallidum (syphilis)* | |

**TETRACYCLINES (CONTINUED)**

| ORGANISMS | Doxycycline | Minocycline | Tetracycline | |
|---|---|---|---|---|
| **GRAM-POSITIVE AEROBES** *(Continued)* | | | | |
| *Streptococcus pneumoniae§§* | + | + | + | |
| *Streptococcus (Group A,B,C,F,G)* | + | + | + | |
| *Streptococcus species* | + | + | + | |
| **MISCELLANEOUS** | | | | |
| *Chlamydia pneumoniae* | +++ | +++ | +++ | |
| *Chlamydia trachomatis* | +++ | +++ | +++ | |
| *Ehrlichia/Anaplasma species* | +++ | | +++ | |
| **MYCOBACTERIA** | | | | |
| *Mycobacterium avium (MAI) (non-HIV)* | | | | |
| Mycoplasma pneumoniae | ++ | ++ | ++ | |
| **SPIROCHETES** | | | | |
| *Leptospira interrogans* | ++ | ++ | ++ | |
| *Treponema pallidum (syphilis)* | ++ | ++ | ++ | |

+++ = excellent activity (1st line recommendation). ++ = good activity (2nd line recommendation). + = moderate activity (acceptable in vitro data suggesting some isolates may be sensitive).

Blank = no or insufficient activity, or unknown.

†† 2nd line against *S. typhi.* † Penicillin sensitive; MIC ≤1.0 mcg/mL. §§ Penicillin resistant; MIC ≥2.0 mcg/mL.

*These are generalizations. There are major differences among countries, areas, and hospitals depending on antibiotic usage patterns.

# ANTIBIOTIC SENSITIVITY – MISCELLANEOUS*

| ORGANISMS | Chloramphenicol | Colistin | Daptomycin | Fosfomycin | Linezolid | Metronidazole | Nitrofurantoin | Quinupristin + Dalfopristin | Rifampin | Vancomycin |
|---|---|---|---|---|---|---|---|---|---|---|
| **ANAEROBES** | | | | | | | | | | |
| *Actinomyces* | | | | | | | | + | | + |
| *Bacillus anthracis* | ++ | | | | | | | | ++ | ++ |
| *Bacteroides fragilis* | ++ | | | | | +++ | | + | | |
| *Clostridium difficile* | | | | | + | +++ | | | + | ++ |
| *Clostridium species* | ++ | | | | + | ++ | | + | | + |
| **GRAM-NEGATIVE AEROBES** | | | | | | | | | | |
| *Aeromonas hydrophila* | + | | | | | | | | | |
| *Bartonella henselae* | + | | | | | | | | ++ | |
| *Bordetella species* | + | | | | | | | | + | |
| *Burkholderia cepacia* | ++ | | | | | | | | + | |
| *Campylobacter jejuni* | ++ | | | | | | | | | |
| *Citrobacter species* | + | + | | + | | | ++ | | | |
| *Coxiella burnetti* | + | | | | | | | | ++ | |
| *Enterobacter species* | | + | | + | | | | | | |
| *Escherichia coli* | + | + | | ++ | | | ++ | | + | |
| *Francisella tularensis* | ++ | | | | | | | | | |

+++ = excellent activity (1st line recommendation). ++ = good activity (2nd line recommendation). + = moderate activity (acceptable in vitro data suggesting some isolates may be sensitive).

Blank = no or insufficient activity, or unknown.

†† 2nd line against *S. typhi.* † Penicillin sensitive; MIC ≤1.0 mcg/mL. §§ Penicillin resistant; MIC ≥2.0 mcg/mL.

*These are generalizations. There are major differences among countries, areas, and hospitals depending on antibiotic usage patterns.

**MISCELLANEOUS (CONTINUED)**

| ORGANISMS | Chloramphenicol | Colistin | Daptomycin | Fosfomycin | Linezolid | Metronidazole | Nitrofurantoin | Quinupristin + Dalfopristin | Rifampin | Vancomycin |
|---|---|---|---|---|---|---|---|---|---|---|
| **GRAM-NEGATIVE AEROBES** *(Continued)* | | | | | | | | | | |
| *Haemophilus influenzae* | ++ | | | | | | | + | + | |
| *Klebsiella species* | + | + | | + | | | | | | |
| *Legionella species* | | | | | | | | + | ++ | |
| *Moraxella catarrhalis* | ++ | | | | | | | + | + | |
| *Morganella morganii* | | | | + | | | + | | | |
| *Neisseria gonorrhoeae* | | | | + | | | | + | ++ | |
| *Neisseria meningitidis* | ++ | | | | | | | + | ++ | |
| *Pasturella multocida* | | | | | | | | | + | |
| *Proteus mirabilis* | | | | ++ | | | ++ | | + | |
| *Proteus vulgaris* | | | | + | | | + | | + | |
| *Providencia stuartii* | + | | | + | | | ++ | | | |
| *Pseudomonas aeruginosa* | | ++ | | | | | | | | |
| *Rickettsia species* | ++ | | | | | | | | + | |
| *Salmonella species* | ++ | + | | | | | | | | |
| *Serratia species* | + | | | + | | | + | | + | |
| *Shigella species* | ++ | + | | | | | | | | |
| *Stenotrophomonas maltophilia* | + | | | | | | | | | |

+++ = excellent activity (1st line recommendation). ++ = good activity (2nd line recommendation). + = moderate activity (acceptable in vitro data suggesting some isolates may be sensitive).
Blank = no or insufficient activity, or unknown.
†† 2nd line against *S. typhi.* † Penicillin sensitive; MIC ≤1.0 mcg/mL. §§ Penicillin resistant; MIC ≥2.0 mcg/mL.
*These are generalizations. There are major differences among countries, areas, and hospitals depending on antibiotic usage patterns.

| ORGANISMS | Chloramphenicol | Colistin | Daptomycin | Fosfomycin | Linezolid | Metronidazole | Nitrofurantoin | Quinupristin + Dalfopristin | Rifampin | Vancomycin |
|---|---|---|---|---|---|---|---|---|---|---|
| **GRAM-NEGATIVE AEROBES** *(Continued)* | | | | | | | | | | |
| *Vibrio vulnificus* | | | | | | | | | | |
| *Yersinia enterocolitica* | ++ | | | | | | | | | |
| *Yersinia pestis* | ++ | | | | | | | | | |
| **GRAM-POSITIVE AEROBES** | | | | | | | | | | |
| *Enterococcus faecalis* | + | | | ++ | ++ | | ++ | | + | ++ |
| *Enterococcus faecium* | ++ | | ++ | ++ | +++ | | ++ | ++ | + | +++ |
| *Enterococcus faecium (VRE)* | ++ | | ++ | + | +++ | | ++ | +++ | + | |
| *Listeria monocytogenes* | ++ | | | | + | | | + | ++ | + |
| *Nocardia* | | | | | + | | | | | |
| *Staphylococcus aureus (MSSA)* | + | | ++ | | ++ | | ++ | ++ | ++ | ++ |
| *Staphylococcus aureus (MRSA)* | + | | ++ | | ++ | | + | ++ | ++ | +++ |
| *Staphylococcus epidermidis* | + | | ++ | | ++ | | ++ | ++ | ++ | +++ |
| *Staphylococcus epidermidis (MRSE)* | + | | ++ | | ++ | | + | ++ | | +++ |
| *Streptococcus pneumoniae†* | + | | ++ | | ++ | | | ++ | ++ | ++ |
| *Streptococcus pneumoniae§§* | + | | ++ | | ++ | | | ++ | ++ | +++ |

+++ = excellent activity (1st line recommendation). ++ = good activity (2nd line recommendation). + = moderate activity (acceptable in vitro data suggesting some isolates may be sensitive).
Blank = no or insufficient activity, or unknown.
†† 2nd line against *S. typhi.* † Penicillin sensitive; MIC ≤1.0 mcg/mL. §§ Penicillin resistant; MIC ≥2.0 mcg/mL.
*These are generalizations. There are major differences among countries, areas, and hospitals depending on antibiotic usage patterns.

**MISCELLANEOUS (CONTINUED)**

| ORGANISMS | Chloramphenicol | Colistin | Daptomycin | Fosfomycin | Linezolid | Metronidazole | Nitrofurantoin | Quinupristin + Dalfopristin | Rifampin | Vancomycin |
|---|---|---|---|---|---|---|---|---|---|---|
| **GRAM-POSITIVE AEROBES** *(Continued)* | | | | | | | | | | |
| *Streptococcus (Group A,B,C,F,G)* | + | | + | | ++ | | | ++ | + | ++ |
| *Streptococcus species* | ++ | | + | | ++ | | | + | + | ++ |
| **MISCELLANEOUS** | | | | | | | | | | |
| *Chlamydia pneumoniae* | | | | | | | | + | + | |
| *Chlamydia trachomatis* | | | | | | | + | | + | |
| *Ehrlichia/Anaplasma species* | ++ | | | | | | | | ++ | |
| **MYCOBACTERIA** | | | | | | | | | | |
| *Mycobacterium avium (MAI) (non-HIV)* | | | | | + | | | | ++ | |
| *Mycoplasma pneumoniae* | | | | | | | | + | | |
| **SPIROCHETES** | | | | | | | | | | |
| *Leptospira interrogans* | | | | | | | | | | |
| *Treponema pallidum (syphilis)* | ++ | | | | | | | | | |

+++ = excellent activity (1st line recommendation). ++ = good activity (2nd line recommendation). + = moderate activity (acceptable in vitro data suggesting some isolates may be sensitive).

Blank = no or insufficient activity, or unknown.

†† 2nd line against *S. typhi*. † Penicillin sensitive; MIC ≤1.0 mcg/mL. §§ Penicillin resistant; MIC ≥2.0 mcg/mL.

*These are generalizations. There are major differences among countries, areas, and hospitals depending on antibiotic usage patterns.

# DRUG TREATMENTS FOR COMMON STDs*

| DISEASE | DRUG | RECOMMENDED DOSAGE |
|---|---|---|
| **Bacterial Vaginosis** | | |
| Nonpregnant Women | Metronidazole (Flagyl) *or*<br>Clindamycin cream (Cleocin) *or*<br>Metronidazole gel (MetroGel) | 500mg PO bid x 7d.<br>2%, 1 full applicator intravaginally qhs x 7d.<br>0.75%, 1 full applicator intravaginally qd x 5d. |
| *Alternative Regimens*<br>(Nonpregnant Women) | Clindamycin *or*<br>Clindamycin ovules | 300mg PO bid x 7d.<br>100g intravaginally qhs x 3d. |
| Pregnant Women | Metronidazole (CI in 1st trimester) *or* Clindamycin | 250mg PO tid x 7d.<br>500mg PO bid x 7d. |
| **Chancroid** | Azithromycin (Zithromax) *or*<br>Ceftriaxone (Rocephin) *or*<br>Ciprofloxacin (Cipro) *or*<br>Erythromycin base | 1g PO single dose.<br>250mg IM single dose.<br>500mg PO bid x 3d.<br>500mg PO tid x 7d. |
| **Chlamydial Infection** | Amoxicillin<br>Azithromycin (Zithromax) *or*<br>Doxycycline (Vibramycin) | 500mg PO tid x 7d.<br>1g PO single dose.<br>100mg PO bid x 7d. |
| *Alternative Regimens* | Erythromycin base or<br>Erythromycin Ethylsuccinate or<br>Ofloxacin (Floxin) *or*<br>Levofloxacin (Levaquin) | 500mg PO qid x 7d or 250mg PO qid x 14d.<br>800mg PO qid x 7d or 400mg PO qid x 14d.<br>300mg PO bid x 7d.<br>500mg PO qd x 7d. |
| **Epididymitis** | | |
| Gonococcal or Chlamydial Infection | Ceftriaxone (Rocephin) *plus*<br>Doxycycline (Vibramycin) | 250mg IM single dose.<br>100mg PO bid x 10d. |
| Enteric Organisms (>35 yrs or allergic to cephalosporins and/or tetracyclines) | Ofloxacin (Floxin) *or*<br>Levofloxacin (Levaquin) | 300mg PO bid x 10d.<br>500mg PO qd x 10d. |
| **Granuloma Inguinale** | Doxycycline (Vibramycin) | 100mg PO bid for at least 3 weeks. |
| *Alternative Regimens* | Ciprofloxacin (Cipro) *or*<br>Erythromycin base (during pregnancy) *or*<br>Azithromycin (Zithromax)<br>plus (if no improvement)<br>Aminoglycoside (ie, gentamicin)<br>Trimethoprim/Sulfamethoxazole (Bactrim, Septra) | 750mg PO bid for at least 3 weeks.<br>500mg PO qid for at least 3 weeks.<br>1g PO once weekly for at least 3 weeks.<br>1mg/kg IV q8h for at least 3 weeks.<br>1 tab (DS) PO bid for at least 3 weeks. |
| **Herpes Simplex Virus (HSV)** | | |
| First Episode | Acyclovir (Zovirax) *or*<br>Famciclovir (Famvir) *or*<br>Valacyclovir (Valtrex) | 400mg PO tid x 7-10d or 200mg PO 5x/d x 7-10d.<br>250mg PO tid x 7-10d.<br>1g PO bid x 7-10d. |
| Recurrent Episodes | Acyclovir *or*<br>Famciclovir *or*<br>Valacyclovir | 400mg PO tid x 5d or 200mg PO 5x/d x 5d or 800mg PO tid x 2d.<br>125mg PO bid x 5d.<br>500mg PO bid x 3-5d or 1g PO bid x 1d. |
| Daily Suppressive Therapy | Acyclovir *or*<br>Famciclovir *or*<br>Valacyclovir | 400mg PO bid.<br>250mg PO bid.<br>500mg PO qd (<10 episodes/yr) or 1g PO qd. |
| **Human Papillomavirus (HPV) Infection** | | |
| External Genital Area | Podofilox (Condylox) *or*<br>Imiquimod (Aldara)<br>Cryotherapy *or*<br>Podophyllum resin<br>Trichloroacetic acid *or*<br>Bichloroacetic acid *or*<br>Surgical removal | 0.5% sol or gel (patient-applied) bid x 3d, wait 4d, repeat as necessary x 4 cycles.<br>5% cre (patient-applied) tiw at bedtime up to 16 wks.<br>Physician-applied every 1-2 wks.<br>10-25% (physician-applied) qwk if necessary.<br>80-90% (physician-applied) qwk if necessary.<br>80-90% (physician-applied) qwk if necessary. |

*(Continued)*

| DISEASE | DRUG | RECOMMENDED DOSAGE |
|---|---|---|
| **HPV Infection**<br>External Genital Area (cont.) | | |
| *Alternative Regimens* | Intralesional interferon *or*<br>laser surgery | |
| Vaginal | Cryotherapy *or*<br>Trichloroacetic acid *or*<br>Bichloroacetic acid | With liquid nitrogen.<br>80-90% (physician-applied) qwk if necessary.<br>80-90% (physician-applied) qwk if necessary. |
| Urethral Meatus | Cryotherapy *or*<br>Podophyllum | With liquid nitrogen.<br>10-25% (physician-applied) qwk if necessary. |
| Anal Area | Cryotherapy<br>Trichloroacetic acid *or*<br>Bichloroacetic acid *or*<br>Surgical removal | With liquid nitrogen.<br>80-90% (physician-applied) qwk if necessary.<br>80-90% (physician-applied) qwk if necessary. |
| **Lymphogranuloma Venereum** | Doxycycline (Vibramycin) | 100mg PO bid x 21d. |
| *Alternative Regimen*<br>(including pregnancy) | Erythromycin base | 500mg PO qid x 21d. |
| **Nongonococcal Urethritis** | Azithromycin (Zithromax) *or*<br>Doxycycline (Vibramycin) | 1g PO single dose.<br>100mg PO bid x 7d. |
| *Alternative Regimens* | Erythromycin base or<br>Erythromycin ethylsuccinate *or*<br>Ofloxacin (Floxin) *or*<br>Levofloxacin (Levaquin) | 500mg PO qid x 7d.<br>800mg PO qid x 7d.<br>300mg PO bid x 7d.<br>500mg PO qd x 7d. |
| Recurrent and Persistent Urethritis | Metronidazole *or*<br>Tinidazole *plus*<br>Azithromycin | 2g PO single dose.<br>2g PO single dose.<br>1g PO single dose (if not used for initial episodes). |
| **Pediculosis Pubis** | Permethrin cream (NIX) | 1% cre: Apply to affected area & wash off after 10 min. |
| | Pyrethrins with piperonyl butoxide (compounded by pharmacist) | Apply to affected area and wash off after 10 min. |
| *Alternative Regimens* | Malathion<br>Ivermectin | 0.5% lotion: Apply for 8-12 hours and wash off.<br>250µg/kg repeat in 2 weeks. |
| **Pelvic Inflammatory Disease**<br>Parenteral Regimen A | Cefotetan (Cefotan) *or*<br>Cefoxitin (Mefoxin) *plus*<br>Doxycycline (Vibramycin) | 2g IV q12h.<br>2g IV q6h.<br>100mg IV/PO q12h. |
| Parenteral Regimen B | Clindamycin (Cleocin) *plus*<br>Gentamicin | 900mg IV q8h.<br>LD: 2mg/kg IM/IV. MD: 1.5mg/kg IM/IV q8h (may substitute single daily dosing). |
| *Alternative Regimen* | Ampicillin/Sulbactam *plus*<br>Doxycycline | 3g IV q6h.<br>100mg IV/PO q12h. |
| Oral Regimen A | Ceftriaxone (Rocephin) *or*<br>Cefoxitin *or*<br>3rd gen cephalosporin (eg ceftizoxime or cefotaxime)<br>*plus* Doxycycline w/ or w/o<br>Metronidazole | 250mg IM single dose.<br>2g IM single dose plus.<br>probenecid 1g PO single dose.<br><br>100mg PO bid x 14d.<br>500mg PO bid x 14d. |
| *Alternative Regimen B (also give presumptive therapy for Chlamydia infection: Doxycycline 100mg PO bid x 7d)* | Levofloxacin *or*<br>Ofloxacin *w/ or w/o*<br>Metronidazole | 500mg PO qd x 14d.<br>400mg PO bid x 14d.<br>500mg PO bid x 14d. |
| Parenteral Regimen | Ampicillin/Sulbactam *plus*<br>Doxycycline | 3g IV q6h.<br>100 mg PO or IV q12h. |
| **Proctitis, Proctocolitis & Enteritis** | Ceftriaxone (Rocephin) *plus*<br>Doxycycline (Vibramycin) | 125mg IM single dose.<br>100mg PO bid x 7d. |
| **Scabies** | Permethrin cream (Elimite)<br><br>Ivermectin | 5% cre: Apply to body from the neck down & wash off after 8-14h; re-evaluate in 1 week.<br>200mcg/kg PO; repeat in 2 weeks. |

*(Continued)*

| DISEASE | DRUG | RECOMMENDED DOSAGE |
|---|---|---|
| **Scabies** (cont.)<br>*Alternative Regimens* | Lindane (Kwell) | 1% lot or cre: Apply 1oz lotion or 30g cream to body from the neck down & wash off after 8h; re-evaluate in 1 wk (not recommended in pregnancy, lactating women or children <2 yrs). |
| **Syphilis**<br>Primary & Secondary Disease | Benzathine Penicillin G | **Adults:** 2.4 MU IM single dose.<br>**Pediatrics:** 50,000 U/kg IM single dose.<br>**Max:** 2.4 MU/dose. |
| Penicillin Allergy | Doxycycline (Vibramycin) *or*<br>Tetracycline | 100mg PO bid x 14d.<br>500mg PO qid x 14d. |
| Early Latent Disease | Benzathine Penicillin G | **Adults:** 2.4 MU IM single dose.<br>**Pediatrics:** 50,000 U/kg IM single dose.<br>**Max:** 2.4 MU/dose. |
| Late Latent, Unknown Duration | Benzathine Penicillin G | **Adults:** 2.4 MU IM qwk x 3 doses.<br>**Pediatrics:** 50,000 U/kg IM qwk x 3 doses.<br>**Max:** 2.4 MU/dose. |
| Tertiary Disease | Benzathine Penicillin G | 2.4 MU IM qwk x 3 doses. |
| Neurosyphilis | Aqueous Crystalline Penicillin G | 3-4 MU IV q4h or continuous infusion x 10-14d. |
| *Alternative Regimen* | Procaine Penicillin *plus*<br>Probenecid | 2.4 MU IM qd x 10-14d.<br>500mg PO qid x 10-14d. |
| **Trichomoniasis** | Metronidazole (Flagyl)<br>Timidazole | 2g PO single dose.<br>2g PO single dose. |
| *Alternative Regimen* | Metronidazole | 500mg PO bid x 7d. |
| Pregnant Women | Metronidazole (CI in 1st trimester) | 2g PO single dose. |
| **Uncomplicated Gonococcal Infections**<br>Cervix, Urethra, and Rectum<br>*Recommended Regimens* | Ceftriaxone or<br>Cefixime Plus<br>*If Chlamydial infection is not ruled out:*<br>Azithromycin (Zithromax) *or*<br>Doxycycline (Vibramycin) | 125 mg IM single dose.<br>400 mg PO single dose.<br><br>1g PO single dose.<br>100mg PO bid x 7d. |
| *Alternative Regimens* | Spectinomycin<br>*Cephalosporin regimens:*<br>Ceftizoxime *or*<br>Cefotaxime *or*<br>Cefoxitin plus<br>Probenecid | 2g IM single dose.<br><br>500mg IM single dose.<br>500mg IM single dose.<br>2g IM.<br>1g PO. |
| Pharynx<br>*Recommended Regimen* | Ceftriaxone *plus*<br>*If Chlamydial infection is not ruled out:*<br>Azithromycin (Zithromax) *or*<br>Doxycycline (Vibramycin) | 125mg IM single dose.<br><br>1g PO single dose.<br>100mg PO bid x 7d. |
| **Vulvovaginal Candidiasis**<br>Intravaginal Agents | Butoconazole *or*<br>Butoconazole *or*<br>Clotrimazole *or*<br>Clotrimazole *or*<br>Miconazole *or*<br>Miconazole *or*<br>Miconazole *or*<br>Miconazole<br>Nystatin *or*<br>Tioconazole *or*<br>Terconazole *or*<br>Terconazole *or*<br>Terconazole | 2% cre, 5g intravaginally x 3d or 5g single dose.<br>2% cre, 5g intravaginally single dose.<br>1% cre, 5g intravaginally x 7-14d.<br>100mg vaginal tab qd x 7 days or 2 tabs qd x 3d.<br>2% cre, 5g intravaginally qd x 7d.<br>200mg vaginal supp qd x 3d.<br>100mg vaginal supp qd x 7d.<br>1,200 mg vaginal supp, intravaginally single dose.<br>100,000-U vaginal tab qd x 14d.<br>6.5% oint, 5g intravaginally single dose.<br>0.4% cre, 5g intravaginally x 7d.<br>0.8% cre, 5g intravaginally x 3d.<br>80mg vaginal supp qd x 3d. |
| Oral Agent | Fluconazole | 150mg tab PO single dose. |

*Adapted from: Centers for Disease Control and Prevention. Sexually Transmitted Diseases Treatment Guidelines 2006. MMWR 2002; 51 (No. RR-6): 1-77.

# HIV/AIDS PHARMACOTHERAPY

| DRUG | BRAND | HOW SUPPLIED | USUAL DOSE | FOOD EFFECT |
|---|---|---|---|---|
| **NUCLEOSIDE REVERSE TRANSCRIPTASE INHIBITORS (NRTIs)** | | | | |
| Abacavir (ABC) | Ziagen | Sol: 20mg/mL [240mL]; Tab: 300mg | *Adults:* >16 yrs: or 600mg qd. *Pediatrics:* 3 months-16 yrs: 8mg/kg bid. Max: 300mg bid. | Take without regard to meals. |
| Didanosine (ddI) | Videx Powder for Oral Sol; Videx EC | Powder for Sol: 2g, 4g; Cap, Delayed Release: (Videx EC) 125mg, 200mg, 250mg, 400mg | *Adults:* ≥60kg: (Cap) 400mg qd; (Sol) 200mg bid or 400mg qd. <60kg: (Cap) 250mg qd. (Sol) 125mg bid. or 250mg qd. *Pediatrics:* 2 weeks-8 months: (Sol) 100mg/m² bid. >8 months: 120mg/m² bid. | Take on empty stomach at least 30 minutes before or 2 hrs after meals. Swallow caps whole. |
| Emtricitabine (FTC) | Emtriva | Cap: 200mg; Sol: 10mg/mL | *Adults:* ≥18 yrs: Cap: 200mg qd. Sol: 240mg (24mL) qd. *Pediatrics:* 0-3 mos: 3mg/kg qd. 3 mos-17 yrs: Cap: >33kg: 200mg qd. Sol: 6mg/kg qd. Max: 240mg (24mL). | Take without regard to meals. |
| Lamivudine | Epivir | Sol: 10mg/mL [240mL]; Tab: 150mg, 300mg | *Adults:* 150mg bid or 300mg qd. *Pediatrics:* 3 months-16 yrs: 4mg/kg bid. Max: 150mg bid. | Take without regard to meals. |
| Stavudine (d4T) | Zerit | Cap: 15mg, 20mg, 30mg, 40mg; Sol: 1mg/mL [200mL] | *Adults:* ≥60kg: 40mg q12h. <60kg: 30mg q12h. *Pediatrics:* ≥60kg: 40mg q12h. 30-59 kg: 30mg q12h. ≥14 days and <30kg: 1mg/kg q12h. Birth-13 days: 0.5mg/kg q12h. | Take without regard to meals |
| Tenofovir Disoproxil Fumarate (TDF) | Viread | Tab: 300mg | *Adults:* 300mg once daily. | Take without regard to meals. |
| Zalcitabine (ddC) | Hivid | Tab: 0.375mg, 0.75mg | *Adults:* 0.75mg q8h. *Pediatrics:* >13 yrs: 0.75mg q8h. | Take without regard to meals. |
| Zidovudine (AZT, ZDV) | Retrovir | Cap: 100mg; Inj: 10mg/mL; Sol: 10mg/mL; Tab: 300mg | *Adults:* (Cap, Tab) 600mg/day in divided doses. (Inj) 1mg/kg IV over 1 hr 5-6 times/day. *Pediatrics:* 6 weeks-12 yrs: 160mg/m² PO q8h. Max: 200mg PO q8h. | Take without regard to meals. |
| **NON NUCLEOSIDE REVERSE TRANSCRIPTATSE INHIBITORS (NNRTIs)** | | | | |
| Delavirdine (DLV) | Rescriptor | Tab: 100mg, 200mg | *Adults:* Usual: 400mg tid. *Pediatrics:* ≥16yrs: Usual: 400mg tid. | Take without regard to meals. |
| Efavirenz (EFV) | Sustiva | Cap: 50mg, 100mg, 200mg; Tab: 600mg | *Adults:* Initial: 600mg qd at bedtime. *Pediatrics:* ≥3 yrs: 10 to <15kg: 200mg qd. 15 to <20kg: 250mg qd. 20 to <25kg: 300mg qd. 25 to <32.5kg: 350mg qd. 32.5 to <40kg: 400mg qd. ≥40kg: 600mg qd at bedtime. | Take on an empty stomach. |

*(Continued)*

| DRUG | BRAND | HOW SUPPLIED | USUAL DOSE | FOOD EFFECT |
|---|---|---|---|---|
| **NON NUCLEOSIDE REVERSE TRANSCRIPTATSE INHIBITORS (NNRTIs)** *(Continued)* | | | | |
| Nevirapine (NVP) | Viramune | Sus: 50mg/5mL [240mL]; Tab: 200mg* *scored | *Adults:* 200mg qd for 14 days (lead-in period), then 200mg bid. *Pediatrics:* 2 months-8 yrs: 4mg/kg qd for 14 days, then 7mg/kg bid. Max: 400mg/day. 8 yrs: 4mg/kg qd for 14 days, then 4mg/kg bid. Max: 400mg/day. | Take without regard to meals. |
| **PROTEASE INHIBITORS (PIs)** | | | | |
| Amprenavir (APV) | Agenerase | Cap: 50mg; Sol: 15mg/mL [240mL] | *Adults:* (Cap) 1200mg bid. (Sol): 1400mg bid. *Pediatrics:* (Cap) 13-16 yrs: 1200mg bid. 13-16 yrs and <50kg or 4-12yrs: 20mg/kg bid or 15mg/kg tid. Max: 2400mg/day. (Sol) >16 yrs or 13-16 yrs and ≥50kg: 1400mg bid. 4-12 yrs or 13-16 yrs and <50kg: 22.5mg/kg bid or 17mg/kg tid. Max: 2800mg/day. | Take without regard to meals but avoid high fat foods. |
| Atazanavir (ATV) | Reyataz | Cap: 100mg, 150mg, 200mg, 300mg | *Adults:* Therapy-naive: 400mg qd. Therapy Experienced: (ATV 300mg + RTV 100mg)qd. | Take with food; avoid taking with antacids. |
| Darunavir (DRV) | Prezista | Tab: 300mg | *Adults:* (DRV 600mg + RTV 100mg) bid. | Take with food. |
| Fosamprenavir (fAPV) | Lexiva | Tab: 700mg | *Adults:* Therapy-naive: 1400mg bid OR 1400mg qd + RTV 200mg qd OR 700mg bid + RTV 100mg bid. PI-Experienced: 700mg bid + RTV 100mg bid. | Take without regard to meals. |
| Indinavir (IDV) | Crixivan | Cap: 100mg, 200mg, 333mg, 400mg | *Adults:* 800mg q8h OR (IDV 800mg + RTV 100 or 200mg) q12h. | Take 1 hr before or 2 hr after meals; may take with skim milk or low-fat meal. RTV-boosted, take with or without food. |
| Nelfinavir (NFV) | Viracept | Sus: (powder) 50mg/g [144g] Tab: 250mg, 625mg | *Adults:* 1250mg bid or 750mg tid. *Pediatrics:* 2-13 yrs: 45-55mg/kg bid; 25-35mg/kg tid. Max: 2500mg/day | Take with meal. |
| Ritonavir (RTV) | Norvir | Cap: 100mg Sol: 80mg/mL [240mL] | *Adults:* Initial: 300mg bid. Titrate: Increase every 2-3 days by 100mg bid. Maint: 600mg bid. *Pediatrics:* >1 month: Initial: 250mg/m² po bid. Titrate: Increase by 50mg/m² every 2-3 days. Maint: 350-400mg/m² po bid or highest tolerated dose. Max: 600mg bid. | Take with food, may improve tolerability. |

*(Continued)*

| DRUG | BRAND | HOW SUPPLIED | USUAL DOSE | FOOD EFFECT |
|---|---|---|---|---|
| **PROTEASE INHIBITORS (PIs)** *(Continued)* | | | | |
| Saquinavir (SQV) | Invirase* | Hard Gel Cap: 200mg<br>Tab: 500mg | *Adults/Pediatrics:* >16 yrs: 1000mg bid with RTV 100mg bid OR 1000mg bid with LPV/RTV 400/100mg bid (no additional RTV). | Take within 2 hrs after a meal when taken with RTV. |
| | Fortovase* | Soft Gelatin Cap: 200mg | *Adults/Pediatrics:* >16 yrs: 1200mg tid OR 1000mg bid with RTV 100mg bid. | Take with a meal or up to 2 hrs after a meal. |
| Tipranavir (TPV) | Aptivus | Cap: 250mg | *Adults:* (500mg + RTV 200mg) bid. | Take with food. |
| **FUSION INHIBITORS** | | | | |
| Enfuvirtide (T20) | Fuzeon | Inj: 90mg/1ml (60s) | *Adults:* 90mg SQ bid.<br>*Pediatrics:* 6-16 yrs: 2mg/kg SQ bid. Max: 90mg bid.<br>11-15.5kg: 27mg bid.<br>15.6-20.0kg: 36mg bid.<br>20.1-24.5kg: 45mg bid.<br>24.6-29.0kg: 54mg bid.<br>29.1-33.5kg: 63mg bid.<br>33.6-38.0kg: 72mg bid.<br>38.1- 42.5kg: 81mg bid.<br>≥42.6kg: 90mg bid. | |
| **COMBINATIONS** | | | | |
| EFV/FTC/TDF | Atripla | Tab: (Efavirenz-Emtricitabine-Tenofovir DF) 600mg-200mg-300mg | *Adults:* ≥18 yrs: 1 tab qd. | Take on empty stomach. |
| 3TC/ZDV | Combivir | Tab: (Lamivudine-Zidovudine) 150mg-300mg | *Adults:* 1 tab bid.<br>*Pediatrics:* ≥12 yrs: 1 tab bid. Do not give if CrCl ≤50mL/min. | Take without regard to meals. |
| ABC/3TC | Epzicom | Tab: (Abacavir Sulfate-Lamivudine) 600mg-300mg | *Adults:* ≥18 yrs: CrCl >50mL min: 1 tab qd. | Take without regard to meals. |
| LPV/RTV | Kaletra | Tab: (Lopinavir-Ritonavir) 200mg-50mg; Sol: (Lopinavir-Ritonavir) 80mg-20mg/mL [160mL] | *Adults:* Therapy-Naive: 400/100mg (2 tabs or 5mL) bid or 800/200mg qd (4 tabs or 10mL). Therapy Experienced: 400/100mg bid (2 tabs or 5mL). | Take without regard to meals.<br>Sol: Take with meal. |
| ABC/ZDV/3TC | Trizivir | Tab: (Abacavir-Lamivudine-Zidovudine) 300mg-150mg-300mg | *Adults:* >40kg and CrCl >50mL/min: 1 tab bid. | Take without regard to meals. |
| FTC/TDF | Truvada | Tab: (Emtricitabine-Tenofovir Disoproxil Fumarate) 200mg-300mg | *Adults:* ≥18 years: CrCl ≥50mL/min: 1 tab qd. CrCl 30-49mL/min: 1 tab q48h. | Take without regard to meals. |

*Invirase and Fortovase are not bioequivalent and cannot be used interchangeably.

Sources: FDA Approved Labeling; Guidelines for the Use of Antiretroviral Agents in HIV-1-Infected Adults and Adolescents - October 10, 2006.

# HIV/AIDS COMPLICATIONS THERAPY

| BRAND | USE | DOSE |
|---|---|---|
| **ANTIBIOTICS** | | |
| Atovaquone (Mepron) | PCP prevention and treatment | **Adults/Pediatrics:** ≥**13yrs:** Prevention: 1500mg qd. Treatment: 750mg bid x 21 days. Take with food. |
| Azithromycin (Zithromax) | MAC prevention and treatment | **Adults: Prevention:** 1200mg once weekly. Treatment: 600mg qd with ethambutol 15mg/kg/day. |
| Clarithromycin (Biaxin) | MAC prevention and treatment | **Adults:** 500mg bid. **Pediatrics:** ≥20 months: 7.5mg/kg bid, up to 500mg bid. |
| Pentamidine (NebuPent) | PCP prevention | **Adults/Pediatrics:** ≥4 months: Prevention: 1500mg qd. Treatment: 750mg bid x 21days. Take with food. |
| Rifabutin (Mycobutin) | MAC prevention | **Adults:** 300mg qd; give 150mg bid with food if intolerant to GI side effects. |
| Sulfamethoxazole/ Trimethoprim (Bactrim, Septra) | PCP prevention and treatment | **Adults/Pediatrics:** Treatment: 15-20mg/kg TMP and 75-100mg/kg SMX divided q6h x 14-21 days. **Adults:** Prevention: 800mg SMX-160mg TMP qd. **Pediatrics:** Prevention: 150mg/m$^2$ TMP and 750mg/m$^2$ SMX divided bid x 3 consecutive days per week. |
| Trimetrexate glucuronate (Neutrexin) | PCP treatment | **Adults:** 45mg/m$^2$ qd x 21 days w/leucovorin x 24 days. |
| **ANTIFUNGALS** | | |
| Amphotericin B (Ambisome) | Aspergillosis, candida, cryptococcal meningitis, visceral leishmaniasis | See complete monograph for full dosing information. |
| Amphotericin B lipid complex (Abelcet) | Invasive fungal infections | **Adults/Pediatrics:** 5mg/kg at 2.5mg/kg/hr. |
| Fluconazole (Diflucan) | Candidiasis, cryptococcal meningitis | See complete monograph for full dosing information. |
| Itraconazole (Sporanox) | Aspergillosis, blastomycosis, candidiasis, histoplasmosis, | See complete monograph for full dosing information. |
| Voriconazole (VFEND) | Aspergillosis, candidiasis, serious fungal infection | See complete monograph for full dosing information. |
| **ANTIVIRALS** | | |
| Cidofovir (Vistide) | CMV retinitis | **Adults: Induction:** 5mg/kg q week x 2 weeks. Maint: 5mg/kg q 2 weeks. |
| Famciclovir (Famvir) | HSV | **Adults:** 500mg bid x 7 days. |
| Foscarnet (Foscavir) | HSV, CMV retinitis | **Adults:** CMV: Induction: 90mg/kg q12h or 60mg/kg q8h. Maint: 90-120mg/kg/day. HSV: 40mg/kg q 8-12h. |
| Ganciclovir (Cytovene) | CMV retinitis | **Adults:** 1000mg tid or 500mg 6 times/day. Take with food. IV: Induction 5mg/kg q12h x 14-21 days. Maint: 5mg/kg x 7 days/week or 6mg/kg qd x 5 days/week. |
| Ganciclovir (Vitrasert) | CMV retinitis | **Adults/Pediatrics:** ≥**9yrs:** One implant q 5-8 months. |
| Interferon alfa-2a (Roferon-A) | Kaposi's sarcoma, HCV | **Adults:** KS: Induction: 36MIU SC/IM qd x 10-12 weeks. Maint: 36MIU SC/IM tiw. HCV: 3MIU SC/IM tiw x 18-24 months or 6MIU tiw x 3 months, then 3MIU tiw x 9 months. |
| Interferon alfa-2b (Intron A) | Kaposi's sarcoma, HCV | **Adults:** KS: 30MIU/m$^2$ SC/IM tiw. HCV: 3MIU IM/SC tiw x 18-24 months. |
| Valganciclovir (Valcyte) | CMV retinitis | **Adults:** Induction: 900mg bid x 21 days. Maint: 900mg qd. |
| **CHEMOTHERAPEUTICS** | | |
| Daunorubicin (DaunoXome) | Kaposi's sarcoma | **Adults:** 40mg/m2 over 60 minutes q 2 weeks. |
| Doxorubicin (Doxil) | Kaposi's sarcoma | **Adults:** 20mg/m2 over 30 minutes q 3 weeks. |
| Paclitaxel (Taxol) | Kaposi's sarcoma | **Adults:** 135mg/m2 over 3h q 3 weeks or 100mg/m2 q 2 weeks. |
| **MISCELLANEOUS** | | |
| Dronabinol (Marinol) | Appetite loss | **Adults:** 2.5mg qhs or bid before meal. Max: 20mg/day in divided doses. |
| Megestrol (Megace) | Appetite/weight loss | **Adults:** Initial: 800mg/d. Usual: 400-800mg/d. |
| Somatropin (Serostim) | Weight loss | **Adults:** >55kg: 6mg SQ qhs. 45-55kg: 5mg SQ qhs. 35-44kg: 4mg SQ qhs. <35kg: 0.1mg/kg SQ qhs. |

Abbreviations: CMV-Cytomegalovirus, HCV-Hepatitis C Virus, HSV-Herpes Simplex Virus, MAC-Mycobacterium avium, PCP-Pneumocystis carinii pneumonia

# Oral Antibiotics

| DRUG | BRAND | FORMULATIONS (mg or mg/5mL)* |
|---|---|---|
| **CEPHALOSPORINS** | | |
| Cefaclor | Ceclor | Cap: 250, 500<br>Sus: 125, 187, 250, 375 |
| | Ceclor CD | Tab, ER: 375, 500 |
| Cefadroxil | Duricef | Cap: 500<br>Sus: 125, 250, 500<br>Tab: 1g |
| Cefdinir | Omnicef | Cap: 300<br>Sus: 125, 250 |
| Cefditoren | Spectracef | Tab: 200 |
| Cefixime | Suprax | Sus: 100, 200 |
| Cefpodoxime | Vantin | Sus: 50, 100<br>Tab: 100, 200 |
| Cefprozil | Cefzil | Sus: 125, 250<br>Tab: 250, 500 |
| Ceftibuten | Cedax | Cap: 400<br>Sus: 90 |
| Cefuroxime | Ceftin | Sus: 125, 250<br>Tab: 125, 250, 500 |
| Cephalexin | Keflex | Cap: 250, 333, 500, 750 |
| **FLUOROQUINOLONES** | | |
| Ciprofloxacin** | Cipro | Sus: 250, 500<br>Tab: 100, 250, 500, 750 |
| | Cipro XR | Tab, ER: 500, 1000 |
| | ProQuin XR | Tab, ER: 500 |
| Levofloxacin** | Levaquin | Sol: 125<br>Tab: 250, 500, 750 |
| Moxifloxacin | Avelox | Tab: 400 |
| Norfloxacin | Noroxin | Tab: 400 |
| Ofloxacin | Floxin | Tab: 200, 300, 400 |
| **MACROLIDES** | | |
| Azithromycin** | Zithromax | Sus: 100, 200, 1g/pkt<br>Tab: 250, 500, 600 |
| | Zmax | Sus, ER: 2g |
| Clarithromycin | Biaxin | Sus: 125, 250<br>Tab: 250, 500 |
| | Biaxin XL | Tab, ER: 500, 1000 |
| Dirithromycin | | Tab: 250 |
| Erythromycin ethylsuccinate | E.E.S. | Granules: 200<br>Sus: 200, 400<br>Tab: 400 |
| | EryPed | Drops: 100mg/2.5mL<br>Granules: 200, 400<br>Sus: 200, 400 |
| | Eryc | Cap, DR: 250 |
| | Ery-Tab | Tab, DR: 250, 333, 500 |
| | PCE | Tab: 333, 500 |
| **PENICILLINS** | | |
| Amoxicillin | Amoxil | Cap: 250, 500<br>Chew, Tab: 200, 400<br>Drops: 50mg/mL<br>Sus: 125, 200, 250, 400<br>Tab: 500, 875 |
| Ampicillin | Principen | Cap: 250, 500<br>Sus: 125, 250 |
| Penicillin V | Veetids | Sus: 125, 250 Tab: 250, 500 |

*(Continued)*

| DRUG | BRAND | FORMULATIONS (mg or mg/5mL)* |
|---|---|---|
| **TETRACYCLINES** | | |
| Doxycycline | Doryx | Cap: 75, 100 |
| | Monodox | Cap: 50, 100 |
| | Vibramycin | Cap: 50, 100<br>Syr: 50<br>Sus: 25 |
| | Vibra-Tabs | Tab: 100 |
| Minocycline** | Minocin | Cap: 50, 100 |
| | Dynacin | Cap: 75, 100 |
| Tetracycline | Sumycin | Cap: 250, 500<br>Sus: 125<br>Tab: 250, 500 |
| **OTHER** | | |
| Loracarbef | Lorabid | Cap: 200, 400<br>Sus: 100, 200 |
| Clindamycin** | Cleocin | Cap: 75, 150, 300<br>Sus: 75 |
| Fosfomycin | Monurol | Powder: 3g/packet |
| Linezolid** | Zyvox | Sus: 100<br>Tab: 600 |
| Metronidazole | Flagyl | Cap: 375<br>Tab: 250, 500 |
| | Flagyl ER | Tab, ER: 750 |
| Nitrofurantoin | Macrobid | Cap: 100 |
| | Macrodantin | Cap: 25, 50, 100 |
| Telithromycin | Ketek | Tab: 300, 400 |
| Trimethoprim | Primsol | Sol: 50 |
| Vancomycin** | Vancocin | Cap: 125, 250 |
| **COMBINATIONS** | | |
| Erythromycin ethylsuccinate/ Sulfisoxazole | Pediazole | Sus: 200/600 |
| Amoxicillin/Clavulanate | Augmentin | Chew, Tab: 125/31.25, 250/62.5, 200/28.5, 400/57<br>Sus: 125/31.2, 200/28.5, 400/57, 250/62.5<br>Tab: 250/125, 500/125, 875/125 |
| | Augmentin ES | Sus: 600/42.9 |
| | Augmentin XR | Tab, ER: 1000/62.5 |
| Sulfamethoxazole/ Trimethoprim | Bactrim, Septra** | Tab: 400/80<br>Sus: (Septra) 200/40 |
| | Bactrim DS, Septra DS | Tab, DS: 800/160 |

* Unless otherwise indicated. **Injection formulation available.

# AMINOGLYCOSIDE DOSING AND MONITORING

*Therapy should be individualized for specific clinical situations in appropriate patients. The following are guidelines for initiating therapy.*

**1. Determine patient's dosing weight**

a. Non-Obese patients:

Use ideal body weight (IBW) unless total body weight (TBW) is less. Non-obese is defined as TBW < 30% over IBW

IBW (males) = 50 kg + (2.3 x height in inches > 60 inches)

IBW (females) = 45 kg + (2.3 x height in inches > 60 inches)

b. Obese patients:

Use adjusted body weight (ABW) in obese patients (TBW > 30% over IBW)

ABW (kg) = IBW + 0.4 (TBW – IBW)

**2. Estimate patient's creatinine clearance (CrCL)**

$$\text{CrCL (male) mL/min} + \frac{(140\text{–age}) \times \text{IBW (kg)}}{72 \times \text{SCr}} \text{ (x 0.85 for females)}$$

**3. Select appropriate loading and maintenance doses based on the drug and estimated CrCL.**

**All patients require a loading dose independent of renal function*

| Drug | Loading dose (mg/kg) | Maintenance Dose | Dosing interval based on estimated CrCL (mL/min) | | | |
|---|---|---|---|---|---|---|
| | | | Age: <60 | Age: >60* | | |
| | | | > 90 | 50-90 | 10-50 | < 10 |
| Amikacin | 7.5mg/kg | 7.5 mg/kg | q12h | q24h | q48 | q48-72h |
| Gentamicin | 2-3mg/kg | 1.5-2mg/kg | q8h | q12h | q24h | q24-48h |
| Tobramycin | 2-3mg/kg | 1.5-2mg/kg | q8h | q12h | q24h | q24-48h |

**Patients >65 years of age should not receive initial aminoglycoside maintenance dosing more often than every 12 hours.*

**4. Serum concentration monitoring**

- Serum peaks for efficacy and troughs for toxicity must be monitored
- Patients who are anticipated to receive aminoglycosides for 7 days should have levels monitored.
  - Obtain levels with the 4th dose after initiation of therapy or after dose adjustment. In patients with low CrCL (<50ml/min) obtain with 3rd dose.
  - Peak serum concentrations should be drawn 30 minutes after the completion of a 30-minute infusion.
  - Trough level should be obtained within 30 minutes of a dose. (Documentation of aminoglycoside administration time and times of the samples obtained are essential in interpreting the results.)
  - In patients with severe renal dysfunction, random levels, taken around the time the subsequent dose is due, should be obtained to determine appropriate dosing interval. In hemodialysis patients, check a level prior to the next scheduled dialysis.

**5. Desired measured serum concentrations**

| | Peak (mcg/mL) | Trough* (mcg/mL) |
|---|---|---|
| Amikacin | 20-30 | <5 |
| Gentamicin | 6-10 | 0.5-2.0 |
| Tobramycin | 6-10 | 0.5-2.0 |

**Periodic trough levels are suggested to ensure low levels in the elderly and those with renal dysfunction.*

Sources:

FDA Approved Product Labeling.

Gonzalez LS, Spencer JP. Aminoglycosides: A Practical Review. Am Fam Physician. 1998;58(8):1811-1820.

TBW= total body weight; IBW= ideal body weight;
ABW= adjusted body weight.

# Systemic Antibiotics

| BRAND NAME (Generic) | DOSAGE FORM/ STRENGTH | INDICATIONS | ADULT DOSE | PEDIATRIC DOSE |
|---|---|---|---|---|
| **AMINOGLYCOSIDES** | | | | |
| Amikin (amikacin sulfate) | Inj: 50mg/mL, 250mg/mL | Short-term treatment of serious infections caused by gram-negative bacteria such as septicemia, and respiratory tract, bone/joint, CNS (including meningitis), skin and soft tissue, and intra-abdominal infections; burns and postoperative infections; complicated and recurrent urinary tract infections (UTI); and staphylococcal disease. | (IM/IV)15mg/kg/day given q8h or q12h. Max: 15mg/kg/day. Heavier Weight Patients: Max: 1.5g/day. Recurrent Uncomplicated UTI: 250mg bid. Duration: 7-10 days. Stop therapy if no response after 3-5 days. Reduce dose if suspect renal dysfunction. Discontinue if azotemia increases or if a progressive decrease in urinary output occurs. | 15mg/kg/day given bid-tid. Newborns: LD: 10mg/kg. MD: 7.5mg/kg q12h. Duration: 7-10 days. |
| Amikin Pediatric (amikacin sulfate) | Inj: 50mg/mL | Short-term treatment of serious infections caused by gram-negative bacteria such as septicemia, and respiratory tract, bone/joint, CNS (including meningitis), skin and soft tissue, and intra-abdominal infections; burns and postoperative infections; complicated and recurrent urinary tract infections (UTI); and staphylococcal disease. | | 15mg/kg/day given bid-tid. Newborns: LD: 10mg/kg. MD: 7.5mg/kg q12h. Duration: 7-10 days. |
| Gentamicin sulfate | Inj: 10mg/mL, 40mg/mL | Treatment of bacterial neonatal sepsis, bacterial septicemia, and serious bacterial infections of the CNS (meningitis), urinary tract, respiratory tract, gastrointestinal tract (including peritonitis), skin, bone and soft tissue (including burns) caused by susceptible strains of microorganisms. | (IM/IV) Serious Infections: 3mg/kg/day given q8h. Life-Threatening Infections: 5mg/kg/day tid-qid; reduce to 3mg/kg/day as soon as clinically indicated. Treat for 7-10 days; may need longer course in difficult and complicated infections. Renal Impairment: Reduced dose given q8h or usual dose given at prolonged intervals based on either CrCl or serum creatinine. Dialysis: 1-1.7mg/kg, depending on severity of infection, at end of each dialysis period. Obese Patients: Calculate dose based on estimated lean body mass. | 6-7.5mg/kg/day (2-2.5mg/kg given q8h). Infants and Neonates: 7.5mg/kg/day (2.5mg/kg given q8h). Premature and Full-Term Neonates 1 week: 5mg/kg/day (2.5mg/kg given q12h). Treat for 7-10 days; may need longer course in difficult and complicated infections. Renal Impairment: Reduced dose given q8h or usual dose given at prolonged intervals based on either CrCl or serum creatinine. Dialysis: 2mg/kg at end of each dialysis period. Obese Patients: Calculate dose based on estimated lean body mass. |

| BRAND NAME (Generic) | DOSAGE FORM/ STRENGTH | INDICATIONS | ADULT DOSE | PEDIATRIC DOSE |
|---|---|---|---|---|
| Nebcin (tobramycin sulfate) | Inj: 10mg/mL, 40mg/mL, 1.2g | Treatment of serious lower respiratory tract, CNS (eg, meningitis), intra-abdominal, bone, skin and skin structure, and complicated/recurrent urinary tract infections; and septicemia. | (IM/IV) Serious Infections: 3mg/kg/day given q8h. Life-Threatening Infections: Up to 5mg/kg/day given tid-qid. Reduce to 3mg/kg/day as soon as clinically indicated. Max: 5mg/kg/day unless serum levels monitored. Treat for 7-10 days; may need longer course in difficult and complicated infections. Severe Cystic Fibrosis: Inital: 10mg/kg/day given qid. Measure levels to determine subsequent doses. Renal Impairment: LD: 1mg/kg followed by reduced doses given q8h or normal doses given at prolonged intervals based on either CrCl or serum creatinine. Do not use either method during dialysis. Obese Patients: Calculate dose based on estimated lean body weight plus 40% of the excess as the basic weight on which to figure mg/kg. ADD-Vantage vials are not for IM use. | >1 week: (IM/IV) 6-7.5mg/kg/day given tid-qid (eg, 2-2.5mg/kg q8h or 1.5-1.89mg/kg q6h). 1 week: Up to 2mg/kg q12h. Treat for 7-10 days; may need longer course in difficult and complicated infections. Severe Cystic Fibrosis: Initial: 10mg/kg/day given qid. Measure levels to determine subsequent doses. Renal Impairment: LD: 1mg/kg, followed by reduced doses given q8h or normal doses given at prolonged intervals based on either CrCl or serum creatinine. Do not use either method during dialysis. Obese Patients: Calculate dose based on estimated lean body weight plus 40% of the excess as the basic weight on which to figure mg/kg. ADD-Vantage vials are not for IM use. |
| Streptomycin sulfate | Inj: 1g | Treatment of moderate to severe infections such as mycobacterium tuberculosis (TB) and non-TB infections (eg, plague, tularemia, chancroid, granuloma inguinale, *H.influenzae* and *K.pneumoniae* infections, UTI, gram-negative bacillary bacteremia, endocardial infections). | IM only. TB: 15mg/kg/day (Max: 1g), or 25-30mg/kg twice weekly (Max: 1.5g), or 25-30mg/kg three times weekly (Max: 1.5g). Do not exceed a total dose of 120g over the course of theraphy unless no other therapeutic options exist. Elderly (>60 yrs): Reduce dose. Treat for minimum of 1 year if possible. Tularemia: 1-2g/day in divided doses for 7-14 days until afebrile for 5-7 days. Plague: 1g bid for minimum of 10 days. Streptococcal Endocarditis: With PCN, 1g bid for week 1, then 500mg bid for week 2. Elderly (>60 yrs): 500mg bid for 2 weeks. Enterococcal Endocarditis: With PCN, 1g bid for 2 weeks, then 500mg bid for 4 weeks. Renal Impairment: Reduce dose. Moderate/Severe Infections: 1-2g/day in divided doses q6-12h. Max: 2g/day. | IM only. TB: 20-40mg/kg/day (Max: 1g), or 25-30 mg/kg twice weekly (Max: 1.5g), or 25-30mg/kg three times weekly (Max: 1.5g). Do not exceed a total dose of 120g over the course of therapy unless no other therapeutic options exist. Treat for minimum of 1 year if possible. Moderate/Severe Infections: 20-40mg/kg/day (8-20mg/lb/day) in divideddoses q6-12h. |

(Continued)

| BRAND NAME (Generic) | DOSAGE FORM/ STRENGTH | INDICATIONS | ADULT DOSE | PEDIATRIC DOSE |
|---|---|---|---|---|
| **AMINOGLYCOSIDES** *(Continued)* | | | | |
| TOBI (tobramycin) | Sol: 60mg/mL (300mg/ampule) | Management of cystic fibrosis patients with *P.aeruginosa*. | Inhale via nebulizer 300mg q12h for 28 days, then stop for 28 days. Resume therapy for next 28-day on/28-day off cycle. | ≥6 yrs: Inhale via nebulizer 300mg q12h for 28 days, then stop for 28 days. Resume therapy for next 28-day on/28-day off cycle. |
| Trobicin (spectinomycin HCl) | Inj: 2g | Treatment of acute gonorrheal urethritis and proctitis in men and acute gonorrheal cervicitis in women due to *Neisseria gonorrhoeae*. Treatment of men and women recently exposed to gonorrhea. | Administer 2g (5mL) IM into upper outer quandrant of gluteal muscle. Use 4g (10mL) for treatment in geographic areas with prevalent antibiotic resistance. Divide dose between 2 gluteal sites. | |
| **CARBAPENEMS** | | | | |
| Invanz (ertapenem sodium) | Inj: 1g | Treatment of complicated intra-abdominal infections; skin and skin structure infections (SSSI), including diabetic foot infections without osteomyelitits; community acquired pneumonia (CAP); complicated urinary tract infections (UTI) including pyelonephritis; acute pelvic infections including postpartum endomyometritis, septic abortion, and post surgical gynecologic infections; prophylaxis of surgical site infection following elective colorectal surgery. | Treatment: 1g IM/IV qd. Duration: Intra-Abdominal Infections: 5-14 days. SSSI: 7-14 days. CAP/UTI: 10-14 days. Pelvic Infection: 3-10 days. May administer IV for up to 14 days and IM for up to 7 days. CrCl ≤30mL/min/1.73m²: 500mg IM/IV qd. Hemodialysis: Give 150mg IM/IV after dialysis only if 500mg dose was given within 6 hrs prior to dialysis. Prophylaxis: 1g IV as single dose given 1 hr prior to surgical incision. | ≥13 yrs: 1g IM/IV qd. 3 mo-12 yrs: 15mg/kg IM/IV bid (not to exceed 1g/day). Treatment Duration: Intra-Abdominal Infections: 5-14 days. SSSI: 7-14 days. CAP/UTI: 10-14 days. Pelvic Infections: 3-10 days. May administer IV for up to 14 days and IM for up to 7 days. CrCl ≤30mL/min/1.73 m²: 500mg IM/IV qd. |
| **CEPHALOSPORINS, FIRST GENERATION** | | | | |
| Duricef (cefadroxil monohydrate) | Cap: 500mg; Sus: 250mg/5mL [50mL, 100mL], 500mg/5mL [50mL, 75mL, 100mL]; Tab: 1g | Skin and skin structure infections (SSSI) and urinary tract infections (UTI), pharyngitis, and tonsillitis. | Uncomplicated Lower UTI: 1-2g/day given qd or bid. Other UTI: 1gm bid. SSSI: 1g qd or 500mg bid. Group A ß-hemolytic Strep Pharyngitis/ Tonsillitis: 1g qd or 500mg bid for 10 days. CrCl ≤50mL/min: Initial: 1g. Maint: CrCl 25-50mL/min: 500mg q12h; CrCl 10-25mL/min: 500mg q24h; CrCl 0-10mL/min: 500mg q36h | UTI/SSSI: 15mg/kg q12h. Pharyngitis/Tonsillitis/ Impetigo: 30mg/kg qd or 15mg/kg q12h. Treat ß-hemolytic strep infections for at least 10 days. |
| Keflex (cephalexin) | Cap: 250mg, 333mg 500mg, 750mg; Sus: 125mg/5mL, 250mg/5mL [100mL, 200mL] | Treatment of otitis media and skin and skin structure infections (SSSI); bone, genitourinary tract, and respiratory tract infections. | Usual: 25-50mg/kg/day in divided doses. Streptococcal Pharyngitis/SSSI/Uncomplicated Cystitis (>15 yrs): 500mg q12h. Treat cystitis for 7-14 days. Max: 4g/day. | Usual: 25-50mg/kg/day in divided doses. Streptococcal Pharyngitis (>1 yr)/SSSI: May divide dose and give q12h. Otitis Media: 75-100mg/kg/day in divided doses. Administer for ≥10 days in, ß-hemolytic streptococcal infections. |

| BRAND NAME (Generic) | DOSAGE FORM/ STRENGTH | INDICATIONS | ADULT DOSE | PEDIATRIC DOSE |
|---|---|---|---|---|
| **CEPHALOSPORINS, SECOND GENERATION** | | | | |
| Cefaclor | Cap: 250mg, 500mg; Sus: 125mg/5mL [75mL, 150mL], 187mg/5mL [50mL, 100mL], 250mg/5mL [75mL, 150mL], 375mg/5mL [50mL, 100mL] | Treatment of otitis media, pharyngitis, tonsillitis, lower respiratory tract, urinary tract, and skin and skin structure infections caused by susceptible strains of microorganisms. | Usual: 250mg q8h. Severe Infections/Pneumonia: 500mg q8h. Treat β-hemolytic strep for 10 days. | ≥1 mo: Usual: 20mg/kg/day given q8h. Otitis Media/Serious Infections: 40mg/kg/day. Max: 1g/day. May administer q12h for otitis media and pharyngitis. Treat β-hemolytic strep for 10 days. |
| Cefaclor ER | Tab, Extended-Release: 375mg, 500mg | Acute bacterial exacerbation of chronic bronchitis (ABECB), secondary bacterial infections of acute bronchitis, pharyngitis, tonsillitis, and uncomplicated skin and skin structure infections (SSSI) caused by susceptible strains of microorganisms. | ABECB/Acute Bronchitis: 500mg q12h for 7 days. Pharyngitis/Tonsillitis: 375mg q12h for 10 days. SSSI: 375mg q12h for 7-10 days. Take with meals. Do not crush, cut or chew tab. | ≥16 yrs: ABECB/Acute Bronchitis: 500mg q12h for 7 days. Pharyngitis/Tonsillitis: 375mg q12h for 10 days. SSSI: 375mg q12h for 7-10 days. Take with meals. Do not crush, cut or chew tab. |
| Cefoxitin (cefoxitin sodium) | Inj: 1g, 1g/50mL, 2g, 2g/50mL, 10g | Treatment of lower respiratory tract, urinary tract, intra-abdominal, gynecological, skin and skin structure, and bone and joint infections, and septicemia. For surgical prophylaxis. | Usual: 1-2g IV q6-8h. Uncomplicated Infections: 1g IV q6-8h. Moderate-Severe: 1g IV q4h or 2g IV q6-8h. Gas Gangrene/Other Infections Requiring Higher Dose: 2g IV q4h or 3g IV q6h. Renal Insufficiency: LD: 1-2g IV. Maint: CrCl 30-50mL/min: 1-2g IV q8-12h. CrCl 10-29mL/min: 1-2g IV q12-24h. CrCl 5-9mL/min: 0.5-1g IV q12-24h. CrCl <5mL/min: 0.5-1g IV q24-48h. Hemodialysis: LD: 1-2g IV after dialysis. Maint: See renal insufficiency doses above. Prophylaxis: Uncontaminated GI Surgery/Hysterectomy: 2g IV 0.5-1 hr prior to surgery, then 2g IV q6h after first dose up to 24 hrs. C-Section: 2g IV single dose after umbilical cord is clamped, or 2g IV after umbilical cordis clamped followed by 2g IV 4 and 8 hrs after initial dose. | ≥3 mo: 80-160mg/kg/day divided into 4-6 equal doses. Max: 12g/day. Prophylaxis: Uncontaminated GI Surgery/Hysterectomy: 30-40mg/kg IV 0.5-1 hr prior to surgery, then 30-40mg/kg IV q6h after first dose up to 24 hrs. |

*(Continued)*

| BRAND NAME (Generic) | DOSAGE FORM/ STRENGTH | INDICATIONS | ADULT DOSE | PEDIATRIC DOSE |
|---|---|---|---|---|
| **CEPHALOSPORINS, SECOND GENERATION** *(Continued)* | | | | |
| Ceftin (cefuroxime axetil) | Sus: 125mg/5mL [100mL], 250mg/5mL [50mL, 100mL]; Tab: 125mg, 250mg, 500mg | (Sus/Tab) Pharyngitis/tonsillitis, acute otitis media, and impetigo. (Tab) Uncomplicated skin and skin structure (SSSI), and urinary tract infection (UTI), gonorrhea, early lyme disease, acute bacterial maxillary sinusitis, acute bacterial exacerbations of chronic bronchitis (ABECB) and secondary bacterial infections of acute bronchitis. | (Tab) Pharyngitis/Tonsillitis/Sinusitis: 250mg bid for 10 days. ABECB/SSSI: 250-500mg bid for 10 days. Acute Bronchitis: 250-500mg bid for 5-10 days. UTI: 125-250mg bid for 7-10 days. Gonorrhea: 1000mg single dose. Lyme Disease: 500mg bid for 20 days. | ≥13 yrs: (Tab) Pharyngitis/Tonsillitis/Sinusitis: 250mg bid for 10 days. ABECB/SSSI: 250-500mg bid for 10 days. Acute Bronchitis: 250-500mg bid for 5-10 days. UTI: 125-250mg bid for 7-10 days Gonorrhea: 1000mg single dose. Lyme Disease: 500mg bid for 20 days. 3 mo-12 yrs: (Sus) Pharyngitis/Tonsillitis: 10mg/kg bid for 10 days. Max: 500mg/day. Otitis Media/Sinusitis/Impetigo: 15mg/kg bid for 10 days. Max: 1000mg/day. (Tab-if can swallow whole) Pharyngitis/Tonsillitis: 125mg bid for 10 days. Otitis Media/Sinusitis: 250mg bid for 10 days. |
| Cefzil (cefprozil) | Sus: 125mg/5mL, 250mg/5mL [50mL, 75mL, 100mL]; Tab: 250mg, 500mg | Mild to moderate pharyngitis/tonsillitis, otitis media, acute sinusitis, secondary bacterial infection of acute bronchitis, acute bacterial exacerbation of chronic bronchitis (ABECB), and uncomplicated skin and skin structure infections (SSSI). | ≥13 yrs: Pharyngitis/Tonsillitis: 500mg q24h for 10 days. Acute Sinusitis: 250-500mg q12h for 10 days. ABECB/Acute Bronchitis: 500mg q12h for 10 days. SSSI: 250-500mg q12h or 500mg q24h. CrCl <30mL/min: 50% of standard dose. | 2-12 yrs: Pharyngitis/Tonsillitis: 7.5mg/kg q12h for 10 days. SSSI: 20mg/kg q24h for 10 days. 6 mos-12 yrs: Otitis Media: 15mg/kg q12h for 10 days. Acute Sinusitis: 7.5-15mg/kg q12h for 10 days. Do not exceed adult dose. CrCl <30mL/min: 50% of standard dose. |
| Mefoxin (cefoxitin sodium) | Inj: 1g, 1g/50mL, 2g, 2g/50mL, 10g | Treatment of lower respiratory tract, urinary tract, intra-abdominal, gynecological, skin and skin structure, and bone and joint infections, and septicemia. For surgical prophylaxis. | Usual: 1-2g IV q6-8h. Uncomplicated Infections: 1g IV q6-8h. Moderate-Severe: 1g IV q4h or 2g IV q6-8h. Gas Gangrene/Other Infections Requiring Higher Dose: 2g IV q4h or 3g IV q6h. Renal Insufficiency: LD: 1-2g IV. Maint: CrCl 30-50mL/min: 1-2g IV q8-12h. CrCl 10-29mL/min: 1-2g IV q12-24h. CrCl 5-9mL/min: 0.5-1g IV q12-24h. CrCl <5mL/min: 0.5-1g IV q24-48h. Hemodialysis: LD: 1-2g IV after dialysis. Maint: See renal insufficiency doses above. Prophylaxis: Uncontaminated GI Surgery/Hysterectomy: 2g IV 0.5-1 hr prior to surgery, then 2g IV q6h after first dose up to 24 hrs. C-Section: 2g IV single dose after umbilical cord is clamped, or 2g IV after umbilical cord is clamped followed by 2g IV 4 and 8 hrs after initial dose. | ≥3 mos: 80-160mg/kg/day divided into 4-6 equal doses. Max: 12g/day. Prophylaxis: Uncontaminated GI Surgery/Hysterectomy: 30-40mg/kg IV 0.5-1 hr prior to surgery, then 30- 40mg/kg IV q6h after first dose up to 24 hrs. |

| BRAND NAME (Generic) | DOSAGE FORM/ STRENGTH | INDICATIONS | ADULT DOSE | PEDIATRIC DOSE |
|---|---|---|---|---|
| **CEPHALOSPORINS, THIRD GENERATION** | | | | |
| Cedax (ceftibuten) | Cap: 400mg; Sus: 90mg/5mL [30mL, 60mL, 90mL, 120mL] | Acute bacterial exacerbations of chronic bronchitis (ABECB), acute bacterial otitis media, pharyngitis and tonsillitis. | ABECB/Otitis Media/Pharyngitis/Tonsillitis: 400mg qd for 10 days. Max: 400mg/day. CrCl 30-49mL/min: 4.5mg/kg or 200mg qd. CrCl 5-29mL/min: 2.25mg/kg or 100mg qd. Take 2 hrs before or at least 1 hr after a meal. | ≥6 mo: Pharyngitis/Tonsillitis/Otitis Media: 9mg/kg qd for 10 days. Max: 400mg. ABECB/Otitis Media/Pharyngitis/Tonsillitis: ≥12 yrs: 400mg qd for 10 days Max: 400mg/day. CrCl 30-49mL/min: 4.5mg/kg or 200mg qd. CrCl 5-29mL/min: 2.25mg/kg or 100mg qd. Take 2 hrs before or at least 1 hr after a meal. |
| Cefizox (ceftizoxime) | Inj: 1g, 2g, 10g | Treatment of lower respiratory tract, skin and skin structure, intra-abdominal, bone and joint, and urinary tract infections (UTI), gonorrhea, pelvic inflammatory disease (PID), meningitis, and septicemia. | Uncomplicated UTI: 500mg q12h IM/IV. Other Sites: 1g q8-12h IM/IV. Severe/Refractory Infections: 1-2g IM/IV q8-12h. PID: 2g IV q8h. Life Threatening Infections: 3-4g IV q8h. Uncomplicated Gonorrhea: 1g IM as single dose. Renal Impairment: LD: 500mg-1g IM/IV. Less Severe Infection: Maint: CrCl 50-79mL/min: 500 mg q8h. CrCl 5-49mL/min: 250-500mg q12h. CrCl 0-4mL/min (Dialysis): 500mg q48h or 250mg q24h. Life Threatening Infection: Maint: CrCl 50-79mL/min: 0.75-1.5g q8h. CrCl 5-49mL/min: 0.5-1g q12h. CrCl 0-4mL/min (Dialysis): 0.5-1g q48h or 0.5g q24h. | ≥6 mos: 50mg/kg IM/IV q6-8h, up to 200mg/kg/day. Max: 6g/day for serious infections. |

*(Continued)*

| BRAND NAME (Generic) | DOSAGE FORM/ STRENGTH | INDICATIONS | ADULT DOSE | PEDIATRIC DOSE |
|---|---|---|---|---|
| **CEPHALOSPORINS, THIRD GENERATION** *(Continued)* | | | | |
| Ceptaz (ceftazidime) | Inj: 10g | Treatment of lower respiratory tract (eg, pneumonia), skin and skin structure (SSSI), bone and joint, gynecologic, CNS (eg, meningitis), intra-abdominal, and urinary tract infections (UTI), and septicemia. For use in sepsis. | Usual: 1g IM/IV q8-12h. Uncomplicated UTI: 250mg IM/IV q12h. Complicated UTI: 500mg IM/IV q8-12h. Bone and Joint Infection: 2g IV q 12h. Uncomplicated Pneumonia/SSSI: 500mg-1g IM/IV q8h. Gynecological/Intra-Abdominal/ Meningitis/Severe Life-Threatening Infection: 2g IV q8h. Lung Infection caused by Pseudomonas spp. in Cystic Fibrosis (normal renal function): 30-50mg/kg IV q8h. Max: 6g/day. CrCl 31-50mL/ min: 1g q12h. CrCl 16-30mL/min: 1g q24h. CrCl 6-15mL/min: 500mg q24h. CrCl <5mL/min: 500mg q48h. For severe infections (6g/day), increase renal impairment dose by 50% or increase dosing interval. Apply reduced dosage recommendations after initial 1g LD is given. Hemodialysis: Give 1g before then 1g after each hemodialysis. Intra-Peritoneal Dialysis/Continuous Peritoneal Dialysis: Ambulatory Peritoneal Dialysis: Give 1g followed by 500mg q24h. | ≥12 yrs: Usual: 1g IM/IV q8-12h. Uncomplicated UTI: 250mg IM/IV q12h. Complicated UTI: 500mg IM/IV q8-12h. Bone and Joint Infection: 2g IV q12h. Uncomplicated Pneumonia/SSSI: 500mg-1g IM/IV q8h. Gynecological/Intra-Abdominal/Meningitis/ Severe Life-Threatening Infection: 2g IV q8h. Lung Infection caused by Pseudomonas spp. in Cystic Fibrosis (normal renal function): 30-50mg/kg IV q8h Max: 6g/day. CrCl 31-50mL/min: 1g q12h. CrCl 16-30mL/min: 1g q24h. CrCl 6-15mL/min: 500mg q24h. CrCl <5mL/min: 500mg q48h. For severe infections (6g/day), increase renal impairment dose by 50% or increase dosing interval. Apply reduced dosage recommendations after initial 1g LD is given. Hemodialysis: Give 1g before then 1g after each hemodialysis. Intra-Peritoneal Dialysis/Continuous Ambulatory Peritoneal Dialysis: Give 1g followed by 500mg q24h. |
| Claforan (cefotaxime sodium) | Inj: 500mg, 1g, 2g, 10g | Treatment of lower respiratory tract, genitourinary, gynecologic, intra-abdominal, skin and skin structure, bone and joint, and CNS infections (eg, meningitis), bacteremia, and septicemia. For surgical prophylaxis. | Gonococcal Urethritis/Cervicitis (Males/Females): 500mg single dose IM. Rectal Gonorrhea: 0.5g (females) or 1g (males) single dose IM. Uncomplicated Infections: 1g IM/IV q12h. Moderate-Severe Infections: 1-2g IM/IV q8h. Septicemia: 2g IV q6-8h. Life-Threatening Infections: 2g IV q4h. Max: 12g/day. Surgical Prophylaxis: 1g IM/IV 30-90 min before surgery. Cesarean Section: 1g IV when umbilical cord is clamped, then 1g IV at 6 and 12 hrs after 1st dose. CrCl <20mL/min/1.73 $m^2$: Give 1/2 of usual dose. | ≥50kg: Use adult dose. Max: 12g/day. 1mo-12 yrs and ≤50kg: 50-180mg/kg/day IM/IV divided in 4-6 doses. 1-4 weeks: 50mg/kg IV q8h. 0-1 week: 50mg/kg IV q12h. CrCl <20mL/min/1.73 $m^2$: Give 1/2 of usual dose. |

| BRAND NAME (Generic) | DOSAGE FORM/ STRENGTH | INDICATIONS | ADULT DOSE | PEDIATRIC DOSE |
|---|---|---|---|---|
| Fortaz (ceftazidime) | Inj: 500mg, 1g, 1g/50mL, 2g, 2g/50mL, 6g | Treatment of lower respiratory tract (eg, pneumonia), skin and skin structure (SSSI), bone and joint, gynecologic, CNS (eg, meningitis), intra-abdominal, and urinary tract infections (UTI), and septicemia. For use in sepsis. | Usual: 1g IM/IV q8-12h. Uncomplicated UTI: 250mg IM/IV q12h. Complicated UTI: 500mg IM/IV q8-12h. Bone and Joint Infection: 2g IV q12h. Uncomplicated Pneumonia/SSSI: 500mg-1g IM/IV q8h. Gynecological/Intra-Abdominal/Meningitis/Severe Life-Threatening Infection: 2g IV q8h. Lung Infection Caused by Pseudomonas spp. in Cystic Fibrosis (Normal Renal Function): 30-50mg/kg IV q8h. Max: 6g/day. CrCl 31-50mL/min: 1g q12h. CrCl 16-30mL/min: 1g q24h. CrCl 6-15mL/min: 500mg q24h. CrCl <5mL/min: 500mg q48h. For severe infections (6g/day), increase renal impairment dose by 50% or increase dosing interval. Apply reduced dosage recommendations after initial 1g LD is given Hemodialysis: Give 1g before then 1g after each hemodialysis. Intra-Peritoneal Dialysis/Continuous Ambulatory Peritoneal Dialysis: Give 1g followed by 500mg q24h, or add to fluid at 250mg/2L. | 1 mo-12 yrs: 30-50mg/kg IV q8h. Max: 6g/day. Neonates (0-4 weeks): 30mg/kg IV q12h. Higher doses for cystic fibrosis or meningitis. CrCl 31-50 mL/min: 1g q12h. CrCl 16-30mL/min: 1g q24h. CrCl 6-15mL/min: 500mg q24h. CrCl <5mL/min: 500mg q48h. For severe infections (6g/day), increase renal impairment dose by 50% or increase dosing interval. Apply reduced dosage recommendations after initial 1g LD is given. Hemodialysis: Give 1g before then 1g after each hemodialysis. Intra-Peritoneal Dialysis/Continuous Ambulatory Peritoneal Dialysis: Give 1g followed by 500mg q24h, or add to fluid at 250mg/2L. |
| Omnicef (cefdinir) | Cap: 300mg; Sus: 125mg/5mL, 250mg/5mL [60mL, 100mL] | Community acquired pneumonia (CAP), acute exacerbations of chronic bronchitis (AECB), acute maxillary sinusitis, pharyngitis/tonsillitis, uncomplicated skin and structure infections (SSSI), and acute bacterial otitis media. | (Cap) SSSI/CAP: 300mg q12h for 10 days. AECB/Pharyngitis/Tonsillitis: 300mg q12h for 5-10 days or 600mg q24h for 10 days. Sinusitis: 300mg q12h or 600mg q24h for 10 days. CrCl <30mL/min: 300mg qd. | (Sus) 6 mo-12 yrs: OtitisMedia/Pharyngitis/Tonsillitis: 7mg/kg q12h for 5-10 days or 14mg/kg q24h for 10 days. Sinusitis: 7mg/kg q12h or 14mg/kg q24h for 10 days. SSSI: 7mg/kg q12h for 10 days. (Cap) ≥13 yrs: CAP/SSSI: 300mg q12h for 10 days. AECB/Pharyngitis/Tonsillitis: 300mg q12h for 5-10 days or 600mg q24h for 10 days. Sinusitis: 300mg q12h or 600mg q24h for 10 days. CrCl <30mL/min/1.73m$^2$: 7mg/kg qd. Max: 300mg qd. |
| Rocephin (ceftriaxone sodium) | Inj: 250mg, 500mg, 1g, 2g, 10g | Treatment of lower respiratory tract infections, skin and skin structure infections, bone and joint infections, intra-abdominal infections, acute otitis media, uncomplicated gonorrhea, pelvic inflammatory disease, UTI, septicemia, and meningitis. For surgical prophylaxis. | Usual: 1-2g/day IV/IM given qd-bid. Max: 4g/day. Gonorrhea: 250mg IM single dose. Surgical Prophylaxis: 1g IV 1/2-2 hrs before surgery. | Skin Infections: 50-75mg/kg/day IV/IM given qd-bid. Max: 2g/day. Otitis Media: 50mg/kg (up to 1g) IM single dose. Serious Infections: 50-75mg/kg/day IM/IV given q12h. Max: 2g/day. Meningitis: Initial: 100mg/kg (up to 4g), then 100mg/kg/day given qd-bid for 7-14 days. Max: 4g/day. |

*(Continued)*

| BRAND NAME (Generic) | DOSAGE FORM/ STRENGTH | INDICATIONS | ADULT DOSE | PEDIATRIC DOSE |
|---|---|---|---|---|
| **CEPHALOSPORINS, THIRD GENERATION** *(Continued)* | | | | |
| Spectracef (cefditoren pivoxil) | Tab: 200mg | Treatment of acute bacterial exacerbations of chronic bronchitis (ABECB), pharyngitis/tonsillitis, community acquired pneumonia (CAP), and uncomplicated skin and skin-structure infections (SSSI). | ABECB: 400mg bid for 10 days. Pharyngitis/Tonsillitis/SSSI: 200mg bid for 10 days. CAP: 400mg bid for 14 days. CrCl 30-49mL/min: 200mg bid. CrCl<30mL/min: 200mg qd. Take with meals. | ≥12 yrs: ABECB: 400mg bid for 10 days. Pharyngitis/Tonsillitis/SSSI: 200mg bid for 10 days. CAP: 400mg bid for 14 days. CrCl 30-49mL/min: 200mg bid. CrCl<30mL/min: 200mg qd. Take with meals. |
| Suprax (cefixime) | Sus: 100mg/5mL [50mL, 75mL, 100mL] | Otitis media, pharyngitis, tonsillitis, acute bronchitis, acute exacerbation of chronic bronchitis, uncomplicated UTIs, and cervical/urethral gonorrhea caused by susceptible strains. | Usual: 400mg qd. Gonorrhea: 400mg single dose. CrCl 21-60mL/min/Hemodialysis: Give 75% of standard dose. CrCl <20mL/min/CAPD: Give 50% of standard dose. | >12 yrs or >50kg: (Tab/Sus) Usual: 400mg qd. ≥6 mos: (Sus) 8mg/kg qd or 4mg/kg bid. Treat for at least 10 days with *S. pyogenes*. CrCl 21-60mL/min/Hemodialysis: Give 75% of standard dose. CrCl <20mL/min/CAPD: Give 50% of standard dose. |
| Tazicef (ceftazidime) | Inj: 1g, 2g, 6g | Treatment of lower respiratory tract (eg, pneumonia), skin and skin structure (SSSI), bone and joint, gynecologic, CNS (eg, meningitis), intra-abdominal, and urinary tract infections (UTI), and septicemia. For use in sepsis. | Usual: 1g IM/IV q8-12h. Uncomplicated UTI: 250mg IM/IV q12h. Complicated UTI: 500mg IM/IV q8-12h. Bone and Joint Infection: 2g IV q12h. Uncomplicated Pneumonia/SSSI: 500mg-1g IM/IV q8h. Gynecological/Intra-Abdominal/Meningitis/Severe Life-Threatening Infection: 2g IV q8h. Lung Infection caused by Pseudomonas in Cystic Fibrosis (normal renal function): 30-50mg/kg IV q8h. Max: 6g/day. Renal Impairment: CrCl 31-50mL/min: 1g q12h. CrCl 16-30mL/min: 1g q24h. CrCl 6-15mL/min: 500mg q24h. CrCl <5mL/min: 500mg q48h. For severe infections (6g/day), increase renal impairment dose by 50% or increase dosing interval. Apply reduced dosage recommendations after initial 1g LD is given. Hemodialysis: Give 1g before and 1g after each hemodialysis. Intra-Peritoneal Dialysis/Continuous Ambulatory Peritoneal Dialysis: Give 1g followed by 500mg q24h, or add to fluid at 250mg/2L. | Neonates (0-4 weeks): 30mg/kg IV q12h. 1 mo-12 yrs: 30-50mg/kg IV q8h. Max: 6g/day. Higher doses for patients with cystic fibrosis or when treating meningitis. Renal Impairment: CrCl 31-50mL/min: 1g q12h. CrCl 16-30mL/min: 1g q24h. CrCl 6-5mL/min: 500mg q24h. CrCl <5mL/min: 500mg q48h. For severe infections (6g/day), increase renal impairment dose by 50% or increase dosing interval. Apply reduced dosage recommendations after initial 1g LD is given. Hemodialysis: Give 1g before and 1g after each hemodialysis. Intra-Peritoneal Dialysis/Continuous Ambulatory Peritoneal Dialysis: Give 1g followed by 500mg q24h, or add fluid at 250mg/2L. |

| BRAND NAME (Generic) | DOSAGE FORM/ STRENGTH | INDICATIONS | ADULT DOSE | PEDIATRIC DOSE |
|---|---|---|---|---|
| Tazidime (ceftazidime) | Inj: 1g, 2g, 6g | Treatment of lower respiratory tract (eg, pneumonia), skin and skin structure (SSSI), bone and joint, gynecologic, CNS (eg, meningitis), intra-abdominal, and urinary tract infections (UTI), and septicemia. For use in sepsis. | Usual: 1g IM/IV q8-12h. Uncomplicated UTI: 250mg IM/IV q12h. Complicated UTI: 500mg IM/IV q8-12h. Bone and Joint Infection: 2g IV q12h. Uncomplicated Pneumonia/Skin and Skin Structure Infection: 500mg-1g IM/IV q8h. Gynecological/Intra-Abdominal/Meningitis/Severe Life-Threatening Infection: 2g IV q8h. Lung Infection caused by Pseudomonas spp. in Cystic Fibrosis (normal renal function): 30-50mg/kg IV q8h. Max: 6g/day. Renal impairment: CrCl 31-50mL/min: 1g q12h. CrCl 16-30mL/min: 1g q24h. CrCl 6-15mL/min: 500mg q24h. CrCl <5mL/min: 500mg q48h. For severe infections (6g/day), increase renal impairment dose by 50% or increase dosing interval. Apply reduced dosage recommendations after initial 1g LD is given. Hemodialysis: Give 1g before then 1g after each hemodialysis. Intra-Peritoneal Dialysis/Continuous Ambulatory Peritoneal Dialysis: Give 1g followed by 500mg q24h, or add to fluid at 250mg/2L. | Neonates (0-4 weeks): 30mg/kg IV q12h. 1 mo-12 yrs: 30-50mg/kg IV q8h. Max: 6g/day. Higher doses for cystic fibrosis and meningitis. Renal Impairment: CrCl 31-50mL/min: 1g q12h. CrCl 16-30mL/min: 1g q24h. CrCl 6-15mL/min: 500mg q24h. CrCl <5mL/min: 500mg q48h. For severe infections (6g/day), increase renal impairment dose by 50% or increase dosing interval. Apply reduced dosage recommendations after initial 1g LD is given. Hemodialysis: Give 1g before then 1g after each hemodialysis. Intra-Peritoneal Dialysis/Continuous Ambulatory Peritoneal Dialysis: Give 1g followed by 500mg q24h, or add to fluid at 250mg/2L. |
| Vantin (cefpodoxime proxetil) | Sus: 50mg/5mL [50mL, 100mL], 100mg/5mL [50mL, 75mL, 100mL]; Tab: 100mg, 200mg | Acute otitis media, pharyngitis/tonsillitis, community acquired pneumonia (CAP), acute bacterial exacerbation of chronic bronchitis (ABECB), acute uncomplicated urethral and cervical gonorrhea, acute uncomplicated ano-rectal infections in women, uncomplicated skin and skin structure infections (SSSI), acute maxillary sinusitis, uncomplicated urinary tract infections (UTI). | Take tabs with food. Pharyngitis/Tonsillitis: 100mg q12h for 5-10 days. CAP: 200mg q12h for 14 days. ABECB: 200mg q12h for 10 days. Uncomplicated Gonorrhea (Men and Women)/Rectal Gonococcal Infections (women): 200mg single dose. SSSI: 400mg q12h for 7-14 days. Sinusitis: 200mg q12h for 10 days. UTI: 100mg q12h for 7 days. CrCl<30mL/min: Increase interval to q24h. Hemodialysis: Dose 3 times weekly after dialysis. | ≥12 yrs: Take tabs with food. Pharyngitis/Tonsillitis: 100mg q12h for 5-10 days. CAP: 200mg q12h for 14 days. ABECB: 200mg q12h for 10 days. Uncomplicated Gonorrhea (men and women)/Rectal Gonococcal Infections (women): 200mg single dose. SSSI: 400mg q12h for 7-14 days. Sinusitis: 200mg q12h for 10 days. UTI: 100mg q12h for 7 days. 2 mos-11 yrs: Otitis Media: 5mg/kg q12h for 5 days. Max: 200mg/dose. Pharyngitis/Tonsillitis: 5mg/kg q12h for 5-10 days. Max: 100mg/dose. Sinusitis: 5mg/kg q12h for 10 days. Max: 200mg/dose. CrCl<30mL/min: Increase interval to q24h. Hemodialysis: Dose 3 times weekly after dialysis. |

*(Continued)*

| BRAND NAME (Generic) | DOSAGE FORM/ STRENGTH | INDICATIONS | ADULT DOSE | PEDIATRIC DOSE |
|---|---|---|---|---|
| **CEPHALOSPORIN, FOURTH GENERATION** | | | | |
| Maxipime (cefepime HCl) | Inj: 500mg, 1g, 2g | Treatment of uncomplicated/complicated urinary tract (UTI), uncomplicated skin and skin structure (SSSI), and complicated intra-abdominal infections, and pneumonia. Emperic therapy for febrile neutropenia. | Moderate-Severe Pneumonia: 1-2g IV q12h for 10 days. Febrile Neutropenia Emperic Therapy: 2g IV q8h for 7 days or until neutropenia resolved. Mild-Moderate UTI: 0.5-1g IM/IV q12h for 7-10 days. Severe UTI/Moderate-Severe SSSI: 2g IV q12h for 10 days. Complicated Intra-Abdominal Infections: 2g IV q12h for 7-10 days. CrCl<60mL/min: Initial: Same dose as normal renal function. Maint: Refer to prescribing information for dose-adjustment. | 2 months-16 yrs: ≤40kg: UTI/SSSI/Pneumonia: 50mg/kg IV q12h. Febrile Neutropenia: 50mg/kg IV q8h. Max: Do not exceed adult dose. CrCl ≤60mL/min: Initial: Same dose as normal renal function. Maint: Refer to prescribing information for dose adjustment. |
| **FLUOROQUINOLONES** | | | | |
| Avelox (moxifloxacin HCl) | Inj: 400mg/250mL; Tab: 400mg [ABC pack, 5 tabs] | Acute bacterial sinusitis, acute bacterial exacerbation of chronic bronchitis (ABECB), uncomplicated skin and skin structure infections (SSSI), complicated skin and skin structure infections (cSSSI), complicated intra-abdominal infections (cIAI), and community acquired pneumonia (CAP), including multi-drug resistant *S.pneumoniae.* | ≥18 yrs: Sinusitis: 400mg PO/IV q24h for 10 days. ABECB: 400mg PO/IV q24h for 5 days. SSSI: 400mg PO/IV q24h for 7 days. cSSSI: 400mg PO/IV q24h for 7-21 days. cIAI: 400mg IV q24h for 5-14 days. CAP: 400mg PO/IV q24h for 7-14 days. | |

| BRAND NAME (Generic) | DOSAGE FORM/ STRENGTH | INDICATIONS | ADULT DOSE | PEDIATRIC DOSE |
|---|---|---|---|---|
| Cipro (ciprofloxacin HCl) | Sus: 250mg/5mL, 500mg/5mL [100mL]; Tab: 250mg, 500mg, 750mg | Treatment of lower respiratory tract (LRTI), complicated intra-abdominal, skin and skin structure (SSSI), bone and joint, and urinary tract infections (UTI), acute exacerbations of chronic bronchitis, acute sinusitis, acute uncomplicated cystitis in females, chronic bacterial prostatitis, infectious diarrhea, typhoid fever, post-exposure inhalational anthrax, uncomplicated cervical and urethral gonorrhea, complicated UTI and pyelonephritis in pediatrics. | ≥18 yrs: Acute Sinusitis/Typhoid Fever: 500mg q12h for 10 days. LRTI/SSSI: Mild-Moderate: 500mg q12h for 7-14 days. Severe/Complicated: 750mg q12h for 7-14 days. Cystitis/Acute Uncompilcated UTI: 250mg q12h for 3 days. Mild-Moderate UTI: 250mg q12h for 7-14 days. Severe/ Complicated UTI: 500mg q12h for 7-14 days. Chronic Bacterial Prostatitis: 500mg q12h for 28 days. Intra-Abdominal: 500mg q12h (w/ metronidazole) for 7-14 days. Bone and Joint: Mild-Moderate: 500mg q12h for ≥4-6 weeks. Severe/Complicated: 750mg q12h for ≥4-6 weeks. Infectious Diarrhea: 500mg q12h for 5-7 days. Uncomplicated Urethral/Cervical Gonococcal: 250mg single dose. Inhalational Anthrax: 500mg q12h for 60 days. CrCl 30-50mL/min: 250-500mg q12h. CrCl 5-29mL/min: 250-500mg q18h. Hemodialysis/Peritoneal Dialysis: 250-500mg q24h (after dialysis). Administer at least 2 hrs before or 6 hrs after magnesium or aluminum containing antacids, sucralfate, Videx (didanosine) chewable/buffered tablets or pediatric powder, or other products containing calcium, iron or zinc. | <18 yrs: Inhalational Anthrax: 15mg/kg q12h for 60 days. Max: 500mg/dose. 1-17 yrs: Complicated UTI/Pyelonephritis: 10-20mg/kg q12h for 10-21 days. Max: 750mg/dose. |

*(Continued)*

| BRAND NAME (Generic) | DOSAGE FORM/ STRENGTH | INDICATIONS | ADULT DOSE | PEDIATRIC DOSE |
|---|---|---|---|---|
| **FLUOROQUINOLONES** *(Continued)* | | | | |
| Cipro IV (ciprofloxacin) | Inj: 10mg/mL, 200mg/100mL, 400mg/200mL | Treatment of skin and skin structure (SSSI), bone and joint, complicated intra-abdominal infections, lower respiratory (LRTI), and urinary tract infections (UTI), nosocomial pneumonia, acute sinusitis, chronic bacterial prostatitis, post-exposure inhalational anthrax, empirical therapy for febrile neutropenia, complicated UTI and pyelonephritis in pediatrics | ≥18 yrs: IV: UTI: Mild-Moderate: 200mg q12h for 7-14 days. Complicated/Severe: 400mg q12h for 7-14 days. LRTI/SSSI: Mild-Moderate: 400mg q12h for 7-14 days. Complicated/Severe: 400mg q8h for 7-14 days. Bone and Joint: Mild-Moderate: 400mg q12h for ≥4-6 weeks. Complicated/Severe: 400mg q8h for ≥4-6 weeks. Nosocomial Pneumonia: 400mg q8h for 10-14 days. Complicated Intra-Abdominal: 400mg q12h (w/metronidazole) for 7-14 days. Acute Sinusitis: 400mg q12h for 10 days. Chronic Bacterial Prostatitis: 400mg q12h for 28 days. Febrile Neutropenia: 400mg q8h (w/piperacillin 50mg/kg q4h) for 7-14 days. Max: 24g/day. Inhalational Anthrax: 400mg q12h for 60 days. Administer over 60 min. CrCl 5-29mL/min: 200-400mg q18-24h. | <18 yrs: Inhalational Anthrax: 10mg/kg q12h for 60 days. Max: 400mg/dose; 800mg/day. 1-17 yrs: Complicated UTI/Pyleonephritis: 6-10mg/kg q8h for 10-21 days. Max: 400mg/dose. |
| Cipro XR (ciprofloxacin) | Tab, Extended-Release: 500mg, 1000mg | Uncomplicated (acute cystitis) and complicated urinary tract infections (UTI), and acute uncomplicated pyelonephritis due to *E.coli.* | ≥18 yrs: Uncomplicated UTI: 500mg qd for 3 days. Complicated UTI: 1000mg qd for 7-14 days. CrCl <30mL/min: 500 mg qd. Acute Uncomplicated Pyelonephritis: 1000mg qd for 7-14 days. CrCl <30mL/min: 500mg qd. Take with fluids. Administer at least 2 hrs before or 6 hrs after magnesium or aluminum containing antacids, sucralfate, Videx (didanosine) chewable/buffered tablets or pediatric powder, metal cations (eg, iron), multivitamins with zinc. Avoid concomitant administration with dairy products alone, or with calcium-fortified products. Space concomitant calcium intake (>800mg) by at least 2 hrs. Do not split, crush, or chew. Swallow tab whole. Dialysis: Give after procedure is completed. | |

| BRAND NAME (Generic) | DOSAGE FORM/ STRENGTH | INDICATIONS | ADULT DOSE | PEDIATRIC DOSE |
|---|---|---|---|---|
| Factive (gemifloxacin mesylate) | Tab: 320mg | Treatment of community-acquired pneumonia (CAP), including multi-drug resistant *Streptococcus pneumoniae* (MDRSP), and acute bacterial exacerbation of chronic bronchitis (ABECB). | ≥18 yrs: ABECB: 320mg qd for 5 days. CAP: 320mg qd for 5 days *S.pneumoniae*, *H.influenzae*, *M. pneumoniae*, or *C.pneumoniae* or 7 days (MDRSP, *K.pneumoniae*, or *M.catarrhalis*. Renal Impairment: CrCl ≤40mL/min or Dialysis: 160mg qd. Take with fluids. | |
| Floxin (ofloxacin) | Tab: 200mg, 300mg, 400mg | Treatment of acute urinary tract (UTI) and uncomplicated skin and skin structure infection (SSSI), acute bacterial exacerbation of chronic bronchitis (ABECB), community acquired pneumonia (CAP), acute uncomplicated urethral and cervical gonorrhea, nongonococcal urethritis and cervicitis, mixed infections of the urethra and cervix, acute pelvic inflammatory disease (PID), uncomplicated cystitis, prostatitis. | ≥18 yrs: ABECB/CAP/SSSI: 400mg q12h for 10 days. Cervicitis/Urethritis: 300mg q12h for 7 days. Gonorrhea: 400mg single dose. PID: 400mg q12h for 10-14 days. Uncomplicated Cystitis: 200mg q12h for 3 days (*E.coli* or *K.pneumoniae*) or 7 days (other pathogens). Complicated UTI: 200mg q12h for 10 days. Prostatitis: (*E.coli*) 300mg q12h for 6 weeks. CrCl 20-50mL/min: Dose q24h. CrCl <20mL/min: After regular initial dose, give 50% of normal dose q24h. Severe Hepatic Impairment: Max: 400mg/day. | |
| Floxin IV (ofloxacin) | Inj: 4mg/mL, 40mg/mL | Treatment of acute bacterial exacerbation of chronic bronchitis, community-acquired pneumonia, uncomplicated skin and skin structure infections, acute uncomplicated urethral and cervical gonorrhea, nongonoccal urethritis and cervicitis, urethral and cervical infections, acute pelvic inflammatory disease (PID), uncomplicated cystitis, urinary tract infections (UTI), prostatitis. | Lower Respiratory Tract Infection/Skin Structure Infections: 400mg q12h for 10 days. Cervicitis/Urethritis: 300mg q12h for 7 days. Gonorrhea: 400mg single dose. PID: 400mg q12h for 10-14 days. Uncomplicated Cystitis: 200mg q12h for 3 days. Other Uncomplicated UTIs: 200mg q12h for 7 days. Complicated UTI: 200mg q12h for 10 days. Prostatitis: 300mg q12h for 6 weeks. Renal Impairment: CrCl 20-50mL/min: increase dosing interval to 24 hrs. CrCl<20mL/min: give normal initial dose then 50% of normal dose and increase dosing interval to 24 hrs. Severe Hepatic Impairment: Max: 400mg qdy. Switch to oral form when appropriate. Max: 10 days IV. | |

*(Continued)*

| BRAND NAME (Generic) | DOSAGE FORM/ STRENGTH | INDICATIONS | ADULT DOSE | PEDIATRIC DOSE |
|---|---|---|---|---|
| **FLUOROQUINOLONES** *(Continued)* | | | | |
| Levaquin (levofloxacin) | Inj: 5mg/mL, 25mg/mL; Sol: 25mg/mL; Tab: 250mg, 500mg, 750mg [Leva-pak, 5[s]] | Uncomplicated and complicated skin and skin structure (SSSI), and urinary tract infections (UTI), acute bacterial sinusitis, acute bacterial exacerbation of chronic bronchitis (ABECB), community acquired pneumonia (CAP), including multi-drug resistant *Streptococcus pneumoniae,* nosocomial pneumonia, chronic bacterial prostatitis (CBP), and acute pyelonephritis caused by susceptible strains of microorganisms. Prevention of inhalational anthrax following exposure to *Bacillus anthracis.* | ≥18 yrs: IV/PO: ABECB: 500mg qd for 7 days. CAP: 500mg qd for 7-14 days or 750mg qd for 5 days.Sinusitis: 500mg qd for 10-14 days or 750mg qd for 5 days. CBP: 500mg qd for 28 days. Uncomplicated SSSI: 500mg qd for 7-10 days. Complicated SSSI/Nosocomial Pneumonia: 750mg qd for 7-14 days. Inhalational Anthrax: 500mg qd for 60 days.Complicated SSSI/Nosocomial Pneumonia/CAP/Sinusitis: CrCl 20-49mL/min: 750mg, then 750mgq48h. CrCl 10-19mL/min/ Hemodialysis/CAPD: 750mg, then 500mg q48h. ABECB/CAP/Sinusitis/Uncomplicated SSSI/CBP/ Inhalational Anthrax:CrCl 20-49mL/min: 500mg, then 250mg q24h. CrCl 10-19mL/min/Hemodialysis/ CAPD: 500mg,then 250mg q48h. Complicated UTI/ Acute Pyelonephritis: 250mg qd for 10 days. CrCl 10-19mL/min: 250mg, then 250mg q48h. Uncomplicated UTI: 250mg qd for 3 days. Take oral solution 1 hr before or 2 hrs after eating. | |
| Maxaquin (lomefloxacin HCl) | Tab: 400mg | Treatment of acute bacterial exacerbation of chronic bronchitis (ABECB) and uncomplicated/complicated urinary tract infections (UTI). Preoperatively for the prevention of infections from transrectal prostate biopsy (TRPB) and in transurethral surgical procedures (TUSP). | ≥18 yrs: ABECB: 400mg qd for 10 days. Uncomplicated Cystitis: 400mg qd for 3 days *E.coli* or 10 days *K.pneumoniae*, *P.mirabilis*, or *S.saprophyticus.* Complicated UTI: 400mg qd for 14 days. Hemodialysis/CrCl>10 to <40mL/min: LD: 400mg. Maint: 200mg qd. Preoperative Prevention: TRPB: 400mg single dose 1-6 hrs before procedure. TUSP: 400mg single dose 2-6 hrs before procedure. | |
| Proquin XR (ciprofloxacin HCl) | Tab, Extended-Release: 500mg | Treatment of uncomplicated urinary tract infections (acute cystitis) caused by *E.coli* and *K.pneumoniae.* | 500mg qd with pm meal for 3 days. Administer at least 4 hrs before or 2 hrs after magnesium or aluminum containing antacids, sucralfate, Videx (didanosine) chewable/buffered tablets of pediatric powder, metal cations (eg, iron), multivitamins with zinc. Do not split, crush, or chew. Swallow tab whole. | |

| BRAND NAME (Generic) | DOSAGE FORM/ STRENGTH | INDICATIONS | ADULT DOSE | PEDIATRIC DOSE |
|---|---|---|---|---|
| **MACROLIDES** | | | | |
| Biaxin (clarithromycin) | Sus: 125mg/5mL, 250mg/5mL [50mL, 100mL]; Tab: 250mg, 500mg | Adults: Pharyngitis/tonsillitis, acute maxillary sinusitis, acute bacterial exacerbation of chronic bronchitis (ABECB), community acquired pneumonia (CAP), uncomplicated skin and skin structure infections (SSSI), disseminated mycobacterial infections, combination therapy for *H.pylori* infection with duodenal ulcers. MAC prophylaxis in advanced HIV. Pediatrics: Pharyngitis/tonsillitis, CAP, acute maxillary sinusitis, acute otitis media, uncomplicated SSSI, disseminated mycobacterial infections. MAC prophylaxis in advanced HIV. | Pharyngitis/Tonsillitis: 250mg q12h for 10 days. Sinusitis: 500mg q12h for 14 days. ABECB: 250-500mg q12h for 7-14 days. SSSI/CAP: 250mg q12h for 7-14 days. MAC Prophylaxis/Treatment: 500mg bid. *H.pylori*: Triple Therapy: 500mg + amoxicillin 1g + omeprazole 20mg, all q12h for 10 days; or 500mg + amoxicillin 1g + lansoprazole 30mg, all q12h for 10-14 days. Give additional omeprazole 20mg qd for 18 days with active ulcer. Dual Therapy: 500mg q8h + omeprazole 40mg qd for 14 days (give additional omeprazole 20mg qd for 14 days with active ulcer); or 500mg q8h or q12h + ranitidine bismuth citrate 400mg q12h for 14 days (give additional ranitidine bismuth citrate 400mg bid for 14 days with active ulcer). Avoid Biaxin and ranitidine bismuth citrate combination with CrCl<25mL/min. | ≥6 mo: Usual: 7.5mg/kg q12h for 10 days. MAC Prophylaxis/Treatment: ≥20 mo: 7.5mg/kg bid, up to 500mg bid. CrCl <30mL/min: Give 50% dose or double interval. |
| Biaxin XL (clarithromycin) | Tab, Extended-Release: 500mg [PAC 14 tabs] | Treatment of acute maxillary sinusitis, community acquired pneumonia (CAP), and acute bacterial exacerbation of chronic bronchitis (ABECB). | Sinusitis: 1000mg qd for 14 days. ABECB/CAP: 1000mg qd for 7 days. CrCl <30mL/min: Give 50% dose or double interval. Take with food. | |
| E.E.S. (erythromycin ethylsuccinate) | Sus: 200mg/5mL, 400mg/5mL (100mL, 480mL); Tab: 400mg | Mild to moderate upper and lower respiratory tract and skin and skin structure infections, listeriosis, pertussis, diphtheria, erythrasma, intestinal amebiasis, acute pelvic inflammatory disease (PID) *N.gonorrhea*, primary syphilis in PCN allergy, Legionnaires' disease, chlamydial infections (eg, newborn conjunctivitis urethral, endocervical, or rectal, etc), and nongonococcal urethritis. Prophylaxis of endocarditis or rheumatic fever. | Usual: 1600mg/day given q6h, q8h or q12h. Max: 4g/day. Treat strep infections for 10 days. Streptococcal Infection Prophylaxis with Rheumatic Heart Disease: 400mg bid. Urethritis *C.trachomatis* or *U. urealyticum*: 800mg tid for 7 days. Primary Syphilis: 48-64g in divided doses over 10-15 days. Intestinal Amebiasis: 400mg qid for 10-14 days. Pertussis: 40-50mg/kg/day in divided doses for 5-14 days. Legionnaires' Disease: 1.6-4g/day in divided doses. | Usual: 30-50mg/kg/day in divided doses q6h, q8h or q12h. Double dose for more severe infections. Treat strep infections for 10 days. Intestinal Amebiasis: 30-50mg/kg/day in divided doses for 10-14 days. Pertussis: 40-50mg/kg/day in divided doses for 5-14 days. |

(Continued)

| BRAND NAME (Generic) | DOSAGE FORM/ STRENGTH | INDICATIONS | ADULT DOSE | PEDIATRIC DOSE |
|---|---|---|---|---|
| **MACROLIDES** *(Continued)* | | | | |
| ERYC (erythromycin) | Cap, Delayed-Release: 250mg | Mild to moderate upper and lower respiratory tract and skin and soft tissue infections, pertussis, diphtheria, erythrasma, intestinal amebiasis, acute pelvic inflammatory disease (PID) (*N. gonorrhea), Listeria monocytogenes* infections, primary syphilis in PCN allergy, Legionnaires' disease, chlamydial infections (eg, newborn conjunctivitis, urethral, endocervical, or rectal, etc), and nongonococcal urethritis. Prophylaxis of endocarditis or rheumatic fever in PCN allergy. | Usual: 250mg q6h or 500mg q12h. Max: 4g/day. Treat strep infections for 10 days. Chlamydial Urogenital Infection During Pregnancy: 500mg qid for at least 7 days or 250mg qid for 14 days. Urethral/Endocervical/Rectal Chlamydial Infections: 500mg qid for 7 days. Primary Syphilis: 30-40g in divided doses for 10-15 days. Acute PID: 500mg (erythromycin lactobionate) IV q6h for 3 days, then 250mg PO q6h for 7 days. Streptococcal Infection Long-Term Prophylaxis of Rheumatic Fever: 250mg bid. Intestinal Amebiasis: 250mg qid for 10-14 days. Pertussis: 40-50mg/kg/day in divided doses for 5-14 days. Legionnaires' Disease: 1-4g/day in divided doses. Bacterial Endocarditis Prophylaxis: 1g 1 hr before procedure, then 500mg 6 hrs later. | Usual: 30-50mg/kg/day in divided doses without food. Max: 4g/day. Severe Infections: Double dose up to 4g/day. Treat strep infections for 10 days. Intestinal Amebiasis: 30-50mg/kg/day in divided doses for 10-14 days. Bacterial Endocarditis Prophylaxis: 20mg/kg 1 hr before procedure, then 10mg/kg 6 hrs later. |
| EryPed (erythromycin ethylsuccinate) | Sus: 100mg/2.5mL [50mL], 200mg/5mL, 400mg/5mL [5mL, 100mL, 200mL]; Tab, Chewable: 200mg | Treatment of mild to moderate upper and lower respiratory tract and skin and skin structure infections, listeriosis, pertussis, diphtheria, erythrasma, intestinal amebiasis, acute pelvic inflammatory disease (PID) *N.gonorrhea,* primary syphilis in PCN allergy, Legionnaires' disease, chlamydial infections (eg, newborn conjunctivitis, urethral, endocervical, or rectal, etc), and nongonococcal urethritis. Prophylaxis of endocarditis or rheumatic fever. | Usual: 1600mg/day given q6h, q8h or q12h. Max: 4g/day. Treat strep infections for 10 days. Streptococcal Infection Prophylaxis with Rheumatic Heart Disease: 400mg bid. Urethritis *C.trachomatis* or *U. urealyticum*: 800mg tid for 7 days. Primary Syphilis:48-64g in divided doses over 10-15 days. Intestinal Amebiasis: 400mg qid for 10-14 days. Pertussis:40-50mg/kg/day in divided doses for 5-14 days. Legionnaires' Disease: 1.6-4g/day in divided doses. | Usual: 30-50mg/kg/day in divided doses q6h, q8h or q12h. Double dose for more severe infections. Treat strep infections for 10 days. Intestinal Amebiasis: 30-50mg/kg/day in divided doses for 10-14 days. Pertussis: 40-50mg/kg/day in divided doses for 5-14 days. |

| BRAND NAME (Generic) | DOSAGE FORM/ STRENGTH | INDICATIONS | ADULT DOSE | PEDIATRIC DOSE |
|---|---|---|---|---|
| Ery-Tab (erythromycin) | Tab, Delayed-Release: 250mg, 333mg, 500mg | Mild to moderate upper and lower respiratory tract and skin and skin structure infections, listeriosis, pertussis, diphtheria, erythrasma, intestinal amebiasis, acute pelvic inflammatory disease (PID) *(N.gonorrhea)*, primary syphilis in PCN allergy, Legionnaires' disease, chlamydial infections (eg, newborn conjunctivitis urethral, endocervical, rectal, etc), and nongonococcal urethritis. Prophylaxis of rheumatic fever. | Usual: 250mg qid, 333mg q8h or 500mg q12h without food. Max: 4g/day. Do not take bid when dose is ≥1g/day. Treat strep infections for 10 days. Chlamydial Urogenital Infection During Pregnancy: 500mg qid or 666mg q8h for 7 days, or 500mg q 12h, 333mg q8h or 250mg qid for 14 days. Urethral/Endocervical/Rectal Chlamydial Infections and Nongonococcal Urethritis: 500mg qid or 666mg q8h for at least 7 days. Primary Syphilis: 30-40g in divided doses for 10-15 days. Acute PID: 500mg (erythromycin lactobionate) IV q6h for 3 days, then 500mg PO q12h or 333mg q8h for 7 days. Streptococcal Infection Long-Term Prophylaxis of Rheumatic Fever: 250mg bid. Intestinal Amebiasis: 500mg q12h, 333mg q8h or 250mg q6h for 10-14 days. Pertussis: 40-50mg/kg/day in divided doses for 5-14 days. Legionnaires' Disease: 1-4g/day in divided doses. | Usual: 30-50mg/kg/day in divided doses without food. Max: 4g/day. Severe Infections: Double dose up to 4g/day. Treat strep infections for 10 days. Chlamydial Conjunctivitis of Newborns and Chlamydial Pneumonia in Infancy: 12.5mg/kg qid for 2 weeks and 3 weeks, respectively. Intestinal Amebiasis: 30-50mg/kg/day in divided doses for 10-14 days. Long-Term Prophylaxis of Rheumatic Fever: 250mg bid. Intestinal Amebiasis: 30-50mg/kg/day in divided doses for 10-14 days. Pertussis: 40-50mg/kg/day in divided doses for 5-14 days. Legionnaire's Disease: 1-4g/day in divided doses. |
| Erythrocin (erythromycin stearate) | Tab: 250mg, 500mg | Mild to moderate upper and lower respiratory tract, and skin and skin structure infections, listeriosis, pertussis, diphtheria, erythrasma, intestinal amebiasis, acute pelvic inflammatory disease (PID) (gonorrhea), primary syphilis in PCN allergy, Legionnaires' disease, chlamydial infections (eg, newborn conjunctivitis urethral, endocervical, or rectal, etc), and nongonococcal urethritis. Prophylaxis of rheumatic fever. | Usual: 250mg q6h or 500mg q12h without food. Max: 4g/day. Treat strep infections for 10 days. Streptococcal Infection Prophylaxis of Rheumatic Fever: 250mg bid. Chlamydial Urogenital Infection During Pregnancy: 500mg qid for 7 days or 250mg qid for 14 days. Urethral/Endocervical/Rectal Chlamydial Infections and Nongonococcal Urethritis: 500mg qid for at least 7 days. Primary Syphilis: 30-40g in divided doses over 10-15 days. Acute PID: 500mg (erythromycin lactobionate) IV q6h for 3 days, then 500mg PO q12h for 7 days. Intestinal Amebiasis: 250mg qid for 10-14 days. Pertussis: 40-50mg/kg/day in divided doses for 5-14 days. Legionnaires' Disease: 1-4g/day in divided doses. | Usual: 30-50mg/kg/day in divided doses without food. Severe Infections: Double dose up to 4g/day. Treat strep infections for 10 days. Streptococcal Infection Prophylaxis of Rheumatic Fever: 250mg bid. Chlamydial Conjunctivitis of Newborns/Chlamydial Pneumonia in Infancy: 12.5mg/kg qid for 2 weeks and 3 weeks, respectively. Intestinal Amebiasis: 30-50mg/kg/day in divided doses for 10-14 days. Pertussis: 40-50mg/kg/day in divided doses for 5-14 days. |

*(Continued)*

| BRAND NAME (Generic) | DOSAGE FORM/ STRENGTH | INDICATIONS | ADULT DOSE | PEDIATRIC DOSE |
|---|---|---|---|---|
| **MACROLIDES** *(Continued)* | | | | |
| Erythromycin | Cap, Delayed-Release: 250mg | Mild to moderate upper and lower respiratory tract and skin and skin structure infections, listeriosis, pertussis, diphtheria, erythrasma, intestinal amebiasis, primary syphilis in PCN allergy, Legionnaires' disease, chlamydial infections (eg, newborn conjunctivitis urethral, endocervical, rectal, etc), and nongonococcal urethritis. Prophylaxis of endocarditis or rheumatic fever. | Usual: 250mg q6h or 500mg q12h without food. Max: 4g/day. Treat strep infections for 10 days. Streptococcal Infection Prophylaxis of Rheumatic Fever: 250mg bid. Chlamydial Urogenital Infection During Pregnancy: 500mg qid for 7 days or 250mg qid for 14 days. Urethral/Endocervical/Rectal Chlamydial Infections: 500mg qid for at least 7 days. Primary Syphilis: 30-40g in divided doses over 10-15 days. Intestinal Amebiasis: 250mg q6h for 10-14 days. Pertussis: 40-50mg/kg/day in divided doses for 5-14 days. Legionnaires' Disease: 1-4g/day in divided doses. Bacterial Endocarditis Prophylaxis: 1g 1 hr before procedure, then 500mg 6 hrs later. | Usual: 30-50mg/kg/day in divided doses without food. Severe Infections: Double dose up to 4g/day. Treat strep infections for 10 days. Streptococcal Infection Prophylaxis of Rheumatic Fever: 250mg bid. Intestinal Amebiasis: 30-50mg/kg/day in divided doses for 10-14 days. Pertussis: 40-50mg/kg/day in divided doses for 5-14 days. Bacterial Endocarditis Prophylaxis: 20mg/kg 1 hr before procedure, then 10mg/kg 6 hrs later. |
| Erythromycin Base | Tab: 250mg | Mild to moderate upper and lower respiratory tract and skin and skin structure infections, listeriosis, pertussis, diphtheria, erythrasma, intestinal amebiasis, acute pelvic inflammatory disease (PID) *(N.gonorrhea)*, primary syphilis in PCN allergy, Legionnaires' disease, chlamydial infections (eg, newborn conjunctivitis urethral, endocervical, rectal, etc), and nongonococcal urethritis. Prophylaxis of rheumatic fever. | Usual: 250mg q6h or 500mg q12h without food. Max: 4g/day. Treat strep infections for 10 days. Streptococcal Infection Prophylaxis of Rheumatic Fever: 250mg bid. Chlamydial Urogenital Infection During Pregnancy: 500mg qid for 7 days or 250mg qid for 14 days. Urethral/Endocervical/Rectal Chlamydial Infections and Nongonococcal Urethritis: 500mg qid for at least 7 days. Primary Syphilis: 30-40g in divided doses over 10-15 days. Acute PID: 500mg (erythromycin lactobionate) IV q6h for 3 days, then 500mg PO q12h for 7 days. Intestinal Amebiasis: 250mg qid for 10-14 days. Pertussis: 40-50mg/kg/day in divided doses for 5-14 days. Legionnaires' Disease: 1-4g/day in divided doses. | Usual: 30-50mg/kg/day in divided doses without food. Severe Infections: Double dose up to 4g/day. Treat strep infections for 10 days. Streptococcal Infection Prophylaxis of Rheumatic Fever: 250mg bid. Chlamydial Conjunctivitis of Newborns and Chlamydial Pneumonia in Infancy: 12.5mg/kg qid for 2 weeks and 3 weeks, respectively. Intestinal Amebiasis: 30-50mg/kg/day in divided doses for 10-14 days. Pertussis: 40-50mg/kg/day in divided doses for 5-14 days. |
| Pediazole (sulfisoxazole acetyl-erythromycin ethysuccinate) | Sus: (Erythromycin Ethylsuccinate-Sulfisoxazole Acetyl) 200 mg-600mg/5mL [100 mL, 150mL, 200mL] | Acute otitis media caused by *H.influenzae.* | | >2 mos: Dose based on 50mg/kg/day erythromycin or 150mg/kg/day sulfisoxazole given tid-qid for 10 days. Max: 6g/day sulfisoxazole. |

| BRAND NAME (Generic) | DOSAGE FORM/ STRENGTH | INDICATIONS | ADULT DOSE | PEDIATRIC DOSE |
|---|---|---|---|---|
| PCE (erythromycin) | Tab, Extended-Release: 333mg, 500mg | Mild to moderate upper and lower respiratory tract and skin and skin structure infections, listeriosis, pertussis, diphtheria, erythrasma, intestinal amebiasis, acute pelvic inflammatory disease (PID) *(N.gonorrhea)*, primary syphilis in PCN allergy, Legionnaires' disease, chlamydial infections (eg, newborn conjunctivitis urethral, endocervical, or rectal, etc), and nongonococcal urethritis. Prophylaxis of rheumatic fever. | Usual: 333mg q8h or 500mg q12h without food. Max: 4g/day. Do not take bid when dose is ≥1g/day. Treat strep infections for 10 days. Chlamydial Urogenital Infection During Pregnancy: 500mg qid or 666mg q8h for 7 days, or 500mg q12h, 333mg q8h or 250mg qid for 14 days. Urethral/Endocervical/ Rectal Chlamydial Infections and Nongonococcal Urethritis: 500mg qid or 666mg q8h for at least 7 days. Primary Syphilis: 30-40g in divided doses for 10-15 days. Acute PID: 500mg (erythromycin lactobionate) IV q6h for 3 days, then 500mg PO q12h or 333mg q8h for 7 days. Streptococcal Infection Long-Term Prophylaxis of Rheumatic Fever: 250mg bid. Intestinal Amebiasis: 500mg q12h, or 333mg q8h or 250mg q6h for 10-14 days. Pertussis: 40-50mg/kg/day in divided doses for 5-14 days. Legionnaires' Disease: 1-4g/day in divided doses. | Usual: 30-50mg/kg/day in divided doses without food. Max: 4g/day. Severe Infections: Double dose up to 4g/day. Treat strep infections for 10 days. Chlamydial Conjunctivitis of Newborns and Chlamydial Pneumonia in Infancy: 12.5mg/kg qid for 2 weeks and 3 weeks, respectively. Intestinal Amebiasis: 30-50mg/kg/day in divided doses for 10-14 days. Long-Term Prophylaxis of Rheumatic Fever: 250mg bid. Pertussis: 40-50mg/kg/day in divided doses for 5-14 days. Legionnaires' Disease: 1-4g/day in divided doses. |
| Zithromax (azithromycin) | Inj: 500mg; Sus: 100mg/5mL [15mL], 200mg/5mL [15mL, 22.5mL, 30mL], 1g/pkt [3[s] 10[s]]; Tab: 250mg [Z-Pak, 6 tabs], 500mg [Tri-Pak, 3 tabs], 600mg | (PO) Treatment of acute bacterial exacerbations of COPD, acute bacterial sinusitis (ABS), community acquired pneumonia (CAP), pharyngitis/tonsillitis, uncomplicated skin and skin structure, urethritis/ cervicitis, genital ulcer disease (men), acute otitis media, prevention of disseminated *Mycobacterium avium* complex (MAC) disease in advanced HIV infection. (IV) Treatment of CAP and pelvic inflammatory disease (PID). | (PO) COPD/CAP/Pharyngitis/Tonsillitis (second line therapy)/SSSI: ≥16 yrs: 500mg on day 1, then 250 mg qd on days 2-5. COPD: 500mg qd for 3 days. ABS: 500mg qd for 3 days. Genital Ulcer Disease and Non-Gonococcal Urethritis/Cervicitis: 1g single dose. Urethritis/Cervicitis due to gonorrhea: 2g single dose. MAC Prophylaxis: 1200mg once weekly. MAC Treatment: 600mg qd with ethambutol 15mg/ kg/day. (IV) ≥16 yrs: CAP: 500mg qd for at least 2 days, then 500mg PO to complete 7-10 day course. PID: 500mg qd for 1-2 days, then 250mg PO to complete 7-day course. | (Sus) Otitis Media: ≥6 mo: 30mg/kg single dose; 10mg/kg qd for 3 days; or 10mg/kg qd on day 1, then 5mg/kg qd on days 2-5. ABS: ≥6 mo: 10mg/kg qd for 3 days. CAP: ≥6 mo: 10mg/kg qd on day 1, then 5mg/kg qd on days 2-5. (Sus, Tab) Pharyngitis/Tonsillitis: ≥2 yrs: 12mg/kg qd for 5 days. 1g suspension is not for pediatric use. |
| Zmax (azithromycin) | Sus, Extended-Release: 2g | Treatment of mild to moderate acute bacterial sinusitis due to *Haemophilus influenzae, Moraxella catarrhalis*, or *Streptococcus pneumoniae*. Treatment of community-acquired pneumonia due to *Chlamydophila pneumoniae, Haemophilus influenzae*, Mycoplasma pneumoniae, or Streptococcus pneumoniae in patients appropriate for oral therapy. | 2g single dose. Take on an empty stomach (1 hr before or 2 hrs after a meal). | |

(Continued)

| BRAND NAME (Generic) | DOSAGE FORM/ STRENGTH | INDICATIONS | ADULT DOSE | PEDIATRIC DOSE |
|---|---|---|---|---|
| **PENICILLINS** | | | | |
| Amoxil (amoxicillin) | Cap: 250mg, 500mg; Sus: 50mg/mL [15mL, 30mL], 125mg/5mL [80mL, 100mL, 150mL], 200mg/5mL [5mL, 50mL, 75mL, 100mL], 250mg/5mL [80mL, 100mL, 150mL], 400mg/5mL [5mL, 50mL, 75mL, 100mL]; Tab: 500mg, 875mg; Tab, Chewable: 200mg, 400mg | Infections of the ear, nose, throat, genitourinary tract, skin and skin structure, lower respiratory tract due to susceptible (beta lactamase negative) organisms; gonorrhea (acute uncomplicated). *H.pylori* eradication to reduce the risk of duodenal ulcer recurrence. | Ear/Nose/Throat/SSSI/GU: (Mild/Moderate): 500mg q12h or 250mg q8h. (Severe): 875mg q12h or 500 mg q8h. LRTI: 875mg q12h or 500mg q8h. Gonorrhea: 3g as single dose. *H.pylori:* (Dual Therapy) 1g + 30mg lansoprazole, both tid for 14 days. (Triple Therapy) 1g + 30mg lansoprazole + 500mg clarithromycin, all q12h X 14 days. CrCl 10-30mL/min: 250-500mg q12h. <10mL/min: 250-500mg q24h. Hemodialysis: 250-500mg or 250mg q24h, additional dose during and at the end. | Neonates: ≤12 weeks: Max: 30mg/kg/day divided q12h. >3 mo: Ear/Nose/Throat/SSSI/GU: (Mild/Moderate): 25mg/kg/day given q12h or 20mg/kg/day given q8h. (Severe): 45mg/kg/day given q12h or 40 mg/kg/day given q8h. LRTI: 45mg/kg/day given q12h or 40mg/kg/day given q8h. Gonorrhea: (Prepubertal) 50mg/kg with 25mg/kg probenecid as single dose. (Not for <2 yrs). >40kg: Dose as adult. |
| Ampicillin (ampicillin sodium) | Inj: 125mg, 250mg, 500mg, 1g, 2g, 10g | Treatment of respiratory tract, urinary tract, and GI infections, bacterial meningitis, septicemia, endocarditis. | IM/IV: Respiratory Tract: ≥40kg: 250-500mg q8h. <40kg: 25-50mg/kg/day given q6-8h. GI/GU Caused by *N.gonorrhea* (Females): ≥40kg: 500mg q6h. <40kg: 50mg/kg/day given q6-8h. Urethritis Caused by *N.gonorrhea* (Males): 500mg q8-12h for 2 doses; may retreat if needed. Bacterial Meningitis: 150-200mg/kg/day given q3-4h. Septicemia: 150-200mg/kg/day IV for 3 days, continue with IM q3-4h. Treat for minimum of 10 days and 48-72 hrs after being asymptomatic. | Bacterial Meningitis: 150-200mg/kg/day given q3-4h. Septicemia: 150-200mg/kg/day IV given q3-4h for 3 days, continue with IM q3-4h. Treat for minimum of 10 days and 48-72 hrs after being asymptomatic. |

| BRAND NAME (Generic) | DOSAGE FORM/ STRENGTH | INDICATIONS | ADULT DOSE | PEDIATRIC DOSE |
|---|---|---|---|---|
| Augmentin (amoxicillin-clavulanate potassium) | (Amoxicillin-Clavulanate) Sus: 125-31.25mg/5mL [75mL, 100mL, 150mL] 200-28.5mg/5mL [50mL, 75mL, 100mL], 250-62.5mg/5mL [75mL, 100mL, 150mL], 400-57mg/5mL [50mL, 75mL, 100mL]; Tab: 250-125mg, 500-125mg, 875-125mg; Tab, Chewable: 200-28.5mg, 250-62.5mg, 400-57mg | Treatment of lower respiratory tract (LRTI), skin and skin structure (SSSI), and urinary tract infections (UTI), otitis media (OM), sinusitis. | (Dose based on amoxicillin) 500mg q12h or 250mg q8h. Severe Infections/RTI: 875mg q12h or 500mg q8h. May use 125mg/5mL or 250mg/5mL sus in place of 500mg tab and 200mg/5mL sus or 400mg/5mL sus in place of 875mg tab. CrCl <30mL/min: Do not give 875mg tab. CrCl 10-30mL/min: 250-500mg q12h. CrCl <10mL/min: 250-500mg q24h. Hemodialysis: 250-500mg q24h, give additional dose during and at the end of dialysis. | (Dose based on amoxicillin) ≥40kg: Use adult dose. ≥12 weeks: Sinusitis/OM/LRTI/Severe Infections: (Sus/Tab, Chewable) 45mg/kg/day given q12h or 40mg/kg/day given q8h. Less Severe Infections: 25mg/kg/day given q12h or 20mg/kg/day given q8h. <12 weeks:15mg/kg q12h (use 125mg/5mL sus). |
| Augmentin ES-600 (amoxicillin-clavulanate potassium) | Sus: (Amoxicillin-Clavulanate) 600mg-42.9mg/5mL [50mL, 75mL, 100mL, 150mL] | Treatment of recurrent or persistent acute otitis media. | | (Dose based on amoxicillin) 3 mo-12 yrs: <40kg: 45mg/kg q12h for 10 days. |
| Augmentin XR (amoxicillin-clavulanate potassium) | Tab, Extended-Release: (Amoxicillin-Clavulanate) 1000 mg-62.5mg | Treatment of community acquired pneumonia (CAP) or acute bacterial sinusitis due to confirmed or suspected ß-lactamase producing pathogens. | Sinusitis: 2 tabs q12h for 10 days. CAP: 2 tabs q12h for 7-10 days. Take at the start of a meal. | ≥16 yrs: Sinusitis: 2 tabs q12h for 10 days. CAP: 2 tabs q12h for 7-10 days. Take at the start of a meal. |
| Bicillin C-R (penicillin G benzathine-penicillin G procaine) | Inj: (Penicillin G Benzathine-Penicillin G Procaine) 300,000-300,000 U/mL | Treatment of moderately severe to severe upper-respiratory tract (URTI) and skin and soft-tissue infections (SSTI), scarlet fever and erysipelas due to streptococci. Treatment of moderately severe pneumonia and otitis media due to pneumococci. | Group A Strep: URTI/SSTI/Scarlet Fever/Erysipelas: 2.4 MU IM. Treat at a single session using multiple IM sites, or use an alternative schedule and give 1/2 of the total dose on Day 1 and 1/2 on Day 3. Pneumococcal Infections (Except Meningitis): 1.2 MU IM, repeat every 2-3 days until temperature is normal for 48 hrs. Administer IM into upper, outer quadrant of buttock. | Group A Strep: URTI/SSTI/Scarlet Fever/Erysipelas: >60 lbs: 2.4 MU IM. 30-60 lbs: 900,000 U-1.2 MU IM. <30 lbs: 600,000 U IM. Treat at a single session using multiple IM sites, or use an alternative schedule and give 1/2 of the total dose on Day 1 and 1/2 on Day 3. Pneumococcal Infections (Except Meningitis): 600,000 U IM, repeat every 2-3 days until temperature is normal for 48 hrs. Administer IM into upper, outer quadrant of buttock. Use the midlateral aspect of thigh in neonates, infants, and small children. |

*(Continued)*

| BRAND NAME (Generic) | DOSAGE FORM/ STRENGTH | INDICATIONS | ADULT DOSE | PEDIATRIC DOSE |
|---|---|---|---|---|
| **PENICILLINS** *(Continued)* | | | | |
| Bicillin C-R 900/300 (penicillin G benzathine-penicillin G procaine) | Inj: (Penicillin G Benzathine-Penicillin G Procaine) 900,000-300,000 U/2mL | Treatment of moderately severe to severe upper-respiratory tract (URTI) and skin and soft-tissue infections (SSTI), scarlet fever and erysipelas due to streptococci. Treatment of moderately severe pneumonia and otitis media due to pneumococci. | | Group A Strep: URTI/SSTI/Scarlet Fever/Erysipelas: 1.2 MU IM single dose. Pneumococcal Infections (Except Meningitis): 1.2 MU IM every 2-3 days until temperature is normal for 48 hrs. Administer IM into upper, outer quadrant of buttock. Use midlateral aspect of thigh in neonates, infants, and small children. |
| Bicillin L-A (penicillin G benzathine) | Inj: 600,000 U/mL | Treatment of mild to moderate upper respiratory tract infections (URTI) due to streptococci and venereal infections (eg, syphilis, yaws, bejel, pinta). Prophylaxis to prevent recurrence of rheumatic fever or chorea. | Group A Strep: URTI: 1.2 MU IM single dose. Primary/Secondary/Latent Syphilis: 2.4 MU IM single dose. Late Syphilis (Tertiary/Neurosyphilis): 2.4 MU IM every 7 days for 3 doses. Yaws/Bejel/Pinta: 1.2 MU IM single dose. Rheumatic Fever/Glomerulonephritis Prophylaxis: 1.2 MU IM once a mo or 600,000 U IM every 2 weeks. Administer IM into upper, outer quadrant of buttock. | Group A Strep: URTI: Older Pediatrics: 900,000 U IM single dose. <60lbs: 300,000-600,000 U IM single dose. Congenital Syphilis: 2-12 yrs: Adjust dose based on adult schedule. <2 yrs: 50,000 U/kg IM single dose. Rheumatic Fever/Glomerulonephritis Prophylaxis: 1.2 MU IM once a mo or 600,000 U every 2 weeks. Administer IM into upper, outer quadrant of buttock. Use the midlateral aspect of thigh in neonates, infants, and small children. |
| Dicloxacillin (dicloxacillin sodium) | Cap: 250mg, 500mg; Sus: 62.5mg/5mL [100mL] | Infections caused by penicillinase-producing staphylococci. | Mild-Moderate Infection: 125mg q6h. Severe Infection: 250mg q6h for at least 14 days. | <40kg: Mild-Moderate Infection: 12.5mg/kg/day in divided doses q6h. Severe Infection: 25mg/kg/day in divided doses q6h for at least 14 days. |
| Geocillin (carbenicillin disodium) | Tab: 382mg | Treatment of acute and chronic infections of the upper and lower urinary tract (UTI) and asymptomatic bacteriuria. | UTI: *E.coli, Proteus,* and *Enterobacter:* 1-2 tabs qid. *Pseudomonas, Enterococcus:* 2 tabs qid. Prostatitis: *E.coli, Proteus, Enterococcus* and *Enterobacter:* 2 tabs qid. CrCl 10-20mL/min: Adjust dose. | |
| Penicillin VK, Veetids (penicillin V potassium) | Sus: 125mg/5mL, 250mg/5mL [100mL, 200mL]; Tab: 250mg, 500mg | Mild to moderately severe bacterial infections including conditions of the respiratory tract, oropharynx, skin and soft tissue. Prevention of recurrence following rheumatic fever and/or chorea. | Usual: Streptococcal Infections (Scarlet Fever, Erysipelas, Upper Respiratory Tract): 125-250mg q6-8h for 10 days. Pneumococcal Infections (Otitis Media, Respiratory Tract): 250-500mg q6h until afebrile for at least 2 days. Staphylococcus Infections (Skin/Soft Tissue): 250-500mg q6-8h. Fusospirochetosis Infections (Oropharnyx): 250-500mg | ≥12 yrs: Usual: Streptococcal Infections (Scarlet fever, Erysipelas, Upper Respiratory Tract): 125-250mg q6-8h for 10 days. Pneumococcal Infections (Otitis media, Respiratory Tract): 250-500mg q6h until afebrile for at least 2 days. Staphylococcus Infections (Skin/Soft Tissue): 250-500mg q6-8h. Fusospirochetosis Infections (Oropharnyx): 250-500mg q6-8h. Rheumatic Fever/Chorea Prevention: 125-250mg bid. |

| BRAND NAME (Generic) | DOSAGE FORM/ STRENGTH | INDICATIONS | ADULT DOSE | PEDIATRIC DOSE |
|---|---|---|---|---|
| Pfizerpen (penicillin G potassium) | Inj: 1 MU, 5 MU, 20 MU | For therapy of severe infections when rapid and high blood levels of penicillin required. Management of streptococcal, pneumococcal, staphylococcal, clostridial, fusospirochetal, listeria, and gram negative bacillary, and pasteurella infections. For anthrax, actinomycosis, diphtheria, erysipeloid, meningitis, endocarditis, bacteremia, rat-bite fever, syphilis, and gonorrheal endocarditis and arthritis. With combined oral therapy, prophylaxis against endocarditis in patients with congenital heart disease, rheumatic, or other acquired valvular heart disease undergoing dental procedures or surgical procedures of upper respiratory tract. | Anthrax/Gonorrheal Endocarditis/Severe Infections (Streptococci, Pneumococci, Staphylococci): Minimum of 5 MU/day. Syphilis: Administer in hospital. Determine dose and duration based on age and weight. Meningococcic Meningitis: 1-2 MU IM q2h or 20-30 MU/day continuous IV. Actinomycosis: 1-6 MU/day for cervicofacial cases; 10-20 MU/day for thoracic and abdominal disease. Clostridial Infections: 20 MU/day (adjunct to antitoxin). Fusospirochetal Severe Infections: 5-10 MU/day for oropharynx, lower respiratory tract, and genital area infection. Rat-bite Fever: 12-15 MU/day for 3-4 weeks. Listeria Endocarditis: 15-20 MU/day for 4 weeks. Pasteurella Bacteremia/Meningitis: 4-6 MU/day for 2 weeks. Erysipeloid Endocarditis: 2-20 MU/day for 4-6 weeks. Gram Negative Bacillary Bacteremia: 20-80 MU/day. Diphtheria (carrier state): 0.3-0.4 MU/day in divided doses for 10-12 days. Endocarditis Prophylaxis: 1 MU IM mixed with 0.6 MU procaine penicillin G 0.5-1 hr before procedure. Renal/Cardiac/Vascular Dysfunction: Consider dose reduction. For streptococcal infection, treat for minimum 10 days. | Listeria Infections: Neonates: 0.5-1 MU/day. Congenital Syphilis: Administer in hospital. Determine dose and duration based on age and weight. Endocarditis Prophylaxis: 30,000 U/kg IM mixed with 0.6 MU procaine penicillin G 0.5-1 hr before procedure. For streptococcal infection, treat for minimum 10 days. |
| Permapen (penicillin G benzathine) | Inj: 600,000 U/mL | Treatment of microorganisms susceptible to low and very prolonged serum levels in upper respiratory tract infections (streptococci group A—without bacteremia), syphilis, yaws, bejel, and pinta. Prophylaxis for rheumatic fever and/or chorea. Follow-up prophylactic therapy for rheumatic heart disease and acute glomerulonephritis. | Streptococcal Infection: 1.2 MU IM single dose. Primary/Secondary/Latent Syphilis: 1 MU IM single dose. Late (Tertiary/Neurosyphilis) Syphilis: 3 MU IM every 7 days for total of 6-9 MU. Yaws/Bejel/Pinta: 1.2 MU IM single dose. Rheumatic Fever/Glomerulonephritis Prophylaxis: 1.2 MU IM once moly or 600,000 U IM twice moly. Use upper outer quadrant of buttock. Rotate injection site. | ≤12 yrs: Adjust dose according to age and weight and severity of infection. Streptococcal Infection: 900,000 U IM single dose in older children. Congenital Syphilis: <2 yrs: 50,000 U/kg IM single dose. 2-12 yrs: Adjust dose based on adult schedule. Use midlateral aspect of thigh in infants and small children. May divide dose between 2 buttocks in peds <2 yrs. Rotate injection site. |

*(Continued)*

| BRAND NAME (Generic) | DOSAGE FORM/ STRENGTH | INDICATIONS | ADULT DOSE | PEDIATRIC DOSE |
|---|---|---|---|---|
| **PENICILLINS** *(Continued)* | | | | |
| Piperacillin | Inj: 2g, 3g, 4g | Treatment of serious intra-abdominal, urinary tract, gynecologic, lower respiratory tract, skin and skin structure, bone and joint, and gonococcal infections, septicemia, and perioperative surgical prophylaxis. | Usual: 3-4g IM/IV q4-6h. Max: 24g/day; IM: 2g/site. Usual: 3-4g IM/IV q4-6h. Max: 24g/day; IM: 2g/site. Serious Infections: 200-300mg/kg/day IV divided q4-6h. Complicated UTI: 125-200mg/kg/day IV divided q6-8h. Uncomplicated UTI/Community Acquired Pneumonia: 100-125mg/kg/day IM/IV divided q6-12h. Uncomplicated Gonorrhea: 2g IM single dose with 1g PO probenecid 1/2 hr before injection. Surgical Prophylaxis: 2g IV 20-30 min just prior to anesthesia (See labeling for follow-up dosing). C-Section: 2g IV after cord is clamped, then 2g 4 hrs and 8 hrs after 1st dose. Renal Impairment: Uncomplicated/Complicated UTI: CrCl<20mL/min: 3g q12h. Complicated UTI: CrCl 20-40mL/min: 3g q8h. Serious Infection: CrCl 20-40mL/min: 4g q8h. CrCl<20mL/min: 4g q12h. Hemodialysis: Give 1g additional dose after each dialysis. Max: 2g q8h. Usual treatment is for 7-10 days; treat gynecologic infections for 3-10 days; treat *S.pyogenes* infections for at least 10 days. | ≥12 yrs: Usual: 3-4g IM/IV q4-6h. Max: 24g/day; IM: 2g/site. Serious Infections: 200-300mg/kg/day IV divided q4-6h. Complicated UTI: 125-200mg/kg/day IV divided q6-8h. Uncomplicated UTI/Community Acquired Pneumonia: 100-125mg/kg/day IM/IV divided q6-12h. Uncomplicated Gonorrhea: 2g IM single dose with 1g PO probenecid 1/2 hr before injection. Surgical Prophylaxis: 2g IV 20-30 minute just prior to anesthesia (See labeling for follow-up dosing). C-section: 2g IV after cord is clamped, then 2g 4 hrs and 8 hrs after 1st dose. Renal Impairment: Uncomplicated/Complicated UTI: CrCl <20mL/min: 3g q12h. Complicated UTI: CrCl 20-40mL/min: 3g q8h. Serious Infection: CrCl 20-40mL/min: 4g q8h. CrCl <20mL/min: 4g q12h. Hemodialysis: Give 1g additional dose after each dialysis. Max: 2g q8h. Usual treatment is for 7-10 days; treat gynecologic infections for 3-10 days; treat *S.pyogenes* nfections for at least 10 days. |
| Timentin (ticarcillin-clavulunate potassium) | Inj: (Ticarcillin-Clavulanate) 3g-100mg, 3g-100mg/100mL, 30g-1g | Treatment of lower respiratory tract, bone and joint, skin and skin structure, urinary tract (UTI), gynecologic, and intra-abdominal infections, and septicemia. | ≥60kg: UTI/Systemic Infection: 3g-100mg (3.1g vial) IV q4-6h. Gynecologic Infections: Moderate: 200mg/kg/day ticarcillin IV given q6h. Severe: 300mg/kg/day ticarcillin IV given q4h.<60kg: Usual: 200-300mg/kg/day ticarcillin IV given q4-6h. UTI: 3g-200mg (3.2g vial) q8h. Renal Impairment (based on ticarcillin): CrCl 60-30mL/min: 2g IV q4h. CrCl 30-10mL/min: 2g IV q8h. CrCl<10mL/min: 2g IV q12h (2g IV q24h with hepatic dysfunction). Peritoneal Dialysis: 3.1g IV q12h. Hemodialysis: 2g IV q12h, and 3.1g after each dialysis. Apply reduced dosage after initial 3.1g LD is given. | ≥3 mo: >60kg: Mild to Moderate: 3g-100mg (3.1g vial) IV q6h. Severe: 3g-100mg (3.1g vial) IV q4h. <60kg: Mild to Moderate: 50mg/kg ticarcillin IV q6h. Severe: 50mg/kg ticarcillin IV q4h. Renal Impairment (based on ticarcillin): CrCl 60-30mL/min: 2g IV q4h. CrCl 30-10mL/min: 2g IV q8h. CrCl<10mL/min: 2g IV q12h (2g IV q24h with hepatic dysfunction). Peritoneal Dialysis: 3.1g IV q12h. Hemodialysis: 2g IV q12h, and 3.1g after each dialysis. Apply reduced dosage after initial 3.1g LD is given. |

| BRAND NAME (Generic) | DOSAGE FORM/ STRENGTH | INDICATIONS | ADULT DOSE | PEDIATRIC DOSE |
|---|---|---|---|---|
| Unasyn (ampicillin sodium/ sulbactam sodium) | Inj: (Ampicillin-Sulbactam) 1g-0.5g, 2g-1g, 10g-5g | Treatment of skin and skin structure (SSSI), intra-abdominal, and gynecological infections caused by susceptible microorganisms. | 1.5-3g (ampicillin + sulbactam) IM/IV q6h. Max: 4g/day sulbactam. Renal Impairment: CrCl ≥30mL/min: 1.5-3g q6-8h. CrCl 15-29mL/min: 1.5-3g q12h. CrCl 5-14mL/min: 1.5-3g q24h. | ≥1 yr: SSSI: 1.5-3g (ampicillin + sulbactam) IM/IV q6h. Max: 4g/day sulbactam. |
| Veetids (penicillin V potassium) | Sus: 125mg/5mL, 250mg/5mL [100mL, 200mL]; Tab: 250mg, 500mg | Mild to moderately severe bacterial infections including conditions of the respiratory tract, oropharynx, skin and soft tissue. Prevention of recurrence following rheumatic fever and/or chorea. | Streptococcal Infections (Scarlet Fever, Erysipelas, Upper Respiratory Tract): 125-250mg q6-8h for 10 days. Pneumococcal Infections (Otitis media, Respiratory Tract): 250-500mg q6h until afebrile for at least 2 days. Staphylococcus Infections (Skin/Soft Tissue): 250-500mg q6-8h. Fusospirochetosis Infections (Oropharnyx): 250-500mg q6-8h. Rheumatic Fever/Chorea Prevention: 125-250mg bid. | Streptococcal Infections (Scarlet fever, Erysipelas, Upper Respiratory Tract): 125-250mg q6-8h for 10 days. Pneumococcal Infections (Otitis media, Respiratory Tract): 250-500mg q6h until afebrile for at least 2 days. Staphylococcus Infections (Skin/Soft Tissue): 250-500mg q6-8h. Fusospirochetosis Infections (Oropharnyx): 250-500mg q6-8h. Rheumatic Fever/Chorea Prevention: 125-250mg bid. |
| Zosyn (piperacillin sodium-tazobactam) | Inj: (Piperacillin-Tazobactam) 40mg-5mg/mL, 60mg-7.5mg/mL, 2g-0.25g, 3g-0.375g, 4g-0.5g, 4g-0.5g/100mL, 36g-4.5g | Treatment of appendicitis, peritonitis, uncomplicated/complicated skin and skin structure infections, postpartum endometritis, pelvic inflammatory disease, moderate severity of community acquired pneumonia, and moderate to severe nosocomial pneumonia. | Usual: 3.375g q6h for 7-10 days. Nosocomial Pneumonia: 4.5g q6h for 7-14 days plus aminoglycoside. CrCl 20-40mL/min: 2.25g q6h. CrCl <20mL/min: 2.25g q8h. Hemodialysis: Max: 2.25g q12h.Give 1 additional 0.75g dose after each dialysis period. | |
| **STREPTOMYCES DERIVATIVES** | | | | |
| Sumycin (tetracycline HCl) | Sus: 125mg/5mL; Tab: 250mg, 500mg | Treatment of respiratory tract, urinary tract, and skin and skin structure infections, lymphogranuloma, psittacosis, trachoma, uncomplicated urethral/endocervical/rectal infection caused by *Chlamydia,* nongonococcal urethritis, chancroid, plague, cholera, brucellosis, and others. When PCN is contraindicated, treatment of uncomplicated gonorrhea, syphilis, listeriosis, anthrax, *Clostridium* species, and others. Adjunct therapy for amebicides and severe acne. | Mild-Moderate: 250mg qid or 500mg bid. Severe: 500mg qid. Continue for 24-48 hrs after symptoms subside (minimum 10 days with Group A hemolytic streptococci). Severe Acne: Initial: 1g/day in divided streptococci). Severe Acne: Initial: 1g/day in divided doses. Maint: After improvement, 125-500mg/day. Brucellosis: 500mg qid for 3 weeks plus streptomycin 1g IM bid for 1 week, then qd for 1 week. Syphilis: 30-40g equally divided over 10-15 days. Gonorrhea: 500mg q6h for 7 days. Chlamydia: 500mg qid for at least 7 days. Renal Dysfunction: Reduce dose or extend dose interval. | Usual: 25-50mg/kg divided bid-qid. Continue for 24-48 hrs after symptoms subside (minimum 10 days with Group A ß-hemolytic streptococci). Severe Acne: Initial: 1g/day in divided doses. Maint: After improve ment, 125-500mg/day. Renal Dysfunction: Reduce dose or extend dose interval. |

(Continued)

| BRAND NAME (Generic) | DOSAGE FORM/ STRENGTH | INDICATIONS | ADULT DOSE | PEDIATRIC DOSE |
|---|---|---|---|---|
| **STREPTOMYCES DERIVATIVES** *(Continued)* | | | | |
| Lincocin (lincomycin HCl) | Inj: 300mg/mL | Treatment of serious infections due to streptococci, pneumococci, and staphylococci. Reserve for PCN allergy or if PCN is inappropriate. | IM: Serious Infection: 600mg q24h. More Severe Infection: 600mg q12h or more often. IV: Dose depends on severity. Serious Infection: 600mg-1g q8-12h. More Severe Infection: Increase dose. Infuse over ≥1 hr. Life-Threatening Situation: Up to 8g/day has been given. Max: 8g/day. Severe Renal Dysfunction: 25-30% of normal dose. | >1 mo: IM: Serious Infection: 10mg/kg q24h. More Severe Infection: 10mg/kg q12h or more often. IV: 10-20mg/kg/day, depending on severity infused in divided doses as described for adults. Severe Renal Dysfunction: 25-30% of normal dose. |
| **TETRACYCLINE DERIVATIVES** | | | | |
| Declomycin (demeclocycline HCl) | Tab: 150mg, 300mg | Treatment of infections due to *rickettsiae, Mycoplasma pneumoniae, B.recurrentis,* agents of psittacosis, ornithosis, lymphomagranuloma venereum or granuloma inguinale. Treatment of gram-negative infections (eg, respiratory, urinary tract ), gram-positive infections (eg, respiratory tract, skin and soft tissue), trachoma, inclusion conjunctivitis. When PCN is contraindicated, treatment of gonorrhea, syphilis, listeriosis, anthrax, *Clostridium* species, and others. Adjunct therapy for amebicides. | Usual: 150mg qid or 300mg bid. Gonorrhea: Initial: 600mg, then 300mg q12h for 4 days. Gonorrhea: 600mg followed by 300mg q12h for 4 days to a total of 3g. Renal/Hepatic Impairment: Reduce dose and/or extend dose intervals. Continue therapy for at least 24-48 hrs after symptoms subside. Treat strep infections for at least 10 days. Take at least 1 hr before or 2 hrs after meals with plenty of fluids. | >8 yrs: Usual: 3-6mg/lb/day given bid-qid. Gonorrhea: 600mg followed by 300mg q12h for 4 days to a total of 3g. Renal/Hepatic Impairment: Reduce dose and/or extend dose intervals. Continue therapy for at least 24-48 hrs after symptoms subside. Treat strep infections for at least 10 days. Take at least 1 hr before or 2 hrs after meals with plenty of fluids. |
| Doryx (doxycycline hyclate) | Cap: 75mg, 100mg | Treatment of susceptible infections including respiratory, urinary, skin and skin structure, lymphogranuloma, psittacosis, trachoma, uncomplicated urethral/endocervical/rectal, nongonococcal urethritis, rickettsiae, chancroid, plague, cholera, brucellosis, anthrax. When penicillin is contraindicated, treatment of syphilis, listeriosis, *Clostridium* species, and others. Adjunct therapy for amebiasis and severe acne. | Usual: 100mg q12h on 1st day, followed by 100mg qd. Severe Infections/Chronic UTI: 100mg q12h. Uncomplicated Gonococcal Infections (Men, except anorectal infections): 100mg bid for 7 days, or 300mg followed in 1 hr by another 300mg dose. Acute Epididymo-Orchitis: 100mg bid for at least 10 days. Primary/Secondary Syphilis: 300mg/day in divided doses for at least 10 days. Nongonococcal Urethritis, Uncomplicated Urethral/Endocervical/Rectal Infection: 100mg bid for at least 7 days. Inhalational Anthrax (post-exposure): 100mg bid for 60 days. Treat Strep infections for 10 days. | >8 yrs: >100 lbs: 100mg q12h on 1st day, followed by 100mg qd. Severe Infections/Chronic UTI: 100mg q12h. ≤100 lbs: 2mg/lb given bid on Day 1, followed by 1mg/lb given qd-bid thereafter. Severe Infections: Up to 2mg/lb. Inhalational Anthrax (post-exposure): <100 lbs: 1mg/lb bid for 60 days. ≤100 lbs: 100mg bid for 60 days. |

| BRAND NAME (Generic) | DOSAGE FORM/ STRENGTH | INDICATIONS | ADULT DOSE | PEDIATRIC DOSE |
|---|---|---|---|---|
| Dynacin (minocycline HCl) | Cap: 50mg, 75mg, 100mg; Tab: 50mg, 75mg, 100mg | Treatment of inclusion conjunctivitis, nongonococcal urethritis, and other infections (eg, respiratory tract, endocervical, rectal, urinary tract, skin and skin structure) caused by susceptible strains of microorganisms. Alternative treatment in certain other infections (eg, urethritis, gonococcal, syphilis, anthrax). Adjunctive therapy in acute intestinal amebiasis and severe acne. Treatment of *Mycobacterium marinum* and asymptomatic carriers of *Neisseria meningitidis.* | Usual: 200mg initially, then 100mg q12h; alternative is 100-200mg initially, then 50mg qid. Uncomplicated Gonococcal Infection (Men, Other Than Urethritis and Anorectal Infections): 200mg initially, then 100mg q12h for minimum 4 days. Uncomplicated Gonococcal Urethritis (Men): 100mg q12h for 5 days. Syphilis: Administer usual dose for 10-15 days. Meningococcal Carrier State: 100mg q12h for 5 days. *Mycobacterium marinum:* 100mg q12h for 6-8 weeks. Uncomplicated urethral, endocervical, or rectal infection: 100mg q12h for at least 7 days. Renal Dysfunction: Reduce dose and/or extend dose intervals. | >8 yrs: 4mg/kg initially followed by 2mg/kg q12h. Take with plenty of fluids. |
| Minocin (minocycline HCl) | Cap: 50mg, 100mg; Inj: 100mg; Sus: 50mg/5mL [60mL] | Treatment of inclusion conjunctivitis, nongonococcal urethritis, and other infections (eg, respiratory tract, endocervical, rectal, urinary tract, skin and skin structure) caused by susceptible strains of microorganisms. Alternative treatment in certain other infections (eg, urethritis, gonococcal, syphilis, anthrax). Adjunctive therapy in acute intestinal amebiasis and severe acne. Treatment of *Mycobacterium marinum* and asymptomatic carriers of *Neisseria meningitidis.* | Usual: 200mg initially, then 100mg q12h; alternative is 100-200mg initially, then 50mg qid. Uncomplicated Gonococcal Infection (Men, other than urethritis and anorectal infections): 200mg initially, then 100mg q12h for minimum 4 days. Uncomplicated Gonococcal Urethritis (Men): 100mg q12h for 5 days. Syphilis: Administer usual dose for 10-15 days. Meningococcal Carrier State: 100mg q12h for 5 days. *Mycobacterium marinum*: 100mg q12h for 6-8 weeks. Uncomplicated Urethral, Endocervical, or Rectal Infection Caused by *Chlamydia trachomatis* or *Ureaplasma urealyticum*: 100mg q12h for at least 7 days. Gonorrhea in Patients Sensitive to PCN: 200mg initially, then 100mg q12h for at least 4 days, with post-therapy cultures within 2-3 days. Take with plenty of fluids. Renal Dysfunction: Max: 200mg/24hrs. | >8 yrs: 4mg/kg initially followed by 2mg/kg q12h. Take with plenty of fluids. Renal Dysfunction: Max: 200mg/24 hrs. |

*(Continued)*

| BRAND NAME (Generic) | DOSAGE FORM/ STRENGTH | INDICATIONS | ADULT DOSE | PEDIATRIC DOSE |
|---|---|---|---|---|
| **TETRACYCLINE DERIVATIVES** *(Continued)* | | | | |
| Monodox (doxycycline monohydrate) | Cap: 50mg, 100mg | Treatment of respiratory tract, urinary tract, skin and skin structure, uncomplicated urethral/endocervical/rectal infection caused by *C.trachomatis,* nongonococcal urethritis caused by *C.trachomatis* and *U.urealyticum,* lymphogranuloma, psittacosis, trachoma, chancroid, plague, cholera, brucellosis. Treatment of uncomplicated gonorrhea, syphilis, listeriosis, anthrax, *Clostridium* species when PCN is contraindicated. Adjunct therapy for amebicides and severe acne. | Usual: 100mg q12h or 50mg q6h for 1 day, then 100 mg/day. Severe Infection: 100mg q12h. Uncomplicated Gonococcal Infections (except anorectal infections in men): 100mg bid for 7 days or 300mg stat, then repeat in 1 hr. Acute Epididymo-Orchitis caused by *N.gonorrhea* or *C.trachomatis:* 100mg bid for at least 10 days. Primary/Secondary Syphilis: 300mg/day in divided dose for at least 10 days. Uncomplicated Urethral/Endocervical/Rectal Infection caused by *C.trachomatis:* 100mg bid for at least 7 days. Nongonococcal Urethritis caused by *C.trachomatis* and *U.urealyticum:* 100mg bid for at least 7 days. Take with full glass of water. Take with food if GI upset occurs. | >8 yrs: ≤100 lbs: 2mg/lb divided in 2 doses for 1 day, then 1mg/lb daily in single or 2 divided doses. Severe Infection: May use up to 2mg/lb/day. >100 lbs; 100mg q12h or 50mg q6h for 1 day, then 100mg/day. Severe Infection: 100mg q12h. Take with a full glass of water. Take with food if GI upset occurs. |
| Oracea (doxycycline) | Cap: 40mg | Treatment of only inflammatory lesions (papules and pustules) of rosacea. | 40mg qd in am. Take on empty stomach. | |
| Periostat (doxycycline hyclate) | Tab: 20mg | Adjunct to scaling and root planing to promote attachment level gain and reduces pocket depth in patients with adult periodontitis. | Following scaling and root planing, 20mg bid, 1 hour prior to morning and evening meals for up to 9 mos. Maintain adequate fluid intake with caps to reduce risk of esophageal irritation and ulceration. | |
| Solodyn (minocycline HCl) | Tab, Extended-Release: 45mg, 90mg, 135mg. | Treatment of inflammatory lesions of non-nodular moderate to severe acne vulgaris in patients ≥12 yrs. | 1mg/kg qd for 12 weeks. Reduce dose with renal impairment. | ≥12 yrs: 1mg/kg qd for 12 weeks. Reduce dose with renal impairment. |
| Vibra-tabs (doxycycline hyclate) | Tab: 100mg | Treatment of susceptible infections including respiratory, urinary, skin and skin structure, lymphogranuloma, psittacosis, trachoma, uncomplicated urethral/endocervical/rectal, nongonococcal urethritis, rickettsiae, chancroid, plague, cholera, brucellosis, anthrax. When penicillin is contraindicated, treatment of uncomplicated gonorrhea, syphilis, listeriosis, *Clostridium species,* and others. Adjunct therapy for amebiasis and severe acne. Prophylaxis of malaria. | Usual: 100mg q12h on day 1, then 100mg qd or 50mg q12h. Severe Infection: 100mg q12h. Treat for 10 days with strep infection. Uncomplicated Gonococcal Infection (Except Anorectal in Men): 100mg bid for 7 days or 300mg followed by 300mg in 1 hr. Uncomplicated Urethral/Endocervical/Rectal Infection and Nongonococcal Urethritis: 100mg bid for 7 days. Syphilis: 100mg bid for 2 weeks. Syphilis for >1 yr: 100mg bid for 4 weeks. Acute Epididymo-orchitis: 100mg bid for at least 10 days. Inhalation Anthrax (Post-Exposure): 100mg bid for 60 days. Malaria Prophylaxis: 100mg qd. Begin 1-2 days before travel and continue for 4 weeks after leaving malarious area. | |

| BRAND NAME (Generic) | DOSAGE FORM/ STRENGTH | INDICATIONS | ADULT DOSE | PEDIATRIC DOSE |
|---|---|---|---|---|
| Vibramycin (doxycycline) | Cap: (Doxycycline Hyclate) 50mg, 100mg; Syrup: (Doxycycline Calcium) 50mg/5mL; Sus: (Doxycycline Monohydrate) 25mg/5mL [60mL] | Treatment of susceptible infections including respiratory, urinary, skin and skin structure, lymphogranuloma, psittacosis, trachoma, uncomplicated urethral/endocervical/rectal, nongonococcal urethritis, rickettsiae, chancroid, plague, cholera, brucellosis, anthrax. When penicillin is contraindicated, treatment of uncomplicated gonorrhea, syphilis, listeriosis, *Clostridium species,* and others. Adjunct therapy for amebiasis and severe acne. Prophylaxis of malaria. | Usual: 100mg q12h on day 1, then 100mg qd or 50mg q12h. Severe Infection: 100mg q12h. Treat for 10 days with strep infection. Uncomplicated Gonococcal Infection (Except Anorectal in Men): 100mg bid for 7 days or 300mg followed by 300mg in 1 hr. Uncomplicated Urethral/Endocervical/Rectal Infection and Nongonococcal Urethritis: 100mg bid for 7 days. Syphilis: 100mg bid for 2 weeks. Syphilis for >1 yr: 100mg bid for 4 weeks. Acute Epididymo-orchitis: 100mg bid for at least 10 days. Inhalation Anthrax (Post-Exposure): 100mg bid for 60 days. Malaria Prophylaxis: 100mg qd. Begin 1-2 days before travel and continue for 4 weeks after leaving malarious area. | >8 yrs: ≤100 lbs: 1mg/lb bid on day 1, then 1mg/lb qd or 0.5mg/lb bid. Severe Infections: Maint: 2mg/lb. >100 lbs: Usual: 100mg q12h on day 1, then 100mg qd or 50mg q12h. Severe Infection: 100mg q12h. Treat for 10 days with strep infection. Inhalation Anthrax (Post-Exposure): <100 lbs: 1mg/lb bid for 60 days. ≥100 lbs: 100mg bid for 60 days. Malaria Prophylaxis: 2mg/kg qd. Max: 100mg/day. Begin 1-2 days before travel and continue for 4 weeks after leaving malarious area. |
| Vibramycin IV (doxycycline hyclate) | Inj: 100mg, 200mg | Treatment of *rickettsiae, Mycoplasma pneumoniae, psittacosis,* ornithosis, lymphogranuloma venereum, granuloma inguinale, relapsing fever, chancroid, *Pasteurella pestis, Pasturella tularensis, Bartonella bacilliformis, Bacteroides* species, *Vibrio comma, Vibrio fetus, Brucella* species, *E.coli, Enterobacter aerogenes, Shigella* species, *Mima* species, *Herellea* species, *Haemophilus influenzae, Klebsiella* species, *Streptococcus* species, *Diplococcus pneumoniae, Staphylococcus aureus,* anthrax, and trachoma. When PCN is contraindicated; treatment of *Neisseria gonorrheae, N.meningitidis,* syphilis, yaws, *Listeria monocytogenes, Clostridium* species, *Fusobacterium fusiforme* and *Actinomyces species.* Adjunct therapy for amebiasis. | Usual: 200mg IV divided qd-bid on Day 1 then 100-200mg/day IV depending on severity, with 200mg administered in 1 or 2 infusions. Primary/Secondary Syphilis: 300mg/day IV for at least 10 days. Inhalational Anthrax (Post-Exposure): 100mg IV bid. Institute oral therapy as soon as possible and continue therapy for a total of 60 days. | >8 yrs: >100 lbs: Usual: 200mg IV divided qd-bid on Day 1 then 100-200mg/day IV depending on severity, with 200mg administered in 1 or 2 infusions. ≤100 lbs: 2mg/lb IV divided qd-bid on Day 1 then 1-2mg/lb/day IV divided qd-bid depending on severity. Inhalational Anthrax (Post-Exposure): <100 lbs: 1mg/lb IV bid. Institute oral therapy as soon as possible and continue therapy for a total of 60 days. |

*(Continued)*

| BRAND NAME (Generic) | DOSAGE FORM/ STRENGTH | INDICATIONS | ADULT DOSE | PEDIATRIC DOSE |
|---|---|---|---|---|
| **MISCELLANEOUS** | | | | |
| Bactrim (trimethoprim-sulfamethoxazole) | (Sulfamethoxazole [SMX]-Trimethoprim [TMP]) Tab: 400mg-80mg; Tab, DS: 800mg-160mg | Treatment of urinary tract infection (UTI), acute otitis media, acute exacerbation of chronic bronchitis (AECB), travelers' diarrhea, Shigellosis, and pneumocystitis carinii pneumonia (PCP). | UTI: 800mg SMX-160mg TMP q12h for 10-14 days. Shigellosis: 800mg SMX-160mg TMP q12h for 5 days. AECB: 800mg SMX-160mg TMP q12h for 14 days. PCP Treatment: 15-20mg/kg TMP and 75-100 mg/kg SMX per 24 hrs given q6h for 14-21 days. PCP Prophylaxis: 800mg SMX-160mg TMP qd. Traveler's Diarrhea: 800mg SMX-160mg TMP q12h for 5 days. CrCl: 15-30mL/min: 50% usual dose. CrCl: <15mL/min: Not recommended. | ≥2 mo: UTI/Otitis Media: 4mg/kg TMP and 20mg/kg SMX q12h for 10 days. Shigellosis: 8mg/kg TMP and 40mg/kg SMX per 24 hrs given q12h for 5 days. PCP Treatment: 15-20mg/kg TMP and 75-100mg/kg SMX per 24 hrs given q6h for 14-21 days. PCP Prophylaxis: 150mg/m2/day TMP with 750mg/m2/day SMX given bid, on 3 consecutive days/week. Max: 320mg TMP/1600mg SMX/day. CrCl: 15-30mL/min: 50% usual dose. CrCl: <15mL/min: Not recommended. |
| Cleocin (clindamycin) | Cap: (HCl) 75mg, 150mg, 300mg; Inj: (Phosphate) 150mg/mL, 300mg/50mL, 600mg/50mL, 900mg/50mL; Sus: (HCl) 75mg/5mL [100g] | Serious infections caused by anaerobes, *streptococci, pneumococci* and *staphylococci*. | Serious Infection: 150-300mg PO q6h or 600-1200 mg/day IM/IV given bid-qid. More Severe Infection: 300-450mg PO q6h or 1200-2700mg/day IM/IV given bid-qid. Life-threatening Infections: Up to 4800mg/day IV. Max: 600mg per IM injection. Take oral form with full glass of water. Treat ß-hemolytic strep for at least 10 days. | Birth-16 yrs: Serious Infection: 8-16mg/kg/day PO. More Severe Infection: 16-20mg/kg/day PO. 1 mo-16 yrs: 20-40mg/kg/day IM/IV given tid-qid; use higher dose for more severe infection. <1 mo: 15-20mg/kg/day IM/IV given tid-qid. Take oral form with full glass of water. Treat ß-hemolytic strep for at least 10 days. |
| Coly-Mycin M (colistimethate sodium) | Inj: 150mg | Treatment of acute or chronic infections due to certain gram-negative bacilli (eg, *Pseudomonas aeruginosa, Enterobacter aerogenes, E.coli, Klebsiella pneumoniae)*. | Usual: 2.5-5mg/kg/day IV/IM in 2-4 divided doses. Max: 5mg/kg/day. SCr 1.3-1.5mg/dL: 2.5-3.8mg/kg/day IV/IM in 2 divided doses. SCr 1.6-2.5mg/dL: 2.5mg/kg/day IV/IM in 1-2 divided doses. SCr 2.6-4mg/dL: 1.5mg/kg/day IV/IM q36h. Obesity: Base dose on IBW. | Usual: 2.5-5mg/kg/day IV/IM in 2-4 divided doses. Max: 5mg/kg/day. SCr 1.3-1.5mg/dL: 2.5-3.8mg/kg/day IV/IM in 2 divided doses. SCr 1.6-2.5mg/dL: 2.5mg/kg/day IV/IM in 1-2 divided doses. SCr 2.6-4mg/dL: 1.5mg/kg/day IV/IM q36h. Obesity: Base dose on IBW. |
| Cubicin (daptomycin) | Inj: 500mg | Susceptible complicated skin and skin structure infections (cSSSI). *Staphylococcus aureus* blood stream infections (bacteremia). | ≥18 yrs: Administer as IV infusion over 30 minutes. cSSSI: 4mg/kg once every 24 hrs for 7-14 days. *S.aureus* Bacteremia: 6mg/kg once every 24 hrs for minimum 2-6 weeks. Renal impairment: CrCl <30 mL/min, Hemodialysis or CAPD: (cSSSI) 4mg/kg or *(S.aureus bacteremia)* 6mg/kg once every 48 hrs. | |
| Flagyl IV (metronidazole HCl) | Inj: 500mg, 500mg (RTU) | Treatment of anaerobic intra-abdominal, skin and skin structure, gynecologic, bone and joint, CNS, lower respiratory tract infections, endocarditis, and septicemia. | LD: 15mg/kg IV. Maint: 6 hrs later, 7.5mg/kg IV q6h for 7-10 days or more. Max: 4g/24 hrs. | |

| BRAND NAME (Generic) | DOSAGE FORM/ STRENGTH | INDICATIONS | ADULT DOSE | PEDIATRIC DOSE |
|---|---|---|---|---|
| Hiprex (methenamine hippurate) | Tab: 1g | Prophylaxis or suppression of recurrent urinary tract infections when long-term therapy is necessary. For use only after infection is eradicated by other appropriate antimicrobials. | 1g bid. | >12 yrs: 1g bid. 6 to 12 yrs: 0.5g-1g bid. |
| Ketek (telithromycin) | Tab: 300mg [20$^S$], 400mg [60$^S$, Ketek Pak, 100$^S$] | Treatment of mild to moderate community-acquired pneumonia (CAP). | 800mg qd for 7-10 days. Severe Renal Impairment (CrCl <30mL/min): 600mg qd. Hemodialysis: Give after dialysis session on dialysis days. Severe Renal Impairment (CrCl <30mL/min) with Hepatic Impairment: 400mg qd. | |
| Macrobid (nitrofurantoin monohydrate) | Cap: 100mg | Treatment of acute uncomplicated urinary tract infections (acute cystitis). | 100mg every 12 hrs for 7 days. Take with food. | >12 yrs: 100mg every 12 hrs for 7 days. Take with food. |
| Macrodantin (nitrofurantoin macrocrystals) | Cap: 25mg, 50mg, 100mg | Treatment of urinary tract infection. | 50-100mg qid for at least 7 days. Take with food. Long-term Suppressive Use: 50-100mg at bedtime. | ≥1 mo: 5-7mg/kg/day given qid for at least 7 days. Take with food. Long-term Suppressive Use: 1mg/kg/day given qd-bid. |
| Monurol (fosfomycin tromethamine) | Pow: 3g/sachet | Uncomplicated urinary tract infection (acute cystitis) in women. | ≥18 yrs: 1 single-dose sachet. Mix with 3-4oz of water before ingesting. | |
| Primsol (trimethoprim HCl) | Sol: 50mg/5mL | Treatment of acute otitis media in pediatrics and urinary tract infection (UTI) in adults. | UTI: Usual: 100mg q12h or 200mg q24h for 10 days. CrCl: 15-30mL/min: Give 50% of usual dose. | Otitis Media: ≥6 mos: 5mg/kg q12h for 10 days. CrCl: 15-30mL/min: Give 50% of usual dose. |
| Rifadin (rifampin) | Cap: 150mg, 300mg; Inj: 600mg | Treatment of all forms of tuberculosis (TB). Treatment of asymptomatic carriers of *Neisseria meningitidis* to eliminate meningococci from the nasopharynx. | TB: 10mg/kg PO/IV qd. Max: 600mg/day. Meningococcal Carriers: 600mg bid for 2 days. Take 1 hrbefore or 2 hrs after a meal with a full glass of water.TB: 10-20mg/kg PO/IV qd. Max: 600mg/day. | Meningococcal Carriers: ≥1 mo: 10mg/kg q12h for 2 days. Max: 600mg/dose. <1 mo: 5mg/kg q12h for 2 days. Take 1 hr before or 2 hrs after a meal with a full glass of water. |
| Rifamate (isoniazid-rifampin) | Cap: (Isoniazid-Rifampin) 150mg-300mg | For pulmonary tuberculosis (TB). Not for initial therapy or prevention of TB. | 2 caps qd. Take 1 hr before or 2 hrs after meals. Give with pyridoxine in the malnourished, those predisposed to neuropathy (eg, alcoholics, diabetics), and adolescents. | |

*(Continued)*

| BRAND NAME (Generic) | DOSAGE FORM/ STRENGTH | INDICATIONS | ADULT DOSE | PEDIATRIC DOSE |
|---|---|---|---|---|
| **MISCELLANEOUS** *(Continued)* | | | | |
| Rifater (isoniazid-rifampin-pyrazinamide) | Tab: (Isoniazid-Pyrazinamide-Rifampin) 50mg-300mg-120mg | For initial phase of pulmonary tuberculosis treatment | ≥44kg: 4 tabs single dose qd. 45-54kg: 5 tabs single dose. ≥55kg: 6 tabs single dose. Give pyridoxine in malnourished, if predisposed to neuropathy (eg, alcoholics, diabetics), and adolescents. Take 1 hr before or 2 hrs after meals with full glass of water. Treatment usually lasts 2 months. | ≥15 yrs: ≤44kg: 4 tabs single dose qd. 45-54kg: 5 tabs qd single dose. ≥55kg: 6 tabs qd single dose. Give pyridoxine in malnourished, if predisposed to neuropathy (eg, alcoholics, diabetics), and adolescents. Take 1 hr before or 2 hrs after meals with full glass of water. Treatment usually lasts 2 months. |
| Septra (sulfamethoxazole-trimethoprim) | (Sulfamethoxazole [SMX]-Trimethoprim [TMP]) Inj: 80mg-16mg/mL; Sus: 200mg-40mg/5mL [100mL, 473mL]; Tab: 400mg-80mg; Tab, DS: 800mg-160mg | (Inj, Sus, Tab) Treatment of urinary tract infection (UTI), pneumocystitis carinii pneumonia (PCP) and enteritis caused by *Shigella*. (Sus, Tab). Treatment of acute exacerbation of chronic bronchitis (AECB), travelers' diarrhea, and acute otitis media. | (Sus, Tab) UTI: 800mg-160mg PO q12h for 10-14 days. Shigellosis/Traveler's Diarrhea: 800mg-160mg PO q12h for 5 days. AECB: 800mg-160mg PO q 12h for 14 days. PCP Treatment: 15-20mg/kg TMP and 75-100mg/kg SMX per 24 hrs given PO q6h for 14-21 days PCP Prophylaxis: 800mg-160mg PO qd. (Inj) Severe UTI: 8-10mg/kg TMP IV given in divided doses q6, 8 or 12h for up to 14 days. PCP Treatment: 15-20mg/kg TMP IV given in divided doses q6-8h for up to 14 days. Shigellosis: 8-10mg/kg TMP IV given in divided doses q6, 8 or 12h for 5 days. (Inj, Sus, Tab) Renal Impairment: CrCl 15-30 mL/min: 50% usual dose. CrCl <15mL/min: Not recommended. | (Sus, Tab) ≥2 mo: UTI/Otitis Media: 4mg/kg TMP and 20mg/kg SMX q12h for 10 days. Shigellosis/ Traveler's Diarrhea: 4mg/kg TMP and 20mg/kg SMX q12h for 5 days. PCP Treatment: 15-20mg/kg TMP and 75-100mg/kg SMX/24 hrs given q6h for 14-21 days. PCP Prophylaxis: 150mg/m2/day TMP and 750mg/m2/day SMX PO given bid, on 3 consecutive days per week. Max: 320mg TMP and 1600mg SMX per day. (Inj) Severe UTI: 8-10mg/kg TMP IV given in divided doses q6, 8 or 12h for up to 14 days. PCP Treatment: 15-20mg/kg TMP IV given in divided doses q6-8h for up to 14 days. Shigellosis: 8-10mg/kg TMP IV given in divided doses q6, 8 or 12h for 5 days. (Inj, Sus, Tab) Renal Impairment: CrCl 15-30mL/min: 50% usual dose. CrCl <15mL/min: Not recommended. |
| Synercid (dalfopristin-quinupristin) | Inj: (Dalfopristin-Quinupristin) 350mg-150mg per 500mg vial | Treatment of serious or life-threatening infections associated with vancomycin-resistant *Enterococcus faecium* (VREF) bacteremia and complicated skin and skin structure infections (SSSI) caused by *Staphylococcus aureus* (methicillin susceptible) or *Streptococcus pyogenes*. | VREF: 7.5mg/kg IV q8h. Duration depends on site and severity of infection. Complicated SSSI: 7.5mg/kg IV q12h for at least 7 days. Hepatic Cirrhosis (Child Pugh A or B): May need dose reduction. | ≥16 yrs: VREF: 7.5mg/kg IV q8h. Duration depends on site and severity of infection. Complicated SSSI: 7.5mg/kg IV q12h for at least 7 days. Hepatic Cirrhosis (Child Pugh A or B): May need dose reduction. |

| BRAND NAME (Generic) | DOSAGE FORM/ STRENGTH | INDICATIONS | ADULT DOSE | PEDIATRIC DOSE |
|---|---|---|---|---|
| Vancocin (vancomycin HCl) | Inj: 500mg/100mL, 1g/200mL | Treatment of severe infections caused by susceptible strains of methicillin-resistant staphylococci. Indicated for penicillin-allergic patients, those who cannot receive or have failed to respond to other drugs, and for vancomycin-susceptible organisms that are resistant to other antimicrobials. | Usual: 500mg IV q6h or 1g IV q12h. Mild to Moderate Renal Impairment: Initial: 15mg/kg/day. Maint: 1.9mg/kg/d. Administer 10mg/min or over at least 60 min, whichever is longer. Renal Dysfunction: Initial: 15mg/kg. Dose is about 15x the GFR in mL/min (refer to table in labeling). Elderly: Require greater dose reduction. Functionally Anephric: Initial: 15mg/kg, then 1.9mg/kg/24hrs. Marked Renal Dysfunction: 250-1000mg every several days. Anuria: 1000mg every 7-10 days. | Usual: 10mg/kg IV q6h. Infants/Neonates: Initial: 15mg/kg, then 10mg/kg q12h for neonates in the 1st week of life and q8h thereafter until 1 mo of age. Administer over at least 60 min. Renal Dysfunction: Initial: 15mg/kg. Dose is about 15x the GFR in mL/min (refer to table in labeling). Premature Infants: Require greater dose reduction. |
| Vancocin Oral (vancomycin HCl) | Cap: 125mg, 250mg | Staphylococcal enterocolitis and antibiotic-associated pseudomembranous colitis caused by *C.difficile.* | 500mg-2g/day given tid-qid for 7-10 days. | 40mg/kg/day given tid-qid for 7-10 days. Max: 2g/day. |
| Zyvox (linezolid) | Inj: 2mg/mL [100mL, 200mL, 300mL]; Sus: 100mg/5mL; Tab: 400mg, 600mg | Vancomycin resistant *Enterococcus faecium* (VRE) infections, nosocomial pneumonia caused by *Staphylococcus aureus* (methicillin-susceptible and-resistant strains) or *Streptococcus pneumoniae* (including multi-drug resistant strains [MDRSP]), complicated skin and skin structure infections (SSSI) including diabetic foot infections without concomitant osteomyelitis caused by *Staphylococcus aureus* (methicillin-susceptible and -resistant strains), *Streptococcus pyogenes,* or *Streptococcus agalactiae,* uncomplicated SSSI caused by *Staphylococcus aureus* (methicillin-susceptible only) or *Streptococcus pyogenes,* community-acquired pneumonia (CAP) caused by *Streptococcus pneumoniae* (MDRSP), including concurrent bacteremia, or *Staphylococcus aureus* (methicillin-susceptible strains only). | Complicated SSSI/CAP/Nosocomial Pneumonia: 600mg IV/PO q12h for 10-14 days. VRE: 600mg IV/PO q12h for 14-28 days. Uncomplicated SSSI: 400mg PO q12h for 10-14 days. | Complicated SSSI/CAP/Nosocomial Pneumonia: Treat for 10-14 days. ≥12 yrs: 600mg IV/PO q12h. Birth-11 yrs: 10mg/kg IV/PO q8h. VRE: Treat for 14-28 days: ≥12 yrs: 600mg IV/PO q12h. Birth-11 yrs: 10mg/kg IV/PO q8h. Uncomplicated SSSI: Treat for 10-14 days: ≥12 yrs: 600mg PO q12h. 5-11 yrs: 10mg/kg PO q12h. <5 yrs: 10mg/kg PO q8h. Neonates <7 days should be initiated with dosing regimen of 10mg/kg q12h; may increase to 10mg/kg q8h if suboptimal response. All neonatal patients should receive 10mg/kg q8h by 7 days of life. |

# SYSTEMIC ANTIFUNGALS

| GENERIC | BRAND | INDICATION | DOSAGE FORM | DOSAGE |
|---|---|---|---|---|
| Amphotericin B lipid complex injection | Abelcet | Invasive fungal infections in patients who are refractory to or intolerant of conventional amphotericin B therapy. | Inj: 5mg/mL | Single infusion 5mg/kg. |
| Amphotericin B liposome injection | AmBisome | Treatment of patients with *Aspergillus* species, *Candida* species and/or *Cryptococcus* species infections refractory to amphotericin B deoxycholate, cryptococcal meningitis in HIV patients, fungal infection in febrile, neutropenic patients, and treatment of visceral leishmaniasis. | Inj: 50mg | 3-6mg/kg/day. |
| Amphotericin B | Amphocin | Progressive, potentially life-threatening fungal infections: Aspergillosis, cryptococcosis, North American blastomycosis, systemic candidiasis, coccidioidomycosis, histoplasmosis, zygomycosis, sporotrichosis, and infections due to *Conidiobolus* and *Basidiobolus* species. | Inj: 50mg | **Initial:** 0.25mg/kg. **Titrate:** Increase by 5-10mg/day, depending on cardio-renal status, up to 0.5-0.7mg/kg/day. |
| Amphotericin B cholesteryl sulfate | Amphotec | Treatment of invasive aspergillosis in patients with renal impairment, unacceptable toxicity, or previous failure to amphotericin deoxycholate. | Inj: 50mg, 100mg | 3-4mg/kg/day IV at 1mg/kg/hr. |
| Caspofungin Acetate | Cancidas | Treatment of candidemia, esophageal candidiasis, fungal infections in febrile, neutropenic patients, invasive aspergillosis in patients who are refractory to or intolerant of other therapies. | Inj: 50mg, 70mg | 70mg loading dose on Day 1 and then 50mg qd. |
| Griseofulvin | Grifulvin V | Indicated for ringworm. | Sus: 125mg/5mL [120mL]; Tab: 500mg | 0.5-1g qd. |
| Griseofulvin | Gris-PEG | Indicated for ringworm. | Tab (ultramicrosize): 125mg, 250mg | 375mg as a single dose or in divided doses. |
| Terbinafine HCl | Lamisil | Onychomycosis of the toenail or fingernail. | Tab: 250mg | 250mg po qd for 6 weeks. |
| Micafungin sodium | Mycamine | Esophageal candidiasis and prophylaxis of *Candida* infection in HSCT patients. | Inj: 50mg | **Candidiasis:** 150mg/day for 5 days; **Prophylaxis:** 150mg/day for 20 days. |
| Voriconazole | Vfend | Invasive aspergillosis, esophageal candidiasis, serious fungal infections caused by *Scedosporium apiospermum* and *Fusarium* spp. including *Fusarium solani,* candidemia in nonneutropenic patients. | Inj: 200mg; Sus: 40mg/mL [100mL]; Tab: 50mg, 200mg | PO 200mg q12h. IV LD: 6mg/kg q12h for first 24h. IV MD: 3-4mg/kg q12h. |
| Fluconazole | Diflucan | Treatment of vaginal, oropharyngeal, esophageal, and systemic candidiasis. Treatment of peritonitis and UTI caused by *Candida.* Treatment of cryptococcal meningitis. Prophylaxis in patients undergoing BMT. | Inj: 200mg/100mL, 400mg/200mL; Sus: 50mg/5mL, 200mg/5mL [35mL];Tab: 50mg, 100mg,150mg, 200mg | **Vaginal *Candida:*** 150mg po x 1 day. **All other:** 100-200mg/day. **Max:** 400mg/day. |

*(Continued)*

| GENERIC | BRAND | INDICATION | DOSAGE FORM | DOSAGE |
|---|---|---|---|---|
| Clotrimazole | Mycelex Troche | Oropharyngeal candidiasis. To prevent oropharyngeal candidiasis in immunocompromised conditions. | Loz/Troche: 10mg | 1 troche in mouth 5 times/day for 14 days. **Prophylaxis:** 1 troche tid. |
| Nystatin | Mycostatin | (Cream, Powder) Treatment of cutaneous or mucocutaneous mycotic infections caused by *Candida.* | Cream: 100,000 U/gm, Powder: 100,000 U/gm | **Powder:** Apply to affected area twice daily or as indicated until healing is complete. **Cream:** Apply to candidal lesions two or three times daily until healing is complete. |
| Flucytosine | Ancobon | Treatment of septicemia, endocarditis, and urinary tract infections caused by *Candida.* Treatment of meningitis and pulmonary infection caused by *Cryptococcus.* | Cap: 250mg, 500mg | 50-150mg/kg/day given q6h. |
| Ketoconazole | Nizoral | Candidiasis, chronic mucocutaneous candidiasis, oral thrush, candiduria, blastomycosis, coccidioidomycosis, histoplasmosis, chromomycosis, and paracoccidioidomycosis. Treatment of patients with severe recalcitrant cutaneous dermatophyte infections. | Tab: 200mg | 200mg qd. **Max:** 400mg qd. |
| Itraconazole | Sporanox | Onychomycosis of the toenail and fingernail, blastomycosis and histoplasmosis. Treatment of aspergillosis if refractory to or intolerant to amphoteracin B. (Sol) Treatment of oropharyngeal and esophageal candidiasis. | Cap: 100mg; Inj: 10mg/mL; Sol: 10mg/mL [150mL] | **(Cap) Blastomycosis:** 200mg once daily (2 capsules). **Aspergillosis:** 200-400mg. **Max:** 400mg/day. **(Inj):** 200 mg b.i.d. for four doses, followed by 200 mg once daily for up to 14 days. **(Sol):** Swish (10 mL at a time) for several seconds and swallow. |
| Anidulafungin | Eraxis | Treatment of candidemia and other forms of *Candida* infections esophageal candidiasis. | Inj: 50mg | **Candidemia:** LD 200mg on Day 1, MD 100mg x 14d. **Esophageal Candidiasis:** 100mg qd x 1 day then 50mg qd x 14 days |
| Posaconazole | Noxafil | Prophylaxis of invasive *Aspergillus* and *Candida,* oropharyngeal candidiasis, including oropharyngeal candidiasis refractory to itraconazole and/or fluconazole. | Susp: 40mg/mL [105mL] | **Prophylaxis:** 200mg tid. **Oropharyngeal Candidiasis:** 100mg bid x 1 day, 100mg qd x 13 days. |

# GYNECOLOGICAL ANTI-INFECTIVES

| DRUG | CLASS | FORMULATION | ROUTE | RECOMMENDED DOSAGE |
|---|---|---|---|---|
| **ANTIBACTERIALS** | | | | |
| **Clindamycin** | | | | |
| Cleocin Vaginal, Clindamax | RX | Cream: 2% | Vaginal | **Bacterial Vaginosis:** *Adults:* 1 applicatorful qhs x 3-7 days (non-pregnant) or x 7 days (2nd or 3rd trimester). |
| Cleocin Vaginal Ovules | RX | Supp: 100mg | Vaginal | **Bacterial Vaginosis:** *Adults:* 1 sup qhs x 3 days. |
| Clindesse | RX | Cream: 2% | Vaginal | **Bacterial Vaginosis:** *Adults:* 1 applicatorful qd (non-pregnant). |
| **Metronidazole** | | | | |
| Flagyl | RX | Cap: 375mg<br>Tab: 250mg, 500mg | Oral | **Trichomoniasis:** *Adults:* 375mg bid or 250mg tid x 7 days. Alternate Regimen (Tab): If non-pregnant, 2g as single or divided dose. Contraindicated in 1st trimester. |
| Flagyl ER | RX | Tab, ER: 750mg | Oral | **Bacterial Vaginosis:** *Adults:* 750mg qd x 7 days. Contraindicated in 1st trimester. |
| MetroGel Vaginal | RX | Gel: 0.75% | Vaginal | **Bacterial Vaginosis:** *Adults:* 1 applicatorful qd-bid x 5 days. |
| **Sulfanilamide** | | | | |
| AVC | RX | Cream: 15% | Vaginal | **Candidiasis:** *Adults:* 1 applicatorful qd-bid x 30 days. |
| **ANTIFUNGALS: CANDIDIASIS TREATMENT** | | | | |
| **Butoconazole** | | | | |
| Gynazole-1 | RX | Cream: 2% | Vaginal | *Adults:* 1 applicatorful single dose. |
| **Clotrimazole** | | | | |
| Mycelex-3 | OTC | Cream: 2% | Vaginal | *Adults/Pediatrics ≥12 yrs:* 1 applicatorful qhs x 3 days. |
| Mycelex-7 | OTC | Cream: 1% | Vaginal | *Adults/Pediatrics ≥12 yrs:* 1 applicatorful qhs x 7 days. |
| Mycelex-7 Combination Pack | OTC | Cream: 1% + Sup: 100mg | Vaginal | *Adults/Pediatrics ≥12 yrs:* 1 sup qhs x 7 days. Apply cream externally qd-bid up to 7 days prn. |
| Gyne-Lotrimin 3 | OTC | Cream: 2%<br>Sup: 200mg | Vaginal | *Adults/Pediatrics ≥12 yrs:* 1 applicatorful or 1 sup qhs x 3 days. |
| Gyne-Lotrimin 3 Combination Pack | OTC | Cream: 1% + Sup: 200mg | Vaginal | *Adults/Pediatrics ≥12 yrs:* 1 sup qhs x 3 days. Apply cream externally qd-bid prn. |
| Gyne-Lotrimin Combination Pack | OTC | Cream: 1% + Sup: 100mg | Vaginal | *Adults/Pediatrics ≥12 yrs:* 1 sup qhs x 7 days. Apply cream externally qd-bid prn. |
| **Fluconazole** | | | | |
| Diflucan | RX | Tab: 150mg | Oral | *Adults:* 150mg single dose. |
| **Miconazole** | | | | |
| Monistat 1 Combination Pack | OTC | Cream: 2% + Sup: 1200mg | Vaginal | *Adults/Pediatrics ≥12 yrs:* 1 sup single dose. Apply cream externally bid up to 7 days prn. |
| Monistat 3 | OTC | Cream: 4% | Vaginal | *Adults/Pediatrics ≥12 yrs:* 1 applicatorful qhs x 3 days. |
| Monistat 3 Combination Pack | OTC | Cream: 2% + Sup: 200mg | Vaginal | *Adults/Pediatrics ≥12 yrs:* 1 applicatorful qhs x 3 days. Apply cream bid externally prn x 7 days. |
| Monistat 7 | OTC | Cream: 2% | Vaginal | *Adults/Pediatrics ≥12 yrs:* 1 applicatorful qhs x 7 days. |
| Monistat 7 Combination Pack | OTC | Cream: 2%<br>Sup: 100mg | Vaginal | *Adults/Pediatrics ≥12 yrs:* 1 sup qhs x 7 days. Apply cream bid externally x 7 days. |

*(Continued)*

| DRUG | CLASS | FORMULATION | ROUTE | RECOMMENDED DOSAGE |
|---|---|---|---|---|
| **ANTIFUNGALS: CANDIDIASIS TREATMENT** *(Continued)* | | | | |
| **Nystatin** | RX | Tab, Vaginal: 100,000U | Vaginal | *Adults:* 1 tablet daily x 14 days. |
| **Terconazole** | | | | |
| Terazol 3 | RX | Cream: 0.8%<br>Supp: 80mg | Vaginal | *Adults:* 1 applicatorful or 1 sup qhs x 3 days. |
| Terazol 7 | RX | Cream: 0.4% | Vaginal | *Adults:* 1 applicatorful qhs x 7 days. |
| **Tioconazole** | | | | |
| Monistat 1, Vagistat 1 | OTC | Oint: 6.5% | Vaginal | *Adults/Pediatrics:* ≥12yrs: 1 applicatorful single dose hs. |

# HORMONE THERAPY

| DRUG | BRAND | DOSAGE (mg) |
|---|---|---|
| **ORAL ESTROGEN PRODUCTS** | | |
| Conjugated equine estrogens | Premarin | 0.3, 0.45, 0.625, 0.9, 1.25 |
| Synthetic conjugated estrogens | Cenestin | 0.3, 0.45, 0.625, 0.9, 1.25 |
| Esterified estrogens | Menest | 0.3, 0.625, 1.25, 2.5 |
| Micronized 17ß-estradiol | Estrace | 0.5, 1, 2 |
| Estropipate (piperazine estrone sulfate) | Ortho-Est | 0.75, 1.5 |
| | Ogen | 0.625, 1.25, 2.5, 5 |
| **TRANSDERMAL ESTROGEN PRODUCTS** | | |
| | | **RELEASE RATE (mg/day)** |
| 17ß-estradiol matrix patch | Alora | 0.025, 0.05, 0.075, 0.1 |
| | Climara | 0.025, 0.0375, 0.05, 0.06, 0.075, 0.1 |
| | Vivelle, Vivelle-Dot | 0.025, 0.0375, 0.05, 0.075, 0.1 |
| 17ß-estradiol reservoir patch | Estraderm | 0.05, 0.1 |
| **VAGINAL ESTROGEN PRODUCTS** | | |
| **Vaginal Creams**<br>17ß-estradiol | Estrace Vaginal Cream | 2-4g/day x 1-2 wks, reduce to 1-2g/day x 1-2 wks, then 1g/day x 1-3x/wk |
| Conjugated equine estrogens | Premarin Vaginal Cream | 0.5-2g/day x 3 wks on 1 wk off |
| **Vaginal Ring**<br>17ß-estradiol | Estring | Releases 0.0075mg/day x 90 days |
| **Vaginal Tablet**<br>Estradiol hemihydrate | Vagifem | 25mcg/day x 2 wks then 25mcg BIW |
| **PROGESTOGEN ONLY PRODUCTS** | | |
| Medroxyprogesterone acetate | Provera | 2.5, 5, 10 |
| Norethindrone acetate | Aygestin | 5 |
| Progesterone USP (in peanut oil) | Prometrium | 100, 200 |
| **ESTROGEN + PROGESTOGEN COMBINATIONS** | | |
| **Oral continuous-cyclic regimen**<br>Conjugated equine estrogens (E) + Medroxyprogesterone acetate (P) | Premphase | 0.625mg (E), 5mg (P) [E alone for days 1-14, followed by E+P on days 15-28] |
| **Oral continuous-combined regimen**<br>Conjugated equine estrogens (E) + Medroxyprogesterone (P) | Prempro | 0.3mg (E) + 1.5mg (P); 0.45mg + 1.5mg; 0.625mg + 2.5 or 5mg |
| Ethinyl estradiol (E) + Norethindrone acetate (P) | femhrt | 2.5mcg (E) + 0.5mg (P);<br>5mcg (E) + 1mg (P) |
| 17ß-estradiol (E) + Norethindrone acetate (P) | Activella | 1mg (E) + 0.5mg (P);<br>0.5mg (E) + 0.1mg (P) |
| **Transdermal continuous-cyclic or continuous-combined regimen**<br>17ß-estradiol (E) + Norethindrone acetate (P) | CombiPatch | 0.05mg/day (E) + 0.14 or 0.25mg/day (P) |
| Estradiol (E) + Levonorgestrel (P) | Climara Pro | 0.045mg/day (E) + 0.015mg/day (P) |
| **ESTROGEN + ANDROGEN COMBINATIONS** | | |
| **Oral cyclic regimen**<br>Esterified estrogens (E) + | Estratest | 1.25 (E) + 2.5 (A) |
| Methyltestosterone (A) | Estratest H.S. | 0.625 (E) + 1.25 (A) |

**NOTE:** This list is not inclusive of all estrogen and progestogen products available. Indications vary among the different products. For more detailed information please refer to the individual monograph listings or the drug's FDA-approved labeling. Unopposed estrogen replacement therapy (ERT) is for use in women without an intact uterus. For women with an intact uterus, progestin must be added to the estrogen (HRT) for protection against estrogen-induced endometrial cancer. As with any therapy, the lowest possible effective dosage should be used. Re-evaluate periodically.

# Oral Contraceptives

| DRUG | ESTROGEN | PROGESTIN | STRENGTH (ESTROGEN/PROGESTIN) |
|---|---|---|---|
| **MONOPHASIC** | | | |
| Alesse, Levlite | Ethinyl Estradiol | Levonorgestrel | 20mcg/0.1mg |
| Brevicon, Modicon | Ethinyl Estradiol | Norethindrone | 35mcg/0.5mg |
| Demulen 1/35 | Ethinyl Estradiol | Ethynodiol Diacetate | 35mcg/1mg |
| Demulen 1/50 | Ethinyl Estradiol | Ethynodiol Diacetate | 50mcg/1mg |
| Desogen, Ortho-Cept | Ethinyl Estradiol | Desogestrel | 30mcg/0.15mg |
| Levlen, Nordette-28 | Ethinyl Estradiol | Levonorgestrel | 30mcg/0.15mg |
| Loestrin 21 1/20, Loestrin Fe 1/20 | Ethinyl Estradiol | Norethindrone Acetate | 20mcg/1mg |
| Loestrin 21 1.5/30, Loestrin Fe 1.5/30 | Ethinyl Estradiol | Norethindrone Acetate | 30mcg/1.5mg |
| Lo/Ovral | Ethinyl Estradiol | Norgestrel | 30mcg/0.3mg |
| Lybrel | Ethinyl Estradiol | Levonorgestrel | 20mcg/90mcg |
| Norinyl 1/35, Ortho-Novum 1/35 | Ethinyl Estradiol | Norethindrone | 35mcg/1mg |
| Norinyl 1/50, Ortho-Novum 1/50 | Mestranol | Norethindrone | 50mcg/1mg |
| Ortho-Cyclen | Ethinyl Estradiol | Norgestimate | 35mcg/0.25mg |
| Ovcon 35 | Ethinyl Estradiol | Norethindrone | 35mcg/0.4mg |
| Ovcon 50 | Ethinyl Estradiol | Norethindrone | 50mcg/1mg |
| Seasonale | Ethinyl Estradiol | Levonorgestrel | 30mcg/0.15mg |
| Seasonique | Ethinyl Estradiol | Levonorgestrel | 0.01mg, 0.15mg/0.03mg |
| Yasmin | Ethinyl Estradiol | Drospirenone | 30mcg/3mg |
| YAZ | Ethinyl Estradiol | Drospirenone | 0.02mg/3mg |
| **BIPHASIC** | | | |
| Ortho-Novum 10/11 | Ethinyl Estradiol | Norethindrone | **Phase 1:** 35mcg/0.5mg<br>**Phase 2:** 35mcg/1mg |
| Mircette | Ethinyl Estradiol | Desogestrel | **Phase 1:** 20mcg/0.15mg<br>**Phase 2:** 10mcg/NONE |
| **TRIPHASIC** | | | |
| Cyclessa | Ethinyl Estradiol | Desogestrel | **Phase 1:** 25mcg/0.1mg<br>**Phase 2:** 25mcg/0.125mg<br>**Phase 3:** 25mcg/0.15mg |
| Estrostep Fe | Ethinyl Estradiol | Norethindrone Acetate | **Phase 1:** 20mcg/1mg<br>**Phase 2:** 30mcg/1mg<br>**Phase 3:** 35mcg/1mg |
| Ortho-Novum 7/7/7 | Ethinyl Estradiol | Norethindrone | **Phase 1:** 35mcg/0.5mg<br>**Phase 2:** 35mcg/0.75mg<br>**Phase 3:** 35mcg/1mg |
| Ortho Tri-Cyclen | Ethinyl Estradiol | Norgestimate | **Phase 1:** 35mcg/0.18mg<br>**Phase 2:** 35mcg/0.215mg<br>**Phase 3:** 35mcg/0.25mg |
| Ortho Tri-Cyclen Lo | Ethinyl Estradiol | Norgestimate | **Phase 1:** 25mcg/0.18mg<br>**Phase 2:** 25mcg/0.215mg<br>**Phase 3:** 25mcg/0.25mg |
| Tri-Levlen, Triphasil, Trivora 28 | Ethinyl Estradiol | Levonorgestrel | **Phase 1:** 30mcg/0.05mg<br>**Phase 2:** 40mcg/0.075mg<br>**Phase 3:** 30mcg/0.125mg |

*(Continued)*

| DRUG | ESTROGEN | PROGESTIN | STRENGTH (ESTROGEN/PROGESTIN) |
|---|---|---|---|
| **TRIPHASIC** *(Continued)* | | | |
| Tri-Norinyl | Ethinyl Estradiol | Norethindrone | **Phase 1:** 35mcg/0.5mg<br>**Phase 2:** 35mcg/1mg<br>**Phase 3:** 35mcg/0.5mg |
| **PROGESTIN ONLY** | | | |
| Nor-Q.D.,<br>Ortho-Micronor | | Norethindrone | 0.35mg |

# CHEMOTHERAPY REGIMENS*†

| CANCER TYPE | DRUGS OF CHOICE | ALTERNATIVE THERAPIES |
|---|---|---|
| Bladder | *Superficial:* Instillation of BCG | *Superficial:* Instillation of mitomycin, doxorubicin, thiotepa, gemcitabine or epirubicin |
| | *Systemic:* MTX + vinblastine + doxorubicin + cisplatin (MVAC); gemcitabine + cisplatin | *Systemic:* Cisplatin + MTX + vinblastine (CMV); cisplatin w/ mesna; gallium nitrate + paclitaxel; cisplatin + docetaxel; gemcitabine + epirubicin; ifosfamide |
| Breast | *Risk reduction:* Tamoxifen | |
| | *Adjuvant*[1]*:* Doxorubicin + cyclophosphamide ± 5-FU (AC or CAF) ± followed by paclitaxel or docetaxel; Cyclophosphamide + MTX + 5-FU (CMF)<br>*For hormone receptor-*(+): Tamoxifen | *Adjuvant*[1]*:* Cyclophosphamide + epirubicin + 5-FU (CEF);<br>*For postmenopausal hormone receptor-*(+): Anastrozole[2] |
| | *Metastatic:* Doxorubicin + cyclophosphamide ± 5-FU (AC or CAFs); cyclophosphamide + MTX + 5-FU (CMF);<br>*For hormone receptor-*(+): Letrozole[3], anastrozole[3], exemestane[3], tamoxifen, toremifene, or fulvestrant | *Metastatic:* Capecitabine; paclitaxel; docetaxel; vinorelbine; mitoxantrone; epirubicin; 5-FU by continuous infusion<br>*For hormone receptor-*(+): megestrol acetate; fluoxymesterone |
| | *For tumors overexpressing HER2 protein:* Trastuzumab[4] + vinorelbine or paclitaxel | *For tumors overexpressing HER2 protein:* Trastuzumab[4] + docetaxel; pegylated liposomal doxorubicin + trastuzumab[4] or gemcitabine |
| Colorectal | *Adjuvant Stage III:* 5-FU + LV; oxaliplatin + 5-FV + LV<br>*Metastatic (Stage IV):* 5-FU + LV + either irinotecan or oxaliplatin | Capecitabine (stage III)<br>*For hepatic metastases:* hepatic intra-arterial (HIA) floxuridine[5] |
| Esophageal | Cisplatin + 5-FU | Cisplatin + either irinotecan or paclitaxel; doxorubicin; MTX; vinorelbine; docetaxel; bleomycin |
| Leukemia<br>Acute lymphocytic leukemia (ALL) | *Induction:* Vincristine + prednisone + daunorubicin or doxorubicin ± asparaginase ± cyclophosphamide<br>*CNS prophylaxis:* Intrathecal MTX (± intrathecal cytarabine ± intrathecal hydrocortisone) ± systemic high-dose MTX with LV<br>*Post induction:* High-dose cytarabine ± other drugs | *Induction:* Same ± high-dose MTX ± cytarabine; pegaspargase substitution for asparaginase; teniposide or etoposide; high-dose cytarabine + mitoxantrone; vincristine + doxorubicin + dexamethasone alternating with high-dose MTX + cytarabine (Hyper-CVAD) |
| | *Maintenance:* Mercaptopurine + MTX<br>*Poor prognosis or relapse:* Allogenic peripheral stem-cell or bone-marrow transplant | *Maintenance:* Same plus monthly vincristine and prednisone |
| Acute myelogenous leukemia (AML) | *Induction:* Cytarabine + either daunorubicin or idarubicin ± etoposide | High-dose cytarabine + daunorubicin or idarubicin<br>*Additional drugs for induction or post-induction include:* Vincristine, cyclophosphamide, MTX, mitoxantrone, fludarabine[6], carboplatin, topotecan, thioguanine, gemtuzumab, doxorubicin |

*(Continued)*

| CANCER TYPE | DRUGS OF CHOICE | ALTERNATIVE THERAPIES |
|---|---|---|
| AML (con't) | *For acute promyelocytic leukemia (APL)*: Tretinoin + further induction therapy<br>*CNS prophylaxis:* intrathecal cytarabine or MTX ± intrathecal hydrocortisone<br>*Post Induction:* High-dose cytarabine ± other drugs<br>*Poor prognosis or relapse:* Allogenic peripheral stem-cell or bone-marrow transplant | *For APL:* arsenic trioxide |
| Chronic lymphocytic leukemia (CLL) | Fludarabine[6] ± cyclophosphamide; chlorambucil or cyclophosphamide ± prednisone | Cyclophosphamide + vincristine + prednisone ± doxorubicin; aletuzumab; cladribine; pentostatin; rituximab |
| Chronic myelogenous leukemia (CML)[7] | | |
| Chronic phase | Imatinib; Interferon alfa ± cytarabine; allogenic peripheral stem-cell or bone-marrow transplant | Hydroxyurea |
| Accelerated | Imatinib; cytarabine + daunorubicin or idarubicin; Allogenic peripheral stem-cell or bone-marrow transplant | Hydroxyurea; interferon alfa |
| Blast phase | *Lymphoid:* Imatinib ± same as for ALL induction<br>*Myeloid:* Imatinib ± same as for AML induction | Allogenic peripheral stem-cell or bonemarrow transplant |
| Hairy cell leukemia | Cladribine; pentostatin | Interferon alfa |
| Liver | Hepatic intra-arterial floxuridine or cisplatin | Doxorubicin; 5-FU; mitomycin |
| Lung | | |
| Non-small cell | Paclitaxel + either carboplatin or cisplatin; cisplatin + vinorelbine; gemcitabine + cisplatin; carboplatin or cisplatin + docetaxel | Docetaxel; irinotecan; cisplatin; vinorelbine; oxaliplatin; mitomycin + vinblastine + cisplatin (MVP); mitomycin + ifosfamide w/mesna + cisplatin (MIC); gemcitabine + paclitaxel |
| Small cell | Cisplatin or carboplatin + etoposide (PE); irinotecan + cisplatin | Topotecan; cyclophosphamide + doxorubicin + vincristine (CAV); paclitaxel; irinotecan; docetaxel; etoposide + ifosfamide w/mesna + cisplatin (VIP); ifosfamide w/mesna + carboplatin + etoposide (ICE) |
| Lymphomas | | |
| Non-Hodgkin's Lymphomas | | |
| High Grade | | |
| Burkitt's | Cyclophosphamide + doxorubicin + vincristine + high-dose MTX + intrathecal MTX (CODOX-M) alternating with ifosfamide with mesna + etoposide + high-dose cytarabine and intrathecal MTX (IVAC) | Autologous or allogenic peripheral stem cell or bone-marrow transplant |
| Lymphoblastic | Cyclophosphamide + doxorubicin + vincristine + prednisone + asparaginase + maintenance with MTX + merceptopurine + intrathecal MTX ± cytarabine | Autologous or allogenic peripheral stem cell or bone-marrow transplant |
| Intermediate Grade[8] | | |
| Diffuse large cell, diffuse small cell, diffused mixed, follicular large cell | Cyclophosphamide + doxorubicin + vincristine + prednisone (CHOP) ± rituximab ± intrathecal MTX or cytarabine | Other combination regimens that may include MTX, etoposide, cytarabine, bleomycin, procarbazine, mechlorethamine, dexamethasone, cisplatin, mitoxantrone, alemtuzumab; autologous or allogenic peripheral stem-cell or bone-marrow transplant |
| Low Grade[9] | | |
| Follicular small cleaved cell, follicular mixed, small cleaved and large cell | Cyclophosphamide or chlorambucil; cyclophosphamide + vincristine + prednisone ± doxorubicin ± rituximab; fludarabine[4] + mitoxantrone ± dexamethasone ± rituximab | Cladribine; interferon alfa; etoposide; ibritumomab; tostumomab; alemtuzumab; autologous or allogenic peripheral stem cell or bone-marrow transplant |

*(Continued)*

| CANCER TYPE | DRUGS OF CHOICE | ALTERNATIVE THERAPIES |
|---|---|---|
| Lymphoblastic (con't) | | |
| Cutaneous T-cell | Topical mechlorethamine or carmustine; PUVA (psoralen + ultraviolet A); topical steroids: clobetasol, diflorasone, halobetasol, betamethasone; *Systemic chemotherapy:* MTX | Bexarotene; denileukin; isotretinoin; pentostatin; fludarabine; cladribine; photophoresis (extra-corporeal photochemotherapy) |
| Ovarian | | |
| Germ Cell Tumor | Bleomycin + etoposide + cisplatin (BEP) | Vincristine + dactinomycin + cyclophosphamide; etoposide + cisplatin or carboplatin |
| Epithelial | Carboplatin ± paclitaxel | Topotecan; cyclophosphamide; ifosfamide w/mesna; tamoxifen; melphalan; altretamine; oral etoposide; docetaxel; liposomal doxorubicin; gemcitabine; interferon gamma, oxaliplatin; megestrol acetate; intra-peritoneal chemotherapy |
| Pancreatic | *Adjuvant and localized unresectable:* 5-FU<br>*Metastatic:* Gemcitabine | Doxorubicin; mitomycin; cisplatin + 5-FU; docetaxel; oxaliplatin + gemcitabine; irinotecan |
| Prostate | Gonadotropin-releasing hormone (GnRH) agonists (leuprolide, goserelin or triptorelin) ± antiandrogen (flutamide, bicalutamide or nilutamide) | Mitoxantrone + prednisone; estra mustine + either docetaxel, vinblastine, paclitaxel or etoposide; ketoconazole ± either doxorubicin or prednisone |

**Abbreviations:** MTX: Methotrexate; 5-FU: Fluorouracil; LV: Leucovorin

* Selected cancers. For more detailed information, refer to the individual monograph listings in the Oncology/Hematology section or the drug's FDA-approved labeling.

† Source: Treatment Guidelines from The Medical Letter. Drugs of Choice for Cancer. March 2003; 1:7.

1. Adjuvant treatment with chemotherapy and/or hormone therapy is generally recommended for node-(+) patients, and for node-(-) patients with tumors ≥1cm in size or other unfavorable prognostic features. Hormone therapy is limited to hormone receptor-(+) or unknown tumors, and should begin after chemotherapy. If radiation therapy is used, it is best to have a similar delay. An anthracycline-containing regimen is preferred with node-(+) disease.
2. Anastrozole may be more effective than tamoxifen as adjuvant therapy in postmenopausal women with hormone receptor-(+) tumors, but longer follow-up is needed.
3. An LHRH agonist should be given with an aromastase inhibitor in premenopausal hormone receptor-(+) women.
4. Concurrent use increases cardiac toxicity of doxorubicin.
5. Intrahepatic regimens may be associated with a higher rate of extrahepatic metastases if given without systemic chemotherapy.
6. May compromise future stem-cell collection.
7. Allogenic HLA-identical sibling bone marrow transplantation may cure 30%-50% of patients with CML in chronic phase, 15%-20% in accelerated phase and <15% in blast phase. Disease-free survival after transplantation is adversely influenced by age >50 yrs, duration of disease >3 yrs from diagnosis, and use of one-antigen-mismatched or matched unrelated donor marrow. Interferon alfa may be curative in patients with chonic phase CML who achieve a complete cytogenic response (about 10%). Chemotherapy alone is palliative.
8. Three cycles of CHOP followed by involved-field irradiation has been shown to be superior to eight cycles of CHOP alone in localized intermediate or high-grade Non-Hodgkin's.
9. Lymphoma of mucosa-associated lymphoid tissue is treated similarly to other low-grade lymphomas. When affecting the stomach, it is often associated with *H. pylori* infection, and treatment with omeprazole, amoxicillin, and metronidazole alone is sufficient to produce a histologic response.

# Opioid Products

| GENERIC | BRAND | DOSAGE FORMS | ORAL EQUI-ANALGESIC DOSE | EQUI-ANALGESIC DOSE | USUAL ADULT DOSE | MAX DOSE | INDICATION | DEA SCHEDULE |
|---|---|---|---|---|---|---|---|---|
| Codeine | | Inj, Oral Sol: (15mg/5mL); Tab: 15mg, 30mg, 60mg | 200mg. | 130mg. | PO, IM, SC, IV 15-60mg q4-6h. | 360mg/24 hrs. | Relief of mild to moderate pain; cough suppression. | Schedule II |
| Codeine phosphate/ Acetaminophen | Tylenol w/Codeine | Elixir: 12mg-120mg/5mL | | | 15mL q4h prn. | Codeine: 360mg/ 24 hrs. Acetaminophen: 4g/day. | Relief of mild to moderately severe pain. | Schedule V |
| | Tylenol #3 | Tab: 30mg/300mg | | | 15-60mg codeine/dose and 300-1000mg APAP. | | | Schedule III |
| | Tylenol #4 | Tab: 60mg/300mg | | | | | | Schedule III |
| Hydrocodone bitartrate/ Acetaminophen | Lortab Elixir | Sol: 7.5mg-500mg/15mL | | | 1 tbs q4-6h prn | 6 tbs. | Relief of moderate to moderately severe pain. | Schedule III |
| | Lortab | Tab: 2.5mg/500mg, 5mg/ 500mg, 7.5mg/500mg, 10mg/500mg | | | (2.5/500, 5/500): 1-2 tabs q4-6h prn. (7.5/500,10/500): 1 tab q4-6h prn. | (2.5/500, 5/500):8 tabs/day. (7.5/500, 10/500): 6 tabs/day. | | |
| | Norco | Tab: 5mg/325mg, 7.5mg/ 325mg, 10mg/325mg | | | (5/325): 1-2 tabs q4-6h prn. (7.5/325, 10/325): 1 tab q4-6h prn. | (7.5/325,10/325): 6 tabs/day. | | |
| | Vicodin | Tab: 5mg/500mg | | | 1-2 tabs q4-6h prn. | 8 tabs/day. | | |
| | Vicodin ES | Tab: 7.5mg/750mg | | | 1 tab q4-6h prn. | 5 tabs/day. | | |
| | Vicodin HP | Tab: 10mg/660mg | | | 1 tab q4-6h prn. | 6 tabs/day. | | |
| | Zydone | Tab: 5mg/400mg, 7.5mg/400mg, 10mg/400mg | | | (5/400): 1-2 tabs q4-6h prn. (7.5/400, 10/400): 1 tab q4-6h prn. | (5/400): 8 tabs/day (7.5/400, 10/400): 6 tabs/day. | | |
| Hydrocodone bitartrate/Ibuprofen | Vicoprofen | Tab: 7.5/200mg | | | 1-2 tabs q4-6h prn. | 5 tabs/day. | Short-term (generally <10 days) management of acute pain. | Schedule III |
| Oxycodone HCl | OxyContin | Tab, ER: 10mg, 20mg, 40mg, 80mg, 160mg | | | 10mg q12h. Titrate: May increase the q12h dose (not the dosing frequency). May increase the total daily dose by 25-50% of the current dose. | | Management of moderate to severe pain when a continuous around the clock analgesic is needed for an extended period. Only for postoperative use in patients already receiving the drug before surgery or those expected to have moderate-severe postoperative pain for an extended period of time. | Schedule II |

| GENERIC | BRAND | DOSAGE FORMS | ORAL EQUI-ANALGESIC DOSE | EQUI-ANALGESIC DOSE | USUAL ADULT DOSE | MAX DOSE | INDICATION | DEA SCHEDULE |
|---|---|---|---|---|---|---|---|---|
| | OxyFast | Sol: 20mg/mL | | | 5mg q6h prn for pain. | | Relief of moderate to moderately severe pain. | |
| | OxyIR | Cap, IR 5mg | | | 5mg q6h prn.. | | | |
| | Roxicodone | Sol: 5mg/5mL; Liq: 20mg/mL; Tab: 5mg,15mg, 30mg | | | Tab: 15mg q4-6h prn; Sol/ Liq: 10-30mg q4h prn. | | | |
| Oxycodone/ Acetaminophen | Percocet | Tab: 2.5mg/325mg, 5mg/325mg, 7.5mg/325mg 7.5mg/500mg, 10mg/325mg,10mg/650mg | | | (2.5/325): 1-2 tabs q6h.<br>(5/325): 1 tab q6h prn.<br>(7.5/500): 1 tab q6h prn.<br>(10-650) 1 tab q6h prn.<br>(7.5/325): 1 tab q6h prn.<br>(10/325): 1 tab q6h prn. | (2.5/325): 12 tabs/day.<br>(5/325):12 tabs/day.<br>(7.5/500): 8 tabs/day.<br>(10-650) 6 tabs/day.<br>(7.5/325):8 tabs/day.<br>(10/325): 6 tabs/day. | Relief of moderate to moderately severe pain. | Schedule II |
| | Tylox | Cap: 5mg/500mg | | | 1 cap q6h prn. | | | |
| Oxycodone/Ibuprofen | Combunox | Tab: 5mg/400mg | | | 1 tab/dose. | 4 tabs/day for 7 days. | Short term (<7 days) management of acute, moderate to severe pain. | Schedule II |
| Oxycodone HCl/ Aspirin | Percodan | Tab: 4.8355mg/325mg | | | 1 tab q6h prn | 12 tabs/day or ASA 4g/day. | Relief of moderate to moderately severe pain. | Schedule II |
| Meperidine HCl | Demerol | Syr: 50mg/5mL; Tab: 50mg; Inj: 25mg/mL, 50mg/mL, 75mg/mL, 100mg/mL | 300mg. | 75mg. | Tab: 50-150mg q3-4h prn. Inj: 50-150mg IM/SC q3-4h prn. | | Moderate to severe pain. Inj: also for preoperative medication, anesthesia support, and obstetrical analgesia. | Schedule II |
| Propoxyphene HCl | Darvon | Cap: 65mg | | | 65mg q4h prn. | 390mg/day. | Relief of mild to moderate pain. | Schedule IV |
| Propoxyphene napsylate | Darvon-N | Tab: 100mg | | | 100mg q4h prn. | 600mg/day. | Relief of mild to moderate pain. | Schedule IV |
| Propoxyphene HCl/ Aspirin/Caffeine | Darvon Compound-65 | Cap: 65mg/389mg/32.4mg | | | 1 cap q4h prn. | 6 caps/day. | Relief of mild to moderate pain. | Schedule IV |

*(Continued)*

| GENERIC | BRAND | DOSAGE FORMS | ORAL EQUI-ANALGESIC DOSE | EQUI-ANALGESIC DOSE | USUAL ADULT DOSE | MAX DOSE | INDICATION | DEA SCHEDULE |
|---|---|---|---|---|---|---|---|---|
| Propoxyphene napsylate/ Acetaminophen | Darvocet-N 50 | Tab: 50mg/325mg | | | 100mg propoxyphene napsylate/650mg APAP q4h prn. | 600mg propoxyphene napsylate/day. Acetaminophen: 4g/day. | Relief of mild to moderate pain. | Schedule IV |
| | Darvocet-N 100 | Tab: 100mg/650mg | | | | | | |
| Tramadol | Ultram | Tab: 50mg; Tab, ER: 100mg, 200mg, 300mg | | | Tab: 50-100mg q4-6h prn. Tab, ER: 100mg/day. Titrate: 100mg q 5 days. | Tab: 400mg/day. Tab, ER: 300mg/day. | Management of moderate to moderately severe pain. | Rx only |
| Morphine sulfate | Astramorph PF | Inj: 0.5mg/mL, 1mg/mL | 40-60mg. | 10mg. | IV: 2-10mg/70kg of body weight. Epidural: 2-4mg/ 24 hrs. IT: 0.2-1mg/24 hrs. | | Management of pain where use of an opioid analgesic by PCA is appropriate. | Schedule II |
| | Duramorph | Inj: 0.5mg/mL, 1mg/mL | | | IV: 2-10mg/70kg of body weight. Epidural: 2-4mg/ 24 hrs. IT: 0.2-1mg/24 hrs. | | Management of pain where use of an opioid analgesic by PCA is appropriate. | |
| | Avinza | Cap, ER: 30mg, 60mg, 90mg, 120mg | | | 30mg q24h. | 1600mg/day. | Relief of moderate to severe pain requiring continuous opioid therapy for an extended period of time. | |
| | Kadian | Cap, ER: 10mg, 20mg, 30mg, 50mg, 60mg, 80mg, 100mg, 200mg | | | Give 50% of daily oral morphine dose q12h or give 100% oral morphine dose q24h. | Do not give more frequently than q12h. | Management of moderate to severe pain. | |
| | MS Contin | Tab, ER: 15mg, 30mg, 60mg, 100mg, 200mg | | | Give 50% of pts 24-hr requirement q12h or $^1/_3$ of pts 24-hr requirement q8h. | | Relief of moderate to severe pain for patients who require repeated dosing with potent opioid analgesics over periods of more than a few days. | |
| | Oramorph SR | Tab, ER: 15mg, 30mg, 60mg, 100mg | | | Single dose is 1/2 of daily morphine requirement q12h. | | Relief of pain in patients who require opioid analgesics for more than a few days. | |

| GENERIC | BRAND | DOSAGE FORMS | ORAL EQUI-ANALGESIC DOSE | EQUI-ANALGESIC DOSE | USUAL ADULT DOSE | MAX DOSE | INDICATION | DEA SCHEDULE |
|---|---|---|---|---|---|---|---|---|
| Hydromorphone HCl | Dilaudid, Dilaudid-HP | Tab: 8mg; Sol: 5mg/5mL; HP: 10mg/mL, 50mg/5mL, 500mg/50mL; Pow: 250mg | 6.5-7.5mg. | 1.3-2mg. | Tab: 2-4mg, PO every 4 to 6 hours. Sol: 2.5-10mL q3-6h as directed. HP: Individualized for each patient. | | Management of pain. (HP) Relief of moderate to severe pain in opioid-tolerant patients who require larger than usual doses of opioids to provide adequate pain relief. | Schedule II |
| Methadone HCl | Dolophine | Tab: 5mg, 10mg; Inj: 10mg/mL | 10-20mg. | 10mg. | Dolophine: 2.5mg to 10mg every 8 to 12 hrs, slowly titrated to effect. Detox: Titrate to a total daily dose of about 40mg in divided doses. Inj: 2.5-10mg q8-12h. Methadose: 2.5mg to 10mg every 3-4 hrs. | 21 days. May not repeat earlier than 4 weeks after completing previous course. | Detoxification and temporary maintenance treatment of narcotic addiction (heroin or other morphine-like drugs). Relief of severe pain. | Schedule II |
| | Methadose | Concentrate: 10mg/mL; Tab: 5mg, 10mg; Tab, Dispersible: 40mg | | | | | | |
| Fentanyl | Duragesic | Patch: 12.5mcg/hr, 25mcg/hr, 50mcg/hr, 75mcg/hr, 100mcg/hr | | | Initial: 25mcg/hr for 72 hrs. Individualize dose. | | Management of moderate to severe chronic pain when continuous opioid analgesia is required and cannot be managed by lesser means. | Schedule II |
| Fentanyl citrate | Actiq | Loz: 200mcg, 400mcg, 600mcg, 800mcg, 1200mcg, 1600mcg | 1000mcg/hr. | 0.1mg. | Six 200mcg units. Individually titrate. | 4 units/day. | Management of breakthrough cancer pain in patients with malignancies who are already receiving and are tolerant to opioid therapy for their underlying persistent cancer pain. | Schedule II |
| | Fentora | Tab, Buccal: 100mcg, 200mcg, 400mcg, 600mcg, 800mcg | | | Initial:100mcg. | Not more than 4 tabs simultaneously. | Management of breakthrough pain in patients with cancer who are already receiving and who are tolerant to opioid therapy for their underlying persistent cancer pain. | |

# ORAL ANTICONVULSANTS

| DRUG (BRAND) | INDICATIONS | USUAL ADULT DOSE* | THERAPEUTIC SERUM LEVELS |
|---|---|---|---|
| **BARBITURATES** | | | |
| **Phenobarbital** | Cortical focal, tonic-clonic | 60-250mg/day | 10-40mcg/mL |
| **Primidone** (Mysoline) | Tonic-clonic, psychomotor, focal | 750-2000mg/day | 5-12mcg/mL |
| **BENZODIAZEPINES** | | | |
| **Clonazepam** (Klonopin) | Absence, myoclonic, akinetic, Lennox-Gastaut syndrome | 1.5-20mg/day | NA |
| **Clorazepate dipotassium** (Tranxene-SD) | Partial | 22.5-90mg/day | NA |
| **Diazepam** (Valium) | Convulsive disorders, all forms | 4-40mg/day | NA |
| **HYDANTOIN** | | | |
| **Phenytoin** (Dilantin, Phenytek) | Tonic-clonic, psychomotor | 300-600mg/day | 10-20mcg/mL |
| **SUCCINIMIDES** | | | |
| **Ethosuximide** (Zarontin) | Absence | 20-30mg/kg/day | 40-100mcg/mL |
| **Methsuximide** (Celontin) | Absence | 300-1200mg/day | 10-40mcg/mL |
| **Zonisamide** (Zonegran) | Partial | 100-400mg/day | NA |
| **MISCELLANEOUS** | | | |
| **Carbamazepine** (Carbatrol, Tegretol) | Tonic-clonic, mixed, psychomotor | 800-1200mg/day | 4-12mcg/mL |
| **Divalproex sodium** (Depakote, Depakote ER) **Valproic acid** (Depakene) | Absence, partial | 10-60mg/kg/day | 50-100mcg/mL |
| **Felbamate** (Felbatol) | Partial (adults), partial/generalized with Lennox-Gastaut syndrome (pediatrics) | 2400mg/day | NA |
| **Gabapentin** (Neurontin) | Partial with and without secondary generalization (adults), partial (pediatrics) | 900-1800mg/day | NA |
| **Lamotrigine** (Lamictal) | Partial (adults), partial/generalized with Lennox-Gastaut syndrome (pediatrics) | 100-400mg/day | NA |
| **Levetiracetam** (Keppra) | Partial | 1000-3000mg/day | NA |
| **Oxcarbazepine** (Trileptal) | Partial | 600-2400mg/day | NA |
| **Pregabalin** (Lyrica) | Partial | 150-600mg/day | NA |
| **Tiagabine** (Gabitril) | Partial | 32-56mg/day | NA |
| **Topiramate** (Topamax) | Partial, tonic-clonic, Lennox-Gastaut syndrome (pediatrics) | 200-400mg/day | NA |

*Please refer to complete monograph for pediatric dosing. NA = Not Available.

# ORAL NARCOTIC ANALGESICS

| DRUG | BRAND | FORMULATION | STRENGTH | FREQUENCY* |
|---|---|---|---|---|
| **SINGLE-SOURCE PRODUCTS** | | | | |
| Butorphanol tartrate | Stadol NS | Nasal Spray | 10mg/mL | 3 to 4 hours |
| Codeine sulfate | | Tablet | 15mg, 30mg, 60mg | 4 to 6 hours |
| Fentanyl | Duragesic | Patch | 12.5mcg/hr, 25mcg/hr, 50mcg/hr, 75mcg/hr, 100mcg/hr | 72 hours |
| Fentanyl citrate | Actiq | Lozenge | 0.2mg, 0.4mg, 0.6mg, 0.8mg, 1.2mg, 1.6mg | 15 minutes (Max: 2 doses) |
| | Fentora | Tablet, Buccal | 100mcg, 200mcg, 300mcg, 400mcg, 600mcg, 800mcg | 30 minutes (Max: 4 tabs/dose) |
| Hydromorphone HCl** | Dilaudid | Solution | 1mg/mL | 3 to 6 hours |
| | | Suppository | 3mg | 6 to 8 hours |
| | | Tablet | 2mg, 4mg, 8mg | 4 to 6 hours |
| Meperidine HCl** | Demerol | Syrup | 50mg/5mL | 3 to 4 hours |
| | | Tablet | 50mg, 100mg | 3 to 4 hours |
| Methadone HCl | Methadose | Tablet | 5mg, 10mg, 40mg | 3 to 4 hours |
| Morphine sulfate** | Avinza | Capsule, Extended-Release | 30mg, 60mg, 90mg, 120mg | 24 hours |
| | Kadian | Capsule, Extended-Release | 10mg, 20mg, 30mg, 50mg, 60mg, 80mg, 100mg, 200mg | 12 or 24 hours |
| | MS Contin | Tablet, Extended-Release | 15mg, 30mg, 60mg, 100mg, 200mg | 12 hours |
| | MSIR | Capsule, Tablet | 15mg, 30mg | 4 hours |
| | | Solution | 10mg/5mL | 4 hours |
| | | Solution, Conc. | 20mg/mL | 4 hours |
| | Oramorph SR | Tablet, Extended-Release | 15mg, 30mg, 60mg, 100mg | 12 hours |
| Oxycodone HCl | OxyContin | Tablet, Extended-Release | 10mg, 15mg, 20mg, 30mg, 40mg, 60mg, 80mg | 12 hours |
| | OxyFast | Solution | 20mg/mL | 6 hours |
| | OxyIR | Capsule | 5mg | 6 hours |
| | Percolone | Tablet | 5mg | 4 hours |
| | Roxicodone | Solution | 5mg/5mL | 4 to 6 hours |
| | | Solution (Intensol) | 20mg/mL | 4 to 6 hours |
| | | Tablet | 5mg, 15mg, 30mg | 4 to 6 hours |
| Propoxyphene HCl | Darvon | Capsule | 65mg | 4 hours |
| Propoxyphene napsylate | Darvon-N | Tablet | 100mg | 4 hours |
| **MULTI-SOURCE PRODUCTS** | | | | |
| Aspirin/Codeine | | Tablet | 325mg/30mg, 325mg/60mg | 4 hours |
| Codeine phosphate/ Acetaminophen | Tylenol w/Codeine | Elixir | 12mg-120mg/5mL | 4 hours |
| | Tylenol #3 | Tablet | 30mg/300mg | 4 hours |
| | Tylenol #4 | Tablet | 60mg/300mg | 4 hours |
| Dihydrocodeine/Aspirin/ Caffeine | Synalgos DC | Capsule | 16mg/356.4mg/30mg | 4 hours |
| Hydrocodone bitartrate/ Acetaminophen | Lorcet-HD | Capsule | 5mg/500mg | 4 to 6 hours |
| | Lorcet Plus | Tablet | 7.5mg/650mg | 4 to 6 hours |
| | Lorcet 10/650 | Tablet | 10mg/650mg | 4 to 6 hours |

*(Continued)*

| DRUG | BRAND | FORMULATION | STRENGTH | FREQUENCY* |
|---|---|---|---|---|
| **MULTI-SOURCE PRODUCTS** *(Continued)* | | | | |
| Hydrocodone bitartrate/ Acetaminophen | Lortab Elixir | Solution | 7.5mg-500mg/15mL | 4 to 6 hours |
| | Lortab 2.5/500 | Tablet | 2.5mg/500mg | 4 to 6 hours |
| | Lortab 5/500 | Tablet | 5mg/500mg | 4 to 6 hours |
| | Lortab 7.5/500 | Tablet | 7.5mg/500mg | 4 to 6 hours |
| | Lortab 10/500 | Tablet | 10mg/500mg | 4 to 6 hours |
| | Norco 5/325 | Tablet | 5mg/325mg | 4 to 6 hours |
| | Norco 7.5/325 | Tablet | 7.5mg/325mg | 4 to 6 hours |
| | Norco 10/325 | Tablet | 10mg/325mg | 4 to 6 hours |
| | Vicodin | Tablet | 5mg/500mg | 4 to 6 hours |
| | Vicodin ES | Tablet | 7.5mg/500mg | 4 to 6 hours |
| | Vicodin HP | Tablet | 10mg/660mg | 4 to 6 hours |
| | Zydone 5/400 | Tablet | 5mg/400mg | 4 to 6 hours |
| | Zydone 7.5/400 | Tablet | 7.5mg/400mg | 4 to 6 hours |
| | Zydone 10/400 | Tablet | 10mg/400mg | 4 to 6 hours |
| Hydrocodone bitartrate/ Ibuprofen | Vicoprofen | Tablet | 7.5mg/200mg | 4 to 6 hours |
| Oxycodone/ Acetaminophen | Percocet 2.5/325 | Tablet | 2.5mg/325mg | 6 hours |
| | Percocet 5/325 | Tablet | 5mg/325mg | 6 hours |
| | Percocet 7.5/325 | Tablet | 7.5mg/325mg | 6 hours |
| | Percocet 7.5/500 | Tablet | 7.5mg/500mg | 6 hours |
| | Percocet 10/325 | Tablet | 10mg/325mg | 6 hours |
| | Percocet 10/650 | Tablet | 10mg/650mg | 6 hours |
| | Tylox | Capsule | 5mg/500mg | 6 hours |
| Oxycodone/ Ibuprofen | Combunox | Tablet | 5mg/400mg | 24 hours |
| Oxycodone (HCl/ Terephthalate)/Aspirin | Percodan | Tablet | 4.5mg/0.38mg/325mg | 6 hours |
| Pentazocine/ Acetaminophen | Talacen | Tablet | 25mg/650mg | 4 hours |
| Pentazocine HCl/ Naloxone | Talwin NX | Tablet | 50mg/0.5mg | 3 to 4 hours |
| Propoxyphene HCl/ Aspirin/Caffeine | Darvon Compound-65 | Capsule | 65mg/389mg/32.4mg | 4 hours |
| Propoxyphene napsylate/ Acetaminophen | Darvocet-N 50 | Tablet | 50mg/325mg | 4 hours |
| | Darvocet-N 100 | Tablet | 100mg/650mg | 4 hours |

*Usual dosage interval.
**Injection formulation available.

# TRIPTANS FOR ACUTE MIGRAINE

| DRUG | BRAND | HOW SUPPLIED | INITIAL & (MAX) DOSE* | HEPATIC/RENAL DOSE ADJUSTMENT* |
|---|---|---|---|---|
| Almotriptan malate | Axert | Tab: 6.25mg, 12.5mg | 6.25-12.5mg. May repeat after 2 hours. (2 doses/24 hours) | Initial: 6.25mg. Max: 12.5mg/24 hours. |
| Eletriptan hydrobromide | Relpax | Tab: 20mg, 40mg | 20-40mg. May repeat after 2 hours. (40mg/dose or 80mg/day) | Severe Hepatic Impairment: Avoid use. |
| Frovatriptan succinate | Frova | Tab: 2.5mg | 2.5mg. May repeat after 2 hours. (7.5mg/day) | No adjustment. |
| Naratriptan hydrochloride | Amerge | Tab: 1mg, 2.5mg | 1-2.5mg. May repeat after 4 hours. (5mg/24 hours) | Severe Renal/Hepatic Impairment: Avoid use. Mild-Moderate Renal/Hepatic Impairment: Use lower dose. Max: 2.5mg/24 hours. |
| Rizatriptan benzoate | Maxalt | Tab: 5mg, 10mg | 5-10mg. May repeat after 2 hours. (30mg/24 hours) | No adjustment. |
| | Maxalt MLT | Tab, Disintegrating: 5mg, 10mg | 5-10mg. May repeat after 2 hours. (30mg/24 hours) | No adjustment. |
| Sumatriptan | Imitrex | Inj**: 6mg/0.5mL | 6mg SQ. May repeat after 1 hour. (12mg/24 hours) | Severe Hepatic Impairment: Avoid use. |
| | | Nasal Spray: 5mg, 20mg | 5mg, 10mg, or 20mg. May repeat after 2 hours. (40mg/24 hours) | Severe Hepatic Impairment: Avoid use. |
| | | Tab: 25mg, 50mg, 100mg | 25-100mg. May repeat after 2 hours. (200mg/24 hours) | Severe Hepatic Impairment: Avoid use. Hepatic Disease: Max: 50mg/single dose. |
| Zolmitriptan | Zomig | Nasal Spray: 5mg | 5mg. May repeat after 2 hours. (10mg/24 hours) | Hepatic Impairment: Use lower dose. |
| | | Tab: 2.5mg, 5mg | 2.5mg or lower. May repeat after 2 hours. (10mg/24 hours) | Hepatic Impairment: Use lower dose. |
| | Zomig-ZMT | Tab, Disintegrating: 2.5mg, 5mg | 2.5mg or lower. May repeat after 2 hours. (10mg/24 hours) | Hepatic Impairment: Use lower dose. |

* Dosages shown are for adults ≥18 yrs. For more detailed information, refer to the individual monograph listings or the drug's FDA-approved labeling.

** Also indicated for acute treatment of cluster headaches.

# ANTIDEPRESSANTS

| DRUG (BRAND) | HOW SUPPLIED | DAILY DOSE Initial (I), Usual (U), Max (M) | TITRATE |
|---|---|---|---|
| **AMINOKETONE** | | | |
| **Bupropion** (Wellbutrin) | **Tab:** 75mg, 100mg | **(I)**200mg **(U)**300mg **(M)**450mg | Increase by 100mg/d q3d. |
| (Wellbutrin SR) | **Tab, SR:** 100mg, 150mg, 200mg | **(I)**150mg **(U)**300mg **(M)**400mg | Increase by 150mg/d q4d. |
| (Wellbutrin XL) | **Tab, ER:** 150mg, 300mg | **(I)**150mg **(U)**300mg **(M)**450mg | Increase by 150mg/d q4d. |
| **MONOAMINE OXIDASE INHIBITORS** | | | |
| **Phenelzine** (Nardil) | **Tab:** 15mg | **(I)**45mg **(U)**15mg qd or qod | Increase rapidly to 60-90mg/d then decrease to maintenance dose. |
| **Tranylcypromine** (Parnate) | **Tab:** 10mg | **(I,U)**30mg **(M)**60mg | Increase by 10mg/d q1-3 weeks. |
| **PHENYLETHYLAMINE** | | | |
| **Venlafaxine** (Effexor) | **Tab:** 25mg*, 37.5mg*, 50mg*, 75mg*, 100mg* | **(I)**75mg **(U)**150-225mg **(M)**375mg | Increase by 75mg/d q4d. |
| (Effexor XR) | **Cap, ER:** 37.5mg, 75mg, 150mg | **(I)**37.5-75mg **(U)**75-225mg **(M)**225mg | Increase by 75mg/d q4d. |
| **PHENYLPIPERAZINE** | | | |
| **Nefazodone** | **Tab:** 50mg, 100mg*, 150mg*, 200mg, 250mg | **(I)**200mg **(U)**300-600mg **(M)**600mg | Increase by 100-200mg/d in no less than 1 week. |
| **SELECTIVE SEROTONIN NOREPINEPHRINE REUPTAKE INHIBITOR** | | | |
| **Duloxetine** (Cymbalta) | **Cap:** 20mg, 30mg, 60mg | **(I,U)**40-60mg **(M)**60mg | N/A |
| **SELECTIVE SEROTONIN REUPTAKE INHIBITORS** | | | |
| **Citalopram** (Celexa) | **Sol:** 10mg/5mL; **Tab:** 10mg, 20mg*, 40mg* | **(I)**20mg **(U)**40mg **(M)**60mg | Increase by 20mg/d q week. |
| **Escitalopram** (Lexapro) | **Sol:** 5mg/5mL; **Tab:** 5mg, 10mg*, 20mg* | **(I)**10mg **(U)**10-20mg | Increase to 20mg/d after 1 week. |
| **Fluoxetine** (Prozac) | **Cap:** 10mg, 20mg, 40mg; **Sol:** 20mg/5mL; **Tab:** 10mg* | **(I)**20mg **(M)**80mg | Consider after several weeks of therapy. |
| **Paroxetine** (Paxil) | **Sus:** 10mg/5mL; **Tab:** 10mg*, 20mg*, 30mg, 40mg | **(I)**20mg **(M)**50mg | Increase by 10mg/d. |
| (Paxil CR) | **Tab, CR:** 12.5mg, 25mg, 37.5mg | **(I)**25mg **(M)**62.5mg | Increase by 12.5mg/d. |
| **Sertraline** (Zoloft) | **Sol:** 20mg/mL; **Tab:** 25mg*, 50mg*, 100mg* | **(I)**50mg **(M)**200mg | Increase at 1-week intervals. |
| **TETRACYCLIC** | | | |
| **Mirtazapine** (Remeron) | **Tab:** 15mg*, 30mg*, 45mg; **Tab, Disintegrating:** 15mg, 30mg, 45mg | **(I)**15mg **(M)**45mg | Increase q 1-2 weeks. |
| **TRIAZOLOPYRIDINE** | | | |
| **Trazodone** (Desyrel) | **Tab:** 50mg*, 100mg*, 150mg*, 300mg* | **(I)**150mg **(M)**400-600mg | Increase by 50mg/d q3-4d. |
| **TRICYCLICS** | | | |
| **Amitriptyline** | **Inj:** 10mg/mL; **Tab:** 10mg, 25mg, 50mg, 75mg, 100mg, 150mg | **(I)**OP: 50-100mg, IP: 100mg **(U)**50-100mg **(M)**OP: 150mg, IP: 300mg | OP: Increase by 25-50mg/d. IP: Increase to 200mg/d. |

*(Continued)*

| DRUG (BRAND) | HOW SUPPLIED | DAILY DOSE Initial (I), Usual (U), Max (M) | TITRATE |
|---|---|---|---|
| **TRICYCLICS** *(Continued)* | | | |
| **Amoxapine** | **Tab:** 25mg*, 50mg*, 100mg*, 150mg* | **(I)**100-150mg **(U)**200-300mg **(M)**OP: 400mg IP: 600mg | Increase to 100mg bid-tid by end of first week. |
| **Clomipramine** (Anafranil) | **Cap:** 25mg, 50mg, 75mg | **(I)**25mg **(U)**100-250mg **(M)**250mg | Increase to 100mg/d in 2 weeks, then increase gradually. |
| **Desipramine** (Norpramin) | **Tab:** 10mg, 25mg, 50mg, 75mg, 100mg, 150mg | **(I,U)**100-200mg **(M)**300mg | N/A |
| **Doxepin** (Sinequan) | **Cap:** 10mg, 25mg, 50mg, 75mg, 100mg, 150mg; **Sol:** 10mg/mL | **(I)**75mg **(U)**75-150mg **(M)**300mg | Increase gradually. |
| **Imipramine** (Tofranil PM) | **Cap:** 75mg, 100mg, 125mg, 150mg | **(I)**OP: 75mg, IP: 100mg **(U)**75-150mg **(M)**OP: 200mg, IP: 250-300mg | OP: Increase to 150mg/d. IP: Increase to 200mg/d. |
| (Tofranil) | **Tab:** 10mg, 25mg, 50mg | **(I)**OP: 75mg, IP: 100mg **(U)**50-150mg **(M)**OP: 200mg, IP: 250-300mg | OP: Increase to 150mg/d. IP: Increase to 200mg/d. |
| **Nortriptyline** (Pamelor, Aventyl) | **Cap:** 10mg, 25mg, 50mg, 75mg; Sol:10mg/5mL | **(I,U)**75-100mg **(M)**150mg | N/A |
| **Protriptyline** (Vivactil) | **Tab:** 5mg, 10mg | **(U)**15-40mg **(M)**60mg | Titrate morning dose. |
| **Trimipramine** (Surmontil) | **Cap:** 25mg, 50mg, 100mg | **(I)**OP: 75mg, IP: 100mg **(U)**50-150mg, IP: 200mg **(M)**OP: 200mg, IP: 250-300mg | OP: Increase to 150mg/d. IP: Increase to 200mg/d. |

**Abbreviations:** IP=Inpatient; OP=Outpatient *Scored.

# ANTIPSYCHOTIC AGENTS

| DRUG (BRAND) | HOW SUPPLIED (mg)* | INITIAL & (MAX) DOSE** | USUAL DOSE RANGE** |
|---|---|---|---|
| **ATYPICAL** | | | |
| **Aripiprazole** (Abilify) | Tab: 5, 10, 15, 20, 30 | 10-15mg qd (30mg/day) | 10-15mg qd |
| **Clozapine** (Clozaril) | Tab: 12.5†, 25, 100 | 12.5mg qd-bid (900mg/day) | 100-900mg/day given tid |
| **Olanzapine** (Zyprexa, Zyprexa Zydis) | Tab: 2.5, 5, 7.5, 10, 15, 20<br>OTD: 5, 10, 15, 20 | Schizophrenia: 5-10mg qd<br>Bipolar Mania: 10-15mg qd<br>(20mg/day for both) | Schizophrenia: 10-15mg qd<br>Bipolar Mania: 5-20mg qd |
| (Zyprexa IntraMuscular) | Inj: 10mg | Agitation: 10mg IM (3 doses) | Agitation: 2.5-10mg IM |
| **Paliperidone** (Invega) | Tab, Extended-Release: 3mg, 6mg, 9mg | 6mg qd (12mg/day) | 3-12mg/day |
| **Quetiapine fumarate** (Seroquel) | Tab: 25, 100, 200, 300 | Schizophrenia: 25mg bid<br>Bipolar Mania: 50mg bid<br>(800mg/day for both) | Schizophrenia: 150-750mg/day<br>Bipolar Mania: 400-800mg/day |
| **Risperidone** (Risperdal) | Sol: 1mg/mL<br>Tab: 0.25, 0.5, 1, 2, 3, 4 | Schizophrenia: 1mg bid (16mg/day) | Schizophrenia: 4-8mg/day<br>Bipolar Mania: 1-6mg/day |
| (Risperdal M-Tab) | OTD: 0.5, 1, 2 (6mg/day) | Bipolar Mania: 2-3mg qd | |
| (Risperdal Consta) | Inj: 25, 37.5, 50 | Schizophrenia: 25mg IM | Schizophrenia: 25-50mg IM q2wks (50mg/dose) q2wks |
| **Ziprasidone HCl** (Geodon) | Cap: 20, 40, 60, 80 | 20mg bid (160mg/day) | 20-80mg bid |
| **Ziprasidone mesylate** (Geodon) for Injection) | Inj: 20mg/mL | 10mg IM q2h or 20mg IM q4h (40mg/day) | Switch to oral for long-term therapy |
| **CONVENTIONAL** | | | |
| **Chlorpromazine** | Tab: 10, 25, 50, 100, 200<br>Inj: 25mg/mL | 10-25mg PO bid-qid or 25mg IM (1000mg/day PO) | PO: 10-800mg/day<br>IM: 25-50mg IM q4-6h‡<br>Switch to PO when controlled |
| **Fluphenazine HCl** (Prolixin) | Elixir: 2.5mg/5mL<br>Sol, Conc: 5mg/mL<br>Tab: 1†, 5, 10<br>Inj: 2.5mg/mL | 2.5mg-10mg/day in divided doses (40mg/day)<br>1.25mg IM q6-8h (10mg/day) | 1-5mg qd |
| **Fluphenazine decanoate** (Prolixin Decanoate) | Inj: 25mg/mL | 12.5-25mg IM/SQ q4-6 wks (100mg/dose) | 2.5-10mg/day in divided doses |
| **Haloperidol** | Sol, Conc: 2mg/mL<br>Tab: 0.5, 1, 2, 5, 10, 20 | Moderate: 0.5-2mg bid-tid<br>Sev/Resist: 3-5mg bid-tid (100mg/day) | 2-20mg/day |
| **Haloperidol lactate** (Haldol) | Inj: 5mg/mL | 2-5mg IM q4-8h or hourly if needed (100mg/day) | Switch to PO 12-24 hours after last injection |
| **Haloperidol decanoate** (Haldol Decanoate) | Inj: 50mg/mL, 100mg/mL | 10-20x daily oral dose up to 100mg/dose (450mg/month) | 10-15x daily oral dose |
| **Loxapine succinate** (Loxitane) | Cap: 5, 10, 25, 50 | 10mg bid, up to 50mg/day (250mg/day) | 60-100mg/day |

*(Continued)*

| DRUG (BRAND) | HOW SUPPLIED (mg)* | INITIAL & (MAX) DOSE** | USUAL DOSE RANGE** |
|---|---|---|---|
| **CONVENTIONAL** *(Continued)* | | | |
| **Molindone** (Moban) | Tab: 5, 10, 25, 50, 100 | 50-75mg/day (225mg/day) | 5-25mg tid/qid |
| **Perphenazine** | Tab: 2, 4, 8, 16 | Non-hospitalized: 4-8mg tid<br>Hospitalized: 8-16mg (64mg/day) | Reduce dose as soon as possible to minimum effective dose. |
| **Prochlorperazine maleate** | Tab: 5, 10 | 5-10mg tid-qid | Moderate/Severe: 50-75mg/day<br>Severe: 100-150mg/day |
| **Thioridazine HCl** (Mellaril) | Sol, Conc: 30mg/mL, 100mg/mL.<br>Tab: 10†, 15, 25†, 50†, 100, 150†, 200 | 50-100mg tid (800mg/day) | 200-800mg/day given bid-qid |
| **Thiothixene** (Navane) | Cap: 2, 5, 10, 20 | Mild: 2mg tid<br>Severe: 5mg bid (60mg/day) | 20-30mg/day |
| **Trifluoperazine HCl** | Tab: 1, 2, 5, 10 | 2-5mg bid (40mg/day or higher if needed) | 15-20mg/day |

Note: This list is not inclusive of all antipsychotic agents. Indications may vary among the different products.

* Unless otherwise indicated.

** Doses shown are for adults. For pediatric dosing and additional information please refer to the individual monograph listings or the drug's FDA-approved labeling. Dosages need to be adjusted by titration to individual patient needs and may need to be reduced in the elderly, debilitated, or with renal/hepatic impairment. Periodically reassess to determine the need for maintenance treatment.

† Available only in generic forms.

‡ Severe cases may require up to 2g/day or 400mg/dose IM.

ODT - Orally disintegrating tablet.

# BIPOLAR DISORDER PHARMACOTHERAPY

| DRUG | BRAND | HOW SUPPLIED | USUAL DOSE | COMMENTS |
|---|---|---|---|---|
| **MOOD STABILIZER** | | | | |
| Lithium | Various | Cap: 150mg, 300mg, 600mg; Tab: 300mg; Tab, Extended-Release: 450mg | **Adults/Pediatrics: ≥12 yrs:** Acute Mania: 600mg tid to achieve effective serum levels of 1-1.5mEq/L; monitor levels twice a week until stabilized. Maintenance Therapy: 300mg tid-qid or (ER) 450mg bid to maintain serum levels of 0.6-1.2 mEq/L; monitor levels every 2 months. | Treatment of manic episodes of bipolar disorder and maintenance treatment of bipolar disorder. |
| **ANTICONVULSANTS** | | | | |
| Carbamazepine | Equetro | Cap, Extended-Release: 100mg, 200mg, 300mg | **Adults:** Initial: 400mg/day, given in divided doses, bid. Titrate: 200mg qd. **Max:**1600mg/day. Do not crush or chew. | Treatment of acute manic and mixed episodes associated with bipolar I disorder. |
| Divalproex sodium | Depakote ER | Tab, Extended-Release: 250mg, 500mg | **Adults:** Mania: Initial: 25mg/kg/day given once daily. Titrate: Increase dose rapidly to clinical effect. **Max:** 60mg/kg/day. Conversion from Depakote: Administer Depakote ER qd using a dose 8-20% higher than the total daily dose of Depakote. If cannot directly convert to Depakote ER, consider increasing to next higher Depakote total daily dose before converting to appropriate total daily Depakote ER dose. Elderly: Give lower initial dose and titrate slowly. Decrease dose or discontinue if decreased food or fluid intake or if excessive somnolence occurs. Swallow whole; do not crush or chew. | Acute manic or mixed episodes associated with bipolar disorder. |
| | Depakote | Tab, Delayed-Release: 125mg, 250mg, 500mg | **Adults:** Mania: 750mg daily in divided doses. Titrate: Increase dose rapidly to clinical effect. **Max:** 60mg/kg/day. Decrease dose or discontinue if decreased food or fluid intake or if excessive somnolence occurs. | Treatment of mania associated with bipolar disorder. |
| Lamotrigine | Lamictal | Tab: 25mg*, 100mg*, 150mg*, 200mg*; Tab, Chewable: (Lamictal CD) 2mg, 5mg, 25mg *scored | **Adults:** Bipolar Disorder: Patients not taking carbamazepine, other enzyme-inducing drugs (EIDs) or VPA: **Weeks 1 and 2:** 25mg qd. **Weeks 3 and 4:** 50mg 50mg qd. **Week 5:** 100mg qd. **Weeks 6 and 7:** 200mg qd. Patients taking VPA: **Weeks 1 and 2:** 25mg every other day. **Weeks 3 and 4:** 25mg qd. **Week 5:** 50mg qd. **Weeks 6 and 7:** 100mg qd. Patients taking carbamazepine (or other EIDs) and not taking VPA: **Weeks 1 and 2:** 50mg qd. **Weeks 3 and 4:** 100mg qd (divided doses). **Week 5:**200mg qd (divided doses). **Week 6:** 300mg qd (divided doses). **Week 7:** Up to 400mg qd (divided doses). After discontinuation of psychotropic drugs excluding VPA, carbamazepine, or other EIDs: Maintain current dose. After discontinuation of VPA and current lamotrigine dose of 100mg qd: **Week 1:** 150mg qd. Week 2 and onward: 200mg qd. After discontinuation of carbamazepine or other EIDs and current lamotrigine dose of 400mg qd: **Week 1:** 400mg qd. **Week 2:** 300mg qd. **Week 3 and onward:** 200mg | Maintenance treatment of bipolar I disorder to the delay the time to occurence of mood episodes (depression, mania, hypomania, mixed episodes) in patients treated for mood episodes with standard therapy. |

*(Continued)*

| DRUG | BRAND | HOW SUPPLIED | USUAL DOSE | COMMENTS |
|---|---|---|---|---|
| **CONVENTIONAL ANTIPSYCHOTIC** | | | | |
| Chlorpromazine HCl | **Thorazine** | Inj: 25mg/mL; Sup: 25mg, 100mg; Syrup: 10mg/5mL; Tab: 10mg, 50mg, 100mg, 200mg | **Adults:** Inpatient: Acute schizophrenic/ Manic state: 25mg IM, then 25-50mg IM in 1 hr if needed. Titrate: Increase over several days up to 400mg q4-6h until controlled then switch to PO. Usual: 500mg/day PO. **Max:** 1000mg/day PO. Less acutely disturbed: 25mg PO tid. Titrate: Increase gradually to 400mg/day. Outpatient: 10mg PO tid-qid or 25mg PO bid-tid. More Severe: 25mg PO tid. Titrate: After 1-2 days, increase by 20-50mg twice weekly until calm. Prompt control of severe symptoms: 25mg IM, may repeat in 1 hr then 25-50mg PO tid. | Control manifestations of manic type of manic-depressive illness. |
| **ATYPICAL ANTIPSYCHOTICS** | | | | |
| Aripiprazole | **Abilify** | Tab: 2mg, 5mg, 10mg, 15mg, 20mg, 30mg; Tab, Disintegrating: 10mg, 15mg Sol: 1mg/mL [50mL, 150mL, 480mL]. Inj: 7.5mg/mL | **Adults:** (PO) Bipolar Mania: Initial: 30mg qd. Titrate: May decrease to 15mg qd based on assessment and tolerability. Oral solution can be given on a mg-per-mg basis up to 25mg. Patients receiving 30mg tablets should receive 25mg of the solution. (Inj) Agitation: 9.75mg IM. Range: 5.25-15mg IM. **Max:** 30mg/ day; initiate PO therapy as soon as possible. Concomitant CYP3A4 inhibitors (eg, ketoconazole): Reduce usual aripiprazole dose by 50%. Concomitant CYP2D6 inhibitors (eg, quinidine, fluoxetine, paroxetine): Reduce usual aripiprazole dose by 50%. Concomitant CYP3A4 inducers (eg, carbamazepine): Double aripiprazole dose (to 20mg or 30mg). Periodically reassess for maintenance therapy. | (PO) Treatment of acute manic and mixed episodes associated with bipolar disorder. (Inj) Treatment of agitation associated with schizophrenia or bipolar disorder, manic or mixed. |
| Olanzapine | **Zyprexa, Zyprexa Zydis** | Inj: 10mg; Tab: 2.5mg, 5mg, 7.5mg, 10mg, 15mg, 20mg; Tab, Disintegrating: (Zydis) 5mg, 10mg, 15mg, 20mg | **Adults:** Bipolar Mania: Initial: 10-15mg qd. Titrate: Increase/decrease by5mg daily. **Max:** 20mg/day. With lithium or valproate: Initial/Usual: 10mg qd. Max: 20mg/day. Debilitated/ Hypotension risk/slow metabolizers/ sensitivity to olanzapine effects: Initial: 5mg qd. Titrate: Increase cautiously. (IM) Agitation: Initial: 10mg IM. Usual: 2.5-10mg IM. **Max:** 3 doses of 10mg q 2-4h. Elderly: 5mg IM. Debilitated/Hypotension risk/ sensitivity to olanzapine effects: 2.5mg IM. May initiate PO therapy when clinically appropriate. | Treatment of acute mixed or manic episodes in bipolar I disorder. (Inj only) Agitation associated with schizophrenia, bipolar I mania. |
| Olanzapine-fluoxetine | **Symbyax** | Cap: (Olanzapine-Fluoxetine): 6-25mg, 6-50mg, 12-25mg, 12-50mg | **Adults:** ≥18 yrs: Initial: 6-25mg cap qpm. Titrate: Adjust dose based on efficacy and tolerability. **Max:** 18mg/75mg. Hypotension risk /hepatic impairment/metabolizers: Initial: 6-25mg cap qpm. Titrate: Increase cautiously. Re-evaluate periodically. | Treatment of depressive episodes associated with bipolar disorder. |

*(Continued)*

| DRUG | BRAND | HOW SUPPLIED | USUAL DOSE | COMMENTS |
|---|---|---|---|---|
| **ATYPICAL ANTISPYCHOTICS** *(Continued)* | | | | |
| Quetiapine | **Seroquel** | Tab: 25mg, 50mg, 100mg, 200mg, 300mg, 400mg | **Adults:** Bipolar mania: monotherapy/adjunctive: Give bid. Initial: 100mg/day on Day 1. Titrate: Increase to 400mg/day on Day 4 in increments of up to 100mg/day in bid divided doses. Adjust doses up to 800mg/day by Day 6 in increments ≤200mg/day. **Max:** 800mg/day. Bipolar depressive episodes: Give once daily hs. Day 1: 50mg/day. Day 2: 100mg/day. Day 3: 200mg/day. Day 4: 300mg/day. Schizophrenia: Initial: 25mg bid. Titrate: Increase by 25-50mg bid-tid on the 2nd and 3rd day to 300-400mg/day given bid-tid by the 4th day. Adjust doses by 25-50mg bid at intervals of at least 2 days. Maint: Lowest effective dose. **Max:** 800mg/day. | Treatment of acute manic episodes associated with bipolar I disorder, as monotherapy or adjunct therapy to lithium or divalproex. Treatment of depressive episodes associated with bipolar disorder. |
| Risperidone | **Risperdal** | Sol: 1mg/mL [30mL]; Tab: 0.25mg, 0.5mg, 1mg, 2mg, 3mg, 4mg; Tab, Disintegrating: (M-Tab) 0.5mg, 1mg, 2mg, 3mg, 4mg | **Adults:** Bipolar mania: Initial: 2-3mg qd. Titrate: Increase/Decrease by 1mg qd. Usual: 1-6mg/day. **Max:** 6mg/day. | Short-term treatment of acute manic or mixed episodes associated with bipolar I disorder as monotherapy or with lithium or valproate. |
| Ziprasidone | **Geodon** | Cap: (HCl) 20mg, 40mg, 60mg, 80mg | **Adults:** Bipolar mania: Initial: 40mg bid with food. Titrate: Increase to 60-80mg bid on 2nd day of treatment. Maint: 40-80mg bid. | Treatment of acute manic or mixed episodes associated with bipolar disorder, with or without psychotic features. |

Source: FDA approved labeling.

# ASTHMA MANAGEMENT

| DRUG (BRAND) | DOSAGE FORM | ADULT DOSE | CHILD DOSE* |
|---|---|---|---|
| **SYSTEMIC CORTICOSTEROIDS** | | | |
| **Methylprednisolone** | Tab: 2, 4, 8, 16, 32mg | 7.5-60mg qd in a single dose or qod prn for control. Short course "burst": 40-60 mg/day as single dose or 2 divided doses for 3-10 days. | 0.25-2mg/kg qd in a single dose or qod prn for control. Short course "burst": 1-2mg/kg/day. Max: 60mg/day for 3-10 days. |
| **Prednisolone** | Tab: 5mg; Liq: 5mg/5mL, 15mg/5mL | | |
| **Prednisone** | Tab: 1, 2.5, 5, 10, 20, 50mg Liq: 5mg/mL, 5mg/5mL | | |
| **CROMOLYN & NEDOCROMIL** | | | |
| **Cromolyn** (Intal) | MDI: 800mcg/puff | 2 puffs qid | 1-2 puffs tid-qid |
| | Neb Sol: 20mg/ampule | 1 ampule tid-qid | 1 ampule tid-qid |
| **Nedocromil** (Tilade) | MDI: 1.75mg/puff | 2-4 puffs bid-qid | 1-2 puffs bid-qid |
| **LONG-ACTING BETA$_2$-AGONISTS** | | | |
| **Salmeterol** (Serevent) | MDI: 21mcg/puff | 2 puffs q 12 hours | 1-2 puffs q 12 hours |
| | DPI: 50mcg/blister | 1 blister q 12 hours | 1 blister q 12 hours |
| **Formoterol** (Foradil) | DPI: 12mcg | 1 cap q 12 hours | 1 cap q 12 hours |
| **COMBINATION AGENTS** | | | |
| **Fluticasone/ Salmeterol** (Advair) | DPI: 100, 250, 500mcg/50mcg | 1 puff bid | (100mcg/50mcg) 1 puff bid |
| **METHYLXANTHINE** | | | |
| **Theophylline** | Liquid, Capsules, Sustained-Release Tabs | Initial: 10mg/kg/day up to 300mg max. Usual Max: 800mg/day. | Initial: 10mg/kg/day. Usual Max: <1 yr: 0.2 x age in weeks + 5 = mg/kg/day. 1 yr: 16mg/kg/day. |
| **LEUKOTRIENE MODIFIERS** | | | |
| **Montelukast** (Singulair) | Tab: 10mg; Chewable: 4mg, 5mg | 10mg qhs | 2-5 yrs: 4mg qhs. 6-14 yrs: 5mg qhs. 15 yrs: 10mg qhs. |
| **Zafirlukast** (Accolate) | Tab: 10mg, 20mg | 20mg bid | ≥12 yrs: 20mg bid. 5-11 yrs: 10mg bid. |
| **Zileuton** (Zyflo) | Tab: 600mg | 600mg qid | ≥12 yr: 600mg qid |

**ESTIMATED COMPARATIVE DAILY DOSAGES FOR INHALED CORTICOSTEROIDS**

| | LOW DAILY DOSE | | MEDIUM DAILY DOSE | | HIGH DAILY DOSE | |
|---|---|---|---|---|---|---|
| DRUG | ADULT | CHILD* | ADULT | CHILD* | ADULT | CHILD* |
| **Beclomethasone HFA** 40, 80mcg/puff (QVAR) | 80-240mcg | 80-160mcg | 240-480mcg | 160-320mcg | >480mcg | >320mcg |
| **Budesonide DPI** 200mcg/inhalation (Pulmicort Turbuhaler) | 200-600mcg | 200-400mcg | 600-1200mcg | 400-800mcg | >1200mcg | >800mcg |
| **Budesonide Neb** Sol: 0.25, 0.5mg/2mL (Pulmicort Respules) | N/A | 0.5mg | N/A | 1.0mg | N/A | 2.0mg |
| **Flunisolide** 250mcg/puff (Aerobid) | 500-1000mcg | 500-750mcg | 1000-2000mcg | 1000-1250mcg | >2000mcg | >1250mcg |
| **Fluticasone MDI** 44, 110, or 220mcg/puff (Flovent) | 88-264mcg | 88-176mcg | 264-660mcg | 176-440mcg | >660mcg | >440mcg |
| **Triamcinolone acetonide** 100mcg/puff (Azmacort) | 400-1000mcg | 400-800mcg | 1000-2000mcg | 800-1200mcg | >2000mcg | >1200mcg |

*Children ≤12 yrs unless otherwise noted. MDI: metered-dose inhaler; DPI: dry powder inhaler.
Adopted from: The NAEPP Expert Panel Report: Guidelines for the Diagnosis and Management of Asthma–Update on Selected Topics 2002. http://www.nhlbi.nih.gov/guidelines/asthma/asthsumm.htm

# ASTHMA TREATMENT PLAN

| CLASSIFICATION | LUNG FUNCTION | STEPWISE APPROACH TO THERAPY IN PATIENTS OVER 5 YEARS OF AGE |
|---|---|---|
| **Mild intermittent**<br>• Symptoms ≤2 times a week<br>• Asymptomatic and normal PEF between exacerbations<br>• Brief exacerbations (from a few hours to a few days); intensity may vary<br>• Nighttime symptoms ≤twice/month | • $FEV_1$ or PEF ≥80% predicted<br>• PEF variability <20% | **Step 1**<br>• **No daily medication required.**<br>• **Short-acting inhaled $\beta_2$-agonists as needed (2-4 puffs prn).**<br>• Severe exacerbations may occur, separated by long periods of normal lung function and no symptoms; a course of systemic corticosteroids is recommended. |
| **Mild persistent**<br>• Symptoms >2 times a week but <1 time a day<br>• Exacerbations may affect activity<br>• Nighttime symptoms >twice/month | • $FEV_1$ or PEF ≥80% predicted<br>• PEF variability 20% to 30% | **Step 2**<br>• **Low-dose inhaled corticosteroids.**<br>• **Short-acting inhaled $\beta_2$-agonists as needed (2-4 puffs prn).**<br>ALTERNATIVE TREATMENT:<br>• Cromolyn, leukotriene modifier, nedocromil OR<br>• Sustained-release theophylline to serum concentration of 5 to 15mcg/mL. |
| **Moderate persistent**<br>• Daily symptoms<br>• Daily use of inhaled short-acting $\beta_2$-agonist<br>• Exacerbations affect activity<br>• Exacerbations ≥2 times a week; may last days<br>• Nighttime symptoms >once/week | • $FEV_1$ or PEF >60% to <80% predicted<br>• PEF variability >30% | **Step 3**<br>• **Low- to medium-dose inhaled corticosteroids**<br>AND<br>• **Long-acting inhaled $\beta_2$-agonists.**<br>• **Short-acting inhaled $\beta_2$-agonists as needed (2-4 puffs prn).**<br>ALTERNATIVE TREATMENT:<br>• Increase inhaled corticosteroids within medium-dose range OR<br>• Low- to medium-dose inhaled corticosteroids and either leukotriene modifier or theophylline.<br>IF NEEDED:<br>• Increase inhaled corticosteroids within medium-dose range, and add long-acting inhaled $\beta_2$-agonists.<br>ALTERNATIVE TREATMENT:<br>Increase inhaled corticosteroids in medium-dose range, and add either leukotriene modifier or theophylline. |
| **Severe persistent**<br>• Continual symptoms<br>• Limited physical activity<br>• Frequent exacerbations<br>• Nighttime symptoms are frequent | • $FEV_1$ or PEF ≤60% predicted<br>• PEF variability >30% | **Step 4**<br>• **High-dose inhaled corticosteroids**<br>AND<br>• **Long-acting inhaled $\beta_2$-agonists.**<br>• **Short-acting inhaled $\beta_2$-agonists as needed (2-4 puffs prn).**<br>AND, IF NEEDED:<br>• Long-term corticosteroid tablets or syrup (2mg/kg/day; Usual Max: 60mg/day). Make repeat attempts to reduce systemic corticosteroids and maintain control with high-dose inhaled corticosteroids. |

**Note: Preferred treatments are in bold.**

**Key Points:**

- Stepwise approach presents general guidelines. Review treatment every 1 to 6 months; a gradual stepwise reduction in treatment may be possible. If control is not maintained, consider step up.
- The presence of one of the features of severity is sufficient to place a patient in that category. An individual should be assigned to the most severe grade in which any feature occurs (PEF is % of personal best; FEV is % predicted).
- Intensity of treatment will depend on severity of exacerbation; up to 3 treatments at 20-minute intervals or a single nebulizer treatment as needed. Course of systemic corticosteroids may be needed.
- Use of short-acting beta$_2$-agonists on a daily basis, or increasing use, indicates the need to initiate or increase long-term control therapy.
- Airflow obstruction is indicated by reduced $FEV_1$ and $FEV_1$/FVC values relative to reference or predicted values.
- Abnormalities of lung function are categorized as restrictive and obstructive defects. A reduced ratio of $FEV_1$/FVC (eg, <65%) indicates obstruction to the flow of air from the lungs, whereas a reduced FVC with a normal $FEV_1$/FVC ratio suggests a restrictive pattern.

**Abbreviations:** $FEV_1$: Forced expiratory volume in one second. FVC: Forced vital capacity.

*Adapted from the *1997 Guidelines for the Diagnosis and Management of Asthma* and the *Update on Selected Topics 2002*. Executive Summary of the NAEPP Expert Panel Report II.

# ANKYLOSING SPONDYLITIS AGENTS

| DRUG (BRAND) | HOW SUPPLIED | USUAL DOSE RANGE | MAX DOSE |
|---|---|---|---|
| **COX-2 INHIBITOR** | | | |
| **Celecoxib** (Celebrex) | Cap: 100mg, 200mg, 400mg | 200mg qd or 100mg bid. | 400mg/day with food. |
| **MONOCLONAL ANTIBODIES** | | | |
| **Infliximab** (Remicade) | Inj: 100mg | 5mg/kg as IV infusion repeat at 2 and 6 wks. | 20mg/kg. |
| **Adalimumab** (Humira) | Inj: 40mg/0.8mL | 40mg SQ every other wk. | n/a |
| **NSAIDs** | | | |
| **Sulindac** (Clinoril) | Tab: 150mg, 200mg* | 150mg bid with food. | 400mg/day with food. |
| **Diclofenac Potassium** (Cataflam) | Tab: 50mg | 50mg tid-qid. | 200mg/day. |
| **Diclofenac Sodium** (Voltaren) | Tab, Delayed-Release: 25mg, 50mg, 75mg | 25mg qid and 25mg qhs prn. | 200mg/day. |
| **Indomethacin** (Indocin) | Cap: 25mg, 50mg; Sus: 25mg/5mL [237mL] | 25mg PO bid-tid. | 200mg/day. |
| **Naproxen** (EC-Naprosyn, Naprosyn) | Sus: 25mg/mL; Tab: 250mg, 375mg, 500mg; Tab, Delayed-Release: 375mg, 500mg | 250mg, 375mg, or 500mg bid; 375mg or 500mg bid. | 1500mg/day. |
| **Naproxen sodium** (Anaprox) | Tab: 275mg | 750mg-1g qd; 275mg bid or 550mg bid. | 1650mg/day. |
| (Anaprox DS) | Tab: 550mg* | 750mg-1g qd; 275mg bid or 550mg bid. | 1g/day. |
| (Naprelan) | Tab, Extended-Release: 375mg, 500mg | 750mg-1g qd; 275mg bid or 550mg bid. | 1g/day. |
| **SALICYLATE** | | | |
| **Aspirin** (Genuine Bayer Aspirin, Bayer Extra Strength) | Tab: 325mg; Tab, Extra-Strength: 500mg | Up to 4g/day in divided doses. | 4g/day. |
| (Ecotrin) | Tab, Delayed-Release: 81mg, 325mg, 500mg | Up to 4g/day in divided doses. | 4g/day. |
| **TNF-RECEPTOR BLOCKER** | | | |
| **Etanercept** (Enbrel) | Inj: 25mg [vial], 50mg/mL [syringe] | 50mg SQ per wk, given as one SQ injection. | 50mg/wk. |

*Scored.

# GOUT AGENTS

| DRUG (BRAND) | HOW SUPPLIED | USUAL DOSE RANGE | MAX DOSE |
|---|---|---|---|
| **ALKALINIZING AGENT** | | | |
| **Citric acid/ Potassium citrate** (Polycitra) | Packet: 1002mg-3300mg/pack [100S]; Sol: (Citric Acid-Potassium Citrate) 334mg-550mg/5mL [480mL] | 15mL or 1 packet qid, pc and hs. Dilute in 6 oz of water or juice. | |
| **CORTICOSTEROID** | | | |
| **Hydocortisone acetate** | Inj: 25mg/mL | **Large joints:** 25-37.5mg. **Small joints:** 10-25mg. **Bursae:** 25-37.5mg. **Tendon Sheaths:** 5-12.5mg. **Soft Tissue Infiltration:** 25-50mg. **Ganglia:** 12.5-25mg. | 50mg/injection. |
| **NSAIDs** | | | |
| **Indomethacin** (Indocin) | Cap: 25mg, 50mg; Sus: 25mg/5mL [237mL] | **Acute Gout:** 50mg PO tid until pain is tolerable, then d/c. | |
| **Naproxen** (Anaprox DS) | Tab: 275mg; 550mg* | **Acute Gout:** 825mg followed by 275mg q8h. | |
| (Naprelan) | Tab, Extended-Release: 375mg, 500mg | **Acute Gout:** 1-1.5g qd x 1 day, then 1g qd until attack subsides. | 1g/day. |
| (Naprosyn) | Sus: 25mg/mL; Tab: 250mg*, 375mg, 500mg*; Tab, Delayed-Release: (EC-Naprosyn) 375mg, 500mg | **Acute Gout:** 750mg followed by 250mg q8h until attack subsides. | 1500mg/day. |
| **PHENANTHRENE DERIVATIVE** | | | |
| **Colchicine** | Inj: 0.5mg/mL; Tab: 0.6mg | **Acute Gout:** 1-1.2mg, then 0.5-0.6mg/hr until pain relief or diarrhea ensues (wait 3 days between courses). **Prophylaxis:** <1 attack/yr: 0.5-0.6mg/day given 3-4x/wk. >1 attack/yr: 0.5-0.6mg qd. | 4-8mg/acute attack. |
| **URICOSURIC AGENTS** | | | |
| **Probenecid** | Tab: 500mg | **Initial:** 250mg bid x 1 wk. **Titrate:** Increase by 500mg every 4 wks. **Maint:** 500mg bid. | 2g/day. |
| **Sulfinpyrazone** | Tab: 100mg, 200mg | **Initial:** 100-200mg bid x 1 wk. **Maint:** 200mg bid, increase to 300mg if needed. | 800mg/day. |
| **XANTHINE OXIDASE INHIBITOR** | | | |
| **Allopurinol** (Zyloprim) | Tab: 100mg*, 300mg* | **Mild Gout:** Usual: 200-300mg/day. **Moderately-Severe Gout:** Usual: 400-600mg/day. | 800mg/day. |
| **COMBINATION** | | | |
| **Colchicine/ Probenecid** | Tab: (Colchicine-Probenecid) 0.5mg-500mg | 1 tab qd x 1 wk, then 1 tab bid. **Titrate:** May increase by 1 tab/day every 4 wks. | 4 tabs/day. |

*Scored.

# OSTEOARTHRITIS AGENTS

| DRUG (BRAND) | HOW SUPPLIED | USUAL DOSE RANGE | MAX DOSE |
|---|---|---|---|
| **NSAIDs** | | | |
| **Diclofenac sodium** (Voltaren) | Tab, Delayed-Release: 25mg, 50mg, 75mg; | 50mg bid-tid or 75mg bid 100mg qd. | 150mg/day. |
| (Voltaren-XR) | Tab, Delayed-Release: 100mg | 50mg bid-tid or 75mg bid 100mg qd. | 150mg/day. |
| **Etodolac** | Cap: 300mg, 400mg, 500mg | 300mg bid-tid or 400-500mg bid. | 1000mg/day. |
| **Flurbiprofen** (Ansaid) | Tab: 50mg, 100mg | 200-300mg/day given bid, tid or qid. | 300mg/day or 100mg/dose. |
| **Ketoprofen** (Oruvail) | Cap, Extended-Release: 200mg | 200mg qd. | 200mg/day. |
| **Ibuprofen** (Motrin, Motrin IB) | Sus: 100mg/5mL [120mL, 480mL]; Tab: 400mg, 600mg, 800mg Tab: 200mg | 300mg qid or 400mg, 600mg or 800mg tid-qid. (Motrin IB) 200mg q4-6h. 400mg with meals/milk. | 3200mg/day. 1200mg/day. (Motrin IB) |
| **Meloxicam** (Mobic) | Sus: 7.5mg/5mL Tab: 7.5mg, 15mg | 7.5mg qd. | 15mg/day. |
| **Nabumetone** (Relafen) | Tab: 500mg, 750mg | 1000mg qd. | 2000mg/day. |
| **Naproxen** (Naprosyn, EC-Naprosyn) | Sus: 25mg/mL Tab: 250mg, 375mg, 500mg; Tab, Delayed-Release: 375 or 500mg bid | 250, 375, or 500mg bid. 375mg, 500mg. | 1500mg/day. |
| **Naproxen sodium** (Anaprox) | Tab: 275mg | 750mg-1g qd, 275mg bid or 550mg bid. | 1650mg/day. |
| (Anaprox DS) | Tab: 550mg* | 750mg-1g qd, 275mg bid or 550mg bid. | 1.5g/day. |
| (Naprelan) | Tab, Extended-Release: 375mg, 500mg | 750mg-1g qd, 275mg bid or 550mg bid. | 1.5g/day. |
| **Oxaprozin** (Daypro) | Tab: 600mg* | 1200mg qd. | 1800mg/day in divided doses (not to exceed 26mg/kg/day). |
| **Piroxicam** (Feldene) | Cap: 10mg, 20mg | 20mg qd or 10mg bid. | |
| **Sulindac** (Clinoril) | Tab: 150mg, 200mg | 150mg bid with food. | 400mg/day with food. |
| **Tolmetin** (Tolectin) | Cap: (DS) 400mg; Tab: 200mg*, 600mg | 400mg tid. | 1800mg/day. |
| **COX-2 INHIBITOR** | | | |
| **Celecoxib** (Celebrex) | Cap: 100mg, 200mg, 400mg | 200mg qd or 100mg bid. | |
| **SALICYLATE** | | | |
| **Aspirin** (Genuine Bayer Aspirin, Bayer Extra Strength, Ecotrin) | Tab: 325mg Tab, Extra Strength: Tab, Delayed-Release: 81mg, 325mg, 500mg | Up to 3g/day in 500mg divided doses. | 4g/day. |
| **NSAID COMBINATION** | | | |
| **Diclofenac sodium/Misoprostol** (Arthrotec) | Tab: 50mg-0.2mg, 75mg-0.2mg | 50mg tid. Do not crush, chew or divide. | |
| **MISCELLANEOUS** | | | |
| **Hyaluronan** (Euflexxa) | Inj: 1% [2mL] | Inject 2mL intra-articularly into the knee weekly for 3 wks. Total 3 injections. | 3 injections. |
| (Orthovisc) | Inj: 30mg/2mL | 30mg intra-articularly once a wk. Total 3-4 injections. | 3-4 injections. |

*Scored

# RHEUMATOID ARTHRITIS AGENTS

| **DRUG** (Brand) | **HOW SUPPLIED** | **USUAL DOSE RANGE** | **MAX DOSE** |
|---|---|---|---|
| **5-AMINOSALICYLIC ACID DERIVATIVE** | | | |
| **Sulfasalazine** (Azulfidine EN) | Tab, Delayed-Release: 500mg | 1g bid. | 4g/day. |
| **COPPER CHELATING AGENT** | | | |
| **Penicillamine** (Cuprimine, Depen) | Cap: (Cuprimine) 125mg, 250mg; Tab: (Depen) 250mg* | 500-750mg/day. | 1.5g/day. |
| **COX-2 INHIBITOR** | | | |
| **Celecoxib** (Celebrex) | Cap: 100mg, 200mg, 400mg | 100-200mg bid. | 400mg/day. |
| **DIHYDROFOLIC ACID REDUCTASE INHIBITOR** | | | |
| **Methotrexate sodium** | Inj: 25mg/mL; Tab: 2.5mg | 7.5mg once weekly. | 20mg/wk. |
| **GOLD AGENT** | | | |
| **Auranofin** (Ridaura) | Cap: 3mg | 6mg qd or 3mg bid. | 9mg/day. |
| **IMMUNOSUPPRESSANTS** | | | |
| **Azathioprine** (Imuran) | Tab: 50mg* | **Initial:** 1mg/kg/day given qd-bid. **Titrate:** Increase by 0.5mg/kg/day after 6-8 wks, then at 4 wk intervals. | 2.5mg/kg/day. |
| **Cyclosporine** (Neoral) | Cap: 25mg, 100mg; Sol: 100mg/mL [50mL] | **Initial:** 1.25mg/kg bid. **Titrate:** Increase by 0.5-0.75mg/kg/day after 8 wks, again after 12 wks. D/C if no benefit by wk 16. | 4mg/kg/day. |
| **INTERLEUKIN-1 RECEPTOR ANTAGONIST** | | | |
| **Anakinra** (Kineret) | Inj: 100mg/0.67mL | 100mg SQ qd | |
| **MONOCLONAL ANTIBODIES/CD20-BLOCKER** | | | |
| **Rituximab** (Rituxan) | Inj: 10mg/mL | Two-1000mg IV infusions separated by 2 wks, with MTX. | |
| **MONOCLONAL ANTIBODIES/TNF-BLOCKERS** | | | |
| **Adalimumab** (Humira) | Inj: 40mg/0.8mL | 40mg SQ every other wk. | 40mg w/o MTX. |
| **Infliximab** (Remicade) | Inj: 100mg | 3mg/kg IV infusion repeat at 2 and 6 wks. **Maint:** 3mg/kg every 8 wks. | 10mg/kg or every 4 wks. |
| **NONSTEROIDAL ANTI-INFLAMMATORY DRUGS (NSAIDs)** | | | |
| **Diclofenac** (Voltaren XR) | Tab, Delayed-Release: (Voltaren) 25mg, 50mg, 75mg; Tab, Extended-Release: (Voltaren-XR) 100mg | 50mg tid-qid or 75mg bid. | 200mg/day. |
| **Etodolac** | Cap: 300mg, 400mg, 500mg | 300mg bid-tid or 400-500mg bid. | 1000mg/day. |
| **Flurbiprofen** (Ansaid) | Tab: 50mg, 100mg | 200-300mg/day bid, tid or qid. | 300mg/day. |
| **Ibuprofen** | | | |
| (Motrin) | Sus: 100mg/5mL; Tab: 400mg, 600mg, 800mg | 300mg qid or 400mg, 600mg or 800mg tid-qid. | 3200mg/day. |
| (Motrin IB) | Tab: 200mg | 200mg q4-6h. 400mg if no response. | 3200mg/day. |
| **Ketoprofen** (Oruvail) | Cap, Extended-Release: 200mg | 200mg qd. | 200mg/day. |

*(Continued)*

| DRUG (Brand) | HOW SUPPLIED | USUAL DOSE RANGE | MAX DOSE |
|---|---|---|---|
| **NONSTEROIDAL ANTI-INFLAMMATORY DRUGS (NSAIDs)** *(Continued)* | | | |
| **Meloxicam** (Mobic) | Sus: 7.5mg/5mL; Tab: 7.5mg, 15mg | 7.5mg qd. | 15mg/day. |
| **Nabumetone** (Relafen) | Tab: 500mg, 750mg | 1000mg qd. | 2000mg/day. |
| **Naproxen** | | | |
| (Anaprox DS) | Tab: 275mg, 550mg* | 275mg bid or 550mg bid. | 1650mg/day. |
| (Naprelan) | Tab, Extended-Release: 375mg, 500mg | 750mg-1g qd. | 1.5g/day. |
| (Naprosyn) | Sus: 25mg/mL; Tab: 250mg*, 375mg, 500mg*; Tab, Delayed-Release: (EC-Naprosyn) 375mg, 500mg | 250, 375, or 500mg bid (EC-Naprosyn) 375 or 500mg bid. | 1500mg/day. |
| **Oxaprozin** (Daypro) | Tab: 600mg* | 1200mg qd. | 1800mg/day. |
| **Piroxicam** (Feldene) | Cap: 10mg, 20mg 20mg qd or 10mg bid. | | 20mg/day. |
| **Sulindac** (Clinoril) | Tab: 150mg, 200mg* | 150mg bid. | 400mg/day. |
| **Tolmetin** (Tolectin) | Cap: (DS) 400mg; Tab: 200mg*, 600mg | 200-600mg tid. | 1800mg/day. |
| **NSAID/PROSTAGLANDIN $E_1$ ANALOGUE** | | | |
| **Diclofenac/Misoprostol** (Arthrotec) | Tab: (Diclofenac-Misoprostol) 50mg-0.2mg, 75mg-0.2mg | 50mg tid-qid. | |
| **SELECTIVE COSTIMULATION MODULATOR** | | | |
| **Abatacept** (Orencia) | Inj: 250mg | **Initial:** <60kg: 500mg; 60-100kg: 750mg; >100kg: 1g. **Maint:** Give at 2 and 4 wks after initial infusion, then q 4 wks thereafter. | |
| **SALICYLATE** | | | |
| **Aspirin** | | | |
| (Bayer Aspirin) | Tab: (Genuine Bayer Aspirin) 325mg Tab: (Bayer Extra Strength) 500mg | **Initial:** 3g/day in divided doses. | 4g/day. |
| (Ecotrin) | Tab, Delayed-Release: 81mg, 325mg, 500mg | 3g qd in divided doses. | 4g/day. |
| **TNF-RECEPTOR BLOCKER** | | | |
| **Etanercept** (Enbrel) | Inj: 25mg [vial], 50mg/mL [syringe] | 50mg SQ per wk. | |
| **MISCELLANEOUS** | | | |
| **Hydroxychloroquine** (Plaquenil) | Tab: 200mg | **Initial:** 400-600mg qd. **Maint:** After 4-12 wks, 200-400mg qd with food or milk. | |

*scored

# UROLOGICAL THERAPIES

| OVERACTIVE BLADDER AGENTS | | | | |
|---|---|---|---|---|
| **DRUG** | **BRAND** | **HOW SUPPLIED** | **DOSING** | **COMMENTS** |
| Darifenacin | Enablex | Tab, ER: 7.5mg, 15mg | Initial: 7.5mg qd. Max: 15mg qd. | Swallow whole. Moderate Hepatic Impairment/ Concomitant Potent CYP3A4 Inhibitors: Do not exceed 7.5mg/d. Severe Hepatic Impairment: Avoid use. |
| Oxybutynin | Ditropan | Syrup: 5mg/5mL Tab: 5mg | Usual: 5mg bid-tid. Max: 5mg qid. | A lower starting dose of 2.5mg bid-tid is recommended for elderly patients. |
| | Ditropan XL | Tab, ER: 5mg, 10mg, 15mg | Initial: 5mg or 10mg qd. Max: 30mg/day. | Swallow whole. Increase dose by 5mg weekly if needed. |
| | Oxytrol | Patch: 3.9mg/day | Usual: Apply twice weekly. | Rotate site of application. |
| Solifenacin | VESIcare | Tab: 5mg, 10mg | Usual: 5mg qd. Max: 10mg qd. | Renal (CrCl <30mL/min)/Hepatic (Child Pugh B)/Concomitant Potent CYP3A4 Inhibitors: Do not exceed 5mg/d. Hepatic (Child Pugh C): Avoid use. |
| Tolterodine | Detrol | Tab: 1mg, 2mg | Initial: 2mg bid. | Decrease dose to 1mg bid if needed. Significant Hepatic/Renal Dysfunction/Concomitant CYP3A4 Inhibitors: 1mg bid. |
| | Detrol LA | Cap, ER: 2mg, 4mg | Initial: 4mg qd. | Swallow whole. Decrease dose to 2mg qd if needed. Significant Hepatic/ Renal Dysfunction/ Concomitant CYP3A4 Inhibitors: 2mg qd. |
| Trospium | Sanctura | Tab: 20mg | Usual: 20mg bid. | CrCl <30mL/min: 20mg qhs. Elderly ≥75 yrs: May titrate to 20mg qd based upon tolerability. |

| BENIGN PROSTATIC HYPERTROPHY AGENTS | | | | |
|---|---|---|---|---|
| **DRUG** | **BRAND** | **HOW SUPPLIED** | **DOSING** | **COMMENTS** |
| **ALPHA-BLOCKERS** | | | | |
| Alfuzosin | Uroxatral | Tab, ER: 10mg | Usual: 10mg qd. | Take dose immediately after the same meal each day. Swallow whole. |
| Doxazosin | Cardura | Tab: 1mg, 2mg, 4mg, 8mg | Initial: 1mg qd. Max: 8mg/day. | Double dose every two weeks if needed. |
| | Cardura XL | Tab, ER: 4mg, 8mg | Initial: 4mg qd. Max: 8mg qd. | Take with breakfast. Swallow whole. |
| Tamsulosin | Flomax | Cap: 0.4mg | Initial: 0.4mg qd. Max: 0.8mg qd. | Take dose 1/2 hour after the same meal each day. Titrate after 2-4 weeks if needed. Restart at initial dose if therapy is interrupted. |
| Terazosin | Hytrin | Cap: 1mg, 2mg, 5mg, 10mg | Initial: 1mg qhs. Usual: 10mg/day. Max: 20mg/day. | Increase stepwise as needed. Restart at initial dose if therapy is interrupted. |
| **5-ALPHA-REDUCTASE INHIBITORS** | | | | |
| Dutasteride | Avodart | Cap: 0.5mg | Usual: 0.5mg qd. | Swallow whole. |
| Finasteride | Proscar | Tab: 5mg | Usual: 5mg qd. | May be administered with doxazosin. |

# RECOMMENDED IMMUNIZATION SCHEDULE FOR PERSONS AGED 0–6 YEARS

| Vaccine ▼ Age ▶ | Birth | 1 month | 2 months | 4 months | 6 months | 12 months | 15 months | 18 months | 19–23 months | 2–3 years | 4–6 years |
|---|---|---|---|---|---|---|---|---|---|---|---|
| Hepatitis B[1] | HepB | HepB | | *see footnote 1* | HepB | | | | HepB Series | | |
| Rotavirus[2] | | | Rota | Rota | Rota | | | | | | |
| Diphtheria, Tetanus, Pertussis[3] | | | DTaP | DTaP | DTaP | | DTaP | | | | DTaP |
| *Haemophilus influenzae* type b[4] | | | Hib | Hib | *Hib*[4] | Hib | | Hib | | | |
| Pneumococcal[5] | | | PCV | PCV | PCV | PCV | | | | PCV<br>PPV | |
| Inactivated Poliovirus | | | IPV | IPV | IPV | | | | | | IPV |
| Influenza[6] | | | | | Influenza (Yearly) | | | | | | |
| Measles, Mumps, Rubella[7] | | | | | | MMR | | | | | MMR |
| Varicella[8] | | | | | | Varicella | | | | | Varicella |
| Hepatitis A[9] | | | | | | HepA (2 doses) | | | | HepA Series | |
| Meningococcal[10] | | | | | | | | | | MPSV4 | |

Range of recommended ages | Catch-up immunization | Certain high-risk groups

This schedule indicates the recommended ages for routine administration of currently licensed childhood vaccines, as of December 1, 2006, for children aged 0–6 years. Additional information is available at **http://www.cdc.gov/nip/recs/child-schedule.htm**. Any dose not administered at the recommended age should be administered at any subsequent visit, when indicated and feasible. Additional vaccines may be licensed and recommended during the year. Licensed combination vaccines may be used whenever any components of the combination are indicated and other components of the vaccine are not contraindicated and if approved by the Food and Drug Administration for that dose of the series. Providers should consult the respective Advisory Committee on Immunization Practices statement for detailed recommendations. Clinically significant adverse events that follow immunization should be reported to the Vaccine Adverse Event Reporting System (VAERS). Guidance about how to obtain and complete a VAERS form is available at **http://www.vaers.hhs.gov** or by telephone, **800-822-7967**.

1. **Hepatitis B vaccine (HepB).** *(Minimum age: birth)*
   **At birth:**
   - Administer monovalent HepB to all newborns before hospital discharge.
   - If mother is hepatitis surface antigen (HBsAg)-positive, administer HepB and 0.5 mL of hepatitis B immune globulin (HBIG) within 12 hours of birth.
   - If mother's HBsAg status is unknown, administer HepB within 12 hours of birth. Determine the HBsAg status as soon as possible and if HBsAg-positive, administer HBIG (no later than age1 week).
   - If mother is HBsAg-negative, the birth dose can only be delayed with physician's order and mother's negative HBsAg laboratory report documented in the infant's medical record.

   **After the birth dose:**
   - The HepB series should be completed with either monovalent HepB or a combination vaccine containing HepB. The second dose should be administered at age 1–2 months. The final dose should be administered at age ≥24 weeks. Infants born to HBsAg-positive mothers should be tested for HBsAg and antibody to HBsAg after completion of ≥3 doses of a licensed HepB series, at age 9–18 months (generally at the next well-child visit).

   **4-month dose:**
   - It is permissible to administer 4 doses of HepB when combination vaccines are administered after the birth dose. If monovalent HepB is used for doses after the birth dose, a dose at age 4 months is not needed.
2. **Rotavirus vaccine (Rota).** *(Minimum age: 6 weeks)*
   - Administer the first dose at age 6–12 weeks. Do not start the series later than age 12 weeks.
   - Administer the final dose in the series by age 32 weeks. Do not administer a dose later than age 32 weeks.
   - Data on safety and efficacy outside of these age ranges are insufficient.
3. **Diphtheria and tetanus toxoids and acellular pertussis vaccine (DTaP).** *(Minimum age: 6 weeks)*
   - The fourth dose of DTaP may be administered as early as age 12 months, provided 6 months have elapsed since the third dose.
   - Administer the final dose in the series at age 4–6 years.
4. **Haemophilus influenzae type b conjugate vaccine (Hib).** *(Minimum age: 6 weeks)*
   - If PRP-OMP (PedvaxHIB® or ComVax® [Merck]) is administered at ages 2 and 4 months, a dose at age 6 months is not required.
   - TriHiBit® (DTaP/Hib) combination products should not be used for primary immunization but can be used as boosters following any Hib vaccine in children aged ≥12 months.

*(Continued)*

5. **Pneumococcal vaccine.** *(Minimum age: 6 weeks for pneumococcal conjugate vaccine [PCV]; 2 years for pneumococcal polysaccharide vaccine [PPV])*
   - Administer PCV at ages 24–59 months in certain high-risk groups. Administer PPV to children aged ≥2 years in certain high-risk groups. See *MMWR* 2000;49(No. RR-9):1–35.
6. **Influenza vaccine.** *(Minimum age: 6 months for trivalent inactivated influenza vaccine [TIV]; 5 years for live, attenuated influenza vaccine [LAIV])*
   - All children aged 6–59 months and close contacts of all children aged 0–59 months are recommended to receive influenza vaccine.
   - Influenza vaccine is recommended annually for children aged ≥59 months with certain risk factors, health-care workers, and other persons (including household members) in close contact with persons in groups at high risk. See *MMWR* 2006;55(No. RR-10):1–41.
   - For healthy persons aged 5–49 years, LAIV may be used as an alternative to TIV.
   - Children receiving TIV should receive 0.25 mL if aged 6–35 months or 0.5 mL if aged ≥3 years.
   - Children aged <9 years who are receiving influenza vaccine for the first time should receive 2 doses (separated by ≥4 weeks for TIV and ≥6 weeks for LAIV).
7. **Measles, mumps, and rubella vaccine (MMR).** *(Minimum age: 12 months)*
   - Administer the second dose of MMR at age 4–6 years. MMR may be administered before age 4–6 years, provided ≥4 weeks have elapsed since the first dose and both doses are administered at age ≥12 months.
8. **Varicella vaccine.** *(Minimum age: 12 months)*
   - Administer the second dose of varicella vaccine at age 4–6 years. Varicella vaccine may be administered before age 4–6 years, provided that ≥3 months have elapsed since the first dose and both doses are administered at age ≥12 months. If second dose was administered ≥28 days following the first dose, the second dose does not need to be repeated.
9. **Hepatitis A vaccine (HepA).** *(Minimum age: 12 months)*
   - HepA is recommended for all children aged 1 year (i.e., aged 12–23 months). The 2 doses in the series should be administered at least 6 months apart.
   - Children not fully vaccinated by age 2 years can be vaccinated at subsequent visits.
   - HepA is recommended for certain other groups of children, including in areas where vaccination programs target older children. See *MMWR* 2006;55(No. RR-7):1–23.
10. **Meningococcal polysaccharide vaccine (MPSV4).** *(Minimum age: 2 years)*
   - Administer MPSV4 to children aged 2–10 years with terminal complement deficiencies or anatomic or functional asplenia and certain other high-risk groups. See MMWR 2005;54(No. RR-7):1–21.

The Recommended Immunization Schedules for Persons Aged 0–18 Years are approved by the Advisory Committee on Immunization Practices **(http://www.cdc.gov/nip/acip)**, the American Academy of Pediatrics **(http://www.aap.org)**, and the American Academy of Family Physicians **(http://www.aafp.org)**.

# RECOMMENDED IMMUNIZATION SCHEDULE FOR PERSONS AGED 7-18 YEARS

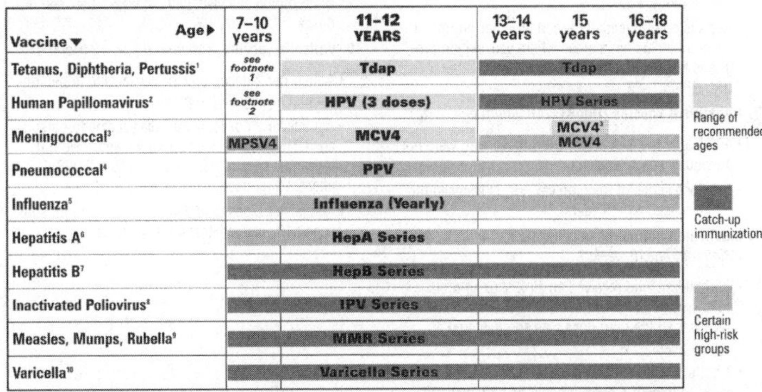

| Vaccine ▼ / Age ▶ | 7–10 years | 11–12 YEARS | 13–14 years | 15 years | 16–18 years |
|---|---|---|---|---|---|
| Tetanus, Diphtheria, Pertussis[1] | see footnote 1 | Tdap | | Tdap | |
| Human Papillomavirus[2] | see footnote 2 | HPV (3 doses) | | HPV Series | |
| Meningococcal[3] | MPSV4 | MCV4 | | MCV4[3] MCV4 | |
| Pneumococcal[4] | | PPV | | | |
| Influenza[5] | | Influenza (Yearly) | | | |
| Hepatitis A[6] | | HepA Series | | | |
| Hepatitis B[7] | | HepB Series | | | |
| Inactivated Poliovirus[8] | | IPV Series | | | |
| Measles, Mumps, Rubella[9] | | MMR Series | | | |
| Varicella[10] | | Varicella Series | | | |



This schedule indicates the recommended ages for routine administration of currently licensed childhood vaccines, as of December 1, 2006, for children aged 7-18 years. Additional information is available at **http://www.cdc.gov/nip/recs/child-schedule.htm**. Any dose not administered at the recommended age should be administered at any subsequent visit, when indicated and feasible. Additional vaccines may be licensed and recommended during the year. Licensed combination vaccines may be used whenever any components of the combination are indicated and other components of the vaccine are not contraindicated and if approved by the Food and Drug Administration for that dose of the series. Providers should consult the respective Advisory Committee on Immunization Practices statement for detailed recommendations. Clinically significant adverse events that follow immunization should be reported to the Vaccine Adverse Event Reporting System (VAERS). Guidance about how to obtain and complete a VAERS form is available at **http://www.vaers.hhs.gov** or by telephone, **800-822-7967**.

1. **Tetanus and diphtheria toxoids and acellular pertussis vaccine (Tdap).** *(Minimum age: 10 years for BOOSTRIX® and 11 years for ADACEL™)*
   - Administer at age 11–12 years for those who have completed the recommended childhood DTP/DTaP vaccination series and have not received a tetanus and diphtheria toxoids vaccine (Td) booster dose.
   - Adolescents aged 13–18 years who missed the 11–12 year Td/Tdap booster dose should also receive a single dose of Tdap if they have completed the recommended childhood DTP/DTaP vaccination series.
2. **Human papillomavirus vaccine (HPV).** *(Minimum age: 9 years)*
   - Administer the first dose of the HPV vaccine series to females at age 11–12 years.
   - Administer the second dose 2 months after the first dose and the third dose 6 months after the first dose.
   - Administer the HPV vaccine series to females at age 13–18 years if not previously vaccinated.
3. **Meningococcal vaccine.** *(Minimum age: 11 years for meningococcal conjugate vaccine [MCV4]; 2 years for meningococcal polysaccharide vaccine [MPSV4])*
   - Administer MCV4 at age 11–12 years and to previously unvaccinated adolescents at high school entry (at approximately age 15 years).
   - Administer MCV4 to previously unvaccinated college freshmen living in dormitories; MPSV4 is an acceptable alternative.
   - Vaccination against invasive meningococcal disease is recommended for children and adolescents aged ≥2 years with terminal complement deficiencies or anatomic or functional asplenia and certain other high-risk groups. See MMWR 2005;54(No. RR-7):1–21. Use MPSV4 for children aged 2–10 years and MCV4 or MPSV4 for older children.
4. **Pneumococcal polysaccharide vaccine (PPV).** *(Minimum age: 2 years)*
   - Administer for certain high-risk groups. See *MMWR* 1997;46(No. RR-8):1–24, and *MMWR* 2000;49(No. RR-9):1–35.
5. **Influenza vaccine.** *(Minimum age: 6 months for trivalent inactivated influenza vaccine [TIV]; 5 years for live, attenuated influenza vaccine [LAIV])*
   - Influenza vaccine is recommended annually for persons with certain risk factors, health-care workers, and other persons (including household members) in close contact with persons in groups at high risk. See *MMWR* 2006;55 (No. RR-10):1–41.
   - For healthy persons aged 5–49 years, LAIV may be used as an alternative to TIV.
   - Children aged <9 years who are receiving influenza vaccine for the first time should receive 2 doses (separated by >4 weeks for TIV and >6 weeks for LAIV).

*(Continued)*

6. **Hepatitis A vaccine (HepA).** *(Minimum age: 12 months)*
   - The 2 doses in the series should be administered at least 6 months apart.
   - HepA is recommended for certain other groups of children, including in areas where vaccination programs target older children. See *MMWR* 2006;55 (No. RR-7):1–23.
7. **Hepatitis B vaccine (HepB).** *(Minimum age: birth)*
   - Administer the 3-dose series to those who were not previously vaccinated.
   - A 2-dose series of Recombivax HB® is licensed for children aged 11–15 years.
8. **Inactivated poliovirus vaccine (IPV).** *(Minimum age: 6 weeks)*
   - For children who received an all-IPV or all-oral poliovirus (OPV) series, a fourth dose is not necessary if the third dose was administered at age ≥4 years.
   - If both OPV and IPV were administered as part of a series, a total of 4 doses should be administered, regardless of the child's current age.
9. **Measles, mumps, and rubella vaccine (MMR).** *(Minimum age: 12 months)*
   - If not previously vaccinated, administer 2 doses of MMR during any visit, with >4 weeks between the doses.
10. **Varicella vaccine.** *(Minimum age: 12 months)*
    - Administer 2 doses of varicella vaccine to persons without evidence of immunity.
    - Administer 2 doses of varicella vaccine to persons aged <13 years at least 3 months apart. Do not repeat the second dose, if administered ≥28 days after the first dose.
    - Administer 2 doses of varicella vaccine to persons aged ≥13 years at least 4 weeks apart.

The Recommended Immunization Schedules for Persons Aged 0–18 Years are approved by the Advisory Committee on Immunization Practices **(http://www.cdc.gov/nip/acip)**, the American Academy of Pediatrics **(http://www.aap.org)**, and the American Academy of Family Physicians **(http://www.aafp.org)**.

# CATCH-UP IMMUNIZATION SCHEDULE FOR PERSONS AGED 4 MONTHS–18 YEARS WHO START LATE OR WHO ARE MORE THAN 1 MONTH BEHIND

| CATCH-UP SCHEDULE FOR PERSONS AGED 4 MONTHS–6 YEARS | | | | | |
|---|---|---|---|---|---|
| **Vaccine** | **Minimum Age for Dose 1** | **Minimum Interval Between Doses** | | | |
| | | **Dose 1 to Dose 2** | **Dose 2 to Dose 3** | **Dose 3 to Dose 4** | **Dose 4 to Dose 5** |
| Hepatitis B[1] | Birth | **4 weeks** | **8 weeks** (and 16 weeks after first dose) | | |
| Rotavirus[2] | 6 wks | **4 weeks** | **4 weeks** | | |
| Diphtheria, Tetanus, Pertussis[3] | 6 wks | **4 weeks** | **4 weeks** | **6 months** | **6 months**[3] |
| *Haemophilus influenzae* type b[4] | 6 wks | **4 weeks** if first dose administered at age <12 months<br>**8 weeks (as final dose)** if first dose administered at age 12-14 months<br>**No further doses needed** if first dose administered at age ≥15 months | **4 weeks**[4] if current age <12 months<br>**8 weeks (as final dose)**[4] if current age ≥12 months and second dose administered at age <15 months<br>**No further doses needed** if previous dose administered at age ≥15 months | **8 weeks (as final dose)** This dose only necessary for children aged 12 months–5 years who received 3 doses before age 12 months | |
| Pneumococcal[5] | 6 wks | **4 weeks** if first dose administered at age <12 months and current age <24 months<br>**8 weeks (as final dose)** if first dose administered at age ≥12 months or current age 24–59 months<br>**No further doses needed** for healthy children if first dose administered at age ≥24 months | **4 weeks** if current age <12 months<br>**8 weeks (as final dose)** if current age ≥12 months<br>**No further doses needed** for healthy children if previous dose administered at age ≥24 months | **8 weeks (as final dose)** This dose only necessary for children aged 12 months–5 years who received 3 doses before age 12 months | |
| Inactivated Poliovirus[6] | 6 wks | **4 weeks** | **4 weeks** | **4 weeks**[6] | |
| Measles, Mumps, Rubella[7] | 12 mos | **4 weeks** | | | |
| Varicella[8] | 12 mos | **3 months** | | | |
| Hepatitis A[9] | 12 mos | **6 months** | | | |
| **CATCH-UP SCHEDULE FOR PERSONS AGED 7–18 YEARS** | | | | | |
| Tetanus, Diphtheria/ Tetanus, Diphtheria, Pertussis[10] | 7 yrs[10] | **4 weeks** | **8 weeks** if first dose administered at age <12 months<br>**6 months** if first dose administered at age ≥12 months | **6 months** if first dose administered at age <12 months | |
| Human Papillomavirus[11] | 9 yrs | **4 weeks** | **12 weeks** | | |
| Hepatitis A[9] | 12 mos | **6 months** | | | |
| Hepatitis B[1] | Birth | **4 weeks** | **8 weeks** (and 16 weeks after first dose) | | |
| Inactivated Poliovirus[6] | 6 wks | **4 weeks** | **4 weeks** | **4 weeks**[6] | |
| Measles, Mumps, Rubella[7] | 12 mos | **4 weeks** | | | |
| Varicella[8] | 12 mos | **4 weeks** if first dose administered at age ≥13 years<br>**3 months** if first dose administered at age <13 years | | | |

The table above provides catch-up schedules and minimum intervals between doses for children whose vaccinations have been delayed. A vaccine series does not need to be restarted, regardless of the time that has elapsed between doses. Use the section appropriate for the child's age.

1. **Hepatitis B vaccine (HepB).** *(Minimum age: birth)*
   - Administer the 3-dose series to those who were not previously vaccinated.
   - A 2-dose series of Recombivax HB® is licensed for children aged 11–15 years.
2. **Rotavirus vaccine (Rota).** *(Minimum age: 6 weeks)*
   - Do not start the series later than age 12 weeks.
   - Administer the final dose in the series by age 32 weeks. Do not administer a dose later than age 32 weeks.
   - Data on safety and efficacy outside of these age ranges are insufficient.
3. **Diphtheria and tetanus toxoids and acellular pertussis vaccine (DTaP).** *(Minimum age: 6 weeks)*
   - The fifth dose is not necessary if the fourth dose was administered at age ≥4 years.
   - DTaP is not indicated for persons aged ≥7 years.
4. **Haemophilus influenzae type b conjugate vaccine (Hib).** *(Minimum age: 6 weeks)*
   - Vaccine is not generally recommended for children aged ≥5 years.
   - If current age <12 months and the first 2 doses were PRP-OMP (PedvaxHIB® or ComVax® [Merck]), the third (and final) dose should be administered at age 12–15 months and at least 8 weeks after the second dose.
   - If first dose was administered at age 7–11 months, administer 2 doses separated by 4 weeks plus a booster at age 12–15 months.
5. **Pneumococcal conjugate vaccine (PCV).** *(Minimum age: 6 weeks)*
   - Vaccine is not generally recommended for children aged ≥5 years.
6. **Inactivated poliovirus vaccine (IPV).** *(Minimum age: 6 weeks)*
   - For children who received an all-IPV or all-oral poliovirus (OPV) series, a fourth dose is not necessary if third dose was administered at age ≥4 years.
   - If both OPV and IPV were administered as part of a series, a total of 4 doses should be administered, regardless of the child's current age.

*(Continued)*

**7. Measles, mumps, and rubella vaccine (MMR).** *(Minimum age: 12 months)*

- The second dose of MMR is recommended routinely at age 4–6 years but may be administered earlier if desired.
- If not previously vaccinated, administer 2 doses of MMR during any visit with ≥4 weeks between the doses.

**8. Varicella vaccine.** *(Minimum age: 12 months)*

- The second dose of varicella vaccine is recommended routinely at age 4–6 years but may be administered earlier if desired.
- Do not repeat the second dose in persons aged <13 years if administered ≥28 days after the first dose.

**9. Hepatitis A vaccine (HepA).** *(Minimum age: 12 months)*

- HepA is recommended for certain groups of children, including in areas where vaccination programs target older children. See *MMWR* 2006;55(No. RR-7):1–23.

**10. Tetanus and diphtheria toxoids vaccine (Td) and tetanus and diphtheria toxoids and acellular pertussis vaccine (Tdap).** *(Minimum ages: 7 years for Td, 10 years for BOOSTRIX®, and 11 years for ADACEL™)*

- Tdap should be substituted for a single dose of Td in the primary catch-up series or as a booster if age appropriate; use Td for other doses.
- A 5-year interval from the last Td dose is encouraged when Tdap is used as a booster dose. A booster (fourth) dose is needed if any of the previous doses were administered at age <12 months. Refer to ACIP recommendations for further information. See *MMWR* 2006;55(No. RR-3).

**11. Human papillomavirus vaccine (HPV).** *(Minimum age: 9 years)*

- Administer the HPV vaccine series to females at age 13–18 years if not previously vaccinated.

Information about reporting reactions after immunization is available online at **http://www.vaers.hhs.gov** or by telephone via the 24-hour national toll-free information line 800-822-7967. Suspected cases of vaccine-preventable diseases should be reported to the state or local health department. Additional information, including precautions and contraindications for immunization, is available from the National Center for Immunization and Respiratory Diseases at **http://www.cdc.gov/nip/default.htm** or telephone, **800-CDC-INFO (800-232-4636).**

# RECOMMENDED ADULT IMMUNIZATION SCHEDULE, BY VACCINE AND AGE GROUP

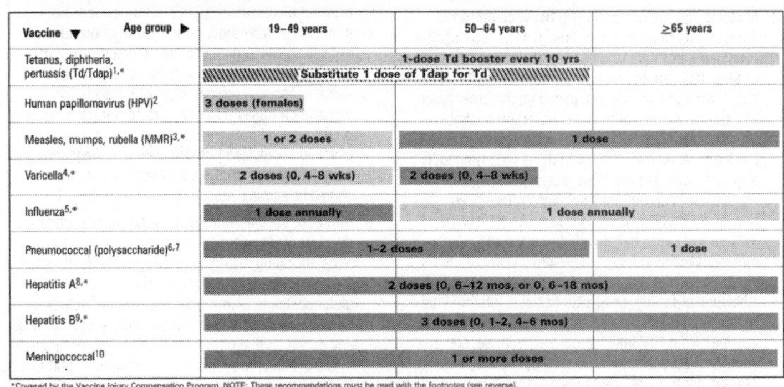

| Vaccine ▼ / Age group ▶ | 19–49 years | 50–64 years | ≥65 years |
|---|---|---|---|
| Tetanus, diphtheria, pertussis (Td/Tdap)[1,*] | 1-dose Td booster every 10 yrs; Substitute 1 dose of Tdap for Td | 1-dose Td booster every 10 yrs; Substitute 1 dose of Tdap for Td | 1-dose Td booster every 10 yrs |
| Human papillomavirus (HPV)[2] | 3 doses (females) | | |
| Measles, mumps, rubella (MMR)[3,*] | 1 or 2 doses | 1 dose | 1 dose |
| Varicella[4,*] | 2 doses (0, 4–8 wks) | 2 doses (0, 4–8 wks) | |
| Influenza[5,*] | 1 dose annually | 1 dose annually | 1 dose annually |
| Pneumococcal (polysaccharide)[6,7] | 1–2 doses | 1–2 doses | 1 dose |
| Hepatitis A[8,*] | 2 doses (0, 6–12 mos, or 0, 6–18 mos) | 2 doses (0, 6–12 mos, or 0, 6–18 mos) | 2 doses (0, 6–12 mos, or 0, 6–18 mos) |
| Hepatitis B[9,*] | 3 doses (0, 1–2, 4–6 mos) | 3 doses (0, 1–2, 4–6 mos) | 3 doses (0, 1–2, 4–6 mos) |
| Meningococcal[10] | 1 or more doses | 1 or more doses | 1 or more doses |

*Covered by the Vaccine Injury Compensation Program. NOTE: These recommendations must be read with the footnotes (see reverse).

For all persons in this category who meet the age requirements and who lack evidence of immunity (e.g., lack documentation of vaccination or have no evidence of prior infection)

Recommended if some other risk factor is present (e.g., on the basis of medical, occupational, lifestyle, or other indications)

This schedule indicates the recommended age groups and medical indications for routine administration of currently licensed vaccines for persons aged ≥19 years, as of October 1, 2006. Licensed combination vaccines may be used whenever any components of the combination are indicated and when the vaccine's other components are not contraindicated. For detailed recommendations on all vaccines, including those used primarily for travelers or that are issued during the year, consult the manufacturers' package inserts and the complete statements from the Advisory Committee on Immunization Practices (*www.cdc.gov/nip/publications/acip-list.htm*).

Report all clinically significant postvaccination reactions to the Vaccine Adverse Event Reporting System (VAERS). Reporting forms and instructions on filing a VAERS report are available at *www.vaers.hhs.gov* or by telephone, *800-822-7967*.

Information on how to file a Vaccine Injury Compensation Program claim is available at *www.hrsa.gov/vaccinecompensation* or by telephone, *800-338-2382*. To file a claim for vaccine injury, contact the *U.S. Court of Federal Claims, 717 Madison Place, N.W., Washington, D.C. 20005*; telephone, *202-357-6400*.

Additional information about the vaccines in this schedule and contraindications for vaccination is also available at *www.cdc.gov/nip* or from the CDC-INFO Contact Center at *800-CDC-INFO (800-232-4636)* in English and Spanish, 24 hours a day, 7 days a week.

1. **Tetanus, diphtheria, and acellular pertussis (Td/Tdap) vaccination.** Adults with uncertain histories of a complete primary vaccination series with diphtheria and tetanus toxoid–containing vaccines should begin or complete a primary vaccination series. A primary series for adults is 3 doses; administer the first 2 doses at least 4 weeks apart and the third dose 6–12 months after the second. Administer a booster dose to adults who have completed a primary series and if the last vaccination was received ≥10 years previously. Tdap or tetanus and diphtheria (Td) vaccine may be used; Tdap should replace a single dose of Td for adults aged <65 years who have not previously received a dose of Tdap (either in the primary series, as a booster, or for wound management). Only one of two Tdap products (Adacel® [sanofi pasteur]) is licensed for use in adults. If the person is pregnant and received the last Td vaccination ≥10 years previously, administer Td during the second or third trimester; if the person received the last Td vaccination in <10 years, administer Tdap during the immediate postpartum period. A one-time administration of 1 dose of Tdap with an interval as short as 2 years from a previous Td vaccination is recommended for postpartum women, close contacts of infants aged <12 months, and all healthcare workers with direct patient contact. In certain situations, Td can be deferred during pregnancy and Tdap substituted in the immediate postpartum period, or Tdap can be given instead of Td to a pregnant woman after an informed discussion with the woman (see *www.cdc.gov/nip/publications/acip-list.htm*). Consult the ACIP statement for recommendations for administering Td as prophylaxis in wound management (*www.cdc.gov/mmwr/preview/mmwrhtml/00041645.htm*).
2. **Human papillomavirus (HPV) vaccination.** HPV vaccination is recommended for all women aged ≤26 years who have not completed the vaccine series. Ideally, vaccine should be administered before potential exposure to HPV through sexual activity; however, women who are sexually active should still be vaccinated. Sexually active women who have not been infected with any of the HPV vaccine types receive the full benefit of the vaccination. Vaccination is less beneficial for women who have already been infected with one or more of the four HPV vaccine types. A complete series consists of 3 doses. The second dose should be administered 2 months after the first dose; the third dose should be administered 6 months after the first dose. Vaccination is not

*(Continued)*

recommended during pregnancy. If a woman is found to be pregnant after initiating the vaccination series, the remainder of the 3-dose regimen should be delayed until after completion of the pregnancy.

3. **Measles, mumps, rubella (MMR) vaccination.** *Measles component:* adults born before 1957 can be considered immune to measles. Adults born during or after 1957 should receive ≥1 dose of MMR unless they have a medical contraindication, documentation of ≥1 dose, history of measles based on healthcare provider diagnosis, or laboratory evidence of immunity. A second dose of MMR is recommended for adults who 1) have been recently exposed to measles or in an outbreak setting; 2) have been previously vaccinated with killed measles vaccine; 3) have been vaccinated with an unknown type of measles vaccine during 1963–1967; 4) are students in postsecondary educational institutions; 5) work in a healthcare facility; or 6) plan to travel internationally. Withhold MMR or other measles-containing vaccines from HIV-infected persons with severe immunosuppression.
*Mumps component:* adults born before 1957 can generally be considered immune to mumps. Adults born during or after 1957 should receive 1 dose of MMR unless they have a medical contraindication, history of mumps based on healthcare provider diagnosis, or laboratory evidence of immunity. A second dose of MMR is recommended for adults who 1) are in an age group that is affected during a mumps outbreak; 2) are students in postsecondary educational institutions; 3) work in a healthcare facility; or 4) plan to travel internationally. For unvaccinated healthcare workers born before 1957 who do not have other evidence of mumps immunity, consider giving 1 dose on a routine basis and strongly consider giving a second dose during an outbreak.
Rubella component: administer 1 dose of MMR vaccine to women whose rubella vaccination history is unreliable or who lack laboratory evidence of immunity. For women of childbearing age, regardless of birth year, routinely determine rubella immunity and counsel women regarding congenital rubella syndrome. Do not vaccinate women who are pregnant or who might become pregnant within 4 weeks of receiving vaccine. Women who do not have evidence of immunity should receive MMR vaccine upon completion or termination of pregnancy and before discharge from the healthcare facility.

4. **Varicella vaccination.** All adults without evidence of immunity to varicella should receive 2 doses of varicella vaccine. Special consideration should be given to those who 1) have close contact with persons at high risk for severe disease (e.g., healthcare workers and family contacts of immunocompromised persons) or 2) are at high risk for exposure or transmission (e.g., teachers of young children; child care employees; residents and staff members of institutional settings, including correctional institutions; college students; military personnel; adolescents and adults living in households with children; nonpregnant women of childbearing age; and international travelers). Evidence of immunity to varicella in adults includes any of the following: 1) documentation of 2 doses of varicella vaccine at least 4 weeks apart; 2) U.S.-born before 1980 (although for healthcare workers and pregnant women, birth before 1980 should not be considered evidence of immunity); 3) history of varicella based on diagnosis or verification of varicella by a healthcare provider (for a patient reporting a history of or presenting with an atypical case, a mild case, or both, healthcare providers should seek either an epidemiologic link with a typical varicella case or evidence of laboratory confirmation, if it was performed at the time of acute disease); 4) history of herpes zoster based on healthcare provider diagnosis; or 5) laboratory evidence of immunity or laboratory confirmation of disease. Do not vaccinate women who are pregnant or might become pregnant within 4 weeks of receiving the vaccine. Assess pregnant women for evidence of varicella immunity. Women who do not have evidence of immunity should receive dose 1 of varicella vaccine upon completion or termination of pregnancy and before discharge from the healthcare facility. Dose 2 should be administered 4–8 weeks after dose 1.

5. **Influenza vaccination.** Medical indications: chronic disorders of the cardiovascular or pulmonary systems, including asthma; chronic metabolic diseases, including diabetes mellitus, renal dysfunction, hemoglobinopathies, or immunosuppression (including immunosuppression caused by medications or HIV); any condition that compromises respiratory function or the handling of respiratory secretions or that can increase the risk of aspiration (e.g., cognitive dysfunction, spinal cord injury, or seizure disorder or other neuromuscular disorder); and pregnancy during the influenza season. No data exist on the risk for severe or complicated influenza disease among persons with asplenia; however, influenza is a risk factor for secondary bacterial infections that can cause severe disease among persons with asplenia. Occupational indications: healthcare workers and employees of long-term–care and assisted living facilities. Other indications: residents of nursing homes and other long-term–care and assisted living facilities; persons likely to transmit influenza to persons at high risk (e.g., in-home household contacts and care-givers of children aged 0–59 months, or persons of all ages with high-risk conditions); and anyone who would like to be vaccinated. Healthy, nonpregnant persons aged 5–49 years without high-risk medical conditions who are not contacts of severely immunocompromised persons in special care units can receive either intranasally administered influenza vaccine (FluMist®) or inactivated vaccine. Other persons should receive the inactivated vaccine.

6. **Pneumococcal polysaccharide vaccination**. Medical indications: chronic disorders of the pulmonary system (excluding asthma); cardiovascular diseases; diabetes mellitus; chronic liver diseases, including liver disease as a result of alcohol abuse (e.g., cirrhosis); chronic renal failure or nephrotic syndrome; functional or anatomic asplenia (e.g., sickle cell disease or splenectomy [if elective splenectomy is planned, vaccinate at least 2 weeks before surgery]); immunosuppressive conditions (e.g., congenital immunodeficiency, HIV infection [vaccinate as close to diagnosis as possible when CD4 cell counts are highest], leukemia, lymphoma, multiple myeloma, Hodgkin disease, generalized malignancy, or organ or bone marrow transplantation); chemotherapy with alkylating agents, antimetabolites, or high-dose, long-term corticosteroids; and cochlear implants. Other indications: Alaska Natives and certain American Indian populations and residents of nursing homes or other long-term–care facilities.

7. **Revaccination with pneumococcal polysaccharide vaccine.** One-time revaccination after 5 years for persons with chronic renal failure or nephrotic syndrome; functional or anatomic asplenia (e.g., sickle cell disease or splenectomy); immunosuppressive conditions (e.g., congenital immunodeficiency, HIV

infection, leukemia, lymphoma, multiple myeloma, Hodgkin disease, generalized malignancy, or organ or bone marrow transplantation); or chemotherapy with alkylating agents, antimetabolites, or high-dose, long-term corticosteroids. For persons aged ≥65 years, one-time revaccination if they were vaccinated ≥5 years previously and were aged <65 years at the time of primary vaccination.

8. **Hepatitis A vaccination.** *Medical indications:* persons with chronic liver disease and persons who receive clotting factor concentrates. Behavioral indications: men who have sex with men and persons who use illegal drugs. Occupational indications: persons working with hepatitis A virus (HAV)–infected primates or with HAV in a research laboratory setting. Other indications: persons traveling to or working in countries that have high or intermediate endemicity of hepatitis A (a list of countries is available at *www.cdc.gov/travel/diseases.htm*) and any person who would like to obtain immunity. Current vaccines should be administered in a 2-dose schedule at either 0 and 6–12 months, or 0 and 6–18 months. If the combined hepatitis A and hepatitis B vaccine is used, administer 3 doses at 0, 1, and 6 months.

9. **Hepatitis B vaccination.** *Medical indications:* persons with end-stage renal disease, including patients receiving hemodialysis; persons seeking evaluation or treatment for a sexually transmitted disease (STD); persons with HIV infection; persons with chronic liver disease; and persons who receive clotting factor concentrates. Occupational indications: healthcare workers and public-safety workers who are exposed to blood or other potentially infectious body fluids. Behavioral indications: sexually active persons who are not in a long-term, mutually monogamous relationship (i.e., persons with >1 sex partner during the previous 6 months); current or recent injection-drug users; and men who have sex with men. *Other indications:* household contacts and sex partners of persons with chronic hepatitis B virus (HBV) infection; clients and staff members of institutions for persons with developmental disabilities; all clients of STD clinics; international travelers to countries with high or intermediate prevalence of chronic HBV infection (a list of countries is available at *www.cdc.gov/travel/diseases.htm*); and any adult seeking protection from HBV infection. Settings where hepatitis B vaccination is recommended for all adults: STD treatment facilities; HIV testing and treatment facilities; facilities providing drug-abuse treatment and prevention services; healthcare settings providing services for injection-drug users or menwho have sex with men; correctional facilities; end-stage renal disease programs and facilities for chronic hemodialysis patients; and institutions and nonresidential daycare facilities for persons with developmental disabilities. Special formulation indications: for adultpatients receiving hemodialysis and other immunocompromised adults, 1 dose of 40 ìg/mL (Recombivax HB®) or 2 doses of 20 ìg/mL (Engerix-B®).

10. **Meningococcal vaccination.** *Medical indications:* adults with anatomic or functional asplenia, or terminal complement component deficiencies. Other indications: first-year college students living in dormitories; microbiologists who are routinely exposed to isolates of *Neisseria meningitidis*; military recruits; and persons who travel to or live in countries in which meningococcal disease is hyperendemic or epidemic (e.g., the "meningitis belt" of sub-Saharan Africa during the dry season [December–June]), particularly if their contact with local populations will be prolonged. Vaccination is required by the government of Saudi Arabia for all travelers to Mecca during the annual Hajj. Meningococcal conjugate vaccine is preferred for adults with any of the preceding indications who are aged ≤55 years, although meningococcal polysaccharide vaccine (MPSV4) is an acceptable alternative. Revaccination after 5 years might be indicated for adults previously vaccinated with MPSV4 who remain at high risk for infection (e.g., persons residing in areas in which disease is epidemic).

11. **Selected conditions for which *Haemophilus influenzae* type b (Hib) vaccine may be used.** Hib conjugate vaccines are licensed for children aged 6 weeks–71 months. No efficacy data are available on which to base a recommendation concerning use of Hib vaccine for older children and adults with the chronic conditions associated with an increased risk for Hib disease. However, studies suggest good immunogenicity in patients who have sickle cell disease, leukemia, or HIV infection or whohave had splenectomies; administering vaccine to these patients is not contraindicated.

# RECOMMENDED ADULT IMMUNIZATION SCHEDULE, BY VACCINE AND MEDICAL AND OTHER INDICATIONS

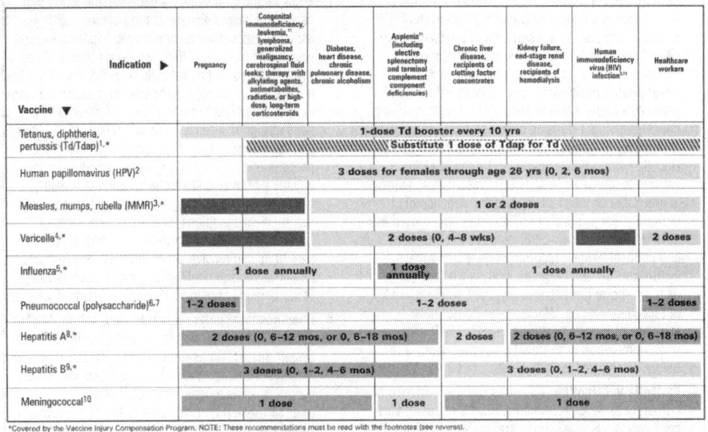

| Indication ▶ / Vaccine ▼ | Pregnancy | Congenital immunodeficiency, leukemia,[11] lymphoma, generalized malignancy, cerebrospinal fluid leaks; therapy with alkylating agents, antimetabolites, radiation, or high-dose, long-term corticosteroids | Diabetes, heart disease, chronic pulmonary disease, chronic alcoholism | Asplenia[11] (including elective splenectomy and terminal complement component deficiencies) | Chronic liver disease, recipients of clotting factor concentrates | Kidney failure, end-stage renal disease, recipients of hemodialysis | Human immunodeficiency virus (HIV) infection[3,11] | Healthcare workers |
|---|---|---|---|---|---|---|---|---|
| Tetanus, diphtheria, pertussis (Td/Tdap)[1,*] | 1-dose Td booster every 10 yrs | | | | | | | |
| | | Substitute 1 dose of Tdap for Td | | | | | | |
| Human papillomavirus (HPV)[2] | | 3 doses for females through age 26 yrs (0, 2, 6 mos) | | | | | | |
| Measles, mumps, rubella (MMR)[3,*] | | | 1 or 2 doses | | | | | |
| Varicella[4,*] | | | 2 doses (0, 4–8 wks) | | | | | 2 doses |
| Influenza[5,*] | 1 dose annually | | | 1 dose annually | 1 dose annually | | | |
| Pneumococcal (polysaccharide)[6,7] | 1–2 doses | 1–2 doses | | | | | | 1–2 doses |
| Hepatitis A[8,*] | 2 doses (0, 6–12 mos, or 0, 6–18 mos) | | | | 2 doses | 2 doses (0, 6–12 mos, or 0, 6–18 mos) | | |
| Hepatitis B[9,*] | 3 doses (0, 1–2, 4–6 mos) | | | | 3 doses (0, 1–2, 4–6 mos) | | | |
| Meningococcal[10] | 1 dose | | | 1 dose | 1 dose | | | |

*Covered by the Vaccine Injury Compensation Program. NOTE: These recommendations must be read with the footnotes (see reverse).

For all persons in this category who meet the age requirements and who lack evidence of immunity (e.g., lack documentation of vaccination or have no evidence of prior infection)

Recommended if some other risk factor is present (e.g., on the basis of medical, occupational, lifestyle, or other indications)

Contraindicated

1. **Tetanus, diphtheria, and acellular pertussis (Td/Tdap) vaccination.** Adults with uncertain histories of a complete primary vaccination series with diphtheria and tetanus toxoid–containing vaccines should begin or complete a primary vaccination series. A primary series for adults is 3 doses; administer the first 2 doses at least 4 weeks apart and the third dose 6–12 months after the second. Administer a booster dose to adults who have completed a primary series and if the last vaccination was received ≥10 years previously. Tdap or tetanus and diphtheria (Td) vaccine may be used; Tdap should replace a single dose of Td for adults aged <65 years who have not previously received a dose of Tdap (either in the primary series, as a booster, or for wound management). Only one of two Tdap products (Adacel® [sanofi pasteur]) is licensed for use in adults. If the person is pregnant and received the last Td vaccination ≥10 years previously, administer Td during the second or third trimester; if the person received the last Td vaccination in <10 years, administer Tdap during the immediate postpartum period. A one-time administration of 1 dose of Tdap with an interval as short as 2 years from a previous Td vaccination is recommended for postpartum women, close contacts of infants aged <12 months, and all healthcare workers with direct patient contact. In certain situations, Td can be deferred during pregnancy and Tdap substituted in the immediate postpartum period, or Tdap can be given instead of Td to a pregnant woman after an informed discussion with the woman (see *www.cdc.gov/nip/publications/acip-list.htm*). Consult the ACIP statement for recommendations for administering Td as prophylaxis in wound management (*www.cdc.gov/mmwr/preview/mmwrhtml/00041645.htm*).

2. **Human papillomavirus (HPV) vaccination.** HPV vaccination is recommended for all women aged ≤26 years who have not completed the vaccine series. Ideally, vaccine should be administered before potential exposure to HPV through sexual activity; however, women who are sexually active should still be vaccinated. Sexually active women who have not been infected with any of the HPV vaccine types receive the full benefit of the vaccination. Vaccination is less beneficial for women who have already been infected with one or more of the four HPV vaccine types. A complete series consists of 3 doses. The second dose should be administered 2 months after the first dose; the third dose should be administered 6 months after the first dose. Vaccination is not recommended during pregnancy. If a woman is found to be pregnant after initiating the vaccination series, the remainder of the 3-dose regimen should be delayed until after completion of the pregnancy.

3. **Measles, mumps, rubella (MMR) vaccination.** *Measles component:* adults born before 1957 can be considered immune to measles. Adults born during or after 1957 should receive ≥1 dose of MMR unless they have a medical contraindication, documentation of ≥1 dose, history of measles based on healthcare provider diagnosis, or laboratory evidence of immunity. A second dose of MMR is recommended for adults who 1) have been recently exposed to measles or in an outbreak setting; 2) have been previously vaccinated with killed measles vaccine; 3) have been vaccinated with an unknown type of measles vaccine during 1963–1967; 4) are students in postsecondary educational institutions; 5) work in a healthcare facility; or 6) plan to travel internationally. Withhold MMR or other measles-containing vaccines from HIV-infected persons with severe immunosuppression.

*(Continued)*

*Mumps component:* adults born before 1957 can generally be considered immune to mumps. Adults born during or after 1957 should receive 1 dose of MMR unless they have a medical contraindication, history of mumps based on healthcare provider diagnosis, or laboratory evidence of immunity. A second dose of MMR is recommended for adults who 1) are in an age group that is affected during a mumps outbreak; 2) are students in postsecondary educational institutions; 3) work in a healthcare facility; or 4) plan to travel internationally. For unvaccinated healthcare workers born before 1957 who do not have other evidence of mumps immunity, consider giving 1 dose on a routine basis and strongly consider giving a second dose during an outbreak. Rubella component: administer 1 dose of MMR vaccine to women whose rubella vaccination history is unreliable or who lack laboratory evidence of immunity. For women of childbearing age, regardless of birth year, routinely determine rubella immunity and counsel women regarding congenital rubella syndrome. Do not vaccinate women who are pregnant or who might become pregnant within 4 weeks of receiving vaccine. Women who do not have evidence of immunity should receive MMR vaccine upon completion or termination of pregnancy and before discharge from the healthcare facility.

4. **Varicella vaccination.** All adults without evidence of immunity to varicella should receive 2 doses of varicella vaccine. Special consideration should be given to those who 1) have close contact with persons at high risk for severe disease (e.g., healthcare workers and family contacts of immunocompromised persons) or 2) are at high risk for exposure or transmission (e.g., teachers of young children; child care employees; residents and staff members of institutional settings, including correctional institutions; college students; military personnel; adolescents and adults living in households with children; nonpregnant women of childbearing age; and international travelers). Evidence of immunity to varicella in adults includes any of the following: 1) documentation of 2 doses of varicella vaccine at least 4 weeks apart; 2) U.S.-born before 1980 (although for healthcare workers and pregnant women, birth before 1980 should not be considered evidence of immunity); 3) history of varicella based on diagnosis or verification of varicella by a healthcare provider (for a patient reporting a history of or presenting with an atypical case, a mild case, or both, healthcare providers should seek either an epidemiologic link with a typical varicella case or evidence of laboratory confirmation, if it was performed at the time of acute disease); 4) history of herpes zoster based on healthcare provider diagnosis; or 5) laboratory evidence of immunity or laboratory confirmation of disease. Do not vaccinate women who are pregnant or might become pregnant within 4 weeks of receiving the vaccine. Assess pregnant women for evidence of varicella immunity. Women who do not have evidence of immunity should receive dose 1 of varicella vaccine upon completion or termination of pregnancy and before discharge from the healthcare facility. Dose 2 should be administered 4–8 weeks after dose 1.
5. **Influenza vaccination.** Medical indications: chronic disorders of the cardiovascular or pulmonary systems, including asthma; chronic metabolic diseases, including diabetes mellitus, renal dysfunction, hemoglobinopathies, or immunosuppression (including immunosuppression caused by medications or HIV); any condition that compromises respiratory function or the handling of respiratory secretions or that can increase the risk of aspiration (e.g., cognitive dysfunction, spinal cord injury, or seizure disorder or other neuromuscular disorder); and pregnancy during the influenza season. No data exist on the risk for severe or complicated influenza disease among persons with asplenia; however, influenza is a risk factor for secondary bacterial infections that can cause severe disease among persons with asplenia. Occupational indications: healthcare workers and employees of long-term–care and assisted living facilities. Other indications: residents of nursing homes and other long-term–care and assisted living facilities; persons likely to transmit influenza to persons at high risk (e.g., in-home household contacts and care-givers of children aged 0–59 months, or persons of all ages with high-risk conditions); and anyone who would like to be vaccinated. Healthy, nonpregnant persons aged 5–49 years without high-risk medical conditions who are not contacts of severely immunocompromised persons in special care units can receive either intranasally administered influenza vaccine (FluMist®) or inactivated vaccine. Other persons should receive the inactivated vaccine.
6. **Pneumococcal polysaccharide vaccination**. Medical indications: chronic disorders of the pulmonary system (excluding asthma); cardiovascular diseases; diabetes mellitus; chronic liver diseases, including liver disease as a result of alcohol abuse (e.g., cirrhosis); chronic renal failure or nephrotic syndrome; functional or anatomic asplenia (e.g., sickle cell disease or splenectomy [if elective splenectomy is planned, vaccinate at least 2 weeks before surgery]); immunosuppressive conditions (e.g., congenital immunodeficiency, HIV infection [vaccinate as close to diagnosis as possible when CD4 cell counts are highest], leukemia, lymphoma, multiple myeloma, Hodgkin disease, generalized malignancy, or organ or bone marrow transplantation); chemotherapy with alkylating agents, antimetabolites, or high-dose, long-term corticosteroids; and cochlear implants. Other indications: Alaska Natives and certain American Indian populations and residents of nursing homes or other long-term–care facilities.
7. **Revaccination with pneumococcal polysaccharide vaccine.** One-time revaccination after 5 years for persons with chronic renal failure or nephrotic syndrome; functional or anatomic asplenia (e.g., sickle cell disease or splenectomy); immunosuppressive conditions (e.g., congenital immunodeficiency, HIV infection, leukemia, lymphoma, multiple myeloma, Hodgkin disease, generalized malignancy, or organ or bone marrow transplantation); or chemotherapy with alkylating agents, antimetabolites, or high-dose, long-term corticosteroids. For persons aged ≥65 years, one-time revaccination if they were vaccinated ≥5 years previously and were aged <65 years at the time of primary vaccination.
8. **Hepatitis A vaccination.** *Medical indications:* persons with chronic liver disease and persons who receive clotting factor concentrates. Behavioral indications: men who have sex with men and persons who use illegal drugs. Occupational indications: persons working with hepatitis A virus (HAV)–infected primates or with HAV in a research laboratory setting. Other indications: persons traveling to or working in countries that have high or intermediate endemicity of hepatitis A (a list of countries is available at *www.cdc.gov/travel/diseases.htm*) and any person who would like to obtain immunity. Current vaccines should be administered in a 2-dose schedule at either 0 and

6–12 months, or 0 and 6–18 months. If the combined hepatitis A and hepatitis B vaccine is used, administer 3 doses at 0, 1, and 6 months.

9. **Hepatitis B vaccination.** *Medical indications:* persons with end-stage renal disease, including patients receiving hemodialysis; persons seeking evaluation or treatment for a sexually transmitted disease (STD); persons with HIV infection; persons with chronic liver disease; and persons who receive clotting factor concentrates. Occupational indications: healthcare workers and public-safety workers who are exposed to blood or other potentially infectious body fluids. Behavioral indications: sexually active persons who are not in a long-term, mutually monogamous relationship (i.e., persons with >1 sex partner during the previous 6 months); current or recent injection-drug users; and men who have sex with men. *Other indications:* household contacts and sex partners of persons with chronic hepatitis B virus (HBV) infection; clients and staff members of institutions for persons with developmental disabilities; all clients of STD clinics; international travelers to countries with high or intermediate prevalence of chronic HBV infection (a list of countries is available at *www.cdc.gov/travel/diseases.htm*); and any adult seeking protection from HBV infection. Settings where hepatitis B vaccination is recommended for all adults: STD treatment facilities; HIV testing and treatment facilities; facilities providing drug-abuse treatment and prevention services; healthcare settings providing services for injection-drug users or menwho have sex with men; correctional facilities; end-stage renal disease programs and facilities for chronic hemodialysis patients; and institutions and nonresidential daycare facilities for persons with developmental disabilities. Special formulation indications: for adultpatients receiving hemodialysis and other immunocompromised adults, 1 dose of 40 ìg/mL (Recombivax HB®) or 2 doses of 20 ìg/mL (Engerix-B®).

10. **Meningococcal vaccination.** *Medical indications:* adults with anatomic or functional asplenia, or terminal complement component deficiencies. Other indications: first-year college students living in dormitories; microbiologists who are routinely exposed to isolates of *Neisseria meningitidis*; military recruits; and persons who travel to or live in countries in which meningococcal disease is hyperendemic or epidemic (e.g., the "meningitis belt" of sub-Saharan Africa during the dry season [December–June]), particularly if their contact with local populations will be prolonged. Vaccination is required by the government of Saudi Arabia for all travelers to Mecca during the annual Hajj. Meningococcal conjugate vaccine is preferred for adults with any of the preceding indications who are aged ≤55 years, although meningococcal polysaccharide vaccine (MPSV4) is an acceptable alternative. Revaccination after 5 years might be indicated for adults previously vaccinated with MPSV4 who remain at high risk for infection (e.g., persons residing in areas in which disease is epidemic).

11. **Selected conditions for which *Haemophilus influenzae* type b (Hib) vaccine may be used.** Hib conjugate vaccines are licensed for children aged 6 weeks–71 months. No efficacy data are available on which to base a recommendation concerning use of Hib vaccine for older children and adults with the chronic conditions associated with an increased risk for Hib disease. However, studies suggest good immunogenicity in patients who have sickle cell disease, leukemia, or HIV infection or whohave had splenectomies; administering vaccine to these patients is not contraindicated.

# ALCOHOL-FREE PRODUCTS

The following is a selection of alcohol-free products grouped by therapeutic category. The list is not comprehensive. Generic and alternate brands may exist. Always check product labeling for definitive information on specific ingredients.

**ANALGESICS**

Acetaminophen Infants Drops
Actamin Maximum Strength Liquid
Addaprin Tablet
Advil Children's Suspension
Aminofen Tablet
Aminofen Max Tablet
APAP Elixir
Aspirtab Tablet
Buffasal Tablet
Demerol Hydrochloride Syrup
Dolono Elixir
Dyspel Tablet
Genapap Children Elixir
Genapap Infant's Drops
Motrin Children's Suspension
Motrin Infants' Suspension
Silapap Children's Elixir
Silapap Infant's Drops
Tylenol Children's Suspension
Tylenol Extra Strength Solution
Tylenol Infant's Drops
Tylenol Infant's Suspension

**ANTIASTHMATIC AGENTS**

Dilor-G Liquid
Dy-G Liquid
Elixophyllin-GG Liquid

**ANTICONVULSANT**

Zarontin Syrup

**ANTIVIRAL AGENT**

Epivir Oral Solution

**COUGH/COLD/ALLERGY PREPARATIONS**

Accuhist Pediatric Drops
Alacol DM Syrup
Allergy Relief Medicine Children's Elixir
Altarussin Syrup
Amerifed DM Liquid
Amerifed Liquid
Anaplex DM Syrup
Anaplex DMX Suspension
Anaplex HD Syrup
Andehist DM Drops
Andehist DM Syrup
Andehist DM NR Liquid
Andehist DM NR Syrup
Andehist NR Syrup
Andehist Syrup
Aquatab DM Syrup
Aridex Solution
Atuss DR Syrup
Atuss EX Liquid
Atuss G Liquid
Atuss HC Syrup
Atuss MS Syrup
Baltussin Solution
Benadryl Allergy Solution
Benadryl Allergy/Sinus Children's Solution
Biodec DM Drops
Bromaline Solution
Bromaline DM Elixir
Bromanate Elixir
Bromatan-DM Suspension
Bromaxefed DM RF Syrup
Bromaxefed RF Syrup
Broncotron Liquid
Bromdec Solution
Bromdec DM Solution
Bromhist Pediatric Solution
Bromhist-DM Pediatric Syrup
Bromhist-DM Solution
Bromphenex HD Solution
Bromplex DM Solution
Bromplex HD Solution
Broncotron-D Suspension
Bron-Tuss Liquid
Brovex HC Solution
B-Tuss Liquid
Carbaphen 12 Ped Suspension
Carbaphen 12 Suspension
Carbatuss Liquid
Carbatuss-CL Solution
Carbaxefed DM RF Liquid
Carbetaplex Solution
Carbihist Solution
Carbofed DM Drops
Carbofed DM Syrup
Carboxine Solution
Carboxine-PSE Solution
Cardec Syrup
Cardec DM Syrup
Cepacol Sore Throat Liquid
Chlordex GP Syrup
Chlor-Mes D Solution
Chlor-Trimeton Allergy Syrup
Codal-DH Syrup
Codal-DM Syrup
Codotuss Liquid
Coldec DS Solution
Coldec-DM Syrup
Coldmist DM Solution
Coldmist DM Syrup
Coldmist S Syrup
Coldonyl Tablet
Coldtuss DR Syrup
Colidrops Pediatric Liquid
Complete Allergy Elixir
Cordron-D Solution
Cordron-DM Solution
Cordron-HC Solution
Corfen DM Solution
Co-Tussin Liquid
Cotuss-V Syrup
Crantex HC Syrup
Crantex Syrup
Creomulsion Complete Syrup
Creomulsion Cough Syrup
Creomulsion For Children Cough Syrup
Creomulsion Pediatric Syrup
Cytuss HC Syrup
Dacex-A Solution
Dacex-DM Solution
Decahist-DM Solution
De-Chlor DM Solution
De-Chlor DR Solution
Dehistine Syrup
Deka Liquid
Deka Pediatric Drops Solution
Deltuss Liquid
Denaze Solution
Despec Liquid
Dex PC Syrup
Dexcon-DM Solution
Diabetic Tussin Allergy Relief Liquid
Diabetic Tussin C Expectorant Liquid
Diabetic Tussin Cold & Flu Tablet
Diabetic Tussin DM Liquid
Diabetic Tussin DM Maximum Strength Liquid

**COUGH/COLD/ALLERGY PREPARATIONS (Continued)**

Diabetic Tussin DM Maximum Strength Capsule
Diabetic Tussin EX Liquid
Dimetapp Allergy Children's Elixir
Dimetapp Cold & Fever Children's Suspension
Dimetapp Decongestant Pediatric Drops
Double-Tussin DM Liquid
Drocon-CS Solution
Duradal HD Plus Syrup
Duratan DM Suspension
Duratuss DM Solution
Dynatuss Syrup
Dynatuss EX Syrup
Dynatuss HC Solution
Dynatuss HCG Solution
Endacof DM Solution
Endacof HC Solution
Endacof XP Solution
Endagen-HD Syrup
Endal HD Solution
Endal HD Syrup
Endal HD Plus Syrup
Endotuss-HD Syrup
Enplus-HD Syrup
Entex Syrup
Entex HC Syrup
Exo-Tuss
Father John's Medicine Plus Drops
Friallergia DM Liquid
Friallergia Liquid
Ganidin NR Liquid
Gani-Tuss NR Liquid
Gani-Tuss-DM NR Liquid
Genahist Elixir
Genebronco-D Liquid
Genecof-HC Liquid
Genecof-XP Liquid
Genecof-XP Syrup
Genedel Syrup
Genedotuss-DM Liquid
Genepatuss Liquid
Genetuss-2 Liquid
Genexpect-DM Liquid
Genexpect-PE Liquid
Genexpect-SF Liquid
Giltuss HC Syrup
Giltuss Liquid
Giltuss Pediatric Liquid
Guai-Co Liquid
Guaicon DMS Liquid
Guai-Dex Liquid
Guaifed Syrup
Guaitussin AC Solution
Guaitussin DAC Solution
Guapetex HC Solution
Guapetex Syrup
Halotussin AC Liquid
Hayfebrol Liquid
H-C Tussive Syrup
Histacol DM Pediatric Solution
Histacol DM Pediatric Syrup
Histex HC Syrup
Histex Liquid
Histex PD Drops
Histex PD Liquid
Histinex HC Syrup
Histinex PV Syrup
Histuss HC Solution
Hi-Tuss Syrup
Hycomal DH Liquid
Hydex-PD Solution
Hydone Liquid
Hydramine Elixir
Hydro PC Syrup
Hydro PC II Plus Solution
Hydro Pro Solution
Hydrocof-HC Solution
Hydro-DP Solution
Hydron CP Syrup
Hydron EX Syrup
Hydron KGS Liquid
Hydron PSC Liquid
Hydro-Tussin DM Elixir
Hydro-Tussin HC Syrup
Hydro-Tussin HD Liquid
Hydro-Tussin XP Syrup
Hyphen-HD Syrup
Jaycof Expectorant Syrup
Jaycof-HC Liquid
Jaycof-XP Liquid
Kita La Tos Liquid
Levall Liquid Andrx
Levall 5.0 Liquid
Lodrane Liquid
Lodrane D Suspension
Lodrane XR Suspension
Lohist D Syrup
Lohist-LQ Solution
Lortuss DM Solution
Lortuss HC Solution
Marcof Expectorant Syrup
Maxi-Tuss HCX Solution
M-Clear Jr Solution
M-Clear Syrup
Medi-Brom Elixir
Mintex Liquid
Mintex PD Liquid
Mintuss DM Syrup
Mintuss EX Syrup
Mintuss G Syrup
Mintuss HD Syrup
Mintuss MR Syrup
Mintuss MS Syrup
Mintuss NX Solution
Motrin Cold Children's Suspension
Mytussin-PE Liquid
Nalex DH Liquid
Nalex-A Liquid
Nalspan Senior DX Liquid
Nasop Suspension
Neotuss S/F Liquid
Neotuss-D Liquid
Norel DM Liquid
Nucofed Syrup
Nycoff Tablet
Orgadin Liquid
Orgadin-Tuss Liquid
Orgadin-Tuss DM Liquid
Organidin NR Liquid
Palgic-DS Syrup
Pancof Syrup
Pancof EXP Syrup
Pancof HC Liquid
Pancof HC Solution
Pancof XP Liquid
Pancof XP Solution
Panmist DM Syrup
Panmist-S Syrup
PediaCare Cold + Allergy Children's Liquid
PediaCare Cough + Cold Children's Liquid
PediaCare Decongestant Infants Drops
PediaCare Decongestant Plus Cough Drops
PediaCare Multi-Symptom Liquid
PediaCare Nightrest Liquid
Pediahist DM Syrup
Pedia-Relief Liquid

Pediatex Liquid
Pediatex Solution
Pediatex-D Liquid
Pediatex D Solution
Pediatex DM Solution
Pediox Liquid
Phanasin Syrup
Phanatuss Syrup
Phanatuss-HC Diabetic
Phena-HC Solution
Phena-S Liquid
Phena-S 12 Suspension
Pneumotussin 2.5 Syrup
Poly Hist DM Solution
Poly Hist PD Solution
Poly-Tussin Syrup
Poly-Tussin DM Syrup
Poly-Tussin HD Syrup
Poly-Tussin XP Syrup
Primsol Solution
Pro-Clear Solution
Pro-Cof Liquid
Pro-Cof D Liquid
Prolex DH Liquid
Prolex DM Liquid
Pro-Red Solution
Protex Solution
Protex D Solution
Protuss Liquid
Protuss-D Liquid
Pyrroxate Extra Strength Tablet
Q-Tussin PE Liquid
Qual-Tussin DC Syrup
Quintex Syrup
Quintex HC Syrup
Relacon-DM Solution
Relacon-HC Solution
Relasin DM Solution
Rescon-DM Liquid
Rescon-GG Liquid
Rhinacon A Solution
Rhinacon DH Solution
Rindal HD Liquid
Rindal HD Plus Solution
Rindal HPD Solution
Robitussin Cough & Congestion Liquid
Robitussin DM Syrup
Robitussin PE Syrup
Robitussin Pediatric Drops
Robitussin Pediatric Cough Syrup
Robitussin Pediatric Night Relief Liquid
Romilar AC Liquid
Romilar DM Liquid
Rondamine DM Liquid
Rondec Syrup
Rondec DM Drops
Rondec DM Syrup
Ru-Tuss A Syrup
Ru-Tuss DM Syrup
Scot-Tussin Allergy Relief Formula Liquid
Scot-Tussin DM Liquid
Scot-Tussin Expectorant Liquid
Scot-Tussin Original Syrup
Scot-Tussin Senior Liquid
Siladryl Allergy Liquid
Siladryl DAS Liquid
Sildec Liquid
Sildec Syrup
Sildec-DM Drops
Sildec-DM Syrup
Sil-Tex Liquiduid Liquid
Siltussin DAS Liquid
Siltussin DM Syrup
Siltussin DM DAS Cough Formula Syrup
Siltussin SA Syrup
Simply Cough Liquid
Simply Stuffy Liquid
S-T Forte 2 Liquid
Statuss DM Syrup
Sudafed Children's Cold & Cough Solution
Sudafed Children's Solution
Sudafed Children's Tablets
Sudanyl Tablets
Sudatuss DM Syrup
Sudatuss-2 Liquid
Sudatuss-SF Liquid
Triaminic Infant Decongestant Drops
Triant-HC Solution
Trispec-PE Liquid
Trituss DM Solution
Trituss Solution
Tri-Vent DM Solution
Tri-Vent DPC Syrup
Tusdec-DM Solution
Tusdec-HC Solution
Tusnel Pediatric Solution
Tusnel Solution
Tussafed Syrup
Tussafed-EX Syrup
Tussafed-EX Pediatric Liquid
Tussafed-HC Syrup
Tussafed-HCG Solution
Tussall Solution
Tussbid Capsule
Tuss-DM Liquid
Tuss-ES Syrup
Tussex Syrup
Tussinate Syrup
Tussi-Organidin DM NR Liquid
Tussi-Organidin NR Liquid
Tussi-Pres Liquid
Tussirex Liquid
Tussirex Syrup
Tylenol Allergy-D Children's Liquid
Tylenol Cold Children's Liquid
Tylenol Cold Children's Suspension
Tylenol Cold Infants' Drops
Tylenol Cold Plus Cough Children's Liquid
Tylenol Cold Plus Cough Infants' Suspension
Tylenol Flu Children's Suspension
Tylenol Flu Night Time Maximum Strength Liquid
Tylenol Sinus Children's Liquid
Uni-Lev 5.0 Solution
Vanex-HD Syrup
Vazol Solution
Vicks 44E Pediatric Liquid
Vicks 44M Pediatric Liquid
Vicks Dayquil Multi-Symptom Liquicap
Vicks Dayquil Multi-Symptom Liquid
Vicks 44 Liquid Capsules Cold, Flu, Cough
Vicks Nyquil Children's Liquid
Vicks Sinex 12-Hour Spray
Vicks Sinex Spray
Vi-Q-Tuss Syrup
V-Tann Suspension
Vitussin Expectorant Syrup
Vortex Syrup
Welltuss EXP Solution
Welltuss HC Solution
Z-Cof DM Syrup
Z-Cof DMX Solution
Z-Cof HC Syrup
Ztuss Expectorant Solution

**EAR/NOSE/THROAT PRODUCTS**

4-Way Saline Moisturizing Mist Spray
Ayr Baby Saline Spray
Bucalcide Solution
Bucalcide Spray

**EAR/NOSE/THROAT PRODUCTS (Continued)**
Bucalsep Solution
Bucalsep Spray
Cepacol Sore Throat Liquid
Cheracol Sore Throat Spray
Fresh N Free Liquid
Gly-Oxide Liquid
Isodettes Sore Throat Spray
Lacrosse Mouthwash Liquid
Larynex Lozenges
Listermint Liquid
Nasal Moist Gel
Orajel Baby Liquid
Orajel Baby Nighttime Gel
Oramagic Oral Wound Rinse Powder for Suspension
Orasept Mouthwash/Gargle Liquid
Tanac Liquid
Tech 2000 Dental Rinse Liquid
Throto-Ceptic Spray
Zilactin Baby Extra Strength Gel

**GASTROINTESTINAL AGENTS**
Axid
Axid Solution
Baby Gasz Drops
Colidrops Pediatric Drops
Colace Solution
Diarrest Tablet
Imogen Liquid
Kaodene NN Suspension
Liqui-Doss Liquid
Mylicon Infants' Suspension
Neoloid Liquid
Neutralin Tablet
Senokot Children's Syrup

**HEMATINIC**
Irofol Liquid

**MISCELLANEOUS**
Cytra-2 Solution
Cytra-K Solution
Emetrol Solution
Fluorinse Solution
Primsol Solution
Rum-K Liquid

**PSYCHOTROPIC**
Thorazine Syrup

**TOPICAL**
Aloe Vesta 2-N-1 Antifungal Ointment
Blistex Complete Moisture Stick
Blistex Fruit Smoothies Stick
Blistex Herbal Answer Gel
Blistex Herbal Answer Stick
Dermatone Lips N Face Protector Ointment
Dermatone Moisturizing Sunblock Cream
Dermatone Outdoor Skin Protection Cream
Dermatone Skin Protector Cream
Eucapsulein Facial Lotion
Evoclin Foam
Fleet Pain Relief Pads
Fresh & Pure Douche Solution
Handclens Solution
Joint-Ritis Maximum Strength Ointment
Neutrogena Acne Wash Liquid
Neutrogena Antiseptic Liquid
Neutrogena Clear Pore Gel
Neutrogena T/Derm Liquid
Neutrogena Toner Liquid
Podiclens Spray
Propa pH Foaming Face Wash Liquid
Sea Breeze Foaming Face Wash Gel
Shade Uvaguard Lotion
Sportz Bloc Cream
Stri-Dex Maximum Strength Pad
Stri-Dex Sensitive Skin Pad
Stri-Dex Super Scrub Pad
Therasoft Anti-Acne Cream
Therasoft Skin Protectant Cream
Tiger Balm Arthritis Rub Lotion

**VITAMINS/MINERALS/ SUPPLEMENTS**
Adaptosode For Stress Liquid
Adaptosode R+R For Acute Stress Liquid
Apetigen Elixir
Biosode Liquid
Detoxosode Liquid
Folbic Tablet
Folplex 2.2 Gel
Genesupp-500 Liquid
Genetect Plus Liquid
Multi-Delyn w/Iron Liquid
Poly-Vi-Sol Drops
Poly-Vi-Sol w/Iron Drops
Poly-Vi-Solution Liquid
Poly-Vi-Solution w/Iron Liquid
Protect Plus Liquid
Soluvite-F Drops
Strovite Forte Syrup
Supervite Liquid
Suplevit Liquid
Tri-Vi-Sol Drops
Tri-Vi-Sol w/Iron Drops
Vitafol Syrup
Vitalize Liquid
Vitamin C/Rose Hips Tablet, Extended-Release

# COMMON LABORATORY TEST VALUES

Listed below are generally accepted normal values for a selection of common laboratory assays conducted on serum, plasma, and blood. Remember that norms may vary from laboratory to laboratory in accordance with the methodology and quality control measures employed by the facility. When in doubt, check with the laboratory that performed the analysis.

"SI range" refers to Système International d'Unités, a uniform system of reporting numerical values that permits interchangeability of information among nations and disciplines.

| TEST | US RANGE | SI RANGE |
|---|---|---|
| Acid phosphatase | ≤2.5 ng/mL | ≤2.5 µg/L |
| Prostatic Total | ≤5.8 U/L | <97 nkat/L |
| Alanine aminotransferase [ALT] (SGPT) | ≤48 U/L | ≤0.8 µkat/L |
| Albumin, serum | 3.5-5.5 g/dL | 35-55 g/L |
| Alkaline phosphatase | 20-125 U/L | 0.33-2.08 µkat/L |
| Ammonia [$NH_3$+] | 10-80 µg/dL | 6-47 µmol/L |
| Amylase, serum | 60-180 U/L | 0.8-3.2 µkat/L |
| Antinuclear antibodies (ANA) | Negative at 1:40 dilution | |
| Aspartate aminotransferase (AST) (SGOT) | ≤42 U/L | ≤0.7 µkat/L |
| Bilirubin | | |
| Total | 0.3-1.0 mg/dL | 5.1-17 µmol/L |
| Direct | 0.1-0.3 mg/dL | 1.7-5.1 µmol/L |
| Indirect | 0.2-0.7 mg/dL | 3.4-12 µmol/L |
| Blood urea nitrogen/ creatinine ratio | 10:1-20:1 | Average 15:1 |
| Calcium, plasma | 9-10.5 mg/dL | 2.2-2.6 mmol/L |
| Calcium, ionized | 4.5-5.6 mg/dL | 1.1-1.4 mmol/L |
| Chloride, serum | 95-108 mEq/L | 95-108 mmol/L |
| Cholesterol (total plasma) | | |
| Desirable level | <200 mg/dL | <5.20 mmol/L |
| Moderate risk | 200-240 mg/dL | 5.2-6.3 mmol/L |
| High risk | >240 mg/dL | >6.3 mmol/L |
| Copper | 70-140 µg/dL | 11-22 µmol/L |
| Cortisol, serum | | |
| 0800 hours | 5-25 µg/dL | 140-690 nmol/L |
| 1600 hours | 3-12 µg/dL | 80-330 nmol/L |
| Creatinine kinase (CK) | | |
| Isoenzymes | CK-MM: 97-100% of total<br>CK-MB: <3% of total<br>CK-BB: 0% of total | CK-MM: 0.97-1.00 of total<br>CK-MB: <0.03 of total<br>CK-BB: 0 of total |
| Total | Male ≤235 U/L<br>Female: ≤190 U/L | Male: ≤3.92 µkat/L<br>Female: ≤3.17 µkat/L |
| Creatinine, serum | <1.5 mg/dL | <133 µmol/L |
| Creatinine clearance | 75-125 mL/min | 1.24-2.08 mL/sec |
| Digoxin | | |
| Therapeutic | 0.5-2.2 ng/mL | 0.6 -2.8 nmol/L |
| Toxic | >2.4 ng/mL | >3.1 nmol/L |
| Erythrocyte count (RBC) | 4.15-4.90 x 106/mm$^3$ | 4.15-4.90 x $10^{12}$/L |
| Erythrocyte sedimentation rate (ESR) | | |
| Male | 0-20 mm/hr | 0-20 mm/hr |
| Female | 0-30 mm/hr | 0-30 mm/hr |
| Ferritin | | |
| Male | 15-400 ng/mL | 15-400 µg/L |
| Female | 10-200 ng/mL | 10-200 µg/L |
| Folic acid | 3-16 ng/mL | 7-36 nmol/L |

## Common Laboratory Test Values

| TEST | US RANGE | SI RANGE |
|---|---|---|
| Follicle-stimulating hormone (FSH) | | |
| Female | 1.4-9.6 mIU/mL | 1.4-9.6 IU/L |
| Ovulation | 2.3-21 mIU/mL | 2.3-21 IU/L |
| Postmenopausal | 34-96 mIU/mL | 34-96 IU/L |
| Male | 0.9-15 mIU/mL | 0.9-15 IU/L |
| Gamma-glutamyl transferase (GGT) | | |
| Male | ≤65 U/L | ≤1.08 μkat/L |
| Female | ≤45 U/L | ≤0.75 μkat/L |
| Gases, arterial blood | | |
| $pO_2$ | 80-100 mmHg | 11-13 kPa |
| $pCO_2$ | 35-45 mmHg | 4.7-6 kPa |
| Glucose, plasma | | |
| Fasting | 75-115 mg/dL | 4.2-6.4 mmol/L |
| Postprandial (2 h) | <140 mg/dL | <7.8 mmol/L |
| Immunoglobulins (Ig) | | |
| IgG | 800-1500 mg/dL | 8.0-15.0 g/L |
| IgA | 90-325 mg/dL | 0.9-3.2 g/L |
| IgM | 45-150 mg/dL | 0.45-1.5 g/L |
| IgD | 0-8 mg/dL | 0-0.08 g/L |
| IgE | <0.025 mg/dL | <0.00025 g/L |
| Iron, serum | 50-150 μg/dL | 9-27 μmol/L |
| Iron binding capacity | 250-370 μg/dL | 45-66 μmol/L |
| Iron saturation | 20-45% | |
| Lactic acid (plasma, venous) | 9-16 mg/dL | 1.0-1.8 mmol/L |
| Lactic dehydrogenase (LDH) | 100-190 U/L | 1.7-3.2 μkat/L |
| Lead | <20 μg/dL | 1.0 μmol/L |
| Leukocyte count (WBC) | 4.3-10.8 x $10^3$ | 4.3-10.8 x $10^9$/L |
| Lipase | 0-160 U/L | 0-2.66 μkat/L |
| Lipoproteins (desirable levels) | | |
| Low density (LDL) | <130 mg/dL | <3.36 mmol/L |
| High density (HDL) | >60 mg/dL | >1.55 mmol/L |
| Lithium ion — therapeutic | 0.6-1.2 mEq/L | 0.6-1.2 mmol/L |
| Luteinizing hormone | | |
| Female | 0.8-26 mIU/mL | 0.8-26 IU/L |
| Ovulation | 25-57 mIU/mL | 25-57 IU/L |
| Postmenopausal | 40-104 mIU/mL | 40-104 IU/L |
| Male | 1.3-13 mIU/mL | 1.3-13 IU/L |
| Osmolality, plasma | 285-295 mOsm/kg | 285-295 mmol/kg |
| Phenytoin | | |
| Therapeutic | 10-20 mg/L | 40-80 μmol/L |
| Toxic | >30 mg/L | >120 μmol/L |
| Phosphorus, serum | 2.5-4.5 mg/dL | 0.8-1.45 mmol/L |
| Potassium, serum | 3.5-5 mEq/L | 3.5-5 mmol/L |
| Prolactin | 2-15 ng/mL | 2-15 μg/L |
| Prostate-specific antigen (PSA) | ≤4 ng/mL | ≤4 μg/L |
| Protein | | |
| Total | 5.5-8.0 g/dL | 55-80 g/L |
| Albumin | 3.5-5.5 g/dL | 35-55 g/L |
| Globulin | 2.0-3.5 g/dL | 20-35 g/L |
| Reticulocyte count | 0.5-2.3% of RBCs | 0.005-0.023 of RBCs |
| Rheumatoid factor | <40 IU/mL | <40 kIU/L |
| Sodium, serum | 136-145 mEq/L | 136-145 mmol/L |
| Theophylline — therapeutic | 10-20 mg/L | 55-110 μmol/L |
| Thyroxine-binding globulin (TBG) | 16-34 mg/L | 16-34 mg/L |

| TEST | US RANGE | SI RANGE |
|---|---|---|
| Thyroid-stimulating hormone (TSH) | 0.4-5 μU/mL | 0.4-5 mU/L |
| Thyroxine ($T_4$) | | |
| Free | 0.8-1.8 ng/dL | 10-23 pmol/L |
| Total | 4.5-12.5 μg/dL | 58-161 nmol/L |
| Transferrin | 230-390 μg/dL | 2.3-3.9 mg/L |
| Triglycerides | <160 μg/dL | <1.8 mmol/L |
| Triiodothyronine ($T_3$) | 70-190 ng/dL | 1.1-2.9 nmol/L |
| $T_3$ uptake | 25-35% | 0.25-0.35 (proportion of 1.0) |
| Urea nitrogen, blood (BUN) | 7-30 mg/dL | 2.5-10.7 mmol/L |
| Uric acid | | |
| Male | 4.0-8.5 mg/dL | 238-506 μmol/L |
| Female | 2.5-7.5 mg/dL | 149-446 μmol/L |
| Vitamin $B_{12}$ | 200-600 pg/mL | 148-443 pmol/L |

**SOURCES:**

Beers MH, Berkow R. *Merck Manual of Diagnosis and Therapy,* ed 17. Whitehouse Station, NJ: Merck Research Laboratories; 1999.

Cahill M. *Illustrated Guide to Diagnostic Tests,* ed 2. Springhouse, PA: Springhouse Corporation; 1998.

Fauci AS, Braunwald E, Isselbacher KJ, et al. *Harrison's Principles of Internal Medicine,* ed 14. New York, NY: McGraw Hill; 1998.

Sacher RA, McPherson RA, Campos JM. *Wildmann's Clinical Interpretation of Laboratory Tests.* Philadelphia, PA: FA Davis Company; 2000.

# DRUGS EXCRETED IN BREAST MILK

The following list is not comprehensive; generic forms and alternate brands of some products may be available. When recommending drugs to pregnant or nursing patients, always check product labeling for specific precautions.

Accolate
Accuretic
Aciphex
Actiq
Activella
Actonel with Calcium
ActoPlus Met
Actos
Adalat
Adderall
Advicor
Aggrenox
Aldactazide
Aldactone
Aldomet
Aldoril
Alesse
Allegra-D
Alfenta
Aloprim
Altace
Ambien
Anaprox
Ancef
Androderm
Antara
Apresoline
Aralen
Arthrotec
Asacol
Ativan
Augmentin
Avalide
Avandia
Avelox
Axid
Axocet
Azactam
Azasan
Azathioprine
Azulfidine
Bactrim
Baraclude
Benadryl
Bentyl
Betapace
Bextra
Bexxar
Bicillin
Blocadren
Boniva
Brethine
Brevicon
Brontex
Byetta
Caduet
Cafergot
Calan
Campral
Capoten
Capozide
Captopril
Carbatrol
Cardizem
Cataflam
Catapres
Ceclor
Cefizox
Cefobid
Cefotan
Ceftin
Celebrex
Celexa
Ceptaz
Cerebyx
Ceredase
Cipro
Ciprodex
Claforan
Clarinex
Claritin
Claritin-D
Cleocin
Climara
Clozaril
Codeine
CombiPatch
Combipres
Combivir
Combunox
Compazine
Cordarone
Corgard
Cortisporin
Corzide
Cosopt
Coumadin
Covera-HS
Cozaar
Crestor
Crinone
Cyclessa
Cymbalta
Cystospaz
Cytomel
Cytotec
Cytoxan
Dapsone
Daraprim
Darvon
Darvon-N
Decadron
Deconsal II
Demerol
Demulen
Depacon
Depakene
Depakote
DepoDur
Depo-Provera
Desogen
Desoxyn
Desyrel
Dexedrine
DextroStat
D.H.E. 45
Diabinese
Diastat
Diflucan
Digitek
Dilacor
Dilantin
Dilaudid
Diovan
Diprivan
Diuril
Dolobid
Dolophine
Doral
Doryx
Droxia
Duraclon
Duragesic
Duramorph
Duratuss
Duricef
Dyazide
Dyrenium
E.E.S.
EC-Naprosyn
Ecotrin
Effexor
Elestat
EMLA
Enduron
Epzicom
Equetro
ERYC
EryPed
Ery-Tab
Erythrocin
Erythromycin
Esgic-plus
Eskalith
Estrogel
Estrostep
Ethmozine
Evista
FazaClo
Felbatol
Feldene
femhrt
Fiorinal
Flagyl
Florinef
Floxin
Foradil
Fortamet
Fortaz
Fosamax Plus D
Furosemide
Gabitril
Galzin
Garamycin
Glucophage
Glyset
Guaifed
Halcion
Haldol
Helidac
Hydrocet
Hydrocortone
HydroDIURIL
Iberet-Folic
Ifex
Imitrex
Imuran
Inderal
Inderide
Indocin
INFeD
Inspra
Invanz
Inversine
Isoptin
Kadian
Keflex
Keppra
Kerlone
Ketek
Klonopin
Kronofed-A
Kutrase
Lamictal
Lamisil
Lamprene
Lanoxicaps
Lanoxin
Lariam
Lescol
Levbid
Levitra
Levlen
Levlite
Levora
Levothroid
Levoxyl
Levsin
Levsinex
Lexapro
Lexiva
Lexxel
Lindane
Lioresal
Lipitor
Lithium
Lithobid
Lo/Ovral
Loestrin
Lomotil
Loniten
Lopressor
Lortab
Lotensin
Lotrel
Luminal
Luvox
Lyrica
Macrobid
Macrodantin
Marinol
Maxipime

Maxzide
Mefoxin
Menostar
Methergine
Methotrexate
MetroCream/Gel/Lotion
Mexitil
Micronor
Microzide
Midamor
Migranal
Miltown
Minizide
Minocin
Mirapex
Mircette
M-M-R II
Mobic
Modicon
Moduretic
Monodox
Monopril
Morphine
MS Contin
MSIR
Myambutol
Mycamine
Mysoline
Namenda
Naprelan
Naprosyn
Nascobal
Necon
NegGram
Nembutal
Neoral
Niaspan
Nicotrol
Niravam
Nizoral
Norco
Nor-QD
Nordette
Norinyl
Noritate
Normodyne
Norpace
Norplant
Novantrone
Nubain
Nucofed
Nydrazid
Oramorph
Oretic
Ortho-Cept
Ortho-Cyclen
Ortho-Novum
Ortho Tri-Cyclen
Orudis
Ovcon
Oxistat
OxyContin
OxyFast
OxyIR
Pacerone
Pamelor
Pancrease
Paxil
PCE
Pediapred
Pediazole
Pediotic
Pentasa
Pepcid
Periostat
Persantine
Pfizerpen
Phenergan
Phenobarbital
Phrenilin
Pipracil
Plan B
Ponstel
Pravachol
Premphase
Prempro
Prevacid
Prevacid NapraPAC
PREVPAC
Prinzide
Procanbid
Prograf
Proloprim
Prometrium
Pronestyl
Propofol
Prosed/DS
Protonix
Provera
Prozac
Pseudoephedrine
Pulmicort
Pyrazinamide
Quinidex
Quinine
Raptiva
Reglan
Relpax
Renese
Requip
Reserpine
Restoril
Retrovir
Rifadin
Rifamate
Rifater
Rimactane
Risperdal
Rocaltrol
Rocephin
Roferon A
Roxanol
Rozerem
Sanctura
Sandimmune
Sarafem
Seconal
Sectral
Semprex-D
Septra
Seroquel
Sinequan
Slo-bid
Soma
Sonata
Spiriva
Sporanox
Stadol
Streptomycin
Stromectol
Symbyax
Symmetrel
Synthroid
Tagamet
Tambocor
Tapazole
Tarka
Tavist
Tazicef
Tazidime
Tegretol
Tenoretic
Tenormin
Tenuate
Tequin
Testoderm
Thalitone
Theo-24
Theo-Dur
Thorazine
Tiazac
Timolide
Timoptic
Tindamax
Tobi
Tofranil
Tolectin
Toprol-XL
Toradol
Trandate
Tranxene
Trental
Tricor
Triglide
Trilafon
Trileptal
Tri-Levlen
Trilisate
Tri-Norinyl
Triostat
Triphasil
Trivora
Trizivir
Trovan
Truvada
Tygacil
Tylenol
Tylenol with Codeine
Ultane
Ultram
Unasyn
Uniphyl
Uniretic
Unithroid
Urimax
Valium
Valtrex
Vanceril
Vancocin
Vantin
Vascor
Vaseretic
Vasotec
Ventavis
Verelan
Vermox
Versed
Vibramycin
Vibra-Tabs
Vicodin
Vigamox
Viramune
Voltaren
Vytorin
Wellbutrin
Xanax
Xolair
Zantac
Zarontin
Zaroxolyn
Zegerid
Zemplar
Zestoretic
Zetia
Ziac
Zinacef
Zithromax
Zocor
Zomig
Zonalon
Zonegran
Zosyn
Zovia
Zovirax
Zyban
Zydone
Zyloprim
Zyprexa
Zyrtec

# DRUGS THAT MAY CAUSE PHOTOSENSITIVITY

The drugs in this table are known to cause photosensitivity in some individuals. Effects can range from itching, scaling, rash, and swelling to skin cancer, premature skin aging, skin and eye burns, cataracts, reduced immunity, blood vessel damage, and allergic reactions. The list is not all-inclusive, and shows only representative brands of each generic. When in doubt, always check specific product labeling. Individuals should be advised to wear protective clothing and to apply sunscreens while taking the medications listed below.

| GENERIC | BRAND |
|---|---|
| Acamprosate | Campral |
| Acetazolamide | Diamox |
| Acitretin | Soriatane |
| Acyclovir | Zovirax |
| Alendronate | Fosamax |
| Alitretinoin | Panretin |
| Almotriptan | Axert |
| Amiloride/ hydrochlorothiazide | Moduretic |
| Aminolevulinic acid | Levulan Kerastick |
| Amiodarone | Cordarone, Pacerone |
| Amitriptyline | Elavil |
| Amitriptyline/ chlordiazepoxide | Limbitrol |
| Amitriptyline/perphenazine | Triavil |
| Amlodipine/atorvastatin | Caduet |
| Amoxapine | |
| Anagrelide | Agrylin |
| Apripiprazole | Abilify |
| Atazanavir | Reyataz |
| Atenolol/chlorthalidone | Tenoretic |
| Atorvastatin | Lipitor |
| Atovaquone/proguanil | Malarone |
| Azatadine/ pseudoephedrine | Rynatan, Trinalin |
| Azithromycin | Zithromax |
| Benazepril | Lotensin |
| Benazepril/ hydrochlorothiazide | Lotensin HCT |
| Bendroflumethiazide/ nadolol | Corzide |
| Bexarotene | Targretin |
| Bismuth/metronidazole/ tetracycline | Helidac |
| Bisoprolol/ hydrochlorothiazide | Ziac |
| Brompheniramine/ dextromethorphan/ phenylephrine | Alacol DM |
| Brompheniramine/ dextromethorphan/ pseudoephedrine | Bromfed-DM |
| Buffered aspirin/ pravastatin | Pravigard PAC |
| Bupropion | Wellbutrin, Zyban |
| Candesartan/ hydrochlorothiazide | Atacand HCT |
| Capecitabine | Xeloda |
| Captopril | Capoten |
| Captopril/ hydrochlorothiazide | Capozide |
| Carbamazepine | Carbatrol, Tegretol, Tegretol-XR |
| Carbinoxamine/ pseudoephedrine | Palgic-D, Palgic-DS, Pediatex-D |
| Carvedilol | Coreg |
| Celecoxib | Celebrex |
| Cetirizine | Zyrtec |
| Cetirizine/pseudoephedrine | Zyrtec-D |
| Cevimeline | Evoxac |
| Chlorhexidine gluconate | Hibistat |
| Chloroquine | Aralen |
| Chlorothiazide | Diuril |
| Chlorpheniramine/ hydrocodone/ pseudoephedrine | Tussend |
| Chlorpheniramine/ phenylephrine/pyrilamine | Rynatan |
| Chlorpromazine | Thorazine |
| Chlorpropamide | Diabinese |
| Chlorthalidone | Thalitone |
| Chlorthalidone/clonidine | Clorpres |
| Cidofovir | Vistide |
| Ciprofloxacin | Cipro |
| Citalopram | Celexa |
| Clemastine | Tavist |
| Clonidine/chlorthalidone | Clorpres |
| Clozapine | Clozaril, Fazaclo |
| Cromolyn sodium | Gastrocrom |
| Cyclobenzaprine | Flexeril |
| Cyproheptadine | Cyproheptadine |
| Dacarbazine | DTIC-Dome |
| Dantrolene | Dantrium |
| Demeclocycline | Declomycin |
| Desipramine | Norpramin |
| Diclofenac potassium | Cataflam |
| Diclofenac sodium | Voltaren |
| Diclofenac sodium/ misoprostol | Arthrotec |
| Diflunisal | Dolobid |
| Dihydroergotamine | D.H.E. 45 |
| Diltiazem | Cardizem, Tiazac |
| Diphenhydramine | Benadryl |
| Divalproex | Depakote |
| Doxepin | Sinequan |
| Doxycycline hyclate | Doryx, Periostat, Vibra-Tabs, Vibramycin |
| Doxycycline monohydrate | Monodox |
| Duloxetine | Cymbalta |
| Enalapril | Vasotec |
| Enalapril/felodipine | Lexxel |
| Enalapril/ hydrochlorothiazide | Vaseretic |
| Enalaprilat | Vasotec I.V. |
| Epirubicin | Ellence |
| Eprosartan mesylate/ hydrochlorothiazide | Teveten HCT |
| Erythromycin/ sulfisoxazole | Pediazole |
| Estazolam | ProSom |
| Estradiol | Gynodiol, Estrogel |
| Eszopiclone | Lunesta |
| Ethionamide | Trecator-SC |
| Etodolac | Lodine |
| Felbamate | Felbatol |
| Fenofibrate | Tricor, Lofibra |
| Floxuridine | Sterile FUDR |
| Flucytosine | Ancobon |
| Fluorouracil | Efudex |
| Fluoxetine | Prozac, Sarafem |
| Fluphenazine | Prolixin |

| GENERIC | BRAND |
|---|---|
| Flutamide | Eulexin |
| Fluvastatin | Lescol |
| Fluvoxamine | Luvox |
| Fosinopril | Monopril |
| Fosphenytoin | Cerebyx |
| Furosemide | Lasix |
| Gabapentin | Neurontin |
| Gatifloxacin | Tequin |
| Gemfibrozil | Lopid |
| Gemifloxacin mesylate | Factive |
| Gentamicin | Garamycin |
| Glatiramer | Copaxone |
| Glimepiride | Amaryl |
| Glipizide | Glucotrol |
| Glyburide | DiaBeta, Glynase, Micronase |
| Glyburide/metformin HCl | Glucovance |
| Griseofulvin | Fulvicin P/G, Grifulvin, Gris-PEG |
| Haloperidol | Haldol |
| Hexachlorophene | pHisoHex |
| Hydralazine/ hydrochlorothiazide | Hydra-zide |
| Hydrochlorothiazide | HydroDIURIL, Microzide, Oretic |
| Hydrochlorothiazide/ fosinopril | Monopril HCT |
| Hydrochlorothiazide/ irbesartan | Avalide |
| Hydrochlorothiazide/ lisinopril | Prinzide, Zestoretic |
| Hydrochlorothiazide/ losartan potassium | Hyzaar |
| Hydrochlorothiazide/ methyldopa | Aldoril |
| Hydrochlorothiazide/ moexipril | Uniretic |
| Hydrochlorothiazide/ propranolol | Inderide |
| Hydrochlorothiazide/ quinapril | Accuretic |
| Hydrochlorothiazide/ spironolactone | Aldactazide |
| Hydrochlorothiazide/ telmisartan | Micardis HCT |
| Hydrochlorothiazide/timolol | Timolide |
| Hydrochlorothiazide/ triamterene | Dyazide, Maxzide |
| Hydrochlorothiazide/ valsartan | Diovan HCT |
| Hydroflumethiazide | Hydroflumethiazide |
| Hydroxychloroquine | Plaquenil |
| Hypericum | Kira, St. John's wort |
| Hypericum/vitamin B1/ vitamin C/kava-kava | One-A-Day Tension & Mood |
| Ibuprofen | Motrin |
| Imatinib mesylate | Gleevec |
| Imipramine | Tofranil |
| Imiquimod | Aldara |
| Indapamide | Lozol |
| Interferon alfa-2b, recombinant | Intron A |
| Interferon alfa-n3 (human leukocyte derived) | Alferon-N |
| Interferon beta-1a | Avonex |
| Interferon beta-1b | Betaseron |
| Irbesartan/hydrochlorothiazide | Avalide |
| Isoniazid/pyrazinamide/ rifampin | Rifater |
| Isotretinoin | Accutane, Amnesteem |
| Itraconazole | Sporanox |
| Ketoprofen | Orudis, Oruvail |
| Lamotrigine | Lamictal |
| Leuprolide | Lupron |
| Levamisole | Levamisole |
| Lisinopril | Prinivil, Zestril |
| Lisinorpil/ hydrochlorothiazide | Prinivil, Zestoretic |
| Lomefloxacin | Maxaquin |
| Loratadine | Claritin |
| Loratadine/ pseudoephedrine | Claritin-D |
| Losartan | Cozaar |
| Losartan/ hydrochlorothiazide | Hyzaar |
| Lovastatin | Altoprev, Mevacor |
| Lovastatin/niacin | Advicor |
| Maprotiline | Maprotiline |
| Mefenamic acid | Ponstel |
| Meloxicam | Mobic |
| Mesalamine | Pentasa |
| Methazolamide | |
| Methotrexate | Trexall |
| Methoxsalen | Uvadex, Oxsoralen, 8-MOP |
| Methyclothiazide | Enduron |
| Methyldopa/ hydrochlorothiazide | Aldoril |
| Metolazone | Mykrox, Zaroxolyn |
| Minocycline | Dynacin, Minocin |
| Mirtazapine | Remeron |
| Moexipril | Univasc |
| Moexipril/ hydrochlorothiazide | Uniretic |
| Moxifloxacin | Avelox |
| Nabumetone | Relafen |
| Nadolol/ bendroflumethiazide | Corzide |
| Nalidixic acid | Nalidixic acid |
| Naproxen | Naprosyn, EC-Naprosyn |
| Naproxen sodium | Anaprox, Naprelan |
| Naratriptan | Amerge |
| Nefazodone | Serzone |
| Nifedipine | Adalat CC, Procardia |
| Nisoldipine | Sular |
| Norfloxacin | Noroxin |
| Nortriptyline | Pamelor |
| Ofloxacin | Floxin |
| Olanzapine | Zyprexa |
| Olanzapine/fluoxetine | Symbyax |
| Olmesartan medoxomil/ hydrochlorothiazide | Benicar HCT |
| Olsalazine | Dipentum |
| Oxaprozin | Daypro |
| Oxcarbazepine | Trileptal |
| Oxycodone | Roxicodone |
| Oxytetracycline | Terramycin |
| Pantoprazole | Protonix |
| Paroxetine | Paxil |
| Pastinaca sativa | Parsnip |
| Pentosan polysulfate | Elmiron |
| Pentostatin | Nipent |
| Perphenazine | Perphenazine |
| Pilocarpine | Salagen |
| Piroxicam | Feldene |

| GENERIC | BRAND |
|---|---|
| Polythiazide | Renese |
| Polythiazide/prazosin | Minizide |
| Porfimer sodium | Photofrin |
| Pravastatin | Pravachol |
| Prochlorperazine | Compazine, Compro |
| Promethazine | Phenergan |
| Protriptyline | Vivactil |
| Pyrazinamide | Pyrazinamide |
| Quetiapine | Seroquel |
| Quinapril | Accupril |
| Quinapril/ hydrochlorothiazide | Accuretic |
| Quinidine gluconate | Quinidine |
| Quinidine sulfate | Quinidex |
| Rabeprazole sodium | Aciphex |
| Ramipril | Altace |
| Riluzole | Rilutek |
| Risperidone | Risperdal, Risperdal Consta |
| Ritonavir | Norvir |
| Rizatriptan | Maxalt |
| Ropinirole | Requip |
| Rosuvastatin | Crestor |
| Ruta graveolens | Rue |
| Saquinavir | Fortovase |
| Saquinavir mesylate | Invirase |
| Selegiline | Eldepryl |
| Sertraline | Zoloft |
| Sibutramine | Meridia |
| Sildenafil | Viagra |
| Simvastatin | Zocor |
| Simvastatin/ezetimibe | Vytorin |
| Somatropin | Serostim |
| Sotalol | Betapace, Betapace AF |
| Sulfamethoxazole/ trimethoprim | Bactrim, Septra |
| Sulfasalazine | Azulfidine |
| Sulindac | Clinoril |
| Sumatriptan | Imitrex |
| Tacrolimus | Prograf, Protopic |
| Tazarotene | Tazorac |
| Telmisartan/ hydrochlorothiazide | Micardis HCT |
| Tetracycline | Sumycin |
| Thalidomide | Thalomid |
| Thioridazine hydrochloride | Mellaril |
| Thiothixene | Navane |
| Tiagabine | Gabitril |
| Tolazamide | Tolazamide |
| Tolbutamide | Tolbutamide |
| Topiramate | Topamax |
| Tretinoin | Retin-A |
| Triamcinolone | Azmacort |
| Triamterene | Dyrenium |
| Triamterene/ hydrochlorothiazide | Dyazide, Maxzide |
| Trifluoperazine | Trifluoperazine |
| Trimipramine | Surmontil |
| Trovafloxacin | Trovan |
| Valacyclovir | Valtrex |
| Valdecoxib | Bextra |
| Valproate | Depacon |
| Valproic acid | Depakene |
| Valsartan/ hydrochlorothiazide | Diovan HCT |
| Vardenafil | Levitra |
| Venlafaxine | Effexor |
| Verteporfin | Visudyne |
| Vinblastine | Vinblastine |
| Voriconazole | Vfend |
| Zalcitabine | Hivid |
| Zaleplon | Sonata |
| Ziprasidone | Geodon |
| Zolmitriptan | Zomig |
| Zolpidem | Ambien |

# DRUGS THAT SHOULD NOT BE CRUSHED

Listed below are various slow-release as well as enteric-coated products that should not be crushed or chewed. Slow-release (sr) represents products that are controlled-release, extended-release, long-acting, or timed-release. Enteric-coated (ec) represents products that are delayed-release.

In general, capsules containing slow-release or enteric-coated particles may be opened and their contents administered on a spoonful of soft food. Instruct patients not to chew the particles, though. (Patients should, in fact, be discouraged from chewing any medication unless it is specifically formulated for that purpose.)

This list should not be considered all-inclusive. Generic and alternate brands of some products may exist. Tablets intended for sublingual or buccal administration (not included in this list) should also be administered only as intended, in an intact form.

| DRUG | FORM |
|---|---|
| Aciphex | ec |
| Adalat CC | sr |
| Adderall XR | sr |
| Advicor | sr |
| Aerohist | sr |
| Aerohist Plus | sr |
| Afeditab CR | sr |
| Aggrenox | sr |
| Aldex | sr |
| Aldex-G | sr |
| Aleve Cold & Sinus | sr |
| Aleve Sinus & Headache | sr |
| Allegra-D 12 Hour | sr |
| Allegra-D 24 Hour | sr |
| Allerx | sr |
| Allerx-D | sr |
| Allfen | sr |
| Allfen-DM | sr |
| Alophen | ec |
| Altex-PSE | sr |
| Altoprev | sr |
| Ambi 1000/55 | sr |
| Ambi 45/800 | sr |
| Ambi 45/800/30 | sr |
| Ambi 60/580 | sr |
| Ambi 60/580/30 | sr |
| Ambi 80/700 | sr |
| Ambi 80/700/40 | sr |
| Ambien CR | sr |
| Ambifed-G | sr |
| Ambifed-G DM | sr |
| Amdry-C | sr |
| Amdry-D | sr |
| Amibid DM | sr |
| Amibid LA | sr |
| Amidal | sr |
| Aminoxin | ec |
| Ami-Tex PSE | sr |
| Anextuss | sr |
| Aquabid-DM | sr |
| Aquatab C | sr |
| Aquatab D | sr |
| Aquatab DM | sr |
| Arthrotec | ec |
| Asacol | ec |
| Ascocid-1000 | sr |
| Ascocid-500-D | sr |
| Ascriptin Enteric | ec |
| ATP | ec |
| Atrohist Pediatric | sr |
| Augmentin XR | sr |
| Avinza | sr |
| Azulfidine Entabs | ec |
| Bayer Aspirin Regimen | ec |
| Bellahist-D LA | sr |
| Bellatal ER | sr |
| Biaxin XL | sr |
| Bidex-DM | sr |
| Bidhist | sr |
| Bidhist-D | sr |
| Biohist LA | sr |
| Bisac-Evac | ec |
| Biscolax | ec |
| Blanex-A | sr |
| Bontril Slow-Release | sr |
| Bromfed | sr |
| Bromfed-PD | sr |
| Bromfenex | sr |
| Bromfenex PD | sr |
| Bromfenex PE | sr |
| Bromfenex PE Pediatric | sr |
| Budeprion SR | sr |
| Buproban | sr |
| Calan SR | sr |
| Campral | ec |
| Carbatrol | sr |
| Cardene SR | sr |
| Cardizem CD | sr |
| Cardizem LA | sr |
| Cardura XL | sr |
| Carox Plus | sr |
| Cartia XT | sr |
| Catemine | ec |
| Cemill 1000 | sr |
| Cemill 500 | sr |
| Certuss-D | sr |
| Cevi-Bid | sr |
| Chlorex-A | sr |
| Chlor-Phen | sr |
| Chlor-Trimeton Allergy | sr |
| Chlor-Trimeton Allergy Decongestant | sr |
| Cipro XR | sr |
| Clarinex-D 24 Hour | sr |
| Coldamine | sr |
| Coldec D | sr |
| Coldec TR | sr |
| Coldex-A | sr |
| ColdMist DM | sr |
| ColdMist Jr | sr |
| ColdMist LA | sr |
| Colfed-A | sr |
| Concerta | sr |
| Contac 12-Hour | sr |
| Correctol | ec |
| Cotazym-S | ec |
| Covera-HS | sr |
| CPM 8/PE 20/MSC 1.25 | sr |
| Crantex ER | sr |
| Crantex LA | sr |
| Crantex Lac | sr |
| Creon 10 | ec |
| Creon 20 | ec |
| Creon 5 | ec |
| Cymbalta | ec |
| Cypex-LA | sr |
| Dacex-PE | sr |
| Dairycare | ec |
| Dallergy | sr |
| Dallergy-Jr | sr |
| D-Amine-SR | sr |
| Deconamine SR | sr |
| Deconex | sr |
| Decongest II | sr |
| De-Congestine | sr |
| Deconsal II | sr |
| Depakote | ec |
| Depakote ER | sr |
| Depakote Sprinkles | ec |
| Despec SR | sr |
| Detrol LA | sr |
| Dexaphen SA | sr |
| Dexcon-PE | sr |
| Dexedrine Spansules | sr |
| D-Feda II | sr |
| Diabetes Trio | sr |

**Enteric-coated= ec** **Slow-release = sr**

## Drugs That Should Not Be Crushed

| DRUG | FORM | DRUG | FORM | DRUG | FORM |
|---|---|---|---|---|---|
| Diamox Sequels | sr | Entex PSE | sr | Gua-SR | sr |
| Dilacor XR | sr | Entocort EC | ec | Guia-D | sr |
| Dilantin Kapseals | sr | Equetro | sr | Guiadex D | sr |
| Dilatrate-SR | sr | ERYC | ec | Guiadex PD | sr |
| Diltia XT | sr | Ery-Tab | ec | Guiadrine DM | sr |
| Dilt-XR | sr | Eskalith-CR | sr | Guiadrine G-1200 | sr |
| Dimetane Extentabs | sr | Exefen-DM | sr | Guiadrine GP | sr |
| Disophrol Chronotab | sr | Exefen-PD | sr | Guiadrine PSE | sr |
| Ditropan XL | sr | Extendryl Jr | sr | H 9600 SR | sr |
| Donnatal Extentabs | sr | Extendryl SR | sr | Halfprin | ec |
| Doryx | ec | Extress-30 | sr | Hemax | sr |
| Drexophed SR | sr | Extuss LA | sr | Histacol LA | sr |
| Drihist SR | sr | Feen-A-Mint | ec | Histade | sr |
| Drixomed | sr | Femilax | ec | Histade MX | sr |
| Drixoral | sr | Fero-Folic-500 | sr | Hista-Vent DA | sr |
| Drixoral Plus | sr | Fero-Grad-500 | sr | Hista-Vent PSE | sr |
| Drixoral Sinus | sr | Ferro-Sequels | sr | Histex CT | sr |
| Drize-R | sr | Ferro-Time | sr | Histex I/E | sr |
| Drysec | sr | Ferrous Fumarate DS | sr | Histex SR | sr |
| Dulcolax | ec | Fetrin | sr | Humavent LA | sr |
| Duomax | sr | Flagyl ER | sr | Humibid DM | sr |
| Duradex | sr | Fleet Bisacodyl | ec | Humibid L.A. | sr |
| Duradryl Jr | sr | Focalin XR | sr | Hydro Pro DM SR | sr |
| Durahist | sr | Folitab 500 | sr | Hyoscyamine TR | sr |
| Durahist D | sr | Fortamet | sr | Iberet-500 | sr |
| Durahist PE | sr | Fumatinic | sr | Iberet-Folic-500 | sr |
| Duraphen DM | sr | G/P 1200/75 | sr | Icar-C Plus SR | sr |
| Duraphen Forte | sr | Genacote | ec | Imdur | sr |
| Duraphen II | sr | GFN 1000/DM 50 | sr | Inderal LA | sr |
| Duraphen II DM | sr | GFN 1200/DM 20/PE 40 | sr | Indocin SR | sr |
| Duratuss | sr | GFN 1200/DM 60/PSE 60 | sr | Innopran XL | sr |
| Duratuss GP | sr | GFN 1200/Phenylephrine 40 | sr | Iobid DM | sr |
| Dynabac | ec | GFN 1200/PSE 50 | sr | Ionamin | sr |
| Dynabac D5-Pak | ec | GFN 500/DM 30 | sr | Iosal II | sr |
| Dynacirc CR | sr | GFN 550/PSE 60 | sr | Iotex PSE | sr |
| Dynahist-ER Pediatric | sr | GFN 550/PSE 60/DM 30 | sr | Isochron | sr |
| Dynex | sr | GFN 595/PSE 48 | sr | Isoptin SR | sr |
| Dytan-CS | sr | GFN 595/PSE 48/DM 32 | sr | Kadian | sr |
| Easprin | ec | GFN 795/PSE 85 | sr | Kaon-Cl 10 | sr |
| EC Naprosyn | ec | GFN 800/DM 30 | sr | K-Dur 10 | sr |
| Ecotrin | ec | GFN 800/PE 25 | sr | K-Dur 20 | sr |
| Ecotrin Adult Low Strength | ec | GFN 800/PSE 60 | sr | Klor-Con 10 | sr |
| Ecotrin Maximum Strength | ec | Gilphex TR | sr | Klor-Con 8 | sr |
| Ecpirin | ec | Giltuss TR | sr | Klor-Con M10 | sr |
| Ed A-Hist | sr | Glucophage XR | sr | Klor-Con M15 | sr |
| Ed-Chlor-Tan | sr | Glucotrol XL | sr | Klor-Con M20 | sr |
| Effexor-XR | sr | GP-1200 | sr | Klotrix | sr |
| Efidac 24 Chlorpheniramine | sr | Guaifed | sr | Kronofed-A | sr |
| Efidac 24 Pseudoephedrine | sr | Guaifed-PD | sr | Kronofed-A-Jr | sr |
| Enablex | sr | Guaifenex DM | sr | K-Tab | sr |
| Endal | sr | Guaifenex GP | sr | K-Tan | sr |
| Entab-DM | sr | Guaifenex PSE 120 | sr | Lescol XL | sr |
| Entercote | ec | Guaifenex PSE 60 | sr | Levall G | sr |
| Entex ER | sr | Guaifenex PSE 80 | sr | Levbid | sr |
| Entex LA | sr | Guaimax-D | sr | Levsinex | sr |

| DRUG | FORM |
|---|---|
| Lexxel | sr |
| Lipram 4500 | ec |
| Lipram-CR10 | ec |
| Lipram-CR20 | ec |
| Lipram-CR5 | ec |
| Lipram-PN10 | ec |
| Lipram-PN16 | ec |
| Lipram-PN20 | ec |
| Lipram-UL12 | ec |
| Lipram-UL18 | ec |
| Lipram-UL20 | ec |
| Liquibid-D | sr |
| Liquibid-D 1200 | sr |
| Liquibid-PD | sr |
| Lithobid | sr |
| Lodine XL | sr |
| Lodrane 12 Hour | sr |
| Lodrane 12D | sr |
| Lodrane 24 | sr |
| Lohist-12 | sr |
| Lohist-12D | sr |
| Lusonex | sr |
| Mag Delay | ec |
| Mag64 | ec |
| Mag-SR | sr |
| Mag-SR Plus Calcium | sr |
| Mag-Tab SR | sr |
| Maxifed | sr |
| Maxifed DM | sr |
| Maxifed DMX | sr |
| Maxifed-G | sr |
| Maxiphen DM | sr |
| Maxovite | sr |
| Medent DM | sr |
| Medent LD | sr |
| Mega-C | sr |
| Melfiat | sr |
| Menopause Trio | sr |
| Mestinon Timespan | sr |
| Metadate CD | sr |
| Metadate ER | sr |
| Methylin ER | sr |
| Micro-K | sr |
| Micro-K 10 | sr |
| Mild-C | sr |
| Mindal | sr |
| Mindal DM | sr |
| Mintab C | sr |
| Mintab D | sr |
| Mintab DM | sr |
| Miraphen PSE | sr |
| Modane | ec |
| MS Contin | sr |
| MSP-BLU | ec |
| Mucinex | sr |
| Mucinex D | sr |
| Muco-Fen DM | sr |
| Multi-Ferrous Folic | sr |
| Multiret Folic-500 | sr |
| Myfortic | ec |
| Nacon | sr |
| Nalex-A | sr |
| Naprelan | sr |
| Nasatab LA | sr |
| Nasex | sr |
| Nd Clear | sr |
| Nescon-PD | sr |
| New Ami-Tex LA | sr |
| Nexium | ec |
| Niaspan | sr |
| Nicomide | sr |
| Nifediac CC | sr |
| Nifedical XL | sr |
| Nitrocot | sr |
| Nitro-Time | sr |
| Nohist | sr |
| Norel SR | sr |
| Norpace CR | sr |
| Obstetrix EC | ec |
| Omnihist L.A. | sr |
| Opana ER | sr |
| Oramorph SR | sr |
| Oracea | sr |
| Oruvail | sr |
| Oxycontin | sr |
| Palcaps 10 | ec |
| Palcaps 20 | ec |
| Palgic-D | sr |
| Pancrease | ec |
| Pancrease MT 10 | ec |
| Pancrease MT 16 | ec |
| Pancrease MT 20 | ec |
| Pancrecarb MS-16 | ec |
| Pancrecarb MS-4 | ec |
| Pancrecarb MS-8 | ec |
| Pangestyme CN-10 | ec |
| Pangestyme CN-20 | ec |
| Pangestyme EC | ec |
| Pangestyme MT16 | ec |
| Pangestyme UL12 | ec |
| Pangestyme UL18 | ec |
| Pangestyme UL20 | ec |
| Panmist DM | sr |
| Panmist Jr | sr |
| Panmist LA | sr |
| Pannaz | sr |
| Panocaps | ec |
| Panocaps MT 16 | ec |
| Panocaps MT 20 | ec |
| Papacon | sr |
| Para-Time SR | sr |
| Paser | sr |
| Pavacot | sr |
| Paxil CR | sr |
| PCE Dispertab | sr |
| PCM LA | sr |
| Pendex | sr |
| Pentasa | sr |
| Pentopak | sr |
| Pentoxil | sr |
| Pharmadrine | sr |
| Phenabid | sr |
| Phenabid DM | sr |
| Phenavent | sr |
| Phenavent D | sr |
| Phenavent LA | sr |
| Phenavent PED | sr |
| Phendiet-105 | sr |
| Phenytek | sr |
| Plendil | sr |
| Poly Hist Forte | sr |
| Poly-Vent | sr |
| Poly-Vent Jr | sr |
| Prehist D | sr |
| Prelu-2 | sr |
| Prevacid | ec |
| Prilosec | ec |
| Prilosec Otc | sr |
| Procanbid | sr |
| Procardia XL | sr |
| Profen Forte | sr |
| Profen Forte DM | sr |
| Profen II | sr |
| Profen II DM | sr |
| Prolex PD | sr |
| Prolex-D | sr |
| Pronestyl-SR | sr |
| Proquin XR | sr |
| Prosed EC | ec |
| Proset-D | sr |
| Protid | sr |
| Protonix | ec |
| Prozac Weekly | ec |
| Pseubrom | sr |
| Pseubrom-PD | sr |
| Pseudatex | sr |
| Pseudocot-C | sr |
| Pseudocot-G | sr |
| Pseudovent | sr |
| Pseudovent 400 | sr |
| Pseudovent DM | sr |
| Pseudovent PED | sr |
| P-Tuss DM | sr |
| Qdall | sr |
| Quibron-T/SR | sr |

**Enteric-coated= ec**

**Slow-release = sr**

## Drugs That Should Not Be Crushed

| DRUG | FORM | DRUG | FORM | DRUG | FORM |
|---|---|---|---|---|---|
| Quindal | sr | Sudafed 12 Hour | sr | Ultrase | ec |
| Ralix | sr | Sudafed 24 Hour | sr | Ultrase MT12 | ec |
| Ranexa | sr | Sudal DM | sr | Ultrase MT18 | ec |
| Razadyne ER | sr | Sudal SR | sr | Ultrase MT20 | ec |
| Reliable Gentle Laxative | ec | Sular | sr | Uniphyl | sr |
| Rescon-Jr | sr | Sulfazine EC | ec | Uni-Tex | sr |
| Rescon-MX | sr | Symax Duotab | sr | Urimax | ec |
| Respa-1ST | sr | Symax-SR | sr | Uritact-EC | ec |
| Respa-AR | sr | Tarka | sr | Urocit-K 10 | sr |
| Respa-DM | sr | Taztia XT | sr | Urocit-K 5 | sr |
| Respahist | sr | Tegretol-XR | sr | Uroxatral | sr |
| Respaire-120 SR | sr | Tenuate Dospan | sr | Utira | sr |
| Respaire-60 SR | sr | Theo-24 | sr | V-Dec-M | sr |
| Respa-PE | sr | Theocap | sr | Veracolate | ec |
| Rhinabid | sr | Theochron | sr | Verelan | sr |
| Rhinabid PD | sr | Theo-Time | sr | Verelan PM | sr |
| Rhinacon A | sr | Thiamilate | ec | Versacaps | sr |
| Ribo-2 | ec | Tiazac | sr | Videx EC | ec |
| Risperdal Consta | sr | Time-Hist | sr | Vivotif Berna | ec |
| Ritalin LA | sr | Toprol XL | sr | Voltaren | ec |
| Ritalin-SR | sr | TotaLDay | sr | Voltaren-XR | sr |
| Rodex Forte | sr | Touro Allergy | sr | Vospire | sr |
| Rondec-TR | sr | Touro CC | sr | Vospire ER | sr |
| Ru-Tuss 800 | sr | Touro CC-LD | sr | We Mist II LA | sr |
| Ru-Tuss 800 DM | sr | Touro DM | sr | We Mist LA | sr |
| Ru-Tuss Jr | sr | Touro HC | sr | Wellbid-D | sr |
| Ryneze | sr | Touro LA | sr | Wellbid-D 1200 | sr |
| Rythmol SR | sr | Touro LA-LD | sr | Wellbutrin SR | sr |
| Sam-E | ec | Tranxene-SD | sr | Wellbutrin XL | sr |
| Sinemet CR | sr | Trental | sr | Wobenzym N | ec |
| Sinutuss DM | sr | Trikof-D | sr | Xanax XR | sr |
| Sinuvent PE | sr | Trinalin Repetabs | sr | Xiral | sr |
| Sitrex | sr | Trituss-ER | sr | XpeCT-At | sr |
| Slo-Niacin | sr | Tussafed-LA | sr | XpeCT-HC | sr |
| Slow Fe | sr | Tussall-ER | sr | Z-Cof LA | sr |
| Slow Fe With Folic Acid | sr | Tussbid | sr | Z-Cof LAX | sr |
| Slow-Mag | ec | Tussi-Bid | sr | Zephrex LA | sr |
| Solodyn | sr | Tussitab | sr | Zmax | sr |
| Spacol T/S | sr | Tylenol Arthritis | sr | Zorprin | sr |
| St. Joseph Pain Reliever | ec | Ultrabrom | sr | Zyban | sr |
| Sta-D | sr | Ultrabrom PD | sr | Zymase | ec |
| Stahist | sr | Ultracaps MT 20 | ec | Zyrtec-D | sr |
| Stamoist E | sr | Ultram ER | sr | | |

**Enteric-coated= ec** **Slow-release = sr**

# GENERIC AVAILABILITY GUIDE

This section allows you to quickly determine which forms and strengths of a brand-name drug are also available generically. The entries are organized alphabetically by brand name and dosage form, with strengths in ascending order. Generic availability is indicated by a mark in the "Yes" column. Included are all prescription products described in *PDR*® and *PDR® for Ophthalmic Medicines* that have generic equivalents. Generic availability information is drawn from the drug database maintained by *Red Book*® affiliate Thomson Micromedex.

**Note: Brand-name products with no generic equivalents have been omitted.**

| STRENGTH | GENERIC YES | GENERIC NO |
|---|---|---|
| **Abelcet Injection** | | |
| 5 mg/ml | ■ | |
| **AccuNeb Inhalation Solution** | | |
| 0.021% | | ■ |
| 0.042% | ■ | |
| **Accutane Capsules** | | |
| 10 mg | ■ | |
| 20 mg | ■ | |
| 40 mg | ■ | |
| **Accuzyme Debriding Ointment** | | |
| 1.1 million u/gm-100 mg/ | ■ | |
| **Acticin Cream** | | |
| 5% | ■ | |
| **Activella Tablets** | | |
| 1 mg-0.5 mg | ■ | |
| **Adalat CC Tablets** | | |
| 30 mg | ■ | |
| 60 mg | ■ | |
| 90 mg | ■ | |
| **Adderall Tablets** | | |
| 5 mg | ■ | |
| 7.5 mg | ■ | |
| 10 mg | ■ | |
| 12.5 mg | ■ | |
| 15 mg | ■ | |
| 20 mg | ■ | |
| 30 mg | ■ | |
| **Adenocard Injection** | | |
| 3 mg/ml | ■ | |
| **Adenoscan** | | |
| 3 mg/ml | ■ | |
| **Adipex-P Capsules** | | |
| 37.5 mg | ■ | |
| **Adipex-P Tablets** | | |
| 37.5 mg | ■ | |
| **Adriamycin for Injection, USP** | | |
| 10 mg | ■ | |
| 20 mg | ■ | |
| 50 mg | ■ | |
| 150 mg | | ■ |
| **Adriamycin Injection, USP** | | |
| 2 mg/ml | ■ | |
| **Agrylin Capsules** | | |
| 0.5 mg | ■ | |
| 1 mg | ■ | |
| **Alacol DM Syrup** | | |
| 2 mg/5 ml-10 mg/5 ml-5 mg/5ml | ■ | |
| **Albalon Ophthalmic Solution** | | |
| 0.1% | ■ | |
| **Aldoclor Tablets** | | |
| 150 mg-250 mg | ■ | |
| 250 mg-250 mg | ■ | |
| **Aldoril Tablets** | | |
| 15 mg-250 mg | ■ | |
| 25 mg-250 mg | ■ | |
| **Alesse-28 Tablets** | | |
| 0.02 mg-0.1 mg | ■ | |
| **Aloprim for Injection** | | |
| 500 mg | ■ | |
| **Alupent Inhalation Aerosol** | | |
| 0.65 mg/actuation | ■ | |
| **Amnesteem Capsules** | | |
| 10 mg | ■ | |
| 20 mg | ■ | |
| 40 mg | ■ | |
| **Amoxil Capsules** | | |
| 250 mg | ■ | |
| 500 mg | ■ | |
| **Amoxil Chewable Tablets** | | |
| 125 mg | ■ | |
| 200 mg | ■ | |
| 250 mg | ■ | |
| 400 mg | ■ | |
| **Amoxil Pediatric Drops for Oral Suspension** | | |
| 50 mg/ml | ■ | |
| 125 mg/5 ml | ■ | |
| 200 mg/5 ml | ■ | |
| 250 mg/5 ml | ■ | |
| 400 mg/5 ml | ■ | |
| **Amoxil Powder for Oral Suspension** | | |
| 125 mg/5 ml | ■ | |
| 200 mg/5 ml | ■ | |
| 250 mg/5 ml | ■ | |
| 400 mg/5 ml | ■ | |
| **Amoxil Tablets** | | |
| 500 mg | ■ | |
| 875 mg | ■ | |
| **Anadrol-50 Tablets** | | |
| 50 mg | ■ | |
| **Analpram HC Cream** | | |
| 1%-1% | ■ | |
| 2.5%-1% | | ■ |
| **Analpram HC Lotion** | | |
| 2.5%-1% | ■ | |
| **Anaprox Tablets** | | |
| 275 mg | ■ | |
| **Anaprox DS Tablets** | | |
| 550 mg | ■ | |
| **Ancef for Injection** | | |
| 1 gm | ■ | |
| 10 gm | ■ | |
| 500 mg | ■ | |
| **AndroGel** | | |
| 1% | ■ | |
| **Anzemet Injection** | | |
| 20 mg/ml | ■ | |
| **Apexicon E Cream** | | |
| 0.05% | ■ | |
| **Appearex Tablets** | | |
| 2.5 mg | ■ | |
| **AquaMEPHYTON Injection** | | |
| 1 mg/0.5 ml | ■ | |
| 10 mg/ml | ■ | |
| **Aralast** | | |
| 1 mg | ■ | |
| **Aredia for Injection** | | |
| 30 mg | ■ | |
| 90 mg | ■ | |
| **Atrovent Inhalation Solution** | | |
| 0.02% | ■ | |
| **Atrovent Nasal Spray** | | |
| 0.03% | ■ | |
| 0.06% | ■ | |
| **Augmentin Chewable Tablets** | | |
| 125 mg-31.25 mg | | ■ |
| 200 mg-28.5 mg | ■ | |
| 250 mg-62.5 mg | | ■ |
| 400 mg-57 mg | ■ | |
| **Augmentin Powder for Oral Suspension** | | |
| 125 mg/5 ml-31.25 mg/5 ml | | ■ |
| 200 mg/5 ml-28.5 mg/5 ml | ■ | |
| 250 mg/5 ml-62.5 mg/5 ml | | ■ |
| 400 mg/5 ml-57 mg/5 ml | ■ | |

| STRENGTH | GENERIC YES | GENERIC NO |
|---|---|---|
| **Augmentin Tablets** | | |
| 250 mg125 mg | | ■ |
| 500 mg-125 mg | ■ | |
| 875 mg-125 mg | ■ | |
| **Augmentin XR Tablets** | | |
| 1000 mg-62.5 mg | | ■ |
| **Augmentin ES-600 Powder for Oral Suspension** | | |
| 600 mg/5 ml-42.9 mg/5 ml | ■ | |
| **Avar Cleanser** | | |
| 10%-5% | ■ | |
| **Avar Gel** | | |
| 10%-5% | ■ | |
| **Avar Green** | | |
| 10%-5% | ■ | |
| **Avita Cream** | | |
| 0.025% | ■ | |
| **Avita Gel** | | |
| 0.025% | ■ | |
| **Axid Oral Solution** | | |
| 150 mg | ■ | |
| 300 mg | ■ | |
| **Aygestin Tablets** | | |
| 5 mg | ■ | |
| **Bactroban Ointment** | | |
| 2% | ■ | |
| **Balamine DM Oral Drops** | | |
| 2 mg/ml-3.5 mg/ml-25 mg/ml | ■ | |
| **Balamine DM Syrup** | | |
| 4 mg/5 ml-12.5 mg/5 ml-60 mg/5 ml | ■ | |
| **Benzaclin Topical Gel** | | |
| 5%-1% | ■ | |
| **Betadine 5% Ophthalmic Solution** | | |
| 5% | ■ | |
| **Betagan Ophthalmic Solution, USP** | | |
| 0.25% | ■ | |
| 0.5% | ■ | |
| **Bleph-10 Ophthalmic Solution** | | |
| 10% | ■ | |
| **Blocadren Tablets** | | |
| 5 mg | ■ | |
| 10 mg | ■ | |
| 20 mg | ■ | |
| **Brevibloc Concentrate** | | |
| 250 mg/ml | ■ | |
| **Brevibloc Injection** | | |
| 10 mg/m | ■ | |
| **Brevibloc Double Strength Injection** | | |
| 20 mg/ml | | ■ |
| **Brevibloc Premixed Injection** | | |
| 10 mg/ml | ■ | |
| **Brevibloc Double Strength Premixed Injection** | | |
| 20 mg/ml | | ■ |
| **Brimonidine Tartrate Ophthalmic Solution** | | |
| 0.2% | ■ | |
| **Bumex Tablets** | | |
| 0.25 mg/ml | ■ | |
| 0.5 mg | ■ | |
| 1 mg | ■ | |
| 2 mg | ■ | |
| **Buminate 5% Solution, USP** | | |
| 5% | ■ | |
| **Buminate 25% Solution, USP** | | |
| 25% | ■ | |
| **Buphenyl Tablets** | | |
| 500 mg | ■ | |
| **Buprenex Injectable** | | |
| 0.3 mg/ml | ■ | |
| **Byetta Injection** | | |
| 250 mcg/ml | ■ | |
| **Calcijex Injection** | | |
| 1 mcg/ml | ■ | |
| **Canasa Rectal Suppositories** | | |
| 500 mg | ■ | |
| **Captopril Tablets** | | |
| 12.5 mg | ■ | |
| 25 mg | ■ | |
| 50 mg | ■ | |
| 100 mg | ■ | |
| **Carafate Suspension** | | |
| 1 gm/10 ml | ■ | |
| **Carafate Tablets** | | |
| 1 gm | ■ | |
| **Carnitor Injection** | | |
| 100 mg/ml | | ■ |
| 200 mg/ml | ■ | |
| 330 mg | ■ | |
| **Carnitor Tablets and Oral Solution** | | |
| 100 mg/ml | | ■ |
| 330 mg | ■ | |
| **Carteolol Hydrochloride Ophthalmic Solution USP** | | |
| 1% | ■ | |
| **Cataflam Tablets** | | |
| 50 mg | ■ | |
| **Catapres Tablets** | | |
| 0.1 mg | | ■ |
| 0.2 mg | | ■ |
| 0.3 mg | | ■ |
| **Catapres-TTS** | | |
| 0.1 mg/24 hr | ■ | |
| 0.2 mg/24 hr | ■ | |
| 0.3 mg/24 hr | ■ | |
| **Caverject Impulse Injection** | | |
| 10 mcg | ■ | |
| 20 mcg | ■ | |
| **Ceftin Tablets** | | |
| 250 mg | ■ | |
| 500 mg | ■ | |
| **Celexa Oral Solution** | | |
| 10 mg/5 ml | ■ | |
| **Celexa Tablets** | | |
| 10 mg | ■ | |
| 20 mg | ■ | |
| 40 mg | ■ | |
| **Centany Ointment** | | |
| 2% | ■ | |
| **Cerubidine for Injection** | | |
| 20 mg | ■ | |
| **Chromagen Soft Gelatin Capsules** | | |
| 150 mg-0.01 mg-70 mg-100 mg | ■ | |
| **Ciloxan Ophthalmic Ointment** | | |
| 0.3% | ■ | |
| **Ciloxan Ophthalmic Solution** | | |
| 0.3% | ■ | |
| **Cipro Oral Suspension** | | |
| 250 mg/5 ml | | ■ |
| 500 mg/5 ml | | ■ |
| **Cipro Tablets** | | |
| 100 mg | | ■ |
| 250 mg | ■ | |
| 500 mg | ■ | |
| 750 mg | ■ | |
| **Cipro XR Tablets** | | |
| 500 mg | | ■ |
| 1000 mg | | ■ |
| **Citracal Prenatal Rx Tablets** | | |
| 120 mg-125 mg-2 mg-50 mg | ■ | |
| **Claripel Cream** | | |
| 4% | ■ | |
| **Cleocin Capsules** | | |
| 75 mg | ■ | |
| 150 mg | ■ | |
| 300 mg | ■ | |
| **Climara Transdermal System** | | |
| 0.025 mg/24 hr | ■ | |
| 0.0375 mg/24 hr | ■ | |
| 0.05 mg/24 hr | ■ | |
| 0.06 mg/24 hr | | ■ |
| 0.075 mg/24 hr | ■ | |
| 0.1 mg/24 hr | ■ | |
| **Clindagel** | | |
| 1% | ■ | |
| **Clindesse Vaginal Cream** | | |
| 2% | ■ | |

| STRENGTH | GENERIC YES | GENERIC NO |
|---|---|---|
| **Clindets Pledgets** | | |
| 1% | ■ | |
| **Clinoril Tablets** | | |
| 150 mg | ■ | |
| 200 mg | ■ | |
| **Clobevate Gel** | | |
| 0.05% | ■ | |
| **Clorpres Tablets** | | |
| 15 mg-0.1 mg | ■ | |
| 15 mg-0.2 mg | ■ | |
| 15 mg-0.3 mg | ■ | |
| **Clozapine Tablets** | | |
| 25 mg | ■ | |
| 100 mg | ■ | |
| **Clozaril Tablets** | | |
| 25 mg | ■ | |
| 100 mg | ■ | |
| **Colyte with Flavor Packs for Oral Solution** | | |
| 4000 ml | ■ | |
| **Coumadin for Injection** | | |
| 5 mg | | ■ |
| **Coumadin Tablets** | | |
| 1 mg | ■ | |
| 2 mg | ■ | |
| 2.5 mg | ■ | |
| 3 mg | ■ | |
| 4 mg | ■ | |
| 5 mg | ■ | |
| 6 mg | ■ | |
| 7.5 mg | ■ | |
| 10 mg | ■ | |
| **Creon 5 Capsules** | | |
| 16600 u-5000 u-18750 u | ■ | |
| **Creon 10 Capsules** | | |
| 33200 u-10000 u-37500 u | ■ | |
| **Creon 20 Capsules** | | |
| 66400 u-20000 u-75000 u | ■ | |
| **Crolom Cromolyn Sodium Sterile Ophthalmic Solution USP** | | |
| 4% | ■ | |
| **Cytovene Capsules** | | |
| 250 mg | ■ | |
| 500 mg | ■ | |
| **Cytovene-IV** | | |
| 500 mg | | ■ |
| **Dalmane Capsules** | | |
| 15 mg | ■ | |
| 30 mg | ■ | |
| **Dantrium Capsules** | | |
| 25 mg | ■ | |
| 50 mg | ■ | |
| 100 mg | ■ | |
| **DDAVP Injection** | | |
| 4 mcg/ml | ■ | |
| **DDAVP Nasal Spray** | | |
| 0.01 mg/actuation | ■ | |
| **DDAVP Tablets** | | |
| 0.1 mg | | ■ |
| 0.2 mg | | ■ |
| **Decadron Phosphate Injection** | | |
| 4 mg/ml | ■ | |
| 24 mg/ml | ■ | |
| **Decadron Tablets** | | |
| 0.5 mg | ■ | |
| 0.75 mg | ■ | |
| 4 mg | ■ | |
| **Delatestryl Injection** | | |
| 200 mg/ml | ■ | |
| **Demadex Tablets** | | |
| 5 mg | ■ | |
| 10 mg | ■ | |
| 10 mg/ml. | | ■ |
| 20 mg | ■ | |
| 100 mg | ■ | |
| **Depacon Injection** | | |
| 100 mg/ml | ■ | |
| Depakene Capsules | | |
| 250 mg | ■ | |
| Depakene Syrup | | |
| 250 mg/5 ml | ■ | |
| **Depo-Medrol Injectable Suspension** | | |
| 20 mg/ml | ■ | |
| 40 mg/ml | ■ | |
| 80 mg/ml | ■ | |
| **Desferal Vials** | | |
| 2 gm | ■ | |
| 500 mg | ■ | |
| **Desmopressin Acetate Injection** | | |
| 4 mcg/m | ■ | |
| **Desmopressin Acetate Rhinal Tube** | | |
| 0.01% | ■ | |
| **Dexedrine Spansule Capsules** | | |
| 5 mg | ■ | |
| 10 mg | ■ | |
| 15 mg | ■ | |
| **Dexedrine Tablets** | | |
| 5 mg | ■ | |
| **DextroStat Tablets** | | |
| 5 mg | ■ | |
| 10 mg | ■ | |
| **Diastat Rectal Delivery System** | | |
| 15 mg | ■ | |
| **Digitek Tablets** | | |
| 0.125 mg | ■ | |
| 0.25 mg | ■ | |
| **Dilaudid Ampules** | | |
| 1 mg/ml | ■ | |
| 2 mg/ml | ■ | |
| 4 mg/ml | ■ | |
| **Dilaudid Multiple Dose Vials** | | |
| 2 mg/ml | ■ | |
| **Dilaudid Oral Liquid** | | |
| 1 mg/ml | ■ | |
| **Dilaudid Rectal Suppositories** | | |
| 3 mg | ■ | |
| **Dilaudid Tablets** | | |
| 2 mg | ■ | |
| 4 mg | ■ | |
| 8 mg | ■ | |
| **Dilaudid-HP Injection** | | |
| 10 mg/ml | ■ | |
| **Dilaudid-HP Lyophilized Powder** | | |
| 250 mg | | ■ |
| **Diprolene Gel** | | |
| 0.05% | ■ | |
| **Diprolene Lotion** | | |
| 0.05% | | ■ |
| **Diprolene Ointment** | | |
| 0.05% | ■ | |
| **Diprolene AF Cream** | | |
| 0.05% | ■ | |
| **Diprosone Cream, USP** | | |
| 0.05% | ■ | |
| **Diuril Oral Suspension** | | |
| 250 mg/5 ml | | ■ |
| **Diuril Tablets** | | |
| 250 mg | ■ | |
| 500 mg | ■ | |
| **Diuril Sodium Intravenous** | | |
| 0.5 gm | | ■ |
| **Dolobid Tablets** | | |
| 250 mg | ■ | |
| 500 mg | ■ | |
| **Drysol Solution** | | |
| 20% | ■ | |
| **Duac Topical Gel** | | |
| 5%-1% | ■ | |
| **Duragesic Transdermal System** | | |
| 12.5 mcg/hr | | ■ |
| 25 mcg/hr | ■ | |
| 50 mcg/hr | ■ | |
| 75 mcg/hr | ■ | |
| 100 mcg/hr | ■ | |
| **Dyazide Capsules** | | |
| 25 mg-37.5 mg | ■ | |
| 25 mg-50 mg | ■ | |

| Strength | Generic Yes | Generic No |
|---|---|---|
| **Dynacin Tablets** | | |
| 50 mg | ■ | |
| 75 mg | ■ | |
| 100 mg | ■ | |
| **Dyrenium Capsules** | | |
| 50 mg | ■ | |
| 100 mg | ■ | |
| **EC-Naprosyn Delayed-Release Tablets** | | |
| 500 mg | ■ | |
| **Edex Injection** | | |
| 10 mcg | ■ | |
| 20 mcg | ■ | |
| 40 mcg | ■ | |
| **E.E.S. 200 Liquid** | | |
| 200 mg/5 ml | ■ | |
| **E.E.S. 400 Liquid** | | |
| 400 mg/5 ml | ■ | |
| **E.E.S. 400 Filmtab Tablets** | | |
| 400 mg | ■ | |
| **E.E.S. Granules** | | |
| 200 mg/5 ml | ■ | |
| **Efudex Topical Cream** | | |
| 5% | | ■ |
| **Efudex Topical Solutions** | | |
| 2% | ■ | |
| 5% | ■ | |
| **Eldepryl Capsules** | | |
| 5 mg | ■ | |
| **Elocon Cream** | | |
| 0.1% | ■ | |
| **Elocon Lotion** | | |
| 0.1% | | ■ |
| **Elocon Ointment** | | |
| 0.1% | ■ | |
| **Epogen for Injection** | | |
| 2000 u/ml | ■ | |
| 3000 u/ml | ■ | |
| 4000 u/ml | ■ | |
| 10000 u/ml | ■ | |
| 20000 u/ml | ■ | |
| 40000 u/ml | ■ | |
| **Erygel Topical Gel** | | |
| 2% | ■ | |
| **EryPed** | | |
| 200 mg/5 ml | ■ | |
| 400 mg/5 ml | | ■ |
| **EryPed Drops** | | |
| 100 mg/2.5 ml | | ■ |
| **EryPed Chewable Tablets** | | |
| 200 mg | | ■ |
| **Ery-Tab Tablets** | | |
| 250 mg | ■ | |
| 333 mg | ■ | |
| 500 mg | ■ | |
| **Erythrocin Stearate Filmtab Tablets** | | |
| 250 mg | ■ | |
| 500 mg | ■ | |
| **Erythromycin Base Filmtab Tablets** | | |
| 250 mg | ■ | |
| 500 mg | ■ | |
| **Erythromycin Delayed-Release Capsules, USP** | | |
| 250 mg | ■ | |
| **Eskalith Capsules** | | |
| 300 mg | ■ | |
| **Eskalith CR Controlled-Release Tablets** | | |
| 450 mg | | ■ |
| **Estratest Tablets** | | |
| 1.25 mg-2.5 mg | ■ | |
| **Estratest H.S. Tablets** | | |
| 0.625 mg-1.25 mg | ■ | |
| **Ethyol for Injection** | | |
| 500 mg | ■ | |
| **Eulexin Capsules** | | |
| 125 mg | ■ | |
| **Feiba VH** | | |
| 1 iu | ■ | |
| **Flexbumin I.V.** | | |
| 25% | ■ | |
| **Flexeril Tablets** | | |
| 5 mg | ■ | |
| 10 mg | ■ | |
| **Fluarix** | | |
| 45 mcg/0.5 ml | ■ | |
| **Flumadine Syrup** | | |
| 50 mg/5 ml | | ■ |
| **Flumadine Tablets** | | |
| 100 mg | ■ | |
| **Fluorescite Injection** | | |
| 10% | ■ | |
| 25% | ■ | |
| **Fluor-I-Strip A.T. Ophthalmic Strips** | | |
| 1 mg | ■ | |
| **Fluor-I-Strip Ophthalmic Strips** | | |
| 9 mg | | ■ |
| **FML Ophthalmic Ointment** | | |
| 0.1% | | ■ |
| **FML Ophthalmic Suspension** | | |
| 0.1% | ■ | |
| **FML Forte Ophthalmic Suspension** | | |
| 0.25% | | ■ |
| **FML-S Liquifilm Sterile Ophthalmic Suspension** | | |
| 0.1%-10% | | ■ |
| **Fortamet Extended-Release Tablets** | | |
| 500 mg | ■ | |
| 1000 mg | ■ | |
| **Fortaz Injection** | | |
| 1 gm | ■ | |
| 2 gm | ■ | |
| 6 gm | ■ | |
| 500 mg | ■ | |
| **Fortaz for Injection** | | |
| 1 gm/50 ml-2.2 gm/50 ml | | ■ |
| 2 gm/50 ml-1.6 gm/50 ml | | ■ |
| **Furosemide Tablets** | | |
| 20 mg | ■ | |
| 40 mg | ■ | |
| 80 mg | ■ | |
| **Gammagard Liquid** | | |
| 100 mg/ml | ■ | |
| **Gammagard S/D** | | |
| 0.5 gm | ■ | |
| 2.5 gm | ■ | |
| 5 gm | ■ | |
| 10 gm | ■ | |
| **Garamycin Injectable** | | |
| 40 mg/ml | ■ | |
| **Gengraf Capsules** | | |
| 25 mg | ■ | |
| 100 mg | ■ | |
| **Genoptic Sterile Ophthalmic Solution** | | |
| 3 mg/ml | ■ | |
| **GlucaGen for Injection** | | |
| 1 mg | ■ | |
| **Glucagon for Injection Vials and Emergency Kit** | | |
| 1 mg | ■ | |
| **Gordochom Solution** | | |
| 3%-25% | ■ | |
| **Grifulvin V Tablets Microsize and Oral Suspension Microsize** | | |
| 125 mg/5 ml | ■ | |
| 500 mg | ■ | |
| **Gris-PEG Tablets** | | |
| 125 mg | ■ | |
| 250 mg | ■ | |
| **Gynazole-1 Vaginal Cream** | | |
| 2% | ■ | |
| **Hemofil M** | | |
| 1 iu | ■ | |
| **HibTITER** | | |
| 10 mcg | ■ | |
| 100 mcg | | ■ |

| STRENGTH | GENERIC YES | GENERIC NO |
|---|---|---|
| **Humatrope Vials and Cartridges** | | |
| 5 mg | ■ | |
| 6 mg | | ■ |
| 12 mg | | ■ |
| 24 mg | | ■ |
| **Humulin 70/30 Pen** | | |
| 70 u/ml-30 u/ml | ■ | |
| **Humulin R (U-500)** | | |
| 500 u/ml | | ■ |
| **Hyalgan Solution** | | |
| 10 mg/ml | ■ | |
| **Hycodan Syrup** | | |
| 1.5 mg/5 ml-5 mg/5 ml | ■ | |
| **Hycodan Tablets** | | |
| 1.5 mg-5 mg | ■ | |
| **Hycotuss Expectorant Syrup** | | |
| 100 mg/5 ml-5 mg/5 ml | ■ | |
| **Hydrocortone Tablets** | | |
| 10 mg | ■ | |
| 20 mg | ■ | |
| **HyperRAB** | | |
| 150 iu/ml | ■ | |
| **Hytrin Capsules** | | |
| 1 mg | ■ | |
| 2 mg | ■ | |
| 5 mg | ■ | |
| 10 mg | ■ | |
| **Idamycin PFS Injection** | | |
| 1 mg/ml | ■ | |
| **Imdur Tablets** | | |
| 30 mg | ■ | |
| 60 mg | ■ | |
| 120 mg | ■ | |
| **Indapamide Tablets** | | |
| 1.25 mg | ■ | |
| 2.5 mg | ■ | |
| **Inderal LA Long-Acting Capsules** | | |
| 60 mg | ■ | |
| 80 mg | ■ | |
| 120 mg | ■ | |
| 160 mg | ■ | |
| **Indocin Capsules** | | |
| 25 mg | ■ | |
| 50 mg | ■ | |
| **Indocin I.V.** | | |
| 1 mg | | ■ |
| **Indocin Oral Suspension** | | |
| 25 mg/5 ml | ■ | |
| **Indocin Suppositories** | | |
| 50 mg | ■ | |
| **Infed Injection** | | |
| 50 mg/ml | ■ | |
| **K-Dur Extended-Relase Tablets** | | |
| 10 meq | ■ | |
| 20 meq | ■ | |
| **Klaron Lotion** | | |
| 10% | ■ | |
| **Klonopin Tablets** | | |
| 0.5 mg | ■ | |
| 1 mg | ■ | |
| 2 mg | ■ | |
| **Klonopin Wafers** | | |
| 0.125 mg | | ■ |
| 0.25 mg | | ■ |
| 0.5 mg | | ■ |
| 1 mg | | ■ |
| 2 mg | | ■ |
| **K-Lor Powder Packets** | | |
| 15 meq | ■ | |
| 20 meq | ■ | |
| **Koate-DVI** | | |
| 1 iu | ■ | |
| **Kogenate FS** | | |
| 1 iu | ■ | |
| **Kogenate FS with Bio-Set** | | |
| 1 iu | ■ | |
| **K-Phos Neutral Tablets** | | |
| 155 mg-852 mg-130 mg | ■ | |
| **K-Phos Original (Sodium Free) Tablets** | | |
| 500 mg | | ■ |
| **K-Tab Filmtab Tablets** | | |
| 10 meq | ■ | |
| **Lanoxin Injection** | | |
| 0.25 mg/ml | ■ | |
| **Lanoxin Tablets** | | |
| 0.125 mg | ■ | |
| 0.25 mg | ■ | |
| 0.5 mg | ■ | |
| **Lanoxin Injection Pediatric** | | |
| 0.1 mg/ml | ■ | |
| **Lariam Tablets** | | |
| 250 mg | ■ | |
| **Leustatin Injection** | | |
| 1 mg/ml | ■ | |
| **Levothroid Tablets** | | |
| 0.025 mg | ■ | |
| 0.05 mg | ■ | |
| 0.075 mg | ■ | |
| 0.088 mg | ■ | |
| 0.1 mg | ■ | |
| 0.112 mg | ■ | |
| 0.125 mg | ■ | |
| 0.137 mg | ■ | |
| 0.15 mg | ■ | |
| 0.175 mg | ■ | |
| 0.2 mg | ■ | |
| 0.3 mg | ■ | |
| **Levoxyl Tablets** | | |
| 0.025 mg | ■ | |
| 0.05 mg | ■ | |
| 0.075 mg | ■ | |
| 0.088 mg | ■ | |
| 0.1 mg | ■ | |
| 0.112 mg | ■ | |
| 0.125 mg | ■ | |
| 0.137 mg | ■ | |
| 0.15 mg | ■ | |
| 0.175 mg | ■ | |
| 0.2 mg | ■ | |
| 0.3 mg | ■ | |
| **Librium Capsules** | | |
| 5 mg | ■ | |
| 10 mg | ■ | |
| 25 mg | ■ | |
| **Lithobid Tablets** | | |
| 300 mg | ■ | |
| **Locoid Cream** | | |
| 0.1% | | ■ |
| **Locoid Lipocream Cream** | | |
| 0.1% | | ■ |
| **Locoid Ointment** | | |
| 0.1% | | ■ |
| **Locoid Topical Solution** | | |
| 0.1% | ■ | |
| **Lofibra Capsules** | | |
| 67 mg | ■ | |
| 134 mg | ■ | |
| 200 mg | ■ | |
| **Lo/Ovral-28 Tablets** | | |
| 30 mcg-0.3 mg | ■ | |
| **Lopressor HCT 50/25 Tablets** | | |
| 25 mg-50 mg | | ■ |
| **Lopressor HCT 100/25 Tablets** | | |
| 25 mg-100 mg | | ■ |
| **Lopressor HCT 100/50 Tablets** | | |
| 50 mg-100 mg | | ■ |
| **Lopressor Injection** | | |
| 1 mg/ml | ■ | |
| **Lopressor Tablets** | | |
| 50 mg | ■ | |
| 100 mg | ■ | |
| **Lortab Elixir** | | |
| 500 mg/15 ml-7.5 mg/15 ml | ■ | |
| **Lotensin Tablets** | | |
| 5 mg | ■ | |
| 10 mg | ■ | |
| 20 mg | ■ | |
| 40 mg | ■ | |

| STRENGTH | GENERIC YES | GENERIC NO |
|---|---|---|
| **Lotensin HCT Tablets** | | |
| 5 mg-6.25 mg | ■ | |
| 10 mg-12.5 mg | ■ | |
| 20 mg-12.5 mg | ■ | |
| 20 mg-25 mg | ■ | |
| **Lotrimin Cream** | | |
| 1% | ■ | |
| **Lotrimin Lotion** | | |
| 1% | ■ | |
| **Lotrimin Topical Solution** | | |
| 1% | ■ | |
| **Lotrisone Cream** | | |
| 0.05%-1% | ■ | |
| **Lustra Cream** | | |
| 4% | ■ | |
| **Lustra-AF Cream** | | |
| 4% | ■ | |
| **Maxzide Tablets** | | |
| 25 mg-37.5 mg | ■ | |
| 50 mg-75 mg | ■ | |
| **Mebaral Tablets, USP** | | |
| 32 mg | ■ | |
| 50 mg | ■ | |
| 100 mg | ■ | |
| **Mefoxin for Injection** | | |
| 1 gm | ■ | |
| 2 gm | ■ | |
| 10 gm | ■ | |
| **Metadate CD Capsules** | | |
| 10 mg | ■ | |
| 20 mg | ■ | |
| 30 mg | ■ | |
| **Mevacor Tablets** | | |
| 10 mg | ■ | |
| 20 mg | ■ | |
| 40 mg | ■ | |
| **Miacalcin Injection** | | |
| 200 iu/ml | ■ | |
| **Miacalcin Nasal Spray** | | |
| 200 iu/actuation | | ■ |
| **Midamor Tablets** | | |
| 5 mg | ■ | |
| **Mivacron Injection** | | |
| 2 mg/ml | ■ | |
| **Moduretic Tablets** | | |
| 5 mg-50 mg | ■ | |
| **MS Contin Tablets** | | |
| 15 mg | ■ | |
| 30 mg | ■ | |
| 60 mg | ■ | |
| 100 mg | ■ | |
| 200 mg | ■ | |
| **Nadolol Tablets** | | |
| 20 mg | ■ | |
| 40 mg | ■ | |
| 80 mg | ■ | |
| **Naprosyn Suspension** | | |
| 25 mg/ml | ■ | |
| **Naprosyn Tablets** | | |
| 250 mg | ■ | |
| 375 mg | ■ | |
| 500 mg | ■ | |
| **Narcan Injection** | | |
| 0.02 mg/ml | ■ | |
| 0.4 mg/ml | ■ | |
| 1 mg/ml | ■ | |
| **Nasarel Nasal Spray** | | |
| 0.025 mg/actuation | ■ | |
| **Naturethroid Tablets** | | |
| 32.4 mg | ■ | |
| 64.8 mg | ■ | |
| 129.6 mg | ■ | |
| 194.4 mg. | | ■ |
| **Navelbine Injection** | | |
| 10 mg/ml | ■ | |
| **Nembutal Sodium Solution, USP** | | |
| 50 mg/ml | ■ | |
| **Neoral Soft Gelatin Capsules** | | |
| 25 mg | ■ | |
| 100 mg | ■ | |
| **Neoral Oral Solution** | | |
| 100 mg/ml | ■ | |
| **Neurontin Capsules** | | |
| 100 mg | ■ | |
| 300 mg | ■ | |
| 400 mg | ■ | |
| **Neurontin Oral Solution** | | |
| 250 mg/5 ml | | ■ |
| **Neurontin Tablets** | | |
| 600 mg | ■ | |
| 800 mg | ■ | |
| **Niaspan Extended-Release Tablets** | | |
| 500 mg | ■ | |
| 750 mg | ■ | |
| 1000 mg | ■ | |
| **Nicomide Tablets** | | |
| 0.5 mg-750 mg-25 mg | ■ | |
| **Nitro-Dur Transdermal Infusion System** | | |
| 0.1 mg/hr | ■ | |
| 0.2 mg/hr | ■ | |
| 0.3 mg/hr | ■ | |
| 0.4 mg/hr | ■ | |
| 0.6 mg/hr | ■ | |
| 0.8 mg/hr | ■ | |
| **Norflex Injection** | | |
| 30 mg/ml | ■ | |
| **Novarel for Injection** | | |
| 10000 u | ■ | |
| **Novolin 70/30 Human Insulin** | | |
| 10 ml Vials | | |
| 70 u/ml-30 u/ml | ■ | |
| **Novolin 70/30 InnoLet** | | |
| 70 u/ml-30 u/ml | ■ | |
| **Novolin 70/30 PenFill 3 ml Cartridges** | | |
| 70 u/ml-30 u/ml | ■ | |
| **Novolin N Human Insulin 10 ml Vials** | | |
| 100 u/ml | ■ | |
| **Novolin N PenFill 3 ml Cartridges** | | |
| 100 u/ml | ■ | |
| **Novolin R Human Insulin** | | |
| 10 ml Vials | | |
| 100 u/ml | ■ | |
| **Novolin R PenFill 1.5 ml Cartridges** | | |
| 100 u/ml | ■ | |
| **Novolin R PenFill 3 ml Cartridges** | | |
| 100 u/ml | ■ | |
| **Nubain Injection** | | |
| 10 mg/ml | ■ | |
| 20 mg/ml | ■ | |
| **Nutropin for Injection** | | |
| 5 mg | ■ | |
| 10 mg | | ■ |
| **Nutropin AQ Injection** | | |
| 5 mg/ml | | ■ |
| **Nutropin AQ Pen Cartridge** | | |
| 5 mg/ml | | ■ |
| **Nystatin Vaginal Tablets, USP** | | |
| 100000 u | ■ | |
| **Nystop Topical Powder USP** | | |
| 100000 u/gm | ■ | |
| **Ocucoat** | | |
| 0.1%-0.8% | ■ | |
| **Ocufen Ophthalmic Solution** | | |
| 0.03% | ■ | |
| **Ophthetic Ophthalmic Solution** | | |
| 0.5% | ■ | |
| **OptiPranolol Metipranolol Ophthalmic Solution** | | |
| 0.3% | ■ | |
| **Ortho-Cept Tablets** | | |
| 0.15 mg-0.03 mg | ■ | |
| **Ortho-Cyclen Tablets** | | |
| 35 mcg-0.25 mg | ■ | |
| **Ortho Micronor Tablets** | | |
| 0.35 mg | ■ | |
| **Ortho Tri-Cyclen** | | |
| 35 mcg-0.180 mg, 0.125 mg, 0.250 mg | ■ | |

| STRENGTH | GENERIC YES | GENERIC NO |
|---|---|---|
| **Ortho Tri-Cyclen Lo Tablets** | | |
| 0.025 mg-0.18 mg | | ■ |
| **OsmoPrep Tablets** | | |
| 0.398 gm-1.102 gm | ■ | |
| **OxyContin Tablets** | | |
| 10 mg | ■ | |
| 20 mg | ■ | |
| 40 mg | ■ | |
| 80 mg | ■ | |
| 160 mg | | ■ |
| **OxyFast Oral Concentrate Solution** | | |
| 20 mg/ml | ■ | |
| **OxyIR Capsules** | | |
| 5 mg | ■ | |
| **Oxytrol Transdermal System** | | |
| 3.9 mg/24 hr | | ■ |
| **Pacerone Tablets** | | |
| 200 mg | ■ | |
| 400 mg | | ■ |
| **Panafil Ointment** | | |
| 0.5%-10%-10% | ■ | |
| 10%-10% | | ■ |
| **Panafil SE Spray Emulsion** | | |
| 0.5%-10% | ■ | |
| **Paxil CR Controlled-Release Tablets** | | |
| 12.5 mg | | ■ |
| 25 mg | | ■ |
| 37.5 mg | | ■ |
| **Paxil Oral Suspension** | | |
| 10 mg/5 ml | | ■ |
| 40 mg | ■ | |
| **Paxil Tablets** | | |
| 10 mg | ■ | |
| 20 mg | ■ | |
| 30 mg | ■ | |
| 40 mg | ■ | |
| **Pediapred Oral Solution** | | |
| 5 mg/5 ml | ■ | |
| **Pentasa Capsules** | | |
| 250 mg | ■ | |
| 500 mg | | ■ |
| **Pepcid Injection** | | |
| 0.4 mg/ml | ■ | |
| 10 mg/ml | ■ | |
| **Pepcid Injection Premixed** | | |
| 0.4 mg/ml | ■ | |
| **Pepcid for Oral Suspension** | | |
| 0.4 mg/ml | ■ | |
| 40 mg/5 ml | | ■ |
| **Pepcid Tablets** | | |
| 20 mg | ■ | |
| 40 mg | ■ | |
| **Percocet Tablets** | | |
| 325 mg-10 mg | ■ | |
| 325 mg-2.5 mg | | ■ |
| 325 mg-5 mg | ■ | |
| 325 mg-7.5 mg | ■ | |
| 500 mg-7.5 mg | ■ | |
| 650 mg -10 mg | ■ | |
| **Percodan Tablets** | | |
| 325 mg-4.5 mg-0.38 mg | ■ | |
| **Permax Tablets** | | |
| 0.05 mg | ■ | |
| 0.25 mg | ■ | |
| **Persantine Tablets** | | |
| 25 mg | ■ | |
| 50 mg | ■ | |
| 75 mg | ■ | |
| **Phenergan Suppositories** | | |
| 12.5 mg | ■ | |
| 25 mg | ■ | |
| 50 mg | ■ | |
| **Phenergan Tablets** | | |
| 12.5 mg | ■ | |
| 25 mg | ■ | |
| 50 mg | ■ | |
| **Plasbumin-5** | | |
| 5% | ■ | |
| **Plasbumin-20** | | |
| 20% | ■ | |
| **Plasbumin-25** | | |
| 25% | ■ | |
| **Plasmanate** | | |
| 5% | ■ | |
| **Plendil Extended-Release Tablets** | | |
| 2.5 mg | ■ | |
| 5 mg | ■ | |
| 10 mg | ■ | |
| **Pletal Tablets** | | |
| 50 mg | ■ | |
| **Plexion Cleanser** | | |
| 10%-5% | ■ | |
| **Plexion Cleansing Cloths** | | |
| 10%-5% | | ■ |
| **Plexion SCT** | | |
| 10%-5% | ■ | |
| **Plexion Topical Suspension** | | |
| 10%-5% | ■ | |
| **Pneumovax 23** | ■ | |
| **Polytrim Ophthalmic Solution** | | |
| 10000 u/ml-1 mg/ml | ■ | |
| **Potaba Envules** | | |
| 2 gm/packet | ■ | |
| **Potaba Tablets** | | |
| 0.5 gm | ■ | |
| **Pramosone Cream** | | |
| 1%-1% | ■ | |
| 2.5%-1% | | ■ |
| **Pramosone Lotion** | | |
| 1%-1% | ■ | |
| 2.5%-1% | ■ | |
| **Pramosone Ointment** | | |
| 1%-1% | | ■ |
| 2.5%-1% | | ■ |
| **PreCare Chewables Tablets** | ■ | |
| **PreCare Prenatal Caplets** | ■ | |
| **Pred Forte Ophthalmic Suspension** | | |
| 1% | ■ | |
| **Pred Mild Sterile Ophthalmic Suspension** | | |
| 0.12% | | ■ |
| **Pred-G Ophthalmic Suspension** | | |
| 0.3%-1% | | ■ |
| **Pred-G Sterile Ophthalmic Ointment** | | |
| 0.12% | ■ | |
| **PremesisRx Tablets** | ■ | |
| **Prenate Elite Tablets** | | |
| 120 mg-0.03 mg-200 mg-6 | ■ | |
| **PrimaCare AM Capsules** | ■ | |
| **PrimaCare PM Tablets** | ■ | |
| **Prinivil Tablets** | | |
| 2.5 mg | ■ | |
| 5 mg | ■ | |
| 10 mg | ■ | |
| 20 mg | ■ | |
| 40 mg | ■ | |
| **Prinzide Tablets** | | |
| 12.5 mg-10 mg | ■ | |
| 12.5 mg-20 mg | ■ | |
| 25 mg-20 mg | ■ | |
| **ProAmatine Tablets** | | |
| 2.5 mg | ■ | |
| 5 mg | ■ | |
| 10 mg | ■ | |
| **Prochieve Gel** | | |
| 4% | ■ | |
| 8% | ■ | |
| **Procrit for Injection** | | |
| 2000 u/ml | ■ | |
| 3000 u/ml | ■ | |
| 4000 u/ml | ■ | |
| 10000 u/ml | ■ | |
| 20000 u/ml | ■ | |
| 40000 u/ml | ■ | |
| **ProctoFoam-HC** | | |
| 1%-1% | ■ | |
| **Prolastin** | | |
| 1 mg | ■ | |

| STRENGTH | GENERIC YES | GENERIC NO |
|---|---|---|
| **Propine Ophthalmic Solution** | | |
| 0.1% | ■ | |
| **Prosed/DS Tablets** | | |
| 0.06 mg-9 mg-0.06 mg-81 | ■ | |
| 9 mg-0.12 mg-81.6 mg-10. | | ■ |
| **ProSom Tablets** | | |
| 1 mg | ■ | |
| 2 mg | ■ | |
| **Proventil Inhalation Aerosol** | | |
| 0.09 mg/actuation | ■ | |
| **Proventil HFA Inhalation Aerosol** | | |
| 0.09 mg/actuation | ■ | |
| **Prozac Pulvules and Liquid** | | |
| 10 mg | ■ | |
| 20 mg | ■ | |
| 20 mg/5 ml | ■ | |
| 40 mg | ■ | |
| **Psoriatec Cream** | | |
| 1% | ■ | |
| **Purinethol Tablets** | | |
| 50 mg | ■ | |
| **Rabies Vaccine RabAvert** | | |
| 2.5 iu | ■ | |
| **Raptiva for Injection** | | |
| 125 mg | ■ | |
| **Rebetol Capsules** | | |
| 200 mg | ■ | |
| **Recombinate** | | |
| 1 iu | ■ | |
| **ReFacto Vials** | | |
| 1 iu | ■ | |
| **Relafen Tablets** | | |
| 500 mg | ■ | |
| 750 mg | ■ | |
| **Renova Cream** | | |
| 0.02% | | ■ |
| 0.05% | ■ | |
| **Repronex for Intramuscular and Subcutaneous Injection** | | |
| 75 iu-75 iu | ■ | |
| **Ritalin Hydrochloride Tablets** | | |
| 5 mg | ■ | |
| 10 mg | ■ | |
| 20 mg | ■ | |
| **Ritalin LA Capsules** | | |
| 20 mg | ■ | |
| 30 mg | ■ | |
| 40 mg | | ■ |
| **Ritalin-SR Tablets** | | |
| 20 mg | ■ | |
| **Rocaltrol Capsules** | | |
| 0.25 mcg | ■ | |
| 0.5 mcg | ■ | |
| **Rocaltrol Oral Solution** | | |
| 1 mcg/ml | ■ | |
| **Roferon-A Injection** | | |
| 3 million iu/0.5 ml | ■ | |
| 3 million u/ml | | ■ |
| 6 million iu/0.5 ml | ■ | |
| 6 million u/ml | | ■ |
| 9 million iu/0.5 ml | ■ | |
| 9 million u/0.9 ml | | ■ |
| 36 million u/ml | | ■ |
| **Romazicon Injection** | | |
| 0.1 mg/ml | ■ | |
| **Rythmol SR Capsules** | | |
| 150 mg | ■ | |
| 225 mg | ■ | |
| 300 mg | ■ | |
| **Sandimmune I.V. Ampuls for Infusion** | | |
| 50 mg/ml | ■ | |
| **Sandimmune Oral Solution** | | |
| 100 mg/ml | | ■ |
| **Sandimmune Soft Gelatin Capsules** | | |
| 25 mg | | ■ |
| 50 mg | | ■ |
| 100 mg | | ■ |
| **Seasonale Tablets** | | |
| 30 mcg-0.15 mg | ■ | |
| **Sedapap Tablets** | | |
| 650 mg-50 mg | ■ | |
| **Skelaxin Tablets** | | |
| 400 mg | ■ | |
| 800 mg | | ■ |
| **Somavert Injection** | | |
| 10 mg | ■ | |
| 15 mg | ■ | |
| 20 mg | ■ | |
| **Soriatane Capsules** | | |
| 30 mg | ■ | |
| **Spectracef Tablets** | | |
| 200 mg | ■ | |
| **Subutex Tablets** | | |
| 2 mg | ■ | |
| 8 mg | ■ | |
| **Symmetrel Syrup** | | |
| 50 mg/5 ml | ■ | |
| **Symmetrel Tablets** | | |
| 100 mg | ■ | |
| **Synthroid Tablets** | | |
| 0.025 mg | ■ | |
| 0.05 mg | ■ | |
| 0.075 mg | ■ | |
| 0.088 mg | ■ | |
| 0.1 mg | ■ | |
| 0.112 mg | ■ | |
| 0.125 mg | ■ | |
| 0.137 mg | ■ | |
| 0.15 mg | ■ | |
| 0.175 mg | ■ | |
| 0.2 mg | ■ | |
| 0.3 mg | ■ | |
| **Tagamet Tablets** | | |
| 200 mg | ■ | |
| 300 mg | ■ | |
| 400 mg | ■ | |
| 800 mg | ■ | |
| **Tambocor Tablets** | | |
| 50 mg | ■ | |
| 100 mg | ■ | |
| 150 mg | ■ | |
| **Tegretol Chewable Tablets** | | |
| 100 mg | ■ | |
| **Tegretol-XR Tablets** | | |
| 100 mg | | ■ |
| 200 mg | | ■ |
| 400 mg | | ■ |
| **Tenormin I.V. Injection** | | |
| 0.5 mg/ml | | ■ |
| **Tenormin Tablets** | | |
| 25 mg | ■ | |
| 50 mg | ■ | |
| 100 mg | ■ | |
| **Tessalon Capsules** | | |
| 100 mg | ■ | |
| **Tessalon Perles** | | |
| 100 mg | ■ | |
| 200 mg | ■ | |
| **Testim Gel** | | |
| 1% | ■ | |
| **Tev-Tropin for Injection** | | |
| 5 mg | ■ | |
| **Thioridazine Hydrochloride Tablets** | | |
| 10 mg | ■ | |
| 25 mg | ■ | |
| 50 mg | ■ | |
| 100 mg | ■ | |
| **Thiothixene Capsules** | | |
| 1 mg | ■ | |
| 2 mg | ■ | |
| 5 mg | ■ | |
| 10 mg | ■ | |
| **Thrombate III** | | |
| 1 iu | ■ | |

| STRENGTH | GENERIC YES | GENERIC NO |
|---|---|---|
| **Thrombin-JMI** | | |
| 1000 u | ■ | |
| 5000 u | ■ | |
| 10000 iu | ■ | |
| 20000 iu | ■ | |
| 50000 u | ■ | |
| **Tiazac Capsules** | | |
| 120 mg | ■ | |
| 180 mg | ■ | |
| 240 mg | ■ | |
| 300 mg | ■ | |
| 360 mg | ■ | |
| 420 mg | | ■ |
| **Ticlid Tablets** | | |
| 250 mg | ■ | |
| **Timoptic in Ocudose** | | |
| 0.25% | ■ | |
| 0.5% | ■ | |
| **Timoptic Sterile Ophthalmic Solution** | | |
| 0.25% | ■ | |
| 0.5% | ■ | |
| **Timoptic-XE Sterile Ophthalmic Gel Forming Solution** | | |
| 0.25% | ■ | |
| 0.5% | ■ | |
| 0.25% | ■ | |
| 0.5% | ■ | |
| **Topicort Gel** | | |
| 0.05% | ■ | |
| **Topicort Cream** | | |
| 0.25% | ■ | |
| **Topicort Ointment** | | |
| 0.25% | ■ | |
| **Topicort LP Cream** | | |
| 0.05% | ■ | |
| **Tranxene T-TAB Tablets** | | |
| 3.75 mg | ■ | |
| 7.5 mg | ■ | |
| 15 mg | ■ | |
| **Triaz Cleanser** | | |
| 3% | | ■ |
| 6% | ■ | |
| 10% | ■ | |
| **Triaz Gel** | | |
| 3% | | ■ |
| 6% | ■ | |
| 10% | ■ | |
| **Triaz Pads** | | |
| 3% | | ■ |
| 6% | | ■ |
| 9% | | ■ |
| **Triglide Tablets** | | |
| 50 mg | | ■ |

| STRENGTH | GENERIC YES | GENERIC NO |
|---|---|---|
| 160 mg | ■ | |
| **Twinject 0.3** | | |
| 1 mg/ml | ■ | |
| **Twinject 0.15** | | |
| 1mg/ml | ■ | |
| **Tylenol with Codeine Elixir** | | |
| 120 mg/5 ml-12 mg/5 ml | ■ | |
| **Tylenol with Codeine Tablets** | | |
| 300 mg-7.5 mg | ■ | |
| 300 mg-15 mg | ■ | |
| 300 mg-30 mg | ■ | |
| 300 mg-60 mg | ■ | |
| **Ultracet Tablets** | | |
| 325 mg-37.5 mg | ■ | |
| **Ultrase Capsules** | | |
| 20000 u-4500 u-25000 u | ■ | |
| **Ultrase MT Capsules** | | |
| 39000 u-12000 u-39000 u | ■ | |
| 58500 u-18000 u-58500 u | ■ | |
| 65000 u-20000 u-65000 u | ■ | |
| **Uniphyl Tablets** | | |
| 400 mg | ■ | |
| 600 mg | ■ | |
| **Univasc Tablets** | | |
| 7.5 mg | ■ | |
| 15 mg | ■ | |
| **Urecholine Tablets** | | |
| 5 mg | ■ | |
| 10 mg | ■ | |
| 25 mg | ■ | |
| 50 mg | ■ | |
| **Vagifem Tablets** | | |
| 25 mcg | ■ | |
| **Vandazole Vaginal Gel** | | |
| 0.75% | ■ | |
| **Vantin Tablets and Oral Suspension** | | |
| 50 mg/5 ml | | ■ |
| 100 mg | ■ | |
| 100 mg/5 ml | | ■ |
| 200 mg | ■ | |
| **Vaseretic Tablets** | | |
| 5 mg-12.5 mg | ■ | |
| 10 mg-25 mg | ■ | |
| **Ventolin HFA Inhalation Aerosol** | | |
| 0.09 mg/actuatio■ | ■ | |
| **Vermox Chewable Tablets** | | |
| 100 mg | ■ | |
| **Vicodin Tablets** | | |
| 500 mg-5 mg | ■ | |
| **Vicodin ES Tablets** | | |
| 750 mg-7.5 mg | ■ | |
| **Vicodin HP Tablets** | | |
| 660 mg-10 mg | ■ | |

| STRENGTH | GENERIC YES | GENERIC NO |
|---|---|---|
| **Vicoprofen Tablets** | | |
| 7.5 mg-200 mg | ■ | |
| **Viokase Powder** | | ■ |
| **Viokase Tablets** | ■ | |
| **Viroptic Ophthalmic Solution** | | |
| 1% | ■ | |
| **Vivactil Tablets** | | |
| 5 mg | ■ | |
| 10 mg | ■ | |
| **Vivelle Transdermal System** | | |
| 0.025 mg/24 hr | ■ | |
| 0.0375 mg/24 hr | ■ | |
| 0.05 mg/24 hr | ■ | |
| 0.075 mg/24 hr | ■ | |
| 0.1 mg/24 hr | ■ | |
| **Vivelle-Dot Transdermal System** | | |
| 0.025 mg/24 hr | ■ | |
| 0.0375 mg/24 hr | ■ | |
| 0.05 mg/24 hr | ■ | |
| 0.075 mg/24 hr | ■ | |
| 0.1 mg/24 hr | ■ | |
| **Voltaren Ophthalmic Solution** | | |
| 0.1% | ■ | |
| **Voltaren Tablets** | | |
| 25 mg | ■ | |
| 50 mg | ■ | |
| 75 mg | ■ | |
| **Voltaren-XR Tablets** | | |
| 100 mg | ■ | |
| **VoSpire Extended-Release Tablets** | | |
| 4 mg | ■ | |
| 8 mg | ■ | |
| **Wellbutrin Tablets** | | |
| 75 mg | ■ | |
| 100 mg | ■ | |
| **Wellbutrin SR Sustained-Release Tablets** | | |
| 100 mg | ■ | |
| 150 mg | ■ | |
| 200 mg | ■ | |
| **Wellbutrin XL Extended-Release Tablets** | | |
| 150 mg | ■ | |
| 300 mg | ■ | |
| **Westhroid Tablets** | | |
| 60 mg | ■ | |
| 64.8 mg | ■ | |
| 129.6 mg | ■ | |
| 180 mg | ■ | |
| 240 mg | ■ | |
| **Zantac 150 Tablets** | | |
| 150 mg | ■ | |

| STRENGTH | GENERIC YES | GENERIC NO |
|---|---|---|
| **Zantac 300 Tablets** | | |
| 300 mg | ■ | |
| **Zantac 25 EFFERdose Tablets** | | |
| 150 mg | | ■ |
| 150 mg/packet | | ■ |
| **Zantac 150 EFFERdose Tablets** | | |
| 150 mg | | ■ |
| **Zantac Injection** | | |
| 25 mg/ml | ■ | |
| **Zantac Injection Premixed** | | |
| 1 mg/ml | | ■ |
| **Zantac Syrup** | | |
| 15 mg/ml | ■ | |
| **Zemaira** | | |
| 1 mg | ■ | |
| **Zestoretic Tablets** | | |
| 12.5 mg10 mg | ■ | |
| 12.5 mg-20 mg | ■ | |
| 25 mg-20 mg | ■ | |
| **Zestril Tablets** | | |
| 2.5 mg | ■ | |
| 5 mg | ■ | |
| 10 mg | ■ | |
| 20 mg | ■ | |
| 30 mg | ■ | |
| 40 mg | ■ | |
| **Zinacef Injection** | | |
| 1.5 gm | ■ | |
| 1.5 gm/50 ml | ■ | |
| 7.5 gm | ■ | |
| 750 mg | ■ | |
| 750 mg/50 ml | ■ | |
| **Zovirax Capsules** | | |
| 200 mg | ■ | |
| **Zovirax Cream** | | |
| 5% | | ■ |
| **Zovirax for Injection** | | |
| 500 mg | ■ | |
| 1000 mg | ■ | |
| **Zovirax Ointment** | | |
| 5% | | ■ |
| **Zovirax Suspension** | | |
| 200 mg/5 ml | ■ | |
| **Zovirax Tablets** | | |
| 400 mg | ■ | |
| 800 mg | ■ | |
| **Zyban Sustained-Release Tablets** | | |
| 150 mg | ■ | |

# LACTOSE- AND GALACTOSE-FREE DRUGS

The following is a selection of lactose- and galactose-free products. The list is not comprehensive. Generic and alternate brands may exist. Always check product labeling for definitive information on specific ingredients.

| TRADE NAME (OTC) | FORM |
|---|---|
| Advil | Tablets |
| Aleve | Caplets, Gelcaps, Tablets |
| Alka-Mints | Tablets |
| Alka-Seltzer | Effervescent Tablets |
| Alka-Seltzer Plus Cold | Effervescent Tablets |
| Anti-Tuss DM | Syrup |
| Ascriptin | Tablets |
| Axid AR | Tablets |
| Benadryl | Liquid, Tablets |
| Benadryl Allergy & Cold | Caplets |
| Benylin Expectorant | Liquid |
| Bufferin | Tablets |
| Caltrate 600 PLUS | Tablets |
| Casec | Powder |
| Cenafed | Syrup |
| Claritin-D | Tablets |
| Colace | Capsules |
| Doxidan Liqui-Gels | Capsules |
| Dramamine | Tablets |
| Elecare | Powder |
| Ensure | Liquid |
| Ensure High Calcium | Liquid |
| Ensure Plus | Liquid |
| Excedrin Extra-Strength | Tablets |
| Excedrin QuickTabs | Tablets |
| Ex-Lax Maximum Strength | Tablets |
| Fergon Iron | Tablets |
| Fibersource | Liquid |
| Fibersource HN | Liquid |
| Gaviscon Regular Strength | Tablets |
| Hytinic | Capsules |
| Iberet | Tablets |
| Imodium A-D | Liquid, Tablets |
| Impact | Liquid |
| Impact with Fiber | Liquid |
| Isosource | Liquid |
| Isosource HN | Liquid |
| Jevity | Liquid |
| Kaopectate Children's | Liquid |
| Konsyl | Powder |
| Lactaid | Tablets |
| Lipisorb | Liquid |
| MCT Oil | Oil |
| Medi-Lyte | Tablets |
| Metamucil | Powder, Wafers |
| Moducal | Powder |
| Motrin IB | Tablets |
| Mylanta Gas | Tablets |
| Mylicon Infants' | Drops |
| Naldecon Senior DX | Liquid |
| Naldecon Senior EX | Liquid |
| Nepro | Liquid |
| NoDoz Maximum Strength | Tablets |
| Ocuvite Vitamin and Mineral Supplement | Tablets |
| One-A-Day Active | Tablets |
| One-A-Day Garlic Softgels | Capsules |
| One-A-Day Maximum | Tablets |
| One-A-Day Men's | Tablets |
| One-A-Day Women's | Tablets |
| Orudis KT | Tablets |
| Osmolite | Liquid |
| Pediasure | Liquid |
| Pepto-Bismol | Suspension, Tablets |
| Pepto-Bismol Max. Strength | Suspension |
| Percy Medicine | Liquid |
| Polycose | Liquid, Powder |
| Poly-Vi-Sol | Drops |
| Poly-Vi-Sol with Iron | Drops |
| Portagen | Powder |
| Prilosec OTC | Tablets |
| Promote | Liquid |
| Pulmocare | Liquid |
| Purge | Oil |
| RCF | Liquid |
| Resource Plus | Liquid |
| Riopan | Suspension |
| Riopan Plus | Suspension |
| Similac with Iron | Concentrate, Powder |
| Simply Sleep | Caplets |
| St. Joseph Adult Low Strength Aspirin | Tablets |
| Sucrets Maximum Strength | Lozenges |
| Sudafed | Tablets |
| Sudafed Children's | Liquid |
| Sudafed Sinus | Tablets |
| Sunkist Vitamin C | Tablets |
| Titralac | Tablets |
| Titralac Plus | Tablets |
| Tri-Vi-Sol | Drops |
| Tri-Vi-Sol with Iron | Drops |
| Tums | Tablets |
| Tylenol | Drops, Liquid, Tablets |
| Unisom SleepTabs | Tablets |
| Vi-Daylin ADC Vitamins Plus Iron | Drops |
| Zantac 75 | Tablets |

| TRADE NAME (RX) | FORM |
|---|---|
| Accutane | Capsules |
| Actigall | Capsules |
| Advicor | Tablets |
| Aldactazide | Tablets |
| Aldactone | Tablets |
| Allegra | Tablets |
| Allegra-D | Tablets |
| Altace | Capsules |
| Amicar | Tablets |
| Antivert | Tablets |
| Aromasin | Tablets |
| Atrohist Pediatric | Capsules |
| Augmentin | Tablets |
| Augmentin XR | Tablets |
| Axid | Capsules |
| Bactrim | Tablets |
| Biaxin Filmtab | Tablets |
| Calan SR | Tablets |
| Carafate | Tablets |
| Cardene | Capsules |
| Cardizem CD | Capsules |
| Cardizem SR | Capsules |
| Ceclor | Capsules |
| Ceftin | Suspension, Tablets |
| Cefzil | Suspension, Tablets |
| Cipro | Tablets |
| Cipro XR | Tablets |
| Clinoril | Tablets |
| Combivir | Tablets |
| Comtan | Tablets |
| Covera-HS | Tablets |
| Creon | Capsules |
| Cytotec | Tablets |
| Darvon-N/Darvocet-N | Tablets |
| Daypro | Tablets |
| Deconsal II | Tablets |
| Demerol | Tablets |
| Depakene | Capsules |
| Depakote | Tablets |
| Depakote Sprinkle | Capsules |
| Desoxyn | Tablets |
| Detrol | Tablets |
| DiaBeta | Tablets |
| Diabinese | Tablets |
| Diovan | Capsules |

|  |  |
|---|---|
| Diovan HCT | Tablets |
| Dolobid | Tablets |
| Donnatal Extentabs | Tablets |
| Duricef | Capsules, Tablets, Suspension |
| E.E.S. | Suspension, Tablets |
| Entex LA | Tablets |
| Epivir | Tablets, Solution |
| Epivir-HBV | Tablets |
| Ery-Tab | Tablets |
| Esgic-Plus | Capsules, Tablets |
| Exelon | Capsules |
| Fero-Folic/Iberet Folic | Tablets |
| Fioricet | Tablets |
| Flomax | Capsules |
| Gleevec | Tablets |
| Glucotrol XL | Tablets |
| Glucovance | Tablets |
| Glyset | Tablets |
| GoLYTELY | Powder |
| Grifulvin V | Suspension, Tablets |
| Guaifed | Capsules |
| Hytrin | Capsules |
| Inderal LA | Capsules |
| Isoptin SR | Tablets |
| Kaletra | Capsules, Solution |
| K-Dur | Tablets |
| Keppra | Tablets |
| K-Lor | Powder |
| K-Phos Neutral | Tablets |
| K-Phos Original Formula | Tablets |
| K-Tab | Tablets |
| Lamisil | Tablets |
| Lanoxicaps | Capsules |
| Lescol | Capsules |
| Lescol XL | Tablets |
| Levaquin | Tablets |
| Levothroid | Tablets |
| Levoxyl | Tablets |
| Lexapro | Tablets |
| Librium | Capsules |
| Lomotil | Tablets |
| Lopid | Tablets |
| Malarone | Tablets |
| Malarone Pediatric | Tablets |
| Materna | Tablets |
| Maxzide | Tablets |
| Methylin ER | Tablets |
| Micardis | Tablets |
| Micro-K | Capsules |
| Micronase | Tablets |
| Minipress | Capsules |
| Minocin | Capsules |
| Motrin | Tablets |
| Mycostatin | Pastilles |
| Niaspan | Tablets |
| Nicomide | Tablets |
| Niferex-150 | Capsules |
| Niferex-150 Forte | Capsules |
| Niferex-PN | Tablets |
| Nolvadex | Tablets |
| Norpramin | Tablets |
| Norvasc | Tablets |
| Omnicef | Capsules |
| Pamelor | Capsules |
| Pamine Forte | Tablets |
| Pancrease | Capsules |
| Pancrease MT | Capsules |
| Paxil | Tablets |
| Pepcid | Suspension, Tablets |
| Percocet | Tablets |
| Percodan | Tablets |
| PhosLo | Tablets |
| Plaquenil | Tablets |
| Pletal | Tablets |
| Prandin | Tablets |
| Precare | Tablets |
| Precose | Tablets |
| Prevacid | Capsules |
| Prinivil | Tablets |
| ProAmatine | Tablets |
| Procardia | Capsules |
| Procardia XL | Tablets |
| Prometrium | Capsules |
| Protonix | Tablets |
| Prozac | Capsules |
| Questran | Powder |
| Relafen | Tablets |
| Remeron SolTab | Tablets |
| Rifadin | Capsules |
| Robaxin | Tablets |
| Sarafem | Pulvules |
| Sectral | Capsules |
| Serzone | Tablets |
| Sinemet | Tablets |
| Sinemet CR | Tablets |
| Soma | Tablets |
| Stalevo | Tablets |
| StrongStart | Caplets |
| Symmetrel | Tablets |
| Tamiflu | Capsules |
| Tegretol/Tegretol-XR | Tablets |
| Tenoretic | Tablets |
| Tenormin | Tablets |
| Tequin | Tablets |
| Tessalon | Capsules |
| Tiazac | Capsules |
| Ticlid | Tablets |
| Tikosyn | Capsules |
| Tofranil-PM | Capsules |
| Toprol-XL | Tablets |
| Trental | Tablets |
| Trileptal | Tablets |
| Trilisate | Tablets |
| Trizivir | Tablets |
| Ultrase | Capsules |
| Uniphyl | Tablets |
| Valcyte | Tablets |
| Valium | Tablets |
| Valtrex | Caplets |
| Vibramycin Hyclate | Capsules |
| Vicodin | Tablets |
| Vicodin ES | Tablets |
| Vicodin HP | Tablets |
| Vicoprofen | Tablets |
| Videx | Tablets |
| Visicol | Tablets |
| Vistaril | Capsules |
| Welchol | Tablets |
| Wellbutrin | Tablets |
| Wellbutrin SR | Tablets |
| Xenical | Capsules |
| Yocon | Tablets |
| Zantac | Syrup, Tablets |
| Zarontin | Capsules |
| Zaroxolyn | Tablets |
| Zebeta | Tablets |
| Zestril | Tablets |
| Ziac | Tablets |
| Ziagen | Tablets |
| Zofran | Solution, Tablets (disintegrating) |
| Zoloft | Tablets |
| Zonegran | Capsules |
| Zyban | Tablets |
| Zyflo Filmtab | Tablets |
| Zymase | Capsules |
| Zyvox | Suspension, Tablets |

# POISON ANTIDOTE CHART

**WARNING:** While every effort has been made to ensure the accuracy of this chart, it is not intended to serve as the sole source of information on antidotes. Guidelines may need to be adjusted based on factors such as anticipated usage in the hospital's local area, the nearest alternate sources of antidotes, and distance to tertiary care institutions. Contact your nearest regional poison control center (1-800-222-1222) for treatment information regarding any exposure, including indications for use of antidote therapy. Directions in this chart assume that all basic life support and decontamination measures have been initiated as needed.

| ANTIDOTE | POISON/DRUG/TOXIN | SUGGESTED MINIMUM STOCK QUANTITY | COMMENTS |
|---|---|---|---|
| N-Acetylcysteine (Acetadote®, Mucomyst®) | Acetaminophen<br>Carbon tetrachloride<br>Other hepatotoxins | Oral product: 600 mL in 10 mL or 30 mL vials of 20% solution<br>IV product: One carton of four 30 mL vials of 20% solution | Acetaminophen is the most common drug involved intentional and unintentional poisonings. 600 mL (120 g) of the oral product provides enough antidote to treat an adult for an entire 3-day course of therapy, or enough to treat three adults for 24 h. Several vials may be stocked in the ED to provide a loading dose and the remaining vials in the pharmacy for the q 4 h maintenance doses. The IV product dose of 120mL (24 g) will treat one adult patient for an entire 20-hour IV protocol. |
| Amyl nitrite, sodium nitrite, and sodium thiosulfate (Cyanide antidote kit) | Acetonitrile<br>Acrylonitrile<br>Bromates (thiosulfate only)<br>Chlorates (thiosulfate only)<br>Cyanide (e.g., HCN, KCN and NaCN)<br>Cyanogen chloride<br>Cyanogenic glycoside natural sources (e.g., apricot pits and peach pits)<br>Hydrogen sulfide (nitrites only)<br>Laetrile<br>Mustard agents (thiosulfate only)<br>Nitroprusside (thiosulfate only)<br>Smoke inhalation (combustion of synthetic materials) | One to two kits | Stock one kit in the ED. Consider also stocking one kit in the pharmacy.<br>Note: This kit has a short shelf life of 24 months. |
| Antivenin, Crotalidae Polyvalent (equine origin) | Pit viper envenomation (e.g., rattlesnakes, cottonmouths, and timber rattlers | Ten vials | Stock in pharmacy. Advised in geographic areas with endemic populations of copperheads, water mocassins, or eastern massasauga ratlesnakes. In low-risk areas, know nearest alternate source of antivenin. Note: 20 to 40 vials or more may be needed for moderate to severe envenomations. The antivenin must be administered in a critical care setting since it is an equine-derived product. Refrigeration is unnecessary. |

*(Continued)*

This chart is adapted from material furnished by the Illinois Poison Center, a program of the Metropolitan Chicago Healthcare Council (MCHC).

| ANTIDOTE | POISON/DRUG/TOXIN | SUGGESTED MINIMUM STOCK QUANTITY | COMMENTS |
|---|---|---|---|
| Antivenin, Crotalidae Polyvalent Immune Fab–Ovine (CroFab®) | Pit viper envenomation (e.g., rattlesnakes, cottonmouths, copperheads, and timber rattlers) | Four to six vials | Stock in pharmacy. This product is a possible alternate to equine product. May have lower risk of hypersensitivity reaction than equine product. Average dose in premarketing trials was 12 vials but more may be needed. Note: Store in refrigerator. See entry above for equine antivenin. |
| Antivenin, *Latrodectus mactans* (Black widow spider) | Black widow spider envenomation | Zero to one vial | Serious *Latrodectus* envenomations are rare. This product is only used for severe envenomations. Antivenin must be given in a critical care setting since it is an equine-derived product. Know the nearest source of antidote. Note: Product must be refrigerated at all times. |
| Atropine sulfate | Alpha$^2$ agonists (e.g., clonidine, guanabenz, and guanfacine)<br>Alzheimer's drugs (e.g., donepezil, galantamine, rivastigmine, tacrine)<br>Antimyesthenic agents (e.g., pyridostigmine)<br>Bradyarrhythmia-producing agents (e.g., beta blockers, calcium channel blockers, and digitalis glycosides)<br>Cholinergic agonists (e.g., bethanechol)<br>Muscarine-containing mushrooms (e.g., Clitocybe and Inocybe)<br>Nerve agents (e.g., sarin, soman, tabun, and VX)<br>Organophosphate and carbamate insecticides | Total 100 mg to 150 mg<br><br>Available in various formulations:<br>0.4 mg/mL (20 mL, 8 mg vials)<br>0.1 mg/mL (10 mL, 1 mg ampules)<br>0.1 mg/mL (10 mL, 1 mg ampules)<br><br>Atropine sulfate military-style auto-injectors: 2mg 2 mg/0.7 mL, 1 mg/0.7 mL, 0.5 mg/0.7 mL, 0.25 mg/0.3 mL | The product should be immediately available in the ED. Some may also be stored in the pharmacy or other hospital sites, but should be easily mobilized if a severely poisoned patient needs treat ment. Note: Product is nec essary for adequate preparedness for a weapon of mass destruction (WMD) incident; the suggested amount may not be sufficient for mass-casualty events. Auto-injectors are available from Bound Tree Medical, Inc. Drug stocked in chempack container is intended only for use in mass-casualty events. |
| Calcium disodium EDTA (Versenate®) | Lead Zinc salts (e.g., zinc chloride) | One 5 mL amp (200 mg/mL) | Stock in pharmacy. One vial provides 1 day of therapy for a child. More may be needed in lead-endemic areas. |
| Calcium chloride and Calcium gluconate | Beta blockers<br>Calcium channel blockers<br>Fluoride salts (e.g., NaF)<br>Hydrofluoric acid (HF)<br>Hyperkalemia (not digoxin-induced)<br>Hypermagnesemia | 10% calcium chloride: fifteen 10 mL vials<br>10% calcium gluconate: five 10 mL vials | Stock in ED. More may be stocked in pharmacy. Many ampules of calcium chloride may be necessary in life-threatening calcium channel blocker or hydrofluoric acid poisoning. |
| Deferoxamine mesylate (Desferal®) | Iron | Twelve 500 mg vials | Stock in pharmacy. Note: Per package insert, the maximum daily dose is 6 g (12 vials). However, this dose may be exceeded in serious poisonigs. |
| Digoxin immune Fab (Digibind®, DigiFab®) | Cardiac glycoside-containing plants (e.g., foxglove and oleander)<br>Digitoxin<br>Digoxin | Ten vials | Stock in ED or pharmacy. This amount (ten vials) may be given to a digoxin-poisoned patient in whom the digoxin level is unknown. This amount would effectively neutralize a steady-state digoxin level of 14.2 ng/mL in a 70-kg patient. More may be necessary in severe intoxications. Know nearest source of additional supply. |

(Continued)

| ANTIDOTE | POISON/DRUG/TOXIN | SUGGESTED MINIMUM STOCK QUANTITY | COMMENTS |
|---|---|---|---|
| Dimercaprol (BAL in oil) | Arsenic<br>Copper<br>Gold<br>Lead<br>Lewisite<br>Mercury | Two 3 mL amps (100 mg/mL) | Stock in pharmacy. This amount provides two doses of 3 to 5 mg/kg/dose given q 4 h to treat one seriously poisoned adult or provides enough to treat a 15-kg child for 24 h. |
| Ethanol | Ethylene glycol<br>Methanol | 6 L of 5% alcohol in D5W<br>10% alcohol in D5W was discontinued in 2004; however, it can be prepared from 5% alcohol in D5W and dehydrated alcohol. Consult Poison Control Center. | Stock in pharmacy. This amount (6 L) provides enough to treat two adults with a loading dose followed by a maintenance infusion for 4 hours each. More alcohol or fomepizole will be needed during dialysis or prolonged treatment. 95% or 40% alcohol diluted in juice may be given po if IV alcohol is unavailable. Note: Ethanol is unnecessary if fomepizole is stocked. |
| Flumazenil (Romazicon®) | Benzodiazepines<br>Zaleplon<br>Zolpidem | Total 1 mg: two 5 mL vials (0.1 mg/mL) | Suggested minimum is for ED stocking. Due to risk of seizures, use with extreme caution, if at all, in poisoned patients. More may be stocked in the pharmacy for use in reversal of conscious sedation. |
| Folic acid and Folinic acid (Leucovorin) | Methanol<br>Methotrexate, trimetrexate<br>Pyrimethamine<br>Trimethoprim | Folic acid: three 50 mg vials<br>Folinic acid: one 50 mg vial | Stock in pharmacy. For methanol-poisoned patients with an acidosis, give 50mg folinic acid initially, then 50mg of folic acid q 4 h for six doses. |
| Fomepizole (Antizol®) | Ethylene glycol<br>Methanol | Two 1.5 g vial<br>Note: Available in a kit of four 1.5 g vials | Stock in pharmacy. Know where nearest alternate supply is located. One vial will provide at least one initial adult dose. Hospitals with critical care and hemodialysis capabilities should consider stocking one kit of four vials (enough to treat one patient for up to several days). Note: Product has a 2-year shelf life; however, the manufacturer offers a credit for unused, expired product. |
| Glucagon | Beta blockers<br>Calcium channel blockers<br>Hypoglycemia<br>Hypoglycemic agents | Fifty 1 mg vials | Stock 20 mg in ED and remainder in pharmacy. The total amount (50 mg) provides approximately 5 to 10 hours of high-dose therapy in life-threatening beta blocker or calcium channel blocker poisoning. A protocol using high doses of insulin/dextrose also may be considered. Consult regional poison center for guidelines. |
| Hyperbaric oxygen (HBO) | Carbon monoxide<br>Carbon tetrachloride<br>Cyanide<br>Hydrogen sulfide<br>Methemoglobinemia | Post the location and phone number of nearest HBO chamber in the ED. | Consult regional poison center to determine if HBO treatment is indicated. |

*(Continued)*

| ANTIDOTE | POISON/DRUG/TOXIN | SUGGESTED MINIMUM STOCK QUANTITY | COMMENTS |
|---|---|---|---|
| Methylene blue | Methemoglobin-inducing agents including:<br>Aniline dyes<br>Dapsone<br>Dinitrophenol<br>Local anesthetics (e.g., benzocaine)<br>Metoclopramide<br>Monomethylhydrazine-containing mushrooms (e.g., Gyromitra)<br>Naphthalene<br>Nitrates and nitrites<br>Nitrobenzene<br>Phenazopyridine | Three 10 mL amps (10 mg/mL) | Stock in pharmacy. This amount provides three doses of 1 to 2 mg/kg (0.1 to 0.2 mL/kg) for an adult patient. |
| Nalmefene (Revex®) and Naloxone (Narcan®) | ACE inhibitors<br>Alpha$^2$ agonists (e.g., clonidine, guanabenz, and guanfacine)<br>Coma of unknown cause<br>Imidazoline decongestants (e.g., oxymetazoline and tetrahydrozoline)<br>Loperamide<br>Opioids (e.g., codeine, dextromethorphan, diphenoxylate, fentanyl, heroin, meperidine, morphine, and propoxyphene) | Nalmefene: none required<br>Naloxone: total 40 mg, any combination of 0.4 mg 1 mg, and 2 mg ampules | Stock 20 mg naloxone in the the institution. Note: Nalmefene has a longer duration of action but it offers no therapeutic advantage over a naloxone infusion. |
| D-penicillamine (Cuprimine®) | Arsenic<br>Copper<br>Lead<br>Mercury | None required as an antidote. Available in bottles of 100 capsules (125 mg or 250 mg/capsule) | D-penicillamine is no longer considered the drug of choice for heavy-metal poisonings. It may be stocked in the pharmacy for other indications such as Wilson's disease or rheumatoid arthritis. |
| Physostigmine salicylate (Antilirium®) | Anticholinergic alkaloid-containing plants (e.g., deadly nightshade and jimson weed)<br>Antihistamines<br>Atropine and other anticholinergic agents<br>Intrathecal baclofen | Two 2 mL ampules (1 mg/mL) | Stock in ED or pharmacy. Usual adult dose is 1 to 2 mg slow IV push. Note: Duration of effect is 30 to 60 min. |
| Phytonadione (Vitamin K1) (AquaMEPHYTON®, Mephyton®) | Indandione derivatives<br>Long-acting anticoagulant rodenticides (e.g., brodifacoum and bromadiolone)<br>Warfarin | Two 0.5 mL ampules (2 mg/mL) and ten 1 mL ampules (10 mg/mL)<br>5 mg tablets available in packages of 10, 14, 20, 30, and 100 | Stock in pharmacy. |
| Pralidoxime chloride (2-PAM) (Protopam®) | Antimyesthenic agents (e.g., pyridostigmine)<br>Nerve agents (e.g., sarin, soman, tabun, and VX)<br>Organophosphate insecticides<br>Tacrine | Six 1 g vials<br>Pralidoxime chloride military-style auto-injectors: 600 mg/2 mL | Stock in ED or pharmacy. Note: Serious intoxications may require 500 mg/h (12 g/day). Product is necessary for adequate preparedness for a weapon of mass destruction (WMD) incident; the suggested amount may not be sufficient for mass-casualty events. Auto-injectors are available from Bound Tree Medical, Inc. Drug stocked in chempack container is intended only for use in mass-casualty events. |

*(Continued)*

| ANTIDOTE | POISON/DRUG/TOXIN | SUGGESTED MINIMUM STOCK QUANTITY | COMMENTS |
|---|---|---|---|
| Protamine sulfate | Enoxaparin<br>Heparin | Variable, consider recommendation of hospital P&T Committee<br>Available as 5 mL ampules (10 mg/mL) and 25 mL vials (250 mg/25 mL) | Stock in pharmacy. |
| Pyridoxine hydrochloride (Vitamin B6) | Acrylamide<br>Ethylene glycol<br>Hydrazine<br>Isoniazid (INH)<br>Monomethylhydrazine-containing mushrooms (e.g., Gyromitra) | Four 30 mL vials (100 mg/mL 3 g/vial) or one hundred 1 mL vials (100 mg/mL vials) | Stock in ED or pharmacy. Usual dose is 1 g pyridoxine HCl for each gram of INH ingested. If amount ingested is unknown, give 5 g of pyridoxine. Repeat dose if seizures are uncontrolled Know nearest source of additional supply. For ethylene glycol, a dose of 100 mg/day enhances the clearance of toxic metabolite. |
| Sodium bicarbonate | Chlorine gas<br>Hyperkalemia<br>Serum alkalinization:<br>Agents producing a quinidine-like effect as noted by widened QRS complex on EKG (e.g., amantadine, carbamazepine, chloroquine, cocaine, diphenhydramine, flecainide, propafenone, propoxyphene, tricyclic antidepressants, quinidine, and related agents)<br>Urine alkalinization: Weakly acidic agents (e.g., chlorophenoxy herbicides, chlorpropamide, phenobarbital, and salicylates) | Twenty 50 mEq vials | Stock 10 vials in the ED and 10 vials elsewhere in the hospital. |
| Succimer (Chemet®) | Arsenic<br>Lead<br>Lewisite<br>Mercury | One bottle of 100 capsules (100 mg/capsule) | Stock in pharmacy. FDA-approved only for pediatric lead poisoning; however, it has shown efficacy for other heavy-metal poisonings. |

# SUGAR-FREE PRODUCTS

Listed below, by therapeutic category, is a selection of drug products that contain no sugar. When recommending these products to diabetic patients, keep in mind that many may contain sorbitol, alcohol, or other sources of carbohydrates. This list should not be considered all-inclusive. Generics and alternate brands of some products may be available. Check product labeling for a current listing of inactive ingredients.

**ANALGESICS**

Actamin Maximum Strength Liquid
Addaprin Tablet
Aminofen Tablet
Aminofen Max Tablet
Aspirtab Tablet
Back Pain-Off Tablet
Backprin Tablet
Buffasal Tablet
Dyspel Tablet
Febrol Liquid
I-Prin Tablet
Medi-Seltzer Effervescent Tablet
Ms.-Aid Tablet
PMS Relief Tablet
Silapap Children's Elixir

**ANTACIDS/ANTIFLATULENTS**

Almag Chewable Tablet
Alcalak Chewable Tablet
Aldroxicon I Suspension
Aldroxicon II Suspension
Baby Gasz Drops
Dimacid Chewable Tablet
Diotame Chewable Tablet
Diotame Suspension
Gas-Ban Chewable
Mallamint Chewable
Mylanta Gelcaplet
Neutralin Tablet
Tums E-X Chewable Tablet

**ANTIASTHMATIC/RESPIRATORY AGENT**

Jay-Phyl Syrup

**ANTIDIARRHEALS**

Diarrest Tablet
Di-Gon II Tablet
Imogen Liquid

**BLOOD MODIFIERS/IRON PREPARATIONS**

I.L.X. B-12 Elixir
Irofel Liquid
Nephro-Fer Tablet

**CORTICOSTEROID**

Pediapred Solution

**COUGH/COLD/ALLERGY PREPARATIONS**

Accuhist DM Pediatric Drops
Accuhist Pediatric Drops
Alacol DM Syrup
Amerifed DM Liquid
Amerifed Liquid
Amerituss AD Solution
Anaplex DM Syrup
Anaplex DMX Syrup
Anaplex HD Syrup
Andehist DM Liquid
Andehist DM NR Liquid
Andehist DM NR Syrup
Andehist DM Syrup
Andehist Liquid
Andehist NR Liquid
Andehist NR Syrup
Andehist Syrup
Aridex Solution
Atuss EX Liquid
Atuss NX Solution
Baltussin Solution
Bellahist-D LA Tablet
Benadryl Allergy/Sinus Children's Solution
Biodec DM Drops
Bromaxefed DM RF Syrup
Bromaxefed RF Syrup
Bromdec Solution
Bromdec DM Solution
Bromhist-DM Solution
Bromhist Pediatric Solution
Bromophed DX Syrup
Bromphenex DM Solution
Bromphenex HD Solution
Bromplex DM Solution
Bromplex HD Solution
Bromtuss DM Solution
Broncotron Liquid
Broncotron-D Suspension
Brovex HC Solution
B-Tuss Liquid
Carbaphen 12 Ped Suspension
Carbaphen 12 Suspension
Carbatuss-CL Solution
Carbetaplex Solution
Carbihist Solution
Carbinoxamine PSE Solution
Carbofed DM Liquid
Carbofed DM Syrup
Carbofed DM Drops
Carboxine Solution
Carboxine-PSE Solution
Cardec DM Syrup
Cetafen Cold Tablet
Cheratussin DAC Liquid
Chlordex GP Syrup
Codal-DM Syrup
Colace Solution
ColdCough EXP Solution
ColdCough HC Solution
ColdCough PD Solution
ColdCough Solution
ColdCough XP Solution
Coldec DS Solution
ColdMist DM Syrup
Coldonyl Tablet
Colidrops Pediatric Liquid
Cordron-D Solution
Cordron-DM Solution
Cordron-HC Solution
Corfen DM Solution
Co-Tussin Liquid
Cotuss-V Syrup
Coughtuss Solution
Crantex HC Syrup
Crantex Syrup
Cypex-LA Tablet
Cytuss HC Syrup
Dacex-A Solution
Dacex-DM Solution
Dacex-PE Solution
Decahist-DM Solution
De-Chlor DM Solution
De-Chlor DR Solution
De-Chlor G Solution
De-Chlor HC Solution
De-Chlor HD Solution
De-Chlor MR Solution

De-Chlor NX Solution
Decorel Forte Tablet
Denaze Solution
Despec Liquid
Despec-SF Liquid
Dexcon-DM Solution
Diabetic Tussin Allergy Relief Liquid
Diabetic Tussin Allergy Relief Gelcaplet
Diabetic Tussin C Expectorant Liquid
Diabetic Tussin Cold & Flu Gelcaplet
Diabetic Tussin DM Liquid
Diabetic Tussin EX Liquid
Dimetapp Allergy Children's Elixir
Diphen Capsule
Double-Tussin DM Liquid
Drocon-CS Solution
Duratuss DM Solution
Dynatuss Syrup
Dynatuss HC Solution
Dynatuss HCG Solution
Dytan-CS Tablet
Emagrin Forte Tablet
Endacof DM Solution
Endacof HC Solution
Endacof XP Solution
Endacof-PD Solution
Endal HD Liquid
Endal HD Plus Liquid
Endotuss-HD Syrup
Enplus-HD Syrup
Entex Syrup
Entex HC Syrup
Exo-Tuss Syrup
Ganidin NR Liquid
Gani-Tuss NR Liquid
Gani-Tuss-DM NR Liquid
Genebronco-D Liquid
Genecof-HC Liquid
Genecof-XP Liquid
Genedel Syrup
Genedotuss-DM Liquid
Genelan Liquid
Genetuss-2 Liquid
Genexpect DM Liquid
Genexpect-PE Liquid
Genexpect-SF Liquid
Gilphex TR Tablet
Giltuss Liquid
Giltuss HC Syrup
Giltuss Pediatric Liquid
Giltuss TR Tablet
Guai-Co Liquid
Guaicon DMS Liquid
Guai-DEX Liquid
Guaitussin AC Solution
Guaitussin DAC Solution
Guapetex HC Solution
Guapetex Syrup
Guiatuss AC Syrup
Guiatuss AC Syrup
Halotussin AC Liquid
Hayfebrol Liquid
Histacol DM Pediatric Solution
Histex PD Liquid
Histex PD 12 Suspension
Histinex HC Syrup
Histinex PV Syrup
Histuss HC Solution
Histuss PD Solution
Hydex-PD Solution
Hydone Liquid
Hydro-DP Solution
Hydro GP Syrup
Hydro PC Syrup
Hydro PC II Plus Solution
Hydro Pro Solution
Hydrocof-HC Solution
Hydron CP Syrup
Hydron EX Syrup
Hydron KGS Liquid
Hydron PSC Liquid
Hydro-Tussin CBX Solution
Hydro-Tussin DM Elixir
Hydro-Tussin HC Syrup
Hydro-Tussin HD Liquid
Hydro-Tussin XP Syrup
Hytuss Tablet
Hytuss 2X Capsule
Jaycof Expectorant Syrup
Jaycof-HC Liquid
Jaycof-XP Liquid
Kita LA Tos Liquid
Lodrane Liquid
Lodrane D Suspension
Lodrane XR Suspension
Lohist-LQ Solution
Lortuss DM Solution
Lortuss HC Solution
Marcof Expectorant Syrup
Maxi-Tuss HCX Solution
M-Clear Syrup
M-Clear Jr Solution
Metanx Tablet
Mintex PD Liquid
Mintuss NX Solution Syrup
Mytussin DAC Syrup
Nalex DH Liquid
Nalex-A Liquid
Nasop Suspension
Neotuss S/F Liquid
Nescon-PD Tablet
Niferex Elixir
Norel DM Liquid
Nycoff Tablet
Onset Forte Tablet
Orgadin Liquid
Orgadin-Tuss Liquid
Orgadin-Tuss DM Liquid
Organidin NR Liquid
Organidin NR Tablet
Palgic-DS Syrup
Pancof Syrup
Pancof EXP Syrup
Pancof HC Solution
Pancof XP Liquid
Pancof XP Solution
Panmist DM Syrup
Pediatex Solution
Pediatex D
Pediatex DM Liquid
Pediatex DM Solution
Pediatex HC Solution
Phanasin Syrup
Phanasin Diabetic Choice Syrup
Phanatuss Syrup
Phanatuss DM Diabetic Choice Syrup
Phanatuss-HC Diabetic Choice Solution
Phena-HC Solution
Phenabid DM Tablet
Phenydryl Solution
Pneumotussin 2.5 Syrup
Poly Hist DM Solution
Poly Hist PD Solution
Poly-Tussin Syrup
Poly-Tussin DM Syrup
Poly-Tussin HD Syrup
Poly-Tussin XP Syrup
Pro-Clear Solution
Pro-Cof D Liquid
Pro-Red Solution

Prolex DH Liquid
Prolex DM Liquid
Protex Solution
Protex D Solution
Protuss Liquid
Quintex Syrup
Quintex HC Syrup
Relacon-DM Solution
Relacon-HC Solution
Rescon-DM Liquid
Rhinacon A Solution
Rhinacon DH Solution
Rindal HD Liquid
Rindal HD Plus Solution
Rindal HPD Solution
Romilar AC Liquid
Romilar DM Liquid
Rondamine DM Liquid
Rondec Syrup
Rondec DM Syrup
Rondec DM Drops
Ru-Tuss A Syrup
Ru-Tuss DM Syrup
Scot-Tussin Allergy
Relief Formula Liquid
Scot-Tussin DM Cough Chasers Lozenge
Scot-Tussin Original Liquid
Siladryl Allergy Liquid
Siladryl DAS Liquid
Sildec Syrup
Sildec Drops
Sildec-DM Syrup
Silexin Syrup
Silexin Tablet
Sil-Tex Liquid Liquid
Siltussin DM DAS Cough Formula Syrup
S-T Forte 2 Liquid
Statuss Green Liquid Sudodrin Tablet
Sudafed Children's Cold & Cough Solution
Sudafed Children's Solution
Sudafed Children's Tablet
Sudanyl Tablet
Sudatuss-SF Liquid
Sudodrin Tablet
Supress DX Pediatric Drops
Suttar-SF Syrup
Triant-HC Solution
Tricodene Syrup
Trispec-PE Liquid
Trituss DM Solution
Trituss Solution
Tri-Vent DM Solution
Tusdec-DM Solution
Tusdec-HC Solution
Tusnel Solution
Tussafed Syrup
Tussafed-EX Pediatric Drops
Tussafed-HC Syrup
Tussafed-HCG Solution
Tussall Solution
Tuss-DM Liquid
Tuss-ES Syrup
Tussi-Organidin DM NR Liquid
Tussi-Organidin NR Liquid
Tussi-Organidin-S NR Liquid
Tussi-Pres Liquid
Tussirex Liquid
Uni Cof EXP Solution
Uni Cof Solution
Uni-Lev 5.0 Solution
Vazol Solution
Vi-Q-Tuss Syrup
Vitussin Expectorant Syrup
Welltuss EXP Solution
Welltuss HC Solution
Z-Cof HC Solution
Z-Cof HC Syrup
Ztuss Expectorant Solution
Zyrtec Syrup

**FLUORIDE PREPARATIONS**
Ethedent Chewable Tablet
Fluor-A-Day Tablet
Fluor-A-Day Lozenge
Flura-Loz Tablet
Lozi-Flur Lozenge
Sensodyne w/Fluoride Gel
Sensodyne w/Fluoride Tartar Control Toothpaste
Sensodyne w/Fluoride Toothpaste

**LAXATIVES**
Citrucel Powder
Colace Solution
Fiber Ease Liquid
Fibro-XL Capsule
Genfiber Powder
Konsyl Easy Mix Formula Powder
Konsyl-Orange Powder
Metamucil Smooth Texture Powder
Reguloid Powder
Senokot Wheat Bran

**MISCELLANEOUS**
Acidoll Capsule
Alka-Gest Tablet
Bicitra Solution
Colidrops Pediatric Drops
Cytra-2 Solution
Cytra-K Solution
Cytra-K Crystals
Melatin Tablet
Methadose Solution
Neutra-Phos Powder
Neutra-Phos-K Powder
Polycitra-K Solution
Polycitra-LC Solution
Questran Light Powder

**MOUTH/THROAT PREPARATIONS**
Aquafresh Triple Protection Gum
Cepacol Maximum Strength Spray
Cepacol Sore Throat Lozenges
Cheracol Sore Throat Spray
Cylex Lozenges
Fisherman's Friend Lozenges
Fresh N Free Liquid
Isodettes Sore Throat Spray
Larynex Lozenges
Listerine Pocketpaks Film
Medikoff Drops
Oragesic Solution
Orasept Mouthwash/Gargle Liquid
Robitussin Lozenges
Sepasoothe Lozenges
Thorets Maximum Strength Lozenges
Throto-Ceptic Spray
Vademecum Mouthwash & Gargle Concentrate

**POTASSIUM SUPPLEMENTS**
Cena K Liquid
Kaon Elixir
Kaon-Cl 20% Liquid
Rum-K Liquid

**VITAMINS/MINERALS/SUPPLEMENTS**
Action-Tabs Made For Men
Adaptosode For Stress Liquid
Adaptosode R+R For Acute Stress Liquid
Alamag Tablet
Alcalak Tablet
Aldroxicon I Suspension
Aldroxicon II Suspension
Aminoplex Powder
Aminostasis Powder

Aminotate Powder
Apetigen Elixir
Apptrim Capsule
Apptrim-D Capsule
B-C-Bid Caplet
Bevitamel Tablet
Biosode Liquid
Biotect Plus Caplet
C & M Caps-375 Capsule
Calbon Tablet
Cal-Cee Tablet
Calcet Plus Tablet
Calcimin-300 Tablet
Cal-Mint Chewable Tablet
Cena K Solution
Cerefolin Tablet
Cevi-Bid Tablet
Choice DM Liquid
Cholestratin Tablet
Chromacaps Tablet
Chromium K6 Tablet
Citrimax 500 Plus Tablet
Combi-Cart Tablet
Delta D3 Tablet
Detoxosode Liquids
Dexfol Tablet
Diabeze Tablet
Diatx Tablet
Diatx ZN Tablet
Diet System 6 Gum
Dimacid Tablet
Diucaps Capsule
Dl-Phen-500 Capsule
Electrotab Tablet
Endorphenyl Capsule
Ensure Nutra Shake Pudding
Enterex Diabetic Liquid
Essential Nutrients Plus Silica Tablet
Evolve Softgel
Ex-L Tablet
Extress Tablet
Eyetamins Tablet
Fem-Cal Tablet
Fem-Cal Plus Tablet
Ferrocite F Tablet
Folacin-800 Tablet
Folbee Plus Tablet
Folplex 2.2 Tablet
Foltx Tablet
Gabadone Capsule
Gram-O-Leci Tablet
Hemovit Tablet
Herbal Slim Complex Capsule
Irofol Liquid
Lynae Calcium/Vitamin C Chewable Tablet
Lynae Chondroitin/Glucosamine Capsule
Lynae Ginse-Cool Chewable Tablet
Mag-Caps Capsule
Mag-Ox 400 Tablet
Mag-SR Tablet
Magimin Tablet
Magnacaps Capsule
Mangimin Capsule
Mangimin Tablet
Medi-Lyte Tablet
Metanx Tablet
Multi-Delyn w/Iron Liquid
Natelle C Tablet
Nephro-Fer Tablet
Neutra-Phos Powder
Neutra-Phos-K Powder
New Life Hair Tablet
Niferex Elixir
Nutrisure OTC Tablet
O-Cal Fa Tablet
Plenamins Plus Tablet
Powervites Tablet
Prostaplex Herbal
Complex Capsule
Prostatonin Capsule
Protect Plus Liquid
Protect Plus NR Softgel
Pulmona Capsule
Quintabs-M Tablet
Re/Neph Liquid
Replace Capsule
Replace w/o Iron Capsule
Resource Arginaid Powder
Ribo-100 T.D. Capsule
Samolinic Softgel
Sea Omega 30 Softgel
Sea Omega 50 Softgel
Sentra AM Capsule
Sentra PM Capsule
Soy Care for Bone Health
Soy Care for Menopause
Span C Tablet
Strovite Forte Syrup
Sunnie Tablet
Sunvite Tablet
Super Dec B100 Tablet
Super Quints 50 Tablet
Supervite Liquid
Suplevit Liquid
Theramine Capsule
Triamin Tablet
Triamino Tablet
Ultramino Powder
Uro-Mag Capsule
Vinatal 600 Kit
Vitalize Liquid
Vitrum Jr. Chewable Tablet
Xtramins Tablet
Yohimbe Power Max 1500 For Women Tablet
Yohimbized 1000 Capsule
Ze-Plus Softgel

# SULFITE-CONTAINING PRODUCTS

The following is a selection of products that contain sulfites, a common allergic trigger. Please remember, however, that the list is not comprehensive. Always check product labeling for definitive information on specific ingredients.

| PRODUCT | GENERIC NAME |
|---|---|
| Alphaquin HP | Hydroquinone |
| Amikacin Sulfate Injection | Amikacin sulfate |
| Amikin Injectable | Amikacin sulfate |
| Apokyn | Apomorphine hydrochloride |
| Aramine Injection | Metaraminol |
| Betagan Liquifilm | Levobunolol |
| Campral (residual traces) | Acamprosate calcium |
| Claripel Cream | Hydroquinone |
| Corlopam Injection | Fenoldopam |
| Cortisporin Otic Solution | Hydrocortisone/neomycin sulfate/polymyxin B |
| Decadron Phosphate Ophthalmic Solution | Dexamethasone sodium phosphate |
| Decadron Phosphate Injection | Dexamethasone sodium phosphate |
| Dilaudid Oral Liquid; Dilaudid Tablets - 2 mg, 4 mg, 8 mg | Hydromorphone |
| Dobutamine | Dobutamine |
| Eldopaque Forte 4% | Hydroquinone |
| Eldoquin Forte 4% | Hydroquinone |
| Enlon | Edrophonium |
| EpiPen Auto-Injector | Epinephrine |
| EpiPen Jr. | Epinephrine |
| EpiQuin Micro | Hydroquinone |
| Etidocaine/epinephrine bitartrate | Etidocaine/epinephrine bitartrate |
| Garamycin Injectable | Gentamicin |
| Innohep Injection | Tinzaparin |
| Isuprel Hydrochloride Injection 1:5000; Inhalation Solution 1:200 & 1:100 | Isoproterenol |
| Ketoconazole Cream | Ketoconazole |
| Klaron Lotion 10% | Sodium sulfacetamide |
| Levophed Bitartrate Injection | Norepinephrine |
| Lustra | Hydroquinone |
| Lustra-AF | Hydroquinone |
| Marcaine Hydrochloride/ Epinephrine 1:200,000 | Bupivacaine/epinephrine bitartrate |
| Melpaque HP | Hydroquinone |
| Melquin HP | Hydroquinone |
| Morphine Sulfate Injection | Morphine |
| Nebcin vials, Hyporets, Add-vantage | Tobramycin |
| NeoStrata | Hydroquinone |
| Nizoral A-D | Ketoconazole |
| Norflex Injection | Orphenadrine |
| Novocain Hydrochloride for Spinal Anesthesia | Procaine |
| Nubain ampules/Multiple-Dose Vial | Nalbuphine |
| Numorphan Injection | Oxymorphone |
| Nuquin HP | Hydroquinone |
| Oxytetracycline Injection | Oxytetracycline |
| Pamelor Capsules | Nortriptyline |
| Perphenazine Injections/Tablets | Perphenazine |
| Phenergan Injection | Promethazine hydrochloride |
| Pred Forte | Prednisolone acetate |
| Pred Mild | Prednisolone acetate |
| Propofol Injectable Emulsion | Propofol |
| ROWASA Suspension Enema | Mesalamine |
| Sensorcaine with Epinephrine Injection | Bupivacaine/epinephrine bitartrate |
| Sensorcaine-MPF with Epinephrine Injection | Bupivacaine/epinephrine bitartrate |
| SMZ-TMP Concentrate | Trimethoprim/sulfamethoxazole |
| Solaquin Forte 4% Cream; 4% Gel | Hydroquinone |
| Soma Compound with Codeine | Carisoprodol/ aspirin/codeine |
| Streptomycin Sulfate Injection | Streptomycin |
| Sulfamylon Cream | Mafenide acetate |
| Sumycin Suspension | Tetracycline hydrochloride |
| Talacen | Pentazocine hydrochloride/ acetaminophen |
| Talwin Lactate Carpuject/ Multi-Dose Vials | Pentazocine lactate |
| Thorazine Ampules/ Multi-Dose Vials | Chlorpromazine |
| Torecan Injection | Triethylperazine maleate |
| Tri-Luma | Fluocinolone acetonide/ hydroquinone/tretinoin |
| Tylenol with Codeine Tablets | Acetaminophen/codeine |
| Tylox Capsules | Acetaminophen/oxycodone |
| Vibramycin Calcium Syrup | Doxycycline calcium |
| Xylocaine with Epinephrine Injection | Lidocaine/epinephrine |

# Top 200 Brand-Name Rx Drugs

The following list contains the top 200 brand-name prescription drugs dispensed through independent, chain, food store, mass merchandiser, and deep-discount pharmacies. Rankings are based on total number of prescriptions for January 2006 to December 2006, as measured by Verispan's Vector One National Reports. Insulin products are included in the tally.

| RANK | PRODUCT | TOTAL UNITS |
|---|---|---|
| 1. | Lipitor | 62,311,328 |
| 2. | Toprol XL | 37,091,023 |
| 3. | Norvasc | 33,498,793 |
| 4. | Synthroid | 27,209,473 |
| 5. | Lexapro | 26,098,362 |
| 6. | Nexium | 25,917,257 |
| 7. | Singulair | 24,611,082 |
| 8. | Prevacid | 21,180,253 |
| 9. | Ambien | 20,344,499 |
| 10. | Zoloft | 18,640,260 |
| 11. | Advair Diskus | 18,190,160 |
| 12. | Zyrtec | 17,217,968 |
| 13. | Effexor XR | 17,101,230 |
| 14. | Fosamax | 16,720,363 |
| 15. | Plavix | 16,248,359 |
| 16. | Protonix | 16,089,111 |
| 17. | Vytorin | 15,764,654 |
| 18. | Zocor | 14,678,037 |
| 19. | Diovan | 14,165,678 |
| 20. | Lotrel | 13,914,437 |
| 21. | Levaquin | 13,907,030 |
| 22. | Premarin Tabs | 13,350,811 |
| 23. | Zetia | 12,271,534 |
| 24. | Wellbutrin XL | 12,264,504 |
| 25. | Klor-Con | 11,915,074 |
| 26. | Diovan HCT | 11,504,189 |
| 27. | Crestor | 11,410,297 |
| 28. | Avandia | 11,331,164 |
| 29. | Actos | 11,329,039 |
| 30. | Altace | 11,108,602 |
| 31. | Celebrex | 11,074,327 |
| 32. | Viagra | 10,588,511 |
| 33. | Levoxyl | 10,552,047 |
| 34. | Coreg | 10,480,302 |
| 35. | Yasmin 28 | 10,473,944 |
| 36. | Nasonex | 10,198,478 |
| 37. | Seroquel | 9,566,472 |
| 38. | Tricor | 9,565,674 |
| 39. | Lantus | 9,519,010 |
| 40. | Flomax | 9,500,998 |
| 41. | Actonel | 9,264,567 |
| 42. | Adderall XR | 8,870,249 |
| 43. | Cymbalta | 8,520,354 |
| 44. | Cozaar | 8,495,920 |
| 45. | Omnicef | 8,434,028 |
| 46. | Concerta | 7,859,118 |
| 47. | Digitek | 7,685,651 |
| 48. | Risperdal | 7,477,241 |
| 49. | Ortho Tri-Cyclen Lo | 7,360,002 |
| 50. | Valtrex | 7,338,331 |
| 51. | Aciphex | 6,992,183 |
| 52. | Topamax | 6,701,854 |
| 53. | Hyzaar | 6,519,545 |
| 54. | Xalatan | 6,519,012 |
| 55. | Ambien CR | 6,278,505 |
| 56. | Avapro | 5,909,965 |
| 57. | Lunesta | 5,893,499 |
| 58. | Benicar | 5,604,071 |
| 59. | Lyrica | 5,595,318 |
| 60. | Lamictal | 5,583,920 |
| 61. | Combivent | 5,463,705 |
| 62. | Detrol LA | 5,455,196 |
| 63. | Benicar HCT | 5,167,559 |
| 64. | Trinessa | 5,104,000 |
| 65. | Aricept | 5,035,909 |
| 66. | Evista | 4,958,370 |
| 67. | Spiriva | 4,741,068 |
| 68. | Zithromax Suspension | 4,690,452 |
| 69. | Glycolax | 4,636,206 |
| 70. | Tri-Sprintec | 4,605,339 |
| 71. | Endocet | 4,601,111 |
| 72. | Coumadin Tabs | 4,580,407 |
| 73. | Imitrex Oral | 4,535,232 |
| 74. | Cialis | 4,516,621 |
| 75. | Ortho Evra | 4,513,704 |
| 76. | Flovent HFA | 4,396,475 |
| 77. | Niaspan | 4,290,026 |
| 78. | Allegra-D 12 Hour | 4,182,223 |
| 79. | Avalide | 4,151,427 |
| 80. | Zyprexa | 4,069,878 |
| 81. | Pravachol | 4,055,758 |
| 82. | Zyrtec Syrup | 3,947,506 |
| 83. | Nasacort AQ | 3,902,271 |
| 84. | Mobic | 3,883,566 |
| 85. | Strattera | 3,851,349 |
| 86. | NuvaRing | 3,774,970 |
| 87. | Clarinex | 3,774,207 |
| 88. | Skelaxin | 3,742,998 |
| 89. | Patanol | 3,731,163 |
| 90. | Depakote | 3,701,698 |
| 91. | Abilify | 3,691,019 |
| 92. | Flonase | 3,668,030 |
| 93. | Avelox | 3,590,442 |
| 94. | Humalog | 3,538,473 |
| 95. | Depakote ER | 3,508,231 |
| 96. | Budeprion SR | 3,317,490 |
| 97. | Vigamox | 3,312,658 |
| 98. | Aviane | 3,278,405 |
| 99. | Paxil CR | 3,229,719 |
| 100. | Boniva | 3,193,972 |
| 101. | Zyrtec-D | 3,184,370 |
| 102. | Rhinocort Aqua | 3,177,683 |
| 103. | Levothroid | 2,987,586 |
| 104. | Tussionex | 2,973,299 |
| 105. | Kariva | 2,909,790 |
| 106. | Lidoderm | 2,887,713 |
| 107. | Prempro | 2,885,129 |
| 108. | Namenda | 2,877,936 |
| 109. | Humulin N | 2,849,724 |
| 110. | Inderal LA | 2,793,902 |
| 111. | Trileptal | 2,738,223 |
| 112. | Zelnorm | 2,664,832 |
| 113. | Requip | 2,661,154 |
| 114. | Astelin | 2,580,451 |
| 115. | Low-Ogestrel | 2,553,503 |
| 116. | Apri | 2,545,972 |
| 117. | Thyroid, Armour | 2,524,374 |
| 118. | Cosopt | 2,516,688 |
| 119. | Levitra | 2,509,878 |
| 120. | Vivelle-DOT | 2,476,194 |
| 121. | Necon 1/35 | 2,442,393 |
| 122. | Atacand | 2,393,300 |
| 123. | Lanoxin | 2,389,175 |
| 124. | Pulmicort Respules | 2,389,162 |
| 125. | Tobradex | 2,371,373 |
| 126. | Trivora-28 | 2,347,606 |
| 127. | Alphagan P | 2,290,785 |

*(Continued)*

| RANK | PRODUCT | TOTAL UNITS |
|---|---|---|
| 128. | Dilantin Kapseals | 2,266,608 |
| 129. | Provigil | 2,234,373 |
| 130. | Estrostep Fe | 2,207,057 |
| 131. | Xopenex | 2,205,393 |
| 132. | Lumigan | 2,192,975 |
| 133. | Humulin 70/30 | 2,189,396 |
| 134. | Keppra | 2,156,651 |
| 135. | Ditropan XL | 2,097,257 |
| 136. | Lescol XL | 2,025,113 |
| 137. | Avodart | 2,021,239 |
| 138. | Caduet | 2,013,933 |
| 139. | Lamisil Oral | 1,997,380 |
| 140. | Ortho Tri-Cyclen | 1,989,013 |
| 141. | Prometrium | 1,970,666 |
| 142. | Geodon Oral | 1,960,134 |
| 143. | Glipizide XL | 1,952,522 |
| 144. | Biaxin XL | 1,944,251 |
| 145. | Micardis | 1,940,921 |
| 146. | Fluzone | 1,915,175 |
| 147. | Zymar | 1,894,005 |
| 148. | Byetta | 1,868,492 |
| 149. | BenzaClin | 1,826,731 |
| 150. | Ciprodex Otic | 1,806,289 |
| 151. | Travatan | 1,797,965 |
| 152. | Roxicet | 1,783,746 |
| 153. | Tamiflu | 1,780,268 |
| 154. | Sprintec | 1,767,136 |
| 155. | Asacol | 1,756,849 |
| 156. | Ovcon-35 | 1,741,666 |
| 157. | Arimidex | 1,740,448 |
| 158. | Bactroban | 1,735,566 |
| 159. | Restasis | 1,671,519 |
| 160. | Micardis HCT | 1,612,957 |
| 161. | Fosamax Plus D | 1,584,550 |
| 162. | Differin | 1,562,015 |
| 163. | Amoxil | 1,543,946 |
| 164. | Proscar | 1,533,585 |
| 165. | Mirapex | 1,523,538 |
| 166. | Relpax | 1,498,547 |
| 167. | ProAir HFA | 1,467,135 |
| 168. | Ketek Pack | 1,459,942 |
| 169. | Novolin 70/30 | 1,456,533 |
| 170. | Premarin Vaginal | 1,452,994 |
| 171. | Levora | 1,444,058 |
| 172. | Augmentin XR | 1,442,545 |
| 173. | Vagifem | 1,438,035 |
| 174. | OxyContin | 1,413,548 |
| 175. | Cardizem LA | 1,393,750 |
| 176. | Focalin XR | 1,387,383 |
| 177. | Elidel | 1,379,153 |
| 178. | Arthrotec | 1,358,970 |
| 179. | Catapres-TTS | 1,355,672 |
| 180. | Zantac | 1,336,948 |
| 181. | NovoLog Mix 70/30 | 1,319,272 |
| 182. | Sular | 1,297,342 |
| 183. | Tarka | 1,295,126 |
| 184. | Climara | 1,291,584 |
| 185. | M-Oxy | 1,282,646 |
| 186. | Allegra | 1,261,992 |
| 187. | Aldara | 1,257,177 |
| 188. | Propecia | 1,252,361 |
| 189. | Epipen | 1,246,228 |
| 190. | AndroGel | 1,245,717 |
| 191. | Necon 0.5/35E | 1,242,506 |
| 192. | Jantoven | 1,235,459 |
| 193. | Methylin | 1,228,704 |
| 194. | Taztia XT | 1,223,351 |
| 195. | Uroxatral | 1,216,543 |
| 196. | Floxin Otic | 1,213,037 |
| 197. | Zovirax Topical | 1,212,986 |
| 198. | Allegra-D 24 Hour | 1,206,697 |
| 199. | Miacalcin Nasal | 1,190,224 |
| 200. | Aggrenox | 1,175,037 |

# Top 200 Generic Rx Drugs

The following list contains the top 200 generic prescription drugs dispensed through independent, chain, food store, mass merchandiser, and deep-discount pharmacies. Rankings are based on total number of prescriptions for January 2006 to December 2006, as measured by Verispan's Vector One National Reports.

| RANK | PRODUCT | TOTAL UNITS |
|---|---|---|
| 1. | Hydrocodone/APAP | 109,651,664 |
| 2. | Lisinopril | 55,038,862 |
| 3. | Amoxicillin | 52,803,027 |
| 4. | Hydrochlorothiazide | 45,123,751 |
| 5. | Atenolol | 42,770,731 |
| 6. | Levothyroxine | 42,512,598 |
| 7. | Alprazolam | 37,327,218 |
| 8. | Furosemide Oral | 36,830,157 |
| 9. | Azithromycin | 36,061,970 |
| 10. | Metformin | 34,814,839 |
| 11. | Albuterol Aerosol | 31,056,555 |
| 12. | Metoprolol Tartrate | 24,797,131 |
| 13. | Ibuprofen | 23,676,962 |
| 14. | Cephalexin | 22,788,769 |
| 15. | Prednisone Oral | 22,657,231 |
| 16. | Triamterene w/HCTZ | 22,436,061 |
| 17. | Propoxyphene-N/APAP | 21,939,637 |
| 18. | Fluoxetine | 21,733,298 |
| 19. | Lorazepam | 19,788,565 |
| 20. | Warfarin | 19,532,700 |
| 21. | Oxycodone w/APAP | 19,013,660 |
| 22. | Amoxicillin/Potassium Clavulanate | 18,346,000 |
| 23. | Clonazepam | 18,151,712 |
| 24. | Cyclobenzaprine | 17,182,989 |
| 25. | Potassium Chloride | 16,449,357 |
| 26. | Paroxetine | 16,242,347 |
| 27. | Fexofenadine | 16,212,785 |
| 28. | Gabapentin | 16,150,288 |
| 29. | Tramadol | 15,906,002 |
| 30. | Ciprofloxacin HCl | 15,814,504 |
| 31. | Acetaminophen w/Codeine | 14,772,996 |
| 32. | Trazodone HCl | 14,628,310 |
| 33. | Lisinopril/HCTZ | 14,037,120 |
| 34. | Amitriptyline | 13,923,965 |
| 35. | Lovastatin | 13,919,952 |
| 36. | Simvastatin | 13,162,021 |
| 37. | Enalapril | 13,015,526 |
| 38. | Omeprazole | 12,974,800 |
| 39. | Naproxen | 12,884,278 |
| 40. | Trimethoprim/Sulfamethoxazole | 12,766,415 |
| 41. | Diazepam | 12,764,201 |
| 42. | Ranitidine HCl | 12,071,017 |
| 43. | Citalopram HBR | 11,985,799 |
| 44. | Fluconazole | 11,842,055 |
| 45. | Fluticasone Nasal | 11,077,819 |
| 46. | Allopurinol | 10,763,136 |
| 47. | Doxycycline | 10,744,691 |
| 48. | Carisoprodol | 10,689,664 |
| 49. | Clonidine | 10,534,233 |
| 50. | Methylprednisolone Tabs | 10,232,813 |
| 51. | Sertraline | 9,420,341 |

| RANK | PRODUCT | TOTAL UNITS |
|---|---|---|
| 52. | Isosorbide Mononitrate | 9,415,689 |
| 53. | Promethazine Tabs | 8,889,539 |
| 54. | Verapamil SR | 8,867,956 |
| 55. | Glyburide | 8,807,927 |
| 56. | Oxycodone | 8,472,421 |
| 57. | Folic Acid | 8,357,036 |
| 58. | Penicillin VK | 8,325,023 |
| 59. | Spironolactone | 7,618,500 |
| 60. | Temazepam | 7,396,286 |
| 61. | Albuterol Nebulizer Solution | 7,256,403 |
| 62. | Glipizide ER | 7,241,849 |
| 63. | Glimepiride | 6,945,682 |
| 64. | Quinapril | 6,870,584 |
| 65. | Clindamycin Systemic | 6,717,167 |
| 66. | Metformin HCl ER | 6,550,943 |
| 67. | Triamcinolone Acetonide, Topical | 6,447,311 |
| 68. | Glipizide | 6,375,707 |
| 69. | Benazepril | 6,311,627 |
| 70. | Metronidazole Tabs | 6,261,544 |
| 71. | Metoclopramide | 5,982,222 |
| 72. | Hydroxyzine | 5,900,811 |
| 73. | Estradiol Oral | 5,784,843 |
| 74. | Diclofenac Sodium | 5,762,416 |
| 75. | Gemfibrozil | 5,703,379 |
| 76. | Clopidogrel | 5,692,591 |
| 77. | Doxazosin | 5,564,871 |
| 78. | Diltiazem CD | 5,344,988 |
| 79. | Meclizine HCl | 5,294,674 |
| 80. | Glyburide/Metformin HCl | 5,232,427 |
| 81. | Nitrofurantoin Monohydrate Macrocrystals | 5,075,672 |
| 82. | Mirtazapine | 4,851,619 |
| 83. | Nabumetone | 4,755,466 |
| 84. | Bisoprolol/HCTZ | 4,612,236 |
| 85. | Propranolol HCl | 4,545,531 |
| 86. | Pravastatin | 4,480,173 |
| 87. | Acyclovir | 4,471,868 |
| 88. | Minocycline | 4,402,288 |
| 89. | Butalbital/APAP/Caffeine | 4,358,563 |
| 90. | Tramadol HCl/APAP | 4,324,285 |
| 91. | Promethazine/Codeine | 4,263,988 |
| 92. | Buspirone HCl | 4,201,099 |
| 93. | Methotrexate | 4,188,012 |
| 94. | Bupropion SR | 4,164,490 |
| 95. | Cartia XT | 4,070,735 |
| 96. | Terazosin | 4,054,673 |
| 97. | Clotrimazole/Betamethasone | 4,035,631 |
| 98. | Amphetamine Salt Combo | 3,953,581 |
| 99. | Quinine Sulfate | 3,945,502 |
| 100. | Fentanyl Transdermal | 3,818,097 |
| 101. | Sulfamethoxazole/Trimethoprim | 3,736,845 |

*(Continued)*

| RANK | PRODUCT | TOTAL UNITS |
|---|---|---|
| 102. | Nifedipine ER | 3,699,211 |
| 103. | Famotidine | 3,598,800 |
| 104. | Phenytoin Sodium Extended-Release | 3,591,440 |
| 105. | Digoxin | 3,590,133 |
| 106. | Ferrous Sulfate | 3,582,285 |
| 107. | Phentermine | 3,523,119 |
| 108. | Lithium Carbonate | 3,416,532 |
| 109. | Atenolol Chlorthalidone | 3,415,292 |
| 110. | Benzonatate | 3,382,506 |
| 111. | Tizanidine HCl | 3,379,214 |
| 112. | Etodolac | 3,353,702 |
| 113. | Methocarbamol | 3,255,750 |
| 114. | Phenazopyridine HCl | 3,243,751 |
| 115. | Nitroquick | 3,184,632 |
| 116. | Morphine Sulfate, Non-Injectable | 3,175,882 |
| 117. | Nortriptyline | 3,173,948 |
| 118. | Nitroglycerin | 3,173,184 |
| 119. | Mupirocin | 3,086,582 |
| 120. | Fosinopril Sodium | 3,003,438 |
| 121. | Chlorhexidine Gluconate | 2,995,841 |
| 122. | Aspirin, Enteric-Coated | 2,985,020 |
| 123. | Colchicine | 2,947,525 |
| 124. | Hyoscyamine | 2,929,535 |
| 125. | Felodipine ER | 2,927,992 |
| 126. | Hydroxychloroquine | 2,924,444 |
| 127. | Dicyclomine HCl | 2,908,842 |
| 128. | Phenobarbital | 2,884,874 |
| 129. | Polyethylene Glycol | 2,860,657 |
| 130. | Clobetasol | 2,829,380 |
| 131. | Nystatin Systemic | 2,826,823 |
| 132. | Prednisolone Sodium Phosphate, Oral | 2,768,053 |
| 133. | Meloxicam | 2,751,844 |
| 134. | Ketoconazole Topical | 2,693,392 |
| 135. | Baclofen | 2,671,958 |
| 136. | Indomethacin | 2,612,771 |
| 137. | Medroxyprogesterone Tablets | 2,597,328 |
| 138. | NovoLog | 2,522,278 |
| 139. | Cefuroxime Axetil | 2,517,671 |
| 140. | Clarithromycin | 2,515,443 |
| 141. | Labetalol | 2,506,593 |
| 142. | Hydrocortisone | 2,491,516 |
| 143. | Carbidopa/Levodopa | 2,478,736 |
| 144. | Nystatin Topical | 2,474,588 |
| 145. | Fluocinonide | 2,469,021 |
| 146. | Oxybutynin Chloride | 2,463,396 |
| 147. | Tetracycline | 2,439,117 |
| 148. | Nifedical XL | 2,394,317 |
| 149. | Hydrocodone/Ibuprofen | 2,388,543 |
| 150. | Captopril | 2,364,281 |
| 151. | Carbamazepine | 2,363,337 |
| 152. | Methadone HCl, Non-Injectable | 2,356,638 |
| 153. | Amiodarone | 2,353,965 |
| 154. | Clindamycin Topical | 2,339,881 |
| 155. | Hydroxyzine Pamoate | 2,301,832 |
| 156. | Benztropine | 2,266,455 |
| 157. | Naproxen Sodium | 2,180,365 |
| 158. | Prednisone Intensol | 2,177,011 |
| 159. | Piroxicam | 2,176,861 |
| 160. | Doxepin | 2,145,202 |
| 161. | Diltiazem SR | 2,051,197 |
| 162. | Nitrofurantoin Macrocrystals | 2,025,615 |
| 163. | Hydralazine | 1,983,977 |
| 164. | Torsemide | 1,929,465 |
| 165. | Prochlorperazine Maleate | 1,906,984 |
| 166. | Methylphenidate | 1,878,781 |
| 167. | Nadolol | 1,874,616 |
| 168. | Benazepril/HCTZ | 1,870,377 |
| 169. | Mometasone Topical | 1,864,461 |
| 170. | Dexamethasone Oral | 1,864,350 |
| 171. | Tamoxifen | 1,827,689 |
| 172. | Erythromycin Ophthalmic | 1,822,384 |
| 173. | Diphenoxylate w/ Atropine Sulfate | 1,816,451 |
| 174. | Indapamide | 1,804,225 |
| 175. | Docusate Sodium | 1,760,105 |
| 176. | Cefprozil | 1,759,018 |
| 177. | Bumetanide, Non-Injectable | 1,738,416 |
| 178. | Cheratussin AC | 1,715,019 |
| 179. | Promethazine DM | 1,711,653 |
| 180. | Prednisolone Acetate, Ophthalmic | 1,690,937 |
| 181. | Nystatin/Triamcinolone | 1,660,521 |
| 182. | Sotalol | 1,630,553 |
| 183. | Imipramine HCl | 1,628,535 |
| 184. | Metolazone | 1,628,159 |
| 185. | Multi-Vita Bets w/ Fluoride | 1,604,047 |
| 186. | Ibuprofen Liquid | 1,595,873 |
| 187. | Diltiazem | 1,589,425 |
| 188. | Nifedipine | 1,586,215 |
| 189. | Methadose | 1,555,177 |
| 190. | Polymyxin B/Trimethoprim Sulfate | 1,499,882 |
| 191. | Timolol Maleate GFS | 1,480,627 |
| 192. | Cilostazol | 1,465,785 |
| 193. | Hycoclear Tuss | 1,437,970 |
| 194. | Timolol Maleate Ophthalmic | 1,434,053 |
| 195. | Penicillin V Potassium | 1,427,196 |
| 196. | Terconazole | 1,410,789 |
| 197. | Cefadroxil | 1,409,787 |
| 198. | Sodium Fluoride | 1,404,177 |
| 199. | Bupropion ER | 1,395,278 |
| 200. | Microgestin Fe 1/20 | 1,393,371 |

# USE-IN-PREGNANCY RATINGS

The U.S. Food and Drug Administration's Use-in-Pregnancy rating system weighs the degree to which available information has ruled out risk to the fetus against the drug's potential benefit to the patient. Below is a listing of drugs (by generic name) for which ratings are available.

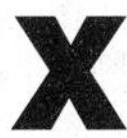

**Contraindicated in pregnancy**

*Studies in animals or humans, or investigational or postmarketing reports, have demonstrated fetal risk which clearly outweighs any possible benefit to the patient.*

Acetohydroxamic Acid
Acitretin
Amlodipine Besylate/
  Atorvastatin Calcium
Amprenavir
Anisindione
Atorvastatin Calcium
Bexarotene
Bicalutamide
Bosentan
Cetrorelix Acetate
Choriogonadotropin Alfa
Chorionic Gonadotropin
Clomiphene Citrate
Desogestrel/Ethinyl Estradiol
Diclofenac Sodium/Misoprostol
Dihydroergotamine Mesylate
Dutasteride
Estazolam
Estradiol
Estradiol Acetate
Estradiol Cypionate/
  Medroxyprogesterone Acetate
Estradiol Valerate
Estradiol/Levonorgestrel
Estradiol/Norethindrone Acetate
Estrogens, Conjugated
Estrogens, Conjugated, Synthetic A
Estrogens, Conjugated/
  Medroxyprogesterone Acetate
Estrogens, Esterified
Estrogens, Esterified/
  Methyltestosterone
Estropipate
Ethinyl Estradiol/Drospirenone
Ethinyl Estradiol/
  Ethynodiol Diacetate
Ethinyl Estradiol/Etonogestrel
Ethinyl Estradiol/Ferrous Fumarate/
  Norethindrone Acetate
Ethinyl Estradiol/Levonorgestrel
Ethinyl Estradiol/Norelgestromin
Ethinyl Estradiol/Norethindrone
Ethinyl Estradiol/Norethindrone
  Acetate
Ethinyl Estradiol/Norgestimate
Ethinyl Estradiol/Norgestrel
Ezetimibe/Simvastatin
Finasteride
Fluorouracil
Fluoxymesterone
Flurazepam Hydrochloride
Fluvastatin Sodium
Follitropin Alfa
Follitropin Beta
Ganirelix Acetate
Goserelin Acetate
Histrelin Acetate
Hydromorphone Hydrochloride
Interferon Alfa-2B,
  Recombinant/Ribavirin
Iodine I 131 Tositumomab/
  Tositumomab
Isotretinoin
Leflunomide
Leuprolide Acetate
Levonorgestrel
Lovastatin
Lovastatin/Niacin
Medroxyprogesterone Acetate
Megestrol Acetate
Menotropins
Mequinol/Tretinoin
Mestranol/Norethindrone
Methotrexate Sodium
Methyltestosterone
Miglustat
Misoprostol
Nafarelin Acetate
Norethindrone
Norethindrone Acetate
Norgestrel
Oxandrolone
Oxymetholone
Plicamycin
Pravastatin Sodium
Pravastatin Sodium/Aspirin Buffered
Raloxifene Hydrochloride
Ribavirin
Rosuvastatin Calcium
Simvastatin
Tazarotene
Testosterone
Testosterone Enanthate
Thalidomide
Tositumomab
Triptorelin Pamoate
Urofollitropin
Warfarin Sodium

# D

**Positive evidence of risk**

*Investigational or postmarketing data show risk to the fetus. Nevertheless, potential benefits may outweigh the potential risk.*

Alitretinoin
Alprazolam
Altretamine
Amiodarone Hydrochloride
Amlodipine Besylate/
  Benazepril Hydrochloride
Anastrozole
Arsenic Trioxide
Aspirin Buffered/Pravastatin Sodium
Aspirin/Dipyridamole
Atenolol
Azathioprine
Azathioprine Sodium
Benazepril Hydrochloride*
Benazepril Hydrochloride/
  Hydrochlorothiazide*
Bortezomib
Busulfan
Candesartan Cilexetil*
Candesartan Cilexetil/
  Hydrochlorothiazide*
Capecitabine
Captopril*
Carbamazepine
Carboplatin
Carmustine (Bcnu)
Chlorambucil
Cladribine
Clofarabine
Clonazepam
Cytarabine Liposome
Dactinomycin
Daunorubicin Citrate Liposome
Daunorubicin Hydrochloride
Demeclocycline Hydrochloride
Diazepam
Divalproex Sodium
Docetaxel
Doxorubicin Hydrochloride
Doxorubicin Hydrochloride Liposome
Doxycycline Calcium
Doxycycline Hyclate
Doxycycline Monohydrate
Efavirenz
Enalapril Maleate*
Enalapril Maleate/Hydrochlorothiazide*
Epirubicin Hydrochloride
Eprosartan Mesylate

* Category C or D depending on the trimester the drug is given.

Erlotinib
Exemestane
Felodipine/Enalapril Maleate
Floxuridine
Fludarabine Phosphate
Flutamide
Fosinopril Sodium*
Fosinopril Sodium/
Hydrochlorothiazide*
Fosphenytoin Sodium
Fulvestrant
Gefitinib
Gemcitabine Hydrochloride
Gemtuzumab Ozogamicin
Goserelin Acetate
Ibritumomab Tiuxetan
Idarubicin Hydrochloride
Ifosfamide
Imatinib Mesylate
Irbesartan*
Irbesartan/Hydrochlorothiazide*
Irinotecan Hydrochloride
Letrozole
Lisinopril*
Lisinopril/Hydrochlorothiazide*
Lithium Carbonate
Losartan Potassium*
Losartan Potassium/
Hydrochlorothiazide*
Mechlorethamine Hydrochloride
Melphalan
Melphalan Hydrochloride
Mephobarbital
Mercaptopurine
Methimazole
Midazolam Hydrochloride
Minocycline Hydrochloride
Mitoxantrone Hydrochloride
Moexipril Hydrochloride*
Moexipril Hydrochloride/
Hydrochlorothiazide*
Nelarabine
Neomycin Sulfate/
Polymyxin B Sulfate
Nicotine
Olmesartan Medoxomil
Oxaliplatin
Pamidronate Disodium
Pemetrexed
Penicillamine
Pentobarbital Sodium
Pentostatin
Perindopril Erbumine*
Phenytoin
Procarbazine Hydrochloride
Quinapril Hydrochloride*
Quinapril Hydrochloride/
Hydrochlorothiazide*
Ramipril*
Sorafenib
Streptomycin Sulfate
Sunitinib
Tamoxifen Citrate
Telmisartan
Telmisartan/Hydrochlorothiazide
Temozolomide
Thioguanine
Tigecycline
Tobramycin
Topotecan Hydrochloride
Toremifene Citrate
Trandolapril*
Trandolapril/Verapamil
Hydrochloride*
Tretinoin
Valproate Sodium
Valproic Acid
Valsartan*
Valsartan/Hydrochlorothiazide*
Vinorelbine Tartrate
Voriconazole
Zoledronic Acid

# C

**Risk cannot be ruled out**

*Human studies are lacking, and animal studies are either positive for risk or are lacking as well. However, potential benefits may outweigh the potential risk.*

Abacavir Sulfate
Abacavir Sulfate/Lamivudine
Abacavir Sulfate/
Lamivudine/Zidovudine
Abciximab
Acamprosate Calcium
Acetaminophen
Acetaminophen/
Butalbital/Caffeine
Acetaminophen/Caffeine/
Chlorpheniramine Maleate/
Hydrocodone Bitartrate/
Phenylephrine Hydrochloride
Acetazolamide
Acetazolamide Sodium
Acyclovir
Adapalene
Adefovir Dipivoxil
Adenosine
Alatrofloxacin Mesylate
Albendazole
Albumin (Human)
Albuterol
Albuterol Sulfate
Albuterol Sulfate/Ipratropium
Bromide
Alclometasone Dipropionate
Aldesleukin
Alemtuzumab
Alendronate Sodium
Alendronate Sodium/Cholecalciferol
Allopurinol Sodium
Almotriptan Malate
Alpha1-Proteinase Inhibitor (Human)
Alprostadil
Alteplase
Amantadine Hydrochloride
Amifostine
Aminocaproic Acid
Aminohippurate Sodium
Aminolevulinic Acid Hydrochloride
Aminosalicylic Acid
Amlodipine Besylate
Amlodipine Besylate/Benazepril
Hydrochloride
Amoxicillin/Clarithromycin/
Lansoprazole
Amphetamine Aspartate/
Amphetamine Sulfate/
Dextroamphetamine Saccharate/
Dextroamphetamine Sulfate
Amprenavir
Anagrelide Hydrochloride
Anthralin
Antihemophilic Factor (Human)
Antihemophilic Factor (Recombinant)
Anti-Inhibitor Coagulant Complex
Anti-Thymocyte Globulin
Apomorphine Hydrochloride
Aripiprazole
Arnica Montana/Herbals, Multiple/
Sulfur
Asparaginase
Atomoxetine Hydrochloride
Atovaquone
Atovaquone/Proguanil Hydrochloride
Atropine Sulfate/Benzoic Acid/
HyoscyamineSulfate/
Methenamine/Methylene Blue/
Phenyl Salicylate
Atropine Sulfate/Hyoscyamine
Sulfate/Scopolamine
Hydrobromide
Azelastine Hydrochloride
Bacitracin Zinc/Neomycin Sulfate/
Polymyxin B Sulfate
Baclofen
Bcg, Live (Intravesical)
Becaplermin
Beclomethasone Dipropionate
Beclomethasone Dipropionate
Monohydrate
Benazepril Hydrochloride*
Benazepril Hydrochloride/
Hydrochlorothiazide*
Bendroflumethiazide
Benzocaine
Benzonatate
Benzoyl Peroxide
Benzoyl Peroxide/Clindamycin
Benzoyl Peroxide/Erythromycin
Betamethasone Dipropionate
Betamethasone Dipropionate/
Clotrimazole
Betamethasone Valerate
Betaxolol Hydrochloride
Bethanechol Chloride

Bevacizumab
Bimatoprost
Bisacodyl/Polyethylene Glycol/ Potassium Chloride/ Sodium Bicarbonate/ Sodium Chloride
Bisoprolol Fumarate
Bisoprolol Fumarate/ Hydrochlorothiazide
Bitolterol Mesylate
Black Widow Spider Antivenin (Equine)
Botulinum Toxin Type A
Botulinum Toxin Type B
Brinzolamide
Brompheniramine Maleate/ Dextromethorphan Hydrobromide/ Phenylephrine Hydrochloride
Budesonide
Bupivacaine Hydrochloride
Bupivacaine Hydrochloride/ Epinephrine Bitartrate
Buprenorphine Hydrochloride
Buprenorphine Hydrochloride/ Naloxone Hydrochloride
Butabarbital/Hyoscyamine Hydrobromide/Phenazopyridine Hydrochloride
Butalbital/Acetaminophen
Butenafine Hydrochloride
Butoconazole Nitrate
Butorphanol Tartrate
Caffeine Citrate
Calcipotriene
Calcitonin-Salmon
Calcitriol
Calcium Acetate
Candesartan Cilexetil*
Candesartan Cilexetil/ Hydrochlorothiazide*
Capreomycin Sulfate
Captopril*
Carbetapentane Tannate/ Chlorpheniramine Tannate
Carbetapentane Tannate/Chlorpheniramine Tannate/Ephedrine Tannate/Phenylephrine Tannate
Carbidopa/Entacapone/Levodopa
Carbidopa/Levodopa
Carbinoxamine Maleate/ Dextromethorphan Hydrobromide/ Pseudoephedrine Hydrochloride
Carteolol Hydrochloride
Carvedilol
Caspofungin Acetate
Celecoxib
Cetirizine Hydrochloride
Cetuximab
Cevimeline Hydrochloride
Chloramphenicol
Chloroprocaine Hydrochloride
Chlorothiazide
Chlorothiazide Sodium
Chlorpheniramine Maleate/ Methscopolamine Nitrate/ Phenylephrine Hydrochloride
Chlorpheniramine Maleate/ Pseudoephedrine Hydrochloride
Chlorpheniramine Polistirex/ Hydrocodone Polistirex
Chlorpheniramine Tannate/ Phenylephrine Tannate
Chlorpropamide
Chlorthalidone/Clonidine Hydrochloride
Choline Magnesium Trisalicylate
Cidofovir
Cilostazol
Cinacalcet Hydrochloride
Ciprofloxacin Hydrochloride
Ciprofloxacin Hydrochloride/ Hydrocortisone
Ciprofloxacin/Dexamethasone
Citalopram Hydrobromide
Clarithromycin
Clobetasol Propionate
Clonidine
Clonidine Hydrochloride
Codeine Phosphate/Acetaminophen
Colistimethate Sodium
Colistin Sulfate/Hydrocortisone Acetate/Neomycin Sulfate/ Thonzonium Bromide
Corticorelin Ovine Triflutate
Cycloserine
Cyclosporine
Cytomegalovirus Immune Globulin
Dacarbazine
Daclizumab
Dantrolene Sodium
Dapsone
Darbepoetin Alfa
Darifenacin
Deferoxamine Mesylate
Delavirdine Mesylate
Denileukin Diftitox
Desloratadine
Desloratadine/Pseudoephedrine Sulfate
Desoximetasone
Dexamethasone
Dexamethasone Sodium Phosphate
Dexmethylphenidate Hydrochloride
Dexrazoxane
Dextroamphetamine Sulfate
Diazoxide
Dichlorphenamide
Diclofenac Potassium
Diclofenac Sodium
Diflorasone Diacetate
Diflunisal
Digoxin
Digoxin Immune Fab (Ovine)
Diltiazem Hydrochloride
Dimethyl Sulfoxide
Dinoprostone
Diphtheria & Tetanus Toxoids and Acellular Pertussis Vaccine Adsorbed
Diphtheria & Tetanus Toxoids and Acellular Pertussis Vaccine Adsorbed/Hepatitis B Vaccine, Recombinant/Poliovirus Vaccine Inactivated
Dirithromycin
Dofetilide
Donepezil Hydrochloride
Dorzolamide Hydrochloride
Dorzolamide Hydrochloride/ Timolol Maleate
Doxazosin Mesylate
Dronabinol
Drotrecogin Alfa (Activated)
Duloxetine Hydrochloride
Echothiophate Iodide
Econazole Nitrate
Efalizumab
Eflornithine Hydrochloride
Eletriptan Hydrobromide
Enalapril Maleate*
Enalapril Maleate/Felodipine*
Enalapril Maleate/Hydrochlorothiazide*
Entacapone
Entecavir
Epinastine Hydrochloride
Epinephrine
Epoetin Alfa
Eprosartan Mesylate
Erythromycin Ethylsuccinate/ Sulfisoxazole Acetyl
Escitalopram Oxalate
Esmolol Hydrochloride
Eszopiclone
Ethionamide
Ethotoin
Etidronate Disodium
Exenatide
Ezetimibe
Factor IX Complex
Felodipine
Fenofibrate
Fentanyl
Fentanyl Citrate
Ferrous Fumarate/Folic Acid/ Intrinsic Factor Concentrate/ Liver Preparations/ Vitamin B12/Vitamin C/ Vitamins with Iron
Fexofenadine Hydrochloride
Fexofenadine Hydrochloride/ Pseudoephedrine Hydrochloride
Filgrastim
Flecainide Acetate
Fluconazole
Flucytosine
Fludrocortisone Acetate
Flumazenil
Flunisolide
Fluocinolone Acetonide
Fluocinolone Acetonide/ Hydroquinone/Tretinoin
Fluocinonide
Fluorometholone

* Category C or D depending on the trimester the drug is given.

Fluorometholone/Sulfacetamide Sodium
Fluoxetine Hydrochloride
Fluoxetine Hydrochloride/Olanzapine
Flurandrenolide
Flurbiprofen Sodium
Fluticasone Propionate
Fluticasone Propionate Hfa
Fluticasone Propionate/ Salmeterol Xinafoate
Fomivirsen Sodium
Formoterol Fumarate
Fosamprenavir Calcium
Foscarnet Sodium*
Fosinopril Sodium*
Fosinopril Sodium/Hydrochlorothiazide*
Frovatriptan Succinate
Furosemide
Gabapentin
Gallium Nitrate
Ganciclovir
Ganciclovir Sodium
Gatifloxacin
Gemfibrozil
Gemifloxacin Mesylate
Gentamicin Sulfate
Gentamicin Sulfate/ Prednisolone Acetate
Glimepiride
Glipizide
Glipizide/Metformin Hydrochloride
Globulin, Immune (Human)
Globulin, Immune (Human)/ Rho (D) Immune Globulin (Human)
Glyburide
Gramicidin/Neomycin Sulfate/ Polymyxin B Sulfate
Guaifenesin/Hydrocodone Bitartrate
Haemophilus B Conjugate Vaccine
Haemophilus B Conjugate Vaccine/ Hepatitis B Vaccine, Recombinant
Halobetasol Propionate
Haloperidol Decanoate
Hemin
Heparin Sodium
Hepatitis A Vaccine, Inactivated
Hepatitis A Vaccine, Inactivated/Hepatitis B Vaccine, Recombinant
Hepatitis B Immune Globulin (Human)
Hepatitis B Vaccine, Recombinant
Homatropine Methylbromide/ Hydrocodone Bitartrate
Homeopathic Formulations
Hydralazine Hydrochloride/Isosorbide Dinitrate
Hydrochlorothiazide
Hydrocodone Bitartrate
Hydrocodone Bitartrate/ Acetaminophen
Hydrocodone Bitartrate/Ibuprofen
Hydrocortisone
Hydrocortisone Acetate
Hydrocortisone Acetate/Neomycin Sulfate/Polymyxin B Sulfate
Hydrocortisone Acetate/Pramoxine Hydrochloride
Hydrocortisone Butyrate
Hydrocortisone Probutate
Hydrocortisone/Neomycin Sulfate/ Polymyxin B Sulfate
Hydromorphone Hydrochloride
Hydroquinone
Hyoscyamine Sulfate
Ibandronate Sodium
Ibutilide Fumarate
Iloprost
Imiglucerase
Imipenem/Cilastatin
Imiquimod
Immune Globulin Intravenous (Human)
Indinavir Sulfate
Indocyanine Green
Influenza Virus Vaccine
Insulin Aspart
Insulin Aspart Protamine,Human/ Insulin Aspart, Human
Insulin Glargine
Insulin Glulisine
Interferon Alfa-2A, Recombinant
Interferon Alfa-2B, Recombinant
Interferon Alfacon-1
Interferon Alfa-N3 (Human Leukocyte Derived)
Interferon Beta-1A
Interferon Beta-1B
Interferon Gamma-1B
Iodoquinol/Hydrocortisone
Irbesartan*
Irbesartan/Hydrochlorothiazide*
Iron Dextran
Isoniazid/Pyrazinamide/Rifampin
Isosorbide Mononitrate
Isradipine
Itraconazole
Ivermectin
Ketoconazole
Ketorolac Tromethamine
Ketotifen Fumarate
Labetalol Hydrochloride
Lamivudine
Lamivudine/Zidovudine
Lamotrigine
Lanthanum Carbonate
Latanoprost
Levalbuterol Hydrochloride
Levalbuterol Tartrate
Levamisole Hydrochloride
Levetiracetam
Levobunolol Hydrochloride
Levofloxacin
Linezolid
Lisinopril*
Lisinopril/Hydrochlorothiazide*
Lopinavir/Ritonavir
Losartan Potassium*
Losartan Potassium/Hydrochlorothiazide*
Loteprednol Etabonate
Mafenide Acetate
Magnesium Salicylate Tetrahydrate
Measles Virus Vaccine, Live
Measles, Mumps & Rubella Virus Vaccine, Live
Mebendazole
Mecamylamine Hydrochloride
Mecasermin [Rdna Origin]
Medrysone
Mefenamic Acid
Mefloquine Hydrochloride
Meloxicam
Meningoccal Polysaccharide Diphtheria Toxoid Conjugate Vaccine
Meningococcal Polysaccharide Vaccine
Meperidine Hydrochloride
Mepivacaine Hydrochloride
Metaproterenol Sulfate
Metaraminol Bitartrate
Metformin Hydrochloride/ Pioglitazone Hydrochloride
Metformin Hydrochloride/ Rosiglitazone Maleate
Methamphetamine Hydrochloride
Methazolamide
Methenamine Mandelate/ Sodium Acid Phosphate
Methocarbamol
Methoxsalen
Methscopolamine Nitrate/ Pseudoephedrine Hydrochloride
Methyldopa/Chlorothiazide
Methyldopa/Hydrochlorothiazide
Methylphenidate Hydrochloride
Metipranolol
Metoprolol Succinate
Metoprolol Tartrate
Metoprolol Tartrate/ Hydrochlorothiazide
Metyrosine
Mexiletine Hydrochloride
Micafungin Sodium
Midodrine Hydrochloride
Mivacurium Chloride
Modafinil
Moexipril Hydrochloride*
Moexipril Hydrochloride/ Hydrochlorothiazide*
Mometasone Furoate
Mometasone Furoate Monohydrate
Morphine Sulfate
Morphine Sulfate, Liposomal
Moxifloxacin Hydrochloride
Mumps Virus Vaccine, Live
Muromonab-Cd3
Mycophenolate Mofetil
Mycophenolate Mofetil Hydrochloride
Mycophenolic Acid
Nabumetone
Nadolol

Nadolol/Bendroflumethiazide
Naloxone Hydrochloride/ Pentazocine Hydrochloride
Naltrexone Hydrochloride
Naphazoline Hydrochloride
Naproxen
Naproxen Sodium
Naratriptan Hydrochloride
Natamycin
Nateglinide
Nefazodone Hydrochloride
Neomycin Sulfate/ Dexamethasone Sodium Phosphate
Neomycin Sulfate/Polymyxin B Sulfate/Prednisolone Acetate
Nesiritide
Nevirapine
Niacin
Nicardipine Hydrochloride
Nifedipine
Nilutamide
Nimodipine
Nisoldipine
Nitroglycerin
Norfloxacin
Ofloxacin
Olanzapine
Olmesartan Medoxomil/ Hydrochlorothiazide
Olopatadine Hydrochloride
Olsalazine Sodium
Omega-3-Acid Ethyl Esters
Omeprazole
Oprelvekin
Orphenadrine Citrate
Oseltamivir Phosphate
Oxcarbazepine
Oxycodone Hydrochloride/ Acetaminophen
Oxycodone Hydrochloride/Ibuprofen
Oxymorphone Hydrochloride
Palifermin
Palivizumab
Pancrelipase
Paricalcitol
Paroxetine Hydrochloride
Paroxetine Mesylate
Peg-3350/Potassium Chloride/ Sodium Bicarbonate/ Sodium Chloride
Pegademase Bovine
Pegaspargase
Pegfilgrastim
Peginterferon Alfa-2A
Peginterferon Alfa-2B
Pemirolast Potassium
Pentazocine Hydrochloride/ Acetaminophen
Pentoxifylline
Perindopril Erbumine*
Phenoxybenzamine Hydrochloride
Phentermine Hydrochloride
Pilocarpine Hydrochloride
Pimecrolimus
Pimozide
Pioglitazone Hydrochloride
Pirbuterol Acetate
Piroxicam
Plasma Fractions, Human/ Rabies Immune Globulin (Human)
Plasma Protein Fraction (Human)
Pneumococcal Vaccine, Diphtheria Conjugate
Pneumococcal Vaccine, Polyvalent
Podofilox
Polyethylene Glycol
Polyethylene Glycol/Potassium Chloride/Sodium Bicarbonate/ Sodium Chloride
Polyethylene Glycol/Potassium Chloride/Sodium Bicarbonate/Sodium Chloride/Sodium Sulfate
Polymyxin B Sulfate/ Trimethoprim Sulfate
Polythiazide/Prazosin Hydrochloride
Porfimer Sodium
Potassium Acid Phosphate
Potassium Chloride
Potassium Citrate
Potassium Phosphate/ Sodium Phosphate
Pralidoxime Chloride
Pramipexole Dihydrochloride
Pramlintide Acetate
Pramoxine Hydrochloride/ Hydrocortisone Acetate
Prazosin Hydrochloride
Prednisolone Acetate
Prednisolone Acetate/ Sulfacetamide Sodium
Prednisolone Sodium Phosphate
Pregabalin
Procainamide Hydrochloride
Promethazine Hydrochloride
Propafenone Hydrochloride
Proparacaine Hydrochloride
Propranolol Hydrochloride
Pseudoephedrine Hydrochloride
Pyrimethamine
Quetiapine Fumarate
Quinapril Hydrochloride*
Quinidine Sulfate
Rabies Vaccine
Ramelteon
Ramipril*
Rasburicase
Remifentanil Hydrochloride
Repaglinide
Reteplase
Rho (D) Immune Globulin (Human)
Rifampin
Rifapentine
Rifaximin
Riluzole
Rimantadine Hydrochloride
Risedronate Sodium
Risedronate Sodium/Calcium Carbonate
Risperidone
Rituximab
Rizatriptan Benzoate
Rocuronium Bromide
Rofecoxib
Ropinirole Hydrochloride
Rosiglitazone Maleate
Rubella Virus Vaccine, Live
Salmeterol Xinafoate
Sargramostim
Scopolamine
Selegiline Hydrochloride
Sertaconazole Nitrate
Sertraline Hydrochloride
Sevelamer Hydrochloride
Sibutramine Hydrochloride Monohydrate
Sirolimus
Sodium Benzoate/ Sodium Phenylacelate
Sodium Phenylbutyrate
Sodium Sulfacetamide/Sulfur
Solifenacin Succinate
Somatropin
Somatropin (rDNA origin)
Stavudine
Streptokinase
Succimer
Sulfacetamide Sodium
Sulfamethoxazole/Trimethoprim
Sulfanilamide
Sumatriptan
Sumatriptan Succinate
Tacrine Hydrochloride
Tacrolimus
Telithromycin
Telmisartan*
Telmisartan/Hydrochlorothiazide*
Tenecteplase
Terazosin Hydrochloride
Teriparatide
Tetanus & Diphtheria Toxoids Adsorbed
Tetanus Immune Globulin (Human)
Theophylline
Theophylline Anhydrous
Thiabendazole
Thrombin
Thyrotropin Alfa
Tiagabine Hydrochloride
Tiludronate Disodium
Timolol Hemihydrate
Timolol Maleate
Timolol Maleate/Hydrochlorothiazide
Tinidazole
Tiotropium Bromide
Tipranavir
Tizanidine Hydrochloride
Tobramycin/Dexamethasone
Tobramycin/Loteprednol Etabonate
Tolcapone
Tolterodine Tartrate
Topiramate

* Category C or D depending on the trimester the drug is given.

Tramadol Hydrochloride
Tramadol Hydrochloride/Acetaminophen
Trandolapril*
Trandolapril/Verapamil Hydrochloride*
Travoprost
Tretinoin
Triamcinolone Acetonide
Triamterene
Triamterene/Hydrochlorothiazide
Trientine Hydrochloride
Triethanolamine Polypeptide Oleate-Condensate
Trifluridine
Trimethoprim Hydrochloride
Trimipramine Maleate
Tropicamide/Hydroxyamphetamine Hydrobromide
Trospium Chloride
Trovafloxacin Mesylate
Tuberculin Purified Protein Derivative, Diluted
Typhoid Vaccine Live Oral Ty21A
Unoprostone Isopropyl
Urea
Valdecoxib
Valganciclovir Hydrochloride
Valsartan*
Valsartan/Hydrochlorothiazide*
Varicella Virus Vaccine, Live
Venlafaxine Hydrochloride
Verapamil Hydrochloride
Verteporfin
Vitamin K1
Yellow Fever Vaccine
Zalcitabine
Zaleplon
Zanamivir
Zidovudine
Zileuton
Ziprasidone Mesylate
Zolmitriptan
Zonisamide

# B

**No evidence of risk in humans**

*Either animal findings show risk while human findings do not, or, if no adequate human studies have been done, animal findings are negative.*

Acarbose
Acrivastine
Acyclovir
Acyclovir Sodium
Adalimumab
Agalsidase Beta
Alefacept
Alfuzosin Hydrochloride
Alosetron Hydrochloride
Amiloride Hydrochloride
Amiloride Hydrochloride/Hydrochlorothiazide
Amoxicillin
Amoxicillin/Clavulanate Potassium
Amphotericin B
Amphotericin B Lipid Complex
Amphotericin B, Liposomal
Amphotericin B/Cholesteryl Sulfate Complex
Ampicillin Sodium/Sulbactam Sodium
Anakinra
Antithrombin III
Aprepitant
Aprotinin
Argatroban
Arginine Hydrochloride
Atazanavir Sulfate
Azelaic Acid
Azithromycin
Azithromycin Dihydrate
Aztreonam
Balsalazide Disodium
Basiliximab
Bivalirudin
Brimonidine Tartrate
Budesonide
Bupropion Hydrochloride
Cabergoline
Carbenicillin Indanyl Sodium
Cefaclor
Cefazolin Sodium
Cefdinir
Cefditoren Pivoxil
Cefepime Hydrochloride
Cefixime
Cefoperazone Sodium
Cefotaxime Sodium
Cefotetan Disodium
Cefoxitin Sodium
Cefpodoxime Proxetil
Cefprozil
Ceftazidime Sodium
Ceftibuten Dihydrate
Ceftizoxime Sodium
Ceftriaxone Sodium
Cefuroxime
Cefuroxime Axetil
Cephalexin
Cetirizine Hydrochloride
Ciclopirox
Ciclopirox Olamine
Cimetidine
Cimetidine Hydrochloride
Cisatracurium Besylate
Clindamycin Hydrochloride/Clindamycin Phosphate
Clindamycin Palmitate Hydrochloride
Clindamycin Phosphate
Clopidogrel Bisulfate
Clotrimazole
Clozapine
Colesevelam Hydrochloride
Cromolyn Sodium
Cyclobenzaprine Hydrochloride
Cyproheptadine Hydrochloride
Dalfopristin/Quinupristin
Dalteparin Sodium
Dapiprazole Hydrochloride
Daptomycin
Desflurane
Desmopressin Acetate
Dicyclomine Hydrochloride
Didanosine
Diphenhydramine Hydrochloride
Dipivefrin Hydrochloride
Dipyridamole
Dolasetron Mesylate
Dornase Alfa
Doxapram Hydrochloride
Doxepin Hydrochloride
Doxercalciferol
Edetate Calcium Disodium
Emtricitabine
Emtricitabine/Tenofovir Disoproxil Fumarate
Enfuvirtide
Enoxaparin Sodium
Eplerenone
Epoprostenol Sodium
Ertapenem
Erythromycin
Erythromycin Ethylsuccinate
Erythromycin Stearate
Esomeprazole Magnesium
Esomeprazole Sodium
Etanercept
Ethacrynate Sodium
Ethacrynic Acid
Famciclovir
Famotidine
Fenoldopam Mesylate
Fondaparinux Sodium
Galantamine Hydrobromide
Glatiramer Acetate
Glucagon
Glyburide/Metformin Hydrochloride
Granisetron Hydrochloride
Hydrochlorothiazide
Ibuprofen
Indapamide
Infliximab
Insulin Lispro Protamine, Human/Insulin Lispro, Human
Insulin Lispro, Human
Ipratropium Bromide
Iron Sucrose
Isosorbide Mononitrate
Lactulose
Lansoprazole
Lansoprazole/Naproxen
Laronidase
Lepirudin
Levocarnitine
Lidocaine
Lidocaine Hydrochloride
Lidocaine/Prilocaine
Lindane
Loperamide Hydrochloride

Loracarbef
Loratadine
Malathion
Meclizine Hydrochloride
Memantine Hydrochloride
Meropenem
Mesalamine
Metformin Hydrochloride
Methohexital Sodium
Methyldopa
Metolazone
Metronidazole
Miglitol
Montelukast Sodium
Mupirocin
Mupirocin Calcium
Naftifine Hydrochloride
Nalbuphine Hydrochloride
Nalmefene Hydrochloride
Naloxone Hydrochloride
Naproxen Sodium
Nedocromil Sodium
Nelfinavir Mesylate
Nitazoxanide
Nitrofurantoin Macrocrystals
Nitrofurantoin Macrocrystals/
Nitrofurantoin Monohydrate
Nizatidine
Octreotide Acetate
Omalizumab
Ondansetron
Ondansetron Hydrochloride
Orlistat
Oxiconazole Nitrate
Oxybutynin
Oxybutynin Chloride
Oxycodone Hydrochloride
Palonosetron Hydrochloride
Pancrelipase
Pantoprazole Sodium
Pegvisomant
Pemoline
Penciclovir
Penicillin G Benzathine
Penicillin G Benzathine/
Penicillin G Procaine
Penicillin G Potassium
Pentosan Polysulfate Sodium
Pergolide Mesylate
Permethrin
Piperacillin Sodium
Piperacillin Sodium/
Tazobactam Sodium
Praziquantel
Progesterone
Propofol
Pseudoephedrine Hydrochloride
Pseudoephedrine Sulfate
Psyllium Preparations
Rabeprazole Sodium
Ranitidine Hydrochloride
Rifabutin
Ritonavir
Rivastigmine Tartrate
Ropivacaine Hydrochloride
Saquinavir
Saquinavir Mesylate
Sevoflurane
Sildenafil Citrate
Silver Sulfadiazine
Sodium Ferric Gluconate
Somatropin
Sotalol Hydrochloride
Sucralfate
Sulfasalazine
Tadalafil
Tamsulosin Hydrochloride
Tegaserod Maleate
Tenofovir Disoproxil Fumarate
Terbinafine Hydrochloride
Ticarcillin Disodium/
Clavulanate Potassium
Ticlopidine Hydrochloride
Tirofiban Hydrochloride
Torsemide
Trastuzumab
Treprostinil Sodium
Urokinase
Ursodiol
Valacyclovir Hydrochloride
Vancomycin Hydrochloride
Vardenafil Hydrochloride
Zafirlukast
Zolpidem Tartrate

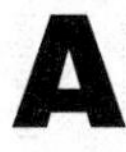

**Controlled studies show no risk**

*Adequate, well-controlled studies in pregnant women have failed to demonstrate risk to the fetus.*

Levothyroxine Sodium
Liothyronine Sodium
Liotrix
Nystatin

* Category C or D depending on the trimester the drug is given.

# VITAMIN COMPARISON TABLE

For easy comparison, the grid below lists the contents of an assortment of widely available vitamin/mineral supplements. It includes entries for all vitamins and minerals—except sodium—assigned a Recommended Dietary Allowance (Daily Value) by the U.S. Food and Drug Administration.

The grid is divided into two parts: the first covers general multivitamin/mineral supplements for adults; the second focuses on supplements sold especially for children.

Many of the brands in the grid include other ingredients that have nutritional importance but lack an official Recommended Dietary Allowance from the government. The presence of additional ingredients is noted in the last column of the grid.

The amounts listed are drawn from the manufacturer's package labeling, primarily as published in the *Physicians' Desk Reference®* and *PDR® for Nonprescription Drugs, Dietary Supplements and Herbs.* For easy comparison, the figures have been converted as necessary from the unit of measure used by the manufacturer to the measurement most frequently employed in the industry. **Amounts listed are those found in a single tablet, capsule, packet, or dose.** Check package labeling for the total daily dose recommended by the manufacturer.

To conserve space, units of measure are not shown in the grid. They are as follows:

| Ingredient | Measure | Ingredient | Measure | Ingredient | Measure |
|---|---|---|---|---|---|
| Vitamin A (retinol, beta-carotene) | International Units | Vitamin B12 (cobalamin) | Micrograms | Iodine | Micrograms |
| Vitamin B1 (thiamin) | Milligrams | Vitamin C (ascorbic acid) | Milligrams | Iron | Milligrams |
| Vitamin B2 (riboflavin) | Milligrams | Vitamin D | International Units | Magnesium | Milligrams |
| Vitamin B3 (niacin) | Milligrams | Vitamin E | International Units | Phosphorus | Milligrams |
| Vitamin B5 (pantothenic acid) | Milligrams | Biotin | Micrograms | Potassium | Milligrams |
| Vitamin B6 (pyridoxine) | Milligrams | Calcium | Milligrams | Zinc | Milligrams |
| Vitamin B9 (folic acid) | Micrograms | Copper | Milligrams | | |

## ADULTS

| BRAND | A | B-1 | B-2 | B-3 | B-5 | B-6 | B-9 | B-12 | C | D | E | BIOTIN | CALCIUM | COPPER | IODINE | IRON | MAGNESIUM | PHOSPHORUS | POTASSIUM | ZINC | OTHER |
|---|---|---|---|---|---|---|---|---|---|---|---|---|---|---|---|---|---|---|---|---|---|
| ACES (Carlson) | 5,000 | — | — | — | — | — | — | — | 500 | — | 200 | — | 50 | — | — | — | — | — | — | — | Y |
| Active Calcium | — | — | — | — | — | — | — | — | — | 100 | — | — | 200 | — | — | — | 100 | — | — | — | Y |
| Anti-Aging Daily Premium Pak | 11,250 | 9 | 9 | 15 | 9 | 9 | 300 | 6 | 575 | 400 | 130 | 375 | 202 | 0.75 | 75 | 7.5 | 80 | — | — | 7.5 | Y |

| BRAND | A | B-1 | B-2 | B-3 | B-5 | B-6 | B-9 | B-12 | C | D | E | BIOTIN | CALCIUM | COPPER | IODINE | IRON | MAGNESIUM | PHOSPHORUS | POTASSIUM | ZINC | OTHER |
|---|---|---|---|---|---|---|---|---|---|---|---|---|---|---|---|---|---|---|---|---|---|
| Caltrate 600 Plus | — | — | — | — | — | — | — | — | — | 400 | — | — | 600 | 1 | — | — | 50 | — | — | 7.5 | Y |
| Centrum | 3,500 | 1.5 | 1.7 | 20 | 10 | 2 | 400 | 6 | 60 | 400 | 30 | 30 | 162 | 2 | 150 | 18 | 100 | 109 | 80 | 15 | Y |
| Centrum Performance | 3,500 | 4.5 | 5.1 | 40 | 10 | 6 | 400 | 18 | 120 | 400 | 60 | 40 | 100 | 2 | 150 | 18 | 40 | 48 | 80 | 15 | Y |
| Centrum Silver | 3,500 | 1.5 | 1.7 | 20 | 10 | 3 | 400 | 25 | 60 | 400 | 45 | 30 | 200 | 2 | 150 | — | 100 | 48 | 80 | 15 | Y |
| Chelated Mineral Tablets | — | — | — | — | — | — | — | — | — | — | — | — | 67.5 | 0.5 | 56.25 | — | 75 | — | — | 5 | Y |
| Chromagen | — | — | — | — | — | — | — | 10 | 150 | — | — | — | — | — | — | 70 | — | — | — | — | — |
| Chromagen FA | — | — | — | — | — | — | 1,000 | 10 | 150 | — | — | — | — | — | — | 70 | — | — | — | — | — |
| Chromagen Forte | — | — | — | — | — | — | 1,000 | 10 | 60 | — | — | — | — | — | — | 151 | — | — | — | — | — |
| Citracal Prenatal Rx | 2,700 | 3 | 3.4 | 20 | — | 20 | 1,000 | — | 120 | 400 | 30 | — | 125 | 2 | 150 | 27 | — | — | — | 25 | — |
| Dexatrim Results, Ephedrine Free | — | — | — | — | 5 | 2 | — | — | 10 | — | 5 | — | 90 | — | — | — | 6.7 | 70 | — | 2.5 | Y |
| Duet by Stuartnatal | 3,000 | 1.8 | 4 | 20 | — | 25 | 1,000 | 12 | 120 | 400 | 30 | — | 200 | 2 | — | 29 | 25 | — | — | 25 | — |
| Duet Chewable by Stuartnatal | 3,000 | 1.8 | 4 | 20 | — | 25 | 1,000 | 12 | 120 | 400 | 30 | — | 100 | 2 | — | 29 | 25 | — | — | 25 | — |
| Eldertonic | — | 0.5 | 0.6 | 7 | 3 | 0.7 | — | 2 | — | — | — | — | — | — | — | — | 0.7 | — | — | 5 | Y |
| Estroven | — | 2 | 2 | 20 | — | 10 | 400 | 6 | — | — | 30 | — | 150 | — | — | — | — | — | — | — | Y |
| Folgard Rx 2.2 | — | — | — | — | — | 25 | 2,200 | 1,000 | — | — | — | — | — | — | — | — | — | — | — | — | — |
| Hep-Forte | 1,200 | 1 | 1 | 10 | 2 | 0.5 | 60 | 1 | 10 | — | 10 | 3.3 | — | — | — | — | — | — | — | 2 | Y |
| Mega Antioxidant | 5,000 | 9 | 9 | 13.3 | 30 | 9 | 333 | 20 | 433 | 150 | 150 | 100 | — | — | — | — | — | — | — | — | Y |

| BRAND | A | B-1 | B-2 | B-3 | B-5 | B-6 | B-9 | B-12 | C | D | E | BIOTIN | CALCIUM | COPPER | IODINE | IRON | MAGNESIUM | PHOSPHORUS | POTASSIUM | ZINC | OTHER |
|---|---|---|---|---|---|---|---|---|---|---|---|---|---|---|---|---|---|---|---|---|---|
| Mega-B | — | 100 | 100 | 100 | 100 | 100 | 100 | 100 | — | — | — | 100 | — | — | — | — | — | — | — | — | Y |
| Megadose | 25,000* | 80 | 80 | 80 | 80 | 80 | 400 | 80 | 250 | 1,000* | 100 | 80 | 50 | 0.5 | 150 | 10 | 7 | — | 10 | 25 | Y |
| NataChew | 1,000 | 2 | 3 | 20 | — | 10 | 1 | 12 | 120 | 400 | 11 | — | — | — | — | 29 | — | — | — | — | — |
| Nephrocaps | — | 1.5 | 1.7 | 20 | 5 | 10 | 1,000 | 6 | 100 | — | — | 150 | — | — | — | — | — | — | — | — | — |
| Nicomide Tablets | — | — | — | 750 | — | — | 500 | — | — | — | — | — | — | — | — | — | — | — | — | 25 | — |
| Niferex-150 Forte | — | — | — | — | — | — | 1,000 | 25 | 60 | — | — | — | — | — | — | 150 | — | — | — | — | — |
| Nu-Iron V | 4,000 | 3 | 3 | 10 | — | 2 | 1 | 3 | 50 | 400 | — | — | 312 | — | — | 60 | — | — | — | — | — |
| Obegyn Prenatal | 5,000 | 1.7 | 2 | 20 | 10 | 10 | 1 | 12 | 120 | 400 | 60 | 300 | 455 | 2 | 150 | 18 | 150 | — | — | 25 | — |
| One-A-Day Active | 5,000 | 4.5 | 5.1 | 40 | 10 | 6 | 400 | 18 | 120 | 400 | 60 | 40 | 110 | 2 | 150 | 9 | 40 | 48 | 200 | 15 | Y |
| One-A-Day Men's Health | 3,500 | 1.2 | 1.7 | 16 | 5 | 3 | 400 | 18 | 90 | 400 | 45 | 30 | 210 | 2 | — | — | 120 | — | 100 | 15 | Y |
| One-A-Day Women's | 2,500 | 1.5 | 1.7 | 10 | 5 | 2 | 400 | 6 | 60 | 400 | 30 | — | 450 | — | — | 18 | 50 | — | — | 15 | — |
| PreCare Chewable | — | — | — | — | — | 2 | 1,000 | — | 50 | 6mcg | 3.5 | — | 250 | 2 | — | 40 | 50 | — | — | 15 | — |
| PreCare Conceive | — | 3 | 3.4 | 20 | — | 50 | 1,000 | 12 | 60 | — | 30 | — | 200 | 2 | — | 30 | 100 | — | — | 15 | — |
| PreCare Prenatal | — | 3 | 3.4 | 20 | — | 50 | 1,000 | 12 | 50 | 6mcg | 3.5 | — | 250 | 2 | — | 40 | 50 | — | — | 15 | — |
| PremesisRx Tablets | — | — | — | — | — | 75 | 1,000 | 12 | — | — | — | — | 200 | — | — | — | — | — | — | — | — |
| Prenate GT. | 2,700 | 3 | 3.4 | 20 | 6 | 20 | 1,000 | 12 | 120 | 400 | 10 | 30 | 200 | 2 | — | 90 | 30 | — | — | 15 | — |
| PrimaCare AM Capsules | — | — | — | — | — | — | — | — | — | 170 | 30 | — | 150 | — | — | — | — | — | — | — | — |
| PrimaCare PM Tablets | — | 3 | 3.4 | 20 | 7 | 50 | 1,000 | 12 | 100 | 230 | — | 35 | 250 | 1.3 | — | 30 | — | — | — | 11 | Y |
| Right Choice AM | 833 | 8.3 | 5 | 16.6 | 16.6 | 8.3 | 266.6 | 66.6 | 200 | — | 66.6 | 100 | — | — | — | — | — | — | — | — | Y |

*USP units.

| BRAND | A | B-1 | B-2 | B-3 | B-5 | B-6 | B-9 | B-12 | C | D | E | BIOTIN | CALCIUM | COPPER | IODINE | IRON | MAGNESIUM | PHOSPHORUS | POTASSIUM | ZINC | OTHER |
|---|---|---|---|---|---|---|---|---|---|---|---|---|---|---|---|---|---|---|---|---|---|
| Right Choice PM | — | — | — | — | — | — | — | — | — | 133.3 | — | — | 166.6 | 0.66 | 50 | — | 83.3 | — | 33 | 5 | Y |
| StrongStart Caplets | 1,000 | 3 | 3.4 | 20 | 7 | 75 | 1,000 | 12 | 50 | 400 | 30 | 35 | 225 | — | — | 40 | 30 | — | — | 15 | Y |
| Strovite Advance | 3,000 | 20 | 5 | 25 | 15 | 25 | 1,000 | 50 | 300 | 400 | 100 | 100 | — | 1.5 | — | — | 50 | — | — | 25 | Y |
| Vicon Forte | 8,000 | 10 | 5 | 25 | 10 | 2 | 1,000 | 10 | 150 | — | 50 | — | — | — | — | — | 70 | — | — | 80 | Y |

## CHILDREN

| BRAND | A | B-1 | B-2 | B-3 | B-5 | B-6 | B-9 | B-12 | C | D | E | BIOTIN | CALCIUM | COPPER | IODINE | IRON | MAGNESIUM | PHOSPHORUS | POTASSIUM | ZINC | OTHER |
|---|---|---|---|---|---|---|---|---|---|---|---|---|---|---|---|---|---|---|---|---|---|
| Centrum, Kids | 3,500 | 1.5 | 1.7 | 20 | 10 | 2 | 400 | 6 | 60 | 400 | 30 | 45 | 108 | 2 | 150 | 18 | 40 | 50 | — | 15 | Y |
| Flintstones | 3,000 | 1.5 | 1.7 | 15 | 10 | 2 | 400 | 6 | 60 | 400 | 30 | 40 | 100 | 2 | 150 | 18 | 20 | 100 | — | 12 | — |
| My First Flintstones | 1,998 | 1.05 | 1.2 | 10 | — | 1.05 | 300 | 4.5 | 60 | 400 | 15 | — | — | — | — | — | — | — | — | — | — |
| One-A-Day Kids Bugs Bunny and Friends | 3,000 | 1.5 | 1.7 | 15 | 10 | 2 | 400 | 6 | 60 | 400 | 30 | 40 | 100 | 2 | 150 | 18 | 20 | 100 | — | 12 | — |
| One-A-Day Kids Scooby-Doo | 3,000 | 1.5 | 1.7 | 15 | 10 | 2 | 400 | 6 | 60 | 400 | 30 | 40 | 100 | 2 | 150 | 18 | 20 | 100 | — | 12 | — |
| One-A-Day Kids Scooby-Doo Plus Calcium | 2,500 | 1.05 | 1.2 | 13.5 | — | 1.05 | 300 | 4.5 | 60 | 400 | 15 | — | 250 | — | — | — | — | — | — | — | — |

# Indices

# BRAND/GENERIC INDEX

Organized alphabetically, this index includes the brand and generic names of each drug described in the Product Information section. Brand-name drug entries are capitalized; generic names are not. If more than one brand name is associated with a generic, each brand can be found under the generic entry.

## A

## D

## E

## F

## G

## H

## I

## N

## O

## S

## T

## W



## X



## Y



## Z

# THERAPEUTIC CLASS INDEX

Organized alphabetically, this index includes the therapeutic class for each drug described in the Product Information section. Therapeutic class headings are based on information provided in the drug monographs. The drug entries listed under each bold therapeutic class are organized alphabetically by brand name or monograph title (shown in capitalized letters), followed by the generic name in parentheses.

## A

**ABORTIFACIENT**
MIFEPREX (Mifepristone) .......... 525

**ACE INHIBITOR**
ACCUPRIL (Quinapril HCl) .......... 6
ACEON (Perindopril Erbumine) .......8
ALTACE (Ramipril) ................ 45
CAPOTEN (Captopril) .............142
CAPTOPRIL (Captopril) ...........142
LOTENSIN (Benazepril HCl) .......479
MAVIK (Trandolapril) .............496
MONOPRIL (Fosinopril Sodium) ... 537
PRINIVIL (Lisinopril) .............. 695
UNIVASC (Moexipril HCl) .........893
VASOTEC (Enalapril Maleate) .....906
VASOTEC I.V. (Enalaprilat) ........907
ZESTRIL (Lisinopril) .............. 965

**ACE INHIBITOR/CALCIUM CHANNEL BLOCKER (DIHYDROPYRIDINE)**
LEXXEL (Felodipine - Enalapril Maleate) .......................464

**ACE INHIBITOR/CALCIUM CHANNEL BLOCKER (NONDIHYDROPYRIDINE)**
TARKA (Trandolapril - Verapamil HCl) ...........................824

**ACE INHIBITOR/THIAZIDE DIURETIC**
ACCURETIC (Hydrochlorothiazide - Quinapril HCl) ..................... 6
CAPOZIDE (Captopril - Hydrochlorothiazide) ............ 141
LOTENSIN HCT (Hydrochlorothiazide - Benazepril HCl) ..................480
MONOPRIL HCT (Hydrochlorothiazide - Fosinopril Sodium) .............. 538
PRINZIDE (Lisinopril - Hydrochlorothiazide) ............696
UNIRETIC (Hydrochlorothiazide - Moexipril HCl) ...................891
VASERETIC (Hydrochlorothiazide - Enalapril Maleate) .............905
ZESTORETIC (Lisinopril - Hydrochlorothiazide) ...........964

**ACETAMIDE LOCAL ANESTHETIC**
EMLA ANESTHETIC DISC (Lidocaine - Prilocaine) .......... 297
EMLA (Lidocaine - Prilocaine) ..... 297
LIDOCAINE OINTMENT (Lidocaine) ...................... 467
LIDODERM PATCH (Lidocaine) .... 467
SYNERA (Lidocaine - Tetracaine)...816
XYLOCAINE JELLY (Lidocaine HCl) ...............................951
XYLOCAINE VISCOUS (Lidocaine HCl) .............................. 952

**ACETAMINOPHEN ANTIDOTE**
ACETADOTE (Acetylcysteine) ....... 9

**ACETAMINOPHEN ANTIDOTE/ MUCOLYTIC**
MUCOMYST (Acetylcysteine) ..... 543

**ACETYLCHOLINESTERASE INHIBITOR**
ARICEPT (Donepezil HCl) .......... 75
ARICEPT ODT (Donepezil HCl) ..... 75
EXELON (Rivastigmine Tartrate) .. 326
RAZADYNE ER (Galantamine Hydrobromide) .................. 726
RAZADYNE (Galantamine Hydrobromide) .................. 726

**ACID-STABLE PENICILLIN**
PENICILLIN VK (Penicillin V Potassium) ..................... 649
VEETIDS (Penicillin V Potassium) .. 649

**ACTINOMYCIN ANTIBIOTIC**
COSMEGEN (Dactinomycin) ....... 207

**ACTIVATED PROTEIN C**
XIGRIS (Drotrecogin alfa) ......... 949

**ACYCLIC NUCLEOTIDE ANALOG**
HEPSERA (Adefovir Dipivoxil) ..... 396

**ADAMANTANE CLASS ANTIVIRAL**
FLUMADINE (Rimantadine HCl) ....351

**ADRENAL CYTOTOXIC AGENT**
LYSODREN (Mitotane) ............ 491

**ADRENERGIC/ANTICHOLINERGIC AGENT**
PAREMYD (Tropicamide - Hydroxyamphetamine HBr) ......640

**ADRENOCORTICAL STEROID SYNTHESIS INHIBITOR**
CYTADREN (Aminoglutethimide)...217

**AGONIST-ANTAGONIST ANALGESIC**
NUBAIN (Nalbuphine HCl) ......... 599

**ALCOHOL DEHYDROGENASE INHIBITOR**
ANTIZOL (Fomepizole) ............. 67

**ALCOHOL OXIDATION INHIBITOR**
ANTABUSE (Disulfiram) ........... 66

**ALDOSTERONE BLOCKER**
INSPRA (Eplerenone) ............. 424

**ALKALINIZING AGENT**
POLYCITRA (Citric Acid - Potassium Citrate) ................671

NEOSPORIN OPHTHALMIC (Bacitracin Zinc - Neomycin Sulfate - Polymyxin B Sulfate).... 568
POLYSPORIN OPHTHALMIC (Bacitracin Zinc - Polymyxin B Sulfate) .......................... 671
TERRAMYCIN/POLYMYXIN B SULFATE (Oxytetracycline HCl - Polymyxin B Sulfate) ........... 836

**ANTIBACTERIAL/ANALGESIC**
NEOSPORIN + PAIN RELIEF MAXIMUM STRENGTH (Neomycin - Bacitracin - Polymyxin B - Pramoxine HCl) ... 567

**ANTIBACTERIAL/ANTIFUNGAL**
DOMEBORO OTIC (Acetic Acid - Aluminum Acetate).............. 269

**ANTIBACTERIAL/ CORTICOSTEROID**
CORTISPORIN (Bacitracin Zinc - Neomycin Sulfate - Polymyxin B Sulfate - Hydrocortisone Acetate) ........................ 203
CORTISPORIN OPHTHALMIC (Hydrocortisone - Bacitracin Zinc - Neomycin Sulfate - Polymyxin B Sulfate) ........... 204

**ANTIBACTERIAL/ CORTICOSTEROID COMBINATION**
ACETASOL HC (Acetic Acid - Hydrocortisone)................ 938
CIPRO HC (Hydrocortisone - Ciprofloxacin HCl) ............... 171
CIPRODEX (Ciprofloxacin - Dexamethasone) ................. 174
CORTISPORIN OTIC (Neomycin - Hydrocortisone - Polymyxin B Sulfate) ........................ 204
CORTISPORIN-TC OTIC (Colistin Sulfate - Neomycin Sulfate - Thonzonium Bromide - Hydrocortisone Acetate) ........ 205
PEDIOTIC (Hydrocortisone - Neomycin Sulfate - Polymyxin B Sulfate) ........................ 647
VOSOL HC (Acetic Acid - Hydrocortisone)................ 938

**ANTIBACTERIAL/KERATOLYTIC**
BENZAC AC (Benzoyl Peroxide).... 112
BENZACLIN (Clindamycin - Benzoyl Peroxide) ............... 112
BENZAGEL (Benzoyl Peroxide)..... 112
BENZAGEL WASH (Benzoyl Peroxide)......................... 112
BENZAMYCIN (Erythromycin - Benzoyl Peroxide)............... 113
BREVOXYL (Benzoyl Peroxide).....132
DUAC (Clindamycin - Benzoyl Peroxide)......................... 277
SULFOXYL LOTION REGULAR (Sulfur - Benzoyl Peroxide) ...... 806
SULFOXYL LOTION STRONG (Sulfur - Benzoyl Peroxide) ...... 806
TRIAZ (Benzoyl Peroxide)......... 869
ZODERM (Benzoyl Peroxide).......971

**ANTIBIOTIC**
BACITRACIN INJECTION (Bacitracin)..................... 103

**ANTICHOLINERGIC**
ATROPINE SULFATE (Atropine Sulfate) .......................... 86
BENTYL (Dicyclomine HCl)..........111
CYSTOSPAZ (Hyoscyamine Sulfate) .........................217
IB-STAT (Hyoscyamine Sulfate) ... 410
LEVBID (Hyoscyamine Sulfate) .... 458
LEVSIN (Hyoscyamine Sulfate) .... 458
LEVSINEX (Hyoscyamine Sulfate) ........................ 458
NULEV (Hyoscyamine Sulfate)..... 601
OXYTROL (Oxybutynin)........... 634
PAMINE FORTE (Methscopolamine Bromide)..... 636
PAMINE (Methscopolamine Bromide)........................ 636
ROBINUL FORTE (Glycopyrrolate)................ 752
ROBINUL (Glycopyrrolate) ........ 752
ROBINUL INJECTION (Glycopyrrolate)................ 753

**ANTICHOLINERGIC AGENT**
ATROVENT NASAL (Ipratropium Bromide)......................... 87
BENZTROPINE (Benztropine Mesylate)......................... 113
COGENTIN (Benztropine Mesylate)......................... 113
DITROPAN (Oxybutynin Chloride) ........................ 266
DITROPAN XL (Oxybutynin Chloride) ........................266
TRANSDERM SCOP (Scopolamine).................. 863

**ANTICHOLINERGIC BRONCHODILATOR**
ATROVENT HFA (Ipratropium Bromide)......................... 87
ATROVENT (Ipratropium Bromide)......................... 87
SPIRIVA (Tiotropium Bromide) .... 793

**ANTICHOLINERGIC/ ANTIBACTERIAL/ANTISEPTIC/ ANALGESIC/ACIDIFIER**
URIMAX (Methenamine - Methylene Blue - Phenyl Salicylate - Sodium Biphosphate - Hyoscyamine Sulfate) .......... 894
UROGESIC BLUE (Methenamine - Methylene Blue - Phenyl Salicylate - Sodium Biphosphate - Hyoscyamine Sulfate) .......... 897

**ANTICHOLINERGIC/ANTISEPTIC/ ANTIBACTERIAL/ANALGESIC**
URISED (Methenamine - Benzoic Acid - Methylene Blue - Phenyl Salicylate - Atropine Sulfate - Hyoscyamine Sulfate) ........... 895

**ANTICHOLINERGIC/ ANTISPASMODIC**
TRIHEXYPHENIDYL HCL (Trihexyphenidyl HCl) .......... 871

**ANTICHOLINERGIC/ BARBITURATE**
DONNATAL EXTENTABS (Phenobarbital - Atropine Sulfate - Hyoscyamine Sulfate - Scopolamine Hydrobromide) .... 270
DONNATAL (Phenobarbital - Atropine Sulfate - Hyoscyamine Sulfate - Scopolamine Hydrobromide) .......... 270

**ANTICHOLINERGIC/ BARBITURATE/ANALGESIC**
PYRIDIUM PLUS (Butabarbital - Phenazopyridine HCl - Hyoscyamine Hydrobromide) ..... 719

**ANTICHOLINERGIC/ERGOT DERIVATIVE/BARBITURATE**
BELLAMINE-S (Phenobarbital - Belladonna Alkaloids - Ergotamine Tartrate) .......... 109

**ANTIDOTE**
CYANIDE ANTIDOTE PACKAGE (Amyl Nitrite - Sodium Nitrite - Sodium Thiosulfate) .......... 214

**ANTIDOTE, DIGOXIN TOXICITY**
DIGIBIND (Digoxin Immune Fab (Ovine)) .......... 259

**ANTIESTROGEN**
SOLTAMOX (Tamoxifen Citrate) ... 787
TAMOXIFEN (Tamoxifen Citrate) ... 821

**ANTIFOLATE**
ALIMTA (Pemetrexed) .......... 38

**ANTIFUNGAL AGENT**
AVC (Sulfanilamide) .......... 94

**ANTIGAS**
MYLANTA GAS MAXIMUM STRENGTH (Simethicone) ....... 550
MYLANTA GAS MAXIMUM STRENGTH SOFTGELS (Simethicone) .......... 550
MYLANTA GAS REGULAR STRENGTH CHEWABLE TABLETS (Simethicone) ......... 550

**ANTIHEMOPHILIC FACTOR (RECOMBINANT)**
KOGENATE FS (Antihemophilic Factor) .......... 446

**ANTIHISTAMINE**
ANTIVERT (Meclizine HCl) .......... 67
ASTELIN (Azelastine HCl) .......... 81
BENADRYL ALLERGY (Diphenhydramine HCl) .......... 110
CHLOR-TRIMETON (Chlorpheniramine Maleate) ...... 168
DIPHENHYDRAMINE HCL INJECTION (Diphenhydramine HCl) .......... 264
TAVIST ALLERGY (Clemastine Fumarate) .......... 825
UNISOM (Doxylamine Succinate) .. 892

**ANTIHISTAMINE/ ANTICHOLINERGIC/ SYMPATHOMIMETIC**
DALLERGY (Phenylephrine HCl - Methscopolamine Nitrate - Chlorpheniramine Maleate) ...... 222

**ANTIHISTAMINE/ ANTICHOLINERGIC/ DECONGESTANT**
ALLERX (Pseudoephedrine HCl - Methscopolamine Nitrate - Chlorpheniramine Maleate) ........ 41

**ANTIHISTAMINE/ ANTICHOLINERGIC/ SYMPATHOMIMETIC**
HISTA-VENT DA (Phenylephrine HCl - Methscopolamine Nitrate - Chlorpheniramine Maleate) ...... 398

**ANTIHISTAMINE/ANTITUSSIVE/ SYMPATHOMIMETIC**
ALACOL DM (Phenylephrine HCl - Dextromethorphan HBr - Brompheniramine Maleate) ........ 31

**ANTIHISTAMINE/COUGH SUPPRESSANT/DECONGESTANT**
BALAMINE DM (Pseudoephedrine HCl - Dextromethorphan HBr - Carbinoxamine Maleate) ......... 105

**ANTIHISTAMINE/DECONGESTANT**
BROMFED (Pseudoephedrine HCl - Brompheniramine Maleate) ...... 132
BROMFED-PD (Pseudoephedrine HCl - Brompheniramine Maleate) .......... 132
BROMFENEX (Pseudoephedrine HCl - Brompheniramine Maleate) .......... 132
BROMFENEX-PD (Pseudoephedrine HCl - Brompheniramine Maleate) ....... 132
DECONAMINE (Pseudoephedrine HCl - Chlorpheniramine Maleate) .......... 232
DECONAMINE SR (Pseudoephedrine HCl - Chlorpheniramine Maleate) ...... 232
DE-CONGESTINE TR (Pseudoephedrine HCl - Chlorpheniramine Maleate) ...... 232
KRONOFED-A (Pseudoephedrine HCl - Chlorpheniramine Maleate) .......... 232
RONDEC ORAL DROPS (Pseudoephedrine HCl - Carbinoxamine Maleate) ......... 757
RONDEC (Pseudoephedrine HCl - Carbinoxamine Maleate) ......... 757
RONDEC SYRUP (Pseudoephedrine HCl - Brompheniramine Maleate) ...... 758
RONDEC-TR (Pseudoephedrine HCl - Carbinoxamine Maleate) ... 757
SEMPREX-D (Acrivastine - Pseudoephedrine HCl) .......... 774
VASOCON-A (Naphazoline HCl - Antazoline Phosphate) .......... 906

TUSSI-ORGANIDIN DM NR (Guaifenesin - Dextromethorphan Hydrobromide) .... 882
TUSSI-ORGANIDIN DM S NR (Guaifenesin - Dextromethorphan Hydrobromide) .... 882

**ANTITUSSIVE/EXPECTORANT/ DECONGESTANT**
MYTUSSIN DAC (Guaifenesin - Codeine Phosphate - Pseudoephedrine HCl) .... 600
NUCOFED PEDIATRIC EXPECTORANT (Guaifenesin - Codeine Phosphate - Pseudoephedrine HCl) .... 600

**ANTIVIRAL**
ABREVA (Docosanol) .... 5

**ARGININE VASOPRESSIN ANTAGONIST**
VAPRISOL (Conivaptan HCl) .... 904

**AROMATASE INACTIVATOR**
AROMASIN (Exemestane) .... 78

**AROMATASE INHIBITOR (NON-STEROIDAL)**
ARIMIDEX (Anastrozole) .... 76

**ARYLOXYACETIC ACID DERIVATIVE**
EDECRIN (Ethacrynic Acid) .... 286
EDECRIN SODIUM (Ethacrynate Sodium) .... 287

**ATTENUATED LIVE BCG CULTURE**
THERACYS (BCG Live) .... 843
TICE BCG (BCG Live) .... 847

**ATYPICAL ANXIOLYTIC**
BUSPAR (Buspirone HCl) .... 134

**AVERMECTINS DERIVATIVE**
STROMECTOL (Ivermectin) .... 801

**AZOLE ANTIFUNGAL**
1-DAY (Tioconazole) .... 1
ERTACZO (Sertaconazole Nitrate) .... 309
GYNAZOLE-1 (Butoconazole Nitrate) .... 387
GYNE-LOTRIMIN 3 (Clotrimazole) .... 387
GYNE-LOTRIMIN 3 COMBINATION PACK (Clotrimazole) .... 387
GYNE-LOTRIMIN (Clotrimazole) .... 387
GYNE-LOTRIMIN COMBINATION PACK (Clotrimazole) .... 387
KETOCONAZOLE TOPICAL (Ketoconazole) .... 441
LOTRIMIN AF (Clotrimazole) .... 481
LOTRIMIN AF SPRAY & POWDER (Miconazole Nitrate) .... 482
LOTRIMIN (Clotrimazole) .... 481
MONISTAT 1 COMBINATION PACK (Miconazole Nitrate) .... 535
MONISTAT 3 (Miconazole Nitrate) .... 535
MONISTAT 7 (Miconazole Nitrate) .... 535
MONISTAT (Miconazole Nitrate) .... 535
MONISTAT-DERM (Miconazole Nitrate) .... 536
MYCELEX-3 (Butoconazole Nitrate) .... 548
MYCELEX-7 (Clotrimazole) .... 548
NIZORAL A-D (Ketoconazole) .... 587
NIZORAL (Ketoconazole) .... 587
NIZORAL SHAMPOO (Ketoconazole) .... 587
OXISTAT (Oxiconazole Nitrate) .... 631
SPECTAZOLE (Econazole Nitrate) .... 793
SPORANOX (Itraconazole) .... 794
TERAZOL 3 (Terconazole) .... 835
TERAZOL 7 (Terconazole) .... 835
VAGISTAT-1 (Tioconazole) .... 899

## B

**BACTERIAL PROTEIN SYNTHESIS INHIBITOR**
BACTROBAN (Mupirocin) .... 105

**BARBITURATE**
MEBARAL (Mephobarbital) .... 499
NEMBUTAL SODIUM (Pentobarbital Sodium) .... 565
PHENOBARBITAL (Phenobarbital) .... 660
SECONAL SODIUM (Secobarbital Sodium) .... 773

**BARBITURATE ANESTHETIC**
BREVITAL (Methohexital Sodium) .... 131

**BARBITURATE/ANALGESIC**
ESGIC (Caffeine - Butalbital - Acetaminophen) .... 315
ESGIC-PLUS (Caffeine - Butalbital - Acetaminophen) .... 316
FIORICET (Caffeine - Butalbital - Acetaminophen) .... 341
FIORICET WITH CODEINE (Caffeine - Butalbital - Acetaminophen - Codeine Phosphate) .... 341
FIORINAL (Aspirin - Caffeine - Butalbital) .... 341
FIORINAL WITH CODEINE (Aspirin - Caffeine - Butalbital - Codeine Phosphate) .... 342
LANORINAL (Aspirin - Caffeine - Butalbital) .... 341
PHRENILIN (Butalbital - Acetaminophen) .... 663
PHRENILIN FORTE (Butalbital - Acetaminophen) .... 663

**B-COMPLEX VITAMIN**
NIASPAN (Niacin) .... 576

**B-COMPLEX VITAMIN/HMG-COA REDUCTASE INHIBITOR**
ADVICOR (Niacin - Lovastatin) .... 26

**BENZISOXAZOLE DERIVATIVE**
GEODON FOR INJECTION (Ziprasidone HCl) .... 376
GEODON (Ziprasidone HCl) .... 376

## D

## E

**EXPECTORANT**



**EXPECTORANT/DECONGESTANT**

## H

## I

**PENICILLIN (PENICILLINASE-RESISTANT)**
DICLOXACILLIN (Dicloxacillin Sodium) .......... 257

***PENICILLIUM*-DERIVED ANTIFUNGAL**
GRIFULVIN V (Griseofulvin) .......... 384
GRIS-PEG (Griseofulvin) .......... 385

**PEPTIDE SYNTHESIS INHIBITOR**
TRECATOR (Ethionamide) .......... 867

**PERIPHERAL VASODILATOR**
MINOXIDIL (Minoxidil) .......... 529

**PHENOTHIAZINE**
CHLORPROMAZINE (Chlorpromazine) .......... 166
PERPHENAZINE (Perphenazine) .......... 657

**PHENOTHIAZINE DERIVATIVE**
COMPRO (Prochlorperazine) .......... 699
PHENERGAN INJECTION (Promethazine HCl) .......... 659
PHENERGAN (Promethazine HCl) .......... 704
PROCHLORPERAZINE (Prochlorperazine) .......... 699
PROMETHAZINE (Promethazine HCl) .......... 704
PROMETHEGAN (Promethazine HCl) .......... 704

**PHENOTHIAZINE DERIVATIVE/ SYMPATHOMIMETIC**
PROMETHAZINE VC (Promethazine HCl - Phenylephrine HCl) .......... 705

**PHENOTHIAZINE DERIVATIVE/ ANTITUSSIVE**
PROMETHAZINE DM (Promethazine HCl - Dextromethorphan HBr) .......... 704
PROMETHAZINE W/CODEINE (Promethazine HCl - Codeine Phosphate) .......... 706

**PHENOTHIAZINE DERIVATIVE/ ANTITUSSIVE/ SYMPATHOMIMETIC**
PROMETHAZINE VC/CODEINE (Promethazine HCl - Codeine Phosphate - Phenylephrine HCl) .......... 705

**PHENYLTRIAZINE**
LAMICTAL CD (Lamotrigine) .......... 449
LAMICTAL (Lamotrigine) .......... 449

**PHOSPHATE BINDER**
FOSRENOL (Lanthanum Carbonate) .......... 364
PHOSLO (Calcium Acetate) .......... 662
RENAGEL (Sevelamer HCl) .......... 735

**PHOSPHATE SUPPLEMENT**
URO KP NEUTRAL (Sodium Phosphate - Disodium Phosphate - Dipotassium Phosphate) .......... 896

**PHOSPHODIESTERASE III INHIBITOR**
PLETAL (Cilostazol) .......... 669

**PHOSPHODIESTERASE TYPE 5 INHIBITOR**
CIALIS (Tadalafil) .......... 169
LEVITRA (Vardenafil HCl) .......... 459
REVATIO (Sildenafil Citrate) .......... 741
VIAGRA (Sildenafil Citrate) .......... 918

**PHOSPHONIC ACID DERIVATIVE**
MONUROL (Fosfomycin Tromethamine) .......... 538

**PHOTOSENSITIZING AGENT**
VISUDYNE (Verteporfin) .......... 932

**PIPERAZINE ANTIHISTAMINE**
ATARAX (Hydroxyzine HCl) .......... 407
HYDROXYZINE HCL (Hydroxyzine HCl) .......... 407
HYDROXYZINE PAMOATE (Hydroxyzine Pamoate) .......... 407
VISTARIL (Hydroxyzine Pamoate) .......... 407

**PIPERAZINE PHENOTHIAZINE**
FLUPHENAZINE (Fluphenazine HCl) .......... 353
PROLIXIN DECANOATE (Fluphenazine HCl) .......... 353
PROLIXIN (Fluphenazine HCl) .......... 353
TRIFLUOPERAZINE HCL (Trifluoperazine HCl) .......... 870

**PIPERAZINE PHENOTHIAZINE/ TRICYCLIC ANTIDEPRESSANT**
TRIAVIL (Perphenazine - Amitriptyline HCl) .......... 868

**PIPERAZINO-AZEPINE**
REMERON (Mirtazapine) .......... 733
REMERON SOLTAB (Mirtazapine) .......... 733

**PIPERIDINE PHENOTHIAZINE**
THIORIDAZINE (Thioridazine HCl) .......... 845

**PITUITARY HORMONE**
DOSTINEX (Cabergoline) .......... 272

**PLATELET AGGREGATION INHIBITOR**
AGGRENOX (Aspirin - Dipyridamole) .......... 29
PLAVIX (Clopidogrel Bisulfate) .......... 668
TICLID (Ticlopidine HCl) .......... 848

**PLATELET INHIBITOR**
PERSANTINE (Dipyridamole) .......... 657

**PLATELET-DERIVED GROWTH FACTOR (RECOMBINANT HUMAN)**
REGRANEX (Becaplermin) .......... 731

**PLATELET-REDUCING AGENT**
AGRYLIN (Anagrelide HCl) .......... 29

**PLATINUM COORDINATION COMPOUND**
CARBOPLATIN (Carboplatin) .......... 144

**PLEUROMUTILIN ANTIBACTERIAL**
ALTABAX (Retapamulin) .......... 45

**PODOPHYLLOTOXIN DERIVATIVE**
ETOPOPHOS (Etoposide Phosphate) .......... 323
ETOPOSIDE (Etoposide) .......... 324

## S

## U



## V

# Visual Identification Guide

# VISUAL PRODUCT IDENTIFICATION GUIDE*

## ABILIFY

RX

(aripiprazole)
**BRISTOL-MYERS SQUIBB/ OTSUKA AMERICA**

2 mg 5 mg 10 mg

15 mg 20 mg 30 mg

## ABILIFY DISCMELT

RX

(aripiprazole)
**BRISTOL-MYERS SQUIBB/ OTSUKA AMERICA**

10 mg 15 mg

## ACCUTANE

RX

(isotretinoin)
**ROCHE**

10 mg 20 mg 40 mg

## ACIPHEX

RX

(rabeprazole sodium)
**EISAI/PRICARA**

20 mg

Delayed-Release Tablets

## ACTONEL

RX

(risedronate sodium)
**PROCTER & GAMBLE**

5 mg 30 mg 35 mg

## ACTOPLUS MET

RX

(pioglitazone HCl/metformin HCl)
**TAKEDA**

15/500 mg 15/850 mg

## ACTOS

RX

(pioglitazone HCl)
**TAKEDA**

15 mg 30 mg 45 mg

## ADDERALL

CII

(amphetamine salt combo)
**SHIRE**

5 mg 7.5 mg 10 mg 12.5 mg

15 mg 20 mg 30 mg

## ADDERALL XR

CII

(amphetamine salt combo)
**SHIRE**

5 mg 10 mg

15 mg 20 mg

25 mg 30 mg

Extended-Release Capsules

## ADVICOR

RX

(niacin extended-release/lovastatin)
**KOS**

500 mg/20 mg 750 mg/20 mg

1000 mg/20 mg 1000 mg/40 mg

## AGGRENOX

RX

(aspirin/extended-release dipyridamole)
**BOEHRINGER INGELHEIM**

25 mg/200 mg

*Other dosage forms and strengths may be available

## ALLEGRA

RX (fexofenadine HCl)
**SANOFI-AVENTIS**

30 mg 60 mg

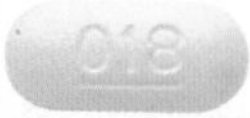

180 mg

## ALLEGRA-D 12 HOUR

RX (fexofenadine HCl/pseudoephedrine HCl)
**SANOFI-AVENTIS**

60 mg/120 mg
Extended-Release Tablets

## ALLEGRA-D 24 HOUR

RX (fexofenadine HCl/pseudoephedrine HCl)
**SANOFI-AVENTIS**

308 AV

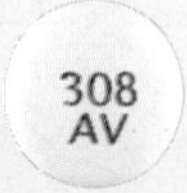

180 mg/240 mg
Extended-Release Tablets

## ALTACE

RX (ramipril)
**KING**

1.25 mg 2.5 mg

5 mg 10 mg

## ALTOPREV

RX (lovastatin)
**SCIELE**

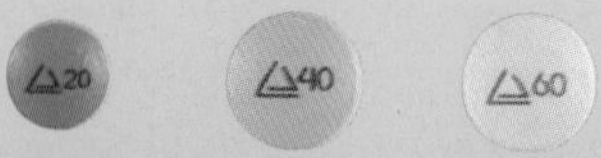

20 mg 40 mg 60 mg
Extended-Release Tablets

## AMARYL

RX (glimepiride)
**SANOFI-AVENTIS**

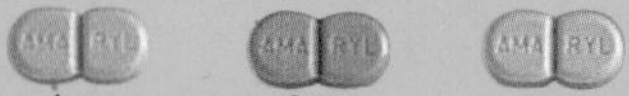

1 mg 2 mg 4 mg

## AMBIEN

CIV (zolpidem tartrate)
**SANOFI-AVENTIS**

5 mg 10 mg

## AMERGE

RX (naratriptan HCl)
**GLAXOSMITHKLINE**

1 mg 2.5 mg

## AMOXIL

RX (amoxicillin)
**GLAXOSMITHKLINE**

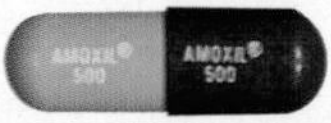

500 mg

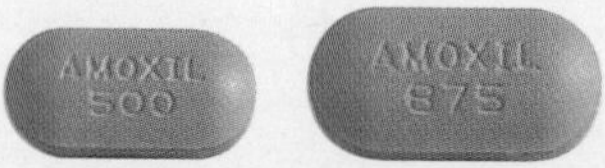

500 mg 875 mg

## ARICEPT

RX (donepezil HCl)
**EISAI**

5 mg 10 mg

## ARICEPT ODT

RX (donepezil HCl)
**EISAI**

5 mg

10 mg
Orally Disintegrating Tablets

## ARIMIDEX

RX (anastrozole)
**ASTRAZENECA**

1 mg

## ATACAND

RX (candesartan cilexetil)
**ASTRAZENECA**

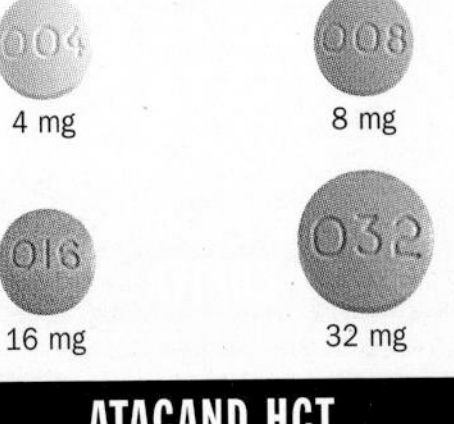

4 mg 8 mg

16 mg 32 mg

## ATACAND HCT

RX (candesartan cilexetil/hydrochlorothiazide)
**ASTRAZENECA**

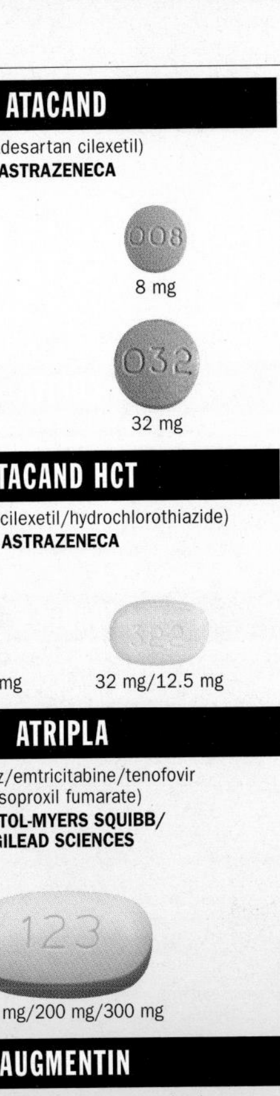

16 mg/12.5 mg 32 mg/12.5 mg

## ATRIPLA

RX (efavirenz/emtricitabine/tenofovir disoproxil fumarate)
**BRISTOL-MYERS SQUIBB/ GILEAD SCIENCES**

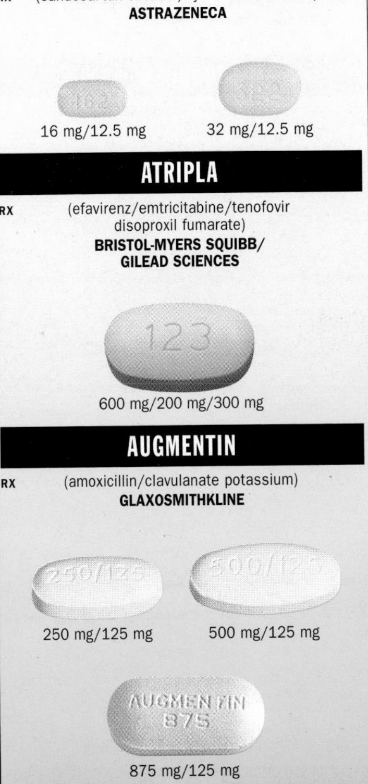

600 mg/200 mg/300 mg

## AUGMENTIN

RX (amoxicillin/clavulanate potassium)
**GLAXOSMITHKLINE**

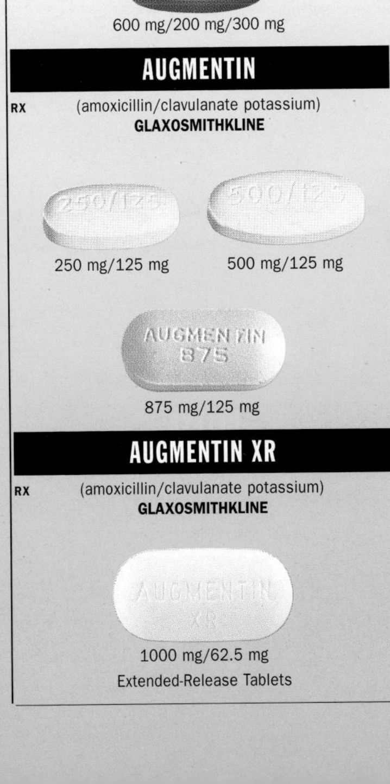

250 mg/125 mg 500 mg/125 mg

875 mg/125 mg

## AUGMENTIN XR

RX (amoxicillin/clavulanate potassium)
**GLAXOSMITHKLINE**

1000 mg/62.5 mg
Extended-Release Tablets

## AVALIDE

RX (irbesartan/hydrochlorothiazide)
**BRISTOL-MYERS SQUIBB**

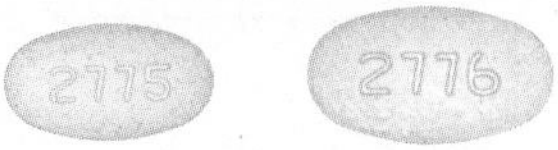

150 mg/12.5 mg 300 mg/12.5 mg

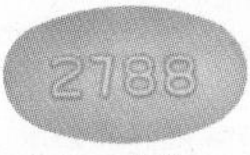

300 mg/25 mg

## AVANDAMET

RX (rosiglitazone maleate/metformin HCl)
**GLAXOSMITHKLINE**

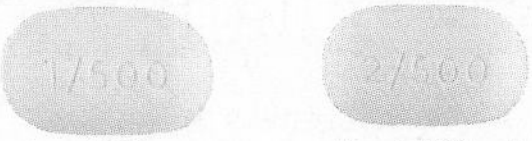

1 mg/500 mg 2 mg/500 mg

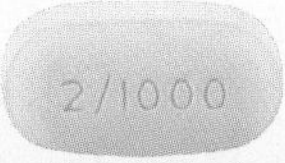

2 mg/1000 mg

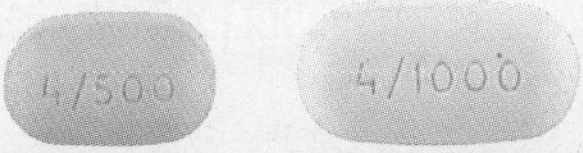

4 mg/500 mg 4 mg/1000 mg

## AVANDARYL

RX (rosiglitazone maleate/glimepiride)
**GLAXOSMITHKLINE**

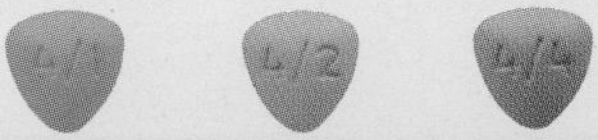

4 mg/1 mg 4 mg/2 mg 4 mg/4 mg

## AVANDIA

RX (rosiglitazone maleate)
**GLAXOSMITHKLINE**

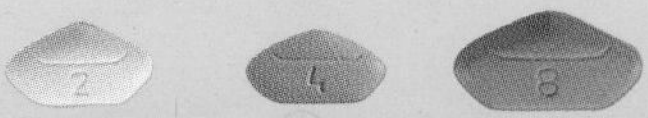

2 mg 4 mg 8 mg

## AVAPRO

RX (irbesartan)
**BRISTOL-MYERS SQUIBB/SANOFI-AVENTIS**

75 mg 150 mg

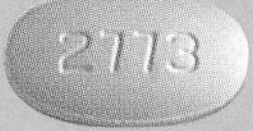

300 mg

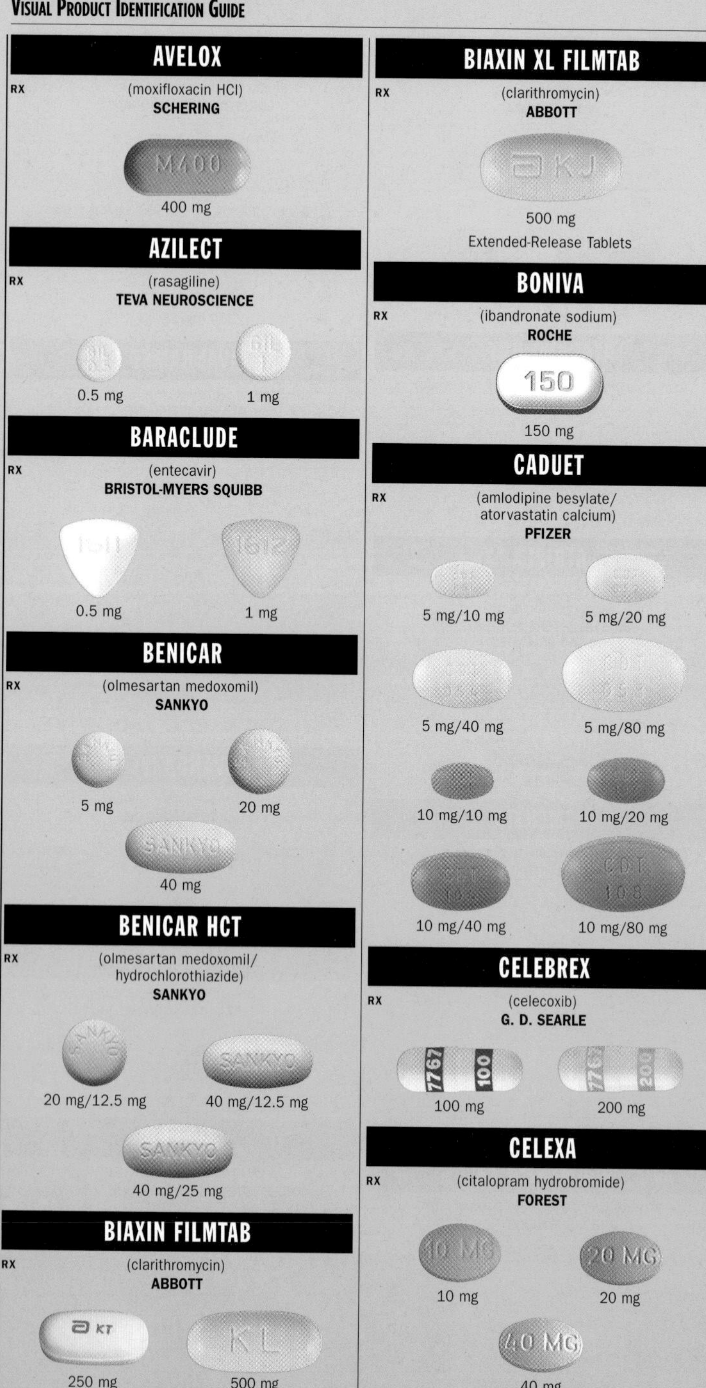

AVELOX
RX
(moxifloxacin HCl)
SCHERING
400 mg
AZILECT
RX
(rasagiline)
TEVA NEUROSCIENCE
0.5 mg
1 mg
BARACLUDE
RX
(entecavir)
BRISTOL-MYERS SQUIBB
0.5 mg
1 mg
BENICAR
RX
(olmesartan medoxomil)
SANKYO
5 mg
20 mg
40 mg
BENICAR HCT
RX
(olmesartan medoxomil/
hydrochlorothiazide)
SANKYO
20 mg/12.5 mg
40 mg/12.5 mg
40 mg/25 mg
BIAXIN FILMTAB
RX
(clarithromycin)
ABBOTT
250 mg
500 mg
BIAXIN XL FILMTAB
RX
(clarithromycin)
ABBOTT
500 mg
Extended-Release Tablets
BONIVA
RX
(ibandronate sodium)
ROCHE
150 mg
CADUET
RX
(amlodipine besylate/
atorvastatin calcium)
PFIZER
5 mg/10 mg
5 mg/20 mg
5 mg/40 mg
5 mg/80 mg
10 mg/10 mg
10 mg/20 mg
10 mg/40 mg
10 mg/80 mg
CELEBREX
RX
(celecoxib)
G. D. SEARLE
100 mg
200 mg
CELEXA
RX
(citalopram hydrobromide)
FOREST
10 mg
20 mg
40 mg

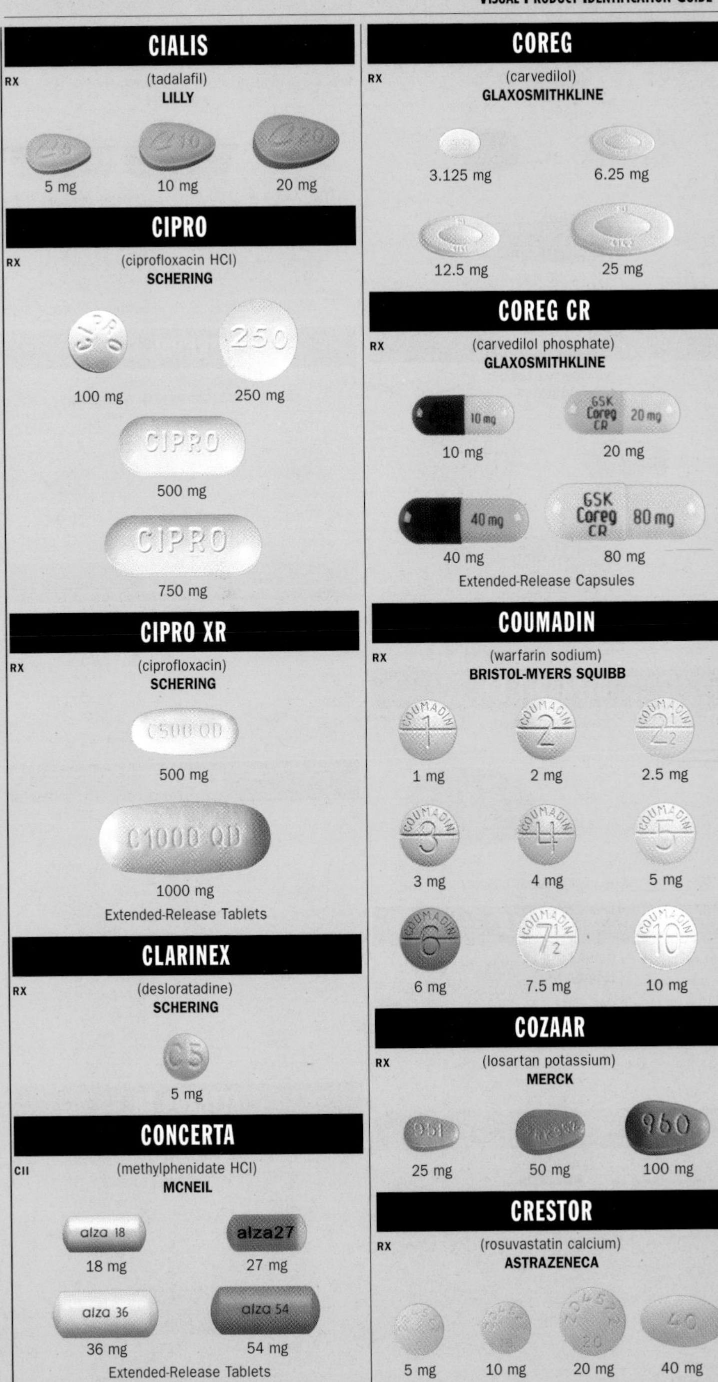
CIALIS
RX
(tadalafil)
LILLY
5 mg
10 mg
20 mg
CIPRO
RX
(ciprofloxacin HCl)
SCHERING
100 mg
250 mg
500 mg
750 mg
CIPRO XR
RX
(ciprofloxacin)
SCHERING
500 mg
1000 mg
Extended-Release Tablets
CLARINEX
RX
(desloratadine)
SCHERING
5 mg
CONCERTA
CII
(methylphenidate HCl)
MCNEIL
18 mg
27 mg
36 mg
54 mg
Extended-Release Tablets
COREG
RX
(carvedilol)
GLAXOSMITHKLINE
3.125 mg
6.25 mg
12.5 mg
25 mg
COREG CR
RX
(carvedilol phosphate)
GLAXOSMITHKLINE
10 mg
20 mg
40 mg
80 mg
Extended-Release Capsules
COUMADIN
RX
(warfarin sodium)
BRISTOL-MYERS SQUIBB
1 mg
2 mg
2.5 mg
3 mg
4 mg
5 mg
6 mg
7.5 mg
10 mg
COZAAR
RX
(losartan potassium)
MERCK
25 mg
50 mg
100 mg
CRESTOR
RX
(rosuvastatin calcium)
ASTRAZENECA
5 mg
10 mg
20 mg
40 mg

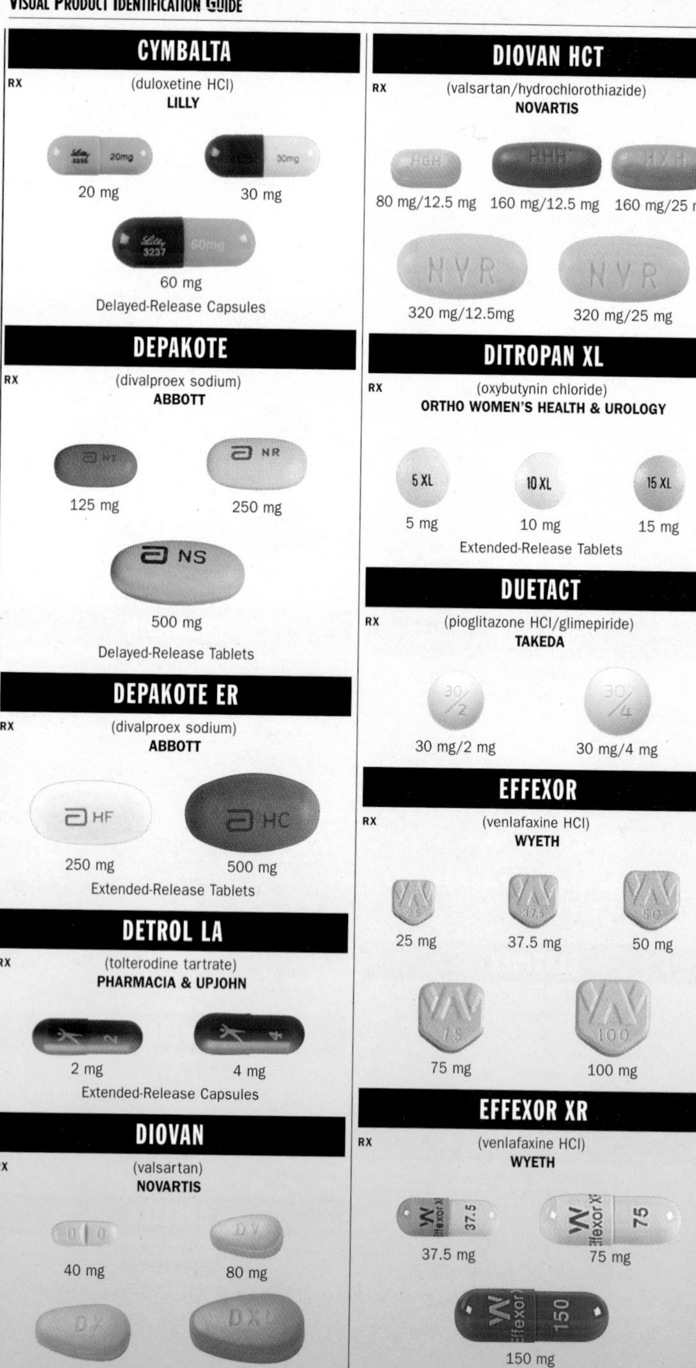
CYMBALTA
RX
(duloxetine HCl)
LILLY
20 mg
30 mg
60 mg
Delayed-Release Capsules
DEPAKOTE
RX
(divalproex sodium)
ABBOTT
125 mg
250 mg
500 mg
Delayed-Release Tablets
DEPAKOTE ER
RX
(divalproex sodium)
ABBOTT
250 mg
500 mg
Extended-Release Tablets
DETROL LA
RX
(tolterodine tartrate)
PHARMACIA & UPJOHN
2 mg
4 mg
Extended-Release Capsules
DIOVAN
RX
(valsartan)
NOVARTIS
40 mg
80 mg
160 mg
320 mg
DIOVAN HCT
RX
(valsartan/hydrochlorothiazide)
NOVARTIS
80 mg/12.5 mg
160 mg/12.5 mg
160 mg/25 mg
320 mg/12.5mg
320 mg/25 mg
DITROPAN XL
RX
(oxybutynin chloride)
ORTHO WOMEN'S HEALTH & UROLOGY
5 mg
10 mg
15 mg
Extended-Release Tablets
DUETACT
RX
(pioglitazone HCl/glimepiride)
TAKEDA
30 mg/2 mg
30 mg/4 mg
EFFEXOR
RX
(venlafaxine HCl)
WYETH
25 mg
37.5 mg
50 mg
75 mg
100 mg
EFFEXOR XR
RX
(venlafaxine HCl)
WYETH
37.5 mg
75 mg
150 mg
Extended-Release Capsules

## ENABLEX

RX

(darifenacin)
**NOVARTIS**

7.5 mg    15 mg
Extended-Release Tablets

## EVISTA

RX

(raloxifene HCl)
**LILLY**

60 mg

## EXELON

RX

(rivastigmine tartrate)
**NOVARTIS**

1.5 mg    3 mg

4.5 mg    6 mg

## FEMARA

RX

(letrozole)
**NOVARTIS**

2.5 mg

## FENTORA

RX

(fentanyl buccal tablet)
**CEPHALON**

100 mcg    200 mcg    400 mcg

600 mcg    800 mcg

## FLOMAX

RX

(tamsulosin HCl)
**BOEHRINGER INGELHEIM**

0.4 mg

## FOCALIN

CII

(dexmethylphenidate HCl)
**NOVARTIS**

2.5 mg    5 mg    10 mg

## FOCALIN XR

CII

(dexmethylphenidate HCl)
**NOVARTIS**

5 mg    10 mg

20 mg
Extended-Release Capsules

## FORTAMET

RX

(metformin HCl)
**SCIELE**

500 mg    1000 mg
Extended-Release Tablets

## FOSAMAX

RX

(alendronate sodium)
**MERCK**

5 mg    10 mg    35 mg

40 mg    70 mg

## FOSAMAX PLUS D

RX

(alendronate sodium/cholecalciferol)
**MERCK**

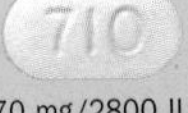

70 mg/2800 IU

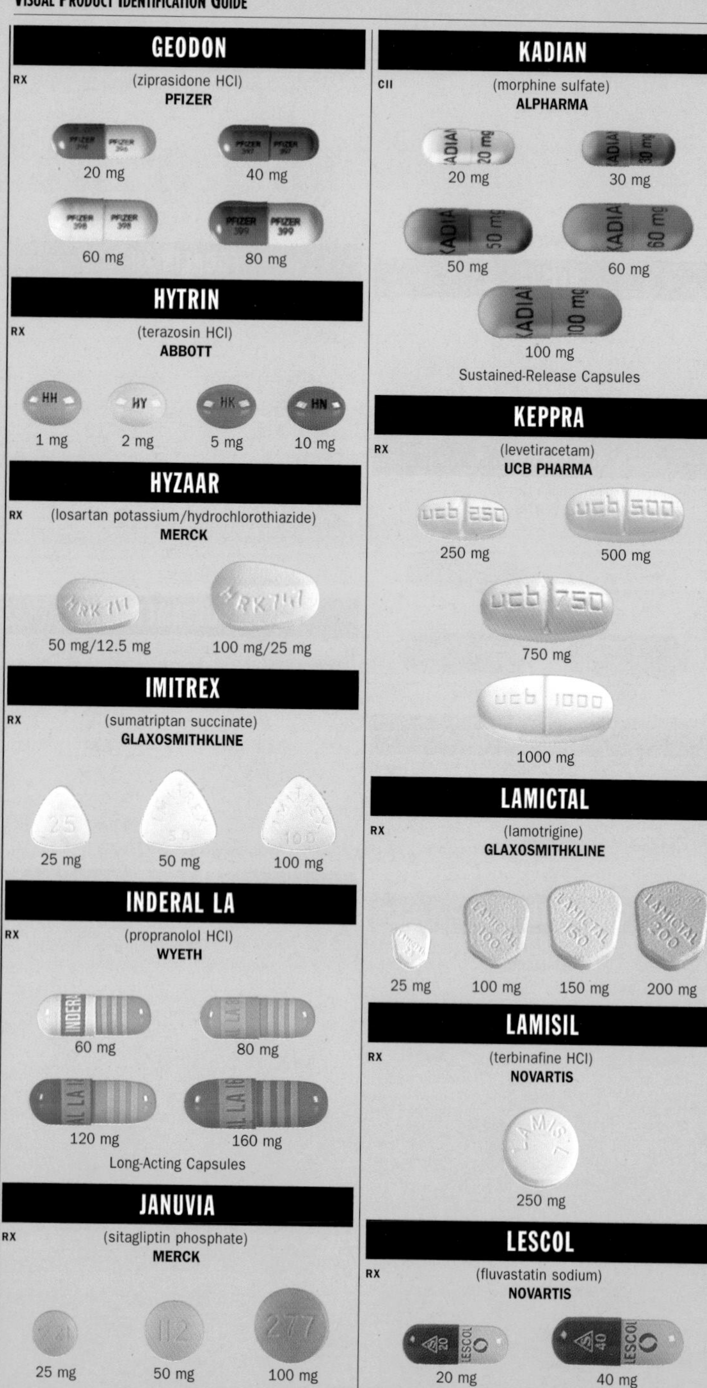
GEODON
RX
(ziprasidone HCl)
PFIZER
20 mg
40 mg
60 mg
80 mg
HYTRIN
RX
(terazosin HCl)
ABBOTT
1 mg
2 mg
5 mg
10 mg
HYZAAR
RX
(losartan potassium/hydrochlorothiazide)
MERCK
50 mg/12.5 mg
100 mg/25 mg
IMITREX
RX
(sumatriptan succinate)
GLAXOSMITHKLINE
25 mg
50 mg
100 mg
INDERAL LA
RX
(propranolol HCl)
WYETH
60 mg
80 mg
120 mg
160 mg
Long-Acting Capsules
JANUVIA
RX
(sitagliptin phosphate)
MERCK
25 mg
50 mg
100 mg
KADIAN
CII
(morphine sulfate)
ALPHARMA
20 mg
30 mg
50 mg
60 mg
100 mg
Sustained-Release Capsules
KEPPRA
RX
(levetiracetam)
UCB PHARMA
250 mg
500 mg
750 mg
1000 mg
LAMICTAL
RX
(lamotrigine)
GLAXOSMITHKLINE
25 mg
100 mg
150 mg
200 mg
LAMISIL
RX
(terbinafine HCl)
NOVARTIS
250 mg
LESCOL
RX
(fluvastatin sodium)
NOVARTIS
20 mg
40 mg

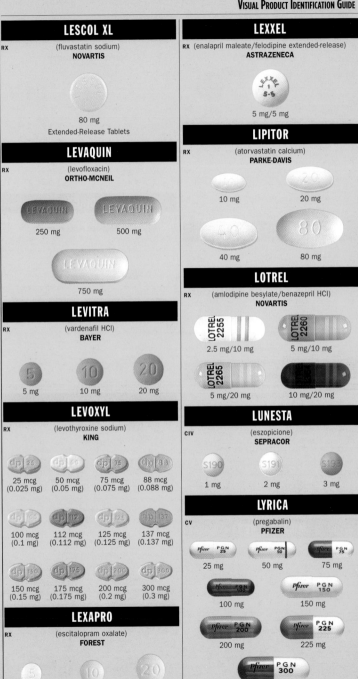

## LESCOL XL

RX (fluvastatin sodium)
**NOVARTIS**

80 mg
Extended-Release Tablets

## LEVAQUIN

RX (levofloxacin)
**ORTHO-MCNEIL**

250 mg | 500 mg

750 mg

## LEVITRA

RX (vardenafil HCl)
**BAYER**

5 mg | 10 mg | 20 mg

## LEVOXYL

RX (levothyroxine sodium)
**KING**

25 mcg (0.025 mg) | 50 mcg (0.05 mg) | 75 mcg (0.075 mg) | 88 mcg (0.088 mg)

100 mcg (0.1 mg) | 112 mcg (0.112 mg) | 125 mcg (0.125 mg) | 137 mcg (0.137 mg)

150 mcg (0.15 mg) | 175 mcg (0.175 mg) | 200 mcg (0.2 mg) | 300 mcg (0.3 mg)

## LEXAPRO

RX (escitalopram oxalate)
**FOREST**

5 mg | 10 mg | 20 mg

## LEXXEL

RX (enalapril maleate/felodipine extended-release)
**ASTRAZENECA**

5 mg/5 mg

## LIPITOR

RX (atorvastatin calcium)
**PARKE-DAVIS**

10 mg | 20 mg

40 mg | 80 mg

## LOTREL

RX (amlodipine besylate/benazepril HCl)
**NOVARTIS**

2.5 mg/10 mg | 5 mg/10 mg

5 mg/20 mg | 10 mg/20 mg

## LUNESTA

CIV (eszopicione)
**SEPRACOR**

1 mg | 2 mg | 3 mg

## LYRICA

CV (pregabalin)
**PFIZER**

25 mg | 50 mg | 75 mg

100 mg | 150 mg

200 mg | 225 mg

300 mg

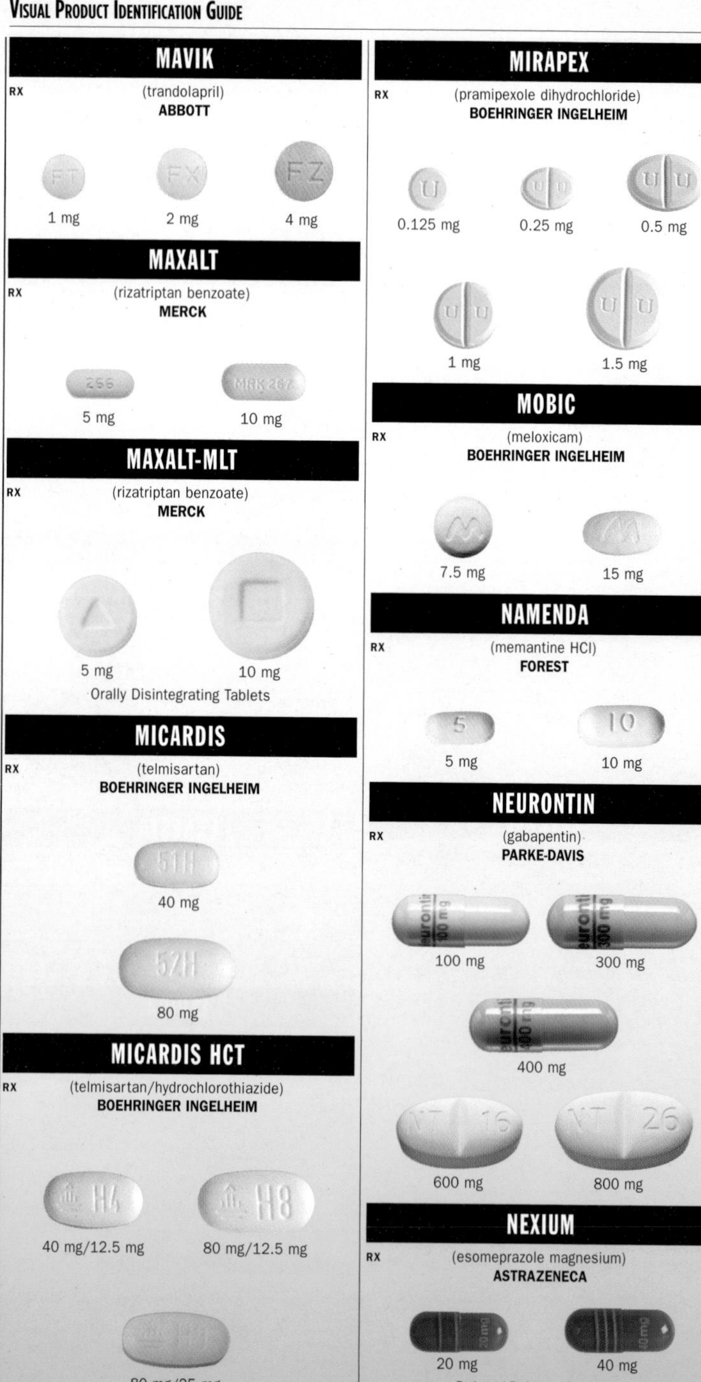
MAVIK
RX
(trandolapril)
ABBOTT
1 mg
2 mg
4 mg
MAXALT
RX
(rizatriptan benzoate)
MERCK
5 mg
10 mg
MAXALT-MLT
RX
(rizatriptan benzoate)
MERCK
5 mg
10 mg
Orally Disintegrating Tablets
MICARDIS
RX
(telmisartan)
BOEHRINGER INGELHEIM
40 mg
80 mg
MICARDIS HCT
RX
(telmisartan/hydrochlorothiazide)
BOEHRINGER INGELHEIM
40 mg/12.5 mg
80 mg/12.5 mg
80 mg/25 mg
MIRAPEX
RX
(pramipexole dihydrochloride)
BOEHRINGER INGELHEIM
0.125 mg
0.25 mg
0.5 mg
1 mg
1.5 mg
MOBIC
RX
(meloxicam)
BOEHRINGER INGELHEIM
7.5 mg
15 mg
NAMENDA
RX
(memantine HCl)
FOREST
5 mg
10 mg
NEURONTIN
RX
(gabapentin)
PARKE-DAVIS
100 mg
300 mg
400 mg
600 mg
800 mg
NEXIUM
RX
(esomeprazole magnesium)
ASTRAZENECA
20 mg
40 mg
Delayed-Release Capsules

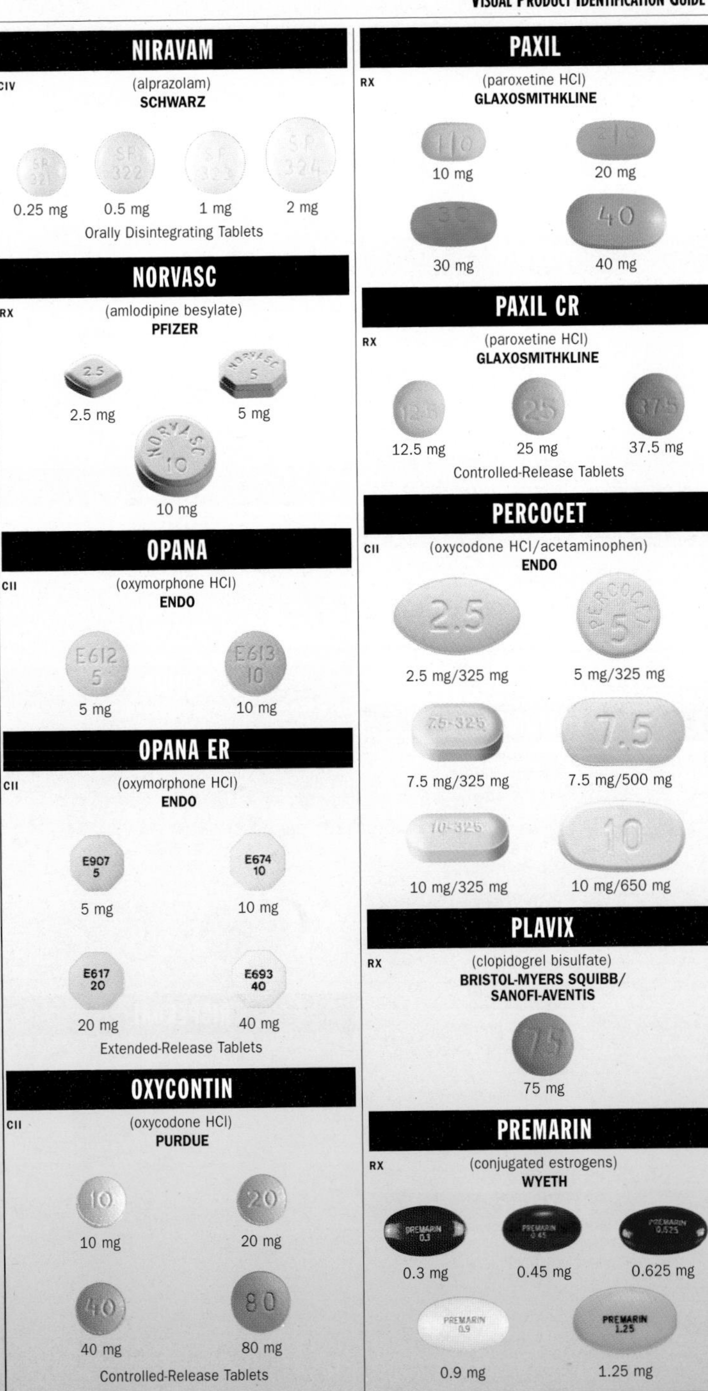

## NIRAVAM

CIV (alprazolam)
**SCHWARZ**

0.25 mg, 0.5 mg, 1 mg, 2 mg

Orally Disintegrating Tablets

## NORVASC

RX (amlodipine besylate)
**PFIZER**

2.5 mg, 5 mg, 10 mg

## OPANA

CII (oxymorphone HCl)
**ENDO**

5 mg, 10 mg

## OPANA ER

CII (oxymorphone HCl)
**ENDO**

5 mg, 10 mg, 20 mg, 40 mg

Extended-Release Tablets

## OXYCONTIN

CII (oxycodone HCl)
**PURDUE**

10 mg, 20 mg, 40 mg, 80 mg

Controlled-Release Tablets

## PAXIL

RX (paroxetine HCl)
**GLAXOSMITHKLINE**

10 mg, 20 mg, 30 mg, 40 mg

## PAXIL CR

RX (paroxetine HCl)
**GLAXOSMITHKLINE**

12.5 mg, 25 mg, 37.5 mg

Controlled-Release Tablets

## PERCOCET

CII (oxycodone HCl/acetaminophen)
**ENDO**

2.5 mg/325 mg, 5 mg/325 mg, 7.5 mg/325 mg, 7.5 mg/500 mg, 10 mg/325 mg, 10 mg/650 mg

## PLAVIX

RX (clopidogrel bisulfate)
**BRISTOL-MYERS SQUIBB/ SANOFI-AVENTIS**

75 mg

## PREMARIN

RX (conjugated estrogens)
**WYETH**

0.3 mg, 0.45 mg, 0.625 mg, 0.9 mg, 1.25 mg

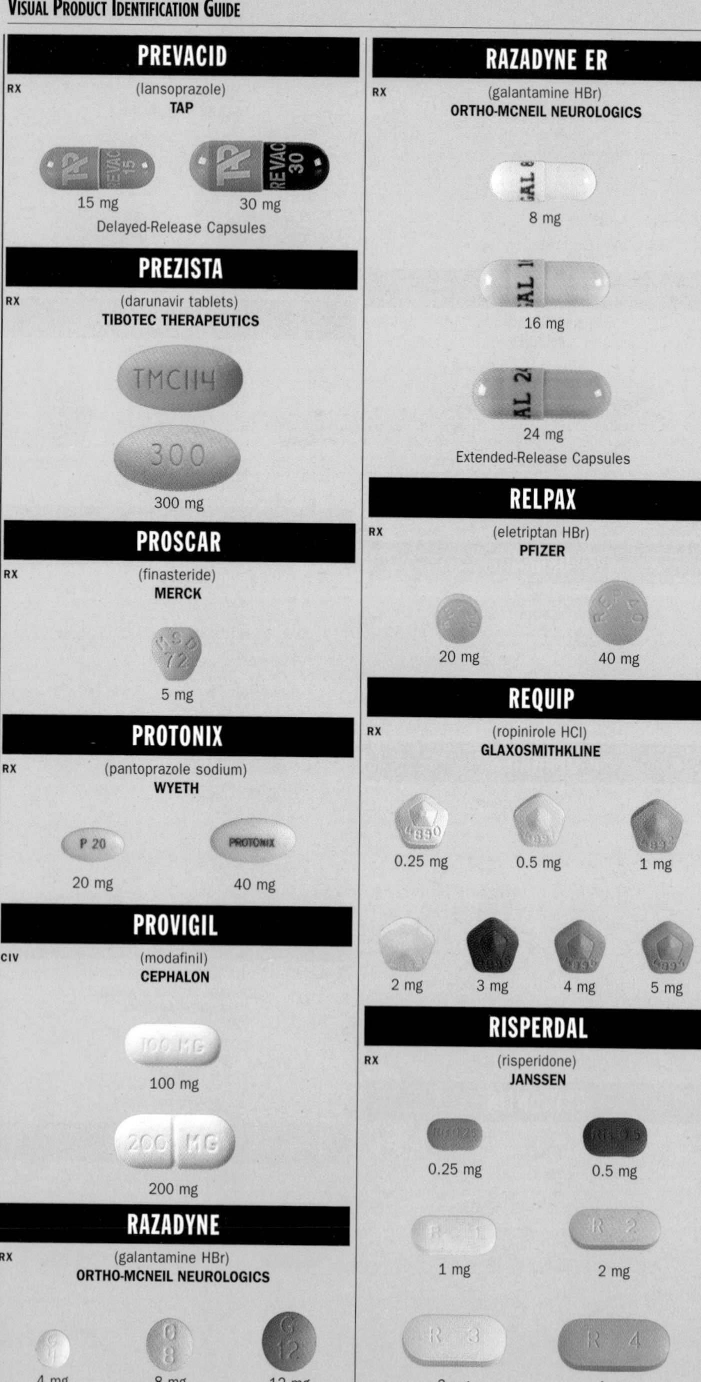

## PREVACID

RX (lansoprazole)
**TAP**

15 mg 30 mg
Delayed-Release Capsules

## PREZISTA

RX (darunavir tablets)
**TIBOTEC THERAPEUTICS**

300 mg

## PROSCAR

RX (finasteride)
**MERCK**

5 mg

## PROTONIX

RX (pantoprazole sodium)
**WYETH**

20 mg 40 mg

## PROVIGIL

CIV (modafinil)
**CEPHALON**

100 mg

200 mg

## RAZADYNE

RX (galantamine HBr)
**ORTHO-MCNEIL NEUROLOGICS**

4 mg 8 mg 12 mg

## RAZADYNE ER

RX (galantamine HBr)
**ORTHO-MCNEIL NEUROLOGICS**

8 mg

16 mg

24 mg
Extended-Release Capsules

## RELPAX

RX (eletriptan HBr)
**PFIZER**

20 mg 40 mg

## REQUIP

RX (ropinirole HCl)
**GLAXOSMITHKLINE**

0.25 mg 0.5 mg 1 mg

2 mg 3 mg 4 mg 5 mg

## RISPERDAL

RX (risperidone)
**JANSSEN**

0.25 mg 0.5 mg

1 mg 2 mg

3 mg 4 mg

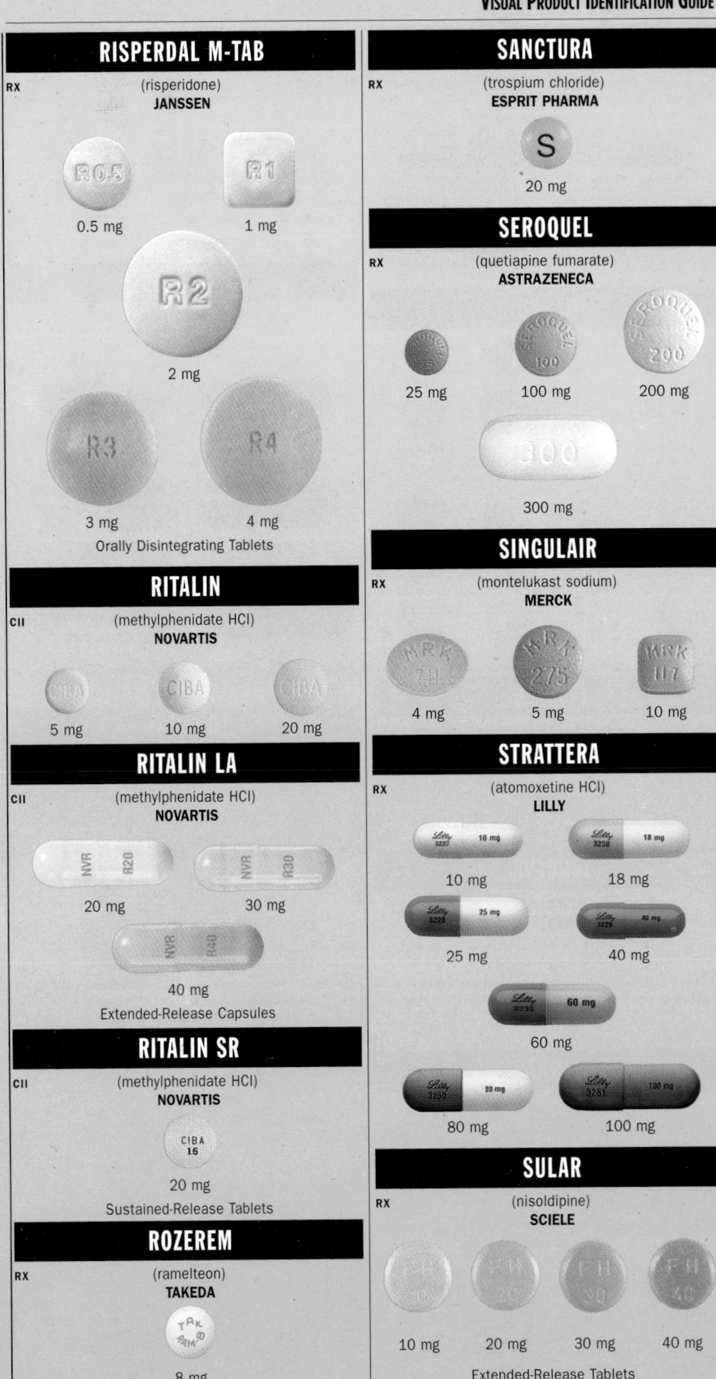
RISPERDAL M-TAB
RX
(risperidone)
JANSSEN
0.5 mg
1 mg
2 mg
3 mg
4 mg
Orally Disintegrating Tablets
RITALIN
CII
(methylphenidate HCl)
NOVARTIS
5 mg
10 mg
20 mg
RITALIN LA
CII
(methylphenidate HCl)
NOVARTIS
20 mg
30 mg
40 mg
Extended-Release Capsules
RITALIN SR
CII
(methylphenidate HCl)
NOVARTIS
20 mg
Sustained-Release Tablets
ROZEREM
RX
(ramelteon)
TAKEDA
8 mg
SANCTURA
RX
(trospium chloride)
ESPRIT PHARMA
20 mg
SEROQUEL
RX
(quetiapine fumarate)
ASTRAZENECA
25 mg
100 mg
200 mg
300 mg
SINGULAIR
RX
(montelukast sodium)
MERCK
4 mg
5 mg
10 mg
STRATTERA
RX
(atomoxetine HCl)
LILLY
10 mg
18 mg
25 mg
40 mg
60 mg
80 mg
100 mg
SULAR
RX
(nisoldipine)
SCIELE
10 mg
20 mg
30 mg
40 mg
Extended-Release Tablets

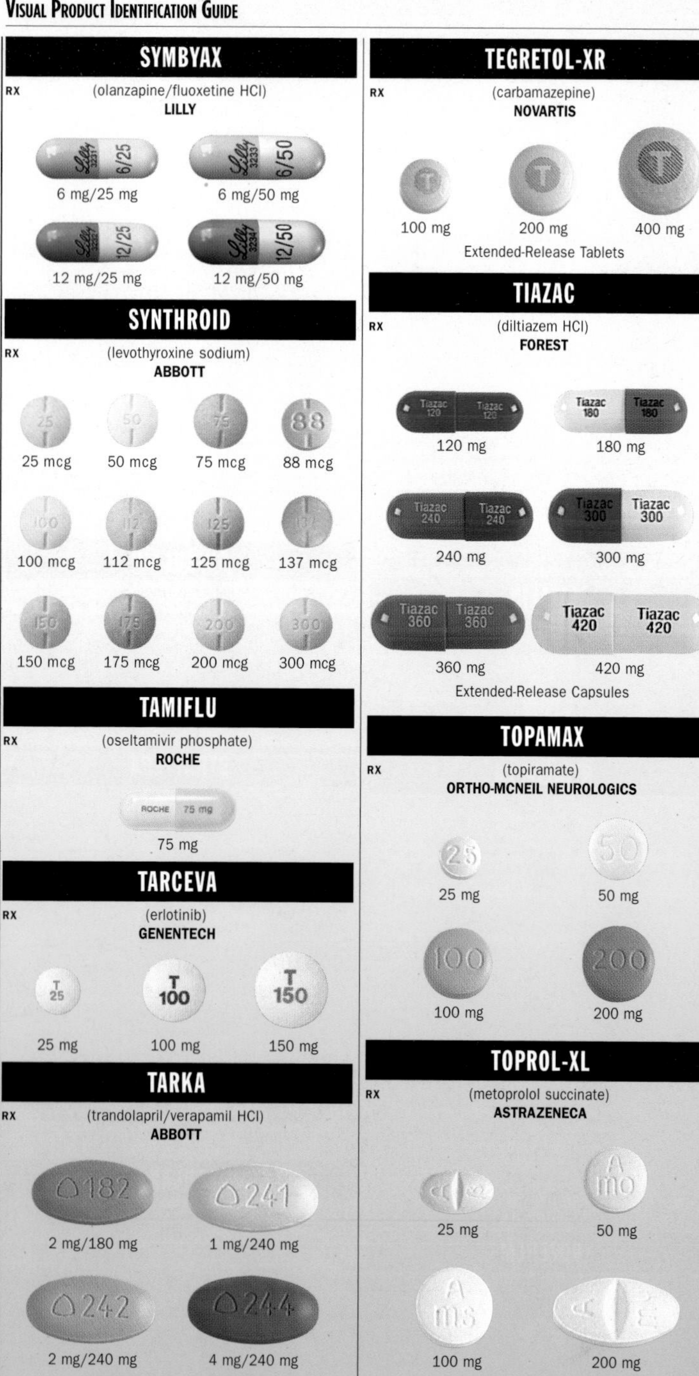
SYMBYAX
RX
(olanzapine/fluoxetine HCl)
LILLY
6 mg/25 mg
6 mg/50 mg
12 mg/25 mg
12 mg/50 mg
SYNTHROID
RX
(levothyroxine sodium)
ABBOTT
25 mcg
50 mcg
75 mcg
88 mcg
100 mcg
112 mcg
125 mcg
137 mcg
150 mcg
175 mcg
200 mcg
300 mcg
TAMIFLU
RX
(oseltamivir phosphate)
ROCHE
ROCHE 75 mg
75 mg
TARCEVA
RX
(erlotinib)
GENENTECH
T 25
T 100
T 150
25 mg
100 mg
150 mg
TARKA
RX
(trandolapril/verapamil HCl)
ABBOTT
182
241
2 mg/180 mg
1 mg/240 mg
242
244
2 mg/240 mg
4 mg/240 mg
Extended-Release Tablets
TEGRETOL-XR
RX
(carbamazepine)
NOVARTIS
100 mg
200 mg
400 mg
Extended-Release Tablets
TIAZAC
RX
(diltiazem HCl)
FOREST
Tiazac 120
120 mg
Tiazac 180
180 mg
Tiazac 240
240 mg
Tiazac 300
300 mg
Tiazac 360
360 mg
Tiazac 420
420 mg
Extended-Release Capsules
TOPAMAX
RX
(topiramate)
ORTHO-MCNEIL NEUROLOGICS
25
50
25 mg
50 mg
100
200
100 mg
200 mg
TOPROL-XL
RX
(metoprolol succinate)
ASTRAZENECA
25 mg
A mo
50 mg
A ms
100 mg
200 mg
Extended-Release Tablets

## TRICOR

RX (fenofibrate)
**ABBOTT**

48 mg 145 mg

## TRILEPTAL

RX (oxcarbazepine)
**NOVARTIS**

150 mg 300 mg

600 mg

## VALTREX

RX (valacyclovir HCl)
**GLAXOSMITHKLINE**

500 mg

1 g

## VERELAN PM

RX (verapamil HCl)
**SCHWARZ**

100 mg 200 mg

300 mg

Extended-Release Capsules Controlled-Onset

## VFEND

RX (voriconazole)
**PFIZER**

50 mg 200 mg

## VIAGRA

RX (sildenafil citrate)
**PFIZER**

25 mg 50 mg 100 mg

## VICODIN

CIII (hydrocodone bitartrate/acetaminophen)
**ABBOTT**

5 mg/500 mg

## VICODIN ES

CIII (hydrocodone bitartrate/acetaminophen)
**ABBOTT**

7.5 mg/750 mg

## VYTORIN

RX (ezetimibe/simvastatin)
**MERCK/SCHERING-PLOUGH**

10 mg/10 mg 10 mg/20 mg

10 mg/40 mg 10 mg/80 mg

## WELLBUTRIN SR

RX (bupropion HCl)
**GLAXOSMITHKLINE**

100 mg 150 mg 200 mg

Sustained-Release Tablets

## WELLBUTRIN XL

RX (bupropion HCl)
**GLAXOSMITHKLINE**

150 mg 300 mg

Extended-Release Tablets

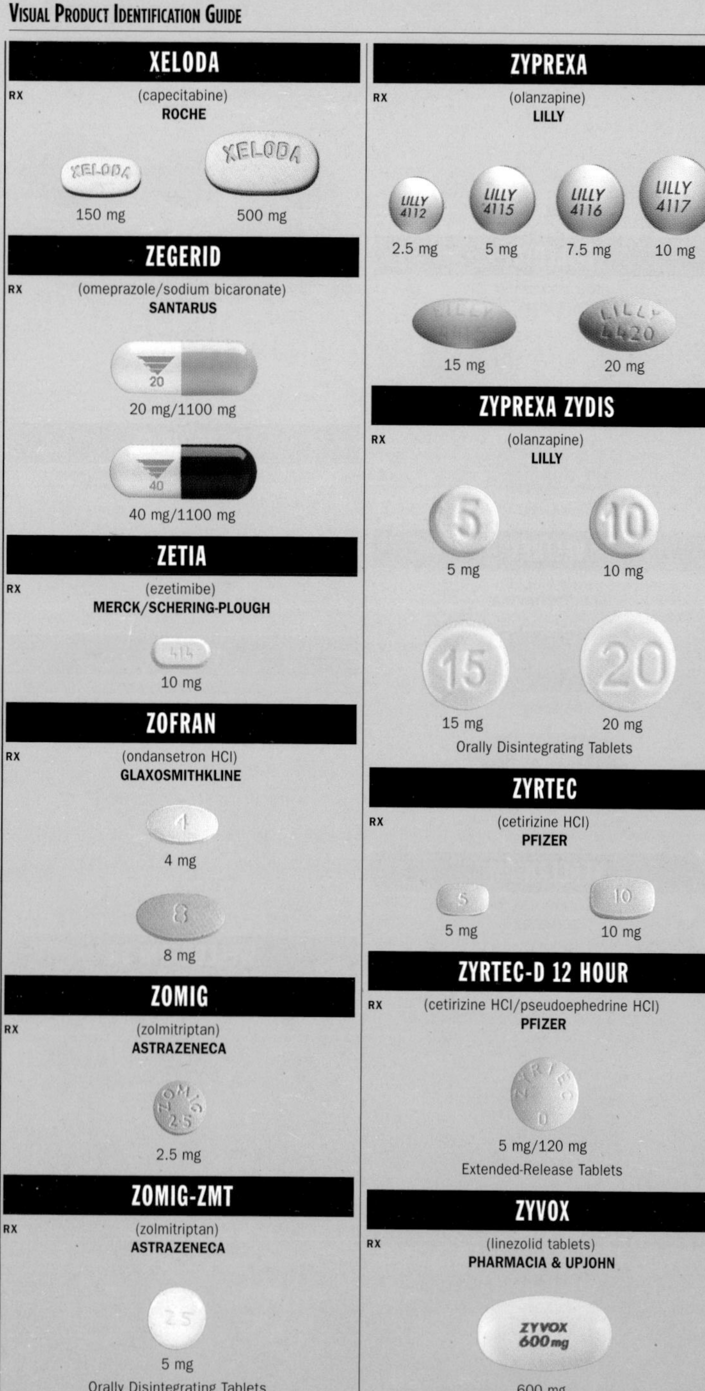
XELODA
RX
(capecitabine)
ROCHE
XELODA
XELODA
150 mg
500 mg
ZEGERID
RX
(omeprazole/sodium bicaronate)
SANTARUS
20
20 mg/1100 mg
40
40 mg/1100 mg
ZETIA
RX
(ezetimibe)
MERCK/SCHERING-PLOUGH
414
10 mg
ZOFRAN
RX
(ondansetron HCl)
GLAXOSMITHKLINE
4
4 mg
8
8 mg
ZOMIG
RX
(zolmitriptan)
ASTRAZENECA
ZOMIG 2.5
2.5 mg
ZOMIG-ZMT
RX
(zolmitriptan)
ASTRAZENECA
2.5
5 mg
Orally Disintegrating Tablets
ZYPREXA
RX
(olanzapine)
LILLY
LILLY 4112
LILLY 4115
LILLY 4116
LILLY 4117
2.5 mg
5 mg
7.5 mg
10 mg
LILLY 4420
15 mg
20 mg
ZYPREXA ZYDIS
RX
(olanzapine)
LILLY
5
10
5 mg
10 mg
15
20
15 mg
20 mg
Orally Disintegrating Tablets
ZYRTEC
RX
(cetirizine HCl)
PFIZER
5
10
5 mg
10 mg
ZYRTEC-D 12 HOUR
RX
(cetirizine HCl/pseudoephedrine HCl)
PFIZER
ZYRTEC D
5 mg/120 mg
Extended-Release Tablets
ZYVOX
RX
(linezolid tablets)
PHARMACIA & UPJOHN
ZYVOX 600mg
600 mg